10th Edition

Abrams' Clinical Drug Therapy

RATIONALES FOR NURSING PRACTICE

Geralyn Frandsen, EdD, RN
Professor of Nursing
School of Health Professions
Maryville University
St. Louis, Missouri

Sandra Smith Pennington, PhD, RN
Provost
Rocky Mountain University of Health Professions
Provo, Utah

Professor Emeritus
Department of Nursing
Berea College
Berea, Kentucky

Wolters Kluwer | Lippincott Williams & Wilkins
Health

Philadelphia • Baltimore • New York • London
Buenos Aires • Hong Kong • Sydney • Tokyo

Executive Editor: Matt Kane
Product Manager: Michelle Clarke
Production Project Manager: Cynthia Rudy
Editorial Assistant: Dan Reilly
Senior Book Designer: Joan Wendt
Art Director: Brett MacNaughton
Manufacturing Coordinator: Karin Duffield
Prepress Vendor: SPi Global

10th edition

9 8 7 6 5 4 3 2 1

Printed in China

Library of Congress Cataloging-in-Publication Data
Frandsen, Geralyn.
    Abrams' clinical drug therapy : rationales for nursing practice / Geralyn Frandsen, Sandra Smith Pennington. — 10th ed.
      p. ; cm.
    Clinical drug therapy
    Rev. ed. of: Clinical drug therapy / Anne Collins Abrams. 9th ed. c2009.
    Includes bibliographical references and index.
    ISBN 978-1-60913-711-3
  I. Pennington, Sandra Smith. II. Abrams, Anne Collins. Clinical drug therapy. III. Title. IV. Title: Clinical drug therapy.
    [DNLM: 1. Pharmaceutical Preparations—Nurses' Instruction. 2. Drug Therapy—Nurses' Instruction. 3. Pharmacological Phenomena—Nurses' Instruction. QV 55]
    615.1'9—dc23

2012034990

LWW.com

I would like to thank my wonderful husband, Gary, for his love, support, and talented contributions to this textbook. I would also like to thank our children Claire and Joe for their love and support through the writing of the book.

GERALYN FRANDSEN

I dedicate this work to my husband, Everett Pennington, whose support is always a constant and his willingness to accept my crazy work schedule a daily gift. Our children (Jennifer, Brad, and Leah) and grandchildren (Laney and Maddie) give balance and joy to my life. Having Jennifer provide a pharmacist's perspective to my many questions has enriched this text.

SANDY PENNINGTON

Contributors

Lisa Albers, MSN, RN
Clinical Assistant Professor of Nursing
Maryville University
St. Louis, Missouri
> Chapter 4: Pharmacology and the Care of the Infant
> and Pediatric Patient

Jacqueline Lee Rosenjack Burchum, DNSc, FNP-BC, CNE
Associate Professor
University of Tennessee Health Science Center
Memphis, Tennessee
> Chapter 13: Inflammation, Infection, and the Use of
> Antimicrobial Agents

Thomas J. Evans, DNP, CRNA
Nurse Anesthetist
Wilford Hall Medical Center
Lackland Air Force Base, Texas
> Chapter 50: Drug Therapy with General Anesthetics

Gary Frandsen, JD, MSN, RN
Assistant Professor of Nursing
University of Missouri
St. Louis, Missouri
> Chapter 20: Drug Therapy for Tuberculosis and
> *Mycobacterium avium* Complex Disease
> Chapter 33: Nutritional Support Products,
> Vitamins, and Mineral Supplements
> Chapter 48: Drug Therapy with Opioids

Cheryl S. Hazen, MSN, BSN, RN
Registered Nurse
Mercy Hospital
St. Louis, Missouri
> Chapter 39: Drug Therapy for Diabetes Mellitus

Nancy Hutt, MSN, RN, NP-C
Nursing Faculty
Portland Community College
Portland, Oregon
> Chapter 10: Drug Therapy: Immunizations
> Chapter 11: Drug Therapy to Suppress Immunity
> Chapter 12: Drug Therapy for the Treatment of Cancer

Brian Koonce, MSN, CRNA
Huntsville, Alabama
Decatur Morgan Hospital
Decatur, Alabama
> Chapter 49: Drug Therapy with Local Anesthetics

Dana Manley, PhD, ARNP
Assistant Professor
Murray State University
School of Nursing
Murray, Kentucky
> Chapter 44: Drug Therapy for Women's Health

Jennifer Binggeli Miles, PharmD, MBA
Clinical Pharmacist
St. Petersburg, Florida
> Chapter 16: Drug Therapy with Beta-Lactam
> Antibacterial Agents
> Chapter 17: Drug Therapy with Aminoglycosides and
> Fluoroquinolones
> Chapter 29: Drug Therapy for Nasal Congestion

Marthe J. Moseley, PhD, RN, CCRN, CCNS, CNL
Associate Director of Clinical Practice
Department of Veterans Affairs
Office of Nursing Services
Washington, District of Columbia
> Chapter 25: Drug Therapy for Dysrhythmias
> Chapter 27: Drug Therapy to Enhance Adrenergic Response

Michele Muraski, PhD, RN
Associate Professor of Nursing
Maryville University
St. Louis, Missouri
> Chapter 6: Pharmacology and the Pregnant or
> Lactating Woman

Pamela Newland, PhD, RN
Assistant Professor
Southern Illinois University Edwardsville
Edwardsville, Illinois
> Chapter 46: Drug Therapy for Myasthenia Gravis and
> Alzheimer's Disease
> Chapter 47: Drug Therapy for Parkinson's Disease and
> Anticholinergics

Jacqueline R. Saleeby, PhD, RN, BCCS
Associate Professor
Mayville University
St. Louis, Missouri
> Chapter 53: Drug Therapy to Reduce Anxiety and
> Produce Hypnosis
> Chapter 55: Drug Therapy for Psychotic Disorders
> Chapter 56: Drug Therapy to Stimulate the Central
> Nervous System
> Chapter 57: Drug Therapy for Substance Abuse Disorders

Reviewers

Debra Backus, PhD, RN, NEA-BC
Associate Professor
State University of New York—Canton
Canton, New York

Roger J.S. Bidwell, RN, MSN, ARNP
Faculty
Penn Valley School of Nursing
Metropolitan Community College
Kansas City, Missouri

Maria Danet Lapiz Bluhm, RN, PhD
Assistant Professor
University of Texas Health Science Center
San Antonio, Texas

Darlene Clark, RN, MS
Senior Lecturer in Nursing
Pennsylvania State University
University Park, Pennsylvania

Wendy Clark, BSN, MSN
Assistant Professor
University of Saint Francis
Fort Wayne, Indiana

Katherine Conrad, MN, RN, CNS
Nursing Instructor
Mt. Hood Community College
Gresham, Oregon

Crystal Dunlevy, EdD
Clinical Associate Professor
Ohio State University
Columbus, Ohio

Janet B. Fox-Moatz, MSN, RN
Assistant Professor
Neumann University
Aston, Pennsylvania

Sophia Gardner, MSN, RN
Professor of Nursing
Community College of Allegheny County—Boyce Campus
Monroeville, Pennsylvania

Melissa J. Geist, EdD, MSN, MEd, FNP-BC, PNP-BC
Assistant Professor
Tennessee Technological University
Cookeville, Tennessee

Eleanor S. Greene, RN, MSN
Professor
Bucks County Community College
Newtown, Pennsylvania

Sheila Grossman, PhD, APRN-BC
Professor and Director
Family Nurse Practitioner Program
Fairfield University School of Nursing
Fairfield, Connecticut

Brenda L. Haile, BA, MSN, DrPH
Associate Professor
Texas Woman's University
Houston, Texas

Gina Hale, MSN, RN, CNE
Instructor
Lamar University
Beaumont, Texas

Mary Jane S. Hanson, PhD, CRNP, CNS, RN
Professor and Director of Graduate Nursing Program
University of Scranton
Scranton, Pennsylvania

Nancy B. Hartel, MS, RN, CNE
Associate Professor
St. Joseph's College of Nursing
Syracuse, New York

Katherine I. Hayes, RN, MSN
Professor of Nursing
San Jacinto College—Central Campus
Pasadena, Texas

Kevin D. Hite, RN, MSN
Assistant Professor
Fairmont State University
Fairmont, West Virginia

Sheri Lynn Jacobson, RN, MS, APRN, ANP
Assistant Professor
Winston-Salem State University
Winston-Salem, North Carolina

Dana Johnson, MSN, RN
Professor of Nursing
Sierra College
Rocklin, California

v

Ellen Ketcherside, RN, MA, CCRN
Nursing Instructor
Mineral Area College
Park Hills, Missouri

Stephen D. Krau, PhD, MSN, MA, BSN, BA
Associate Professor
Vanderbilt University
Nashville, Tennessee

Yolanda Lonsford, RN, MS, MSN
Professor of Nursing
San Jacinto College—Central Campus
Pasadena, Texas

Christa MacLean, RN, BSN, MN
Faculty
Saskatchewan Institute of Applied Science and Technology
Regina, Saskatchewan, Canada

Alice L. March, PhD, RN, FNP-C, CNE
Assistant Professor
The University of Alabama
Tuscaloosa, Alabama

Patricia Martin, MSN, APRN, CNE
Associate Professor
West Kentucky Community and Technical College
Paducah, Kentucky

Kimberly Mau, RN, MSN
Director of Nursing Programs
Kankakee Community College
Kankakee, Illinois

Jane Mighton, RN, BSN, MSN
Nurse Educator
Langara College
Vancouver, British Columbia, Canada

James D. Mendez, MSN, CRNP
Instructor
Villanova University
Villanova, Pennsylvania

Jo Ann L. Nicoteri, PhD, CRNP, FNP-BC
Family Nurse Practitioner
Student Health Services
University of Scranton
Scranton, Pennsylvania

Jeanne Marie Papa, MBE, MSN, CRNP, CCRN
Senior Instructor
Neumann University
Aston, Pennsylvania

VaLinda Pearson, PhD, MS, RN, CNE
Professor of Nursing and Associate Degree Nursing Program
   Director
St. Catherine University
Minneapolis, Minnesota

Donna Peters, MA, BS, AAS
Professor of Nursing
Rockland Community College
Suffern, New York

Wanda Pierson, RN, BSN, MN, MA, PhD
Nursing Department Chair
Langara College
Vancouver, British Columbia, Canada

Cynthia L. Pins, MS, RN
Nursing Instructor
North Hennepin Community College
Brooklyn Park, Minnesota

Julia R. Popp, RN, MSN
Professor of Nursing
Owens Community College
Toledo, Ohio

Judith Swanson, RN, MSN
Assistant Professor
Minot State University
Minot, North Dakota

Mary Tan, PhD, RN
Project Director Allied Health and Research
Holmes Community College
Ridgeland, Mississippi

Elizabeth A. VandeWaa, PhD
Associate Professor
University of South Alabama
Mobile, Alabama

Ina Warboys, MS, RN
Clinical Assistant Professor
The University of Alabama—Huntsville
Huntsville, Alabama

Laura White, BSN, RN
Vocational Nursing Instructor
North Central Texas College
Gainesville, Texas

Thomas Worms, MSN, RN
Professor of Nursing
Truman College
Chicago, Illinois

Foreword

Administering medication safely is a multifaceted, complex, team-based patient intervention. From the manufacturing process to patient administration, many errors can occur. Nurses have significant and independent roles in medication administration, and it is essential that they understand the risks associated with inaccurate administration. Recent data from the Institute of Medicine reveal disturbing quality issues in medication administration across all health care settings in the United States (Aspen, Walcott, Bootman, & Cronenwett, 2007). On average, there is one medication error per day per hospitalized patient. Quality varies in different facilities; some have higher error rates than others. At least 1.5 million preventable adverse drug events occur each year. Why are patients so vulnerable to medication errors? What are nurses' roles and responsibilities in improving quality and safety in clinical drug therapy?

In caring for patients, nurses are accountable for current knowledge of a particular patient's medication regimen and what is involved in the safe and reliable administration of drugs to that particular patient. How do nurses ensure that the right medication is administered in the right dose, by the right route, at the right time, to the right patient? New safety science concepts are changing how nurses view safe medication administration so that health providers have organizational resources for reporting errors and "near misses." In "just culture" organizations, trained risk management personnel analyze reported mistakes to determine the root cause of critical errors and "near misses" by questioning decisions made at every juncture along the medication pathway. With this method of system analysis, lessons learned help prevent the same mistake from happening again.

This new edition of *Abrams' Clinical Drug Therapy* by Frandsen and Pennington integrates the quality and safety competencies defined by the national award-winning Quality and Safety Education for Nurses (QSEN) (Cronenwett et al., 2007) project. Redesigned to incorporate disease characteristics as well as clinical drug knowledge, the text provides a comprehensive approach to safe medication administration. The first step in safe medication administration is knowledge of the medications, including evidence-based standards for administration. The second step is recognition of the organizational challenges and opportunities for careful medication administration. Faculty in schools of nursing have mastered the many steps in the skill of administering and documenting medications in clinical learning laboratories. The learning actions included in this text guide students to look beyond medication administration and think of related actions in the total process that affect accuracy and reflect safety science.

To help define a new paradigm in nursing to integrate quality and safety into the daily work of nurses, the QSEN project has identified the knowledge, skills, and attitudes that make up the six competencies required to deliver quality, safe care—patient-centered care, teamwork and collaboration, evidence-based practice, quality improvement, safety, and informatics. To apply the new safety framework to medication administration, nurses must consider patient-centered preferences and situations, collaborate across interprofessional teams, apply evidence-based standards for the medication and within the patient's context, participate in continuous quality improvement, apply safety science concepts, and use informatics in planning and managing the pharmacology needs of their patients. These six competencies are integrated into the national curriculum standards for nursing so that all nurses are accountable for integrating safety and quality responsibilities into their daily work.

How do nurses apply these competencies in medication administration?

- Patient-centered care means basing care decisions on knowledge of patient values and preferences. It is important for health care professionals (1) to treat all patients and families with respect and honor and (2) to include patients and families as partners in care and as safety allies. For example, if a patient and the patient's spouse are familiar with the treatment plan, they have an opportunity to participate as important team members by determining when medications are not providing the patient with the desired therapeutic effects.
- Teamwork and collaboration use the health professional's personal strengths to foster effective team functioning. A medical team working with the patient may include a nurse, a physician, a nurse practitioner, and a physician assistant, as well as a pharmacist, social worker, dietitian, physical therapist, occupational therapist, and speech language pathologist. To help coordinate the complexities of safe medication administration, teamwork behaviors include flexible leadership, standardized communication, mutual support, and constant environmental scans.
- Evidence-based practice involves using new information in pharmacotherapeutics, which appears in the Evidence-Based Practice boxes throughout the text. Safe medication administration uses evidence-based practice standards to ensure that appropriate precautions are taken to assess for adverse effects.
- Quality improvement is integral to safe medication administration. Nurses must develop skills to measure care in their own setting to compare with benchmark data to determine areas to improve and to use quality improvement tools to raise performance.

- Safety is based on constantly asking how actions affect patient risk, where the next error is likely to occur, and what actions can prevent near misses. Safety science positions individual accountability within the context of the system so that mistakes are analyzed to identify ways to change actions in future situations.
- Informatics is the thread in all the competencies for managing care, documentation, and decision support tools. Knowledge, skills, and attitudes in informatics enable the nurse to seek evidence and measure care outcomes as well as to benchmark data to assess current practice.

As noted throughout this text with its QSEN Safety Alerts, nurses must develop a spirit of inquiry in which they reflect before they act, reflect during action, and reflect on action. This leads to questions to determine current evidence and best practices, and this spirit of inquiry promotes a practice attitude of continuously improving care.

As you, the nurse, use this text, several central questions guide your development.

- What are the roles and responsibilities for each team member in the complex steps in medication administration? Maintaining awareness of the scope of responsibility for each discipline involved is critical, particularly in transitions in care.

- How do I ensure medication safety during transitions in care when I turn over my patient to another provider?
- What do I need to know about this medication for safe administration? With the wide range of pharmacologic agents available, each nurse must acknowledge and ask questions about his or her own limitations in knowledge and skills to be able to seek expert advice and current clinical information before administering medications.
- What communication skills will help me understand my patient's preferences and values related to medications?

Asking these questions, developing these quality and safety competencies, and following the guidance in this book will ensure that the next national medication safety measures will show improvement.

Gwen Sherwood, PhD, RN, FAAN
Professor and Associate Dean for Academic Affairs
University of North Carolina at Chapel Hill School of Nursing

References

Aspen, P., Walcott, J., Bootman, L., & Cronenwett, L. (Eds.) and the Committee on Identifying and Preventing Medication Errors. (2007). *Identifying and preventing medication errors.* Washington, DC: National Academies Press.

Cronenwett, L., Sherwood, G., Barnsteiner, J., Disch, J., Johnson, J., Mitchell, P., et al. (2007). Quality and safety education for nurses. *Nursing Outlook,* 55(3), 122–131.

Preface

Abrams' Clinical Drug Therapy has a long tradition of guiding students and instructors through the practice of safe and effective medication administration. The 10th edition has expanded on this tradition with the inclusion of Quality and Safety Education for Nurses (QSEN) content in each chapter. Each chapter also includes new information about the pathophysiology of disease and associated drug therapy for prevention and treatment of disease.

Goals and Responsibilities of Nursing Care Related to Drug Therapy

Varied goals and responsibilities inherent in safe medication administration are identified in each chapter. The following information will guide you in developing your own goals and responsibilities inherent to safe and effective nursing practice.

- Preventing the need for drug therapy, when possible, by promoting health and preventing conditions that require drug therapy
- Using nonpharmacological interventions alone or in conjunction with drug therapy. When used with drugs, such interventions may promote lower drug dosage, less frequent administration, and fewer adverse effects.
- Administering drugs accurately and taking into consideration patient characteristics such as age, weight, and hepatic function, which can influence drug response
- Preventing or minimizing adverse effects by knowing the major adverse effects associated with particular drugs. It is important to assess patients with impaired hepatic and renal function closely for adverse effects. The early recognition of adverse effects allows for the implementation of interventions to minimize their severity. All drugs cause adverse effects, and nurses must maintain a high index of suspicion that the development of new signs and symptoms may be drug induced.
- Teaching patients and families about the effects of medications. The nurse must instruct patients and families about the role and importance of their medications in treating particular illnesses, accurate administration of medications, nonpharmacologic treatments to use with or instead of pharmacologic treatments, and when to contact their health care provider.

Organizational Framework

Eleven sections of the textbook provide the reader with basic information about drug therapy as well as the administration of medications for the prevention and treatment of disease. The first section introduces the safeguards in place to promote drug safety, the Institute of Medicine Core Competencies, and medication administration. It also describes the nursing process and explains the application of the nursing process in the care of patients receiving drug therapy. The second section addresses the effect medications have throughout the lifespan. The text introduces the effects of drugs on infants, children, older adults, and pregnant and lactating women. The remaining sections provide information on drug therapy related to systems, infections, and disease processes.

Each chapter opens with a case study, and its use throughout the chapter helps the reader integrate information about a particular disease and its drug therapy so he or she can apply it. The chapters also have NCLEX-style questions distributed throughout to test knowledge of the content and its application to patient care. This approach will help the reader prepare for class examinations as well as the NCLEX itself.

The chapters that focus on drug treatment for specific diseases use the prototype approach, allowing the reader to see the similarity in medications within each broad drug classification. Introduction and Overview sections provide the basis for understanding the drug therapy that prevents or treats the disease. The presentation of disease pathophysiology helps the reader understand the effect of a particular medication on the prevention and treatment of disease. Drug therapy sections summarize the medications, identifying the pharmacokinetics, action, use, adverse effects, contraindications, and nursing implications—including administration, assessment, and patient teaching. Many chapters discuss the effect of herbal supplements on prescribed medications. This information has become crucial for the maintenance of patient safety. Boxes containing patient teaching guidelines for a drug or class of drugs highlight crucial information the nurse should teach to the patient and family.

Recurring Features

This thoroughly updated edition includes new and revised features to enhance learning.

Chapter Opening Features

- **Learning Objectives** summarize what the student should learn while reading the chapter and answering both the Clinical Application Case Study Questions and NCLEX Success questions, described below.
- A **Clinical Application Case Study** opens each chapter with a patient-focused clinical scenario. Throughout the chapter, the reader is asked **critical thinking questions**

to apply chapter content, emphasizing a patient-centered and interdisciplinary approach to pharmacology.

- **Key Terms** with definitions help the reader understand the chapter's content.

Special Features

- **NEW! QSEN Safety Alerts**, presented in the context of the chapter discussion, alert the reader to important safety considerations and emphasize safety as a primary objective in patient care.
- **Black Box Warnings** highlight serious or life-threatening adverse effects identified by the FDA as being associated with a drug.
- **Drugs at a Glance Tables** summarize the routes and dosage ranges (for adults and for children), as well as the pregnancy category, for each drug in the class. The prototype drug is indicated with an icon.
- **NEW! Drug Interactions** and **Herb and Dietary Interactions** boxes highlight the risk of interactions as well as increased or decreased drug effects when drugs are combined with other medications, food, or herbal supplements.
- **Evidence-Based Practice** boxes provide information about current research and its integration into nursing practice. Updated for the 10th edition, these boxes present a summary of a recent study followed by implications for nursing.
- **Patient Teaching Guidelines** list specific information for the education of the patient and family.
- **Nursing Process** sections provide an overview of drug therapy in terms of assessment, nursing diagnosis, planning/goals, nursing interventions, and evaluation. Located at the end of the chapters, the nursing process provides the guidelines for nursing care specific to the disease process and related drug therapy.
- **NEW! NCLEX Success** sections interspersed throughout the chapter ask the student to answer NCLEX-style questions that pertain to the learning objectives and the information just presented. This feature helps students check and apply their knowledge as they read and helps them prepare for patient care and for the NCLEX.

Chapter Ending Features

- **Key Concepts** summarize the most salient content that appears in each chapter.
- **Critical Thinking Questions**, pertaining to one or two case studies, enhance the reader's understanding of chapter content.
- **References and Resources** provide sources on which content is based and direction for further reading.

Teaching/Learning Package

To facilitate mastery of this text's foundational content, a comprehensive teaching/learning package has been developed to assist faculty and students.

Resources for Instructors

Tools to assist with teaching this text are available upon its adoption on thePoint at http://thePoint.lww.com/Abrams10e.

- An **e-Book** on thePoint gives you access to the book's full text and images online.
- The **Test Generator** lets you put together exclusive new tests from a bank containing more than 1000 questions to help assess students' understanding of the material. Test questions are mapped to chapter learning objectives and page numbers.
- An extensive collection of materials is provided for each book chapter:
  - **Pre-Lecture Quizzes** (and answers) are quick, knowledge-based assessments that allow you to check students' reading comprehension.
  - **PowerPoint Presentations** provide an easy way for you to integrate the textbook with your students' classroom experience, either via slide shows or handouts. Multiple-choice and true/false questions are integrated into the presentations to promote class participation and allow you to use i-clicker technology.
  - **Guided Lecture Notes** walk you through the chapters, objective by objective, and provide you with corresponding PowerPoint slide numbers.
  - **Discussion Topics** (and suggested answers) can be used as conversation starters or in online discussion boards.
  - **Assignments** (and suggested answers) include group, written, clinical, and Web assignments.
  - **Case Studies** with related questions (and suggested answers) give students an opportunity to apply their knowledge to a client case similar to one they might encounter in practice.
- An **Image Bank** lets you use the photographs and illustrations from this textbook in your PowerPoint slides or as you see fit in your course.
- A sample **Syllabus** provides guidance for structuring your nursing pharmacology course.

Resources for Students

An exciting set of free resources is available to help students review material and become even more familiar with vital concepts. Students can access all these resources on thePoint at http://thePoint.lww.com/Abrams10e, using the codes printed in the front of their textbooks.

- An **e-Book** on thePoint allows access to the book's full text and images online.
- **NCLEX-Style Review Questions** for each chapter help students review important concepts and practice for NCLEX.
- **Concepts in Action Animations** bring physiologic and pathophysiologic concepts to life and enhance student comprehension.
- **Watch & Learn Video Clips** demonstrate nursing skills and appeal to visual and auditory learners.
- **Practice & Learn Activities** present case scenarios and offer interactive exercises and questions to help students apply what they have learned.

- **Journal Articles** for each book chapter offer access to current research available in Lippincott Williams & Wilkins journals.
- **Dosage Calculation Quizzes** provide opportunities for students to practice math skills and calculate drug dosages.
- A **Spanish–English Audio Glossary** provides helpful terms and phrases for communicating with patients who speak Spanish.

In addition, for on-the-go access to monographs for 100 of the most commonly prescribed drugs, students can download the free **Lippincott Nursing Drug Handbook App**, available for both Apple and Android devices. Based on the best-selling *Nursing2013 Drug Handbook*, this app is reviewed by pharmacists and nurses and updated weekly to provide the most current, relevant information that students and practicing nurses need.

Study Guide

Developed to complement this textbook, the *Study Guide for Abrams' Clinical Drug Therapy* engages students' interest and active participation by providing a variety of learning exercises and opportunities to practice cognitive skills. Each chapter of the Study Guide is organized into three sections. **Assessing Your Understanding** promotes the learning of concepts, principles, and characteristics and uses of major drug groups, and can be completed independently or by small groups as in-class learning activities. **Applying Your Knowledge** scenarios promote appropriate data collection, critical analysis of both drug- and patient-related data, and application of the data in patient care. **Practicing for NCLEX** provides NCLEX-style review questions to help students apply and retain the key information from each chapter.

Acknowledgments

This 10th edition builds on the decades of work and commitment by Anne Collins Abrams. We thank her for her legacy as we continue with the book's tradition. We acknowledge Mark Greaves, RPh, Jill Davidson, RPh, and Bisma Khan, PharmD, for answering numerous questions throughout the writing of this edition. We would like to thank Joy Harriman, MBA, MLS, DM/AHIP, for her assistance in organizing multiple chapters in the text and for providing evidence to support best practice in clinical drug therapy. We also wish to thank Martha Cushman, Developmental Editor, for her gifted expertise in editing. Her ability to put words together in a meaningful way is masterful.

Contents

SECTION 4
Drugs Affecting Inflammation and Infection

AVAILABLE ON thePoint

SECTION **1**

The Conceptual Framework of Pharmacology

1 Introduction to Pharmacology

Clinical Application Case Study

Joan Clark, a senior nursing student, is preparing for the NCLEX-RN examination. As she reviews material, she examines safeguards in place to protect the public from injury due to medication administration.

KEY TERMS

Biotechnology: process that may involve manipulating deoxyribonucleic acid (DNA) and ribonucleic acid (RNA) and recombining genes into hybrid molecules that can be inserted into living organisms (often *Escherichia coli* bacteria) and repeatedly reproduced

Brand (trade) name: manufacturer's chosen name for a drug, which is protected by a patent

Controlled substances: drugs that are categorized by federal law according to therapeutic usefulness and potential for abuse; also known as scheduled drugs

Drug classifications: groups of medications that are classified according to their effects on particular body systems, their therapeutic uses, and their chemical characteristics

Generic name: chemical or official name of the drug that is independent of the manufacturer and often indicates the drug group

Over-the-counter (OTC) drugs: medications available for purchase without a prescription

Pharmacoeconomics: costs of drug therapy, including costs of purchasing, dispensing, storage, administration, and laboratory and other tests used to monitor patient responses; also considers losses due to expiration

Pharmacotherapy: use of drugs to prevent, diagnose, or treat signs, symptoms, and disease processes

Placebo: inert substance containing no medication and given to reinforce a person's expectation to improve

Prescription drugs: medications that are ordered in writing by a licensed health care provider

Prototype: often the first drug of a particular drug class to be developed; usually the standard against which newer, similar drugs are compared

Introduction

Pharmacology is the study of drugs (chemicals) that alter functions of living organisms. **Pharmacotherapy**, also known as drug therapy, is the use of drugs to prevent, diagnose, or treat signs, symptoms, and diseases. When prevention or cure is not a reasonable goal, relief of symptoms can greatly improve a patient's quality of life and ability to perform activities of daily living. Contemporary nursing guidelines require that nurses keep safety issues in mind when involved in the practice of pharmacotherapy.

Drugs given for therapeutic purposes are also called medications. These substances may be given for their local or systemic effects. Drugs with local effects, such as sunscreen lotions and local anesthetics, act mainly at the site of application. Those with systemic effects are taken into the body, circulated through the bloodstream to their sites of action in various body tissues, and eventually eliminated from the body. Most drugs are given for their systemic effects. Drugs may also be given for acute disorders, such as pain or infection, or to relieve signs and symptoms of long-term disease processes, such as hypertension or diabetes.

Drug Sources

Historically, drugs came from plants, animals, and minerals. Now, most drugs are synthetic compounds manufactured in laboratories. Chemists, for example, often create useful new drugs by altering the chemical structure of existing drugs. Such techniques and other technologic advances have enabled the production of new drugs as well as synthetic versions of many drugs originally derived from plants and animals. Synthetic drugs are more standardized in their chemical characteristics, more consistent in their effects, and less likely to produce allergic reactions. Semisynthetic drugs (e.g., many antibiotics) are naturally occurring substances that have been chemically modified.

Biotechnology is also an important source of drugs. This process may involve manipulating deoxyribonucleic acid (DNA) and ribonucleic acid (RNA) and recombining genes into hybrid molecules that can be inserted into living organisms (*Escherichia coli* bacteria are often used), which can be repeatedly reproduced. Each hybrid molecule produces a genetically identical molecule, called a clone. Cloning makes it possible to identify the DNA sequence in a gene and to produce the protein product encoded by a gene, such as insulin. Cloning also allows production of adequate amounts of the drug for therapeutic or research purposes. Biotechnology drugs constitute an increasing percentage of drugs now undergoing development, and this trend is expected to continue into the foreseeable future.

Drug Classifications and Prototypes

Drugs are classified according to their effects on particular body systems, their therapeutic uses, and their chemical characteristics. For example, morphine can be classified as a central nervous system depressant and a narcotic or opioid analgesic. The names of therapeutic classifications usually reflect the conditions for which the drugs are used (e.g., antidepressants, antihypertensives). However, the names of many drug groups reflect their chemical characteristics rather than their therapeutic uses (e.g., adrenergics, benzodiazepines). Many drugs fit into multiple groups because they have wide-ranging effects on the human body.

An individual drug that represents groups of drugs is called a **prototype**. The prototype, often the first drug of a particular drug class to be developed, is usually the standard with which newer drugs in the class are compared. For example, morphine is the prototype of the opioid analgesics and penicillin is the prototype of the beta-lactam antibacterial drugs.

Drug classifications and prototypes are quite settled, and most new drugs can be assigned to a group and compared with an established prototype. However, some groups lack a universally accepted prototype, and some prototypes are replaced over time by newer, more commonly used drugs. In this text, information about the prototype is provided for each drug class.

Drug Names

Individual drugs may have several different names, but the two that are most commonly used are the generic (official) name and the brand (trade) name. The **generic name** (e.g., amoxicillin) is related to the chemical or official name and is independent of the manufacturer. The generic name often indicates the drug group (e.g., drugs with generic names ending in "cillin" are penicillins). In the United States, the United States Adopted Names Council assigns the generic name. The **brand (trade) name** is designated and patented by the manufacturer. For example, amoxicillin is manufactured by several pharmaceutical companies, some of which assign a specific trade name (e.g., Amoxil, Trimox) and several of which use only the generic name. In drug literature, trade names are capitalized and generic names are presented in lowercase unless in a list or at the beginning of a sentence. Drugs may be prescribed and dispensed by generic or trade name. Generic equivalents are available for the majority of drugs and can be substituted for trade-named drugs unless the prescriber requests the trade-named medication by writing "do not substitute" on the prescription. Generic drugs are required to be therapeutically equivalent and are less expensive than trade name drugs.

NCLEX Success

1. The nurse is caring for a woman who has strong beliefs about not putting anything unnatural into her body. It is most accurate to say that most modern medications are
   A. natural products derived from plants
   B. natural products derived from minerals
   C. synthetic products manufactured in laboratories
   D. synthetic modifications of natural products

2. The nurse is taking care of a man who is confused about the different medications he is prescribed. He notes that some of the drug names have changed over the course of time he has been taking them. When counseling him, it is most important to keep the following statement in mind:
   A. A drug can belong to only one group or classification.
   B. A prototype drug is the standard by which similar drugs are compared.
   C. Drug groups and prototypes change frequently, and knowledge about a prototype cannot guide knowledge about other drugs in the same class.
   D. The generic name of a drug changes among manufacturers.

Drug Marketing

A patent protects a new drug for several years, during which time only the pharmaceutical manufacturer that developed it can market it. The company views this protection as a return on its investment in developing the drug, which might have required years of work and millions of dollars, and as

an incentive to develop other drugs. Other pharmaceutical companies cannot manufacture and market the drug until the patent expires. However, for new drugs that are popular and widely used, other companies often produce similar drugs, with different generic and trade names.

Pharmacoeconomics

Pharmacoeconomics involves the costs of drug therapy, including costs of purchasing, dispensing (i.e., salaries of pharmacists, pharmacy technicians), storage, administration (i.e., salaries of nurses, costs of supplies), and laboratory and other tests used to monitor patient responses, as well as losses due to expiration. Length of illness or hospitalization is also a consideration. The goal of most pharmacoeconomic research is to identify drug therapy regimens that provide the desired benefits at the lowest cost.

Access to Drugs

Prescription and Nonprescription Drugs

Legally, American consumers have two ways to access therapeutic drugs. They can obtain them as **prescription drugs**, which require a written order. A licensed health care provider such as a physician, dentist, or nurse practitioner writes the prescription. Alternatively, they can purchase **over-the-counter (OTC) drugs**, which do not require a prescription. Various laws regulate these routes. Acquiring and using prescription drugs for nontherapeutic purposes by people who are not authorized to have the drugs or for whom they are not prescribed is illegal.

American Drug Laws and Standards

Current drug laws and standards have evolved over many years. Their main goal is to protect the public by ensuring that drugs marketed for therapeutic purposes are safe and effective. Table 1.1 further describes and summarizes the main provisions.

TABLE 1.1
American Drug Laws and Amendments

Year	Name	Main Provision(s)
1906	Pure Food and Drug Act	Established official standards and requirements for accurate labeling of drug products Established the forerunner of U.S. Food and Drug Administration (FDA)
1912	Shirley Amendment	Prohibited fraudulent claims of drug effectiveness
1914	Harrison Narcotic Act	Restricted the importation, manufacture, sale, and use of opium, cocaine, marijuana, and other drugs that the Act defined as narcotics
1938	Food, Drug, and Cosmetic Act	Revised and broadened FDA powers and responsibilities; gave the FDA control over drug safety Required proof of safety from the manufacturer before a new drug could be marketed Authorized factory inspections Established penalties for fraudulent claims and misleading labels

(Continued on page 6)

TABLE 1.1

American Drug Laws and Amendments (Continued)

Year	Name	Main Provision(s)
1945	Amendment	Required governmental certification of biologic products, such as insulin and antibiotics
1951	Durham-Humphrey Amendment	Designated drugs that must be prescribed by a physician and dispensed by a pharmacist (e.g., controlled substances, drugs considered unsafe for use except under supervision by a health care provider, and drugs limited to prescription use under a manufacturer's new drug application)
1962	Kefauver-Harris Amendment	Required a manufacturer to provide evidence (from well-controlled research studies) that a drug was effective for claims and conditions identified in the product's labeling Gave the federal government the authority to standardize drug names
1970	Comprehensive Drug Abuse Prevention and Control Act; Controlled Substance Act	Regulated distribution of narcotics and other drugs of abuse Categorized these drugs according to therapeutic usefulness and potential for abuse Title II, Controlled Substances Act Updated or replaced all previous laws regarding narcotics and other dangerous drugs
1978	Drug Regulation Reform Act	Established guidelines for research studies and data to be submitted to the FDA by manufacturers Shortened the time required to develop and market new drugs
1983	Orphan Drug Act	Decreased taxes and competition for manufacturers who would produce drugs to treat selected serious rare diseases
1987		Established new regulations designed to speed up the approval process for high-priority medications
1992	Prescription Drug User Fee Act	Allowed the FDA to collect user fees from pharmaceutical companies, with each new drug application, to shorten the review time (e.g., by hiring more staff) Specified a review time of 12 mo for standard drugs and 6 mo for priority drugs
1993	NIH Revitalization Act	Requires inclusion of women and minorities in NIH-funded research studies, including Phase III clinical drug trials
1997	FDA Modernization Act	Updated regulation of biologic products Increased patient access to experimental drugs and medical devices Accelerated review of important new drugs Allowed drug companies to disseminate information about off-label (non–FDA-approved) uses and costs of drugs Extended user fees
2002	Best Pharmaceuticals for Children Act	Encouraged pharmaceutical companies to conduct studies and label drugs for use in children Provided funds for 5 y for pediatric drug studies
2003	Medicare Prescription Drug Improvement and Modernization Act	Afforded the largest overhaul of Medicare in the 38-y history of the program Provided entitlement benefit for prescription drugs and other benefits for seniors and those with medical disabilities
2005	Combat Methamphetamine Epidemic Act	Established federal law that regulates retail over-the-counter sales of ephedrine, pseudoephedrine, and phenylpropanolamine products due to their use in the manufacturing of illegal drugs. Specifically, these drugs are: • Kept behind the counter or in a locked case • Limited in purchase to no more than 3.6 g a day and 9 g a month • Dispensed after purchasers produce identification and sign a sales log • Handled by employees who are properly trained Geared at curtailing clandestine production of methamphetamine
2008	Ryan Haight Online Pharmacy Consumer Protection Act	Applies to all controlled substances in all schedules Established federal law that it is illegal to deliver, distribute, or dispense a controlled substance by means of the Internet unless the online pharmacy holds a modification of DEA registration authorizing it to operate as an online pharmacy

DEA, Drug Enforcement Administration; FDA, U.S. Food and Drug Administration; NIH, National Institutes of Health.

The Food, Drug, and Cosmetic Act of 1938 and its amendments regulate the manufacture, distribution, advertising, and labeling of drugs. The law also requires that official drugs (i.e., those listed in the United States Pharmacopeia and designated USP) must meet standards of purity and strength as determined by chemical analysis or by animal response to specified doses (bioassay). The Durham-Humphrey Amendment designates drugs that must be prescribed by a licensed physician or nurse practitioner and dispensed by a pharmacist. The U.S. Food and Drug Administration (FDA) is charged with enforcing the law. In addition, the Public Health Service regulates vaccines and other biologic products, and the Federal Trade Commission can suppress misleading advertisements of nonprescription drugs.

The Comprehensive Drug Abuse Prevention and Control Act was passed in 1970. Title II of this law, called the Controlled Substances Act, regulates the manufacture and distribution of narcotics, stimulants, depressants, hallucinogens, and anabolic steroids and requires the pharmaceutical industry to maintain physical security and strict recordkeeping for these drugs and substances. These drugs are categorized according to therapeutic usefulness and potential for abuse (Box 1.1) and are labeled as **controlled substances** (e.g., morphine is a C-II or Schedule II drug).

The Drug Enforcement Administration (DEA) enforces the Controlled Substances Act. Individual people and companies legally empowered to handle controlled substances must be registered with the DEA, keep accurate records of all transactions, and provide for secure storage. The DEA assigns prescribers a number, which they must include on all prescriptions they write for a controlled substance. Prescriptions for Schedule II drugs cannot be refilled; a new prescription is required. Nurses are responsible for storing controlled substances in locked containers, administering them only to people for whom they are prescribed, recording each dose given on agency narcotic sheets and on the patient's medication administration record, maintaining an accurate inventory, and reporting discrepancies to the proper authorities.

In addition to federal laws, state laws also regulate the sale and distribution of controlled drugs. These laws may be more stringent than federal laws; if so, the stricter laws usually apply.

Drug Approval Processes: Food and Drug Administration

The FDA is responsible for ensuring that new drugs are safe and effective before approving the drugs and allowing them to be marketed. The FDA reviews research studies (usually conducted or sponsored by pharmaceutical companies) about proposed new drugs; the organization does not test the drugs.

Testing Procedure

Since 1962, newly developed drugs undergo extensive testing before being marketed for general use. Initially, drug testing occurs in animals, and the FDA reviews the test results. Next, researchers perform clinical trials in humans, usually with a randomized, controlled experimental design that involves selection of subjects according to established criteria, random assignment of subjects to experimental groups, and administration of the test drug to one group and a control substance to another group.

Testing proceeds through several phases if there is continuing evidence of drug safety and effectiveness. In Phase I, a few doses are given to a certain number of healthy volunteers to determine safe dosages, routes of administration, absorption, metabolism, excretion, and toxicity. In Phase II, a few doses are given to a certain number of subjects with the disease or symptom for which the drug is being studied, and responses are compared with those of healthy subjects. In Phase III, the drug is given to a larger and more representative group of subjects. In double-blind, placebo-controlled designs, half of the subjects receive the new drug and half receive a **placebo** (an inactive

---

BOX 1.1   Categories of Controlled Substances

Schedule I
Drugs that have no accepted medical use, lack of accepted safety, and have high abuse potentials: heroin, lysergic acid diethylamide (LSD), marijuana, methaqualone (Quaalude), 3,4-methylenedioxy-methamphetamine (MDMA or ecstasy), mescaline, peyote, tetrahydrocannabinol.

Schedule II
Drugs that are used medically and have high abuse potentials: opioid analgesics (e.g., codeine, hydromorphone, methadone, meperidine, morphine, oxycodone), central nervous system (CNS) stimulants (e.g., cocaine, methamphetamine, methylphenidate), and barbiturate sedative-hypnotics (amobarbital, pentobarbital, secobarbital).

Schedule III
Drugs with less potential for abuse than those in Schedules I and II, but abuse may lead to psychological or physical dependence: androgens and anabolic steroids, some depressants (e.g., ketamine, pentobarbital, zolazepam), some CNS stimulants (e.g., benzphetamine,

chlorphentermine), and mixtures containing small amounts of controlled substances (e.g., codeine, barbiturates not listed in other schedules). These drugs and substances have an accepted medical use in the United States.

Schedule IV
Drugs with an accepted medical use in the United States but with some potential for abuse: benzodiazepines (e.g., diazepam, lorazepam, temazepam), other sedative-hypnotics (e.g., phenobarbital, chloral hydrate), and some prescription appetite suppressants (e.g., mazindol, phentermine).

Schedule V
Products containing moderate amounts of controlled substances. They may be dispensed by the pharmacist without a physician's prescription but with some restrictions regarding amount, recordkeeping, and other safeguards. Included are cough suppressants containing small amounts of codeine and antidiarrheal drugs, such as diphenoxylate and atropine (Lomotil).

substance similar in appearance to the actual drug), with neither subjects nor researchers knowing who receives which formulation. In crossover studies, subjects serve as their own control; each subject receives the experimental drug during half of the study and a placebo during the other half. Other research methods include control studies in which some patients receive a known drug rather than a placebo; in subject matching, patients are paired with others of similar characteristics. Phase III studies help determine whether the potential benefits of the drug outweigh the risks. Testing may be stopped during any of the early phases if inadequate effectiveness or excessive toxicity becomes evident. In Phase IV, the FDA evaluates the data from the first three phases for drug safety and effectiveness, allows the drug to be marketed for general use, and requires manufacturers to continue monitoring the drug's effects.

Historically, drug research involved mainly young, white males. In 1993, Congress passed the National Institutes of Health (NIH) Revitalization Act, which formalized a policy of the NIH that women and minorities be included in human subject research studies funded by the NIH and that women and minorities be included in clinical drug trials. Now, major drug trials must recruit female subjects and include outcome data on women. In addition, all newly developed drugs must include gender-related effectiveness and safety information in the initial FDA application. Knowledge about the drug effects in women has increased but is still relatively limited because many commonly used drugs were developed before enactment of these regulations.

Subsequent withdrawal of some approved and marketed drugs (e.g., Vioxx) may occur, usually because of serious adverse effects that become evident only when the drugs are used in a large, diverse population. In addition, in recent years, the FDA has issued warnings about several drugs that can cause serious adverse effects (e.g., antidepressants, nonsteroidal anti-inflammatory drugs [NSAIDs] such as aspirin and ibuprofen, and oseltamivir [Tamiflu], an antiflu drug). As a result, the FDA has received criticism for approving these and other drugs and allowing them to be marketed in the first place. Some authorities are urging major reforms in the drug approval process, the methods of reporting adverse drug effects, and postmarketing surveillance procedures.

Drug Approval

The FDA approves many new drugs annually. New drugs are categorized according to their review priority and therapeutic potential. A status of "1P" indicates a new drug reviewed on a priority (accelerated) basis and with some therapeutic advantages over drugs already available. A status of "1S" indicates standard review and drugs with few, if any, therapeutic advantages (i.e., the new drug is similar to one or more older drugs currently on the market). Most new drugs are "1S" prescription drugs.

The FDA also approves drugs for OTC availability, including the transfer of drugs from prescription to OTC status, and may require additional clinical trials to determine the safety and effectiveness of OTC use. For prescription drugs taken orally, transfer to OTC status may mean different indications for use and lower doses. FDA approval of a drug for OTC availability involves evaluation of evidence that the consumer can use the drug safely, using information on the product label, and

shifts primary responsibility for safe and effective drug therapy from health care professionals to consumers. With prescription drugs, a health care professional diagnoses the condition, often with the help of laboratory and other diagnostic tests, and determines a need for the drug. With OTC drugs, the patient must make these decisions, with or without consultation with a health care provider.

Having drugs available over the counter has potential advantages and disadvantages for consumers. Advantages include greater autonomy, faster and more convenient access to effective treatment, possibly earlier resumption of usual activities of daily living, fewer visits to a health care provider, and possibly increased efforts by consumers to learn about their symptoms/conditions and recommended treatments. Disadvantages include inaccurate self-diagnoses and potential risks of choosing a wrong or contraindicated drug, delayed treatment by a health care professional, and development of adverse drug reactions and interactions. When a drug is switched from prescription to OTC status, sales and profits of pharmaceutical companies increase and costs of insurance companies decrease. Costs to consumers increase because health insurance policies do not cover OTC drugs.

Clinical Application 1-1

Ms. Clark analyzes drug safety, including the national organizations charged with ensuring it.

- What is the role of the U.S. Food and Drug Administration (FDA) in the drug approval process?
- What is the role of the Drug Enforcement Administration (DEA) and the nurse with regard to controlled substances?

NCLEX Success

3. In understanding the use of controlled substances for patients, it is important that the nurse knows that controlled drugs are
   A. categorized according to prescription or nonprescription status
   B. regulated by state and local laws more than federal laws
   C. those that must demonstrate high standards of safety
   D. scheduled according to medical use and potential for abuse

4. A patient is asking what the difference is between a prescription for 800 mg of a medication that can be purchased on an OTC basis as a 200-mg tablet. To address this issue, it is important that the nurse knows that OTC drugs
   A. are considered safe for any consumer to use
   B. are not available for treatment of most commonly occurring symptoms
   C. often differ in indications for use and recommended dosages from their prescription versions
   D. are paid for by most insurance policies

Safety in Drug Administration

At least 1.5 million preventable adverse drug events costing more than four billion dollars occur in the health care system each year (Institute of Medicine [IOM]). As described previously, multiple safeguards to promote drug safety in packaging, drug laws, and approval processes are in place. Just as critical are safeguards to promote the safe administration of drugs at the point of care.

Rights of Medication Administration

Patient safety with medication administration begins by adhering to the rights of medication administration. The 7 traditional rights of medication administration (right drug, right dose, right patient, right route, right time, right reason, and right documentation) now include additional rights that should also be

considered (right education, right evaluation, and right to refuse the medication). These rights are goals of the medication administration process, and discussion of the effort to reduce medication errors and harm has expanded over the years. However, the focus on rights has been on the nurse and not the system in which medication administration takes place. Chapter 3 discussed the medication rights and their application to the nursing process.

New technology in medication administration has expanded required competencies for safe medication administration. Electronic charting, automated drug dispensing systems, and barcode medication administration have required enhanced nursing skills to manage these complex systems. The entire process of medication administration in a hospital is distracting, causing the nurse to lose focus on the task at hand; multiple interruptions and the extended hours that nurses work inevitably lead to the possibility of unintended consequences.

EVIDENCE-BASED PRACTICE

Shaping Systems for Better Behavioral Choices: Lessons Learned from a Fatal Medication Error

by J. SMETZER, C. BAKER, F. D. BYRNE, M. R. COHEN

Joint Commission Journal on Quality and Patient Safety/Joint Commission Resources
2010, 36(4), 152–163.

The researchers reported on an infusion intended exclusively for the epidural route, which was connected to a pregnant woman's peripheral intravenous line and infused by pump in a birthing suite. Complications developed, and although cesarean section resulted in the delivery of a healthy infant, the mother died from cardiovascular collapse. Media publicity called attention to the error when a nurse was charged with a criminal offense. The hospital's medication and safety procedures were analyzed using a root cause analysis. An external review team evaluated the organization's medication system and processes, patterns of staffing, leadership, and institutional culture; identified problems; and suggested improvements. Enhance safety initiatives included team training for staff working in the birthing suites, implementing consistent procedures for scanning-adherence tracking, and streamlining the barcode scanning tracking of medications.

IMPLICATIONS FOR NURSING PRACTICE: This incident identified system gaps and process failures within an organization that led to the death of a patient. Prudent nursing actions support an organization's culture of safety by complying with processes (safety nets and fail-safe mechanisms) that are aimed at preventing and/or reducing environmental effects to prevent medication errors.

QSEN Safety Alert

Error-reduction strategies during medication administration include

- *Having a "quiet zone" to prepare medications*
- *Placing "quiet zone" signs at the entrance to the medication room or above the automated medication dispensing system*
- *Following protocols and checklist outlining medication administration*
- *Wearing a sash or vest to signal others to avoid interrupting the nurse during medication administration*
- *Educating staff to reduce interruptions of nurses administering medications*

Multiple national strategies have been implemented to reduce medication errors since the seminal work of the IOM (1999), which highlighted the breadth of preventable medical errors in the U.S. Examining human factors and the response of nurses to workflow changes and technology have led to more successful system design, operation, and usability.

Quality and Safety Education for Nurses Project

The Quality and Safety Education for Nurses (QSEN) project, sponsored by the Robert Wood Johnson Foundation, is committed to the continuous improvement in the quality and safety of health care systems by focusing on the needed knowledge, skills, and attitudes (KSA) required in the preparation of future nurses in six areas: patient-centered care, teamwork and collaboration, evidence-based practice, quality improvement, safety, and informatics. Using the IOM competencies for nursing, QSEN faculty outlined prelicensure and graduate quality and safety competencies for nursing. Additionally, recommended targets for the KSA that need to be developed in prelicensure nursing students for each competency have been established. The QSEN competencies are highlighted throughout the text as they relate to medication administration.

Two of the QSEN competencies, safety and patient-centered care, are frequently emphasized. Safety factors reduce risk of

TABLE 1.2

Quality and Safety Education for Nurses (QSEN) Safety Competency

Knowledge	Skills	Attitudes
Examines human factors and other basic safety design principles as well as commonly used unsafe practices (such as work-arounds and dangerous abbreviations) Describes the benefits and limitations of selected safety-enhancing technologies (such as, barcodes, computer provider order entry, medication pumps, and automatic alerts/alarms) Discusses effective strategies to reduce reliance on memory	Demonstrates effective use of technology and standardized practices that support safety and quality Demonstrates effective use of strategies to reduce risk of harm to self or others Uses appropriate strategies to reduce reliance on memory (such as forcing functions, checklists)	Values the contributions of standardization/reliability to safety Appreciates the cognitive and physical limits of human performance
Delineates general categories of errors and hazards in care Describes factors that create a culture of safety (such as, open communication strategies and organizational error reporting systems)	Communicates observations or concerns related to hazards and errors to patients, families, and the health care team Uses organizational error reporting systems for near miss and error reporting	Values own role in preventing errors
Describes processes used in understanding causes of error and allocation of responsibility and accountability (such as root cause analysis and failure mode effects analysis)	Participates appropriately in analyzing errors and designing system improvements Engages in root cause analysis rather than blaming when errors or near misses occur	Values vigilance and monitoring (even of own performance of care activities) by patients, families, and other members of the health care team
Discusses potential and actual impact of national patient safety resources, initiatives, and regulations	Uses national patient safety resources for own professional development and to focus attention on safety in care settings	Values relationship between national safety campaigns and implementation in local practices and practice settings

Reprinted from Cronenwett, L., Sherwood, G., Barnsteiner, J., Disch, J., Johnson, J., Mitchell, P., et al. (Copyright 2007) Quality and safety education for nurses. *Nursing Outlook, 55*(3), 122–131, with permission from Elsevier.

harm to patients and providers through individual performance and system effectiveness. Patient-centered care engages the patient or designee as a full partner and source of control in administering coordinated, compassionate care; the care is based on respect for patient's preferences, values, and needs. Tables 1.2 and 1.3, respectively, outline these competencies.

National Patient Safety Goals

The Joint Commission is also concerned with implementing strategies to enhance safety and annually updates targeted patient safety goals related to medication safety. Outlined below are two areas of particular interest to medication administration safety.

"Do Not Use" List of Abbreviations

QSEN Safety Alert

The Joint Commission published a Sentinel Event Alert in 2001 regarding medical abbreviations. Since then, this organization has developed a standardized list of abbreviations, acronyms, dose designations, and symbols that are not to be used in a health care organization.

Table 1.4 lists these terms. This list was developed as part of the requirements for meeting one of the National Patient Safety goals.

Targeted High-Risk Activities

The Joint Commission also requires performance measures related to safety in drug administration. Specifically, a health care facility must demonstrate safe medication management using risk-reduction activities with medication labeling and use of anticoagulant medications.

In the perioperative area and other procedural settings, all medications must be labeled in syringes and basins if transferred from the original packaging. This practice focuses on an identified risk point in medication administration.

Health care institutions that provide anticoagulant therapy must establish a defined process that has a positive impact on patient safety with this class of medications (see Chap. 7) and leads to better outcomes. It is necessary to develop a process for anticoagulant use related to education, standardized ordering,

TABLE 1.3

Quality and Safety Education for Nurses (QSEN) Patient-Centered Care Competency

Knowledge	Skills	Attitudes
Integrate understanding of multiple dimensions of patient-centered care: • patient/family/community preferences, values • coordination and integration of care • information, communication, and education • physical comfort and emotional support • involvement of family and friends • transition and continuity Describe how diverse cultural, ethnic, and social backgrounds function as sources of patient, family, and community values	Elicit patient values, preferences, and expressed needs as part of clinical interview, implementation of care plan, and evaluation of care Communicate patient values, preferences, and expressed needs to other members of health care team Provide patient-centered care with sensitivity and respect for the diversity of human experience	Value seeing health care situations "through patients' eyes" Respect and encourage individual expression of patient values, preferences, and expressed needs Value the patient's expertise with own health and symptoms Seek learning opportunities with patients who represent all aspects of human diversity Recognize personally held attitudes about working with patients from different ethnic, cultural, and social backgrounds Willingly support patient-centered care for individuals and groups whose values differ from own
Demonstrate comprehensive understanding of the concepts of pain and suffering, including physiologic models of pain and comfort	Assess the presence and extent of pain and suffering Assess levels of physical and emotional comfort Elicit expectations of patient and family for relief of pain, discomfort, or suffering Initiate effective treatments to relieve pain and suffering in light of patient values, preferences, and expressed needs	Recognize personally held values and beliefs about the management of pain or suffering Appreciate the role of the nurse in relief of all types and sources of pain or suffering Recognize that patient expectations influence outcomes in management of pain or suffering
Examine how the safety, quality, and cost-effectiveness of health care can be improved through the active involvement of patients and families Examine common barriers to active involvement of patients in their own health care processes Describe strategies to empower patients or families in all aspects of the health care process	Remove barriers to presence of families and other designated surrogates based on patient preferences Assess level of patient's decisional conflict and provide access to resources Engage patients or designated surrogates in active partnerships that promote health, safety and well-being, and self-care management	Value active partnership with patients or designated surrogates in planning, implementation, and evaluation of care Respect patient preferences for degree of active engagement in care process Respect patient's right to access to personal health records
Explore ethical and legal implications of patient-centered care Describe the limits and boundaries of therapeutic patient-centered care	Recognize the boundaries of therapeutic relationships Facilitate informed patient consent for care	Acknowledge the tension that may exist between patient rights and the organizational responsibility for professional, ethical care Appreciate shared decision making with empowered patients and families, even when conflicts occur
Discuss principles of effective communication Describe basic principles of consensus building and conflict resolution Examine nursing roles in ensuring coordination, integration, and continuity of care	Assess own level of communication skill in encounters with patients and families Participate in building consensus or resolving conflict in the context of patient care Communicate care provided and needed at each transition in care	Value continuous improvement of own communication and conflict resolution skills

TABLE 1.4

Official "Do Not Use" List*

Do Not Use	Potential Problem	Use Instead
U (unit)	Mistaken for "0" (zero), the number "4" (four), or "cc"	Write "unit"
IU (International Unit)	Mistaken for IV (intravenous) or the number 10 (ten)	Write "International Unit"
Q.D., QD, q.d., qd (daily)	Mistaken for each other	Write "daily"
Q.O.D., QOD, q.o.d, qod (every other day)	Period after the Q mistaken for "I" and the "O" mistaken for "I"	Write "every other day"
Trailing zero (X.0 mg)† Lack of leading zero (.X mg)	Decimal point is missed	Write X mg Write 0.X mg
MS	Can mean morphine sulfate or magnesium sulfate	Write "morphine sulfate"
MSO_4 and $MgSO_4$	Confused with one another	Write "magnesium sulfate"

*This list applies to all orders and all medication-related documentation that is handwritten (including free-text computer entry) or on preprinted forms.

†**Exception:** A "trailing zero" may be used only where required to demonstrate the level of precision of the value being reported, such as for laboratory results, imaging studies that report size of lesions, or catheter/tube sizes. It may not be used in medication orders or other medication-related documentation.

Source: Copyright 2011, The Joint Commission. http://www.jointcommission.org. © The Joint Commission, 2011. Reprinted with permission.

dispensing, administration, and monitoring. Routine short-term use of anticoagulants for prevention of venous thromboembolism is not included as an element of performance when it is expected that the patient's laboratory values will remain within or close to normal limits with the therapy.

High-Alert Medications

The Institute for Safe Medication Practices (ISMP) identifies drugs that when used in error have a heightened risk of causing significant patient harm.

QSEN Safety Alert ❗

To reduce the chance of errors, strategies such as automatic alerts, limited access, expanded education related to the drugs, and standardizations of processes are important.

Box 1.2 lists drug classes and specific drugs that appear on the ISMP high-alert list.

Pregnancy Categories for Safety

As discussed in detail in Chapter 2, pregnancy categories identify risk of fetal injury due to drug therapy if used as directed by the mother during pregnancy. Each drug in this text contains the associated pregnancy category in the Drugs at a Glance tables. The categories range from A (safest) to X (known danger). The categories do not account for potential harm from drugs or their metabolites found in breast milk.

Beers Criteria

The Beers Criteria, a list of medications that are generally considered inappropriate when given to elderly people, confirms

that toxic medication effects and drug-related problems affect the safety of the elderly. For a wide variety of reasons, the medications listed tend to cause adverse effects in the elderly due to the physiologic changes of aging. Thirty percent of hospital admissions by older adults are linked to drug reactions. Further discussion of the Beers Criteria, including the medications on the list and strategies used to identify age-related changes associated with drug administration, is found in Chapter 5.

NCLEX Success

5. A man is very upset with a drug recall of a medication he has been taking for a long time. He states that he feels like he can no longer trust anyone to protect him. In response to his questions about the process of drug development, it is important to know that with a new drug, the U.S. Food and Drug Administration (FDA) is responsible for

   A. testing the drug with animals
   B. testing the drug with healthy people
   C. marketing the drug to health care providers
   D. evaluating the drug for safety and effectiveness

6. Error-reduction strategies during medication administration include (choose all that apply)

   A. quiet zone signs at entrance to the medication room
   B. protocols and checklist outlining medication administration
   C. wearing of a sash or vest to signal others to avoid interruptions of the nurse during medication administration
   D. carrying several patients' prescanned medications on a tray

---

BOX 1.2   High-Alert Medications

Classes/Categories of Medications

Adrenergic agonists, IV (e.g., epinephrine, phenylephrine, norepinephrine)

Adrenergic antagonists, IV (e.g., propranolol, metoprolol, labetalol)

Anesthetic agents, general, inhaled and IV (e.g., propofol, ketamine)

Antidysrhythmics, IV (e.g., lidocaine, amiodarone)

Antithrombotic agents (anticoagulants), including warfarin, low-molecular-weight heparin, IV unfractionated heparin, factor Xa inhibitors (fondaparinux), direct thrombin inhibitors (e.g., argatroban, lepirudin, bivalirudin), thrombolytics (e.g., alteplase, reteplase, tenecteplase), and glycoprotein IIb/IIIa inhibitors (e.g., eptifibatide)

Cardioplegic solutions

Chemotherapeutic agents, parenteral and oral

Dextrose, hypertonic, 20% or greater

Dialysis solutions, peritoneal and hemodialysis

Epidural or intrathecal medications

Hypoglycemics, oral

Inotropic medications, IV (e.g., digoxin, milrinone)

Insulin, subcutaneous and IV

Liposomal forms of drugs (e.g., liposomal amphotericin B)

Moderate sedation agents, IV (e.g., midazolam)

Moderate sedation agents, oral, for children (e.g., chloral hydrate)

Narcotics/opiates, IV, transdermal, and oral (including liquid concentrates, immediate and sustained-release formulations)

Neuromuscular blocking agents (e.g., succinylcholine, rocuronium, vecuronium)

Radiocontrast agents, IV

Sodium chloride for injection, hypertonic (greater than 0.9% concentration)

Sterile water for injection, inhalation, and irrigation (excluding pour bottles) in containers of 100 mL or more

Total parenteral nutrition solutions

Specific Medications

Epoprostenol (Flolan), IV

Magnesium sulfate injection

Methotrexate, oral, nononcologic use

Opium tincture

Oxytocin, IV

Nitroprusside sodium for injection

Potassium chloride for injection concentrate

Potassium phosphate injection

Promethazine, IV

Vasopressin, IV or intraosseous

From the Institute for Safe Medication Practices (ISMP). ISMP's List of High-Alert Medications. http://www.ismp.org/Tools/highalert-medications.pdf

---

Sources of Drug Information

Sources of drug information include pharmacology and other textbooks, drug reference books, journal articles, and Internet sites. Textbooks provide information regarding groups of drugs in relation to therapeutic uses. Drug reference books are most helpful concerning individual drugs. Two authoritative sources are (1) the *American Hospital Formulary Service*, published by the American Society of Health-System Pharmacists and updated periodically and (2) *Drug Facts and Comparisons*, published by the Facts and Comparisons division of Lippincott Williams & Wilkins and updated monthly (loose-leaf edition) or annually (hardbound edition). A less authoritative source is the *Physicians' Desk Reference* (PDR), published yearly, which compiles manufacturers' package inserts for selected drugs.

Numerous drug handbooks (e.g., *Lippincott's Nursing Drug Guide*, published annually) and pharmacologic, medical, and nursing journals also contain information about drugs. Textbook chapters and journal articles often present information about drug therapy for patients with specific disease processes and may thereby facilitate application of drug knowledge in clinical practice.

Internet sites also contain drug information, but it is essential to assess their quality. A wide variety of information, ranging in accuracy, reliability, and value, is easily accessible. The website for Lippincott's *Nursing Drug Guide* is a reliable clinical resource for drug information (see *References and Resources*).

Clinical Application 1-2

Ms. Clark also reviews additional strategies to promote the system safety in the administration of drugs at the point of care.

- What systemic issues in a hospital or nursing home have an impact on safe medication administration?

- What can the nurse do to avoid medication errors while dispensing medications?

Strategies for Studying Pharmacology

- Concentrate on therapeutic classifications and their prototypes. For example, morphine is the prototype of opioid analgesics (see Chap. 48). Understanding morphine makes learning about other opioid analgesics easier because they are compared with morphine.

- Compare a newly encountered drug with a prototype or similar drug when possible. Relating the unknown to the known aids learning and retention of knowledge.

- Try to understand how the drug acts in the body. This understanding allows prediction of therapeutic effects and prediction, prevention, or minimization of adverse effects by early detection and treatment.

- Concentrate study efforts on major characteristics. Such characteristics include the main indications for use, common and potentially serious adverse effects, conditions in which the drug is contraindicated or must be used cautiously, and related nursing care needs.
- Keep an authoritative, up-to-date drug reference readily available. A drug reference is a more reliable source of drug information than memory, especially for dosage ranges. Use the reference freely when learning about an unfamiliar drug or when answering a question about a familiar one. Also, nurses have access to computerized databases of drug information through multiple electronic sources, and these can provide a ready source of up-to-date information.

- Use your own words when taking notes or writing drug information cards. Also, write notes, answers to review questions, definitions of new terms, and trade names of drugs encountered in clinical practice settings directly into your pharmacology textbook. The mental processing required for these activities helps in both initial learning and later retention and application of knowledge.
- Rehearse applying drug knowledge in nursing care by asking (yourself), "What if I have a patient who is receiving this drug? What must I do to safely administer the drug? For what must I assess the patient before giving the drug and for what must I observe in the patient after drug administration? What if my patient is an elderly person or a child?"

Key Concepts

- Drug therapy or pharmacotherapy is the use of drugs to prevent, diagnose, or treat signs, symptoms, and disease processes.
- Drugs given for therapeutic purposes are called medications.
- Drugs may be given for local or systemic effects; most are given for systemic effects.
- A prototype is an example of a group of drugs, often the first one of the group to be developed.
- Trade names of drugs are determined by manufacturers; generic names are independent of manufacturers.
- Controlled drugs are categorized according to therapeutic usefulness and potential for abuse.
- Electronic charting, automated drug dispensing systems, and barcode medication administration require enhanced nursing skills to manage administration of drugs in the clinical setting.
- Observe for the 7 rights of medication administration (right drug, right dose, right patient, right route, right time, right reason, and right documentation).
- Error-reduction strategies that prevent and/or reduce environmental effects can assist in preventing medication errors.

Critical Thinking Questions

1-1. A discussion in the first day of a pharmacology class concerns developing strategies for studying pharmacology.

- Why is it important to concentrate on therapeutic classifications and their prototypes?
- Why is it important to understand the physiology related to a drug's action?

References and Resources

Cronenwett, L., Sherwood, G., Barnsteiner J., Disch, J., Johnson, J., Mitchell, P., et al. (2007). Quality and safety education for nurses. *Nursing Outlook, 55*(3), 122–131.

DiPiro, J., Talbert, R. Yee, G., Matzke, G., Wells, B., & Posey. L. M. (Eds.). (2011). *Pharmacotherapy: A pathophysiologic approach* (8th ed.). New York, NY: McGraw-Hill.

Fick, D. M., Cooper, J. W., Wade, W. E., Waller, J. L., Maclean, J. R., & Beers, M. (2003). Updating the Beers criteria for potentially inappropriate medication use in older adults results of a US panel of experts. *Archives of Internal Medicine, 10,* 761–768. Available at http://archinte.ama-assn.org/cgi/reprint/163/22/2716

Furberg, C. D., Levin, A. A., Gross, P. A., Shapiro, R. S., & Strom, B. L. (2006). The FDA and drug safety: A proposal for sweeping changes. *Archives of Internal Medicine, 166,* 1938–1942.

Institute for Safe Medication Practices. http://www.ismp.org

Institute of Medicine. (2003). *Health professions education: A bridge to quality.* Washington, DC: National Academies Press.

Institute of Medicine. (2007). *Preventing medication errors.* Washington, DC: National Academies Press.

The Joint Commission. http://www.jointcommission.org

Karch AM. *2011 Lippincott's Nursing Drug Guide*. Philadelphia, PA: Lippincott Williams & Wilkins. http://www.NursingDrugGuide.com

Quality and Safety Education for Nurses (QSEN). http://www.qsen.org

Smetzer, J., Baker, C., Byrne, F. D., & Cohen, M. R. (2010). Shaping systems for better behavioral choices: Lessons learned from a fatal medication error. *Joint Commission Journal on Quality and Patient Safety/Joint Commission Resources*, 36(4), 152–163.

The Joint Commission. (2011). *National patient safety goals*. Retrieved May 12, 2011, from http://www.jointcommission.org/standards_information/npsgs.aspx

U.S. Food and Drug Administration. *Frequently asked questions*. Retrieved January 1, 2011, from http://www.fda.gov/opacom/faqs/faqs.html

2 Basic Concepts and Processes

LEARNING OBJECTIVES

After studying this chapter, you should be able to:

1. Discuss cellular physiology in relation to drug therapy.
2. Describe the main pathways and mechanisms by which drugs cross biologic membranes and move through the body.
3. Explain each process of pharmacokinetics.
4. Discuss the clinical usefulness of measuring serum drug levels.
5. Describe major characteristics of the receptor theory of drug action.
6. Differentiate between agonist drugs and antagonist drugs.
7. List drug-related and patient-related variables that affect drug actions.
8. Discuss mechanisms and potential effects of drug–drug interactions.
9. Identify signs and symptoms that may occur with adverse drug effects on major body systems.
10. Discuss general management of drug overdose and toxicity.
11. Discuss selected drug antidotes.

Clinical Application Case Study

Doris Green, an 89-year-old widow with cardiovascular and renal disease, takes a number of medications, including three medications to control her hypertension. She has recently switched to a new antihypertensive medication. She prides herself on being independent and able to manage on her own, despite failing memory and failing health.

You, as a home health nurse, visit Mrs. Green to assess the therapeutic and adverse effects of her antihypertensive medications and her adherence to the prescribed medical regimen. You plan to measure her blood pressure to check that it is within normal limits (for Mrs. Green), as well as assess her understanding of her antihypertensive medications and dosing regimen.

KEY TERMS

Absorption: process that occurs from the time a drug enters the body to the time it enters the bloodstream to be circulated

Agonist: drug that produces effects similar to those produced by naturally occurring hormones, neurotransmitters, and other substances

Antagonist: drug that inhibits cell function by occupying receptor sites

Antidote: substance that relieves, prevents, or counteracts the effect of a poison

Bioavailability: portion of a drug dose that reaches the systemic circulation and is available to act on body cells

Biotransformation: when drugs are altered from their original form into a new form by the body; also referred to as metabolism

Distribution: transport of drug molecules within the body; after a drug is injected or absorbed into the bloodstream, it is carried by the blood and tissue fluids to its sites of action, metabolism, and excretion

Enterohepatic recirculation: drugs or metabolites that are excreted in bile, reabsorbed from the small intestine, returned to the liver, metabolized, and eventually excreted in urine.

Enzyme induction: production of larger amounts of drug-metabolizing enzymes by liver cells; process accelerates drug metabolism because larger amounts of the enzymes (and more binding sites) allow larger amounts of a drug to be metabolized during a given time

Enzyme inhibition: process in which a molecule binds to enzymes and inhibits their activity

Excretion: elimination of a drug from the body; effective excretion requires adequate functioning of the circulatory system and of the organs of excretion (kidneys, bowel, lungs, and skin)

First-pass effect: initial metabolism of some oral drugs as they are carried from the intestine to the liver by the portal circulatory system prior to reaching the systemic circulation for distribution to site of action

Hypersensitivity: immune-mediated reaction to a drug

Loading dose: dose larger than the regular prescribed daily dosage of a medication; used to attain a therapeutic blood level

Maintenance dose: quantity of drug that is needed to keep blood levels and/or tissue levels at a steady state or constant level

Nephrotoxicity: toxic or damaging effect of a substance on the kidney; potentially serious because renal damage interferes with drug excretion, causing drug accumulation and increased adverse effects

Pharmacodynamics: reactions between living systems and drugs; drug actions on target cells and the resulting alterations in cellular biochemical reactions and functions

Pharmacokinetics: drug movement through the body to reach sites of action, metabolism, and excretion

Prodrugs: initially inactive drugs that exert no pharmacologic effects until they are metabolized

Serum drug level: laboratory measurement of the amount of a drug in the blood at a particular time

Serum half-life: time required for the serum concentration of a drug to decrease by 50%; also called elimination half-life

Introduction

All body functions, disease processes, and most drug actions occur at the cellular level. Drugs are chemicals that alter basic processes in body cells. They can stimulate or inhibit normal cellular functions; however, they cannot change the type of function that occurs normally. To act on body cells, drugs given for systemic effects must reach adequate concentrations in the blood and other tissue fluids surrounding the cells. Thus, they must enter the body and be circulated to their sites of action (target cells). After they act on cells, they must be eliminated from the body.

How do systemic drugs reach, interact with, and leave body cells? How do people respond to drugs? The answers to these questions are derived from cellular physiology, pathways and mechanisms of drug transport, pharmacokinetics, pharmacodynamics, and other basic concepts and processes that form the foundation of rational drug therapy and the content of this chapter.

Cellular Physiology

Cells are dynamic, busy "factories" (Box 2.1, Fig. 2.1) that take in raw materials, manufacture products required to maintain bodily functions, and deliver those products to their appropriate destinations in the body. Although cells differ from one tissue to another, their common characteristics include the ability to

- Exchange materials with their immediate environment
- Obtain energy from nutrients
- Synthesize hormones, neurotransmitters, enzymes, structural proteins, and other complex molecules
- Reproduce
- Communicate with one another via various biologic chemicals, such as neurotransmitters and hormones

BOX 2.1	Cell Structures and Functions

Protoplasm, which constitutes the internal environment of body cells, is composed of water, electrolytes (potassium, magnesium, phosphate, sulfate, bicarbonate), proteins, lipids, and carbohydrates. **Water** makes up 70% to 85% of most cells; cellular enzymes, electrolytes, and other chemicals are dissolved or suspended in the water. **Electrolytes** provide chemicals for cellular reactions and are required for some processes (e.g., transmission of electrochemical impulses in nerve and muscle cells). **Proteins** consist of "physical" proteins that form the structure of cells and "chemical" proteins that function mainly as enzymes within the cell. **Lipids**, mainly phospholipids and cholesterol, form the membranes that separate structures inside the cell and the cell itself from surrounding cells and body fluids. **Carbohydrates** play a major role in cell nutrition. Glucose is present in extracellular fluid and is readily available to supply the cell's need for energy. In addition, a small amount of carbohydrate is stored within the cell as glycogen, which can be rapidly converted back to glucose when needed.

The **nucleus** regulates the types and amounts of proteins, enzymes, and other substances to be produced. The **cytoplasm** surrounds the nucleus and contains the working units of the cell. The **cytosol**, the clear fluid portion of the cytoplasm, contains dissolved proteins, electrolytes, and glucose. The **endoplasmic reticulum (ER)** contains ribosomes, which synthesize proteins, including enzymes that synthesize glycogen, triglycerides, and steroids and those that metabolize drugs and other chemicals. The ER is also important in the production of hormones by glandular cells and the production of plasma proteins by liver cells. Most proteins produced by the ribosomes are released into the cytosol where they act as enzymes or structural proteins of the cell. The **Golgi complex** stores the substances produced by the ER. It also packages these substances into secretory granules, which then move out of the Golgi complex into the cytoplasm and, after a stimulus, are released from the cell. **Mitochondria** generate energy for cellular activities and require oxygen. **Lysosomes** are membrane-enclosed vesicles that contain enzymes capable of digesting nutrients (proteins, carbohydrates, fats), damaged cellular structures, foreign substances (e.g., bacteria), and the cell itself. When

a cell becomes worn out or damaged, the membrane around the lysosome breaks and the enzymes (hydrolases) are released. However, lysosomal contents also are released into extracellular spaces and may destroy surrounding cells. Normally, the enzymes are inactivated by enzyme inhibitors, and excessive tissue destruction is prevented.

The **cell membrane**, a complex structure of phospholipids, proteins, cholesterol, and carbohydrates, separates intracellular contents from the extracellular environment; provides receptors for hormones and other biologically active substances; participates in electrical events that occur in nerve and muscle cells; and helps regulate growth and proliferation.

The cell membrane covers the entire surface of the cell and consists of a thin, double layer of lipids interspersed with proteins. The lipid layer is composed of phospholipid (fatty acid and phosphate) molecules. The proteins are usually combined with a carbohydrate and called glycoproteins. Some proteins provide structural pores through which water and water-soluble substances (e.g., sodium, potassium, and calcium ions) can diffuse between extracellular and intracellular fluids. Other proteins act as carriers to transport substances through the cell membrane. Still others act to regulate intracellular function or as enzymes to catalyze chemical reactions within the cell.

Carbohydrates in the cell membrane occur mainly in combination with proteins (glycoproteins) or lipids (glycolipids). Glycoproteins (composed of carbohydrate around a small, inner core of protein and called proteoglycans) often are attached to and cover the entire outside surface of the cell. As a result, the carbohydrate molecules are free to interact with extracellular substances and perform several important functions. First, many have a negative electrical charge that repels other negatively charged substances. Second, the "carbohydrate coat" of some cells attaches to the carbohydrate coat of other cells and thereby connects cells to each other. Third, many of the carbohydrates act as receptor molecules for binding hormones (e.g., insulin). The receptor–hormone combination then activates the attached inner core of protein to perform its enzymatic or other functions in the cell.

Drug Transport Through Cell Membranes

Drugs must reach and interact with or cross the cell membrane to stimulate or inhibit cellular function. Most drugs are given to affect body cells that are distant from the sites of administration (i.e., systemic effects). To move through the body and reach their sites of action, metabolism, and excretion (Fig. 2.2), drug molecules must cross numerous cell membranes. For example, molecules of most oral drugs must cross the membranes of cells in the gastrointestinal (GI) tract, liver, and capillaries to reach the bloodstream, circulate to their target cells, leave the bloodstream and attach to receptors on cells, perform their action, return to the bloodstream, circulate to the liver, reach drug-metabolizing enzymes in liver cells, reenter the bloodstream (usually as

metabolites), circulate to the kidneys, and be excreted in urine. Box 2.2 and Figure 2.3 describe the transport pathways and mechanisms used to move drug molecules through the body.

Pharmacokinetics

Pharmacokinetics involves drug movement through the body (i.e., "what the body does to the drug") to reach sites of action, metabolism, and excretion. Specific processes are absorption, distribution, metabolism, and excretion. Metabolism and excretion are often grouped together as drug elimination or clearance mechanisms. Overall, these processes largely determine serum drug levels; onset, peak, and duration of drug actions; therapeutic and adverse effects; and other important aspects of drug therapy.

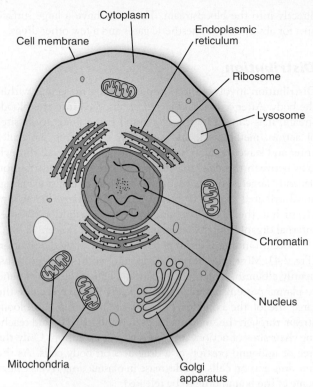

Figure 2.1 Cytoplasmic organelles of the cell.

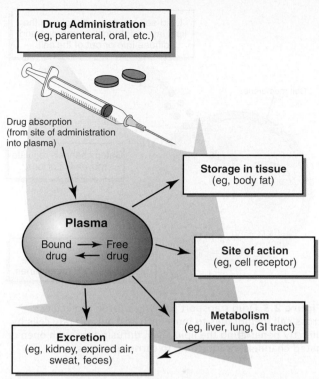

Figure 2.2 Entry and movement of drug molecules through the body to sites of action, metabolism, and excretion.

Absorption

Absorption is the process that occurs from the time a drug enters the body to the time it enters the bloodstream to be circulated. Onset of drug action is largely determined by the rate of absorption; intensity is determined by the extent of absorption.

Numerous factors affect the rate and extent of drug absorption, including dosage form, route of administration, blood flow to the site of administration, GI function, the presence of food or other drugs, and other variables. Dosage form is a major determinant of a drug's **bioavailability** (the portion of a dose that

---

BOX 2.2	Drug Transport Pathways and Mechanisms

Pathways

There are three main pathways of drug movement across cell membranes. The most common pathway is **direct penetration** of the membrane by lipid-soluble drugs, which are able to dissolve in the lipid layer of the cell membrane. Most systemic drugs are formulated to be lipid soluble so they can move through cell membranes, even oral tablets and capsules that must be sufficiently water soluble to dissolve in the aqueous fluids of the stomach and small intestine.

A second pathway involves passage through **protein channels** that go all the way through the cell membrane. Only a few drugs are able to use this pathway because most drug molecules are too large to pass through the small channels. Small ions (e.g., sodium and potassium) use this pathway, but their movement is regulated by specific channels with a gating mechanism (a flap of protein that opens briefly to allow ion movement and then closes).

The third pathway involves **carrier proteins** that transport molecules from one side of the cell membrane to the other. All of the carrier proteins are selective in the substances they transport; a drug's chemical structure determines which carrier will transport it.

Mechanisms

Once absorbed into the body, drugs are transported to and from target cells by passive diffusion, facilitated diffusion, and active transport.

Passive diffusion, the most common mechanism, involves movement of a drug from an area of higher concentration to one of lower concentration. For example, after oral administration, the initial concentration of a drug is higher in the gastrointestinal tract than in the blood. This promotes movement of the drug into the bloodstream. When the drug is circulated, the concentration is higher in the blood than in body cells, so that the drug moves (from capillaries) into the fluids surrounding the cells or into the cells themselves. Passive diffusion continues until a state of equilibrium is reached between the amount of drug in the tissues and the amount in the blood.

Facilitated diffusion is a similar process, except that drug molecules combine with a carrier substance, such as an enzyme or other protein.

In **active transport**, drug molecules are moved from an area of lower concentration to one of higher concentration. This process requires a carrier substance and the release of cellular energy.

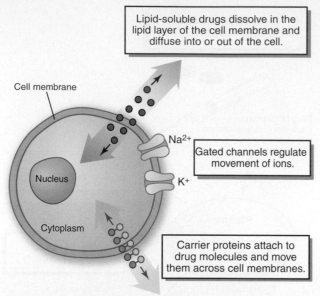

Lipid-soluble drugs dissolve in the lipid layer of the cell membrane and diffuse into or out of the cell.

Cell membrane

Na²⁺

Gated channels regulate movement of ions.

Nucleus

K⁺

Cytoplasm

Carrier proteins attach to drug molecules and move them across cell membranes.

Figure 2.3 Drug transport pathways. Drug molecules cross cell membranes to move into and out of body cells by directly penetrating the lipid layer, diffusing through open or gated channels, or attaching to carrier proteins.

reaches the systemic circulation and is available to act on body cells). An intravenous (IV) drug is virtually 100% bioavailable. In contrast, an oral drug is virtually always less than 100% bioavailable because some of it is not absorbed from the GI tract and some goes to the liver and is partially metabolized before reaching the systemic circulation.

Most oral drugs must be swallowed, dissolved in gastric fluid, and delivered to the small intestine (which has a large surface area for absorption of nutrients and drugs) before they are absorbed. Liquid medications are absorbed faster than tablets or capsules because they need not be dissolved. Rapid movement through the stomach and small intestine may increase drug absorption by promoting contact with absorptive mucous membrane; it also may decrease absorption because some drugs may move through the small intestine too rapidly to be absorbed. For many drugs, the presence of food in the stomach slows the rate of absorption and may decrease the amount of drug absorbed.

Drugs injected into subcutaneous (subcut) or intramuscular (IM) tissues are usually absorbed more rapidly than oral drugs because they move directly from the injection site to the bloodstream. Absorption is rapid from IM sites because muscle tissue has an abundant blood supply. Drugs injected intravenously do not need to be absorbed because they are placed directly into the bloodstream.

Other absorptive sites include the skin, mucous membranes, and lungs. Most drugs applied to the skin are given for local effects (e.g., sunscreens). Systemic absorption is minimal from intact skin but may be considerable when the skin is inflamed or damaged. Also, some drugs are formulated in adhesive skin patches for absorption through the skin (e.g., clonidine, fentanyl, nitroglycerin). Some drugs applied to mucous membranes also are given for local effects. However, systemic absorption occurs from the mucosa of the oral cavity, nose, eye, vagina, and rectum. Drugs absorbed through mucous membranes pass

directly into the bloodstream. The lungs have a large surface area for absorption of anesthetic gases and a few other drugs.

Distribution

Distribution involves the transport of drug molecules within the body. After a drug is injected or absorbed into the bloodstream, it is carried by the blood and tissue fluids to its sites of action, metabolism, and excretion. Most drug molecules enter and leave the bloodstream at the capillary level, through gaps between the cells that form capillary walls. Distribution depends largely on the adequacy of blood circulation. Drugs are distributed rapidly to organs receiving a large blood supply, such as the heart, liver, and kidneys. Distribution to other internal organs, muscle, fat, and skin is usually slower.

Protein binding is an important factor in drug distribution (Fig. 2.4). Most drugs form a compound with plasma proteins, mainly albumin, which act as carriers. Drug molecules bound to plasma proteins are pharmacologically inactive because the large size of the complex prevents their leaving the bloodstream through the small openings in capillary walls and reaching their sites of action, metabolism, and excretion. Only the free or unbound portion of a drug acts on body cells. As the free drug acts on cells, the decrease in plasma drug levels causes some of the bound drug to be released.

Protein binding allows part of a drug dose to be stored and released as needed. Some drugs also are stored in muscle, fat, or other body tissues and released gradually when plasma drug levels fall. These storage mechanisms maintain lower, more consistent blood levels and reduce the risk of toxicity. Drugs that are highly bound to plasma proteins or stored extensively in other tissues have a long duration of action.

Drug distribution into the central nervous system (CNS) is limited because the blood–brain barrier, which is composed of capillaries with tight walls, limits movement of drug molecules into brain tissue. This barrier usually acts as a selectively permeable membrane to protect the CNS. However, it also can make drug therapy for CNS disorders more difficult because drugs must pass through cells of the capillary wall rather than

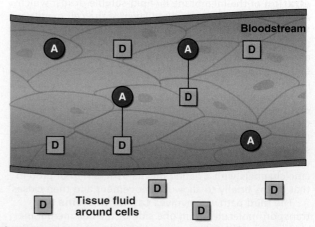

Figure 2.4 Plasma proteins, mainly albumin (A), act as carriers for drug molecules (D). Bound drug (A–D) stays in the bloodstream and is pharmacologically inactive. Free drug (D) can leave the bloodstream and act on body cells.

between cells. As a result, only drugs that are lipid soluble or have a transport system can cross the blood–brain barrier and reach therapeutic concentrations in brain tissue.

Drug distribution during pregnancy and lactation is also an important consideration (see Chap. 6). During pregnancy, most drugs cross the placenta and may affect the fetus. During lactation, many drugs enter breast milk and may affect the nursing infant.

Metabolism

Metabolism, or **biotransformation,** is the method by which drugs are inactivated or biotransformed by the body. Most often, an active drug is changed into inactive metabolites, which are then excreted. Some active drugs yield metabolites that are also active and that continue to exert their effects on body cells until they are metabolized further or excreted. Other drugs (called **prodrugs**) are initially inactive and exert no pharmacologic effects until they are metabolized. Most drugs are lipid soluble, a characteristic that aids their movement across cell membranes. However, the kidneys can excrete only water-soluble substances. Therefore, one function of metabolism is to convert fat-soluble drugs into water-soluble metabolites. Hepatic drug metabolism or clearance is a major mechanism for terminating drug action and eliminating drug molecules from the body.

Most drugs are metabolized by cytochrome P450 (CYP) enzymes in the liver. Red blood cells, plasma, kidneys, lungs, and GI mucosa also contain drug-metabolizing enzymes. The CYP system consists of several groups of enzymes, some of which metabolize endogenous substances and some of which metabolize drugs. The drug-metabolizing groups are labeled CYP1, CYP2, and CYP3. Individual members of the groups usually metabolize specific drugs; more than one enzyme participates in the metabolism of some drugs. In terms of importance in drug metabolism, the CYP3A4 enzymes are thought to metabolize about 50% of drugs; CYP2D6 enzymes about 25%; CYP2C8/9 about 15%; and CYP1A2, 2C19, 2A6, and 2E1 in decreasing order for the remaining 10%.

CYP enzymes are complex proteins with binding sites for drug molecules (and endogenous substances). They catalyze the chemical reactions of oxidation, reduction, hydrolysis, and conjugation with endogenous substances, such as glucuronic acid or sulfate. With chronic administration, some drugs stimulate liver cells to produce larger amounts of drug-metabolizing enzymes. This **enzyme induction** accelerates drug metabolism because larger amounts of the enzymes (and more binding sites) allow larger amounts of a drug to be metabolized during a given period. As a result, larger doses of the rapidly metabolized drug may be required to produce or maintain therapeutic effects. Rapid metabolism may also increase the production of toxic metabolites with some drugs (e.g., acetaminophen). Drugs that induce enzyme production also may increase the rate of metabolism for endogenous steroidal hormones (e.g., cortisol, estrogens, testosterone, vitamin D). However, enzyme induction does not occur for 1 to 3 weeks after an inducing agent is started, because new enzyme proteins must be synthesized.

Metabolism also can be decreased or delayed in a process called **enzyme inhibition**, which most often occurs with concurrent administration of two or more drugs that compete for the same metabolizing enzymes. In this case, smaller doses of the slowly metabolized drug may be needed to avoid adverse effects and toxicity from drug accumulation. Enzyme inhibition occurs within hours or days of starting an inhibiting agent. Cimetidine, a gastric acid suppressor, inhibits several CYP enzymes (e.g., 1A, 2C, 2D, 3A) and can greatly decrease drug metabolism. The rate of drug metabolism also is reduced in infants (their hepatic enzyme system is immature), in people with impaired blood flow to the liver or severe hepatic or cardiovascular disease, and in people who are malnourished or on low-protein diets.

When drugs are given orally, they are absorbed from the GI tract and carried to the liver through the portal circulation. Some drugs are extensively metabolized in the liver, with only part of a drug dose reaching the systemic circulation for distribution to sites of action. This is called the **first-pass effect** or presystemic metabolism.

Excretion

Excretion refers to elimination of a drug from the body. Effective excretion requires adequate functioning of the circulatory system and of the organs of excretion (kidneys, bowel, lungs, and skin). Most drugs are excreted by the kidneys and eliminated (unchanged or as metabolites) in the urine. Some drugs or metabolites are excreted in bile and then eliminated in feces; others are excreted in bile, reabsorbed from the small intestine, returned to the liver (called **enterohepatic recirculation**), metabolized, and eventually excreted in urine. Some oral drugs are not absorbed and are excreted in the feces. The lungs mainly remove volatile substances, such as anesthetic gases. The skin has minimal excretory function. Factors impairing excretion, especially severe renal disease, lead to accumulation of numerous drugs and may cause severe adverse effects if dosage is not reduced.

NCLEX Success

1. A nurse practitioner (NP) has just changed a patient's medication from an oral form to a patch formulation to avoid the first-pass effect. The NP has explained it to the patient, but the patient still has questions and asks the nurse to explain again what is meant by the first-pass effect. The NP would be most correct in explaining that this has to do with how
   A. drugs initially bind to plasma proteins
   B. initial renal function is involved in drug excretion
   C. the way drugs first reach their target cells
   D. initial metabolism of an oral drug occurs before it reaches the systemic circulation

2. A nurse is reading a research report about use of a medication that describes the pharmacokinetics of a particular medication that a patient is taking. Pharmacokinetics involves
   A. drug effects on human cells
   B. drug binding with receptors
   C. drug absorption, distribution, metabolism, and elimination
   D. drug stimulation of normal cell functions

3. **A nurse is caring for a man who has worsening liver disease. In monitoring his medication, it is important to know that a patient with liver disease may have impaired drug**

   A. absorption
   B. distribution
   C. metabolism
   D. excretion

Serum Drug Levels

A **serum drug level** is a laboratory measurement of the amount of a drug in the blood at a particular time (Fig. 2.5). It reflects dosage, absorption, bioavailability, half-life, and the rates of metabolism and excretion. A minimum effective concentration (MEC) must be present before a drug exerts its pharmacologic action on body cells; this is largely determined by the drug dose and how well it is absorbed into the bloodstream. A toxic concentration is a level at which toxicity occurs; what is toxic for some patients is not toxic for others (see subsequent discussion). Toxic concentrations may stem from a single large dose, repeated small doses, or slow metabolism that allows the drug to accumulate in the body. Between these low and high concentrations is the therapeutic range, which is the goal of drug therapy—that is, enough drug to be beneficial but not enough to be toxic.

For most drugs, serum levels indicate the onset, peak, and duration of drug action. When a single dose of a drug is given, onset of action occurs when the drug level reaches the MEC. The drug level continues to climb as more of the drug is absorbed, until it reaches its highest concentration and peak drug action occurs. Then, drug levels decline as the drug is eliminated (i.e., metabolized and excreted) from the body. Although there may still be numerous drug molecules in the body, drug action stops when drug levels fall below the MEC. The duration of action is the time during which serum drug levels are at or above the MEC. When multiple doses of a drug are given (e.g., for chronic conditions), the goal is usually to give sufficient doses often enough to maintain serum drug levels in the therapeutic range and avoid the toxic range.

In clinical practice, measuring serum drug levels is useful in several circumstances:

- When drugs with a narrow margin of safety are given, because their therapeutic doses are close to their toxic doses (e.g., digoxin, aminoglycoside antibiotics, lithium)
- To document the serum drug levels associated with particular drug dosages, therapeutic effects, or possible adverse effects
- To monitor unexpected responses to a drug dose such as decreased therapeutic effects or increased adverse effects
- When a drug overdose is suspected

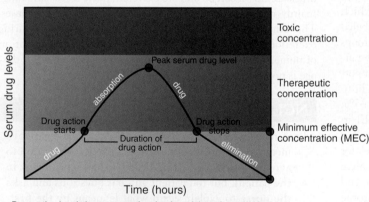

Drug action in relation to serum drug levels and time after a single dose.

A

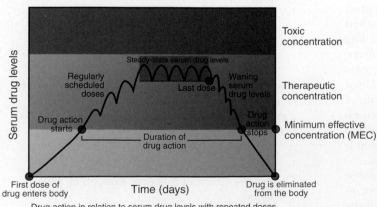

Drug action in relation to serum drug levels with repeated doses.

B

Figure 2.5 Serum drug levels with single (**A**) and multiple (**B**) oral drug doses. Drug action starts when enough drug is absorbed to reach the minimum effective concentration (MEC), continues as long as the serum level is above the MEC, wanes as drug molecules are metabolized and excreted (if no more doses are given), and stops when the serum level drops below the MEC. The goal of drug therapy is to maintain serum drug levels in the therapeutic range.

Serum Half-Life

Serum half-life, also called elimination half-life, is the time required for the serum concentration of a drug to decrease by 50%. It is determined primarily by the drug's rates of metabolism and excretion. A drug with a short half-life requires more frequent administration than one with a long half-life.

When a drug is given at a stable dose, four or five half-lives are required to achieve steady-state concentrations and to develop equilibrium between tissue and serum concentrations. Because maximal therapeutic effects do not occur until equilibrium is established, some drugs are not fully effective for days or weeks. To maintain steady-state conditions, the amount of drug given must equal the amount eliminated from the body. When a drug dose is changed, an additional four to five half-lives are required to reestablish equilibrium; when a drug is discontinued, it is eliminated gradually over several half-lives.

Pharmacodynamics

Pharmacodynamics involves drug actions on target cells and the resulting alterations in cellular biochemical reactions and functions (i.e., "what the drug does to the body").

Receptor Theory of Drug Action

Like the physiologic substances (e.g., hormones, neurotransmitters) that normally regulate cell functions, most drugs exert their effects by chemically binding with receptors at the cellular level (Fig. 2.6). Most receptors are proteins located on the surfaces of cell membranes or within cells. Specific receptors include enzymes involved in essential metabolic or regulatory processes (e.g., dihydrofolate reductase, acetylcholinesterase); proteins involved in transport (e.g., sodium–potassium adenosine triphosphatase) or structural processes (e.g., tubulin); and

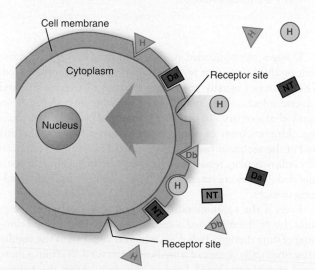

Figure 2.6 Cell membrane contains receptors for physiologic substances such as hormones (H) and neurotransmitters (NT). These substances stimulate or inhibit cellular function. Drug molecules (Da and Db) also interact with receptors to stimulate or inhibit cellular function.

nucleic acids (e.g., DNA) involved in cellular protein synthesis, reproduction, and other metabolic activities.

When drug molecules bind with receptor molecules, the resulting drug–receptor complex initiates physiochemical reactions that stimulate or inhibit normal cellular functions. One type of reaction involves activation, inactivation, or other alterations of intracellular enzymes. Because enzymes catalyze almost all cellular functions, drug-induced changes can markedly increase or decrease the rate of cellular metabolism. For example, an epinephrine–receptor complex increases the activity of the intracellular enzyme adenyl cyclase, which then causes the formation of cyclic adenosine monophosphate (cAMP). In turn, cAMP can initiate any one of many different intracellular actions, the exact effect depending on the type of cell.

A second type of reaction involves changes in the permeability of cell membranes to one or more ions. The receptor protein is a structural component of the cell membrane, and its binding to a drug molecule may open or close ion channels. In nerve cells, for example, sodium or calcium ion channels may open and allow movement of ions into the cell. This movement usually causes the cell membrane to depolarize and excite the cell. At other times, potassium channels may open and allow movement of potassium ions out of the cell. This action inhibits neuronal excitability and function. In muscle cells, movement of the ions into the cells may alter intracellular functions, such as the direct effect of calcium ions in stimulating muscle contraction.

A third reaction may modify the synthesis, release, or inactivation of the neurohormones (e.g., acetylcholine, norepinephrine, serotonin) that regulate many physiologic processes. Box 2.3 describes additional elements and characteristics of the receptor theory.

Nonreceptor Drug Actions

Relatively few drugs act by mechanisms other than combination with receptor sites on cells. Drugs that do not act on receptor sites include the following:

- Antacids, which act chemically to neutralize the hydrochloric acid produced by gastric parietal cells and thereby raise the pH of gastric fluid
- Osmotic diuretics (e.g., mannitol), which increase the osmolarity of plasma and pull water out of tissues into the bloodstream
- Drugs that are structurally similar to nutrients required by body cells (e.g., purines, pyrimidines) and that can be incorporated into cellular constituents, such as nucleic acids, which interfere with normal cell functioning. Several anticancer drugs act by this mechanism.
- Metal chelating agents, which combine with toxic metals to form a complex that can be more readily excreted

Variables that Affect Drug Actions

Historically, expected responses to drugs were based on those occurring when a particular drug was given to healthy adult men (18–65 years of age) of average weight (150 lb [70 kg]). However, other groups (e.g., women, children, older adults,

---

BOX 2.3   Additional Elements of the Receptor Theory of Drug Action

■ The site and extent of drug action on body cells are determined primarily by specific characteristics of receptors and drugs. Receptors vary in type, location, number, and functional capacity. For example, many different types of receptors have been identified. Most types occur in most body tissues, such as receptors for epinephrine (whether received from stimulation of the sympathetic nervous system or administration of drug formulations) and receptors for growth hormone, thyroid hormone, and insulin. Some occur in fewer body tissues, such as receptors for opioids in the brain and subgroups of receptors for epinephrine in the heart (beta$_1$-adrenergic receptors) and lungs (beta$_2$-adrenergic receptors). Receptor type and location influence drug action. The receptor is often described as a lock into which the drug molecule fits as a key, and only those drugs able to bond chemically to the receptors in a particular body tissue can exert pharmacologic effects on that tissue. Thus, all body cells do not respond to all drugs, even though virtually all cell receptors are exposed to any drug molecules circulating in the bloodstream.

The number of receptor sites available to interact with drug molecules also affects the extent of drug action. Drug molecules must occupy a minimal number of receptors to produce pharmacologic effects. Thus, if many receptors are available but only a few are occupied by drug molecules, few drug effects occur. In this instance, increasing the drug dosage increases the pharmacologic effects. Conversely, if only a few receptors are available for many drug molecules, receptors may be saturated. In this instance, if most receptor sites are occupied, increasing the drug dosage produces no additional pharmacologic effect.

Drugs vary even more widely than receptors. Because all drugs are chemical substances, chemical characteristics determine drug actions and pharmacologic effects. For example, a drug's chemical structure affects its ability to reach tissue fluids around a cell and bind with its cell receptors. Minor changes in drug structure may pro-

duce major changes in pharmacologic effects. Another major factor is the concentration of drug molecules that reach receptor sites in body tissues. Drug-related and patient-related variables that affect drug actions are further described later in this chapter.

■ When drug molecules chemically bind with cell receptors, pharmacologic effects result from agonism or antagonism. **Agonists** are drugs that produce effects similar to those produced by naturally occurring hormones, neurotransmitters, and other substances. Agonists may accelerate or slow normal cellular processes, depending on the type of receptor activated. For example, epinephrine-like drugs act on the heart to increase the heart rate, and acetylcholine-like drugs act on the heart to slow the heart rate; both are agonists. **Antagonists** are drugs that inhibit cell function by occupying receptor sites. This strategy prevents natural body substances or other drugs from occupying the receptor sites and activating cell functions. After drug action occurs, drug molecules may detach from receptor molecules (i.e., the chemical binding is reversible), return to the bloodstream, and circulate to the liver for metabolism and the kidneys for excretion.

■ Receptors are dynamic cellular components that can be synthesized by body cells and altered by endogenous substances and exogenous drugs. For example, prolonged stimulation of body cells with an excitatory agonist usually reduces the number or sensitivity of receptors. As a result, the cell becomes less responsive to the agonist (a process called receptor desensitization or down-regulation). Prolonged inhibition of normal cellular functions with an antagonist may increase receptor number or sensitivity. If the antagonist is suddenly reduced or stopped, the cell becomes excessively responsive to an agonist (a process called receptor up-regulation). These changes in receptors may explain why some drugs must be tapered in dosage and discontinued gradually if withdrawal symptoms are to be avoided.

---

different ethnic or racial groups, patients with diseases or symptoms that the drugs are designed to treat) receive drugs and respond differently from healthy adult men. As a result, newer clinical trials include more representatives of these groups. In any patient, however, responses may be altered by both drug-related and patient-related variables.

Drug-Related Variables

Dosage

Dosage refers to the frequency, size, and number of doses; it is a major determinant of drug actions and responses, both therapeutic and adverse. If the amount is too small or administered infrequently, no pharmacologic action occurs because the drug does not reach an adequate concentration at target cells. If the amount is too large or administered too often, toxicity (poisoning) may occur. Overdosage may occur with a single large dose or with chronic ingestion of smaller doses.

Dosages recommended in drug literature are usually those that produce particular responses in 50% of the people tested. These dosages usually produce a mixture of therapeutic and adverse effects. The dosage of a particular drug depends on many characteristics of the drug (reason for use, potency, pharmacokinetics, route of administration, dosage form, and so on) and of the recipient (age; weight; state of health; and function of cardiovascular, renal, and hepatic systems). Thus, recommended dosages are intended only as guidelines for individualizing dosages.

Even if the recommended dose controls a patient's symptoms, he or she may need a special **loading dose** at the beginning of drug therapy. This dose, which is larger than the regular prescribed daily dosage of a medication, is used to attain a more rapid therapeutic blood level of the drug. After the patient has been taking the drug for a few days, a **maintenance dose,** or quantity of drug that is needed to keep blood levels and/or tissue levels at a steady state, or constant level, is usually sufficient.

Route of Administration

Routes of administration affect drug actions and patient responses largely by influencing absorption and distribution. For rapid drug action and response, the IV route is most effective because the drug is injected directly into the bloodstream. For some drugs, the IM route also produces drug action within a few minutes because muscles have a large blood supply. The oral route usually produces slower drug action than parenteral routes. Absorption and action of topical drugs vary according to the drug formulation, whether the drug is applied to skin or mucous membranes, and other factors.

Drug–Diet Interactions

A few drugs are used therapeutically to decrease food absorption in the intestinal tract. For example, orlistat (Xenical) decreases absorption of fats from food and is given to promote weight loss, and ezetimibe (Zetia) decreases absorption of cholesterol from food and is given to lower serum cholesterol levels. However, most drug–diet interactions are undesirable because food often slows absorption of oral drugs by slowing gastric emptying time and altering GI secretions and motility.

QSEN Safety Alert

Giving medications 1 hour before or 2 hours after a meal can minimize interactions that decrease drug absorption.

In addition, some foods contain certain substances that react with certain drugs. One such interaction occurs between tyramine-containing foods and monoamine oxidase (MAO) inhibitor drugs. Tyramine causes the release of norepinephrine, a strong vasoconstrictive agent, from the adrenal medulla and sympathetic neurons. Normally, norepinephrine is quickly inactivated by MAO. However, because MAO inhibitor drugs prevent inactivation of norepinephrine, ingesting tyramine-containing foods with an MAO inhibitor may produce severe hypertension or intracranial hemorrhage. MAO inhibitors include the antidepressants isocarboxazid and phenelzine and the antiparkinson drugs rasagiline and selegiline.

QSEN Safety Alert

Tyramine-rich foods to be avoided by patients taking MAO inhibitors include aged cheeses, sauerkraut, soy sauce, tap or draft beers, and red wines.

Another interaction may occur between warfarin (Coumadin), an oral anticoagulant, and foods containing vitamin K. Because vitamin K antagonizes the action of warfarin, large amounts of spinach and other green leafy vegetables may offset the anticoagulant effects and predispose the person to thromboembolic disorders.

A third interaction occurs between tetracycline, an antibiotic, and dairy products, such as milk and cheese. The drug combines with the calcium in milk products to form a nonabsorbable compound that is excreted in the feces.

Still another interaction involves grapefruit. Grapefruit contains a substance that strongly inhibits the metabolism of drugs normally metabolized by the CYP3A4 enzyme. This effect greatly increases the blood levels of some drugs (e.g., the widely used "statin" group of cholesterol-lowering drugs) and the effect lasts for several days. Patients who take medications metabolized by the 3A4 enzyme should be advised against eating grapefruit or drinking grapefruit juice.

Drug–Drug Interactions

The action of a drug may be increased or decreased by its interaction with another drug in the body. Most interactions occur whenever the interacting drugs are present in the body; some, especially those affecting the absorption of oral drugs, occur when the interacting drugs are taken at or near the same time. The basic cause of many drug–drug interactions is altered drug metabolism. For example, drugs metabolized by the same enzymes compete for enzyme binding sites, and there may not be enough binding sites for two or more drugs. Also, some drugs induce or inhibit the metabolism of other drugs. Protein binding is also the basis for some important drug–drug interactions.

Interactions that can increase the therapeutic or adverse effects of drugs include the following:

- Additive effects, which occur when two drugs with similar pharmacologic actions are taken (e.g., ethanol + sedative drug increases sedative effects)
- Synergism, which occurs when two drugs with different sites or mechanisms of action produce greater effects when taken together (e.g., acetaminophen [nonopioid analgesic] + codeine [opioid analgesic] increases analgesic effects)
- Interference by one drug with the metabolism of a second drug, which may result in intensified effects of the second drug. For example, cimetidine inhibits CYP1A, 2C, and 3A drug-metabolizing enzymes in the liver and therefore interferes with the metabolism of many drugs (e.g., benzodiazepine antianxiety and hypnotic drugs, several cardiovascular drugs). When these drugs are given concurrently with cimetidine, they are likely to cause adverse and toxic effects because blood levels of the drugs are higher. The overall effect is the same as taking a larger dose of the drug whose metabolism is inhibited or slowed.
- Displacement (i.e., a drug with a strong attraction to protein-binding sites may displace a less tightly bound drug) of one drug from plasma protein-binding sites by a second drug, which increases the effects of the displaced drug. This increase occurs because the displaced drug, freed from its bound form, becomes pharmacologically active. The overall effect is the same as taking a larger dose of the displaced drug. For example, aspirin displaces warfarin and increases the drug's anticoagulant effects.

Interactions in which drug effects are decreased include the following:

- An **antidote** drug, which can be given to antagonize the toxic effects of another drug. For example, naloxone is commonly used to relieve respiratory depression caused by morphine and related drugs. Naloxone molecules displace morphine molecules from their receptor sites on nerve cells in the brain so that the morphine molecules cannot continue to exert their depressant effects.

- Decreased intestinal absorption of oral drugs, which occurs when drugs combine to produce nonabsorbable compounds. For example, drugs containing aluminum, calcium, or magnesium bind with oral tetracycline (if taken at the same time) to decrease its absorption and therefore its antibiotic effect.
- Activation of drug-metabolizing enzymes in the liver, which increases the metabolism rate of any drug metabolized mainly by that group of enzymes and therefore decreases the drug's effects. Several drugs (e.g., phenytoin, rifampin) and cigarette smoking are known enzyme inducers.

Patient-Related Variables

Age

The effects of age on drug action are especially important in neonates, infants, and older adults. In children, drug action depends largely on age and developmental stage.

During pregnancy, drugs cross the placenta and may harm the fetus. Fetuses have no effective mechanisms for eliminating drugs because their liver and kidney functions are immature. Newborn infants (birth to 1 month) also handle drugs inefficiently. Drug distribution, metabolism, and excretion differ markedly in neonates, especially premature infants, because their organ systems are not fully developed. Older infants (1 month to 1 year) reach approximately adult levels of protein binding and kidney function, but liver function and the blood–brain barrier are still immature.

Children (1–12 years) have a period of increased activity of drug-metabolizing enzymes so that some drugs are rapidly metabolized and eliminated. Although the onset and duration of this period are unclear, a few studies have been done with particular drugs. Theophylline, for example, is eliminated much faster in a 7-year-old child than in a neonate or adult (18–65 years). After about 12 years of age, healthy children handle drugs similarly to healthy adults.

In older adults (65 years and older), physiologic changes may alter all pharmacokinetic processes. Changes in the GI tract include decreased gastric acidity, decreased blood flow, and decreased motility. Despite these changes, however, there is little difference in drug absorption. Changes in the cardiovascular system include decreased cardiac output and therefore slower distribution of drug molecules to their sites of action, metabolism, and excretion. In the liver, blood flow and metabolizing enzymes are decreased. Thus, many drugs are metabolized more slowly, have a longer action, and are more likely to accumulate with chronic administration. In the kidneys, there is decreased blood flow, decreased glomerular filtration rate, and decreased tubular secretion of drugs. All these changes tend to slow excretion and promote accumulation of drugs in the body. Impaired kidney and liver function greatly increase the risks of adverse drug effects. In addition, older adults are more likely to have acute and chronic illnesses that require the use of multiple drugs or long-term drug therapy. Thus, possibilities for interactions among drugs and between drugs and diseased organs are greatly multiplied.

Body Weight

Body weight affects drug action mainly in relation to dose. The ratio between the amount of drug given and body weight influences drug distribution and concentration at sites of action.

In general, people who are heavier than average may need larger doses, provided that their renal, hepatic, and cardiovascular functions are adequate. Recommended doses for many drugs are listed in terms of grams or milligrams per kilogram of body weight.

Genetic and Ethnic Characteristics

Drugs are given to cause particular effects in recipients. However, when given the same drug in the same dose, by the same route, and in the same time interval, some people experience inadequate therapeutic effects and others experience unusual or exaggerated effects, including increased toxicity. These variations in drug response are often attributed to genetic or ethnic differences in drug metabolism.

Genetics

Genes determine the types and amounts of proteins produced in body cells and thereby control both the physical and chemical functions of the cells. When most drugs enter the body, they interact with proteins (e.g., in plasma, tissues, cell membranes, drug receptor sites) to reach their sites of action, and they interact with other proteins (e.g., drug-metabolizing enzymes in the liver and other organs) to be biotransformed and eliminated from the body. Genetic characteristics that alter any of these proteins can alter drug responses. For example, metabolism of isoniazid, an antitubercular drug, requires the enzyme acetyltransferase. People may metabolize isoniazid rapidly or slowly, depending largely on genetic differences in acetyltransferase activity. Clinically, rapid metabolizers may need larger-than-usual doses to achieve therapeutic effects, and slow metabolizers may need smaller-than-usual doses to avoid toxic effects.

In addition, several genetic variations (called polymorphisms) of the CYP450 drug-metabolizing enzymes have been identified. Specific variations may influence any of the chemical processes by which drugs are metabolized. For example, CYP2D6 metabolizes several antidepressant, antipsychotic, and beta-blocker drugs. Some Caucasians (about 7%) metabolize these drugs poorly and are at increased risk for drug accumulation and adverse effects. CYP2C19 metabolizes diazepam, omeprazole, and some antidepressants. As many as 15% to 30% of Asians may metabolize these drugs poorly and develop adverse effects if dosage is not reduced.

Still another example of genetic variation in drug metabolism is that some people are deficient in glucose-6-phosphate dehydrogenase, an enzyme normally found in red blood cells and other body tissues. These people may have hemolytic anemia when given antimalarial drugs, sulfonamides, analgesics, antipyretics, and other drugs.

The study of genetic variations (e.g., gene mutations that produce changes in structure and function of drug-metabolizing enzymes) that result in interindividual differences in drug response is called pharmacogenetics. Research has increased with awareness that genetic and ethnic characteristics are important factors and that diverse groups must be included in clinical trials. There is also increased awareness that each person is genetically unique and must be treated as an individual rather than as a member of a particular ethnic group. Research is ongoing toward improving drug safety and "personalized medicine," in which prescribers can use a patient's genetic characteristics to design a drug therapy regimen to maximize the therapeutic effects and minimize the adverse effects.

Genetic testing to determine a person's reaction to drug therapy is increasing, but clinical use is limited. Much research is being done in this area, especially related to cardiovascular and anticancer drugs (see the discussion of pharmacogenetics).

Ethnicity

Most drug information has been derived from clinical drug trials using white men. Interethnic variations became evident when drugs and dosages developed for Caucasians produced unexpected responses, including toxicity, when given to people from other ethnic groups. One common variation is that African Americans respond differently to some cardiovascular drugs. For example, for African Americans with hypertension, angiotensin-converting enzyme (ACE) inhibitors and beta-adrenergic blocking drugs are less effective and diuretics and calcium channel blockers are more effective. Also, African Americans with heart failure seem to respond better to a combination of hydralazine and isosorbide than do Caucasian patients with heart failure.

Another variation is that Asians usually require much smaller doses of some commonly used drugs, including beta-blockers and several psychotropic drugs (e.g., alprazolam, an antianxiety agent, and haloperidol, an antipsychotic). Some documented interethnic variations are included in later chapters.

Gender

Most drug-related research has involved men, and the results have been extrapolated to women, sometimes with adjustment of dosage based on the usually smaller size and weight of women. Historically, gender was considered a minor influence on drug action except during pregnancy and lactation. Now, differences between men and women in responses to drug therapy are being increasingly identified, and since 1993, regulations require that major clinical drug trials include women. However, data on drug therapy in women are still limited. Some identified differences include the following:

- Women who are depressed are more likely to respond to the selective serotonin reuptake inhibitors (SSRIs), such as fluoxetine (Prozac), than to the tricyclic antidepressants (TCAs), such as amitriptyline (Elavil).
- Women with anxiety disorders may respond less well than men to some antianxiety medications.
- Women with schizophrenia seem to need smaller doses of antipsychotic medications than men. If given the higher doses required by men, women are likely to have adverse drug reactions.
- Women may obtain more pain relief from opioid analgesics (e.g., morphine) and less relief from nonopioid analgesics (e.g., acetaminophen, ibuprofen), compared with men.

Different responses in women are usually attributed to anatomic and physiologic differences. In addition to smaller size and weight, for example, women usually have a higher percentage of body fat, less muscle tissue, smaller blood volume, and other characteristics that may influence responses to drugs. In addition, women have hormonal fluctuations during the menstrual cycle. Altered responses have been demonstrated in some women taking clonidine, an antihypertensive; lithium, a mood-stabilizing agent; phenytoin, an anticonvulsant; propranolol, a beta-adrenergic blocking drug used in the management of hypertension, angina pectoris, and migraine; and antidepressants. In addition, a significant percentage of women with arthritis, asthma, depression, diabetes mellitus, epilepsy, and migraine experience increased symptoms premenstrually. The increased symptoms may indicate a need for adjustments in their drug therapy regimens. Women with clinical depression, for example, may need higher doses of antidepressant medications premenstrually, if symptoms exacerbate, and lower doses during the rest of the menstrual cycle.

There may also be differences in pharmacokinetic processes, although few studies have been done. With absorption, it has been noted that women absorb a larger percentage of an oral dose of two cardiovascular medications than men (25% more verapamil and 40% more aspirin). With distribution, women may have higher blood levels of medications that distribute into body fluids (because of the smaller amount of water in which the medication can disperse) and lower blood levels of medications that are deposited in fatty tissues (because of the generally higher percentage of body fat), compared with men. With metabolism, the CYP3A4 enzyme metabolizes more medications than other enzymes, and women are thought to metabolize the drugs processed by this enzyme 20% to 40% faster than men (and therefore may have lower blood levels than men of similar weight given the same doses). The CYP1A2 enzyme is less active in women so that women who take the cardiovascular drugs clopidogrel or propranolol may have higher blood levels than men (and possibly greater risks of adverse effects if given the same doses as men). With excretion, renally excreted medications may reach higher blood levels because a major mechanism of drug elimination, glomerular filtration, is approximately 20% lower in women.

In general, women given equal dosages or equal weight-based dosages are thought to be exposed to higher concentrations of medications compared to men. Although available data are limited, the main reasons postulated for the gender differences are that women have a lower volume of distribution, lower glomerular filtration, and lower hepatic enzyme activity (except for the medications metabolized by the CYP3A4 enzyme system, which is more active in women). As a result, all women should be monitored closely during drug therapy because they are more likely to experience adverse drug effects than are men.

Other Considerations
Preexisting Conditions

Various pathologic conditions may alter some or all pharmacokinetic processes and lead to decreased therapeutic effects or increased risks of adverse effects. Examples include the following:

- Cardiovascular disorders (e.g., myocardial infarction, heart failure, hypotension), which may interfere with all pharmacokinetic processes, mainly by decreasing blood flow to sites of drug administration, action, metabolism (liver), and excretion (kidneys)

- GI disorders (e.g., vomiting, diarrhea, inflammatory bowel disease, trauma or surgery of the GI tract), which may interfere with absorption of oral drugs
- Hepatic disorders (e.g., hepatitis, cirrhosis, decreased liver function), which mainly interfere with metabolism. Severe liver disease or cirrhosis may interfere with all pharmacokinetic processes.
- Renal disorders (e.g., acute or chronic renal failure), which mainly interfere with excretion. Severe kidney disease may interfere with all pharmacokinetic processes.
- Thyroid disorders, which mainly affect metabolism. Hypothyroidism slows metabolism, prolonging drug action and slowing elimination. Hyperthyroidism accelerates metabolism, shortening drug action and hastening elimination.

Psychological Factors

Psychological considerations influence individual responses to drug administration, although specific mechanisms are unknown. An example is the placebo response. A placebo is a pharmacologically inactive substance. Placebos are used in clinical drug trials to compare the medication being tested with a "dummy" medication. Recipients often report both therapeutic and adverse effects from placebos.

Attitudes and expectations related to drugs in general, a particular drug, or a placebo influence patient response. They also influence compliance or the willingness to carry out the prescribed drug regimen, especially with long-term drug therapy.

Tolerance and Cross-Tolerance

Drug tolerance occurs when the body becomes accustomed to a particular drug over time so that larger doses must be given to produce the same effects. Tolerance may be acquired to the pharmacologic action of many drugs, especially opioid analgesics, alcohol, and other CNS depressants. Tolerance to pharmacologically related drugs is cross-tolerance. For example, a person who regularly drinks large amounts of alcohol becomes able to ingest even larger amounts before becoming intoxicated—this is tolerance to alcohol. If the person is then given sedative-type drugs or a general anesthetic, larger-than-usual doses are required to produce a pharmacologic effect—this is cross-tolerance.

Tolerance and cross-tolerance are usually attributed to activation of drug-metabolizing enzymes in the liver, which accelerates drug metabolism and excretion. They also are attributed to decreased sensitivity or numbers of receptor sites.

Adverse Effects of Drugs

As used in this book, the term "adverse effects" refers to any undesired responses to drug administration, as opposed to therapeutic effects, which are desired responses. Most drugs produce a mixture of therapeutic and adverse effects; all drugs can produce adverse effects. Adverse effects may produce essentially any symptom or disease process and may

---

EVIDENCE-BASED PRACTICE

Preventing Potentially Inappropriate Medication Use in Hospitalized Older Patients With a Computerized Provider Order Entry Warning System
by MATTISON, M. L., AFONSO, K. A., NGO, L. H., PHD; KENNETH J. MUKAMAL, K. J.

Archives of Internal Medicine 2010, 170(15), 1331–1336.

A list of drugs that should be avoided in older adults is available (Beers medications; see Chap. 5). Nevertheless, older patients continue to experience significant use of potentially inappropriate medications (PIMs). Implementation of a medication-specific warning system within a hospital's computerized provider order entry (CPOE) system alerted providers regarding PIM ordered for elders. The alert reduced the number of medications ordered in patients ages 65 years and older by offering recommendations regarding lowering the dose or suggesting an alternative medication.

IMPLICATIONS FOR NURSING PRACTICE: Older adults are at significant risk for adverse drug events, especially when hospitalized. Prompts, such as an alert in the CPOE system, allows for increased awareness of the risk associated with PIM and leads to safer drug therapy in elderly patients.

---

involve any body system or tissue. They may be common or rare, mild or severe, localized or widespread—depending on the drug and the recipient. Some adverse effects occur with usual therapeutic doses of drugs (often called side effects); most are more likely to occur and to be more severe with high doses. Box 2.4 describes common or serious adverse effects. Although adverse effects may occur in anyone who takes medications, they are especially likely to occur with some drugs (e.g., insulin, warfarin) and in older adults, who often take multiple drugs.

Black Box Warnings

For some drug groups and individual drugs that may cause serious or life-threatening adverse effects, the Food and Drug Administration (FDA) requires drug manufacturers to place a **BLACK BOX WARNING (BBW)** ◆ on the label of a prescription drug or in the literature describing it. A BBW is usually added after a significant number of serious adverse effects have occurred, often several years after a drug is first marketed and after it has been used in large numbers of people. The BBW is the strongest warning that the FDA can give consumers and often includes prescribing or monitoring information intended to improve the safety of using the particular drug or drug group. In recent years, BBWs have been added

| BOX 2.4 | **Common or Serious Adverse Drug Effects** |

Central Nervous System Effects

Central nervous system (CNS) effects may result from CNS stimulation (e.g., agitation, confusion, disorientation, hallucinations, psychosis, seizures) or CNS depression (e.g., impaired level of consciousness, sedation, coma, impaired respiration and circulation). CNS effects may occur with many drugs, including most therapeutic groups, substances of abuse, and over-the-counter preparations.

Gastrointestinal Effects

Gastrointestinal (GI) effects (e.g., nausea, vomiting, constipation, diarrhea) commonly occur. Nausea and vomiting occur with many drugs as a result of local irritation of the GI tract or stimulation of the vomiting center in the brain. Diarrhea occurs with drugs that cause local irritation or increase peristalsis. More serious effects include bleeding or ulceration (most often with nonsteroidal anti-inflammatory agents such as ibuprofen) and severe diarrhea/colitis (most often with antibiotics).

Hematologic Effects

Hematologic effects (excessive bleeding, clot formation [thrombosis], bone marrow depression, anemias, leukopenia, agranulocytosis, thrombocytopenia) are relatively common and potentially life threatening. Excessive bleeding is often associated with anticoagulants and thrombolytics; bone marrow depression is associated with anticancer drugs.

Hepatic Effects

Hepatic effects (hepatitis, liver dysfunction or failure, biliary tract disorders) are potentially life threatening. The liver is especially susceptible to drug-induced injury because most drugs are circulated to the liver for metabolism and some drugs are toxic to liver cells. Hepatotoxic drugs include acetaminophen (Tylenol), isoniazid (INH), methotrexate (Trexall), phenytoin (Dilantin), and aspirin and other salicylates. In the presence of drug- or disease-induced liver damage, the metabolism of many drugs is impaired. Besides hepatotoxicity, many drugs produce abnormal values in liver function tests without producing clinical signs of liver dysfunction.

Nephrotoxicity

Nephrotoxicity (nephritis, renal insufficiency or failure) occurs with several antimicrobial agents (e.g., gentamicin and other aminoglycosides), nonsteroidal anti-inflammatory agents (e.g., ibuprofen and related drugs), and others. It is potentially serious because it may interfere with drug excretion, thereby causing drug accumulation and increased adverse effects.

Hypersensitivity

Hypersensitivity or allergy may occur with almost any drug in susceptible patients. It is largely unpredictable and unrelated to dose. It occurs in those who have previously been exposed to the drug or a similar substance (antigen) and who have developed antibodies. When readministered, the drug reacts with the antibodies to cause cell damage and the release of histamine and other substances. These substances produce reactions ranging from mild skin rashes to anaphylactic shock. Anaphylactic shock is a life-threatening hypersensitivity reaction characterized by respiratory distress and cardiovascular collapse. It occurs within a few minutes after drug administration and requires emergency treatment with epinephrine. Some allergic reactions (e.g., serum sickness) occur 1 to 2 weeks after the drug is given.

Drug Fever

Drugs can cause fever by several mechanisms, including allergic reactions, damaging body tissues, interfering with dissipation of body heat, or acting on the temperature-regulating center in the brain. The most common mechanism is an allergic reaction. Fever may occur alone or with other allergic manifestations (e.g., skin rash, hives, joint and muscle pain, enlarged lymph glands, eosinophilia). It may begin within hours after the first dose if the patient has taken the drug before or within about 10 days of continued administration if the drug is new to the patient. If the causative drug is discontinued, fever usually subsides within 48 to 72 hours unless drug excretion is delayed or significant tissue damage has occurred (e.g., hepatitis). Many drugs have been implicated as causes of drug fever, including most antimicrobials.

Idiosyncrasy

Idiosyncrasy refers to an unexpected reaction to a drug that occurs the first time it is given. These reactions are usually attributed to genetic characteristics that alter the person's drug-metabolizing enzymes.

Drug Dependence

Drug dependence may occur with mind-altering drugs, such as opioid analgesics, sedative-hypnotic agents, antianxiety agents, and CNS stimulants. Dependence may be physiologic or psychological. Physiologic dependence produces unpleasant physical symptoms when the dose is reduced or the drug is withdrawn. Psychological dependence leads to excessive preoccupation with drugs and drug-seeking behavior.

Carcinogenicity

Carcinogenicity is the ability of a substance to cause cancer. Several drugs are carcinogens, including some hormones and anticancer drugs. Carcinogenicity apparently results from drug-induced alterations in cellular DNA.

Teratogenicity

Teratogenicity is the ability of a substance to cause abnormal fetal development when taken by pregnant women. Drug groups considered teratogenic include antiepileptic drugs and "statin" cholesterol-lowering drugs.

---

to antidepressant drugs, nonopioid analgesics, and the antiflu drug oseltamivir (Tamiflu).

Pregnancy Categories

In 1979, the FDA assigned pregnancy categories to identify risk of fetal injury from drugs used as directed by the mother during pregnancy. The categories range from A (safest) to X (known danger). The categories do not account for potential harm from drugs or their metabolites found in breast milk.

Five categories are identified:

- Category A. Risk to the fetus in the first trimester (and in later trimesters) has not been demonstrated in well-controlled studies in pregnant women.
- Category B. Animal reproduction studies have not demonstrated risk to the fetus, and there are no well-controlled studies in pregnant women.
- Category C. Animal reproduction studies have not demonstrated risk to the fetus, and there are no well-controlled

studies in pregnant women; however, potential benefits may outweigh potential risk in use of drug in pregnant women.

- Category D. Evidence of risk to the fetus has been demonstrated. However, the benefits may outweigh risk in pregnant women if the drug is needed in a life-threatening situation and other safer drugs cannot be used or are ineffective.
- Category X. Studies in humans or animals have demonstrated fetal abnormalities or evidence of fetal risk, and the risk clearly outweighs the benefit. The drug is contraindicated in women who are pregnant or in those who may become pregnant.

The Drugs at a Glance tables in this book give the pregnancy category for each listed drug.

Clinical Application 2-1

- During your most recent visit (3 days ago), you instructed Mrs. Green to take her medication with a large glass of water and set up a daily pill calendar. You also checked her vital signs; her blood pressure was 148/70 mm Hg. Today, you recheck her vital signs, and her blood pressure is 96/60 mm Hg. You ask her about her medication, and she tells you she has been taking each medication according to the calendar three times a day. What future actions should the home health nurse take?

Toxicology: Drug Overdose

Drug toxicity (also called poisoning or overdose) results from excessive amounts of a drug and may damage body tissues. It is a common problem in both adult and pediatric populations. It may result from a single large dose or prolonged ingestion of smaller doses. Toxicity may involve alcohol or prescription, over-the-counter, or illicit drugs. Clinical manifestations are often nonspecific and may indicate other disease processes. Because of the variable presentation of drug intoxication, health care providers must have a high index of suspicion so that toxicity can be rapidly recognized and treated.

When toxicity occurs in a home or outpatient setting and the victim is collapsed or not breathing, call 911 for emergency aid. If the victim is responsive, someone needs to contact the National Poison Control Center by phone at 1-800-222-1222. The caller is connected to a local Poison Control Center and, if possible, needs to tell the responding pharmacist or physician the name of the drug or substance that was taken as well as the amount and time of ingestion. The poison control consultant may recommend treatment measures over the phone or taking the victim to a hospital emergency department.

It is possible that the patient or someone else may know the toxic agent (e.g., accidental overdose of a therapeutic drug, use of an illicit drug, a suicide attempt). Often, however, multiple drugs have been ingested, the causative drugs are unknown, and the circumstances may involve traumatic injury or impaired mental status that make the patient unable to provide useful information. The main goals of treatment are starting

treatment as soon as possible after drug ingestion, supporting and stabilizing vital functions, preventing further damage from the toxic agent by reducing absorption or increasing elimination, and administering antidotes when available and indicated. Box 2.5 describes general aspects of care, Table 2.1 lists selected antidotes, and relevant chapters discuss specific aspects of care.

Most overdosed patients are treated in emergency departments and discharged to their homes. A few are admitted to intensive care units (ICUs), often because of unconsciousness and the need for endotracheal intubation and mechanical ventilation. Unconsciousness is a major toxic effect of several commonly ingested substances such as benzodiazepine antianxiety and sedative agents, TCAs, ethanol, and opioid analgesics. Serious cardiovascular effects (e.g., cardiac arrest, dysrhythmias, circulatory impairment) are also common and warrant admission to an ICU.

Clinical Application 2-2

- You see Mrs. Green again in a few days. She is taking three antihypertensive medications, and her blood pressure is 128/72 mm Hg. She tells you that she has been feeling better and that she is moving in with her daughter. What suggestions could you provide Mrs. Green's daughter regarding her mother's medication management?

NCLEX Success

4. A nurse is looking up information about the effects of a drug on different receptors. Characteristics of receptors include which of the following?

   A. They are carbohydrates located in cell membranes or inside cells.
   B. They are constantly synthesized and degraded in the body.
   C. They bind with molecules of any drug circulating in the bloodstream.
   D. They regulate the actions of all drugs.

5. A patient with an overdose of an oral drug usually receives which of the following?

   A. specific antidote
   B. activated charcoal
   C. syrup of ipecac
   D. strong laxative

6. The mother of a 14-month old girl calls a nurse working in a pediatric clinic and reports that her daughter ingested an unknown number of sleeping pills about four hours ago and is now drowsy. The mother asks what she should do. The best response to give the mother is

   A. "Administer a dose of syrup of ipecac to ensure vomiting"
   B. "Call the Poison Control Center immediately"
   C. "Administer a strong laxative and observe for a response"
   D. "Call 911 to transport your daughter to the nearest emergency department"

BOX 2.5   General Management of Toxicity

■ The first priority is support of vital functions, as indicated by rapid assessment of vital signs and level of consciousness. In serious poisonings, an electrocardiogram is indicated, and findings of severe toxicity (e.g., dysrhythmias, ischemia) justify aggressive treatment. Standard cardiopulmonary resuscitation (CPR) measures may be needed to maintain breathing and circulation. An intravenous (IV) line is usually needed to administer fluids and drugs, and invasive treatment or monitoring devices may be inserted.

Endotracheal intubation and mechanical ventilation are often required to maintain breathing (in unconscious patients), correct hypoxemia, and protect the airway. Hypoxemia must be corrected quickly to avoid brain injury, myocardial ischemia, and cardiac dysrhythmias.

Serious cardiovascular manifestations often require drug therapy. Hypotension and hypoperfusion may be treated with inotropic and vasopressor drugs to increase cardiac output and raise blood pressure. Dysrhythmias are treated according to Advanced Cardiac Life Support (ACLS) protocols.

Recurring seizures or status epilepticus requires treatment with anticonvulsant drugs.

■ For unconscious patients, as soon as an IV line is established, some authorities recommend a dose of naloxone (2 mg IV) for possible narcotic overdose and thiamine (100 mg IV) for possible brain dysfunction due to thiamine deficiency. In addition, a fingerstick blood glucose test should be done, and if hypoglycemia is indicated, a 50% dextrose solution (50 mL IV) should be given.

■ After the patient is out of immediate danger, a thorough physical examination and efforts to determine the drug(s), the amounts, and the time lapse since exposure are needed. If the patient is unable to supply needed information, anyone else who may be able to do so should be interviewed. It is necessary to ask about the use of prescription and over-the-counter drugs, alcohol, and illicit substances.

■ There are no standard laboratory tests for poisoned patients, but baseline tests of liver and kidney function are usually indicated. Screening tests for toxic substances are not very helpful because test results may be delayed, many substances are not detected, and the results rarely affect initial treatment. Specimens of blood, urine, or gastric fluids may be obtained for laboratory analysis. Serum drug levels are needed when acetaminophen, alcohol, aspirin, digoxin, lithium, or theophylline is known to be an ingested drug, to assist with treatment.

■ For most orally ingested drugs, the initial and major treatment is a single dose of activated charcoal. Sometimes called the "universal antidote," it is useful in many poisonings because it adsorbs many toxins and rarely causes complications. When given within 30 minutes of drug ingestion, it decreases absorption of the toxic drug by about 90%; when given an hour after ingestion, it decreases absorption by about 37%. Activated charcoal (1 g/kg of body weight or 50–100 g) is usually mixed with 240 mL of water (25–50 g in 120 mL of water for children) to make a slurry, which is gritty and unpleasant to swallow. It is often given by nasogastric tube. The charcoal blackens subsequent bowel movements. If used with whole bowel irrigation (WBI; see below), activated charcoal should be given

before the WBI solution is started. If given during WBI, the binding capacity of the charcoal is decreased. Activated charcoal does not significantly decrease absorption of some drugs (e.g., ethanol, iron, lithium, metals).

Multiple doses of activated charcoal may be given in some instances (e.g., ingestion of sustained-release drugs). One regimen is an initial dose of 50 to 100 g, then 12.5 g every 1, 2, or 4 to 6 hours for a few doses.

Adverse effects of activated charcoal include pulmonary aspiration and bowel obstruction from impaction of the charcoal–drug complex.

QSEN Safety Alert

To prevent these effects, unconscious patients should not receive activated charcoal until the airway is secure against aspiration, and many patients are given a laxative (e.g., sorbitol) to aid removal of the charcoal–drug complex.

Ipecac-induced vomiting and gastric lavage are no longer routinely used because of minimal effectiveness and potential complications. Ipecac is no longer recommended to treat poisonings in children in home settings; parents should call a poison control center or a health care provider. Gastric lavage may be beneficial in serious overdoses if performed within an hour of drug ingestion. If the ingested agent delays gastric emptying (e.g., drugs with anticholinergic effects), the 1-hour time limit for gastric lavage may be extended. When used after ingestion of pills or capsules, the tube lumen should be large enough to allow removal of pill fragments.

■ WBI with a polyethylene glycol solution (e.g., Colyte) may be used to remove toxic ingestions of long-acting, sustained-release drugs (e.g., many beta-blockers, calcium channel blockers, and theophylline preparations); enteric-coated drugs; and toxins that do not bind well with activated charcoal (e.g., iron, lithium). It may also be helpful in removing packets of illicit drugs, such as cocaine or heroin. When used, 500 to 2000 mL/h are given orally or by nasogastric tube until bowel contents are clear. Vomiting is the most common adverse effect. WBI is contraindicated in patients with serious bowel disorders (e.g., obstruction, perforation, ileus), hemodynamic instability, or respiratory impairment (unless intubated).

■ Urinary elimination of some drugs and toxic metabolites can be accelerated by changing the pH of urine (e.g., alkalinizing with IV sodium bicarbonate for salicylate overdose), diuresis, or hemodialysis. Hemodialysis is the treatment of choice in severe lithium and aspirin (salicylate) poisoning.

■ Specific antidotes can be administered when available and as indicated by the patient's clinical condition. Available antidotes vary widely in effectiveness. Some are very effective and rapidly reverse toxic manifestations (e.g., naloxone for opioids, specific Fab fragments for digoxin).

When an antidote is used, its half-life relative to the toxin's half-life must be considered. For example, the half-life of naloxone, a narcotic antagonist, is relatively short compared with the half-life of the longer-acting opioids such as methadone, and repeated doses may be needed to prevent recurrence of the toxic state.

TABLE 2.1

Antidotes for Overdoses of Selected Therapeutic Drugs

Overdosed Drug (Poison)	Antidote	Route and Dosage Ranges	Comments
Acetaminophen (see Chap. 14)	Acetylcysteine (Mucomyst 10% or 20% oral solution, Acetadote 20% [200 mg/mL] injection solution)	PO 140 mg/kg initially, then 70 mg/kg every 4 h for 17 doses. IV (Acetadote only): loading dose 150 mg/kg, diluted in 200 mL 5% dextrose, infused over 15 min Maintenance dose one: 50 mg/kg, diluted in 500 mL 5% dextrose, infused over 4 h Maintenance dose two: 100 mg/kg, diluted in 1000 mL 5% dextrose, infused over 16 h	Dilute oral solution to a 5% solution with a cola or other soft drink for oral administration. Follow instructions carefully and note that doses, amounts of diluent, and infusion times are different for the three total IV infusions.
Anticholinergics (atropine; see Chap. 58)	Physostigmine	IV, IM 2 mg; give IV slowly, over at least 2 min	Infrequently used because of its toxicity; should not be given to patients with a seizure disorder, overdose of unknown drugs, or overdose of drugs known to cause seizures in overdose (e.g., cocaine, lithium). In such circumstances, the risks of seizures outweigh drug benefits.
Benzodiazepines (see Chap. 52)	Flumazenil	IV 0.2 mg over 30 s; if no response, may give additional 0.3 mg over 30 s Additional doses of 0.5 mg may be given at 1-min intervals up to a total amount of 3 mg	Should not be given to patients with overdose of unknown drugs or drugs known to cause seizures in overdose (e.g., cocaine, lithium)
Beta-blockers (see Chap. 29)	Glucagon	IV 50–150 mcg/kg (5–10 mg for adults) over 1 min initially, then 2–5 mg/h by continuous infusion as needed	Glucagon increases myocardial contractility and raises blood pressure. It does not act on beta-adrenergic receptors and is therefore not affected by beta-blocking drugs.
Calcium channel blockers (see Chap. 26)	Calcium gluconate 10%	IV 1 g over 5 min; may be repeated	Increases myocardial contractility
Cholinergics (see Chap. 58)	Atropine	Adults: IV 2 mg, repeated as needed Children: IV 0.05 mg/kg, up to 2 mg	If poisoning is due to organophosphates (e.g., insecticides), pralidoxime may be given with the atropine.
Digoxin (see Chap. 24)	Digoxin immune Fab (Digibind)	IV 40 mg (one vial) for each 0.6 mg of digoxin ingested Reconstitute each vial with 4 mL Water for Injection, then dilute with sterile isotonic saline to a convenient volume and give over 30 min, through a 0.22-micron filter. If cardiac arrest seems imminent, may give the dose as a bolus injection.	Recommended for severe toxicity; reverses cardiac and extracardiac symptoms in a few minutes *Note:* Serum digoxin levels increase after antidote administration, but the drug is bound and therefore inactive.

Table 2.1

Antidotes for Overdoses of Selected Therapeutic Drugs (Continued)

Overdosed Drug (Poison)	Antidote	Route and Dosage Ranges	Comments
Heparin (see Chap. 7)	Protamine sulfate	IV 1 mg/100 units of heparin, slowly, over at least 10 min; a single dose should not exceed 50 mg	
Iron (see Chap. 34)	Deferoxamine	IM 1 g every 8 h PRN IV 15 mg/kg/h if hypotensive	Indicated for serum iron levels >500 mg/dL or serum levels >350 mg/dL with GI or cardiovascular symptoms. Can bind and remove a portion of an ingested dose; urine becomes red as iron is excreted
Isoniazid (INH) (see Chap. 20)	Pyridoxine	IV 1 g per gram of INH ingested, at rate of 1 g every 2–3 min. If amount of INH unknown, give 5 g; may be repeated.	Indicated for management of seizures and correction of acidosis
Lead	Succimer (Chemet)	Children: PO 10 mg/kg every 8 h for 5 d	
Opioid analgesics (see Chap. 48)	Naloxone (Narcan)	Adults: IV 0.4–2 mg PRN Children: IV 0.1 mg/kg per dose	Can also be given IM, subcutaneously, or by endotracheal tube
Phenothiazine antipsychotic agents (see Chap. 53)	Diphenhydramine (Benadryl)	Adults: IV 50 mg Children: IV 1–2 mg/kg, up to a total of 50 mg	Given to relieve extrapyramidal symptoms (movement disorders)
Thrombolytics (see Chap. 7)	Aminocaproic acid (Amicar)	PO, IV infusion, 5 g initially, then 1–1.25 g/h for 8 h or until bleeding is controlled; maximum dose, 30 g/24 h	
Tricyclic antidepressants (see Chap. 54)	Sodium bicarbonate	IV 1–2 mEq/kg initially, then continuous IV drip to maintain serum pH of 7.5	To treat cardiac dysrhythmias, conduction disturbances, and hypotension
Warfarin (see Chap. 7)	Vitamin K_1	PO 5–10 mg daily IV (severe overdose) continuous infusion at rate no faster than 1 mg/min	

Key Concepts

- Drugs can stimulate or inhibit normal cellular activities; however, they cannot change the type of function that occurs normally.
- Most drugs exert their effects by chemically combining with receptors at the cellular level.
- Receptor proteins can be altered by endogenous substances and exogenous drugs.
- Pharmacokinetic processes involve absorption, distribution, metabolism, and excretion.
- Serum drug levels reflect dosage, absorption, bioavailability, elimination half-life, and the rate of elimination.
- Drug-related variables that affect drug action include dosage, route, and drug–diet and drug–drug interactions.
- Patient-related variables that affect drug action include age, body weight, genetic and ethnic characteristics, gender, pathologic conditions, and psychological status.

- All drugs can produce adverse effects; adverse effects may produce essentially any symptom or disease process and may involve any body system.

- Drug toxicity results from excessive amounts of a drug, whether received in a single large dose or multiple smaller doses.

- Activated charcoal is considered the "universal" antidote; most drugs do not have specific antidotes for overdoses.

- Ipecac-induced vomiting and gastric lavage are no longer routinely used because of minimal effectiveness and potential complications.

- Pregnancy categories identify risk of fetal injury due to drug therapy when used as directed by the mother during pregnancy.

Critical Thinking Questions

2-1. You are a new nurse exploring the causes of both therapeutic and adverse drug effects and are asked to consider the following:

- What are some factors that decrease absorption of an oral drug?

- Does protein binding speed or slow drug distribution to sites of action? Why?

- What are the implications of hepatic enzyme induction and inhibition in terms of drug metabolism and elimination from the body?

References and Resources

Bamshad, M. (2005). Genetic influences on health: Does race matter? *Journal of the American Medical Association, 294,* 937–946.

DiPiro, J. T., Talbert, R. L., Yee, G. C., Matzke, G. R., Wells B., & Posey, L. M. (Eds.). (2011). *Pharmacotherapy: A pathophysiologic approach* (8th ed.). New York: McGraw-Hill.

Facts and Comparisons. *Drug facts and comparisons.* (Updated monthly). St. Louis, MO: Facts and Comparisons.

Hall, J. E. (2011). *Guyton and Hall textbook of medical physiology* (12th ed.). Philadelphia, PA: Elsevier.

Karch, A. M. (2010). *2010 Lippincott's nursing drug guide.* Philadelphia, PA: Lippincott Williams & Wilkins.

Lacy, C. F., Armstrong, L. L., Goldman, M. P., & Lance, L. L. (2010). *Lexi-Comp's drug information handbook* (19th ed.). Hudson, OH: American Pharmaceutical Association.

Manno, M. S. (2006). Preventing adverse drug events. *Nursing, 36,* 56–61.

Munoz, C., & Hilgenberg, C. (2005). Ethnopharmacology. *American Journal of Nursing, 105,* 40–48.

Olson, K. R. (2007). Poisoning. In S. J. McPhee, M. A. Papadakis, & L. M. Tierney, Jr. (Eds.), *Current medical diagnosis & treatment 2007* (46th ed., pp. 1639–1669). New York: McGraw-Hill.

Shannon, M. W., Borron, S. W., & Burns, M. J. (2007). *Haddad and Winchester's Clinical Management of Poisoning and Drug Overdose* (4th ed.). Philadelphia, PA: Saunders Elsevier.

Smeltzer, S. C., Bare, B. G., Hinkle, J. L., & Cheever, K. H. (2009). *Brunner & Suddarth's textbook of medical-surgical nursing* (12th ed.). Philadelphia, PA: Lippincott Williams & Wilkins.

3 Medication Administration and the Nursing Process of Drug Therapy

Clinical Application Case Study

Jacqueline Baranski has been admitted to the hospital for a total abdominal hysterectomy. This is the first postoperative day. She is currently taking lisinopril 10 mg PO daily and estradiol 1 mg PO. She is also receiving morphine sulfate by patient-controlled analgesia and heparin 5000 units subcutaneously every 12 hours for 7 days.

KEY TERMS

Assessment: collection of patient data that affects drug therapy

Controlled-release: oral tablet or capsule formulations that maintain consistent serum drug levels

Dosage form: form in which drugs are manufactured; includes elixirs, tablets, capsules, suppositories, parenteral drugs, and transdermal systems

Enteric-coated: coating of a tablet or capsule that makes it insoluble in stomach acid

Evaluation: determining a patient's status in relation to stated goals and expected outcomes

Evidence-based practice: scientific evidence that yields the best practice in patient care

Interventions: planned nursing activities performed on a patient's behalf, including assessment, promotion of adherence to drug therapy, and solving problems related to drug therapy

Medication history: list of prescription medications, over-the-counter medications, herbal supplements, or illegal substances taken by the patient (both current and past)

Nursing diagnosis: description of patient problems based on assessment data

Nursing process: systematic way of gathering and using information to plan and provide individualized patient care

Parenteral: injected administration; subcutaneous, intramuscular, or intravenous route

Planning/goals: expected outcomes of prescribed drug therapy

Rights of medication administration: assist to ensure accuracy in drug therapy; rights include right drug, right dose, right patient, right route, right time, right reason, and right documentation

Topical: application of drugs (e.g., solutions, ointments, creams, or suppositories) to skin or mucous membranes

Transdermal: absorption of drugs (e.g., skin patches) through the skin

This chapter discusses the administration of medications and the implementation of the nursing process with medication administration. The purpose of administering medications is to evoke a therapeutic response. Giving medications to a patient is an important nursing responsibility in many health care settings, including ambulatory clinics, hospitals, long-term care facilities, schools, and in homes. The basic requirements for accurate drug administration are the **rights of medication administration**, which are:

- Right drug
- Right dose
- Right patient
- Right route
- Right time
- Right reason
- Right documentation

These "rights" require knowledge of the drugs to be given and the patients who are to receive them as well as specific nursing skills and interventions. The implementation of the **nursing process** in the administration of medications provides a systematic way of gathering and using information to plan and provide individualized patient care as well as to evaluate the outcomes of that care. It involves both cognitive and psychomotor skills. Knowledge of, and skill in, the nursing process is required for drug therapy as in other aspects of patient care. The five steps of the nursing process are assessment, nursing diagnosis, planning and establishing goals for care, interventions, and evaluation as it is applied to medication administration.

General Principles of Accurate Drug Administration

The nurse adheres to the following principles:

- Follow the "rights" associated with medication administration consistently.
- Learn essential information about each drug to be given (e.g., indications for use, contraindications, therapeutic effects, adverse effects, any specific instructions about administration).
- Interpret the prescriber's order accurately (i.e., drug name, dose, frequency of administration). Question the prescriber if any information is unclear or if the drug seems inappropriate for the patient's condition.
- In the event a verbal or telephone order is given by a prescriber, write down the order or enter it in the computer and then read the order back to the prescriber.
- Read labels of drug containers for the drug name and concentration (usually in milligrams per tablet, capsule, or milliliter of solution). Many medications are available in different dosage forms and concentrations, and it is extremely important to use the correct ones.
- Use only approved abbreviations for drug names, doses, routes of administration, and times of administration. For example, do not use U to refer to units. Instead, write out *units*. This promotes safer administration and reduces errors. Consult the "Do Not Use" list, the safety guidelines published by the Joint Commission (see Table 1.4). Check the organization's Web site for details.
- Calculate doses accurately. Current nursing practice requires few dosage calculations (most are done by pharmacists). However, when they are needed, accuracy is essential. For medications with a narrow safety margin or potentially serious adverse effects, ask a pharmacist or a colleague to do the calculation also and compare the results. This is especially important when calculating children's dosages.
- Measure doses accurately. Ask a colleague to double-check measurements of insulin and heparin, unusual doses (i.e., large or small), and any drugs to be given intravenously.
- Use the correct procedures and techniques for all routes of administration. For example, use appropriate anatomic landmarks to identify sites for intramuscular (IM) injections, follow the manufacturers' instructions for preparation and administration of intravenous (IV) medications, and use sterile materials and techniques for injectable and eye medications.
- Seek information about the patient's medical diagnoses and condition in relation to drug administration (e.g., ability to swallow oral medications; allergies or contraindications to ordered drugs; new signs or symptoms that may

indicate adverse effects of administered drugs; heart, liver, or kidney disorders that may interfere with the patient's ability to distribute, metabolize, or eliminate drugs).

- Verify the identity of all patients before administering medications; check identification bands on patients who have them (e.g., in hospitals or long-term care facilities).
- Omit or delay doses as indicated by the patient's condition and report or record omissions appropriately.
- Be especially vigilant when giving medications to children because there is a high risk of medication errors. One reason is children's great diversity in age, from birth to 18 years, and in weight, from 2 to 3 kg to 100 kg or more. A second reason is that most drugs have not been tested in children. A third reason is that many drugs are marketed in dosage forms and concentrations suitable for adults. This often requires dilution, calculation, preparation, and administration of very small doses. A fourth reason is that children have limited sites for administration of IV drugs, and several may be given through the same site. In many cases, the need for small volumes of fluid limits flushing between drugs (which may produce undesirable interactions with other drugs and IV solutions).

Clinical Application 3-1

- Prior to administering the medications to Ms. Baranski, how does the nurse incorporate the rights of medication administration into the patient's care?
- Why is the Joint Commission's "Do Not Use" list so important in the prevention of medication administration errors?

NCLEX Success

1. A physician writes an order using the abbreviation MS. The order states "MS 10 mg IV push every 6 hours as needed for pain." According to the Joint Commission's "Do Not Use" list, what is the potential problem in this order?

   A. The order does not include a dosage.
   B. The drug could be magnesium sulfate or morphine sulfate.
   C. The potential problem is minimal, and the order is clear.
   D. The order does not include the route.

2. A prescriber has written an order for an oral medication to a patient following a cerebrovascular accident (stroke). Prior to administering the medication, which of the following nursing interventions is most important?

   A. allowing the patient to take the medication with thickened liquids
   B. placing the patient in the sitting position
   C. assessing the patient's blood pressure and pulse
   D. assessing the patient's ability to swallow

Legal Responsibilities

Registered and licensed practical nurses are legally empowered, under state nurse practice acts, to give medications ordered by licensed physicians and dentists. In some states, nurse practitioners may prescribe medications.

When giving medications, the nurse is legally responsible for safe and accurate administration. This means that the nurse may be held liable for not giving a drug or for giving a wrong drug or a wrong dose. In addition, the nurse is expected to have sufficient drug knowledge to recognize and question erroneous orders. If, after questioning the prescriber and seeking information from other authoritative sources, the nurse considers that giving a drug is unsafe, the nurse must refuse to give the drug. The fact that a physician wrote an erroneous order does not excuse the nurse from legal liability if he or she carries out that order.

The nurse also is legally responsible for actions delegated to people who are inadequately prepared for or legally barred from administering medications (e.g., nursing assistants). However, certified medical assistants (CMAs) may administer medications in physicians' offices, and certified medication aides (nursing assistants with a short course of training, also called CMAs) often administer medications in long-term care facilities.

The nurse who consistently follows safe practices in giving medications does not need to be excessively concerned about legal liability. The basic techniques and guidelines described in this chapter are aimed at safe and accurate preparation and administration. Most errors result when these practices are not followed.

Legal responsibilities in other aspects of drug therapy are less clear-cut. However, in general, nurses are expected to monitor patients' responses to drug therapy (e.g., therapeutic and adverse effects) and to teach patients safe and effective self-administration of drugs when indicated.

Medication Errors and their Prevention

Medication errors continue to receive increasing attention from numerous health care organizations and agencies. Much of this interest stems from a 1999 report of the Institute of Medicine (IOM), which estimated that 44,000 to 98,000 deaths occur each year in the United States because of medical errors, including medication errors. The 2004 report of the IOM, *Keeping Patients Safe: Transforming the Work Environment of Nurses,* reported that the extended hours nurses work contributes to medication errors. Potential adverse patient outcomes of medication and other errors include serious illness, conditions that prolong hospitalization or require additional treatment, and death. Medication errors commonly reported include giving an incorrect dose, not giving an ordered drug, and giving an unordered drug. Specific drugs often associated with errors and adverse drug events (ADEs) include insulin, heparin, and warfarin. The risk of ADEs increases with the number of drugs a patient uses.

Medication errors may occur at any step in the drug distribution process, from the manufacturer to the patient, including prescribing, transcribing, dispensing, and administering. Many steps and numerous people are involved in giving the correct dose of a medication to the intended patient; each step or person has a potential for contributing to a medication error or preventing a medication error. All health care providers involved in drug therapy need to recognize risky situations, intervene to prevent errors when possible, and be extremely vigilant in all phases of drug administration. Recommendations for prevention of

medication errors have been developed by several organizations, including the IOM, the Agency for Healthcare Research and Quality (AHRQ), the Joint Commission, the Institute for Safe Medication Practices (ISMP), and the National Coordinating Council for Medication Error Reporting and Prevention (NCCMERP). Some sources of medication errors and recommendations to prevent them are summarized in Table 3.1.

TABLE 3.1

Medication Errors: Sources and Prevention Strategies

Sources of Errors	Recommendation to Prevent Errors
Drug Manufacturers • Drugs may have similar names that can lead to erroneous prescribing, dispensing, or administration. • For example, the antiseizure drug Lamictal (lamotrigine) has been confused with Lamisil, an antifungal drug; lamivudine, an antiviral drug; and others. • The FDA estimates that 10% of all reported medication errors result from drug name confusion. • In addition to similar names, many drugs, especially those produced by the same manufacturer, have similar packaging. This can lead to errors if container labels are not read carefully, especially if the products are shelved or stored next to each other. • Long-acting oral dosage forms with various, sometimes unclear, indicators (e.g., LA, XL, XR) may be crushed, chewed, or otherwise broken so that the long-acting feature is destroyed. This can cause an overdose.	• FDA evaluation of proposed trade names in manufacturers' new drug applications in seeking FDA approval for marketing • When choosing a trade name for a new drug, avoid names that are similar to drugs already on the market. • Design packaging so that all drugs from an individual manufacturer do not look alike in terms of color, appearance, etc. • Clearly designate long-acting drug formulations. • Use "Tall Man" lettering on drug labels to distinguish between generic drug with similar names (e.g., NICARdipine; NIFEdipine; vinBLAstine, VinCristine).
Health Care Agencies • Prescribers, pharmacists, and nurses have a heavy workload, with resultant rushing of prescribing, dispensing, and administering medications. • They may also experience distractions by interruptions, noise, and other events in the work environment that make it difficult to pay needed attention to the medication-related task.	• Provide prescribers with CPOE technology and standardized drug order sheets; discourage handwritten drug orders; minimize verbal orders and state procedures to follow when verbal orders are necessary. • Provide computerized technology (e.g., bar coding for patients; handheld scanning devices for nursing staff) to verify the drug, the dose, and the patient identity before administration of a dose and to record administration after a dose. • Provide sufficient pharmacy staff to dispense medications. • Provide sufficient nursing staff to administer medications. • Try to provide a quiet and orderly work environment, with limited traffic, telephones, and other distractions. • Provide adequate equipment for the required medication-related tasks. For pharmacies, this includes an adequate computer system for accessing databases of drug information and for detecting risks of adverse drug effects and drug–drug interactions. • Standardize drug administration materials and equipment (e.g., infusion pumps) throughout the agency. • Be sure that all professional staff members know and follow safety standards and medication reconciliation processes mandated by The Joint Commission.
Prescribers • May write orders illegibly • Order a drug that is not indicated by the patient's condition	• Use CPOE when available. • Be sure that any handwritten drug order is legible (e.g., printed in block letters if necessary), clear, and unambiguous.

TABLE 3.1

Medication Errors: Sources and Prevention Strategies (Continued)

Sources of Errors	Recommendation to Prevent Errors
• Fail to order a drug that is indicated • Fail to consider the patient's age, size, kidney function, liver function, and disease process when selecting a drug or dosage • Fail to consider other medications the patient is taking, including prescription, over-the-counter, and herbal drugs • Lack sufficient knowledge about the drug • Fail to monitor for, or instruct others to monitor for, effects of administered drugs • Fail to discontinue drugs appropriately	• Avoid or minimize the use of abbreviations. Consult the Joint Commission's "Do Not Use" list. • Use generic names of medications rather than brand names and include the purpose of the drug. • Avoid verbal orders when possible. If a verbal order is necessary, have the person taking the order write the order and read it back, spelling drug names, dosages, routes, and so forth when indicated. • Review the patient's health status and other drugs being taken before ordering any new drug. Also, discontinue drugs appropriately when no longer needed. • Maintain a current knowledge base about new drugs and changes in uses of drugs for the relevant area of clinical practice.
Nurses • May have inadequate knowledge about a drug or about the patient receiving the drug • Not follow the rights to medication administration • Fail to question the medication order when indicated	• Be aware of agency policies and procedures about medication use, storage, administration, and recording. • Maintain an up-to-date knowledge base about drugs and their administration. • Make a diligent effort to learn about patients' health status and the drugs they are receiving. • Question or clarify any unclear drug orders. • Verify medication calculations with another nurse or a pharmacist, especially for children. • Recheck a single dose any time the amount seems unusually large or small. • Verify settings on drug infusion pumps with another nurse, when indicated. • Follow the rights of medication administration consistently. • Recheck the original drug order when a patient questions whether a particular drug dose should be taken. • Report errors, so that preventive efforts can be designed. • Discuss patients' medications during change-of-shift reports, including new and discontinued drugs, patients' responses to their medications, patient teaching about medications, and medications given 1–2 h before or after shift report.
Patients and Consumers • Outpatients may take drugs from several prescribers. • Fail to inform one prescriber about drugs prescribed by another health care provider • Get prescriptions filled at more than one pharmacy • Fail to get prescriptions filled or refilled • Underuse or overuse an appropriately prescribed drug • Take drugs left over from a previous illness or prescribed for someone else • Fail to follow instructions for drug administration or storage • Fail to keep appointments for follow-up care • Fail to ask for information when needed	• Inform all health care providers about health status, any drug allergies, and all medications being taken (e.g., prescription, over-the-counter, herbal, and dietary supplements). • Ask prescribers to include the purpose of a drug on the label of all prescription medications. • If able, know names, strengths, doses, and the reason for use of all medications. • Follow instructions about when and how to take medications; do not increase amount or frequency of any medication without checking with a health care provider. Ask questions or request written instructions if needed. • If unable to take medications or if problems occur, discuss with a health care provider. Do not stop taking prescribed medications. • Maintain a current list of all medications being taken. Take the list or the medications to each visit to a health care provider. • Keep all medications in their original containers. • Read labels of medication containers every time a dose is taken. • Do not chew, crush, or break any tablets or capsules unless a health care provider says it is okay to do so.

CPOE, computerized provider order entry; FDA, U.S. Food mend Drug Administration.

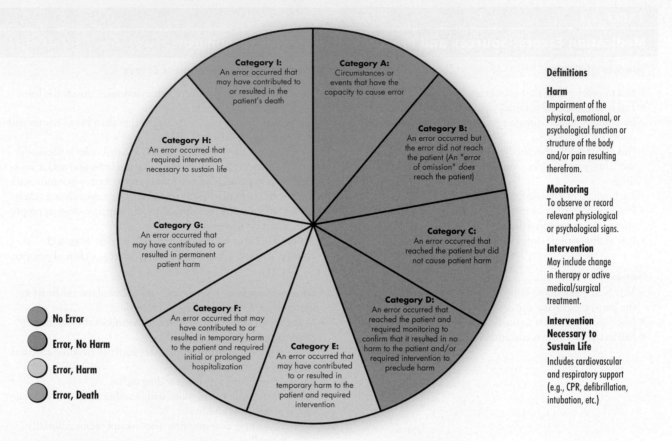

Figure 3.1 Index for categorizing medication errors, National Coordinating Council for Medication Error Reporting and Prevention. http://www.nccmerp.org/pdf/index-Color2001-06-12.pdf ©2001 National Coordinating Council for Medication Error Reporting and Prevention. All rights reserved.

The NCCMERP has developed an index for categorizing medication errors (Fig. 3.1) and an algorithm (Fig. 3.2). This categorization of medication errors can be adopted by health care institutions. Using the A through I, this system ranks medication errors according to the severity of their outcomes. Category A identifies circumstances that have the capacity to cause an error, and category I identifies an error that contributed to a patient's death. This system gives health care institutions the ability to track the rate of medication errors.

Medication Systems

Each health care facility has a system for distributing drugs. The unit–dose system, in which most drugs are dispensed in single-dose containers for individual patients, is widely used. The pharmacist or pharmacy technician checks drug orders and stocks the medication in the patient's medication drawer. When a dose is due to be taken, the nurse removes the medication and gives it to the patient. Unit–dose wrappings of oral drugs should be left in place until the nurse is in the presence of the patient and ready to give the medication. It is essential that each dose of a drug be recorded on the patient's medication administration record (MAR) as soon as possible after administration.

Increasingly, institutions are using automated, computerized, locked cabinets for which each nurse on a unit has a password or code for accessing the cabinet and obtaining a drug dose. The pharmacy maintains the medications and replaces the drug when needed.

Controlled drugs, such as opioid analgesics, are usually kept as a stock supply in a locked drawer or automated cabinet and replaced as needed. The nurse must sign for each dose and record it on the patient's MAR. He or she must comply with legal regulations and institutional policies for dispensing and recording controlled drugs.

Changes to Prevent Medication Errors

Changes in medication systems are being increasingly implemented, largely in efforts to decrease medication errors and improve patient safety. These include the following:

- Computerized provider order entry (CPOE). In this system, a prescriber types a medication order directly into a computer. This decreases errors associated with illegible handwriting and erroneous transcription or dispensing. CPOE, which is already used in many health care facilities, is widely recommended as the preferred alternative to error-prone handwritten orders.

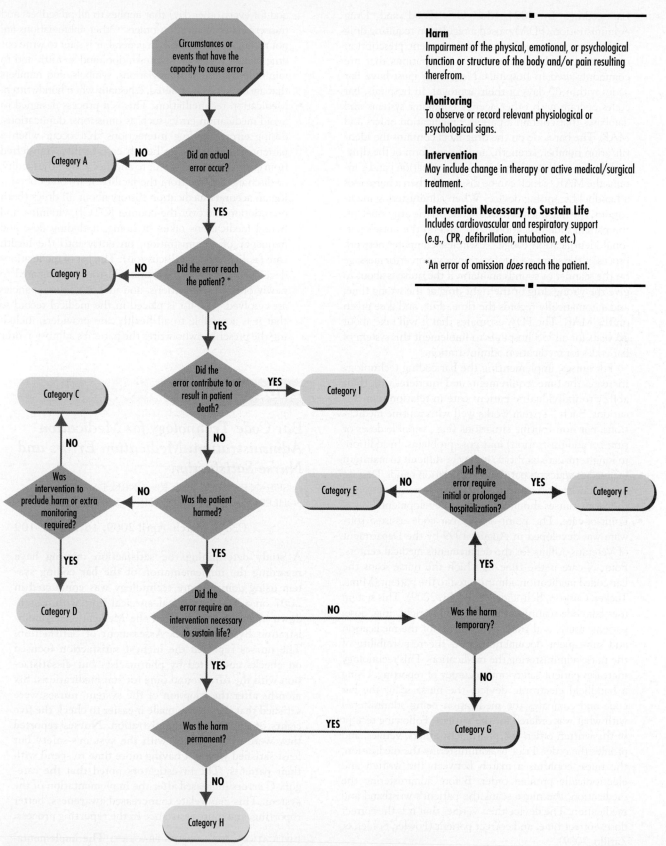

Harm
Impairment of the physical, emotional, or psychological function or structure of the body and/or pain resulting therefrom.

Monitoring
To observe or record relevant physiological or psychological signs.

Intervention
May include change in therapy or active medical/surgical treatment.

Intervention Necessary to Sustain Life
Includes cardiovascular and respiratory support (e.g., CPR, defibrillation, intubation, etc.)

*An error of omission *does* reach the patient.

Figure 3.2 Algorithm for categorizing medication errors, National Coordinating Council for Medication Error Reporting and Prevention. http://www.nccmerp.org/pdf/algor-Color2001-06-12.pdf ©2001 National Coordinating Council for Medication Error Reporting and Prevention. All rights reserved.

- Bar coding. In 2004, the U.S. Food and Drug Administration (FDA) passed a regulation requiring drug manufacturers to put bar codes on current prescription medications and nonprescription medications that are commonly used in hospitals. New drugs must have bar codes within 60 days of their approval. In hospitals, bar codes operate with other agency computer systems and databases that contain a patient's medication orders and MAR. The bar code on the drug label contains the identification number, strength, and dosage form of the drug, and the bar code on the patient's identification band contains the MAR, which can be displayed when a nurse uses a handheld scanning device. When administering medications, the nurse scans the bar code on the drug label, on the patient's identification band, and on the nurse's personal identification badge. A wireless computer network processes the scanned information; gives an error message on the scanner or sounds an alarm if the nurse is about to give the wrong drug or the right drug at the wrong time; and automatically records the time, drug, and dose given on the MAR. The FDA estimates that it will take about 20 years for all US hospitals to implement this system of bar codes for medication administration.

  For nurses, implementing the bar coding technology increases the time requirements and interferes with their ability to individualize patient care in relation to medications. Such a system works well with routine medications, but non-routine situations (e.g., variable doses or times of administration) may pose problems. In addition, in long-term care facilities, it may be difficult to maintain legible bar codes on patient identification bands. Despite some drawbacks, bar coding increases patient safety, and therefore, nurses should support its development.

- Point-of-care. The point-of-care bar code–assisted software was developed in August 1999 by the Department of Veterans Affairs for the department's medical centers. Point-of-care is the time in which the nurse scans the bar-coded medication administered to the patient (Mims, Tucker, Carlson, Schneider, & Bagby, 2009). This system uses bar code scanning that verifies the right drug, dose, patient, route, and time. The reason for the medication and subsequent documentation is the responsibility of the nurse administering the medication. This technology increases patient safety and accuracy of reporting. Using a handheld electronic device, the nurse scans the bar code and compares the medication being administered with what was ordered for the patient. Following receipt of the written order, the pharmacist enters, verifies, and profiles the order. Prior to administering the medication, the nurse confirms a match between the written and electronically profiled order. Before administering the medication, the nurse scans the patient's wristband and medication. The device then verifies that it is the correct dose, correct time, and correct patient (Fowler, Sohler, & Zarillo, 2009).

- Limiting use of abbreviations. The ISMP has long maintained a list of abbreviations that are often associated with medication errors, and the Joint Commission requires accredited organizations to maintain a "Do Not Use" list (e.g., u or U for units, IU for international units, qd for daily, qod for every other day) that applies to all prescribers and transcribers of medication orders. Other abbreviations are not recommended as well. In general, it is safer to write out drug names, routes of administration, and so forth and to minimize the use of abbreviations, symbols, and numbers that are often misinterpreted, especially when handwritten.

- Medication reconciliation. This is a process designed to avoid medication errors such as omissions, duplications, dosing errors, or drug interactions that occur when a patient is admitted to a health care facility, transferred from one department or unit to another within the facility, or discharged home from the facility. It involves obtaining an accurate medication history about all drugs (both prescription and over-the-counter [OTC]), vitamins, and herbal medications taken at home, including dose and frequency of administration, on entry into the health care facility (see later discussion). The list of medications developed from the medication history is compared to newly ordered medications, and identified discrepancies are resolved. The list is placed in the medical record so that it is accessible to all health care providers, including the prescriber who writes the patient's admission drug

EVIDENCE-BASED PRACTICE

Bar Code Technology for Medication Administration: Medication Errors and Nurse Satisfaction

by SUSAN FOWLER, PHD, RN, CNRN, PATRICIA SOHLER, MA, RN, & DOROTHY ZARILLO, MSN, RN

CNAA March–April 2009, 18(2):103–109

A study determining the satisfaction nursing have regarding the implementation of the bar coding system using point-of-care technology was conducted in 2007 on a 53-bed medical–surgical unit with a step-down area. The study used the Medications Administration System–Nurses Assessment of Satisfaction. The nurses reported the highest satisfaction focused on checks completed by pharmacists but dissatisfaction with the turnaround time for stat medications. Six months after the adoption of the system, nurses were satisfied that the system made it easier to check the five rights of medication administration. Nurses reported they were most satisfied with the system's safety but least satisfied with not having more time to spend with their patients. The investigators noted that the category C errors increased after the implementation of the system. This may relate to increased awareness, better reporting, and more assistance in the reporting process.

IMPLICATIONS FOR NURSING PRACTICE: The implementation of point-of-care medication administration systems using bar codes allows for greater safety in medication administration. However, the profiling step in the process delays the administration of "stat" medications.

orders. When the patient is transferred, the updated list must be communicated to the next health care provider. When a patient is discharged, an updated list should be given to the next provider and to the patient. The patient should be encouraged to keep the list up-to-date when changes are made in the medication regimen and to share the list with future health care providers.

Clinical Application 3-2

- The nurse is checking Ms. Baranski's patient-controlled analgesia of morphine sulfate. The medication cartridge is empty and needs to be changed. What are the nurse's legal responsibilities when changing an opioid medication?

- What nursing interventions prevent medication errors?

NCLEX Success

3. **A prescriber has written an order for levothyroxine sodium (Synthroid) 50 mg per day by mouth. The nurse knows that the standard dose is 50 mcg. What action should the nurse take?**

   A. Call the prescriber and question the order.
   B. Administer 50 mcg instead.
   C. Consult the pharmacist about the order.
   D. Ask the patient what he or she usually takes.

4. **The nurse is administering the first dose of an anti-infective agent. Which of the following assessments should the nurse make prior to administering the anti-infective agent?**

   A. Assess the patient's temperature.
   B. Assess the patient's level of consciousness.
   C. Assess if the patient is allergic to any anti-infective agent.
   D. Assess if the patient has taken the medication previously.

5. **Which of the following nursing actions will prevent adverse drug events?**

   A. Use only the trade name when documenting medications.
   B. Crush long-acting medications if the patient has dysphagia.
   C. After receiving a verbal order, administer the medication and then write down the order.
   D. Use bar code technology according to institutional policy.

Medication Orders

Medication orders should include the full name of the patient; the name of the drug (preferably the generic name); the dose, route, and frequency of administration; and the date, time, and signature of the prescriber.

Orders in a health care facility may be typed into a computer (the preferred method) or handwritten on an order sheet in the patient's medical record. Occasionally, verbal or telephone orders are acceptable. When taken, they should be written on the patient's order sheet, signed by the person taking the order, and later countersigned by the prescriber. After the order is written, a copy is sent to the pharmacy, where the order is recorded and the drug is dispensed to the appropriate patient care unit. In many facilities, pharmacy staff prepares a computer-generated MAR for each 24-hour period.

For patients in ambulatory care settings, the procedure is essentially the same for drugs to be given immediately. For drugs to be taken at home, written prescriptions are given. In addition to the previous information, a prescription should include instructions for taking the drug (e.g., dose, frequency) and whether the prescription can be refilled. Prescriptions for Schedule II controlled drugs cannot be refilled.

To interpret medication orders accurately, the nurse must know commonly used abbreviations for routes, dosages, and times of drug administration (Table 3.2). As a result of medication errors that occurred because of incorrect or misinterpreted abbreviations, many abbreviations that were formerly commonly used are now banned or are no longer recommended by The Joint Commission, the ISMP, and other organizations concerned with increasing patient safety. Thus, it is safer to write out such words as "daily" or "three times daily," "at bedtime,"

TABLE 3.2	
Common Abbreviations	
Routes of Drug Administration	
IM	intramuscular
IV	intravenous
PO	by mouth, oral
SL	sublingual
Sub-Q, subcut	subcutaneous
Drug Dosages	
cc	cubic centimeter
g	gram
mg	milligram
mcg	microgram
mL	milliliter
oz	ounce
tbsp	tablespoon
tsp	teaspoon
Times of Drug Administration	
ad lib	as desired
PRN	as needed
q4h	every 4 h
stat	immediately

"ounce," "teaspoon" or "tablespoon," or "right," "left," or "both eyes" rather than using abbreviations, in both medication orders and in transcribing orders to the patient's MAR. If the nurse cannot read the physician's order or if the order seems erroneous, he or she must question the order before giving the drug.

NCLEX Success

6. A nurse is administering an elixir. Which of the following measures is appropriate?

A. microgram
B. milligram
C. milliliter
D. kilogram

7. The nurse has administered lacosamide (Vimpat) to the wrong patient. What is the first action the nurse should take?

A. Assess the patient's vital signs and level of consciousness.
B. Notify the physician.
C. Fill out an incident report.
D. Call the respiratory therapist for administration of oxygen.

Drug Preparations and Dosage Forms

Drug preparations and dosage forms vary according to the drug's chemical characteristics, reason for use, and route of administration. Some drugs are available in only one dosage form, and others are available in several forms. Table 3.3 and the following section describe characteristics of various dosage forms.

Dosage forms of systemic drugs include liquids, tablets, capsules, suppositories, and transdermal and pump delivery systems. Systemic liquids are given orally, or PO (Latin *per os*, "by mouth"), or by injection. Those given by injection must be sterile.

Administration of tablets and capsules is PO. Tablets contain active drug plus binders, colorants, preservatives, and other substances. Capsules contain active drug enclosed in a gelatin capsule. Most tablets and capsules dissolve in the acidic fluids of the stomach and are absorbed in the alkaline fluids of the upper small intestine. **Enteric-coated** tablets and capsules are coated with a substance that is insoluble in stomach acid. This delays dissolution until the medication reaches the intestine, usually to avoid gastric irritation or to keep the drug from being destroyed by gastric acid. Tablets for sublingual (under the tongue) or buccal (held in cheek) administration must be specifically formulated for such use.

Several **controlled-release** dosage forms and drug delivery systems are available, and more continue to be developed. These formulations maintain more consistent serum drug levels and allow less frequent administration, which is more convenient for patients. Controlled-release oral tablets and capsules are called by a variety of names (e.g., timed release, sustained release, extended release), and their names usually include CR, SR, XL, or other indications that they are long-acting formulations. Most of these formulations are given once or twice daily. Some drugs (e.g., alendronate for osteoporosis, fluoxetine for major depression) are available in formulations that deliver a full week's dosage in one oral tablet. Because controlled-release

TABLE 3.3

Drug Dosage Forms

Dosage Forms and Their Routes of Administration	Characteristics	Considerations/Precautions
Tablets		
Regular: PO, gastrointestinal (GI) tube (crushed and mixed with water)	• Contain active drug plus binders, dyes, and preservatives • Dissolve in gastric fluids	8 oz of water recommended, to promote dissolution and absorption
Chewable: PO	Colored and flavored, mainly for young children	Children may think tablets are candy; keep out of reach to avoid accidental overdose
Enteric-coated: PO	Dissolve in small intestine; mainly used for medications that cause gastric irritation	Do not crush; instruct patients not to chew or crush.
Extended release (XL) (also called sustained release [SR], long acting [LA], and other names): PO	Slowly absorbed; effects prolonged, usually 12–24 h Contain relatively large amounts of active drug	**Warning:** Crushing to give orally or through a GI tube administers an overdose, with potentially serious adverse effects or death!! *Never crush*; instruct patients not to chew or crush.
Sublingual: Under the tongue	Dissolve quickly	
Buccal: Held in cheek	Medication absorbed directly into the bloodstream and exerts rapid systemic effects	Few medications formulated for administration by SL or buccal routes

TABLE 3.3

Drug Dosage Forms (Continued)

Dosage Forms and Their Routes of Administration	Characteristics	Considerations/Precautions
Capsules *Regular:* PO	Contain active drug, fillers, and preservatives Gelatin capsules dissolve in gastric fluid and release medication.	8 oz of fluid recommended to promote dissolution and absorption
Extended release (XL); sustained release (SR); long acting (LA): PO	Slowly absorbed; effects prolonged, usually 12–24 h Contain relatively large amounts of active drug	**Warning:** Emptying a capsule to give the medication orally or through a GI tube administers an overdose, with potentially serious adverse effects or death!! Instruct patients not to bite, chew, or empty these capsules.
Solutions *Oral:* PO, GI tube	Absorbed rapidly because they do not need to be dissolved	Use of appropriate measuring devices and accurate measurement is extremely important.
Parenteral: IV, IM, Sub-Q, intradermal	Medications and all administration devices must be sterile. IV produces rapid effects; Sub-Q is used mainly for insulin and heparin; IM is used for only a few drugs; intradermal is used mainly to inject skin test material.	Use of appropriate equipment and accurate measurement is extremely important. Insulin syringes should always be used for insulin, and tuberculin syringes are recommended for measuring small amounts of other drugs.
Suspensions PO, Sub-Q (e.g., NPH, Lente insulins)	Particles of active drug are suspended in a liquid; the liquid must be rotated or shaken before measuring a dose.	Drug particles settle to the bottom on standing. If not remixed, the liquid vehicle is given rather than the drug dose.
Dermatologic Creams, Lotions, Ointments Topically to Skin	Most are minimally absorbed through skin and exert local effects at the site of application; some (e.g., skin patches) are absorbed and exert systemic effects.	*Formulations vary with intended uses and are not interchangeable.* When removed from the patient, skin patches must be disposed of properly to prevent someone else from being exposed to the active drug remaining in the patch.
Solutions and Powders for Oral or Nasal Inhalation, Including Metered-dose Inhalers (MDIs)	Oral inhalations are used mainly for asthma; nasal sprays for nasal allergies (allergic rhinitis). Effective with less systemic effect than oral drugs Deliver a specified dose per inhalation	Several research studies indicate that patients often do not use MDIs correctly; correct use is essential to obtaining therapeutic effects and avoiding adverse effects.
Eye Solutions and Ointments	*Should be sterile* Packaged in small amounts for individual use	Can be systemically absorbed and cause systemic adverse effects
Throat Lozenges	Used for cough and sore throat	
Ear Solutions	Used mainly for ear infections	
Vaginal Creams and Suppositories	Used to treat vaginal infections	
Rectal Suppositories and Enemas	Suppositories may be used to administer sedatives, analgesics, and laxatives. Medicated enemas may be used for constipation or inflammatory bowel diseases.	Effects somewhat unpredictable because absorption is erratic

tablets and capsules contain high amounts of drug intended to be absorbed slowly and act over a prolonged period of time, they should never be broken, opened, crushed, or chewed. Such an action allows the full dose to be absorbed immediately and constitutes an overdose, with potential organ damage or death. **Transdermal** (skin patch) formulations include systemically absorbed clonidine, estrogen, fentanyl, and nitroglycerin. These medications are slowly absorbed from the skin patches over varying periods of time (e.g., 1 week for clonidine and estrogen). Pump delivery systems may be external or implanted under the skin and refillable or long acting without refills. Pumps are used to administer insulin, opioid analgesics, antineoplastics, and other drugs.

Solutions, ointments, creams, and suppositories are applied topically to skin or mucous membranes. They are formulated for the intended route of administration. For example, several drugs are available in solutions for nasal or oral inhalation; they are usually self-administered as a spray into the nose or mouth.

Many combination products containing fixed doses of two or more drugs are also available. Commonly used combinations include analgesics, antihypertensive drugs, and cold remedies. Most are oral tablets, capsules, or solutions.

Calculating Drug Dosages

When calculating drug dosages, the importance of accuracy cannot be overemphasized. Accuracy requires basic skills in mathematics, knowledge of common units of measurement, and methods of using data in performing calculations.

Systems of Measurement

The most commonly used system of measurement is the metric system, in which the meter is used for linear measure, the gram for weight, and the liter for volume. One milliliter (mL) equals 1 cubic centimeter (cc), and both equal 1 gram (g) of water. The household system, with units of drops, teaspoons, tablespoons, and cups, is infrequently used in health care agencies but may be used at home. Table 3.4 lists some commonly used equivalent measurements.

A few drugs are ordered and measured in terms of units or milliequivalents (mEq). Units express biologic activity in animal tests (i.e., the amount of drug required to produce a particular response). Units are unique for each drug. For example, concentrations of insulin and heparin are both expressed in units, but there is no relation between a unit of insulin and a unit of heparin. These drugs are usually ordered in the number of units per dose (e.g., NPH insulin 30 units subcutaneously every morning, or heparin 5000 units subcutaneously every 12 hours) and labeled in number of units per milliliter (U 100 insulin contains 100 units/mL; heparin may have 1000, 5000, or 10,000 units/mL). Milliequivalents express the ionic activity of a drug. Drugs such as potassium chloride are ordered and labeled in the number of milliequivalents per dose, tablet, or milliliter.

TABLE 3.4

Selected Equivalent Measurements

Metric	Household
Weights	
1000 mcg = 1 mg	
1000 mg = 1 g	
30 g	1 oz
454 g	1 lb
1000 g = 1 kg	2.2 lb
Liquids	
1 mL = 1 cc	
5 mL	1 tsp
30 mL	2 tbsp or 1 oz
250 mL	1 cup or 8 oz
500 mL	1 pint
1000 mL = 1 L	1 quart

Mathematical Calculations

Most drug orders and labels are expressed in metric units of measurement. If the amount specified in the order is the same as that on the drug label, no calculations are required, and preparing the right dose is a simple matter. For example, if the order reads "ibuprofen 400 mg PO" and the drug label reads "ibuprofen 400 mg per tablet," it is clear that one tablet is to be given.

What happens if the order calls for a 400-mg dose and 200-mg tablets are available? The question is, "How many 200-mg tablets are needed to give a dose of 400 mg?" In this case, the answer can be readily calculated mentally to indicate two tablets. This is a simple example that also can be used to illustrate mathematical calculations. This problem can be solved by several acceptable methods; the following formula is presented because of its relative simplicity for students lacking a more familiar method:

$$\frac{D}{H} = \frac{X}{V}$$

D = desired dose (dose ordered, often in milligrams)
H = on hand or available dose (dose on the drug label; often in mg per tablet, capsule, or milliliter)
X = unknown (number of tablets, in this example)
V = volume or unit (one tablet, in this example)

$$\frac{400\,mg}{200\,mg} = \frac{X\,tablet}{1\,tablet}$$

Cross multiply:

$$200X = 400$$

$$X = \frac{400}{200} = 2\,tablets$$

What happens if the order and the label are written in different units? For example, the order may read "amoxicillin 0.5 g" and the label may read "amoxicillin 500 mg/capsule." To calculate the number of capsules needed for the dose, the first step is to convert 0.5 g to the equivalent number of milligrams, or convert 500 mg to the equivalent number of grams. *The desired or ordered dose and the available or label dose must be in the same units of measurement.* Using the equivalents (i.e., 1 g = 1000 mg) listed in Table 3.4, an equation can be set up as follows:

$$\frac{1g}{1000\,mg} = \frac{0.5g}{X\,mg}$$
$$X = 0.5 \times 1000 = 500\,mg$$

The next step is to use the new information in the formula, which then becomes

$$\frac{D}{H} = \frac{X}{V}$$
$$\frac{500\,mg}{500\,mg} = \frac{X\,capsules}{1\,capsule}$$
$$500X = 500$$
$$X = \frac{500}{500} = 1\,capsule$$

The same procedure and formula can be used to calculate portions of tablets or doses of liquids. These are illustrated in the following problems:

1. Order: 25 mg PO
   Label: 50-mg tablet

$$\frac{25\,mg}{50\,mg} = \frac{X\,tablet}{1\,tablet}$$
$$50X = 25$$
$$X = \frac{25}{50} = 0.5\,tablet$$

2. Order: 25 mg IM
   Label: 50 mg in 1 cc

$$\frac{25\,mg}{50\,mg} = \frac{X\,cc}{1\,cc}$$
$$50X = 25$$
$$X = \frac{25}{50} = 0.5\,cc$$

3. Order: 4 mg IV
   Label: 10 mg/mL

$$\frac{4\,mg}{10\,mg} = \frac{X\,mL}{1\,mL}$$
$$10X = 4$$
$$X = \frac{4}{10} = 0.4\,mL$$

Routes of Administration

Routes of administration depend on drug characteristics, patient characteristics, and desired responses. The major routes are oral (by mouth), **parenteral** (injected), and **topical** (applied to skin or mucous membrane). Each has advantages, disadvantages, indications for use, and specific techniques of administration (Table 3.5). Common parenteral routes are subcutaneous, IM, and IV injections. Injections require special drug preparations, equipment, and techniques. The following section discusses general characteristics of the IV route, and Box 3.1 presents specific considerations.

Drugs for Injection

Injectable drugs must be prepared, packaged, and administered in ways to maintain sterility. Vials are closed containers with rubber stoppers through which a sterile needle can be inserted for withdrawing medication. Single-dose vials usually do not contain a preservative and must be discarded after a dose is withdrawn. Multiple-dose vials contain a preservative and may be reused if aseptic technique is maintained.

Ampules are sealed glass containers, the tops of which must be broken off to allow insertion of a needle and withdrawal of the medication. Broken ampules and any remaining medication are discarded. When vials or ampules contain a powder form of the drug, a sterile solution of water or 0.9% sodium chloride must be added and the drug dissolved before withdrawal. When available, a filter needle is used to withdraw the medication from an ampule or vial because broken glass or rubber fragments may need to be removed from the drug solution. The filter needle is replaced with a regular needle before injecting the patient.

Many injectable drugs (e.g., morphine, heparin) are available in prefilled syringes with attached needles. These units are inserted into specially designed holders and used like other needle–syringe units.

QSEN Safety Alert

It is important to note that many such units, especially those from the same manufacturer, are similar, and their use may lead to medication errors if the label is not read carefully.

Equipment for Injections

Sterile needles and syringes are used to measure and administer parenteral medications; they may be packaged together or separately. Needles are available in various gauges and lengths. The term *gauge* refers to lumen size, with larger numbers indicating smaller lumen sizes. For example, a 25-gauge needle is smaller than an 18-gauge needle. Choice of needle gauge and length depends on the route of administration, the viscosity (thickness) of the solution to be given, and the size of the patient. Usually, a 25-gauge, 5/8-inch needle is used for subcutaneous injections, and a 22- or 20-gauge, 1½-inch needle is used for IM injections. Other needle sizes are available for special uses,

TABLE 3.5

Routes of Drug Administration

Route and Description	Advantages	Disadvantages	Comments
Oral	Simple and can be used by most people Convenient; does not require complex equipment Relatively inexpensive	Dosage is unknown because some drug is not absorbed and some is metabolized in the liver before reaching the bloodstream. Slow drug action Irritation of GI mucosa by some drugs	The oral route should generally be used when possible, considering the patient's condition and ability to take or tolerate oral drugs.
GI tubes (e.g., nasogastric, gastrostomy)	Allows use of GI tract in patients who cannot take oral drugs Can be used over long periods of time, if necessary May avoid or decrease injections	With nasogastric tubes, medications may be aspirated into the lungs. Small-bore tubes often become clogged. Requires special precautions to give correctly and avoid complications	Liquid preparations are preferred over crushed tablets and emptied capsules, when available. Tube should be rinsed before and after instilling medication.
Subcutaneous (Sub-Q) injection—injection of drugs under the skin, into the underlying fatty tissue	Relatively painless Very small needles can be used. Insulin and heparin, commonly used medications, can be given Sub-Q.	Only a small amount of drug (up to 1 mL) can be given. Drug absorption is relatively slow. Only a few drugs can be given Sub-Q.	Sub-Q route is commonly used for only a few drugs because many drugs are irritating to Sub-Q tissues. Such drugs may cause pain, necrosis, and abscess formation if injected Sub-Q.
Intramuscular (IM) injection—injection of drugs into selected muscles	May be used for several drugs Drug absorption is rapid because muscle tissue has an abundant blood supply.	A relatively small amount of drug (up to 3 mL) can be given. Risks of damage to blood vessels or nerves if needle is not positioned correctly	It is very important to use anatomic landmarks when selecting IM injection sites.
Intravenous (IV) injection—injection of a drug into the bloodstream	Allows medications to be given to a patient who cannot take fluids or drugs by GI tract Bypasses barriers to drug absorption that occur with other routes Rapid drug action Larger amounts can be given than by Sub-Q and IM routes. Allows slow administration when indicated	Time and skill required for venipuncture and maintaining an IV line After it is injected, drug cannot be retrieved if adverse effects or overdoses occur. High potential for adverse reactions due to rapid drug action and possible complications of IV therapy (i.e., bleeding, infection, fluid overload, extravasation) Phlebitis and thrombosis may occur and cause discomfort or pain, take days or weeks to subside, and limit the veins available for future therapy.	The nurse should wear latex gloves to start IV infusions, for protection against exposure to blood-borne pathogens. Phlebitis and thrombosis result from injury to the endothelial cells that form the inner lining (intima) of veins and may be caused by repeated venipunctures, the IV catheter, hypertonic IV fluid, or irritating drugs.

TABLE 3.5

Routes of Drug Administration (Continued)

Route and Description	Advantages	Disadvantages	Comments
Topical administration—application to skin or mucous membranes. Application to mucous membranes includes drugs given by nasal or oral inhalation; by instillation into the lungs, eyes, or nose; and by insertion under the tongue (sublingual), into the cheek (buccal), and into the vagina or rectum.	With application to intact skin, most medications act at the site of application, with little systemic absorption or systemic adverse effects. Some drugs are given topically for systemic effects (e.g., medicated skin patches). Effects may last several days, and the patches are usually convenient for patients. With application to mucous membranes, most drugs are well and rapidly absorbed.	Some drugs irritate skin or mucous membranes and cause itching, rash, or discomfort. With inflamed, abraded, or damaged skin, drug absorption is increased and systemic adverse effects may occur. Application to mucous membranes may cause systemic adverse effects (e.g., beta-blocker eye drops, used to treat glaucoma, can cause bradycardia just as oral beta-blockers can). Specific drug preparations must be used for application to skin, eyes, sublingual, buccal, vaginal, and rectal sites.	When available and effective, topical drugs are often preferred over oral or injected drugs because of fewer and/or less severe systemic adverse effects.

BOX 3.1   Principles and Techniques With Intravenous Drug Therapy

Methods

Intravenous (IV) injection or **IV** push is the direct injection of a medication into the vein. The drug may be injected through an injection site on IV tubing or an intermittent infusion device. Most IV push medications should be injected slowly. The time depends on the particular drug but is often 2 minutes or longer for a dose. Rapid injection should generally be avoided because the drug produces high blood levels and is quickly circulated to the heart and brain, where it may cause adverse or toxic effects. Although IV push may be useful with a few drugs or in emergency situations, slower infusion of more dilute drugs is usually preferred.

Intermittent infusion is administration of intermittent doses, often diluted in 50 to 100 mL of fluid and infused over 30 to 60 minutes. The drug dose is usually prepared in a pharmacy and connected to an IV administration set that controls the amount and flow rate. Intermittent infusions are often connected to an injection port on a primary IV line, through which IV fluids are infusing continuously. The purpose of the primary IV line may be to provide fluids to the patient or to keep the vein open for periodic administration of medications. The IV fluids are usually stopped for the medication infusion, then restarted. Drug doses may also be infused through an intermittent infusion device (e.g., a heparin lock) to conserve veins and allow freedom of motion between drug doses. The devices decrease the amount of IV fluids given to patients who do not need them (i.e., those who are able to ingest adequate amounts of oral fluids) and those who are at risk of fluid overload, especially children and older adults.

An intermittent infusion device may be part of an initial IV line or used to adapt a continuous IV for **intermittent** use. The devices include a heparin lock or a resealable adapter added to a peripheral or central IV catheter. These devices must be flushed routinely to maintain patency. If the IV catheter has more than one lumen, all must be flushed, whether being used or not. Saline is probably the most commonly used flushing solution; heparin may also be used if recommended by the device's manufacturer or required by institutional policy.

Continuous infusion indicates medications mixed in a large volume of IV fluid and infused continuously, over several hours. For example, vitamins and minerals (e.g., potassium chloride) are usually added to liters of IV fluids. Greater dilution of the drug and administration over a longer time decreases risks of accumulation and toxicity, as well as venous irritation and thrombophlebitis.

Equipment

Equipment varies considerably from one health care agency to another. Nurses must become familiar with the equipment available in their work setting, including IV catheters, types of IV tubing, needles and needleless systems, types of volume control devices, and electronic infusion devices (IV pumps).

Catheters vary in size (both gauge and length), design, and composition (e.g., polyvinyl chloride, polyurethane, silicone). The most common design type is over the needle; the needle is used to start the IV, then it is removed. When choosing a catheter to start an IV, one that is much smaller than the lumen of the vein is recommended. This allows good blood flow and rapidly dilutes drug solutions as they enter the vein. This, in turn, prevents high drug

(*Continued on page 50*)

BOX 3.1	**Principles and Techniques With Intravenous Drug Therapy** (Continued)

concentrations and risks of toxicity. Also, after a catheter is inserted, it is very important to tape it securely so that it does not move around. Movement of the catheter increases venous irritation and risks of thrombophlebitis and infection. If signs of venous irritation and inflammation develop, the catheter should be removed and a new one inserted at another site. Additional recommendations include application of a topical antibiotic or antiseptic ointment at the IV site after catheter insertion, a sterile occlusive dressing over the site, and limiting the duration of placement to a few days.

Many medications are administered through peripherally inserted central catheters (PICC lines) or central venous catheters, in which the catheter tips are inserted into the superior vena cava, next to the right atrium of the heart. Central venous catheters may have single, double, or triple lumens. Other products, which are especially useful for long-term IV drug therapy, include a variety of implanted ports, pumps, and reservoirs.

If a catheter becomes clogged, do not irrigate it. Doing so may push a clot into the circulation and result in a pulmonary embolus, myocardial infarction, or stroke. It may also cause septicemia, if the clot is infected.

Needleless systems are products with a blunt-tipped plastic insertion device and an injection port that opens. These systems greatly decrease needlestick injuries and exposure to blood-borne pathogens.

Electronic infusion devices allow amounts and flow rates of IV drug solutions to be set and controlled by a computer. Although the devices save nursing time because the nurse does not need to continually adjust flow rates, the biggest advantage is the steady rate of drug administration. The devices are used in most settings where IV drugs and IV fluids are administered, but they are especially valuable in pediatrics, where very small amounts of medication and IV fluid are needed, and in intensive care units, where strong drugs and varying amounts of IV fluid are usually required. Several types of pumps are available, even within the same health care agency. It is extremely important that nurses become familiar with the devices used in their work setting, so that they can program them accurately and determine whether or not they are functioning properly (i.e., delivering medications as ordered).

Site Selection

IV needles are usually inserted into a vein on the hand or forearm; IV catheters may be inserted in a peripheral site or centrally. In general, recommendations are

- Start at the most distal location. This conserves more proximal veins for later use, if needed. Veins on the back of the hand and on the forearm are often used to provide more comfort and freedom of movement for patients.
- Use veins with a large blood volume flowing through them when possible. Many drugs cause irritation and phlebitis in small veins.
- When possible, avoid the antecubital vein on the inner surface of the elbow, veins over or close to joints, and veins on the inner aspect of the wrists. Reasons include the difficulty of stabilizing and maintaining an IV line at these sites and inner wrist venipunctures are very painful. *Do not perform venipuncture in foot or leg veins.* The risks of serious or fatal complications are too high.

- Rotate sites when long-term use (more than a few days) of IV fluid or drug therapy is required. Venous irritation occurs with longer duration of site use and with the administration of irritating drugs or fluids. When it is necessary to change an IV site, use the opposite arm if possible.
- Most IV drugs are prepared for administration in pharmacies, and this is the safest practice. When a nurse must prepare a medication, considerations include the following.
- Only drug formulations manufactured for IV use should be given IV. Other formulations contain various substances that are not sterile, pure enough, or soluble enough to be injected into the bloodstream. *In recent years, there have been numerous reports of medication errors resulting from IV administration of drug preparations intended for oral use!!* Such errors can and should be prevented. For example, when liquid medications intended for oral use are measured or dispensed in a syringe (as they often are for children, adults with difficulty in swallowing tablets and capsules, or for administration through a gastrointestinal [GI] tube), the syringe should have a blunt tip that will not connect to or penetrate IV tubing injection sites.
- Use sterile technique during all phases of IV drug preparation.
- Follow the manufacturer's instructions for mixing and diluting IV medications. Some liquid IV medications need to be diluted prior to IV administration, and powdered medications must be reconstituted with the recommended diluent. The diluent recommended by the drug's manufacturer should be used because different drugs require different diluents. In addition, be sure any reconstituted drug is completely dissolved to avoid particles that may be injected into the systemic circulation and lead to thrombus formation or embolism. A filtered aspiration needle should be used when withdrawing medication from a vial or ampule, to remove any particles in the solution. The filter needle should then be discarded, to prevent filtered particles from being injected when the medication is added to the IV fluid. Filters added to IV tubing also help to remove particles.
- Check the expiration date on all IV medications. Many drugs have a limited period of stability after they are reconstituted or diluted for IV administration.
- IV medications should be compatible with the infusing IV fluids. Most are compatible with 5% dextrose in water or saline solutions.
- If adding a medication to a container of IV fluid, invert the container to be sure the additive is well mixed with the solution.
- For any IV medication that is prepared or added to an IV bag, label the medication vial or IV bag with the name of the patient, drug, dosage, date, time of mixing, expiration date, and the preparer's signature.
- Most IV medications are injected into a self-sealing site in any of several IV setups, including a scalp–vein needle and tubing; a plastic catheter connected to a heparin lock or other intermittent infusion device; or IV tubing and a plastic bag containing IV fluid.

| **BOX 3.1** | **Principles and Techniques With Intravenous Drug Therapy** (Continued) |

■ Before injecting any IV medication, be sure the IV line is open and functioning properly (e.g., catheter not clotted, IV fluid not leaking into surrounding tissues, phlebitis not present). If leakage occurs, some drugs are very irritating to subcutaneous tissues and may cause tissue necrosis.

■ Maintain sterility of all IV fluids, tubings, injection sites, drug solutions, and equipment coming into contact with the IV system. Because medications and fluids are injected directly into the bloodstream, breaks in sterile technique can lead to serious systemic infection (septicemia) and death.

■ When two or more medications are to be given one after the other, flush the IV tubing and catheter (with the infusing IV fluid or with sterile 0.9% sodium chloride injection) so that the drugs do not come into contact with each other.

■ In general, administer slowly to allow greater dilution of the drug in the bloodstream. Most drugs given by IV push (direct injection) can be given over 2 to 5 minutes, and most drugs diluted in 50 to 100 mL of IV fluid can be infused in 30 to 60 minutes.

■ When injecting or infusing medications into IV solutions that contain other additives (e.g., vitamins, insulin, minerals such as potassium or magnesium), be sure the medications are compatible with the other substances. Consult compatibility charts (usually available on nursing units) or pharmacists when indicated.

■ IV flow rates are usually calculated in mL/hour and drops per minute.

such as for insulin or intradermal injections. When needles are used, avoid recapping them and dispose of them in appropriate containers. Such containers are designed to prevent accidental needlestick injuries to health care and housekeeping personnel.

In many settings, needleless systems are used. These systems involve a plastic tip on the syringe that can be used to enter vials and injection sites on IV tubing. Openings created by the tip reseal themselves. Needleless systems were developed because of the risk of injury and spread of blood-borne pathogens, such as the viruses that cause acquired immunodeficiency syndrome and hepatitis B.

Syringes also are available in various sizes. The 3-mL size is often used. It is usually plastic and is available with or without an attached needle. Syringes are calibrated so that drug doses can be measured accurately. However, the calibrations vary according to the size and type of syringe.

Insulin and tuberculin syringes are used for specific purposes. Insulin syringes are calibrated to measure up to 100 units of insulin. Safe practice requires that *only* insulin syringes be used to measure insulin and that they be used for no other drugs. Tuberculin syringes have a capacity of 1 mL. They should be used for small doses of any drug because measurements are more accurate than with larger syringes.

Sites for Injections

Common sites for subcutaneous injections are the upper arms, abdomen, back, and thighs (Fig. 3.3). Sites for IM injections are the deltoid, dorsogluteal, ventrogluteal, and vastus lateralis muscles. It should be noted that many health care agencies do not allow the administration of IM injections in the dorsogluteal site. It is important to review the policies and procedures of the institution before administering medications utilizing that site. To select the proper injection sites, the anatomical landmarks are identified. (Fig. 3.4). Common sites for IV injections are the veins on the back of the hands and on the forearms (Fig. 3.5). Less common sites include intradermal (into layers of the skin), intra-arterial (into arteries), intra-articular (into joints), and intrathecal (into spinal fluid). Nurses may perform intradermal and intra-arterial injections (if an established arterial line is present); physicians perform intra-articular and intrathecal injections.

Clinical Application 3-3

- Ms. Baranski's IV line has infiltrated and will not be restarted. Her physician has ordered hydrocodone/acetaminophen (Vicodin) 500 mg by mouth every 6 hours PRN for pain as well as ketorolac. In the event the pain is severe, the nurse can administer ketorolac 15 mg IM every 6 hours PRN. Five hours after receiving the Vicodin, the patient rates her pain as 9 on a scale of 1 to 10. The nurse decides to administer the ketorolac. The only ketorolac available is 30 mg/1 mL. How much ketorolac should be administered?

NCLEX Success

8. A patient is to receive lamotrigine (Lamictal) 300 mg by mouth two times per day. The pharmacy has delivered 50-mg tablets. How many tablets should the nurse administer each time?

    A. 2 tablets
    B. 4 tablets
    C. 6 tablets
    D. 8 tablets

9. A nurse is preparing to administer a subcutaneous injection. What size needle should the nurse use to administer the injection?

    A. 18 gauge
    B. 20 gauge
    C. 23 gauge
    D. 25 gauge

10. A patient is to receive an IM injection of ketorolac. Which of the following muscles should be avoided?

    A. deltoid
    B. dorsogluteal
    C. ventrogluteal
    D. vastus lateralis

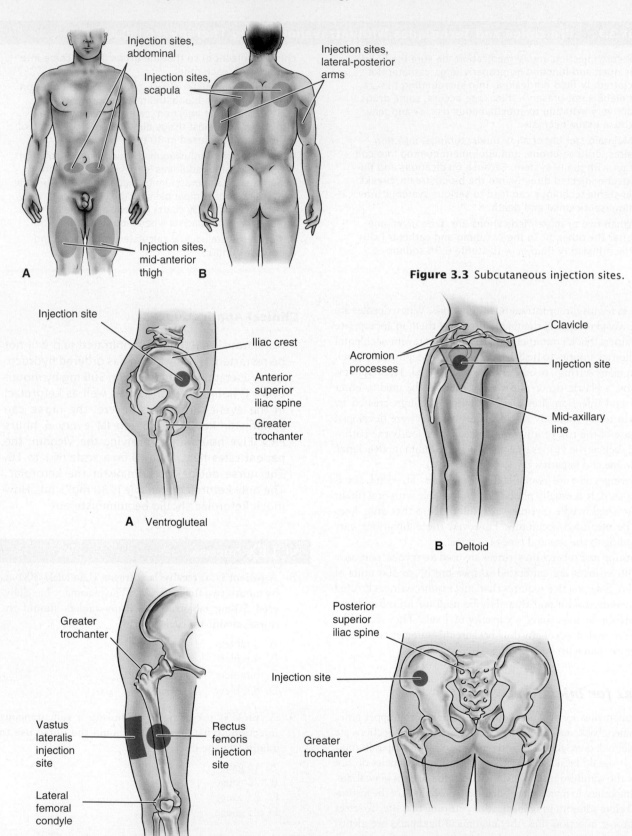

A

Injection sites, abdominal

Injection sites, scapula

Injection sites, mid-anterior thigh

B

Injection sites, lateral-posterior arms

Figure 3.3 Subcutaneous injection sites.

Injection site

Iliac crest

Anterior superior iliac spine

Greater trochanter

A   Ventrogluteal

Clavicle

Acromion processes

Injection site

Mid-axillary line

B   Deltoid

Greater trochanter

Vastus lateralis injection site

Rectus femoris injection site

Lateral femoral condyle

C   Vastus lateralis and rectus femoris

Posterior superior iliac spine

Injection site

Greater trochanter

D   Dorsogluteal

Figure 3.4 Anatomic landmarks and intramuscular (IM) injection sites. **A.** Ventrogluteal muscle. **B.** Deltoid muscle **C.** Vastus lateralis and rectus femoris muscle. **D.** Dorsogluteal muscle.

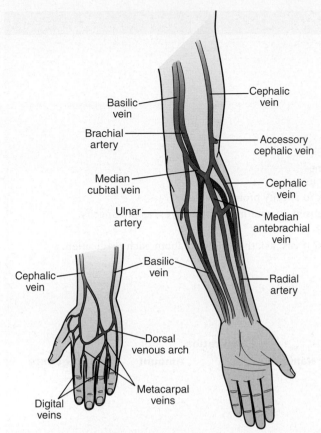

Figure 3.5 Veins of the hand and forearm that may be used to administer intravenous (IV) fluids and medications.

Nursing Process in Drug Therapy

As previously stated, the nursing process involves assessment, nursing diagnosis, planning and establishing goals for nursing care, interventions, and evaluation. Assessment and intervention are "action" phases, whereas analyzing assessment data, establishing nursing diagnoses and goals, and performing evaluations are "thinking" phases. However, knowledge and informed, rational thinking should underlie all data collection, decision making, and interventions.

Assessment

Assessment involves collecting data about patient characteristics known to affect drug therapy. This includes observing and interviewing the patient, interviewing family members or others involved in patient care, completing a physical assessment, reviewing medical records for pertinent laboratory and diagnostic test reports, and other methods. Initially (before drug therapy is started or on first contact), the nurse assesses age, weight, vital signs, health status, pathologic conditions, and ability to function in usual activities of daily living. In addition, the nurses assess for previous and current use of prescription, nonprescription, and nontherapeutic (e.g., alcohol, caffeine, nicotine, cocaine, marijuana) drugs. A **medication history** (Box 3.2) is useful; it is possible to incorporate the information

into any data collection tool. Specific questions and areas of assessment include the following:

- What are current drug orders?
- What does the patient know about current drugs? Is teaching needed?
- What drugs has the patient taken before? Include any drugs taken regularly, such as those for hypertension, diabetes mellitus, or other chronic conditions. Ask the patient about OTC drugs for colds, headaches, or indigestion, because some people do not think of these preparations as drugs.
- Has the patient ever had an allergic reaction to a drug? If so, what signs and symptoms occurred and how were they managed?
- Is the patient able to communicate verbally; can he or she swallow oral medications?
- Does the patient have pathologic conditions that influence drug therapy? For example, all seriously ill patients should be assessed for impaired function of vital organs.
- Assess for current use of herbal or dietary supplements (e.g., echinacea, glucosamine/chondroitin, vitamins). If so, ask for names, how much is taken and how often, for how long, their reason for use, and perceived benefits or adverse effects.

In addition to assessment data, the nurse uses progress notes (of any other health care providers), laboratory reports, and other sources to obtain baseline data for monitoring therapeutic or adverse drug effects. Laboratory tests of liver, kidney, and bone marrow function are often helpful because some drugs may damage these organs. Also, if liver or kidney damage exists, drug metabolism or excretion may be altered. The nurses consult authoritative sources for information about the patient's disease processes and ordered drugs, if needed.

After assessment data are obtained, they need to be analyzed to determine the patient's nursing care needs. Although listed as the first step in the nursing process for discussion purposes, assessment is a component of all steps and occurs with every contact with the patient. Ongoing assessment of a patient's health status and response to treatment is needed to determine whether nursing care requirements have changed. In general, nurses must provide care based on available information while knowing that assessment data are always relatively incomplete.

Nursing Diagnosis

A **nursing diagnosis,** as developed by the North American Nursing Diagnosis Association, describes patient problems or needs. It is based on assessment data and individualized according to the patient's condition and the drugs prescribed. Thus, the number of nursing diagnoses needed to adequately reflect the patient's condition varies considerably. Because almost any nursing diagnosis may apply in specific circumstances, this text emphasizes those diagnoses that generally apply to drug therapy.

- Deficient knowledge: drug therapy regimen (e.g., drug ordered; reason for use; expected effects; monitoring of response by health care providers, including diagnostic tests and office visits)
- Deficient knowledge: safe and effective self-administration (when appropriate)

BOX 3.2	Medication History

Name _____ Age _____
Health problems, acute and chronic
Are you allergic to any medications?
If yes, describe specific effects or symptoms.

Part 1: Prescription Medications

1. Do you take any prescription medications on a regular basis?

2. If yes, ask the following about each medication.

Name	Dose
Frequency	Specific times
How long taken	Reason for use

3. Do you have any difficulty in taking your medicines? If yes, ask to specify problem areas.

4. Have you had any symptoms or problems that you think are caused by your medicines? If yes, ask to specify.

5. Do you need help from another person to take your medicines?

6. Do you take any prescription medications on an irregular basis? If yes, ask the following about each medication.

Name	Dose
Frequency	Reason
How long taken	

Part 2: Nonprescription Medications

Do you take over-the-counter medications?

		Medication		
Problem	**Yes/No**	**Name**	**Amount**	**Frequency**
Pain				
Headache				
Sleep				
Cold				
Indigestion				
Heartburn				
Diarrhea				
Constipation				
Other				

Part 3: Social Drugs

	Yes/No	**Amount/day**
Coffee		
Tea		
Cola drinks		
Alcohol		
Tobacco		

Part 4: Herbal or Dietary Supplements

Do you take any herbal or dietary supplements (e.g., gingko, glucosamine/chondroitin)? If so, ask for names, how much and how often taken, reason for use, perceived effectiveness, and any adverse effects.

- Risk for injury related to adverse drug effects
- Noncompliance: overuse
- Noncompliance: underuse

Planning/Goals

The **planning/goals** phase describes the expected outcomes of prescribed drug therapy. As a general rule, goals are stated in terms of patient behavior, not nurse behavior. For example, the patient will

- Receive or take drugs as prescribed
- Experience relief of signs and symptoms
- Avoid preventable adverse drug effects
- Self-administer drugs safely and accurately
- Verbalize essential drug information

- Keep appointments for monitoring and follow-up
- Use any herbal and dietary supplements with caution and report such use to health care providers

Interventions

Interventions involve implementing planned activities and include any task performed directly with a patient or indirectly on a patient's behalf. Areas of intervention are broad and may include assessment, promoting adherence to prescribed drug therapy, and solving problems related to drug therapy, among others.

General interventions related to drug therapy include promoting health, preventing or decreasing the need for drug therapy, using nondrug measures to enhance therapeutic effects or decrease adverse effects, teaching, individualizing care, administering drugs, and observing patient responses. Some examples include

- Promoting healthful lifestyles in terms of nutrition, fluids, exercise, rest, and sleep
- Performing hand hygiene and other measures to prevent infection
- Ambulating, positioning, and exercising
- Assisting to cough and deep breathe
- Applying heat or cold
- Increasing or decreasing sensory stimulation
- Scheduling activities to promote rest or sleep
- Recording vital signs, fluid intake, urine output, and other assessment data

The intervention of teaching patients and caregivers about drug therapy is essential because most medications are self-administered and patients need information and assistance to use therapeutic drugs safely and effectively. Adequate knowledge, skill, and preparation are required to fulfill teaching responsibilities. Teaching aids to assist the nurse in this endeavor are included in Boxes 3.3, 3.4, and 3.5. Future chapters will address the patient teaching guidelines for medications discussed in each chapter.

Certain interventions exist with the administration of medications based on the route. No matter which route of medication administration is being implemented, it is important for the nurse to be uninterrupted during the time. According to Biron, Lavoie-Tremblay, and Loiselle (2009), the most frequent source of interruptions experienced by the nurse comes from the nurse's coworkers. Also, failures within the medication administration system lead to interruptions in administration.

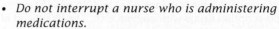

QSEN Safety Alert

It is necessary to observe the following safety alerts relating to medication administration:

- *Do not interrupt a nurse who is administering medications.*
- *Instruct staff members about the risk of medication administration error when a nurse is interrupted during medication administration.*
- *Implement all rights of medication administration.*
- *Do not use creative "work-arounds" with medication administration. Examples include:*
- *Printing multiple copies of patients' wristbands to scan the medication before or after administering them*
- *Carrying multiple prescanned pills on the tray (Diconsiglio, 2008)*

BOX 3.3 Preparing to Teach a Patient or Caregiver

■ Assess learning needs, especially when new drugs are added or new conditions are being treated. This includes finding out what the person already knows about a particular drug. Do not assume that teaching Is unneeded, even if the patient has been taking a drug for a while.

■ Assess ability to manage a drug therapy regimen (i.e., read printed instructions and drug labels, remember dosage schedules, self-administer medications by ordered routes). A medication history (see Box 3.2) helps assess the patient's knowledge about drug therapy.

■ From assessment data, develop an individualized teaching plan. This saves time for both nurse and patient by avoiding repetition of known material. It also promotes adherence to prescribed drug therapy.

■ Try to decrease anxiety. Patients and caregivers may feel overwhelmed by complicated medication regimens. Provide positive reinforcement for effort.

■ Choose an appropriate time (e.g., when the patient is mentally alert and not in acute distress from pain or other symptoms) and a place with minimal noise and distractions, when possible.

■ Proceed slowly, in small steps; emphasize essential information; and provide opportunities to express concerns or ask questions.

■ Provide a combination of verbal and written instructions, which is more effective than either alone. Minimize medical jargon and be aware that patients may have difficulty understanding and retaining the material being taught because of the stress of the illness.

■ When explaining a drug to a hospitalized patient, describe the name (preferably both the generic and a trade name), purpose, expected effects, and so on. The purpose can usually be stated in terms of symptoms to be relieved or other expected benefits. In many instances, the drug is familiar and can be described from personal knowledge. If the drug is unfamiliar, use available resources (e.g., drug reference books, computer drug databases, pharmacists) to learn about the drug and provide accurate information to the patient.

■ When teaching a patient about medications to be taken at home, provide specific information and instructions about each drug, including how to take them and how to observe for beneficial and adverse effects. If adverse effects occur, teach them how to manage minor ones and which ones to report to a health care provider. In addition, discuss ways to develop a convenient routine for taking medications, so that usual activities of daily living are minimally disrupted. Allow time for questions and try to ensure that the patient understands how, when, and why to take the medications.

■ When teaching a patient about potential adverse drug effects, the goal is to provide needed information without causing unnecessary anxiety. Most drugs produce undesirable effects; some are minor, and some are potentially serious. Many people stop taking a drug rather than report adverse reactions. If reactions are reported, it may be possible to continue the drug by reducing dosage, changing the time of administration, or other measures. If severe reactions occur, the drug should be stopped and the prescriber should be notified.

■ Emphasize the importance of taking medications as prescribed throughout the teaching session and perhaps at times of other contacts. Common patient errors include taking incorrect doses, taking doses at the wrong times, omitting doses, and stopping a medication too soon. Treatment failure can often be directly traced to these errors.

■ Reassess learning needs when medication orders are changed (e.g., when medications are added because of a new illness or stopped).

BOX 3.4 | **Patient Teaching Guidelines for Safe and Effective Use of Prescription Medications**

General Considerations

■ Use drugs cautiously and only when necessary because all drugs affect body functions and may cause adverse effects.

■ Use nondrug measures, when possible, to prevent the need for drug therapy or to enhance beneficial effects and decrease adverse effects of drugs.

■ Do not take drugs left over from a previous illness or prescribed for someone else, and do not share prescription drugs with anyone else. The likelihood of having the right drug in the right dose is remote, and the risk of adverse effects is high in such circumstances.

■ Keep all health care providers informed about all the drugs being taken, including over-the-counter (OTC) products and herbal or dietary supplements.

■ Take drugs as prescribed and for the length of time prescribed; notify a health care provider if unable to take a medication. Therapeutic effects greatly depend on taking medications correctly. Altering the dose or time may cause underdosage or overdosage. Stopping a medication may cause a recurrence of the problem for which it was given or withdrawal symptoms. Some medications need to be tapered in dosage and gradually discontinued. If problems occur with taking a drug, report them to a health care provider. An adjustment in dosage or other aspect of administration may solve the problem.

■ Follow instructions for follow-up care (e.g., office visits, laboratory or other diagnostic tests that monitor therapeutic or adverse effects of drugs). Some drugs require more frequent monitoring than others. However, safety requires periodic checks with essentially all medications. With long-term use of a medication, responses may change over time with aging, changes in kidney function, and so on.

■ Take drugs in current use (or an up-to-date list) to appointments with a health care provider.

■ Get all prescriptions filled at the same pharmacy, when possible. This is an important safety factor in helping to avoid multiple prescriptions of the same or similar drugs and to minimize undesirable interactions of newly prescribed drugs with those already in use.

■ Report any drug allergies to all health care providers, and wear a medical identification emblem that lists allergens.

■ Ask questions (and write down the answers) about newly prescribed medications, such as:

  ■ What is the medicine's name?

  ■ What is it supposed to do (i.e., what symptoms or problems will it relieve)?

  ■ How and when do I take it and for how long?

  ■ Should it be taken with food or on an empty stomach?

■ While taking this medicine, should I avoid certain foods, beverages, other medications, and certain activities? (For example, alcoholic beverages and driving a car should be avoided with medications that cause drowsiness or decrease alertness.)

  ■ What side effects are likely and what do I do if they occur?

  ■ Will the medication affect my ability to sleep or work?

  ■ What should I do if I miss a dose?

  ■ Is there a drug information sheet I can have?

■ Store medications out of reach of children, and to prevent accidental ingestion, never refer to medications as "candy."

■ When taking prescription medications, talk to a doctor, pharmacist, or nurse before starting an OTC medication or herbal or dietary supplement. This is a safety factor to avoid undesirable drug interactions.

■ Inform health care providers if you have diabetes or kidney or liver disease. These conditions require special precautions with drug therapy.

■ If pregnant, consult your obstetrician before taking any medications prescribed by another physician.

■ If breast-feeding, consult your obstetrician or pediatrician before taking any medications prescribed by another health care provider.

Self-Administration

■ Develop a routine for taking medications (e.g., at the same time and place each day). A schedule that minimally disrupts usual activities is more convenient and more likely to be followed accurately.

■ Take medications in a well-lighted area and read labels of containers to ensure taking the intended drug. Do not take medications if you are not alert or cannot see clearly.

■ Most tablets and capsules should be taken whole. If unable to take them whole, ask a health care provider before splitting, chewing, or crushing tablets or taking the medication out of capsules. Some long-acting preparations are dangerous if altered so that the entire dose is absorbed at the same time.

■ As a general rule, take oral medications with 6 to 8 ounces of water, in a sitting or standing position. The water helps tablets and capsules dissolve in the stomach, "dilutes" the drug so that it is less likely to upset the stomach, and promotes absorption of the drug into the bloodstream.

■ Take most oral drugs at evenly spaced intervals around the clock. For example, if ordered once daily, take about the same time every day. If ordered twice daily or morning and evening, take about 12 hours apart.

■ Follow instructions about taking a medication with food, on an empty stomach, or with other medications.

■ If a dose is missed, most authorities recommend taking the dose if remembered soon after the scheduled time and omitting the dose if it is not remembered for several hours. If a dose is omitted, the next dose should be taken at the next scheduled time. Do not double the dose.

BOX 3.4 **Patient Teaching Guidelines for Safe and Effective Use of Prescription Medications** (Continued)

■ If taking a liquid medication (or giving one to a child), measure with a calibrated medication cup or measuring spoon. A dose cannot be measured accurately with household teaspoons or tablespoons because they are different sizes and deliver varying amounts of medication. If the liquid medication is packaged with a measuring cup that shows teaspoons or tablespoons, that should be used to measure doses, for adults or children.

■ Use oral or nasal inhalers, eye drops, and skin medications according to instructions. If not clear how a medication is to be used, be sure to ask a health care provider. Correct use is essential for therapeutic effects.

■ Report problems or new symptoms to a health care provider.

■ Store medications safely, in a cool, dry place. Do not store them in a bathroom; heat, light, and moisture may cause them to decompose. Do not store them near a dangerous substance, which could be taken by mistake. Keep medications in the container in which they were dispensed by the pharmacy, where the label identifies it and gives directions. Do not mix different medications in a single container.

■ Discard outdated medications; do not keep drugs for long periods. Drugs are chemicals that may deteriorate over time, especially if exposed to heat and moisture.

BOX 3.5 **Patient Teaching Guidelines for Safe and Effective Use of Over-the-Counter Medications**

■ Read product labels carefully. The labels contain essential information about the name, ingredients, indications for use, usual dosage, when to stop using the medication or when to see a health care provider, possible adverse effects, and expiration dates.

■ Use a magnifying glass, if necessary, to read the fine print. If you do not understand the information on labels, ask a physician, pharmacist, or nurse.

■ Do not take over-the-counter (OTC) medications longer or in higher doses than recommended.

■ Note that all OTC medications are not safe for everyone. Many OTC medications warn against use with certain illnesses (e.g., hypertension). Consult a health care provider before taking the product if you have a contraindicated condition. If taking any prescription medications, consult a health care provider before taking any OTC drugs to avoid undesirable drug interactions and adverse effects. Some specific precautions include the following:

  ■ Avoid alcohol if taking sedating antihistamines, cough or cold remedies containing dextromethorphan, or sleeping pills. Because all these drugs cause drowsiness alone, combining any of them with alcohol may result in excessive and potentially dangerous sedation.

  ■ Avoid OTC sleeping aids if you are taking a prescription sedative-type drug (e.g., for anxiety or nervousness).

  ■ Ask a health care provider before taking products containing aspirin if you are taking an anticoagulant (e.g., Coumadin).

  ■ Ask a health care provider before taking other products containing aspirin if you are already taking a regular dose of aspirin to prevent blood clots, heart attack, or stroke. Aspirin is commonly used for this purpose, often in doses of 81 mg (a child's dose) or 325 mg.

■ Do not take a laxative if you have stomach pain, nausea, or vomiting, to avoid worsening the problem.

■ Do not take a nasal decongestant (e.g., Sudafed); a multisymptom cold remedy containing phenylephrine products, that is, formulated to remove pseudoephedrine (e.g., Actifed); or an antihistamine–decongestant combination (e.g., Claritin D) if you are taking a prescription medication for high blood pressure. Such products can raise blood pressure and decrease or cancel the blood pressure–lowering effect of the prescription drug. This could lead to severe hypertension and stroke.

■ Store OTC drugs in a cool, dry place, in their original containers; check expiration dates periodically and discard those that have expired.

■ If pregnant, consult your obstetrician before taking any OTC medications.

■ If breast-feeding, consult your pediatrician or family doctor before taking any OTC medications.

■ For children, follow any age limits on the label.

■ Measure liquid OTC medications with the measuring device that comes with the product (some have a dropper or plastic cup calibrated in milliliters, teaspoons, or tablespoons). If such a device is not available, use a measuring spoon. It is not safe to use household teaspoons or tablespoons because they are different sizes and deliver varying amounts of medication.

■ Do not assume continued safety of an OTC medication you have taken for years. Older people are more likely to have adverse drug reactions and interactions because of changes in the heart, kidneys, and other organs that occur with aging and various disease processes.

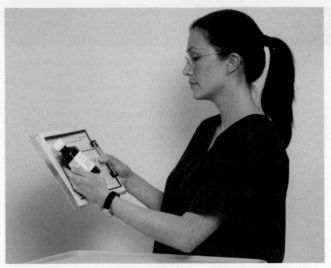

Figure 3.6 The nurse assesses the medication using the medication administration record.

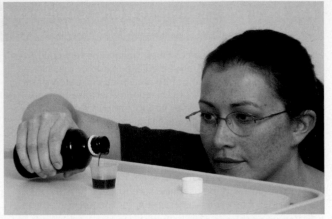

Figure 3.8 The nurse pours the liquid medication at eye level.

The following sections present a list of guidelines for each route of medication administration. The process begins by checking the medication against the MAR (Fig. 3.6) and ends with the nurse documenting the medication administration (Fig. 3.7).

Oral Medication Administration

- Position the patient to prevent aspiration (Fig. 3.8).
- Open the unit-dose package at the patient's bedside and place the capsule or tablet in a medicine cup.
- For liquid medications, place the cup at eye level and pour the desired amount of solution (Fig. 3.9). (Shake the elixir before measuring, if recommended by the manufacturer.)
- Administer medications with or without food as indicated to enhance absorption.
- For infants and children, administer liquid medications with a syringe or dropper.

- Hold liquid medications if the patient cannot take anything orally (Latin *nil per os*, or nothing by mouth [NPO]), vomiting, sedated, or unconscious.

Nasogastric or Gastrostomy Tube Medication Administration

- Administer liquid medications when available.
- Crush pills and dissolve in 30 mL of water. (Do not crush enteric-coated or extended-release medications, and do not empty the powdered medication in extended-release capsules.)
- Using a large catheter-tipped syringe, aspirate gastric fluid and assess pH.
- Rinse the tube and instill medication by gravity flow, and rinse the tube again with 50 mL of water. Do not allow the syringe to empty completely between additions of medication or water.
- Clamp off the tube from suction or drainage for at least 30 minutes.

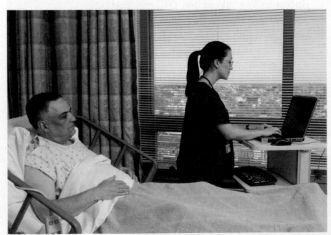

Figure 3.7 The nurse documents the administration of the medication in the electronic medical record.

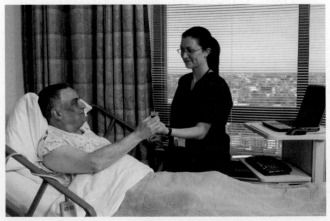

Figure 3.9 The nurse administers the oral medication with the patient positioned to prevent aspiration.

Subcutaneous Medication Administration

- Use only sterile drug preparations labeled or commonly used for subcutaneous injections.
- Use a 25-gauge, 5/8-inch needle for most subcutaneous injections.
- Select an appropriate injection site, based on patient preferences, drug characteristics, and visual inspection of possible sites. In long-term therapy, such as insulin, rotate injection sites. Avoid areas with lumps, bruises, or other lesions.
- Cleanse the site with an alcohol sponge.
- Tighten the skin or pinch a fold of skin and tissue between the thumb and fingers.
- Hold the syringe like a pencil, and insert the needle quickly at a 45- or 90-degree angle. Use enough force to penetrate the skin and subcutaneous tissue in one smooth motion.
- Release the skin so that both hands are free to manipulate the syringe. Pull back gently on the plunger to aspirate. If blood does not appear in the syringe, administer the medication. If blood appears, remove the needle and prepare a new medication for administration. *Never aspirate when giving heparin subcutaneously.*
- Remove the needle quickly and apply pressure for a few seconds.

Intramuscular Medication Administration

- Use only drug preparations labeled or commonly used for IM injections. Check label instructions for mixing drugs in powder form.
- Use a 1½-inch needle for most adults and 5/8-inch to 1½-inch needle for children, depending on the size of the patient.
- Use the smallest gauge needle that accommodates the medication. A 22-gauge is satisfactory for most drugs; a 20-gauge may be used for viscous medications.
- Select an appropriate injection site, based on the patient preferences, drug characteristics, anatomic landmarks, and visual inspection of possible sites. Rotate sites if frequent injections are being given, and avoid areas with lumps, bruises, or other lesions. *If the patient has had a mastectomy, do not administer any injection in the arm on the affected side.*
- Cleanse the site with an alcohol sponge.
- Tighten the skin, hold the syringe like a pencil, and insert the needle quickly at a 90-degree angle. Use enough force to penetrate the skin and subcutaneous tissue into the muscle in one smooth motion.
- Remove the needle quickly and apply pressure for several seconds.

Clinical Application 3-4

- Ms. Baranski's pain is not controlled with the Vicodin, and administration of ketorolac is necessary. What is the proper procedure for giving an IM injection?

Intravenous Medication Administration

- Use only drug preparations that are labeled for IV use.
- Check label instructions for the type and amount of fluid to use for dissolving or diluting the drug.
- Prepare drugs just before use, as a general rule. Also add drugs to IV fluids just before use.
- For venipuncture and direct injection into a vein, apply a tourniquet, select a site in the arm, cleanse the skin with an antiseptic (e.g., povidone-iodine or alcohol), insert the needle, and aspirate a small amount of blood into the syringe to be sure that the needle is in the vein. (*If the patient has had a mastectomy, do not administer any injection in the arm on the affected side.*) Remove the tourniquet, and inject the drug slowly. Remove the needle and apply pressure until there is no evidence of bleeding.
- For administration by an established IV line:
  1. Check the infusion for patency and flow rate. Check the venipuncture site for signs of infiltration and phlebitis before each drug dose.
  2. For direct injection, cleanse an injection site on the IV tubing, insert the needle, and inject the drug slowly.
  3. To use a volume control set, fill it with 50 to 100 mL of IV fluid and clamp it so that no further fluid enters the chamber and dilutes the drug. Inject the drug into the injection site after cleansing the site with an alcohol sponge and infuse, usually in 1 hour or less. After the drug is infused, add solution to maintain the infusion.
  4. To use a "piggyback" method, add the drug to 50 to 100 mL of IV solution in a separate container. Attach the IV tubing and needle. Insert the needle in an injection site on the main IV tubing after cleansing the site. Infuse the drug over 15 to 60 minutes, depending on the drug.
- When more than one drug is to be given, flush the line between drugs. Do not mix drugs in syringes or in IV fluids unless the drug literature states that the drugs are compatible.

NCLEX Success

11. **The patient receives regular insulin 5 units subcutaneously. To what degree is the syringe held for the injection? (Select all that apply.)**

    A. 30 degrees
    B. 45 degrees
    C. 60 degrees
    D. 90 degrees

12. **How is a medication delivered by piggyback administered?**

    A. It is pushed into the IV line.
    B. It is retrograded into the IV line.
    C. It is injected intramuscularly after another medication.
    D. It is mixed with 50 to 100 mL of IV fluid in a separate container.

Medication Administration to the Skin

- Use only drug preparations labeled for dermatologic use.
- Cleanse the skin, remove any previously applied medication, and apply the drug in a thin layer. For broken skin or open lesions, use sterile gloves, a tongue blade, or a cotton-tipped applicator to apply the drug.

Medication Administration to the Eye

- Use drug preparations labeled for ophthalmic use. Wash hands, open the eye to expose the conjunctival sac, and drop the medication into the sac, without touching the dropper tip to anything. Provide tissue for blotting any excess drug. If two or more eye drops are scheduled at the same time, wait 1 to 5 minutes before instillations.
- With children, prepare the medication, place the child in a head-lowered position, steady the hand holding the medication against the child's head, gently retract the lower lid, and instill the medication in the conjunctival sac.

Medication Administration to the Nose

- Have the patient hold his or her head back and drop the medication into the nostrils. Give the amount ordered.
- With children, place in a supine position with the head lowered, instill the medication, and maintain the position for 2 to 3 minutes. Then place the child in the prone position.

Medication Administration to the Ear

- Open the ear canal in adults by pulling the ear up and back for adults.
- Open the ear canal in children by pulling the ear down and back for children.
- Drop the medication on the side of the ear canal.

Medication Administration to the Rectum

- Lubricate the end with a water-soluble lubricant, wear a glove or finger cot, and insert into the rectum the length of the finger. Place the suppository next to the mucosal wall.
- If the patient prefers and is able, provide supplies for self-administration.

Medication Administration to the Vagina

- Use gloves or an applicator for insertion. If an applicator is used, wash thoroughly with soap and water after each use.
- If the patient prefers and is able, provide supplies for self-administration.

Evaluation

Evaluation involves determining the patient's response in relation to stated goals and expected outcomes. Some outcomes can be evaluated within a few minutes of drug administration (e.g., relief of acute pain after administration of an analgesic), but most require longer periods of time. Over time, the patient is likely to experience brief contacts with many health care providers, which increase the difficulty of evaluating outcomes

of drug therapy. However, it is possible to manage difficulties by using appropriate techniques and criteria of evaluation.

General techniques include directly observing the patient's status, interviewing the patient or others about the patient's response to drug therapy, and checking appropriate medical records, including medication records and diagnostic test reports.

General criteria include progress toward stated outcomes, such as relief of symptoms, accurate administration, avoidance of preventable adverse effects, and compliance with instructions for follow-up monitoring by a health care provider. Specific criteria indicate the parameters that must be measured to evaluate responses to particular drugs (e.g., blood sugar with antidiabetic drugs, blood pressure with antihypertensive drugs).

Integrating Evidence-Based Practice with the Nursing Process

Evidence-based nursing practice requires a conscientious and continuing effort to provide high-quality care to patients by obtaining and analyzing the best available scientific evidence from research. Then, the scientific evidence is integrated with the nurse's clinical expertise and the patient's preferences and values to yield "best practices" for a patient with a particular disease process or health problem.

Evidence-based practice (EBP) may include any step of the nursing process, and it does not accept tradition or "that's the way we've always done it" as sufficient rationale for any aspect of nursing care. Requirements for implementing EBP include

- Using research. Although professional nurses have always been encouraged to use research, EBP structures and formalizes the process. The nurse must use computer skills to search for the best evidence in making decisions about patient care. The search needs to be systematic; obtained data need to be critically analyzed for quality and relevance to the clinical situation.
- Keeping up-to-date in regard to research studies related to one's area of clinical practice. This includes reading research reports and analyzing them to determine their applicability.
- Considering levels of evidence to support clinical decision making. Level A is the strongest level.
- Interpreting research evidence in relation to one's clinical expertise and patient choices to provide a scientific rationale for one's clinical decisions
- Applying the available information to improve nursing care of a patient or group of patients
- Evaluating the effectiveness of application—did the intervention improve the patient's condition?

Herbal and Dietary Supplements

Complementary and alternative therapies, including herbal and dietary supplements, can be helpful in patient care. However, they can potentiate or negate the effects of prescribed medications, and it is important that the nurse evaluate the effects in a particular patient. Herbal and dietary supplements are commonly used, and patients who take them are likely to be encountered in any clinical practice setting. Herbal medicines, also called botanicals, phytochemicals, and nutraceuticals, are derived from plants. Other dietary supplements may be derived from a variety of sources. The 1994 Dietary Supplement Health and Education Act (DSHEA) defined a dietary supplement as "a vitamin, a mineral, an herb or other botanical used to supplement the diet." Under this law, herbs can be labeled according to their possible effects on the human body, but the products cannot claim to diagnose, prevent, relieve, or cure specific human diseases unless approved by the FDA.

It has become evident that nurses need to know about their patient's use of herbal and dietary supplements to provide safe care. An additional impetus came from the IOM, which released a report on complementary and alternative medicine (CAM) in 2005 in which it recommended that "health profession schools incorporate sufficient information about … CAM into the standard curriculum at all levels to enable licensed professionals to competently advise their patients about CAM" (cited in Hughes, Jacobs, & Berman., 2007). Recent qualitative studies have identified patients who use CAM because they view the therapies as having fewer adverse side effects (Bishop, Yardley, & Lewith, 2010). The National Center for Complementary and Alternative Medicine (2009) asserts that nurses should be the first to discuss CAM with their patients.

More specifically, there are five major concerns associated with the nursing role in relation to herbal products and drug therapy, as follows:

1. Many of the products may not be safe because active ingredients and effects on humans are often unknown. Some contain heavy metals (e.g., lead) and other contaminants (e.g., pesticides); some contain prescription or nonprescription drugs. In addition, ingredients are not standardized and often differ from those listed on the product label.
2. Use of supplements may keep the patient from seeking treatment from a health care provider when indicated. This may allow disease processes to worsen and be more difficult to treat.
3. The products may interact with prescription drugs to decrease therapeutic effects or increase adverse effects. Dangerous interactions have been identified with St. John's wort and some herbs that affect blood clotting mechanisms.
4. Most products have not been studied sufficiently to evaluate their safety or effectiveness. In many studies, the products have not been standardized in terms of types or amounts of active ingredients. In addition, most reported studies have been short-term and with few subjects.
5. Many patients who use supplements do not tell their health care providers. This omission can lead to dangerous interactions when the supplements are combined with prescription or OTC drugs.

In general, nurses need to have an adequate knowledge base to assess and assist patients who use herbal products to do so safely. To develop and maintain a knowledge base, nurses (and patients) need to seek information from authoritative, objective sources rather than product labels, advertisements, or personal testimonials from family members, friends, or celebrities. Some resources are listed as follows:

- Commonly used supplements, some of which are described in Table 3.6. Later chapters describe selected supplements with some scientific support for their use in more detail. For example, Chapter 14 discusses some products reported to be useful in relieving pain, fever, inflammation, or migraines.
- Basic teaching guidelines about herbal and dietary supplements, which are presented in Box 3.6. This chapter provides general information. Later chapters have guidelines that may emphasize avoidance or caution in using supplements thought to interact adversely with prescribed drugs or particular patient conditions.
- Assessment guidelines. This chapter presents general information about the use or nonuse of supplements. Later chapters discuss specific supplements that may interact with particular drug group(s). For example, some supplements are known to increase blood pressure or risk of excessive bleeding.

Clinical Application 3-5

- Ms. Baranski says that a friend suggested that she take black cohosh for the hot flashes she is experiencing with menopause instead of the estrogen preparation her prescriber ordered. What information should the nurse teach Ms. Baranski regarding black cohosh in menopause?

NCLEX Success

13. During an initial nursing assessment, the patient reports that he is allergic to a particular medicine. What should the nurse ask the patient?

   A. What symptoms occurred when you had the allergic reaction?
   B. Did you need to take epinephrine (Adrenaline)?
   C. Did your physician think this information needed to be communicated?
   D. Have you ever overdosed on this medication?

14. How do nursing interventions increase safety and effectiveness of drug therapy?

   A. By avoiding the use of nondrug measures during drug therapy
   B. By using multiple drugs to relieve most symptoms or problems
   C. By teaching patients about their drug therapy
   D. By avoiding excessive instructions

15. What should the nurse keep in mind when evaluating a patient's response to drug therapy?

   A. Few drugs cause adverse effects.
   B. Drugs may cause virtually any symptom or problem.
   C. Patients always report adverse effects.
   D. Therapeutic effects are more important than adverse effects.

TABLE 3.6

Herbal and Dietary Supplements

Name/Uses	Characteristics	Remarks
Black Cohosh Most often used to relieve symptoms of menopause (e.g., flushes, vaginal dryness, irritability) May also relieve premenstrual syndrome (PMS) and dysmenorrhea	Well tolerated; in overdose may cause nausea, vomiting, dizziness, visual disturbances, and reduced pulse rate Most clinical trials done with Remifemin, in small numbers of women; other trade names include Estroven and Femtrol	There is no convincing evidence that black cohosh has a therapeutic role in the treatment of menopausal symptoms (Palacio, Masari, & Mooradian, 2009). Not recommended for use longer than 6 mo
Capsaicin Used to treat pain associated with neuralgia, neuropathy, and osteoarthritis Self-defense as the active ingredient in "pepper spray"	A topical analgesic that may inhibit the synthesis, transport, and release of substance P, a pain transmitter Derived from cayenne pepper Adverse effects include skin irritation, itching, redness, and stinging	Applied topically
Chamomile Used mainly for antispasmodic effects in the GI tract; may relieve abdominal cramping	Usually ingested as a tea; may delay absorption of oral medications May cause contact dermatitis and severe hypersensitivity reactions, including anaphylaxis, in people allergic to ragweed, asters, and chrysanthemums May increase risks of bleeding	Few studies and little data to support use and effectiveness in GI disorders
Chondroitin Arthritis	Derived from the trachea cartilage of slaughtered cattle Usually taken with glucosamine Adverse effects may include GI upset, nausea, and headache	Several studies support use
Creatine Athletes take creatine supplements to gain extra energy, to train longer and harder, and to improve performance.	An amino acid produced in the liver and kidneys and stored in muscles Causes weight gain, usually within 2 wk of starting use Legal and available in health food stores as a powder to be mixed with water or juice, as a liquid, and as tablets and capsules	Not recommended for use by children because studies have not been done and effects are unknown Nurses and parents need to actively discourage children and adolescents from using creatine supplements.
Echinacea Most often used for the common cold but also advertised for many other uses (immune system stimulant, anti-infective)	Many species but *E. purpurea* most often used medicinally Effects on immune system include stimulation of phagocytes and monocytes. Contraindicated in persons with immune system disorders Hepatotoxic with long-term use	Hard to interpret validity of claims because various species and preparations used in reported studies Some evidence (level B) to support use in patients with the common cold, with possibly shorter durations and less severe symptoms

TABLE 3.6

Herbal and Dietary Supplements (Continued)

Name/Uses	Characteristics	Remarks
Feverfew Migraines, menstrual irregularities, arthritis	May increase risk of bleeding May cause hypersensitivity reactions in people allergic to ragweed, asters, daisies, or chrysanthemums May cause a withdrawal syndrome if use is stopped abruptly	Some studies support use in patients with migraine
Garlic Used to lower serum cholesterol and for other uses	Active ingredient thought to be allicin Has antiplatelet activity and may increase risk of bleeding Adverse effects include allergic reactions (asthma, dermatitis), dizziness, nausea, vomiting.	Some evidence that garlic has a small cholesterol-lowering effect; no reliable evidence to support other uses
Ginger Used mainly to treat nausea, including motion sickness and postoperative nausea	Inhibits platelet aggregation; may increase clotting time Gastroprotective effects in animal studies	Should not be used for morning sickness associated with pregnancy—may increase risk of miscarriage
Ginkgo Biloba Used mainly to improve memory and cognitive function in people with Alzheimer's disease; may be useful in treating peripheral arterial disease	May increase blood flow to the brain and legs, improve memory, and decrease intermittent claudication (leg pain with walking) Inhibits platelet aggregation; may increase risks of bleeding with any drug that has antiplatelet effects (e.g., aspirin) Adverse effects include GI upset, headache, bleeding, and allergic skin reaction.	Good evidence (level A) for small effects in treating dementia and claudication NIH is conducting a clinical trial with more than 3000 volunteers to see if ginkgo prevents the onset of dementia (specifically, Alzheimer's disease), slows cognitive decline and functional disability, and reduces the incidence of cardiovascular disease.
Ginseng Used to increase stamina, strength, endurance, and mental acuity	Has various pharmacologic effects that vary with dose and duration of use Adverse effects include hypertension, nervousness, depression, insomnia, skin rashes, epistaxis, palpitations, and vomiting. May increase risks of bleeding with any drug that has antiplatelet effects (e.g., aspirin) Increases risk of hypoglycemic reactions if taken with antidiabetic drugs Should not be taken with other herbs or drugs that inhibit monoamine oxidase (e.g., St. John's wort, selegiline); headache, mania, and tremors may occur	Insufficient evidence to support use for any indication A ginseng abuse syndrome, with insomnia, hypotonia, and edema, has been reported. Caution patients to avoid ingesting excessive amounts. Instruct patients with cardiovascular disease, diabetes mellitus, or hypertension to check with their health care provider before taking ginseng. Instruct any patient taking ginseng to avoid long-term use. Siberian ginseng should not be used longer than 3 wk.

(Continued on page 64)

TABLE 3.6

Herbal and Dietary Supplements (Continued)

Name/Uses	Characteristics	Remarks
Glucosamine Osteoarthritis	Usually used with chondroitin Has beneficial effects on cartilage Adverse effects mild, may include GI upset, drowsiness	Several studies support use
Melatonin Used mainly for treatment of insomnia and prevention and treatment of jet lag	Several studies of effects on sleep, energy level, fatigue, mental alertness, and mood indicate some improvement, compared with placebo. Contraindicated in persons with hepatic insufficiency or a history of cerebrovascular disease, depression, or neurologic disorders Adverse effects include altered sleep patterns, confusion, headache, sedation, and tachycardia.	Patients with renal impairment should use cautiously
St. John's Wort Used for treatment of depression, advertised as an "herbal Prozac"	Active component may be hypericin or hyperforin Adverse effects include confusion, dizziness, GI upset, and photosensitivity. Interacts with many drugs; can decrease effectiveness of birth control pills, anticancer drugs, antivirals used to treat acquired immunodeficiency syndrome (AIDS), and organ transplant drugs (e.g., cyclosporine)	Good evidence (level A) for improvement in mild to moderate depression; not effective in major or serious depression Should not be combined with monoamine oxidase inhibitors or selective serotonin reuptake inhibitor antidepressants Use has declined since serious herb–drug interactions reported.
Saw Palmetto Used to prevent and treat urinary symptoms in men with benign prostatic hyperplasia	May have antiandrogenic effects Adverse effects may include GI upset and headache; diarrhea may occur with high doses.	Some evidence (Level B) of small beneficial effects with doses of 320 mg/d
Valerian Used mainly to promote sleep and allay anxiety and nervousness; also has muscle relaxant effects	Adverse effects with acute overdose or chronic use include blurred vision, drowsiness, dizziness, excitability, hypersensitivity reactions, and insomnia; also, risk of liver damage from combination products containing valerian and from overdoses averaging 2.5 g Additive sedation if taken with other CNS depressants	Should not be combined with sedative drugs and should not be used regularly Many extract products contain 40%–60% alcohol. Insufficient evidence to support use for treatment of insomnia

GI, gastrointestinal; NIH, National Institutes of Health.

| BOX 3.6 | Patient Teaching Guidelines for General Information About Herbal and Dietary Supplements |

■ Herbal and dietary products are chemicals that have drug-like effects in people. Unfortunately, their effects are largely unknown and may be dangerous for some people because there is little reliable information about them. For most products, little research has been done to determine either their benefits or their adverse effects.

■ The safety and effectiveness of these products are not regulated by laws designed to protect consumers, as are pharmaceutical drugs. As a result, the types and amounts of ingredients may not be identified on the product label. In fact, most products contain several active ingredients, and it is often not known which ingredient, if any, has the desired pharmacologic effect. In addition, components of plants can vary considerably, depending on the soil, water, and climate where the plants are grown. Quality is also a concern, as heavy metals (e.g., lead), pesticides, and other contaminants have been found in some products.

■ These products can be used more safely if they are manufactured by a reputable company that states the ingredients are standardized (meaning that the dose of medicine in each tablet or capsule is the same).

■ The product label should also state specific percentages, amounts, and strengths of active ingredients. With herbal medicines especially, different brands of the same herb vary in the amounts of active ingredients per recommended dose. Dosing is also difficult because a particular herb may be available in several different dosage forms (e.g., tablet, capsule, tea, extract) with different amounts of active ingredients.

■ These products are often advertised as "natural." Many people interpret this to mean the products are safe and better than synthetic products. This is not true; "natural" does not mean safe, especially when taken concurrently with other herbals, dietary supplements, or drugs.

■ When taking herbal or dietary supplements, follow the instructions on the product label. Inappropriate use or taking excessive amounts may cause dangerous side effects.

■ Inform health care providers when taking any kind of herbal or dietary supplement to reduce risks of severe adverse effects or drug–supplement interactions.

■ Most herbal and dietary supplements should be avoided during pregnancy or lactation and in young children.

■ The American Society of Anesthesiologists recommends that all herbal products be discontinued 2 to 3 weeks before any surgical procedure. Some products (e.g., echinacea, feverfew, garlic, ginkgo, ginseng, valerian, and St. John's wort) can interfere with or increase the effects of some drugs, affect blood pressure or heart rhythm, or increase risks of bleeding; some have unknown effects when combined with anesthetics, other perioperative medications, and surgical procedures.

■ Store herbal and dietary supplements out of the reach of children.

Key Concepts

• The rights of safe and accurate medication administration are the right drug, right dose, right patient, right route, right time, right reason, and right documentation.

• Basic knowledge and techniques for accurate medication administration include knowledge of the medication, knowledge of the patient, interpretation of the prescriber orders, and labels of medication container, calculations and measurements of doses, and correct techniques for all dosage forms and routes of administration.

• Each health care facility has a system for distributing drugs.

• Each nurse must follow the legal aspects of medication administration and the policies of the health care institution for the administration of medications.

• The nurse must accurately calculate dosages to be administered to prevent medications errors that are harmful to the patient.

• The nurse must identify potential sources of medication errors and intervene to prevent errors when possible.

• The nurse needs to apply the nursing process in drug therapy and all aspects of nursing care.

• The nurse is responsible for safe and effective administration of medications and the observation of the medication's response.

• Instructing patients and caregivers about medications is imperative for safe and effective patient care.

- Evidence-based nursing practice requires continued searching for and using best practice interventions, as based on research and other authoritative evidence.
- It is important for the nurse to understand the effect herbal remedies and dietary supplements have and the related interactions with medications.

Critical Thinking Questions

3-1. A 3-year-old child is admitted to the pediatric neurological division following his first seizure. The prescriber has ordered phenytoin (Dilantin) orally. The recommended loading dose is 15 mg/kg. The patient weighs 36 pounds. The medication is an elixir in a 125 mg/5 mL suspension.

- How much phenytoin does the nurse administer to this patient in a loading dose?
- How does the nurse administer the medication to a 3-year-old child?
- The patient eventually takes 5 mg/kg orally in two divided doses. How much phenytoin (Dilantin) is the nurse then administering?

3-2. An 84-year-old woman lives alone, but her daughter lives approximately one mile away. The daughter sets the medications up weekly and checks on her mother either by visiting or by phone daily. The elderly woman takes the following medications: ibuprofen (Motrin) 600 mg three times per day, hydrochlorothiazide (HCTZ) 50 mg every day, and captopril (Capoten) 25 mg three times per day.

- During the first home visit, what assessments will be made by the nurse regarding the patient's medications?
- What conditions are these medications used to treat?
- What nursing interventions are appropriate to implement?

References and Resources

Biron, A., Lavoie-Tremblay, M., & Loiselle, C. G. (2009). Characteristics of work interruptions during medication administration. *Journal of Nursing Scholarship, 41*(4), 330–336.

Bishop, F. L., Yardley, L., & Lewith, G. T. (2010). Why consumers maintain complementary and alternative medicine use: A qualitative study. *Journal of Alternative and Complementary Medicine, 16*(2), 175–182.

Consiglio, J. (2008). Creative 'work-arounds' defeat barcoding safeguard for meds. *Materials Management in Health Care, 17*(9), 26–29.

Fowler, S. B., Sohler, P., & Zarillo, D. F. (2009). Bar-code technology for medication administration: Medication errors and nurse satisfaction. *Medsurg Nursing, 18*(2), 103–109.

Helmons, P. J., Wargel, L. N., & Daniels, C. E. (2009). Effect of bar-code-assisted medication administration on medication administration errors and accuracy in multiple patient areas. *American Journal of Health-System Pharmacy, 66*(12), 1202–1210.

Hughes, E. F., Jacobs, B. P., & Berman, B. M. (2007). Complementary and alternative medicine. In S. J. McPhee, M. A. Papadakis, & L. M. Tierney Jr (Eds.), *Current medical diagnosis and treatment 2007* (pp. 1743–1766). New York, NY: McGraw-Hill.

Institute of Medicine of the National Academies. (2007). *Preventing medications errors.* Washington, DC: National Academies Press.

Institutes of Medicine of the National Academies. (2004). *Keeping patients safe: Transforming the work environment of nurses.* Washington, DC: National Academies Press.

Karch, A. M. (2010). *2010 Lippincott's nursing drug guide.* Philadelphia, PA: Lippincott Williams & Wilkins.

Mims, E., Tucker, C., Carlson, R., Schneider, R., & Bagby, J. (2009). Quality-monitoring program for bar-code-assisted medication administration. *American Journal of Health-System Pharmacy, 66*(12), 1125–1131.

National Center for Complementary and Alternative Medicine. (2009). *Time to talk: Ask your patients about their use of complementary and alternative medicine.* Retrieved July 29, 2010, from http://www.nccam.nih.gov/timetotalk/forphysicians.htm

Olsen, C. G., Tindall, W. N., & Clasen, M. E. (2007). *Geriatric pharmacotherapy a guide to the helping professional.* Washington, DC: American Pharmacists Association.

Palacio, C., Masri, G., & Mooradian, A. D. (2009). Black cohosh for the management of menopausal symptoms. *Drugs and Aging, 26*(1), 23–36.

The Joint Commission National Patient Safety Guidelines Do Not Use List. (2009). Retrieved July 21, 2010, from http://www.jointcommission.org/patientsafety/donotuselist/

The Joint Commission National Patient Safety Guidelines Read Back Orders. (2009). Retrieved July 21, 2010, from http://www.jointcommission.org/AccreditationPrograms/HomeCare/standards/FAQ/NPSG/Communication/NPSG.02.010/

Smeltzer, S. C., Bare, B. G., Hinkle, J. H., & Cheever, K. H. (2008). *Brunner & Suddarth's textbook of medical-surgical nursing* (11th ed.). Philadelphia, PA: Lippincott Williams & Wilkins.

Taylor, C., Lillis, C., LeMone, P., & Lynn, P. (2008). *Fundamentals of nursing: The art and science of nursing care* (6th ed.). Philadelphia, PA: Lippincott Williams & Wilkins.

SECTION 2

Drug Therapy Throughout the Lifespan

4

Pharmacology and the Care of the Infant and Pediatric Patient

LEARNING OBJECTIVES

After studying this chapter, you should be able to:

1. Identify the characteristics of pediatric pharmacotherapy in children from birth to 18 years of age.

2. Describe the evolution of pediatric pharmacotherapy and the purpose of federal legislation in the development of current practice standards.

3. Describe methods for determining accurate pediatric dosing.

4. Explain differences in pharmacodynamic variables between children and adults.

5. Explain pharmacokinetic differences between children and adults.

6. Describe nursing interventions that include caregivers to help ensure safe and effective medication administration to children.

Clinical Application Case Study

Billy Lee, a 4-year-old Native American boy, complains of shortness of breath. He is restless with expiratory wheezes. His mother reports that her son has a 2-day history of cold-like symptoms, with a productive cough and fever.

KEY TERMS

Blood–brain barrier: barrier in the central nervous system composed of capillaries with tight bonds, which acts to prevent the passage of most ions and large-molecular-weight compounds, including some drugs, from the blood to the brain

Body surface area: surface of a human body expressed in square meters

Child(ren): person(s) between birth and 18 years of age

Total body water: amount of water within the body (both intracellular and extracellular)

Introduction

Children naturally differ from adults. However, therapeutic indications and effects of drug therapy are similar in many ways. It is essential that nurses and other health care professionals understand the many ways they differ because this presents a challenge in medication dosing, administration, and management for children. For example, physiological changes throughout development influence both the pharmacodynamic and pharmacokinetic actions of medications. A child's immature organ systems mean that molecular binding, receptor reactions, and intended actions of medications may not mimic those known for adults. Variables in absorption, distribution, metabolism, and excretion further complicate the medication process, and taken together, these differences indicate a need for vigilance in nursing management of pediatric pharmacotherapy.

Pediatrics includes the evaluation and management of all **children**—patients from birth to age 18. This group is further divided into five subgroups (Table 4.1), and each developmental group is characterized by a select set of physiological changes that affect pharmacotherapy. The younger the patient, the greater the variation in medication action. Of course, many pediatric patients cannot verbalize adverse effects, and good assessment skills are crucial. It is also important to remember that as patients go through puberty, they begin to respond more like adults physiologically, but they are still immature psychologically and may lack the ability to dose, administer, or evaluate the effectiveness of medications.

Drug Safety in Pediatrics

Legislation and Drug Testing

Many challenges in pediatric medication management involve both the known physical differences in pediatric patients and the unknown action of drugs; these problems often relate to the lack of adequate information. Historically, researchers used only adults to test medications, and prescribers simply assumed that smaller doses would elicit the same results in smaller patients. However, since 1994, the process began to change. In 1994, the U.S. Food and Drug Administration (FDA) enacted the Pediatric Rule, which compelled the pharmaceutical industry to submit all known data about the pharmacokinetics, safety,

and efficacy of medications used for children (Zajicek, 2009). The FDA continued the trend toward safer medication management for children when it passed the U.S. *Food and Drug Administration Modernization Act of 1997* (FDAMA) followed by the *2002 Best Pharmaceuticals for Children Act* (BPCA). These acts provide incentives to companies who perform research to determine the safety, efficacy, dosage, and unique risks associated with medications for children (USFDA, 2009).

The FDA continued to press for more research and better practice standards by issuing the *Pediatric Research Equity Act of 2003* and renewing the BPCA in 2007. Since these measures were put in place, all the research has now uncovered other gaps in pediatric studies, including a need for pediatric formulations, preclinical studies, and pediatric outcome measures. With the current emphasis on increased patient safety and decreased medication-related adverse events, it is especially important for pediatric practitioners to be at the forefront of current research and practice standards in pediatric pharmacotherapy. Prescribers must continue to treat pediatric patients with drugs for which they lack information; therefore, they must practice good assessment, dosing, and evaluation during the administration of any medication to a pediatric patient.

Clinical Application 4-1

- Are Billy's medications chosen based on empiric evidence obtained from solid research performed on other 4-year-old Native American boys?

Calculating Drug Dosages

The basis of pediatric drug dosing is weight, and determining drug dosages is highly dependent on the growth and development changes that occur across the lifespan. The prescriber uses weight alone to calculate pediatric dosages in an expression such as gentamicin 5 mg/kg/24 hours or determines the **body surface area** (BSA), the surface of a human body expressed in square meters, using the child's weight (Mosteller, 1987) (Table 4.2).

TABLE 4.1

Pediatric Age Groups

Group	Age
Premature infant	<38 wk gestational age
Neonate	From full-term newborn 0 to 4 wk of age
Infant	From >4 wk to 1 y of age
Child	From >1 to 12 y of age
Adolescent	13 to 18 y of age

TABLE 4.2

Body Surface Area (BSA)*

Age	Average BSA (m²)
Neonate (newborn)	0.25
Child, 2 y	0.50
Child, 9 y	1.07
Child, 10 y	1.14
Child, 12–13 y	1.33
Man (older than 18 y)	1.90
Woman (older than 18 y)	1.60

*The following formula is used to calculate BSA:

$$\text{BSA (m}^2) = \sqrt{\frac{\text{body weight (kg)} - \text{body height (cm)}}{3600}}$$

Then the prescriber calculates the dose based on a known adult dose by using the following equation: pediatric dose = BSA/1.73 × adult dose.

Pharmacodynamics in Pediatrics

Pharmacodynamics involves drug actions on target cells and the resulting alterations in cellular reactions and functions. These actions occur because of chemicals that bind with receptors at the cellular level. Most of these receptors are proteins on the surface or within cells. Therefore, pharmacodynamic variables in pediatric patients are related to differences in target cell sites and changing numbers of protein receptors. Immature organ systems and changing body compositions mean that drugs affect children differently. Causes of pharmacodynamic variability across the lifespan include differences in body composition, immature systems, and genetic makeup. Total body water, fat stores, and protein amounts change throughout childhood and greatly influence the effectiveness of drugs in the pediatric population.

One example of a drug that has different pharmacodynamic actions in adults and children is the fetal disaster caused by the drug thalidomide in the 1960s. Thalidomide worked wonders for decreasing morning sickness in pregnant women. However, it was soon apparent that it had severe teratogenic (adverse) effects on the fetus. This antiemetic drug, which was used to prevent vomiting in pregnant women, resulted in tragic limb abnormalities and often death for the fetus. Pharmacodynamic differences between drug action in adult females and their unborn fetuses illustrate one of the many differences between medication management in adults and children.

Another example of pharmacodynamic problems in younger patients involves antidepressants. Initially, prescribers assumed that these drugs, widely used successfully in treating adults, could be safely used therapeutically in adolescents and children. However, by October 2004, the FDA had found that these medications needed a **BLACK BOX WARNING ◆** stating that antidepressants may play a causal role in inducing suicidality in pediatric patients (Singh et al., 2009, p. 30).

Clinical Application 4-2

- What nursing interventions would take priority in Billy's care?

NCLEX Success

1. Billy's medications should be individualized to ensure the best outcome. Individualizing drug therapy for a child involves which one of the following?
   A. Assessing the child's age and development level
   B. Administering an adult drug selection and dosage and observing for adverse reactions
   C. Deferring treatment until definitive pediatric dosing can be determined
   D. Determining the child's diet and exercise needs

2. Billy is unable to tolerate montelukast (Singulair) for his asthma, although this drug works well for his father. Billy's physician is aware that the boy's reaction is most likely a reflection of his
   A. inability to understand the purpose of the drug
   B. hope that he will not have to take the drug
   C. inability to swallow pills
   D. genetic variability

Pharmacokinetics in Pediatrics

Pharmacokinetics refers to the processes of drug absorption, distribution, metabolism, and elimination. The organ systems in pediatric patients vary widely in their growth and maturation compared with adult patients, and this, in turn, greatly affects a prescriber's ability to dose pediatric drugs effectively. Newborn infants are a prime example, because they process drugs inefficiently. However, by age 12, children have grown and matured sufficiently to develop pharmacokinetic responses that resemble those of adults. Older children tolerate many drugs reasonably well. To account for immature or impaired body systems in neonates and infants, it is often necessary to change drug dosages.

Absorption

Drug absorption in pediatrics is affected by the age of the child, gastric emptying, intestinal motility, routes of administration, and skin permeability. Careful thought to proper route, good monitoring, and anticipation of potential adverse effects can help ensure intended outcomes are seen with administered drugs.

Age is one important factor. During pregnancy, most drugs cross the placenta, and they may harm the fetus. The possible teratogenic risk is coded for each medication as a pregnancy risk category from A to X, with A being the safest and X known to be dangerous ("do not use"). Also, during infancy, neonates have delayed, irregular gastric emptying and reduced gastric acidity. This delay potentially leads to greatly increased drug levels. The decreased acidity results in greater absorption of acid-labile medications or reduced absorption of weakly acidic medications.

In addition, the route of administration affects absorption. Prescribers avoid the use of intramuscular (IM) injections in pediatric patients because of the associated pain and unpredictable absorption. Low blood flow to skeletal muscles and weak muscle contractions also contribute to the erratic absorption of IM injections. Thin and highly permeable skin increases the rate of absorption of topical drugs, and careful administration is important to avoid toxicity.

Distribution

Distribution of drugs in pediatric patients is dependent on percentage of body water, liver function and degree of protein binding, and the development of the blood–brain barrier. Children differ from adults in the percentages of **total body water**, or the amount of water within the body, including in the intracellular and extracellular compartments, plus the water in the gastrointestinal and urinary tracts (Bianchetti et al., 2009)

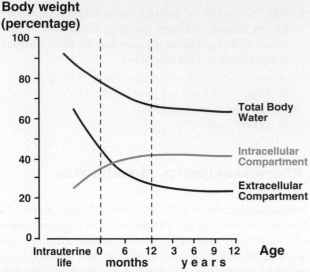

Figure 4.1 Total body water. Winters diagram with the subdivision of total body water, intracellular fluid, and extracellular fluid as a function of age. For clinical purpose, the use of "the rule of 3" is recommended: (1) total body water makes up two thirds of the body mass; (2) the intracellular compartment contains two thirds of the total body water, and the remaining amount (one third) is held in the extracellular compartment; and (3) the extracellular compartment is further subdivided into the interstitial and the intravascular compartments (blood volume), which contain two thirds and one third of the extracellular fluid, respectively. After puberty, males generally have 2% to 10% higher water content than females.

(Fig. 4.1). In adults, total body water is approximately 60%, whereas in newborns, it is 80%. This difference means that water-soluble drugs such as atenolol (Tenormin) and penicillin (Penicillin-G) are diluted easily and readily moved into intercellular tissue. As a result, serum drug concentrations are lower, and increased dosages of water-soluble drugs may be necessary to maintain therapeutic drug levels in neonates and premature infants.

In infants, immature liver function leads to very low plasma protein levels, which limits the amount of protein binding by drugs. Consequently, the serum concentrations of highly protein-bound drugs, including phenytoin (Dilantin), warfarin (Coumadin), ampicillin (Omnipen), and morphine (Duramorph), may be higher. Toxicity may occur. By the end of the first year, protein-binding ability is at the adult level, and its effect on drug distribution is no longer a concern.

The **blood–brain barrier**, which is composed of capillaries with tight bonds in the central nervous system (CNS), prevents the passage of most ions and large-molecular-weight compounds—including certain drugs—from the blood to the brain. Although this barrier protects the CNS, it can make drug delivery to the neurons more difficult. In neonates, the blood–brain barrier is poorly developed; thus, drugs and other chemicals easily affect the CNS in young infants. The nurse must assess for increased drug effects or toxic results from drug administration and must be alert for other chemicals or drugs that may cause unwanted CNS effects such as dizziness, sedation, and seizures.

Metabolism

The enzyme cytochrome P450 (CYP450) in the liver metabolizes most drugs. In neonates, the ability to metabolize drugs is very low because of the immaturity of the liver and the resultant inability to break down drugs. To avoid toxicity, the prescriber needs to calculate drug doses carefully, and the nurse must monitor infants and young children closely until the liver matures—by the end of the second year.

Elimination

Excretion of most drugs occurs via the kidneys, and elimination in the urine follows. Young children have immature kidneys, a reduced glomerular filtration rate, and slower renal clearance. Neonates are especially prone to increased levels of drugs that are eliminated primarily by the kidneys; the prescriber should give smaller doses until renal function reaches that of an adult—between 1 and 2 years of age.

Clinical Application 4-3

- How does the nurse know whether interventions designed to help Billy have been successful? What assessment data are warranted?

NCLEX Success

3. For Billy's asthma, a prescriber has ordered albuterol (Proventil). Which one of the following important factors related to growth and development is most likely to affect absorption of this beta$_2$-adrenergic agonist?

   A. The ability of Billy to cough up his secretions
   B. The need to decrease the dose as Billy's age increases
   C. The need to monitor Billy for hypotension
   D. The ability of Billy and his caregivers to understand the inhaler and how to use it to administer the albuterol

4. A 3-month-old infant who receives fosphenytoin (Cerebyx) for a seizure disorder does not process this drug in the same way as an adult. Alterations in infant pharmacokinetics that influence their action include which of the following concepts?

   A. Drug response in infants is slower and less rapid than in adults.
   B. Neonates have a decreased response to drugs that affect the CNS.
   C. Infants have a decreased response to water-soluble drugs and an increased response to protein-bound drugs.
   D. By 3 months of age, drug response in infants is similar to that of adults.

Medication Administration in Pediatrics

Administering medications to infants and children presents its own set of challenges because of difficulties in communication, cooperation, and adherence. Trends in growth and development serve as the basis for care across different age groups, and the nurse must continue to focus on safety in all activities involving drug administration.

Infants

The focus in this age group is aimed at calculation of correct dosages, safety in administration, and teaching parents how to deliver medications correctly. This includes a few key points related to infant growth and development.

- Oral medications are administered with a dropper or oral syringe into the inner aspect of the cheek, giving children time to swallow the medication as it is instilled.
- Some practitioners prefer giving oral medications through a nipple with a small amount of formula or breast milk, but this is controversial. Some authorities believe that infants may then refuse feedings if they associate food with the taste of the medication.
- Infants lack well-developed muscles. Thus, care is practiced with IM injections, using the smallest needle, preferably in the vastus lateralis.
- Many medications come in suppository form, which makes administration easier.
- Comfort care is important with infants. They need holding and cuddling and are offered a pacifier with, or shortly after, medication administration.
- Intravenous (IV) sites are often found in the scalp, hands, or feet.

Toddlers and Preschoolers

Toddlers are mobile and curious. Preschoolers are inquisitive and controlling. They love investigating but have short attention spans and want to exert their independence. The nurse involves toddlers and preschoolers in medication administration by having them hold items or choose the self-adhesive bandage or cup, but explanations should be short and simple, and adults need to control administration.

- To make oral medications more palatable, the nurse often mixes them with flavored syrups or fruit purees. Children may receive their favorite drink afterward.
- As the toddlers develop bigger muscle mass, IM injections can move from the vastus lateralis to the ventrogluteal area.
- Reaction to suppositories is strong. Therefore, explanations should be short, and for successful administration, an assistant may be necessary.
- For toddlers, IV sites in the scalp are still occasionally appropriate, but for older toddlers and preschoolers, the feet, the hands, or antecubital are more often preferable.

School-Aged Children and Adolescents

These children are able to participate more in medication administration. They develop an ability to reason and as they mature, the nurse can explain medication use in more detail. Often, these patients want to take medications independently, but they need supervision to make sure they take all of their medications at the correct times. Adolescents may try to self-medicate if medications are available in the home, so the nurse stresses safe medication practices for these children.

- Some medications are available as chewable tablets. These work well for children who cannot swallow tablets or capsules.
- IM injections are frightening for older children, and they need praise and encouragement. They often respond well to rewards after the injections have been completed.
- It is necessary to assess adolescents for risky behavior related to use of laxatives in eating disorders; drug experimentation; and the use of illicit, prescription, or over-the-counter medications. Teaching and monitoring for alcohol use and abuse is also important.
- Important information about self-care related to medication administration are good teaching points for this age group. Adolescents need explanations about the use of acne medications and antibiotics, including adverse effects. The nurse should tell teenage girls who are taking birth control medications about possible adverse effects and drug interactions. The nurse should also discuss the importance for sun protection. Adolescents should be aware of all such information.

Clinical Application 4-4

- What is the best way to teach Billy about his discharge plan, teach him how to use his inhaler, and review how to take his medications?

QSEN Safety Alerts for Pediatric Patients

- *Ensure that medications are dosed based on weight and calculated individually for each child.*
- *Use adequate measuring devices, graduated to tenths, for pediatric patients and help make sure that these devices are available to caregivers.*
- *Administer oral medications only in oral syringes.*
- *Order, dispense, and administer medications based on individual dosages in milligrams, micrograms, units, and so on, not on variables such as tablets or milliliters, for which the concentration may vary.*
- *Administer IV medications using smart pump technology with safety systems enabled.*
- *Administer IV fluids and medications with syringe pump technology for smaller amounts over set times or at set rates.*
- *Ensure a double-check system in prescribing, dispensing, and administering high-risk pediatric medications.*
- *Collaborate with interdisciplinary team members on best practice solutions to pediatric medication management problems.*
- *Have access to current, pediatric focused medication references.*
- *Administer medications using a caring approach, involving knowledge of pediatric growth and development.*
- *Involve family or caregivers in the management of a child's medications.*

Key Concepts

- Medications are dosed, administered, and their effectiveness evaluated differently in pediatric patients because of physiologic differences across developmental levels.

- Federal legislation has resulted in increased testing, improved surveillance, and attention to medication effectiveness in the various pediatric age groups.

- The FDA has issued a **BLACK BOX WARNING** ◆ stating that antidepressants may play a causal role in inducing suicidality in pediatric patients.

- Pharmacodynamic variability is related to total body water, fat stores, and protein-carrying ability.

- Dosages of pediatric medications are calculated based on weight.

- Effects of drugs are longer and stronger in infants than in adults because of delayed gastric emptying and reduced gastric acidity.

- The risk of CNS effects related to drugs is higher in infants than in adults because of the immature blood–brain barrier.

- Water-soluble drugs lead to lower drug levels in infants than in adults. In contrast, protein-bound drugs lead to increased drug levels.

- Drug metabolism and excretion is decreased in infants compared with adults because of immature hepatic and renal function.

Critical Thinking Questions

4-1. Megan is a 7-month-old infant with a 2-day history of vomiting and fever. She has only had one wet diaper today and just 8 oz of formula. Her mother is concerned that this illness may have started with an ear infection and is concerned about giving her daughter any medications. Megan lies on the examination table without crying but does smile and interact with her mother. Vital signs are temperature 102.4°F, heart rate 160 beats per minute, and respiratory rate 34 per minute. In addition, she is pulling at her ears.

- What nursing interventions take priority?

- What medications does the nurse anticipate having to administer to Megan?

- What challenges are there in administering medications to Megan?

- What are key teaching points to address with Megan's mother?

- What outcomes will be expected from these nursing interventions?

References and Resources

Berlin, C. M. (2009). Pharmacokinetics in children. *The Merck Manual For Health Professionals* [On line version]. Retrieved from http://www.merck.com/mmpe/sec19/ch270/ch270b.html

Bianchetti, M., Simonetti, G., & Bettinelli, A. (2009). Body fluids and salt metabolism: Part I. *Italian Journal of Pediatrics, 35*(36). doi: 10.1186/1824-7288-35-36

Hockenberry, M., & Wilson, D. (2011). *Wong's nursing care of infants and children.* St. Louis, MO: Mosby Elsevier.

Kishore, R., & Tabor, E. (2010). Overview of the FDA Amendments Act of 2007: Its effect on the drug development landscape. *Drug Information Journal, 44*(4), 469–475.

Mosteller, R. D. (1987). Simplified calculation of body surface area. *The New England Journal of Medicine, 317*(17), 1098.

Singh, T., Prakash, A., Rais, T., & Kumari, N. (2009). Decreased use of antidepressants in youth after U.S. Food and Drug Administration black box warning. *Psychiatry, 6*(10), 30–34.

U.S. Food and Drug Administration (USFDA). (2009). FDAAA Implementation: Highlights two years after enactment. *Regulatory Information: FDAAA Implementation.* Retrieved from http://www.fda.gov/RegulatoryInformation/Legislation/FederalFoodDrugandCosmeticActFDCAct/SignificantAmendmentstotheFDCAct/FoodandDrugAdministrationAmendmentsActof2007/ucm184271.htm

Vargesson, N. (2009). Thalidomide-induced limb defects: Resolving a 50-year-old puzzle. *Bioessays: News and Reviews in Molecular, Cellular and Developmental Biology, 31*(12), 1327–1336.

Wong, I. C. (2009). Minimising medication errors in children. *Archives of Disease in Childhood, 94*(2), 161–164.

Zajicek, A. (2009). The National Institutes of Health and the Best Pharmaceuticals for Children Act. *Pediatric Drugs, 11*(1), 45–47.

5 Pharmacology and the Care of the Adult and Geriatric Patient

Clinical Application Case Study

Charles Franklin is a 75-year-old African American man with a diagnosis of an enlarged prostate. He has been experiencing insomnia for the past month and has begun taking acetaminophen in the form of Tylenol PM.

KEY TERMS

Adult: person who ranges in age from 19 to 64 years

Age-related changes: physiological events due to increasing age, which affect drug responses

Older adult: person who is 65 years of age or older

Polypharmacy: use of several drugs during the same period

Risk-to-benefit ratio: poor outcome (adverse effects of medications) in relation to good outcome (desired medication effects); increases with increasing age

Introduction

Aging is a natural process that begins at birth. The most significant **age-related changes** begin in the **adult** years (19 to 64 years of age). These physiological events, which can affect drug responses, are due to increasing age. Most commonly, they occur in middle age and are related to heart disease, pulmonary insufficiency, cancer, arthritis, diabetes mellitus, obesity, substance abuse, and depression.

Older adults, people who are 65 years of age or older, are the largest consumers of health care. According to the National Institutes of Health (2010), chronic conditions have roots in the aging process. The most common health problems in older adults include arthritis, heart disease, decreased sensory perception, bone disorders, and diabetes mellitus. Older adults are also more prone to antibiotic resistant infections. The treatment of chronic illnesses and associated comorbidities results in **polypharmacy,** the use of multiple medications. The interactions of medications can lead to greater complications and diminished mental status. In addition, the **risk-to-benefit ratio,** the relationship between the negative effects and the positive effects of a medication, increases as the patient ages. The nurse and the prescriber must consider the risk of associated adverse effects of those medications as well as possible benefits these medications might have in changing physiological processes related to disease. As Howland (2009) states, older patients are more sensitive to the pharmacological effects of medication.

Pharmacodynamics in Older Adults

Pharmacodynamics involves drug actions on target cells and the resulting alterations in cellular biochemical reactions and functions. In older adults, physiological changes such as a reduced number of receptor sites for medications or affinity to receptors alter the medication's ability to produce the desired effect. Older adults are prone to adverse drug reactions because of a decrease in the number of receptors needed for drug distribution. Beta-adrenergic agonists are less effective as a result of the decreased function of the beta-receptor system.

Cardiovascular disease is the number one cause of death in adults, including older adults. In patients with hypertension, the control of blood pressure is key to the prevention of cardiovascular disease. The administration of thiazide diuretics is the most effective treatment of hypertension in older adults (Olsen, Tindall, & Clasen, 2007). The use of digoxin (Lanoxin) in heart disease should not exceed 0.125 mg per day except when treating atrial dysrhythmias (Aschenbrenner & Venable, 2009; Fick et al., 2003). Digoxin has a low therapeutic index, placing patients at risk for adverse effects. Thus, administration of the medication with a reduced dose assists in maintaining safety.

Beers Criteria

Dr. Mark Beers initially developed the Beers Criteria list of potentially inappropriate medications used by the older adult population in 1997. Updated in 2003 (Fick et al., 2003), the list confirms that toxic medication effects and drug-related problems affect the safety of older adults and names drugs that cause problems in this population. Thirty percent of elderly hospital admissions are linked to drug reactions.

In nursing practice, it is vital to implement strategies to identify age-related changes associated with medication administration.

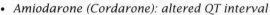

QSEN Safety Alert

Drugs that produce adverse effects in older adults include

- *Amiodarone (Cordarone): altered QT interval*
- *Amitriptyline hydrochloride: anticholinergic effects, sedation*
- *Cimetidine (Tagamet): confusion*
- *Cyclobenzaprine (Flexeril): anticholinergic effects, weakness*
- *Digoxin (Lanoxin): digoxin toxicity*
- *Diphenhydramine hydrochloride (Benadryl): urinary retention*
- *Flurazepam hydrochloride (Dalmane): sedation*
- *Hydroxyzine hydrochloride (Vistaril): confusion, sedation*
- *Ketorolac: gastrointestinal (GI) bleeding*
- *Meperidine hydrochloride (Demerol): confusion*
- *Methocarbamol (Robaxin): anticholinergic effects, weakness*
- *Methyldopa (Apo-Methyldopa; Aldomet): bradycardia, depression*
- *Nitrofurantoin (Macrodantin): renal toxicity*
- *Propoxyphene hydrochloride (Darvon): respiratory depression*

Prevention of Adverse Effects

Strategies to prevent adverse drug reactions include the following:

- Assess a patient's health history and list of medications taken by the patient, including prescription medications, over-the-counter medications, and herbal supplements.
- Assess blood urea nitrogen and creatinine clearance (CrCl) levels to determine the patient's ability to excrete the medications.
- Assess the ratio of alanine aminotransferase to aspartate aminotransferase to determine the patient's liver function and ability to metabolize drugs.
- Assess therapeutic drug levels as ordered by the prescriber to determine the medication effectiveness and prevention of toxicity.
- Educate the patient and family about all medications and possible drug–drug, drug–herb, and drug–diet interactions.
- Educate the patient and family about the generic and trade names of medications to prevent overmedication.
- Assess the patient's adherence to the prescribed medications.
- Provide the patient with medication administration aids to increase adherence.

NCLEX Success

1. **When administering a beta-adrenergic agonist to a patient older than 65 years of age, what response do you anticipate?**

   A. The drug will work very rapidly to decrease blood pressure.

   B. The dosage will need to be increased to provide an effective response.

   C. The drug should be combined with atropine to enhance effectiveness.

   D. The dosage will need to be titrated over 20 minutes to increase blood pressure.

2. **A 75-year-old woman is having difficulty remembering to take all of her medications. Which of the following nursing interventions will assist her to improve adherence to the medication schedule?**

   A. Have her daughter administer the medications.

   B. Decrease the number of medications administered.

   C. Evaluate her ability to care for herself.

   D. Provide a medication administration aid.

Pharmacokinetics in Older Adults

Aging results in physiological changes that affect the absorption, distribution, metabolism, and excretion of medications. The most relevant physiologic change is the decreased function of vital organs needed for the pharmacokinetic processes. Frail, elderly adults are at greatest risk for altered drug responses. The more physically active older adults are, the less likely they will experience altered drug responses.

Absorption

In older adults, changes in the GI tract include decreased gastric acidity, with an increase in the gastric pH, and delayed absorption or lack of absorption of medications that require this decreased pH. Other changes in the GI tract responsible for affecting drug absorption in older adults are decreased blood flow and decreased surface area to support absorption. Diminished gastric emptying also plays a role by causing the medication to be in the stomach for a longer period. This factor increases the risk of developing nausea and vomiting, thus causing elimination of the medication in emesis and promoting fluid volume deficit.

In older patients, decreased circulation means that parenteral medications are also slowly absorbed. Decreased muscle mass and altered circulation can result in abnormal blood concentrations of medications administered intramuscularly.

In all cases, a slow rate of absorption can result in changes in peak serum drug levels. This factor may require greater dosages to be administered to produce therapeutic results.

Distribution

In older adults, physiological factors that contribute to alterations in distribution of medications include diminished cardiac output, increased body fat, decreased body mass and body fluid, and decreased serum albumin. Aging results in changes in body mass changes; the proportion of body fat increases while lean body mass decreases. These changes may have the following consequences:

- Lipid-soluble drugs such as the anesthetic agents stay in the fat tissue for a longer period of time. This places older adults at risk for respiratory depression following surgery.
- The amount of body fluid decreases in proportion to total body weight. Water-soluble drugs such as antibiotics are distributed in smaller volumes due to the decrease in total body fluid volume. This increases the risk of toxicity because drug concentrations are greater.
- Many medications require serum albumin to bind, transport, and distribute the medication to the target organ. In the event that the amount of serum albumin is insufficient, the amount of free drug rises and the effect of the drug is more intense.
- Medications are not distributed adequately due to the decreased circulation and diminished cardiac output.

Metabolism

Age-related physiological changes of the liver affect the metabolism of medications. At approximately 60 years of age, the liver begins to decrease in size and mass. There is also a decrease in the hepatic circulation, lowering the rate of metabolism. The hepatic enzymes of the liver are decreased, altering the ability to remove metabolic by-products. It is important to understand that because older adults have a reduced metabolism, medications with a long half-life will remain in the body for a greater amount of time.

Some responses to drug therapy are genetically determined and may differ in various ethnic and racial populations. Caucasian Americans and African Americans are poor metabolizers of medication compared with Asian Americans; Asian Americans have the ability to metabolize and excrete medications more quickly than those of Caucasian and African descent. Circulating levels of medications in Caucasian Americans and African Americans are higher. For example, beta-blockers are less effective in African Americans, whereas Asian Americans require a smaller dose due to the ethnic variation in medication response.

Excretion

The elimination of medications is vital in the prevention of adverse drug reactions. In older adults, physiologic changes associated with alterations in medication excretion include diminished renal blood flow, number of functioning nephrons, glomerular filtration rate, and tubular secretion. The assessment of the patient's CrCl is an important indicator of the ability of the renal system to eliminate the medication and prevent adverse drug effects. Dosages of medications should be lower in medications with an increased half-life. In most older adults, the serum creatinine remains within the normal range due to decreasing creatinine levels in association with a decrease in muscle mass. The glomerular filtration rate is the most reliable measure for evaluation of renal function. However, this value is very costly to obtain and is often unavailable. An alternative to the 24-hour CrCl and the glomerular filtration rate is the Cockroft-Gault method. This method estimates the CrCl (Launay-Vacher et al., 2007; Porth, 2009).

$$\text{Estimated CrCl (mL/min)} = \frac{(140-\text{age})\times(\text{body weight in kilograms})}{(72\times\text{serum creatinine in mg/dL})}$$

The result should be multiplied by 0.85 for women.

Prior to the administration of a medication excreted by the renal system, the nurse assesses the patient's glomerular filtration rate and hydration status by using the serum creatinine value to calculate the estimated CrCl. With a decreased CrCl, it is necessary to reduce the dosage of the medication. According to the National Kidney Foundation, the average estimated glomerular filtration rate is 116 mL/min/1.73 m² for males 20 to 29 years of age. The average estimated glomerular filtration rate declines with every decade of life; by 70 years of age, the average estimated glomerular filtration rate is 75 mL/min/1.73 m². The glomerular filtration rate is an overestimation of the CrCl, because creatinine is secreted by the proximal tubule and filtered by the kidneys. The glomerular filtration rate is lower in females as a result of their decreased muscle mass, and it is higher in African Americans, both males and females, because of their increased muscle mass (National Kidney Foundation, 2010).

Clinical Application 5-2

- What is the suspected effect of Mr. Franklin's race on his creatinine clearance and excretion of medications?

NCLEX Success

3. A 68-year-old woman has been prescribed digoxin (Lanoxin) 0.125 mg. Based on her age, what condition is she at risk for developing?
   A. diarrhea
   B. digoxin toxicity
   C. edema
   D. pulmonary embolism

4. An 85-year-old woman is administered a general anesthetic for repair of a hip fracture. Which of the following properties of the anesthetic place her at risk for respiratory depression?
   A. solubility in lipids
   B. solubility in water
   C. binding to cytochrome P450
   D. binding to muscle tissue

Clinical Application 5-3

Mr. Franklin has developed herpes zoster (shingles) and is complaining of severe neuropathic pain. His physician has ordered gabapentin (Neurontin) 300 mg twice daily by mouth. The recommended dosage with renal impairment is 200 to 700 mg twice daily if the creatinine clearance (CrCl) is greater than 30 to 59 mL per minute. Mr. Franklin's serum creatinine is 2.2 mg/dL.

- What is the patient's estimated CrCl?
- Is this dosage of gabapentin appropriate?

Medication Adherence and Aging

As patients increase in age, they use a greater number of medications, both prescription and over the counter, along with alternative therapies such as vitamins or herbal supplements. (As previously mentioned, the use of increased medications is known as polypharmacy.) It is often difficult to remember medications or maintain appropriate administration schedules. Altered mental status and diminished visual acuity also contribute to improper medication use. Patients who have decreased vision may not be able to discriminate the dosing instructions or may not be able to see the amount of insulin drawn up in an insulin syringe.

Economic factors also contribute to nonadherence. Some older adults may have to choose between the cost of their medications and the ability to purchase food or pay for utilities. A multidisciplinary team approach is used to assist patients in obtaining medications. It is important for the prescriber to use generic medications and to order small quantities of medications initially so that an individual patient's reaction to the medication can be determined. In the event the medication needs to be changed, the great financial burden on the patient will not be too great.

Starting slow and with low doses improves adherence to the medication regime. Patients may describe not feeling well after using the prescribed medications. Starting with smaller doses minimizes these adverse effects. The administration of several medications concurrently can result in adverse effects. When adverse effects are experienced by older patients, they may not adhere to the recommended administration guidelines.

Being asymptomatic may contribute to nonadherence to a medication regimen. Many patients begin to feel better with the initiation of therapy and then discontinue medications altogether or miss individual doses. Patients and their families should be educated about adherence to medication regimens. This is particularly evident in patients being treated for hypertension. Kaplan, Bakris, and Sheridan (2010) state that patients who do not take antihypertensives as prescribed have an increased risk of a cardiovascular event. These investigators encourage health care providers to educate the patient and family about medications and their use. To improve adherence, nurses and other health care providers should keep the care inexpensive, using generic preparations, and easy to follow, using the fewest number of doses required.

EVIDENCE-BASED PRACTICE

Challenges of Treatment Adherence in Older Patients with Parkinson's Disease

by J. L. BAINBRIDGE; J. M. RUSCIN

Drugs and Aging
2009, 26(2), 145–155.
Retrieved July 15, 2010.

This review of literature revealed that adherence to medications in the treatment of Parkinson's disease was crucial to quality of life. The lack of adherence to medication administration was a result of the patient's age, cost of medication, and number of medications required for treatment, along with the complicated dosage and titrations. The patient's diminished cognition also played a role in nonadherence.

IMPLICATIONS FOR NURSING PRACTICE: It is important to assist the patient and family with strategies to maintain adherence. These strategies include the provision of medication administration aids or pill set-up boxes and patient and family education on medication actions and adverse effects. The nurse must also communicate with the prescriber to encourage simplified dosing and administration schedules.

The Nursing Process

Assessment

- **Assess the patient's knowledge of medication regimen.**
  - Medication's action and use
  - Adverse effects
  - Dosage and administration
  - Goal of therapy
  - Guidelines for administration (e.g., with or without meals, hold if pulse is less than 60 bpm)
  - Drug–drug; drug–diet; drug–herb interactions
- **Assess the patient's physiological status with regard to the medication's pharmacokinetics.**
  - Renal function
  - Liver function
  - Cardiovascular function
  - Physiological changes (e.g., change in body mass, ability to swallow)
- **Assess the patient's ability to maintain adherence to medications.**
  - Memory
  - Ability to care for self
  - Caregivers' ability to assist in care

Nursing Diagnoses

- Effective therapeutic regimen management
- Risk for falls
- Ineffective health maintenance
- Readiness for enhanced knowledge

Planning/Goals

The patient will

- Take medications as prescribed.
- Tolerate medications based on renal and liver function.
- Report any adverse effects, such as falls.
- Understand all aspects of medication administration, including action, uses, and adverse effects.
- Maintain medication adherence.

Nursing Interventions

The nurse will

- Assess the patient's liver and renal function.
- Assess the patient's circulation and changes in body mass affecting pharmacokinetics.
- Assess the patient's response to medication regimen.
- Assess the patient's ability to maintain medication administration.
- Assess for adverse effects of medications.
- Assess for the patient's adherence to medications.
- Instruct the patient and family about the use of medication administration aids.
- Instruct the patient and family about the administration of medications.
- Instruct the patient and family about the action, use, and adverse effects of medications.

Evaluation

- Evaluate the patient's response to the medication regimen.
- Evaluate the patient's and family's understanding of the medication regimen.
- Evaluate the patient's adherence to the medication regimen.

Clinical Application 5-4

Mr. Franklin's primary health care provider has prescribed the following medications for him:

- Gabapentin (Neurontin) 300 mg twice daily by mouth
- Famciclovir (Famvir) 500 mg every 12 hours by mouth
- Meperidine (Demerol) 50 mg every 6 hours PRN by mouth
- Which of the following medications is inappropriate for this patient?
- How will you assist this patient to maintain medication adherence?

NCLEX Success

5. A 68-year-old woman is receiving chemotherapy. What is the rationale for teaching her to drink eight glasses of water throughout the day following the administration of chemotherapy?

A. Chemotherapy is toxic to the liver, and the water will reduce the adverse effects.
B. The water will prevent the body from rejecting the medication.
C. Chemotherapy is excreted in the kidneys and urine. The water will help eliminate it from the body.
D. The water will prevent dehydration, an adverse effect of the medication.

6. A 78-year-old man is receiving treatment for hypertension. He has been having persistent headaches and difficulty with the medications he has been prescribed. This is the third prescription he has received. He states, "I can't afford to get this filled and then stop it in a few days." Which statement is most appropriate for the nurse to communicate to the patient?

A. Have the pharmacist give you a few pills to start.
B. Take your other medication and then switch.
C. Take the other medications back to the pharmacy for a refund.
D. Save all your pills; you may need them again.

Key Concepts

- Pharmacodynamics involves drug actions on target cells and the resulting alterations in cellular biochemical reactions and functions.
- In older adults, physiological changes alter the ability for the medication to provide the desired effect for which it is intended.
- In nursing practice, it is vital to implement strategies to identify age-related changes associated with medication administration.
- Aging results in physiological changes affecting the absorption, distribution, metabolism, and excretion of medications.
- The most relevant physiologic change is the decreased function of vital organs needed for the pharmacokinetic processes.
- The GI tract changes affecting drug absorption include an increase in the gastric pH.
- A decrease in blood flow to the GI tract, a decrease in surface area to support absorption, and diminished gastric emptying also limit absorption.
- Alterations in distribution of medications include diminished cardiac output; increased body fat; and decreased body mass, body fluid, and serum albumin.
- Physiologic changes associated with alterations in medication excretion include diminished renal blood flow, number of functioning nephrons, glomerular filtration rate, and tubular secretion.
- The nurse implements strategies to increase medication adherence such as educating the patient about medication administration and adverse effects, providing medication administration aids, and assessing for adverse effects.

Critical Thinking Questions

5-1. A 70-year-old woman is being treated with chemotherapy for breast cancer. She recently has developed neuropathic pain related to the chemotherapy agents. Her health care provider has ordered amitriptyline hydrochloride to decrease the neuropathic pain.

- What effect is most noted in the older adult when administered amitriptyline?
- What measures can the nurse instruct the patient to reduce the adverse effects of amitriptyline?

5-2. An 83-year-old woman is admitted to the emergency department following a fall in her home. She has sustained a fractured left femur. She is complaining of severe pain, of 9 to 10 on the pain scale. The physician in the emergency department orders ketorolac for pain. The patient remains on ketorolac for 3 postoperative days. On the 3rd day, she begins to complain of severe abdominal pain. Her blood pressure is 96/50 mm Hg and her pulse rate is 116 beats per minute.

- What type of medication is ketorolac?
- Why is the patient complaining of abdominal pain?

References and Resources

Aschenbrenner, D. S., & Venable, S. J. (2009). *Drug therapy in nursing* (3rd ed.). Philadelphia, PA: Lippincott Williams & Wilkins.

Bainbridge, J. L., & Ruscin, J. M. (2009). Challenges of treatment adherence in older patients with Parkinson's Disease. *Drugs and Aging, 36*(2), 145–155.

Duke Clinical Research Institute. Beers Criteria (Medication List). Available at https://www.dcri.org/trial-participation/the-beers-list/

Fick, D. M., Cooper, J. W., Wade, W. E., Waller, J. L., Maclean, J. R., & Beers, M. (2003). Updating the Beers criteria for potentially inappropriate medication use in older adults results of a US panel of experts. *Archives of Internal Medicine, 10*, 761–768. Available at http://archinte.ama-assn.org/cgi/reprint/163/22/2716

Howland, R. H. (2009). Effects of aging on pharmacokinetic and pharmacodynamic drug processes. *Journal of Psychosocial Nursing, 47*(10), 15–18.

Kaplan, N. M., Bakris, G. L., & Sheridan, A. M. (2010). Patient adherence and the treatment of hypertension. Available at www.uptodate.com

Karch, A. M. (2010). *2010 Lippincott's nursing drug guide.* Philadelphia, PA: Lippincott Williams & Wilkins.

Launay-Vacher, V., Chatelut, E., Lichtman, S. M., Wilders, H., Steer, C., & Aapro, M. (2007). Renal insufficiency in elderly cancer patients; International Society of Geriatric Oncology clinical practice recommendations. *Annals of Oncology, 18*, 1314–1321.

National Institutes of Health. (2010). Fiscal Budget Request. Department of Health and Human Services. Retrieved July 10, 2010, from http://www.nih.gov/about/director/budgetrequest/fy2011testimony.pdf

National Kidney Foundation. (2010). Frequently asked questions about GFR estimates. Retrieved July 15, 2010, from http://www.kidney.org/professionals/kls/pdf/faq_gfr.pdf

Olsen, C. G., Tindall, W. N., & Clasen, M. E. (2007). *Geriatric pharmacotherapy: a guide for the helping professional.* Washington, DC: American Pharmacists Association.

Porth, C. M. (2009). *Pathophysiology: Concepts of altered health status* (8th ed.). Philadelphia, PA: Lippincott Williams & Wilkins.

Smela, T. P., Belzer, J. L., & Higbee, M. D. (2010). *Geriatric dosage handbook* (15th ed.). Washington, DC: American Pharmacists Association.

6 Pharmacology and the Pregnant or Lactating Woman

LEARNING OBJECTIVES

After studying this chapter, you should be able to:

1. Describe the etiology of infertility.
2. Describe the drugs used for infertility.
3. Identify the pregnancy-associated changes that affect drug pharmacokinetics.
4. Analyze the effect of teratogens on the fetus during development.
5. Identify the effects of herbal and dietary supplements on the mother and fetus during pregnancy.
6. Identify pharmacological strategies to manage pregnancy-associated symptoms.
7. Identify the prototype drugs that alter uterine motility and describe these drugs.
8. Identify the prototype drugs used during labor and delivery and describe these drugs.
9. Discuss the use of drugs and herbs during lactation, including their effect on the infant.
10. Implement the nursing process in the care of the women of childbearing age.

Clinical Application Case Study

Lauren Ross is in the 35th week of pregnancy with her fourth child. During her weekly visit to the certified nurse midwife, her blood pressure is elevated, 150/100 mm Hg, on two consecutive readings. The nurse midwife checks her urine for protein and determines that she is spilling protein in her urine. Ms. Ross has facial swelling with edema around the eyes and nose and complains of a headache, with mild epigastric pain. Also, her vaginal culture is positive for perinatal group B streptococcus (GBS). In addition, during her pregnancy, she has been taking the antidepressant escitalopram (Lexapro) 10 mg per day and has continued to smoke. The nurse midwife admits her to the labor and delivery unit.

KEY TERMS

Abortifacients: drugs used to terminate pregnancy up to 20 weeks after the last menstrual period

Eclampsia: characterized by the onset of seizures; occurs in some women with preeclampsia

Galactagogues: a category of herbs known to induce lactation or stimulate the production of breast milk in postpartal women

Organogenesis: formation of organs during development

Oxytocics: drugs that initiate uterine contractions, thus inducing childbirth

Preeclampsia: pregnancy-induced hypertension and proteinuria

Preterm labor: uterine contractions with cervical changes before 37 weeks of gestation, resulting in birth

Prostaglandins: chemical mediators, such as uterotonics, that help initiate uterine contractions

Teratogenic: causing abnormal embryonic or fetal development

Tocolytics: drugs used to stop preterm labor

Uterotonics: drugs to control postpartum bleeding

Introduction

Drug use before and during pregnancy and lactation requires special consideration. Women of childbearing age may become pregnant, and they may ingest drugs that may cause fetal harm before they know they are pregnant. In general, pregnant or lactating women should avoid or minimize use of medications whenever possible. This chapter discusses drugs related to pregnancy and lactation, including infertility drugs, vaccines, tocolytics (drugs used to stop preterm labor), oxytocics (drugs used to initiate uterine contractions), drugs used to stop postpartum hemorrhage (uterotonics), and selected teratogenic drugs (agents causing abnormal embryonic or fetal development). Description of many of these drugs appears elsewhere in the text.

Drug Therapy for Infertility

A woman who has been unable to conceive for at least 1 year of sexual intercourse without the use of any form of birth control is infertile. In women, the most common causes are ovulation disorders, blocked fallopian tubes, endometriosis, and advanced maternal age, which affects egg quality and quantity. In men, causes include absence of sperm, declining sperm counts, testicular abnormalities, and ejaculatory dysfunction. Factors such as implantation, uterine and hormonal environment, and embryo integrity may also play a role. They are critical to fetal viability and a normally progressing pregnancy.

Drug therapy is an integral part of treating infertility. Drugs prescribed for a woman experiencing infertility increase follicular maturation and promote ovulation. It is necessary to take the total dose at the same time each day to enhance effects of a particular medication. Also, coitus every other day enhances fertility due to increased sperm counts.

Table 6.1 presents the routes and dosage ranges for the infertility drugs.

Clomiphene Citrate

Ⓟ **Clomiphene citrate** (Clomid) is an ovarian stimulator and selective estrogen receptor. This drug increases the amount of follicle-stimulating hormone (FSH) secreted by the pituitary gland, thus inducing ovulation for women who have infrequent or absent menstrual periods. Health care providers use it for the treatment of ovulatory failure in women who have tried to become pregnant but have failed. Ovulation occurs 5 to 10 days after the course of clomiphene treatment has been completed. Prior to beginning

the drug regimen, the nurse instructs the woman about taking her basal temperature 5 to 10 days following administration. An incremental rise in temperature is an indication of ovulation.

Clomiphene is a mixture of zuclomiphene and enclomiphene. Metabolized by the liver, the drug has a half-life of 5 to 7 days. It is excreted in the feces and urine.

Possible adverse effects of clomiphene include hot flashes, breast pain and tenderness, and uterine bleeding. Some women have reported blurred vision, visual changes, and headaches. Contraindications include liver disease, thyroid or adrenal disease, ovarian cysts, and abnormal uterine bleeding.

Menotropin

Ⓟ **Menotropin** (Menopur, Repronex) is a gonadotropin given to women who have been diagnosed with anovulation. The drug stimulates FSH and luteinizing hormone (LH) to promote the development and maturation of ovarian follicles. Administration may be subcutaneous, in alternating sides of the abdomen, or intramuscular, in large muscles. Following its administration, the woman receives human chorionic gonadotropin (hCG) (see later discussion). Menotropin is well absorbed and excreted in the urine.

During menotropin therapy, it is necessary to monitor both hCG and serum estradiol measurements. The adverse effects and contraindications of menotropin are similar to those of clomiphene citrate.

Follitropins

Ⓟ **Follitropin alfa** (Gonal-F) and follitropin beta (Follistim AQ) are drugs used to stimulate follicle development and thus promote fertility. Administration is subcutaneous, in calibrated syringes provided by the manufacturer. It is important that the drugs not be shaken before administration. After receiving follitropins, as with menotropins, women should also receive hCG (see later discussion)—1 day after the last dose of follitropin.

The adverse effects of the follitropins are similar to those of clomiphene. Contraindications include hypersensitivity as well as the presence of tumors in the ovary, breast, pituitary gland, uterus, or hypothalamus. It is necessary to monitor serum estradiol levels to determine the medication response.

Human Chorionic Gonadotropin

Ⓟ **Human chorionic gonadotropin,** or hCG, is manufactured as Novarel or Pregnyl. This drug is a human formulation of hCG that is obtained from the urine of pregnant women.

TABLE 6.1

DRUGS AT A GLANCE: Infertility Drugs*

Drug	Routes and Dosage Ranges
Ⓟ **Clomiphene citrate** (Clomid)	50 mg PO once daily for 5 d; begin on the 5th day of the cycle if progestin-induced bleeding is scheduled or spontaneous uterine bleeding occurs prior to therapy; subsequent doses may be increased to 100 mg once daily for 5 d only if ovulation does not occur at the initial dose; maximum dosage: 100 mg PO once daily for 5 d for six cycles; discontinue if ovulation does not occur after three courses of treatment or if ovulatory responses occur but pregnancy is not achieved
Ⓟ **Menotropin** (Menopur, Repronex)	150 international units daily IM or Sub-Q for the first 5 d of treatment; dosage adjustments may occur once every 2 d; maximum daily dose should not exceed 450 international units and dosing should not extend to 12 d
Ⓟ **Follitropin alfa** (Gonal-F)	75 international units Sub-Q daily; dose adjustment up to 37.5 international units after 14 d; if necessary it can be increased every 7 d (maximum dosage: 300 international units); if response to follitropin is appropriate; hCG is given 1 d following the last dose
Follitropin beta (Follistim AQ)	75 international units Sub-Q or IM for the first 7 d; increase by 25–50 international units at weekly intervals; if response to follitropin is appropriate; hCG is given 1 d following the last dose
Ⓟ **Human chorionic gonadotropin (hCG)**	5000–10,000 units 1 d following menotropins or follitropins
Ⓟ **Leuprolide** (Eligard, Lupron)	3.75 mg IM every month for up to 6 mo

*Pregnancy category of all infertility drugs is X.

It is usually used as a replacement for LH. After administration of this form of hCG (after administration of menotropin or follitropin), the LH stimulates ovulation.

Adverse effects of hCG include edema, depression, breast enlargement, ovarian cyst, and ovarian hypersensitivity. Contraindications include neoplasms or known hypersensitivity to the hormone.

Leuprolide

Ⓟ **Leuprolide** (Lupron) is a gonadotropin-releasing hormone that has an unlabeled use in the treatment of infertility. Administered subcutaneously, it prevents premature ovulation and enhances the production of a larger quantity of quality eggs.

Potential adverse effects of leuprolide include hot flashes, headache, mood swings, insomnia, vaginal dryness, decreased breast size, painful intercourse, and bone loss.

NCLEX Success

1. A couple has been trying to conceive for the past 8 months without success. Which of the following medications is the first drug of choice?

   A. leuprolide (Lupron)
   B. human chorionic gonadotropin (hCG) (Novarel)
   C. follitropin beta (Follistim AQ)
   D. clomiphene citrate (Clomid)

2. A woman diagnosed with anovulation receives a prescription for menotropin (Menopur, Repronex) to be administered subcutaneously. The nurse is teaching her about the administration of the medication. The nurse should teach the woman to

   A. massage the area prior to administering the drug
   B. administer the drug at a 90-degree angle
   C. alternate the sides of the abdomen for the injection sites
   D. take human chorionic gonadotropin before the menotropin

Drugs Used in Pregnancy

During pregnancy, mother and fetus undergo physiologic changes that influence drug effects. In pregnant women, physiologic changes alter drug pharmacokinetics (Table 6.2). In general, drug effects are less predictable because plasma volume expansion decreases plasma drug concentrations, and increased metabolism by the liver and increased elimination by the kidneys shorten the duration of drug actions and effects.

Maternal–Placental–Fetal Circulation

Drugs ingested by the pregnant woman reach the fetus through the maternal–placental–fetal circulation, which is completed about the 3rd week after conception. On the maternal side,

TABLE 6.2	
Pregnancy: Physiologic and Pharmacokinetic Changes	
Physiologic Change	**Pharmacokinetic Change**
Increased plasma volume and body water, ~50% in a normal pregnancy Increased cardiac output (30%–50%) and increased blood flow to the uterus, kidneys, skin, and breasts	After it is absorbed into the bloodstream, a drug (especially if water soluble) is distributed and "diluted" more than in the nonpregnant state. Drug dosage requirements may increase. However, this effect may be offset by other pharmacokinetic changes of pregnancy
Increased weight (average 25 lb) and body fat	Drugs (especially fat-soluble ones) are distributed more widely. Drugs that are distributed to fatty tissues stay in the body longer because they are slowly released from storage sites into the bloodstream
Decreased serum albumin. The rate of albumin production is increased. However, serum levels fall because of plasma volume expansion. Also, many plasma-protein binding sites are occupied by hormones and other endogenous substances that increase during pregnancy.	The decreased capacity for drug binding leaves more free drug available for therapeutic or adverse effects on the mother and for placental transfer to the fetus. Thus, a given dose of a drug may produce greater effects than it would in the nonpregnant state
During most of a pregnancy, increased renal blood flow and glomerular filtration rate secondary to increased cardiac output	Increased excretion of drugs by the kidneys, especially those excreted primarily unchanged in the urine (e.g., lithium, penicillins)
In late pregnancy, renal blood flow may decrease when the woman assumes a supine position, secondary to the increased size and weight of the uterus	Decreased renal blood flow may result in delayed excretion and prolonged effects of renally excreted drugs
Increased hormones (e.g., estrogen, progesterone) induce drug-metabolizing enzymes in the liver	Increased metabolism and clearance of many drugs

arterial blood pressure carries blood and drugs to the placenta. In the placenta, maternal and fetal blood are separated by a few thin layers of membrane, which drugs can readily cross. Placental transfer begins about the 5th week after conception. After drugs enter the fetal circulation, relatively large amounts are pharmacologically active because the fetus has low levels of serum albumin and thus low levels of drug binding. Most drug molecules are transported to the fetal liver, where they are metabolized. Metabolism occurs slowly because the liver is immature in quantity and quality of drug-metabolizing enzymes. Drugs metabolized by the fetal liver are excreted by fetal kidneys into amniotic fluid. Excretion also is slow and inefficient due to immature development of fetal kidneys. Other drug molecules are transported directly to the heart, which then distributes them to the brain and coronary arteries. Drugs enter the fetal brain easily because the blood–brain barrier is poorly developed. Approximately half of the drug-containing blood is then transported through the umbilical arteries to the placenta, where it reenters the maternal circulation. The mother can metabolize and excrete some drug molecules for the fetus.

Drug Effects on the Fetus

Drug effects are determined mainly by the type and amount of drug, duration of exposure, and level of fetal growth and development during exposure. The fetus is sensitive to drug effects because it is small, has few plasma proteins that can bind drug molecules, and has a weak capacity for metabolizing and excreting drugs. In addition, the fetus is exposed to any drugs circulating in maternal blood. Molecular size, weight, and lipid solubility determine which substances (chemicals, drugs, and antibodies) are readily absorbed into the fetal circulation from the maternal circulation. When drugs are taken on a regular schedule, fetal blood usually contains 50% to 100% of the amount in maternal blood. This means that any drug that stimulates or depresses the central nervous, cardiovascular, respiratory, or other body system in the mother has the potential to stimulate or depress those systems in the fetus. In some cases, fetotoxicity occurs. Drugs that may be **teratogenic** (causing abnormal embryonic or fetal development) are a major concern. Drug-induced teratogenicity is most likely to occur when drugs are taken during the first 3 months of pregnancy—during **organogenesis** (formation of embryonic organs during the first 3 to 8 weeks after conception) (Fig. 6.1). Malformations that occur during the preembryonic period (first and second week of pregnancy postconception) rarely result in a viable fetus (fetal stage starts after completion of week 8 of embryonic life). During the embryonic and fetal stages, teratogenic insult and timing result in the targeting of specific organ growth during organogenesis and subsequent maturation and refinement of an organ's physiologic purpose.

For drugs taken during the second and third trimesters, adverse effects are usually manifested in the neonate (birth to 1 month) or infant (1 month to 1 year) as growth retardation, respiratory problems, infection, or bleeding. It should be emphasized, however, that drugs taken at any time during pregnancy can affect the baby's brain because brain development continues throughout pregnancy and after birth. The U.S. Food and Drug Administration (FDA) requires manufacturers to assign new drugs a pregnancy risk category to indicate

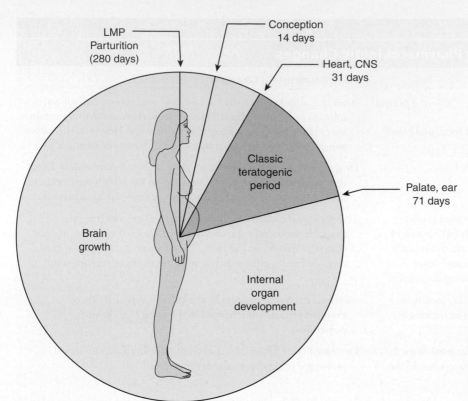

Figure 6.1 The gestational clock showing the classic teratogenic risk assessment. (Adapted from Niebyl, J. (1999). Drugs and related areas in pregnancy. In J. Sciarra (Ed.). *Obstetrics and gynecology*. Philadelphia, PA: Lippincott Williams & Wilkins.)

their potential for causing birth defects (see Chap. 2 for more information). Box 6.1 is a list of teratogenic drugs.

Principles of Drug Therapy in Pregnancy

Before administering a drug to a pregnant woman, it is the responsibility and obligation of all health care providers, including nurses, to conduct a risk–benefit assessment—a comprehensive analytic comparison of the benefits to the mother and the risks to the fetus. Inclusion of family in a decision regarding drug exposure during pregnancy and lactation to obtain informed consent is critical. Ideally, the risk to the fetus should be small compared with the potential maternal benefit. It is necessary to consider the consequences with and without drug therapy. Important factors are gestational age; drug route, dosage, and concentration; and duration of exposure.

BOX 6.1   Selected Teratogenic Drugs

Risk Category D

- Angiotensin-converting enzyme (ACE) inhibitors (e.g., captopril and others) (second and third trimesters)
- Angiotensin II receptor blockers (ARBs; e.g., losartan and others) (second and third trimesters)
- Antibacterials (aminoglycosides, tetracyclines, tigecycline, trimethoprim in third trimester)
- Antiepileptics (carbamazepine, phenytoin, valproic acid)
- Antifungals (voriconazole)
- Antineoplastics (ibritumomab, idarubicin, ifosfamide, imatinib, irinotecan)
- Antithyroid agents (e.g., propylthiouracil)
- Antivirals (efavirenz)
- Benzodiazepine (e.g., alprazolam, diazepam, lorazepam)
- Bisphosphonates (pamidronate, zoledronic acid)
- Mood stabilizer (lithium)

- Nicotine replacement products (oral inhaler, nasal spray, transdermal patch)
- Opioid analgesics (with prolonged use or high doses at term)

Risk Category X

- Anticoagulant (warfarin)
- Antineoplastics (e.g., cyclophosphamide, methotrexate)
- Antirheumatoid arthritis drug (leflunomide)
- Antiviral (ribavirin)
- Benzodiazepine sedative/hypnotics (e.g., flurazepam)
- Female sex hormones (estrogens, progestins, oral contraceptives)
- Male sex hormones (androgens, anabolic steroids)
- Nicotine replacement product, chewing gum
- Retinoids (e.g., acitretin, isotretinoin, and several topical preparations)
- Statin cholesterol-lowering drugs (e.g., atorvastatin, others)

General guidelines for drug therapy in pregnancy include the following:

- Pregnant women should take no drugs, regardless of their pregnancy risk category. It is essential that no drug be used during pregnancy unless it is clearly needed and the potential benefit to the mother outweighs the risk of potential harm to the fetus.
- However, although the teratogenicity of many drugs is unknown, most medications required by pregnant women can be used safely and most children are born healthy.
- When drug therapy is necessary, the choice of drug depends on the stage of pregnancy and available drug information. During the first trimester, for example, an older drug that has not been associated with fetotoxic or teratogenic effects is usually preferred over a newer drug of unknown fetotoxicity or teratogenicity.
- It is important to give any drug used during pregnancy at the lowest effective dose for the shortest possible time.

- Some immunizations are safe in pregnancy, although live-virus vaccines (e.g., measles, mumps, rubella) should be avoided because of possible harmful effects to the fetus. Vaccines against pneumococcal pneumonia, meningococcal meningitis, and hepatitis A can be used if indicated. Influenza vaccine is indicated in all women who are pregnant during influenza season. (However, FluMist, a live virus vaccine given by nasal spray, should *not* be given to pregnant women.) In addition, hepatitis B vaccine (if the mother is high risk and negative for hepatitis B antigen) and toxoids (e.g., diphtheria, tetanus) are considered safe for use. Hyperimmune globulins can be given to pregnant women who are exposed to hepatitis B, tetanus, or varicella (chickenpox).
- It is essential that pregnant women know how these principles affect them. Box 6.2 summarizes patient teaching guidelines regarding the use of drugs during pregnancy (and lactation).

BOX 6.2   Patient Teaching Guidelines: Drug Use During Pregnancy and Lactation

■ Any systemic drug ingested by a pregnant woman reaches the fetus and may interfere with fetal growth and development. For most drugs, safety during pregnancy has not been established, and all drugs are relatively contraindicated. Therefore, any drug use must be cautious and minimal to avoid potential harm to the fetus.

■ Avoid drugs when possible and use them very cautiously when necessary. If women who are sexually active and not using effective contraception take any drugs, there is a high risk that potentially harmful agents may be ingested before pregnancy is suspected or confirmed. It is estimated that 50% or more of pregnancies are unplanned.

■ Lifestyle or nontherapeutic drugs associated with problems during pregnancy include alcohol, caffeine, and cigarette smoking. Women should completely avoid alcohol when trying to conceive and throughout pregnancy; no amount is considered safe. Caffeine intake should be limited to about three caffeinated beverages per day; excessive intake should be avoided. Women who smoke should quit if possible during pregnancy to avoid the effects of nicotine, carbon monoxide, and other chemicals on the fetus. However, the use of nicotine replacement products during pregnancy/lactation is recommended with behavioral interventions.

■ Herbal supplements are not recommended; their effects during pregnancy are unknown.

■ Measures to prevent the need for drug therapy include a healthful lifestyle (adequate nutrition, exercise, rest, and sleep; avoiding alcohol and cigarette smoking) and avoiding infection (personal hygiene, avoiding contact with people known to have infections, maintaining indicated immunizations).

■ Inform any health care provider from whom treatment is sought if there is a possibility of pregnancy.

■ Many drugs are excreted in breast milk to some extent and reach the nursing infant. The infant's health care provider should be informed about medications taken by the nursing mother and consulted

about potential drug effects on the infant. Before taking over-the-counter medications, consult a health care provider. In regard to nontherapeutic drugs, recommendations include the following:

■ Alcohol should be used in moderation and nursing should be withheld temporarily after alcohol consumption (1 to 2 hours per drink). Alcohol reaches the baby through breast milk, with the highest concentration about 30 to 60 minutes after drinking (60 to 90 minutes if taken with food). The effects of alcohol on the baby are directly related to the amount of alcohol the mother consumes. Moderate-to-heavy drinking (two or more drinks per day) can interfere with the ability to breast-feed, harm the baby's motor development, and slow the baby's weight gain. If you plan to drink (e.g., wine with dinner), you can avoid breast-feeding for a few hours (until the alcohol has time to leave your system) or you can pump your milk before drinking alcohol and give it to the baby after you have had the alcohol. You can also pump and discard the milk that is most affected by the ingested alcohol.

■ Caffeine is considered compatible with breast-feeding. However, large amounts should be avoided because infants may be jittery and have difficulty sleeping.

■ Cigarette smoking is contraindicated. Nicotine and an active metabolite are concentrated in milk, and the amounts reaching the infant are proportional to the number of cigarettes smoked by the mother. Ideally, the mother who smokes would stop. If unable or unwilling to stop, she should decrease the number of cigarettes as much as possible, avoid smoking before nursing, and avoid smoking (or allowing other people to smoke) in the same room with the infant. The risk of sudden infant death syndrome (SIDS) is greater when a mother smokes or when the baby is around secondhand (passive) smoke. Maternal smoking and passive smoke may also increase respiratory and ear infections in infants.

■ All drugs of abuse (e.g., cocaine, heroin, marijuana, methamphetamine, and phencyclidine) are contraindicated.

Fetal Therapeutics

Although the major concern about drugs ingested during pregnancy is adverse effects on the fetus, a few drugs are given to the mother for therapeutic effects on the fetus. These include digoxin for fetal tachycardia or heart failure, levothyroxine for hypothyroidism, penicillin for exposure to maternal syphilis and GBS, and prenatal betamethasone to promote surfactant production, thus improving to improve fetal lung function and decreasing respiratory distress syndrome in preterm infants. Also, pregnant women who are rhesus factor (Rh)–negative receive Rh immune globulin (RhoGAM) for antenatal and postpartal prevention of sensitization to the Rh factor and hemolytic disease of the newborn.

Maternal Therapeutics

Thus far, the main emphasis on drug use during pregnancy has related to actual or potential adverse effects on the fetus. Despite the general principle that drug use should be avoided whenever possible, pregnant women may require drug therapy for immunizations, various illnesses, increased nutritional needs, pregnancy-associated problems, chronic disease processes, treatment of preterm labor, induction of labor, pain management during labor, and prevention of postpartum hemorrhage.

To meet the increased nutritional needs of pregnancy, health care providers order prenatal vitamins and mineral supplements for pregnant women. Folic acid supplementation is especially important to prevent neural tube birth defects, primarily spina bifida. Such abnormalities occur early in pregnancy, often before a woman realizes she is pregnant. For this reason, it is recommended that all women of childbearing potential ingest 400 or 600 mcg, of folic acid daily, either from food and/or a supplement. (A supplement is usually necessary to ensure adequate

amounts.) Also, recent research has shown that prenatal vitamins taken during the first 3 months prior to conception and the first month after conception may decrease the risk of autism.

The use of natural herbs as a supplement and as treatment for common ailments has greatly increased in popularity. Although herbs are natural, some may be poisonous. Not all herbs are safe for consumption during pregnancy and lactation. Box 6.3 summarizes information on the use of herbs in pregnancy.

Clinical Application 6-1

- What issues relating to teratogenic substances are of concern in Ms. Ross' pregnancy?

Management of Pregnancy-Associated Symptoms

Anemias

Three types of anemia are common during pregnancy. One is physiologic anemia (often defined as a hemoglobin below 10 g/dL or hematocrit below 30%), which results from expanded blood volume. A second is iron-deficiency anemia, which is often related to long-term nutritional deficiencies. A third type is folic acid–deficiency anemia. The recommended daily intake of folic acid doubles during pregnancy, from 400 to 800 mcg, and a folic acid supplement is often necessary.

For many years, it was considered "best practice" to routinely prescribe daily iron supplements for pregnant women to prevent or treat iron-deficiency anemia. More recently, studies indicate that use of the supplements in women who are not anemic may lead to excessive levels of hemoglobin, iron overload, and hypertension in the mother and premature birth or low birth weight in the infant.

Constipation

Constipation often occurs during pregnancy, probably from decreased peristalsis. Preferred treatment is to increase exercise and intake of fluids and high-fiber foods. If a laxative is required, the bulk-producing agent psyllium (Metamucil) is the most physiologic for the mother and safest for the fetus because it is not absorbed systemically. A stool softener such as docusate (Colace) or an occasional saline laxative (milk of magnesia) may also be used. Mineral oil should be avoided because it interferes with absorption of fat-soluble vitamins. Reduced absorption of vitamin K can lead to bleeding in newborns. Castor oil, all strong laxatives, and excessive amounts of any laxative should be avoided because they can cause uterine contractions and initiate labor.

Gastroesophageal Reflux Disease

Gastroesophageal reflux disease (GERD), of which heartburn (pyrosis) is the main symptom, occurs in one third or more of pregnant women. Hormonal changes relax the lower esophageal sphincter, and the growing fetus increases abdominal pressure. These developments allow gastric acid to splash into the esophagus and cause discomfort and esophagitis. In addition, GERD may trigger asthma attacks in pregnant women with asthma.

BOX 6.3	Use of Herbs During Pregnancy

■ Some herbs may contain ingredients that are contra-indicated in pregnancy and lactation. Many herbs can interfere with blood clotting, glucose metabolism, have a diuretic effect on the body, or induce labor.

■ As remedies, herbs are not subjected to rigorous testing and evaluation because they are not prescription drugs. Consequently, the quality and strength of such supplements may vary significantly, reducing safety for use during pregnancy and lactation.

■ However, some experts recommend raspberry leaf tea to combat morning sickness, help prevent miscarriage, and as a uterine tonic to prevent contractions. They use ginger and peppermint to relieve nausea and vomiting during pregnancy.

■ The U.S. Food and Drug Administration (FDA) urges pregnant and lactating women to discuss the use of herbs or essential oils with their health care provider. Many women may take herbal supplements without informing their obstetrician or nurse midwife, thus complicating and increasing the likelihood of drug interactions with herbal supplements.

■ In an effort to make herbal supplements safe, some organizations specializing in herbal remedies have performed extensive testing and evaluations on herbs to devise a safety rating scale for the general population as well as pregnant and breast-feeding women. However, the safety ratings can often be controversial and vague. For instance, some herbs may be safe when used orally in amounts found in food but considered unsafe or contraindicated when used in medicinal or concentrated amounts, especially in pregnancy.

■ The following herbal supplements are to be avoided during pregnancy:

Black cohosh

Blue cohosh

Cascara sagrada

Dong quai

Ephedra

Fenugreek

Ginseng

Goldenseal

Lovage

Passion flower

Pau d'arco

Pennyroyal

Roman chamomile

Senna leaf

Yohimbe

Nonpharmacologic interventions include eating small meals; not eating for 2 to 3 hours before bedtime; avoiding caffeine, gas-producing foods, and constipation; and sitting in an upright position. For patients who do not obtain adequate relief with these measures, drug therapy may be needed. Antacids may be used if necessary. Because little systemic absorption occurs, the drugs are unlikely to harm the fetus if used in recommended doses. A histamine$_2$ (H$_2$) receptor antagonist such as ranitidine (Zantac) may also be effective. Proton pump inhibitors such as esomeprazole (Nexium) are thought to be safe, but some clinicians reserve them for patients for whom H$_2$ blockers are ineffective.

Gestational Diabetes Mellitus

Gestational diabetes mellitus (GDM) is glucose intolerance that first occurs during pregnancy. Women with risk factors (obesity, age older than 35 years, family history of diabetes, being Hispanic, Native American, Asian, or African American, previous pregnancy with stillbirth, spontaneous abortion, fetal anomalies, or large baby) should be screened at the first prenatal visit. Most women without risk factors, or with a normal initial test, should have a glucose tolerance test between 24 and 28 weeks of gestation because of the maternal peripheral resistance of insulin due to hormones after the 24th week. The criterion for a diagnosis of GDM, based on the results of a 100-g oral glucose tolerance test, is a fasting plasma glucose level of more than 95 mg/dL or a 2-hour glucose level of more than 155 mg/dL (Mattson & Smith, 2011).

Women with GDM are at higher risk for complications of pregnancy and possible fetal harm. Poor glycemic control, primarily hyperglycemia in early gestation resulting in fetal hyperinsulinemia, increases the likelihood of structural defects in the fetus, particularly during organogenesis. Congenital deformities in the fetus often involve the heart and the central nervous system (CNS), leading to multiorgan malformations. Hyperinsulinemia increases the amount of growth factor causing macrosomia. Additionally, hyperinsulinemia interferes with the production of surfactant, which contributes to fetal lung maturity. Lack of surfactant results in respiratory distress syndrome in the neonate. Infants of mothers with GDM who had been under close diabetic monitoring during pregnancy have complications of hypoglycemia, hyperbilirubinemia, hypocalcemia, and polycythemia.

The goal of treatment during pregnancy is to keep blood glucose levels as nearly normal as possible because even mild hyperglycemia is detrimental to the fetus; it stimulates the fetal pancreas to secrete high levels of insulin. Insulin (see Chap. 39) does not cross the placenta and has a long history of safe usage. Thus, it is the drug of choice for treatment of diabetes during pregnancy. Oral antidiabetics have generally been contraindicated. However, several studies indicate that glyburide is acceptable to use when insulin therapy is not feasible (needle phobia or other instances where insulin injection is problematic). It is important to consider the question of maternal adherence regarding subcutaneous insulin or oral hypoglycemic therapy when making a decision regarding maternal and fetal well-being.

When the pregnancy ends, blood glucose levels usually return to a normal range within a few weeks. Women may breast-feed, and hypoglycemics are safe during lactation. Nearly 70% of GDM mothers will have gestational diabetes in subsequent pregnancies, and as many as 50% will develop overt diabetes within 15 years.

NCLEX Success

5. What is the rationale for administering folic acid supplements?

    A. prevent hydrocele
    B. increase absorption
    C. prevent neural tube deformity
    D. decrease blood glucose

6. A nurse is providing prenatal teaching in the obstetric clinic. Which of the following herbal supplements helps in the prevention of nausea and vomiting?

    A. St. John's wort
    B. ginger
    C. black cohosh
    D. garlic

Nausea and Vomiting

Nausea and vomiting often occur during early pregnancy due to high levels of hCG and estrogen. Low blood sugar, as well as magnesium deficiency, can exacerbate nausea and vomiting. Intractable vomiting with subsequent weight loss and its effect on fetal growth and development must be assessed when considering antiemetic drug therapy.

Pregnant women should take antiemetic drugs only if nausea and vomiting are severe enough to threaten maternal and fetal nutritional or metabolic status (hyperemesis gravidarum). Ondansetron (Zofran) (see Chap. 36) is the drug of choice. In severe cases, in which oral medication is not tolerated, metoclopramide (Reglan) can be administered via subcutaneous infusion pump to provide continuous therapy. If drug therapy is unsuccessful in controlling nausea and vomiting, or weight loss and electrolyte imbalance persists, total parenteral nutrition may be necessary until oral fluids are tolerated.

Pregnancy-Induced Hypertension

Pregnancy-induced hypertension (PIH) includes preeclampsia and eclampsia, conditions that endanger the lives of mother and fetus. **Preeclampsia** is manifested by hypertension and proteinuria—a diastolic blood pressure above 90 mm Hg and proteinuria greater than 300 mg in 24 hours or urine dipstick of 2+. It occurs after 20 weeks of gestation and may continue for up to 6 weeks postpartum. Preeclampsia most often occurs during a first pregnancy, but it may affect women with chronic hypertension, diabetes mellitus, or multiple fetuses.

Management of PIH varies. Outpatient observation, with frequent monitoring of mother and fetus, may be sufficient. Women with mild to moderate PIH may take nifedipine (Procardia) (see Chap. 26) orally. Women who are nonresponsive to oral antihypertensives or who have severe preeclampsia require hospitalization. Drug therapy for severe preeclampsia includes intravenous hydralazine (Apresoline) (see Chap. 28) or labetalol (Normodyne) for blood pressure control as well as magnesium sulfate (see Chap. 52) for treatment of severe hypertension and the prevention of seizures.

TABLE 6.3

Magnesium Levels with Associated Signs and Symptoms in Pregnancy*

Magnesium Value (mg/dL)	Signs and Symptoms
8–12	Loss of patellar reflexes
9–12	Sensation of warmth, flushing
10–12	Lethargy
12–16	Respiratory difficulty
14–17	Muscular paralysis
>18	Cardiac dysrhythmia
30–35	Cardiac arrest

*Normal adult values for magnesium: 1.7–2.4 mg/dL; therapeutic serum magnesium level: 4.8–9.6 mg/dL.

QSEN Safety Alert

Magnesium sulfate requires special precautions for administration and monitoring because of potentially severe adverse effects.

Safety measures include a unit protocol that standardizes drug concentration, flow rate, type of infusion pump, and frequency and type of maternal–fetal assessment data to be documented (serum magnesium levels, respiratory status, reflexes, uterine activity, urine output, and fetal heart rate). This therapy reduces perinatal deaths and severe maternal hypertension.

If not effectively treated, preeclampsia may progress to **eclampsia**, which is characterized by potentially fatal seizures. Women who suffer from eclampsia have a 30% chance of maternal mortality due to cerebral hemorrhage, renal failure, or circulatory collapse.

Overdoses of magnesium sulfate may lead to hypotension, muscle paralysis, respiratory depression, and cardiac arrest. Close monitoring of serum levels and signs of hypermagnesemia is necessary (Table 6.3). Calcium gluconate, the antidote for magnesium sulfate, should be readily available for use if hypermagnesemia occurs. Administration is slow IV push over 3 minutes. It is important to observe for signs of pulmonary edema, especially if it is used in combination with tocolytic therapy and/or antenatal steroids. Neonates born to mothers who received magnesium sulfate require assessment for hypermagnesemia and respiratory depression at birth.

Clinical Application 6-2

- What assessments reveal that Ms. Ross is at risk for preeclampsia?

- Why would administration of antiepileptic drugs not be appropriate for Ms. Ross because she is at risk for seizures related to the diagnosis of preeclampsia?

• The protein in Lauren's 24-hour urine collection is 500 mg. Her blood pressure continues to be high, with evidence of hyperreflexia (3+ reflexes). A magnesium sulfate drip is initiated with a loading dose of 4 g over 20 minutes per infusion pump. Oxytocin (Pitocin) infusion is started to induce labor. What are critical nursing assessments in this situation?

Management of Selected Infections in Pregnancy

Group B Streptococcus

An estimated 30% to 50% of pregnant women are infected with GBS. Without intrapartum antibiotic prophylaxis, rates of transmission to the neonate during delivery range from 50% to 75%, resulting in neonatal GBS (sepsis, meningitis, and pneumonia). Maternal outcomes include urinary tract infection (UTI), chorioamnionitis, postcesarean wound infection, and postpartum endometritis.

Because of the potentially serious consequences of infection with GBS, pregnant women should have a rectovaginal culture at 35 to 37 weeks of gestation. A positive culture indicates infection that should be treated with an intravenous antibiotic that is effective against GBS. Penicillin (see Chap. 16) is the drug of choice, with ampicillin as an alternate.

Clinical Application 6-3

• Explain the risk associated with perinatal GBS.

Human Immunodeficiency Virus

Human immunodeficiency virus (HIV) infection in pregnant women requires antiretroviral drug therapy for the mother. This helps prevent transmission to the infant. Almost all HIV infections are transmitted perinatally, either in utero, during labor and delivery, or in breast milk. The goal of treatment is to achieve an HIV plasma RNA load of less than 400 copies per mL. Antiretroviral drug therapy for the pregnant woman reduces perinatal transmission by about two thirds. In general, highly active antiretroviral therapy, or HAART, is safe, with recommended dosage the same as for nonpregnant women (see Chap. 21).

When labor starts, the HIV-positive pregnant woman should receive zidovudine IV. The dosage is 2 mg/kg infused over 1 hour, then 1 mg/kg/h, until the umbilical cord is clamped.

Urinary Tract Infections

UTIs commonly occur during pregnancy and may include asymptomatic bacteriuria, cystitis, and pyelonephritis. Asymptomatic bacteriuria should be treated in pregnant women because of its association with cystitis and pyelonephritis. If untreated, symptomatic cystitis occurs in approximately 30% of pregnant women. Asymptomatic bacteriuria and UTIs are also associated with increased preterm births and infants with low birth weights. Hospitalization and intravenous antibiotics may be needed for management of pyelonephritis.

Influenza

Influenza poses a substantial risk for pregnant women and their fetuses. Serious complications include bacterial pneumonia and dehydration, which can be fatal. Pregnant women are more likely to be hospitalized with influenza-related complications than nonpregnant women. Flu vaccine provides immunity to the fetus because the vaccine crosses the placenta. The immunity protects infants until they are old enough to be vaccinated.

Tetanus, Diphtheria, and Pertussis

The tetanus-diphtheria-pertussis (Tdap) vaccine, licensed in 2005, is the first vaccine for adolescents and adults that protects against all three diseases—tetanus, diphtheria, and pertussis. Experts recommend it for women who may become pregnant. New mothers who have never received Tdap should receive a dose as soon as possible after delivery. If the tetanus vaccination is needed during pregnancy, authorities prefer tetanus-diphtheria (Td) over Tdap. It is important not to administer Tdap after recent blood transfusion or RhoGAM (Karch, 2011).

NCLEX Success

7. A woman has been diagnosed with gestational diabetes. What effect does hyperglycemia have on the fetus?
   A. It results in fetal hyperinsulinemia.
   B. It produces seizures in the newborn.
   C. It increases the mother's risk of preterm labor.
   D. It decreases the birth weight.

8. A woman is receiving intravenous (IV) magnesium sulfate IV to control symptoms of preeclampsia. Which of the following signs or symptoms indicates a need for the administration of IV calcium gluconate?
   A. urine ketosis
   B. respiratory rate of 36 breaths/min
   C. anuria
   D. diminished deep tendon reflexes

9. A pregnant woman is walking through the woods and steps on a rusty nail. She goes to the emergency department. She should receive which of the following vaccines?
   A. tetanus-diphtheria
   B. tetanus-diphtheria-pertussis
   C. influenza A
   D. measles, mumps, and rubella

Drugs that Alter Uterine Motility: Tocolytics

Drugs given to inhibit labor and maintain the pregnancy are called **tocolytics**. Uterine contractions with cervical changes before 37 weeks of gestation are considered **preterm labor**. Preterm labor may occur spontaneously or premature rupture of membranes, infection, preeclampsia, multiple gestation, cigarette smoking, or alcohol may precipitate it. Newborns born after 32 weeks gestation have a high survival rate. Drug therapy is most effective when the

TABLE 6.4

DRUGS AT A GLANCE: Tocolytics

Drug	Pregnancy Category	Route and Dosage
(P) **Magnesium sulfate**	A	IV infusion, loading dose 4–6 g mixed in 5% dextrose in water solution and administered over 20–30 min; maintenance dose 1–2 g/h, according to serum magnesium levels and deep tendon reflexes, respiratory rate, blood pressure, and urinary output
(P) **Nifedipine** (Procardia)	C	10 mg PO every 20 min for 3 or 4 doses; maximum dose 40 mg in 1 h; then 10–20 mg every 4–6 h
(P) **Terbutaline sulfate** (Brethine)	B	IV push 0.25 mg (rapid onset) Sub-Q 0.25 mg PO 2.5 mg every 4–6 h (as maintenance therapy)
(P) **Indomethacin** (Aleve)	B (D third trimester)	50–100 mg rectally, then 25–50 mg PO every 4–8 h for 2–3 d

cervix is minimally dilated and amniotic membranes are intact. Tocolytics do not reduce the number of preterm births, but they may prolong pregnancy from 2 to 7 days. The goal of treatment is to postpone birth long enough to reduce problems associated with prematurity (e.g., respiratory distress, bleeding in the brain, infant death). For example, the delay may allow antenatal administration of a corticosteroid such as betamethasone (Celestone) to the mother to improve pulmonary maturity and function in fetal lungs by the increased production of surfactant, as well as diminish intraventricular hemorrhage in preterm infants. Magnesium sulfate, nifedipine, some nonsteroidal anti-inflammatory drugs (NSAIDs), and terbutaline are used as tocolytics. Table 6.4 presents route and dosage information for the tocolytics.

Magnesium Sulfate

(P) **Magnesium sulfate**, which has neuromuscular blocking activity, has long been given intravenously as a first-line drug to prevent preterm birth. Adjuvant use includes treatment for preeclampsia and eclampsia. Unlike some anticonvulsants, it is safe in pregnancy and lactation. Guidelines for administration of the drug are the same in tocolysis as in PIH. In women with renal insufficiency, it is necessary to decrease the dosage or use an alternative treatment. Contraindications include myasthenia gravis.

Nifedipine

(P) **Nifedipine** (Procardia) is a calcium channel–blocking drug that decreases uterine contractions and lowers blood pressure. Use of nifedipine during pregnancy is controversial. A common adverse effect is maternal hypotension, which may reduce blood flow between the placenta and the uterus and thus compromise the fetus. Prolonged events of this nature can lead to adverse fetal outcomes, and severe adverse reactions have occurred when nifedipine is used in conjunction with IV magnesium sulfate. Women with heart failure or dysfunction of the left ventricle should not receive nifedipine.

EVIDENCE-BASED PRACTICE

Smoking in Pregnancy and Lactation: a Review of Risks and Cessation Strategies

by ADRIENNE EINARSON, SARA RIORDAN

European Journal of Clinical Pharmacology 2009, 65, 325.

The prevalence of smoking by women increased significantly in the 1960s and 1970s. In recent years, smoking prevalence has declined in relation to advertising campaigns informing women of the dangers of smoking. However, 12% to 15% of young women continue to smoke during pregnancy. Nicotine crosses readily through the placenta to the fetus, and as a result fetal growth restriction, preterm delivery, oral–facial cleft, and sudden infant death syndrome are the major results. This study has determined that a combination of behavioral interventions such as biofeedback, telephone quit lines, financial incentives, and the use of nicotine replacement increases a woman's success for the cessation of smoking. The most effective therapy documented is bromocriptine. In a study of 2437 women treated with bromocriptine during pregnancy and subsequent follow-up of 988 infants, there were no recorded birth defects. Thus, the administration of bromocriptine appears safe and useful for the promotion of smoking cessation.

IMPLICATIONS FOR NURSING PRACTICE: It is important that public health nurses, advanced practice nurses, and obstetric nurses encourage the use of bromocriptine along with behavioral interventions to decrease smoking in women of childbearing age.

Terbutaline Sulfate

 Terbutaline sulfate (Brethine) is a beta-adrenergic agent that inhibits uterine contractions by reducing intracellular calcium levels. Adverse effects may include hyperkalemia, hyperglycemia, cardiac dysrhythmias, hypotension, and pulmonary edema. Women commonly experience hand tremors, palpitations, and shortness of breath with chest tightness. Terbutaline crosses the placenta, producing fetal tachycardia and neonatal hypoglycemia. Contraindications include hyperthyroidism and diabetes as well as placenta previa or placental abruption.

Nonsteroidal Anti-Inflammatory Drugs

The NSAID 🅟 **indomethacin** (Aleve) acts as a tocolytic by inhibiting uterine prostaglandins that initiate the uterine contractions of normal labor. Maternal adverse effects include nausea, heartburn, dizziness, and gastrointestinal (GI) bleeding.

NCLEX Success

10. **A woman experiencing preterm labor receives terbutaline tartrate (Brethine). Which of the following adverse effects should the nurse tell her to expect?**

    A. headache
    B. edema
    C. hand tremors
    D. shortness of breath

11. **A woman is admitted to the labor and delivery unit in preterm labor. The woman was diagnosed with hyperthyroidism 3 years ago. Which tocolytic is contraindicated?**

    A. magnesium sulfate
    B. terbutaline tartrate (Brethine)
    C. nifedipine (Procardia)
    D. indomethacin (Aleve)

Drugs Used During Labor and Delivery at Term

Labor usually begins spontaneously and proceeds through delivery of the newborn and placenta. If labor does not occur spontaneously, it may be induced using an oxytocic, a drug that stimulates uterine contractions. Drugs often used during labor, delivery, and the immediate postpartum period include prostaglandins as well.

Labor Induction

Most common reasons for induction include gestation longer than 40 weeks, intrauterine growth restriction, maternal hypertension, and premature rupture of membranes. Labor can also be initiated for the termination of a pregnancy. An **abortifacient** is used to terminate pregnancy up to 20 weeks after the last menstrual period.

Prostaglandins

Prostaglandins have three significant uses in pregnancy: to promote cervical ripening so the cervix becomes thinner, which facilitates labor and induces delivery of the full-term infant; to promote uterine contractility for the expulsion of the fetus and placenta in an abortion; and to increase uterine contractility and decrease uterine bleeding in the postpartum period. The prostaglandin used for the third use is carboprost tromethamine and will be discussed as the prototype for the uterotonic medications later in the chapter. Table 6.5 summarizes the routes of administration and dosage information for prostaglandin medications.

🅟 **Dinoprostone** (Cervidil, Prepidil, Prostin E2) is a synthetic prostaglandin E_2 that stimulates uterine contractions, like the ones in labor. The drug is available as an endocervical gel, a vaginal insert, and a vaginal suppository. The first two forms enhance cervical ripening so the fetus can pass easily through the birth canal. The vaginal suppository is an abortifacient.

TABLE 6.5

DRUGS AT A GLANCE: Prostaglandins

Drug	Pregnancy Category	Routes and Dosages
🅟 **Dinoprostone** (Prostin E₂ Gel, Prepidil, Cervidil)	C	Intravaginally, repeated every 6 h; maximum dose 3 applications in 24 h; not for VBAC
Misoprostol (Cytotec)	X	Intravaginally 25 mcg (1/4 of a 100-mcg tablet) every 3–6 h; maximum dose is 4 doses at 3- to 6-h intervals within 24 h; not for VBAC
🅟 **Carboprost tromethamine** (Hemabate)	C	IM 0.25 mg every 15–90 min, depending on uterine response; maximum 8 doses in 24 h

VBAC, vaginal birth after cesarean.

Adverse effects of dinoprostone include back pain, abnormal uterine contractions, GI upset, diarrhea, and fever. Contraindications are use of other prostaglandins, as well as previous cesarean section, uterine surgery, cephalopelvic disproportion, fetal distress, and vaginal bleeding. Administration to patients with asthma, glaucoma, or ruptured membranes warrants caution. There is a **BLACK BOX WARNING** ◆ stating that women older than 30 years of age have an increased risk of disseminated intravascular coagulation with dinoprostone.

Misoprostol (Cytotec), a synthetic prostaglandin E$_1$, inhibits gastric acid secretion and increases bicarbonate to protect the lining of the stomach. An unlabeled use of the drug is to increase cervical ripening and induce labor. If the course of treatment changes and oxytocin is to be given, it is essential to wait 4 hours from the last administration of misoprostol before starting oxytocin. The nurse assesses for hyperstimulation of the uterus and monitors for a nonreassuring fetal heart rate. Contraindications include prior cesarean section or uterine surgery.

Oxytocics

Ⓟ **Oxytocin** (Pitocin), a synthetic form of oxytocin, is the most commonly used **oxytocic** drug. Use of this manufactured hormone induces labor or augments weak, irregular uterine contractions during labor. Physiologic doses produce a rhythmic uterine contraction–relaxation pattern that approximates the normal labor process. It cannot be combined with fibrinolysin or heparin. It also activates oxytocin and is contraindicated in the presence of fetal distress, preterm labor, previous uterine surgery, and severe preeclampsia. Table 6.6 summarizes the dosage and route of administration for oxytocin.

Maternal adverse effects include cardiac dysrhythmias, hypertension, nausea, vomiting, excessive uterine stimulation, and uterine rupture. If hypertension develops, it is necessary to notify the primary care provider and discontinue the drug. Close monitoring of uterine activity and fetal response every 15 minutes is essential. Fetal adverse effects include fetal bradycardia, neonatal jaundice, and low Apgar scores. If a labor and delivery nurse is not available to monitor the fetal–maternal effects of oxytocin, it is necessary to suspend the infusion.

NCLEX Success

12. A woman is admitted to labor and delivery following the spontaneous rupture of membranes. Labor has lasted for 5 hours without significant ripening of the cervix. Which of the following medications promotes cervical ripening?

    A. dinoprostone (Cervidil, Prepidil, Prostin E2)
    B. nifedipine (Procardia)
    C. naproxen sodium (Naprosyn)
    D. oxytocin (Pitocin)

13. The certified nurse midwife administers misoprostol (Cytotec) in the posterior fornix of a woman's vagina to increase cervical ripening. The cervix ripens, but the contractions are not significant for the fetus to pass through the birth canal. Oxytocin (Pitocin) is ordered. Which of the following is most important with regard to the administration of oxytocin?

    A. Begin the oxytocin immediately.
    B. Begin the oxytocin in 2 hours.
    C. Begin the oxytocin in 4 hours.
    D. Begin the oxytocin in 8 hours.

Pain Management

During early labor, pain occurs with uterine contractions. During later stages of labor, pain occurs with perineal stretching.

Analgesics

Intravenous opioid analgesics nalbuphine (Nubain) and meperidine (Demerol) (see Chap. 48) are commonly used to control pain during labor and delivery. They may prolong labor and cause sedation and respiratory depression in the mother and neonate. Meperidine may cause less neonatal depression than other opioid analgesics. Butorphanol tartrate (Stadol) is an opioid agonist–antagonist analgesic. It is also widely used to relieve severe pain by acting as an opioid agonist in the CNS to produce analgesia, sedation, and induce hallucinations. If neonatal respiratory depression occurs, naloxone (Narcan) can be given.

Regional analgesia may be more effective than IV analgesics. Epidural analgesia involves administration of the opioid

TABLE 6.6		
DRUGS AT A GLANCE: Oxytocics		
Drug	**Pregnancy Category**	**Routes and Dosage**
Ⓟ **Oxytocin** (Pitocin)	X	Induction/augmentation: IV by infusion pump, 0.5–1 milliunits/min, in 30–60 min intervals gradually increased by 1–2 milliunits/min until desired contractions Postpartum hemorrhage: IV 10–40 units added to 1000 mL of IV fluids infused at a bolus rate
Methylergonovine maleate (Methergine)	C	0.2 mg IM after delivery of the placenta or neonate's anterior shoulder, or during puerperium; may be repeated every 2–4 h 0.2 mg IV; infuse slowly over at least 60 s

fentanyl through a catheter placed in the epidural space for that purpose. With regional anesthesia, the mother is alert and comfortable. The neonate is rarely depressed. Fentanyl may be combined with a small amount of a local anesthetic for both analgesia and anesthesia. Following a cesarean section, a long-acting form of morphine, Duramorph, or fentanyl can be injected into the epidural catheter to provide analgesia up to 24 hours. Possible adverse effects include maternal hypotension and urinary retention (bladder distention). No significant effects on the fetus or neonate have been reported.

Anesthetics

Local anesthetics are less commonly used to control discomfort and pain due to their short duration. They are injected by physicians for regional anesthesia in the pelvic area. Bupivacaine (see Chap. 49) is commonly used. Fetal bradycardia may briefly occur after administration but is usually not significant.

Clinical Application 6-4

- An oxytocin (Pitocin) infusion begins to induce Ms. Ross's labor after her fetus is treated with betamethasone (Celestone) to promote lung maturity. What effect might magnesium sulfate have on her labor progress?

Uterotonics for Postpartum Hemorrhage

Uterotonics are drugs used to stop postpartum hemorrhage. After delivery of the placenta, oxytocin is the drug of choice for prevention or control of postpartum uterine bleeding. It is delivered IV through a bolus rate using an infusion pump. The drug reduces uterine bleeding by contracting the uterine muscle. It also plays a role in the letdown of breast milk to the nipples during lactation.

In the event of postpartum hemorrhage, other drugs (uterotonics) may be indicated for immediate use, such as Ⓟ **carboprost tromethamine** (Hemabate). This drug stimulates the uterus to contract. Contraindications include known allergy to prostaglandins, acute pelvic inflammatory disease, and renal or cardiac insufficiency. Caution is warranted in asthma; hypertension; hypotension; anemia; uterine abnormalities; and diseases of the heart, kidneys, or liver. The use of antiemetic drugs reduces GI upset. To control postpartum bleeding, multiple carboprost injections may be necessary. Adequate hydration during administration and throughout the postpartum phase is necessary. Table 6.5 provides route and dosage information for carboprost.

Methylergonovine (Methergine) is an oxytocic drug that increases the strength, duration, and frequency of the uterine contractions. Indications for use include the treatment of postpartum atony and hemorrhage as well as for uterine stimulation during the second stage of labor. Contraindications include known allergy to methylergonovine. Patients with hypertension and toxemia should not receive the methylergonovine. It is important to monitor patients for hypertension, headache, dizziness, palpitations, and GI upset. Table 6.6 provides route and dosage information for methylergonovine.

Clinical Application 6-5

- Why is Ms. Ross at high risk for postpartum hemorrhage?
- What preventive measure is taken immediately after delivery of the placenta?

Lactation

Lactation Induction

Metoclopramide (Reglan) stimulates hormone prolactin after delivery, thus inducing lactation. Clinicians have found that doses of 30 to 45 mg per day, for no longer than 3 weeks, are effective. Higher doses of the drug in the postpartum period have been associated with depression, and use in women with a history of depression warrants caution.

The herbs fenugreek, anise seed, and fennel seed are **galactagogues**, herbs known to induce lactation or stimulate the production of breast milk in postpartal women.

Drug Use During Lactation

Antidepressants (selective serotonin reuptake inhibitors and serotonin-norepinephrine reuptake inhibitors) disturb the serotonin balance and can impair milk production in the lactating mother. Long-term effects of antidepressants during breast-feeding have not been adequately studied. The recommendation for breast-feeding states that human data are limited, with a risk of potential toxicity for the newborn. The American Academy of Pediatrics (AAP) advises that the risk of antidepressants during breast-feeding is unknown and is of concern.

Box 6.4 presents a list of medications contraindicated during lactation. Box 6.2 summarizes patient teaching guidelines regarding the use of drugs during lactation, as well as pregnancy.

Lactation and Birth Control

Exclusive breast-feeding (no formula supplementation) causes a woman to have an absence of menstrual periods. The potential for ovulation is reduced but does not offer total protection against pregnancy. The use of birth control during lactation is safe for the newborn. The concern is related to the quantity of milk production due to the presence of additional hormones in the maternal system.

Progesterone (progestin)-only birth control pills are the contraceptive of choice because they are unlikely to cause a decrease in milk production. The "mini-pill" is safe during lactation. It is a good choice for exclusively breast-feeding mothers because of the already decreased fertility with continuous lactation. A higher dose of progesterone is obtained with Depo-Provera injection, which offers protection for 3 months. Estrogen-containing contraceptives such as NuvaRing and transdermal patches estradiol (Climara) have been associated with decreasing breast milk production.

BOX 6.4	Selected Drugs That Are Contraindicated or Not Recommended During Lactation

Angiotensin-converting enzyme (ACE) inhibitors (e.g., captopril, others)

Angiotensin receptor blockers (ARBs; e.g., losartan, others)

Antibacterials (aminoglycosides, fluoroquinolones, tetracyclines, sulfamethoxazole/trimethoprim)

Antidepressants (e.g., amitriptyline, bupropion, citalopram, fluoxetine, venlafaxine)

Antidiabetic drugs (oral) (e.g., glimepiride, glipizide, pioglitazone, rosiglitazone)

Antiepileptics (carbamazepine, lamotrigine, levetiracetam, phenytoin, tiagabine, topiramate, zonisamide)

Antifungals (e.g., itraconazole, terbinafine)

Antihistamines (cetirizine, clemastine, desloratadine, diphenhydramine, loratadine)

Antimanic agent (lithium)

Antipsychotics (e.g., clozapine, olanzapine, risperidone, others)

Antirheumatic immunosuppressant drugs (e.g., etanercept, infliximab)

Antivirals (e.g., famciclovir)

Benzodiazepine antianxiety and sedative/hypnotic drugs (e.g., alprazolam, diazepam, triazolam, others)

Beta blockers (e.g., metoprolol, others)

Calcium channel blockers (e.g., amlodipine, diltiazem, others)

Diuretics (e.g., hydrochlorothiazide)

Histamine$_2$ receptor antagonists (e.g., cimetidine, ranitidine)

Nonbenzodiazepine sedative/hypnotics (e.g., ramelteon, zolpidem)

Nonsteroidal anti-inflammatory drugs (e.g., naproxen, tolmetin)

Opioid analgesics (codeine, hydromorphone, methadone)

Proton pump inhibitors (e.g., esomeprazole, omeprazole, others)

Retinoids (e.g., isotretinoin)

Statin cholesterol-lowering drugs (e.g., atorvastatin, simvastatin, others)

The Nursing Process

Assessment

- Assess each female patient of childbearing age for possible pregnancy.
- If the patient is known to be pregnant, assess status in relation to pregnancy:
  - Length of gestation
  - Use of prescription, over-the-counter, herbal, nontherapeutic, and illegal drugs. If used, assess specifically for those drugs known to be fetotoxic or teratogenic.
  - Acute and chronic health problems that may influence pregnancy or require drug therapy.
  - With preterm labor, assess length of gestation, the frequency and quality of uterine contractions, the amount of vaginal bleeding or discharge, and the length of labor. Also determine whether any tissue has been expelled from the vagina. When abortion is inevitable, an oxytocic drug may be given. When stopping labor is possible or desired, a tocolytic drug may be given.
  - When spontaneous labor occurs in normal, full-term pregnancy, assess frequency and quality of uterine contractions, amount of cervical dilatation, fetal heart rate and quality, and maternal blood pressure.
  - Assess antepartum women for intention to breast-feed.

Nursing Diagnoses

- Risk for injury: harm to mother, fetus, or neonate from maternal ingestion of drugs
- Noncompliance related to ingestion of nonessential drugs during pregnancy
- Risk for injury related to possible harm to mother or infant during the birth process
- Deficient knowledge: drug and herbal effects during pregnancy and lactation

Planning/Goals

The patient will

- Avoid unnecessary drug ingestion when pregnant or likely to become pregnant.
- Use nonpharmacologic measures to relieve symptoms associated with pregnancy or other health problems, when possible.
- Obtain optimal care during pregnancy, labor and delivery, and the postpartum period.
- Avoid behaviors that may lead to complications of pregnancy and labor and delivery.
- Breast-feed safely and successfully, if desired

Nursing Interventions

The nurse will

- Use nondrug measures to prevent or minimize the need for drug therapy during pregnancy.
- Promote or provide optimal prenatal care to promote a healthy pregnancy (regular monitoring of blood pressure, weight, blood sugar, urine protein; counseling about nutrition and other healthful activities).
- Assist women with chronic health problems (asthma, diabetes, hypertension) to manage the disorders effectively and decrease risks of harm to themselves and their babies.
- Help patients and families cope with complications of pregnancy and newborn attachment.

Evaluation

- Observe and interview regarding actions taken to promote reproductive and general health.
- Observe and interview regarding compliance with instructions for promoting and maintaining a healthy pregnancy and exclusive breast-feeding.

- Interview regarding ingestion of therapeutic and nontherapeutic drugs during prepregnant, pregnant, and lactating states.
- Observe and interview regarding the health status of the mother and neonate.

Key Concepts

- Regardless of the designated pregnancy risk category or presumed safety, no drug should be used during pregnancy unless it is clearly needed and potential benefit to the mother outweighs the risk of potential harm to the fetus.

- A folic acid supplement is recommended for women who may become pregnant and during pregnancy to prevent neural tube defects, especially if a woman is epileptic.

- Depression immediately postpartum ("baby blues") may occur but should not extend past 21 days after birth. Counseling is recommended, with possible antidepressant therapy.

- The AAP supports breast-feeding as optimal nutrition, and not a lifestyle choice, for infants during the first year of life and does not recommend stopping maternal drug therapy unless necessary.

- Prostaglandins promote cervical ripening to facilitate labor and delivery.

- There is a **BLACK BOX WARNING** ◆ stating that women older than 30 years of age are at risk for disseminated intravascular coagulation with the administration of dinoprostone (Cervidil, Prepidil, Prostin E2).

- Oxytocin induces labor or augments weak, irregular uterine contractions during labor.

- Uterotonic agents prevent or control postpartum hemorrhage.

- Most systemic drugs taken by the mother reach the infant in breast milk. For some, the amount of drug is too small to cause significant effects; for others, effects on the nursing infant are unknown or potentially adverse.

- Most over-the-counter and prescription drugs should be taken only with physician approval during breast-feeding.

- Women with HIV infection should not breast-feed. The virus can be transmitted to the nursing infant.

Critical Thinking Questions

6-1. A 33-year-old woman and her husband have been trying to get pregnant for the past 18 months without success. The certified nurse midwife has ordered clomiphene citrate (Clomid) 50 mg PO once daily for 5 days (for the woman).

- What are the action, adverse effects, and contraindications of clomiphene citrate?

- What patient teaching should the nurse provide regarding medication administration and strategies to enhance fertility?

References and Resources

Briggs, G. R., Freeman, R. K., & Yaffe, S. J. (2011). *Drugs in pregnancy and lactation* (9th ed.). Philadelphia, PA: Wolters Kluwer Health/Lippincott Williams & Wilkins.

Einarson, A., & Riordan, S. (2009). Smoking in pregnancy and lactation: A review of risks and cessation strategies. *European Journal of Clinical Pharmacology, 65,* 325–330.

Guyton, A. C., & Hall, J. E. (2006). *Textbook of medical physiology* (11th ed.). Philadelphia, PA: Elsevier Saunders.

Hale, T. (2011). *Safe Use of Birth Control While Breastfeeding.* Retrieved March 26, 2012, from www.infantrisk.com/content/safe-use-birth-control-while-breastfeeding

Hogge, W., & Prosen, T. (2012). *Principles of teratology.* Up-To-Date, Lexi Comp, Inc.

Hurley, J. B. (1995). *The good herb.* New York, NY: William Morrow.

Karch, A. M. (2011). *Lippincott's nursing drug guide.* Philadelphia, PA: Wolters Kluwer Health/Lippincott Williams & Wilkins.

March of Dimes (2010). *Pregnant women need flu vaccine.* Retrieved February 26, 2012, from http://www.marchofdimes.com/news/sept15_2010.html.

Mattson, S., & Smith, J. E. (2011). *Core curriculum for maternal-newborn nursing* (4th ed.). Missouri: Elsevier Saunders.

Porth, C. M. (2009). *Pathophysiology: Concepts of altered health states* (7th ed.). Philadelphia, PA: Lippincott Williams & Wilkins.

Rodriquez-Thompson, D. (2012). *Smoking and pregnancy.* Up-To-Date. Lexi-Comp Inc.

Simhan, H. N., & Caritis, S. (2012). *Inhibition of acute preterm labor.* Up-To-Date. Lexi Comp, Inc.

Simpson, K. R. (2009). Cervical ripening and induction and augmentation of labor (AWHONN Practice Monograph). Washington, DC: Association of Women's Health Obstetric and Neonatal Nursing.

Up-To-Date. (2012). *Carboprost tromethamine: Drug information.* Lexi Comp Inc.

Up-To-Date. (2012). *Dinoprostone: Drug information.* Lexi Comp Inc.

Up-To-Date. (2012). *Clomiphene: Drug information.* Lexi Comp.

Up-To-Date. (2012). *Follitropin alfa (recombinant human follicle stimulating hormone): Drug information.* Lexi Comp Inc.

Up-To-Date. (2012). *Follitropin beta (recombinant human follicle stimulating hormone): Drug information.* Lexi Comp Inc.

Up-To-Date. (2012). *Human chorionic gonadotropin: Drug information.* Lexi Comp Inc.

Up-To-Date. (2012). *Leuprolide: Drug information.* Lexi Comp.

Up-To-Date. (2012). *Menotropins: Drug information.* Lexi Comp.

U.S. Department of Health and Human Services (2011). *Guidance for industry: Reproductive and Developmental Toxicities-Integrating study results to assess concerns.* Retrieved February 27, 2012, from http://www.fda.gov/durgs/guidance complianceregulatoryinformation/guidelines/default.htm

U.S. Department of Health and Human Services (2007). *Use of codeine products in nursing mothers: FDA alert.* Retrieved February 27, 2012, from http://www.fdagov/ drugs/drugsafety/postmarketdrugsafetyinformationforpatientsandproviders/ucm118108.htm

U.S. Department of Health and Human Services (2009). *Tetanus, diphtheria (Td) or tetanus, diphtheria, pertussis (tdap) vaccine: What you need to know.* Vaccine Information Statement form #2432.

U.S. Department of Health and Human Services (2011). *Pregnancy and lactation labeling.* Retrieved February 27, 2012, from http://www.fda.gov/drugs/developmentapprovalprocess/developmentresources/labeling/ucm093307.htm

Drugs Affecting the Hematopoietic and Immune Systems

CHAPTER OUTLINE

7 Drug Therapy for Coagulation Disorders

LEARNING OBJECTIVES

After studying this chapter, you should be able to:

1. Describe important elements in the physiology of hemostasis and thrombosis.

2. Discuss possible consequences of blood clotting disorders.

3. Compare and contrast heparin and warfarin in terms of indications for use, onset and duration of action, route of administration, blood tests used to monitor effects, and nursing process implications.

4. Discuss antiplatelet agents in terms of indications for use and effects on blood coagulation.

5. Discuss direct thrombin inhibitors in terms of indications and contraindications for use, routes of administration, and major adverse effects.

6. Describe thrombolytic agents in terms of indications and contraindications for use, routes of administration, and major adverse effects.

7. Identify the prototype drug for each drug class.

8. Describe systemic hemostatic agents for treating overdoses of anticoagulant and thrombolytic drugs.

9. Understand how to use the nursing process in the care of patients receiving anticoagulant, antiplatelet, and thrombolytic agents.

Clinical Application Case Study

Andrew Oliver is a 45-year-old man who works as a mental health counselor. He presents to a small community emergency department with an acute anterior ST elevation myocardial infarction. Within 20 minutes of arrival, he receives alteplase by continuous intravenous (IV) infusion over 3 hours. He also simultaneously receives an IV bolus of heparin and is started on a heparin drip. You are the nurse assigned to his care.

KEY TERMS

Anticoagulants: drugs that prevent formation of new clots and extension of clots already present; do not dissolve formed clots

Antiplatelets: drugs that prevent one or more steps in the prothrombotic activity of platelets

Embolus: object that migrates through the circulation until it lodges in a blood vessel, causing occlusion; may be a thrombus, fat, air, amniotic fluid, a bit of tissue, or bacterial debris

Essential thrombocythemia: chronic blood disorder characterized by the overproduction of platelets by megakaryocytes in the absence of another cause

Fibrinolysin: enzyme that breaks down the fibrin meshwork that stabilizes blood clots; also referred to as plasmin

Hemostasis: prevention or stoppage of blood loss from an injured blood vessel and is the process that maintains the integrity of the vascular compartment

Heparin-induced thrombocytopenia (HIT): immune-mediated prothrombotic reaction resulting in a decrease in platelet count associated with heparin administration in patients with detectable HIT antibodies

Plasmin: enzyme that breaks down the fibrin meshwork that stabilizes blood clots; also referred to as fibrinolysin

Plasminogen: inactive protein found in many body tissues and fluids

Prothrombotic reaction: adverse effect that leads to thrombogenesis

Thrombogenesis: formation of a blood clot

Thrombolysis: breakdown or dissolution of blood clots

Thrombolytics: drugs that dissolve blood clots

Thrombosis: formation of a blood clot

Thrombus: blood clot

Introduction

Anticoagulant, antiplatelet, and thrombolytic drugs are used in the prevention and management of thrombotic and thromboembolic disorders. **Thrombogenesis (or thrombosis)**, the formation of blood clots, is a normal body defense mechanism to prevent blood loss. Thus, this process may be lifesaving when it occurs as a response to hemorrhage; however, it may be life-threatening when it occurs at other times, because the **thrombus**, or blood clot, can obstruct a blood vessel and block blood flow to tissues beyond the clot either at the site of clot formation or to another part of the body. To aid understanding of drug therapy for thrombotic disorders, normal hemostasis, endothelial functions in relation to blood clotting, platelet functions, blood coagulation, and characteristics of arterial and venous thrombosis are described.

Overview of Coagulation Disorders

Physiology

Hemostasis

Hemostasis is the process that maintains the integrity of the vascular compartment. It involves activation of several mechanisms, including vasoconstriction, formation of a platelet plug (a cluster of aggregated platelets), sequential activation of clotting factors in the blood (Fig. 7.1), and growth of fibrous tissue (fibrin) into the blood clot to make it more stable and to repair the tear (opening) in the damaged blood vessel. Overall, normal hemostasis is a complex process involving numerous interacting activators and inhibitors, including endothelial factors, platelets, and blood coagulation factors (Box 7.1).

Clot Lysis

When a blood clot is being formed, **plasminogen**, an inactive protein present in many body tissues and fluids, is bound to fibrin and becomes a component of the clot. After the outward blood flow is stopped and the tear in the blood vessel is repaired, plasminogen is activated by plasminogen activator (produced by endothelial cells or the coagulation cascade) to produce plasmin. **Plasmin** (also called **fibrinolysin**) is an enzyme that breaks down the fibrin meshwork that stabilizes the clot; this fibrinolytic or thrombolytic action dissolves the clot.

Etiology

Normally, thrombi are constantly being formed and dissolved, but the blood remains fluid and flow is not significantly obstructed. If the balance between thrombogenesis and **thrombolysis**, dissolution of blood clots, is upset, thrombotic or bleeding disorders ensue. Thrombosis may occur in both arteries and veins. Arterial thrombosis is usually associated with atherosclerotic plaque, hypertension, and turbulent blood flow. These conditions damage arterial endothelium and activate platelets to initiate the coagulation process. Arterial thrombi cause disease by obstructing blood flow. If the obstruction is incomplete or temporary, local tissue ischemia (deficient blood supply) occurs. If the obstruction is complete or prolonged, local tissue death (infarction) occurs.

Venous thrombosis is usually associated with venous stasis. When blood flows slowly, thrombin and other procoagulant substances present in the blood become concentrated in local areas and initiate the clotting process. With a normal rate of blood flow, these substances are rapidly removed from the blood, primarily by Kupffer's cells in the liver. A venous thrombus is less cohesive than an arterial thrombus, and an **embolus** can easily become detached and travel to other parts of the body. This embolus may be a thrombus, fat, air, amniotic fluid, tissue, or bacterial debris.

Venous thrombi cause disease by two mechanisms. First, thrombosis causes local congestion, edema, and perhaps inflammation by impairing normal outflow of venous blood (e.g., thrombophlebitis, deep vein thrombosis [DVT]). Second, embolization obstructs the blood supply when the embolus becomes lodged. The pulmonary arteries are common sites of embolization.

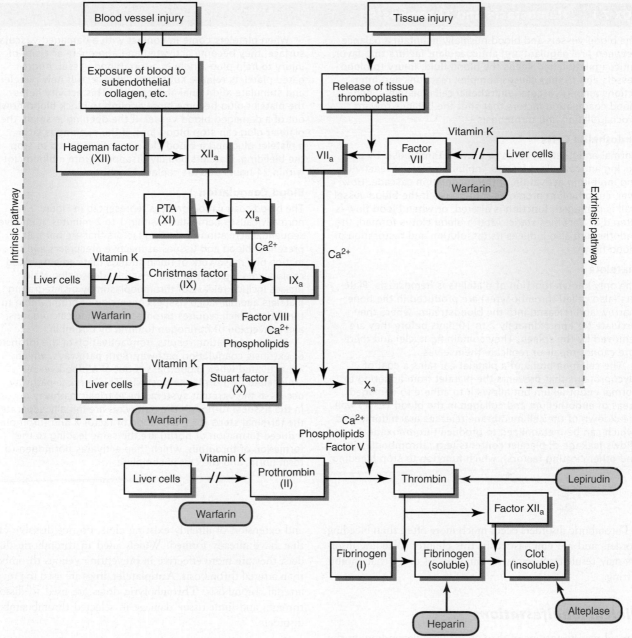

Figure 7.1 Details of the intrinsic and extrinsic clotting pathways. The sites of action of some of the drugs that can influence these processes are shown in *red*.

Pathophysiology

Atherosclerosis is the basic disease process that often leads to pathologic thrombosis. Atherosclerosis begins with accumulation of lipid-filled macrophages (i.e., foam cells) on the inner lining of arteries. Foam cells develop in response to elevated blood lipid levels and eventually become fibrous plaques (i.e., foam cells covered by smooth muscle cells and connective tissue). Advanced atherosclerotic lesions also contain hemorrhages, ulcerations, and scar tissue.

Atherosclerosis can affect any organ or tissue but often involves the arteries supplying the heart, brain, and legs. Over time, plaque lesions become larger and extend farther into

the lumen of the artery. Eventually, a thrombus may develop at plaque sites and partially or completely occlude an artery. In coronary arteries, a thrombus may precipitate myocardial ischemia (angina or infarction) (see Chap. 26); in carotid or cerebral arteries, a thrombus may precipitate a stroke; in peripheral arteries, a thrombus may cause intermittent claudication (pain in the legs with exercise) or acute occlusion. Thus, serious impairment of blood flow may occur with a large atherosclerotic plaque or a relatively small plaque with superimposed vasospasm and thrombosis. Consequences and clinical manifestations of thrombi and emboli depend primarily on their location and size.

BOX 7.1   Hemostasis and Thrombosis

The blood vessels and blood normally maintain a balance between procoagulant and anticoagulant factors that favor anticoagulation and keeps the blood fluid. Injury to blood vessels and tissues causes complex reactions and interactions among vascular endothelial cells, platelets, and blood coagulation factors that shift the balance toward procoagulation and thrombosis.

Endothelial Cells

Normal endothelium helps to prevent thrombosis by producing anticoagulant factors, inhibiting platelet reactivity, and inhibiting activation of the coagulation cascade. However, endothelium promotes thrombosis if the blood vessel wall is damaged, function is altered, or when blood flow is altered or becomes static. After a blood clot is formed, the endothelium also induces its dissolution and restoration of blood flow.

Platelets

The only known function of platelets is hemostasis. Platelets (also called thrombocytes) are produced in the bone marrow and released into the bloodstream, where they circulate for approximately 7 to 10 days before they are removed by the spleen. They contain no nuclei and therefore cannot repair or replicate themselves.

The cell membrane of a platelet contains a coat of glycoproteins that prevents the platelet from adhering to normal endothelium but allows it to adhere to damaged areas of endothelium and collagen in the blood vessel wall. Breakdown of the cell membrane releases arachidonic acid (which can be metabolized to produce thromboxane A_2) and allows leakage of platelet contents (e.g., thromboplastin and other clotting factors), which function to stop bleeding.

When platelets come in contact with a damaged vascular surface, they become activated and aggregate at a site of injury to help plug a hole in a torn blood vessel. Aggregated platelets release substances that recruit new platelets and stimulate additional aggregation. This activity helps the platelet plug become large enough to block blood flow out of a damaged blood vessel. If the opening is small, the platelet plug can stop blood loss. If the opening is large, a platelet plug and a blood clot are both required to stop the bleeding. Platelets usually disappear from a blood clot within 24 hours and are replaced by fibrin.

Blood Coagulation

The blood coagulation process represented in Figure 7.1 normally causes hemostasis within 1 to 2 minutes. It involves sequential activation of clotting factors that are normally present in blood and tissues as inactive precursors and formation of a meshwork of fibrin strands that cements blood components together to form a stable, dense clot. Major phases include release of thromboplastin by disintegrating platelets and damaged tissue; conversion of prothrombin to thrombin, which requires thromboplastin and calcium ions; and conversion of fibrinogen to fibrin by thrombin.

Blood coagulation results from activation of the intrinsic or extrinsic coagulation pathway. Both pathways, which are activated when blood passes out of a blood vessel, are needed for normal hemostasis. The intrinsic pathway occurs in the vascular system; the extrinsic pathway occurs in the tissues. Although the pathways are initially separate, the terminal steps (i.e., activation of factor X and thrombin-induced formation of fibrin) are the same leading to the formation of thrombin, which then activates fibrinogen to form fibrin, and the clot is complete.

Thrombotic disorders occur much more often than bleeding disorders and are emphasized in this chapter. Bleeding disorders may result from excessive amounts of drugs that inhibit clotting.

Clinical Manifestations

Clinical manifestations of thrombosis vary depending on the size and location (arterial or venous system) of the thrombus. Symptoms are the result of decreased perfusion to an area due to the restriction or cessation of blood flow. Arterial blood clots in the cerebral, pulmonary, or cardiac system can produce a cerebrovascular accident, pulmonary embolism, or myocardial infarction, respectively. Venous blood clots may lead to DVT; classic symptoms include leg swelling and pain on palpation in the calf or thigh. However, half of all affected patients do not have any symptoms of DVT. Additional discussion of clinical manifestations is found in The Nursing Process, Assessment.

Drug Therapy

Drugs given to prevent or treat thrombosis alter some aspect of the blood coagulation process (Table 7.1; see Fig. 7.1). **Anticoagulant** drugs, which prevent formation of new clots and extension of already existing clots, do not dissolve clots that have already formed. Widely used in thrombotic disorders, they are more effective in preventing venous thrombosis than arterial thrombosis. **Antiplatelet** drugs are used to prevent arterial thrombosis. **Thrombolytic** drugs are used to dissolve thrombi and limit tissue damage in selected thromboembolic disorders.

Anticoagulant Drugs

There are three types of anticoagulants: heparins, vitamin K antagonists, and direct thrombin inhibitors (DTIs).

Heparins

ⓟ **Heparin** is a pharmaceutical preparation of the natural anticoagulant produced primarily by mast cells in pericapillary connective tissue, and it is the prototype anticoagulant. Endogenous heparin is found in various body tissues, most abundantly in the liver and lungs. Exogenous heparin is obtained from bovine lung or porcine intestinal mucosa and standardized in units of biologic activity. See below for a discussion of low-molecular-weight heparins (LMWHs).

TABLE 7.1

Drugs Administered for the Treatment of Coagulation Disorders

Drug Class	Prototype(s)	Other Drugs in the Class
Anticoagulant Drugs		
Heparins	Heparin	Dalteparin Enoxaparin Fondaparinux*
Vitamin K antagonists	Warfarin	
Direct thrombin inhibitors	Lepirudin	Argatroban Bivalirudin Dabigatran etexilate Desirudin Rivaroxaban
Antiplatelet Drugs		
Adenosine diphosphate receptor antagonists	Clopidogrel	Prasugrel Ticlopidine Tirofiban
Other antiplatelet drugs		Abciximab Anagrelide Aspirin Cilostazol Dipyridamole Eptifibatide
Thrombolytic Drugs	Alteplase	Drotrecogin alfa, activated Reteplase, recombinant Streptokinase Tenecteplase
Drugs Used to Control Bleeding		Aminocaproic acid Protamine sulfate Tranexamic acid Vitamin K

*Chemically related to low molecular weight heparins.

Pharmacokinetics

It is necessary to give heparin intravenously or subcutaneously, because the gastrointestinal (GI) tract does not absorb the drug. After intravenous (IV) injection, it acts immediately. After subcutaneous injection, it acts within 20 to 30 minutes. Metabolism takes place in the liver and the reticuloendothelial system. Excretion, primarily in the form of inactive metabolites, occurs in the urine. Hemodialysis does not remove it.

Action

Heparin combines with antithrombin III (a natural anticoagulant in the blood) to inactivate clotting factors IX, X, XI, and XII; inhibit the conversion of prothrombin to thrombin; and prevent thrombus formation (see Fig. 7.1). After thrombosis has developed, heparin can inhibit additional coagulation by inactivating thrombin, preventing the conversion of fibrinogen to fibrin and inhibiting factor XIII (fibrin-stabilizing factor). Other effects include inhibition of factors V and VIII and platelet aggregation.

Use

Prophylactically, patients at risk for certain disorders take low doses of heparin prophylactically to prevent DVT and pulmonary embolism. These disorders include

- Major illnesses (e.g., acute myocardial infarction, heart failure, serious pulmonary infections, stroke)
- Major abdominal or thoracic surgery
- A history of thrombophlebitis or pulmonary embolism, including pregnant women
- Gynecologic surgery, especially in patients who have been taking estrogens or oral contraceptives or have other risk factors for DVT
- Restrictions such as bed rest or limited activity expected to last longer than 5 days

Therapeutically, patients receive heparin for management of acute thromboembolic disorders (e.g., DVT, thrombophlebitis, pulmonary embolism). In these conditions, the aim of therapy is to prevent further thrombus formation and embolization. Another use is in disseminated intravascular coagulation (DIC), a life-threatening condition characterized by widespread clotting, which depletes the blood of coagulation factors. The depletion of coagulation factors then produces widespread bleeding. The goal of heparin therapy in DIC is to prevent blood coagulation long enough for clotting factors to be replenished and thus be able to control hemorrhage. In addition, clinicians use heparin to prevent clotting during cardiac and vascular surgery, extracorporeal circulation, hemodialysis, and blood transfusions, and in blood samples to be used in laboratory tests. Heparin does not cross the placental barrier and is not secreted in breast milk,

making it the anticoagulant of choice for use during pregnancy and lactation.

Table 7.2 presents the dosage information for the heparins.

Use in Children

Little information about the use of anticoagulants in children is available. When children take heparin for systemic anticoagulation, weight is the basis for determination of dosage (~50 units/kg). It is essential to use extreme caution to ensure that the vial concentration of heparin is correct. Fatalities in

TABLE 7.2

DRUGS AT A GLANCE: Anticoagulants

Drug	Pregnancy Category	Indications for Use	Routes and Dosage Ranges (Adults, Unless Specified)
Heparins Ⓟ **Heparin**	C	Prevention and management of thromboembolic disorders (e.g., DVT, pulmonary embolism, atrial fibrillation with embolization)	Adults: IV injection, 5000 units initially, followed by 5000–10,000 units every 4 to 6 h, to a maximum dose of 25,000 units/d; IV infusion, 5000 units (loading dose), then 15–25 units/kg/h DIC, IV injection, 50–100 units/kg every 4 h; IV infusion, 20,000–40,000 units/d at initial rate of 0.25 units/kg/min, then adjusted according to aPTT; Sub-Q 10,000–12,000 units every 8 h, or 14,000–20,000 units every 12 h Low-dose prophylaxis, Sub-Q 5000 units 2 h before surgery, then every 12 h until discharged from hospital or fully ambulatory Children: DIC, IV injection, 25–50 units/kg every 4 h; IV infusion, 50 units/kg initially, followed by 100 units/kg every 4 h or 20,000 units/m² over 24 h
Dalteparin (Fragmin)	B	Prophylaxis of DVT in patients having hip replacement surgery; also patients at high risk for thromboembolic disorders who are having abdominal surgery	Abdominal surgery, Sub-Q 2500 international units 1–2 h before surgery and then once daily for 5–10 d after surgery Hip replacement surgery, Sub-Q 2500 international units 1–2 h before surgery and the evening of surgery (at least 6 h after first dose) and then 5000 international units once daily for 5 d
Enoxaparin (Lovenox)	B	Prevention and management of DVT and PE Management of unstable angina, to prevent myocardial infarction	DVT prophylaxis in patients having hip or knee replacement surgery, Sub-Q 30 mg twice daily, with first dose within 12–24 h after surgery and continued until risk of DVT diminished or until adequately anticoagulated on warfarin Abdominal surgery, Sub-Q 40 mg once daily with first dose given 2 h before surgery, for 7–10 d DVT/PE management, outpatients, Sub-Q 1 mg/kg every 12 h; inpatients, 1 mg/kg every 12 h or 1.5 mg/kg every 24 h Unstable angina 1 mg/kg every 12 h in conjunction with oral aspirin (100–325 mg once daily)
Fondaparinux (Arixtra)	B	Prevention of DVT following hip fracture surgery or knee or hip replacement	Sub-Q 2.5 mg daily, with first dose 6–8 h after surgery and continuing for a maximum of 11 d

TABLE 7.2

DRUGS AT A GLANCE: Anticoagulants (Continued)

Drug	Pregnancy Category	Indications for Use	Routes and Dosage Ranges (Adults, Unless Specified)
Vitamin K Antagonist			
℗ **Warfarin** (Coumadin)	D	Long-term prevention or management of venous thromboembolic disorders, including DVT, PE, and embolization associated with atrial fibrillation and prosthetic heart valves. May also be used after myocardial infarction to decrease reinfarction, stroke, venous thromboembolism, and death	PO 2–5 mg/d for 2–3 d, then adjusted according to the INR; average maintenance daily dose, 2–5 mg
Direct Thrombin Inhibitors			
℗ **Lepirudin** (Refludan)	B	Heparin alternative for anticoagulation in patients with heparin-induced thrombocytopenia and associated thromboembolic disorders	IV injection, 0.4 mg/kg over 15–20 sec, followed by continuous IV infusion of 0.15 mg/kg for 2–10 d or longer if needed
Argatroban (Argatroban)	B	Thrombosis prophylaxis or management in heparin-induced thrombocytopenia; adjunct to PTCA	IV continuous infusion 2 mcg/kg/min
Bivalirudin (Angiomax)	B	Patients with unstable angina undergoing PTCA; acute coronary syndrome; used concomitantly with aspirin therapy	IV bolus dose of 0.75 mg/kg followed by 4-h infusion at rate of 1.75 mg/kg/min
Dabigatran etexilate (Pradaxa)	C	Decrease the risk of stroke and systemic embolism with nonvalvular atrial fibrillation	PO 150 mg twice daily; in severe renal failure 75 mg twice daily
Desirudin (Iprivask)	C	Prophylaxis of DVT in patients having hip replacement surgery	Sub-Q, 15 mg every 12 h; first dose should be given 5–15 min before surgery and may be administered for up to 12 d post surgery
Rivaroxaban (Xarelto)	C	Prophylaxis of DVT, which may lead to PE in patients having knee or hip replacement surgery	PO 10 mg once daily; may be administered for up to 12 d postsurgery for knee replacement and 35 d postsurgery for hip replacement

aPTT, activated partial thromboplastin time; DIC, disseminated intravascular coagulation; DVT, deep vein thrombosis; INR, international normalized ratio; PE, pulmonary embolism; PTCA, percutaneous transluminal coronary angioplasty or atherectomy; sec, seconds.

infants involving heparin overdoses have occurred. In addition, premature infants should not take heparin solutions containing benzyl alcohol as a preservative; fatal reactions have resulted.

QSEN Safety Alert

Several major adverse events have resulted from the use of heparin, and it is classified as a high-alert drug. Nurses demonstrate consistent practice in administrating heparin by their heightened individual awareness of the risks and by advocating for systems to account for human error such as bar coding and "smart" pumps. Effective standardized practices to support safety and quality include special safeguards to reduce the risk of errors that may harm the patient.

Use in Older Adults

Older adults often have atherosclerosis and thrombotic disorders, including myocardial infarction, thrombotic stroke, and peripheral arterial insufficiency, for which they receive an anticoagulant drug. They are more likely than younger adults to experience bleeding and other complications associated with this therapy. With standard heparin, general principles for safe and effective use apply. With LMWHs, elimination may be delayed in older adults with renal impairment, and the drugs should be used cautiously.

Use in Patients With Renal Impairment

People with renal impairment may take heparin in usual dosages. However, the half-life of the drug may increase.

Use in Patients With Hepatic Impairment

Likewise, people with hepatic impairment may take heparin in usual dosages. However, the half-life of the drug may increase or decrease.

Use in Patients With Critical Illness

Heparin is often used in patients who are critically ill. However, the risk of bleeding is increased in the presence of other coexisting conditions. People who are critically ill have a high risk of DVT and pulmonary embolism, as well as a higher morbidity and mortality, including an increase in length of hospital stay, the need and duration of mechanical ventilation, and death. Effective prevention and treatment of thrombosis is necessary and typically includes LMWHs. In addition, it is essential to consider intermittent pneumatic compression devices and other measures to prevent DVT or pulmonary embolism.

Use in Patients Receiving Home Care

Patients may take standard heparin at home using the subcutaneous route, and use of LMWHs for home management of venous thrombosis has become standard practice. Daily visits by a home care nurse may be necessary if the patient or a family member is unable or unwilling to inject the medication. It is essential to take platelet counts before therapy begins and every 2 to 3 days during heparin therapy. If the platelet count falls below 100,000 platelets per microliter of blood or to less than half the baseline value, it is necessary to discontinue the heparin.

Adverse Effects

Hemorrhage is the major side effect of heparin therapy, hypersensitivity to the drug has occurred, and local irritation with subcutaneous injections of heparin can cause erythema and mild pain. **Heparin-induced thrombocytopenia (HIT)** (type II) is a potentially life-threatening complication of heparin administration, leading to a decrease in platelet count and detectable HIT antibodies. This condition occurs in 1% to 3% of people receiving heparin at therapeutic levels for 4 to 14 days, sometimes sooner in those who have previously received heparin. HIT is one of the most common immune-mediated adverse drug reactions. All patients exposed to any heparin at therapeutic or prophylactic doses or minute amounts in heparin flushes or on heparin-coated catheters, as well as those receiving LMWH, are at risk. If HIT occurs, it is necessary to discontinue all heparin and manage anticoagulation with a DTI such as argatroban.

Contraindications

Contraindications include GI ulcerations (e.g., peptic ulcer disease, ulcerative colitis), intracranial bleeding, dissecting aortic aneurysm, blood dyscrasias, severe kidney or liver disease, severe hypertension, polycythemia vera, and recent surgery of the eye, spinal cord, or brain. Caution is necessary in patients with hypertension, renal or hepatic disease, alcoholism, history of GI ulcerations, drainage tubes (e.g., nasogastric tubes, indwelling urinary catheters), threatened abortion, endocarditis, and any occupation with high risks of traumatic injury.

BOX 7.2   Drug Interactions: Heparin

Drugs That Increase the Effects of Heparin

- Alteplase
  Increases the risk of bleeding
- Antithrombin
  Increases pharmacologic effects
- Cephalosporins
  Lead to potential coagulopathies and risk of bleeding
- Direct thrombin inhibitors
  Increase the risk of bleeding
- Drotrecogin alfa
  Increases the risk of bleeding
- Penicillins (parenteral)
  Lead to altered platelet aggregation and increased risk of bleeding.
- Platelet inhibitors
  Increase the risk of bleeding
- Warfarin
  May prolong and possibly invalidate the PT; if receiving both heparin and warfarin, draw blood for the PT at least 5 hours after the last IV heparin dose

Drugs That Decrease the Effects of Heparin

- Antihistamines
  Decrease the anticoagulant effect
- Digoxin
  Decreases the anticoagulant effect
- Nicotine
  Decreases the anticoagulant effect
- Nitroglycerin (IV)
  Decreases the anticoagulant effect
- Streptokinase
  Leads to relative resistance to anticoagulation
- Tetracycline
  Decreases the anticoagulant effect

IV, intravenous; PT, prothrombin time.

Nursing Implications

Preventing Interactions

Many medications interact with heparin, increasing or decreasing its effect (Box 7.2). Some herbs and foods increase the effects of the drug (Box 7.3). No herbs or foods that decrease the effects of heparin have been identified.

BOX 7.3 **Herb and Dietary Interactions: Heparin**

Herbs and Foods That Increase the Effects of Heparin

- Chamomile, garlic, ginger, ginkgo, ginseng, high-dose vitamin E

Administering the Medication

Traditional anticoagulants have two major limitations: a narrow therapeutic window of adequate anticoagulation without bleeding and a highly variable individual dose–response that requires monitoring by laboratory testing. Prescribers use the activated partial thromboplastin time (aPTT), which is sensitive to changes in blood clotting factors, except factor VII, to regulate heparin dosage. Thus, normal or control values of aPTT indicate normal blood coagulation, and therapeutic values of adequate anticoagulation indicate low levels of clotting factors and delayed blood coagulation. During heparin therapy, the aPTT should be maintained at approximately 1.5 to 2.5 times the control or baseline value. The normal control value is 25 to 35 seconds; therefore, therapeutic values of adequate anticoagulation are 45 to 70 seconds, approximately. With continuous IV infusion, blood for the aPTT may be drawn at any time; with intermittent administration, blood for the aPTT should be drawn approximately 1 hour before a dose of heparin is scheduled. It is not necessary to monitor aPTT with low-dose standard heparin given subcutaneously for prophylaxis of thromboembolism or with the LMWHs (e.g., enoxaparin).

The nurse should be aware that heparin has disadvantages: parenteral injection is necessary, and the drug has a short duration of action, which means that there is a need for frequent administration.

Assessing for Therapeutic Effects

The nurse assesses for the absence or reduction of signs and symptoms of thrombotic disorders (e.g., less edema and pain with DVT, less chest pain and respiratory difficulty with pulmonary embolism, absence of uncontrolled bleeding). It is also necessary to ensure that aPTT values are within the therapeutic range.

Assessing for Adverse Effects

The nurse assesses the patient for signs of overt bleeding or HIT. Protamine sulfate, which is discussed in more detail later in the chapter, is an antidote for standard heparin and LMWHs. Protamine is typically given for bleeding that may not respond to merely withdrawing the heparin.

Patient Teaching

Education related to bleeding risk is essential for patients receiving heparin. The nurse reinforces instructions for safe use of the drug and related anticoagulants, reminding patients to obtain laboratory tests, and teaching how to observe for signs and symptoms of bleeding. Additional patient teaching guidelines for anticoagulants, including heparins, are outlined in Box 7.4.

Other Drugs in the Class

Standard heparin is a mixture of high and low molecular weight fractions, but most anticoagulant activity is attributed to the low molecular weight portion. LMWHs contain the low molecular weight fraction and are as effective as IV heparin in treating thrombotic disorders. Indications for their use include prevention or management of thromboembolic complications associated with surgery or ischemic complications of unstable angina and myocardial infarction. Currently available LMWHs (dalteparin, enoxaparin) differ from standard heparin and each other and are not interchangeable.

LMWHs are given subcutaneously and do not require close monitoring of blood coagulation. These characteristics allow outpatient anticoagulant therapy, an increasing standard. The drugs are also associated with less thrombocytopenia than standard heparin. However, monitoring of platelet counts during therapy is necessary.

EVIDENCE-BASED PRACTICE

A Meta-Analysis of Effects of Heparin Flush and Saline Flush: Quality and Cost Implications

by GOODE, C. J., TITLER, M. RAKEL B, ET AL.

Nursing Research 1991, 40(6), 324–330

An important component of intravenous (IV) care is maintaining line patency. Until recently, heparin solutions had been used to flush catheters despite existence of evidence obtained 20 years ago demonstrating that saline flushes are as effective as heparin for maintaining patency and preventing phlebitis in peripheral devices. The use of saline prevents complications associated with use of an anticoagulant such as hemorrhage and heparin-induced thrombocytopenia. This seminal meta-analysis indicated that there is no statistical difference between the incidence of clotting and phlebitis and the duration of IV patency in saline and heparin flushes.

IMPLICATIONS FOR NURSING PRACTICE: Saline flushes are as effective as heparin solutions for maintaining patency of peripheral devices and are associated with decreased risks compared with heparin. Practice decisions must be supported by the best available evidence and not merely tradition.

Clinical Application 7-1

- To regulate the amount of heparin Mr. Oliver receives, his aPTT is measured. What is the therapeutic value for aPTT?

Vitamin K Antagonists

Ⓟ **Warfarin** (Coumadin) is the most commonly used oral anticoagulant and is the prototype vitamin K antagonist. Table 7.2 presents dosage information for warfarin.

Pharmacokinetics

Warfarin is well absorbed after oral administration. Administration with food may delay the rate but not the extent of absorption. The drug is highly bound to plasma proteins (98%), mainly albumin. Metabolism takes place in the liver. Excretion, primarily as inactive metabolites, occurs in the

---

BOX 7.4   **Patient Teaching Guidelines for Anticoagulants**

General Considerations

■ Anticoagulant drugs are given to people who have had, or who are at risk of having, a heart attack, stroke, or other problems from blood clots. For home management of deep vein thrombosis, which usually occurs in the legs, you are likely to be given heparin injections for a few days, followed by warfarin for long-term therapy. These medications help prevent the blood clot from getting larger, traveling to your lungs, or recurring later.

■ All anticoagulants can increase the risk of bleeding, so you need to take safety precautions to prevent injury.

■ To help prevent blood clots from forming and decreasing blood flow through your arteries, you need to reduce risk factors that contribute to cardiovascular disease. This can be done by a low-fat, low-cholesterol diet (and medication if needed) to lower total cholesterol to below 200 mg/dL and low-density lipoprotein cholesterol to below 130 mg/dL; weight reduction if overweight; control of blood pressure if hypertensive; avoidance of smoking; stress-reduction techniques; and regular exercise.

■ To help maintain a steady level of anticoagulation with warfarin, do not change your intake of foods that are high in vitamin K, which decreases the effects of warfarin. These foods include broccoli, brussels sprouts, cabbage, cauliflower, chives, collard greens, kale, lettuce, mustard greens, peppers, spinach, tomatoes, turnips, and watercress.

■ To help prevent blood clots from forming in your leg veins, avoid or minimize situations that slow blood circulation, such as wearing tight clothing, crossing the legs at the knees, prolonged sitting or standing, and bed rest. For example, on automobile trips, stop and walk around every 1 to 2 hours; on long plane trips, exercise your feet and legs at your seat and walk around when you can.

■ Following instructions regarding these medications is extremely important. Too little medication increases your risk of problems from blood clot formation; too much medication can cause bleeding.

■ While taking any of these medications, you need regular medical supervision and periodic blood tests. The blood tests can help your health care provider regulate drug dosage and maintain your safety.

■ Notify your health care provider if you suddenly stop tobacco smoking, because this may result in a reduced clearance of warfarin. A dosage change may be necessary.

■ With enoxaparin, you need an injection, usually every 12 hours. You or someone close to you may be instructed in injecting the medication, or a visiting nurse may do the injections, if necessary.

■ You need to take the drugs as directed. Avoid taking other drugs without the health care provider's knowledge and consent, inform any health care provider (including dentists) that you are taking an anticoagulant drug before any invasive diagnostic tests or treatments are begun, and keep all appointments for continuing care.

■ With warfarin therapy, you need to avoid walking barefoot; avoid contact sports; use an electric razor; avoid injections when possible; and carry an identification card, necklace, or bracelet (e.g., MedicAlert) stating the name of the drug and the health care provider's name and telephone number.

■ A routine blood test is necessary to ensure that your warfarin dose is appropriate. The results of this test determine your daily dose of warfarin. Once the warfarin dose stabilizes, the blood tests are done less often (e.g., every 2 weeks).

■ Report any sign of bleeding (e.g., excessive bruising of the skin, blood in urine or stool). If superficial bleeding occurs, apply direct pressure to the site for 3 to 5 minutes or longer if necessary.

Self-Administration

■ With enoxaparin, wash hands and cleanse skin to prevent infection; inject deep under the skin, around the navel, upper thigh, or buttocks; and change the injection site daily. If excessive bruising occurs at the injection site, rubbing an ice cube over an area before the injection may be helpful.

■ With warfarin as with all medications, take as prescribed. Because the prescriber may set a dosing schedule that could vary from 1 day to the next, do not rely on memory but keep a written record of the date and the amount of medication taken.

---

kidneys. Renal impairment does not affect drug metabolism but may decrease excretion of the drug.

Action

Warfarin acts in the liver to prevent synthesis of vitamin K–dependent clotting factors (i.e., factors II, VII, IX, and X). Similar to vitamin K in structure, warfarin therefore acts as a competitive antagonist to hepatic use of vitamin K. Conversely, vitamin K serves as the antidote for warfarin. Warfarin has no effect on circulating clotting factors or on platelet function, so the anticoagulant effects do not occur for 3 to 5 days after warfarin is started because clotting factors already in the blood follow their normal pathway of elimination.

Use

Warfarin is most useful in long-term prevention or management of venous thromboembolic disorders, including DVT, pulmonary embolism, and embolization associated with atrial fibrillation and prosthetic heart valves. In addition, warfarin therapy after myocardial infarction may decrease reinfarction, stroke, venous thromboembolism, and death. The smaller doses used now are equally effective as ones used formerly, with similar antithrombotic effects and decreased risks of bleeding.

Use in Children

After cardiac surgery, children receive warfarin to prevent thromboembolism, but there are no established doses and guidelines for safe, effective use. Accurate drug administration, close monitoring of blood coagulation tests, safety measures to prevent trauma and bleeding, avoiding interacting drugs, and informing others in the child's environment (e.g., teachers, babysitters, health care providers) are necessary.

Use in Older Adults

Warfarin metabolism may be altered in older adults. As patient age increases, a lower dose of warfarin is usually required to produce a therapeutic effect.

Use in Patients With Hepatic Impairment

Warfarin is more likely to cause bleeding in patients with hepatic disease because of decreased synthesis of vitamin K and decreased plasma proteins. In addition, only the liver eliminates warfarin; thus, it may accumulate in people with hepatic impairment, and dosage adjustment may be necessary.

Use in Patients With Critical Illness

Because the anticoagulant and antithrombotic effects of warfarin take several days to occur, patients who are critically ill require concurrent treatment with other anticoagulants, such as heparin or LMWHs. Heparin is usually continued until the international normalized ratio (INR) is the therapeutic range.

Use in Patients Receiving Home Care

For prevention of DVT, warfarin is usually self-administered at home, with periodic office or clinic visits for blood tests and other follow-up care. For home management of DVT, warfarin may be self-administered, but a nurse usually visits, performs a fingerstick INR, and notifies the prescriber, who then prescribes the appropriate dose of warfarin. Precautions to decrease risks of bleeding are necessary. However, the risk of bleeding has decreased in recent years because lower doses of warfarin are now used. In addition, medical conditions other than anticoagulation may cause bleeding during warfarin therapy.

Adverse Effects

The primary adverse effect associated with warfarin therapy is hemorrhage. Additionally, nausea, vomiting, abdominal pain, alopecia, urticaria, dizziness, and joint or muscle pain may occur.

Contraindications

Contraindications to warfarin include GI ulcerations, blood disorders associated with bleeding, severe kidney or liver disease, severe hypertension, and recent surgery of the eye, spinal cord, or brain. Caution is warranted in patients with mild hypertension, renal or hepatic disease, alcoholism, history of GI ulcerations, drainage tubes (e.g., nasogastric tubes, indwelling urinary catheters), and occupations with high risks of traumatic injury. Warfarin, a pregnancy category X medication, is contraindicated during pregnancy because it crosses the placenta and may produce fatal fetal hemorrhage. The Food and Drug Administration (FDA) has issued a **BLACK BOX WARNING** ◆ for warfarin due to its risk of causing major or fatal bleeding.

Nursing Implications

Preventing Interactions

Many medications and herbs interact with warfarin, increasing or decreasing its effect (Boxes 7.5 and 7.6).

Administering the Medication

Vitamin K antagonists such as warfarin have a narrow therapeutic window of adequate anticoagulation without bleeding and a highly variable individual dose–response that requires monitoring by laboratory testing.

BOX 7.5	Drug Interactions: Warfarin

Drugs That Increase the Effects of Warfarin
- Acetaminophen (high dose), allopurinol, amiodarone
  Increase the anticoagulant effect
- Alteplase, androgens, aspirin and other nonsteroidal anti-inflammatory drugs, azithromycin, bismuth subsalicylate, carbamazepine, chloral hydrate, chloramphenicol, cimetidine, ciprofloxacin and other quinolone antibiotics, cisapride, clarithromycin, clofibrate, cotrimoxazole, direct thrombin inhibitors, drotrecogin alfa, heparin, macrolide antibiotics, omeprazole, pravastatin, propranolol, quinidine, ranitidine, ritonavir, sertraline, simvastatin, streptokinase, sulfinpyrazone, sulfonamide, tamoxifen, tetracyclines, thyroid hormones, tricyclic antidepressants, vancomycin , vitamin E
  Increase the risk of bleeding
- Antithrombin
  Increases the pharmacologic effect
- Cephalosporins
  Result in potential coagulopathies and risk of bleeding

Drugs That Decrease the Effects of Warfarin
- Chlordiazepoxide, haloperidol, intravenous lipid emulsions (contains soybean oil), isotretinoin, meprobamate, spironolactone
  Cause effects by various mechanisms
- Chlorthalidone
  May diminish warfarin's ability to cause blood clots to form
- Ethchlorvynol, trazodone
  Cause effects by unknown mechanism
- Etretinate
  May induce anticoagulant's hepatic microsomal enzyme

BOX 7.6 · Herb and Dietary Interactions: Warfarin

Herbs and Foods That Increase the Effects of Warfarin

- Angelica
- Cat's claw
- Chamomile
- Chondroitin
- Cranberry juice
- Feverfew
- Garlic
- Ginkgo
- Goldenseal
- Grape seed extract
- Green tea
- Psyllium
- Turmeric

Herbs and Foods That Decrease the Effects of Warfarin

- Ginseng
- St. John's wort
- Vitamin K
- Foods high in vitamin K (broccoli, brussels sprouts, cabbage, cauliflower, chives, collard greens, kale, lettuce, mustard greens, peppers, spinach, tomatoes, turnips, and watercress)

QSEN Safety Alert ❗

When warfarin therapy begins, daily evaluation of INR is necessary until a stable daily dose is reached (the dose that maintains the prothrombin time [PT] and INR within therapeutic ranges and does not cause bleeding). A therapeutic PT value is approximately 1.5 times control, or 18 seconds. Thereafter, a patient's INR values require checking every 2 to 4 weeks for the duration of oral anticoagulant drug therapy. If a prescriber changes the warfarin dose, more frequent INR measurements are necessary until a stable daily dose is again established.

The nurse administers warfarin after ensuring that laboratory values are within therapeutic parameters.

QSEN Safety Alert ❗

Institutions often have protocol for the therapeutic range of INR. In the absence of a protocol, the nurse holds the dose if the INR is above 3.0 and notifies the health care provider.

Assessing for Therapeutic Effects

As with heparin, the nurse assesses for the absence or reduction of signs and symptoms of thrombotic disorders (e.g., less edema and pain with DVT, less chest pain and respiratory difficulty with pulmonary embolism, absence of uncontrolled bleeding, hematuria or blood in the stools). It is also necessary to ensure that PT and INR values are within the therapeutic range.

Assessing for Adverse Effects

The nurse assesses for signs of bleeding, including excessive bruising of the skin, bleeding from IV sites or the gum line, and blood in urine or stool. As previously stated, vitamin K is the antidote for warfarin and may be administered if the INR level is 5 or more and signs of bleeding are present.

Patient Teaching

The nurse reinforces instructions for safe use of warfarin, assists patients to obtain required laboratory tests, and teaches how to observe for signs and symptoms of bleeding. Additional patient teaching guidelines for anticoagulant medications, including vitamin K antagonists, are outlined in Box 7.4.

Other Drugs in the Class

Fondaparinux is a synthetic pentasaccharide that binds to antithrombin administered for prophylaxis of DVT in people undergoing hip or knee surgery. The drug selectively inhibits factor Xa by mechanisms identical to LMWHs but without affecting thrombin activity. It is administered subcutaneously and has a longer half-life than LMWHs, necessitating only a once-daily dose. The Institute for Safe Medication Practices (ISMP) classifies fondaparinux as a high-alert drug because there is a possible risk of significant harm when the drug is used in error. It does not require routine coagulation monitoring, except in patients with renal dysfunction, because fondaparinux is primarily eliminated by the kidneys. Currently, no agents for reversal of fondaparinux are available.

Clinical Application 7-2

- Mr. Oliver's prescriber adds warfarin to his treatment regimen. The order is for warfarin 5 mg PO daily and for evaluation of baseline PT and INR. The nurse administers the warfarin and order the blood work for the next morning. What therapeutic INR value indicates that the warfarin dosage is appropriate?

NCLEX Success

1. The nurse is reviewing the laboratory results of a hospitalized patient receiving intravenous heparin therapy for pulmonary embolism. The activated partial thromboplastin time (aPTT) is 38 seconds (control 28 seconds). The nurse should

   A. not give the next dose because the level is too high
   B. continue the present order because the level is appropriate
   C. notify the health care provider that the aPTT is low and anticipate orders to increase the dose
   D. request an order for warfarin now that the patient is heparinized

2. In explaining the use of warfarin to a female patient, the nurse is correct in telling her all of the following regarding warfarin (choose all that apply):

   A. is a vitamin K antagonist
   B. does not cross the placenta
   C. is used for long-term anticoagulation therapy
   D. is metabolized by the liver

3. In developing a safe plan of care, the nurse recognizes that which of the following agents is the antidote for heparin?

   A. protamine zinc
   B. vitamin K
   C. protamine sulfate
   D. vitamin D

Direct Thrombin Inhibitors

DTIs have benefits compared with agents such as heparin and warfarin, including the inhibition of both circulating and clot-bound thrombin. Other advantages of DTIs include a more predictable dose–response anticoagulant effect, inhibition of thrombin-induced platelet aggregation, and the lack of production of immune-mediated thrombocytopenia. Heparin and warfarin are indirect inhibitors of thrombin. The DTIs exert their effect by interacting directly with the thrombin molecule without the need of a cofactor, such as heparin cofactor II or antithrombin. As such, they inhibit thrombin's ability to convert soluble fibrinogen to fibrin and to activate the fibrin-generating factors V, VIII, and IX. Because thrombin also stimulates platelets, DTIs also have antiplatelet activity.

There are two types of DTIs (bivalent and univalent), depending on their interaction with the thrombin molecule. The original prototype of the bivalent type, hirudin, is not commercially available; however, its discovery led to the development through recombinant technology of its derivatives, lepirudin, desirudin, and bivalirudin. In this discussion, ⓟ **lepirudin** (Refludan) is the prototype.

Table 7.2 presents dosage information for the DTIs.

Pharmacokinetics

Lepirudin, which cannot be absorbed by the GI tract, is administered intravenously and is distributed to the extracellular fluids. The metabolic pathway has not been established. The drug is excreted in the urine, and the systemic elimination is proportional to the glomerular filtration rate. Typically, the elimination half-life is 60 minutes.

Action

Lepirudin is a highly specific direct inhibitor of thrombin, but unlike heparin, its mechanism of action is independent of antithrombin III. DTIs have no known antagonists. Given

intravenously, the drug has an onset within 30 to 90 minutes and has a duration of action for up to 24 hours. Safety and efficacy in children have not been established.

Use

Lepirudin is available for HIT, acute coronary syndrome, prophylaxis and treatment of venous thromboembolism, and management of atrial fibrillation. This drug and the other DTIs are less suitable for long-term treatment because administration by injection is necessary, therapeutic drug monitoring is not widely available, and no pharmacologic antidote to reverse the effects is available.

Use in Older Adults

Renal clearance is decreased in older adults. Therefore, dosage adjustment may be necessary.

Use in Patients With Renal Impairment

Because the drug is cleared by the kidneys, it accumulates in patients with renal insufficiency. The typical elimination half-life of 60 minutes can be prolonged up to 2 days in patients with renal failure.

Adverse Effects

The most common adverse effects associated with the administration of lepirudin are bleeding, injection site reactions, nausea, vomiting, stomach upset, anemia, hematoma, elevated liver function tests (LFTs), hematuria, epistaxis, pain, headache, fever, bradycardia, hypotension or hypertension, insomnia, and anxiety.

Contraindications

Contraindications include a known hypersensitivity to hirudins or to any of the components of lepirudin. Lepirudin is a pregnancy category C medication, and because the drug is found in breast milk, use in pregnancy and lactation requires caution.

Nursing Implications

The ISMP classifies lepirudin as a high-alert drug because of the possible risk of significant harm that result when it is used in error.

Preventing Interactions

Many medications and herbs interact with lepirudin, increasing its effect (Boxes 7.7 and 7.8). No drugs appear to decrease its effects. Similarly, no herbs and foods seem to decrease its effects.

Administering the Medication

Product information recommends that lepirudin be given as an initial IV bolus followed by a continuous IV infusion. However, because of concerns about possible anaphylaxis, a bolus dose is now only recommended when life-threatening thrombosis is present. During continuous IV infusion, the solution remains stable for up to 24 hours at room temperature. Monitoring lepirudin values typically requires using the aPTT and adjusting the dose to maintain an aPTT of 1.5 to 2.5 times the control. To decrease the risk of a **prothrombotic reaction** (an effect leading to thrombogenesis) when beginning oral anticoagulation, administration of lepirudin should overlap with warfarin for 4 to 5 days and stop when the INR reaches the therapeutic range.

Assessing for Therapeutic Effects

The nurse assesses for the absence of signs and symptoms of thrombotic disorders, including HIT, and for laboratory values within the therapeutic range.

Assessing for Adverse Effects

The most common adverse effect associated with the administration of lepirudin is bleeding; therefore, assessing for signs of bleeding is a priority. Additionally, the nurse assesses injection sites for reactions. He or she should watch for other adverse effects, including GI and hematologic effects, as well as elevated LFTs, pain, headache, fever, bradycardia, hypotension or hypertension, insomnia, and anxiety.

Patient Teaching

Because lepirudin requires IV infusion, health care professionals, including nurses, administer the drug in a hospital or clinic setting. Additional general patient teaching guidelines for anticoagulants, including the DTIs, are outlined in Box 7.4.

Other Drugs in the Class

In comparison to heparin, which binds only circulating thrombin, DTIs such as bivalirudin and desirudin block circulating

thrombin and clot-bound thrombin. Bivalirudin is given intravenously as a specific and reversible DTI approved for the treatment of patients with unstable angina undergoing percutaneous transluminal coronary angioplasty (PTCA), as an anticoagulant in patients undergoing PTCA, and as an alternative to heparin in patients with or at risk of developing HIT. Desirudin has been shown to be more effective than enoxaparin in preventing DVT following total hip replacement. Desirudin is administered subcutaneously, and highly protein bound drugs do not modify its effects. The new anticoagulant rivaroxaban is the first available orally active direct factor Xa inhibitor for use in preventing DVT following total knee or hip replacement. The drug is given once daily in the postoperative period, and no routine monitoring of INR or other coagulation parameters is required.

Argatroban is the second agent, after lepirudin, to be indicated for HIT. But unlike lepirudin, argatroban is eliminated in the liver and can be used in people with end-stage renal disease. Administered intravenously, argatroban is very short acting due to its reversible binding to thrombin and differs from lepirudin, which irreversibly binds to thrombin.

Dabigatran etexilate is administered orally and is approved for the prevention of stroke in people with nonvalvular atrial fibrillation. Unlike warfarin, the drug provides predictable and consistent anticoagulation and does not require routine coagulation monitoring. Additionally, dabigatran has few drug–drug interactions and no food interactions, unlike warfarin.

Antiplatelet Drugs

Antiplatelet drugs prevent one or more steps in the prothrombotic activity of platelets. As described previously, platelet activity is very important in both physiologic hemostasis and pathologic thrombosis. Arterial thrombi, which are composed primarily of platelets, may form on top of atherosclerotic plaque and block blood flow in the artery. They may also form on heart walls and valves and embolize to other parts of the body.

Drugs used clinically for antiplatelet effects act by a variety of mechanisms to inhibit platelet activation, adhesion, aggregation, or procoagulant activity. These include drugs that block platelet receptors for thromboxane A_2, adenosine diphosphate (ADP), glycoprotein (GP) IIb/IIIa, and phosphodiesterase. Figure 7.2 describes the mechanism of action of some of the antiplatelet drugs. Aspirin, a cyclooxygenase inhibitor that has potent antiplatelet effects, is well described in Chapter 14.

Adenosine Diphosphate Receptor Antagonists

The antiplatelet drug Ⓟ **clopidogrel** (Plavix) is the prototype ADP receptor antagonist. Other ADP receptor antagonists, prasugrel and ticlopidine, are also used for their antiplatelet activity. Clopidogrel has three shortcomings: delayed onset

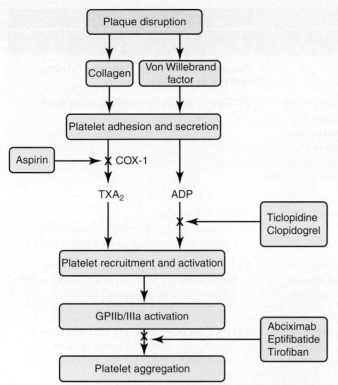

Figure 7.2 Details of the site of action of antiplatelet drugs on the process of platelet aggregation.

of action, irreversible inhibitory effects on platelets with no reversing agent or antidote, and significant individual variability in platelet response.

Pharmacokinetics

Clopidogrel is rapidly absorbed after oral administration and undergoes extensive first-pass metabolism in the liver. Platelet inhibition may occur 2 hours after a single dose, but the onset of action is slow, so that an initial loading dose is usually administered. The drug has a half-life of about 8 hours. The drug is excreted in the urine and feces.

Action

Clopidogrel irreversibly block the ADP receptor on platelet cell membranes. Effective dose-dependent prevention of platelet aggregation can be seen within 2 hours of a single oral dose, but the onset of action is slow, so that a loading dose of 300 to 600 mg is usually administered. Platelet inhibition essentially lasts for the lifespan of the platelet. With repeated doses of 75 mg/d, maximum inhibition of platelet aggregation is achieved within 3 to 7 days. Platelet aggregation progressively returns to baseline about 5 days after discontinuing clopidogrel.

Use

Indications for use include reduction of myocardial infarction, stroke, and vascular death in patients with atherosclerosis and

in those after placement of coronary stents. Specific uses include prevention of vascular ischemic events in patients with symptomatic atherosclerosis or with acute coronary syndrome (with or without ST-segment elevation). In addition, after placement of an intracoronary stent for the prevention of thrombosis, patients may take clopidogrel in conjunction with aspirin (dual antiplatelet therapy). The absolute risk reduction from clopidogrel and other thienopyridines is greater in patients at higher cardiovascular risk—specifically, in patients with acute coronary syndromes or those who have had a coronary stent implanted. The addition of an oral anticoagulation agent to a thienopyridine and aspirin is necessary in some patients with cardiovascular disease; this is termed triple oral antithrombotic therapy.

People with atrial fibrillation who are unable to take vitamin K antagonists take clopidogrel instead. Adding clopidogrel to aspirin in people with atrial fibrillation reduces the rate of major vascular events compared with aspirin alone but is associated with a greater risk of bleeding. Prescribers also order clopidogrel as an alternative antiplatelet drug for patients who cannot tolerate aspirin.

Table 7.3 presents dosages for clopidogrel and other antiplatelet drugs.

Use in Children

The safety and efficacy of clopidogrel in children have not been established.

Use in Older Adults

Older adults are more likely than younger ones to experience bleeding and other complications of antiplatelet drugs. Clopidogrel is commonly used to prevent thrombotic stroke but can increase the risk of hemorrhagic stroke. A loading dose for patients 75 years of age and older has not yet been established.

Use in Patients With Hepatic Impairment

Because clopidogrel is metabolized in the liver, it may accumulate in people with hepatic impairment. Caution is necessary.

Adverse Effects

The most common adverse effects associated with clopidogrel are pruritus, rash, purpura, and diarrhea. Thrombotic thrombocytopenic purpura, hemorrhage, and severe neutropenia have also occurred.

Contraindications

Contraindications to clopidogrel include hypersensitivity to the drug or any other component. It should not be used in patients with active bleeding in conditions such as intracranial hemorrhage or peptic ulcer disease. A category B medication, the drug requires cautious use in pregnant and lactating women.

Nursing Implications

The FDA has issued a **BLACK BOX WARNING** ◆ concerning the use of clopidogrel in the 2% to 14% of the US

TABLE 7.3

DRUGS AT A GLANCE: Antiplatelets

Drug	Pregnancy Category	Indications for Use	Routes and Dosage Ranges (Adults, Unless Specified)
Clopidogrel (Plavix)	B	Reduction of atherosclerotic events (myocardial infarction, stroke, vascular death) in patients with atherosclerosis documented by recent stroke, recent myocardial infarction, or established peripheral artery disease	PO 75 mg once daily with or without food
Aspirin	D (if full dose aspirin is taken in the third trimester)	Prevention of myocardial infarction	PO 81–325 mg daily Prevention of thromboembolic disorders in patients with prosthetic heart valves or TIAs
Abciximab (ReoPro)	C	Used with PTCA to prevent rethrombosis of treated arteries Intended for use with aspirin and heparin	IV bolus injection, 0.25 mg/kg 10–60 min before starting PTCA, then a continuous IV infusion of 10 mcg/min for 12 h
Anagrelide (Agrylin)	C	Essential thrombocythemia, to reduce the elevated platelet count, the risk of thrombosis, and associated symptoms	PO 0.5 mg 4 times daily or 1 mg twice daily initially, then titrate to lowest dose effective in maintaining platelet count <600,000/mm³
Cilostazol (Pletal)	C	Intermittent claudication, to increase walking distance (before leg pain occurs)	PO 100 mg twice daily, 30 min before or 2 h after breakfast and dinner; reduce to 50 mg twice daily with concurrent use of fluconazole, itraconazole, erythromycin, or diltiazem
Dipyridamole (Persantine)	B	Prevention of thromboembolism after cardiac valve replacement, given with warfarin	PO 25–75 mg 3 times per day, 1 h before meals
Dipyridamole and aspirin (Aggrenox)	D	Reduction of stroke risk in patients with previous TIA or thrombotic event	PO 1 capsule (200 mg extended-release dipyridamole/25 mg aspirin) twice daily
Eptifibatide (Integrilin)	B	Acute coronary syndromes, including patients who are to be managed medically and those undergoing PTCA	IV bolus injection, 180 mcg/kg, followed by continuous infusion of 2 mcg/kg/min. See manufacturer's instructions for preparation and administration.
Prasugrel (Effient)	B	Acute coronary syndromes	PO: Adults ≥60 kg: loading dose: 60 mg; maintenance dose: 10 mg once daily (in combination with aspirin 81–325 mg/d).
Ticlopidine (Ticlid)	B	Prevention of thrombosis in patients with coronary artery or cerebral vascular disease (e.g., patients who have had stroke precursors or a completed thrombotic stroke)	PO 250 mg twice daily with food
Tirofiban (Aggrastat)	B	Acute coronary syndromes, with heparin, for patients who are to be managed medically or those undergoing PTCA Acute myocardial infarction Pulmonary embolism	IV infusion, 0.4 mcg/kg/min for 30 min, then 0.1 mcg/kg/min. Patients with severe renal impairment (creatinine clearance <30 mL/min) should receive half the usual rate of infusion. See manufacturer's instructions for preparation and administration.

PTCA, percutaneous transluminal coronary angioplasty or atherectomy; TIA, transient ischemic attack.

BOX 7.9 — Drug Interactions: Clopidogrel

Drugs That Increase the Effects of Clopidogrel

■ Aspirin
Increases the risk of bleeding
■ Atorvastatin
May affect antiplatelet activity
■ Barbiturates, carbamazepine, rifampin, rifapentine
Enhances antiplatelet effect
■ Nonsteroidal anti-inflammatory drugs
Increase the risk of bleeding
■ Platelet inhibitors
Increase the risk of bleeding
■ Rifabutin
May increase metabolism of clopidogrel
■ Thrombolytics
Increases the risk of bleeding

Drugs That Decrease the Effects of Clopidogrel

■ Amiodarone, dalfopristin, delavirdine, diltiazem, quinupristin, Vaprisol, zafirlukast
Affect cytochrome 450 3A4 enzymes, which play a role in clopidogrel metabolism
■ Clarithromycin, erythromycin, ketoconazole, verapamil
Reduce antiplatelet activity
■ Omeprazole
May lead to inadequate platelet response
■ Selective serotonin reuptake inhibitors
May increase the risk of bleeding

BOX 7.10 — Herb and Dietary Interactions: Clopidogrel

Herbs and Foods That Increase the Effects of Clopidogrel

■ Garlic
■ Ginkgo biloba
■ Ginger
■ Green tea
■ Horse chestnut

Clinicians have demonstrated that dual antiplatelet therapy with aspirin and clopidogrel reduces stent thrombosis following percutaneous coronary intervention. It is recommended that patients who receive implants with a bare-metal stent take clopidogrel for at least 1 month and that patients who receive a drug-eluting stent take dual antiplatelet therapy for at least 12 months.

Assessing for Therapeutic Effects

The nurse assesses for the absence of vascular ischemic events (e.g., pain, cyanosis, coolness of extremities). In addition, he or she ensures that hemoglobin and hematocrit levels are within normal limits.

Assessing for Adverse Effects

The nurse assesses for common adverse effects, including pruritus, rash, purpura, and diarrhea; thrombotic thrombocytopenic purpura and hemorrhage; and severe neutropenia.

Patient Teaching

The nurse instructs patients to take medication as directed and not to double the medication if a dose is missed. Additional patient teaching guidelines are outlined in Box 7.11.

Other Drugs in the Class

Prasugrel is indicated to reduce thrombotic cardiovascular events, including stent thrombosis, in persons with acute coronary syndrome being managed with percutaneous coronary intervention. Although the drug requires hepatic conversion to an active metabolite, similar to clopidogrel, it is about 10 times more potent and has a more rapid onset of action. However, unlike clopidogrel, this activation is a rapid single-step process.

In a clinical trial comparing prasugrel with clopidogrel, prasugrel showed a greater reduction in myocardial infarction, a small difference in cardiovascular death, and no difference in stroke reduction (Wiviott, 2007). The risk of bleeding was greater with prasugrel.

Ticlopidine is indicated for prevention of thrombotic stroke in people who have had stroke precursor events (e.g., transient ischemic attacks [TIAs]) or a completed thrombotic stroke. Ticlopidine is considered a second-line

---

population who are reduced metabolizers of the drug. As a result of genetic variations in CYP2C19 function, the drug may be less effective in altering platelet activity in these people. These "poor metabolizers" may remain at risk for heart attack, stroke, and cardiovascular death, and alternate dosing of the clopidogrel or the use of other antiplatelet drugs should be considered. Tests are available to determine if a patient is a poor metabolizer.

Preventing Interactions

Many medications interact with clopidogrel, increasing or decreasing its effect (Box 7.9). Although certain herbs and foods increase the effects of clopidogrel, none seem to decrease the effects of the drug (Box 7.10).

Administering the Medication

Patients take clopidogrel once daily without regard to food intake. As previously stated, although the drug may be effective 2 hours after a single dose, the onset of action is slow, and an initial loading dose is usually administered. The FDA has approved a 300-mg tablet as a loading dose for appropriate patients. The effect of the drug is apparent as soon as 2 hours after the 300-mg dose.

BOX 7.11 **Patient Teaching Guidelines for Antiplatelet Drugs**

General Considerations

■ Antiplatelet drugs are given to people who have had, or who are at risk of having, a heart attack, stroke, or other problems from blood clots. For prevention of a heart attack or stroke, you are most likely to be given an antiplatelet drug (e.g., aspirin, clopidogrel).

■ All antiplatelet drugs can increase your risk of bleeding, so you need to take safety precautions to prevent injury.

■ Following instructions regarding these medications is extremely important. Too little medication increases your risk of problems from blood clot formation; too much medication can cause bleeding.

■ While taking any of these medications, you need regular medical supervision and periodic blood tests. The blood tests can help your health care provider regulate drug dosage and maintain your safety.

■ You need to take the drugs as directed, avoid taking other drugs without the health care provider's knowledge and consent, inform any health care provider (including dentists) that you are taking an antiplatelet before any invasive diagnostic tests or treatments are begun, and keep all appointments for continuing care.

This drug should be withheld 5 to 7 days prior to a planned surgical procedure.

■ Report any sign of bleeding (e.g., excessive bruising of the skin, blood in urine or stool) to your health care provider. If superficial bleeding occurs, apply direct pressure to the site for 3 to 5 minutes or longer if necessary. In addition, notify your prescriber promptly if you develop fever, chills, or a sore throat.

Self-Administration

■ Take aspirin with food or after meals, with 8 ounces of water, to decrease stomach irritation. However, stomach upset is uncommon with the small doses used for antiplatelet effects. Do not crush or chew coated tablets (long-acting preparations).

■ Take cilostazol (Pletal) 30 minutes before or 2 hours after morning and evening meals for better absorption and effectiveness.

■ Take ticlopidine (Ticlid) with food or after meals to decrease GI upset. Clopidogrel (Plavix) may be taken with or without food.

---

drug for patients who cannot take aspirin. Ticlopidine requires routine hematologic monitoring, unlike clopidogrel. The adverse effects (e.g., neutropenia, diarrhea, skin rashes) and greater cost make it prohibitive for use by many patients. Contraindications include active bleeding disorders (e.g., GI bleeding from peptic ulcer, intracranial bleeding), neutropenia, thrombocytopenia, severe hepatic disease, and hypersensitivity to the drug. Neutropenia and thrombocytopenia are more likely to occur with ticlopidine than clopidogrel. No antidote exists for the effects of the ADP receptor antagonists as they produce irreversible platelet effects. Platelet transfusion should be considered in patients who take these drugs and have hemorrhagic complications.

Other Antiplatelet Drugs

Thromboxane A2 Inhibitors

Aspirin exerts pharmacologic actions by inhibiting synthesis of prostaglandins. In this instance, it acetylates cyclooxygenase, the enzyme in platelets that normally synthesizes thromboxane A_2, a prostaglandin product that causes platelet aggregation. Thus, aspirin prevents formation of thromboxane A_2, thromboxane A_2–induced platelet aggregation, and thrombus formation. A single dose of 300 to 600 mg or multiple doses of 30 mg (e.g., daily for several days) of the drug inhibit the cyclooxygenase in circulating platelets almost completely. These antithrombotic effects persist for the life

of the platelet (7–10 days). Aspirin may be used long term for prevention of myocardial infarction or stroke and in patients with prosthetic heart valves. It is also used for the immediate treatment of suspected or actual acute myocardial infarction, for TIAs, and for evolving thrombotic strokes. Adverse effects are uncommon with the small doses used for antiplatelet effects. However, there is an increased risk of bleeding, including hemorrhagic stroke. Because approximately 85% of strokes are thrombotic, the benefits of aspirin or other antiplatelet agents are thought to outweigh the risks of hemorrhagic strokes (~15%). No antidote exists for the effects of aspirin because it produces irreversible platelet effects; platelet transfusion may be required.

Nonsteroidal anti-inflammatory drugs (NSAIDs), including ibuprofen and many other aspirin-related drugs, inhibit cyclooxygenase reversibly. Their antiplatelet effects subside when the drugs are eliminated from the circulation and the drugs usually are not used for antiplatelet effects. However, patients who take an NSAID daily (e.g., for arthritis pain) may not need to take additional aspirin for antiplatelet effects. Acetaminophen does not affect platelets in usual doses (see Chap. 14).

Glycoprotein IIb/IIIa Receptor Antagonists

Abciximab is a monoclonal antibody that prevents the binding of fibrinogen, von Willebrand factor, and other molecules to GP IIb/IIIa receptors on activated platelets. This action inhibits platelet aggregation. This drug is used with PTCA or removal of atherosclerotic plaque to prevent rethrombosis of treated arteries. It is used with aspirin and heparin and is contraindicated in patients who have recently received an oral anticoagulant or IV dextran. Other contraindications include active bleeding, thrombocytopenia, history of a serious stroke, surgery or major trauma within the previous 6 weeks, uncontrolled hypertension, or hypersensitivity to drug components.

Eptifibatide and tirofiban inhibit platelet aggregation by preventing activation of GP IIb/IIIa receptors on the platelet surface and the subsequent binding of fibrinogen and von Willebrand factor to platelets. Antiplatelet effects occur during drug infusion and stop when the drug is stopped. The drugs are indicated for acute coronary syndrome (e.g., unstable angina, myocardial infarction) in patients who are to be treated medically or by angioplasty or atherectomy. Drug half-life is approximately 2.5 hours for eptifibatide and 2 hours for tirofiban; the drugs are cleared mainly by renal excretion. With tirofiban, plasma clearance is approximately 25% lower in older adults and approximately 50% lower in patients with severe renal impairment (creatinine clearance less than 30 mL/min). The drugs are contraindicated in patients with hypersensitivity to any component of the products; current or previous bleeding (within previous 30 days); a history of thrombocytopenia after previous exposure to tirofiban; a history of stroke within 30 days or any history of hemorrhagic stroke; major surgery or severe physical trauma within the previous month; severe hypertension (systolic blood pressure greater than 180 mm Hg with tirofiban or greater than 200 mm Hg with eptifibatide, or diastolic blood pressure greater than 110 mm Hg with either drug); a history of intracranial hemorrhage, neoplasm, arteriovenous malformation, or aneurysm; a platelet count less than 100,000 per cubic millimeter; serum creatinine 2 mg/dL or above (for the 180-mcg/kg bolus and the 2-mcg/kg/min infusion) or 4 mg/dL or above (for the 135-mcg/kg bolus and the 0.5-mcg/kg/min infusion); or dependency on dialysis (eptifibatide).

Bleeding is the most common adverse effect, with most major bleeding occurring at the arterial access site for cardiac catheterization. If bleeding occurs and cannot be controlled with pressure, the drug infusion and heparin should be discontinued. These drugs should be used cautiously if given with other drugs that affect hemostasis (e.g., warfarin, thrombolytics, other antiplatelet drugs).

Phosphodiesterase Inhibitor

Cilostazol inhibits phosphodiesterase, an enzyme that metabolizes cyclic adenosine monophosphate (cAMP). This inhibition increases intracellular cAMP, which then inhibits platelet aggregation and produces vasodilation. The inhibition of platelet aggregation induced by various stimuli (e.g., thrombin, ADP, collagen, arachidonic acid, epinephrine, shear stress) is reversible. The drug is highly protein bound (95%–98%), mainly to albumin; extensively metabolized by hepatic cytochrome P450 enzymes; and excreted in urine (74%) and feces. Cilostazol and its two active metabolites

accumulate with chronic administration and reach steady state within a few days.

The drug is indicated for management of intermittent claudication. Symptoms usually improve within 2 to 4 weeks but may take as long as 12 weeks. The most common adverse effects are diarrhea and headache. The drug is contraindicated in patients with heart failure.

Other Agents

Anagrelide inhibits platelet aggregation induced by cAMP phosphodiesterase, ADP, and collagen. However, it is indicated only to reduce platelet counts for patients with **essential thrombocythemia** (a disorder characterized by excessive numbers of platelets). Doses to reduce platelet production are smaller than those required to inhibit platelet aggregation.

Dipyridamole inhibits platelet adhesion, but its mechanism of action is unclear. It is used for prevention of thromboembolism after cardiac valve replacement and is given with warfarin. The combination of dipyridamole and aspirin is indicated for prevention of stroke in those who have had stroke precursors (TIAs) or a previously completed thrombotic stroke.

NCLEX Success

4. In developing a safe plan of care, the nurse should recognize that the antidote for warfarin is
   A. protamine zinc
   B. vitamin K
   C. protamine sulfate
   D. vitamin D

5. The nurse explains to a patient that aspirin suppresses blood clotting by
   A. inactivating thrombin
   B. promoting fibrin degradation
   C. decreasing synthesis of clotting factors
   D. decreasing platelet aggregation

Thrombolytic Drugs

The purpose of giving thrombolytic agents is to dissolve thrombi. These drugs stimulate conversion of plasminogen to plasmin, a proteolytic enzyme that breaks down fibrin, the framework of a thrombus. The main use of thrombolytic agents is for management of acute, severe thromboembolic disease, such as myocardial infarction, pulmonary embolism, and iliofemoral thrombosis.

The goal of thrombolytic therapy is to reestablish blood flow as quickly as possible and prevent or limit tissue damage. In coronary circulation, restoration of blood flow reduces morbidity and mortality by limiting myocardial infarction size. In cerebral circulation, rapid thrombus dissolution minimizes neuronal death and brain infarction that produce irreversible brain injury. For people with massive pulmonary embolism, the goal of fibrinolytic therapy is to restore pulmonary artery perfusion. Drugs with shorter half-lives increase the risk of rethrombosis or infarction. Anticoagulant drugs, such as heparin and warfarin, and antiplatelet agents are given following thrombolytic therapy to decrease reformation of a thrombus. Thrombolytic drugs are also used to dissolve clots in arterial or venous cannulas or catheters. Ⓟ **Alteplase** (Activase) is the prototype recombinant tissue plasminogen activator (rtPA).

EVIDENCE-BASED PRACTICE

Part 10: Acute Coronary Syndromes: 2010 American Heart Association Guidelines for Cardiopulmonary Resuscitation and Emergency Cardiovascular Care

by O'CONNOR, R.E., BRADY, W., BROOKS, S.C., DIERCKS, D., EGAN, J., GHAEMMAGHAMI, C., MENON, V., O'NEIL, B.J., TRAVERS, A.H., & YANNOPOULOS, D.

Circulation 2010, 122, S787–S817

Clinical trials have demonstrated the benefit of initiating fibrinolysis as soon as possible after onset of ischemic chest discomfort in people with confirmed ST-segment elevation myocardial infarctions (STEMI) or new or presumably new left bundle branch block. The American Heart Association (AHA) recommends that if fibrinolytic drugs are selected, they should be administered ideally within 30 minutes (door to needle) of the first medical contact. Additionally, when fibrinolytic drugs are administered in the prehospital setting, the AHA recommends that the system should include the following features: protocols using fibrinolytic checklists, 12-lead electrocardiogram acquisition and interpretation, experience in advanced life support, communication with the receiving institution, medical director with training and experience in STEMI management, and continuous quality improvement.

IMPLICATIONS FOR NURSING PRACTICE: Prompt treatment of cardiac symptoms of a heart attack can limit the infarction size and improve the patient's health outcome. Teaching of high-risk patients should emphasize the importance of seeking professional help at soon as possible after signs and symptoms of a heart attack.

Pharmacokinetics

Administration of alteplase is by IV infusion. Metabolism occurs predominately in the liver. Following discontinuation of the infusion, more than 50% of the drug is cleared, with more than 80% clearance within 10 minutes. Excretion takes place in the urine. Whether alteplase crosses the placenta or is excreted into breast milk is unknown.

Action

Alteplase is a protein that lyses unwanted fibrin blood clots by catalyzing the conversion of plasminogen to plasmin.

Use

Indications for alteplase include lysis of acute coronary arterial thromboembolism associated with evolving transmural myocardial infarction or acute pulmonary thromboembolism. Clinicians also considered it as first-line therapy for the treatment of acute ischemic stroke in selected people.

Table 7.4 presents dosage information for alteplase and other thrombolytic drugs.

Use in Older Adults

Caution is warranted in older patients (65–80 years of age). Alteplase is not recommended in people older than 80 years of age.

Use in Patients With Hepatic Impairment

Caution is necessary in patients with significant hepatic impairment.

Adverse Effects

As with other anticoagulants and antiplatelet agents, bleeding is the main adverse effect of alteplase. To minimize this risk, it is important to select recipients carefully, avoid invasive procedures when possible, and omit anticoagulant or antiplatelet drugs while thrombolytics are being given. The major risk of rtPA therapy is symptomatic brain hemorrhage, and when rtPA treatment is chosen, the prescriber should obtain informed consent signed by the stroke patient or family member. There is a 3% mortality rate and a 6% to 8% risk of symptomatic hemorrhage associated with its use. In rtPA overdose, aminocaproic acid serves as an antidote.

Contraindications

Due to an increased risk of bleeding, alteplase is contraindicated in patients with uncontrolled severe hypertension, aneurysm, arteriovenous malformation, known coagulopathy or internal bleeding, intracranial or intraspinal surgery or trauma within the past 3 months, intracranial mass, recent major surgery, or current use of oral anticoagulants. Alteplase can increase the risk of cerebral embolism in people with atrial fibrillation or atrial flutter.

TABLE 7.4

DRUGS AT A GLANCE: Thrombolytics

Drug	Pregnancy Category	Indications for Use	Routes and Dosage Ranges (Adults, Unless Specified)
℗ **Alteplase** (Activase)	C	Acute ischemic stroke Acute myocardial infarction Acute PE	Ischemic stroke: IV infusion, 0.9 mg/kg total dose administered (not to exceed 90 mg), with 10% of the total dose administered as an initial IV loading dose over 1 min, and the remainder administered over 60 min. Myocardial infarction or PE: IV infusion, 100 mg over 3 h (first hour, 60 mg with a bolus of 6–10 mg over 1–2 min initially; second hour, 20 mg; third hour, 20 mg) Myocardial infarction: accelerated IV infusion, 100 mg total dosage administered as a 15 mg IV bolus, followed by 50 mg IV infused over 30 min, and then 35 mg IV infused over the next 60 min. IV infusion, 100 mg over 3 h (first hour, 60 mg with a bolus of 6–10 mg over 1–2 min initially; second hour, 20 mg; third hour, 20 mg)
Drotrecogin alfa, activated (Xigris)	C	Reduction of mortality in severe sepsis	IV infusion of 24 mcg/kg/h for 96 h
Reteplase, recombinant (Retavase)	C	Acute myocardial infarction	IV injection, 10 units over 2 min, repeated in 30 min. Inject into a flowing IV infusion line that contains no other medications.
Streptokinase (Streptase)	C	Management of acute, severe pulmonary emboli or iliofemoral thrombophlebitis Used to dissolve clots in arterial or venous cannulas or catheters May be injected into a coronary artery to dissolve a thrombus if done within 6 h of onset of symptoms	IV 250,000 units over 30 min, then 100,000 units/h for 24–72 h
Tenecteplase (TNKase)	C	Acute myocardial infarction	IV bolus dose based on weight, 30 mg (for <60 kg) not to exceed 50 mg (>90 kg)
Urokinase (Abbokinase)	B	Coronary artery thrombi Pulmonary emboli Clearance of clogged IV catheters	IV 4400 units/kg over 10 min, followed by continuous infusion of 4400 units/kg/h for 12 h For clearing IV catheters, see manufacturer's instructions.

PE, pulmonary embolism.

Expansion of the Time Window for Treatment of Acute Ischemic Stroke With Intravenous Tissue Plasminogen Activator

by GJ DEL ZOPPO, JL SAVER., JAUCH, E.C., & ADAMS, H.P. ON BEHALF OF THE AMERICAN HEART ASSOCIATION STROKE COUNCIL

Stroke 2009, 40, 2945–2948

Although the chance of for improved neurological outcomes is greater with earlier treatment of an acute ischemic stroke, the majority of patients are not treated with intravenous recombinant tissue plasminogen activator (rtPA) because they do not seek professional help within the currently recommended 3-hour time limit for administration of the medication set by the 2007 guidelines of the American Heart Association Stroke Council. An advisory from the group now recommends an extended window of 3 to 4 and one-half hours after ischemic stroke for treatment with rtPA.

IMPLICATIONS FOR NURSING PRACTICE: Prompt treatment of acute ischemic stroke can maximize a patient's return to baseline neurologic function. Teaching of high-risk patients should emphasize the importance of seeking professional help as soon as neurologic symptoms develop.

Nursing Implications

Only experienced personnel in a critical care or diagnostic/interventional setting with cardiac and other monitoring devices in place should perform thrombolytic therapy. It is necessary to minimize intramuscular injections in patients who are receiving systemic thrombolytic therapy, because bleeding, bruising, or hematomas may develop.

The nurse assesses patients for cardiac dysrhythmias, including sinus bradycardia, premature ventricular contractions, and ventricular tachycardia resulting from reperfusion following coronary thrombolysis. He or she must promptly identify and report any evidence of bleeding.

Preventing Interactions

Many medications and herbs interact with alteplase, increasing its effect (Boxes 7.12 and 7.13). No herbs or foods appear to decrease its effect.

Administering the Medication

Before a thrombolytic agent is begun, it is essential to check INR, aPTT, platelet count, and fibrinogen to establish baseline values and to determine whether a blood coagulation disorder is present. Two or three hours after thrombolytic therapy is started, the nurse ensures that the fibrinogen level is measured to determine that fibrinolysis is occurring. Alternatively, he or she can check INR or aPTT for increased values because the breakdown products of fibrin exert anticoagulant effects. During and following alteplase administration, the nurse monitors blood pressure frequently and ensures that it is well controlled. The ISMP lists alteplase as a high-alert drug because of its potential risk of causing significant harm when used in error.

Administration is IV as a bolus injection or infusion. The nurse administers all infusions using an IV infusion device. It is necessary to reconstitute alteplase as indicated and not to shake it.

Assessing for Therapeutic Effects

The goal is to minimize total ischemic time and restore blood flow. Therapeutic effects include

- For cardiac revascularization—stabilization of the patient, reversal of symptoms, stabilization of cardiac rhythm, decrease of the ST-segment elevations by 50% of the initial height, and absence of bleeding complications
- For cerebral revascularization—stabilization of the patient, reversal of symptoms, normal mentation, and absence of bleeding complications

---

BOX 7.12 Drug Interactions: Alteplase

Drugs That Increase the Effects of Alteplase

■ Aspirin or other salicylates, abciximab, cilostazol, clopidogrel, dalteparin, dipyridamole, enoxaparin, eptifibatide, fondaparinux, heparin, nonsteroidal anti-inflammatory drugs, tinzaparin, tirofiban, warfarin

Increase the risk of bleeding

BOX 7.13 Herb and Dietary Interactions: Alteplase

Herbs and Foods That Increase the Effects of Alteplase

■ Cat's claw
■ Dong quai
■ Evening primrose
■ Feverfew
■ Garlic
■ Ginkgo
■ Ginseng
■ Green tea
■ Horse chestnut
■ Red clover

Assessing for Adverse Effects

The nurse assesses for evidence of bleeding. In addition, it is necessary to determine that the condition leading to initiation of thrombolytic therapy is reversed and that there is a return of function. If bleeding does occur, it is most likely from a venipuncture or invasive procedure site, and local pressure may control it. If bleeding cannot be controlled or involves a vital organ, it is necessary to stop the thrombolytic drug and replace fibrinogen with whole blood plasma or cryoprecipitate. Giving aminocaproic acid or tranexamic acid may also be appropriate. When the drugs are used in acute myocardial infarction, cardiac dysrhythmias may occur when blood flow is reestablished. Therefore, antidysrhythmic drugs should be readily available.

Patient Teaching

The nurse instructs patients and significant others regarding the purpose of the drug, the underlying condition, and the increased risk of bleeding. Patients should take special care brushing their teeth to reduce bleeding at the gum line. Discharge planning emphasizes managing the complications of the underlying disease (myocardial infarction or stroke) and seeking timely professional help if symptoms recur.

Other Drugs in the Class

All of the available agents are effective with recommended uses. Thus, the choice of a thrombolytic agent depends mainly on risks of adverse effects and costs. All of the drugs may cause bleeding. Reteplase and tenecteplase are additional rtPA drugs used mainly in acute myocardial infarction to dissolve clots obstructing coronary arteries and reestablish perfusion of tissues beyond the thrombotic area. The most common adverse effect is bleeding, which may be internal (e.g., intracranial, GI, genitourinary) or external (e.g., venous or arterial puncture sites, surgical incisions).

In acute evolving myocardial infarction, streptokinase is given intravenously as soon as possible after the onset of a myocardial infarction to dissolve clots and to enhance coronary artery blood flow, thereby reducing the amount of damage to the heart muscle. Streptokinase may also be used to dissolve clots in vascular catheters and to treat acute, severe pulmonary emboli or iliofemoral thrombophlebitis. Streptokinase, the least expensive thrombolytic agent, may cause allergic reactions because it is a foreign protein. Combination therapy (e.g., alteplase and streptokinase) may also be used. Urokinase is recommended for use in patients who are allergic to streptokinase.

Drotrecogin alfa is a recombinant version of human activated protein C that inhibits factors Va and VIIIa. It is indicated for use in adults with severe sepsis as defined by an Acute Physiology and Chronic Health Evaluation (APACHE) score greater than 25 or multiorgan dysfunction. Severe sepsis is characterized by an excessive inflammatory reaction to infection, inappropriate blood clot formation, and impaired breakdown of clots. Drotrecogin alfa is given for its thrombolytic effects, along with other therapies for inflammation and infection. The major adverse effect is bleeding.

Clinical Application 7-3

Before providing care for Mr. Oliver, the nurse reviews his chart (medical diagnosis and medication orders).

- What is the main reason why patients such as Mr. Oliver receive alteplase and heparin?
- What laboratory values should be obtained before a thrombolytic is administered?
- For what adverse effects should the nurse monitor?
- What nursing assessments and patient care goals are necessary in this case?

Drugs Used to Control Bleeding

Anticoagulant, antiplatelet, and thrombolytic drugs profoundly affect hemostasis, and their major adverse effect is bleeding. As a result, systemic hemostatic agents (antidotes) may be needed to prevent or treat bleeding episodes. Antidotes should be used cautiously because overuse can increase risks of recurrent thrombotic disorders.

Aminocaproic acid and tranexamic acid are used to stop bleeding caused by overdoses of thrombolytic agents. Aminocaproic acid also may be used in other bleeding disorders caused by hyperfibrinolysis (e.g., in cardiac surgery, blood disorders, hepatic cirrhosis, prostatectomy, neoplastic disorders). Tranexamic acid also is used for short periods (2–8 days) in patients with hemophilia to prevent or decrease bleeding from tooth extraction. Dosage of tranexamic acid should be reduced in the presence of moderate or severe renal impairment.

Protamine sulfate is an antidote for standard heparin and LMWHs. Because heparin is an acid and protamine sulfate is a base, protamine neutralizes heparin activity. Protamine dosage depends on the amount of heparin administered during the previous 4 hours. Each milligram of protamine neutralizes approximately 100 units of heparin or dalteparin and 1 mg of enoxaparin. **BLACK BOX WARNING ◆** A single dose should not exceed 50 mg due to the risk of severe hypotension, cardiovascular collapse, noncardiogenic pulmonary edema, catastrophic pulmonary vasoconstriction, and pulmonary hypertension with its use. The drug is given by slow IV infusion over at least 10 minutes (to prevent or minimize adverse effects of hypotension, bradycardia, and dyspnea). Its effects occur immediately and last for approximately 2 hours. A second dose may be required because heparin activity lasts approximately 4 hours. Severe hypotensive and anaphylactoid reactions may result from protamine administration. Thus, the drug should be given in settings with equipment and personnel for resuscitation and management of anaphylactic shock.

Vitamin K is the antidote for warfarin overdosage. An oral dose of 10 to 20 mg usually stops minor bleeding and returns the INR to a normal range within 24 hours. INR serum levels less than 5 with no significant bleeding may

TABLE 7.5

DRUGS AT A GLANCE: Drugs Used to Control Bleeding

Drug	Pregnancy Category	Indications for Use	Dosage (Adults, Unless Specified)
Aminocaproic acid (Amicar)	C	Control bleeding caused by overdoses of thrombolytic agents or bleeding disorders caused by hyperfibrinolysis (e.g., cardiac surgery, blood disorders, hepatic cirrhosis, prostatectomy, neoplastic disorders); antidote for tPA	PO, IV infusion, 5 g initially, followed by 1.0 to 1.25 g/h for 8 h or until bleeding is controlled; maximum dose, 30 g/24 h
Protamine sulfate	C	Treatment of heparin overdosage	Depends on the amount of heparin given within the previous 4 h
Tranexamic acid (Cyklokapron)	B	Control bleeding caused by overdoses of thrombolytic agents Prevent or decrease bleeding from tooth extraction in patients with hemophilia	PO 25 mg/kg 3–4 times daily, starting 1 d before surgery, or IV 10 mg/kg immediately before surgery, followed by 25 mg/kg PO 3–4 times daily for 2–8 d
Vitamin K (Mephyton)	C	Antidote for warfarin overdosage	PO 10–20 mg in a single dose

be managed with withholding of the warfarin based on protocols; INR levels greater than 5 may require the use of oral vitamin K. Decisions about management of a patient with an INR above the therapeutic range is based on the degree of elevation of the INR serum level, the clinical status of the patient with regard to bleeding, thrombogenic potential, as well as risk factors such as age and presence of concurrent disease.

Table 7.5 presents the dosage information for the drugs used to control bleeding.

NCLEX Success

6. A patient's Port-A-Cath has become occluded with thrombus. Which of the following agents will likely be used to lyse the clot?

A. protamine sulfate
B. tirofiban
C. streptokinase
D. enoxaparin

7. Clopidogrel is indicated for which of the following?

A. reduction of myocardial infarction, stroke, and vascular death in patients with atherosclerosis
B. adjunctive therapy to warfarin for deep vein thrombosis
C. heparin-induced thrombocytopenia
D. patients in whom bleeding is a consideration

The Nursing Process

Assessment

Assess the patient's status in relation to thrombotic and thromboembolic disorders.

- **Risk factors for thromboembolism include**
  - Immobility (e.g., limited activity or bed rest for more than 5 days)
  - Obesity
  - Cigarette smoking
  - History of thrombophlebitis, DVT, or pulmonary emboli
  - Heart failure
  - Pedal edema
  - Lower limb trauma
  - Myocardial infarction
  - Atrial fibrillation
  - Mitral or aortic stenosis
  - Prosthetic heart valves
  - Abdominal, thoracic, pelvic, or major orthopedic surgery
  - Atherosclerotic heart disease or peripheral vascular disease
  - Use of oral contraceptives
- **Signs and symptoms of thrombotic and thromboembolic disorders depend on the location and size of the thrombus.**
  - DVT and thrombophlebitis usually occur in the legs. The conditions may be manifested by edema (the

affected leg is often measurably larger than the other) and pain. Homans' sign (pain in the calf when the foot is dorsiflexed) is generally unreliable as a clinical sign of DVT. If thrombophlebitis is superficial, it may be visible as a red, warm, tender area following the path of a vein.

- Pulmonary embolism, if severe enough to produce symptoms, is manifested by chest pain, cough, hemoptysis, tachypnea, and tachycardia. Massive emboli cause hypotension, shock, cyanosis, and death.
- DIC is usually manifested by bleeding, which may range from petechiae or oozing from a venipuncture site to massive internal bleeding or bleeding from all body orifices.

Nursing Diagnoses

- Ineffective tissue perfusion related to thrombus or embolus or drug-induced bleeding
- Acute pain related to tissue ischemia
- Impaired physical mobility related to bed rest and pain
- Ineffective coping related to the need for long-term prophylaxis of thromboembolic disorders or fear of excessive bleeding
- Anxiety related to fear of myocardial infarction or stroke
- Deficient knowledge related to anticoagulant or antiplatelet drug therapy
- Risk for injury related to drug-induced impairment of blood coagulation

Planning/Goals

The patient will

- Receive or take anticoagulant and antiplatelet drugs correctly
- Be monitored closely for therapeutic and adverse drug effects, especially when drug therapy is started and when changes are made in drugs or dosages
- Use nondrug measures to decrease venous stasis and prevent thromboembolic disorders
- Act to prevent trauma from falls and other injuries
- Inform any health care provider when taking an anticoagulant or antiplatelet drug
- Avoid or report adverse drug reactions
- Verbalize or demonstrate knowledge of safe management of anticoagulant drug therapy
- Keep follow-up appointments for tests of blood coagulation and drug dosage regulation
- Avoid preventable bleeding episodes

Nursing Interventions

The nurse will

- **Use measures to prevent thrombotic and thromboembolic disorders.**
  - Have the patient ambulate and exercise legs regularly, especially after surgery.
  - For patients who cannot ambulate or do leg exercises, do passive range-of-motion and other leg exercises

several times daily when changing the patient's position or performing other care.
- Have the patient wear elastic stockings. Elastic stockings should be removed every 8 hours and replaced after inspecting the skin. Improperly applied elastic stockings can impair circulation rather than aid it. For patients on bed rest, intermittent pneumatic compression devices can also be used.
- Avoid trauma to lower extremities.
- Maintain adequate fluid intake (1500–3000 mL/d) to avoid dehydration and hemoconcentration.
- Assist patients to promote good blood circulation (e.g., exercise) and avoid situations that impair circulation (e.g., wearing tight clothing, crossing the legs at the knees, prolonged sitting or standing, bed rest, placing pillows under the knees when in bed).

- **For the patient receiving anticoagulant therapy, implement safety measures to prevent trauma and bleeding.**
  - For patients who cannot ambulate safely because of weakness, sedation, or other conditions, keep the call light within reach, keep bed rails elevated, and assist in ambulation.
  - Provide an electric razor for shaving.
  - Avoid intramuscular injections, venipunctures, and arterial punctures when possible.
  - Avoid intubations when possible (e.g., nasogastric tubes, indwelling urinary catheters).

  For the patient receiving tirofiban or eptifibatide:
  - Monitor the femoral artery access site closely. This is the most common site of bleeding.
  - Avoid invasive procedures as much as possible (e.g., arterial and venous punctures, intramuscular injections, urinary catheters, nasotracheal suction, nasogastric tubes). If venipuncture must be done, avoid sites where pressure cannot be applied (e.g., subclavian or jugular veins).
  - While the vascular sheath is in place, keep patients on complete bed rest with the head of the bed elevated 30 degrees and the affected limb restrained in a straight position.
  - Discontinue heparin for 3 to 4 hours and be sure the activated clotting time is less than 180 seconds or the aPTT is less than 45 seconds before removing the vascular sheath.
  - After the vascular sheath is removed, apply pressure to the site and observe closely. For outpatients, be sure there is no bleeding for at least 4 hours before hospital discharge.

- **For the patient receiving a thrombolytic drug or a revascularization procedure for acute myocardial infarction:**
  - Monitor closely for bleeding.
  - Assist the patient and family to understand the importance of diligent efforts to reverse risk factors contributing to coronary artery disease (e.g., diet and perhaps medication to lower serum cholesterol to less than 200 mg/dL and low-density lipoprotein cholesterol to less than 130 mg/dL, weight reduction if

overweight, control of blood pressure if hypertensive, avoidance of smoking, stress-reduction techniques, exercise program designed and supervised by a health care provider).
- Assist the patient and family to understand the importance of complying with medication orders to prevent reinfarction and other complications and continued medical supervision (see Boxes 7.4 and 7.11).

Evaluation
- Observe for signs and symptoms of thromboembolic disorders or bleeding.
- Check blood coagulation tests for therapeutic ranges.
- Observe and interview regarding compliance with instructions about drug therapy.
- Observe and interview regarding adverse drug effects.

Key Concepts

- Anticoagulant drugs are given to prevent formation of new clots and extension of clots already present.
- Antiplatelet drugs are used to prevent arterial thrombosis.
- Thrombolytic agents are used to dissolve thrombi and limit tissue damage in selected thromboembolic disorders.
- Heparin is the anticoagulant of choice in acute venous thromboembolic disorders because the anticoagulant effect begins immediately with IV administration.
- When anticoagulation is required during pregnancy, heparin is used because it does not cross the placenta.
- Currently available LMWHs (dalteparin, enoxaparin) differ from standard heparin and each other and are not interchangeable.
- During heparin therapy, the aPTT should be maintained at approximately 1.5 to 2.5 times the control or baseline value.
- Monitoring of aPTT is not necessary with low-dose standard heparin given subcutaneously for prophylaxis of thromboembolism or with the LMWHs.
- Protamine sulfate is the antidote for standard heparin and LMWHs.
- The FDA has issued a **BLACK BOX WARNING** ◆ with the use of protamine sulfate because of the risk of severe hypotension, cardiovascular collapse, noncardiogenic pulmonary edema, catastrophic pulmonary vasoconstriction, and pulmonary hypertension with its use.
- Warfarin dosage is regulated according to the INR (derived from prothrombin time [PT]), for which a therapeutic value is between 2.0 to 3.0 in most conditions; a therapeutic PT value is approximately 1.5 times the control, or 18 seconds.
- Vitamin K (Mephyton) is the antidote for warfarin.
- The FDA has issued a **BLACK BOX WARNING** ◆ with warfarin because of its risk of causing major or fatal bleeding.
- Aspirin has long been the most widely used antiplatelet drug for prevention of myocardial reinfarction and arterial thrombosis in patients with TIAs and prosthetic heart valves. However, clopidogrel may be more effective than aspirin.
- No antidote exists for the effects of aspirin or the adenosine diphosphate receptor antagonists because both produce irreversible platelet effects; platelet transfusion may be required.
- The FDA has issued a **BLACK BOX WARNING** ◆ with the use of clopidogrel in people who are reduced metabolizers of the drug; in these people, the drug has a reduced effect on platelet function.
- When the thrombolytic agents are used in acute myocardial infarction, cardiac dysrhythmias may occur when blood flow is reestablished; antidysrhythmic drugs should be readily available.

Critical Thinking Questions

7-1. Jane Carter, a 67-year-old retired college faculty member, has a history of TIAs and takes ticlopidine because she cannot tolerate aspirin. She presents for a routine clinic visit. Her complete blood count (CBC) results are as follows: white blood cells 3000 cells/mcL; red blood cells 4.2 to 5.4 million cells/mcL; hemoglobin 12 to 16 g/dL; hematocrit 42%; platelets 100,000/mm³.

- What are the benefits of ticlopidine in patients with a history of TIA?
- How would you interpret her CBC results?
- Given Ms. Carter's laboratory results, what adverse effects would you need to observe for and instruct her about?

References and Resources

Albers, G. W., Amarenco, P., Easton, J. D., et al. (2008). Antithrombotic and thrombolytic therapy for ischemic stroke: American College of Chest Physicians Evidence-Based Clinical Practice Guidelines (8th Edition). *Chest, 133*(6 Suppl), 630S–669S.

Bonnefoy, E., Steg, P. G., Boutitie, F., Dubien, P. Y., Lapostolle, F., Roncalli, J., et al. (2009). Comparison of primary angioplasty and pre-hospital fibrinolysis in acute myocardial infarction (CAPTIM) trial: A 5-year follow-up. *European Heart Journal, 30*, 1598–1606.

Combescure, C. (2010). Clinical implications of clopidogrel non-response in cardiovascular patients: A systematic review and meta-analysis. *Journal of Thrombosis and Haemostasis, 8*(5), 923–933.

del Zoppo, G. J., Saver, J. L., Jauch, E. C., & Adams, H. P., on behalf of the American Heart Association Stroke Council. (2009). Expansion of the time window for treatment of acute ischemic stroke with intravenous tissue plasminogen activator. *Stroke, 40*, 2945–2948.

Goode, C. J., Titler, M. Rakel, B., et al. (1991). A meta-analysis of effects of heparin flush and saline flush: Quality and cost implications. *Nursing Research, 40*(6), 324–330.

Karch, A. M. (2010). *2010 Lippincott's nursing drug guide.* Philadelphia, PA: Lippincott Williams & Wilkins.

Kiernan, T. J. (2007). Thrombolysis in acute myocardial infarction: Current status. *Medical Clinics of North America, 91*, 617–637.

Lacy, C. F., Armstrong, L. L., Goldman, M. P., & Lance, L. L. (2010). *Lexi-Comp's drug information handbook* (19th ed.). Hudson, OH: American Pharmaceutical Association.

Nutescu, E. A., Shapiro, N. L., & Chevalier, A. (2008). New anticoagulant agents: Direct thrombin inhibitors. *Cardiology Clinics, 26*(2), 169–87, v–vi.

O'Connor, R. E., Brady, W., Brooks, S. C., Diercks, D., Egan, J., Ghaemmaghami, C., et al. (2010). Part 10: Acute coronary syndromes: 2010 American Heart Association guidelines for cardiopulmonary resuscitation and emergency cardiovascular care. *Circulation, 122*, S787–S817.

Porth, C. M. (2009). *Pathophysiology: Concepts of altered health status.* (8th ed.). Philadelphia, PA: Lippincott Williams & Wilkins.

Shorr, A. F. (2007). The pharmacoeconomics of deep vein thrombosis treatment. *American Journal of Medicine, 120*(10 Suppl 2), S35–S41.

Squizzato, A. (2009). New direct thrombin inhibitors. *Internal and Emergency Medicine, 4*(6), 479–484.

Warkentin, T. E. (2010). Agents for the treatment of heparin-induced thrombocytopenia. *Hematology/Oncology Clinics of North America, 24*(4), 755–775, ix.

Wiviott, S. D., Braunwald, E., McCabe, C. H., Horvath, I., Keltai, M., Herrman, J. P., et al., for the TRITONTIMI 38 Investigators. (2007). Prasugrel versus clopidogrel in patients with acute coronary syndromes. *The New England Journal of Medicine, 357*, 2001–2015.

8 Drug Therapy for Dyslipidemia

Clinical Application Case Study

Edward Watkins, a 62-year-old man, has had elevated cholesterol and triglyceride levels at his two previous visits to the nurse practitioner. He has tried diet modification and increasing exercise; however, he remains overweight and his lipid values remain elevated. His latest laboratory findings at this visit are total serum cholesterol 239 mg/dL, low-density lipoprotein cholesterol 162 mg/dL, high-density lipoprotein cholesterol 40 mg/dL, and triglycerides 220 mg/dL. His nurse practitioner decides to prescribe atorvastatin 10 mg PO once daily and gemfibrozil 600 mg PO twice a day.

KEY TERMS

Central adiposity: accumulation of abdominal fat, resulting in an increased waist circumference

Cholesterol: component of cell membrane that is produced and processed in the liver; a fat essential for the formation of steroid hormones that is produced in cells and taken in by dietary sources

Dyslipidemia: abnormal lipid levels in the blood; associated with atherosclerosis and its many pathophysiologic effects (e.g., myocardial ischemia and infarction, stroke, peripheral arterial occlusive disease)

Lipoproteins: specific proteins in plasma that transport blood lipids; contain cholesterol, phospholipid, and triglyceride bound to protein. They vary in density and amounts of lipid and protein

Metabolic syndrome: cluster of several cardiovascular risk factors linked with obesity: increased waist circumference, elevated triglycerides, reduced high-density lipoprotein cholesterol, elevated blood pressure, and elevated fasting glucose

Introduction

Although therapeutic lifestyle changes are the cornerstone of population-based interventions to manage dyslipidemia, they are often insufficient in achieving recommended treatment targets. When lifestyle changes alone do not reduce blood lipids, dyslipidemic drugs are used in the management of patients with elevated blood lipids, a major risk factor for atherosclerosis and vascular disorders such as coronary artery disease, strokes, and peripheral arterial insufficiency. These drugs have proven efficacy and are increasingly being used to reduce morbidity and mortality from coronary heart disease and other atherosclerosis-related cardiovascular disorders. Dyslipidemic drugs are used to decrease blood lipids, prevent or delay the development of atherosclerotic plaque, promote the regression of existing atherosclerotic plaque, and reduce morbidity and mortality from cardiovascular disease. To understand the clinical use of these drugs, it is necessary to understand characteristics of blood lipids, metabolic syndrome, and types of blood lipid disorders.

Overview of Dyslipidemia

Etiology

Blood lipids, which include **cholesterol**, phospholipids, and triglycerides, are derived from the diet or synthesized by the liver and intestine. Most cholesterol is found in body cells, where it is a component of cell membranes and performs other essential functions. In cells of the adrenal glands, ovaries, and testes, cholesterol is required for the synthesis of steroid hormones (e.g., cortisol, estrogen, progesterone, testosterone). In liver cells, cholesterol is used to form cholic acid, which is conjugated with other substances to form bile salts; these salts promote absorption and digestion of fats. In addition, a small amount of cholesterol is found in blood serum. Serum cholesterol is the portion of total body cholesterol involved in formation of atherosclerotic plaques. Unless a person has a genetic disorder of lipid metabolism, the amount of cholesterol in the blood is strongly related to dietary intake of saturated fat. Phospholipids are essential components of cell membranes, and triglycerides provide energy for cellular metabolism.

Blood lipids are transported in plasma by specific proteins called **lipoproteins**. Each lipoprotein contains cholesterol, phospholipid, and triglyceride bound to protein. The lipoproteins vary in density and amounts of lipid and protein. Density is determined mainly by the amount of protein, which is more dense than fat. Thus, density increases as the proportion of protein increases. The lipoproteins are differentiated according to these properties, which can be measured in the laboratory. For example, high-density lipoprotein (HDL) cholesterol contains larger amounts of protein and smaller amounts of lipid; low-density lipoprotein (LDL) cholesterol contains less protein and larger amounts of lipid. Other plasma lipoproteins are chylomicrons and very-low-density lipoproteins (VLDLs). Additional characteristics of lipoproteins are described in Box 8.1.

Pathophysiology

Dyslipidemia (also called hyperlipidemia because increased blood levels of lipoproteins accompany increased blood lipid levels), abnormal lipid levels in the blood, is associated with atherosclerosis and its many pathophysiologic effects (e.g., myocardial ischemia and infarction, stroke, peripheral arterial occlusive disease). (Because increased blood levels of lipoproteins accompany increased blood lipid levels, dyslipidemia is also called hyperlipidemia.) Ischemic heart disease has a high rate of morbidity and mortality. Elevated total cholesterol and LDL cholesterol and reduced HDL cholesterol are the abnormalities that are major risk factors for coronary artery disease. Elevated triglycerides also play a role in cardiovascular disease. For example, high blood levels reflect excessive caloric intake (excessive dietary fats are stored in adipose tissue; excessive proteins and carbohydrates are converted to triglycerides and also stored in adipose tissue) and obesity. High caloric intake also increases the conversion of VLDL to LDL cholesterol, and high dietary intake of triglycerides and saturated fat decreases the activity of LDL receptors and increases synthesis of cholesterol. Very high triglyceride levels are associated with acute pancreatitis.

Dyslipidemia may be primary (i.e., genetic or familial) or secondary to dietary habits, other diseases (e.g., diabetes mellitus, alcoholism, hypothyroidism, obesity, obstructive liver disease), and medications (e.g., beta-blockers, cyclosporine, oral estrogens, glucocorticoids, sertraline, thiazide diuretics, anti–human immunodeficiency virus [HIV] protease inhibitors).

Metabolic syndrome is a group of cardiovascular risk factors linked with obesity. The Third Report of the National Cholesterol Education Program Expert Panel on Detection, Evaluation, and Treatment of High Blood Cholesterol in Adults (NCEP III) clustered several elements of metabolic syndrome: **central adiposity** (increased waist circumference), elevated triglycerides, reduced HDL cholesterol, elevated blood pressure, and elevated fasting glucose. These risk factors frequently have an additive effect in the development of cardiovascular, cerebrovascular, and peripheral vascular disease, and they are principal contributors to the significant morbidity and mortality of these conditions. Improvements in insulin resistance and lipid profiles are essential lifestyle modifications and constitute first-line treatment of metabolic syndrome. This chapter specifically addresses management of components of metabolic syndrome related to dyslipidemia; an additional discussion of other factors is found in Chapters 26 and 39.

Clinical Manifestations

A lipid profile consists of a total cholesterol, HDL cholesterol, LDL cholesterol, and triglycerides. For accurate interpretation, blood samples for laboratory testing of triglycerides should be drawn after the patient has fasted for 12 hours. Fasting is not required for cholesterol testing. Normal lipid levels in adults and children are outlined in Table 8.1. Types of dyslipidemias are described in Box 8.2. Although hypercholesterolemia is usually emphasized, hypertriglyceridemia is also associated with most types of hyperlipoproteinemia.

BOX 8.1	Types of Lipoproteins

Chylomicrons, the largest lipoprotein molecules, are synthesized in the wall of the small intestine. They carry recently ingested dietary cholesterol and triglycerides that have been absorbed from the gastrointestinal tract. Hyperchylomicronemia normally occurs after a fatty meal, reaches peak levels in 3 to 4 hours, and subsides within 12 to 14 hours. Chylomicrons carry triglycerides to fat and muscle cells, where the enzyme lipoprotein lipase breaks down the molecule and releases fatty acids to be used for energy or stored as fat. This process leaves a remnant containing cholesterol, which is then transported to the liver. Thus, chylomicrons transport triglycerides to peripheral tissues and cholesterol to the liver.

Low-density lipoprotein (LDL) cholesterol, sometimes called "bad cholesterol," transports approximately 75% of serum cholesterol and carries it to peripheral tissues and the liver. LDL cholesterol is removed from the circulation by receptor and nonreceptor mechanisms. The receptor mechanism involves the binding of LDL cholesterol to receptors on cell surface membranes. The bound LDL molecule is then engulfed into the cell, where it is broken down by enzymes and releases free cholesterol into the cytoplasm.

Most LDL cholesterol receptors are located in the liver. However, nonhepatic tissues (e.g., adrenal glands, smooth muscle cells, endothelial cells, and lymphoid cells) also have receptors by which they obtain the cholesterol needed for building cell membranes and synthesizing hormones. These cells can regulate their cholesterol intake by adding or removing LDL receptors.

Approximately two thirds of the LDL cholesterol is removed from the bloodstream by the receptor-dependent mechanism. The number of LDL receptors on cell membranes determines the amount of LDL degradation (i.e., the more receptors on cells, the more LDL is broken down). Conditions that decrease the number or function of receptors (e.g., high dietary intake of cholesterol, saturated fat, or calories) increase blood levels of LDL.

The remaining one third is removed by mechanisms that do not involve receptors. Nonreceptor uptake occurs in various cells, especially when levels of circulating LDL cholesterol are high. For example, macrophage cells in arterial walls can attach LDL, thereby promoting accumulation of cholesterol and the development of atherosclerosis. The amount of LDL cholesterol removed by nonreceptor mechanisms is increased with inadequate numbers of receptors or excessive amounts of LDL cholesterol.

A high serum level of LDL cholesterol is atherogenic and a strong risk factor for coronary heart disease. The body normally attempts to compensate for high serum levels by inhibiting hepatic synthesis of cholesterol and cellular synthesis of new LDL receptors.

Very-low-density lipoprotein (VLDL) contains approximately 75% triglycerides and 25% cholesterol. It transports endogenous triglycerides (those synthesized in the liver and intestine, not those derived exogenously, from food) to fat and muscle cells. There, as with chylomicrons, lipoprotein lipase breaks down the molecule and releases fatty acids to be used for energy or stored as fat. The removal of triglycerides from VLDL leaves a cholesterol-rich remnant, which returns to the liver. Then the cholesterol is secreted into the intestine, mostly as bile acids, or it is used to form more VLDL and recirculated.

High-density lipoprotein (HDL) cholesterol, often referred to as "good cholesterol," is a small but very important lipoprotein. It is synthesized in the liver and intestine, and some is derived from the enzymatic breakdown of chylomicrons and VLDL. It contains moderate amounts of cholesterol. However, this cholesterol is transported from blood vessel walls to the liver for catabolism and excretion. This reverse transport of cholesterol has protective effects against coronary heart disease.

The mechanisms by which HDL cholesterol exerts protective effects are unknown. Possible mechanisms include clearing cholesterol from atheromatous plaque, increasing excretion of cholesterol so less is available for reuse in the formation of LDL cholesterol, and inhibiting cellular uptake of LDL cholesterol. Regular exercise and moderate alcohol consumption are associated with increased levels of HDL cholesterol; obesity, diabetes mellitus, genetic factors, smoking, and some medications (e.g., steroids and beta-blockers) are associated with decreased levels. HDL cholesterol levels are not directly affected by diet.

Additionally, the total cholesterol–to–HDL cholesterol ratio is a number that is useful in predicting the risk of developing atherosclerosis (total cholesterol value is divided by the value of the HDL cholesterol). The ideal ratio is less than 4. Even with a favorable ratio, it is still important to try to obtain an LDL of less than 80 to 100 mg/dL, particularly in the presence of multiple other risk factors for coronary artery disease.

Management

Overall, the most effective blood lipid profile for prevention or management of metabolic syndrome and its sequelae is high HDL cholesterol, low LDL cholesterol, and low total cholesterol. A low triglyceride level is also desirable. NCEP III classified blood lipid levels and has summarized the current recommendations for the management of dyslipidemia based on a person's blood levels of total and LDL cholesterol and risk factors for cardiovascular disease (Table 8.2). Note that therapeutic lifestyle changes, including exercise, smoking cessation, changes in diet, and drug therapy, are recommended at lower serum cholesterol levels in patients who already have cardiovascular disease or diabetes mellitus. Also, the target LDL serum level is lower in these patients.

Lifestyle Changes

The NCEP III proposed the following guidelines as treatment goals for patients with lipid abnormalities:

- Assess for, and treat, if present, conditions known to increase blood lipids (e.g., diabetes mellitus, hypothyroidism).
- Stop medications known to increase blood lipids, if possible.

TABLE 8.1

Plasma Cholesterol and Triglyceride Levels

	Adults	Children (More Than 3 Y of Age)
Total serum cholesterol (mg/dL)	Normal or desirable = <200 Borderline high = 200 to 239 High = 240 or above	Normal or desirable = <170 Borderline high = 170–199 High = 200 or above
LDL cholesterol (mg/dL)	Optimal = <100 Near or above optimal = 100–129 Borderline high = 130–159 High = 160–189 Very high = 190 or above	Protective level 40–60 Optimal level = <100 Borderline high = 100–129 Elevated = >130
HDL cholesterol (mg/dL)	High = more than 60 Protective level = 40–60 Low = <40	Optimal level = more than 60 Protective level = 40–60 Low = <40
Triglycerides (mg/dL)	Normal or desirable = <150 Borderline high = 150–199 High = 200–499 Very high = 500 or above	Optimal level = <100 Borderline = 100–200 Elevated = >200

BOX 8.2 Types of Dyslipidemias

Type I is characterized by elevated or normal serum cholesterol, elevated triglycerides, and chylomicronemia. This rare condition may occur in infancy and childhood.

Type IIa (familial hypercholesterolemia) is characterized by a high level of low-density lipoprotein (LDL) cholesterol, a normal level of very-low-density lipoprotein (VLDL), and a normal or slightly increased level of triglycerides. It occurs in children and is a definite risk factor for development of atherosclerosis and coronary artery disease.

Type IIb (combined familial hyperlipoproteinemia) is characterized by increased levels of LDL, VLDL, cholesterol, and triglycerides and lipid deposits (xanthomas) in the feet, knees, and elbows. It occurs in adults.

Type III is characterized by elevations of cholesterol and triglycerides plus abnormal levels of LDL and VLDL. This type usually occurs in middle-aged adults (40–60 years)

and is associated with accelerated coronary and peripheral vascular disease.

Type IV is characterized by normal or elevated cholesterol levels, elevated triglycerides, and increased levels of VLDL. This type usually occurs in adults and may be the most common form of hyperlipoproteinemia. Type IV is often secondary to obesity, excessive intake of alcohol, or other diseases. Ischemic heart disease may occur at 40 to 50 years of age.

Type V is characterized by elevated cholesterol and triglyceride levels with an increased level of VLDL and chylomicronemia. This uncommon type usually occurs in adults. Type V is not associated with ischemic heart disease. Instead, it is associated with fat and carbohydrate intolerance, abdominal pain, and pancreatitis, which are relieved by lowering triglyceride levels.

TABLE 8.2

National Cholesterol Education Program Recommendations for Treatment of Dyslipidemia

Patient's Cardiovascular Disease Status	Therapeutic Lifestyle Changes	Drug Therapy	Goal of Therapy
	Low-Density Lipoprotein Cholesterol (mg/dL)		
None or one risk factor	≥160	≥190	<160
Two or more risk factors	≥130	≥160	<130
Presence of cardiovascular disease	≥100	≥130	<100

- Start a low-fat diet. A step I diet contains no more than 30% of calories from fat, less than 10% of calories from saturated fats (e.g., meat, dairy products), and less than 300 mg of cholesterol per day. A step II diet contains no more than 30% of calories from fat, less than 7% of calories from saturated fat, and less than 200 mg of cholesterol per day. The step II diet is more stringent and may be used initially in patients with more severe dyslipidemia, cardiovascular disease, or diabetes mellitus. It can decrease LDL cholesterol levels by 8% to 15%. Diets with more stringent fat restrictions than the step II diet are not recommended because they produce little additional reduction in LDL cholesterol, raise serum triglyceride levels, and lower HDL cholesterol concentrations.
- Use the "Mediterranean diet," which includes moderate amounts of monounsaturated fats (e.g., canola, olive oils) and polyunsaturated fats (e.g., safflower, corn, cottonseed, sesame, soybean, sunflower oils), to also decrease risks of cardiovascular disease.
- Increase dietary intake of soluble fiber (e.g., psyllium preparations, oat bran, pectin, fruits, and vegetables). This diet lowers serum LDL cholesterol by 5% to 10%.
- Dietary supplements (e.g., Cholestin) and cholesterol-lowering margarines (e.g., Benecol, Take Control) can help reduce cholesterol levels. These products are considered to be foods, not drugs, and are costly.
- Start a weight-reduction diet if the patient is overweight or obese. Weight loss can increase HDL and decrease LDL.
- Emphasize regular aerobic exercise (usually 30 minutes at least three times weekly). This strategy increases blood levels of HDL.
- If the patient smokes, help develop a cessation plan. In addition to numerous other benefits, HDL levels are higher in nonsmokers.
- If the patient is postmenopausal, hormone replacement therapy can raise HDL and lower LDL.
- If the patient has elevated serum triglycerides, initial management includes efforts to achieve desirable body weight, ingest low amounts of saturated fat and cholesterol, exercise regularly, stop smoking, and reduce alcohol intake, if indicated. The goal is to reduce serum triglyceride levels to 200 mg/dL or less.
- Unless lipid levels are severely elevated, 6 months of intensive diet therapy and lifestyle modification may be undertaken before drug therapy is considered. It is essential that therapeutic lifestyle changes continue during drug therapy because the benefits of diet, exercise, and drug therapy are additive.

Box 8.3 identifies some herbs and foods that have a known effect on cholesterol.

Clinical Application 8-1

- What is the purpose of attempting weight reduction and increasing activity for Mr. Watkins before starting dyslipidemic medications?
- How would the nurse interpret the current laboratory values of Mr. Watkins?

NCLEX Success

1. The primary focus for prevention and management of metabolic syndrome and its sequelae is
   A. elevated high-density lipoprotein (HDL) cholesterol, depressed low-density lipoprotein (LDL) cholesterol, low total cholesterol
   B. low HDL cholesterol, low LDL cholesterol, low total cholesterol
   C. low triglycerides
   D. high HDL cholesterol, low LDL cholesterol, low triglycerides

2. A person with type 1 diabetes mellitus and hypertension has the following lipid profile: total serum cholesterol 288 mg/dL, low-density lipoprotein (LDL) cholesterol 200 mg/dL, high-density lipoprotein (HDL) cholesterol 48 mg/dL, and triglycerides 200 mg/dL. The patient's total cholesterol–to–HDL cholesterol ratio and relative cardiac risk is
   A. 4.0, with an increased risk of developing atherosclerosis, particularly in the presence of multiple other risk factors for coronary artery disease
   B. 4.5, with no risk of developing atherosclerosis
   C. 5.0, with no risk of developing atherosclerosis
   D. 6.0, with an increased risk of developing atherosclerosis, particularly in the presence of multiple other risk factors for coronary artery disease

3. A 48-year-old man visits his health care provider for his annual checkup. He is otherwise in good health, but assessment findings reveal the new onset of a slight increase in blood pressure and a total serum cholesterol of 240 mg/dL. What can the nurse anticipate as the preferred treatment for this patient?
   A. a low-lipid diet and an exercise program
   B. a low-lipid diet and a cholesterol synthesis inhibitor
   C. an exercise program and a fibrate
   D. a low-lipid diet, an exercise program, and niacin

Drug Therapy

Clinical data suggest that drug therapy may be efficacious even for those with mild to moderate elevations of LDL cholesterol. Dyslipidemic drugs act by altering the production, absorption, metabolism, or removal of lipids and lipoproteins. Drug therapy is initiated when 6 months of dietary and other lifestyle changes fail to decrease dyslipidemia to an acceptable level. It is also recommended for patients with signs and symptoms of coronary heart disease, a strong family history of coronary heart disease or dyslipidemia, or other risk factors for atherosclerotic vascular disease (e.g., hypertension, diabetes mellitus, cigarette smoking). Although several dyslipidemic drugs are available, none is effective in all types of dyslipidemia.

Drug selection is based on the type of dyslipidemia and its severity. To lower cholesterol using a single drug, a statin is preferred. To lower cholesterol and triglycerides, a statin, a cholesterol absorption inhibitor, gemfibrozil, a fibrate, or the vitamin niacin may be used. To lower triglycerides, gemfibrozil,

BOX 8.3	Herbs and Foods Known to Have an Effect on Cholesterol and Triglyceride Levels

■ **Garlic**, an herb, may lower cholesterol and triglycerides. However, there is little scientific support for this therapy. Bleeding may be increased when garlic is combined with anticoagulants, and insulin doses may need to be decreased as a result of the hypoglycemic effect of garlic.

■ **Flax or flax seed**, used internally as a laxative and a dyslipidemic agent. Absorption of all medications may be decreased when taken with flax, resulting in a less than therapeutic effect.

■ **Soy**, used as a food source and has been researched extensively. Use of soy to lower total and LDL cholesterol has been documented. Additionally, it is possible that an intake of soy proteins may have other beneficial vascular effects.

■ **Plant-derived stanol and sterol esters**, which are added to margarine and other food products. These substances may also help lower total and LDL cholesterol. However, cholesterol-lowering margarines containing plant sterols cost approximately two to five times that of ordinary margarine. (Products such as orange juice and other beverages containing lecithin emulsified plant stanols have reduced total and LDL cholesterol to a similar degree as the margarines.) In addition, little is known about their long-term effects, and researchers have shown that plant sterol supplementation may have caused harmful vascular effects in animals.

■ **Theaflavin**, found in green tea, which has been shown to lower total cholesterol and low-density lipoprotein–cholesterol complex

■ **Red yeast rice**, which has been shown to lower cholesterol. However, dosage standardization is a concern, and information about long-term safety is unavailable.

ezetimibe, a cholesterol absorption inhibitor, or niacin may be given. Gemfibrozil, rather than niacin, is usually preferred for people with diabetes because niacin increases blood sugar.

Categories of drugs are described in upcoming sections. Table 8.3 and the DRUGS AT A GLANCE tables list individual drugs used in the treatment of dyslipidemia. Figure 8.1 shows the sites of action of dyslipidemic drugs.

HMG-CoA Reductase Inhibitors

Ⓟ **Atorvastatin** (Lipitor), one of the most widely used drugs in the United States, is the prototype of the class of drugs called the hydroxymethylglutaryl-coenzyme A (HMG-CoA) reductase inhibitors, or statins. By decreasing production of cholesterol, the statins decrease total serum cholesterol, LDL cholesterol, VLDL cholesterol, and triglycerides. They reduce LDL cholesterol within 2 weeks and reach maximal effects in approximately 4 to 6 weeks. HDL cholesterol levels remain unchanged or may increase.

The most commonly prescribed statin, atorvastatin, is useful for treating dyslipidemia and is an overall tool in the primary prevention of cardiovascular disease. Lack of evidence or inconsistent findings concerning the use of statins in women, in people older than 65 years of age, and in people with diabetes mellitus without known cardiovascular disease have led to much controversy concerning the role of statins in primary cardiovascular prevention. The Justification for the Use of Statins in Primary Prevention: an Intervention Trial Evaluating Rosuvastatin (JUPITER) supported the use of the dyslipidemic agents in these clinically defined groups. Atorvastatin and other statins also reduce the risk of angina pectoris and peripheral arterial disease as well as the need for angioplasty and coronary artery grafting to increase or restore blood flow to the myocardium.

Several studies have suggested that atorvastatin may possess some benefits that other statins do not. Research has focused on multiple outcomes, including intimal thickness, results of imaging studies, mortality, incidence of stroke, and progression

TABLE 8.3		
Drugs Administered for the Treatment of Dyslipidemia		
Drug Class	**Prototype**	**Other Drugs in the Class**
HMG-CoA reductase inhibitors (statins)	Atorvastatin (Lipitor)	Fluvastatin (Lescol) Lovastatin (Mevacor) Pitavastatin (Livalo) Pravastatin (Pravachol) Rosuvastatin (Crestor) Simvastatin (Zocor)
Bile acid sequestrants	Cholestyramine (Prevalite, Questran)	Colesevelam (WelChol) Colestipol (Colestid)
Fibrates	Fenofibrate (TriCor)	Gemfibrozil (Lopid)
Cholesterol absorption inhibitor	Ezetimibe (Zetia)	
Miscellaneous dyslipidemic agent	Niacin	

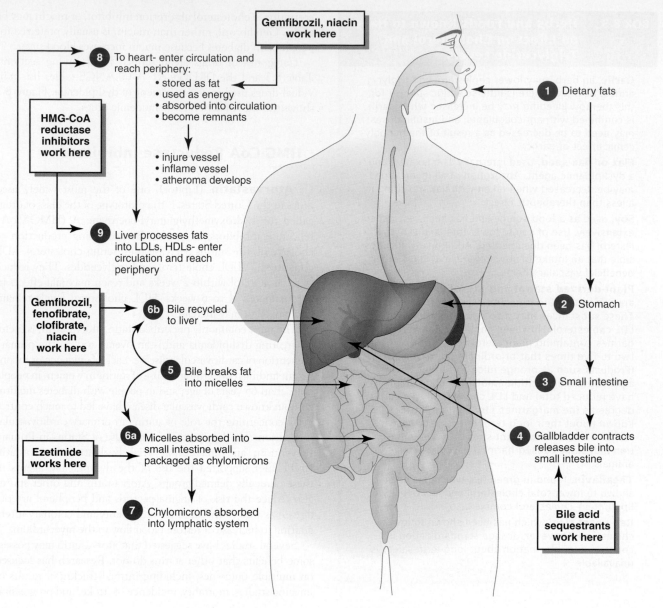

Figure 8.1 Sites of action of dyslipidemic drugs.

of lesions, but there continue to be questions about the benefit profiles of individual drugs.

Pharmacokinetics

Atorvastatin is rapidly absorbed following oral administration and undergoes extensive first-pass metabolism by the liver, which results in low levels of drug available for general circulation. Peak effect occurs in 1 to 2 hours. Food decreases the rate and extent of absorption. Metabolism occurs in the liver, with 80% to 85% of drug metabolites excreted in feces and the remaining products excreted in urine.

Action

The statins inhibit an enzyme (HMG-CoA reductase) required for hepatic synthesis of cholesterol. In part, metabolism involves one or more hepatic cytochrome P450 enzymes (including CYP2D6), leading to an increased risk of drug

interactions and problems with certain foods (e.g., grapefruit juice). Additionally, some of the variability in the response to statins and associated adverse effects statins may relate to genetic differences in the rate of drug metabolism. For example, a CYP2D6 functional deficiency is present in about seven percent of Caucasians and African Americans, and this deficiency is rare in people of Asian descent.

Use

Atorvastatin and the other statins are indicated for the treatment of hypercholesterolemia and reducing cardiovascular events in people with multiple risk factors. The statins are the most powerful drug class for reduction of LDL cholesterol but are expensive. These drugs also decrease triglyceride levels and raise HDL levels. In renal impairment, plasma levels are not affected, and dosage reductions are not necessary.

Table 8.4 presents dosage information for atorvastatin and other statins.

EVIDENCE-BASED PRACTICE

Statin Prescription in Men and Women at Cardiovascular Risk: To Whom and When?

by J. J BRUGTS

Current Opinions in Cardiology
2010, 25(5):484–489.

The Justification for the Use of Statins in Primary Prevention: an Intervention Trial Evaluating Rosuvastatin (JUPITER) demonstrated reduced cardiovascular risk and mortality in people older than 65 years of age, in females, and in people with diabetes mellitus without established cardiovascular disease. Emerging treatment guidelines in primary prevention have yet to include the precise threshold of baseline cardiovascular disease risk associated with the use of beginning statin therapy.

IMPLICATIONS FOR NURSING PRACTICE: Critical primary and secondary prevention strategies include therapeutic lifestyle changes, such as exercise, smoking cessation, changes in diet, as well as drug therapy.

Use in Children

Evidence indicates that atherosclerotic lesions can begin in childhood, and recommendations support selectively screening for children and adolescents starting at age 2 who have a parent with a total cholesterol of 240 mg/dL or higher or a family history of premature cardiovascular disease (age 55 years or younger). Screening children between 5 and 8 years of age using blood testing provides an opportunity to teach health behaviors. Currently, there are no recommendations for the universal screening of children or adolescents. The Food and Drug Administration (FDA) has approved atorvastatin for treatment of high cholesterol levels in children aged 10 to 17 years. Management of younger children with hypercholesteremia focuses on lifestyle modifications.

Use in Older Adults

As in younger adults, diet, exercise, and weight control should be tried first to reduce cholesterol levels. When drug therapy is required, statins are effective for lowering LDL cholesterol and usually are well tolerated by older adults. (As previously mentioned, statins are expensive.)

Use in Patients With Hepatic Impairment

Atorvastatin and other statins, which are metabolized in the liver, may accumulate in patients with impaired hepatic

TABLE 8.4

DRUGS At A GLANCE: HMG-CoA Reductase Inhibitors (Statins)

Drug	Pregnancy Category	Types of Dyslipidemia	Routes and Dosage Ranges	
			Adults	**Children**
Ⓟ **Atorvastatin** (Lipitor)	X	IIa and IIb	PO 10–80 mg daily in a single dose	*10–17 y:* 10 mg once daily to maximum of 20 mg/d
Fluvastatin (Lescol, Lescol XL)	X	IIa and IIb	PO 20–80 mg daily in 1 or 2 doses	*10–16 y:* 20 mg once daily to maximum of 80 mg in 1 or 2 doses
Lovastatin (Mevacor, Altocor, Altoprev)	X	IIa and IIb	PO 20 mg daily with evening meal to 80 mg/d	*10–17 y:* 10–40 mg once daily with evening meal
Pitavastatin (Livalo)	X	IIa and IIb	PO 1–4 mg once daily with or without food	*<18 y:* not recommended
Pravastatin (Pravachol)	X	IIa and IIb	PO 40–80 mg once daily Elderly, PO 10 mg once daily initially	*8–13 y:* 20 mg/d *14–18 y:* 40 mg/d
Rosuvastatin (Crestor)	X	IIa and IIb, IV	PO 5–40 mg once daily	*<18 y:* not recommended
Simvastatin (Zocor)	X	IIa and IIb, IV, V	PO 5–40 mg once daily in the evening Elderly, PO 5–20 mg once daily in the evening	*10–17 y:* 5 mg once daily in the evening to maximum of 40 mg/d

function. Thus, they are contraindicated in patients with active liver disease or unexplained elevations of serum aspartate aminotransferase or alanine aminotransferase. These drugs should be used cautiously, in reduced dosages, for patients who ingest substantial amounts of alcohol or who have a history of liver disease.

Use in Patients Receiving Home Care

Because liver enzymes may be elevated during atorvastatin use, patients need liver function tests and repeat lipid profile testing on a routine basis. Increasing availability of home cholesterol-monitoring devices will require additional patient teaching about technique and interpretation of the results. Patients should notify their health care provider if unexplained muscle pain or tenderness occurs.

Adverse Effects

Statins are usually well tolerated; the most common adverse effects (nausea, constipation, diarrhea, abdominal cramps or pain, headache, skin rash) are usually mild and transient. Hepatic dysfunction has been a source of concern, although the actual risk appears to be small. Myopathy is an important adverse effect. Statins can injure muscle tissue, resulting in muscle ache or weakness. Factors that increase the risk of myopathy include advanced age, frail or small body frame, high dosage of statins, concomitant use of fibrates, hypothyroidism, and multiple systemic diseases such as renal insufficiency secondary to diabetic nephropathy.

QSEN Safety Alert

When women of childbearing age are treated with drug therapy for dyslipidemia, adequate patient education is critical to minimize complications associated with pregnancy. Although the absolute risk of teratogenicity with the use of statins appears relatively small, the use of birth control measures with statin use is essential in sexually active women. Careful consideration should be given if potential benefits warrant use of the drug class in pregnant women despite potential risks. The nurse advocates in the patient's care.

Clinical Application 8-2

- Why is the combination of atorvastatin and gemfibrozil prescribed for Mr. Watkins?

- A nurse is counseling Mr. Watkins about his medication. He asks when he will need to have his laboratory work completed. What is the nurse's response?

- When educating Mr. Watkins about his new medication, the nurse teaches him about common adverse effects. What should be included in teaching about the adverse effects of atorvastatin? What signs and symptoms of complications does the nurse discuss with him?

Contraindications

Statins are potentially teratogenic (pregnancy category X). Careful consideration is necessary if potential benefits warrant use of these drugs in pregnant women. Additional contraindications include lactation, because the drugs are secreted in breast milk, and hypersensitivity to statins.

Nursing Implications

The statins are the most effective dyslipidemic agents for improving clinical outcomes when used for primary and secondary prevention of cardiovascular disease. The choice and use of statins are based on a number of factors, including the degree of dyslipidemia, a specific drug's actions, drug interactions, the presence of renal or liver impairment, and cost.

Preventing Interactions

Many medications and herbs interact with atorvastatin, increasing or decreasing its effect (Boxes 8.4 and 8.5).

Administering the Medication

Because the bulk of cholesterol synthesis appears to occur at night, administration of statins normally takes place in the evening or at bedtime. However, atorvastatin has a long half-life, and evidence suggests that the drug can be given without regard to time of day. There is no definitive global recommendation for the entire class; thus, the timing of administration of statins should be based on manufacturer recommendations.

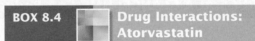

BOX 8.4   Drug Interactions: Atorvastatin

Drugs That Increase the Effects of Atorvastatin

- Magnesium- and aluminum-containing antacids
  Interferes with absorption; administer atorvastatin 2 hours before or after antacids
- Amiodarone, colchicine
  Decrease metabolism
- Azole antifungals
  Increase the risk of myopathy; it is recommended that statin therapy be interrupted temporarily if systemic azole antifungals are needed.
- Cyclosporine, CYP3A inhibitors, diltiazem, fibric acid derivatives, niacin, verapamil
  Increase the risk of severe myopathy or rhabdomyolysis
- Erythromycin, macrolide antibiotics, nefazodone, protease inhibitors
  Decrease elimination

Drugs That Decrease the Effects of Atorvastatin

- Cholestyramine
  Decreases rate of bioavailability; administer atorvastatin at least 4 hours after this bile acid sequestrant
- Colestipol
  Decreases plasma levels

BOX 8.5 Herb and Dietary Interactions: Atorvastatin

Herbs and Foods That Increase the Effects of Atorvastatin

- Grapefruit juice
- Pomegranate juice
- Red yeast rice
- Sitostanol
- Vitamin B_3

Herbs and Foods That May Decrease the Effects of Atorvastatin

- Fibers such as oat bran and pectin

Assessing for Therapeutic Effects

The nurse monitors lipid response to therapy, looking for decreased levels of total serum cholesterol, LDL cholesterol, and triglycerides, as well as increased levels of HDL cholesterol. Effects occur in 1 to 2 weeks, with maximum effects in 4 to 6 weeks.

Assessing for Adverse Effects

Common adverse effects include nausea, diarrhea, abdominal pain, dyspepsia, and elevated liver function tests. The nurse monitors for signs or symptoms of muscle pain or weakness, mainly during the first months of therapy and when dosages are adjusted upward.

Patient Teaching

Women of childbearing age should receive contraceptive counseling to enhance awareness of the risks associated with statin use. In addition, education should focus on the importance of monitoring liver function on a regular basis. Liver function tests are recommended before starting a statin, at 12 weeks after starting the drug, at every increase in dose, and then periodically. The nurse monitors patients with increased serum aminotransferases until the abnormal values resolve. If the increases are more than three times the upper limit of normal levels and persist, it is necessary to reduce the dose or change the drug.

The general teaching guidelines presented in Box 8.6 are a good reference.

Other Drugs in the Class

Table 8.4 lists the other statins. Absorption following oral administration varies depending on the drug. Lovastatin and pravastatin are poorly absorbed, and fluvastatin has the highest rate of absorption. Most of the statins undergo extensive first-pass metabolism by the liver, which results in low levels of drug available for general circulation.

Patients may take pravastatin or simvastatin with or without food in the evening. They may take fluvastatin on an empty stomach or at bedtime. It is important to avoid taking them with grapefruit juice. It should be noted that concurrent use of cimetidine, ranitidine, and omeprazole increases the effects of fluvastatin.

NCLEX Success

4. A man has not been able to decrease his low-density lipoprotein (LDL) cholesterol levels with lifestyle management, and his nurse practitioner has prescribed atorvastatin, a hydroxymethylglutaryl-coenzyme A (HMG-CoA) reductase inhibitor. The nurse explains to him that atorvastatin is best administered

   A. without regard for time of day
   B. at noon, taken with grapefruit juice
   C. with a snack in the early afternoon
   D. every other day with a dose of red yeast rice

5. A 36-year-old woman has been taking atorvastatin 20 mg PO daily for 6 months to treat mild dyslipidemia. At a clinic appointment, she tells the nurse she is 6 weeks pregnant. The nurse counsels the patient that it is likely that her midwife will counsel her

   A. to increase the dose of prenatal vitamins
   B. to reduce the dosage of her lovastatin to 20 mg PO daily
   C. to increase the dosage to 40 mg PO twice daily
   D. about discontinuing the drug during pregnancy

Bile Acid Sequestrants

Ⓟ **Cholestyramine** (Prevalite, Questran), the prototype bile acid sequestrant, has the ability to reduce LDL cholesterol. It has little or no effect on HDL cholesterol and either no effect or an increased effect on triglyceride levels. There is no evidence that cholestyramine can be used as monotherapy, but it can play a role as an add-on drug with statins or niacin in combination therapy.

Pharmacokinetics

Cholestyramine is not absorbed when taken orally. Therefore, the drug is excreted in feces essentially unchanged.

Action

Cholestyramine binds bile acids in the intestinal lumen, causing the bile acids to be excreted in feces, preventing recirculation to the liver. Loss of bile acids stimulates hepatic synthesis of more bile acids from cholesterol. As more hepatic cholesterol is used to produce bile acids, more serum cholesterol moves into the liver to replenish the supply, thereby lowering serum cholesterol (primarily LDL). LDL cholesterol levels decrease within a week of starting cholestyramine and other bile acid sequestrants and reach maximal reductions within a month. When the drugs are stopped, pretreatment LDL cholesterol levels return within a month.

Use

Cholestyramine reduces LDL cholesterol levels and also produces a minimal elevation in HDL cholesterol. Table 8.5 presents dosage information for cholestyramine and other bile acid sequestrants.

BOX 8.6 **Patient Teaching Guidelines for Dyslipidemic Drugs**

■ As you probably know, heart and blood vessel disease causes a great deal of illness and many deaths. The basic problem is usually atherosclerosis, in which the arteries are partly blocked by cholesterol deposits. Cholesterol, a waxy substance made in the liver, is necessary for normal body functioning. However, excessive amounts in the blood increase the likelihood of having a heart attack, stroke, or leg pain from inadequate blood flow. One type of cholesterol (low-density lipoprotein [LDL] or "bad") attaches to artery walls, where it can enlarge over time and block blood flow. The other type (high-density lipoprotein [HDL] or "good") carries cholesterol away from the artery and back to the liver, where it can be broken down. Thus, the healthiest blood cholesterol levels in adults are low total cholesterol (less than 200 mg/dL), low LDL (less than 130 mg/dL), and high HDL (greater than 35 mg/dL). High levels of blood triglycerides, another type of fat, are also unhealthy.

■ Dyslipidemic drugs are given to lower high concentrations of fats (total cholesterol, LDL cholesterol, and triglycerides) in your blood. The goal of management is to prevent heart attack, stroke, and peripheral arterial disease. If you already have heart and blood vessel disease, the drugs can improve your symptoms, activity level, and quality of life.

■ Eat a low-fat diet can help. This is often the first step in treating high cholesterol or triglyceride levels and may be prescribed for 6 months or longer before drug therapy is begun. When drug therapy is prescribed, the diet should be continued. An important part is reducing the amount of saturated fat (from meats, dairy products). In addition, eating a bowl of oat cereal daily can help lower cholesterol by 5% to 10%. Diet counseling by a dietitian or nutritionist can be helpful in developing guidelines that fit your needs and lifestyle. Overeating or gaining weight may decrease or cancel the lipid-lowering effects of the drugs.

■ Make other lifestyle changes to help improve cholesterol levels that include regular aerobic exercise (raises HDL), losing weight (raises HDL, lowers LDL, lowers triglycerides), and not smoking (HDL levels are higher in nonsmokers).

■ As an adult, have measurements of total cholesterol and HDL cholesterol at least once ever every 5 years. People with a personal or family history of dyslipidemia or other risk factors for cardiovascular disease should be tested more often.

■ Techniques for home monitoring of cholesterol levels are improving and are more available for self-use. You may receive instructions about performing self-monitoring and reporting your results to your health care provider.

Use in Children

Experience with cholestyramine in children younger than 10 years of age is limited, and an optimal dosing schedule has not been established. The drug is given in two to three divided doses; dosing is based on 240 mg/kg/d not to exceed 8 g/d.

Use in Older Adults

Cholestyramine and other bile acid sequestrants are effective in older adults, but these patients do not tolerate the adverse effects well.

Use in Patients With Renal Impairment

Extended use of cholestyramine in patients with renal impairment requires caution because the drug releases chloride. This effect can increase the risk of hyperchloremic metabolic acidosis.

Use in Patients With Hepatic Impairment

Cholestyramine can further raise serum cholesterol. Therefore, its use in people with primary biliary cirrhosis warrants caution.

Adverse Effects

Cholestyramine is not absorbed systemically, so the main adverse effects are gastrointestinal (GI) ones (abdominal fullness, flatulence, diarrhea, and constipation). Constipation is especially common, and a bowel program may be necessary to control this problem.

Contraindications

Cholestyramine is contraindicated in people with complete biliary obstruction, because bile is not secreted into the intestine.

The drug can bind with vitamin K; thus, use in people with any coagulopathy requires caution.

Nursing Implications

Preventing Interactions

Cholestyramine may decrease absorption of many oral medications (e.g., digoxin, folic acid, glipizide, propranolol, tetracyclines, thiazide diuretics, thyroid hormones, fat-soluble vitamins, and warfarin). Apparently, no drugs significantly affect cholestyramine. Herbs and foods that increase the effects of cholestyramine include fibers such as oat bran and pectin. No herbs and foods seem to decrease the effects of cholestyramine.

In a patient who is taking cholestyramine in addition to other drugs, dosage of the interactive drug may need to be changed when the bile acid sequestrant is added or withdrawn. Also, because cholestyramine binds bile acids, cholestyramine may interfere with normal fat digestion and absorption and therefore may prevent absorption of the fat-soluble vitamins A, D, E, and K.

Administering the Medication

It is necessary to mix cholestyramine powder with water or other fluids, soups, cereals, or fruits such as applesauce and to follow with more fluid. The nurse ensures that the drug is not taken in a dry form. It is essential that cholestyramine not be given with other drugs; to minimize altered absorption, people should take the other drugs 1 hour before or 4 to 6 hours after cholestyramine. Patients who take colestipol should swallow tablets whole, without cutting, crushing, or chewing.

TABLE 8.5

DRUGS AT A GLANCE: Bile Acid Sequestrants

Drug	Pregnancy Category	Type of Dyslipidemia	Routes and Dosage Ranges	
			Adults	**Children**
Ⓟ **Cholestyramine** (Prevalite, Questran)	C	IIa	PO tablets, 4 g once or twice daily initially, gradually increased at monthly intervals to 8–16 g daily in 2 divided doses. Maximum daily dose, 24 g PO powder, 4 g 1–6 times daily	240 mg/kg/d in 3 divided doses
Colesevelam (WelChol)	B	IIa	PO 3.75 g daily in 1 or 2 doses with meals. Maximum daily dose, 4.375 g	
Colestipol (Colestid)	C	IIa	PO tablets, 2 g once or twice daily initially, gradually increased at 1- to 2-mo intervals, up to 16 g daily PO granules, 5 g daily initially, gradually increased at 1- to 2-mo intervals, up to 30 g daily in single or divided doses	

Assessing for Therapeutic Effects

The nurse observes for decreased levels of total serum cholesterol, LDL cholesterol, and triglycerides and increased levels of HDL cholesterol. Maximum effects occur in approximately 1 month.

Assessing for Adverse Effects

The most common adverse effect is constipation. Other conditions relate to GI effects: abdominal discomfort or pain, nausea, vomiting, flatulence, diarrhea, anorexia, and steatorrhea. Increased bleeding tendencies may result from vitamin K malabsorption.

Patient Teaching

The nurse assesses the adequacy of levels of fat-soluble vitamins A, D, E, and K; supplementation may be required. Good dental hygiene is important because holding the mixture in the mouth can damage the teeth. Some products may contain aspartamine or sugar, so caution is necessary in patients with phenylketonuria or diabetes mellitus.

Also, the nurse teaches patients that these drugs are used mainly to reduce LDL cholesterol further in those who are already taking a statin drug. The inhibition of cholesterol synthesis by a statin drug makes bile acid–binding drugs more effective. In addition, the combination increases HDL cholesterol and can further reduce the risk of cardiovascular disorders. Box 8.6 contains more patient teaching information.

Other Drugs in the Class

In patients with elevated LDL cholesterol, colestipol may be used to reduce serum cholesterol. In digoxin toxicity, the drug may be used to decrease the serum half-life of digoxin. (This is an off-label use.)

Fibrates

Fibrates are derivatives of fibric acid and are similar to endogenous fatty acids. The first fibrate to be developed, clofibrate, has essentially been replaced by other fibrates and is not discussed. Therefore, Ⓟ **fenofibrate** (TriCor) serves as the prototype in this discussion.

Pharmacokinetics

Fenofibrate is administered orally and is highly protein-bound, primarily to albumin. Time to peak effect is 6 to 8 hours. Metabolism occurs in the liver and excretion is by urinary elimination.

Action

Fenofibrate and other fibrates increase the oxidation of fatty acids in liver and muscle tissue. Thus, they decrease hepatic production of triglycerides, decrease VLDL cholesterol, and increase HDL cholesterol.

Use

Fibrates are the most effective drugs for reducing serum triglyceride values, and their main indication for use is high serum triglyceride (greater than 500 mg/dL). They are also helpful for patients with low HDL cholesterol levels. Additionally, fibrates are the drug of choice for hypertriglyceridemia associated with diabetes, gout, gastritis, or ulcer disease (niacin may worsen these conditions). Investigators have not yet established the safety and efficacy of fibrates in children. There are no specific recommendations for use of these drugs in patients who are critically ill; drug interactions and adverse effects may restrict their use in critical illness.

TABLE 8.6

DRUGS AT A GLANCE: Fibrates

Drug	Pregnancy Category	Types of Dyslipidemia	Routes and Dosage Ranges Adults	Children
℗ **Fenofibrate** (TriCor)	C	IV, V (hypertriglyceridemia)	PO 48 mg once daily with meals increased if necessary to a maximum dose of 201 mg daily	
Gemfibrozil (Lopid)	C	IV, V (hypertriglyceridemia)	PO 1200 mg daily, in 2 divided doses, 30 min before morning and evening meals	

Table 8.6 presents dosage information for the fibrates.

Use in Older Adults

Caution is warranted with dosage determination. For fenofibrate, lower starting dosages are recommended (67 mg/d).

Use in Patients With Renal Impairment

As previously stated, fibrates are excreted mainly by the kidneys; therefore, they accumulate in the serum of patients with renal impairment. Fenofibrate is contraindicated in patients with severe renal impairment, and the recommended starting dose is 67 mg/d in patients with a creatinine clearance of less than 50 mL/min. It is necessary to evaluate the effects of this dose effects on renal function and to check triglyceride levels before increasing this dose. Fibrates may cause a reversible elevated serum creatinine. Patients with diabetes mellitus require close monitoring because renal disease is a serious complication in this population.

Use in Patients With Hepatic Impairment

Fibrates may cause hepatotoxicity. Abnormal elevations of serum aminotransferases have occurred with both gemfibrozil and fenofibrate, but they usually subside after the drug is discontinued. Contraindications to fenofibrate include severe hepatic impairment, including primary biliary cirrhosis, and persistent elevations in liver function tests and preexisting gallbladder disease. In addition, hepatitis (hepatocellular, chronic active, and cholestatic) has reportedly occurred after use of fenofibrate from a few weeks to several years. It is necessary to monitor liver function during the first year of drug administration. Discontinuation of the drug is warranted if elevated enzyme levels persist at more than three times the normal limit.

Use in Patients Receiving Home Care

Because liver enzyme tests are recommended, patients who are housebound may need assistance in obtaining blood tests (e.g., lipids, liver function tests). The nurse advises patients to notify their health care provider if unexplained muscle pain or tenderness occurs. Increasing availability of home cholesterol-monitoring devices will require additional patient teaching about technique and interpretation of the results.

Adverse Effects

The main adverse effects are GI discomfort and diarrhea, which may occur less often with fenofibrate than with other fibrates. Fibrates may also increase cholesterol concentration in the biliary tract and formation of gallstones.

Contraindications

Contraindications include a hypersensitivity to fibrates, hepatic or (severe) renal impairment, preexisting gallbladder disease, primary biliary cirrhosis, or persistent liver function abnormalities of unknown origin.

Nursing Implications

Preventing Interactions

Fenofibrate and other fibric acid derivatives may enhance the hypoprothrombinemic effect of warfarin-type oral anticoagulants, increasing the risk of bleeding. Patients receiving warfarin require a substantially decreased dosage of warfarin because fibrates displace warfarin from binding sites on serum albumin. Other drug–drug interactions are outlined in Box 8.7. No herbal interactions have been identified.

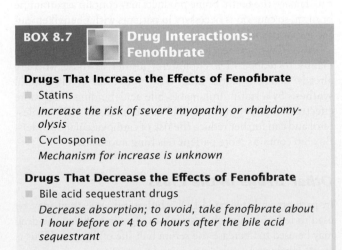

BOX 8.7 **Drug Interactions: Fenofibrate**

Drugs That Increase the Effects of Fenofibrate
- Statins
  Increase the risk of severe myopathy or rhabdomyolysis
- Cyclosporine
  Mechanism for increase is unknown

Drugs That Decrease the Effects of Fenofibrate
- Bile acid sequestrant drugs
  Decrease absorption; to avoid, take fenofibrate about 1 hour before or 4 to 6 hours after the bile acid sequestrant

Administering the Medication

It is necessary to give fenofibrate with food to increase drug absorption.

Assessing for Therapeutic Effects

The nurse assesses for decreased levels of total serum cholesterol, LDL cholesterol, and triglycerides and increased levels of HDL cholesterol. With fibrates, effects occur in approximately 1 month.

Assessing for Adverse Effects

GI disturbances as well as elevated liver function tests are common. Reportedly, hypersensitivity reactions, myopathy, rhabdomyolysis, blood dyscrasias, hepatotoxicity, cholelithiasis, cholestatic jaundice, pancreatitis, and reduced libido also occur, although these effects are rare. Risk of myopathy increases with concomitant use of statins.

Patient Teaching

The nurse instructs patients to report signs and symptoms of adverse effects to the health care provider. Throughout drug therapy, patients should have periodic blood tests. See Box 8.6 for general patient information.

Other Drugs in the Class

Gemfibrozil, rather than niacin, is usually preferred for people with diabetes because niacin increases blood sugar. It is necessary to give gemfibrozil on an empty stomach, about 30 minutes before the morning and evening meal.

Cholesterol Absorption Inhibitor

Ⓟ **Ezetimibe** (Zetia) is the prototype of the newest class of dyslipidemic drugs, which act in the small intestine to inhibit absorption of cholesterol and decrease the delivery of intestinal cholesterol to the liver, resulting in reduced hepatic cholesterol stores and increased clearance of cholesterol from the blood. This distinct mechanism is complementary to that of HMG-CoA reductase inhibitors, producing synergistic cholesterol-lowering effects when these drugs are used in combination. Ezetimibe reduces total cholesterol and triglycerides and increases HDL cholesterol.

Pharmacokinetics

Ezetimibe is significantly protein-bound, is metabolized in the small intestine and liver, and is excreted predominately in feces. The time to peak effect is 4 to 12 hours.

Action

Ezetimibe blocks biliary and dietary cholesterol absorption at the brush border of the intestine without affecting absorption of fat-soluble vitamins and triglycerides.

Use

Ezetimibe is used together with dietary management for treatment of primary dyslipidemia. It can be used as monotherapy on in combination with a statin. When given as monotherapy (without a statin), ezetimibe does not require dosage reduction in geriatric patients. Table 8.7 presents dosage information for the drug.

Use in Children

Safety and efficacy in children younger than 10 years of age have not been established.

Use in Patients With Hepatic Impairment

Dosage adjustment of ezetimibe is necessary in patients with mild hepatic impairment. The drug is not recommended in patients with moderate to severe hepatic impairment.

Adverse Effects

The most common adverse effects of ezetimibe include headache, diarrhea, hypersensitivity reactions such as rash, and nausea.

Contraindications

Contraindications include pregnancy and lactation. Additional contraindications are hypersensitivity to ezetimibe or concomitant use with a statin in people with active hepatic disease.

Nursing Implications

The nurse instructs patients to maintain a low-cholesterol diet during ezetimibe therapy. Patients should report side effects to their health care providers.

Preventing Interactions

Some medications interact with ezetimibe, increasing or decreasing its effect (Box 8.8). Apparently, no herbs interact with this drug.

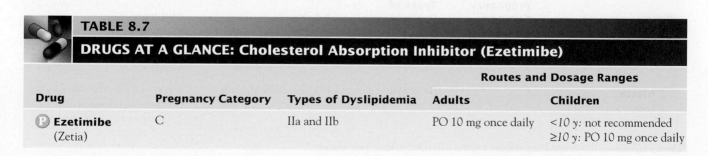

	TABLE 8.7				
	DRUGS AT A GLANCE: Cholesterol Absorption Inhibitor (Ezetimibe)				
				Routes and Dosage Ranges	
Drug	**Pregnancy Category**	**Types of Dyslipidemia**	**Adults**	**Children**
Ⓟ **Ezetimibe** (Zetia)	C	IIa and IIb	PO 10 mg once daily	<10 y: not recommended ≥10 y: PO 10 mg once daily

---

BOX 8.8   **Drug Interactions: Ezetimibe**

Drugs That Increase the Effects of Ezetimibe
- Cyclosporine
  Increases blood levels

Drugs That Decrease the Effects of Ezetimibe
- Bile acid sequestrant drugs
  Mechanism for decrease is unknown.

Administering the Medication

Ezetimibe may be administered with or without food. The patient takes the drug:

- At the same time each day
- At night if used in combination with a statin. (Ezetimibe may be given at the same time as a statin.)
- Either 2 hours before or 4 hours after bile sequestrants to prevent altered absorption

Assessing for Therapeutic Effects

The nurse monitors lipid response to therapy with ezetimibe. Desired results include decreases in total cholesterol, LDL cholesterol, and triglycerides, with increases in HDL cholesterol. A therapeutic response occurs within 2 weeks of initiation of therapy and lasts as long as the drug is continued.

Assessing for Adverse Effects

The nurse observes for headache, dizziness, fatigue, diarrhea, and abdominal pain.

Patient Teaching

The nurse instructs patients to report signs and symptoms of adverse effects to the health care provider. Throughout drug therapy, patients should have periodic blood tests. See Box 8.6 for general patient information.

Miscellaneous Dyslipidemic Agent

(P) **Niacin** (nicotinic acid) is a vitamin that decreases LDL and increases HDL cholesterol, and it serves as the prototype. Nicotinamide, another common form of niacin, does not have the lipid-lowering properties of nicotinic acid.

Pharmacokinetics

Niacin is rapidly absorbed from the GI tract, with peak effect in about 45 minutes. Minimal metabolism occurs through the liver, and the majority of the drug is excreted unchanged in the urine.

Action

Niacin inhibits mobilization of free fatty acids from peripheral tissues, thereby reducing hepatic synthesis of triglycerides and secretion of VLDL, which leads to decreased production of LDL cholesterol. The drug also raises HDL levels by reducing lipid transfer of cholesterol from HDL to VLDL and by delaying clearance of HDL.

Use

Niacin, the most effective drug for increasing the concentration of HDL cholesterol, is most helpful in preventing heart disease when used in combination with another dyslipidemic drug such as a bile acid sequestrant or a fibrate. Its use with a statin lowers serum LDL cholesterol more than either drug alone, but there are no studies of the niacin–statin combination for prevention of cardiovascular disease. No specific recommendations exist for use of niacin in patients who are critically ill, although drug interactions and adverse effects may restrict its use in these patients. Table 8.8 presents dosage information for this oral drug.

Use in Children

Niacin is a form of vitamin B_3. Although dose recommendations are available for children for the treatment of dyslipidemia, use of niacin in children is often aimed at preventing vitamin B_3 deficiency and related conditions such as pellagra.

TABLE 8.8

DRUGS AT A GLANCE: Miscellaneous Dyslipidemic Agent (Niacin)

			Routes and Dosage Ranges	
Drug[*]	**Pregnancy Category**	**Types of Dyslipidemia**	**Adults**	**Children**
(P) **Niacin** (immediate release)	C	II, III, IV, V	PO 2–6 g daily, in 3 or 4 divided doses, with or just after meals	PO 55–87 mg/kg/d, in 3 or 4 divided doses, with or just after meals
(P) **Niacin** (extended release)	C	IIa and IIb	PO 500–2000 mg daily	Safety and effectiveness of extended-release niacin therapy not established

[*]Do *not* substitute the immediate-release for the extended-release preparation.

Use in Older Adults

Although niacin is effective in older adults, these patients do not tolerate the adverse effects of the drug well.

Use in Patients With Renal Impairment

Niacin should be used with caution in patients with renal impairment.

Use in Patients With Hepatic Impairment

Niacin may cause hepatotoxicity; thus, it is contraindicated in patients with hepatic impairment.

Adverse Effects

Disadvantages of niacin are the high doses required for dyslipidemic effects and the subsequent adverse effects. Niacin commonly causes skin flushing, pruritus, and gastric irritation, and it may lead to tachycardia, hypotension, dizziness, hyperglycemia, hyperuricemia, elevated liver aminotransferases, and hepatitis.

Contraindications

Contraindications include hypersensitivity to niacin, active hepatic disease or unexplained hepatic dysfunction, or an active peptic ulcer.

Nursing Implications

Preventing Interactions

The efficacy of oral hypoglycemic agents and insulin may be diminished by niacin, which may affect glucose control. Box 8.9 outlines drug–drug interactions. Herbs and foods that increase the effects of niacin include red yeast rice, which increases the risk of severe myopathy or rhabdomyolysis.

Administering the Medication

Formulations of niacin (immediate release, timed release) are not interchangeable. It is necessary to give immediate-release niacin with meals because it may cause gastric irritation. In contrast, patients may take timed-release niacin without regard to meals.

Flushing may occur with niacin administration. This reaction can be reduced by starting with small doses, gradually increasing doses, taking doses with meals, and taking 325 mg of

aspirin about 30 minutes before or 200 mg of ibuprofen about 60 minutes prior to administering niacin.

Assessing for Therapeutic Effects

The nurse assesses for decreased levels of total serum cholesterol, LDL cholesterol, and triglycerides, as well as increased levels of HDL cholesterol. Effects occur in approximately 1 month.

Assessing for Adverse Effects

Flushing of the face and neck, pruritus, and skin rash may occur. Other adverse effects include tachycardia, hypotension, and dizziness.

Patient Teaching

The nurse tells patients that tablet strengths are not interchangeable and not to substitute immediate-release forms with long-acting ones. Patients should swallow sustained-release preparations whole. See Box 8.6 for general patient information.

Combination Therapy Used to Treat Dyslipidemia

When monotherapy is not effective in attaining target LDL cholesterol levels, combination therapies with lipid-lowering drugs that have different mechanisms of action are recommended. The combination drugs, which include a dyslipidemic agent, are listed in Table 8.9. In general, the drug combinations that are most effective in reducing total and LDL cholesterol are (1) a statin with a cholesterol absorption inhibitor or a bile acid sequestrant or (2) niacin with a bile acid sequestrant. When a goal of therapy is to increase the level of HDL cholesterol, a fibrate, cholesterol absorption inhibitor, or niacin may be used. However, a fibrate–statin combination should be avoided because of increased risks of severe myopathy, and a niacin–statin combination increases the risks of hepatotoxicity. Adverse reactions from combination statin and cholesterol absorption inhibitor therapy are reported to be similar to those from statins alone. Combination preparations are not intended

---

BOX 8.9   Drug Interactions: Niacin

Drugs That Increase the Effects of Niacin
- Alcohol
  Increases flushing
- Leflunomide
  Increases hepatotoxicity
- Statins, zidovudine
  Increase the risk of severe myopathy or rhabdomyolysis

Drugs That Decrease the Effects of Niacin
- Bile acid sequestrant drugs
  Mechanism for decrease is unknown.

TABLE 8.9

Fixed-Combination Dyslipidemic Agents

Trade Name	Fixed-Combination Drug
Advicor	Extended-release niacin (500, 750, and 1000 mg) and lovastatin (20 mg)
Pravigard	Buffered aspirin (81 or 325 mg) and pravastatin (20, 40, 80 mg)
Caduet	Amlodipine (5 or 10 mg) and atorvastatin (10, 20, 40, 80 mg)
Vytorin	Ezetimibe (10 mg) and simvastatin (10, 20, 40, 80 mg)
Simcor	Simvastatin (20 mg) and niacin (500, 750, and 1000 mg)

for initial therapy. The adverse effects and contraindications associated with individual drugs also apply when they are used in combination. All combinations, like individual preparations, should be used in conjunction with a cholesterol-reducing diet.

NCLEX Success

6. John Jones, a 47-year-old teacher, now takes cholestyramine, and the nurse teaches him about the medication and its use. The nurse should be concerned if after the teaching session, Mr. Jones states

   A. "I should take the medicine with a full glass of water when I take my other medications."

   B. "I am taking this medication to decrease my LDL cholesterol level."

   C. "I should swallow the tablets whole."

   D. "I may need to supplement my intake of the fat-soluble vitamins A, D, E, and K."

7. Karen James, a 32-year-old accountant with type 1 diabetes mellitus, is taking gemfibrozil to reduce her serum triglyceride level. She asks why she could not take niacin, as her husband does. The nurse responds

   A. "Either drug reduces triglycerides. Why don't you ask your nurse practitioner if the drug therapy could be changed?"

   B. "Gemfibrozil is the only drug recommended for use to lower cholesterol."

   C. "Niacin therapy is not recommended for use in women."

   D. "Niacin increases blood glucose levels and is not preferred for people with diabetes."

8. A woman is taking niacin (nicotinic acid) to decrease both her cholesterol and her triglycerides. In counseling her about taking this medication, the nurse explains that flushing, a common adverse effect of niacin therapy, can be decreased by

   A. taking half the dose in the morning and half the dose at night

   B. taking 325 mg aspirin 30 minutes before the niacin

   C. taking the drug on an empty stomach

   D. taking niacin as monotherapy for dyslipidemia

The Nursing Process

Assessment

Assess the patient's status in relation to atherosclerotic vascular disease.

- **Identify risk factors:**
  - Hypertension
  - Diabetes mellitus
  - High intake of dietary fat and refined sugars
  - Obesity
  - Inadequate exercise
  - Cigarette smoking
  - Family history of atherosclerotic disorders
  - Dyslipidemia

- **Signs and symptoms depend on the specific problem:**
  - Dyslipidemia is manifested by elevated serum cholesterol (>200 mg/100 mL), triglycerides (>150 mg/100 mL), or both.
  - Coronary artery atherosclerosis is manifested by myocardial ischemia (angina pectoris, myocardial infarction).
  - Cerebrovascular insufficiency may be manifested by syncope, memory loss, transient ischemic attacks (TIAs), or strokes. Impairment of blood flow to the brain is caused primarily by atherosclerosis in the carotid, vertebral, or cerebral arteries.
  - Peripheral arterial insufficiency is manifested by impaired blood flow in the legs (weak or absent pulses; cool, pale extremities; intermittent claudication; leg pain at rest; and development of gangrene, usually in the toes because they are most distal to blood supply). This condition results from atherosclerosis in the distal abdominal aorta, the iliac arteries, and the femoral and smaller arteries in the legs.

Nursing Diagnoses

- Ineffective tissue perfusion related to interruption of arterial blood flow
- Imbalanced nutrition: more than body requirements of fats and calories
- Anxiety related to risks of atherosclerotic cardiovascular disease
- Disturbed body image related to the need for lifestyle changes
- Noncompliance related to dietary restrictions and adverse drug reactions
- Deficient knowledge related to drug and diet therapy of dyslipidemia

Planning/Goals

The patient will:

- Take lipid-lowering drugs as prescribed
- Decrease dietary intake of saturated fats and cholesterol
- Lose weight if obese and maintain the lower weight
- Have periodic measurements of blood lipids
- Avoid preventable adverse drug effects
- Receive positive reinforcement for efforts to lower blood lipid levels
- Feel less anxious and more in control as risks of atherosclerotic cardiovascular disease are decreased

Nursing Interventions

The nurse will:

- Help patients control risk factors. Ideally, primary prevention begins in childhood with healthful eating habits (e.g., avoiding excessive fats, meat, and dairy products; obtaining adequate amounts of all nutrients, including dietary fiber; avoiding obesity), exercise, and avoiding cigarette smoking. However, changing habits to a more healthful lifestyle is helpful at any time, before or after disease manifestations appear. Weight loss often reduces blood lipids and lipoproteins to a normal range. Changing habits is difficult for most people, even those with severe symptoms.
- Use measures to increase blood flow to tissues:

- Exercise is helpful in developing collateral circulation in the heart and legs. Collateral circulation involves use of secondary vessels in response to tissue ischemia related to obstruction of the principal vessels. Patients with angina pectoris or previous myocardial infarction require a carefully planned and supervised program of progressive exercise. Those with peripheral arterial insufficiency usually can increase exercise tolerance by walking regularly. Distances should be determined by occurrence of pain and must be individualized.
- Posture and position may be altered to increase blood flow to the legs in patients with peripheral arterial insufficiency. Elevating the head of the bed and having the legs horizontal or dependent may help. Elevating the feet is usually contraindicated unless edema is present or likely to develop.
- Although drug therapy is being increasingly used to prevent or manage atherosclerotic disorders, a major therapeutic option for management of occlusive vascular disease is surgical removal of atherosclerotic plaque or revascularization procedures. Thus, severe angina pectoris may be relieved by a coronary artery bypass procedure that detours blood flow around occluded vessels. This procedure also may be done after a myocardial infarction. The goal is to prevent infarction or reinfarction. TIAs may be relieved by carotid endarterectomy; the goal is to prevent a stroke. Peripheral arterial insufficiency may be relieved by aortofemoral, femoropopliteal, or other bypass grafts that detour around occluded vessels. Although these procedures increase blood flow to ischemic tissues, they do not halt progression of atherosclerosis.
- The nursing role in relation to these procedures is to provide excellent preoperative and postoperative nursing care to promote healing, prevent infection, maintain patency of grafts, and help the patient to achieve optimum function.
- Provide appropriate teaching related to drug therapy (see Box 8.6).
- Any dyslipidemic drug therapy must be accompanied by an appropriate diet; refer patients to a nutritionist. Overeating or gaining weight may decrease or cancel the lipid-lowering effects of the drugs.
- Encourage adult patients to have their serum cholesterol level measured at least once every 5 years. Adults and children with a personal or family history of dyslipidemia or other risk factors should be tested more often.
- The most effective measures for preventing dyslipidemia and atherosclerosis are those related to a healthful lifestyle (e.g., diet low in cholesterol and saturated fats, weight control, exercise).
- Help patients and family members understand the desirability of lowering high blood lipid levels before serious cardiovascular diseases develop.

Evaluation

- Observe for decreased blood levels of total and LDL cholesterol and triglycerides; observe for increased levels of HDL cholesterol.
- Observe and interview regarding compliance with instructions for drug, diet, and other therapeutic measures.
- Observe and interview regarding adverse drug effects.
- Validate the patient's ability to identify foods high and low in cholesterol and saturated fats.

Key Concepts

- Unless a person has a genetic disorder of lipid metabolism, the amount of cholesterol in the blood is strongly related to dietary intake of saturated fat.
- For accurate interpretation of a patient's lipid profile, blood samples for laboratory testing of triglycerides should be drawn after the patient has fasted for 12 hours. Fasting is not required for cholesterol testing.
- Metabolic syndrome is a group of cardiovascular risk factors linked with obesity that include elevated waist circumference (central adiposity), elevated triglycerides, reduced high-density lipoprotein cholesterol, elevated blood pressure, and elevated fasting glucose.
- Lifestyle changes that can help improve cholesterol levels include a low-fat diet, regular aerobic exercise, losing weight, and not smoking.
- The HMG-CoA reductase inhibitors (statins) are the most effective dyslipidemic agents for improving clinical outcomes when used for primary and secondary prevention of cardiovascular disease.
- Take lovastatin with food; take fluvastatin, pravastatin, or simvastatin in the evening, with or without food; atorvastatin can be taken with or without food and without regard to time of day.
- Skin flushing may occur with niacin.
- Fibrates are the most effective drugs for reducing serum triglyceride levels.

Critical Thinking Questions

8-1. Jason Smith is recently seen in college health services with the following lipid profile: total serum cholesterol 278 mg/dL, LDL cholesterol 210 mg/dL, HDL cholesterol 38 mg/dL, and triglycerides 150 mg/dL.

* What are the main nonpharmacologic measures to decrease total and LDL cholesterol and serum triglycerides and increase HDL cholesterol?
* What is the goal of management of dyslipidemia?

References and Resources

The ACCORD investigators. (2010). Effects of combination lipid therapy in type 2 diabetes mellitus. *The New England Journal of Medicine, 362,* 1563–1574.

American Academy of Pediatrics. (1992). National Cholesterol Education Program: Report of the Expert Panel on Blood Cholesterol Levels in Children and Adolescents. *Pediatrics, 89,* 525–584.

Brugts, J. J. (2010). Statin prescription in men and women at cardiovascular risk: To whom and when? *Current Opinions in Cardiology, 25*(5), 484–489.

Elesber, A. A. (2007). Coronary endothelial dysfunction and hyperlipidemia are independently associated with diastolic dysfunction in humans. *American Heart Journal, 153,* 1081–1087.

Johnston, N. (2006). Improved identification of patients with coronary artery disease by the use of new lipid and lipoprotein biomarkers. *American Journal of Cardiology, 97,* 640–645.

Kasiske, B. L. (2006). An assessment of statin safety by nephrologists. *American Journal of Cardiology, 97,* 82C–85C.

Magnussen, C. G., Raitakari, O. T., Thomson, R., Juonala, M., Patel, D. A., Viikari, J. S. A., et al. (2008). Utility of currently recommended pediatric dyslipidemia classifications in predicting dyslipidemia in adulthood: Evidence from the Childhood Determinants of Adult Health (CDAH) Study, Cardiovascular Risk in Young Finns Study, and Bogalusa Heart Study. *Circulation, 117,* 32–42.

McCrindle, B. W., Urbina, E. M., Dennison, B. A., et al. (2007). Drug therapy of high-risk lipid abnormalities in children and adolescents: a scientific statement from the American Heart Association atherosclerosis, hypertension,

and obesity in youth committee, council of cardiovascular disease in the young, with the council on cardiovascular nursing. *Circulation, 115,* 1948–1967.

McCrindle, B. W., Urbina, E. M., Dennison, B. A., Jacobson, M. S., Steinberger, J., Rocchini, A. P., et al. (2007). Drug therapy of high-risk lipid abnormalities in children and adolescents: A scientific statement from the American Heart Association Atherosclerosis, Hypertension, and Obesity in Youth Committee, Council of Cardiovascular Disease in the Young, with the Council on Cardiovascular Nursing. *Circulation, 115,* 1948–1967.

National Institutes of Health Expert Panel. (2001). Third report of the National Cholesterol Education Program (NCEP) Expert Panel on Detection, Evaluation, and Treatment of High Blood Cholesterol in Adults (Adult Treatment Panel III) (NIH Publication No. 01-3670). Bethesda, MD: National Institutes of Health.

Porth, C. M. (2009). *Pathophysiology: Concepts of altered health status* (8th ed.). Philadelphia, PA: Lippincott Williams & Wilkins.

Ray, K. K., Seshasai, S. R., Erqou, S., Sever, P., Julema, J. W., Ford, I., et al. (2010). Statins and all-cause mortality in high-risk primary prevention: A meta-analysis of 11 randomized controlled trials involving 65,229 participants. *Archives of Internal Medicine, 170*(12), 1024–1031.

Reilly, T., King, G., Park, J. H., & Tracy, A. (2010). Pitavastatin (Livalo) for hyperlipidemia and mixed dyslipidemia a novel therapeutic agent, or a 'Me-Too' drug? *Pharmacy and Therapeutics. 35*(4), 197–198, 204–207.

Zappalla, F. R. (2009). Lipid Management in Children. *Endocrinology and Metabolism Clinics of North America, 38*(1), 171–183.

9

Drug Therapy for Hematopoietic Disorders and to Enhance Immunity

LEARNING OBJECTIVES

After studying this chapter, you should be able to:

1. Briefly describe hematopoietic and immune functions.

2. Identify common clinical manifestations of inadequate erythropoiesis and diminished host defense mechanisms.

3. Discuss characteristics of hematopoietic drugs in terms of the prototype, mechanism of action, indications for use, adverse effects, principles of therapy, and nursing implications.

4. Describe the characteristics of colony-stimulating factors in terms of the prototype, mechanism of action, indications for use, adverse effects, principles of therapy, and nursing implications.

5. Discuss interferons in terms of the prototype, mechanism of action, indications for use, adverse effects, principles of therapy, and nursing implications.

6. Implement the nursing process in the care of patients who take drugs to enhance hematopoietic and immune system function.

Clinical Application Case Study

Alice Paul is a 76-year-old woman who is being treated with chemotherapy for inoperable liver cancer. She receives a combination chemotherapy regimen every 6 weeks. She is in the oncologist's office for routine laboratory work 10 days after chemotherapy and complains of severe fatigue. The results of her blood work are: hemoglobin 10.9 g/dL, hematocrit 32%, white blood cell count 2000 cells/mm^3, absolute neutrophil count 800 cells/mm^3, and platelet count 120,000/microliter.

KEY TERMS

Biologic response modifiers: intrinsic and extrinsic substances in the body that enhance the body's response to infection, for example, interferons

Cytokines: small proteins released by cells that specifically affect cell-to-cell communication; these include colony-stimulating factors, interleukins, and interferons

Erythropoiesis: production of red blood cells

Erythropoietin: hormone secreted by the kidneys that stimulates bone marrow production of red blood cells

Hematopoiesis: formation of blood cells

Immunostimulants: drugs that stimulate immune function to fight infection and disease

Neutropenia: low neutrophil count

Pegylation: process of modifying a protein drug by treatment with polyethylene glycol

Introduction

Adequate blood cell production, or **hematopoiesis**, and normal immune system function, or immunocompetence, are vital processes in the human body's ability to fight harmful invaders. Inadequate or impaired hematopoiesis or immune function (immunodeficiency) leads to high risks of infection and cancer. Efforts to enhance a person's own body systems to fight disease include the development of drugs to stimulate hematopoiesis and immune function. People take these drugs to restore normal function or to increase the ability of the immune system to eliminate potentially harmful invaders. This chapter discusses several drugs that affect hematopoietic function and the immune system.

Overview of Hematopoiesis and Immune Function

Hematopoietic and immune blood cells originate in bone marrow in stem cells, which are often called pluripotent stem cells because they are capable of becoming different types of cells. As these stem cells reproduce, some cells are exactly like the original cells and are retained in the bone marrow to maintain a continuing supply. However, most reproduced stem cells differentiate to form other types of cells. The early offspring are committed to become a particular type of cell, and a committed stem cell that produces a cell type in a specific cell line is called a colony-forming unit (CFU). Figure 9.1 illustrates the process of hematopoiesis in red and white cells. Hematopoietic growth factors or cytokines control the reproduction, growth, and differentiation of stem cells and CFUs. They also initiate the processes required to produce fully mature cells. Overall, cytokines are involved in numerous physiologic responses, including hematopoiesis, cellular proliferation and differentiation, inflammation, wound healing, and cellular and humoral immunity.

Physiology

Hematopoietic Cytokines

To understand the effects of drug therapy to enhance hematopoiesis or immune function, it is necessary to appreciate the physiologic effects of the endogenous hematopoietic **cytokines**. The following section discusses the three major groups of cytokines, and it briefly considers erythropoiesis and immune function as well.

Hematopoietic cytokines are diverse substances produced mainly by bone marrow and white blood cells (WBCs). They regulate many cellular activities by acting as chemical messengers among cells and as growth factors for blood cells. Cytokines act by binding to receptors on target cells. After binding, the cytokine–receptor complexes trigger signal-transduction pathways that alter gene expression in the target cells.

Several factors affect cytokine actions and functions. First, cytokines affect any cells they encounter that have cytokine receptors and are able to respond; they do not act in response to specific antigens. However, cytokine receptors are often expressed on a cell only after that cell has interacted with an antigen, so that cytokine activation is limited to antigen-activated lymphocytes. Second, researchers have determined the actions of most cytokines in laboratories by analyzing the effects of recombinant cytokines, often at nonphysiologic concentrations, and then adding them individually to in vitro systems. Within the human body, however, cytokines rarely, if ever, act alone. Several cytokines, which may have synergistic or antagonistic effects on each other, may affect a target cell. Third, cytokines often induce the synthesis of other cytokines. The resulting interactions may profoundly alter physiologic responses. Fourth, proteins that act as cytokine antagonists are found in the bloodstream and other extracellular fluids. These proteins may bind directly to a cytokine and inhibit its activity or bind to a cytokine receptor but fail to activate the cell.

Colony-Stimulating Factors

The name *colony-stimulating factor* (CSF) comes from the cluster pattern derived when hemopoietic stem cells are cultured. There are various types of CSFs based on the different types of colonies that grow in the presence of different factors. For example, the substance found to stimulate formation of colonies of granulocytes is called granulocyte colony-stimulating factor (G-CSF) and for macrophages, it is called macrophage colony-stimulating factor (M-CSF). The exposure of pluripotent (progenitor) cells to CSFs controls the production, growth, and differentiation of specific blood cell types. CSFs pertinent to this discussion include those related to the production of red blood cells (RBCs) and leukocyte stem cells.

Interferons

Interferons "interfere" with the ability of viruses in infected cells to replicate and spread to uninfected cells. They also inhibit reproduction and growth of other cells, including tumor cells, and activate natural killer (NK) cells. Interferons enhance communication between cells when antigens or tumors are identified. These antiproliferative and immunomodulatory activities are important in normal host defense mechanisms. Interferons also combat bacterial and parasitic infections.

Interleukins

Interleukins (ILs) initially received their name because scientists thought they were produced by and acted only on leukocytes. However, body cells other than leukocytes can produce

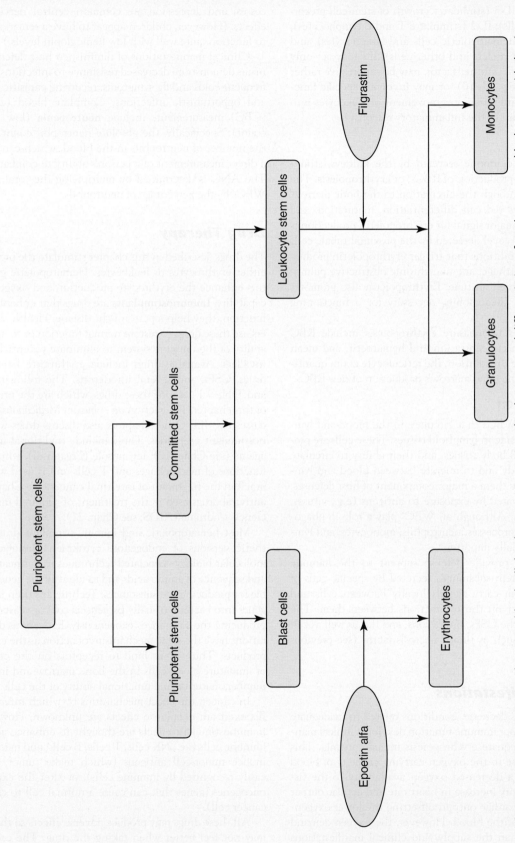

Figure 9.1 Hematopoietic and immune blood cell development. Formation, development, and differentiation of erythrocytes and leukocytes, with the site of effects of selected prototype drugs.

them, and they can act on nonhematopoietic cells. Researchers have characterized 18 ILs and identified more. Especially important ILs are IL-3 (stimulates growth of stem-cell precursors of all blood cells), IL-2 (stimulates T and B lymphocytes), IL-12 (stimulates hematopoietic cells and lymphocytes), and IL-11 (stimulates platelets and other cells). ILs may act only in combination with another factor, may be suppressive rather than stimulatory (e.g., IL-10), or may involve a specific function (e.g., IL-8 mainly promotes movement of leukocytes into injured tissues as part of the inflammatory response).

Erythropoiesis

Erythropoietin, a hormone secreted by the kidneys, stimulates bone marrow production of RBCs, or **erythropoiesis**. The hormone travels through the circulation to the bone marrow, where it stimulates red cell differentiation, maturation, and proliferation. The major signal for erythropoietin production is a decreased oxygen level detected by the proximal tubule cells in the kidneys. Conditions that trigger erythropoietin production include hemorrhage, anemia, chronic obstructive pulmonary disease, and high altitude. Erythropoietin also promotes the production of hemoglobin, necessary for a functioning erythrocyte.

Parameters used to measure erythropoiesis include RBC count, hemoglobin concentration and hematocrit, and mean corpuscular volume. In addition, the reticulocyte count quantitatively measures the bone marrow's production of new RBCs.

Immune Function

Immune cells are WBCs that circulate in the blood and lymphatic vessels or reside in lymphoid tissues. These cells are present in virtually all body tissues, and their ability to circulate throughout the body and to migrate between blood and lymphoid tissues makes them a major component of host defenses. The cells are activated by exposure to antigens (e.g., viruses, bacteria, parasites). Although all WBCs play a role in phagocytic and immune processes, neutrophils, monocytes, and lymphocytes are especially important.

Cytokines also provide defense support to the immune system. These protein substances secreted by specific cells of the immune system carry signals locally between cells and thus have an effect on the interactions between them. The cytokines include the CSFs, interferons, and ILs, as well as cell signal molecules, such as tumor necrosis factor (see previous discussion).

Clinical Manifestations

As RBCs or WBCs decrease, conditions related to inadequate hematopoiesis or poor immune function develop. Clinical manifestations of inadequate erythropoiesis include anemia. This results in a decrease in the oxygen-carrying capacity of blood and consequently a decreased oxygen availability to the tissues. A compensatory increase in heart rate and cardiac output initially increases cardiac output, offsetting the lower oxygen-carrying capacity of the blood. However, the oxygen demand becomes greater than the supply, and clinical manifestations are directly attributable to tissue hypoxia. Muscle weakness and easy fatigability are common. In severe anemia, the skin is usually pale to a waxy pallor, and cyanosis is typically absent. Headache, irritability, light-headedness, slowed thought processes, and depression are common central nervous system effects. (However, children appear to have a remarkable ability to function quite well with low hemoglobin levels.)

Clinical manifestations of diminished host defense mechanisms demonstrate decreased resistance to infections, including frequent colds and flu symptoms, recurring parasitic infections, and opportunistic infections. Complete blood (cell) count (CBC) measurements include **neutropenia** (low neutrophil count). Specifically, the absolute neutrophil count (ANC) is the number of neutrophils in the blood, which can be used as a direct measurement of a person's ability to combat infection. The ANC is determined by multiplying the total number of WBCs by the percentage of neutrophils.

Drug Therapy

The drugs described in this chapter stimulate the production of either erythrocytes or leukocytes. Hematopoietic growth factors enhance the erythrocyte production and oxygen-carrying capability. **Immunostimulants** are drugs that enhance immune function; they help a person fight disease. Health care providers use these drugs to restore normal function or to increase the ability of the immune system to eliminate potentially harmful invaders. Available drugs include erythrocyte hematopoietic drugs, CSFs, and several interferons. The following sections and Table 9.1 describe these drugs, which are the primary focus of this chapter. The section on *Adjuvant Medications* briefly discusses two ILs. Other chapters also discuss drugs with immunostimulant properties. These include traditional immunizing agents (see Chap. 10); levamisole (Ergamisol), which restores functions of macrophages and T cells and is used with fluorouracil in the treatment of intestinal cancer (see Chap. 12); and antiviral drugs used in the treatment of acquired immunodeficiency syndrome (AIDS; see Chap. 21).

Most hematopoietic and immunostimulant drugs are synthetic versions of endogenous cytokines. Manufacturers use molecular biology–associated techniques to delineate the type and sequence of amino acids and to identify the genes responsible for producing the substances. Technicians then insert these genes into bacteria (usually *Escherichia coli*) or yeasts capable of producing the substances exogenously. Exogenous drug preparations have the same mechanisms of action as the endogenous products. Thus, CSFs bind to receptors on the cell surfaces of immature blood cells in the bone marrow and increase the number, maturity, and functional ability of the cells.

In cancer, the exact mechanisms by which interferons and ILs exert antineoplastic effects are unknown. However, their immunostimulant effects are thought to enhance activities of immune cells (i.e., NK cells, T cells, B cells, and macrophages), induce tumor-cell antigens (which make tumor cells more easily recognized by immune cells), or alter the expression of oncogenes (genes that can cause a normal cell to change to a cancer cell).

All these drugs may produce adverse effects so that patients may not feel better when taking the drug. The combination of injections and adverse effects may lead to nonadherence in taking the drugs as prescribed.

TABLE 9.1

Drugs Administered for Hematopoiesis and Immunostimulation

Drug Class	Prototype(s)	Other Drugs in the Class
Erythrocyte hematopoietic drugs	Epoetin alfa (Epogen, Procrit)	Darbepoetin alfa (Aranesp)
Colony-stimulating factors	Filgrastim (G-CSF) (Neupogen)	Pegfilgrastim (G-CSF) (Neulasta) Sargramostim (GM-CSF) (Leukine)
Interferons	Interferon alfa-2b (Intron A)	Peginterferon alfa-2a (Pegasys) Peginterferon alfa-2b (PEG-Intron) Interferon alfa-2a (Roferon-A) Interferon alfacon-1 (Infergen) Interferon beta-1a (Avonex, Rebif) Interferon beta-1b (Betaseron) Interferon gamma-1b (Actimmune)

G-CSF, granulocyte–colony-stimulating factor; GM-CSF, granulocyte macrophage–colony-stimulating factor.

Erythrocyte Hematopoietic Drugs

The hematopoietic growth factor ℗ **epoetin alfa** (Epogen, Procrit) is the prototype recombinant form of human erythropoietin that helps the body make more RBCs. The clinical benefit of erythropoiesis-stimulating drug therapy is to reduce the cost of blood transfusions, lessen the risk of infectious diseases from transfusions, and enhance the overall quality of life as anemia is relieved.

Pharmacokinetics

Both subcutaneous and intravenous (IV) administration lead to good absorption (digestive enzymes would destroy the drug if it were given orally). The distribution is unknown, and metabolism occurs in the plasma. Excretion of a small amount occurs in the kidneys. The onset of action is 11 to 14 days. Whether the drug crosses the placenta or is excreted in breast milk is not known.

Action

Epoetin induces erythropoiesis by stimulating erythroid progenitor cells. This causes the release of reticulocytes from the bone marrow, leading to an increase in hemoglobin and hematocrit levels.

Use

Uses of epoetin include the prevention and treatment of anemia associated with chronic renal failure, hepatic impairment, or anticancer chemotherapy. Prescribers also may order the drug to reduce the need for blood transfusions in patients with anemia undergoing elective noncardiac, nonvascular surgery. Table 9.2 presents route and dosage information for the hematopoietic drugs.

Use in Children

The basis for epoetin dosing in children is body weight and hemoglobin level.

TABLE 9.2

DRUGS AT A GLANCE: Erythrocyte Hematopoietic Drugs

Drug	Pregnancy Category	Routes and Dosage Ranges*
℗ **Epoetin alfa** (Epogen, Procrit)	C	Chronic renal failure: Adults, 50–100 units/kg IV, Sub-Q 3 times weekly to achieve or maintain hemoglobin level of no more than 12 g/dL 1 mo to 12 y, 50 units/kg IV, Sub-Q 3 times a week Cancer chemotherapy: Adults, 150–300 units/kg Sub-Q 3 times weekly 1 mo to 12 y, 600 units/kg IV, Sub-Q once a week Surgery: 300 units/kg/d Sub-Q for 10 d before surgery, on the day of surgery, and for 4 d after surgery
Darbepoetin alfa (Aranesp)	C	Sub-Q, IV 0.45 mcg/kg once weekly, adjusted to achieve and maintain hemoglobin level no >12 g/dL

*Adult dosage unless age is specified.

Use in Older Adults

In general, hematopoietic drugs have the same uses and responses in older adults as in younger adults. However, older adults may be at greater risk of adverse effects, especially if large doses are used.

Use in Patients With Critical Illness

Patients with cancer often take epoetin to prevent or treat anemia. Studies indicate that patients with cancer-related anemia feel better and require fewer blood transfusions when hemoglobin is maintained at 10 g/dL or less. Despite the benefits, evidence indicates that this drug may stimulate tumor growth, mainly when it is used to achieve normal hemoglobin levels of 12 to 14 g/dL. As a result, authorities warn prescribers to avoid dosages that increase hemoglobin to above 12 g/dL. In addition, because cancer-related anemia may have numerous causes, some experts recommend a return to the original indication for use of these drugs in cancer (i.e., for anemia induced by chemotherapy that depresses bone marrow function).

Use in Patients Receiving Home Care

Patients often take epoetin in the home, whether self-administered or given by a caregiver. The home health nurse may need to teach patients or caregivers how to accurately administer the drug and provide assistance in obtaining appropriate laboratory tests (e.g., CBC, platelet count, tests of renal or hepatic function) to monitor the responses to the drug.

Adverse Effects

The most common adverse effect of epoetin is hypertension; raising the hemoglobin slowly minimizes this. Other adverse effects include nausea, vomiting, diarrhea, and arthralgias.

In addition, injection of epoetin alfa increases the risk of thrombus formation. The U.S. Food and Drug Administration (FDA) has issued a **BLACK BOX WARNING** ◆ advising prescribers to avoid using hematopoietic growth factors in patients with hemoglobin values of 12 g/dL or above. In addition, it is important to prescribe epoetin at the lowest dose effective in raising hemoglobin levels just enough to avoid the need for blood transfusion. Regular monitoring of hemoglobin levels is necessary until they stabilize.

Contraindications

Contraindications to epoetin include known hypersensitivity to the drug or to albumin (or other cell-derived products from mammals). Also, people with uncontrolled hypertension should not take epoetin because it may further increase blood pressure.

EVIDENCE-BASED PRACTICE

Efficacy and Safety of Epoetin Alfa in Critically Ill Patients

by CORWIN, H. L., GETTINGER, A., FABIAN, T. C., MAY, A., PEARL, R. G., HEARD, S., AN, R., BOWERS, P. J., BURTON, P., KLAUSNER, M. A., AND CORWIN, M. J., FOR THE EPO CRITICAL CARE TRIALS GROUP

New England Journal of Medicine
2007, 357, 965–976

In this prospective, randomized, double blind, placebo-controlled, multicenter trial, investigators evaluated the efficacy of epoetin alfa in reducing the need of packed red blood cell (PRBC) transfusions in critically ill trauma patients. Patients in the study group received epoetin alfa 40,000 units subcutaneously on study days 1, 8, and 15 (if the hemoglobin level was greater than 12 gm/dL at the time of administration). Those in the placebo group received a placebo injection on the same schedule. All patients received iron supplements. The amount of ordered blood products, which was not reduced, did not reflect the transfusion benefit previously demonstrated with the use of epoetin alfa in other randomized control trials. However, hemoglobin levels at day 29 and again at day 140 were greater in the epoetin alfa group than in the placebo group. An increased risk of blood clots was present in the study group receiving epoetin alfa.

IMPLICATIONS FOR NURSING PRACTICE: The use of epoetin alfa does not reduce the incidence of PRBC transfusions in critically ill patients but may reduce mortality in patients with trauma. Because the risk of thrombosis is greater with the use of epoetin alfa, measures to prevent and assess the risk of thrombosis should be a nursing intervention in patients who receive the drug.

Nursing Implications

Preventing Interactions

No significant interactions with drugs or herbs with epoetin have been reported.

Administering the Medication

For patients with chronic renal failure on hemodialysis, the nurse gives epoetin by bolus injection at the end of dialysis. For other patients with an IV line, IV administration is appropriate. For patients without an IV line or who are ambulatory, subcutaneous administration is suitable. The nurse ensures that the remainder of a multidose vial is discarded 21 days after opening.

Assessing for Therapeutic Effects

The nurse observes for increased RBCs, hemoglobin, and hematocrit; increased energy and exercise capacity; and improved quality of life. Therapeutic effects depend on the dose and the patient's underlying condition. The goal is usually to achieve and maintain a hemoglobin level of no more than 12 g/dL. With epoetin, it is necessary to measure iron stores (transferrin saturation and serum ferritin) before and periodically during treatment. The nurse ensures that hemoglobin levels are measured twice weekly until stabilized and maintenance drug doses are established.

Assessing for Adverse Effects

The nurse ascertains that blood pressure remains within a safe range and also assesses for nausea, vomiting, diarrhea, or joint pain. Because there is an increased risk of myocardial infarction and stroke, assessment of mental status changes and chest pain or decreased cardiac perfusion is necessary.

QSEN Safety Alert

In addition, it is important to assess for signs of deep-vein thrombus formation (e.g., swelling, pain, and redness of the affected limb) in patients taking epoetin.

Patient Teaching

QSEN Safety Alert

Epoetin is not effective unless sufficient iron is present; therefore, patient teaching may need to emphasize the importance of taking an iron supplement.

Box 9.1 presents additional patient teaching guidelines for this drug.

Other Drugs in the Class

Darbepoetin alfa (Aranesp) is another erythrocyte hematopoietic agent. Uses include the prevention or treatment of anemia associated with several conditions, including chronic renal failure and myelosuppressive (depressed bone marrow function) anticancer chemotherapy. The absorption of this drug is slow via the subcutaneous route, and in renal failure, peak plasma levels occur in adults in about 48 hours (36 hours in children). In cancer, the time to peak plasma levels is 74 hours (49 hours in children). Hemoglobin levels increase after 2 to 6 weeks of therapy with darbepoetin. Studies indicate that a patient with cancer-related anemia and hemoglobin of 10 g/dL or less feels better and requires fewer blood transfusions with use of the drug. No significant interactions have reportedly occurred with this drug. As with epoetin, an adequate intake of iron is required for drug effectiveness, and an iron supplement is usually necessary.

Clinical Application 9-1

- What is the significance of Mrs. Paul's laboratory results?

NCLEX Success

1. Patients with chronic renal failure benefit from epoetin alfa (Epogen, Procrit) because the drug
   A. metabolizes the hormone that interferes with red blood cell (RBC) production
   B. neutralizes accumulating waste products in the kidney that destroy circulating RBCs
   C. replaces erythropoietin no longer produced in the proximal tubules of the kidney
   D. increases the kidney's excretion of toxic substances that decrease RBC production

2. The expected outcome of administering epoetin alfa (Epogen, Procrit) or darbepoetin alfa (Aranesp) to a patient with chronic renal failure is
   A. decreased bleeding
   B. increased white blood cell production
   C. increased red blood cell production
   D. improved renal function

3. The nurse who is administering epoetin alfa (Epogen, Procrit) knows that most patients who take epoetin alfa or darbepoetin alfa (Aranesp) also need to take
   A. iron
   B. potassium
   C. antacids
   D. analgesics

Granulocyte Colony-Stimulating Factors

The drug Ⓟ **filgrastim** (Neupogen) is the prototype G-CSF used to stimulate blood cell production by the bone marrow in patients with bone marrow transplantation or chemotherapy-induced neutropenia. This drug can help prevent infection by reducing the incidence, severity, and duration of neutropenia associated with several chemotherapy regimens. Health care providers also use it to collect stem cells for transplantation. Experts believe that filgrastim promotes the growth of arterioles around blocked areas in coronary arteries. It may be more effective than drugs that stimulate capillary growth, because arterioles are larger and can carry more blood.

Pharmacokinetics

Filgrastim is completely absorbed. The duration of action of the drug is 4 days. It is systemically degraded, and the nature of its excretion is unknown. There is no evidence of drug accumulation over a period of 11 to 20 days. Filgrastim crosses the placenta and may enter breast milk.

Action

Filgrastim stimulates the production, maturation, and activation of neutrophils within bone marrow.

BOX 9.1   Patient Teaching Guidelines for Hematopoietic Drugs and Immunostimulants

General Considerations

■ Help your body maintain immune mechanisms and other defenses by healthy lifestyle habits, such as a nutritious diet, adequate rest and sleep, and avoidance of tobacco and alcohol.

■ Practice meticulous personal hygiene and avoid people and circumstances in which you are exposed to infection.

■ Keep appointments with health care providers for follow-up care, blood tests, and so forth.

■ Inform any other physician, dentist, or health care provider about your condition and the medications you are taking.

■ It is possible to administer several of these medications at home, even though they are given by injection. If you are going to self-inject a medication at home, allow sufficient time to learn and practice the techniques under the supervision of a health care provider. Correct preparation and injection are necessary to increase beneficial effects and decrease adverse effects. Be sure to dispose of needles and syringes properly.

■ With interferons, report the occurrence of depression or thoughts of suicide, dizziness, hives, itching, chest tightness, cough, difficulty breathing or wheezing, or visual problems. These symptoms may require that the drug be stopped or the dosage reduced. In addition, avoid pregnancy (use effective contraceptive methods), avoid prolonged exposure to sunlight, wear protective clothing, and use sunscreens.

Self- or Caregiver Administration

■ Take the drugs as prescribed. Although this is important with all medications, it is especially important with these. Obtaining beneficial effects and decreasing adverse effects depend to a great extent on how the drugs are taken.

■ Use correct techniques to prepare and inject the medications. Instructions for mixing the drugs should be followed exactly.

■ With epoetin alfa, follow these instructions:
  □ Do not freeze or shake the drug vial.
  □ Obtain appropriate laboratory tests to monitor the responses to the drug.
  □ Take an iron supplement, if instructed, to ensure absorption of the drug.
  □ Consume foods that contain vitamin C (e.g. fruit juice, strawberries, cantaloupe) to increase the absorption of iron.

■ With filgrastim, follow these instructions:
  □ Take acetaminophen (e.g., Tylenol, others), if desired, to decrease bone pain.
  □ Notify your prescriber if pain not relieved, especially if taking high-dose IV therapy, because opioids may be necessary
  □ Recognize that dosage modification may be necessary if your white blood cell count greater than 100,000 cells/mm³.

■ With interferons, follow these instructions:
  □ Store the drug in the refrigerator.
  □ Do not freeze or shake the drug vial.
  □ Do not change brands (changes in dosage may result).
  □ Take at bedtime to reduce some common adverse effects (e.g., flu-like symptoms such as fever, headache, fatigue, anorexia, nausea, and vomiting).
  □ Take acetaminophen (e.g., Tylenol, others), if desired, to prevent or decrease fever and headache.
  □ Maintain a fluid intake of 2 to 3 quarts daily.

Use

Indications for filgrastim include (1) preventing infection in patients with neutropenia induced by cancer chemotherapy or bone marrow transplantation or (2) mobilizing stem cells from bone marrow to peripheral blood, where they can be collected and reinfused after chemotherapy that depresses bone marrow function. Most patients who take the drug have fewer days of fever, infection, and antimicrobial drug therapy. In addition, by promoting bone marrow recovery after a course of cytotoxic antineoplastic drugs, it also may allow higher doses or more timely administration of subsequent antitumor drugs. Table 9.3 presents route and dosage information for the CSFs.

Use in Children

The therapeutic and adverse effects of filgrastim in children are similar to those in adults. In clinical trials, filgrastim produced a greater incidence of subclinical spleen enlargement in children than in adults, but whether this affects growth and development or has other long-term consequences is unknown.

Use in Older Adults

In general, filgrastim has the same uses and responses in older adults as in younger adults. Older adults may be at greater risk for adverse effects, especially if large doses are used. Older adults are more likely to develop infections (including reactivation of tuberculosis and herpes zoster) and less able to recover from them. Therefore, older adults need protective measures, such as rigorous personal hygiene; good nutrition; adequate exercise, rest, and sleep; minimal exposure to potential pathogens, when possible; and appropriate immunizations (e.g., influenza, pneumonia, tetanus). When an infection develops in older adults, signs and symptoms (e.g., fever, drainage) may be absent or less pronounced than in younger adults.

Use in Patients With Renal Impairment

Little information about the use of filgrastim in patients with renal impairment is available. Authorities recommend that patients with preexisting impairment have renal function tests every 2 weeks.

TABLE 9.3
DRUGS AT A GLANCE: Colony-Stimulating Factors

Drug	Pregnancy Category	Routes and Dosage Ranges (Adults)
Ⓟ **Filgrastim** (G-CSF) (Neupogen)	C	Myelosuppressive chemotherapy: 5 mg/kg/d Sub-Q injection, IV infusion over 15–30 min, or continuous Sub-Q or IV infusion, up to 2 wk until ANC reaches 10,000/mm^3 Bone marrow transplantation: 10 mcg/kg/d IV or Sub-Q infusion initially, then titrated according to neutrophil count (5 mcg/kg/d if ANC over 1000/mm^3 for 3 consecutive days; stop drug if over 1000/mm^3 for 6 d; if ANC drops below 1000/mm^3, restart filgrastim at 5 mcg/kg/d). Collection of peripheral stem cells: 10 mcg/kg/d Sub-Q for 6–7 d, with collection on the last 3 d of drug administration Severe, chronic neutropenia: 5 or 6 mcg/kg Sub-Q, once or twice daily, depending on clinical response and ANC
Pegfilgrastim (G-CSF) (Neulasta)	C	6 mg Sub-Q once per chemotherapy cycle; do not give between 14 d before and 24 h after cytotoxic chemotherapy
Sargramostim (GM-CSF) (Leukine)	C	Bone marrow reconstitution: 250 mcg/m^2/d IV infusion over 2 h, starting 2–4 h after bone marrow infusion and continuing for 21 d Graft failure or delay: 250 mcg/m^2/d IV infusion over 2 h for 14 d; course of treatment may be repeated after 7 d of therapy if engraftment has not occurred Mobilization of stem cells: 250 mcg/m^2/d Sub-Q or IV over 24 h

ANC, absolute neutrophil count; G-CSF, granulocyte–colony-stimulating factor; GM-CSF, granulocyte macrophage–colony-stimulating factor.

Use in Patients With Hepatic Impairment

Close monitoring may be necessary, because the dose, regimen, or timing of administration may need to be altered with hepatic impairment.

Use in Patients With Critical Illness

Critically ill patients may be given filgrastim to restore, promote, or accelerate bone marrow function.

QSEN Safety Alert

Patients should not receive the filgrastim within 24 hours before or 24 hours after cytotoxic chemotherapy because it may act as a growth factor for any tumor, particularly of the myeloid type.

Patients in a hospital setting are most vulnerable to infection, particularly nosocomial organisms, especially if their neutrophil count falls below 500/mm^3.

Use in Patients Receiving Home Care

The home care nurse needs to assess patients who take filgrastim while at home for sign of an infection and to teach them measures to reduce exposure to infection. The nurse also needs to assess for accurate administration of the drug as well as for ability of the patient to obtain appropriate laboratory tests (e.g., CBC, platelet count, tests of renal or hepatic function) (see Box 9.1).

Adverse Effects and Contraindications

The most common adverse effects of filgrastim are drowsiness, fatigue, flu-like symptoms, nausea, and bone pain. Contraindications include a known sensitivity to the drug and *E. coli*–derived proteins.

Nursing Implications

Preventing Interactions

No medications reportedly increase or decrease the effects of filgrastim. Likewise, no herbs or foods appear to increase or decrease the drug's effects.

Administering the Medication

The nurse administers filgrastim by subcutaneous or IV injection according to indication per the manufacturer's recommendation:

- For cancer chemotherapy: subcutaneous bolus injection, IV infusion over 15 to 30 minutes, or continuous subcutaneous or IV infusion
- For bone marrow transplantation, give by IV infusion over 4 hours or by continuous IV or subcutaneous infusion
- For collection of stem cells, give as a bolus or a continuous infusion
- For chronic neutropenia, give as a subcutaneous injection

It is important not to shake a vial of filgrastim and to use it only once.

Assessing for Therapeutic Effects

The nurse assesses for a decreased incidence of infection and a maintenance of the ANC within a target range of 1500 to 10,000 cells/mm³.

Assessing for Adverse Effects

The nurse observes for drowsiness, fatigue, flu-like symptoms, nausea, and bone pain. In addition, it is necessary to assess for erythema at subcutaneous injection sites.

QSEN Safety Alert

The nurse should check the ANC and report to the prescriber if it is 10,000 cells/mm³ or greater.

Patient Teaching

The nurse teaches the patient and family about accurate drug preparation and injection techniques as well as proper disposal of needles and syringes. Box 9.1 contains additional patient teaching guidelines.

Other Drugs in the Class

Pegfilgrastim (Neulasta), which stays in the body longer and can be given less often than filgrastim, is another CSF, a G-CSF. (Conjugation of filgrastim with polyethylene glycol produces pegfilgrastim.) Uses for pegfilgrastim include prevention of infection in neutropenia induced by cancer chemotherapy as well as treatment of bone marrow transplantation for Hodgkin's disease, non-Hodgkin's lymphoma, or acute lymphoblastic leukemia. It is important to note that after transplantation, it takes 2 to 4 weeks for the engrafted bone marrow cells to mature and begin producing blood cells. During this time, patients have virtually no functioning granulocytes and are at high risk for infection. Pegfilgrastim helps reduce the incidence, severity, and duration of neutropenia associated with several chemotherapy regimens and restore, promote, or accelerate bone marrow function.

Most patients who take pegfilgrastim, like those who take filgrastim, have fewer days of fever, infection, and antimicrobial drug therapy. The drug also may allow higher doses or more timely administration of subsequent antitumor drugs by promoting bone marrow recovery after a course of cytotoxic antineoplastic drugs. Patients should not take it 14 days before and 24 hours after cytotoxic chemotherapy. Like filgrastim, the most common adverse effects are drowsiness, fatigue, flu-like symptoms, nausea, and bone pain. Additionally, lithium may potentially cause a drug interaction with pegfilgrastim; lithium increases the production of WBCs, increasing the risk of a stroke or heart attack.

Sargramostim (Leukine) is a granulocyte macrophage–CSF (GM-CSF) used to treat patients who undergo bone marrow transplantation for Hodgkin's disease, non-Hodgkin's lymphoma, or acute lymphoblastic leukemia. Like pegfilgrastim, it takes 2 to 4 weeks after transplantation for the engrafted bone marrow cells to mature and begin producing blood cells. During this time, there are essentially no functioning granulocytes, and there is a high risk of infection. Sargramostim promotes engraftment and function of the transplanted bone marrow, thereby decreasing the risk of infection. If the graft is successful, the granulocyte count starts to rise in approximately 2 weeks.

Health care providers also use sargramostim in stem cell transplantation to stimulate the movement of hematopoietic stem cells from the bone marrow to circulating blood, where they can be readily collected. Indications for use are after bone marrow transplantation to promote bone marrow function or to treat graft failure or delayed function. Transplantation of large numbers of stem cells can lead to more rapid engraftment and recovery, with less risk of transplant failure and complications. When giving sargramostim to patients with cancer who have had bone marrow transplantation, it is necessary to start the drug 2 to 4 hours after the bone marrow infusion and at least 24 hours after the last dose of antineoplastic chemotherapy or 12 hours after the last radiotherapy treatment. The nurse should ensure that CBCs are performed twice weekly during therapy; the neutrophil count should not exceed approximately 20,000/mm³.

In some patients with preexisting renal impairment, sargramostim increases serum creatinine. Values decline to baseline levels when the drug is stopped or its dosage reduced. With preexisting hepatic impairment, sargramostim also can increase serum bilirubin and liver enzymes. Values return to baseline when the drug is stopped or its dosage reduced.

Corticosteroids and lithium are known to increase effects of sargramostim. These drugs have myeloproliferative (bone-marrow stimulating) effects of their own, which may add to those of sargramostim.

Adverse effects occur more often with sargramostim than filgrastim and include bone pain, fever, headache, muscle aches, generalized maculopapular skin rash, and fluid retention (peripheral edema, pleural effusion, pericardial effusion). Bone pain occurs in approximately 33% to 50% of patients. Other effects occur in more than 10% of patients. Pleural and pericardial effusions are more likely at doses greater than 20 mcg/kg/d.

Clinical Application 9-2

- Mrs. Paul has a great risk of infection, with a low white blood cell count and low absolute neutrophil count. What should the nurse teach the patient about preventing infection?

NCLEX Success

4. Which of the following adverse effects should the nurse discuss with a patient receiving filgrastim (Neupogen)?

   A. fatigue
   B. bleeding
   C. headache
   D. bone pain

5. The nurse is administering filgrastim (Neupogen) to a patient who has received a bone barrow transplant. Which laboratory parameter should the nurse monitor to determine if the drug is effective?

   A. hemoglobin
   B. basophils
   C. hematocrit
   D. neutrophils

6. The nurse is caring for a patient who is undergoing chemotherapy for cancer. The physician orders filgrastim (Neupogen). The nurse explains to the patient that an expected outcome after the administration of filgrastim is

A. fewer infections
B. decreased anemia
C. longer life expectancy
D. less nausea and vomiting

Interferons

Interferons, called alfa, beta, or gamma, according to specific characteristics, are **biologic response modifiers** that bind to specific cell-surface receptors and alter intracellular activities. In viral infections, these immunostimulants induce enzymes that inhibit protein synthesis and degrade viral RNA. As a result, viruses are less able to enter uninfected cells, reproduce, and release new viruses. In addition to their antiviral effects, interferons also have antiproliferative and immunoregulatory activities. They can increase expression of major histocompatibility complex molecules, augment the activity of NK cells, increase the effectiveness of antigen-presenting cells in inducing the proliferation of cytotoxic T cells, aid the attachment of cytotoxic T cells to target cells, and inhibit angiogenesis (formation of blood vessels).

Synthetically produced interferons have the same capabilities as endogenous interferons. Thus, indications include treatment of viral infections and certain cancers (for specific details, see *Use*). Ⓟ **Interferon alfa-2b** (Intron-A) is the prototype for this class of drugs and is a product of recombinant DNA technology using *E. coli*.

Pharmacokinetics

Interferon alfa-2b is about 80% absorbed and widely distributed but does not cross the blood–brain barrier. There is minimal hepatic metabolism. Excretion is primarily renal. Peak onset of action is 3 to 12 hours. The elimination half-life is approximately 2 to 3 hours.

Action

Interferon alpha-2b has both antiviral and antineoplastic activities. It exerts its cellular activities by binding to specific membrane receptors on the cell surface enhancing immune response, inhibiting viral replication in virus-infected cells. The drug enhances the overall function of the immune system by increasing phagocytic activity of macrophages and monocytes, which augments cytotoxicity against cancer cells. Additionally, it suppresses the growth and reproduction of similar cells by cell division.

Use

Indications for use of interferon alfa-2b in adults 18 years of age and older include hairy cell leukemia, chronic hepatitis B and C, AIDS-related Kaposi's sarcoma, malignant melanoma, and condylomata. Table 9.4 presents route and dosage information for the interferons.

Use in Children

> **QSEN Safety Alert** ❗
>
> *Neonates and infants should not receive interferon alfa-2b because it contains benzyl alcohol, which could increase the risk of neurologic complications.*

Use in Patients With Hepatic Impairment

Hepatic enzymes may become elevated during treatment, especially in people with preexisting liver disease. Such an increase may require discontinuing the drug. Known hepatic impairment is a contraindication.

Use in Patients Receiving Home Care

The interferon is often self-administered or given by a caregiver to chronically ill patients. The home care nurse may need to teach patients or caregivers accurate drug preparation and injection techniques as well as proper disposal of needles and syringes. It may also be necessary to provide assistance in obtaining appropriate laboratory tests (e.g., CBC, platelet count, tests of renal or hepatic function) to monitor patients' responses to the medications.

Adverse Effects

In the majority of patients, flu-like symptoms (e.g., fever, chills, fatigue, muscle aches, headache, tachycardia) develop within 2 hours of administration of interferon alfa-2b and last up to 24 hours. Other symptoms include chest pain and alopecia. Adverse hematologic effects include neutropenia, anemia, and thrombocytopenia. Additionally, researchers have reported the occurrence of psychiatric complications such as severe depression, psychosis, and suicidal behavior with interferons. Persistently severe or worsening effects usually lead to permanent discontinuation of interferon alfa. In many cases, these disorders resolve after the drug is stopped.

Contraindications

Contraindications to interferon alfa-2b include known sensitivity to the drug as well as signs and symptoms of liver disease (e.g., jaundice, ascites, bleeding disorders, or decreased serum albumin), autoimmune hepatitis, a history of autoimmune disease, or posttransplantation immunosuppression.

Nursing Implications

Preventing Interactions

Some medications interact with interferon alfa-2b, increasing its effects (Box 9.2). Apparently, no herbs interact with this drug.

Administering the Medication

The nurse may administer interferon alfa-2b intravenously, subcutaneously, intramuscularly, or intralesionally. Administration is three times weekly, on a regular schedule (e.g., Monday,

TABLE 9.4

DRUGS AT A GLANCE: Interferons

Drug	Pregnancy Category	Routes and Dosage Ranges (Adults)
℗ **Interferon alfa-2b** (Intron A)	C	Hairy cell leukemia: induction and maintenance, 2 million international units/m² Sub-Q, IM 3 times weekly up to 6 mo Kaposi's sarcoma: induction and maintenance, 30 million IU/m² Sub-Q, IM 3 times weekly Hepatitis B: 5 million international units Sub-Q, IM daily or 10 million international units 3 times weekly (total of 30–35 million international units per week) for 16 wk Hepatitis C: 3 million international units Sub-Q, IM 3 times weekly for 16 wk–24 mo Malignant melanoma: induction, 20 million international units/m² IV on 5 consecutive days per week for 4 wk; maintenance, 10 million international units/m² Sub-Q 3 times per week for 48 wk Condylomata: 1 million international units/lesion (maximum of 5 lesions) 3 times weekly for 3 wk
Interferon alfa-2b with ribavirin (Rebetron)	X	Hepatitis C: interferon alfa-2b Sub-Q, 3 million international units 3 times weekly and ribavirin capsules PO 1000–1200 mg 2 times daily for 24 wk.
Interferon alfa-2a (Roferon-A)	C	Hepatitis C: 3 million international units Sub-Q, IM 3 times weekly for 12 mo Hairy cell leukemia: Sub-Q, IM; induction, 3 million international units daily for 16–24 wk; maintenance, 3 million international units 3 times weekly Kaposi's sarcoma: Sub-Q, IM; induction, 36 million international units daily for 10–12 wk; maintenance, 36 million international units 3 times weekly Chronic myelogenous leukemia: 9 million Sub-Q, IM international units daily
Peginterferon alfa-2a (Pegasys)	C	Sub-Q, 180 mcg (1 mL) once weekly for 48 wk Sub-Q, 180 mcg once weekly for 24 wk for viral genotypes 2 and 3; for 48 wk for viral strains 1 and 4
Peginterferon alfa-2b (PEG-Intron)	C	1 mcg Sub-Q once weekly for 1 y
Interferon alfacon-1 (Infergen)	C	9 mcg Sub-Q 3 times weekly for 24 wk, with at least 48 h between doses
Interferon beta-1a (Avonex, Rebif)	C	Avonex, 30 mcg IM once per week Rebif, 8.8 mcg Sub-Q for 2 wk, then 22 mcg for 2 wk, then 44 mcg; give all doses 3 times weekly, with at least 48 h between doses
Interferon beta-1b (Betaseron)	C	0.25 mg Sub-Q every other day
Interferon gamma-1b (Actimmune)	C	50 mcg/m² Sub-Q if body surface area (BSA) is over 0.5 m²; 1.5 mcg/kg if BSA is under 0.5 m², 3 times weekly

Wednesday, and Friday), at about the same time of day, at least 48 hours apart, per manufacturer's recommendation. To treat condylomata intralesionally, it is important to inject the drug into the base of each wart with a small-gauge needle. For large warts, injections may occur at several points per the manufacturer's recommendation.

Assessing for Therapeutic Effects

With parenteral interferons, the nurse observes for improvement in signs and symptoms. With hairy cell leukemia, hematologic tests may improve within 2 months, but optimal effects may require 6 months of drug therapy. With Kaposi's sarcoma, skin

lesions may resolve or stabilize over several weeks. With chronic hepatitis, liver function tests may improve within a few weeks.

Assessing for Adverse Effects

The nurse observes for acute flu-like symptoms with interferon alfa-2b and assesses patient response through evaluation of liver function tests and WBC, RBC, and platelet values.

Patient Teaching

The nurse teaches the patient about accurate drug preparation and injection techniques as well as proper disposal of needles and syringes.

Drugs That Increase the Effects of Interferon Alfa-2b

- Bowel-cleansing phosphate and sulfate preparations
  Increase the risk of seizure activity
- Clozapine
  Increases the risk and/or severity of hematologic toxicity
- Deferiprone
  Increases the risk of severe bone marrow toxicity
- Iopamidol, metrizamide, and other iodinated contrast media
  Increase the risk of seizure activity
- Leflunomide
  Increases the risk of infections
- Zidovudine
  Increases the risk of severe bone marrow toxicity

QSEN Safety Alert ❗

A pregnancy when either partner is taking interferon alfa-2b and ribavirin (Rebetron; pregnancy category X) may result in a child with birth defects; therefore, patient teaching must include the use of birth control measures to prevent pregnancy during treatment and for at least 6 months after stopping the drug.

Box 9.1 contains other patient teaching guidelines.

Other Drugs in the Class

Interferon alfa-2a (Roferon-A) is structurally the same as interferon alfa-2b except for one amino acid. Uses for this interferon include hairy cell leukemia and AIDS-related Kaposi's sarcoma in adults. The drug is also used to treat chronic myelogenous leukemia in adults and children. Its adverse effect profile is similar to that of interferon alfa-2b.

Peginterferon alfa has largely replaced the older preparations of interferon alfa for some clinical uses. **Pegylation** is a process of modifying an interferon by treatment with polyethylene glycol, changing the pharmacokinetics of interferons so that they act longer and can be given less often. Peginterferons also produce steady blood levels, whereas unpegylated interferons provide fluctuating levels.

Peginterferon alfa-2a (Pegasys), with ribavirin, is the current drug therapy of choice for hepatitis C. Alternative treatment involves a combination of an interferon (alfa-2b, pegylated alfa-2b, alfacon-1, or pegylated alfa-2a) and ribavirin; interferon monotherapy is warranted only when there are specific reasons not to use ribavirin. The particular strain of the causative virus determines the duration of drug therapy. Peginterferon alfa-2b (PEG-Intron) is also indicated for use in chronic hepatitis C, alone or with ribavirin.

Interferon alfacon-1(Infergen) is approved for treatment of chronic hepatitis C, a condition that can lead to liver failure and liver cancer.

Interferon beta-1a (Avonex, Rebif) and interferon beta-1b (Betaseron) are used for multiple sclerosis, an autoimmune neurologic disorder in which the drug slows progression of neurologic dysfunction, prolongs remissions, and reduces the severity of relapses. Flu-like symptoms are common adverse effects.

Interferon gamma-1b (Actimmune) is used to treat chronic granulomatous disease, which involves impaired phagocytosis of ingested microbes and frequent infections. Drug therapy reduces the incidence and severity of infections.

Adjuvant Medications Used to Stimulate the Immune System: Interleukins

Aldesleukin (Proleukin) is a recombinant DNA version of IL-2. It activates cellular immunity; produces tumor necrosis factor (IL-1) and interferon gamma; and inhibits tumor growth. Its uses include treatment of metastatic kidney cancer and metastatic melanoma skin cancer. Only health professionals (e.g., oncologists, oncology nurses) who are experienced in the use of the drug should prescribe and administer aldesleukin; administration should occur only in the hospital setting. Few nurses are likely to give this drug; therefore, this chapter omits details about administration and patient monitoring.

Oprelvekin (Neumega) is recombinant IL-11, which stimulates platelet production. This drug is used to prevent thrombocytopenia and reduce the need for platelet transfusions in patients with cancer who are receiving myelosuppressive chemotherapy. However, its usefulness is limited because it is ineffective in severe thrombocytopenia and is highly toxic. Nurses use oprelvekin infrequently; therefore, this chapter omits details relating to administration and patient monitoring.

NCLEX Success

7. Mrs. Thomas, a 60-year-old woman with cancer who started on interferon alfa-2b (Intron A) today, calls the clinic and reports that she has been having fever, chills, fatigue and muscle aches since she has returned home. For relief of these symptoms, the nurse teaches the patient to take

   A. aspirin
   B. codeine
   C. ibuprofen
   D. acetaminophen

8. Interferons may be used to treat

   A. most types of cancer
   B. chronic hepatitis C
   C. chronic anemia
   D. mental depression

The Nursing Process

Assessment

- Assess the patient's status in relation to conditions for which hematopoietic and immunostimulant drugs are used (e.g., infection, neutropenia, cancer)
- Assess nutritional status, including appetite and weight
- Assess functional abilities in relation to activities of daily living (ADLs)
- Assess adequacy of support systems for outpatients (e.g., transportation for clinic visits)
- Assess ability and attitude toward planned drug therapy and associated monitoring and follow-up
- Assess coping mechanisms of patient and significant others in stressful situations
- Assess patient for factors predisposing to infection (e.g., skin lesions, invasive devices, cigarette smoking)
- Assess environment for factors predisposing to infection (e.g., family or health care providers with infections)
- Assess baseline values of laboratory and other diagnostic test reports to aid monitoring of responses to hematopoietic and immunostimulant drug therapy

Nursing Diagnoses

- Risk for injury: infection related to drug-induced neutropenia, immunosuppression, malnutrition, chronic disease; bleeding related to anemia or thrombocytopenia
- Risk for injury: adverse drug effects
- Activity intolerance related to weakness, fatigue from debilitating disease, or drug therapy
- Anxiety related to the diagnosis of cancer, hepatitis, multiple sclerosis, or human immunodeficiency virus (HIV) infection
- Deficient knowledge: disease process; hematopoietic and immunostimulant drug therapy

Planning/Goals

The patient will

- Participate in interventions to prevent or decrease infection
- Remain afebrile during immunostimulant therapy
- Experience increased immunocompetence as indicated by increased white blood cell (WBC) count (if initially leukopenic) or tumor regression
- Avoid preventable infections
- Experience relief or reduction of disease symptoms
- Maintain independence in ADLs when able; be assisted appropriately when unable
- Maintain adequate levels of nutrition and fluids, rest and sleep, and exercise
- Maintain or increase appetite and weight if initially anorexic and underweight
- Learn to self-administer medications accurately when indicated

Nursing Interventions

The nurse will

- Practice and promote good hand hygiene techniques by patients and all others in contact with the patient
- Use sterile technique for all injections, IV site care, wound dressing changes, and any other invasive diagnostic or therapeutic measures
- Screen staff and visitors for signs and symptoms of infection; if infection is noted, do not allow contact with the patient
- Allow patients to participate in self-care and decision making when feasible
- Use isolation procedures when indicated, usually when the neutrophil count is less than 500/mm^3
- Promote adequate nutrition, with nutritious fluids, supplements, and snacks when indicated
- Promote adequate rest, sleep, and exercise (e.g., schedule frequent rest periods, avoid interrupting sleep when possible, individualize exercise or activity according to the patient's condition)
- Inform patients about diagnostic test results, planned changes in therapeutic regimens, and evidence of progress
- Allow family members or significant others to visit patients when feasible
- Monitor the complete blood (cell) count (CBC) and other diagnostic test reports for normal or abnormal values, reporting test results to prescribers when indicated. It is essential that darbepoetin and epoetin be stopped when the hemoglobin level approaches 12 g/dL and filgrastim and sargramostim be stopped when WBC counts normalize.
- Schedule drug administration, diagnostic tests, and other elements of care to conserve patients' energy
- Consult other health care providers (e.g., physician, dietitian, social worker) on the patient's behalf when indicated
- Assist patients to learn ways to prevent or reduce the incidence of infections (e.g., meticulous personal hygiene, avoiding contact with infected people)
- Assist patients to learn ways to enhance immune mechanisms and other body defenses by healthy lifestyle habits, such as a nutritious diet, adequate rest and sleep, and avoidance of tobacco and alcohol
- Assist patients or caregivers in learning how to prepare and inject darbepoetin alfa, epoetin alfa, filgrastim, or an interferon, when indicated

Evaluation

- Determine the number and type of infections that have occurred in neutropenic patients.
- Compare current CBC reports with baseline values for changes toward normal levels (e.g., WBC count 5000–10,000/mm^3).
- Compare weight and nutritional status with baseline values for maintenance or improvement.
- Observe and interview for decreased numbers or severity of disease symptoms.
- Observe for increased energy and ability to participate in ADLs.
- Observe and interview outpatients regarding adherence to follow-up care.
- Observe and interview regarding the mental and emotional status of the patient and family members.

Clinical Application 9-3

- Epoetin alfa is prescribed for Mrs. Paul's anemia. What dietary considerations should the nurse communicate to Mrs. Paul?

Key Concepts

- Patients with anemia associated with chronic renal failure or bone marrow–damaging anticancer drug therapy may take a drug formulation of erythropoietin to increase their RBC count.

- This use led the FDA to issue a **BLACK BOX WARNING** ◆ advising prescribers to avoid using hematopoietic growth factors in patients with hemoglobin values of 12 g/dL or above. In addition, it is important to prescribe these drugs at the lowest dose effective in raising hemoglobin levels just enough to avoid the need for blood transfusion; the nurse helps ensure that hemoglobin levels are monitored regularly until they stabilize.

- Adverse effects of epoetin and darbepoetin include increased risks of hypertension, myocardial infarction, and stroke, especially when used to increase hemoglobin above 12 g/dL.

- Filgrastim and other CSFs are used to increase WBCs and decrease risks of infection in patients with or at high risk of severe neutropenia.

- Interferons are used mainly for viral hepatitis and certain types of cancer.

- Some interferons, as well as filgrastim, are conjugated with polyethylene glycol, in a process called pegylation, to prolong drug actions.

- Because peginterferon can be given once per week and keeps blood levels constant, it has largely replaced other interferons for both monotherapy and combination therapy for hepatitis C.

Critical Thinking Questions

9-1. John Thomas, a 51-year-old man who has been diagnosed with Hodgkin's disease, has completed a course of antineoplastic chemotherapy. He is currently in the hospital for a bone marrow transplant. His physician orders a colony-stimulating factor (CSF).

- As a nurse, discuss the plan of care.

- Mr. Thomas receives the bone marrow transplant and questions the need for the CSF, stating, "I have new bone marrow now. Won't that make all the bone cells I need?" How should the nurse respond?

References and Resources

Corwin, H. L., Gettinger, A., Fabian, T. C., May, A., Pearl, R. G., Heard, S., et al., for the EPO Critical Care Trials Group. (2007). Efficacy and safety of epoetin alfa in critically ill patients. *The New England Journal of Medicine, 357,* 965–976.

DiPiro, J. T., Talbert, R. L., Yee, G. C., Matzke, G. R., Wells, B. G., & Posey, L. M. (Eds.). (2011). *Pharmacotherapy: A pathophysiologic approach* (8th ed.). New York: McGraw-Hill.

Drug facts and comparisons. (Updated monthly). St. Louis, MO: Facts and Comparisons.

Elliott, S. (2011). Erythropoiesis-stimulating agents. *Cancer Treatment Research, 157,* 55–74.

Karch, A. M. (2010). *2010 Lippincott's nursing drug guide.* Philadelphia, PA: Lippincott Williams & Wilkins.

Lacy, C. F., Armstrong, L. L., Goldman, M. P., & Lance, L. L. (2010). *Lexi-Comp's drug information handbook* (19th ed.). Hudson, OH: American Pharmaceutical Association.

McPhee, S. J., Papadakis, M. A., & Tierney, L. M., Jr. (2012). *Current medical diagnosis and treatment* (51st ed.). New York: McGraw-Hill.

Porth, C. M. (2010). *Pathophysiology: Concepts of altered health states* (8th ed.). Philadelphia, PA: Lippincott Williams & Wilkins.

Rizzo, J. D., Brouwers, M., Hurley, P., Seidenfeld, J., Arcasoy, M. O., Spivak, J. L., et al. (2010). American Society of Hematology/American Society of Clinical Oncology clinical practice guideline update on the use of epoetin and darbepoetin in adult patients with cancer. *Blood, 116*(20), 4045–4059.

Smeltzer, S. C., Bare, B. G., Hinkle, J. L., & Cheever, K. H. (Eds.). (2010). *Brunner & Suddarth's textbook of medical-surgical nursing* (12th ed.). Philadelphia, PA: Lippincott Williams & Wilkins.

10 Drug Therapy: Immunizations

LEARNING OBJECTIVES

After studying this chapter, you should be able to:

1. Describe the types of immunity and the agents that produce them.
2. Identify immunizations recommended for children and adolescents.
3. Identify immunizations recommended for adults.
4. Identify authoritative sources for immunization information.
5. Be able to teach parents (and their children) about the importance of immunizations to public health.
6. Be able to teach people about recommended immunizations and record keeping.

Clinical Application Case Study

Cynthia Williams, a 26-year-old college student, brings her 15-month-old son Riley to a family practice clinic for a well-child checkup. Mrs. Williams says that Riley has had his previous immunizations at the county health department every 2 months until the age of 6 months but that he has not had any immunizations since then.

KEY TERMS

Active immunity: antigenic immune response with antibody formation to an infection through administration of a vaccine or toxoid or through natural exposure to the disease

Antigenicity: ability of an antigen to bind specifically with certain products to promote better antibody formation

Immunization: bolstering a person's immune system by inducing antibody formation, thereby providing active protection against a specific infectious disease

Passive immunity: temporary state of immunity produced in a person who is susceptible to an infectious organism by administering serum containing antibodies to the disease

Toxoids: altered bacterial toxins that are administered to stimulate antitoxin production and protect against the harmful effects of the toxin

Vaccines: microorganisms or components of microorganisms that are administered to stimulate antibody production against the microorganism prior to a natural infection

Introduction

Immunization, which involves bolstering a person's immune system by inducing antibody formation, thereby providing active protection against a specific infectious disease, has greatly improved human health and life expectancy. Immunizations are one of the key factors in reducing mortality and improving life expectancy in the United States over the past century. Worldwide, some infections such as smallpox and polio have almost been eradicated as a result of effective immunization programs. The nurse plays a pivotal role in this process of assessing, teaching, administering immunizations, and evaluating patients who have received them for adverse effects.

Overview of Immunization

Types of Immunity

There are two main types of immunity. **Active immunity** results from administering a dead or weakened microorganism or piece of the microorganism to a person. The person's immune system responds by producing immunoglobulins (antibodies) specific for that microorganism, providing protection against disease with later exposure. **Passive immunity** results from parenteral administration of immune serum containing disease-specific antibodies to a nonimmune person. Passive immunity is only temporary, and the person still needs a vaccine against a specific disease to develop antibodies that provide long-term immunity. Preparations used for immunization are biologic products prepared by pharmaceutical companies and are regulated by the U.S. Food and Drug Administration (FDA). Widespread use of these products in the United States has dramatically decreased the incidence of many infectious diseases, such as polio, influenza, pneumococcal disease, and hepatitis B.

Kinds of Immunizing Agents

Agents for Active Immunity

The biologic products used for active immunity are vaccines and toxoids. For maximum effectiveness, both of these products must be given before exposure to the pathogenic microorganism. Administration by the recommended route helps ensure the desired immunologic response.

Vaccines are suspensions of microorganisms or their antigenic products that have been killed (inactivated) or attenuated (weakened or reduced in virulence) so they can induce antibody formation while preventing infection altogether or causing only a very mild form of it. Many vaccines produce long-lasting immunity. Attenuated live vaccines produce active immunity, usually lifelong, that is similar to that produced by natural infection. There is a small risk that live vaccines may produce disease in people with severely impaired immune function, but this risk is very low with new vaccines developed using recombinant DNA technology.

Toxoids are bacterial toxins or products that have been modified to destroy toxicity while retaining antigenic properties (i.e., ability to induce antibody formation). Immunization with toxoids is not permanent, and scheduled repeat doses (boosters) are required to maintain immunity.

Additional components, such as aluminum or calcium phosphate, are added to some vaccines and toxoids, to slow absorption and increase **antigenicity** (ability of an antigen to bind specifically with certain products to promote better antibody formation). Products containing aluminum can only be given intramuscularly because greater tissue irritation occurs with subcutaneous injections of the immunizing agent.

In general, vaccines and toxoids are quite safe, and risks of the diseases they prevent are significantly greater than the risks of the vaccines. However, risks and benefits of vaccination are always considered individually, because no vaccine is completely effective or completely safe. A few people may still develop a disease after being immunized against it. However, if this happens, symptoms are usually less severe and complications are fewer than if the person had not been immunized. Adverse vaccine effects are usually mild and of short duration. The FDA evaluates vaccine safety before and after a vaccine is marketed, although some adverse effects become apparent only after a vaccine is used in a large population.

Agents for Passive Immunity

Immune serums are the biologic products used for passive immunity. They act rapidly to provide temporary immunity lasting about 1 to 3 months in people exposed to or experiencing an infectious disease. The goal of therapy is to prevent or modify the disease process (i.e., decrease the incidence and severity of symptoms).

Immune globulin products are made from the serum of people with high concentrations of the specific antibody or immunoglobulin required. These products may consist of whole serum or only contain the immunoglobulin portion of serum in which the specific antibodies are concentrated. Immunoglobulin fractions are preferred over whole serum because they are more likely to be effective in disease prevention. All plasma used to prepare these products is screened for hepatitis B surface antigen (HBsAg). Hyperimmune serums are available for cytomegalovirus, hepatitis B, rabies, rubella, tetanus, varicella-zoster (shingles), and respiratory syncytial virus infections.

Individual Immunizing Agents

Box 10.1 provides information about current recommendations for immunizations. Table 10.1 lists vaccines and toxoids that are used routinely in the United States, and Table 10.2 lists immune serums that are used regularly in this country.

Use

Clinical indications for vaccines and toxoids include the following:

- Routine immunization of children against diphtheria, *Haemophilus influenzae* type b infection, hepatitis A and B, influenza, measles (rubeola), mumps, pertussis, pneumococcal infection, poliomyelitis, rotavirus, rubella (German measles), tetanus, and varicella (chickenpox)

BOX 10.1	Recommended Immunizations by Age Group

Children and Adolescents

■ Rotavirus vaccine (RotaTeq) or (Rotarix) started at age 6 weeks through 14 weeks of age to protect infants against rotavirus gastroenteritis. RotaTeq consists of two vaccine doses 2 months apart, with a third dose of Rotarix is recommended at age 6 months.

■ A single booster dose of tetanus and diphtheria toxoids and acellular pertussis vaccine (Tdap) for adolescents and adults because protection against pertussis declines a few years after initial immunization with pertussis vaccine during early childhood. The Tdap booster is recommended 5 years after the last Td immunization. Boostrix is used for people 10 to 18 years of age, and Adacel is used for people 11 to 64 years of age.

■ Four doses of pneumococcal vaccine (PCV13, Prevnar) for healthy young children

■ Two doses of chickenpox vaccine (e.g., Varivax), with the first dose at 12 to 15 months and the second dose at 4 to 6 years of age. Chickenpox vaccine is also recommended for adolescents and nonpregnant adults who have never had chickenpox or been vaccinated previously with a single dose; two doses of vaccine are required for full immunity.

■ A combined vaccine for measles, mumps, rubella, and chickenpox (ProQuad) for children aged 12 months to 12 years. Another vaccine combination (Pentacel), which contains diphtheria, tetanus, pertussis, polio, and *H. influenzae* type b (Hib), can be used for primary immunization in infancy as well as for booster doses. Combination vaccines are recommended for use in children who need multiple vaccines at a single visit.

■ Hepatitis A vaccination for all children in the United States, with the first of two doses between 1 and 2 years of age

■ Annual flu vaccination for all people older than 6 months of age. Infants younger than 2 years of age and all children and adults with underlying medical conditions should receive the trivalent inactive vaccine (TIV). The live attenuate influenza vaccine (LAIV; FluMist) should be used only for nonpregnant people between 2 and 49 years of age who are healthy and not at high risk for influenza complications. Two vaccine doses at least 4 weeks apart should be given to children younger than 9 years of age.

■ Human papillomavirus (HPV) vaccine (Gardasil) for all adolescents 11 or 12 years of age (can be given as early as 9 years) or up to 26 years of age if not received earlier. Bivalent HPV2 vaccine (Cervarix) can be given to females 9 through 26 years of age. Both vaccines are most effective if given before the person becomes sexually active.

■ Meningococcal vaccine administration at 11 or 12 years of age with a booster dose at age 16 years. If not received earlier, two doses at least 8 weeks apart are recommended for adolescents up to age 21.

Adults

■ Chickenpox vaccine for adults who never had the disease or vaccine; a second dose of vaccine for adults who previously received a single dose

■ HPV vaccine in adults up to age 26 years, if not previously received

■ Tdap booster vaccine (e.g., Adacel) once for all adults younger than 65 years of age, especially health professionals and those who have close contact with infants (younger than 1 year of age)

■ The pneumococcal vaccine, Pneumovax, for smokers and people with asthma or other chronic conditions who are between 19 and 64 years of age

■ Zoster vaccine (Zostavax) (to prevent herpes zoster [shingles]) in adults 60 years and older

---

- Routine immunization of adolescents and adults against diphtheria, tetanus, and pertussis (Tdap); varicella, if immunity not established; as well as influenza annually
- Immunization of prepubertal girls or women of childbearing age against rubella.

QSEN Safety Alert ❗

Rubella during the first trimester of pregnancy is associated with a high incidence of birth defects in the newborn.

- Immunization of people at high risk for serious morbidity or mortality from a chronic condition. For example, pneumococcal vaccine is recommended in people 65 years of age and older, as well as in people younger than 65 years of age with chronic diseases.
- Immunization of adults and children at high risk for a particular disease. For example, pneumococcal vaccine is recommended for people older than 2 years of age who

have chronic respiratory disease or have had a splenectomy. Also, administration of quadrivalent human papillomavirus (HPV) vaccine is recommended in young adolescents to prevent genital warts and the risk of cervical cancer.

Use in Children

Routine immunization of children has reduced the prevalence of many common childhood diseases (listed previously; e.g., diphtheria, measles [rubeola], mumps, pertussis, and varicella [chickenpox]), and immunization rates have increased in recent years. By 4 to 6 years of age, children should have received vaccinations against these diseases. Because some vaccines are administered more than once, a child may receive more than 20 injections by 2 years of age. Two strategies to increase immunizations are the use of combination vaccines and the administration of multiple vaccines (in separate syringes and at different sites) at one visit to a health care provider whenever feasible. Combination vaccines decrease the number of injections, and giving multiple vaccines at one visit decreases the number

TABLE 10.1

DRUGS AT A GLANCE: Vaccines and Toxoids for Active Immunity

Name/Characteristics	Pregnancy Category	Indications for Use	Routes and Dosage Ranges	
			Adults	Children
Vaccines				
H. influenzae type b (Hib) (ActHIB, PedvaxHIB, Hiberix) May be given at the same time as DTaP; measles, mumps, rubella (MMR); injected polio vaccine (IPV)	C	Routine immunization of children 6 wk–15 mo of age born to HBsAg-negative mothers		0.5 mL IM at 2, 4, and 12–15 mo of age
Hepatitis A (Havrix, Vaqta) More than 90% effective within 4 wk after first dose; contraindicated during febrile illness, immunosuppression; Havrix and Vaqta are interchangeable.	C	All children at age 1 y; workers in day care centers, laboratories, food-handling establishments; men who have sex with men; IV drug users; military personnel and travelers to areas where hepatitis A is endemic; community residents during an outbreak; people with chronic liver disease (e.g., hepatitis B or C, cirrhosis) or who receive transfusions for clotting disorders	Havrix (1440 units in 1 mL), 1 mL IM initially and 6–12 mo later (2 doses) Vaqta (50 units/mL), IM in deltoid, 1 mL initially and 6–12 mo later (2 doses)	Havrix (360 or 720 units in 0.5 mL), 1–18 y, 360 units IM initially, then 1 and 6–12 mo later (3 doses) or 720 units initially and 6–12 mo later (total of 2 doses) Vaqta (25 units/ 0.5 mL), 25 units IM initially and 6–18 mo later (2 doses)
Hepatitis B (Engerix-B, Recombivax HB) Approximately 96% effective in children and young adults and 88% in adults older than 40 y; duration of protection unknown; serum antibody levels can be obtained.	C (contraindicated)	All infants and children up to age 18; people with occupational exposure to blood (health care and emergency workers); household contacts or sexual partners of people with hepatitis B infection; people with HIV, end-stage renal disease, on hemodialysis; people with multiple sexual partners; men who have sex with men; IV drug users; residents and staff of institutions for developmentally disabled people; residents of correctional facilities	20 y and older Engerix-B, 1 mL IM initially, then 1 mo and 6 mo later (3 doses); predialysis and dialysis patients, 2 mL IM initially and 1, 2, and 6 mo later (4 doses) Recombivax HB, 1 mL IM initially and 1 mo and 6 mo later (3 doses); predialysis and dialysis patients, 1 mL IM initially and 1 mo and 6 mo later (3 doses)	Neonates to 19 y Engerix-B, 0.5 mL IM initially and 1 mo and 6 mo later (3 doses) Recombivax HB, 0.5 mL IM initially and 1 mo and 6 mo later (3 doses)
Human papillomavirus (HPV) (Gardasil, Cervarix) Because HPV is a common sexually transmitted infection, the vaccine is most effective when taken before becoming sexually active.	B	Gardasil, prevention of diseases caused by HPV types 6, 11, 16, and 18 (cervical, vaginal, and vulvar cancer; genital warts) in people ages 9–26 y Cervarix, prevention of HPV types 16 and 18; recommended for girls and women from ages 9 to 26	0.5 mL IM initially, 2 mo after first dose, and 6 mo after first dose (3 doses)	9 y and older; same as adults

(Continued on page 166)

TABLE 10.1

DRUGS AT A GLANCE: Vaccines and Toxoids for Active Immunity (Continued)

Name/Characteristics	Pregnancy Category	Routes and Dosage Ranges		
		Indications for Use	**Adults**	**Children**
Influenza TIV (Afluria, Agriflu, FluLaval, Fluarix, Fluvirin, Fluzone) LAIV (FluMist) Formulated annually to include current strains; provides protective antibody concentrations for about 6 mo	C	Annual immunization for all people older than 6 mo of age; FluMist live intranasal influenza vaccine is indicated for healthy, nonpregnant people aged 2 through 49 y.	0.5 mL IM in a single dose; immunization, then 1 dose each season	6–35 mo, 0.25 mL IM, 1 dose if previously vaccinated; 2 doses at least 1 mo apart if first vaccination 3–8 y, 0.5 mL IM, 1 dose if previously vaccinated 6 mo–8 y, two IM doses of inactivated influenza vaccine (administered a minimum of 4 wk apart) if first vaccination 9 y and older, 0.5 mL IM in a single dose Intranasal spray 5–8 y (not previously vaccinated with FluMist), 0.5 mL per dose, 60 d apart for a total of 2 doses 5–8 y (previously vaccinated with FluMist), 0.5 mL in a single dose per season 9 y and older, 0.6 mL in a single dose per season
Measles, mumps, and rubella (MMR) Preferred and more commonly used than single immunizing agents; contains live, attenuated viruses that cause measles, mumps, and rubella; protects more than 95% of recipients for many years	C	Immunization at 12–15 mo and a second dose at 4–6 y	0.5 mL IM	Same as adults
Pneumococcal polyvalent (Pneumovax 23) Contains 23 strains of pneumococci, which cause most of the serious pneumococcal infections in the United States; protection begins about 3 wk after vaccination and lasts for years	C	Adults 65 y and older who are otherwise healthy; people ages 2 to 64 y who have chronic conditions that cause increased risk of pneumococcal infection (e.g., cardiovascular or respiratory disease; asthma, diabetes mellitus, Hodgkin's disease, multiple myeloma, cirrhosis, alcohol dependence, renal failure, immunosuppression) or who smoke	0.5 mL Sub-Q, IM as a single dose; may be repeated after 5 y if given before age 65	Not recommended for children under 2 y 2 y and older, same dose as adults; may be repeated after 5 y

TABLE 10.1

DRUGS AT A GLANCE: Vaccines and Toxoids for Active Immunity (Continued)

Name/Characteristics	Pregnancy Category	Indications for Use	Routes and Dosage Ranges	
			Adults	**Children**
Pneumococcal 13-valent (Prevnar) Contains 13 *Streptococcus pneumoniae* antigens conjugated to a protein to increase antigenicity	C	All children up to age 6 y to prevent systemic pneumococcal infections (e.g., bacteremia, meningitis, pneumonia, otitis media) in young children		Birth–6 mo, 0.5 mL IM at 2, 4, 6, and 12–15 mo (4 doses) 7–11 mo, 0.5 mL IM initially, at least 4 wk later, and after 1 y birthday (3 doses) 12–23 mo, 0.5 ml IM initially and at least 2 mo later (2 doses) 24 mo–9 y, 0.5 mL IM in a single dose
Poliomyelitis, inactivated (IPV) (IPOL)	C	Routine immunization of infants; immunization of adults not previously immunized and at risk for exposure (e.g., health care or laboratory workers)	0.5 mL Sub-Q monthly for 2 doses, then a third dose 6–12 mo later	0.5 mL Sub-Q at 2, 4, and 6–18 mo, and 4–6 y of age (4 doses) or at 2 and 4 mo (2 doses)
Rabies vaccine (Imovax, RabAvert) Immunity develops in 7–10 d and lasts 1 y or longer	C	Preexposure immunization in people at high risk for exposure (e.g., veterinarians, animal handlers); postexposure prophylaxis in people who have been bitten by potentially rabid animals or who have skin scratches or abrasions exposed to animal saliva (e.g., animal licking of wound), urine, or blood	Preexposure: 1.0 mL IM for 3 doses; second dose is given 1 wk after the first; third dose is given 3–4 wk after the first; then, booster doses (1 mL) every 2–5 y based on antibody titers Postexposure: 1 mL IM for 5 doses; after the initial dose, other doses are given 3, 7, 14, and 28 d later	Same as adults
Rotavirus (RotaTeq; Rotarix) Can be given with most other childhood vaccines; adverse effects are usually mild (e.g., diarrhea); a few cases of intussusception have been reported after administration of RotaTeq.	C	Prevention of rotavirus gastroenteritis in infants between 6 and 32 wk of age	Individual doses administered orally	RotaTeq, 1 dose PO between 6 and 12 wk of age; a second and third dose at 4 to 10 wk intervals; third dose not after 32 wk of age Rotarix, 1 dose PO between 6 and 12 wk of age; second dose at least 4 wk later but no later than 24 wk of age

(*Continued on page 168*)

TABLE 10.1

DRUGS AT A GLANCE: Vaccines and Toxoids for Active Immunity (Continued)

Name/Characteristics	Pregnancy Category	Indications for Use	Routes and Dosage Ranges	
			Adults	**Children**
Varicella (Varivax) Contains live, attenuated varicella virus; contraindicated in hematologic or lymphatic malignancy, immunosuppression, febrile illness, or pregnancy	C (contraindicated)	Immunization of children 12 mo and older; immunization of adults who have not had chickenpox	0.5 mL Sub-Q, followed by a second dose of 0.5 mL 4–8 wk after the first dose	12–15 mo, 0.5 mL Sub-Q followed by a second dose at 4–6 y of age
Zoster vaccine (Zostavax) Not indicated for prevention or treatment of chickenpox or treatment of shingles; duration of protection unknown	C (contraindicated)	Prevention of herpes zoster in adults 50 y and older	0.65 mL Sub-Q (entire single-dose vial)	
Toxoids				
Diphtheria and tetanus toxoids (pediatric type) (DT) Contains a larger amount of diphtheria antigen than "tetanus and diphtheria toxoids, adult type (Td)"		Routine immunization of infants and children 6 y and younger in whom pertussis vaccine is contraindicated (those who have adverse reactions to initial doses of DTaP vaccine); not recommended for use in adults		Infants and children 6 y and younger, 0.5 mL IM for 2 doses at least 4 wk apart, followed by a booster dose 1 y later and when the child starts school
Tetanus and diphtheria toxoids (adult type) (Td) Contains a smaller amount of diphtheria antigen than "diphtheria and tetanus toxoids, pediatric type (DT)"	C	Primary immunization or booster doses in adults and children older than 6 y	0.5 mL IM for 2 doses, at least 4 wk apart, followed by a booster dose 6–12 mo later and every 10 y thereafter	Older than 6 y, same as adults
Tetanus toxoid Protects about 100% of recipients for 10 y or more; for primary immunization of infants and children 6 y of age or older, usually given in combination (e.g., DTaP or DT); for primary immunization of adults usually given or alone or combined with diphtheria toxoid (e.g., Td adult type)	C	Routine immunization of infants and young children; primary immunization of adults; prevention of tetanus in previously immunized people who sustain a potentially contaminated wound Prophylaxis, 0.5 mL IM if wound contaminated and no booster dose was received for 5 y; 0.5 mL if wound is clean and no booster dose was received for 10 y	Primary immunization in adults not previously immunized, 0.5 IM mL for 3 doses: initially, 4–8 wk later, then at 6–12 mo; then, 0.5-mL booster dose every 10 y	Same as adults

TABLE 10.2

DRUGS AT A GLANCE: Immune Serums for Passive Immunity

Serum/Characteristics	Pregnancy Category	Indications for Use	Routes and Dosage Ranges
CMV immune globulin, intravenous, human (CMV-IGIV) (CytoGam) Contains antibodies against CMV	C	Prevention of CMV infection in heart, kidney, liver, lung, and pancreas transplant recipients	Posttransplantation: infusion, 150 mg/kg IV within 72 h, then 100–150 mg/kg at 2, 4, 6, and 8 wk, then 50–100 mg/kg at 12 and 16 wk
Hepatitis B immune globulin, human (HBIG) (BayHep B, Nabi-HB) Solution of immunoglobulins that contains antibodies to HBsAg	C (contraindicated)	To prevent hepatitis after exposure; neonates born to HBsAg-positive or unknown-status mothers are given HBIG and the first dose of hepatitis B vaccine within 12 h of birth.	Adults and children 0.06 mL/kg (usual adult dose, 3–5 mL) IM as soon as possible after exposure, preferably within 7 d; repeat dose in 1 mo.
Immune globulin (human) (IG; IGIM) (BayGam) Given IM only; commonly called "gamma globulin"; obtained from pooled plasma of normal donors; consists primarily of IgG, which contains concentrated antibodies; produces adequate serum levels of IgG in 2–5 d	C	To decrease the severity of hepatitis A, measles, and varicella after exposure; to treat immunoglobulin deficiency	Adults and children Exposure to hepatitis A: 0.02 mL/kg IM Exposure to measles: 0.25 mL/kg IM within 6 d of exposure Exposure to varicella: 0.6–1.2 mL/kg IM Exposure to rubella (pregnant women only): 0.55 mL/kg IM Immunoglobulin deficiency: 1.3 mL/kg IM initially, then 0.6 mL/kg every 3–4 wk
Immune globulin intravenous (IGIV) (Polygam S/D, Panglobulin, Venoglobulin-S) Given IV only; provides immediate antibodies; half-life about 3 wk; mechanism of action in ITP is unknown **BLACK BOX WARNING ◆**—IGIV has been associated with renal dysfunction and failure and death; it should be used cautiously in patients with renal impairment or at risk for developing the condition.	C	Immunodeficiency syndrome; idiopathic thrombocytopenic purpura (ITP)	See manufacturers' instructions
Rabies immune globulin (human) RIG (HyperRAB S/D, Imogam) Gamma globulin obtained from plasma of people hyperimmunized with rabies vaccine; not useful in treatment of clinical rabies infection	C	Postexposure prevention of rabies, in conjunction with rabies vaccine	Adults and children 20 units/kg IM (half the dose may be injected around the wound) as soon as possible after possible exposure (e.g., animal bite)

(*Continued on page 170*)

TABLE 10.2

DRUGS AT A GLANCE: Immune Serums for Passive Immunity (Continued)

Serum/Characteristics	Pregnancy Category	Indications for Use	Routes and Dosage Ranges
Respiratory syncytial virus immune globulin intravenous (human) (RSV-IGIV) (RespiGam) Reduces severity of RSV illness and the incidence and duration of hospitalization in high-risk infants; may cause fluid overload; not established as safe and effective in children with congenital heart disease	C	Prevention of serious RSV infections in high-risk children younger than 2 y of age (i.e., those with bronchopulmonary dysplasia or history of premature birth [gestation of 35 wk or less]); treatment of RSV lower respiratory tract infections in hospitalized infants and young children	Children IV infusion via infusion pump, 1.5 mL/kg/h for 15 min, then 3 mL/kg/h for 15 min, then 6 mL/kg/h until the infusion is completed, then once monthly, if tolerated; max monthly dose, 750 mg/kg
Rh₀(D) immune globulin (human) (RhoGAM) Prepared from fractionated human plasma A sterile concentrated solution of specific immunoglobulin (IgG) containing anti-Rh₀(D)	C	To prevent sensitization in a subsequent pregnancy to the Rh₀(D) factor in an Rh-negative mother who has given birth to an Rh-positive infant by an Rh-positive father	*Obstetric use:* Inject contents of 1 vial IM for every 15 mL fetal packed red cell volume within 72 h after delivery, miscarriage, or abortion. Consult package instructions for blood typing and drug administration procedures.
Tetanus immune globulin (human) (BayTet) Solution of globulins from plasma of people hyperimmunized with tetanus toxoid Tetanus toxoid (Td) should also be given to initiate active immunization if minor wound and more than 10 y since Td, if major wound and more than 5 y since Td, or if Td primary immunization series was incomplete	C	To prevent tetanus in patients with wounds possibly contaminated with *Clostridium tetani* and whose immunization history is uncertain or incomplete Treatment of tetanus infection	Adults and children Prophylaxis: 250 units IM as a single dose Treatment of clinical disease: 3000–6000 units IM in a single dose
Varicella-zoster immune globulin (human) (VZIG) The globulin fraction of human plasma Antibodies last 1 mo or longer.	C	Postexposure to chickenpox or shingles, to prevent or decrease severity of infections in children under 15 y of age who have not been immunized or who are immunodeficient because of illness or drug therapy Infants born to mothers who develop varicella 5 d before or 2 d after delivery and premature infants of less than 28 wk gestation	IM 125 units/10 kg up to a maximum of 625 units within 48 h after exposure if possible; may be given up to 96 h after exposure. Minimal dose, 125 units

CMV, cytomegalovirus; IgG, immunoglobulin G; RSV, respiratory syncytial virus; HBsAg, hepatitis B surface antigen.

EVIDENCE-BASED PRACTICE

Vaccine-preventable Diseases, Immunizations, and MMWR 1961–2011.

by HINMAN, A. R., ORENSTEIN, W. A., & SCHICHAT, A.

Morbidity and Mortality Weekly Report
2011, 60(4 Suppl), 49–57

In the 50 years since the Centers for Disease Control (CDC) has been reporting morbidity and mortality reports, the awareness of diseases now prevented by vaccines has been expanded, new vaccines have been introduced, the incidence of most of these diseases has been dramatically reduced, and some unanticipated challenges have emerged. Three periods (1961–1988, 1989–1999, and 2000–2010) categorize the improvements from immunizations have brought to the United States.

- 1961 to 1988: A nationwide immunization program was initiated. Children in the United States at the start of 1961 received vaccines to prevent five diseases: diphtheria, tetanus, pertussis, poliomyelitis, and smallpox. In this period, increased development of new vaccines lead to a reduction of disease.
- 1989 to 1999: A measles outbreak fundamentally changed the immunization program in the United States and prompted efforts to initiate comprehensive state- and community-based immunization action plans that identified the steps needed during the first 2 years of life. The goal was to achieve at least 90% immunization coverage of preschool-aged children for all recommended vaccines at the recommended ages. This led to immunization schedules that included the addition of several new vaccines, resulting in fewer outbreaks of vaccine-preventable diseases.
- 2000 to 2010: During this decade, disease was substantially reduced within the vaccination-targeted age groups, plus within unvaccinated populations. Immunization coverage for the infant vaccination series (DTaP—inactivated polio vaccine—MMR—Hib—hepatitis B—varicella) neared the Healthy People 2010 target of 80%. Vaccine-preventable diseases declined. The CDC reported that direct and indirect savings to society are estimated to total $69 billion. Advances in immunization information systems (IIS, immunization registries) enhanced confidentiality and coordination with population-based, computerized databases that record all vaccine doses administered by participating providers to people residing within a given geopolitical area; these systems are now in place in 48 of 50 states. Now children receive vaccines to prevent 16 conditions: diphtheria; *H. influenzae* type b, hepatitis A, hepatitis B, and human papillomavirus infections; and influenza, measles, meningococcal disease, mumps, pertussis, pneumococcal disease, poliomyelitis, rotavirus infections, rubella, tetanus, and varicella.

IMPLICATIONS FOR NURSING PRACTICE: The past 50 years of immunization have led to elimination or near elimination of several vaccine-preventable diseases in the United States. Sustaining a well-developed vaccine delivery system and adequate surveillance of disease and of vaccine coverage can continue to significantly decrease the incidence of deaths, disabilities, and illness.

of visits to a health care provider. Several combination vaccines are now available (Box 10.2), and others continue to be developed. Studies indicate that these strategies are effective in improving rates of immunizations. Children's health care providers should implement the recommended childhood immunization schedule issued in January of each year by the Centers for Disease Control and Prevention (CDC). Also, they should refer to current guidelines about immunizations for children with chronic illnesses (e.g., asthma, heart disease, diabetes) or immunosuppression (e.g., from cancer, organ transplantation, or human immunodeficiency virus [HIV] infection).

Use in Adolescents, Young Adults, and Middle-Aged Adults

Adolescents who received all primary immunizations as infants and young children should have a second dose of varicella (chickenpox) vaccine, hepatitis A and B vaccines (if not received earlier), a tetanus–diphtheria–pertussis booster (Tdap) between ages 11 and 18 years if 5 years have passed since a prior tetanus–diphtheria (Td) booster, as well as meningococcal vaccine at age 11 or 12 with a booster dose at age 16. Adolescents of both genders should receive two doses of the quadrivalent HPV vaccine if not received earlier. Young adults who are health care workers, sexually active, or belong to a high-risk group should receive varicella vaccine (or a second dose if they previously received a single dose), hepatitis A and hepatitis B vaccines if not previously received,

BOX 10.2	Combination Vaccines Used for Routine Childhood Immunizations

DTaP–IPV (Kinrix)
DTaP–Hep B–IPV (Pediarix)
DTaP–IPV–Hib (Pentacel)
DTaP–Hib (TriHIBit)
Hib–Hep B (Comvax)
Hep A–Hep B (Twinrix)
MMR–Var (ProQuad)

and Tdap, as well as measles–mumps–rubella (MMR) if they are not pregnant and rubella titer is inadequate or if proof of immunization is unavailable. In addition, annual influenza vaccine is recommended for adolescents as well as children and infants older than 6 months of age. Middle-aged adults should maintain immunizations against tetanus–diphtheria with one booster dose of Tdap and influenza vaccine annually. High-risk groups (e.g., those with chronic illness and health care providers) should receive the hepatitis B vaccine series (if not previously received). Middle-aged adults born after 1956 should have at least one dose of MMR vaccine unless they have had either the vaccine or each of the three diseases.

Use in Older Adults

Older adults become more susceptible to some diseases, and influenza, pneumococcal infections, tetanus, and shingles can be especially serious in this population. The varicella-zoster virus, the same virus that causes chickenpox, can cause shingles later in life. An additional varicella vaccine to prevent zoster infections (shingles) is available for adults 60 years and older who have had chickenpox.

Recommended immunizations for older adults 65 years of age and older include a tetanus–diphtheria (Td) booster every 10 years, annual influenza vaccine, and a one-time administration of pneumococcal vaccine at 65 years of age. A second dose of pneumococcal vaccine may be given at 65 years if the first dose was given 5 years previously. As with younger adults, immunization for most other diseases is recommended for older adults at high risk for exposure due to occupation or travel.

Use in Patients With Specific Health Problems

Use in Patients With Immunosuppression

Compared with healthy people who are immunocompetent, patients with immunosuppression usually have an adequate, but reduced, antibody response to immunization. They require individualized immunizations. In general, patients with diabetes mellitus or chronic pulmonary, renal, or hepatic disorders who are not receiving immunosuppressant drugs may receive both live attenuated and killed vaccines and toxoids to induce active immunity. However, they may need higher doses or more frequent administration to achieve adequate immunity. With hepatitis B vaccine, for example, larger initial doses may be required and booster doses may be needed later, if antibody concentrations fall.

Patients with active malignant disease may receive killed vaccines or toxoids but not live vaccines (an exception is people with leukemia who have not received chemotherapy for at least 3 months). When patients receive vaccines, it is important to give them at least 2 weeks before the start of chemotherapy or 3 months after chemotherapy is completed. Health care providers may give immune serum, which provides passive temporary immunity, to immunocompromised people who are exposed to an infectious disease, such a rubella or varicella, to reduce the risk of a person developing a serious infection.

Patients receiving a systemic corticosteroid in high doses (e.g., prednisone 20 mg or equivalent daily) or for longer than 2 weeks should wait at least 3 months before being receiving a live-virus vaccine. Short-term use (less than 2 weeks) or low to moderate doses (less than 20 mg of prednisone daily) of corticosteroids are not contraindications to immunizations. In addition, long-term alternate-day therapy with short-acting agents; maintenance physiologic replacement doses; and the use of topical, inhaled, or intra-articular injections of corticosteroids are not contraindications.

Patients with HIV infection have less-than-optimal responses to immunizing agents because this viral infection produces major defects in both cell-mediated and humoral immunity. Live bacterial (bacillus Calmette-Guérin [BCG], oral typhoid) or viral (MMR, varicella) vaccines should not be given, because the bacteria or viruses may be able to reproduce and cause active infection. People with asymptomatic HIV infection should receive inactivated vaccines; those exposed to measles or varicella may be given immune globulin or varicella-zoster immune globulin for passive immunization.

For children with HIV infection, most routine immunizations (DTaP, inactivated polio vaccine, MMR, *H. influenzae* type b [Hib], influenza) are recommended. MMR is not recommended in children with severe immunosuppression from HIV. Varicella vaccine is recommended only for children with no evidence of immunosuppression. Pneumococcal vaccine is recommended for HIV-infected people older than 2 years of age.

Use in Patients With Cancer

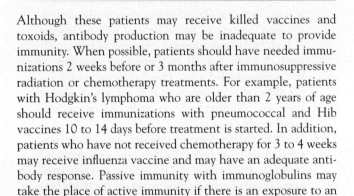

QSEN Safety Alert

Patients with active malignant disease should not receive live vaccines.

Although these patients may receive killed vaccines and toxoids, antibody production may be inadequate to provide immunity. When possible, patients should have needed immunizations 2 weeks before or 3 months after immunosuppressive radiation or chemotherapy treatments. For example, patients with Hodgkin's lymphoma who are older than 2 years of age should receive immunizations with pneumococcal and Hib vaccines 10 to 14 days before treatment is started. In addition, patients who have not received chemotherapy for 3 to 4 weeks may receive influenza vaccine and may have an adequate antibody response. Passive immunity with immunoglobulins may take the place of active immunity if there is an exposure to an active infection (e.g., varicella) during chemotherapy.

Clinical Application 10-1

- Mrs. Williams asks if Riley, who is getting over "a cold" and has some clear nasal discharge, should wait before having his scheduled immunizations. What is the nurse's best response?

- Mrs. Williams reports the last time she had any immunizations was at 14 years of age. Based on her age and gender, what vaccines do authorities recommend?

Adverse Effects

Mild reactions to vaccines, such as injection site soreness and redness, fever, and muscle aches, are common, whereas severe and serious reactions, such as anaphylaxis or serum sickness, are rare. Adverse reactions to individual immunizing agents include the following:

- DTaP: soreness, erythema, edema at injection sites, anorexia, nausea, severe fever, encephalopathy, and seizures
- Hib vaccine: pain and erythema at injection sites
- Hepatitis B vaccine: injection site soreness, erythema, induration, fever, and anaphylaxis
- Influenza vaccine: via injection—pain, induration, and erythema at injection sites and flu-like symptoms such as chills, fever, malaise, muscle aches; via intranasal spray—runny nose, headache, cough, sore throat, and irritability in children
- MMR vaccine: mild symptoms of measles—cough, fever up to 39.4°C (102°F), headache, malaise, photophobia, skin rash, sore throat, febrile seizures, arthralgia (joint pain), and anaphylaxis in recipients who are allergic to eggs
- Pneumococcal vaccine: local effects—soreness, induration, and erythema at injection sites; systemic effects—chills, fever, headache, muscle aches, nausea, photophobia, and weakness
- Polio vaccine: soreness at injection sites, fever, and anaphylaxis
- Varicella vaccine: early effects—transient soreness or erythema at injection sites; late effect—a mild, maculopapular skin rash with a few lesions
- Immune globulin intravenous (IGIV): chills; dizziness; dyspnea; fever; flushing; headache; nausea; urticaria; vomiting; tightness in chest; pain in chest, hip, or back, renal dysfunction, acute renal failure, and death

Contraindications

Contraindications to most vaccines and toxoids include the following:

- Acute febrile illness
- Immunosuppressive drug therapy
- Immunodeficiency states such as congenital immunodeficiency or active HIV disease
- Hematological cancers (leukemia or lymphoma) or generalized malignancy
- Pregnancy

Preventing Interactions

Immunosuppressant drug therapy and interferon administration may interfere with vaccine response to live vaccines. Antiviral drugs may also interfere with the immune response to a live viral vaccine and should not be given 48 hours before and for 14 days after viral vaccine administration. Likewise, passive immunization with immune globulin for exposure to a viral infection (e.g., measles, hepatitis A, varicella) can likewise interfere with active immunity, and it is necessary to delay administration of the viral vaccine for 2 to 6 months or more, depending on the person's immune status.

QSEN Safety Alert

Measles vaccine can interfere with the activity of meningococcal vaccine, and it is essential to separate these two vaccines by at least a month.

Measles vaccine can also interfere with the response to tuberculosis (TB) skin testing. Patients should have the TB skin test either simultaneously with the measles vaccine, or they should delay it for 4 to 6 weeks after the test.

QSEN Safety Alert

In addition, salicylates may increase the risk of Reye's syndrome with administration of the varicella vaccine.

Administering the Medication

Following package insert instructions for storing, reconstituting, and safely administering combination vaccines is essential for effectiveness of all immunizations. To maintain effectiveness of vaccines and other biologic preparations, the nurse helps ensure that immunization products are stored properly. Most products require refrigeration at 2°C to 8°C (35.6°–46.4°F). It is important to follow manufacturer's instructions for storage strictly. The nurse reconstitutes vaccines only with the supplied diluent and then uses them within the time frame recommended after reconstitution to maintain vaccine effectiveness.

Box 10.3 summarizes administration considerations for immunizations.

Assessing for Therapeutic Effects

Most vaccines take about 2 weeks for full antibody response and protection against the disease. A fourfold increase in

BOX 10.3 Administering Immunizing Agents

Accurate administration includes the following:

- Reading the package insert and check the expiration date on all biologic products (e.g., vaccines, toxoids, human immune serums)
- Following instructions for administering each vaccine
- Checking the patient's temperature before giving a vaccine
- Giving intramuscular (IM) human immune serum globulin with an 18- to 20-gauge needle, preferably in the gluteal muscles. If the dose is 5 mL or more, divide it and inject it into two or more IM sites. Follow manufacturer's instructions for preparation and administration of intravenous (IV) formulations.
- Having aqueous epinephrine 1:1000 readily available before administering any vaccine
- After administration of an immunizing agent in a clinic or office setting, having the patient stay in the area for at least 30 minutes
- Providing patients with a Vaccine Information Statement (VIS)

immunoglobulin titer levels indicates an adequate antibody response. It is necessary to obtain antibody titer levels during pregnancy to determine immunity to viral infections such as measles and rubella because the fetus may be affected by active maternal infection during the pregnancy.

Assessing for Adverse Effects

Careful screening of people for contraindications and observing vaccine precautions minimize serious adverse vaccine events.

QSEN Safety Alert

By law, health care providers must report potentially serious adverse effects using the Vaccine Adverse Event Reporting System (VAERS).

The National Vaccine Injury Compensation Program, established in 1986 in the United States, covers injury, disability, or death that may occur due to vaccine administration in cases where significant adverse effects are linked directly to immunization.

Patient Teaching

The nurse ensures that the patient or parent receives current vaccine information about the benefits and risks of immunization—a Vaccine Information Statement (VIS)—for each vaccine dose given. Current VIS forms for all recommended vaccines, along with indications, contraindications, and the timing of immunizations doses, are available for downloading at the CDC Web site (see "References and Resources"). Box 10.4 presents additional patient teaching information.

NCLEX Success

1. **A nurse is explaining to a parent how vaccines work. Vaccines provide**

   A. active immunity
   B. passive immunity
   C. innate immunity
   D. nonspecific immunity

2. **The nurse is caring for a patient with severe immunosuppression. This condition is a contraindication to**

   A. all injectable immunizations
   B. the use of live bacterial or viral vaccines
   C. the use of immune globulins for passive immunity
   D. annual influenza vaccine

3. **A child is receiving an immunization. The nurse should inform the parents that common aftereffects may include which of the following?**

   A. skin rash and itching
   B. redness and soreness at the injection site
   C. muscle weakness and difficulty in walking
   D. nausea, vomiting, and diarrhea

BOX 10.4 — Patient Teaching Guidelines for Immunizations

■ Appropriate vaccinations should be maintained for adults as well as for children. Consult the Centers for Disease Control and Prevention Web site or a health care provider for current information because recommendations for particular groups may change.

■ Maintain immunization records for yourself and all members of your family. This is important because immunizations are often obtained at different places and over a period of many years. Written, accurate, up-to-date records help to prevent diseases and reduce unnecessary immunizations.

■ If a health care provider recommends an immunization and you do not know whether you have had the immunization or the disease, it is probably safer to be immunized than to risk having the disease. Immunization after a previous immunization or after having the disease usually is not harmful.

■ Most vaccines can cause fever and soreness at the site of injection. Acetaminophen (e.g., Tylenol) can be taken two to three times daily for 24 to 48 hours if needed to decrease fever and discomfort. Routine premedication with acetaminophen is not recommended. Lower antibody levels may occur and it may not be necessary.

■ Women of childbearing age who receive a rubella (German measles) or a varicella (chickenpox) immunization must avoid becoming pregnant (i.e., use effective contraception) for 3 months afterward.

■ If skin lesions develop after receiving live varicella vaccine (to prevent chickenpox), avoid skin contact with newborns, pregnant women, and anyone whose immune system is impaired. Skin lesions from a newly immunized person may transmit the vaccine virus to susceptible close contacts.

■ After receiving a vaccine, stay in the area for approximately 30 minutes. If an allergic reaction is going to occur, it will usually do so within that time.

Keeping Up-to-Date with Immunization Recommendations

Recommendations regarding immunizations change periodically as additional information and new immunizing agents become available. Experts review and update vaccine recommendations in the United States on a frequent basis. Consequently, health care providers need to update their knowledge of vaccine recommendations at least annually. The best source of information for current recommendations is the CDC. The most current immunization schedules for all age groups are available at the CDC Web site (see "References and Resources" for Web site addresses). The main source of CDC recommendations is the Advisory Committee on Immunization Practices (ACIP), which consists of experts appointed to advise the CDC on strategies to eliminate vaccine-preventable diseases. Information on vaccines needed for travel to foreign countries (e.g., Japanese encephalitis, typhoid, yellow fever) is also available at the CDC Web site and is frequently updated.

Other sources of information about immunizations include the American Academy of Pediatrics and the American Academy of Family Physicians. Local health departments may also be a source of information about immunizations, whether routine or necessary for foreign travel. Immunization sources can also provide information on new vaccine releases, vaccine availability, and usage of specific vaccines.

The Nursing Process

Assessment

- Determine the patient's previous history of diseases for which immunizing agents are available (e.g., measles, influenza).
- Ask the patient about previous immunizations.
  - For which diseases have immunizations been received?
  - Which immunizing agent was used and how long ago was it given?
  - Were any adverse effects experienced? If so, what symptoms occurred, and how long did they last?
  - Has tetanus toxoid been given for any cuts or wounds?
  - Has any foreign travel required immunizations?
- Determine whether the patient has any conditions that contraindicate administration of immunizing agents (e.g., malignancy, pregnancy, immunosuppressive drug therapy).
- For pregnant women not known to be immunized against rubella, a serum antibody titer should be measured to determine resistance or susceptibility to the disease.
- For patients with wounds, assess the type of wound and determine how, when, and where it was sustained. Such information may reveal whether tetanus immunization is needed.
- For patients exposed to infectious diseases, assess the extent of exposure (e.g., household or brief, casual contact) and when it occurred.

Nursing Diagnoses

- Deficient knowledge: importance of maintaining immunizations for both children and adults
- Readiness for enhanced immunization status related to self-care efficacy
- Noncompliance in obtaining recommended immunizations related to fear of adverse effects
- Risk for injury related to hypersensitivity, fever, and other adverse effects

Planning/Goals

The patient will

- Avoid diseases for which immunizations are available and recommended
- Obtain recommended immunizations for self and children
- Keep immunization appointments and maintain immunization records

Nursing Interventions

The nurse will

- Use measures to prevent infectious diseases. General measures include those that promote health and resistance to disease (e.g., nutrition, rest, exercise).
- Provide information about the availability of immunizing agents.
- Take additional measures, including the following:
  - Educate the public, especially parents of young children, regarding the importance of immunizations to personal and public health. Include information about the diseases that can be prevented and where immunizations can be obtained.
  - Assist patients in developing a system to maintain immunization records for themselves and their children. This is important because immunizations are often obtained at different places and over a period of years. Written, accurate, up-to-date records help to prevent diseases and unnecessary immunizations.
  - Prevent disease transmission, using the following measures:
    - Hand hygiene (probably the most effective method)
    - Avoiding contact with people who have known or suspected infectious diseases, when possible
    - Using appropriate isolation techniques with infection exposure
    - Using medical and surgical aseptic techniques
    - For someone exposed to rubeola, administration of measles vaccine within 48 hours can help prevent the disease.
    - For someone with a puncture wound or a dirty wound, administration of tetanus immune globulin will prevent tetanus, a life-threatening disease.
    - For someone with an animal bite, wash the wound immediately with large amounts of soap and water, then seek prompt health care. Administration of rabies immune globulin and vaccine may be needed to prevent rabies, a life-threatening disease.
    - Explain to the patient that contracting rubella or undergoing rubella immunization during pregnancy, especially during the first trimester, may cause severe birth defects in the infant. The goal of immunization is to prevent congenital rubella syndrome. Current recommendations are to immunize children against rubella at 12 to 15 months of age. It is also recommended that previously unimmunized girls 11 to 13 years of age be immunized against rubella. Furthermore, nonpregnant women of childbearing age should have rubella antibody tests. If antibody concentrations are low, the woman should be immunized. Pregnancy should be avoided for 3 months after rubella immunization.

Evaluation

- Interview and observe for symptoms.
- Interview and observe for adverse drug effects.
- Check immunization records when indicated.

Clinical Application 10-2

- Mrs. Williams does not have a personal immunization record for Riley. When administering the immunizations, the nurse records Riley's immunization information on both the clinic record and on a personal immunization record. Is there any way that the nurse can obtain Riley's previous vaccine record?

NCLEX Success

4. A nurse is caring for a 74-year-old man. The nurse recognizes that he would most likely to have a decreased immune response to the influenza vaccine if he is taking which of the following medications?

   A. levothyroxine (Synthroid)
   B. prednisone (Deltasone)
   C. metoprolol (Lopressor)
   D. lovastatin (Mevacor)

5. A nurse is preparing to administer an unfamiliar vaccine. To obtain current information and provide patient teaching about vaccine recommendations and contraindications, it is best to do which of the following?

   A. Ask a coworker about the vaccine—when and how it should be administered.
   B. Use a drug guide to look up the vaccine information.
   C. Access an Internet search engine to find vaccine information.
   D. Obtain vaccine information and a Vaccine Information Statement (VIS) from the Centers for Disease Control and Prevention (CDC) Web site.

Key Concepts

- Many infectious diseases can be prevented by immunizations.
- Immunizations are needed for all age groups.
- Children in the United States are much more likely to receive recommended immunizations than are adolescents and adults.
- Active immunity is achieved through administration of a vaccine or toxoid or through natural exposure to the disease.
- Passive immunity is a temporary state of immunity produced in a person who is susceptible to an infectious organism by administering serum containing antibodies to the disease.
- Women of childbearing age who receive a rubella (German measles) or a varicella (chickenpox) immunization must avoid becoming pregnant (i.e., use effective contraception) for 3 months after they receive the vaccine.
- A **BLACK BOX WARNING** ◆ exists for intravenous immune globulin (IGIV) because it has been associated with renal dysfunction, renal failure, and death.
- Health care providers who provide or participate in immunizations need to keep their knowledge base current with annual updates regarding recommendations from the CDC.
- Health care providers need to assess and inform patients about recommended immunizations.
- A patient or parent must receive a VIS for each recommended vaccines, along with indications, contraindications, and the timing of immunizations doses with each vaccine dose.
- New immunizing products continue to be developed.

Critical Thinking Questions

10-1. Deborah Little is a 22-year-old mother of 6-month-old twin girls. She has brought the girls into the pediatric clinic for well-child checkups and immunizations. She is questioning the need for the immunizations, stating that she does not understand why some require multiple doses. She states that she is concerned that "all of these shots will be traumatic for the girls."

- Discuss the difference between vaccines and toxoids, including the reason that booster doses are necessary.
- Describe strategies to increase the likelihood that Ms. Little will complete the required immunizations for her daughters.

References and Resources

American Academy of Family Physicians (AAFP). Homepage—http://www.aafp.org

American Academy of Pediatrics (AAP). Homepage—http://www.aap.org

Berberich, F. R., & Landman, Z. (2009). Reducing immunization discomfort in 4- to 6-year-old children: A randomized clinical trial. *Pediatrics, 124,* 203–209.

Burns, J. L., Walsh, L. J., & Popovich, J. M. (2010). Practical pediatric and adolescent immunization update. *The Journal for Nurse Practitioners,* 6(4), 254–266.

Centers for Disease Control and Prevention. Recommendations and Guidelines: Advisory Committee on Immunization Practices (ACIP). http://www.cdc.gov/vaccines/recs/acip/default.htm

Centers for Disease Control and Prevention. Travelers' health. http://www.cdc.gov/travel

Centers for Disease Control and Prevention. Vaccines and immunizations. Immunization schedules. http://www.cdc.gov/vaccines/recs/schedules

Cortese, M. M., & Parashar, U. D. (2009). Prevention of rotavirus gastroenteritis among infants and children: recommendations of the Advisory Committee on Immunization Practices (ACIP). *Morbidity and Mortality Weekly Report,* 58(5), 1–25.

Daley, M. F., O'Leary, S.T., & Nyquist, A. C. (2012). *Current Diagnosis and Treatment in Pediatrics* (21st ed.). Chapter 10, Immunization. New York City: McGraw Hill.

Fiore, A. E., Uyeki, T. M., Broder, K., Finelli, L. Euler, G. L., Singleton, J. A., et al. (2010). Prevention and control of influenza with vaccines: Recommendations of the advisory committee on immunization practices (ACIP). *Morbidity and Mortality Weekly Report,* 59(37), 1–62.

Hinman, A. R., Orenstein, W. A., & Schichat, A. (2011). Vaccine-preventable diseases, immunizations, and MMWR-1961–2011. *Morbidity and Mortality Weekly Report,* 60(4 Suppl), 49–57.

McElligott, J. T., & Darden, P. M. (2010). Are patient held vaccine records associated with improved vaccination recovery rates? *Pediatrics,* 125(3), 467–472.

Miller, B. L., Ahmed, F., Lu, P. J., Euler, G. L., & Kretsinger, K. (2010). Tetanus and pertussis vaccination coverage among adults aged 18 years and older-United States, 1999 and 2008. *Morbidity and Mortality Weekly Report,* 59(40), 1302–1306.

Nuori, J. L. (2010). Updated recommendations for prevention of invasive pneumococcal disease among adults using the 23-valent pneumococcal polysaccharide vaccine (PPSV23). *Morbidity and Mortality Weekly Report,* 59(34), 1102–1106.

Porth, C. M. (2010). *Pathophysiology: Concepts of altered health states* (8th ed.). Philadelphia, PA: Lippincott Williams & Wilkins.

Prymula, R., Siegrist, C. A., Chilbek, R., Zemlickova, H., Vackova, M., Smetana, J., et al. (2009). Effect of prophylactic paracetamol administration at time of vaccination on febrile reactions and antibody responses in children: Two open-label, randomised controlled trials. *Lancet,* 374(9698), 1339–1350.

Vaccine Adverse Event Reporting System (VAERS). Homepage—http://www.vaers.hhs.gov

11 Drug Therapy to Suppress Immunity

Clinical Application Case Study

Sam Jones, a 35-year-old mechanic with type 1 diabetes mellitus and end-stage renal disease, received a renal transplant from a living donor 2 years ago. To prevent organ rejection, he is currently taking cyclosporine, mycophenolate mofetil, and prednisone daily. He has monthly appointments at the nephrology clinic and has serum trough levels for cyclosporine measured before each visit. A month ago, Mr. Jones was hospitalized and received four infusions of muromonab-CD3 for an acute organ rejection reaction.

KEY TERMS

Autoantigens: protein complexes on a person's own tissue that stimulate an abnormal immune reaction

Autoimmune disorders: conditions associated with an abnormal immune response to self-antigens (autoantigens) on body tissue, resulting in ongoing inflammation and damage to body tissues

Cytotoxic: causing cell death

Graft rejection reaction: activated immunological response by the recipient to graft donor organ cells resulting in graft tissue damage and loss of graft organ function

Graft-versus-host disease: complication of bone marrow or stem cell transplantation where activated T cells in donor bone marrow attack host tissues producing inflammatory changes in the skin, liver, and gastrointestinal tract; also can occur infrequently with a blood transfusion

Immunosuppression: suppression of the immune system

Monoclonal antibody: immunoglobulin therapeutically replicated in laboratory cells to react with a specific cell antigen altering the immune response to that antigen

Murine antibodies: immunoglobulins created in mouse cells for use as therapeutic treatment for human diseases

Polyclonal antibody: mixtures of antibodies (IgA, IgD, IgE, IgG, and IgM) produced by several clones of B lymphocytes

Introduction

The immune response, normally a protective process, recognizes and destroys potentially harmful outside substances, helping the body defend itself against disease. However, disease processes can also develop when the immune system perceives a harmless substance, such as an antigen or the person's own body tissues, as foreign and tries to eliminate them. This inappropriate activation of the immune response is a major factor in allergic conditions (e.g., allergic asthma) and **autoimmune disorders** (e.g., rheumatoid arthritis, Crohn's disease, psoriasis). Autoimmune disorders occur when a person's immune system loses its ability to differentiate self from nonself. As a result, an immune response against host tissues occurs.

An appropriate, but undesirable, immune response also occurs when foreign tissue from another organism is transplanted into the body. With transplant therapy, if the immune response is not suppressed, a **graft rejection reaction** occurs, where the body reacts to the implanted cells as with other antigens and attempts to destroy the foreign tissue. Although numerous advances have been made in transplantation technology, the ability to modulate the immune response remains a major factor in determining the success or failure of transplant therapy.

Immunosuppressant drugs are used to decrease an undesirable immune response by interfering with the production or function of immune cells and cytokines that contribute to tissue inflammation and damage. Drugs used therapeutically as immunosuppressants constitute a diverse group, some of which also are used for other purposes. Drug groups that are used to reduce the immune response include corticosteroids (see Chap. 15) and some **cytotoxic** (causing cell death) antineoplastic drugs (see Chap. 12). Health care providers use these drugs, discussed here in relation to their effects in modulating the body's response to autoimmune disorders or organ transplantation, to treat inflammatory autoimmune disorders or to prevent or treat transplant rejection reactions. These drugs are the main focus of this chapter. To aid in the understanding of immunosuppressant drugs, descriptions of selected inflammatory autoimmune disorders, tissue transplantation, and rejection reactions appear below.

Overview of Altered Immune Function

Etiology

In healthy people, the immune system's ability to inherently differentiate between cell surface proteins on its own cells (called self-antigens or **autoantigens**) and antigens on foreign cells provides protection against disease. However, in people

who have received an organ transplant, this protective mechanism must be altered to avoid damage to the transplant and organ rejection. Drug therapy to suppress the body's ability to recognize self from nonself is a major part of transplantation protocols.

Tissue and organ transplantation involves replacing diseased host tissue with healthy donor tissue. The goal of such treatment is to save and enhance the quality of the recipient's life. Skin grafts and kidney transplants are commonly performed, and heart, lung, liver, pancreas, and bone marrow/stem cell transplants are increasing. The use of biological agents, which stimulate the production of hematopoietic stem cells from bone marrow and mobilize them into circulating blood, has helped improve the availability of stem cells for transplant, reducing the need for bone marrow transplants.

Although many factors affect graft survival, including the degree of matching between donor tissues and recipient tissues, drug-induced **immunosuppression** is a major part of transplantation protocols. The goal is to provide adequate immunosuppression while minimizing adverse effects on normal body tissue. If immunosuppression is inadequate, a graft rejection reaction will occur with solid organ transplantation, and **graft-versus-host disease** (GVHD) will develop with bone marrow/stem cell transplantation. If immunosuppressive drug therapy is excessive, serious infection may occur, some malignancies such as lymphomas and skin cancers may develop, and organ damage related to the proliferation of activated lymphocytes in normal body cells may result.

Pathophysiology

After self-antigens develop, the tissue containing them is perceived as foreign and antigenic, triggering an inappropriate immune response that may involve T lymphocytes in direct destruction of tissue, as well as the production of proinflammatory cytokines, chemical messengers that attract and activate phagocytes contributing to the inflammatory immune process. Stimulation of B lymphocytes to produce antibodies leads to further inflammation and tissue damage.

Knowledge about the role of inflammatory cells and cytokines in the immune response to tissue injury continues to expand. This has led to the development of biological agents that can modulate inflammatory cytokine production by activated lymphocytes. Cytokines act as messengers between different types of lymphocytes to increase or decrease the immune response, modifying the production and activity of different white blood cells. Attachment of an antigen to an antigen-presenting cell activates macrophages to produce interleukin-1 (IL-1) and T cells to produce IL-2. Lymphocyte activation by IL-1 causes the activated lymphocytes and other immune cells to produce more IL-2 receptors, amplifying the immune response. IL-2 activates production and promotes the activity of cytotoxic T cells, macrophages, natural killer (NK) cells, and B lymphocytes. Hence, decreasing IL-2 production induces lymphocyte apoptosis, reducing the numbers of T lymphocytes available to participate in an immune response.

Another inflammatory mediator mediating the inflammatory process of autoimmune disease is tumor necrosis factor (TNF)-alpha, a cytokine that plays a major role in the response to infection. Functions of TNF include activation of monocytes, macrophages, and cytotoxic T cells; enhancement of NK cell functions; increased leukocyte movement into areas of tissue injury; increased phagocytosis by neutrophils; and stimulation of B and T lymphocytes. Although TNF can be beneficial in helping to fight infection, an excessive TNF response has been associated with the pathogenesis of autoimmune disorders. Overproduction of cytokines, such as IL-2 and TNF, contributes to prolonged tissue inflammation and damage in autoimmune disease.

In addition to the factors that activate an immune response, there are also factors that prevent the immune system from "turning off" an abnormal immune or inflammatory process. One of these factors may be a decrease in the number of suppressor T cells, which help modulate the immune response. Another factor may be inadequate amounts of anti-inflammatory cytokines (e.g., IL-10) to modulate the immune reaction.

A transplant rejection reaction occurs when the host's immune system is stimulated to destroy the transplanted organ. The immune cells of the transplant recipient attach to the donor cells of the transplanted organ and react against the antigens in the donor organ. The rejection process involves T and B lymphocytes, antibodies, multiple cytokines, and inflammatory mediators. In most cases, T-cell activation and proliferation are more important initially in the rejection reaction than B-cell activation and the presence of active antibodies. Typically, during an organ rejection reaction, helper T cells become activated by donor antigen attachment to an antigen-presenting cell; the activated helper T cells then stimulate B cells to produce antibodies, leading to a delayed hypersensitivity reaction weeks or months later. The antibodies injure the transplanted organ by activating complement, producing antigen–antibody complexes or causing antibody-mediated tissue destruction. This reaction can destroy the solid organ graft within 2 weeks if the recipient's immune system is not adequately suppressed by immunosuppressant drugs. Immunosuppressive drug therapy begins either immediately before or at the time of the transplant procedure to prevent antibody formation, and it must continue for life to prevent organ rejection.

Clinical Manifestations

Allergic Disorders

Allergic asthma is characterized by increased production of IgE in response to inhaled allergens. The IgE–allergen complexes trigger inflammation, producing airway edema and increasing mucus production. People use immunosuppressants to reduce the airway edema and excessive vascular permeability that accompany this type of asthma.

EVIDENCE-BASED PRACTICE

Barriers to Immunosuppressive Medication Adherence in High-Risk Adult Renal Transplant Recipients
by M. CONSTATINER, D. CUKOR

Dialysis and Transplantation
2011, 2, 60–65

Investigators identified two sets of barriers to adherence in a convenience sample of 94 postrenal transplant patients: (1) intentional omissions (too many pills or doses daily; perceived adverse effects related to the drugs) and (2) unintentional omission (forgetting doses, getting out of daily administration routine, lack of money to buy medications). Nurses can intervene to help patients improve adherence to posttransplant immunosuppressant medication by:

- Helping patients organize and set up a scheduled medication routine that is integrated with activities of daily living (e.g., meals, activities, bedtime)
- Using individualized cues and reminders to help the patient maintain their routine; a special medication container, prefilled by a pharmacist with a week of medications (e.g., Medisets); pill bottle alarm caps; environmental cues
- Making use of support by family and significant others to encourage ongoing compliance
- Helping the patient develop a plan to cope with and address common adverse effects
- Helping the patient to complete application forms for drug company assistance programs, as needed, to pay for medications

IMPLICATIONS FOR NURSING PRACTICE: Lack of adherence to immunosuppressant medication is a major factor in rejection reactions after transplant therapy. Nursing measures to assist patients with medication adherence can prevent organ loss and reduce patient morbidity and mortality after transplant therapy.

Immune Disorders

Crohn's disease is a chronic, recurrent, inflammatory bowel disorder that can affect any area of the gastrointestinal (GI) tract. The chronic inflammation is attributed to a mixture of inflammatory mediators (e.g., IL-1 and -6, TNF-alpha) produced by overactivated macrophages in the lining of the bowel, which contribute to GI ulceration, bleeding, and diarrhea. The goal of treatment is to decrease inflammation and promote healing of bowel lesions.

Psoriasis, a hyperproliferative skin disorder, is characterized by an abnormal overproduction of skin cells, forming plaque lesions. Activated T lymphocytes producing cytokines are believed to stimulate the abnormal growth of the affected skin cells with accompanying inflammation from tissue infiltration of neutrophils and monocytes. Some medications (e.g., beta-blockers, lithium) may precipitate or aggravate psoriasis.

Psoriatic arthritis is a type of arthritis associated with psoriasis that is similar to rheumatoid arthritis. It may be characterized by extensive and disabling joint damage, especially in the hand and finger joints.

Rheumatoid arthritis occurs when an abnormal immune response leads to chronic inflammation and damage of joint cartilage and bone. It is thought to involve the activation of T lymphocytes, release of inflammatory cytokines, and formation of antibodies in the joint tissue as well as other organs. Research in recent years has delineated the roles of TNF-alpha and IL-1 in the pathophysiology of rheumatoid arthritis. Symptoms may include fatigue, loss of energy, lack of appetite, low-grade fever, muscle and joint aches, and stiffness. Joints frequently become red, swollen, painful, and tender.

Rejection Reactions With Solid Organ Transplantation

Rejection reactions may be either acute or chronic. Acute reactions may occur from 10 days to a few months after transplantation and mainly involve cellular immunity and proliferation of T lymphocytes. Characteristics include signs of organ failure and inflammation of blood vessels, leading to arterial narrowing or obliteration. Treatment with immunosuppressant drugs is usually effective in ensuring short-term survival of the transplant but does not prevent chronic rejection. Chronic reactions, which occur after months or years of normal function, are caused by both cellular and humoral immunity and do not respond to increasing immunosuppressive drug therapy. Characteristics include fibrosis of blood vessels and progressive failure of the transplanted organ.

Rejection reactions produce both general manifestations of inflammation and specific organ manifestations, depending on the organ involved. With renal transplantation, for example, acute rejection reactions produce fever, flank tenderness over the graft organ site, and symptoms of renal failure (e.g., increased serum creatinine, decreased urine output, edema, weight gain, hypertension). Chronic renal rejection reactions are characterized by a gradual increase in serum creatinine levels over 4 to 6 months. Along with observing for symptoms of decline in organ function, periodic organ tissue biopsies are often required to diagnose a chronic organ rejection process.

Bone Marrow/Stem Cell Transplantation and Graft-Versus-Host Disease

With bone marrow/stem cell transplantation, the donor marrow or stem cells, which contain T lymphocytes, develop an active immune response against antigens on the host's tissues, producing GVHD. Tissue damage is produced directly by the action of cytotoxic T cells and indirectly through the release of inflammatory mediators (e.g., complement) and cytokines (e.g., TNF-alpha and ILs).

Acute GVHD occurs in 30% to 50% of patients, usually within 6 weeks of transplant. Signs and symptoms include delayed recovery of blood cell production in the bone marrow, skin rash, liver dysfunction (indicated by increased alkaline phosphatase, aminotransferases, and bilirubin), and diarrhea. The skin reaction is usually a pruritic maculopapular rash that begins on the palms and soles and may progress to cover the entire body. Liver involvement can lead to bleeding disorders and the development of hepatic encephalopathy.

Chronic GVHD occurs when symptoms persist or occur 100 days or more after transplantation. It is characterized by abnormal humoral and cellular immunity, severe skin disorders, and liver disease. Chronic GVHD appears to be an autoimmune disorder in which activated donor T cells continue to respond to the recipient's surface proteins as if they are foreign antigens.

Drug Therapy

Immunosuppressant drugs compose several groups of pharmacological agents, with often overlapping mechanisms and sites of action (Table 11.1; Fig. 11.1). Older groups of immunosuppressant drugs often depress the immune system of the recipient nonspecifically. Therapeutic use of these drugs increases the risk of serious infections with bacteria, viruses, fungi, or protozoa. In addition, most cytotoxic immunosuppressant drugs that slow the proliferation of activated lymphocytes also produce damage to rapidly dividing cells in other tissues (e.g., mucosal cells, intestinal cells, hematopoietic stem cells). As a result, serious, life-threatening complications can occur with the use of immunosuppressant agents. For example, patients with autoimmune disorders or organ transplants, who are receiving long-term immunosuppressant drug therapy, are at increased risk for serious infections, cancer (especially lymphoma), hypertension, renal and hepatic disease, and metabolic bone disease.

Ongoing research has helped develop drugs that modify the immune response more specifically in response to excessive levels of cytokines and T-cell activity that cause tissue damaging inflammation and autoimmune reactions. These drugs, called immunomodulators or biologic response modifiers, are part of the growing number of drugs with more specific immunosuppressive actions that have been developed through monoclonal antibody cloning technology. Most are used in combination with older immunosuppressants for synergistic effects with lower doses that minimize drug toxicities, whereas some are replacing the older, nonspecific immunosuppressants.

Immunosuppressants discussed here are cytotoxic immunosuppressant agents; conventional antirejection agents; and adjuvant medications, including antibody preparations, cytokine inhibitors, and corticosteroids.

NCLEX Success

1. **After organ transplantation, immunosuppressants are given to prevent which of the following?**

   A. nephrotoxicity
   B. hepatotoxicity
   C. rejection reaction
   D. bleeding disorders

2. **The most common cancers that develop with long-term immunosuppression after organ transplant are**

   A. skin cancers and lymphomas
   B. cancers of the gastrointestinal tract
   C. renal and liver cancers
   D. brain and spinal cord cancers

TABLE 11.1

Drugs Administered to Suppress Immunity

Drug Class	Prototype(s)	Other Drugs in the Class
Cytotoxic Immunosuppressive Agents		
	Mycophenolate mofetil IV (CellCept)	Azathioprine (Azasan, Imuran)
	Mycophenolate sodium PO (Myfortic)	Leflunomide (Arava) Methotrexate (MTX) (Rheumatrex)
Conventional Antirejection Agents		
	Cyclosporine	Everolimus (Zortress, Afinitor)
		Sirolimus (Rapamune)
		Tacrolimus (Prograf)
Adjuvant Medications Used to Suppress Immune Function		
Antibody preparations	Muromonab-CD3 (Orthoclone OKT3)	*Monoclonal*
		Basiliximab (Simulect) Daclizumab (Zenapax)
		Omalizumab (Xolair)
		Polyclonal
		Antithymocyte globulin (Atgam, Thymoglobulin)
		Others
Tumor necrosis factor-alpha–blocking agents	Infliximab (Remicade)	Adalimumab (Humira)
		Certolizumab (Cimzia)
		Etanercept (Enbrel)
Interleukin-blocking agents	Anakinra (Kineret)	Alefacept (Amevive)
		Tocilizumab (Actemra)
		Ustekinumab (Stelara)
Fusion protein inhibitors	Abatacept (Orencia)	Belatacept (Nulojix)

Cytotoxic Immunosuppressive Agents

Cytotoxic immunosuppressive drugs damage or kill dividing cells, such as immunologically competent lymphocytes. Health care providers use these drugs primarily in cancer chemotherapy (see Chap. 12). However, in smaller doses, some cytotoxic drugs also exhibit immunosuppressive activities and are useful in the treatment of autoimmune disorders and the prevention of rejection reactions in organ transplantation. For many years, azathioprine was the drug selected to induce immunosuppression and prevent rejection reactions to transplanted organs. Now, Ⓟ **mycophenolate mofetil** (CellCept), the prototype in this discussion, has essentially replaced it.

Pharmacokinetics

Mycophenolate mofetil is a prodrug that, after oral or intravenous (IV) administration, is rapidly broken down to mycophenolic acid, the active component. Metabolism to an active metabolite occurs in the liver, finally resulting in inactive metabolites. Excretion takes place in the urine.

Action

Mycophenolate is an antimetabolite agent that interferes with the production of cellular deoxyribonucleic acid (DNA) and

ribonucleic acid (RNA) and thus blocks cellular reproduction, growth, and development. As its active component, mycophenolic acid inhibits an enzyme needed for DNA synthesis and reduces the proliferation of lymphocytes.

Use

Uses of mycophenolate mofetil include the prophylaxis of organ rejection after cardiac, hepatic, and renal transplants, as well as immunosuppression after other solid organ transplant procedures involving the lung, pancreas, and small intestine. Mycophenolate sodium (Myfortic), an oral formulation, has received U.S. Food and Drug Administration (FDA) approval for use after kidney transplant to prevent organ rejection. Table 11.2 gives route and dosage information for mycophenolate and other cytotoxic immunosuppressant agents.

Use in Children

A few children undergoing renal transplantation have taken mycophenolate. In children with impaired renal function, recommended doses of mycophenolate may cause a high incidence of adverse effects. Thus, it is necessary to adjust the dosage for the renal function of the individual child.

Use in Older Adults

Mycophenolate has similar therapeutic and adverse effects in older adults compared with younger adults. However, because

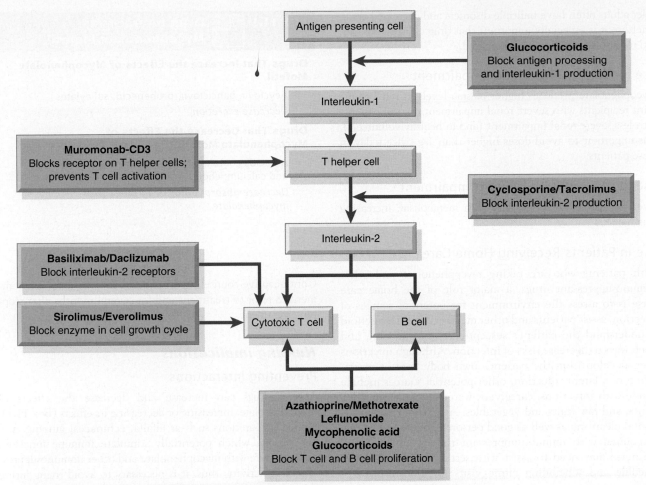

Figure 11.1 Activity of immunosuppressant drugs. Available immunosuppressants inhibit the immune response by blocking that response at various sites.

TABLE 11.2

DRUGS AT A GLANCE: Cytotoxic Immunosuppressive Agents

Drug	Pregnancy Category	Routes and Dosage Ranges	
		Adults	*Children*
ⓟ **Mycophenolate mofetil** (CellCept, Myfortic)	D	Renal transplantation: PO, IV 1 g twice daily Cardiac and hepatic transplantation: PO, IV 1.5 g twice daily Extended-release tablets (Myfortic), PO 720 mg twice daily	Safety and efficacy not established
Azathioprine (Azasan, Imuran)	D	PO, IV 3–5 mg/kg/d initially; may be able to decrease to 1–3 mg/kg/d	Safety and efficacy not established
Leflunomide (Arava)	X	PO 100 mg once daily for 3 d, then 20 mg once daily	Not recommended for children younger than 18 y of age
Methotrexate (MTX) (Rheumatrex)	X	PO 7.5 mg/wk as single dose, or 2.5 mg every 12 h for 3 doses once weekly	Safe for children 2–16 y of age with juvenile rheumatoid arthritis

older adults often have multiple disorders and decreased organ function, it is especially important that drug choices, dosages, and monitoring tests be individualized.

Use in Patients With Renal Impairment

Mycophenolate produces higher plasma levels in renal transplant recipients with severe renal impairment than in patients with less severe renal impairment (and in healthy volunteers). It is important to avoid doses higher than 1 g twice a day in these patients.

Use in Patients With Hepatic Impairment

Liver impairment may interfere with metabolism, increasing drug half-life.

Use in Patients Receiving Home Care

With patients who are taking mycophenolate and other immunosuppressant drugs, a major role of the home care nurse is to assess the environment for potential sources of infection, assist patients and other members of the household to understand the patient's susceptibility to infection, and teach ways to decrease risks of infection. Although infections often develop from the patient's own body flora or reactivation of a latent infection, other potential sources include people with infections, caregivers, water or soil around live plants, and raw fruits and vegetables. Attention to environmental cleansing as well as good personal and hand hygiene is required with immunosuppressant therapy. In addition, the nurse may need to assist with setting up a medication schedule and scheduling clinic visits for monitoring and follow-up care.

The home care nurse also assesses the patient's ability to safely self-administer the medications as prescribed, monitors for adverse drug effects, and observes for signs of drug toxicity. Drug interactions with drugs from multiple prescribers as well as drug–nutrient and drug–herbal interactions can all have an impact on the patient's response to immunosuppressant drug therapy.

Adverse Effects

Common GI adverse effects of mycophenolate include nausea, vomiting, and diarrhea. The most serious risks associated with the use of this drug and some other immunosuppressant drugs are infection and increased risk of malignancy. Latent infections with the tuberculosis bacillus or hepatitis B virus may become active infections during immunosuppressant therapy.

Contraindications

Use of cytotoxic immunosuppressant drugs is not recommended during pregnancy or lactation. The FDA has issued a **BLACK BOX WARNING** ◆ for mycophenolate mofetil regarding the risk of fetal loss and malformations. Women of childbearing age must use contraception. A negative pregnancy test for such women is required prior to starting therapy.

BOX 11.1 **Drug Interactions: Mycophenolate Mofetil**

Drugs That Increase the Effects of Mycophenolate Mofetil

- Acyclovir, ganciclovir, probenecid, salicylates
  Decrease excretion

Drugs That Decrease the Effects of Mycophenolate Mofetil

- Antacids containing magnesium, aluminum, and calcium; cholestyramine
  Decrease absorption as drug binds with mycophenolate

Contraceptive counseling for patients of both sexes is recommended prior to treatment and for several months after stopping treatment.

Nursing Implications

Preventing Interactions

Several drugs can increase and decrease the effects of mycophenolate, increasing or decreasing its effects (Box 11.1). Herbal preparations such as alfalfa, echinacea, ginseng, and bee venom, which potentially stimulate immune function, may interfere with mycophenolate and other immunosuppressant drug activity; thus, it is necessary to avoid them during therapy.

Administering the Medication

QSEN Safety Alert

It is necessary to handle immunosuppressant drugs such as mycophenolate with care to avoid direct contact with skin or mucous membranes. Such contacts have produced teratogenic effects in animals. Patients should swallow oral tablets or capsules whole, without crushing or altering them. They should avoid inhaling the powder from the capsules.

For best absorption, it is important to take oral mycophenolate on an empty stomach.

To ensure correct dosing, it is important to measure oral mycophenolate solution carefully using an accurate measuring device.

Assessing for Therapeutic Effects

After organ transplant, the absence of signs and symptoms of a rejection reaction is evidence of the therapeutic effects of mycophenolate immunosuppressive therapy. (Inflammatory changes in the organ tissue along with laboratory evidence of organ impairment usually accompany acute rejection reactions.) Periodic organ tissue biopsy is used to evaluate for signs of chronic rejection reaction.

Assessing for Adverse Effects

A primary focus for nursing assessment is evidence of signs of infection, including fever, chills, sore throat, headache, swollen glands, cough, and urinary burning or frequency. Following organ transplant surgery, patients often take prophylactic antimicrobials for the first 3 to 6 months to prevent opportunistic infections. Wound healing may be slower during cytotoxic drug therapy with suppression of the normal inflammatory response.

Nursing care includes assessment of GI symptoms, oral intake, elimination pattern, fluid and electrolyte balance, and weight changes. Skin assessment for signs of rash, bruising, petechiae, and color changes such as pallor or jaundice of the skin or sclera offers important clues to allergic or hematological complications and hepatotoxicity. Laboratory monitoring of the complete blood count (CBC), renal function tests, and liver function tests performed prior to therapy and periodically during treatment limits the potential for bone marrow suppression and potential hepatotoxicity.

Clinical Application 11-1

At his office visit, Mr. Jones tells the nurse he has been regularly attending his son's Little League baseball games at a local park. What self-care measures related to his long-term need for immunosuppressive drug therapy should the nurse recommend?

Patient Teaching

Box 11.2 lists patient teaching guidelines for the cytotoxic immunosuppressant drugs.

Other Drugs in the Class

Health care providers have long used methotrexate (Rheumatrex) for the treatment of cancer (higher doses), as well as for the treatment of autoimmune disorders, such as severe rheumatoid arthritis, juvenile rheumatoid arthritis, and severe psoriasis (lower doses). It is also useful in combination with cyclosporine in the prevention of GVHD after bone marrow transplantation.

Excretion of methotrexate is mainly in the urine, so the drug's half-life is prolonged in patients with renal impairment, with risks of accumulation to toxic levels and additional renal damage. However, the risks are less with the small doses used for treatment of rheumatoid arthritis than for the high doses used in cancer chemotherapy. To decrease these risks, it is important to document adequate renal function using the drug. Patients should be well hydrated.

The lower doses of methotrexate used for autoimmune disorders and transplant therapy reduce the incidence and severity of adverse effects. Oral mucositis can occur with methotrexate therapy, interfering with nutritional intake and contributing to the risk of infection. However, even in the low doses used in rheumatoid arthritis and psoriasis, methotrexate may cause hepatotoxicity. Prior to and during therapy, monitoring the CBC, renal function, and liver function is essential. Liver function tests help guide methotrexate dosage. In general, dosage warrants decreasing if bilirubin is between 3 and 5 mg/dL or aspartate aminotransferase (AST) is above 180 International Units per liter, and the drug should be omitted if bilirubin is above 5 mg/dL. Many clinicians recommend serial liver biopsies for patients on long-term, low-dose methotrexate.

Administration of methotrexate is weekly for rheumatoid arthritis or psoriasis, and patients should keep an accurate record of the date and time of each dose. To reduce gastric upset, they may take the drug with food. However, daily dosing for cytotoxic immunosuppressants should be consistent with regard to time and food (i.e., at the same time of day, with the same meal).

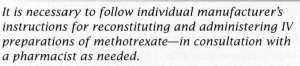

QSEN Safety Alert

It is necessary to follow individual manufacturer's instructions for reconstituting and administering IV preparations of methotrexate—in consultation with a pharmacist as needed.

Leflunomide (Arava), an anti-inflammatory immunosuppressant, is useful only in the treatment of adults with rheumatoid arthritis. Authorities do not recommend the drug for children younger than 18 years of age. Contraindications include the presence of active hepatitis B or C infection or if the alanine aminotransferase (ALT) level is greater than two times normal. With leflunomide, hepatotoxicity is a concern; hence, it is essential to obtain liver function tests before starting therapy. Also, patients should have renal function tests, as well as liver function tests, every month for the first 6 months then every 6 to 8 weeks thereafter. The FDA has issued a **BLACK BOX WARNING ◆** for leflunomide regarding the risk of fetal loss and malformations. Women of childbearing age must use contraception. A negative pregnancy test for such women of childbearing age is necessary prior to starting therapy. Contraceptive counseling for both genders is recommended prior to treatment and for several months after stopping treatment.

Azathioprine (Azasan, Imuran) is sometimes used for the prevention of kidney rejection and treatment of rheumatoid arthritis. Health care providers have used azathioprine after organ transplant in children, but safety data are limited. Contraindications to use include pregnancy and lactation, and it is essential to use extreme caution with hepatic disease or hepatic impairment. The drug is metabolized in the liver and erythrocytes. Researchers have reported genetic variation in the rate of metabolism.

Adverse effects of azathioprine include bone marrow suppression with neutropenia, thrombocytopenia, and anemia; hepatotoxicity with increased risk of posttransplant venoocclusive liver disease; GI upset, nausea, vomiting, and diarrhea; fever and muscle aches; and skin rash. It is necessary to obtain baseline liver function tests and a pregnancy test prior to therapy. Lower doses are required in the presence of renal disease to prevent drug toxicities such as myelosuppression and hepatotoxicity. Patients should have CBCs and liver function tests on a set schedule. Azathioprine has a high potential for toxicity, so regular assessments for adverse effects are critical.

General Considerations

- People taking medications that suppress the immune system are at high risk for development of infections. As a result, patients, caregivers, and others in the patient's environment need to wash their hands often and thoroughly, practice meticulous personal hygiene (e.g., take good care of the mouth, gums, and skin), avoid contact with infected people, and practice other methods of preventing infection.

- Understand that lifelong drug treatment to prevent potential organ rejection is required after transplant therapy. Obtain complete instructions about all the medications used to prevent rejection, including the purpose and activity of the drug; dose; route of administration (e.g., oral, injection); frequency and timing, potential adverse effects and their management; and signs of complications and drug toxicity. Poor adherence and missed medication doses are an important cause of organ rejection and need for a subsequent transplant.

- Report adverse drug effects (e.g., signs or symptoms of infection such as sore throat or fever, decreased urine output if taking cyclosporine, easy bruising or bleeding if taking methotrexate) to a health care provider. If you have had a transplant, know the signs of transplant rejection.

- Try to maintain healthy lifestyle habits, such as a nutritious diet, adequate rest and sleep, and avoiding tobacco and alcohol. These measures enhance immune mechanisms and other body defenses.

- Carry identification that lists the drugs being taken; the dosage; the prescriber's name, address, and telephone number; and instructions for emergency treatment. Use of a Medic-Alert bracelet is recommended in case of an accident or other emergency situation.

- Inform all health care providers that you are taking immunosuppressant drugs.

- Maintain regular supervision by a health care provider. This is extremely important for evaluating health status, evaluating drug responses and indications for dosage change, detecting adverse drug reactions, and having blood tests or other monitoring tests when indicated.

- Take no other drugs, prescription or nonprescription, without notifying the prescriber who is managing immunosuppressant therapy. Immunosuppressant drugs may influence reactions to other drugs, and other drugs may influence reactions to the immunosuppressants. Thus, taking other drugs may decrease therapeutic effects or increase adverse effects. In addition, some vaccinations should be avoided while taking immunosuppressant drugs.

- People of reproductive capability who are sexually active should practice effective contraceptive techniques during immunosuppressive drug therapy. With methotrexate, use contraception during and for at least 3 months (men) or one ovulatory cycle (women) after stopping the drug. With mycophenolate, effective contraception should be continued for 6 weeks after the drug is stopped. With sirolimus, effective contraception must be used before, during, and for 12 weeks after drug therapy.

- Wear protective clothing and use sunscreens to decrease exposure of skin to sunlight and risks of skin cancers. Also, methotrexate and sirolimus increase sensitivity to sunlight and may increase sunburn. Have cancer screening for early detection if you take immunosuppressant drugs.

Self-Administration

- Follow instructions about taking the drugs. This is vital to achieving beneficial effects and decreasing adverse effects. If unable to take a medication, report to the prescriber or other health care provider; do not stop unless advised to do so. For transplant recipients, missed doses may lead to transplant rejection; for patients with autoimmune diseases, missed doses may lead to acute flare-ups of symptoms. Take medications at approximately the same time each day to maintain consistent drug levels in the blood.

- With cyclosporine oral solution, use the same solution consistently. The available cyclosporine solutions (Neoral, Gengraf, Sandimmune) are not equivalent and cannot be used interchangeably. If a change in formulation is necessary, the dispensing pharmacy should consult the prescriber.

- Measure oral cyclosporine solution with the dosing syringe provided; add to orange or apple juice that is at room temperature (avoid grapefruit juice) into a glass container, stir well, and drink at once (do not allow diluted solution to stand before drinking). Rinse the glass with more juice to ensure the total dose is taken. Do not rinse the dosing syringe with water or other cleaning agents. Take on a consistent schedule with regard to time of day and meals.

These are the manufacturer's recommendations.

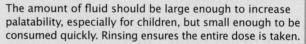

QSEN Safety Alert

Mixing with orange or apple juice improves taste; do not use grapefruit juice because it inhibits the metabolism of cyclosporine.

The amount of fluid should be large enough to increase palatability, especially for children, but small enough to be consumed quickly. Rinsing ensures the entire dose is taken.

- Take mycophenolate on an empty stomach; food decreases drug absorption by approximately 40%. Do not crush mycophenolate tablets and do not open or crush the capsules.

- Take sirolimus consistently with or without food; do not mix or take the drug with grapefruit juice. Grapefruit juice inhibits metabolism and increases adverse effects. If also taking cyclosporine, take the sirolimus 4 hours after a dose of cyclosporine.

- If taking the oral solution, use the syringe that comes with the medication to measure and withdraw the dose from the bottle. Empty the dose into a glass or plastic container with at least 2 oz (1/4 cup or 60 mL) of water or orange juice. *Do not use any other liquid to dilute the drug.* Stir the mixture vigorously, and drink it immediately. Refill the container with at least 4 oz (1/2 cup or 120 mL) of water or orange juice, stir vigorously, and drink at once.

- Take tacrolimus with food to decrease stomach upset.

- If giving or taking an injected drug, be sure you understand how to mix and inject the medication correctly. With Enbrel, for example, rotate injection sites, give a new injection at least 1 inch from a previous injection site, and do not inject the medication into areas where the skin is tender, bruised, red, or hard. When possible, practice the required techniques and perform at least the first injection under supervision of a qualified health care professional.

Conventional Antirejection Agents

Ⓟ Cyclosporine (Neoral, Gengraf, Sandimmune), the first antirejection drug used to prevent transplant rejection reactions, is the prototype antirejection agent. Cyclosporine and related drugs are fungal metabolites with strong immunosuppressive effects. By selectively inhibiting proliferation of helper T cells and expression of cytokines, these antirejection drugs reduce the activity of other immune cells involved in graft rejection. Consequently, they are widely used in transplant therapy to prevent or reduce the graft rejection response.

Pharmacokinetics

Absorption of cyclosporine is highly variable. After oral administration, absorption is rather poor. The drug is highly bound to plasma proteins, and approximately 50% is distributed in erythrocytes, so drug levels in whole blood are higher than those in plasma. Peak plasma levels occur 4 to 5 hours after a dose. Metabolism of cyclosporine involves the CYP3A4 liver enzyme system, and elimination occurs mainly in the bile.

Action

Cyclosporine inhibits calcineurin, a protein needed for the synthesis of IL-2 and the subsequent proliferation of T cells and B cells. The drug binds with calcineurin on T lymphocytes and interferes with the production of IL-2. As previously described, activated T cells produce a cytokine, IL-2, which in turn activates other lymphocytes, amplifying the immune response and producing the damaging inflammatory changes in tissue that occur with organ rejection and autoimmune disease.

Use

Health care providers use cyclosporine to prevent rejection reactions and prolong graft survival after solid organ transplantation (e.g., kidney, liver, heart, lung) or to treat chronic rejection in patients previously treated with other immunosuppressive agents. The drug inhibits both cellular and humoral immunity but affects T lymphocytes significantly more than B lymphocytes. With cyclosporine-induced deprivation of IL-2, T cells stimulated by the graft antigen are unable to multiple and differentiate, and graft organ destruction is inhibited. In addition to its use in solid organ transplantation, cyclosporine is useful in the prevention and treatment of GVHD, a complication of bone marrow transplantation. In GVHD, T lymphocytes from the transplanted marrow of the donor mount an immune response against the tissues of the recipient. Cyclosporine may inhibit donor T-cell activity, reducing the risk of GVHD. Other indications for use include treatment of psoriasis and rheumatoid arthritis.

Cyclosporine dosing is weight based in both adults and children, with higher doses given immediately before and after the transplant and then tapered over several months to minimize adverse effects and avoid excessive immunosuppression. Table 11.3 outlines the routes and dosages for cyclosporine and related drugs.

Use in Children

Children as young as 6 months of age may receive cyclosporine. Experience with this drug indicates that children require relatively high doses because they metabolize the drug rapidly.

TABLE 11.3

DRUGS AT A GLANCE: Conventional Antirejection Agents

Drug	Pregnancy Category	Routes and Dosage Ranges	
		Adults	*Children*
Ⓟ Cyclosporine (Sandimmune, Neoral)	C	Sandimmune, PO 15 mg/kg 4–12 h before transplantation, then 15 mg/kg once daily for 1–2 wk, then decrease by 5% per week to a maintenance dose of 5–10 mg/kg/d; IV 5–6 mg/kg infused over 2–6 h Neoral, PO, the first dose in patients with new transplants is the same as the first oral dose of Sandimmune; later doses are titrated according to cyclosporine blood levels	Same as in adults with caution
Everolimus (Zortress, Afinitor)	D	PO 10 mg once daily	Limited research and little experience
Sirolimus (Rapamune)	C	PO 6 mg as soon after kidney transplantation as possible, then 2 mg daily	Older than 13 y of age: PO 3 mg/m² as loading dose, then 1 mg/m² daily
Tacrolimus (Prograf)	C	IV infusion, 25–50 mcg/kg/d, starting 6 h after transplantation or later, until the patient can tolerate oral drug; PO 150–200 mcg/kg/d, in two divided doses every 12 h, with the first dose 8–12 h after stopping the IV infusion	IV 50–100 mcg/kg/d; PO 200–300 mcg/kg/d

Use in Older Adults

Due to an increased incidence of infection and a greater risk of malignancy, it is necessary to monitor older adults carefully during antirejection drug therapy. Doses are individualized, considering age, function, and concurrent conditions. More frequent assessment and therapeutic blood level monitoring are essential in older adults after organ transplantation because of the increased risk of organ toxicity.

Use in Patients With Renal Impairment

Patients with kidney and other organ transplants commonly use cyclosporine, but there is an increased risk of nephrotoxicity associated with the drug. Nephrotoxicity has occurred in 25% of kidney, 38% of heart, and 37% of liver transplant recipients, especially with high doses of cyclosporine. Monitoring serum blood levels can help reduce this risk, and nephrotoxicity usually subsides after decreasing the dosage or stopping the drug. In kidney transplant recipients, when serum creatinine and blood urea nitrogen (BUN) levels remain elevated, an evaluation of the patient and tissue biopsy is often necessary to differentiate cyclosporine-induced nephrotoxicity from a transplant rejection reaction.

Use in Patients With Hepatic Impairment

With cyclosporine, it is important to check serum bilirubin and liver enzymes prior to and during treatment. Cyclosporine reportedly causes hepatotoxicity (e.g., elevated serum aminotransferases and bilirubin) in approximately 4% of kidney and liver transplant recipients and in 7% of cardiac transplant recipients. This is most likely to occur during the first month of therapy, when high doses of cyclosporine are usually given, and usually subsides with dosage reduction.

Use in Patients With Critical Illness

Use of immunosuppressants during critical illness requires individualized risk versus benefit decision making. It is necessary to balance the need to prevent transplant organ rejection against the risk of infection and associated drug toxicities, which may lead to loss of the engrafted organ.

Use in Patients Receiving Home Care

Survival rates are now longer in transplant recipients, and multiple organ transplants and retransplants occur. Thus, there are challenges in managing chronic rejection and minimizing drug toxicities in the home setting. Promoting correct medication use is critical to maintaining therapeutic blood levels after transplantation and preventing organ rejection. Due to the variable bioavailability of cyclosporine when taken orally, patients should consistently take the drug at the same time each day. In addition to monitoring medication use, the home care nurse provides self-care teaching, monitors for sources of infection, obtains and monitors blood work, and implements health maintenance measures.

Adverse Effects

Nephrotoxicity, hirsutism, gingival hypertrophy, hypertension, and hyperlipidemia are significant adverse effects of cyclosporine. The FDA has issued a **BLACK BOX WARNING** ◆ for cyclosporine regarding risks of hypertension and nephrotoxicity. After solid organ transplantation, with the need to continue lifelong immunosuppression to avoid graft rejection, serious infection is an ongoing concern.

As previously stated, transplant recipients are living longer, and this has led to the recognition that there are long-term adverse effects associated with immunosuppressant drug therapy. As a consequence of long-term survival and chronic immunosuppression, patients have an increased risk of developing a malignancy. The incidence of malignancy is unknown, but after 10 years of immunosuppression, authorities often estimate it to be 20% or more. The most common malignancies in transplant recipients are skin cancers and lymphomas, and solid organ tumors may also occur. Regular screening tests for breast, cervical, colon, and prostate cancer, along with annual skin examinations, are recommended. The FDA has issued a **BLACK BOX WARNING** ◆ limiting all long-term use of antirejection drugs to prescribers experienced in transplant therapy because of the increased risk of infections and certain malignancies such as lymphoma and skin cancer.

Contraindications

Contraindications to cyclosporine include the combined use of antirejection drugs that have the same mechanism of action and toxicities (e.g., tacrolimus and cyclosporine). Prescribers usually avoid such use after organ transplant.

Nursing Implications

Preventing Interactions

Numerous potential drug interactions affect the blood levels of cyclosporine, increasing or decreasing its effects (Box 11.3). Because these drugs are metabolized mainly by CYP3A4 enzymes and have a low therapeutic index, any drugs that increase or decrease levels of these enzymes have the potential to alter blood levels of cyclosporine. The herb St. John's wort may reduce this drug's therapeutic effects.

BOX 11.3	**Drug Interactions: Cyclosporine**

Drugs That Increase the Effects of Cyclosporine

■ Aminoglycoside antibiotics, amphotericin B
Increase nephrotoxic effects
■ Azithromycin, fluconazole, and related antifungals
Increase blood levels and toxic effects
■ Macrolide antibiotics
Increase blood levels and toxic effects

Drugs That Decrease the Effects of Cyclosporine

■ Carbamazepine, phenytoin, rifampin
Decreases therapeutic effects

Administering the Medication

It is necessary to initiate antirejection drugs several hours prior to the transplant procedure. Administration is by IV infusion only until the patient can take the drug by the oral route. The risk of a severe allergic reaction is significantly higher following IV administration. Dilution of an oral cyclosporine solution should follow package instructions.

To improve bioavailability, cyclosporine preparations were once prepared in alcohol and olive oil for oral administration and in alcohol and castor oil for IV administration. Anaphylactic reactions, attributed to the castor oil, have occurred with the IV formulation. Neoral and Gengraf are oral microemulsion formulations that are better absorbed than oral Sandimmune. These different drug formulations are not equivalent in their absorption and cannot be used interchangeably.

Assessing for Therapeutic Effects

The nurse assesses therapeutic effects by monitoring for organ function and signs of rejection with solid organ transplants, assessing serum blood levels, and monitoring and managing adverse drug effects. Cyclosporine has a very narrow therapeutic index; therefore, prescribers use serum drug levels to regulate cyclosporine dosing, and close monitoring is necessary. They use blood levels measured 2 hours after a dose for dosage adjustments. Subtherapeutic levels may lead to organ transplant rejection, whereas high levels increase adverse effects.

Assessing for Adverse Effects

Acute nephrotoxicity can occur, progressing to chronic nephrotoxicity and kidney failure. It is essential to monitor renal function tests (serum creatinine and BUN) and urine protein throughout cyclosporine therapy. To check for hepatotoxicity, it is necessary to conduct liver function tests (bilirubin, ALT, and AST) regularly. Periodic monitoring of fasting lipid levels (cholesterol, high- and low-density lipoproteins, and triglycerides) should also occur.

Patient Teaching

Box 11.2 presents patient teaching information for the conventional antirejection drugs.

Other Drugs in the Class

Everolimus (Zortress, Afinitor) reduces T-cell activation to decrease the immune response after kidney transplant and rejection. This drug, generally combined with cyclosporine and prednisone, allows lower posttransplant doses of both cyclosporine and the steroid; this minimizes adverse effects. Everolimus is available only as an oral formulation, and patients should take the drug consistently, with or without food, to maintain consistent therapeutic blood levels. It has been associated with an increased incidence of angioedema, early kidney graft thrombosis, delayed wound healing, elevated lipid levels, new-onset diabetes, and an increased risk of nephrotoxicity and proteinuria when combined with cyclosporine. It is necessary to obtain therapeutic blood levels of both cyclosporine and everolimus to minimize the risks of renal toxicity when the drugs are used concurrently.

Sirolimus is an immunosuppressant used to prevent organ rejection in kidney transplants. Often, it is given concomitantly with a corticosteroid and cyclosporine. Sirolimus may have synergistic effects with cyclosporine because it has a different mechanism of action, and prescribers may order both drugs in combination. However, because the two drugs are metabolized by the same liver CYP3A4 enzymes, cyclosporine can increase blood levels of sirolimus, potentially to toxic levels. Consequently, it is essential that the drugs not be given at the same time; patients should take sirolimus 4 hours after a dose of cyclosporine.

Extensive metabolism of sirolimus occurs in the liver, and the drug may accumulate in the presence of hepatic impairment. If this occurs, reducing the maintenance dose by 35% may be warranted; changing the loading dose is not necessary. Monitoring using serum drug levels in patients who are likely to have altered drug metabolism due to age, concurrent disease, or other drugs is important. Use of sirolimus in children after renal transplant to reduce the risk of nephropathy from cyclosporine or tacrolimus allows these other drugs to be given at lower doses or discontinued. Contraindications to use of sirolimus include recent lung and liver transplantation due to an increased incidence of delayed healing and graft failure in the transplanted organs. The FDA has issued a **BLACK BOX WARNING** ◆ that use of sirolimus in lung and liver transplant patients has been associated with increased morbidity and mortality.

Tacrolimus is similar to cyclosporine in its mechanisms of action, pharmacokinetic characteristics, and adverse effects. It prevents transplant rejection by inhibiting proliferation of T lymphocytes. Some transplant centers now use tacrolimus rather than cyclosporine, mainly because cyclosporine is given with corticosteroids. Using tacrolimus may allow corticosteroids to be reduced or stopped, thereby decreasing the adverse effects of long-term corticosteroid therapy. Tacrolimus, like cyclosporine, is not well absorbed orally, so it is necessary to give higher oral doses than IV doses to obtain similar blood levels. With IV administration, onset of action is rapid, but with oral administration, onset varies. It is essential that patients take the oral drug on a consistent time schedule because its bioavailability may vary. Dosing of tacrolimus is individualized according to clinical response, adverse effects, and serum blood levels.

Metabolism of tacrolimus takes place in the liver and intestine, and excretion of the several metabolites occurs in bile and urine. Dosage reduction is necessary with impaired liver function. The drug also has the potential to cause nephrotoxicity.

Clinical Application 11-2

- Mr. Jones calls the nephrology clinic to report shortness of breath and fatigue. Despite a decrease in appetite, he reports his weight has increased by 2 kg over the last week. The nurse recognizes that he is most likely experiencing which adverse effects from one of his immunosuppressant medications?

Adjuvant Medications Used to Suppress Immune Function

A significant number of adjuvant medications are used as immunosuppressants. Table 11.4 summarizes indications for use and dosages for these drugs.

Corticosteroids

Corticosteroids are potent anti-inflammatory agents that suppress the systemic immune response. Chapters 15 and 31 contain information about specific agents, including effects of therapeutic doses of corticosteroids. Used in a wide variety of inflammatory and allergic disorders, pharmacological doses of corticosteroids block the production of IL-1, relieving signs and symptoms of inflammation by decreasing the accumulation of lymphocytes and macrophages and reducing levels of other cell-damaging cytokines. Corticosteroids, used in pharmacological doses, suppress inflammation by suppressing activation and growth of lymphoid T cells and decreasing the formation and function of antibodies by B cells. For patients with transplanted tissues, corticosteroids are usually given with other agents to prevent acute graft rejection. Increasingly, in autoimmune

TABLE 11.4

DRUGS AT A GLANCE: Adjuvant Medications Used as Immunosuppressants

Drug	Pregnancy Category	Routes and Dosage Ranges	
		Adults	Children
Antibody Preparations			
Ⓟ **Muromonab-CD3** (Orthoclone OKT3)	C	5 mg bolus IV injection once daily for 10–14 d	By weight, IV ≤30 kg, 2.5 mg/d for 10–14 d > 30 kg, 5 mg/d for 10–14 d; may increase 2.5 mg/d increments if needed
Monoclonal antibodies			
Basiliximab (Simulect)	B	20 mg IV within 2 h before transplantation and 20 mg 4 d after transplantation (total of two doses)	2–15 y, IV 12 mg/m² up to a maximum of 20 mg for two doses, as for adults
Daclizumab (Zenapax)	C	IV 1 mg/kg IV over 15 min; first dose within 24 h before transplantation, then a dose every 14 d for four doses (total of five doses)	11 mo to 17 y of age, same as adults
Omalizumab (Dipentum)	B	150–375 mg Sub-Q every 2–4 wk	Not for use in patients 11 y of age and younger
Polyclonal antibodies			
Antithymocyte globulin (Atgam, equine; Thymoglobulin, rabbit)	C	Atgam, 15 mg/kg/d IV for 14 d, then every other day for 14 d (total of 21 doses) Thymoglobulin, 1.5 mg/kg/d IV for 7–14 d	Optimal dose still under debate
Tumor Necrosis Factor-Alpha–Blocking Agents			
Ⓟ **Infliximab** (Remicade)	B	IV infusion, 3–5 mg/kg initially, 2 and 6 wk later, then every 8 wk	≥ 6 y: same as adults
Adalimumab (Humira)	B	40 mg Sub-Q every other week	Ages 4–17 y 15 to <30 kg, 20 mg Sub-Q every other wk; 30 kg or more, 40 mg Sub-Q every other week
Certolizumab (Cimzia)	B	400 mg Sub-Q every 2 wk for 3 doses then every 4 wk	Safety and efficacy not established
Etanercept (Enbrel)	B	25 mg Sub-Q twice weekly, 72–96 h apart	4–17 y, 0.4 mg/kg Sub-Q up to a maximum of 25 mg per dose, twice weekly, 72–96 h apart

TABLE 11.4

DRUGS AT A GLANCE: Adjuvant Medications Used as Immunosuppressants (Continued)

Drug	Pregnancy Category	Routes and Dosage Ranges	
		Adults	Children
Interleukin-Blocking Agents			
Ⓟ **Anakinra** (Kineret)	B	100 mg Sub-Q once daily	Safety and efficacy not established
Alefacept (Amevive)	B	15 mg IM once weekly for 12 wk; 7.5 mg IV once weekly for 12 wk	Safety and efficacy not established
Tocilizumab (Actemra) (given with or without methotrexate)	C	8 mg/kg IV, diluted in 100 mL normal saline infused over 1 h every 4 wk	<25 kg, 8 mg/kg dilute in 50 mL normal saline infused over 1 h every 2–4 wk
Ustekinumab (Stelara)	B	Sub-Q by weight <100 kg, 45-mg dose >100 kg, 90-mg dose Initial dose repeated in 4 wk, then every 12 wk thereafter	Not used in children
Fusion Protein Inhibitors			
Ⓟ **Abatacept** (Orencia)	B	IV, according to body weight, initially at 2 and 4 wk after initial dose, then every 4 wk; weight below 60 kg, 500 mg; 60–100 kg, 750 mg; above 100 kg, 1000 mg	IV, according to body weight, initially at 2 and 4 wk after initial dose, then every 4 wk; <75 kg, 10 mg/kg; 75–100 kg, 750 mg; more than 100 kg, 1000 mg
Belatacept (Nulojix)	C	IV infusion over 30 min; initially 10 mg/kg before transplant; repeated in 96 h then at wk 2, 4, 8, and 12; 5 mg/kg at week 16 and every 4 wk thereafter	Safety and efficacy not established

disease, health care providers use biological response modifiers, combined with a cytotoxic immunosuppressant (or alone), as primary therapy. These disease-modifying anti-inflammatory drugs, known as DMARDs, more specifically address the underlying autoimmune tissue process and can slow the destructive changes. Currently, prescribers order corticosteroids for episodic use during acute exacerbations of autoimmune disease and then taper or discontinue them as soon as possible.

The important adverse effects of corticosteroids have led many transplant centers to try to minimize or eliminate the use of these drugs as part of chronic immunosuppressive therapy when possible. Methods such as gradually tapering doses after transplant to no more than 10 mg daily in adults and using alternate-day therapy in children are strategies used to minimize the long-term adverse effects of corticosteroids.

Antibody Preparations

Antibody (immunoglobulin) preparations are produced in the laboratory or derived from animals injected with human lymphoid tissue to stimulate an immune response. Health care providers use such preparations in inflammatory autoimmune disorders, transplantation rejection reactions, and cancer

treatment to block cell receptors that are part of the abnormal inflammation or cell proliferation process. The antibodies produced may be polyclonal or monoclonal.

Polyclonal antibodies are mixtures of antibodies (IgA, IgD, IgE, IgG, and IgM) produced by several clones of B lymphocytes. Polyclonal immune globulin preparations contain a mixture of immunoglobulins. Each lymphocyte clone produces structurally and functionally different antibodies, even though a single antigen induces the humoral immune response.

Monoclonal antibodies, on the other hand, originate from a single B-cell source. The isolation and cloning of individual B lymphocytes result in the production of biologically identical antibody molecules. To produce a monoclonal antibody, the human antigen to which the desired antibody will respond is first injected into a mouse or hamster. The animal mounts an immune response in which its B lymphocytes are stimulated to produce a specific antibody against that antigen. These B lymphocytes are then recovered from the spleen of the animal and fused with immortal myeloma cells (a cell line that can live forever in culture). This produces an antibody-secreting hybridoma, a cellular "antibody factory" able to produce large amounts of the desired identical antibody. The antibodies can then be isolated from the culture and prepared for clinical use.

Because the antibodies are proteins and would be destroyed if taken orally, immunoglobulins must always be given by parenteral injection.

Because monoclonal antibodies are derived from one single cell line or clone, it is possible to design them to suppress the specific components of the immune system that cause tissue damage in particular disorders. These antibodies are able to block cellular growth receptors or inhibit proinflammatory cytokines that mediate inflammatory tissue damage associated with autoimmune disorders or transplant organ rejection. The generic names of drugs that are monoclonal antibodies end in "-mab," which identifies their origin and classification.

Older animal-derived immunoglobulin antibody preparations (e.g., antithymocyte globulin [ATG], muromonab-CD3) are themselves antigenic. They usually elicit human antibodies against the animal cells within 2 weeks; hence, their use is appropriate only for short periods. Newer mouse-derived **murine antibodies** (e.g., basiliximab) are humanized, have parts of human antibodies added by recombinant DNA technology, and are less likely to elicit an immune response. However, because antibodies are proteins, there is a risk of hypersensitivity reactions with administration of all biological antibody products.

Polyclonal Antibodies

ATG (Atgam, Thymoglobulin) is a nonspecific immune globulin preparation used for immunosuppression. Health care providers use ATG equine (Atgam) obtained from horse serum to treat rejection reactions after kidney transplants and aplastic anemia in patients who are not considered candidates for bone marrow transplantation. They also use ATG rabbit (Thymoglobulin) to treat these rejection reactions. ATG contains antibodies that destroy lymphoid tissues and decrease the number of circulating T cells, thereby suppressing acute cellular and humoral immune responses. In addition to its high concentration of antibodies against T lymphocytes, the preparation contains low concentrations of antibodies against other blood cells. With Atgam, it is necessary that potential recipients have skin tests before administration to determine if they are allergic to horse serum. Because there is a high risk of anaphylactic reactions in recipients previously sensitized to horse serum, patients with positive skin tests require desensitization before drug therapy is begun. It is essential that emergency equipment for airway and allergy management be immediately available when ATG is administered. The FDA has issued a **BLACK BOX WARNING ◆** for ATG urging that its use be restricted to experienced prescribers.

Monoclonal Antibodies

The monoclonal antibody ℗ **muromonab-CD3** (Orthoclone OKT3) acts against an antigenic receptor called CD3, which is found on the surface membrane of most T cells in blood and body tissues. CD indicates clusters of differentiation or groups of cells with the same surface markers (antigenic receptors). The drug's name derives from its source (murine or mouse cells) and its action (monoclonal antibody against the CD3 antigen). The CD3 molecule is associated with the antigen recognition structure of T cells and is essential for T-cell activation. Muromonab-CD3 binds with its antigen (CD3) and therefore

blocks all known functions of T cells containing the CD3 molecule. Because rejection reactions are mainly T-cell–mediated immune responses against antigenic engrafted tissues, the drug's ability to suppress such reactions accounts for its therapeutic effects in treating renal, cardiac, and hepatic transplant rejection.

Both basiliximab (Simulect) and daclizumab (Zenapax) are humanized IgG monoclonal antibodies that act as IL-2 receptor antagonists. By binding to IL-2 receptors on the surface of activated lymphocytes, they inhibit lymphocyte proliferation and cytokine production, critical components of the cellular immune response involved in rejection reactions. Uses include prevention of rejection of kidney transplants. Prescribers order the drugs to be given in combination with cyclosporine and a corticosteroid. Common adverse effects include constipation, diarrhea, edema, fever, headache, hypertension, infection, nausea, and vomiting.

Omalizumab (Xolair) is a humanized monoclonal IgE antibody used to treat allergic asthma that is not relieved by inhaled corticosteroids. Chapters 11 and 31 contain a further discussion of omalizumab, including dosage, route, and frequency of administration. Because of the risk of anaphylaxis, the FDA has issued a **BLACK BOX WARNING ◆** for omalizumab. Administration should occur only in a health care setting under direct medical supervision by provider who can initiate treatment of life-threatening anaphylaxis.

Cytokine Inhibitors

Two major cytokines in chronic, inflammatory autoimmune disorders are TNF-alpha and IL-1. Knowledge of the role of these cytokines in autoimmune disease along with advances in monoclonal antibody production has led to the development of biologic agents directed against TNF and IL-1. Several monoclonal cytokine-inhibiting antibodies, which block either block receptors for or reduce production of these cytokines, are used therapeutically in disorders such as rheumatoid arthritis, Crohn's disease, and psoriasis to suppress inflammation and promote tissue healing.

Tumor Necrosis Factor-Alpha–Blocking Agents

The TNF-alpha–blocking agents act more rapidly than cytotoxic immunosuppressants (e.g., methotrexate) for autoimmune disorders and greatly improve the quality of life for patients with rheumatoid arthritis and Crohn's disease. However, their use is also associated with significant risks of serious infections, especially with opportunistic organisms. Tuberculosis characterized by increased extrapulmonary and/or disseminated disease may occur. Other serious infections include pneumococcal infections, necrotizing fasciitis, *Pneumocystis* pneumonia, and systemic fungal infections such as aspergillosis and cryptococcosis.

℗ **Infliximab** (Remicade) is a humanized IgG monoclonal antibody used to treat rheumatoid arthritis and Crohn's disease. The drug inhibits TNF-alpha from binding to its receptors and thus neutralizes its actions. Its ability to neutralize TNF-alpha accounts for its anti-inflammatory effects. Adverse effects of infliximab include formation of autoimmune antibodies and hypersensitivity reactions. Infections reportedly developed in approximately 21% of patients in clinical trials. In addition, dyspnea, hypotension, and urticaria have occurred.

It is important (1) to administer infliximab in settings in which personnel and supplies (e.g., epinephrine, antihistamines, corticosteroids) are available for treatment of hypersensitivity reactions and (2) to discontinue the drug if severe reactions occur. The drug may aggravate congestive heart failure.

Adalimumab (Humira) is a recombinant monoclonal antibody that binds to TNF-alpha receptor sites and prevents endogenous TNF-alpha from binding to the sites and exerting its injurious effects. Used to treat moderate to severe rheumatoid arthritis, the drug reduces the elevated levels of TNF-alpha in synovial fluid that are thought responsible for pain and joint destruction. Common adverse effects include injection site reactions, upper respiratory tract infections, headache, nausea, and skin rash.

Certolizumab (Cimzia), a TNF-alpha monoclonal antibody, has recently received approval for treating refractory Crohn's disease. As with the other TNF-alpha blockers, risk of infection and allergic reactions are the major adverse effects of this drug. In addition, caution is advised when using certolizumab in patients with heart failure. Other common adverse effects include upper respiratory or bladder infection, rash, GI upset, headache, and injection site reactions.

Etanercept (Enbrel) is a synthetic TNF receptor that binds with TNF and prevents it from binding with its "normal" receptors on cell surfaces. This action inhibits TNF activity in inflammatory and immune responses. The drug is indicated for the treatment of moderate to severe rheumatoid arthritis in adults and children. In this condition, the TNF increases in joint synovial fluid are considered important in joint inflammation and destruction. Etanercept may be effective in combination with methotrexate in patients who do not respond adequately to methotrexate alone. Common adverse effects include headache, injection site reactions, and infections.

Limited information is available about the use of many of the newer immunosuppressants in children. The FDA has approved three TNF-alpha blockers, etanercept, infliximab, and adalimumab, for use in children 4 to 17 years of age who have severe juvenile rheumatoid arthritis that has not responded to conventional therapy.

Interleukin-Blocking Agents

(P) **Anakinra** (Kineret) is a recombinant IL-receptor antagonist. The drug binds to the IL-1 receptor and thereby blocks the inflammatory effects of IL-1. Indications for use include moderate to severe rheumatoid arthritis in adults. It may be used alone or in combination with cytotoxic immunomodulators but not with TNF-alpha–blocking agents or the fusion protein inhibitor abatacept because of increased risk of infection when these biological agents are combined. Common adverse effects include headache, injection site reactions (redness, bruising, inflammation, pain), infection, nausea, diarrhea, decreased white blood cells, sinusitis, and flu-like symptoms.

Alefacept (Amevive) is a monoclonal antibody used to treat moderate to severe psoriasis. This drug binds to receptors on the surface of T lymphocytes, preventing the receptors from interacting with particular antigens, and thereby inhibiting activation of T lymphocytes. Common adverse effects include lymphopenia and injection site reactions (e.g., edema, inflammation, pain).

Tocilizumab (Actemra), a humanized monoclonal antibody that blocks IL-6 receptors, recently received approval for use in adults and children with severe rheumatoid arthritis that has not responded to conventional immunosuppressants. IL-6, an inflammatory cytokine, is found in higher than normal concentrations in joints of patients with rheumatoid arthritis and contributes to chronic inflammation and joint destruction in the disorder. Tocilizumab may be combined with methotrexate. Common adverse effects include upper respiratory infection, hyperlipidemia, hypertension, leukopenia, and elevated liver enzymes. Screening for tuberculosis prior to treatment and monitoring of lipid levels and liver enzymes every 3 months during therapy is recommended.

Ustekinumab (Stelara) is another monoclonal antibody used to treat psoriasis. It blocks IL-12 and IL-23, reducing the inflammatory response and overactivity of T cells. Common adverse effects include headache; infection; lymphocytosis; and a first-dose reaction characterized by chills, fever, muscle aches, and nausea.

Fusion Protein Inhibitors

(P) **Abatacept** (Orencia) is a fusion protein inhibitor synthesized from an IgG antibody fused to a cell protein that binds to antigen-presenting molecules. This action prevents the activation of T lymphocytes and the production of inflammatory cytokines. It inhibits activation of T lymphocytes in synovial membranes of joints affected by rheumatoid arthritis and decreases inflammation and joint destruction. It may be used alone or with other antirheumatoid arthritis drugs except anakinra and TNF-alpha–blocking agents. Common adverse effects include dizziness, headache, infections, and nausea. Evidence does not suggest the need for dose adjustment in the presence of liver or renal disease.

Belatacept (Nulojix), a new fusion protein inhibitor, recently received approval for use in the prevention of organ rejection after kidney transplant. The drug binds to a receptor protein on antigen-presenting cells and prevents T-cell activation and cytokine production, thus reducing the risk of transplant organ rejection. There is an increased risk of lymphoma in people who develop Epstein-Barr virus infection during belatacept therapy. Because of that risk, the FDA has issued a **BLACK BOX WARNING** ◆ that limits belatacept use to people who test positive for Epstein-Barr virus prior to transplant. Authorities do not recommend the drug for use after liver transplant because of increased risk of graft loss and associated mortality. Adverse effects include anemia, peripheral edema, hypertension, vomiting, diarrhea, constipation, fever, bladder and kidney infection, and leukopenia.

NCLEX Success

3. **The nurse should instruct the patient taking cyclosporine or tacrolimus that toxic levels of the drug may be reached if taken with**

   A. orange juice
   B. coffee
   C. grapefruit juice
   D. milk

4. **A nurse is caring for a patient who is taking immunosuppressant drugs. The most critical information to teach the patient is ways**

   A. to decrease infection
   B. to avoid weight gain
   C. to maintain a good fluid intake
   D. to increase rest and decrease exercise

5. **A patient in an outpatient clinic is taking mycophenolate after a kidney transplant. Which of the following over-the-counter products is likely to interfere with the activity of this immunosuppressant?**

   A. diphenhydramine (Benadryl), used for itchy mosquito bites
   B. acetaminophen (Tylenol), used for a tension headache
   C. magnesium/aluminum hydroxide (Maalox), used for heartburn
   D. benzocaine/dextromethorphan (Chloraseptic) throat lozenges, used for throat irritation

6. **A woman is taking leflunomide (Arava) for rheumatoid arthritis, and her provider monitors her laboratory results on a regular basis. Which of the following laboratory findings indicates that the patient is experiencing an adverse effect?**

   A. increased red blood cell count
   B. decreased creatinine
   C. increased white blood cell count
   D. decreased liver enzymes

The Nursing Process

Assessment

- Assess patients receiving or anticipating immunosuppressant drug therapy for signs and symptoms of current infection or factors predisposing them to potential infection (e.g., impaired skin integrity, invasive devices, cigarette smoking)
- Assess the environment for factors predisposing to infection (e.g., family or health care providers with infections, contact with young children, potential exposure to childhood infectious diseases).
- Assess nutritional status, including appetite and weight.
- Assess baseline values of laboratory and other diagnostic test results to aid monitoring of responses to immunosuppressant drug therapy. With pretransplantation patients, this includes assessing for impaired function of the diseased organ and for abnormalities that need treatment before surgery.
- Assess adequacy of support systems for transplant recipients.
- Assess patients after transplant for surgical wound healing, signs of organ rejection, and adverse effects of immunosuppressant drugs.
- Assess patients with autoimmune disorders (e.g., rheumatoid arthritis, Crohn's disease) for manifestations of the disease process and responses to drug therapy.

Nursing Diagnoses

- Risk for injury: adverse drug effects
- Risk for injury: infection and cancer related to immunosuppression and increased susceptibility
- Deficient knowledge: disease process and immunosuppressant drug therapy
- Anxiety related to the diagnosis of serious disease or need for organ transplantation
- Social isolation related to activities to reduce exposure to infection

Planning/Goals

The patient will

- Participate in decision making about the treatment plan.
- Take immunosuppressant drugs according to treatment plan.
- Verbalize or demonstrate essential drug information.
- Participate in interventions to prevent infection (e.g., maintain personal hygiene, avoid known sources of infection) while immunosuppressed.
- Experience relief or reduction of disease symptoms.
- Maintain adequate levels of nutrition and fluids, rest and sleep, and exercise.
- Cope with anxiety related to the disease process and drug therapy.
- Keep appointments for follow-up care.
- Have adverse drug effects prevented or recognized and treated promptly.
- Maintain diagnostic test values within acceptable limits.
- Maintain family and other emotional/social support systems.
- Receive optimal instructions and information about the treatment plan, self-care in activities of daily living, report adverse drug effects, and other concerns.
- Receive appropriate care before and after tissue or organ transplantation, including prevention or early recognition and treatment of rejection reactions.

Nursing Interventions

The nurse will

- Practice and teach good hand and personal hygiene to patient and to others in contact with the patient.
- Use protective isolation techniques according to institutional policies after transplantation and/or when the neutrophil count is less than 500 per mm^3.
- Use sterile technique for all injections, IV site care, wound dressing changes, and all invasive diagnostic tests or therapeutic procedures.
- Screen staff and visitors for signs and symptoms of infection; persons with signs of infection should not have patient contact.
- Allow family members or significant others to visit patient when feasible.
- Teach patient to report fever and other signs of infection immediately.
- Assist patient to maintain adequate nutrition, rest, sleep, and exercise patterns.
- Inform patient about diagnostic test results, changes in therapeutic regimen, and evidence of progress.

- Monitor renal function (creatinine, BUN), liver function (serum bilirubin, AST, ALT, alkaline phosphatase, albumin), CBC, and other diagnostic test results related to organ function throughout drug therapy.
- Schedule drug administration to maximize therapeutic effects and minimize adverse effects.
- Consult other health care team members (e.g., physician, dietitian, social worker) on the patient's behalf when indicated. Multidisciplinary consultation is essential for transplantation patients and desirable for patients with autoimmune disorders.
- Assist patients in learning strategies to manage day-to-day activities during long-term immunosuppression.

Evaluation

- Interview and observe for accurate drug administration.
- Interview and observe for personal hygiene practices and infection-avoiding maneuvers.
- Interview and observe for therapeutic and adverse drug effects with each patient contact.

- Interview regarding knowledge and attitude toward the drug therapy regimen, including follow-up care and symptoms to report to health care providers.
- Determine the number and types of infections that have occurred in the neutropenic patient.
- Compare current CBC and other reports with baseline values for acceptable levels, according to the patient's condition.
- Observe and assess outpatients regarding ability to comply with follow-up care.
- Interview and observe for organ function and absence of rejection reactions in posttransplantation patients.

Clinical Application 11-3

What are the specific teaching points to be covered with Mr. Jones regarding proper self-administration of his medication (cyclosporine, mycophenolate, and prednisone)?

Key Concepts

- Immunosuppressants are used to decrease the immune response in allergic and autoimmune disorders and to avoid graft rejection after transplantation.
- With current treatments, most transplant patients must continue to take immunosuppressive drugs the rest of their lives.
- When caring for patients who are taking immunosuppressant drugs, it is critical for the home care nurse to assess the environment for potential sources of infection, assist patients and other members of the household to understand the patient's susceptibility to infection, and teach ways to decrease risks of infection.
- Mycophenolate mofetil is used for prophylaxis of organ rejection after cardiac, hepatic, and renal transplants, as well as immunosuppression after transplant procedures involving the lung, pancreas, and small intestine.
- The FDA has issued a **BLACK BOX WARNING** ◆ for mycophenolate mofetil regarding the risk of fetal loss and malformations. Women of childbearing age must use contraception.
- The FDA has issued a **BLACK BOX WARNING** ◆ for leflunomide, another cytotoxic immunosuppressant, regarding the risk of fetal loss and malformations. Women of childbearing age must use contraception.
- Cyclosporine and tacrolimus, immunosuppressants widely used in organ transplantation, often cause nephrotoxicity and are subject to numerous drug interactions (enzyme-inhibiting drugs increase blood levels and enzyme-inducing drugs decrease blood levels).
- The FDA has issued a **BLACK BOX WARNING** ◆ for cyclosporine regarding the risk of hypertension and associated nephrotoxicity.
- The FDA has issued a **BLACK BOX WARNING** ◆ that use of sirolimus in lung and liver transplant patients has been associated with increased morbidity and mortality.
- Immunosuppressant drugs greatly increase risks of infection and some kinds of cancer such as lymphoma and skin cancer.
- The FDA has issued a **BLACK BOX WARNING** ◆ limiting all antirejection drugs use to prescribers experienced in transplant therapy, because of the increased risk of infection as well as malignancies such as lymphoma and skin cancer with their long-term use.
- Immunoglobulins (e.g., ATG, muromonab-CD3) are often used to prevent and suppress an acute rejection reaction after transplant therapy.

- The FDA has issued a **BLACK BOX WARNING** ◆ for ATG, urging that its use be restricted to experienced prescribers.
- Newer monoclonal antibody therapies have more specific effects on specific immune system receptors and may cause fewer or less severe adverse effects than traditional drugs.
- Due to the risk of anaphylaxis, the FDA has issued a **BLACK BOX WARNING** ◆ for omalizumab. The drug should only be administered to patients in a health care setting under direct medical supervision by provider who can initiate treatment of life-threatening anaphylaxis.
- The FDA has issued a **BLACK BOX WARNING** ◆ that limits belatacept use to people who test positive for Epstein-Barr virus prior to transplant due to the significant risk of lymphoma with an initial Epstein-Barr virus infection during belatacept therapy.

Critical Thinking Questions

11-1. Mary Johnson is a 31-year-old elementary school teacher who has been diagnosed with rheumatoid arthritis. She is currently taking methotrexate for this condition but has continued to experience significant joint pain, particularly in her hands. She tells the nurse during her office visit today that her pain and joint stiffness are making it difficult for her to work and to care for her two young children. Her primary care provider has prescribed etanercept (Enbrel) to be given in addition to the methotrexate.

- Ms. Johnson asks the nurse to explain how the etanercept and methotrexate work and asks why she is to continue taking the methotrexate when it has not helped. How should the nurse respond?
- Discuss the nursing assessments and interventions that the nurse should implement to reduce Ms. Johnson's risk of infection.
- What additional precautions should the nurse take to minimize adverse effects from Ms. Johnson's medications?

References and Resources

Constatiner, M. & Cukor, D. (2011). Barriers to immunosuppressive medication adherence in high-risk adult renal transplant recipients. *Dialysis and Transplantation*, 40(2), 60–65.

Gabardi, S. & Baroletti, S. A. (2010). Everolimus: a proliferation signal inhibitor with clinical applications in organ transplantation, oncology, and cardiology. *Pharmacotherapy*, 30, 1044–1056.

Lundsford, K. E., Barbas, A. S., & Brennan, T. V. (2011). Recent advances in immunosuppressive therapy for prevention of renal allograft rejection. *Current Opinion in Organ Transplantation*, 16(4), 390–397.

Martin, S. T., Tichy, E. M., & Gabardi, S. (2011). Belatacept: a novel biologic for maintenance immunosuppression after renal transplantation. *Pharmacotherapy*, 31, 394–407.

Porth, C. M. (2010). *Pathophysiology: Concepts of altered health states* (8th ed.). Philadelphia, PA: Lippincott Williams & Wilkins.

Smeltzer, S. C., Bare, B. G., Hinkle, J. L., & Cheever, K. H. (2010). *Brunner and Suddarth's textbook of medical-surgical nursing* (12th ed.). Philadelphia, PA: Lippincott Williams & Wilkins.

12 Drug Therapy for the Treatment of Cancer

Clinical Application Case Study

Julia Gardner, a 60-year-old school secretary, has stage 2b breast cancer and is receiving adjuvant chemotherapy after a mastectomy. Mrs. Gardner has finished her fourth cycle of doxorubicin (Adriamycin) and cyclophosphamide (Cytoxan) treatment. She will be receiving subsequent chemotherapy in 3 weeks with paclitaxel (Taxol) and trastuzumab (Herceptin).

KEY TERMS

Alopecia: hair loss

Cell cycle: series of intracellular events occurring from one cell division to the next

Chemotherapy: in oncology, the treatment of cancer with an antineoplastic drug or with a combination of such drugs typically given in cycles

Mucositis: inflammation of mucous membranes

Mutation: structural change in the genetic material of a cell

Myelosuppression: bone marrow depression

Neutropenia: low neutrophil count

Oncogenes: genes that have the potential to cause a normal cell to become cancerous

Palliation: alleviation of pain and symptoms without expecting to eliminate the cause

Proto-oncogenes: genes that have the potential to change into active oncogenes

Remission: period when symptoms of a disease have subsided ("remitted")

Thrombocytopenia: low platelet count

Tumor lysis syndrome: life-threatening condition that occurs when large numbers of cancer cells are killed or damaged simultaneously and release their intracellular contents into the bloodstream

Tumor suppressor genes: genes that inhibit unrestrained cell growth; when inactivated, mutant abnormal cells may be allowed to proliferate; also called antioncogenes

Introduction

The term *cancer* is used to describe many disease processes with the common characteristics of uncontrolled cell growth, invasiveness, and metastasis as a result of intracellular genetic changes that allow new cells to grow in an unregulated manner. Oncology is the study of cancer and its treatment. Drugs used in oncologic disorders include cytotoxic medications that kill, damage, or slow the growth of cancer cells as well as those that prevent or treat adverse drug effects. **Chemotherapy** is a major treatment modality for cancer, along with surgery and radiation therapy. Major groups of anticancer drugs include traditional cytotoxic agents (e.g., alkylating agents, antimetabolites, antitumor antibiotics, plant alkaloids); newer cytotoxic "biologic targeted therapies" (e.g., monoclonal antibodies, growth factor inhibitors); and hormone inhibitors, which are not cytotoxic. In addition, several drugs play a role in ameliorating the adverse effects of cytotoxic drugs (e.g., cytoprotectants), including some immunostimulants. This chapter describes the characteristics of cancer etiology, pathophysiology, clinical manifestations, and the drugs used in the treatment of this disease. A nurse who has additional training in chemotherapy use administers these drugs. The focus of this chapter is on the nursing management of patients receiving the medication and not on dosing and administration of individual drugs. The general considerations for chemotherapy management are outlined for each major drug group.

Overview of Cancer

Etiology

Normal cells reproduce in response to a need for tissue growth or repair and stop reproduction in response to growth regulation signals. The normal **cell cycle** is the interval between the "birth" of a cell and its subsequent division into two daughter cells. This cycle involves the orderly stages of growth as well as protein, deoxyribonucleic acid (DNA), and ribonucleic acid (RNA) synthesis (Fig. 12.1). Newly formed daughter cells may then enter the resting phase (G_0) or proceed through the reproductive cycle to form more new cells. Normal cells regulated by normal growth genes are well differentiated in appearance and function, and they have a characteristic lifespan.

In contrast, malignant cells have lost the normal genetic regulation that controls cell growth, invading normal tissues and taking blood and nutrients away from these tissues. They grow in an uncontrolled fashion without regard to growth regulation signals (e.g., contact with other cells) that stop the

growth of normal cells. Also, they are undifferentiated, having lost the structural and functional characteristics of the cells from which they originated. In addition, they lack cell adhesion; hence, as well as invading normal tissue, malignant cells enter blood and lymph vessels, circulate through the body, and can produce additional neoplasms at sites distant from the primary tumor.

A malignant cell develops from a damaged normal cell, beginning with a random **mutation** (abnormal structural change in the genetic material of a cell) that occurs in conjunction with acquired damage to genes that regulate normal cell growth. Usually, body defenses (e.g., an immune response) destroy a mutated cell if the DNA damage cannot be repaired by normal cell enzymes. However, if the mutated cell eludes destruction by the immune system and additional mutations

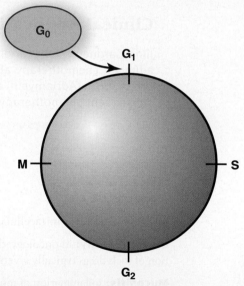

Figure 12.1 Normal cell cycle. The normal cell cycle (the interval between the birth of a cell and its division into two daughter cells) involves several phases. During the resting phase (G_0), cells perform all usual functions except replication; that is, they are not dividing but are capable of doing so when stimulated. Different types of cells spend different lengths of time in this phase, after which they either reenter the cell cycle and differentiate or die. During the first active phase (G_1), ribonucleic acid (RNA) and enzymes required for production of deoxyribonucleic acid (DNA) are developed. During the next phase (S), DNA is synthesized for chromosomes. During G_2, RNA is synthesized, and the mitotic spindle is formed. Mitosis occurs in the final phase (M). The resulting two daughter cells may then enter the resting phase (G_0) or proceed through the reproductive cycle.

develop without repair or apoptosis (programmed cell death) during succeeding cell divisions, malignant transformation may occur. Underlying the failure to repair or destroy these abnormal cells is damage to genes that regulate cell growth; the cells have lost their ability to effectively regulate cell growth. Additional changes allow cells with progressively more malignant characteristics to survive despite their abnormalities. It often takes years for malignant cells to be able to grow into a clinically detectable neoplasm.

Cancer is a heterogeneous disease and has multiple causes, such as environmental factors (tobacco) and genetic factors that may combine to contribute to the progression of malignancy. Genetic causes include mutation of genes, abnormal activation of genes that regulate cell growth and mitosis, and damage to tumor suppressor genes.

Pathophysiology

Abnormal genes, called **oncogenes**, which are involved in cancer growth, are mutations of normal growth-regulating genes, called **proto-oncogenes**, which are present in all body cells. When proto-oncogenes are exposed to carcinogens and genetically altered to become oncogenes, they may stimulate cell growth continuously, allowing abnormal, disordered, and unregulated cell replication. The unregulated cell growth and proliferation promoted by oncogenes contributes to neoplastic transformation of the cell. Tumors of the breast, colon, lung, and bone have all been linked to activation of oncogenes.

Tumor suppressor genes (antioncogenes) normally function to inhibit inappropriate cellular growth and proliferation. Abnormal tumor suppressor genes (i.e., absent, damaged, mutated, or inactivated) may be inherited or result from exposure to carcinogens. When a tumor suppressor gene inside a cell is inactivated, abnormal cells can begin unregulated cell growth. One tumor suppressor gene, p53, is present in virtually all normal tissues. When cellular DNA is damaged, the p53 gene allows time for DNA repair and restricts proliferation of cells with abnormal DNA. Mutations of the p53 gene, a common genetic change in cancer, are associated with more than 90% of small cell lung cancers and more than 50% of breast and colon cancers. Mutant p53 proteins can also form complexes with normal p53 proteins and inactivate the function of the normal suppressor gene.

Thus, activation of oncogenes and inactivation of antioncogenes probably both play roles in cancer development. Multiple genetic abnormalities are characteristic of cancer cells and may occur concurrently or sequentially. Overall, evidence indicates that neoplastic transformation is a progressive process involving both a series of cellular mutations and damage to growth-regulating genes, which allows abnormal cells to replicate without normal immune destruction. Malignancy probably results from a combination of genetic and environmental factors experienced over a person's lifetime, including random cell mutations, exposure to carcinogens, and host genetic or tissue characteristics, that increase susceptibility to cancer development.

Once a cancer develops, factors influencing its continued growth include blood and nutrient supply, immune response, and hormonal stimulation (e.g., in tumors of the breast, uterus, ovary, and prostate). Malignant tumors are able to form new blood vessels, a process called angiogenesis, to support their growth and escape immune destruction as a result of their similarity to other normal cells.

Types of Malignant Neoplasms

Malignant neoplasms are classified according to the type of tissue involved and other characteristics. With the exception of the acute leukemias, they are considered chronic diseases.

Hematologic malignancies involve the bone marrow and lymphoid tissues; they include leukemias, lymphomas, and multiple myeloma. Leukemias are cancers of the bone marrow characterized by overproduction of abnormal white blood cells. The four main types are acute lymphocytic, acute myelogenous, chronic lymphocytic, and chronic myelogenous. Lymphomas are tumors of lymphoid tissue characterized by abnormal proliferation of the white blood cells normally found in lymphoid tissue. They usually develop within lymph nodes and may occur anywhere, because virtually all body tissues contain lymphoid structures. The two main types are Hodgkin's disease and non-Hodgkin's lymphoma. Multiple myeloma is a tumor of the bone marrow in which abnormal plasma cells proliferate. Because normal plasma cells produce antibodies and abnormal plasma cells cannot fulfill this function, the body's immune system is impaired. As the malignant cells expand, they crowd out normal cells, interfere with other bone marrow functions, infiltrate and destroy bone, and eventually metastasize to other tissues, such as the spleen, liver, and lymph nodes.

Solid neoplasms are composed of a mass of malignant cells (parenchyma) and a supporting structure of connective tissue, blood vessels, and lymphatics (stroma). The two major classifications are carcinomas and sarcomas. Carcinomas are derived from epithelial tissues (skin, mucous membrane, linings and coverings of viscera) and are the most common type of malignant tumors. They are further classified by cell type, such as adenocarcinoma or basal cell carcinoma. Sarcomas are derived from connective tissue (muscle, bone, cartilage, fibrous tissue, fat, blood vessels). They are subclassified by cell type (e.g., osteogenic sarcoma, angiosarcoma).

Grading and Staging of Malignant Neoplasms

When a malignant neoplasm is identified, it is further "graded" according to the degree of malignancy and "staged" according to tissue involvement. Grades 1 and 2 are similar to the normal tissue of origin and show cellular differentiation. Grades 3 and 4 are unlike the normal tissue of origin, less differentiated, and more malignant. Staging indicates whether the neoplasm is localized or metastasized and which organs are involved. These characteristics assist in treatment decision-making (e.g., localized tumors are usually amenable to surgery, radiation, or chemotherapy combined with radiation [concurrent] therapy, whereas metastatic disease requires systemic chemotherapy).

Clinical Manifestations

Clinical manifestations vary according to the location and extent of the disease process. There are few effects initially. However, local effects occur as the tumor grows; it becomes

BOX 12.1	General Characteristics of Cytotoxic Antineoplastic Drugs

- Most of these drugs kill malignant cells by interfering with cell replication, with the supply and use of nutrients (e.g., amino acids, purines, pyrimidines), or with the genetic materials in the cell nucleus (DNA or RNA).

- The drugs act during the cell's reproductive cycle. Some, called cell cycle–specific, act mainly during specific phases such as DNA synthesis or formation of the mitotic spindle. Others act during any phase of the cell cycle and are called cell cycle–nonspecific.

- The drugs are most active against rapidly dividing cells, both normal and malignant. Commonly damaged normal cells are those of the bone marrow, the lining of the gastrointestinal tract, and the hair follicles. Healthy cells usually recover fairly soon. However, malignant cells have lost normal genetic growth regulation and continue to actively divide in an unregulated way; thus, more of them are susceptible to the effects of cytotoxic drugs.

- Each drug dose kills a specific percentage of cells. To achieve a cure, all malignant cells must be killed or reduced to a small number that can be killed by the person's immune system.

- Most cytotoxic antineoplastic drugs are potential teratogens, and women should not become pregnant during drug therapy and for several months after the therapy stops.

- Weight-based dosing is used to individualize dosing with all cytotoxic drugs due to their potential to cause significant toxicities to normal cells as well as cancer cells.

- Oncologists combine various cytotoxic drugs with different cell cycle activities and different organ toxicities in treatment plans called "regimens" to more effectively kill the cancer cells while minimizing damage to normal tissues.

- Most cytotoxic drugs are water soluble rather than lipid soluble; thus, they do not cross cell membranes readily and must be administered by intravenous injection or infusion.

- Many of the cytotoxic drugs are prodrugs that are metabolized by liver enzymes to active metabolites, which then have cytotoxic activity affecting protein, DNA, or RNA synthesis or cell division.

- Because cytotoxic drugs are primarily metabolized in the liver and then excreted in urine, they can also have toxic effects on the liver and kidney, especially at higher doses.

- Many cytotoxic antineoplastic drugs have U.S. Food and Drug Administration (FDA)–issued **BLACK BOX WARNINGS** ◆ about potentially serious adverse effects, and all have special precautions for safe usage.

---

large enough to cause pressure, distort or affect blood supply in surrounding tissues, interfere with organ function, or obstruct ducts and organ outlets. Systemic conditions such as cachexia, anorexia, and weight loss occur from the effects of the growing tumor increasing overall metabolic demands and altering glucose utilization at the cellular level. Other symptoms and signs may include anemia, malnutrition, pain, immunosuppression, infection, hemorrhagic tendencies, thromboembolism, and hypercalcemia, as well as various symptoms related to impaired function of affected organs and tissues.

Drug Therapy

Chemotherapy is most often used to indicate the use of traditional cytotoxic antineoplastic drugs for the treatment of cancer. Except for hormone inhibitors that slow the growth of cancer cells stimulated by hormones, the purpose of all antineoplastic drugs is to damage or kill cancer cells (i.e., be cytotoxic). The goal of treatment with cytotoxic antineoplastic drugs is cure, **remission** (period when symptoms of a disease have subsided) or **palliation** (alleviation of pain and symptoms without expecting to eliminate the cause). In hematologic malignancies such as leukemias, drug therapy is the treatment of choice because the disease is disseminated and must be treated systemically rather than locally, with surgery or radiation. In solid tumors, drug therapy may be used, before (neoadjuvant) or after (adjuvant) surgery or radiation therapy and when there is metastasis that is not surgically resectable.

Antineoplastic drugs are also sometimes used in the treatment of nonmalignant conditions. For example, smaller doses of methotrexate (MTX) are used as an immunosuppressant for treating the inflammation of rheumatoid arthritis and psoriasis.

Traditional chemotherapeutic drugs share common general characteristics (Box 12.1). Most chemotherapy regimens contain a combination of drugs with actions at different places in the cell cycle process of cell growth and replication (Fig. 12.2), destroying a greater number of cancer cells and reducing the risk of the emergence of drug resistance. Drug resistance may emerge when (1) cancer cells overexpress target genes that

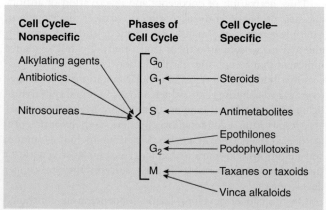

Figure 12.2 Cell cycle effects of cytotoxic antineoplastic drugs.

prevent the drug's being absorbed by the malignant cells, (2) tumor cells are able to inactivate the drug, or (3) apoptosis occurs in tumor cells is defective. Oncologists order many newer drugs for use after initial cytotoxic drug therapy to prevent drug resistance from affecting the tumor response.

Chemotherapy administration usually occurs in cycles, depending on the type of cancer and which drugs are used. Cyclic administration involves taking the drugs for a specific period, with a recovery period following each treatment cycle. The recovery period allows time for the patient to produce new, healthy cells to replace the normal rapidly dividing cells that have been affected by the drugs. Chemotherapy is often continued as long as it is effective and does not produce unacceptable toxicity or until there is no longer any evidence of malignancy. Table 12.1 outlines the drugs used in cancer treatment.

Cytotoxic Antineoplastic Drugs Used to Treat Cancer

The consequences of inappropriate or erroneous chemotherapy may be fatal for patients (from the disease or from the treatment); thus, medical oncologists experienced in use of cancer drugs manage chemotherapy regimens.

QSEN Safety Alert

Because of the toxicity of these drugs, nurses who administer intravenous (IV) cytotoxic chemotherapy receive special training and are certified in handling and administering the chemotherapy drugs safely and accurately.

TABLE 12.1
Drugs Administered for the Treatment of Cancer

Drug Class	Prototype(s)	Other Drugs in the Class
Alkylating Drugs		
	Cyclophosphamide (Cytoxan) (nitrogen mustard derivative)	*Nitrogen mustard derivatives* Chlorambucil (Leukeran) Ifosfamide (Ifex) Melphalan (Alkeran) *Nitrosoureas* Carmustine (BiCNU, Gliadel) Lomustine (CCNU) *Platinum compounds* Carboplatin (Paraplatin) Cisplatin (Platinol) Oxaliplatin (Eloxatin) *Triazene* Dacarbazine (DTIC-Dome)
Antimetabolites		
	Methotrexate (Trexall)	Capecitabine (Xeloda) Cladribine (Leustatin) Cytarabine (Cytosar-U) Fludarabine (Fludara) Fluorouracil (5-FU) (Adrucil, Efudex, Fluoroplex) Gemcitabine (Gemzar) Mercaptopurine (Purinethol) Pemetrexed (Alimta)
Antitumor Antibiotics		
	Daunorubicin conventional Daunorubicin liposomal (DaunoXome) (anthracycline agents) Bleomycin (Blenoxane) (polypeptide antibiotic)	*Anthracycline agents* Doxorubicin conventional Doxorubicin liposomal (Doxil) Epirubicin (Ellence) Idarubicin (Idamycin) Mitoxantrone (Novantrone) Valrubicin (Valstar) *Polypeptide antibiotics* Dactinomycin (Actinomycin D, Cosmegen) Mitomycin (Mutamycin) Pentostatin (Nipent)

(Continued on page 202)

TABLE 12.1

Drugs Administered for the Treatment of Cancer (Continued)

Drug Class	Prototype(s)	Other Drugs in the Class
Plant alkaloids		
	Vincristine (Oncovin) (vinca alkaloid)	*Camptothecins* Irinotecan (Camptosar) Topotecan (Hycamtin) *Podophyllotoxins* Etoposide (VePesid) Teniposide (Vumon) *Taxanes* Docetaxel (Taxotere) Paclitaxel (Taxol) *Vinca alkaloids* Vinblastine (Velban) Vinorelbine (Navelbine)
Miscellaneous agents		
		L-Asparaginase (Elspar) Hydroxyurea (Hydrea) Ixabepilone (Ixempra) Levamisole (Ergamisol) Procarbazine (Matulane)
Biologic Antineoplastic Drugs		
Monoclonal antibodies		Alemtuzumab (Campath IH) Bevacizumab (Avastin) Cetuximab (Erbitux) Gemtuzumab ozogamicin (Mylotarg) Ibritumomab tiuxetan (Zevalin) Panitumumab (Vectibix) Rituximab (Rituxan) Tositumomab and I-131-tositumomab (Bexxar) Trastuzumab (Herceptin)
Growth factor and tyrosine kinase inhibitors		Dasatinib (Sprycel) Erlotinib (Tarceva) Imatinib (Gleevec) Lapatinib (Tykerb) Pazopanib (Votrient) Sorafenib (Nexavar) Sunitinib (Sutent) Temsirolimus (Torisel)
Proteasome inhibitor	Bortezomib (Velcade)	
Antineoplastic Hormone Inhibitors		
	Tamoxifen (Nolvadex) (antiestrogen)	*Antiestrogens* Fulvestrant (Faslodex) Toremifene (Fareston) *Aromatase inhibitors* Anastrozole (Arimidex) Exemestane (Aromasin) Letrozole (Femara) *Antiandrogens* Bicalutamide (Casodex) Flutamide (Eulexin) Nilutamide (Nilandron) *LHRH analogs* Goserelin (Zoladex) Leuprolide (Eligard, Lupron, Viadur) Triptorelin (Trelstar LA, Trelstar Depot)

TABLE 12.1		
Drugs Administered for the Treatment of Cancer (Continued)		
Drug Class	**Prototype(s)**	**Other Drugs in the Class**
Cytoprotectant Drugs (see Chap. 9)		Amifostine (Ethyol) Dexrazoxane (Zinecard) Erythropoietin (Epogen, Procrit) Filgrastim (Neupogen) Leucovorin (Wellcovorin) Mesna (Mesnex) Oprelvekin (Neumega) Palifermin (Kepivance) Sargramostim (Leukine)

LHRH, luteinizing hormone–releasing hormone.

This chapter focuses on the overall nursing considerations for caring for patients receiving chemotherapy, not the administration of particular drugs. Therefore, information is not presented in a prototype format.

Pharmacokinetics

Most cytotoxic drugs are water soluble rather than lipid soluble and require administration by IV injection or infusion. Some, such as cyclophosphamide, are better absorbed and are available as oral formulations. A few, such as MTX, are also given intrathecally. The nitrosoureas (e.g., carmustine, lomustine) are unique in being lipid soluble and able to cross the blood–brain barrier; hence, they are widely used in the treatment of brain tumors. Carmustine is also formulated as a dissolving wafer, which can be implanted in the brain tissue at the time of surgical tumor resection.

Liposomal preparations of some cytotoxic drugs (e.g., doxorubicin) use a lipid membrane to encase the drug molecules. Liposomal preparations can increase drug concentration in malignant tissues that are more permeable, allowing the lipid vesicle to more easily concentrate in the tumor, while lowering the concentration in normal tissues that are less permeable, thereby increasing effectiveness and decreasing toxicity (e.g., cardiotoxicity).

Action

Cytotoxic antineoplastic drugs are usually classified in terms of their mechanisms of action (alkylating agents, antimetabolites) or their sources (plant alkaloids, antibiotics).

Alkylating Drugs

Alkylating drugs include nitrogen mustard derivatives, nitrosoureas, platinum compounds, and triazenes.

- Nitrogen mustard derivatives are cell cycle–nonspecific agents, causing cross-linking of DNA and RNA and interfering with subsequent cell division. The most widely used alkylating drug, a nitrogen mustard derivative, is ℗ **cyclophosphamide** (Cytoxan, Neosar).

- Nitrosoureas also interfere with DNA replication and RNA synthesis and may inhibit essential enzymatic reactions in cancer cells. Carmustine and lomustine are both cell cycle–nonspecific, and they are lipid soluble. These features allow them to enter the brain and cerebrospinal fluid more readily than other antineoplastic drugs, which make them useful for treating lymphomas and brain tumors.

- Platinum compounds are cell cycle–nonspecific agents that cross-link DNA inhibiting DNA, RNA, and protein synthesis. Cisplatin (Platinol) is the most widely used of the platinum compounds.

- Triazene compounds are cell cycle–nonspecific agents with antitumor and mutagenic properties. The drugs are effective for metastatic malignant melanoma, Hodgkin's disease, and various sarcomas. The most widely used drug in the class is dacarbazine (DTIC-Dome).

Antimetabolites

Antimetabolites are drugs that are similar to metabolites or nutrients needed by cells for reproduction. These drugs replace normal metabolites or inhibit essential enzymes, inside the cell, depriving the cell of substances needed for DNA formation or causing abnormal DNA formation. The drugs are cell cycle–specific because they exert their cytotoxic effects only during the S phase of the cell's reproductive cycle, when DNA is being synthesized. Antimetabolites that are used in cancer treatment are folate antagonists, such as ℗ **methotrexate** (Trexall), or MTX; purine antagonists (e.g., mercaptopurine, cladribine, fludarabine); or pyrimidine antagonists (e.g., fluorouracil, capecitabine, cytarabine). These drugs are most effective against rapidly growing tumors, and individual drugs vary in their effectiveness with different kinds of cancer.

Antitumor Antibiotics

℗ **Bleomycin** (Blenoxane) inhibits DNA, RNA, and protein synthesis in susceptible cells, preventing cell division. The anthracycline agents (e.g., doxorubicin, daunorubicin, epirubicin) bind to DNA so that DNA and RNA transcription is blocked. They are active in all phases of the cell cycle, and their cytotoxic effects are similar to those of the alkylating agents. Mitomycin causes DNA cross-linking and inhibits DNA synthesis.

Plant Alkaloids

Plant alkaloids include several types of drugs.

- Camptothecins (also called DNA topoisomerase inhibitors) inhibit an enzyme required for DNA replication and repair.
- Podophyllotoxins act mainly in the G_2 phase of the cell cycle and prevent mitosis.
- Taxanes (e.g., paclitaxel, docetaxel) interfere with the ability of the chromosomes to separate during cell division.
- Vinca alkaloids (e.g., Ⓟ **vincristine** [Oncovin], vinblastine (Velban), vinorelbine (Navelbine)) are cell cycle–specific agents that interfere with cell mitosis. Despite having similar structures, they have different antineoplastic activities and adverse effects.

Miscellaneous Drugs

Miscellaneous agents vary in their sources, mechanisms of action, indications for use, and toxic effects. L-Asparaginase (Elspar) is an enzyme that inhibits protein synthesis and reproduction by depriving cells of required amino acids. Pegaspargase (Oncaspar) is a modified formulation for people who are hypersensitive to L-asparaginase. Hydroxyurea (Hydrea) acts in the S phase of the cell cycle to impair DNA synthesis. Ixabepilone (Ixempra) is the first of a new class of antineoplastic drugs called epothilones. Obtained from bacteria, epothilones stop growth of tumor cells by preventing cell division (antimitotic effects). Ixabepilone is a semisynthetic analog of epothilone. Procarbazine (Matulane), a monoamine oxidase inhibitor, inhibits DNA, RNA, and protein synthesis.

Use

Researchers have found that certain combinations of cytotoxic drugs with different cytotoxic activities in the cell cycle and different organ toxicities are most effective in certain types of cancer. Hence, concurrent administration of multiple drugs based on the patient's type of malignancy may be necessary. When both cytotoxic and hormone inhibitor drug therapies are required, however, concurrent administration is not appropriate, because hormone antagonists decrease malignant cell growth and cytotoxic agents are most effective when the cells are actively dividing. Patients with breast cancer usually receive a hormone-inhibiting drug before a cytotoxic drug in metastatic disease and after chemotherapy when used for adjuvant treatment.

It is important to use weight-based dosing to individualize dosing of all cytotoxic drugs to minimize toxicity of normal cells. In addition, some cytotoxic drugs have a cumulative maximum dose that can be given for cancer treatment without risk of irreversible vital organ damage (e.g., heart failure with doxorubicin, pulmonary fibrosis with carmustine and bleomycin). Table 12.2 provides route and dosage information for some cytotoxic antineoplastic drugs.

TABLE 12.2

DRUGS AT A GLANCE: Cytotoxic Antineoplastic Drugs

Drug/Pregnancy Category	Routes and Dosage Ranges*	Clinical Uses	Adverse Effects
Alkylating Drugs			
Nitrogen Mustard Derivatives			
Ⓟ **Cyclophosphamide** (Cytoxan)/D	Induction therapy, PO 1–5 mg/kg/d; IV 20–40 mg/kg in divided doses over 2–5 d Maintenance therapy, PO 1–5 mg/kg daily	Hodgkin's disease; non-Hodgkin's lymphomas; leukemias; cancer of head and neck, breast, lung, or ovary; multiple myeloma; neuroblastoma	Bone marrow depression, nausea, vomiting, alopecia, hemorrhagic cystitis, hypersensitivity reactions, secondary leukemia or bladder cancer
Chlorambucil (Leukeran)/D	PO 0.1–0.2 mg/kg/d for 3–6 wk Maintenance therapy, 0.03–0.1 mg/kg/d	Chronic lymphocytic leukemia, Hodgkin's and non-Hodgkin's lymphomas	Bone marrow depression, hepatotoxicity, secondary leukemia
Ifosfamide (Ifex)/D	IV 1.2 g/m²/d for 5 consecutive d; repeat every 3 wk or after white blood cell and platelet counts return to normal after a dose	Germ cell testicular cancer	Bone marrow depression, hemorrhagic cystitis, nausea and vomiting, alopecia, CNS depression, seizures
Melphalan (Alkeran)/D	PO, 6 mg/d for 2–3 wk, then 28 drug-free days, then 2 mg daily IV, 16 mg/m² every 2 wk for 4 doses, then every 4 wk	Multiple myeloma, ovarian cancer	Bone marrow depression, nausea and vomiting, hypersensitivity reactions

TABLE 12.2

DRUGS AT A GLANCE: Cytotoxic Antineoplastic Drugs (Continued)

Drug/Pregnancy Category	Routes and Dosage Ranges*	Clinical Uses	Adverse Effects
Nitrosoureas			
Carmustine (BiCNU, Gliadel)/D	IV 150–200 mg/m² every 6 wk Wafer, implanted in brain after tumor resection	Hodgkin's disease, non-Hodgkin's lymphomas, multiple myeloma, brain tumors	Bone marrow depression, nausea, vomiting
Lomustine (CCNU)/D	PO 130 mg/m² every 6 wk	Hodgkin's disease, brain tumors	Nausea and vomiting, bone marrow depression
Platinum Compounds			
Carboplatin (Paraplatin)/D	IV infusion 360 mg/m² on d 1 every 4 wk	Palliation of ovarian cancer, endometrial cancer	Bone marrow depression, nausea and vomiting, nephrotoxicity
Cisplatin (Platinol)/D	IV 100 mg/m² once every 4 wk	Advanced carcinomas of testes, bladder, ovary	Nausea, vomiting, anaphylaxis, nephrotoxicity, bone marrow depression, ototoxicity, peripheral neuropathy
Oxaliplatin (Eloxatin)/D	IV infusion 85 mg/m² every 2 wk	Advanced colon cancer (with 5-fluorouracil and leucovorin)	Anaphylaxis, anemia, increased risk of bleeding or infection, cold-induced acute neurotoxicities
Antimetabolites			
ⓟ **Methotrexate** (Trexall)/X	Acute leukemia in children: induction, PO, IV 3 mg/m²/d; maintenance, PO 30 mg/m² twice weekly Choriocarcinoma: PO, IM 15 mg/m² daily for 5 d	Leukemias; non-Hodgkin's lymphomas; osteosarcoma; choriocarcinoma of testes; cancers of breast, lung, head, and neck	Bone marrow depression, nausea, vomiting, mucositis, diarrhea, fever, alopecia
Capecitabine (Xeloda)/D	PO 1250 mg/m² every 12 h for 2 wk, then a rest period of 1 wk, then repeat cycle	Metastatic breast cancer, colorectal cancer	Bone marrow depression, nausea, vomiting, diarrhea, mucositis, hand–foot syndrome
Cladribine (Leustatin)/D	IV infusion 0.09 mg/kg/d for 7 consecutive d	Hairy cell leukemia	Bone marrow depression, nausea, vomiting
Cytarabine (Cytosar-U)/D	IV infusion 100 mg/m²/d for 7 d	Leukemias of adults and children	Bone marrow depression, nausea, vomiting, anaphylaxis, mucositis, diarrhea
Fludarabine (Fludara)/D	IV 25 mg/m²/d for 5 consecutive d; repeat every 28 d	Chronic lymphocytic leukemia	Bone marrow depression, nausea, vomiting, diarrhea
Fluorouracil (5-FU) (Adrucil, Efudex, Fluoroplex)/D	IV 12 mg/kg/d for 4 d, then 6 mg/kg every other day for 4 doses Topical, apply to skin cancer lesion twice daily for several weeks	Carcinomas of the breast, colon, stomach, and pancreas; solar keratoses, basal cell carcinoma	Bone marrow depression, nausea, vomiting, mucositis; pain, pruritus, burning at site of application

(*Continued on page 206*)

TABLE 12.2

DRUGS AT A GLANCE: Cytotoxic Antineoplastic Drugs (Continued)

Drug/Pregnancy Category	Routes and Dosage Ranges*	Clinical Uses	Adverse Effects
Gemcitabine (Gemzar)/D	IV 1000 mg/m² once weekly up to 7 wk or toxicity, withhold for 1 wk, then once weekly for 3 wk and withhold for 1 wk	Lung and pancreatic cancer	Bone marrow depression, nausea, vomiting, flu-like symptoms, skin rash
Mercaptopurine (Purinethol)/D	PO 2.5 mg/kg/d (100–200 mg for average adult)	Acute and chronic leukemias	Bone marrow depression, nausea, vomiting, mucositis
Pemetrexed (Alimta)/D	IV infusion 500 mg/m² over 10 min, every 21 d	Non–small cell lung cancer	Mucositis, skin rash
Antitumor Antibiotics			
ⓟ **Bleomycin** (Blenoxane)/D	IV, IM, Sub-Q 0.25–0.5 units/kg once or twice weekly	Squamous cell carcinoma, Hodgkin's and non-Hodgkin's lymphomas, testicular carcinoma	Pulmonary toxicity, mucositis, alopecia, nausea, vomiting, hypersensitivity reactions, hypotension
Dactinomycin (Actinomycin D, Cosmegen)/D	IV 15 mcg/kg/d for 5 d and repeated every 2–4 wk	Rhabdomyosarcoma, Wilms' tumor, choriocarcinoma, testicular carcinoma, Ewing's sarcoma	Bone marrow depression, nausea, vomiting; extravasation may lead to tissue necrosis.
Daunorubicin conventional/D	IV 25–45 mg/m² daily for 3 d every 3–4 wk	Acute leukemias, lymphomas	Same as doxorubicin
Daunorubicin liposomal (DaunoXome)/D	IV infusion, 40 mg/m² every 2 wk	AIDS-related Kaposi's sarcoma	Bone marrow depression, nausea, vomiting
Doxorubicin conventional (Adriamycin)/D	Adults, IV 60–75 mg/m² every 21 d Children, IV 30 mg/m² daily for 3 d, repeated every 4 wk	Acute leukemias; lymphomas; carcinomas of breast, lung, and ovary	Bone marrow depression, alopecia, mucositis, gastrointestinal (GI) upset, cardiomyopathy; extravasation may lead to tissue necrosis.
Doxorubicin liposomal (Doxil)/D	IV infusion, 20 mg/m², once every 3 wk	AIDS-related Kaposi's sarcoma	Bone marrow depression, nausea, vomiting, fever, alopecia
Epirubicin (Ellence)/D	IV infusion 120 mg/m² every 3–4 wk	Breast cancer	Cardiotoxicity
Idarubicin (Idamycin)/D	IV injection 12 mg/m²/d for 3 d, with cytarabine	Acute myeloid leukemia	Same as doxorubicin
Mitomycin (Mutamycin)/D	IV 20 mg/m² every 6–8 wk	Metastatic carcinomas of stomach and pancreas	Bone marrow depression, nausea, vomiting; extravasation may lead to tissue necrosis.
Mitoxantrone (Novantrone)/D	IV infusion 12 mg/m² on d 1–3, for induction of remission in leukemia	Acute nonlymphocytic leukemia, prostate cancer	Bone marrow depression, heart failure, nausea
Pentostatin (Nipent)/D	IV 4 mg/m² every other week	Hairy cell leukemia unresponsive to interferon alfa	Bone marrow depression, hepatotoxicity, nausea, vomiting

TABLE 12.2

DRUGS AT A GLANCE: Cytotoxic Antineoplastic Drugs (Continued)

Drug/Pregnancy Category	Routes and Dosage Ranges*	Clinical Uses	Adverse Effects
Valrubicin (Valstar)/D	Intravesically, 800 mg once weekly for 6 wk	Bladder cancer	Dysuria, urgency, frequency, bladder spasms, hematuria
Plant Alkaloids			
Camptothecins			
Irinotecan (Camptosar)/D	IV infusion, 125 mg/m² once weekly for 4 wk, then a 2-wk rest period; repeat regimen	Metastatic cancer of colon or rectum	Bone marrow depression, diarrhea
Topotecan (Hycamtin)/D	IV infusion 1.5 mg/m² daily for 5 consecutive d every 21 d	Advanced ovarian cancer, small cell lung cancer	Bone marrow depression, nausea, vomiting, diarrhea
Podophyllotoxins			
Etoposide (VePesid)/D	IV, 50–100 mg/m²/d on d 1–5, or 100 mg/m²/d on d 1, 3, and 5, every 3–4 wk PO, 2 times the IV dose	Testicular cancer, small cell lung cancer	Bone marrow depression, allergic reactions, nausea, vomiting, alopecia
Teniposide (Vumon)/D	IV infusion 165 mg/m² twice weekly for 8–9 doses	Acute lymphocytic leukemia in children	Same as etoposide
Taxanes			
Docetaxel (Taxotere)/D	IV infusion 60–100 mg/m², every 3 wk	Advanced breast cancer, non–small cell lung cancer	Bone marrow depression, nausea, vomiting, hypersensitivity reactions, peripheral neuropathy
Paclitaxel (Taxol)/D	IV infusion 135 mg/m² every 3 wk	Advanced ovarian cancer, advanced breast cancer, non–small cell lung cancer, AIDS-related Kaposi's sarcoma	Bone marrow depression, allergic reactions, hypotension, bradycardia, nausea, vomiting, peripheral neuropathy
Vinca Alkaloids			
Ⓟ **Vincristine** (Oncovin)/D	Adults, IV 1.4 mg/m² weekly Children, IV 2 mg/m² weekly	Hodgkin's and other lymphomas, acute leukemia, neuroblastoma, Wilms' tumor	Peripheral neuropathy; extravasation may lead to tissue necrosis.
Vinblastine (Velban)/D	Adults, IV 3.7–11.1 mg/m² (average 5.5–7.4 mg/m²) weekly Children, IV 2.5–7.5 mg/m² weekly	Metastatic testicular carcinoma, Hodgkin's disease, choriocarcinoma	Bone marrow depression, nausea, vomiting; extravasation may lead to tissue necrosis.
Vinorelbine (Navelbine)/D	IV injection 30 mg/m² once weekly	Non–small cell lung cancer	Bone marrow depression, peripheral neuropathy; extravasation may lead to tissue necrosis.
Miscellaneous Drugs			
L-Asparaginase (Elspar)/C	IV 1000 IU/kg/d for 10 d	Acute lymphocytic leukemia	Hypersensitivity reactions, including anaphylaxis

(Continued on page 208)

TABLE 12.2

DRUGS AT A GLANCE: Cytotoxic Antineoplastic Drugs (Continued)

Drug/Pregnancy Category	Routes and Dosage Ranges*	Clinical Uses	Adverse Effects
Hydroxyurea (Hydrea)/D	PO 80 mg/kg as a single dose every third day or 20–30 mg/kg as a single dose daily	Chronic myelocytic leukemia, melanoma, ovarian cancer, head and neck cancer	Bone marrow depression, nausea, vomiting, peripheral neuritis
Ixabepilone (Ixempra)/D	IV infusion 40 mg/m² over 3 h, every 3 wk	Advanced breast cancer	Bone marrow suppression, peripheral neuropathy, nausea, vomiting, diarrhea, mucositis, hypersensitivity
Levamisole (Ergamisol)/D	PO 50 mg every 8 h for 3 d every 2 wk	Colon cancer, with fluorouracil	Nausea, vomiting, diarrhea
Procarbazine (Matulane)/D	PO 2–4 mg/kg/d for 1 wk, then 4–6 mg/kg/d	Hodgkin's disease	Bone marrow depression, mucositis, CNS depression, hypertension

*Dosages may vary significantly or change often, according to use in different types of cancer and in different combinations.
AIDS, acquired immunodeficiency syndrome; CNS, central nervous system.

Use in Children

Children are at risk for certain types of malignancies, including acute leukemias, lymphomas, brain tumors, Wilms' tumor, and sarcomas of muscle and bone. In recent years, there have been rapid advances in cancer care for children and high cure rates for many pediatric malignancies. Many of the advances have resulted from the systematic enrollment of children in well-designed clinical trials.

Pediatric oncologists should design, order, and supervise chemotherapy for children. To determine dosage of cytotoxic drugs, prescribers should use body surface area, because this takes overall size into account. Special efforts are necessary to maintain nutrition, organ function, psychological support, growth and development, and other aspects of health status during and after therapy. Long-term follow-up care is important for childhood cancer survivors because they have an increased risk of health problems. For example, children who receive an anthracycline drug (e.g., doxorubicin) are at increased risk for cardiotoxic effects (e.g., heart failure) during treatment or after receiving the drug. Efforts to reduce cardiotoxicity include using alternative drugs (if effective), giving smaller cumulative doses of the anthracycline, and observing patients closely so that early manifestations can be recognized and treated before heart problems occur. In addition, after successful cytotoxic chemotherapy, children are at increased risk for developing cancers in later life (e.g., leukemia). Children treated for Hodgkin's disease seem to have the highest risk of developing a new cancer.

Use in Older Adults

Increasing age is a risk factor for development of cancer, and the number of new cancer cases is about 10 times greater in people 65 years of age and older. Although elderly people are more likely to have chronic cardiovascular, renal, and other disorders (comorbidities) that increase their risks of serious adverse effects, age alone should not be the reason for denying them the potential benefits of traditional cytotoxic chemotherapy. However, it is important to consider several factors when treating older adults for cancer. Physiologic age-related changes that may add to the challenge of managing cancer include decreased renal function, reduced hepatic blood flow, and diminished cardiac reserve. Psychosocial issues that may affect treatment include access to care, financial and transportation issues, functional status, need for independence, and social support.

For example, older adults are more sensitive to the neurotoxic effects of vincristine and need reduced dosages of some drugs (e.g., cyclophosphamide, MTX) if they have impaired renal function. It is necessary to monitor creatinine clearance (CrCl), because serum creatinine is not a reliable indicator of renal function in older adults due to decreased muscle mass. Most antineoplastic drugs are metabolized by the liver; thus, decreased liver blood flow and decreased liver size can lead to accumulation of drug due to decreased clearance, resulting in increased toxicity in the elderly adult.

Use in Patients With Renal Impairment

Some antineoplastic drugs are nephrotoxic (e.g., cisplatin, MTX), and the kidneys play a large role in their excretion. The presence of impaired renal function increases the risk of further impairment or accumulation of toxic drug levels. Thus, it is necessary to monitor renal function carefully during therapy and reduce drug dosages according to CrCl levels. The following paragraphs describe the renal effects of selected cytotoxic chemotherapy drugs and precautions to reduce nephrotoxicity.

The alkylating drugs may be nephrotoxic. These effects usually subside when the drug is stopped. For example, cisplatin, an alkylating agent, has multiple active metabolites that are renally excreted, causing renal tubular damage. When a patient already has significant renal dysfunction, oncologists avoid using this drug.

The antimetabolites may also be nephrotoxic. MTX use in patients with impaired renal function may lead to accumulation of toxic amounts or additional renal damage. Evaluation of the patient's renal status should take place before and during MTX therapy. If significant renal impairment occurs, it is necessary to discontinue the drug or to reduce the dosage until renal function improves. In patients who receive high doses of MTX for treatment of osteosarcoma, the drug may cause renal damage resulting in acute renal failure. Nephrotoxicity is attributed to precipitation of MTX and a metabolite in renal tubules. Reducing renal impairment involves monitoring renal function closely, ensuring adequate hydration, alkalinizing the urine, and measuring serum drug levels. With mercaptopurine, dosage reduction is necessary to prevent nephrotoxicity. With irinotecan, dosage reduction is necessary in patients with moderate renal impairment (CrCl, 20–39 mL/min).

Caution is warranted with many other drugs when used in patients with renal impairment. Cytarabine is detoxified mainly by the liver. However, patients with renal impairment may have more central nervous system–related adverse effects, and dosage reduction may be necessary. Gemcitabine has resulted in mild proteinuria and hematuria during clinical trials, and hemolytic–uremic syndrome has been reported in a few patients. Signs of this syndrome may include anemia, elevated bilirubin and reticulocyte counts, and renal failure. If this condition occurs, it is essential to stop gemcitabine immediately; hemodialysis may be required. Bleomycin is rarely associated with nephrotoxicity, but its elimination half-life is prolonged in patients with a CrCl of less than 35 mL perminute. L-Asparaginase often increases blood urea nitrogen; acute renal failure and fatal renal insufficiency have been reported. Procarbazine may cause more severe adverse effects if given to patients with impaired renal function. Hospitalization is recommended for the first course of treatment.

Use in Patients With Hepatic Impairment

Some antineoplastic drugs are hepatotoxic, and the liver is the site of the metabolism of many. Patients with metastatic cancer often have impaired liver function, and their risk of further impairment or accumulation of toxic drug levels increase. It is necessary to monitor hepatic function with most drugs. However, abnormal values for the usual liver function tests (e.g., serum aspartate aminotransferase [AST] and alanine aminotransferase [ALT], bilirubin, alkaline phosphatase) may indicate liver injury but do not indicate decreased ability to metabolize drugs. Dosage reduction may be necessary in some cases. The following paragraphs describe the hepatic effects of selected cytotoxic chemotherapy drugs and precautions to reduce hepatotoxicity.

Alkylating drugs may lead to hepatotoxicity.

Antimetabolites also have hepatotoxic effects. MTX may cause acute hepatotoxicity (increased serum ALT and AST, hepatitis) as well as chronic hepatotoxicity (fibrosis and cirrhosis). Chronic toxicity is potentially fatal. It is more likely to occur after prolonged use (e.g., 2 years or longer) and after a total dose of at least 1.5 g. It is essential that liver function tests be closely monitored in patients with preexisting liver damage or impaired hepatic function. Gemcitabine has increased serum ALT and AST in most patients during clinical trials. Mercaptopurine causes hepatotoxicity, especially with higher doses (above 2.5 mg/kg/d) and in combination with doxorubicin. Encephalopathy and fatal liver necrosis have occurred. It is essential to stop the drug if signs of hepatotoxicity (e.g., jaundice, hepatomegaly) occur. Serum aminotransferases, alkaline phosphatase, and bilirubin should be monitored weekly initially, then monthly.

Antitumor antibiotics may be hepatotoxic as well. Daunorubicin (liposomal formulation) requires dosage reduction according to serum bilirubin (e.g., bilirubin 1.2–3 mg/dL, three fourths the normal dose; bilirubin above 3 mg/dL, one half the normal dose). Doxorubicin toxicity increases with impaired hepatic function. It is necessary to perform liver function tests before drug administration and to reduce the dosage of both regular and liposomal formulations according to the serum bilirubin. Idarubicin is not appropriate for patients with a serum bilirubin above 5 mg/dL.

Some plant alkaloids have hepatic effects. Irinotecan may cause abnormal liver function tests in patients with liver metastases. Paclitaxel may cause more toxicity in patients with impaired hepatic function. Hospitalization is recommended for the first course of therapy. Topotecan is cleared from plasma more slowly in patients with hepatic impairment. Vinblastine and vincristine may cause more toxicity with hepatic impairment, and dosage should be reduced 50% for patients with a direct serum bilirubin value above 3 mg/dL.

L-Asparaginase is hepatotoxic in most patients; it may increase preexisting hepatic impairment and hepatotoxicity of other medications. Signs of liver impairment, which usually subside when the drug is discontinued, include increased AST, ALT, alkaline phosphatase, and bilirubin and decreased serum albumin, cholesterol, and plasma fibrinogen. Procarbazine may cause increased hepatotoxicity in cases of impaired hepatic function.

Use in Patients With Critical Illness

Cytotoxic drug treatment is often significantly dose reduced or discontinued in the setting of critical illness when there is compromised perfusion to the liver and kidneys, which can increase toxicity. However, palliative chemotherapy, which can alleviate pain or obstruction in critically ill patients with advanced cancer, is used on a case-by-case basis with consideration of therapeutic benefits versus the risks of treatment toxicities.

Use in Home Care

Although administration of cytotoxic drug therapy occurs most frequently in a clinic or hospital setting, people often self-administer oral cytotoxic drugs, and some give themselves IV infusions at home. All cytotoxic drugs are hazardous substances and require special handling and disposal, according to safety guidelines, in the home. The home care nurse may be involved in a wide range of activities associated with antineoplastic drug therapy, including administering the anticancer drugs,

American Society of Clinical Oncology Provisional Clinical Opinion: The integration of Palliative Care into Standard Oncology Care

by SMITH, T. J., TEMIN, S., ALESI, E. R., ABERNETHY, A. P., BALBONI, T. A., BASCH, E. M., FERRELL, B. R., LOSCALZO, M., MEIER, D. E., PAICE, J. A., PEPPERCORN, J. M., SOMERFIELD, M., STOVALL, E & VON ROENN, J. H.

The Journal of Clinical Oncology
2012, 880–887.

Palliative care is a specialized area of health care that focuses on the pain, symptoms, and stress of serious illness. It is frequently misinterpreted as synonymous with end-of-life care. Data from randomized controlled trials have demonstrated that integration of palliative care into the standard oncology care earlier in the disease course has demonstrated an improvement in symptoms, patient satisfaction, and quality of life with reduced caregiver burden. Earlier involvement of palliative care also leads to more appropriate referral to and use of hospice as well as decreased use of futile intensive care.

IMPLICATIONS FOR NURSING PRACTICE: Nurses can play a key role in facilitating referrals to palliative care in health care setting beyond the hospice setting. The American Society of Clinical Oncology has provided a provisional clinical opinion regarding the benefit of integration of palliative care services into standard oncology practice at the time a person receives a diagnosis of metastatic or advanced cancer. Future priorities include developing aligned health policy and reimbursement mechanisms to facilitate early implementation of best-practice palliative care models of care delivery.

administering other drugs to prevent or manage adverse effects, and assessing patient and family responses to therapy.

In addition, a major nursing role involves teaching about the disease process, management of pain and other symptoms, information about the specific anticancer drugs being given, prevention or management of adverse drug effects, preventing infection, maintaining adequate food and fluid intake, and self-care measures. Referral to palliative care early in the disease trajectory has demonstrated improved quality of life, cost of care, and even survival in patients with metastatic cancer.

Adverse Effects

Common adverse effects of the cytotoxic chemotherapy agents include **alopecia** (hair loss), anemia, bleeding, fatigue, **mucositis** (inflammation and erosion of oral mucous membranes), nausea and vomiting, **neutropenia** (low neutrophil count), **myelosuppression** (bone marrow depression), and **thrombocytopenia** (low platelet count). The dose-limiting toxicity for most of the cytotoxic drugs is myelosuppression.

QSEN Safety Alert

When cytotoxic drugs are combined, it is essential to monitor the complete blood (cell) count (CBC) before and after each treatment to allow time for bone marrow recovery before the next treatment.

Other problems may include damage to the heart, liver, lungs, kidneys, or nerves. In general, adverse effects depend on the specific drugs used and the patient's health status. Baseline liver and kidney function testing is necessary before all cytotoxic drug treatment, and the presence of preexisting disease may contraindicate use of a drug that is associated with serious liver or renal toxicity. Box 12.2 describes the adverse effects of treatment with antineoplastic drugs.

With treatment of leukemias and lymphomas, a serious, life-threatening adverse effect called **tumor lysis syndrome** may occur. This condition develops when large numbers of cancer cells are killed or damaged simultaneously and release their intracellular contents into the bloodstream. As a result, hyperkalemia, hyperphosphatemia, hyperuricemia, hypomagnesemia, hypocalcemia, and acidosis develop. Signs and symptoms depend on the severity of the metabolic imbalances but may include gastrointestinal (GI) upset, fatigue, altered mental status, hypertension, muscle cramps, paresthesias (numbness and tingling), tetany, seizures, electrocardiographic changes (e.g., dysrhythmias), cardiac arrest, reduced urine output, and acute renal failure. To prevent or minimize tumor lysis syndrome, aggressive hydration with IV normal saline, alkalinization with IV sodium bicarbonate, and administration of allopurinol (e.g., 300 mg daily for adults and 10 mg/kg/d for children) to reduce uric acid levels is necessary. Treatment of hyperkalemia may include IV dextrose and regular insulin (to drive potassium into cells) or Kayexalate to eliminate potassium in feces. Treatment of hyperphosphatemia may include administration of aluminum hydroxide or another phosphate-binding agent. Maintenance of urine pH of 7 or higher prevents renal failure due to precipitation of uric acid crystals in the kidneys. Hemodialysis may be necessary if the other measures are ineffective in maintaining urinary elimination.

Contraindications

There are several contraindications to the use of cytotoxic antineoplastic drugs.

- Generally, pregnancy and lactation preclude their use.

QSEN Safety Alert

Cytotoxic drugs are potentially embryotoxic, teratogenic, and carcinogenic.

BOX 12.2   Complications of Chemotherapy and Their Management

Complications of anticancer drug therapy range from minor to life-threatening. Vigilant efforts toward prevention or early detection and treatment are needed.

■ **Nausea** and **vomiting** commonly occur and are treated with antiemetics (see Chap. 36). With traditional cytotoxic chemotherapy, the drugs are most effective when started before drug administration and continued on a regular schedule for 24 to 48 hours afterward. An effective regimen is a serotonin receptor antagonist (e.g., ondansetron) and a corticosteroid (e.g., dexamethasone), given orally or intravenously. Other measures include a benzodiazepine (e.g., lorazepam) for anticipatory nausea and vomiting and limiting oral intake for a few hours. Guidelines have not been developed for managing nausea and vomiting with the biologic antineoplastic drugs.

■ **Anorexia** interferes with nutrition. Well-balanced meals, with foods the patient is able and willing to eat, and nutritional supplements, to increase intake of protein and calories, are helpful.

■ **Fatigue** is often caused or aggravated by anemia and can be treated with administration of erythropoietin. Alternating periods of activity and rest and an adequate diet may also be helpful.

■ **Alopecia** (hair loss) occurs with cyclophosphamide, doxorubicin, methotrexate, and vincristine. Counsel patients taking these drugs that hair loss is temporary and that hair may grow back a different color and texture; suggest the purchase of wigs, hats, and scarves before hair loss is expected to occur; and instruct women to use a mild shampoo and avoid rollers, permanent waves, hair coloring, and other treatments that damage the hair.

■ **Mucositis** (also called stomatitis) often occurs with the antimetabolites, antibiotics, plant alkaloids, and growth factor/tyrosine kinase inhibitors. It usually lasts 7 to 10 days and may interfere with nutrition; lead to oral ulcerations, infections, and bleeding; and cause pain. Nurse or patient interventions to minimize or treat this mucositis include the following:

  ■ Brush the teeth after meals and at bedtime with a soft toothbrush and floss once daily. Stop brushing and flossing if the platelet count drops below 20,000/mm³ because gingival bleeding is likely. Teeth may then be cleaned with soft, sponge-tipped or cotton-tipped applicators.

  ■ Rinse the mouth several times daily, especially before meals (to decrease unpleasant taste and increase appetite) and after meals (to remove food particles that promote growth of microorganisms). One suggested solution is 1 tsp of table salt and 1 tsp of baking soda in 1 quart of water. Commercial mouthwashes are not recommended, because their alcohol content causes drying of oral mucous membranes.

  ■ Encourage the patient to drink fluids. Systemic dehydration and local dryness of the oral mucosa contribute to the development and progression of mucositis. Pain and soreness contribute to dehydration. Fluids usually tolerated include tea, carbonated beverages, ices (e.g., popsicles), and plain gelatin desserts. Fruit juices may be diluted

with water, ginger ale, Sprite, or 7-Up to decrease pain, burning, and further tissue irritation. Drinking fluids through a straw may be more comfortable, because this decreases contact of fluids with painful ulcerations.

  ■ Encourage the patient to eat soft, bland, cold, nonacidic foods. Although individual tolerances vary, it is usually better to avoid highly spiced or rough foods.

  ■ Remove dentures entirely or for at least 8 hours daily because they may irritate oral mucosa.

  ■ Inspect the mouth daily for signs of inflammation and lesions.

  ■ Give medications for pain. Local anesthetic solutions, such as viscous lidocaine, can be taken a few minutes before meals. Because the mouth and throat are anesthetized, swallowing and detecting the temperature of hot foods may be difficult, and aspiration or burns may occur. Doses should not exceed 15 mL every 3 hours or 120 mL in 24 hours. If systemic analgesics are used, they should be taken 30 to 60 minutes before eating.

  ■ For oral infections resulting from mucositis, local or systemic antimicrobial drugs are used. Fungal infections with *Candida albicans* can be treated with antifungal tablets, suspensions, or lozenges. Severe infections may require systemic antibiotics, depending on the causative organism as identified by cultures of mouth lesions.

■ **Infection** is common because the disease and its treatment lower host resistance to infection.

  ■ If fever occurs, especially in a neutropenic patient, possible sources of infection are usually cultured, and antibiotics are started immediately.

  ■ Severe neutropenia can be prevented or its extent and duration minimized by administering filgrastim or sargramostim to stimulate the bone marrow to produce leukocytes. A protective environment may be needed to decrease exposure to pathogens.

  ■ Instruct the patient to avoid exposure to infection by avoiding crowds, anyone with a known infection, and contact with fresh flowers, soil, animals, or animal excrement. Frequent and thorough hand hygiene by the patient and everyone involved in his or her care is necessary to reduce exposure to pathogenic microorganisms.

  ■ The patient should take a bath daily and put on clean clothes. In addition, the perineal area should be washed with soap and water after each urination or defecation.

  ■ When venous access devices are used, take care to prevent them from becoming sources of infection. For implanted catheters, inspect and cleanse around exit sites according to agency policies and procedures. Use strict sterile technique when changing dressings or flushing the catheters. For peripheral intravenous lines, the same principles of care apply, except that sites should be changed every 3 days or if signs of phlebitis occur.

(Continued on page 212)

BOX 12.2	**Complications of Chemotherapy and Their Management** (Continued)

■ Avoid indwelling urinary catheters when possible. When they are necessary, cleanse the perineal area with soap and water at least once daily and provide sufficient fluids to ensure an adequate urine output.

■ Help the patient maintain a well-balanced diet. Oral hygiene and analgesics before meals may increase food intake. High-protein, high-calorie foods and fluids can be given between meals. Nutritional supplements can be taken with or between meals. Provide fluids with high nutritional value (e.g., milkshakes or nutritional supplements) if the patient can tolerate them and has an adequate intake of water and other fluids.

■ **Bleeding** may be caused by thrombocytopenia and may occur spontaneously or with minor trauma. Precautions should be instituted if the platelet count drops to 50,000/mm³ or below. Measures to avoid bleeding include giving oprelvekin to stimulate platelet production and prevent thrombocytopenia; avoiding trauma, including venipuncture and injections, when possible; using an electric razor for shaving; checking skin, urine, and stool for blood; and for platelet counts less than 20,000/mm³, stop brushing and flossing the teeth.

■ **Extravasation**. Several drugs (called vesicants) cause severe inflammation, pain, ulceration, and tissue necrosis if they leak into soft tissues around veins. Thus, efforts are needed to prevent extravasation or to minimize tissue damage if it occurs.

  ■ Identify patients at risk for extravasation, including those who are unable to communicate (e.g., sedated patients, infants), have vascular impairment (e.g., from multiple attempts at venipuncture), or have obstructed venous drainage after axillary node surgery.

  ■ Be especially cautious with the anthracyclines (e.g., doxorubicin) and the vinca alkaloids (e.g., vincristine). Choose peripheral IV sites carefully, avoiding veins that are small or located in an edematous extremity or near a joint. Inject the drugs slowly (1–2 mL at a time) into the tubing of a rapidly flowing IV infusion, for rapid dilution and detection of

extravasation. Observe the venipuncture site for swelling and ask the patient about pain or burning. After a drug has been injected, continue the rapid flow rate of the IV fluid for 2 to 5 minutes to flush the vein.

  ■ If using a central IV line, do not give the drug unless patency is indicated by a blood return. Using a central line does not eliminate the risk of extravasation.

  ■ When extravasation occurs, the drug should be stopped immediately. Techniques to decrease tissue damage include aspirating the drug (about 5 mL of blood, if able) through the IV catheter before it is removed, elevating the involved extremity, and applying warm (with dacarbazine, etoposide, vinblastine, and vincristine) or cold (with daunorubicin and doxorubicin) compresses. Nurses involved in cytotoxic chemotherapy must know the procedure to be followed if extravasation occurs so that it can be instituted immediately.

■ **Hyperuricemia** from rapid breakdown of malignant cells can lead to kidney damage. Risks of nephropathy can be decreased by high fluid intake, high urine output, alkalinizing the urine with sodium bicarbonate, and giving allopurinol to inhibit uric acid formation.

■ **Hand–foot syndrome** (also called palmar–plantar erythrodysesthesia or erythema) is a sunburn type of skin reaction with redness, tenderness, and possibly peeling, numbness, and tingling of palms and soles. It is associated with some traditional cytotoxic drugs (e.g., capecitabine, doxorubicin, fluorouracil) and some growth factor/tyrosine kinase inhibitors (e.g., lapatinib, sorafenib, sunitinib). It is attributed to leakage of drug from capillaries into the palms and soles; heat and friction increase leakage. Management efforts involve decreasing heat and friction (e.g., minimizing exposure of hands and feet to hot water), avoiding increased pressure (e.g., from long walks, squeezing small implements in cooking, gardening), or applying ice packs for 15 or 20 minutes at a time. Acetaminophen may be taken for discomfort.

- Myelosuppression may be a factor.

QSEN Safety Alert ❗

Use of the cytotoxic agents that cause bone marrow suppression is not appropriate in people with a white blood count less than 2000 cells/mm³, a neutrophil count less than 1500 cells/mm³, and/or platelet count less than 50,000/mm³.

Hematological monitoring prior to and after each treatment is necessary to limit the risk of infection and serious bleeding.

- As previously stated, specific cytotoxic drugs may lead to certain adverse effects, and these drugs may be contraindicated in individual patients. Severe hepatic or renal impairment is also a contraindication to the use of

specific cytotoxic agents that cause significant toxicities to the liver and kidney, respectively.

Nursing Implications

The nurse should be aware that each antineoplastic drug is used in the schedule, route, and dosage judged to be most effective for a particular type of cancer. With combinations of drugs, it is necessary to adhere to the recommended schedule precisely because safety and effectiveness may be schedule dependent.

Preventing Interactions

Interactions involving changes in hepatic metabolism are the most common reason for cytotoxic drug interactions. Cytochrome P450 (CYP) 3A4 enzymes in the liver metabolize a number of cytotoxic drugs, including taxanes, vinca alkaloids, and irinotecan. Drugs that inhibit these enzymes such as the azole antifungals, erythromycins, and protease inhibitors may increase blood levels and toxicities of a cytotoxic drug. CYP3A4 enzyme inducers, on the other hand (e.g., carbamazepine, griseofulvin, phenytoin, St. John's wort) can decrease blood levels and cytotoxic drug effects. In addition, use of noncancer drugs that have the same toxicities can cause drug interactions. Antimicrobials with renal toxicity, such as amphotericin B and aminoglycosides, can increase the nephrotoxicity of cisplatin and carboplatin. The chemotherapy nurse and a pharmacist should evaluate the potential for drug interactions.

Administering the Medication

A certified chemotherapy nurse administers IV cytotoxic drugs. He or she verifies free flow of IV fluid into the vein and assesses adequate blood return. Peripheral infusion of cytotoxic drugs occurs through a newly initiated IV catheter in a large, upper-extremity vein. Whenever possible, it is necessary to avoid the veins of the antecubital fossa, wrist, dorsum of the hand, and the arm where an axillary lymph node dissection has been performed. Insertion of an indwelling central venous catheter is often appropriate for patients who have poor peripheral venous access, who require many doses of chemotherapy, or who require continuous infusions. When multiple drugs are given, administration of the drug most likely to cause venous irritation occurs first. Some of the cytotoxic drugs given by IV infusion are potential tissue irritants or vesicants and cause tissue necrosis if they leak outside the vein into surrounding tissue (extravasation).

Established infusion guidelines aid nurses who administer these drugs and increase the safety of both patients and nurses. These guidelines include the following:

- Ensure appropriate orders (e.g., be sure the prescriber is qualified to write chemotherapy orders; do not accept verbal or telephone orders).
- Do not give injectable drugs unless certified to administer chemotherapy.

QSEN Safety Alert

Check all IV drug preparations for appropriate dilution, dosage that corresponds to the prescriber's order, absence of precipitates, expiration dates, and so forth.

QSEN Safety Alert

Avoid direct contact with solutions for injection by wearing gloves, face shields, and protective clothing (e.g., disposable, liquid-impermeable gowns).

- If handling a powdered form of a drug, avoid inhaling the powder.
- Do not prepare the drugs in eating areas (to decrease risk of oral ingestion).

QSEN Safety Alert

Dispose of contaminated materials (e.g., needles, syringes, ampules, vials, IV tubing and bags) in puncture-proof containers labeled "Warning: Hazardous Material."

QSEN Safety Alert

Wear gloves when handling patients' clothing, bed linens, or excreta. Blood and body fluids are contaminated with drugs or metabolites for about 3 to 5 days after a dose.

- Ensure adequate hydration before and after administration, frequent voiding, and use of a protective medication (e.g., mesna) to help prevent hemorrhagic cystitis.

QSEN Safety Alert

Wash hands thoroughly after exposure or potential exposure and after removing gloves.

Assessing for Therapeutic Effects

The nurse helps evaluate treatment effects by assessing for

- Absence of or reduction in tumor size on physical examination, radiograph, computed tomography scan, magnetic resonance imaging scan, or bone scan
- Laboratory testing, which demonstrates decrease in malignant cells, normalization of serum chemistry levels, and decrease in abnormal tumor serum (tumor marker) protein levels
- Improved functional status, appetite, weight gain, and energy
- Decrease in cancer-related symptoms (e.g., pain, fatigue, dyspnea, cough, anorexia, nausea, vomiting)

Assessing for Adverse Effects

The nurse assesses for the many adverse effects the cytotoxic drugs have on body tissues. Box 12.2 summarizes common adverse effects of these drugs and their management.

Patient Teaching

Box 12.3 presents patient teaching guidelines for anticancer drugs.

NCLEX Success

1. A priority nursing diagnosis to include in the care plan for a patient receiving cytotoxic chemotherapy is
   A. Risk for Impaired Skin Integrity
   B. Risk for Injury: Infection
   C. Body Image Disturbance related to alopecia
   D. Ineffective Family Coping

2. For a patient receiving a cytotoxic drug that will likely result in bone marrow depression, which of the following teaching considerations should be the priority for the nurse with the patient and family members or caregivers?
   A. Wash hands often and avoid people with colds, flu, or other infections.
   B. Do not expect fatigue and weakness, which are uncommon.
   C. Expect gastrointestinal upset. More nausea and vomiting may occur when the blood cell counts are low.
   D. Take acetaminophen for fever.

BOX 12.3 — Patient Teaching Guidelines for Drugs Used for the Treatment of Cancer

■ There are many different chemotherapy drugs, and the ones used for a particular patient depend on the type of malignancy, its location, and other factors. Some are taken orally at home; many are given intravenously, in outpatient clinics, by nurses who are specially trained to administer the medications and monitor your condition. The medications are usually given in cycles such as every few weeks.

■ The goal of chemotherapy is to be as effective as possible with tolerable side effects. Particular side effects vary with the medications used; some increase risks of infection, and some cause anemia, nausea, or hair loss. All of these can be managed effectively, and several medications can help prevent or minimize side effects. In addition, some helpful activities are listed below.

■ Keep all appointments for chemotherapy, blood tests, and check-ups. This is extremely important. Chemotherapy effectiveness depends on its being given on time; blood tests help to determine when the drugs should be given and how the drugs affect your body tissues.

■ Do everything you can to avoid infection, such as avoiding other people who have infections and washing your hands frequently and thoroughly. If you have a fever, chills, sore throat, or cough, notify your oncologist.

■ Try to maintain or improve your intake of nutritious food and fluids; this will help you feel better and maintain your weight at a more optimal level to promote healing. A dietitian can be helpful in designing a diet to meet your needs and preferences.

■ If your chemotherapy may cause bleeding, decrease the likelihood by shaving with an electric razor; avoiding aspirin and other nonsteroidal antiinflammatory drugs (including over-the-counter Advil, Aleve, and others); and avoiding injections, cuts, and other injuries when possible. If you notice excessive bruising, bleeding gums when you brush your teeth, or blood in your urine or bowel movement, notify your oncologist immediately.

■ If hair loss is expected with the medications you take, use wigs, scarves, and hats. Purchase them before starting chemotherapy, if possible. Hair loss is temporary; your hair will grow back!

■ Inform any other physician, dentist, or health care provider that you are taking chemotherapy before any diagnostic test or treatment begins. Some procedures may be contraindicated or require special precautions.

■ If you are of childbearing age, use effective contraceptive measures during and a few months after chemotherapy.

■ For medications taken at home, instructions for taking the drugs should be followed exactly for the most beneficial effects.

■ Although specific instructions vary depending on the drugs you are taking, the following are a few precautions with some commonly used drugs:

■ With cyclophosphamide, take the tablets on an empty stomach. If severe stomach upset occurs, take with food. Also, drink 2 or 3 quarts of fluid daily, if possible, and urinate often, especially at bedtime. If blood is seen in the urine or signs of cystitis occur (e.g., burning with urination), report to a health care provider. The drug is irritating to the bladder lining and may cause cystitis. High fluid intake and frequent emptying of the bladder help to decrease bladder damage.

■ With doxorubicin, the urine may turn red for 1 to 2 days after drug administration. This discoloration is harmless; it does not indicate bleeding. Also, report to a health care provider if you have edema, shortness of breath, and excessive fatigue. Doxorubicin may need to be stopped if these symptoms occur.

■ With fluorouracil, drink plenty of liquids while taking.

■ With methotrexate, avoid alcohol, aspirin, and prolonged exposure to sunlight.

■ With oxaliplatin, avoid exposure to cold during, and for 3 to 5 days after, drug administration. This helps prevent or minimize nerve damage that may cause numbness, tingling, and pain in the throat or hands. Swallowing and daily activities that require hand grasping may be impaired.

■ With vincristine, eat high-fiber foods, such as whole cereal grains, if you are able, to prevent constipation. Also try to maintain a high fluid intake. A stool softener or bulk laxative may be prescribed for daily use.

---

3. In explaining antineoplastic therapy to a family member of a patient who is to receive treatment with a cytotoxic drug, the nurse explains that it

   A. damages both malignant and nonmalignant cells
   B. causes few adverse effects
   C. stimulates growth of cancer cells
   D. must be given daily

4. A female patient with chronic lymphocytic leukemia is beginning to receive an oral cyclophosphamide. The nurse instructs the patient that the best way to take the drug is

   A. with food
   B. on an empty stomach
   C. at bedtime
   D. one hour after a meal

Clinical Application 12-1

■ Mrs. Gardner returns to the clinic, complaining of nausea, vomiting, and fatigue. She is most concerned about the blood in her urine. What strategies to minimize the hemorrhagic cystitis should the nurse consider and share with Mrs. Gardner?

Adjuvant Medications Used to Treat Cancer

Biologic Antineoplastic Drugs

Two factors promoting carcinogenesis are (1) failure of the immune system to eliminate mutant and malignant cells and

(2) failure of growth-regulating processes to control the proliferation of premalignant and malignant cells. Biologic agents target cellular differences between the malignant and normal cells. By doing this, they stimulate the immune system to fight cancer cells and inhibit their growth and proliferation.

Treatment of cancer with biologic agents continues to expand, as more of these agents are designed to interact with proteins overexpressed on the surface of cancer cells. The ability to test individual tumor tissues for the presence of altered cell surface proteins and growth factors has become feasible. Thus, these drugs inhibit malignant cell growth and in some cases stimulate the immune system to destroy tumor cells. Biologic drugs are useful both alone and combined with cytotoxic drug treatment, reducing the adverse effects of traditional cytotoxic chemotherapy. Others, such as imatinib, which is used for chronic myeloid leukemia (it targets the tyrosine

kinase enzyme involved in leukemia cell growth), are effective as monotherapy treatment for malignancy.

Biologic antineoplastic drugs include immunotherapy drugs and drugs that "target" biologic processes of malignant cells. Some immunologic anticancer drugs are discussed in Chapter 9 (e.g., interferon alfa for acquired immunodeficiency syndrome [AIDS]–related Kaposi's sarcoma, selected leukemias, malignant melanoma, and non-Hodgkin's lymphoma and interleukin-2 for renal cell carcinoma). Newer biologic agents (targeted therapies) are commonly used to treat lung, colorectal, breast, and hematologic malignancies in older adults. Table 12.3 presents the route and dosage information of biologic agents used in cancer treatment plus the use and adverse effects information for the currently approved biologic antineoplastic drugs—the monoclonal antibodies, tyrosine kinase inhibitors, and proteasome inhibitors.

TABLE 12.3

DRUGS AT A GLANCE: Biologic Antineoplastic Drugs

Drug/Pregnancy Category	Routes and Dosage Ranges	Clinical Uses	Adverse Effects
Monoclonal Antibodies			
Alemtuzumab (Campath IH)/C	IV infusion, initially, 3 mg/d as a 2-h infusion; increase to 10 mg/d, then to 30 mg/d as tolerated Maintenance, 30 mg/d 3 times weekly on alternate days for up to 12 wk	Chronic lymphocytic leukemia in patients previously treated with alkylating agents and fludarabine	Allergic infusion reactions (dyspnea, fever, chills, skin rash), immunosuppression, hypotension, hypertension, peripheral edema, nausea, vomiting, diarrhea, mucositis
Bevacizumab (Avastin)/C	IV infusion, 5 mg/kg once every 14 d until disease progression is detected	Breast, colorectal, renal cell cancer; refractory glioblastoma	Heart failure, hemorrhage, hypertension, diarrhea, leukopenia, pain, dyspnea, dermatitis, stomatitis, vomiting
Cetuximab (Erbitux)/C	IV infusion, initially, 400 mg/m² over 2 h; maintenance, 250 mg/m² over 1 h once weekly	Metastatic colorectal cancer	Anemia, leukopenia, infusion reaction, nausea, diarrhea, stomatitis, vomiting, dyspnea, fever
Gemtuzumab ozogamicin (Mylotarg)/D	IV infusion, 9 mg/m², for 2 doses, 14 d apart	Acute myeloid leukemia	Chills, fever, nausea, vomiting, diarrhea
Ibritumomab tiuxetan (Zevalin)/D	See literature	Non-Hodgkin's lymphoma, with rituximab	Severe or fatal infusion reaction, severe bone marrow depression
Panitumumab (Vectibix)/C	IV infusion, 6 mg/kg over 60 min every 14 d; doses over 1000 mg should be given over 90 min.	Metastatic colorectal cancer	Infusion reactions, skin rash, pulmonary fibrosis, nausea, vomiting, diarrhea
Rituximab (Rituxan)/C	IV infusion, 375 mg/m² once weekly for 4 doses	Non-Hodgkin's lymphoma	Hypersensitivity reactions, cardiac dysrhythmias
Tositumomab and iodine 131-tositumomab (Bexxar)/X	See literature	Non-Hodgkin's lymphoma	Fever, chills, nausea, vomiting, skin rash, headache, cough, infection, pain

(Continued on page 216)

TABLE 12.3

DRUGS AT A GLANCE: Biologic Antineoplastic Drugs (Continued)

Drug/Pregnancy Category	Routes and Dosage Ranges	Clinical Uses	Adverse Effects
Trastuzumab (Herceptin)/D	IV infusion, 4 mg/kg initially, then 2 mg/kg once weekly	Metastatic breast cancer	Cardiotoxicity (dyspnea, edema, heart failure)
Growth Factor and Tyrosine Kinase Inhibitors			
Dasatinib (Sprycel)/D	PO 70 mg twice daily	Chronic myelogenous leukemia, acute lymphoblastic leukemia	Anemia, diarrhea, dyspnea, edema, fever, infection, nausea, pain, skin rash
Erlotinib (Tarceva)/D	PO 150 mg daily	Non–small cell lung cancer, brain glioma	Nausea, vomiting, diarrhea, skin rash
Imatinib (Gleevec)/D	Adults, PO 400–800 mg/d; children, 3 y and older, PO 260–340 mg/m²/d	Chronic myeloid leukemia, GIST	Dyspnea, edema, heart failure, hemorrhage, nausea, vomiting, diarrhea, neutropenia, thrombocytopenia
Lapatinib (Tykerb)/D	PO 1250 mg (5 tablets) once daily on d 1–21, with capecitabine PO 2000 mg/m²/d (in 2 doses, 12 h apart) on d 1–14 in a repeating 21-d cycle	Advanced breast cancer, chronic myeloid leukemia	Diarrhea, dyspnea, insomnia, nausea, vomiting, stomatitis
Pazopanib (Votrient)/D	PO 800 mg daily, 1 h before eating	Advanced renal cell cancer	Hepatotoxicity, hypertension, diarrhea, GI upset, fatigue
Sorafenib (Nexavar)/D	PO 400 mg twice daily	Advanced renal cell cancer, advanced liver cell cancer	Hypertension, skin rash, alopecia, anemia, nausea, vomiting, diarrhea
Sunitinib (Sutent)/D	PO 50 mg daily for 4 wk, followed by 2 wk off drug	Advanced renal cell cancer, GIST	Hypertension, skin rash, diarrhea, anemia, neutropenia, nausea and vomiting
Ⓟ **Temsirolimus** (Torisel)/D	IV infusion, 25 mg over 30–60 min once per week	Advanced renal cell cancer	Anorexia, diarrhea, edema, mucositis, nausea, skin rash
Proteasome Inhibitor			
Bortezomib (Velcade)/D	IV injection, 1.3 mg/m², twice weekly for 2 wk, followed by a 10-d rest period	Multiple myeloma	Edema, nausea, vomiting, diarrhea, anemia, neutropenia, thrombocytopenia, peripheral neuropathy

GIST, gastrointestinal stromal tumor.

Monoclonal Antibodies

Monoclonal antibodies, which may be used alone or in combination with traditional cytotoxic antineoplastic drugs and other treatment modalities, have become an integral part of treatment plans for a variety of cancers. Metabolic pathways for many of the monoclonal antibodies are incompletely identified, but experts believe that the drugs are processed mainly in the reticuloendothelial system.

The monoclonal antibodies act in various ways:

- Bevacizumab (Avastin), cetuximab (Erbitux), panitumumab (Vectibix), and trastuzumab (Herceptin) all bind to growth factor receptors found on blood vessels, colorectal cancer cells, and breast cancer cells, respectively, to prevent intracellular growth factors from becoming activated and stimulating cell growth.
- Alemtuzumab (Campath) and rituximab (Rituxan) bind to an antigen on both normal T and B lymphocytes and malignant lymphoid cells to activate antibody- and complement-mediated cytotoxicity. The malignant lymphoid cells are more susceptible to immune destruction while the normal lymphocytes can later repopulate in the bloodstream.
- Gemtuzumab ozogamicin (Mylotarg) consists of a cytotoxic antibiotic molecule attached to a monoclonal

antibody that targets leukemia cells and is used for treating refractory acute myelogenous leukemia.

- Ibritumomab tiuxetan (Zevalin) as well as tositumomab and iodine I-131 tositumomab (Bexxar) are monoclonal antibodies conjugated with radioisotopes that target receptors on B lymphocytes.

Fewer adverse effects are associated with monoclonal antibody therapy than those of cytotoxic drugs. However, although some adverse effects are rare, they are serious (e.g., heart failure, bleeding problems, electrolyte imbalances) and vary with a particular drug.

Significant drug interactions with the monoclonal antibodies are few. Enzymes in the liver do not metabolize the monoclonal antibodies; hence, they do not compete with other drugs for these enzymes. However, when combined with cytotoxic agents in the same treatment regimen, dosage reductions are often advisable.

Administration of monoclonal antibodies is by IV infusion because all preparations would be destroyed by GI enzymes if taken orally. The infusion occurs over a given period, generally 90 to 120 minutes initially, in a monitored health care setting. Premedication may be necessary, and frequent observation of the patient for signs of a hypersensitivity infusion reaction is important. In cases of acute hypersensitivity (urticaria, hypotension, dyspnea, wheezing), it is essential that the infusion be stopped and emergency measures implemented promptly (oxygen, epinephrine, bronchodilators, IV diphenhydramine, and dexamethasone). Mild infusion reactions require slowing or temporarily stopping the infusion and administering IV diphenhydramine 50 mg and acetaminophen 650 to 1000 mg orally.

Clinical Application 12-2

- Mrs. Gardner has begun to receive intravenous trastuzumab (Herceptin) as part of her chemotherapy treatment. During her infusion, the clinic nurse should ensure that certain items are available. What should these include?

Growth Factor and Tyrosine Kinase Inhibitors

Growth factors such as epidermal growth factor (EGF, which stimulates the growth of epithelial cells in the skin and other organs) and platelet-derived growth factor (PDGF, which stimulates the proliferation of vascular smooth muscle and endothelial cells) bind to transcellular membrane receptors and initiate intracellular events that result in cell growth. EGF, which is normally produced in the kidneys and salivary glands, is found in almost all body fluids. When EGF binds to the external portion of the EGF receptor, also called the tyrosine kinase receptor, it sends signals to intracellular kinase enzymes stimulating cell proliferation and angiogenesis. Intracellular tyrosine kinases play an important role in the proliferation and differentiation of cells; thus, blocking these receptors can decrease intracellular protein synthesis and lead to cell death (Fig. 12.3).

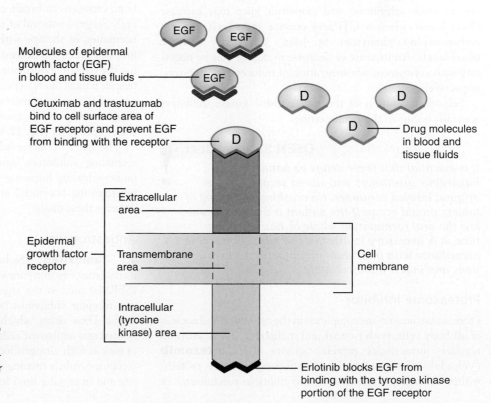

Figure 12.3 Actions of selected biologic targeted drugs. These drugs prevent epidermal growth factor (EGF) from combining with its receptors and thereby prevent or decrease cell growth. Cetuximab and trastuzumab bind with the extracellular portion of the EGF receptor. Erlotinib blocks the intracellular (tyrosine kinase) portion of the EGF receptor.

Molecules of epidermal growth factor (EGF) in blood and tissue fluids

Cetuximab and trastuzumab bind to cell surface area of EGF receptor and prevent EGF from binding with the receptor

Drug molecules in blood and tissue fluids

Extracellular area

Epidermal growth factor receptor

Transmembrane area

Cell membrane

Intracellular (tyrosine kinase) area

Erlotinib blocks EGF from binding with the tyrosine kinase portion of the EGF receptor

Erlotinib (Tarceva) is a growth inhibitor that blocks the tyrosine kinase portion of the EGF receptor, inhibiting cell proliferation and inducing cell death. Other similarly acting tyrosine kinase inhibitors include sorafenib (Nexavar) and sunitinib (Sutent). The tyrosine kinase inhibitor imatinib inhibits several tyrosine kinases that are essential to the growth of some cancer cells, including an abnormal type of tyrosine kinase thought to be the main cause of chronic myelogenous leukemia and the tyrosine kinases activated by PDGF and stem cell factor. This action inhibits cell proliferation and leads to cell death. Dasatinib (Sprycel) and lapatinib (Tykerb), newer tyrosine kinase inhibitors, are recommended for use in chronic myeloid leukemia after disease progression with imatinib or other treatment.

Tyrosine kinase inhibitors, including imatinib, dasatinib, and sorafenib, are available orally, and they are readily absorbed from the GI tract. For example, imatinib is well absorbed with oral administration, and peak serum levels are reached in 2 to 4 hours. It is highly protein bound, its elimination half-life is 18 hours, it is metabolized in the liver, and it is excreted mainly in feces. The other kinase inhibitors are metabolized in the liver as well, primarily by CYP3A4 liver enzymes, and they are largely eliminated in bile with very little renal excretion.

Common adverse effects of the tyrosine kinase inhibitors include leukopenia, thrombocytopenia, skin rashes, and diarrhea. Skin care, maintaining adequate hydration and nutrition, and monitoring for signs of dehydration and electrolyte imbalances are priorities with use of these antineoplastic drugs.

With the tyrosine kinase inhibitors, drugs also metabolized by the CYP3A4 liver enzyme system may affect tyrosine kinase inhibitors. Enzyme inhibitors (azole antifungals, erythromycin, protease inhibitors) and grapefruit juice may increase blood levels, whereas CYP3A4 enzyme inducers (rifampin, carbamazepine, phenytoin, St. John's wort) may decrease blood levels. An increase or decrease in dosage may be necessary with concurrent administration of inducers or inhibitors, respectively.

Self-administration of the oral tyrosine kinase inhibitors generally occurs in the home setting.

QSEN Safety Alert

It is essential that these drugs be handled as hazardous substances and stored securely in the original labeled container. No crushing or cutting of tablets should occur. If the patient is unable to swallow the oral formulation whole or has a feeding tube, it is necessary to dissolve the tablet in water in accordance with individual manufacturer's instructions and ingest it immediately.

Proteasome Inhibitor

Proteasomes are enzyme complexes in the cytoplasm and nucleus of all body cells, both normal and malignant. These enzymes regulate intracellular protein activity. ℗ **Bortezomib** (Velcade) inhibits proteasomes, affecting multiple proteins within cells. Experts believe it has multiple mechanisms of cytotoxicity (e.g., preventing formation of new blood vessels in tumors and accelerating death of malignant cells). The drug is moderately protein bound (83%) and is metabolized by several CYP450 enzyme systems in the liver. Administration leads to cell cycle arrest, delayed tumor growth, and cell death. With bortezomib, which can cause myelosuppression, it is necessary to determine the blood cell count at baseline and periodically during therapy.

Antineoplastic Hormone Inhibitor Drugs

The main hormonal agents used in the treatment of cancer are the corticosteroids (see Chap. 15) and drugs that block the production of activity of estrogens and androgens. Pharmacological doses of corticosteroids suppress lymphocyte production, causing lymphocyte apoptosis and regression of lymphoid tissue. Other uses for these drugs include treatment of the complications of cancer, including nausea and vomiting, intracerebral edema from brain metastases, and hypercalcemia. However, adverse effects may occur. Chronic use of oral glucocorticoids during the maintenance phase of leukemia treatment can contribute to the development of long-term adverse effects such as osteoporosis, myopathy, hypertension, glucose intolerance, cataracts, and decreased growth rate in children. Hence, intermittent long-term therapy with glucocorticoids is generally used to maximize cytotoxic effects on lymphoid tissue while minimizing adverse long-term consequences. Prednisone and dexamethasone are the preparations most commonly used for cancer treatment. Sex hormone–blocking drugs are used mainly to control tumor growth and relieve symptoms. They are not cytotoxic, and adverse effects are usually mild.

Sex hormones act as growth factors in some malignancies (e.g., estrogens in breast cancer, testosterone in prostate cancer). Surgical removal of the ovaries or testes, which produce hormones, or therapy with hormone receptor–blocking drugs may be effective in decreasing hormonal stimulation and slowing the growth of hormone-dependent cancers. Removal of the ovaries is most likely in premenopausal women with breast cancer and the testes in men with prostate cancer. Currently used drugs interfere with hormone production or hormone action at the cellular level (Fig. 12.4).

The main hormone inhibitor drugs are the antiestrogens, aromatase inhibitors, antiandrogens, and luteinizing hormone–releasing hormone (LHRH; also known as gonadotropin-releasing hormone) analogs. Chapter 44 and Table 12.4 describe these drugs.

Antiestrogens

℗ **Tamoxifen** (Nolvadex), raloxifene (Evista), and toremifene (Fareston) are selective estrogen receptor modulators (SERMs) used in the treatment of breast cancer. One estrogen receptor antagonist, fulvestrant (Faslodex), may also be useful. These drugs, which bind to estrogen receptors in both normal and malignant cells, are effective only in the treatment of tumors with estrogen receptors. SERMs block some estrogen receptors while activating others (increasing bone mineral density and improving lipid levels). Fulvestrant is a pure estrogen

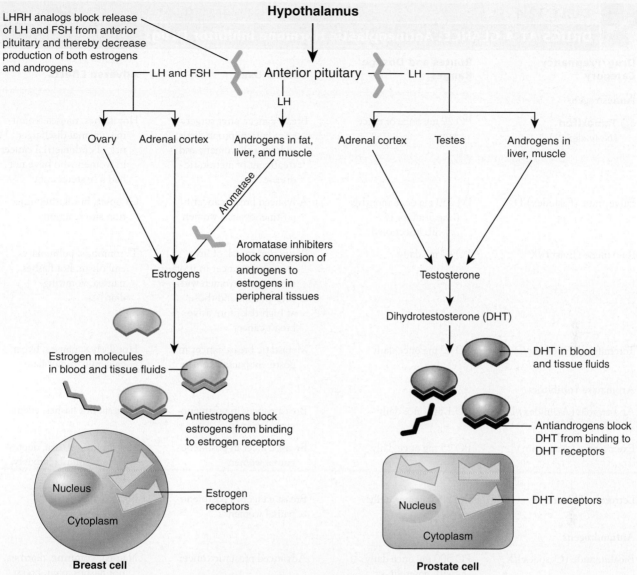

Figure 12.4 Actions of hormone inhibitor drugs. Drugs used to treat breast cancer block the production of estrogens (e.g., luteinizing hormone–releasing hormone [LHRH] analogs, aromatase inhibitors) or prevent estrogens from binding to receptors in breast cancer cells (antiestrogens). Drugs used to treat prostate cancer block the production of androgens (e.g., LHRH analogs) or prevent DHT, the active from of testosterone, from binding to receptors in prostate cancer cells (antiandrogens). FSH, follicle-stimulating hormone; LH, luteinizing hormone.

antagonist, blocking all estrogen receptors. In breast cancer, all of these drugs compete with estrogen for receptor binding sites and thereby decrease estrogen-mediated growth stimulation of malignant cells.

Tamoxifen is an antiestrogen that has been widely used to prevent recurrence of breast cancer after surgical excision in women ages 40 and older and to treat metastatic breast cancer in postmenopausal women with estrogen receptor–positive disease. It is usually necessary to take the drug for 2 to 5 years to prevent tumor recurrence. Some studies indicate greater effectiveness when an aromatase inhibitor (see below) is used instead of tamoxifen after 2 to 5 years of therapy. Although both antiestrogens and aromatase inhibitors

block the growth of breast tumors that respond to estrogen, their mechanisms of action are different. Tamoxifen inhibits the ability of breast cancer cells to use estrogen for growth by blocking receptors, whereas an aromatase inhibitor inhibits the production of estrogen in the ovaries, fat, muscle, and other tissues.

QSEN Safety Alert ❗

Sexually active premenopausal women who take tamoxifen should use effective nonhormonal barrier contraception during therapy and for 2 months after the drug is discontinued.

TABLE 12.4

DRUGS AT A GLANCE: Antineoplastic Hormone Inhibitor Drugs

Drug/Pregnancy Category	Routes and Dosage Ranges	Clinical Uses	Adverse Effects
Antiestrogens			
Ⓟ **Tamoxifen** (Nolvadex)/D	PO 20 mg once or twice daily	Breast cancer, after surgery or radiation; prophylaxis in high-risk women; and treatment of metastatic disease	Hot flashes, nausea, vomiting, vaginal discharge, risk of endometrial cancer in women who have not had a hysterectomy
Fulvestrant (Faslodex)/D	IM 250 mg once monthly (one 5-mL or two 2.5-mL injections)	Advanced breast cancer in postmenopausal women	GI upset, hot flashes, injection site reactions
Raloxifene (Evista)/X	PO 60 mg daily	Reduction in risk of invasive breast cancer in postmenopausal women with osteoporosis and those at high risk of invasive breast cancer	Thrombosis, pulmonary embolism, hot flashes, nausea, vomiting, diarrhea
Toremifene (Fareston)/D	PO 60 mg once daily	Metastatic breast cancer in postmenopausal women	Hot flashes, nausea, hypercalcemia, tumor flare
Aromatase Inhibitors			
Anastrozole (Arimidex)/D	PO 1 mg once daily	Breast cancer in postmenopausal women	Nausea, hot flashes, edema
Exemestane (Aromasin)/D	PO 25 mg once daily	Breast cancer in postmenopausal women	Hot flashes, nausea, depression, insomnia, anxiety, dyspnea, pain
Letrozole (Femara)/X	PO 2.5 mg once daily	Breast cancer in postmenopausal women	Nausea, hot flashes
Antiandrogens			
Bicalutamide (Casodex)/X	PO 500 mg once daily (with goserelin or leuprolide)	Advanced prostatic cancer	Nausea, vomiting, diarrhea, hot flashes, pain, breast enlargement
Flutamide (Eulexin)/X	PO 250 mg every 8 h	Advanced prostatic cancer	Nausea, vomiting, diarrhea, hot flashes, hepatotoxicity
Nilutamide (Nilandron)/C	PO 300 mg daily for 30 d, then 150 mg daily	Advanced breast cancer in postmenopausal women	Diarrhea, GI bleeding, heart failure, hyperglycemia
LHRH Analogs			
Goserelin (Zoladex)/X	Sub-Q implant, 3.6 mg every 28 d or 10.8 mg every 12 wk	Advanced prostatic or breast cancer, endometriosis	Hot flashes, transient increase in bone pain
Leuprolide (Eligard, Lupron, Viadur)/X	Sub-Q 7.5 mg/mo IM 7.5 mg/mo, 22.5 mg/3 mo, or 30 mg/4 mo	Advanced prostatic cancer	Same as for goserelin
Triptorelin (Trelstar LA, Trelstar Depot)/X	IM implant 65 mg/12 mo IM 3.75 mg/28 d or 11.25 mg/3 mo	Advanced prostatic cancer	Same as for goserelin and leuprolide

GI, gastrointestinal.

Aromatase Inhibitors

Anastrozole (Arimidex), exemestane (Aromasin), and letrozole (Femara) are aromatase inhibitors used to prevent or treat recurrence of estrogen-responsive breast cancer in postmenopausal women. Aromatase is an enzyme that catalyzes the production of estrogen in the ovaries of premenopausal women and in fat, liver, and muscle cells of postmenopausal or women who have had an oophorectomy. Thus, inhibiting aromatase reduces estrogen levels in the blood and target tissues, including the breast.

Studies with letrozole or exemestane indicate that changing to an aromatase inhibitor after 2 or 3 years of tamoxifen therapy is more effective in decreasing recurrent breast cancer. Tumors may become resistant to tamoxifen because of mutations in receptors that alter drug binding. Letrozole, following tamoxifen, is the current standard of care, and exemestane is also used (instead of tamoxifen) for metastatic breast cancer in postmenopausal women.

Antiandrogens

Bicalutamide (Casodex), flutamide (Eulexin), and nilutamide (Nilandron) are antiandrogens used to treat advanced prostate cancer, usually with an LHRH analog. The drugs bind to androgen receptors in cells of the prostate gland and thereby block the effects of the active form of testosterone, dihydrotestosterone, on malignant prostate cell growth. Antiandrogens are also able to block the effects of adrenal testosterone production, which accounts for about 10% of testosterone and is not affected by the LHRH analogs.

All of the androgen receptor antagonists are administered orally. Nilutamide is approved specifically for use in prostate cancer after surgical orchiectomy to reduce bone pain, slow progression, and increase survival time.

Luteinizing Hormone–Releasing Hormone Analogs

Goserelin (Zoladex), leuprolide (Eligard, Lupron, Viadur), and triptorelin (Trelstar) are synthetic versions of the hypothalamic LHRH that initiates hormonal stimulation for production of both estrogens and androgens. Therapeutic doses of LHRH analogs initially increase the release of luteinizing hormone (LH) and follicle-stimulating hormone (FSH) from the anterior pituitary. However, with continued administration, the LHRH analog decreases the release of FSH and LH by down-regulating receptor response. Inhibiting the release of LH and FSH blocks the production of ovarian estrogen in women to postmenopausal levels and testicular testosterone in men to castration levels. These effects occur within 2 to 4 weeks after drug therapy is started.

In premenopausal women with estrogen receptor–positive breast cancer, one of these drugs is increasingly being used instead of surgical excision of the ovaries. The LHRH drug is usually combined with a SERM to prevent initial stimulation of cancer cells.

In men with prostate cancer, these drugs reduce androgens to the levels seen with surgical excision of the testes.

In metastatic prostate cancer, an LHRH analog is often given with an antiandrogen to increase effectiveness and to prevent an initial flair in symptoms such as bone pain and urinary outlet obstruction when testosterone production initially increases.

Cytoprotectant Drugs

Cytoprotectant agents reduce the adverse effects of cytotoxic drugs, some of which can be severe, debilitating, or life-threatening (see Box 12.2). Severe adverse effects of cytotoxic drugs may also limit drug dosage or frequency of administration, thereby limiting the effectiveness of chemotherapy. Several cytoprotective drugs are available to protect body tissues from one or more adverse effects and allow for a more optimal dose and schedule of cytotoxic agents. To be effective, it is necessary to time administration in relation to administration of the cytotoxic agent. Table 12.5 lists cytoprotective agents and their clinical uses.

Clinical Application 12-3

- Mrs. Gardner develops some mouth ulcerations (oral mucositis) after her last dose of chemotherapy. To help reduce her risk of oral mucositis with this next cycle of chemotherapy, what interventions should the nurse discuss with Mrs. Gardner?

NCLEX Success

5. **Antineoplastic hormone inhibitor drugs used in the treatment of cancer**

   A. are highly cytotoxic to both cancer cells and normal cells
   B. target specific antigens or vital processes of cancer cells
   C. slow the growth of some cancer cells
   D. protect normal cells from cytotoxic drugs

6. **Hormone inhibitor drugs used in the treatment of cancer are most effective in**

   A. treating breast or prostate cancer
   B. preventing hematological malignancies
   C. treating thyroid and pituitary tumors
   D. protecting normal cells from cytotoxic drugs

7. **A vesicant antineoplastic drug does which of the following?**

   A. It causes minor skin irritation.
   B. It causes extensive tissue damage.
   C. It requires administration only through a central IV line.
   D. It requires deep intramuscular injection if diluted with normal saline.

TABLE 12.5

DRUGS AT A GLANCE: Cytoprotectant Drugs

Drug/Pregnancy Category	Routes and Dosage Ranges	Clinical Use
Amifostine (Ethyol)/C	IV infusion 910 mg/m² once daily within 30 min of starting chemotherapy	Reduction of cisplatin-induced renal toxicity
Dexrazoxane (Zinecard)/C	IV 10 times the amount of doxorubicin (e.g., dexrazoxane 500 mg/m² per doxorubicin 50 mg/m²), then give doxorubicin within 30 min of completing dexrazoxane dose	Reduction of doxorubicin-induced cardiomyopathy in women with metastatic breast cancer who have received a cumulative dose of 300 mg/m² and need additional doxorubicin
Erythropoietin (Epogen, Procrit)/C	Sub-Q 150–300 units/kg 3 times weekly, adjusted to maintain desired hematocrit	Treatment of chemotherapy-induced anemia
Filgrastim (Neupogen)/C	Sub-Q, IV 5 mcg/kg/d, at least 24 h after cytotoxic chemotherapy, up to 2 wk or an absolute neutrophil count of 10,000/mm³	Treatment of chemotherapy-induced neutropenia
Leucovorin (Wellcovorin)/C	"Rescue," PO, IV, IM 15 mg every 6 h for 10 doses, starting 24 h after methotrexate (MTX) begun Colorectal cancer, IV 20 mg/m² or 200 mg/m², followed by 5-fluorouracil, daily for 5 d, repeated every 28 d	"Rescue" after high-dose MTX for osteosarcoma Advanced colorectal cancer, with 5-fluorouracil
Mesna (Mesnex)/B	IV, 20% of ifosfamide dose for 3 doses (at time of ifosfamide dose, then 4 h and 8 h after ifosfamide dose)	Prevention of cyclophosphamide and ifosfamide-induced hemorrhagic cystitis
Oprelvekin (Neumega)/C	Sub-Q 50 mcg/kg once daily, usually for 10–21 d	Prevention of thrombocytopenia
Palifermin (Kepivance)/C	IV bolus, 60 mcg/kg daily for 6 total doses 3 consecutive days before and 3 d after high-dose chemotherapy (fourth dose at least one day before stem cell infusion)	Prevent oral mucositis in hematological malignancies before stem cell transplant
Sargramostim (Leukine)/C	IV infusion, 250 mcg/m²/d until absolute neutrophil count is above 1500/mm³ for 3 d, up to 42 d	Myeloid reconstitution after bone marrow transplant; to decrease chemotherapy-induced neutropenia

The Nursing Process

Assessment

- Assess all patients for risk factors, screening behaviors, and/or manifestations of cancer, to prevent cancer, if possible, or recognize and seek treatment for cancer as early as possible. Risk factors include use of tobacco products (including inhalation of secondhand cigarette smoke in home or work environments), drinking more than one drink a day (for women) or two drinks a day (for men), being overweight, damage to skin unprotected by sunscreen, and unsafe sexual behaviors. Screening behaviors include the use of breast self-examinations, regular mammograms, Papanicolaou (Pap) testing, colonoscopy when indicated, measurement of prostate-specific antigen (PSA), and skin examination.
- Assess the patient's condition before chemotherapy is started and often during treatment. Useful information includes the type, grade, and stage of the tumor as well as

the signs and symptoms of cancer. General manifestations include anemia, malnutrition, weight loss, pain, and infection; specific manifestations depend on the organs affected.

- Assess for other diseases and organ dysfunctions (e.g., cardiac, pulmonary, renal, hepatic) that can influence individual response to chemotherapy.
- Assess emotional status, coping mechanisms, family relationships, financial resources, and social support mechanisms. Anxiety and depression are common features during cancer diagnosis and treatment.
- Assess laboratory test results before chemotherapy to establish baseline data and during chemotherapy to monitor drug effects.
- Blood tests for tumor markers (tumor-specific antigens on cell surfaces). Alpha-fetoprotein is a fetal antigen normally present during intrauterine and early postnatal life but absent in adulthood. Increased amounts may indicate hepatic or testicular cancer. Carcinoembryonic antigen (CEA) is secreted by several types of malignant cells (e.g.,

colorectal cancer). A rising level may indicate tumor progression and levels that are elevated before surgery and disappear after surgery indicate adequate tumor excision. If CEA levels rise later, it probably indicates tumor recurrence. With chemotherapy, falling CEA levels indicate effectiveness. Other tumor markers are immunoglobulins (elevated levels may indicate multiple myeloma) and prostate-specific antigens (elevated levels may indicate prostatic cancer).

- CBC to check for anemia, leukopenia, and thrombocytopenia because most cytotoxic antineoplastic drugs cause bone marrow depression. It is necessary to perform a CBC and white blood cell differential before each cycle of chemotherapy to determine dosage and frequency of drug administration, to monitor bone marrow function so fatal bone marrow depression does not occur, and to assist in planning nursing care. For example, the patient is very susceptible to infection when the leukocyte count is low, and bleeding is likely when the platelet count is low.
- Other tests. These include tests of kidney and liver function, serum calcium, uric acid, and others, depending on the organs affected by the cancer or its treatment.

Nursing Diagnoses

- Pain, nausea and vomiting, weakness, and activity Intolerance related to disease process or chemotherapy
- Imbalanced nutrition: less than body requirements related to disease process or chemotherapy
- Anxiety related to the disease, its possible progression, and its treatment
- Ineffective family coping related to illness and treatment of a family member
- Deficient fluid volume related to chemotherapy-induced nausea, vomiting, and diarrhea
- Risk for injury: infection related to drug-induced neutropenia; bleeding related to drug-induced thrombocytopenia; stomatitis related to damage of GI mucosal cells
- Deficient knowledge about cancer chemotherapy and managing adverse drug effects

Planning/Goals

The patient will

- Receive assistance in coping with the diagnosis of cancer
- Experience reduced anxiety and fear
- Receive chemotherapy accurately and safely
- Experience reduction of tumor size, change of laboratory values toward normal, or other therapeutic effects of chemotherapy
- Experience minimal bleeding, infection, nausea and vomiting, and other consequences of chemotherapy
- Maintain adequate food and fluid intake and body weight
- Receive assistance in activities of daily living when needed
- Be informed about community resources for cancer care (e.g., hospice, Reach to Recovery, other support groups)

Nursing Interventions

The nurse will

- Participate in and promote efforts to prevent cancer.
- Follow and promote the diet recommended by the American Cancer Society (i.e., decrease fat, eat at least five servings of fruits and vegetables daily, increase intake of dietary fiber, minimize intake of salt-cured or smoked foods).
- Promote weight control. Obesity may contribute to the development of several cancers, including breast and endometrial cancer in women.
- Identify cancer-causing agents in homes and workplaces and strategies to reduce exposure to them when possible.
- Strengthen host defenses by promoting a healthful lifestyle (e.g., good nutrition, adequate rest and exercise, stress management techniques, avoiding or minimizing alcohol and tobacco use).
- Avoid smoking cigarettes and being around smokers. Passive smoking increases risk of lung cancer in spouses of smokers and risks of brain cancer, lymphomas, and acute lymphogenous leukemia in children of smokers.
- Minimize exposure to sunlight, use sunscreens liberally, and wear protective clothing to prevent skin cancer.
- Participate in and promote cancer screening tests in nonsymptomatic people, especially those at high risk, to detect cancer before signs and symptoms occur. These tests include regular examination of breasts, cervix (Pap test), testicles, and skin and tests for colon cancer such as Hemoccult tests on stool and colonoscopy. Early recognition of risk factors, premalignant tissue changes (dysplasia), biochemical tumor markers, and beginning malignancies may be lifesaving; early treatment can greatly reduce the suffering and problems associated with advanced cancer.
- For patients receiving cytotoxic anticancer drugs, try to prevent or minimize the incidence and severity of adverse reactions (see Box 12.2).
- Provide supportive care to patients and families. Physiologic care includes pain management, comfort measures, and assistance with nutrition, hygiene, ambulation, and other activities of daily living as needed. Psychological care includes allowing family members or significant others to be with the patient and participate in care when desired and keeping patients and families informed.

Evaluation

- Monitor drug administration for accuracy.
- Observe and interview for therapeutic effects of chemotherapy.
- Compare current laboratory reports with baseline values for changes toward normal values.
- Compare weight and nutritional status with baseline values for maintenance or improvement.
- Observe and interview for adverse drug effects and interventions to prevent or manage them.
- Observe and interview for effective pain management and other symptom control.

Key Concepts

- Traditional cytotoxic antineoplastic drugs are nonselective in their effect on proliferating cells; therefore, bone marrow toxicity is a common adverse effect of many cytotoxic drugs. These drugs kill the same fraction of cells with each cycle of chemotherapy treatment; repeated cycles of cytotoxic drugs potentially lower the number of cancer cells to a level where a person's immune responses are able to take over and destroy the remaining cancer cells.

- Cytoprotectant agents protect body tissues from one or more adverse effects of cytotoxic drugs and allow for a more optimal dose and schedule of cytotoxic agents.

- Biologic targeted antineoplastic agents are designed to specifically attack a target that is expressed exclusively, or disproportionally, by the cancer cell.

- Hormonal therapies that block the effects of estrogen (in an estrogen-responsive tumor) and androgen (in an androgen-responsive tumor), respectively, are essential in the treatment of breast and advanced prostate cancers.

- LHRH analogs decrease the release of FSH and LH by down-regulating receptor response, thus inhibiting the release of LH and FSH. This action blocks the production of ovarian estrogen in women to postmenopausal levels and testicular testosterone in men to castration levels.

- Cancer in older adults presents a unique challenge, due in part to the presence of comorbidities and the physical, biologic, and physiologic changes that occur with normal aging. Until recently, older adults were excluded from participating in clinical trials.

Critical Thinking Questions

12-1. Tim Fox, a 42-year-old man with a history of mild renal insufficiency, has received a diagnosis of Hodgkin's disease. He has completed a course of radiation therapy and is preparing to begin adjuvant chemotherapy, with a drug regimen that includes doxorubicin, bleomycin, vinblastine, and dacarbazine.

- Mr. Fox asks the nurse why he has to take so many different chemotherapeutic drugs. How should the nurse respond?

- Discuss the major adverse effects of chemotherapy that Mr. Fox may expect. What nursing interventions may mitigate these effects?

References and Resources

Abraham, J., Gulley, J. L., & Allegra, C. J. (2010). *The Bethesda handbook of clinical oncology* (3rd ed.). Philadelphia, PA: Lippincott Williams & Wilkins.

Drug facts and comparisons. (Updated monthly). St. Louis, MO: Facts and Comparisons.

Files, J. A., Ko, M. G., & Pruthi, S. (2010). Managing aromatase inhibitors in breast cancer survivors: not just for oncologists. *Mayo Clinic Proceedings.* Published on-line 2010. doi: 10.4065/mcp.2010.0137.

Goodin, S., Griffin, N., Chen, B., Chuk, K., Daouphars, M., Doreau, C., et al. (2011). Safe handling of oral chemotherapeutic agents in clinical practice: Recommendations from an international pharmacy panel. *Journal of Oncology Practice, 7*(1), 7–12.

Harandi, A., Zaida, A. S., Stocker, A. M., & Laber, D. A. (2009). Clinical efficacy and toxicity of anti-EGFR therapy in common cancers. *Journal of Oncology, 14*(4), 337–349.

Karch, A. M. (2010). *2010 Lippincott's nursing drug guide.* Philadelphia, PA: Lippincott Williams & Wilkins.

Lacy, C. F., Armstrong, L. L., Goldman, M. P., & Lance, L. L. (2010). *Lexi-Comp's drug information handbook* (19th ed.). Hudson, OH: American Pharmaceutical Association.

Polovich, M., Whitford, J. M., & Olsen, M. M. (2009). *Chemotherapy and biotherapy guidelines and recommendations for practice* (3rd ed.). Pittsburgh, PA: Oncology Nursing Society.

Porth, C. M. (2010). *Pathophysiology: Concepts of altered health states* (8th ed.). Philadelphia, PA: Lippincott Williams & Wilkins.

Rudek, M.A., Flexner, C., & Ambinder, R. F. (2011). Use of antineoplastic agents in patients with cancer who have HIV/AIDs. *The Lancet Oncology, 12*(9), 905–912.

Smith, T. J., Temin, S., Alesi, E. R., Abernethy, A. P., Balboni, T. A., Basch, E. M., et al. (2012). American Society of Clinical Oncology Provisional Clinical Opinion: The integration of palliative care into standard oncology care. *The Journal of Clinical Oncology, 30*(8), 880–887.

Steward, C. (2010). Oncology: Nursing management in cancer care. In: S. C. Smeltzer, & B. G. Bare (Eds.), *Brunner & Suddarth's textbook of medical-surgical nursing* (12th ed., pp. 336–394). Philadelphia, PA: Lippincott Williams & Wilkins.

Schulmeister, L. (2011). Extravasation management: clinical update. *Seminars in Oncology Nursing, 27*(1), 82–90.

Drugs Affecting Inflammation and Infection

CHAPTER OUTLINE

13 Inflammation, Infection, and the Use of Antimicrobial Agents

LEARNING OBJECTIVES

After studying this chapter, you should be able to:

1. Identify the common etiologies of inflammation.
2. Discuss the pathophysiology of inflammation.
3. Describe, in general, the groups of drugs used to treat inflammation.
4. Identify the common pathogens and methods of infection control.
5. Discuss the pathophysiology of infection.
6. Discuss ways to minimize emergence of drug-resistant microorganisms.
7. Discuss ways to increase the benefits and decrease the risk associated with antimicrobial drug therapy.
8. Know how to apply the nursing process to the care of the patient who is receiving antimicrobial therapy.

Clinical Application Case Study

Alisa Warren is a 25-year-old woman with early-onset rheumatoid arthritis who works as a social worker in a pediatric hospital. She has a heavy caseload, and her lunch often consists of a soda, chips, and a sweet roll from the snack machine. She and her husband spend most evenings watching movies and television because her pain prevents her from participating in many activities. Recently, her practitioner prescribed methylprednisolone, a corticosteroid, to help manage the inflammation associated with the arthritis.

KEY TERMS

Antibacterial: ability to kill bacteria or interfere with the ability of bacteria to grow and replicate

Antibiotic: drug that has the ability to kill or inhibit bacterial growth and replication

Antibiotic resistance: ability of certain bacteria to survive and multiply in the presence of antibiotics

Anti-infective: agent or substance with antibacterial, antiviral, and antifungal properties

Anti-inflammatory agent: drug indicated when the inflammatory response is inappropriate, abnormal, or persistent, or destroys tissue

Antimicrobial agent: drug used to prevent or treat infections caused by pathogenic (disease-producing) microorganisms such as bacteria, fungi, viruses, and parasites

Bacteria: single-celled microorganisms that do not have nuclei and reproduce by fission or splitting

Bactericidal: agent that kills bacteria

Bacteriostatic: agent that inhibits bacterial growth and replication

Broad spectrum: effective against a wide range of bacteria

Colonization: presence and growth of microorganisms on host tissues

Community-acquired infection: infection caused by microorganisms that originated in a setting outside of a health care facility

Detection of antigens: technique to identify pathogens that uses features of culture and serology but reduces the time required for diagnosis

Fungi: plant-like microorganisms that live as parasites on living tissue or as saprophytes on decaying organic matter

Inflammation: immunological response to allergy, infection, or injury that increases the migration of leukocytes and blood flow to assist in repairing tissues

Nosocomial infection: infection acquired from microorganisms in hospitals and other health care facilities

Opportunistic: microorganisms in normal flora that become pathogenic under conditions that are favorable for their (over)growth

Penicillin-binding proteins: proteins in bacteria that serve as target sites for penicillin to bind

Serology: method of identifying infectious agents by measuring the antibody level (titer) in the serum of an infected host

Susceptibility: vulnerability of the bacteria to an antibiotic's effects

Viruses: intracellular parasites that survive only in living tissues

Introduction

This chapter is an introduction to the pathophysiological effects of inflammation and infection. Readers should note that the format of this chapter is different from previous chapters. This chapter presents an overview of the anti-inflammatory and antimicrobial therapy to allow an understanding of a broad classification of the drugs involved and their impact on decreasing inflammation associated with infection and the infective process.

To help prevent **inflammation** caused by allergy, injury, or infection, the nurse should be familiar with **anti-inflammatory agents**. The anti-inflammatory agents administered to reduce the inflammatory process include aspirin, nonsteroidal anti-inflammatory drugs (NSAIDs), and corticosteroids. These drugs are indicated when the inflammatory response is inappropriate, abnormal, or persistent, or in the presence of tissue destruction. Health care providers use medicines known as **antimicrobial agents** to prevent or treat infections caused by pathogenic (disease-producing) microorganisms such as bacteria, fungi, viruses, and parasites. They treat inflammation resulting from infectious processes with antimicrobial drugs.

Most microorganisms live in equilibrium with the human host and do not cause disease; however, even beneficial bacteria may cause infections in certain conditions. When the balance

is upset and infection occurs, characteristics of the infecting microorganisms and the adequacy of host defense mechanisms are major factors in determining the severity of the infection and the person's ability to recover. In addition, overuse of antimicrobial agents may lead to serious infections caused by drug-resistant microorganisms. To help prevent infectious diseases and participate effectively in antimicrobial drug therapy, the nurse must be knowledgeable about microorganisms, host responses to microorganisms, and antimicrobial drugs.

Overview of Inflammation

To adequately understand the pharmacologic treatment of inflammation, it is important to understand the causes, pathophysiology, and clinical manifestations of inflammation. This will make it easier to understand the drug therapy associated with the treatment of inflammation, as addressed in Chapters 14 and 15.

Etiology

Inflammation is the cellular response of the body to injury. The cells and tissues of the body are killed or injured by chemical, physical, or infectious agents. The immunological response of the body produces increased migration of leukocytes and flow of blood to the cells and tissues affected to help repair the tissues.

Pathophysiology

There are two types of inflammation. Acute inflammation is the immediate response to injury of local tissues. The body responds by attempting to remove the offending agent to limit the amount of damage to the tissues affected. Chronic inflammation occurs over longer periods, even years. An acute inflammatory response may become chronic.

Acute Inflammation

The process of acute inflammation occurs in three stages. The first stage is the vascular stage; notable changes occur in the small blood vessels at the site of the cellular and tissue injury. At the time of the injury, vasoconstriction results, followed by vasodilation of the capillaries and venules to increase capillary blood flow, increasing temperature and redness at the site. The body then increases protein exudates into the extravascular spaces. As protein exudates occupy the extravascular spaces, the capillary osmotic pressure diminishes and the interstitial osmotic pressure increases, resulting in increasing amounts of fluid in the tissue spaces causing swelling, pain, and diminished function or mobility. In the event that the inflammation is caused by an infectious agent, the localizing effects increase the risk of the spread of infection (Fig. 13.1).

The second stage of acute inflammation is also known as the cellular stage. At this time, there is an influx of leukocytes, primarily neutrophils, to the injury site. As the leukocytes invade, there is a slowing of the blood flow and margination, which is the adhesion of the leukocytes to the wall of the blood vessels. The leukocytes then transmigrate from the vascular space to the extravascular tissue. They travel to the tissue injury site by chemotaxis (Fig. 13.2).

The third stage involves opsonization, which facilitates phagocytosis. During opsonization, a substance coats the foreign antigens, producing inflammation. This inflammation makes the antigens more susceptible to the macrophages and leukocytes, thus increasing phagocytic activity. The two opsonins are complement factor C3b and antibodies (Fig. 13.3).

Chronic Inflammation

There are two kinds of chronic inflammation. Nonspecific chronic inflammation is a diffuse accumulation of macrophages and lymphocytes in the area of tissue destruction, yielding fibroblast proliferation and scarring. Granulomatous chronic inflammation generates 1 to 2 mm granulomas made up of macrophages surrounded by lymphocytes. The granulomatous process results from foreign bodies that have not been controlled by the acute inflammatory process.

Clinical Manifestations

In acute inflammation, pain, redness, and swelling are apparent. Breaks in the integumentary system result in the drainage of exudate. In the event of a viral or bacterial infection associated with the inflammation, fever and general malaise sometimes occur. In chronic inflammation, tissue destruction and scarring may develop, resulting in diminished mobility. As previously stated, granulomas may occur because of an uncontrolled acute inflammatory process.

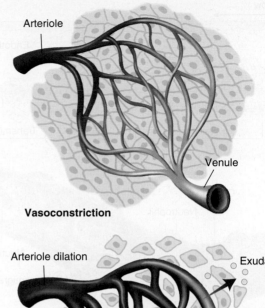

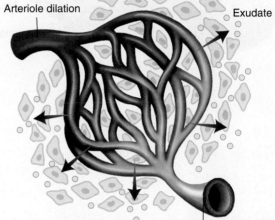

Vasoconstriction

Vasodilation   Venule dilation

Figure 13.1 Stage 1: vascular stage. The vascular stage of acute inflammation, which is characterized by changes in the small blood vessels at the site of injury. It begins with vasoconstriction followed rapidly by vasodilation. Vasodilation results in an increase in capillary blood flow, causing heat and redness, which are two of the cardinal signs of inflammation. This is accompanied by an increased in vascular permeability with outpouring of protein-rich fluid (exudate) into the extravascular spaces. The loss of proteins reduces the capillary osmotic pressure and increases the interstitial osmotic pressure. This, coupled with an increase in capillary pressure, causes a marked outflow of fluid and its accumulation in the tissue spaces, producing the swelling, pain, and impaired function that represent the other cardinal signs of acute inflammation. As fluid moves out of the vessels, stagnation of flow and clotting of blood occur. This aids in localizing the spread of infectious microorganisms.

Drug Therapy

Aspirin, NSAIDs, and corticosteroids are administered to decrease inflammation (see Chaps. 14 and 15). Aspirin and NSAIDs block the synthesis of prostaglandin in the central and peripheral nervous systems. The anti-inflammatory response produced by the administration of corticosteroids occurs through the inhibition of interleukin-1, cytokines, and the tumor necrosis factor. Corticosteroids also impair phagocytosis by preventing phagocytic cells from leaving the bloodstream.

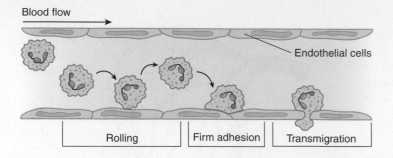

Blood flow

Endothelial cells

Rolling Firm adhesion Transmigration

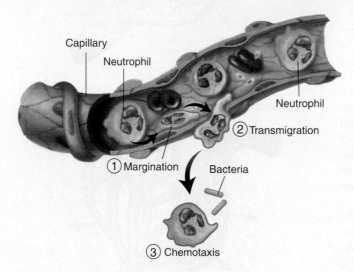

Capillary

Neutrophil

Neutrophil

② Transmigration

① Margination

Bacteria

③ Chemotaxis

Figure 13.2 Stage 2: leukocyte margination, adhesion, and transmigration. The cellular stage of acute inflammation, which involves the delivery of leukocytes, mainly neutrophil, to the site of injury so they can perform their normal functions of host defense. The delivery and activation of leukocytes can be divided into the following steps: adhesion and margination, transmigration, and chemotaxis. The recruitment of leukocytes to the precapillary venules, where they exit the circulation, is facilitated by the slowing of blood flow and margination along the vessel surface. Leukocyte adhesion and transmigration from the vascular space into the extravascular tissue is facilitated by adhesion molecules on the leukocyte and endothelial surfaces. After extravasation, leukocytes migrate in the tissues toward the site of injury by chemotaxis, or locomotion oriented along a chemical gradient.

They decrease the amount of lymphocytes, fibroblasts, and collagen needed for tissue repair.

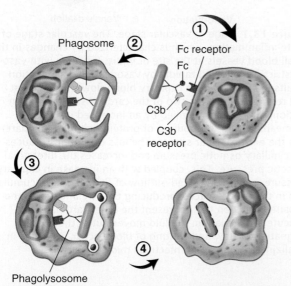

Phagosome ②

①

Fc receptor

Fc

C3b

C3b
receptor

③

④

Phagolysosome

Figure 13.3 Stage 3: opsonization and phagocytosis. Once at the site of injury, the products generated by tissue injury trigger a number of leukocyte responses, including phagocytosis and cell killing. Opsonization of microbes (1) by complement factor C3b and antibody facilitates recognition by neutrophil C3b and the antibody Fc receptor. Receptor activation (2) triggers intracellular signaling and actin assembly in the neutrophil, leading to formation of pseudopods that enclose the microbe within a phagosome. The phagosome (3) then fuses with an intracellular lysosome to form a phagolysosome into which lysosomal enzymes and oxygen radicals (4) are released to kill and degrade the microbe.

> ### Clinical Application 13-1
>
> ■ Now that Ms. Warren has been given a corticosteroid to decrease the inflammation of her joints, what is she at risk for developing?

Overview of Microorganisms

Infections occur when microorganisms invade a host, attach to host cell receptors, and multiply in sufficient numbers to cause injury. The infection stimulates the body's immune response. In many instances, this immune response is sufficient to contain an infection. However, most microorganisms have characteristics that allow them to adapt to ensure their survival, and these adaptations help protect them from normal body defense mechanisms.

Antimicrobial drugs are an important intervention to treat infections that could otherwise cause significant injury and harm to the human host. To understand antimicrobial drug use, it is important to have a basic understanding of the microorganisms that they target. The following sections provide information about microorganisms and how they interact with human hosts.

Microorganisms that cause infectious disease include bacteria, viruses, fungi, and parasites. **Bacteria** are single-celled microorganisms without nuclei that reproduce by fission or splitting. They are classified according to whether they are aerobic (require oxygen) or anaerobic (cannot live in the presence of oxygen, their ability to retain Gram's stain [gram positive] or to reject Gram's stain [gram negative], and their shape [e.g., cocci, rods]). **Antibiotics** are antimicrobial drugs used to treat bacterial infections. **Viruses** are intracellular parasites that survive only in living tissues. They are officially classified according to their structure but are more commonly described according to origin and the disorders or symptoms they produce. Human pathogens include adenoviruses, herpesviruses, and retroviruses (see Chap. 21). **Fungi** are plant-like microorganisms that live as parasites on living tissue or as saprophytes on decaying organic matter. Approximately 50 species are pathogenic in humans (see Chap. 22). Parasites are microorganisms in the animal kingdom that infect other animals. Parasites that infect human hosts include arthropods, protozoa, and helminths (see Chap. 23).

Etiology

Normal Flora

Colonization is the presence and growth of microorganisms. The microorganisms do not necessarily cause tissue injury or elicit an immune response in the human body. The human body also has sterile areas, in which microorganisms do not live. Sterile areas that do not communicate directly with the external environment include organs such as the heart and liver, the musculoskeletal system, and body fluids such as urine. Areas typically populated by microorganisms include the skin, upper respiratory tract, and colon.

Normal skin flora includes staphylococci, streptococci, diphtheroids, and transient environmental microorganisms. The upper respiratory tract contains staphylococci, streptococci, pneumococci, and diphtheroids, as well as *Haemophilus influenzae*. The external genitalia contain skin organisms, and the vagina contains lactobacilli, *Candida*, and *Bacteroides*. The colon contains *Escherichia coli*, *Klebsiella*, *Enterobacter*, *Proteus*, *Pseudomonas*, *Bacteroides*, clostridia, lactobacilli, streptococci, and staphylococci.

Normal flora protects the human host in a variety of ways. For example, normal bowel flora synthesizes vitamin K and vitamin B complex. The intestinal flora also plays a role in digestion. Furthermore, by competing with potential pathogens for nutrients and by preventing adhesion and growth of pathogens, beneficial microorganisms interfere with the ability of potential pathogens to cause infections.

In certain instances, normal flora can become pathogenic. For example, microorganisms that are part of the normal flora and nonpathogenic in one area of the body may be pathogenic in other parts of the body; for example, *E. coli* is part of the normal intestinal flora but it is a common cause of urinary tract infections.

Host Defense Mechanisms

Although the numbers and virulence of microorganisms help determine whether a person acquires an infection, another major factor is the host's ability to defend itself against the would-be invaders.

Major defense mechanisms of the human body are intact skin and mucous membranes, various anti-infective secretions, mechanical movements, phagocytic cells, and the immune and inflammatory processes. The skin prevents penetration of foreign particles, and its secretions and normal bacterial flora inhibit growth of pathogenic microorganisms. Secretions of the gastrointestinal, respiratory, and genitourinary tracts (e.g., gastric

acid, mucus) kill, trap, or inhibit growth of microorganisms. Coughing, swallowing, and peristalsis help remove foreign particles and pathogens trapped in mucus, as does the movement of cilia. Phagocytic cells in various organs and tissues engulf and digest pathogens and cellular debris. The immune system produces lymphocytes and antibodies. The inflammatory process is the body's response to injury by microorganisms, foreign particles, chemical agents, or physical irritation of tissues. Inflammation localizes, destroys, dilutes, or removes the injurious agents so tissue healing can occur (see previous discussion).

Many factors impair host defense mechanisms and predispose to infection by disease-producing microorganisms. These factors include the following:

- Breaks in the skin and mucous membranes related to trauma, inflammation, open lesions, or insertion of prosthetic devices, tubes, and catheters for diagnostic or therapeutic purposes
- Impaired blood supply
- Neutropenia and other blood disorders
- Malnutrition
- Poor personal hygiene
- Suppression of normal bacterial flora by antimicrobial drugs
- Suppression of the immune system and the inflammatory response by immunosuppressive drugs, cytotoxic antineoplastic drugs, and adrenal corticosteroids
- Diabetes mellitus and other chronic diseases
- Advanced age

Clinical Application 13-2

- Which alteration in Ms. Warren's defense mechanisms places her at risk for the development of an infection?

NCLEX Success

1. A college student is seen in the campus health center with a sore throat. Examination of the throat reveals redness and swelling but no sign of infection. Which of the following is an accurate description of the inflammatory process?

   A. A granuloma will develop if the inflammation is unresolved.

   B. The student is not at risk for the development of an infection.

   C. There is an influx of leukocytes to the throat.

   D. Scarring will result from phagocytic action.

2. A sputum specimen report from the laboratory states, "Contamination with typical oral flora." Which interpretation is correct?

   A. Bacteria in the mouth are growing in the lungs.

   B. The normal flora has become pathogenic.

   C. The patient has a pulmonary infection.

   D. The sputum from the lungs has mixed with bacteria in the mouth.

Pathophysiology

Infection begins with colonization by microorganisms. Infectious disease occurs when growth of microbial pathogens results in injury and is accompanied by clinical signs and symptoms indicative of an infection. Box 13.1 describes common bacterial pathogens of humans. Accurate assessment and documentation of symptoms can aid in early detection and diagnosis of infectious disease.

Opportunistic Pathogens

Opportunistic microorganisms are usually normal endogenous or environmental flora and nonpathogenic. However, they become pathogens in hosts whose defense mechanisms are impaired. Opportunistic infections are likely to occur in people with severe burns, cancer, human immunodeficiency virus (HIV) infection, indwelling intravenous or urinary catheters, and antibiotic or corticosteroid drug therapy. Opportunistic bacterial

---

BOX 13.1	Common Bacterial Pathogens

Gram-Positive Bacteria

Staphylococci

Staphylococcus aureus bacteria are part of the normal microbial flora of the skin and upper respiratory tract and also are common pathogens. Some people carry (are colonized with) *S. aureus* in the anterior nares. The bacteria are spread mainly by direct contact with people who are infected or who are carriers. The hands of health care workers are considered a major source of indirect spread and nosocomial infections. The bacteria also survive on inanimate surfaces for long periods of time.

    S. aureus organisms can cause skin infections such as boils and carbuncles. When burns or surgical wounds become contaminated with *S. aureus*, they often produce endotoxins that destroy erythrocytes, leukocytes, platelets, fibroblasts, and other human cells. These bacteria may also cause infections of the respiratory tract and urinary tract. Also, when many strains are ingested, they produce enterotoxins that cause food poisoning. The enterotoxins survive heating at temperatures high enough to kill the bacteria, so reheating foods does not prevent food poisoning.

    High-risk groups for staphylococcal infections include newborns, older adults, and people who are malnourished or obese, or who have diabetes. In children, staphylococcal infections of the respiratory tract are most common in those younger than 2 years of age. In adults, staphylococcal pneumonia often occurs in people with chronic lung disease or as a secondary bacterial infection after influenza. The influenza virus destroys the ciliated epithelium of the respiratory tract and thereby aids bacterial invasion.

    Staphylococcus species, non*aureus* (SSNA) describes a group of bacteria that are also part of the normal microbial flora of the skin and mucosal surfaces and are increasingly common pathogens. The most common member of this group involved in infections is *S. epidermidis*.

    Infections due to SSNA are often associated with the use of treatment devices such as intravascular catheters, prosthetic heart valves, cardiac pacemakers, orthopedic prostheses, cerebrospinal fluid shunts, and peritoneal catheters. SSNA infections include endocarditis, bacteremia, and other serious infections and are especially hazardous to immunocompromised patients. Treatment usually requires removal of any infected medical device as well as appropriate antibiotic therapy.

Streptococci

Certain streptococci are part of the normal microbial flora of the throat and nasopharynx in many healthy people. These bacteria do not usually cause disease unless the mucosal barrier is damaged by trauma, previous infection, or surgical manipulation. Such damage allows the bacteria

to enter the bloodstream and gain access to other parts of the body where they colonize and then cause an infection.

    S. pneumoniae bacteria, often called "pneumococci," are common bacterial pathogens. They cause pneumonia, sinusitis, otitis media, and meningitis. Pneumococcal pneumonia usually develops when the mechanisms that normally expel inhaled microorganisms (i.e., the mucociliary blanket and cough reflex) are impaired by viral infection, smoking, immobility, or other insults. When *S. pneumoniae* reach the alveoli, they proliferate, cause acute inflammation, and spread rapidly to involve one or more lobes. Alveoli fill with proteinaceous fluid, neutrophils, and bacteria. Older adults have high rates of illness and death from pneumococcal pneumonia, which can often be prevented by pneumococcal vaccine (see Chap. 10). Pneumococcal sinusitis and otitis media usually follow a viral illness, such as the common cold. The viral infection injures the protective ciliated epithelium and fills the air spaces with nutrient-rich tissue fluid, in which the pneumococci thrive. *S. pneumoniae* is a common pathogen in bacterial sinusitis. In young children, upper respiratory tract infections may be complicated by acute sinusitis. Many children have repeated episodes of pneumococcal otitis media by 6 years of age. Recurrent otitis media during early childhood may result in reduced hearing acuity. Pneumococcal meningitis may develop from sinus or middle ear infections or an injury that allows pneumococcal bacteria from the nasopharynx to enter the meninges. *S. pneumoniae* infection is a common cause of bacterial meningitis in adults. Other potential secondary complications include septicemia, endocarditis, pericarditis, and empyema.

    Streptococcus pyogenes (beta-hemolytic streptococcus) bacteria are often part of the normal flora of the skin and oropharynx that may become pathogenic in other body regions. The bacteria spread from person to person by direct contact with oral or respiratory secretions. They cause severe streptococcal pharyngitis ("strep throat"), scarlet fever, and rheumatic fever. Endocarditis and glomerulonephritis may occur as sequelae following untreated or inadequately treated streptococcal pharyngitis.

Enterococci

Enterococci are normal flora in the human intestine but are also found in soil, food, water, and animals. Although the genus *Enterococcus* contains approximately 12 species, the main pathogens are *Enterococcus faecalis* and *Enterococcus faecium*. Most enterococcal infections occur in hospitalized patients, especially those in critical care units. Risk factors for nosocomial infections include serious underlying disease, prior surgery, renal impairment, and the presence of urinary or vascular catheters. These bacteria, especially *E. faecalis*, are usually secondary invaders in urinary tract

BOX 13.1   Common Bacterial Pathogens (Continued)

or wound infections. Enterococci may also cause endocarditis. This serious infection occurs most often in people with underlying heart disease, such as an injured valve. When the bacteria reach a heart valve, they multiply and release emboli of foreign particles into the bloodstream. Symptoms of endocarditis include fever, heart murmurs, enlarged spleen, and anemia. This infection is diagnosed by isolating enterococci from blood cultures. If not treated promptly and appropriately, enterococcal endocarditis may be fatal.

Gram-Negative Bacteria

Bacteroides

Bacteroides are anaerobic bacteria normally found in the digestive, respiratory, and genital tracts. They are the most common bacteria in the colon. *Bacteroides fragilis,* the major human pathogen, causes intraabdominal and pelvic abscesses (e.g., after surgery or trauma that allows fecal contamination of these tissues), brain abscesses (e.g., from bacteremia or spread from a middle ear or sinus infection), and bacteremia, which may spread the bacteria throughout the body.

Escherichia coli

E. coli inhabit the intestinal tract of humans. They are normally nonpathogenic in the intestinal tract where they serve a beneficial role by synthesizing vitamins and by competitively discouraging growth of potential pathogens. In other parts of the body, however, they act as pathogens.

E. coli cause most urinary tract infections. They also cause pneumonia and sepsis in immunocompromised hosts and meningitis and sepsis in newborns. *E. coli* pneumonia often occurs in debilitated patients after colonization of the oropharynx. In healthy people, the normal gram-positive bacteria of oral cavities attach to material that coats the surface of oral mucosa and prevents transient *E. coli* from establishing residence. Debilitated or severely ill people produce an enzyme that destroys the material that allows gram-positive flora to adhere to oral mucosa. This allows *E. coli* (and other gram-negative enteric bacteria) to compete successfully with the normal gram-positive flora and colonize the oropharynx. Then, droplets of the oral flora are aspirated into the respiratory tract, where impaired protective mechanisms allow survival of the aspirated bacteria.

E. coli also cause enteric gram-negative sepsis, which is acquired from the normal enteric bacterial flora. When *E. coli* and other gram-negative bacteria reach the bloodstream of healthy people, host defenses eliminate the organisms; however, when the organisms reach the bloodstream of people with severe illnesses or immunocompromised status, the host is unable to mount adequate defenses and sepsis occurs. In newborns, *E. coli* are the most common gram-negative bacteria causing nosocomial septic shock and meningitis.

E. coli often cause diarrhea and dysentery. One strain, called *O157:H7,* causes hemorrhagic colitis, a disease characterized by severe abdominal cramps, copious bloody diarrhea, and hemolytic-uremic syndrome (hemolytic anemia, thrombocytopenia, and acute renal failure). Hemolytic-uremic syndrome occurs most often in children. The main reservoir of this strain is the intestinal tract of animals, especially cattle, and several epidemics have been associated with ingestion of undercooked ground beef. Other sources include contaminated water and milk and person-to-person spread.

Klebsiella

Klebsiella bacteria, which are normal bowel flora, may infect the respiratory tract, urinary tract, bloodstream,

burn wounds, and meninges, most often as opportunistic infections in debilitated persons. *Klebsiella pneumoniae* are a common cause of pneumonia, especially in people with pulmonary disease, bacteremia, and sepsis.

Proteus

Proteus bacteria are normally found in the intestinal tract and in decaying matter. They most often cause urinary tract and wound infections but may infect any tissue, especially in debilitated people. Infection often occurs with antibiotic therapy, which decreases drug-sensitive bacteria and allows drug-resistant *Proteus* bacteria to proliferate.

Pseudomonas

Pseudomonas bacteria are found in water, soil, skin, and intestines. They are found in the stools of some healthy people and possibly 50% of inpatients. *Pseudomonas aeruginosa,* the species most often associated with human disease, can cause infections of the respiratory tract, urinary tract, wounds, burns, meninges, eyes, and ears. Because of its resistance to many antibiotics, it can cause severe infections in people receiving antibiotic therapy for burns, wounds, and cystic fibrosis. *P. aeruginosa* colonizes the respiratory tract of most patients with cystic fibrosis and infects approximately 25% of burn patients. Infection is more likely to occur in hosts who are very young or very old or who have an impaired immune system. Sources of infection include catheterization of the urinary tract, trauma or procedures involving the brain or spinal cord, and contamination of respiratory ventilators.

Serratia

Serratia marcescens bacteria are found in infected people, water, milk, feces, and soil. They cause serious nosocomial infections of the urinary tract, respiratory tract, skin, burn wounds, and bloodstream. They also may cause hospital epidemics and produce drug-resistant strains. High-risk patients include newborns, the debilitated, and the immunosuppressed.

Salmonella

Approximately 1400 *Salmonella* species have been identified; several are pathogenic to humans. The bacteria cause gastroenteritis, typhoid fever, septicemia, and a severe, sometimes fatal type of food poisoning. The primary reservoir is the intestinal tract of many animals. Humans become infected through ingestion of contaminated water or food. Water becomes polluted by introduction of feces from any animal excreting salmonellae. Infection via food usually results from ingestion of contaminated meat or by hands transferring organisms from an infected source. In the United States, undercooked poultry and eggs are common sources.

Salmonella enterocolitis is a common cause of foodborne outbreaks of gastroenteritis. Diarrhea usually begins several hours after ingesting contaminated food and may continue for several days, along with nausea, vomiting, headache, and abdominal pain.

Shigella

Shigella species cause gastrointestinal problems ranging from mild diarrhea to severe bacillary dysentery. Humans, who seem to be the only natural hosts, become infected after ingestion of contaminated food or water. Effects of shigellosis are attributed to loss of fluids, electrolytes, and nutrients and to the ulceration that occurs in the colon wall.

infections, often caused by drug-resistant microorganisms, are usually serious and may be life threatening. Fungi of the *Candida* genus, especially *C. albicans*, may cause life-threatening bloodstream or deep-tissue infections, such as abdominal abscesses. Viral infections may cause fatal pneumonia in people with renal or cardiac disorders, in those with HIV infection, and in those who have received bone marrow transplants.

Clinical Application 13-3

- Although Ms. Warren realizes that she has an increased risk of infection, she enjoys her work. What factors other than the administration of corticosteroid medications place her at risk for contracting an infection?

- What teaching can a nurse provide to decrease Ms. Warren's risk of infection?

Laboratory Identification of Pathogens

Laboratory tests of infected fluids or tissues can identify the pathogen that is responsible for an infection. Bacteria and fungi can be differentiated by simple microscopy. In this test, a specimen is applied to a slide and examined under a microscope. Various dyes, such as Gram's stain, and solutions, such as potassium hydroxide, are often applied to help differentiate or further classify microorganisms.

In some cases, there are insufficient microbes in a specimen to identify a causative organism. To obtain a sufficient amount of microbes, laboratory personnel resort to culturing microorganisms from a specimen sample. Culture involves growing a microorganism in the laboratory. Identification of some microorganisms (e.g., intracellular pathogens such as chlamydiae and viruses) requires different techniques. **Serology** identifies infectious agents indirectly by measuring the antibody level (titer) in the serum of an infected host. A tentative diagnosis can be made if the antibody level against a specific pathogen rises

during the acute phase of the disease and falls during convalescence. The **detection of antigens** is a technique to identify pathogens that uses features of culture and serology but reduces the time required for diagnosis. Microbial deoxyribonucleic acid (DNA) and ribonucleic acid (RNA) can also be used to identify pathogenic microorganisms. Examples of these tests include DNA probe hybridization and polymerase chain reaction, which can detect whether DNA for a specific organism is present in a sample.

Community-Acquired Versus Nosocomial Infections

Infections are often categorized as community acquired or nosocomial. **Community-acquired infections** are infections caused by microorganisms that originated in a community setting outside of a health care facility. In contrast, **nosocomial infections** are infections acquired from microorganisms in hospitals and other health care facilities. As a general rule, community-acquired infections are less severe and easier to treat. Nosocomial infections are usually more severe and difficult to manage because they are often caused by microorganisms that are less susceptible to the effects of antimicrobial drugs. These microorganisms are discussed in the next section.

Antibiotic-Resistant Microorganisms

Antibiotic resistance is the ability of certain bacteria to survive and multiply despite antibiotic therapy. Bacteria that have this ability to live in the presence of antibiotics are said to be antibiotic resistant.

Infections that are often associated with high rates of resistance include lower respiratory tract infections and those infections associated with cystic fibrosis or osteomyelitis. These infections are often difficult to treat because they tend to recur, involve multiple or resistant organisms, or, in the case of osteomyelitis, involve anatomic locations where antibiotics do not penetrate well. The increasing prevalence of antibiotic-resistant bacteria is a major public health concern (Box 13.2). Infections caused by antibiotic-resistant organisms

---

BOX 13.2   Antibiotic-Resistant Staphylococci, Streptococci, and Enterococci

Methicillin-Resistant and Vancomycin-Intermediate/Resistant *Staphylococcus* Species

Penicillin-resistant staphylococci developed in the early days of penicillin use because these bacteria produced beta-lactamase enzymes (penicillinases) that destroyed penicillin. Methicillin was one of five drugs developed to resist the action of beta-lactamase enzymes; however, eventually strains of *Staphylococcus aureus* became resistant to these drugs as well. The mechanism of resistance in methicillin-resistant *S. aureus* (MRSA) is alteration of penicillin-binding proteins (PBPs). PBPs, the target sites of penicillins and other beta-lactam antibiotics, are proteins required for maintaining integrity of bacterial cell walls. Beta-lactam antibiotics bind to these PBPs and produce defective bacterial cell walls, which kill the bacteria. MRSA have an additional altered PBP. Methicillin cannot bind effectively to this PBP, and so it is unable to inhibit bacterial cell wall synthesis except with very high drug concentrations. Consequently, minimum inhibitory concentrations

(MICs) of methicillin increased to high levels that were difficult to achieve.

The term "MRSA" is commonly used but misleading because the bacteria are widely resistant to many antibiotics other than just methicillin. MRSA frequently colonize nasal passages of health care workers and are increasing as a cause of nosocomial infections, especially in critical care units. In addition, the incidence of methicillin-resistant *Staphylococcus epidermidis* [MRSE, often reported as methicillin-resistant Staphylococcus species, non*aureus* (SSNA)] isolates is increasing.

A major reason for concern about infections caused by MRSA and MRSE is that bacteria are now developing resistance to vancomycin, an antibiotic previously used extensively to treat or prevent infections caused by *S. aureus*, *S. epidermidis*, and enterococci. Options to treat these infections are limited and measures to reduce the incidence and prevent spread of methicillin- and vancomycin-resistant organisms are of paramount importance.

| **BOX 13.2** | **Antibiotic-Resistant Staphylococci, Streptococci, and Enterococci** (Continued) |

Penicillin-Resistant *Streptococcus pneumoniae* (Pneumococci)

Penicillin has long been the drug of choice for treating pneumococcal infections caused by *S. pneumoniae* (e.g., community-acquired pneumonia, bacteremia, meningitis, and otitis media). However, penicillin-resistant strains and multidrug-resistant strains are being identified with increasing frequency. Risk factors for the development of resistant strains include frequent antibiotic use and prophylactic use of antibiotics. After resistant strains have developed, they spread to other people, especially in areas where people are in close contact such as in children's daycare centers and in hospital settings.

S. pneumoniae are thought to develop resistance to penicillin by decreasing the ability of their PBPs to bind with penicillin. Bacteria displaying high-level penicillin resistance may also be cross-resistant to drugs from the same or similar antibiotic classes. To decrease the spread of resistant *S. pneumoniae,* the Centers for Disease Control and Prevention (CDC) have proposed:

- Improved surveillance to delineate prevalence by geographic area and assist clinicians in choosing appropriate antimicrobial therapy.
- Rational use of antibiotics to reduce exposures to drug-resistant pneumococci. For example, prophylactic antibiotic therapy for otitis media may increase colonization and infection of young children with drug-resistant organisms.
- Pneumococcal vaccination for people older than 2 years of age with increased risk of pneumococcal infection, and for all people older than 65 years of age.

Vancomycin-Resistant Enterococci (VRE)

Enterococci are a component of normal intestinal flora that can act as pathogens if they infect other areas of the body. Vancomycin is an antibiotic that was commonly used to treat these bacteria; however, in large part to the widespread use of vancomycin to treat other drug-resistant staphylococcal infections such as MRSA and MRSE, VRE have emerged. Additionally, some strains of enterococci have developed additional resistance to other antibiotics. The incidence of multidrug-resistant enterococci and VRE has increased in recent years.

To decrease the spread of VRE, the CDC recommends limiting the use of vancomycin. Specific recommendations include avoiding or minimizing its use in routine surgical prophylaxis, empiric therapy for febrile patients with neutropenia (unless the prevalence of MRSA or MRSE is high), systemic or local prophylaxis for intravascular catheter infection or colonization, selective decontamination of the gastrointestinal tract, eradication of MRSA colonization, primary treatment of antibiotic-associated colitis, and routine prophylaxis for very low-birth-weight infants or patients on continuous ambulatory peritoneal dialysis. Thorough hand hygiene and environmental cleaning are also important, because VRE can survive for long periods on hands, gloves, stethoscopes, and environmental surfaces. Personnel must remove or change gloves after contact with patients known to be colonized or infected with VRE. Ideally, designated stethoscopes are restricted for use only with VRE-infected patients. If stethoscopes must be used for both VRE-infected and uninfected patients, it is important to thoroughly clean stethoscopes between patients.

---

often require more toxic and expensive drugs, leading to prolonged illness or hospitalization and increased mortality rates.

Interestingly, antibiotic overuse can contribute to antibiotic resistance. Resistant organisms are especially likely to emerge in critical care units and large hospitals where seriously ill patients often require extensive antibiotic therapy. The constant presence of antibiotics provides an environment conducive to the survival of the fittest bacteria, which is facilitated by killing of microorganisms that might ordinarily serve to keep these bacteria in check. Furthermore, because pathogenic microorganisms are often spread by contaminated hands or objects, patients in critical care units are more at risk for infection with antibiotic-resistant organisms resulting from person-to-person transmission by health care workers or equipment.

Resistant organisms and the antibiotics to which they develop resistance vary in geographic areas, communities, and hospitals according to the use of particular antibiotics. Nationally, resistant bacterial strains of major concern include penicillin-resistant *Streptococcus pneumoniae*, methicillin-resistant *Staphylococcus aureus* (MRSA) and *Staphylococcus epidermidis*, vancomycin-resistant enterococcus (VRE), extended-spectrum beta-lactamase (ESBL)-producing gram-negative bacilli, and multidrug-resistant tuberculosis (MDR-TB). All of these organisms are resistant to multiple antibiotics. The first four are described in Box 13.2, and MDR-TB is discussed in Chapter 20. Viruses and fungi also develop resistance to antimicrobial drugs, as discussed in Chapters 21 and 22, respectively.

QSEN Safety Alert

It is essential to monitor patients receiving antibiotics closely for evidence of improvement. A failure to improve within 24 to 36 hours could indicate antibiotic resistance.

NCLEX Success

3. When a woman who is taking an antibiotic develops a thick, white, curd-like vaginal discharge with pruritus, the nurse suspects that the patient has a vaginal yeast infection. What would explain this development?

   A. A drug for a fungal infection should have been prescribed instead of a drug for bacterial infection.
   B. The antibiotic has altered the normal vaginal environment.
   C. The antibiotic that was prescribed was not effective.
   D. Yeast infections are side effects of antibiotics.

4. A health care worker has nasal colonization of methicillin-resistant *Staphylococcus aureus* (MRSA). Which interpretation of this finding by the nurse is correct?

   A. The health care worker has a nasal infection caused by MRSA.
   B. The health care worker poses a danger to patients.
   C. The health care worker is immune to MRSA.
   D. The health care worker produces beta-lactamase.

Clinical Application 13-4

- Despite taking care to prevent an infection, Ms. Warren becomes ill and develops a fever with other signs and symptoms of an infection. The family nurse practitioner asks her what infectious illnesses her assigned patients have had and whether she has had direct contact with these patients. The nurse also asks if any of her friends or family members have been ill. What rationale underlies the nurse's questions?

Mechanisms of Antibiotic Resistance in Bacteria

Bacterial resistance to antimicrobial drugs may be either intrinsic or acquired.

The five main processes of intrinsic mechanisms of resistance are outlined below:

1. Bacteria may inactivate the antibiotic. For example, some bacteria produce enzymes that change the chemical structure of certain antibiotics, thus rendering them ineffective.
2. Bacteria may modify target sites for the antibiotic. For example, **penicillin-binding proteins** (PBPs) are bacterial proteins that function in cell wall synthesis. Penicillin typically binds to these bacterial proteins. By altering the PBPs, the bacteria prevent the antibiotic from recognizing and engaging this target.
3. Bacteria may alter metabolic pathways or substitute the usual enzymes needed to carry out activities involved with growth and reproduction. In doing this, bacteria develop resistance to antibiotics that exert their effect by interfering with enzymes needed for growth and reproduction.
4. Bacteria may alter their cell wall structure to reduce permeability. This confers resistance to antibiotics that must enter the bacterial cell to attach to a target.
5. Some bacteria have the ability to pump drug molecules out of the cell (efflux). By removing the antibiotic, the bacteria prevent the antibiotic from engaging the target site and exerting an effect.

The mechanisms of acquired resistance include genetic alterations. The three processes of acquired resistance are as follows:

1. In gene transfer, bacteria are in close approximation to then transfer to genetic content. For example, bacteria with inherent mechanisms for antibiotic resistance may transfer genetic content material that confers this antibiotic resistance to other species of bacteria. When these genetically altered bacteria replicate, the resistance is passed on to subsequent generations of bacteria.
2. In transfer mutations, the mutations often develop during bacterial replication. If the mutation provides antibiotic resistance, the mutated bacteria can continue to multiply and thus produce billions of copies of resistant microorganisms.
3. Selective pressure, or natural selection, refers to the survival of the fittest bacteria. When antibiotic therapy is initially begun, the weakest bacteria are killed first while the strongest bacteria, which are best able to withstand

the effects of antibiotic therapy, remain. If antibiotic therapy is stopped prematurely before these more resistant microorganisms are overcome, the more resistant organisms predominate. These mechanisms explain why, when a new antibiotic is used, resistance may rapidly appear and be disseminated to multiple bacteria.

Clinical Manifestations

The clinical manifestations of infections are outlined in Box 13.2.

Drug Therapy

Several terms are used to describe drugs that are used to treat infections caused by microorganisms. **Anti-infective**, like antimicrobial, is a general descriptive terms that designate agents with antibacterial, antiviral, and antifungal properties. **Antibacterial** is a term that designates agents that kill bacteria or interfere with the ability of bacteria to grow and replicate. An antibiotic is a drug that has the ability to kill or inhibit bacterial growth and replication; therefore, an antibiotic is an antibacterial drug. Antibiotics are used to treat bacterial infections.

Both antiviral and antifungal drugs are agents that have the ability to destroy or inhibit the replication of viruses or fungi, respectively. Antiviral drugs are used to treat viral infections, and antifungal drugs are used to treat fungal infections.

Additional terms are used to describe properties of antibacterial drugs. **Broad-spectrum** antibiotics are antibacterial drugs that are effective against a wide range of bacteria (e.g., both gram-positive and gram-negative bacteria), whereas narrow-spectrum antibiotics are those that are effective against a limited range or a specific type of bacteria. Generally, a narrow-spectrum antibiotic is preferred over a broad-spectrum antibiotic when possible because broad-spectrum drugs are more likely to kill some normal flora, which disrupts the microbial balance. As a result, the patient is at greater risk for an opportunistic infection when taking a broad-spectrum antibiotic. The action of an antibacterial drug is usually described as **bactericidal** (kills the bacteria) or **bacteriostatic** (inhibits growth of the bacteria). Whether a drug is bactericidal or bacteriostatic often depends on its concentration at the infection site and the sensitivity of the bacteria to the drug. Because successful treatment with bacteriostatic antibiotics depends on the ability of the host's immune system to eliminate the inhibited bacteria, bactericidal drugs are preferred in serious infections, especially in people with impaired immune function.

Antimicrobials are among the most frequently used drugs worldwide. Their success in saving lives and decreasing severity and duration of infectious diseases has encouraged their extensive use. Unfortunately, these same attributes have led to antibiotic overuse, misuse, or abuse. Inappropriate use of antibiotics is responsible for unnecessary adverse drug effects, emergence of drug-resistant microorganisms, and increases in health care costs. All health care professionals should note that the goal of treatment with antibiotics is to eradicate the causative microorganism and return the host to full physiologic functioning. This differs from the goal of most drug therapy, which is

BOX 13.3   Patient Teaching Guidelines for Antimicrobial Drugs

General Considerations

■ Wash hands often and thoroughly, especially before preparing food or eating and after exposure to body secretions (e.g., urine, feces, sputum, nasal secretions). This is probably the most effective way to prevent infection and to avoid spreading an infection to others.

■ Eat a balanced diet and get adequate fluid intake, rest, and exercise. This helps the body fight infection, prevents further infection, and increases the effectiveness of antimicrobial drugs by optimizing body processes.

■ Take all prescribed doses of an antimicrobial drug. This prevents recurrence of the infection. Also, stopping antimicrobial drugs when symptoms are relieved can lead to the development of antibiotic-resistant microorganisms that cause infections that are more severe and harder to treat.

■ Report any problems that occur when taking an antimicrobial drug. This allows identification of important adverse effects that can be managed through interventions or through substitution by another equally effective antimicrobial drug.

■ Discard all discontinued antimicrobial drugs. This is important because antimicrobial drugs are carefully selected to treat specific illnesses, so taking inadequate amounts of an inappropriate drug can cause greater harm than benefit.

■ Report any other drugs being taken to the prescriber. This is necessary in order to avoid drug interactions that could have harmful consequences.

■ Report any drug allergies to all health care providers and wear a medical identification emblem that lists allergens. This is necessary to ensure that the antimicrobial drug ordered is safe.

■ Notify the prescriber if you are pregnant. This is important because some antimicrobial drugs can cause problems for the developing fetus.

■ Be aware that antibiotics are not indicated for treatment of viral infections. If an antibiotic is not indicated, taking it may result in more harm than good.

Self-Administration

■ Take antimicrobial drugs at evenly spaced intervals around the clock, unless instructed otherwise. This helps maintain adequate blood levels.

■ Ask if the antimicrobial drug can be taken with food. This is important because food may decrease drug absorption for some oral antimicrobials; therefore, these are taken on an empty stomach, approximately 1 hour before or 2 hours after meals.

■ Store most liquid preparations in the refrigerator, check expiration dates, and discard any that remains after all prescribed doses have been taken. This is important to ensure that the medicine remains stable and is evenly dispersed in solution.

■ Take the medications with a full glass of water. This helps tablets and capsules to dissolve better in the stomach and decreases stomach irritation.

■ Report nausea, vomiting, diarrhea, skin rash, recurrence of symptoms for which the antimicrobial drug was prescribed, or signs of new infection (e.g., fever, cough, sore mouth, drainage) to a health care professional. These problems may indicate adverse effects of the drug, lack of therapeutic response to the drug, or another infection. Any of these requires evaluation and may indicate changes in drug therapy.

---

to relieve signs and symptoms rather than cure the underlying disorder.

Guidelines to promote more appropriate use of antimicrobial drugs include

- Avoid the use of antibacterial drugs to treat viral infections; antibacterial drugs are ineffective in viral infections.
- Give antibacterial drugs only when a significant bacterial infection is diagnosed or strongly suspected or when there is an established indication for prophylaxis.
- Use a narrow-spectrum antibacterial drug instead of a broad-spectrum drug, whenever possible, in order to decrease the risk of a superinfection.
- Collect specimens (e.g., sputum, urine) for culture and Gram's stain before giving the first dose of an antibiotic. For best results, specimens must be collected accurately and taken directly to the laboratory. If analysis is delayed, contaminants may overgrow pathogenic microorganisms.
- Minimize antimicrobial drug therapy for fever unless other clinical manifestations or laboratory data indicate infection.
- Follow recommendations of the Centers for Disease Control and Prevention (CDC) for prevention and treatment of infections, especially those caused by drug-resistant organisms (e.g., gonorrhea, penicillin-resistant streptococcal infections, MRSA, VRE, MDR-TB).

- Consult infectious disease physicians, infection control nurses, and infectious disease pharmacists about local patterns of drug-resistant organisms and treatment of complicated infections.

Box 13.3 presents patient teaching guidelines for antimicrobials.

Empiric Therapy

Because laboratory tests used to definitively identify causative organisms and to determine susceptibility to antibiotics usually require 48 to 72 hours, the prescriber usually initiates treatment with an antimicrobial drug that is likely to be effective. Drug therapy undertaken prior to obtaining a definite diagnosis is called empiric therapy. This empiric therapy is based on an informed estimate of the most likely pathogen(s) given the patient's signs and symptoms and the site of infection, as well as knowledge of communicable diseases currently infecting other people in the community. For example, urinary tract infections are often caused by *E. coli*; thus, an antibiotic that is effective against this microorganism is indicated.

Culture and Sensitivity Studies

Culture identifies the causative microorganism. Once a specific microorganism is identified by laboratory culture, it is important to determine **susceptibility**, which is the vulnerability of the bacteria to the effects of an antibiotic. Susceptibility tests determine which drugs are likely to be effective against the organism. Laboratory reports indicate whether the organism is susceptible (S) or resistant (R) to the tested drugs. It is then possible to "match the drug to the bug."

One indication of susceptibility is the minimum inhibitory concentration (MIC). The MIC is the lowest concentration of an antibiotic that prevents visible growth of microorganisms. Some laboratories report MIC instead of, or in addition to, S or R.

Susceptible organisms have low or moderate MICs that can be attained by giving usual doses of an antimicrobial agent. For the drug to be effective, its serum and tissue concentrations should usually exceed the MIC of an organism for a certain period. By how much and for how long drug concentrations need to exceed the MIC depend on the drug class and the bacterial species. Some antibiotics may be given for shorter lengths of time as a result of a postantibiotic effect, a persistent effect of an antimicrobial on bacterial growth after brief exposure of the organisms to a drug.

Resistant organisms have high MICs and may require higher concentrations of drug than can be achieved in the body. In some cases, the minimum bactericidal concentration (MBC) is reported, indicating no growth of the organism in the presence of a particular antibiotic. The MBC is especially desirable for infected hosts with impaired immune functions.

A patient's response to antimicrobial therapy cannot always be correlated with the MIC of an infecting pathogen. Thus, reports of drug susceptibility testing must be applied in the context of the site of infection, the characteristics of the drug, and the clinical status of the patient.

NCLEX Success

5. **When a patient fails to respond to an antibiotic, the nurse suspects antibiotic resistance. Which mechanism of resistance does the nurse recognize as an example of acquired antibiotic resistance?**

   A. Alterations are made in the bacterial cell wall structure to make it less permeable.
   B. Bacteria exchange genetic content that transfers resistance from one bacterial strain to another.
   C. Efflux is used to extrude bacteria from within the bacterial cell.
   D. Metabolic pathways are altered so bacteria targeting a specific enzyme of the metabolic pathway are ineffective.

6. **A patient who is taking an antibiotic for an infection shows no signs of improvement. When a laboratory report indicates that the causative organism is not susceptible to the prescribed antibiotic, what is the priority nursing action?**

   A. Notify the pharmacist to provide a different antibiotic.
   B. Notify the prescriber of the laboratory results.
   C. Stop the current antibiotic and use the susceptible antibiotic.
   D. Inform the patient that the antibiotic is ineffective.

7. **What is the best action a nurse can take to prevent infection?**

   A. Instruct patients with respiratory illnesses on proper pulmonary hygiene.
   B. Recommend influenza and pneumococcal vaccines to patients older than 65 years of age.
   C. Teach a patient the importance of adequate nutrition and rest.
   D. Wash hands before and after each patient contact.

Clinical Application 13-5

- Ms. Warren has been exposed to numerous infections both in the community and in the hospital setting. The nurse practitioner decides to treat her initially with a broad-spectrum antibiotic until it is possible to determine the causative agent. Why does the nurse select a broad-spectrum antibiotic?

Patterns of Antibiotic Resistance

Over time, patterns of antibiotic resistance change in the community and in health care facilities; therefore, continuing efforts must be made to identify which antibiotics are most effective. Bacteria that are resistant to certain antibiotics are typically susceptible to others. Infectious disease specialists and laboratory personnel are helpful resources to identify resistance patterns and trends in these instances, and this information may be considered when deciding empiric therapy.

Ability to Penetrate Infected Tissues

Several antimicrobials are effective in urinary tract infections because they concentrate in the urine. However, the choice of an effective antimicrobial drug may be limited in infections of the brain, eyes, gallbladder, or prostate gland because many drugs are unable to reach therapeutic concentrations in these tissues. For infection in these areas, the prescriber will consider the ability of the drug to penetrate the affected region rather than deciding therapy based solely on susceptibility testing.

Toxicity and Risk-to-Benefit Ratio

In general, the least toxic drug is used; however, for serious infections, drugs with an increased risk of toxicity may be necessary. In these instances, the prescriber will weigh the benefits of treatment versus the risks of adverse effects when determining therapy.

Cost

It is always necessary to take the cost of the medication into account. If a less expensive drug is likely to be effective in a given infection, it is recommended instead of a more expensive agent. For hospitals and nursing homes, personnel costs relating to preparation and administration are also important to consider. For example, for the patient who cannot swallow tablets, a liquid preparation may be less expensive to prepare than a tablet that needs to be crushed.

Combination Therapy

Antimicrobial drugs are often used in combination. Indications for combination therapy may include

- Infections caused by multiple microorganisms (e.g., abdominal and pelvic infections)
- Nosocomial infections, which may be caused by many different organisms
- Serious infections in which a combination of antimicrobial drugs is synergistic
- Likely emergence of drug-resistant organisms if a single drug is used (e.g., in tuberculosis)
- Fever or other signs of infection in patients whose immune system is suppressed. Combinations of antibacterial plus antiviral and/or antifungal drugs may be needed

EVIDENCE-BASED PRACTICE

General Principles of Antimicrobial Therapy

by SURBHI LEEKHA, MBBS, CHRISTINE L. TERRELL, MD, RANDALL S. EDSON, MD

http://www.mayoclinicproceedings.com
Mayo Clinic Proceedings
February 2011, 86(2), 156–167
Retrieved March 29, 2011

The judicious use of antimicrobial therapy is a key factor in the prevention of bacterial resistance. The Infectious Disease Society of America has established evidence-based practice guidelines that stipulate what therapy is appropriate for specific infectious disease syndromes as well as infections. The prescriber must collect diagnostic specimens, including culture and sensitivity, prior to beginning antimicrobial therapy. If a community-acquired or nosocomial infection is suspected, the patient should be administered a broad-spectrum antimicrobial agent until the culture and sensitivity reports are available. The broad-spectrum antimicrobial agent is the initial step in empiric therapy. When the etiologic pathogen and susceptible drug are identified, it is important to narrow the spectrum of antimicrobial therapy. Thus, it is imperative for the prescriber to obtain an accurate diagnosis, determine the need and timing of the antimicrobial therapy, understand the effects of antimicrobial activity, utilize narrow-spectrum agents with the shortest duration, and switch from parenteral to oral agents as soon as possible.

IMPLICATIONS FOR NURSING PRACTICE: The nurse's familiarity with these treatment guidelines enhances patient safety and assists in preventing bacterial resistance.

The Nursing Process

Assessment

- Assess for inflammation and infection.
- The general signs and symptoms of infection are the same as for inflammation. Local signs of inflammation include redness, heat, edema, and pain; systemic signs include fever and leukocytosis.
- Inflammation is the normal response to any injury and infection requires the presence of a microorganism. The two often occur together. Inflammation may weaken the tissue, allowing microorganisms to invade and cause infection. Infection (tissue injury by microorganisms) arouses inflammation.
- Assess for the presence of factors that increase the risk for infection.
- Assess culture and sensitivity reports for appropriate antibacterial therapy.
- Assess for drug allergies. If the patient has allergies, assess for the specific signs and symptoms.
- Assess baseline renal and hepatic function.

Nursing Diagnoses

- Fatigue related to infection
- Pain related to inflammation
- Activity intolerance related to infection
- Diarrhea related to antimicrobial therapy
- Imbalanced nutrition: less than body requirements related to anorexia, nausea, and vomiting associated with antimicrobial therapy
- Risk of injury related to infection or adverse drug effects
- Risk of infection related to emergence of drug-resistant microorganisms
- Deficient knowledge related to strategies to prevent infection

Planning/Goals

The patient will

- Adhere to anti-inflammatory medication regime as ordered.
- Receive antimicrobial drugs accurately when given by health care providers or caregivers.
- Take drugs as prescribed and for the length of time prescribed when self-administered as an outpatient.
- Experience decreased inflammation, fever, white blood cell (WBC) count, and other signs and symptoms of infection.
- Be monitored regularly for therapeutic and adverse drug effects.
- Receive prompt recognition and treatment of potentially serious adverse effects.
- Verbalize and practice measures to prevent future infections.
- Be safeguarded against nosocomial infections by health care providers.

Nursing Interventions

The nurse will

- Instruct the patient regarding the administration of anti-inflammatory agents and risk for infection with corticosteroid therapy.
- Use measures to prevent and minimize the spread of infection.

- Implement good hand hygiene. This is probably the most effective method of preventing infections.
- Support natural defense mechanisms by promoting general health measures (e.g., nutrition, adequate fluid intake, rest, exercise).
- Keep the patient's skin clean and dry because the skin harbors large numbers of microorganisms. Also, take care to prevent trauma to the skin and mucous membranes because damaged tissues are susceptible to infection.
- Treat all body fluids (e.g., blood, aspirates from abdomen or chest) and body substances (e.g., sputum, feces, urine, wound drainage) as infectious. Major elements of standard precautions to prevent transmission of pathogens include wearing gloves when likely to be exposed to body fluids and thorough hand hygiene when the gloves are removed. Wear protective eyewear when a risk of spatter is present.
- Implement isolation procedures appropriately, when indicated.
- To prevent spread of respiratory infections, teach patients to cough into the bend of their elbow instead of covering their mouth or nose with hands or tissues. Advise patients to avoid crowds when they are ill.
- To prevent the likelihood that patients will acquire infections, advise them to avoid crowds during influenza season (approximately November through February) and when other communicable diseases are spreading through the local community. Recommend an annual influenza vaccine and pneumococcal vaccine (see Chap. 10) to high-risk populations (e.g., people with chronic diseases such as diabetes and heart, lung, or renal problems; older adults; health care personnel who are likely to be exposed).
- Assist or instruct patients at risk about pulmonary hygiene measures to prevent accumulation or promote removal of respiratory secretions. These measures include ambulating, turning, coughing and deep-breathing exercises, and incentive spirometry.
- Use sterile technique when changing any dressing. If a wound is not infected, sterile technique helps prevent infection. If the wound is already infected, sterile technique avoids introducing new bacteria. Remove dressings with clean gloves, discard them in a moisture-proof bag, and wash hands before putting on sterile gloves to apply the new dressing.
- To minimize the spread of infections, adhere to current established guidelines published by the CDC for isolation precautions to prevent transmission of infectious agents in health care settings.
- For patients with infections, monitor temperature for increased or decreased fever and monitor the WBC count for changes.
- For patients receiving antimicrobial therapy, maintain an adequate fluid intake to assist with renal clearance to decrease drug toxicity.
- Assist the patient with hand hygiene, maintaining nutrition and fluid balance, getting adequate rest, and handling secretions correctly. These measures help the body to fight the infection, prevent further infection, and enhance the effectiveness of antimicrobial medications.
- Assist patients in using antimicrobial drugs safely and effectively.
- Instruct patient on all aspects of medication administration.

Evaluation

- Assess the patient's adherence to medication administration.
- Assess for adverse drug effects.
- Assess for decreasing signs and symptoms of infection and inflammation.
- Assess patient's understanding of patient teaching regarding antimicrobial medications and anti-inflammatory agents.

Key Concepts

- Inflammation is the cellular response of the body to injury by chemicals, physical trauma, or infectious agent.
- Aspirin, NSAIDs, and corticosteroids are administered to decrease inflammation.
- Aspirin and NSAIDs block the synthesis of prostaglandin in the central and peripheral nervous system.
- Corticosteroids inhibit interleukin-1, cytokines, and the tumor necrosis factor.
- Normal flora has a beneficial role in the human host but can become pathogenic if they invade a normally sterile part of the body or if environmental controls fail to limit their growth.
- Infection occurs when growth of microbial pathogens causes injury to host tissues.
- Opportunistic infections occur when harmless microorganisms in normal flora become pathogenic under conditions that are favorable for their overgrowth.
- Community-acquired infections are infections caused by microorganisms from a community setting outside of a health care facility, whereas nosocomial infections are infections acquired from microorganisms in hospitals and other health care facilities.
- Hospitals and other health care facilities are places where there is an increased prevalence of antibiotic-resistant bacteria, which are increasing in prevalence, are associated with prolonged illness and hospitalization and increased mortality rates, have become a public concern.
- Bacterial mechanisms of antibiotic resistance include inactivation of an antibiotic, modification of target cells for antibiotics, alteration of metabolic pathways, alteration of bacterial cell wall

structure, and efflux. These mechanisms may be passed to other classes of bacterial through gene transfer.

- Human defenses against infection include intact skin and mucous membranes, secretions that inhibit bacterial growth, mechanical movements such as coughing, and immune and inflammatory responses; when defenses are compromised, the risk of infection increases.

- Antimicrobial drugs are an important intervention to treat infections that could otherwise cause significant injury and harm to the human host.

- Antibacterial drugs are a type of antimicrobial drug that is used to treat bacterial infections; these are commonly called antibiotics.

- Antibiotics are generally not indicated for viral infections, fungal infections, and other infections not caused by bacteria.

- Broad-spectrum antibiotics are effective against a wide range of bacteria. Narrow-spectrum antibiotics are effective against a limited range of bacteria.

- Bactericidal antibiotics kill bacteria, and bacteriostatic antibiotics inhibit bacterial growth and reproduction.

- Antibiotics exert an effect by inhibiting bacterial metabolism, inhibiting cell wall synthesis, inhibiting protein synthesis, or inhibiting nucleic acid function or synthesis.

- Decisions regarding antimicrobial selection are based on several factors, including the causative organism, site of infection, risk-to-benefit ratio, and cost.

- Combination therapy is used to treat multiple microorganism

Critical Thinking Questions

13-1. A 3-year-old boy is diagnosed with streptococcal pharyngitis ("strep throat"). An antibiotic suspension of 125 mg/5 mL is prescribed at a dose of 125 mg twice a day for 7 days. You are providing patient teaching to the parents. They are to administer 5 mL every 8 hours.

- The mother states she does not know what milliliters are. How will you instruct her on the medication administration?

- You instruct the parents on the importance of finishing the entire amount of medication and to never skip a dose. What is the purpose of this teaching?

- The mother asks if she can give the medication to the child's sister for prevention of a "strep throat." What patient teaching will need to be implemented with the mother?

- The parents return in 1 week and say that because the child was feeling better after 3 days, they stopped the medication. What is the child at risk for developing?

References and Resources

Aspinall, S. L., Good, C. B., Metlay, J. P., Mor, M. K., & Fine, M. J. (2009). Antibiotic prescribing for presumed nonbacterial acute respiratory tract infections. *American Journal of Emergency Medicine, 27*(5), 544–551.

Centers for Disease Control and Resistance (CDC). (2010, March 12). *Antimicrobial resistance in healthcare settings.* Retrieved from http://www.cdc.gov/ncidod/dhqp/ar.html

Emanuele, P. (2010). Antibiotic resistance. *American Association of Occupational Health Nurses (AAOHN) Journal, 58*(9), 363–365.

Harvey, R. A., & Champe, P. C. (2008). *Lippincott's illustrated reviews: Pharmacology.* Philadelphia, PA: Lippincott Williams & Wilkins.

Jolobe, O. M. (2010). Timely identification of bacterial pathogens may reduce inappropriate antibiotic prescription. *American Journal of Emergency Medicine, 28*(4), 519–520.

Karch, A. M. (2009). *Focus on nursing pharmacology* (5th ed.). Philadelphia, PA: Lippincott Williams & Wilkins.

Karch, A. M. (2011). *2011 Lippincott's nursing drug guide.* Philadelphia, PA: Lippincott Williams & Wilkins.

Katzung, B. G., Masters, S. B., & Trevor, A. J. (2009). *Basic and clinical pharmacology* (11th ed.). New York, NY: McGraw Hill.

Leekha, S., Terrell, C. L., & Edson, R. S. (2011). General principles of antimicrobial therapy, *Mayo Clinic Proceedings, 86*(2), 156–167. Retrieved March 29, 2011 www.mayoclinicproceedings.com

Maclean, R. C., Hall, A. R., Perron, G. G., & Buckling, A. (2010). The evolution of antibiotic resistance: Insight into the roles of molecular mechanisms of resistance and treatment context. *Discovery Medicine, 51.* Retrieved from http://www.discoverymedicine.com/R-Craig-MacLean/2010/08/04/the-evolution-of-antibiotic-resistance-insight-into-the-roles-of-molecular-mechanisms-of-resistance-and-treatment-context

Musher, D. M. (2010). Resistance of Streptococcus pneumonia to the fluoroquinolones, doxycycline, and trimethoprim-sulfamethoxazole. In: A. R. Thorner (Ed.), *UpToDate.* Retrieved from http://www.uptodateonline.com

National Institute of Allergy and Infectious Diseases. (2009, February 18). *Antimicrobial drug resistance.* Retrieved from http://www.niaid.nih.gov/topics/antimicrobialResistance/Understanding/Pages/causes.aspx

Niederman, M. S. (2009). Treatment options for nosocomial pneumonia due to MRSA. [Supplement]. *Journal of Infection, 59,* S25–S31.

Porth, C. M., & Matfin, G. (2009). *Pathophysiology: Concepts of altered health states.* Philadelphia, PA: Lippincott Williams & Wilkins.

14 Drug Therapy to Decrease Pain, Fever, and Inflammation

Clinical Application Case Study

Audrey Mason is a 72-year-old retired physical education teacher and housewife, who is being seen by her primary care provider for bilateral hip and knee pain. She has been taking a minimum of eight 325 mg aspirins per day without pain relief. Her physician orders x-rays of her hips and knees, which reveal osteoarthritis in both joints. She begins taking ibuprofen (Motrin) 600 mg three times per day. In addition, she receives a diagnosis of degenerative joint disease related to osteoarthritis and a referral to an orthopedic surgeon. The surgeon schedules Mrs. Mason for a right total knee replacement in 1 month. Because she is 40 pounds overweight, the surgeon places her on a calorie reduction diet.

Antiprostaglandin: drug that inhibits the synthesis of prostaglandins

Antipyretic: drug that has the ability to lower body temperature

Arachidonic acid: phospholipid released in the cell membrane in response to cellular injury

Cyclooxygenase: enzyme that produces prostaglandins from arachidonic acids

Hyperuricemia: elevated levels of uric acid in the blood resulting from accelerated generation of uric acid through purine metabolism or impaired renal excretion of uric acid

Nonsteroidal anti-inflammatory drug (NSAID): medication that inhibits the synthesis of prostaglandins; used to prevent and treat mild to moderate pain and inflammation

Prostaglandin: chemical mediator found in most body tissues; helps regulate many cell functions and participate in the inflammatory response as well as initiate uterine contractions in labor

Pyrogen: fever-producing agent

Reye's syndrome: potentially fatal disease characterized by encephalopathy and fatty liver accumulations; associated with the use of aspirin and NSAIDs after viral infections such as chickenpox or influenza in children and adolescents

Salicylism: toxic effects of a salicylate drug; may occur with an acute overdose or with chronic use of therapeutic doses, especially the higher doses take for anti-inflammatory effects

Tophi: deposits of uric acid crystals in the joints, kidneys, and soft tissues

Uricosuric: drug that increases urinary excretion of uric acid

Introduction

This chapter provides an introduction to the pharmacological care of the patient who is experiencing pain, fever, or inflammation. The pharmacological agents administered for inflammation can also diminish fever and relieve pain. Acetaminophen also decreases fever and relieve pain, but it does not reduce inflammation. Other topics of discussion will be osteoarthritis and gout, which allows the nurse to apply the knowledge of disease that produces inflammation and the related administration of anti-inflammatory agents to reduce pain. The drugs discussed in this chapter include aspirin (acetylsalicylic acid), acetaminophen, and the **nonsteroidal anti-inflammatory drugs** (NSAIDs), as well as those drugs used to prevent or treat gout.

It is important to note that aspirin, acetaminophen, and NSAIDs can also be called **antiprostaglandins** because they inhibit the synthesis of **prostaglandins**. Prostaglandins are chemical mediators found in most body tissues; they help regulate many cell functions and participate in the inflammatory response. They are formed when cellular injury occurs and phospholipids in cell membranes respond by releasing **arachidonic acid**. Cyclooxygenase (COX) enzymes then metabolize arachidonic acid to produce prostaglandins, which act briefly in the area where they are produced and are then inactivated. The enzyme COX-1 is normally synthesized continuously and is present in all tissues and cell types, especially in platelets and endothelial cells as well as in the gastrointestinal (GI) tract and the kidneys. Prostaglandins produced by COX-1 are important in numerous homeostatic functions and have protective effects on the stomach and kidneys. In the stomach, prostaglandins decrease gastric acid secretion, increase mucus secretion, and regulate blood circulation. In the kidneys, they help maintain adequate blood flow and function. In the cardiovascular system, they help regulate vascular tone (i.e., vasoconstriction and vasodilation) and platelet function. Drug-induced inhibition of these prostaglandins results in the adverse effects associated with aspirin and related nonselective NSAIDs, especially gastric irritation, ulceration, and bleeding. Inhibition of COX-1 activity in platelets may be more responsible for GI bleeding than inhibition of COX-1 activity in gastric mucosa.

COX-2 is also normally present in several tissues (e.g., brain, bone, kidneys, GI tract, female reproductive system). However, it is thought to occur in small amounts or to be inactive until stimulated by pain and inflammation. In inflamed tissues, COX-2 is induced by inflammatory chemical mediators such as interleukin-1 and tumor necrosis factor–alpha. In the GI tract, trauma and *Helicobacter pylori* infection, a common cause of peptic ulcer disease, also induce COX-2. Overall, prostaglandins produced by COX-2 are associated with pain and other signs of inflammation. Inhibition of COX-2 results in the therapeutic effects of analgesia and anti-inflammatory activity. The COX-2 inhibitor drugs are NSAIDs designed to selectively inhibit COX-2 and relieve pain and inflammation with fewer adverse effects than those that inhibit both COX-1 and COX-2, especially stomach damage. However, with long-term use, adverse effects still occur in the GI, renal, and cardiovascular systems.

As indicated in Table 14.1 and Figure 14.1, prostaglandins exert various and opposing effects in different body tissues.

TABLE 14.1		
Prostaglandins		
Prostaglandin	**Locations**	**Effects**
PGD$_2$	Airways, brain, mast cells	Bronchoconstriction
PGE$_2$	Brain, kidneys, vascular smooth muscle, platelets	Bronchodilation Gastroprotection Increased activity of GI smooth muscle Increased sensitivity to pain Increased body temperature Vasodilation
PGF$_2$	Airways, eyes, uterus, vascular smooth muscle	Bronchoconstriction Increased activity of GI smooth muscle Increased uterine contraction (e.g., menstrual cramps)
PGI$_2$ (prostacyclin)	Brain, endothelium, kidneys, platelets	Decreased platelet aggregation Gastroprotection Vasodilation
PGA$_2$ (thromboxane A$_2$)	Kidneys, macrophages, platelets, vascular smooth muscle	Increased platelet aggregation Vasoconstriction

GI, gastrointestinal.

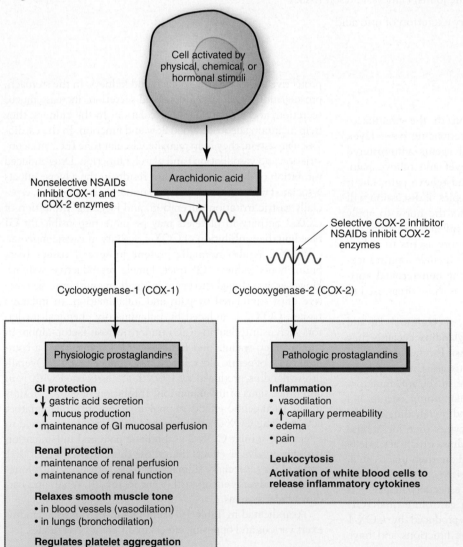

Figure 14.1 Metabolic pathways for arachidonic acid result in production of physiologic and pathologic (i.e., inflammatory prostaglandins). Nonselective and selective nonsteroidal anti-inflammatory drugs (NSAIDs) inhibit production of prostaglandins by inhibiting steps in the arachidonic acid pathway. GI, gastrointestinal.

Overview of Pain, Fever, and Inflammation

To adequately understand the administration of aspirin, acetaminophen, and NSAIDs, it is important to understand the role prostaglandins play in mediating pain, fever, and inflammation.

Pain

Pain is the sensation of discomfort, hurt, or distress. It is a common human ailment and may occur with tissue injury and inflammation. Prostaglandins sensitize pain receptors and increase the pain associated with other chemical mediators of inflammation and immunity, such as bradykinin, histamine, and leukotrienes (Box 14.1).

Fever

Fever is an elevation of body temperature above the normal range. Body temperature is controlled by a regulating center in the hypothalamus. Normally, there is a balance between heat production and heat loss so that a constant body temperature is maintained. When there is excessive heat production, mechanisms to increase heat loss are activated. As a result, blood vessels dilate, more blood flows through the skin, sweating occurs, and body temperature usually stays within normal range.

Fever occurs when the set point of the hypothalamus is raised in response to the presence of **pyrogens** (fever-producing agents). Endogenous pyrogens include cytokines such as interleukin-1, interleukin-6, and tumor necrosis factor (see Box 14.1). Exogenous pyrogens include bacteria and their toxins or other by-products. The upward adjustment of the hypothalamic set point in response to the presence of a pyrogen is mediated by prostaglandin E_2 (see Table 14.1). The body responds to the higher hypothalamic set point by vasoconstriction of blood vessels and shivering, raising the core body temperature to the higher set point. Fever may accompany conditions such as dehydration, inflammation, infectious processes, some drug use, brain injury, or diseases involving the hypothalamus.

Inflammation

Inflammation is the normal body response to tissue damage from any source, and it may occur in any tissue or organ. It is an attempt by the body to remove the damaging agent and repair the damaged tissue. The signs and symptoms of inflammation are the work of a variety of chemical mediators (see Box 14.1). Prostaglandin E_2 and others induce inflammation and also enhance the effects of other mediators of the inflammatory response. Local manifestations are redness, heat, edema, and pain. Redness and heat result from vasodilation and increased blood supply. Edema results from leakage of blood plasma into the area. Pain occurs when pain receptors on nerve endings are stimulated by heat, edema, and pressure; chemicals released by the damaged cells; and prostaglandins. Systemic manifestations include leukocytosis, increased erythrocyte sedimentation rate, fever, headache, loss of appetite, lethargy or malaise, and weakness. Both local and systemic manifestations vary according to the cause and extent of tissue damage. In addition, inflammation may be acute or chronic. See Chapter 13 for more information.

Inflammation may be a component of virtually any illness. Inflammatory conditions affecting organs or systems are often named by adding the suffix "itis" to the involved organ or system (e.g., hepatitis). Current research findings suggest that inflammation may be important in the pathology of disorders (not previously identified as inflammatory conditions) such as heart disease and Alzheimer's disease. Anti-inflammatory drugs are indicated when the inflammatory response is inappropriate, abnormal or persistent, or destroys tissue.

Table 14.2 lists the medications administered in the reduction of pain, fever, and inflammation.

Specific Conditions

OSTEOARTHRITIS

Osteoarthritis produces inflammation and degeneration of joints. To adequately understand the pharmacologic treatment of osteoarthritis, it is important to understand the etiology, pathophysiology, and clinical manifestations of the disease.

Etiology

Aging plays a significant role in the destruction of joints. The degeneration of the articular cartilage begins at approximately 30 years of age and peaks between 50 and 60 years. Primary osteoarthritis occurs without a history of an injury or disease. Secondary osteoarthritis results from a previous injury or the presence of an inflammatory process. Other factors that contribute to the development of osteoarthritis include obesity, repetitive use of a joint, and congenital predisposition.

Pathophysiology

The articular cartilage is the smooth weight-bearing surface at the ends of long bones. The main function of cartilage is to absorb shock and decrease friction during movement and weight-bearing activities. The cartilage transmits the load down to the subchondral bone, dissipating the mechanical stress at the joint. Along with the synovial fluid in the joint, the articular cartilage reduces friction when the joint moves. Osteoarthritis is the degradation of the cartilage, bone, and synovium. Repetitive movement of a joint causes the articular cartilage to be worn down, leading to joint failure. Chondrocytes develop in the joint with the release of enzymes, causing the joint to degenerate. Progressively the articular cartilage is lost, and inflammation develops in the synovial fluid.

Clinical Manifestations

Osteoarthritis produces joint pain, stiffness, and instability, possibly with some degree of immobility. The joints commonly

BOX 14.1   Chemical Mediators of Inflammation and Immunity

Bradykinin is a kinin in body fluids that becomes physiologically active with tissue injury. When tissue cells are damaged, white blood cells (WBCs) increase in the area and ingest damaged cells to remove them from the area. When the WBCs die, they release enzymes that activate kinins. The activated kinins increase and prolong the vasodilation and increased vascular permeability caused by histamine. They also cause pain by stimulating nerve endings for pain in the area. Thus, bradykinin may aggravate and prolong the erythema, heat, and pain of local inflammatory reactions. It also increases mucous gland secretion.

Complement is a group of plasma proteins essential to normal inflammatory and immunologic processes. More specifically, complement destroys cell membranes of body cells (e.g., red blood cells, lymphocytes, platelets) and pathogenic microorganisms (e.g., bacteria, viruses). The system is initiated by an antigen–antibody reaction or by tissue injury. Components of the system (called C1 through C9) are activated in a cascade type of reaction in which each component becomes a proteolytic enzyme that splits the next component in the series. Activation yields products with profound inflammatory effects. C3a and C5a, also called anaphylatoxins, act mainly by liberating histamine from mast cells and platelets, and their effects are therefore similar to those of histamine. C3a causes or increases smooth muscle contraction, vasodilation, vascular permeability, degranulation of mast cells and basophils, and secretion of lysosomal enzymes by leukocytes. C5a performs the same functions as C3a and also promotes movement of WBCs into the injured area (chemotaxis). In addition, it activates the lipoxygenase pathway of arachidonic acid metabolism in neutrophils and macrophages, thereby inducing formation of leukotrienes and other substances that increase vascular permeability and chemotaxis.

In the immune response, the complement system breaks down antigen–antibody complexes, especially those in which the antigen is a microbial agent. It enables the body to produce inflammation and localize an infective agent. More specific reactions include increased vascular permeability, chemotaxis, and opsonization (coating a microbe or other antigen so it can be more readily phagocytized).

Cytokines may act on the cells that produce them, on surrounding cells, or on distant cells if sufficient amounts reach the bloodstream. Thus, cytokines act locally and systemically to produce inflammatory and immune responses, including increased vascular permeability and chemotaxis of macrophages, neutrophils, and basophils. Two major types of cytokines are interleukins (produced by leukocytes) and interferons (produced by T lymphocytes or fibroblasts). Interleukin-1 (IL-1) mediates several inflammatory responses, including fever; IL-2 (also called T-cell growth factor) is required for the growth and function of T lymphocytes. Interferons are cytokines that protect nearby cells from invasion by intracellular microorganisms, such as viruses and rickettsiae. They also limit the growth of some cancer cells.

Histamine is formed (from the amino acid histidine) and stored in most body tissue, with high concentrations in mast cells, basophils, and platelets. Mast cells, which are abundant in skin and connective tissue, release histamine into the vascular system in response to stimuli (e.g., antigen–antibody reaction, tissue injury, and some drugs). After it is released, histamine is highly vasoactive, causing vasodilation (increasing blood flow to the area and producing hypotension) and increasing permeability of capillaries and venules (producing edema). Other effects include contracting smooth muscles in the bronchi (producing bronchoconstriction and respiratory distress), gastrointestinal (GI) tract, and uterus; stimulating salivary, gastric, bronchial, and intestinal secretions; stimulating sensory nerve endings to cause pain and itching; and stimulating movement of eosinophils into injured tissue. Histamine is the first chemical mediator released in the inflammatory response and immediate hypersensitivity reactions (anaphylaxis).

When histamine is released from mast cells and basophils, it diffuses rapidly into other tissues. It then acts on target tissues through both histamine-1 (H_1) and histamine-2 (H_2) receptors. H_1 receptors are located mainly on smooth muscle cells in blood vessels and the respiratory and GI tracts. When histamine binds with these receptors, resulting events include contraction of smooth muscle, increased vascular permeability, production of nasal mucus, stimulation of sensory nerves, pruritus, and dilation of capillaries in the skin. H_2 receptors are also located in the airways, GI tract, and other tissues. When histamine binds to these receptors, there is increased secretion of gastric acid by parietal cells in the stomach mucosal lining, increased mucus secretion and bronchodilation in the airways, contraction of esophageal muscles, tachycardia, inhibition of lymphocyte function, and degranulation of basophils (with additional release of histamine and other mediators) in the bloodstream. In allergic reactions, both types of receptors mediate hypotension (in anaphylaxis), skin flushing, and headache. The peak effects of histamine occur within 1 to 2 minutes of its release and may last as long as 10 minutes, after which it is inactivated by histaminase (produced by eosinophils) or N-methyltransferase.

Leukotrienes, like prostaglandins, are derived from arachidonic acid metabolism. Leukotrienes, identified as LTB_4, LTC_4, LTD_4, and LTE_4, mediate inflammation and immune responses. LTB_4 plays a role in chemotaxis, mediating the aggregation of leukocytes at sites of injury. LTC_4, LTD_4, and LTE_4 produce smooth muscle contractility, bronchospasm, and increased vascular permeability.

Nitric oxide (NO) is synthesized by a variety of cells by the enzyme NO synthase from the amino acid arginine. It readily diffuses across cell membranes, where it reacts with a wide variety of molecules and is inactivated. NO inhibits aggregation of platelets, preventing formation of blood clots. NO relaxes smooth muscles in blood vessels, producing vasodilation. It inhibits inflammation in the walls of blood vessels. NO also plays a role in protecting against invading microbes. Helper T lymphocytes, active in the inflammatory response, secrete NO. NO also enhances the killing of phagocytized microbes within the lysosomes of cells.

Platelet-activating factor (PAF), like prostaglandins and leukotrienes, is derived from arachidonic acid metabolism and has multiple inflammatory activities. It is produced by mast cells, neutrophils, monocytes, and platelets. Because these cells are widely distributed, PAF effects can occur in virtually every organ and tissue. Besides causing platelet aggregation, PAF activates neutrophils, attracts eosinophils, increases vascular permeability, causes vasodilation, and causes IL-1 and tumor necrosis factor–alpha (TNF-alpha) to be released. PAF, IL-1, and TNF-alpha can induce each other's release.

TABLE 14.2

Medications Administered for Pain, Fever, and Inflammation

Drug Class	Prototype	Other Drugs in the Class
Salicylate	Aspirin (acetylsalicylic acid)	Choline magnesium trisalicylate Diflunisal Salicylsalicylic acid (salsalate)
Nonnarcotic analgesic antipyretic	Acetaminophen (Tylenol, paracetamol)	
Nonsteroidal anti-inflammatory drugs (NSAIDs) Propionic acid derivatives	Ibuprofen (Motrin)	Flurbiprofen (Ansaid) Ketoprofen (Oruvail) Naproxen (Naprosyn) Naproxen Sodium (Aleve, Anaprox, Naprelan) Oxaprozin (Daypro)
Oxicam derivatives	Meloxicam (Mobic)	Piroxicam (Feldene)
Acetic acids	Indomethacin (Indocin, Indocin SR)	Diclofenac potassium (Cataflam) Diclofenac sodium (Voltaren, Voltaren XR) Etodolac Ketorolac (Toradol) Nabumetone Sulindac (Clinoril)
Selective COX-2 inhibitor	Celecoxib (Celebrex)	

COX-2, cyclooxygenase-2.

affected by osteoarthritis are the carpometacarpal joint (the distal joint of the hand), metatarsophalangeal joint of the feet, knees, hips, and cervical or lumbar vertebrae. The pain experienced by the patient is related to the inflammation of the synovium. As the synovial fluid increases, the joint capsule becomes stretched and causes irritation to the nerve endings of the periosteum. Joint stiffness is most common on arising, especially on awaking in the morning, and decreases with movement. An impaired joint can limit mobility and cause structural changes.

Drug Therapy

Medications used in the treatment of osteoarthritis include aspirin, acetaminophen, and NSAIDs (see Table 14.2). As previously mentioned, all of these medications produce an analgesic effect and reduce fever. However, only aspirin and the NSAIDs reduce inflammation. As the medications are discussed, their properties will be explained in detail, identifying their use and implications for administration.

Clinical Application 14-1

- In an education session with Mrs. Mason, the nurse employed by Mrs. Mason's insurance provider is instructing her about the pathophysiology of osteoarthritis. What information should the nurse provide?

- What is the rationale for placing Mrs. Mason on a calorie reduction diet?

NCLEX Success

1. A man arrives in the emergency department with a swollen right ankle from a fall. He is complaining of pain and limited mobility. What factor is contributing to the pain in the right ankle?

   A. blocking of cyclooxygenase-1 (COX-1)
   B. blocking of COX-1 and COX-2
   C. release of prostaglandin E_2
   D. release of cytochrome P450

2. A home care nurse is visiting an 88-year-old man, who is taking acetaminophen for arthritic pain in his knees. Which of the following patient teaching statements is most appropriate to implement?

   A. "Acetaminophen will only relieve pain but not the inflammation from arthritis."
   B. "Acetaminophen is appropriate for the treatment of inflammation from arthritis."
   C. "Your primary health care provider should consider a prescription of Vicodin (acetaminophen/hydrocodone)."
   D. "The acetaminophen should be administered on an empty stomach."

3. A patient is admitted to the emergency department with dehydration. Which of the following assessments of the patient's vital signs does the nurse expect to assess?

   A. elevated blood pressure
   B. diminished pulse
   C. diminished respirations
   D. elevated temperature

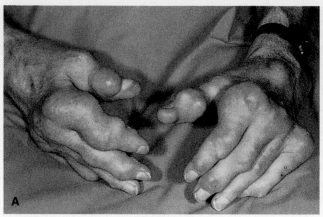
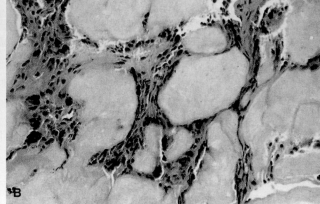

Figure 14.2 Gouty tophi projections.

GOUT

Gout is an arthritic condition characterized by an over-production of uric acid or an inability to excrete uric acid, resulting in **hyperuricemia**. Uric acid is a by-product of purine metabolism. Hyperuricemia occurs when the serum uric acid level exceeds 6.8 mg/dL, the saturation point at which urate crystallizes in biological fluids at normal body temperature (Hilaire & Wozniak, 2010). According to Schub & Pravikoff (2011), there are three stages of gout. Acute gouty arthritis or gouty attack, the first stage, is characterized by hyperuricemia, pain, and swelling of the joints. The pain usually begins at night and persists for 10 days. The most commonly affected joint is the great toe. Intercritical gout, the second stage, is characterized by a symptom-free period of several years followed by the recurrence of symptoms. Chronic tophaceous gout, the third stage, is characterized by the presence of solid deposits of urate crystals, known as **tophi**, in the joints and elsewhere (Fig. 14.2). In the kidneys, urate deposits may form renal calculi or cause other damage. After the first attack of acute gouty arthritis, up to 10 years may pass before permanent damage to the joints and kidneys occurs.

The treatment of gout involves the administration of NSAIDs and corticosteroids (see Chap. 15) to reduce inflammation as well as **uricosuric** agents to increase the elimination of uric acid. Table 14.3 lists the antigout medications and uricosuric agents. These drugs will be discussed later in this chapter.

TABLE 14.3

Medications Administered for Gout

Drug Class	Prototype	Other Drugs in the Class
Mitotic agent	Colchicine (Colcrys)	
Uricosuric	Allopurinol (Zyloprim)	Febuxostat (Uloric) Probenecid

Salicylates

The salicylates, of which ℗ **aspirin** is the prototype, relieve pain by acting both centrally and peripherally to block the transmission of pain impulses. They act peripherally to prevent the sensation of pain receptors to various chemical substances releases by damaged cells. These **antipyretic** agents also reduce fever by acting on the hypothalamus to decrease its response to pyrogens and resetting the body temperature at a lower level. In addition, these drugs diminish inflammation by preventing prostaglandins from increasing the pain and edema produced by other substances released by damaged cells.

Aspirin and other salicylates also have the ability to suppress platelet aggregation. Low-dose aspirin is indicated for patients who have experienced an ischemic stroke, transient ischemic attack, angina, and acute myocardial infarction (or any myocardial infarction), reducing the risk of death and/or a recurrent event (level A recommendations). This indication stems from its antiplatelet activity and resultant effects on blood coagulation (i.e., decreased clot formation). Low-dose aspirin is also be used for primary prevention of myocardial infarction or stroke in healthy adults.

Pharmacokinetics

Aspirin is administered orally or rectally with an onset of action of 5 to 30 minutes orally and 1 to 2 hours rectally. The oral preparation peaks in 15 to 120 minutes, and the duration of action is 3 to 6 hours. The rectal preparation peaks in 4 to 5 hours, and the duration of action is 6 to 8 hours. The drug is metabolized in the liver and has a half-life of 15 minutes to 12 hours. Excretion takes place in the urine. The drug crosses the placenta and enters the breast milk.

Action

The ability of aspirin to inhibit prostaglandins produces the inflammatory effects needed for analgesia and antirheumatic effects. Its antipyretic effects are less well understood. Authorities believe that the drug acts on the thermoregulatory center of the hypothalamus, thus blocking the effects of the endogenous pyrogens and inhibiting the synthesis of prostaglandins. Aspirin also has antiplatelet effects. At low doses, it blocks the synthesis of thromboxane A_2 to inhibit platelet aggregation; this lasts for the life of the platelet.

Use

As an analgesic agent, aspirin is used to relieve mild to moderate pain. As an antipyretic agent, it is used only in adults (see "Use in Children"). As an anti-inflammatory agent, it is used to decrease inflammation in patients with osteoarthritis, juvenile rheumatoid arthritis, and spondyloarthropathies. In addition, aspirin is used for its antiplatelet effects to reduce the risk of transient ischemic attacks and cerebrovascular accidents as well as the risk of death from myocardial infarction. Aspirin, 625 mg, is given to patients who have undergone coronary artery bypass grafting 6 hours after the procedure and daily for 1 year afterward. Table 14.4 presents specific dosage information for aspirin and other salicylates.

Use in Children

Aspirin is not recommended because of its association with **Reye's syndrome**, a life-threatening illness characterized by encephalopathy, hepatic damage, and other serious problems. This syndrome usually occurs after a viral infection, such as influenza or chickenpox, during which aspirin was given for fever.

Use in Older Adults

Aspirin is safe in therapeutic doses for analgesic and antipyretic use. In addition, it is usually safe in the low doses prescribed for prevention of myocardial infarctions and cerebrovascular accidents.

Use in Patients With Renal Impairment

Aspirin is nephrotoxic in high doses, and protein binding of aspirin is reduced in patients with renal failure, which means that blood levels of the active drug are higher than they would be otherwise. Aspirin can also decrease the blood flow in the kidneys by inhibiting the synthesis of prostaglandins that dilate renal

TABLE 14.4

DRUGS AT A GLANCE: Salicylates

Drug	Pregnancy Category	Routes and Dosage Ranges	
		Adults	*Children*
Ⓟ **Aspirin** (acetylsalicylic acid)	D	Pain, fever: PO 325–650 mg every 4 h PRN; usual single dose, 650 mg Osteoarthritis or rheumatoid arthritis: PO 2–6 g/d in divided doses Prophylaxis of myocardial infarction, transient ischemic attack, and cerebrovascular accident: PO 81–325 mg/d Acute rheumatic fever: PO 5–8 g/d, in divided doses Transient ischemic attack: PO 1300 mg/d in divided doses (650 mg twice a day or 325 mg four times a day)	**Do not administer to children with chickenpox or influenza.** **Recommended daily doses by weight:** 24–35 lb (10.6–15.9 kg), 162 mg; 36–47 lb (16–21.4 kg), 243 mg; 48–59 lb (21.5–26.8 kg), 324 mg; 60–71 lb (26.9–32.3 kg), 405 mg; 72–95 lb (32.4–43.2 kg), 486 mg; 96 lb or above (43.3 kg or above), 648 mg Pain, fever: PO 10–15 mg/kg every 4 h, up to 60–80 mg/kg/d Juvenile rheumatoid arthritis: PO 60–110 mg/kg/d, divided doses, every 6–8 h Acute rheumatic fever: PO 100 mg/kg/d, divided doses, for 2 wk, then 75 mg/kg/d for 4–6 wk
Choline magnesium trisalicylate (Tricosal)	C	Arthritis: PO 1.5–2.5 g/d in divided doses; do not exceed 4.5 g/d Pain or fever: PO 2–3 g/d in divided doses	PO 217.5–652.5 mg every 4 h as needed
Diflunisal	C	Osteoarthritis and rheumatoid arthritis: PO 500–1000 mg/d in two divided doses, increased to a maximum of 1500 mg/d if necessary Pain: PO 500–1000 mg initially, then 250–500 mg every 8–12 h	Not recommended for children <12 y of age
Salicylsalicylic acid (salsalate)	C	Osteoarthritis or rheumatoid arthritis: PO 20 mg/d or 10 mg twice daily	Dosage not established

blood vessels. When renal blood flow is normal, these prostaglandins have limited activity. However, when renal blood flow is decreased, synthesis of these prostaglandins is increased, and they protect the kidneys from ischemia and hypoxia by antagonizing the vasoconstrictive effects of angiotensin II, norepinephrine, and other substances. Thus, in patients who depend on prostaglandins to maintain an adequate renal blood flow, the prostaglandin-blocking effects of aspirin result in constriction of renal arteries and arterioles, decreased renal blood flow, decreased glomerular filtration rate, and retention of salt and water.

Adverse Effects

GI adverse effects of aspirin include nausea, dyspepsia, heartburn, and epigastric discomfort. Decreased platelet aggregation results in GI blood loss and hemorrhage. In addition, petechiae and bruising may also occur. Aspirin toxicity occurs at levels above 300 mcg/mL. Acute toxicity results in respiratory alkalosis, hyperpnea, tachypnea, hemorrhage, confusion, pulmonary edema, seizures, tetany, metabolic acidosis, fever, coma, and cardiovascular collapse. Renal and respiratory failure occurs with doses of 20 to 25 g in adults and 4 g in children. **Salicylism**, toxicity due to salicylates that may be associated with chronic use, is characterized by dizziness, tinnitus, difficulty hearing, and mental confusion.

Contraindications

Aspirin is contraindicated in patients with a known sensitivity to aspirin; in those who are allergic to tartrazine, due to a cross-sensitivity; and in those with a known risk of bleeding. The U.S. Food and Drug Administration (FDA) has issued a **BLACK BOX WARNING** ◆ stating that children or teenagers should not take aspirin to treat chickenpox or flu-like symptoms because of the risk of **Reye's syndrome**. This condition is a potentially fatal disease characterized by encephalopathy and fatty liver accumulations. It is associated with the use of aspirin and NSAIDs in children and adolescents after viral infections such as chickenpox or influenza.

Aspirin should be administered cautiously to patients with impaired renal function. Teratogenic effects of aspirin have been reported, and the drug should not be administered during pregnancy. Low-birth-weight infants, increased intracranial bleeding, and stillbirth have been reported in infants of mothers who took aspirin late in pregnancy.

Nursing Implications

Preventing Interactions

Medications and herbs interact with aspirin, increasing or decreasing its effects (Boxes 14.2 and 14.3).

Administering the Medication

Aspirin should be taken with a full glass of water or other fluid and with food or just following food. Administering the medication with food decreases gastric irritation. Although the crushing of tablets or capsules results in faster absorption, this action destroys the long-acting feature and increases the risk of adverse effects and toxicity.

BOX 14.2 **Drug Interactions: Aspirin**

Drugs That Increase the Effects of Aspirin

- Acidifying agents (e.g., vitamin C)
  Acidify urine and thereby decrease the urinary excretion rate of salicylates
- Anticoagulants, oral
  Increase the risk of bleeding; patients taking anticoagulants should not take aspirin.
- Codeine, hydrocodone, oxycodone
  Have additive analgesic effects due to mechanism of action
- Corticosteroids
  Have additive gastric irritation and possible ulcerogenic effects

Drugs That Decrease the Effects of Aspirin

- Alkalinizing agents (e.g., sodium bicarbonate)
  Increase the rate of renal excretion
- Ibuprofen
  Competes with aspirin for COX-1 inhibition
  Negates the cardioprotective benefits of low-dose aspirin
- Misoprostol
  Prevents aspirin-induced gastric ulcers

The dose of aspirin given depends mainly on the condition being treated. Low doses (325 mg initially and 80 mg daily) are used for the drug's antiplatelet effects in preventing arterial thrombotic disorders such as myocardial infarction and stroke. Because aspirin is highly protein bound, lower-than-average doses are needed for patients with low serum albumin levels, because a larger proportion of each dose is free to exert pharmacologic activity. Larger doses are needed for anti-inflammatory effects (maximum daily dosage, 8000 mg) than for analgesic and antipyretic effects (325–650 mg every 4 hours). In general, patients taking low-dose aspirin to prevent myocardial infarction or stroke should continue to take the aspirin if their prescribers order a COX-2–inhibiting NSAID because the COX-2 inhibitors have little effect on platelet function.

Assessing for Therapeutic Effects

When administering aspirin, the nurse assesses for the therapeutic effects of the drug. If aspirin is given for pain, the nurse uses a pain scale to assess the intensity of the patient's pain,

---

BOX 14.3 **Herb and Dietary Interactions: Aspirin**

Herbs and Foods That Increase the Effects of Aspirin

- Alcohol
- Gingko

which should decrease. If the drug is given for fever, the nurse records the patient's temperature every 2 to 4 hours and should see a reduction in temperature. If the drug is given for inflammation, the nurse assesses for signs of inflammation, which should decrease. Patients receiving aspirin as a preventive agent for myocardial infarction or transient ischemic attack should be without chest pain or confusion.

Assessing for Adverse Effects

The nurse assesses the patient for bleeding tendencies, GI irritation, nausea, vomiting, and diarrhea, which all may result from aspirin use. The nurse assesses the skin for signs of decreased coagulation. The nurse performs a thorough pulmonary and integumentary assessment, looking for signs of hypersensitivity to aspirin, including dyspnea, bronchospasm, and rash.

Toxicity: Recognition and Management

Salicylate intoxication (salicylism) may occur with an acute overdose or with chronic use of therapeutic doses, especially the higher doses taken for anti-inflammatory effects. Chronic ingestion of large doses saturates a major metabolic pathway, thereby slowing drug elimination, prolonging the serum half-life, and causing drug accumulation. The therapeutic serum level of salicylate is 100 to 300 mcg/mL for the treatment of arthritis and rheumatic fever. Toxicity occurs at levels above 300 mcg/mL.

As previously stated, salicylism is characterized by dizziness, tinnitus, difficulty hearing, and mental confusion. Additional manifestations include nausea, vomiting, fever, fluid and electrolyte deficiencies, visual changes, drowsiness, hyperventilation, and other conditions. Severe central nervous system (CNS) dysfunction (e.g., delirium, stupor, coma, seizures) indicates life-threatening toxicity.

Treatment of Overdose

In mild salicylate toxicity, stopping the drug or reducing the dose is usually sufficient. In severe salicylate overdose, treatment is symptomatic and aimed at preventing further absorption from the GI tract, increasing urinary excretion, and correcting fluid, electrolyte, and acid–base imbalances. When the drug may still be in the GI tract, gastric lavage and activated charcoal help reduce absorption. Intravenous (IV) sodium bicarbonate produces an alkaline urine in which salicylates are more rapidly excreted, and hemodialysis effectively removes salicylates from the blood. IV fluids are indicated when high fever or dehydration is present. The specific content of IV fluids depends on the serum electrolyte and acid–base status.

Patient Teaching

Box 14.4 presents patient teaching guidelines for aspirin.

Other Drugs in the Class

Diflunisal is a salicylic acid derivative that differs chemically from aspirin. It is reportedly equal or superior to aspirin for mild to moderate pain, rheumatoid arthritis, and osteoarthritis. Compared with aspirin, diflunisal has less antipyretic effect, causes less gastric irritation, and has a longer duration of action.

BOX 14.4   Patient Teaching Guidelines for Aspirin

- Keep aspirin out of the reach of children.
- Use the drug as directed and do not overadminister the medication due to the risk of toxicity.
- Take the medication with food or after meals to prevent stomach upset.
- Do not crush or chew enteric-coated or sustained-release tablets.
- Aspirin is as effective as more costly medication.
- Watch for bleeding, ringing in the ears, or diminished hearing.
- Understand that fever is one way the body fights infection. Taking the medication for fever is not usually recommended unless the fever is high or is accompanied by other symptoms.
- Avoid aspirin for approximately 2 weeks before and after major surgery or dental procedures to decrease the risk of excessive bleeding. If pregnant, do not take aspirin for approximately 2 weeks before the estimated delivery date.
- Inform a health care provider if you have ever had an allergic reaction (e.g., asthma, difficulty breathing, hives), severe gastrointestinal symptoms (e.g., ulcer, bleeding), or rash or other skin disorder after taking aspirin.
- Avoid and minimize ingestion of alcohol due to gastric irritation and risk of bleeding.

Salsalate is a salicylate with antipyretic, analgesic, antirheumatic, and anti-inflammatory properties. It is indicated for relief of pain and fever as well as treatment of rheumatic fever, rheumatoid arthritis, and osteoarthritis. It is absorbed in the small intestine rather than in the stomach and is reported to cause fewer GI adverse effects than aspirin. Onset, peak, and duration of action are similar to aspirin. The drug is metabolized in the liver and excreted in the urine.

Clinical Application 14-2

- Mrs. Mason is taking eight 325 mg aspirin tablets per day without adequate pain relief. She is at risk for what adverse effects associated with aspirin?

NCLEX Success

4. A nurse is teaching a child care class to prospective grandparents. Which of the following medications is contraindicated in children?

   A. ibuprofen
   B. acetaminophen
   C. amoxicillin
   D. aspirin

5. An automobile worker visits an occupational health nurse. He has pain in his right hand due to repetitive movements, for which he has been taking aspirin 650 mg every 2 hours. Which of the following symptoms is indicative of salicylate toxicity?

   A. ringing in the ears
   B. halos around lights
   C. edema
   D. dysrhythmia

6. A physician tells a patient to take aspirin for back pain. It is most important to instruct the patient to

   A. Take the medication on an empty stomach to enhance absorption.
   B. Take the medication after a meal to prevent gastric irritation.
   C. Crush the enteric-coated tablet for increased effectiveness.
   D. Take the medication 2 hours after a meal to enhance absorption.

Nonnarcotic Analgesic Antipyretic: Acetaminophen

Ⓟ **Acetaminophen** (also called APAP, an abbreviation of N-acetyl-p-aminophenol) is a nonprescription drug commonly used as an aspirin substitute because it does not cause nausea, vomiting, or GI bleeding and it does not interfere with blood clotting. It is equivalent to aspirin in analgesic and antipyretic effects; however, it does not have the anti-inflammatory activity of aspirin.

Pharmacokinetics

Acetaminophen is well absorbed with oral administration, and peak plasma concentrations are reached within 30 to 120 minutes. Duration of action is 3 to 4 hours. Acetaminophen is metabolized in the liver (Fig. 14.3). Approximately 94% is excreted in the urine as nontoxic glucuronate and sulfate conjugates, and 2% is excreted unchanged. The remaining 4% is metabolized by cytochrome P450 enzymes to a toxic metabolite, which is normally inactivated by conjugation with glutathione and excreted in the urine. With usual therapeutic doses, a sufficient amount of glutathione is available in the liver to detoxify acetaminophen.

Action

To reduce fever, acetaminophen acts directly on the hypothalamus to increase vasodilation and sweating. To diminish pain, it acts via an unknown mechanism of action.

Use

Acetaminophen is used to reduce fever and decrease minor pain. The drug is sometimes given to children and patients at risk for seizures who are receiving the diphtheria, pertussis, and tetanus immunization to reduce pain and fever; this is an unlabeled use. Table 14.5 presents specific dosage for acetaminophen.

Use in Children

Acetaminophen is usually the drug of choice for pain or fever in children. Children seem less susceptible to liver toxicity than adults, apparently because they form less of the toxic metabolite during metabolism of acetaminophen. However, there is a risk of overdose and hepatotoxicity because acetaminophen is a very common ingredient in over-the-counter (OTC) cold, flu, fever, and pain remedies. An overdose can occur with large doses of one product or smaller amounts of several different products. In addition, toxicity has occurred when parents or caregivers have given the liquid concentration intended for children to infants. The concentrations are different and cannot be given interchangeably. It is necessary to measure infant doses using a dropper and child doses using a teaspoon. The nurse should caution parents and caregivers to ask pediatricians

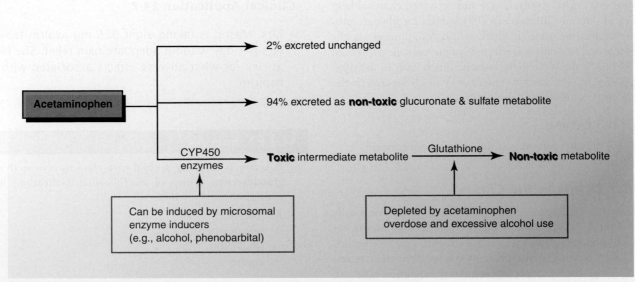

Figure 14.3 Metabolic pathway for acetaminophen. CYP450, cytochrome P450.

TABLE 14.5

DRUGS AT A GLANCE: Acetaminophen

Drug	Pregnancy Category	Routes and Dosage Ranges	
		Adults	Children
(P) **Acetaminophen** (Tylenol)	B	PO or rectal suppository: 325–650 mg every 4–6 h Extended release: 1300 mg every 8 h	Recommended doses by age: PO: 0–3 mo: 40 mg; 4–11 mo: 80 mg; 12–23 mo: 120 mg; 2–3 y: 160 mg; 4–5 y: 240 mg; 6–8 yr: 320 mg; 9–10 y: 400 mg; 11 y: 480 mg Rectal: 3–11 mo: 80 mg every 6 h; 12–36 mo: 80 mg every 4 h; 3–6 y: 120 mg every 4–6 h; 6–12 y: 325 mg every 4–6 h

for written instructions on giving acetaminophen to their children, to read the labels of all drug products very carefully, and to avoid giving children acetaminophen from multiple sources.

Ibuprofen also has antipyretic properties (see subsequent discussion). Alternating acetaminophen and ibuprofen every 4 hours over a 3-day period to control fever in young children (6–36 months of age) has been shown to be more effective than monotherapy with either agent.

Use in Older Adults

The American Geriatric Society recommends acetaminophen be the initial consideration for treatment of middle to moderate pain of musculoskeletal origin (level B). Acetaminophen is usually safe in recommended doses unless liver damage is present or the person is a chronic alcohol abuser.

Use in Patients With Renal Impairment

Acetaminophen is normally metabolized in the liver to metabolites that are excreted by the kidneys, and these metabolites may accumulate in patients with renal failure. In addition, acetaminophen is nephrotoxic in overdose because it forms a metabolite that attacks kidney cells and may cause necrosis.

Use in Patient With Hepatic Impairment

Acetaminophen can cause fatal liver necrosis in overdose because it forms a metabolite that can destroy liver cells. The hepatotoxic metabolite is formed more rapidly when drug-metabolizing enzymes in the liver have been stimulated by ingestion of alcohol, cigarette smoking, and drugs such as antiseizure medications and others. Thus, patients who consume large quantities of alcohol, smoke, and take antiseizure medications are at high risk for hepatotoxicity with usual therapeutic doses.

Use in Patients Receiving Home Care

Home care nurses are responsible for monitoring patients' use of acetaminophen. The drug does have hepatic and renal adverse effects.

Adverse Effects

Hepatotoxicity and renal failure are the most common adverse effects of acetaminophen. Hypersensitivity reactions marked by rash and fever may occur in patients who have developed an allergy to the drug. Myocardial damage may develop in patients

when doses of 5 to 8 g/d are ingested over several weeks or when 4 g/d have been ingested over 1 year.

Contraindications

Contraindications to acetaminophen use include known hypersensitivity to the drug. Caution is necessary with administration in impaired hepatic and renal function. The drug crosses the placenta and enters the breast milk; therefore, caution is also required in pregnancy and lactation.

Nursing Implications

Preventing Interactions

Medications and herbs interact with acetaminophen, increasing or decreasing its effects (Boxes 14.5 and 14.6). It is important to be aware of the interaction of herbal supplements with acetaminophen. Although they do not increase or decrease the effects of acetaminophen, they do place the patient at risk for adverse effects.

Administering the Medication

Acetaminophen is administered orally or by rectal suppository. It is important that the recommended dosage not be exceeded. Acetaminophen should be given with food to reduce GI upset. The recommended maximum daily dose of acetaminophen is 4 g for adults; additional amounts constitute an overdose. Ingestion of an overdose may be accidental or intentional. One contributing factor may be that some people think the drug is so safe that they can take any amount without harm. Another may

BOX 14.5 Drug Interactions: Acetaminophen

Drugs That Increase the Effects of Acetaminophen
■ Carbamazepine, phenytoin, rifampin
  Increase the risk of hepatotoxicity

Drugs That Decrease the Effects of Acetaminophen
■ Carbamazepine, phenytoin, rifampin
  Delay absorption

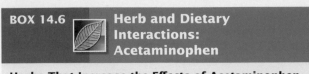

BOX 14.6 **Herb and Dietary Interactions: Acetaminophen**

Herbs That Increase the Effects of Acetaminophen

■ Willow, meadow root
■ Gingko

be that people take the drug in several formulations without calculating or realizing that they are taking potentially harmful amounts. For example, numerous brand names of acetaminophen are available OTC, and acetaminophen is an ingredient in many prescription and OTC combination products (e.g., Percocet; OTC cold, flu, headache, and sinus remedies). For chronic alcohol abusers, short-term ingestion of usual therapeutic doses may cause hepatotoxicity, and it is recommended that these persons ingest no more than 2 g daily. The FDA has issued a warning advising people who ingest three or more alcoholic drinks daily to avoid acetaminophen or to ask a physician before taking even small doses. The FDA also recommends limiting the duration of use (5 days or less in children, 10 days or less in adults, and 3 days in both adults and children when used to reduce fever) unless directed by a physician.

Assessing for Therapeutic Effects

When administering acetaminophen as an antipyretic agent, the nurse assesses for reduced fever. The nurse records the patient's temperature every 2 to 4 hours. When administering the drug as an analgesic, the nurse assesses for decreased pain.

Assessing for Adverse Effects

The most common and severe adverse effect associated with acetaminophen use is hepatotoxicity and hepatic failure. The nurse assesses for jaundice. It is also important to assess urinary output, blood urea nitrogen, and creatinine because of the risk of renal toxicity. In addition, it is critical to assess for a rash or fever because these are the first signs of a hypersensitivity reaction. The nurse assesses a patient who has a past history of myocardial damage and takes acetaminophen daily for chest pain and dyspnea. If the patient develops a rash, he or she should stop taking the drug.

Toxicity: Recognition and Management

Acetaminophen poisoning may occur with a single large dose (possibly as little as 6 g, but usually 10–15 g) or with chronic ingestion of excessive doses (5–8 g/d for several weeks or 3–4 g/d for 1 year). Potentially fatal hepatotoxicity is the main concern and is most likely with doses of 20 g or more. Metabolism of acetaminophen produces a toxic metabolite that is normally inactivated by combining with glutathione. In overdose situations, the supply of glutathione is depleted and the toxic metabolite accumulates and directly damages liver cells (see Fig. 14.1). Acute renal failure may also occur.

Early symptoms (12–24 hours after ingestion) of toxicity are nonspecific (e.g., anorexia, nausea, vomiting, diaphoresis) and may not be considered serious or important enough to report or seek treatment. At 24 to 48 hours, symptoms may subside, but tests of liver function (e.g., aspartate aminotransferase, alanine aminotransferase, bilirubin, prothrombin time) begin to show

increased levels. Later manifestations may include jaundice, vomiting, and CNS stimulation with excitement and delirium, followed by vascular collapse, coma, and death. Peak hepatotoxicity occurs in 3 to 4 days; recovery in nonfatal overdoses occurs in 7 to 8 days.

It is important to obtain plasma acetaminophen levels when an overdose is known or suspected, preferably within 4 hours after ingestion and every 24 hours for several days. Minimal hepatotoxicity is associated with plasma levels of less than 120 µg/mL at 4 hours after ingestion or less than 30 µg/mL at 12 hours after ingestion. With blood levels greater than 300 µg/ milliliter at 4 hours after ingestion, about 90% of patients develop liver damage.

Treatment of Overdose

Gastric lavage is recommended if acetaminophen overdose is detected within 4 hours after ingestion, and activated charcoal can be given to inhibit absorption. In addition, the specific antidote is acetylcysteine (Mucomyst, Acetadote), a mucolytic agent given by inhalation in respiratory disorders. Acetylcysteine may be given orally or intravenously (dosages are listed with other antidotes in Chap. 2). The drug supplies cysteine, a precursor substance required for the synthesis of glutathione. The synthesized glutathione combines with a toxic metabolite and decreases hepatotoxicity. Acetylcysteine is most beneficial if given within 8 to 10 hours of acetaminophen ingestion but may be helpful within 36 hours. It does not reverse damage that has already occurred.

Patient Teaching

Box 14.7 presents patient teaching guidelines for acetaminophen.

NCLEX Success

7. **A toddler is running a fever of 103°F. Which of the following medications is alternated to treat the fever?**

   A. aspirin and acetaminophen
   B. acetaminophen and ibuprofen
   C. naproxen sodium and ibuprofen
   D. aspirin and ibuprofen

8. **Which of the following medications is contraindicated with acetaminophen?**

   A. Percocet
   B. furosemide
   C. phenytoin
   D. ampicillin

BOX 14.7   Patient Teaching Guidelines for Acetaminophen

■ Do not exceed the recommended dosage and do not take any other medications containing acetaminophen.
■ Inform the health care provider of the development of a rash or fever.
■ For better absorption, chew "chewable" tablets and do not swallow them whole.

Nonsteroidal Anti-Inflammatory Drugs

PROPIONIC ACID DERIVATIVES

The propionic acid derivatives are NSAIDs that inhibit prostaglandin synthesis in both the central and peripheral nervous systems. The prototype is Ⓟ **ibuprofen** (Motrin, Advil). The NSAIDs block two enzymes, COX-1 and COX-2.

Pharmacokinetics

Ibuprofen is 80% absorbed in the GI tract. Its onset of action is 1 hour, producing antipyretic effects, reaching a peak in 1 to 2 hours. The duration of action is 6 to 8 hours. Ibuprofen is metabolized in the liver and eliminated in the urine. A small amount of the medication is eliminated in biliary excretion.

Action

Ibuprofen blocks prostaglandin synthesis and modulates T-cell production. It inhibits the inflammatory cells by the process of chemotaxis to destroy the cells of inflammation. It blocks COX-1 and COX-2 but is more selective with COX-1.

Use

Ibuprofen is used to relieve mild to moderate pain, including dysmenorrhea (painful menstruation). It is also used to treat inflammation related to rheumatoid arthritis and osteoarthritis. In addition, it is effective in reducing fever. During initial attacks of acute gout, NSAIDs such as ibuprofen may be administered. Table 14.6 gives dosage information for ibuprofen and the other propionic acid derivatives.

Use in Children

Ibuprofen is recommended for reduction of fever for children older than 6 months of age. As previously stated, it can be alternated with acetaminophen to reduce fever. Children who sustained arm fractures received significant pain relief with ibuprofen compared with those who received acetaminophen with codeine (Medical College of Wisconsin, 2009).

Use in Older Adults

Ibuprofen is relatively safe in therapeutic doses for occasional use as an analgesic or antipyretic in older people. The incidence of musculoskeletal disorders such as osteoarthritis is higher in older adults. However, the nurse should ensure that older adults taking ibuprofen on a long-term basis are evaluated for GI blood loss, renal dysfunction, edema, hypertension, and drug–drug or drug–drug disease interactions. A gastroprotective agent is recommended for patients at risk for upper GI bleeding.

Use in Patients With Renal Impairment

Ibuprofen can cause or aggravate renal impairment even though it is eliminated mainly by hepatic metabolism. By inhibiting prostaglandins that dilate renal blood vessels, it can decrease the blood flow in the kidneys. When renal blood flow is normal, the activity of these prostaglandins is limited.

However, when renal blood flow is decreased, synthesis of these prostaglandins is increased, and they protect the kidneys from ischemia and hypoxia by antagonizing the vasoconstrictive effects of angiotensin II, norepinephrine, and other substances. Thus, in patients who depend on prostaglandins to maintain an adequate renal blood flow, the prostaglandin-blocking effects of ibuprofen result in constriction of renal arteries and arterioles, decreased renal blood flow, decreased glomerular filtration rate, and retention of salt and water. Ibuprofen can also cause kidney damage by other mechanisms, including a hypersensitivity reaction that leads to acute renal failure, manifested by proteinuria, hematuria, and pyuria. Biopsy reports usually indicate inflammatory reactions such as glomerulonephritis or interstitial nephritis.

People at highest risk from the use of ibuprofen and related drugs are those with preexisting renal impairment; those older than 50 years of age; those taking diuretics; and those with hypertension, diabetes, or heart failure. Measures to prevent or minimize renal damage include avoiding nephrotoxic drugs when possible, treating the disorders that increase risk of renal damage, stopping the ibuprofen if renal impairment occurs, monitoring renal function, reducing dosage, and maintaining hydration.

Use in Patients With Hepatic Impairment

Ibuprofen is metabolized in the liver, requiring that the dosage of the medication be decreased in patients with hepatic problems. The maximum daily dosage of ibuprofen in patients with hepatitis is 2 g.

Use in Patients With Critical Illness

The FDA has issued a **BLACK BOX WARNING** ◆ Ibuprofen is contraindicated for the treatment of perioperative pain after coronary artery bypass graft.

Use in Patients Receiving Home Care

It is important for the home care nurse to instruct the patient about all aspects of administration of ibuprofen. Because the medication is available in OTC preparations with many trade names, patients may not realize that they are taking an ibuprofen-containing drug. Overdosing may occur.

Adverse Effects

The GI adverse effects of ibuprofen are many: dry mouth, gingival hyperplasia, dyspepsia, heartburn, nausea, epigastric pain, constipation, and GI ulceration with occult blood loss. The genitourinary effects include nephrotoxicity, elevated blood urea nitrogen and creatinine, and edema. The respiratory adverse effects include dyspnea, bronchospasm, hemoptysis, and pharyngitis. In addition, anaphylactic reactions may also occur.

Contraindications

Ibuprofen is contraindicated in patients with a known allergy to NSAIDs and salicylates. Allergic reactions are more common in patients with rhinitis, asthma, chronic urticaria, and nasal polyps (Karch, 2011).

TABLE 14.6

DRUGS AT A GLANCE: Propionic Acid Derivatives

Drug	Pregnancy Category	Routes and Dosage Ranges	
		Adults	*Children*
Ⓟ Ibuprofen (Motrin, Advil)	B, D in the third trimester	Osteoarthritis, rheumatoid arthritis: PO 300–600 mg 3 or 4 times per day; maximum, 3200 mg/d Pain, dysmenorrhea: PO 400 mg every 4–6 h PRN; max 3200 mg/d IV 400–800 mg every 6 h Migraine: PO 400 mg at onset of headache	6 mo to 12 y: fever, initial temperature 39.2°C (102.5°F) or less, PO 5 mg/kg every 6–8 h; initial temperature above 39.2°C (102.5°F), PO 5–10 mg/kg every 6–8 h; max dose 40 mg/kg/d Juvenile arthritis: PO 20–40 mg/kg/d, in three or four divided doses
Flurbiprofen (Ansaid)	B (oral) C (ophthalmic)	Osteoarthritis, rheumatoid arthritis: PO 200–300 mg/d in two, three, or four divided doses Inhibition of intraoperative miosis: 1 drop every 30 min, beginning 2 h before surgery (total of 4 drops)	Dosage not established
Ketoprofen (Oruvail)	B D in the third trimester	Pain, dysmenorrhea: PO 25–50 mg every 6–8 h PRN Osteoarthritis, rheumatoid arthritis: PO 150–300 mg/d in three or four divided doses Extended release; 200 mg once daily Maximum; 300 mg/d for regular formulation; 200 mg/d for extended release; 100–150 mg/d for patients with impaired renal function	Do not give to children <16 y unless directed by a physician.
Naproxen (Naprosyn) Naproxen sodium (Aleve, Anaprox, Naprelan)	C	Naproxen: PO 250–500 mg twice daily Gout: PO 750 mg initially, then 250 mg every 8 h until symptoms subside Max, 1250 mg/d Naproxen sodium: Pain, dysmenorrhea, acute tendonitis, bursitis: PO 550 mg every 12 h or 275 mg every 6–8 h Maximum, 1375 mg/d OA, RA, AS: PO 275–550 mg twice a day Acute gout: PO 825 mg initially, then 275 mg every 8 h until symptoms subside Controlled release (Naprelan); 750–1000 mg once daily	Juvenile arthritis (naproxen only): PO 10 mg/kg/d in two divided doses. Oral suspension (125 mg/5 mL) twice daily according to weight: 13 kg (29 lb), 2.5 mL; 25 kg (55 lb), 5 mL; 39 kg (84 lb), 7.5 mL OTC preparation not recommended for children <12 y
Oxaprozin (Daypro)	C	PO 600–1200 mg once daily Max, 1800 mg/d or 26 mg/kg/d, whichever is lower, in divided doses	Dosage not established

Nursing Implications

Preventing Interactions

Medications and herbs interact with ibuprofen, increasing or decreasing its effects (Boxes 14.8 and 14.9).

Administering the Medication

Ibuprofen is administered orally, and the total daily dose should not exceed 3200 mg. When administered intravenously, it should be diluted in a concentration of 4 mg/mL or less using 0.9% sodium chloride, 5% dextrose, or lactated Ringer's. The dilution remains stable for 24 hours. Researchers have reported that the rapid infusion of ibuprofen intravenously was safe and

effective treating pain. The maximum total serum amount of IV ibuprofen was twice that of oral ibuprofen (Pavliv, Voss, and Rock, 2011).

Assessing for Therapeutic Effects

When ibuprofen is administered for pain, the nurse assesses for pain. The patient should report diminished pain on a pain scale. When the drug is administered for fever, the nurse records the patient's temperature every 2 to 4 hours. Reduced fever should occur. When the drug is administered for inflammation, the nurse notes anti-inflammatory effects, particularly in the joints related to arthritis. Decreased inflammation should occur.

BOX 14.8   Drug Interactions: Ibuprofen

Drugs That Increase the Effects of Ibuprofen

■ Anticoagulants
Increase the risk of bleeding
■ Codeine, oxycodone, hydrocodone
Have an additive analgesic effect
■ Corticosteroids
Have additive gastric irritant and possible ulcero-genic effects

Assessing Adverse Effects

The nurse assesses the patient for dyspepsia or GI bleeding, including hemoptysis or melena. He or she also assesses complete blood count and clotting times for signs of anticoagulation. In addition, the nurse assesses for signs and symptoms of hypersensitivity to ibuprofen, including rash and bronchospasm.

Patient Teaching

Box 14.10 presents patient teaching guidelines for ibuprofen.

EVIDENCE-BASED PRACTICE

Periorbital Edema Associated With Separate Courses of Ibuprofen and Naproxen

by MORAD BALAS, RODA PLAKOGIANNIS, AND MARK SINNETT

American Journal of Health-System Pharmacy
2010, 66, 906–909

Periorbital edema is an acute vascular reaction that involves the dermis and subcutaneous tissue in the periorbital area, leading to edema. The researchers discussed an 80-year-old woman with a history of osteoarthritis and hypertension who was prescribed 375 mg of naproxen every 8 hours as needed for pain. Following two doses of the naproxen, itching, swelling, and erythema developed at the left eye; her symptoms and signs became progressively worse and spread to the right eye. Her primary care provider discontinued the naproxen. She reported to the physician that several months prior to this incident she had a similar reaction when she took ibuprofen.

IMPLICATIONS FOR NURSING PRACTICE: Although the occurrence of a nonsteroidal anti-inflammatory drug–induced periorbital edema is uncommon, the nurse should be aware that it might develop. Also, it is important to note that patients who take drugs within the broad classification of propionic acid derivatives are at risk for the development of similar adverse effects.

BOX 14.9   Herb and Dietary Interactions: Ibuprofen

Herbs and Foods That Increase the Effects of Ibuprofen

■ Alcohol
■ Garlic, ginger, gingko
■ Feverfew

BOX 14.10   Patient Teaching Guidelines for Ibuprofen

■ Take this drug with food or liquid to decrease gastric irritation.
■ Drink 2 to 3 quarts of fluid daily when taking this drug regularly.
■ Report any signs of bleeding (e.g., nose bleed, vomiting blood, bruising, blood in the urine or stool), difficulty breathing, severe stomach upset, swelling, or weight gain to your health care provider.

Clinical Application 14-3

• When teaching to Mrs. Mason about ibuprofen, what is it necessary to say about the action of the medication?
• What are the adverse reactions of ibuprofen?
• What specific patient teaching should be provided to Mrs. Mason?

OXICAM DERIVATIVES

Oxicam derivatives are another type of NSAID. They include **Ⓟ meloxicam** (Mobic), the prototype drug, and piroxicam (Feldene).

Pharmacokinetics

Meloxicam is metabolized by the liver and excreted in the feces and urine. The onset of action is 1 hour, and peak serum concentrations occur in 5 to 6 hours. The drug crosses the placenta and enters breast milk.

Action

Meloxicam is a COX-1 and COX-2 inhibitor, producing anti-inflammatory, analgesic, and antipyretic effects. It is more selective for COX-2 inhibition in the brain, kidney, ovary, uterus, cartilage, bone, and sites of inflammation (Karch, 2011).

Use

Meloxicam is administered for the treatment of osteoarthritis and rheumatoid arthritis. It is used in children 2 years of age and older for relief of signs and symptoms of pauciarticular or

TABLE 14.7

DRUGS AT A GLANCE: Oxicam Derivatives

Drug	Pregnancy Category	Routes and Dosage Ranges	
		Adults	Children
Ⓟ **Meloxicam** (Mobic)	C, D in the third trimester	PO 7.5 mg daily Max dosage 15 mg	0.125 mg/kg once daily Max dosage 7.5 mg, using oral suspension
Piroxicam (Feldene)	C	PO 20 mg daily; dosage may be divided.	Safety and efficacy not established

polyarticular juvenile rheumatoid arthritis. Table 14.7 gives the dosage information for meloxicam and piroxicam.

Use in Patients With Renal Impairment

Likewise, the dosage of meloxicam does not require adjustment in mild to moderate renal impairment. The use of the drug in patients with creatinine clearance less than 20 mL per minute has not been studied and is not recommended in these patients. Patients undergoing hemodialysis should receive a maximum of 7.5 mg per day (Up-to-Date, 2011).

Use in Patients With Hepatic Impairment

The use of meloxicam in patients with hepatic impairment has not adequately been studied (Up-to-Date, 2011). The dosage of the drug does not appear to be necessary in patients with mild to moderate hepatic impairment.

Adverse Effects

Meloxicam is associated with several adverse effects. Respiratory effects include dyspnea, hemoptysis, bronchospasm, pharyngitis, and rhinitis. Hematological effects consist of bleeding, platelet inhibition, and decreased hemoglobin and hematocrit, along with bone marrow depression and edema. GI effects include nausea, dyspepsia, diarrhea, vomiting, and diarrhea. The FDA has issued a **BLACK BOX WARNING ◆** stating that patients who take meloxicam are at risk for cardiovascular events and GI bleeding. In addition, headache, dizziness, drowsiness, and insomnia may occur.

Contraindications

Meloxicam should not be administered to patients with a known aspirin allergy. It is also contraindicated postoperatively in patients who have just undergone coronary artery bypass surgery.

BOX 14.11 Drug Interactions: Meloxicam

Drugs That Increase the Effects of Meloxicam
- Angiotensin-converting enzyme inhibitors and diuretics
  Increase the risk of renal failure
- Aspirin and anticoagulants
  Increase the risk of gastrointestinal bleeding

Nursing Implications

Preventing Interactions

Some medications interact with meloxicam, increasing its effects (Box 14.11). As with all NSAIDs, alcohol, garlic, ginseng, and ginger increase the risk of bleeding. Giving meloxicam with lithium increases the risk of lithium toxicity.

Administering the Medication

Administration of meloxicam with food or fluids reduces gastric irritation. It is necessary to shake the oral suspension gently before use.

Assessing for Therapeutic Effects

When giving meloxicam for pain, the nurse assesses the pain level using a pain scale to determine that analgesic effects are attained. When giving it for fever, the nurse records the patient's temperature every 2 to 4 hours to check for diminished body temperature. When giving it for inflammation, the nurse assesses for diminished redness and swelling.

Assessing for Adverse Effects

The nurse assesses the patient for signs and symptoms of hypersensitivity reactions such as shortness of breath and bronchospasm. It is also necessary to assess for hemoptysis as well as blood in the stool or urine. In addition, the nurse must assess for signs and symptoms of cardiovascular events.

Patient Teaching

Box 14.12 presents patient teaching guidelines for meloxicam.

BOX 14.12 Patient Teaching Guidelines for Meloxicam

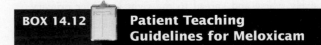

- Take these drugs with food to decrease gastric irritation.
- Take only the prescribed dose.
- Do not operate machinery until you know how these drugs affect you. Dizziness and drowsiness may occur.
- Report sore throat, dyspnea, edema, and tarry stools to your health care provider.

9. A child who is diagnosed with pneumonia is taking ibuprofen for a fever. The nurse observes a rash. Which of the following reactions does the nurse suspect?

   A. hypersensitivity to antimicrobial agents
   B. streptococcal reaction
   C. hypersensitivity to ibuprofen
   D. viral infection

10. A prescriber in an orthopedic care practice orders meloxicam for the treatment of osteoarthritis. Which of the following medications when combined with meloxicam places the patient at greatest risk?

   A. antimicrobials
   B. lithium
   C. selective serotonin inhibitors
   D. hydrochlorothiazide

ACETIC ACID DERIVATIVES

The prototype NSAID of the acetic acid derivative group is ⓟ **indomethacin** (Indocin, Indocin SR). The acetic acid derivatives have strong anti-inflammatory effects and more severe adverse effects than the propionic acid derivatives.

Pharmacokinetics

With oral administration of indomethacin, the onset of action is 30 minutes, with a peak in 1 to 2 hours and a duration of 4 to 6 hours. With IV administration, onset of action is immediate, with an unknown peak and a duration of 15 to 30 minutes. The drug is metabolized in the liver and has a half-life of 4.5 to 6 hours. It is excreted by the kidneys. Indomethacin has the ability to cross the placenta and enter the breast milk.

Action

Indomethacin provides anti-inflammatory, analgesic, and antipyretic activities by inhibiting the prostaglandin synthesis. The exact mechanism is unknown, but it inhibits COX-1 and COX-2. It is mainly a selective COX-1 inhibitor.

Use

Indomethacin is administered to relieve pain associated with rheumatoid arthritis, osteoarthritis, ankylosing spondylitis, bursitis, tendonitis, and gouty arthritis. During initial attacks of acute gout, the drug may be given. Parenteral, but not oral, administration is used to produce closure of patent ductus arteriosus in premature infants who weigh 500 to 1750 g. Unlabeled uses include treatment of juvenile rheumatoid arthritis, premature labor, and macular edema, as well as reduction of the incidence of patent ductus arteriosus in patients at risk for this condition. Table 14.8 gives dosage information for indomethacin and the other acetic acid derivatives.

Use in Children

The safety and efficacy of indomethacin have not been established in children. As previously stated, the FDA has approved IV indomethacin for treatment of patent ductus arteriosus in premature infants. (The ductus arteriosus joins the pulmonary artery to the aorta in the fetal circulation. When it fails to close at the time of birth, blood is shunted from the aorta to the pulmonary artery, causing severe cardiopulmonary problems.) If anuria or oliguria occurs after premature infants receive the IV form, no further doses should be given. If the ductus reopens, the drug is repeated in 12 to 24 hours. Indications that the ductus has reopened would be the signs and symptoms of heart failure such as dyspnea and a heart murmur. The reader should note that oral administration for closure of patent ductus arteriosus in premature infants is an unlabeled use of the drug.

Use in Older Adults

The Beers Criteria indicate that indomethacin is inappropriate in the geriatric population and is associated with a high risk of severity. When an older adult must take indomethacin, it is necessary to use the lowest recommended dose and frequency (Up-to-Date, 2011).

Use in Patients With Renal Impairment

Caution is also required with administration of indomethacin to patients with renal impairment. (Severe renal impairment is a contraindication.)

Use in Patients With Hepatic Impairment

Caution is necessary with administration of indomethacin to patients with hepatic impairment. Dosage reduction is appropriate.

Adverse Effects

Indomethacin and all acetic acid derivatives result in a risk of GI bleeding and bleeding ulcer. Abdominal pain, distention, vomiting, and transient ileus may occur. CNS adverse effects include headache, dizziness, somnolence, and insomnia. Patients are at risk for renal impairment and decreased clotting time. With IV preparations, the most severe respiratory adverse effect is pulmonary hemorrhage.

Contraindications

Indomethacin should not be administered to patients with a known history of salicylate hypersensitivity. Patients with a past history of GI bleeding should not take the drug. It should not be administered to postoperatively to patients who have just had a coronary artery bypass graft. The parenteral formulations are contraindicated in infection, bleeding, thrombocytopenia, coagulation defects, and necrotizing enterocolitis. As stated earlier, indomethacin is contraindicated in severe renal impairment.

TABLE 14.8

DRUGS AT A GLANCE: Acetic Acid Derivatives

Drug	Pregnancy Category	Routes and Dosage Ranges	
		Adults	Children
℗ **Indomethacin** (Indocin, Indocin SR)	B, D in the third trimester	PO, rectal suppository: 75 mg/d initially, increased by 25 mg/d at weekly intervals to a maximum of 150–200 mg/d, if necessary Acute gouty arthritis, acute painful shoulder: PO 75–150 mg/d in three or four divided doses until pain and inflammation are controlled (e.g., 3–5 d for gout; 7–14 d for painful shoulder), then discontinued	In special circumstances, such as juvenile rheumatoid arthritis, children older than 2 y of age may receive the drug. Initial dose is 2 mg/kg/d in divided doses, not to exceed 4 mg/kg/d. Premature infants with patent ductus arteriosus: IV 0.2–0.3 mg/kg every 12 h for a total of three doses
Diclofenac potassium (Cataflam) Diclofenac sodium (Voltaren, Voltaren XR, Cambria, Zipsor, Solaraze, Flector)	C, D in the third trimester	Osteoarthritis: PO 100–150 mg/d in divided doses (e.g., 50 mg two or three times or 75 mg twice or 100 mg once daily) Rheumatoid arthritis: PO 150–200 mg/d in two, three, or four divided doses Ankylosing spondylitis: PO 100–125 mg/d in four or five divided doses (e.g., 25 mg four or five times daily) Pain, dysmenorrhea: (diclofenac potassium only) PO 50 mg three times daily Acute migraine: 50 mg packet mixed in 30–60 mL water as a single dose at the onset of a headache (Cambia) Mild to moderate pain: 25 mg liquid capsule PO 4 times daily Actinic keratosis Topical: Cover lesion with gel and smooth into skin; do not cover with dressing (Solaraze) Transdermal patch: Apply to most painful area 2 times daily (Flector) Ophthalmic: 1 drop to affected eye starting 24 h after cataract surgery for 2 wk	Dosage not established
Etodolac	C	Pain: 200–400 mg PO every 6–8 h Osteoarthritis: 600–1200 mg/d PO in 2–4 divided doses Rheumatoid arthritis: 500 mg PO twice daily	Dosage not established
Ketorolac (Toradol)	C, D in the third trimester	Single dose: IV 30 mg, IM 60 mg Multiple dose: IM or IV 30 mg every 6 h PRN to a maximum of 120 mg/d PO 20 mg as the first dose for patients who received 60 mg IM or 30 mg IV as a single dose or 30 mg in a multiple dose followed by 10 mg every 4–6 h to a maximum of 40 mg/d Older adults (>65 y), those with renal impairment, those with weight <50 kg (110 lb; IV, IM 15 mg every 6 h to a maximum of 60 mg/d) Itching from allergic conjunctivitis: Ophthalmic Acular PF: for cataract surgery, 1 drop every 4 times daily after surgery and continue for 2 wk Acular LS: 1 drop 4 times daily PRN for burning and stinging for up to 4 d after surgery Pain and photophobia: use for 3 d	Use one single-dose injection 1 mg/kg IM up to a maximum of 30 mg or 0.5 mg/kg IV up to a maximum of 15 mg

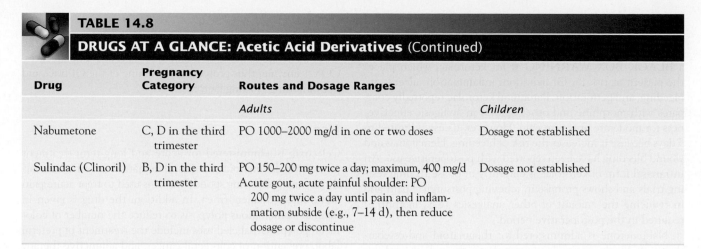

TABLE 14.8

DRUGS AT A GLANCE: Acetic Acid Derivatives (Continued)

Drug	Pregnancy Category	Routes and Dosage Ranges	
		Adults	Children
Nabumetone	C, D in the third trimester	PO 1000–2000 mg/d in one or two doses	Dosage not established
Sulindac (Clinoril)	B, D in the third trimester	PO 150–200 mg twice a day; maximum, 400 mg/d Acute gout, acute painful shoulder: PO 200 mg twice a day until pain and inflammation subside (e.g., 7–14 d), then reduce dosage or discontinue	Dosage not established

Nursing Implications

Preventing Interactions

Certain drugs interact with indomethacin (Box 14.13). The administration of alcohol, feverfew, garlic, ginger, and gingko also increases the bleeding potential.

Administering the Medication

It is important to administer oral indomethacin after meals or with an antacid to decrease GI irritation. Patients with gouty arthritis should not take the sustained-release preparation. Patients with a history of proctitis or rectal bleeding should not use rectal suppositories. IV administration requires dilution of 1 mg with 1 mL of sterile water or normal saline. It is necessary to administer the dose over 5 to 10 seconds. Good IV access is imperative to prevent extravasation of the drug into the tissues. Storage of the oral preparation of indomethacin in a light-protected container is essential.

Assessing for Therapeutic Effects

Before administering indomethacin, it is important to assess patients for salicylate allergy, which can cause bronchospasm, dyspnea, and rash. After the drug has had time to work, it is imperative to assess for diminished pain and inflammation. The nurse observes the patient's mobility in response to diminished inflammation. When administering indomethacin for gout, inflammation is generally relieved in 24 to 36 hours.

Assessing for Adverse Effects

A careful assessment of the cardiac and CNS effects is imperative. The nurse assesses for bleeding, vomiting, and abdominal pain. The FDA has issued a **BLACK BOX WARNING** ◆ stating that an increased risk for adverse cardiovascular thrombotic

effects, including myocardial infarction and cerebrovascular accident, has been noted with indomethacin. Because of the risk of hypersensitivity, the nurse assesses for dyspnea, bronchospasm, and hemoptysis. In addition, if the patient complains of abdominal pain that is indicative of transient ileus, the nurse notifies the physician immediately.

QSEN Safety Alert

Assessment for GI pain, rapid pulse, and diaphoresis is essential in patients who receive ketorolac. These symptoms are indicative of GI perforation.

Patient Teaching

Box 14.14 lists patient teaching guidelines for indomethacin.

Other Drugs in the Class

The acetic acid derivative etodolac reportedly causes less gastric irritation, especially in older adults at high risk for GI bleeding.

Ketorolac, an injectable NSAID often used for pain, is contraindicated in patients at risk for excessive bleeding. Thus, ketorolac should not be administered during labor and

---

BOX 14.13 | **Drug Interactions: Indomethacin**

Drugs That Increase the Effects of Indomethacin
- Phenytoin, salicylates, sulfonamides, sulfonylureas
  Result in displacement of protein-binding activities
- Salicylates, anticoagulants, lithium
  Increase the risk of bleeding

BOX 14.14 | **Patient Teaching Guidelines for Indomethacin**

- If you are the parents or another member of a family of an infant being treated for patent ductus arteriosus, be sure you receive and understand the action, adverse effects, and therapeutic effects of indomethacin, as well as its administration guidelines.
- Administer the oral preparation with food or immediately after a meal.
- If necessary, take the medication with an antacid to decrease gastric irritation.
- Report adverse effects such as chest pain, weakness, or disorientation to your health care provider.
- Do not operate machinery due to dizziness or somnolence.
- Report sore throat, fever, rash, weight gain, or tarry stools to your health care provider.

delivery, before or during any major surgery, with suspected or confirmed cerebrovascular bleeding, or to patients who are currently taking aspirin or other NSAIDs. The FDA has issued a **BLACK BOX WARNING ◆** for ketorolac, which places the patient at risk for GI irritation, inflammation, ulceration, bleeding, and perforation. Parenteral ketorolac reportedly compares with morphine and other opioids in analgesic effectiveness for moderate or severe pain. However, its use is limited to 5 days because it increases the risk of bleeding. Hematomas and wound bleeding have been reported with postoperative use. An intranasal form of ketorolac is currently in phase III drug testing trials and shows promise in relieving postsurgical pain and in reducing the amount of other analgesics (e.g., morphine) required in the postoperative period.

Nabumetone is administered for rheumatoid and osteoarthritis. It blocks prostaglandin synthesis through the inhibition of cyclooxygenase. Prior to administering nabumetone, a baseline hemoglobin and hematocrit should be assessed. The patient should be instructed to report any signs or symptoms of abdominal pain or black tarry stools.

Selective COX-2 Inhibitor: Celecoxib

Ⓟ **Celecoxib** (Celebrex) is the only selective COX-2 inhibitor on the market in the United States. The selective COX-2 inhibitors etoricoxib and parecoxib, which are available in the United Kingdom and other countries, are currently under review by the FDA. COX-2 inhibitors were designed to selectively block production of prostaglandins associated with pain and inflammation without blocking those associated with protective effects on gastric mucosa, renal function, and platelet aggregation. Thus, they produce less gastric irritation and renal impairment than aspirin and other NSAIDs.

Pharmacokinetics

Celecoxib, which is administered orally, has a slow onset of action. The drug reaches its peak in 3 hours. It is highly protein bound (97%), and the serum half-life is 11 hours. It is metabolized by the cytochrome P450 enzymes in the liver to inactive metabolites that are then excreted in the urine. A small amount is excreted unchanged in the urine. Celecoxib crosses the placenta and enters the breast milk.

Action

COX-2 is activated with inflammation. Celecoxib inhibits the COX-2 enzyme to decrease inflammation. It does not affect the COX-1 enzyme, thus protecting the lining of the GI tract and not inhibiting clotting factors.

Use

Celecoxib is administered for acute and long-term treatment of juvenile rheumatoid arthritis, rheumatoid arthritis, osteoarthritis, and ankylosing spondylitis. It is used to treat acute pain and primary dysmenorrhea. In addition, the drug is given in familial adenomatous polyposis to reduce the number of colorectal polyps. Unlabeled uses include the treatment of preterm labor, prevention of colorectal cancer, and adjunctive therapy in schizophrenia (Karch, 2011). Table 14.9 presents specific dosage and pregnancy information for celecoxib.

Use in Children

Celecoxib is recommended only for children ages 2 and older to treat juvenile rheumatoid arthritis. In children, the median peak serum concentration is 3 hours. The range of peak serum concentration is 3 to 6.2 hours.

Use in Patients With Renal Impairment

In patients with significant renal impairment, celecoxib should not be administered.

Use in Patients With Hepatic Impairment

In patients with hepatic impairment, the dosage of celecoxib should be reduced by 50%.

Adverse Effects

The CNS adverse reactions of celecoxib include headache, dizziness, somnolence, and insomnia. Some patients have noted ophthalmic changes with administration of the drug. Patients taking celecoxib are at increased risk for myocardial infarction and cerebrovascular accident. The FDA has issued a **BLACK BOX WARNING ◆** for celecoxib concerning its cardiac and vascular risks. Dermatologic adverse effects include rash, pruritus, sweating, dry mucous membranes, and stomatitis.

TABLE 14.9

DRUGS AT A GLANCE: Celecoxib

Drug	Pregnancy Category	Routes and Dosage Ranges	
		Adults	Children
Ⓟ **Celecoxib** (Celebrex)	C, D in the third trimester	PO 100 mg 2 times daily may be increased to 200 mg/d 2 times daily Acute pain, dysmenorrhea: 400 mg, then 200 mg 2 times daily Familial adenomatous polyposis: 400 mg 2 times daily Ankylosing spondylitis: 200 mg/d after 6 wk, a trial of 400 mg/d may be tried for 6 wk; if not effect is seen another therapy is recommended	Children older than 2 y of age PO 10 or 25 kg or less: 50 mg capsule BID More than 25 kg: 100 mg capsule B.I.D.

Dyspepsia and GI bleeding can occur with the administration of prolonged high doses of celecoxib, but the risk is not as profound as the COX-1 and COX-2 inhibitors. Anaphylactic reactions can also occur if the patient is allergic to celecoxib or has an aspirin or NSAID-related allergy.

Contraindications

Celecoxib is contraindicated in patients who have a known allergy to sulfonamides, NSAIDs, and aspirin. It is also contraindicated in patients with renal impairment. It should not be administered to patients with perioperative pain or to those who have just undergone coronary artery bypass graft surgery.

Nursing Implications

Preventing Interactions

The administration of anticoagulants or aspirin with celecoxib increases the risk of bleeding. Patients taking lithium and celecoxib are at risk for lithium toxicity. Celecoxib combined with alcohol or smoking increases the patient's risk of GI bleeding.

Administering the Medication

When administering celecoxib, the nurse should be certain to administer it 2 hours before or after an antacid to ensure absorption. Prior to administering celecoxib, assess the patient for allergic reactions to NSAIDs. It is necessary to store the medication in a light-protected container.

Assessing for Therapeutic Effects

The nurse assesses for diminished pain and swelling associated with inflammation. The nurse assesses joints for redness, heat, and stiffness. Mobility should increase with the administration of celecoxib.

Assess for Adverse Effects

The nurse assesses the patient for signs and symptoms of chest pain, shortness of breath, confusion, or numbness of the extremities. These symptoms are indicative of cardiac event such as myocardial infarction or cerebrovascular accident. Also, it is necessary to assess for dyspepsia, GI irritation, and GI bleeding. In addition, the nurse assesses for CNS depression and ophthalmic changes. Finally, he or she assesses for anaphylactic reactions, including sore throat, itching, weight gain, and edema.

Patient Teaching

Box 14.15 presents patient teaching guidelines for celecoxib.

BOX 14.15	**Patient Teaching Guidelines for Celecoxib**

- Administer the medication with food or meals to prevent gastric upset.
- Take the medication as prescribed.
- Do not operate machinery if you have central nervous system depression.
- Report sore throat, rash, itching, weight gain, swelling of fee and ankles, and changes in vision to your health care provider.

NCLEX Success

11. A newborn infant has been treated with parenteral indomethacin for treatment of patent ductus arteriosus. Which of the following symptoms would be indicative of a reopening of the ductus arteriosus in 12 hours after the original dosage?

   A. dyspnea
   B. pain
   C. elevated creatinine level
   D. hepatic failure

12. A 76-year-old woman is taking celecoxib for arthritic pain in her back. When administering celecoxib, which of the following patient teaching points is most important?

   A. Any chest pain should be reported to the prescriber immediately.
   B. Celecoxib can be administered with warfarin.
   C. Increased mobility should be reported to the prescriber.
   D. Celecoxib can be administered with aspirin during periods of infection.

Antigout Medication

MITOTIC AGENT: COLCHICINE

Ⓟ **Colchicine** (Colcrys), the prototype agent for the treatment and prevention of gout, is the most commonly administered antigout medication.

Pharmacokinetics

Colchicine is absorbed rapidly in the GI tract, with a slow onset of action; it reaches its peak in 1 to 2 hour. The drug is metabolized in the liver and has a half-life of 26 to 31 hours. It is primarily eliminated in the feces, with a smaller amount excreted in the urine. Colchicine crosses the placenta and enters breast milk.

Action

Colchicine inhibits the migration of white blood cells into the body tissues containing urate crystals. The phagocytic action of the drug decreases the inflammatory reaction to the urate crystals deposited in the tissues.

Use

Colchicine is administered for the treatment and prophylaxis of acute gout in adults. Table 14.10 gives the dosage and pregnancy information for this drug.

Use in Children

Colchicine is only administered to children 4 years of age and older to treat familial Mediterranean fever.

			TABLE 14.10

DRUGS AT A GLANCE: Colchicine

Drug	Pregnancy Category	Routes and Dosage Ranges	
		Adults	Children
Ⓟ Colchicine (Colcrys)	C	Acute gout: PO 1.2 mg at the first sign of gout flare Prophylaxis of gout flares: PO 0.6 mg/d to a maximum of 1.2 mg/d	Safety and efficacy not established

Use in Older Adults

Colchicine is administered cautiously in older adults, and the dosage should be reduced by half in people 70 years of age and older (Up-To-Date, 2011).

Use in Patients With Renal Impairment

For mild to moderate renal impairment, a regular dosage of colchicine is administered. If the creatinine clearance is less than 30 mL per minute, a dosage adjusted is not necessary, but the drug should not be given more often than once every 2 weeks. For patients on dialysis, 0.6 mg is given as a single dose no more than once every 2 weeks.

Use in Patients With Hepatic Impairment

In mild to moderate hepatic impairment, colchicine should be administered cautiously. The patient should be assessed closely for adverse effects. In severe hepatic impairment, the dosage should be the same, but the drug should not be given more often than once every 2 weeks.

Adverse Effects

GI adverse effects are the most common due to the absorption and elimination in the GI tract. These GI conditions include nausea, vomiting, and abdominal pain and dyspepsia. Hematologic adverse effects such as bone marrow depression and aplastic anemia may occur. Hepatotoxicity is also an adverse effect of colchicine. Other adverse effects include peripheral neuropathy, alopecia, rash, purpura, dermatoses, myopathy, muscle pain, and weakness.

Contraindications

Colchicine is contraindicated in patients who have a known hypersensitivity to the medication. It should not be administered concurrently with cyclosporines or ranolazine or with a strong to moderate CYP3A4 inhibitor in the presence of hepatic or renal impairment. It is administered cautiously in pregnancy or in the presence of renal or hepatic impairment.

Nursing Implications

Preventing Interactions

Several medications, when combined with colchicine, result in toxicity and severe adverse effects. These agents increase the serum level of colchicine and the risk of toxicity. They are atazanavir, clarithromycin, indinavir, itraconazole, ketoconazole, nefazodone, nelfinavir, ritonavir, saquinavir, telithromycin, diltiazem, erythromycin, fluconazole, and verapamil. In addition, colchicine should not be combined with grapefruit juice or alcohol. It also decreases cyanocobalamin (vitamin B_{12}) absorption.

Administering the Medication

It is necessary to administer colchicine with food to reduce gastric distress.

Assess for Therapeutic Effects

Therapeutic effects occur within 24 to 48 hours after oral administration. The nurse assesses for decreased pain, swelling, and inflammation of affected joints. Edema may not decrease for several days.

Assess for Adverse Effects

The nurse assesses for severe GI adverse effects such as vomiting and diarrhea, which may lead to an alteration in fluid and electrolytes with dehydration. The nurse also assesses for numbness, tingling, or muscle weakness. In addition, it is important to assess for bone marrow depression. The nurse also monitors liver enzymes.

Patient Teaching

Box 14.16 presents patient teaching guidelines for the mitotic agent colchicine.

URICOSURIC AGENTS

Several uricosuric agents are used to reduce serum uric acid levels. Ⓟ **Allopurinol** (Zyloprim), a xanthine oxidase inhibitor, is the prototype uricosuric drug.

Pharmacokinetics

Allopurinol is absorbed in the GI tract, with an onset of action of 24 to 48 hours and a peak of action of 2 to 6 hours. The drug's half-life is 1 to 3 hours. It is metabolized as an active metabolite oxypurinol and is eliminated slowly in the urine. It is also excreted in the breast milk.

BOX 14.16	Patient Teaching Guidelines for Colchicine

- Take colchicine as prescribed and at the onset of acute gouty symptoms.
- For acute gouty flare-ups, take one dose and the second dose 1 hour later.
- Do not drink grapefruit juice or alcohol.
- Gastrointestinal adverse effects are common with colchicine; call your prescriber if the abdominal pain is too severe.
- Report severe diarrhea and muscle weakness to your health care provider.
- Understand that the resulting bone marrow depression may cause fatigue, increased risk of bleeding, or increased risk of infection.
- See your primary health provider with persistent gouty attacks.
- Follow a low-purine diet by avoiding beer, alcohol, organ and game meats, sardines, anchovies, scallops, asparagus, spinach, and peas.

Action

Allopurinol inhibits the enzyme that is responsible for the conversion of purines to uric acid. This action reduces the purines to uric acid and thus reduces the uric acid production to decrease the serum and urinary uric acid levels. The result of this action is the reduction of the symptoms of gout.

Use

Allopurinol and uricosuric agents are administered for the management of the signs and symptoms of primary and secondary gout or stages of gout. It is also given in acute and chronic tophaceous gout to reduce uric acid concentrations. Other indications include leukemia, lymphoma, and malignancies that result in elevated serum uric acid levels. Table 14.11 gives the specific dosage information and the pregnancy categories for these drugs.

Use in Children

Allopurinol is not routinely administered to children, except to those with hyperuricemia secondary to cancer and

TABLE 14.11

DRUGS AT A GLANCE: Uricosuric Agents

Drug	Pregnancy Category	Routes and Dosage Ranges	
		Adults	Children
Ⓟ **Allopurinol** (Zyloprim)	C	Gout and hyperuricemia: PO 100–800 mg/k/d in divided doses, depending on the severity of the disease (200–300 mg/d is usual dose) Maintenance: Establish dose that maintains serum uric acid levels within normal limits Hyperuricemia: PO 200–300 mg/d; adjust the dose based on urate levels Prevention of uric acid nephropathy in certain malignancies: PO 600–800 mg/d for 203 d with a high fluid intake; maintenance dose as above Recurrent calcium oxalate stones: PO 200–300 mg/d; adjust dose based on 24-h urinary urate determinations Parenteral administration: IV 200–400 mg/m²/d as a continuous infusion or at 6, 8, or 12 h intervals Dosage based on creatinine clearance: 140 mL/min–400 mg 120 mL/min–350 mg 100 mL/min–300 mg 80 mL/min–250 mg 60 mL/min–200 mg 40 mL/min–150 mg	Secondary hyperuricemia associated with various malignancies: 6–10 y: PO 300 mg/d; adjust dose based on serum uric acid levels <6 y: PO 150 mg/d; adjust dose after 48 h of treatment based on serum uric acid level Parenteral: 200 mg/m²/d IV as continuous infusion or at 6, 8, or 12 h intervals
Febuxostat (Uloric)	C	PO 40 mg/d; if serum uric acid level is not <6 mg/dL in 2 wk, dosage should be increased to 80 mg/d.	Safety and efficacy not established
Probenecid	B	PO 0.25 g BID for 1 wk; then 0.5 g BID; maintenance, continue dosage that maintains the normal serum uric acid levels. When no attacks occur for 6 mo or longer, decrease the dose to 0.5 g every 6 mo	Safety and efficacy not established

chemotherapy treatment. When administering allopurinol intravenously, it is essential to ensure that the child is hydrated to maintain an neutral or slightly alkaline urine output.

Use in Older Adults

Allopurinol may be used in geriatric patients. The initial dose is 100 mg/d, which can be increased until the desired uric acid level is obtained. It is necessary to maintain fluid intake to produce a urine output of at least 2000 mL per day. The dosage should be reduced in the event of diminished renal function.

Use in Patients With Renal Impairment

The dosage of allopurinol is reduced based on the patient's creatinine clearance. See Table 14.11 for the specific dosage information.

Use in Patients With Hepatic Impairment

Allopurinol is administered cautiously in patients with hepatic impairment. The dosage does not need to be adjusted, but it is important to monitor liver function.

Adverse Effects

Allopurinol has several adverse effects. CNS adverse effects include drowsiness, headache, and vertigo. Hematologic adverse effects are agranulocytosis, aplastic anemia, and bone marrow depression. The most common GI effects are nausea, vomiting, diarrhea, abdominal pain, and indigestion. Hepatotoxicity and renal insufficiency are risk factors with the use of allopurinol.

Contraindications

Patients with a known hypersensitivity to allopurinol should not take allopurinol. Also, patients with a family history or history of idiopathic hemochromatosis should not receive the drug.

Nursing Implications

Preventing Interactions

Several medications, including azathioprine, mercaptopurine, cyclophosphamide, cyclosporine, and thiazide diuretics, increase the risk of uricosuric-associated toxicity. The administration of ampicillin and amoxicillin with allopurinol increases the risk of developing a rash. Anticoagulation effects are increased when combined with warfarin and aspirin. Alcohol combined with allopurinol decreases the excretion of uric acid.

Administering the Medication

It is necessary to administer allopurinol after meals to ensure absorption.

Assess for Therapeutic Effects

The nurse assesses for decreased pain, inflammation, and joint swelling. In patients with tophi (see Fig. 14.2), it is important to assess for increased joint mobility and decrease in tophi prominence. It is vital to assess serum uric acid levels. The normal serum uric acid level is 3.0 to 7.0 mg/dL.

BOX 14.17 Patient Teaching Guidelines for Allopurinol

- Take fluid to yield at least 2000 mL of urine output per day.
- Report decreased urine output or cloudy urine, which could be indicative of uric acid stone formation, to your health care provider.
- Report any rashes or skin eruptions to your health care provider.
- Do not drive or operate machinery until the central nervous system effects are known.
- Maintain appointments for serum uric acid levels, liver enzymes, and creatinine clearance to be drawn.

Assess for Adverse Effects

The nurse assesses for diminished urine output or cloudy urine, which may be indicative of the development of uric acid kidney stones. It is also important to assess for GI effects such as nausea, vomiting, diarrhea, and abdominal pain. The nurse assesses for bruising, bleeding, and anemia. Finally, the nurse assesses aspartate aminotransferase and alanine aminotransferase levels for hepatotoxicity and creatinine clearance for renal insufficiency.

Patient Teaching

Box 14.17 presents patient teaching guidelines for the uricosuric medications, including allopurinol.

Other Drugs in the Class

Febuxostat (Uloric) is the first medication for the treatment of gout to be developed in 40 years. A chemically engineered nonpurine agent, it selectively inhibits xanthine oxidase. Clinical studies have indicated that it is more effective in lowering serum uric acid levels than allopurinol. The most common adverse effect is hepatotoxicity. It is also necessary to assess patients who take febuxostat for the development of cardiovascular events such as myocardial infarction (Gray & Walters-Smith, 2011).

Probenecid (Benemid) increases the urinary excretion of uric acid. This uricosuric action means that it can be used therapeutically to treat hyperuricemia and gout. It is not effective in acute attacks of gouty arthritis but prevents hyperuricemia and tophi associated with chronic gout. Probenecid may cause acute gout until serum uric acid levels are within the normal range; concomitant administration of colchicine prevents this effect. (Probenecid also is used with penicillin, most often in treating sexually transmitted diseases. It increases blood levels and prolongs the action of penicillin by decreasing the rate of urinary excretion.)

Sulfinpyrazone (Anturane) is a uricosuric agent similar to probenecid. It is not effective in acute gout but prevents or decreases tissue changes of chronic gout. Colchicine is routinely administered during initial sulfinpyrazone therapy to prevent acute gout.

NCLEX Success

13. **A patient is being treated with colchicine for acute gouty flare-up. Which of the following statements indicates the need for increased patient education?**

    A. "I am going to stop taking the colchicine because of the diarrhea I am having."

    B. "The gastrointestinal effects are difficult to deal with but I know they will decrease my gouty symptoms."

    C. "I will continue my colchicine just as it has been prescribed for me."

    D. "The diarrhea I am experiencing can result in dehydration. If I have lethargy I will call my prescriber."

14. **A man with an acute gouty flare-up is taking allopurinol. Which of the following subjective statements indicates that he has developed uric acid kidney stones?**

    A. "I have pain in my right toe and left elbow."

    B. "I am dizzy and feel like I am going to faint."

    C. "I am urinating every hour—approximately 8 ounces."

    D. "I have excruciating pain in my lower abdomen."

15. **A man is taking allopurinol for acute gout. He has also been also receiving anticoagulant therapy since having a myocardial infarction. What is the priority assessment?**

    A. diminished pain in the inflamed joint

    B. adherence to the medication regimen

    C. bleeding

    D. abdominal pain

The Nursing Process

Assessment

- Assess for signs and symptoms of pain, site of pain, type and duration of pain, and factors that relieve or increase pain.
  - In patients with arthritis or musculoskeletal disorders, assess for pain and limitations in activity or mobility.
  - In patients with gout, assess the joint for pain and limitation of mobility.
  - In patients with gout, assess for abdominal pain.
- Assess for fever (thermometer readings above 99.6°F or 37.3°C). Signs and symptoms include:
  - Hot, dry skin
  - Flushed face
  - Reduced urine output
  - Dehydration
- Assess the use of OTC analgesic, antipyretic, or anti-inflammatory agents and drugs or herbal supplements.
- Assess for past allergic reactions to aspirin or NSAIDs.
- Assess for history of peptic ulcer disease, GI bleeding, liver, and kidney disease.

Nursing Diagnoses

- Acute pain
- Chronic pain
- Activity intolerance related to pain or fever
- Risk for poisoning: acetaminophen overdose
- Risk for injury related to adverse drug effects (GI bleeding, renal insufficiency, hepatotoxicity)
- Readiness for enhanced knowledge: therapeutic and adverse effects of commonly used medications
- Readiness for enhanced knowledge: correct use of OTC drugs for pain, fever, inflammation

Planning/Goals

The patient will

- Experience relief of discomfort with minimal adverse drug effects
- Experience increased mobility and activity tolerance
- Inform health care providers if taking aspirin, an NSAID, or acetaminophen regularly.
- Self-administer the drugs safely
- Avoid overuse of the drugs
- Use measures to prevent accidental ingestion or overdose, especially in children

Nursing Interventions

The nurse will

- Implement measures to prevent or minimize pain, fever, and inflammation
- Treat the disease processes (e.g., infection, arthritis) or circumstances (e.g., impaired blood supply, lack of physical activity, poor positioning or body alignment) thought to be causing pain, fever, or inflammation
- Treat pain as soon as possible; early treatment may prevent severe pain and anxiety and allow the use of milder analgesic drugs. Use distraction, relaxation techniques, or other nonpharmacologic techniques along with drug therapy, when appropriate.
- With acute musculoskeletal injuries (e.g., sprains), think RICE: Rest, Ice, Compression, Elevation to decrease pain, swelling, and inflammation. Cold therapy should be applied for 20 minutes every 3 to 4 hours for 48 hours.
- Assist patients to drink 2 to 3 L of fluid daily when taking an NSAID regularly. This strategy decreases gastric irritation and helps to maintain good kidney function. With long-term use of aspirin, fluids help prevent precipitation of salicylate crystals in the urinary tract. With antigout drugs, fluids help prevent precipitation of urate crystals and formation of urate kidney stones. Fluid intake is especially important initially when serum uric acid levels are high and large amounts of uric acid are being excreted.
- Provide appropriate teaching for any drug therapy

Evaluation

- Interview and observe regarding relief of symptoms.
- Interview and observe regarding mobility and activity levels.
- Interview and observe regarding safe, effective use of the drugs.
- Select drugs appropriately.

Key Concepts

- Aspirin, other NSAIDs, and acetaminophen inhibit COX enzymes, which are required for prostaglandin formation.

- Aspirin and other nonselective NSAIDs inhibit both COX-1 and COX-2. The COX-2 inhibitor, celecoxib, is more selective for the COX-2 enzyme. The exact mechanism of action of acetaminophen is unclear.

- The FDA has issued a **BLACK BOX WARNING** ◆ for aspirin stating that children or teenagers should not take aspirin to treat chickenpox or flu-like symptoms because of the risk of Reye's syndrome.

- Prostaglandins produced by COX-1 are important in regulating homeostasis and are associated with platelet aggregation and protective effects on the stomach and kidneys. Drug-induced inhibition results in gastric ulceration, renal dysfunction, and diminished blood clotting.

- Prostaglandins produced by COX-2 are associated with pain and inflammation. Drug-induced inhibition results in therapeutic effects of analgesia and anti-inflammatory activity.

- People with hypersensitivity to aspirin should not take NSAIDs due to the risk of cross-sensitivity to other antiprostaglandin drugs.

- The use of gastroprotective drugs such as antacids, H_2 blockers, and proton pump inhibitors may be indicated to prevent upper GI bleeding with chronic use of aspirin and other nonselective NSAIDs.

- Acetaminophen is the drug of choice for fever in children. Acetaminophen and ibuprofen may be alternated in the treatment of children with fever.

- The major drawback of acetaminophen use is the potentially fatal liver damage with overdose. Acetylcysteine is the specific antidote to acetaminophen overdose.

- The FDA has issued a **BLACK BOX WARNING** ◆ stating that ibuprofen is contraindicated for the treatment of perioperative pain after coronary artery bypass graft.

- A **BLACK BOX WARNING** ◆ states that patients who take meloxicam are at risk for cardiovascular events and GI bleeding.

- Another **BLACK BOX WARNING** ◆ states that an increased risk for adverse cardiovascular thrombotic effects, including myocardial infarction and cerebrovascular accident, may occur with indomethacin.

- Drugs related to indomethacin are etodolac, ketorolac (Toradol), and nabumetone (Relafen). Etodolac reportedly causes less gastric irritation, especially in older adults at high risk for GI bleeding.

- The FDA has issued a **BLACK BOX WARNING** ◆ for ketorolac, which places the patient at risk for GI irritation, inflammation, ulceration, bleeding, and perforation.

- The FDA has issued a **BLACK BOX WARNING** ◆ for celecoxib concerning its cardiac and vascular risks.

- Allopurinol, which inhibits the synthesis of uric acid, is the drug of choice for people with gout due to "overproduction" of uric acid.

- Colchicine is the only antigout drug with anti-inflammatory effects; it is useful for treating acute attacks.

- Febuxostat, probenecid, and sulfinpyrazone are uricosuric drugs effective in treating people with gout who "underexcrete" uric acid.

- During treatment for gout, the nurse encourages patients to increase fluid intake to 2000 mL per day to prevent renal calculi.

Critical Thinking Questions

14-1. A 76-year-old woman is seen by her neurosurgeon for severe low back pain radiating down her left leg. Magnetic resonance imaging (MRI) reveals spinal stenosis. She has refused epidural injections and is prescribed celecoxib (Celebrex).

- What is the action of celecoxib?
- What patient education should be implemented regarding celecoxib?
- What adverse effects is the patient at risk for developing?

References and Resources

Balas, M., Plakogiannis, R., & Sinnett, M. (2010). Periorbital edema associated with separate courses of ibuprofen and naproxen. *American Journal of Health System Pharmacy, 67,* 906–909.

Carpenito-Moyet, L. J. (2011). *Nursing diagnosis: Application to clinical practice.* (13th ed.). Philadelphia, PA: Lippincott Williams and Wilkins.

Gray, C. L., & Walters-Smith, N. E. (2011). Febuxostat for treatment of chronic gout. *American Journal of Health System Pharmacy, 68,* 389–398.

Hilarie, M. L., & Wozniak, J. (2010). Gout: Overview and newer therapeutic developments. *Formulary, 45.* Retrieved: April 17, 2011, www.formularyjournal.com

Karch, A. M. (2011). *2011 Lippincott's nursing drug guide.* Philadelphia, PA: Lippincott Williams & Wilkins.

Medical College of Wisconsin. (2009). Drug update: Ibuprofen as effective as acetaminophen with codeine to treat pain in children. *Healthcare Traveler, 21.*

Nursing 2011 Drug Handbook. (2011). Philadelphia, PA: Lippincott Williams & Wilkins.

Pavliv, L., Voss, B., & Rock, A. (2011). Pharmacokinetics, safety, and tolerability of a rapid infusion of I.V. ibuprofen in healthy adults. *American Journal of Health System Pharmacy, 68,* 47–51.

Porth, C. M., & Matfin, (2009). *Pathophysiology concepts of altered health states.* Philadelphia, PA: Lippincott Williams & Wilkins.

Schub, T. & Pravikoff, D. (2011). Gout. *Quick Lesson: Cinahl Information System.*

Smeltzer, S. C., Bare, B. G., Hinkle, J. H., & Cheever, K. H. (2010). *Brunner & Suddarth's textbook of medical-surgical nursing* (12th ed.). Philadelphia, PA: Lippincott Williams & Wilkins.

Up-To-Date. (2011). *Allopurinol: Drug information.* Lexi-Comp Inc.

Up-To-Date. (2011). *Colchicine: Drug information.* Lexi-Comp Inc.

Up-To-Date. (2011). *Etodolac: Patient drug information.* Lexi-Comp Inc.

Up-To-Date, (2011). *Febuxostat: Drug information.* Lexi-Comp Inc.

Up-To-Date, (2011). *Indomethacin: Drug information.* Lexi-Comp Inc.

Up-To-Date, (2011). Meloxicam: Drug information. Lexi-Comp Inc.

Up-To-Date, (2011). *Treatment of Acute Gout.* Lexi-Comp Inc.

Up-To-Date, (2011). *Prevention of Recurrent Gout.* Lexi-Comp Inc.

Up-To-Date, (2011). *Treatment of Gout.* Lexi-Comp Inc.

Yang, L. P. H. (2010). *Oral colchicine (Colcrys) in the treatment and prophylaxis of gout. Drugs and Aging,* 27(10), 855–857.

15 Drug Therapy With Corticosteroids

After studying this chapter, you should be able to:

1. Understand the physiologic effects of endogenous corticosteroids.

2. Identify the pathophysiology of adrenal cortex disorders.

3. Describe the action and the clinical indications for use of exogenous corticosteroids.

4. Understand the contraindications and adverse effects of corticosteroids as well as the nursing implications of their use.

5. Analyze how other drugs and substances as well as other factors may affect the need for corticosteroids.

6. Apply the nursing process when a patient is administered a corticosteroid.

Clinical Application Case Study

Emma Mae Thompson is a 65-year-old African American woman who lives alone. Since she was 15 years old, she has smoked one pack of unfiltered cigarettes per day. When she was diagnosed with chronic obstructive pulmonary disease 5 years ago, she quit smoking. She takes albuterol sulfate 1 inhalation per nebulizer every 12 hours and beclomethasone dipropionate 160 mcg every 12 hours. Recently, she was treated for pneumonia. Mrs. Thompson's physician prescribes prednisone orally in a tapering dose, according to the following schedule:

Day 1: 10 mg before breakfast, 5 mg before lunch, 5 mg before supper, 10 mg at bedtime
Day 2: 5 mg before breakfast, 5 mg before lunch, 5 mg before supper, 10 mg at bedtime
Day 3: 5 mg before breakfast, 5 mg before lunch, 5 mg before supper, 5 mg at bedtime
Day 4: 5 mg before breakfast, 5 mg before supper, 5 mg at bedtime
Day 5: 5 mg before breakfast, 5 mg at bedtime
Day 6: 5 mg before breakfast

KEY TERMS

Addison's disease: primary adrenocortical insufficiency with inadequate production of cortisol and aldosterone

Addisonian crisis: condition that mimics hypovolemic and septic shock; also known as adrenocortical insufficiency

Aldosterone: mineralocorticoid hormone secreted by the adrenal cortex to increase sodium reabsorption by the kidneys and indirectly regulate blood levels of potassium, sodium, and bicarbonate; also regulates pH, blood volume, and blood pressure

Corticosteroid: steroid hormones produced by the adrenal cortex; examples include androgens, glucocorticoids, and mineralocorticoids

Cortisol: the main glucocorticoid secreted as part of the body's response to stress

Cushing's disease: adrenocortical hyperfunction; may result from excessive corticotropin or primary adrenal tumor

Glucocorticoid: adrenal cortical hormone that protects the body against stress and affects protein and carbohydrate metabolism

Immunosuppression: suppression of the immune system

Mineralocorticoid: steroid hormone released by the adrenal cortex to promote sodium and water retention and potassium excretion

Negative feedback mechanism: when the output of a system affects the stimulus for the system (e.g., hormone secretion produces an effect that shuts off the stimulus for further hormone secretion)

Steroid: lipid-soluble hormone produced by the gonadal organs or the adrenal cortex

Introduction

This chapter provides an introduction to the **corticosteroids**, also known as the **glucocorticoids** or **steroids**. These lipid-soluble hormones are produced by the gonadal organs or the adrenal cortex, part of the adrenal glands. These hormones affect almost all body organs and are extremely important in maintaining homeostasis when secreted in normal amounts. Disease results from inadequate or excessive secretion. Exogenous corticosteroids are used as drugs in a variety of disorders. Their use must be closely monitored, because they have profound therapeutic and adverse effects. To understand the effects of corticosteroids used as drugs (exogenous corticosteroids), it is necessary to understand the physiologic effects and other characteristics of the endogenous hormones.

Physiology of Endogenous Corticosteroids

Corticosteroid secretion is controlled by the hypothalamus, the anterior pituitary, and adrenal cortex (the hypothalamic–pituitary–adrenal, or HPA, axis). Various stimuli (e.g., low plasma levels of corticosteroids, pain, anxiety, trauma, illness, anesthesia) activate the system. These stimuli cause the hypothalamus of the brain to secrete corticotropin-releasing hormone or factor (known as CRH or CRF), which stimulates the anterior pituitary gland to secrete corticotropin, and corticotropin then stimulates the adrenal cortex to secrete corticosteroids.

The rate of corticosteroid secretion is usually maintained within relatively narrow limits but changes according to need. When plasma corticosteroid levels rise to an adequate level, secretion of corticosteroids slows or stops. The mechanism by which the hypothalamus and anterior pituitary "learn" that no more corticosteroids are needed is called a **negative feedback mechanism**.

This negative feedback mechanism is normally very important, but it does not work during stress responses. The stress response activates the sympathetic nervous system (SNS) to produce more epinephrine and norepinephrine and the adrenal cortex to produce as much as 10 times the normal amount of cortisol. The synergistic interaction of these hormones increases the person's ability to respond to stress. However, the increased SNS activity continues to stimulate **cortisol** production (the main glucocorticoid secreted as part of the body's response to stress) and overrules the negative feedback mechanism. Excessive and prolonged corticosteroid secretion damages body tissues.

Corticosteroids are secreted directly into the bloodstream. Cortisol is approximately 90% bound to plasma proteins, and this high degree of protein binding slows cortisol movement out of the plasma, so that it has a relatively long plasma half-life of 60 to 90 minutes. The remaining 10% is unbound and biologically active. In contrast, aldosterone is only 60% bound to plasma proteins and has a short half-life of 20 minutes. In general, protein binding functions as a storage area from which the hormones are released as needed. This promotes more consistent blood levels and more uniform distribution to the tissues.

The adrenal cortex produces approximately 30 steroid hormones, which are divided into glucocorticoids, mineralocorticoids, and adrenal sex hormones. Chemically, all corticosteroids are derived from cholesterol and have similar chemical structures. However, despite their similarities, slight differences cause them to have different functions.

Glucocorticoids

Although the term "corticosteroids" actually refers to all secretions of the adrenal cortex, it is most often used to designate the glucocorticoids, which are important in metabolic, inflammatory, and immune processes. Glucocorticoids include cortisol, corticosterone, and cortisone. Cortisol accounts for at least 95% of glucocorticoid activity; corticosterone and cortisone accounts for a small amount of activity. Glucocorticoids are secreted cyclically, with the largest amount being produced in the early morning and the smallest amount during the evening hours (in people with a normal day–night schedule). At the cellular level, glucocorticoids account for most of the characteristics and physiologic effects of the corticosteroids (Box 15.1).

BOX 15.1 Effects of Glucocorticoids on Body Processes and Systems

Carbohydrate Metabolism

■ ↑Formation of glucose (gluconeogenesis) by breaking down protein into amino acids. The amino acids are then transported to the liver, where they are acted on by enzymes that convert them to glucose. The glucose is then returned to the circulation for use by body tissues or storage in the liver as glycogen.

■ ↓Cellular use of glucose, especially in muscle cells. This is attributed to a ↓effect of insulin on the proteins that normally transport glucose into cells and by ↓numbers and functional capacity of insulin receptors.

■ Both the ↑production and ↓use of glucose promote higher levels of glucose in the blood (hyperglycemia) and may lead to diabetes mellitus. These actions also increase the amount of glucose stored as glycogen in the liver, skeletal muscles, and other tissues.

Protein Metabolism

■ Breakdown of protein into amino acids (catabolic effect); ↑rate of amino acid transport to the liver and conversion to glucose

■ ↓Rate of new protein formation from dietary and other amino acids (antianabolic effect)

■ The combination of ↑breakdown of cell protein and ↓protein synthesis leads to protein depletion in virtually all body cells except those of the liver. Thus, glycogen stores in the body are ↑ and protein stores are ↓.

Lipid Metabolism

■ ↑Breakdown of adipose tissue into fatty acids; the fatty acids are transported in the plasma and used as a source of energy by body cells.

■ ↑Oxidation of fatty acids within body cells.

Inflammatory and Immune Responses

■ ↓Inflammatory response. Inflammation is the normal bodily response to tissue damage and involves three stages. First, a large amount of plasma-like fluid leaks out of capillaries into the damaged area and becomes clotted. Second, leukocytes migrate into the area. Third, tissue healing occurs, largely by growth of fibrous scar tissue. Normal or physiologic amounts of glucocorticoids probably do not significantly affect inflammation and healing, but large amounts of glucocorticoids inhibit all three stages of the inflammatory process.

More specifically, corticosteroids stabilize lysosomal membranes (and thereby prevent the release of inflammatory proteolytic enzymes); ↓capillary permeability (and thereby ↓leakage of fluid and proteins into the damaged tissue); ↓the accumulation of neutrophils and macrophages at sites of inflammation (and thereby impair phagocytosis of pathogenic microorganisms and waste products of cellular metabolism); and ↓production of inflammatory chemicals, such as interleukin-1, prostaglandins, and leukotrienes, by injured cells.

■ ↓Immune response. The immune system normally protects the body from foreign invaders, and several immune responses overlap inflammatory responses, including phagocytosis. In addition, the immune response stimulates the production of antibodies and activated lymphocytes to destroy the foreign substance. Glucocorticoids impair protein synthesis, including the production of antibodies; ↓the numbers of circulating lymphocytes, eosinophils, and macrophages; and ↓amounts of lymphoid tissue. These effects help account for the immunosuppressive and antiallergic actions of the glucocorticoids.

Cardiovascular System

■ Help regulate arterial blood pressure by modifying vascular smooth muscle tone by modifying myocardial contractility and by stimulating renal mineralocorticoid and glucocorticoid receptors

■ ↑The response of vascular smooth muscle to the pressor effects of catecholamines and other vasoconstrictive agents

Nervous System

■ Physiologic amounts help to *maintain normal nerve excitability;* pharmacologic amounts ↓ nerve excitability, slow activity in the cerebral cortex, and alter brain wave patterns.

■ ↓Secretion of CRH by the hypothalamus and of corticotropin by the anterior pituitary gland. This results in suppression of further glucocorticoid secretion by the adrenal cortex (negative feedback system).

Musculoskeletal System

■ Maintain muscle strength when present in physiologic amounts but cause muscle atrophy (from protein breakdown) when present in excessive amounts.

■ ↓Bone formation and growth and ↑bone breakdown. Glucocorticoids also ↓ intestinal absorption and ↑ renal excretion of calcium. These effects contribute to bone demineralization (osteoporosis) in adults and to ↓linear growth in children.

Respiratory System

■ Maintain open airways. Glucocorticoids do not have direct bronchodilating effects, but help maintain and restore responsiveness to the bronchodilating effects of endogenous catecholamines, such as epinephrine.

■ Stabilize mast cells and other cells to inhibit the release of bronchoconstrictive and inflammatory substances, such as histamine.

Gastrointestinal System

■ ↓Viscosity of gastric mucus. This effect may ↓ protective properties of the mucus and contribute to the development of peptic ulcer disease.

↑, increase/increased; ↓, decrease/decreased.

Mineralocorticoids

Mineralocorticoids are a class of steroids that play a vital role in the maintenance of fluid and electrolyte balance through their influence on salt and water metabolism. **Aldosterone** is the main mineralocorticoid and is responsible for approximately 90% of mineralocorticoid activity. Characteristics and physiologic effects of mineralocorticoids are summarized in Box 15.2.

BOX 15.2	Effects of Mineralocorticoids on Body Processes and Systems

- The overall physiologic effects are to conserve sodium and water and eliminate potassium. Aldosterone increases sodium reabsorption from kidney tubules, and water is reabsorbed along with the sodium. When sodium is conserved, another cation must be excreted to maintain electrical neutrality of body fluids; thus, potassium is excreted. This is the only potent mechanism for controlling the concentration of potassium ions in extracellular fluids.

- Secretion of aldosterone is controlled by several factors, most of which are related to kidney function. In general, secretion is increased when the potassium level of extracellular fluid is high, the sodium level of

extracellular fluid is low, the renin–angiotensin system of the kidneys is activated, or the anterior pituitary gland secretes corticotropin.

- Inadequate secretion of aldosterone causes hyperkalemia, hyponatremia, and extracellular fluid volume deficit (dehydration). Hypotension and shock may result from decreased cardiac output. Absence of mineralocorticoids causes death.

- Excessive secretion of aldosterone produces hypokalemia, hypernatremia, and extracellular fluid volume excess (water intoxication). Edema and hypertension may result.

Adrenal Sex Hormones

The adrenal cortex secretes male (androgens) and female (estrogens and progesterone) sex hormones. Compared with the effect of hormones produced by the testes and ovaries, the adrenal sex hormones have an insignificant effect on normal body function. Adrenal androgens, secreted continuously in small quantities by both sexes, are responsible for most of the physiologic effects exerted by the adrenal sex hormones. They increase protein synthesis (anabolism), which increases the mass and strength of muscle and bone tissue; they affect development of male secondary sex characteristics; and they increase hair growth and libido in women. Excessive secretion of adrenal androgens in women causes masculinizing effects (e.g., hirsutism, acne, breast atrophy, deepening of the voice, amenorrhea). Female sex hormones are secreted in small amounts and normally exert few physiologic effects. Excessive secretion may produce feminizing effects in men (e.g., breast enlargement, decreased hair growth, voice changes).

Pathophysiology of Adrenal Cortex Disorders

Disorders of the adrenal cortex involve increased or decreased production of corticosteroids, especially cortisol as the primary glucocorticoid and aldosterone as the primary mineralocorticoid. These disorders include the following:

- **Primary adrenocortical insufficiency (Addison's disease)** is associated with destruction of the adrenal cortex by disorders such as tuberculosis, cancer, or hemorrhage; with atrophy of the adrenal cortex caused by autoimmune disease or prolonged administration of exogenous corticosteroids; and with surgical excision of the adrenal glands. In primary adrenocortical insufficiency, there is inadequate production of both cortisol and aldosterone.

- **Secondary adrenocortical insufficiency,** produced by inadequate secretion of corticotropin, is most often caused by prolonged administration of corticosteroids. This condition is largely a glucocorticoid deficiency; mineralocorticoid secretion is not significantly impaired.

- **Congenital adrenogenital syndromes and adrenal hyperplasia** result from deficiencies in one or more enzymes required for cortisol production. Low plasma levels of cortisol lead to excessive corticotropin secretion, which then leads to excessive adrenal secretion of androgens and hyperplasia (abnormal increase in number of cells).

- **Androgen-producing tumors** of the adrenal cortex, which are usually benign, produce masculinizing effects.

- **Adrenocortical hyperfunction (Cushing's disease)** may result from excessive corticotropin or a primary adrenal tumor. Adrenal tumors may be benign or malignant. Benign tumors often produce one corticosteroid normally secreted by the adrenal cortex, but malignant tumors often secrete several corticosteroids.

- **Hyperaldosteronism** is a rare disorder caused by adenoma (a benign tissue from glandular tissue) or hyperplasia of the adrenal cortex cells that produce aldosterone. It is characterized by hypokalemia, hypernatremia, hypertension, thirst, and polyuria.

Drug Therapy with Exogenous Corticosteroids

Exogenous corticosteroids, or glucocorticoids, are administered to treat disorders of the adrenal cortex or endocrine system. The administration of corticosteroids decreases the inflammatory symptoms and alters the immune response produced by nonendocrine disorders. People once viewed hydrocortisone, a short-acting corticosteroid and an exogenous equivalent of endogenous cortisol, as the prototype corticosteroid drug. Now they consider ℗ **prednisone**, an intermediate acting corticosteroid, to be the prototype corticosteroid. Table 15.1 lists the glucocorticoids and mineralocorticoids.

Pharmacokinetics

The rate of absorption of corticosteroids depends on the route of administration. Oral administration results in rapid absorption by the gastrointestinal (GI) tract, with rapid

TABLE 15.1

Adrenal Corticosteroid Drugs

Drug Class	Prototype	Other Drugs in the Class
Glucocorticoid	Prednisone (Apo-Prednisone, Deltasone)	Beclomethasone (QVAR, Beconase AQ)
		Betamethasone (Celestone)
		Betamethasone acetate and betamethasone sodium phosphate (Celestone Soluspan)
		Budesonide (Pulmicort, Rhinocort, Entocort EC)
		Cortisone
		Dexamethasone (Decadron)
		Dexamethasone acetate
		Dexamethasone sodium phosphate (Decadron Phosphate)
		Flunisolide (AeroBid, Nasarel)
		Fluticasone (Flovent, Flonase)
		Hydrocortisone (Cortaid)
		Hydrocortisone (Cortef)
		Hydrocortisone sodium phosphate
		Hydrocortisone sodium succinate (Solu-Cortef)
		Hydrocortisone retention enema (Cortenema)
		Hydrocortisone acetate (Cortifoam)
		Methylprednisolone (Medrol)
		Methylprednisolone sodium succinate (Solu-Medrol)
		Methylprednisolone acetate (Depo-Medrol)
		Mometasone (Nasonex)
		Prednisolone (Prelone)
		Prednisolone acetate (Pred Forte)
		Triamcinolone
		Triamcinolone acetonide (Azmacort, Nasacort)
		Triamcinolone hexacetonide (Aristospan)
Mineralocorticoid	Fludrocortisone (Florinef)	

distribution to the intestines, muscles, liver, and kidneys. The corticosteroid is metabolized by the liver by cytochrome P450 3A4 enzymes, and the medication is conjugated to inactive metabolites. About 25% of the metabolites are excreted in the bile and then in the feces. The other 75%, which enter the circulation, are excreted in the kidneys. Plasma binding affects metabolism of corticosteroids, which means that patients with serum albumin levels less than 3.5 g/dL are prone to increased effects of corticosteroids and symptoms of hypercorticism.

The administration of exogenous corticosteroids suppresses the HPA axis. As a result, secretion of corticotropin decreases, causing atrophy of the adrenal cortex and decreased production of endogenous adrenal corticosteroids.

Action

Like endogenous glucocorticoids, exogenous corticosteroids act at the cellular level by binding to drug receptors in target tissues. The lipid-soluble drugs easily diffuse through the cell membranes of target cells. Inside the cell, they bind with receptors in intracellular cytoplasm. The drug–receptor complex then moves to the cell nucleus, where it interacts with DNA to stimulate or suppress gene transcription.

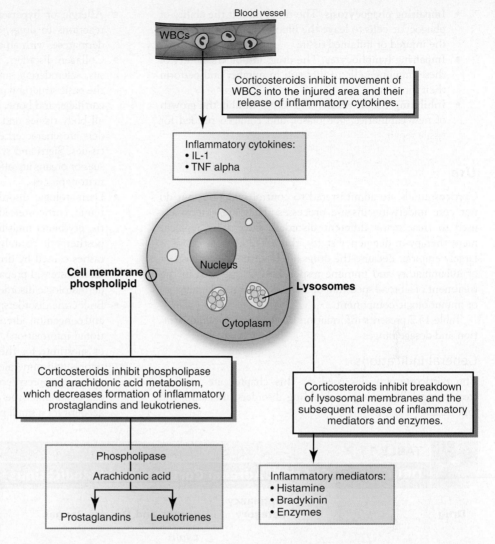

Figure 15.1 Inflammatory processes and anti-inflammatory actions of corticosteroids. Cellular responses to injury include the following: phospholipid in the cell membrane is acted on by phospholipase to release arachidonic acid, metabolism of arachidonic acid produces the inflammatory mediators prostaglandins and leukotrienes, lysosomal membrane breaks down and releases inflammatory chemicals (e.g., histamine, bradykinin, intracellular digestive enzymes), and white blood cells (WBCs) are drawn to the area and release inflammatory cytokines (e.g., interleukin-1 [IL-1] alpha). Overall, corticosteroid drugs act to inhibit the release, formation, or activation of various inflammatory mediators.

Corticosteroids can increase or decrease the transcription of many genes to alter the synthesis of proteins. These proteins regulate many physiologic effects, such as the transportation of proteins. Metabolic effects do not occur for at least 45 to 60 minutes because of the time required for protein synthesis. Several hours or days may be needed for full production of proteins.

Because the genes vary in different types of body cells, corticosteroid effects also vary, depending on the specific cells being targeted. For example, supraphysiologic concentrations of glucocorticoids induce the synthesis of lipolytic and proteolytic enzymes and other specific proteins in various tissues. Overall, corticosteroids have multiple mechanisms of action and effects (Fig. 15.1), including the following:

- **Inhibiting arachidonic acid metabolism.** Normally, when a body cell is injured or activated by various stimuli, the enzyme phospholipase A_2 causes the phospholipids in cell membranes to release arachidonic acid. Free arachidonic acid is then metabolized to produce proinflammatory prostaglandins (see Chap. 14) and leukotrienes. At sites of tissue injury or inflammation, corticosteroids induce the synthesis of proteins that suppress

the activation of phospholipase A_2. This action, in turn, decreases the release of arachidonic acid and the formation of prostaglandins and leukotrienes.

- **Strengthening or stabilizing biologic membranes.** Two biologic membranes are especially important in inflammatory processes. Stabilization of cell membranes inhibits the release of arachidonic acid and production of prostaglandins and leukotrienes, as described above. Stabilization of lysosomal membranes inhibits release of bradykinin, histamine, enzymes, and perhaps other substances from lysosomes. (Lysosomes are intracellular structures that contain inflammatory chemical mediators and enzymes that destroy cellular debris and phagocytized pathogens.) This reduces capillary permeability and thus prevents leakage of fluid into the injured area and development of edema. It also reduces the chemicals that normally cause vasodilation and tissue irritation.

- **Inhibiting the production of interleukin-1, tumor necrosis factor, and other cytokines.** This action also contributes to the anti-inflammatory and immunosuppressant effects of corticosteroids.

- **Impairing phagocytosis.** The drugs inhibit the ability of phagocytic cells to leave the bloodstream and move into the injured or inflamed tissue.
- **Impairing lymphocytes.** The drugs inhibit the ability of these immune cells to increase in number and perform their functions.
- **Inhibiting tissue repair.** The drugs inhibit the growth of new capillaries, fibroblasts, and collagen needed for tissue repair.

Use

Corticosteroids are administered to control symptoms but do not cure underlying disease processes. They are extensively used to treat many different disorders. Except for replacement therapy in deficiency states, the use of corticosteroids is largely empiric. Because the drugs affect virtually every aspect of inflammatory and immune responses, they are used in the treatment of a broad spectrum of diseases with an inflammatory or immunologic component.

Table 15.2 presents information about routes of administration and dosage ranges.

General Indications

The corticosteroids discussed in this chapter are used to treat potentially serious or disabling disorders, including the following:

- Allergic or hypersensitivity disorders, such as allergic reactions to drugs, serum and blood transfusions, and dermatoses with an allergic component
- Collagen disorders, such as systemic lupus erythematosus, scleroderma, and periarteritis nodosa. Collagen is the basic structural protein of connective tissue, tendons, cartilage, and bone, and it is therefore present in almost all body tissues and organ systems. The collagen disorders are characterized by inflammation of various body tissues. Signs and symptoms depend on which body tissues or organs are affected and the severity of the inflammatory process.
- Dermatologic disorders that may be treated with systemic corticosteroids include acute contact dermatitis, erythema multiforme, herpes zoster (prophylaxis of postherpetic neuralgia), lichen planus, pemphigus, skin rashes caused by drugs, and toxic epidermal necrolysis. Corticosteroid preparations that are applied topically in dermatologic disorders are discussed in Chapter 60.
- Endocrine disorders, such as adrenocortical insufficiency and congenital adrenal hyperplasia (see Chap. 43 for additional information). Corticosteroids are given to replace or substitute for the natural hormones (both glucocorticoids and mineralocorticoids) in cases of insufficiency and to suppress corticotropin when excess secretion causes adrenal hyperplasia. These conditions are rare and account for a small percentage of corticosteroid use.

TABLE 15.2

DRUGS AT A GLANCE: Adrenal Corticosteroid Medications

Drug	Pregnancy Category	Routes and Dosage Ranges	
		Adults	*Children*
Glucocorticoids			
Ⓟ **Prednisone** (Apo-Prednisone, Deltasone)	C	5–60 mg PO daily initially, adjusted for maintenance	0.25–2 mg/kg/dose PO every 6–48 h, then 1–2 mg/kg/24 h (maximum 60 mg/24 h)
Beclomethasone (QVAR) Oral inhalation	C	1–2 inhalations (40–80 mcg) 2 times daily (maximum daily dose 320 mcg)	
(Beconase AQ) Nasal inhalation	C	1–2 inhalations (42–84 mcg in each nostril) 2 times daily; as maintenance, 1 inhalation each nostril	Older than 6 y: 1–2 inhalations (42–84 mcg) each nostril daily
Betamethasone (Celestone)	C	0.6–7.2 mg PO daily initially, gradually reduced to lowest effective dose	
Betamethasone acetate and sodium phosphate (Celestone Soluspan)	C	0.5–9 mg IM daily; 0.25–2 mL intraarticular injection	
Budesonide (Pulmicort Flexhaler, Turbuhaler, Pulmicort Respules) Oral inhalation		Pulmicort Flexhaler 360 mcg twice daily; maximum dose 720 mcg twice daily	Pulmicort Respules 12 mo–8 y: 0.5–1 mg once daily or in 2 divided doses using jet nebulizer Pulmicort Flexhaler 180 mcg twice daily; maximum dose 360 mcg twice daily

TABLE 15.2

DRUGS AT A GLANCE: Adrenal Corticosteroid Medications (Continued)

Drug	Pregnancy Category	Routes and Dosage Ranges	
		Adults	Children
Budesonide (Rhinocort) Nasal inhalation		256 mcg daily (2 sprays each nostril morning and evening or 4 sprays each nostril every morning). When symptoms are controlled, reduce dosage to lowest effective maintenance dose	
Budesonide (Entocort EC) Oral capsule		Crohn's disease: 9 mg PO once daily in the morning, for up to 8 wk	
Cortisone	C	25–300 mg PO daily, individualized for condition and response	
Dexamethasone (Decadron)	C	0.75–9 mg PO daily in 2–4 doses; higher range for serious diseases	
Dexamethasone acetate	C	8–16 mg (1–2 mL) IM in single dose, repeated every 1–3 wk if necessary	
Dexamethasone sodium phosphate (Decadron Phosphate)	C	0.5–9 mg IM or IV depending on the severity of disease	
Flunisolide (AeroBid) Oral inhalation	C	2 inhalations (500 mcg) twice daily	6–15 y: same as adults
Flunisolide (Nasarel) Nasal inhalation	C	2 sprays in each nostril twice daily; maximum daily dose 8 sprays in each nostril	6–14 y: 1 spray in each nostril 3 times daily or 2 sprays in each nostril 2 times daily; maximum daily dose 4 sprays in each nostril
Fluticasone (Flovent) Oral inhalation	C	2 inhalations (88 mcg) 2 times daily (maximum daily dose 440 mcg inhaled 2 times daily)	Under 12 y: not recommended
Fluticasone (Flonase) Nasal inhalation		200 mcg daily initially (2 sprays each nostril once daily or 1 spray each nostril twice daily). After a few days, reduce dosage to 100 mcg daily (1 spray each nostril once daily) for maintenance therapy	≥12 y: 100 mcg daily (1 spray per nostril once daily)
Hydrocortisone (Cortaid)	C	Apply sparingly to skin 2–4 times daily	Same as adults
Hydrocortisone (Cortef)	C	20–240 mg PO daily, depending on condition and response	
Hydrocortisone (Cortenema) Retention enema	C	100 mg enema rectally every night for 21 d or until optimal response	
Hydrocortisone acetate (Cortifoam) Intrathecal	C	1 applicator rectally 1–2 times per day for 2–3 wk, then once every 2–3 d if needed	
Methylprednisolone (Medrol)	C	4–48 mg daily PO initially, gradually reduced to lowest effective level	
Methylprednisolone sodium succinate (Solu-Medrol)	C	10–40 mg IM or IV initially, adjusted to condition and response	Infants and children: not <0.5 mg/kg/24 h IM or IV
Methylprednisolone acetate (Depo-Medrol)	C	40–120 mg IM once daily	

(Continued on page 278)

TABLE 15.2

DRUGS AT A GLANCE: Adrenal Corticosteroid Medications (Continued)

Drug	Pregnancy Category	Routes and Dosage Ranges	
		Adults	Children
Mometasone (Nasonex)	C	2 sprays (50 mcg/spray) in each nostril once daily (200 mcg/d)	>12 y: same as adults 3–11 y: 1 spray (50 mcg) in each nostril once daily (100 mcg/d)
Prednisolone (Prelone)	C	5–60 mg PO daily initially, adjusted for maintenance	0.1–2 mg/kg/d PO in divided doses
Prednisolone acetate (Pred Forte)	C	1–2 drops in conjunctival sac every hour during the day; then every 2 h during the night; may decrease to 3–4 times per day	
Triamcinolone	C	4–48 mg daily PO initially, reduced for maintenance	
Triamcinolone acetonide (Azmacort) Oral inhalation	C	2 inhalations (200 mcg) 3–4 times daily or 4 inhalations (400 mcg) 2 times daily	6–12 y: 1–2 inhalations (100–200 mcg) 3–4 times daily or 2–4 inhalations (200–400 mcg) 2 times daily. Maximum daily dose 12 inhalations (1200 mcg)
Triamcinolone acetonide (Nasacort) Nasal inhalation	C	2 sprays (110 mcg) in each nostril once daily (total dose 220 mcg/d); may increase to maximal daily dose of 440 mcg if indicated	≥6 y: 2 sprays (110 mcg) in each nostril once daily (220 mcg/d) initially; reduce to 1 spray per nostril once daily (110 mcg/d)
Triamcinolone hexacetonide (Aristospan)	C	Up to 0.5 mg/in^2 of skin Intraarticular 2–20 mg every 3–4 wk	
Mineralocorticoid			
Fludrocortisone (Florinef)	C	Chronic adrenocortical insufficiency, 0.1 mg PO daily Salt-losing adrenogenital syndromes, 0.1–0.2 mg daily	0.05–0.1 mg PO daily

- GI disorders, such as ulcerative colitis and regional enteritis (Crohn's disease)
- Hematologic disorders, such as idiopathic thrombocytopenic purpura or acquired hemolytic anemia
- Hepatic disorders characterized by edema, such as cirrhosis and ascites
- Neoplastic disease, such as acute and chronic leukemias, Hodgkin's disease, other lymphomas, and multiple myeloma (see later discussion)
- Neurologic conditions, such as cerebral edema, brain tumor, acute spinal cord injury (see later discussion), and myasthenia gravis
- Ophthalmic disorders, such as optic neuritis, sympathetic ophthalmia, and chorioretinitis. Corticosteroid preparations that are applied topically in ophthalmologic disorders are discussed in Chapter 58.

- Organ or tissue transplants and grafts (e.g., kidney, heart, bone marrow). Corticosteroids suppress cellular and humoral immune responses (see Chap. 11) and help prevent rejection of transplanted tissue. Drug therapy is usually continued as long as the transplanted tissue is in place.
- Renal disorders characterized by edema, such as the nephrotic syndrome
- Respiratory disorders, such as asthma, status asthmaticus, chronic obstructive pulmonary disease (COPD), and inflammatory disorders of nasal mucosa (rhinitis)
- Rheumatic disorders, such as ankylosing spondylitis, acute and chronic bursitis, acute gouty arthritis, rheumatoid arthritis, and osteoarthritis
- Shock. Corticosteroids are clearly indicated only for shock resulting from **Addisonian crisis** (also known

as adrenal or adrenocortical insufficiency), which may mimic hypovolemic or septic shock. The use of corticosteroids in septic shock has been highly controversial, and randomized studies and meta-analyses have indicated that corticosteroids are not beneficial in treating septic shock. However, more recent small studies indicate possible clinical usefulness in septic shock, because this form of shock may be associated with relative adrenal insufficiency. In anaphylactic shock resulting from an allergic reaction, corticosteroids may increase or restore cardiovascular responsiveness to adrenergic drugs.

Clinical Application 15-1

- What is the purpose of administering prednisone to Mrs. Thompson?
- What is the purpose of tapering the dose?
- Could prednisone be discontinued without tapering the dose?

NCLEX Success

1. A woman is experiencing periods of increased anxiety and panic attacks over her illness and that of her family members. Epinephrine and norepinephrine are released. What glucocorticoid is released by the adrenal cortex in response to stress?
   A. insulin
   B. glucose
   C. thyroid hormone
   D. cortisol

2. A boy has contracted a rash caused by poison ivy over a large portion of his arms and legs following a camping trip. His health care provider has prescribed oral prednisone, which is to be administered in a tapering dose over the next 10 days. What effect does the medication have on the rash?
   A. It decreases the accumulation of neutrophils and macrophages at the site, thus reducing inflammation.
   B. It eliminates the itching associated with the allergy.
   C. It increases the white blood cell count to assist in healing.
   D. It increases the protein metabolism to allow for the rejuvenation of tissue.

3. A patient is receiving prednisone 10 mg orally every day to reduce symptoms of Crohn's disease. Which of the following effects is associated with daily administration of prednisone?
   A. atrophy of the adrenal cortex
   B. decreased serum glucose
   C. weight loss
   D. fluid volume deficit

4. A patient with chronic obstructive pulmonary disease is being administered a corticosteroid by nebulizer. What effect does the corticosteroid have?
   A. decrease in blood pressure
   B. decrease in mucus secretion
   C. decrease in edema
   D. increase in immunity

5. A patient is admitted to the emergency department in anaphylactic shock following numerous bee stings. The prescriber orders parenteral administration of corticosteroids. What effect is expected from the administration of these agents?
   A. decreased heart rate and blood pressure
   B. increased circulation to the lower extremities
   C. increased or restored cardiovascular responsiveness
   D. decreased production of aldosterone

Specific Uses

Allergic Rhinitis

Allergic rhinitis (also called seasonal rhinitis, hay fever, and perennial rhinitis) is a common problem for which corticosteroids are given by nasal spray, once or twice daily. The drugs decrease mucus secretion and inflammation. Therapeutic effects usually occur within a few days with regular use. Systemic adverse effects are minimal with recommended doses but may occur with higher doses, including adrenocortical insufficiency from HPA suppression.

Arthritis

Corticosteroids are the most effective drugs for rapid relief of the pain, edema, and restricted mobility associated with acute episodes of joint inflammation. They are usually given on a short-term basis. When inflammation is limited to three or fewer joints, the preferred route of drug administration is by injection directly into the joint. Intraarticular injections relieve symptoms in approximately 2 to 8 weeks, and several formulations are available for this route. However, corticosteroids do not prevent disease progression and joint destruction. As a general rule, a joint should not be injected more often than three times yearly because of risks of infection and damage to intraarticular structures from the injections and from overuse when pain is relieved.

Asthma

Corticosteroids are commonly used in the treatment of asthma because of their anti-inflammatory effects. In addition, corticosteroids increase the effects of adrenergic bronchodilators to prevent or treat bronchoconstriction and bronchospasm. The drugs increase the number of beta-adrenergic receptors and increase or restore responsiveness of beta receptors to beta-adrenergic bronchodilating drugs. Research indicates that responsiveness to beta-adrenergic bronchodilators increases within 2 hours and that numbers of beta receptors increase within 4 hours.

In acute asthma or status asthmaticus unrelieved by inhaled beta-adrenergic bronchodilators, high doses of systemic corticosteroids are given orally or intravenously along with bronchodilators for approximately 5 to 10 days. Although these high doses suppress the HPA axis, the suppression lasts for only 1 to 3 days, and other serious adverse effects are avoided. Thus, systemic corticosteroids are used for short-term therapy, as needed, and not for long-term treatment. People who regularly use inhaled corticosteroids also require high doses of systemic drugs during acute attacks because aerosols are not effective. As soon as acute symptoms subside, it is necessary to taper the dose; people should take the lowest effective maintenance dose or discontinue the drug. In chronic asthma, inhaled corticosteroids are the drugs of first choice. This recommendation evolved from increased knowledge about the importance of inflammation in the pathophysiology of asthma and the development of aerosol corticosteroids that are effective with minimal adverse effects.

Inhaled drugs may be given alone or with systemic drugs. In general, inhaled corticosteroids can replace oral drugs when daily dosage of the oral drug has been tapered to 10 to 15 mg of prednisone or the equivalent. When a patient is being switched from an oral to an inhaled corticosteroid, the inhaled drug should be started during tapering of the oral drug, approximately 1 or 2 weeks before discontinuing or reaching the lowest anticipated dose of the oral drug. When a patient requires a systemic corticosteroid, coadministration of an aerosol allows smaller doses of the systemic corticosteroid. Although the inhaled drugs can cause suppression of the HPA axis and adrenocortical function, especially at higher doses, they are much less likely to do so than systemic drugs. However, the U.S. Food and Drug Administration (FDA) has issued a **BLACK BOX WARNING** ◆ for people who are transferred from systemically active corticosteroids to flunisolide inhaler because deaths have occurred from adrenal insufficiency.

EVIDENCE-BASED PRACTICE

Inhaled corticosteroids for Asthma: Are They All the Same?
by A.P. BAPTIST, R.C. REDDY

Journal of Clinical Pharmacy
2009, 34, 1–12

Inhaled corticosteroid therapy provides long-term control of symptoms without serious systemic side effects. Treatment with inhaled corticosteroids is recommended as the first-line therapy for persistent asthma of all severities for patients of all ages. However, the development of adverse effects is significant when the dose is increased beyond the usual recommended dosage. Cataracts and demineralization of bone may develop. The suppression of the hypothalamic–pituitary–adrenal axis is clinically significant in adults receiving large doses.

IMPLICATIONS FOR NURSING PRACTICE: The nurse instructs patients receiving inhaled corticosteroids to have an annual ophthalmologic examination to rule out the development of cataracts.

Cancer

Corticosteroids are commonly used in the treatment of lymphomas, lymphocytic leukemias, and multiple myeloma. In these disorders, corticosteroids inhibit cell reproduction and are cytotoxic to lymphocytes. In addition to their anticancer effects in hematologic malignancies, corticosteroids are beneficial in treatment of several signs and symptoms that often accompany cancer, although the mechanisms of action are unknown and drug/dosage regimens vary widely. Corticosteroids are used to treat anorexia, nausea and vomiting, cerebral edema and inflammation associated with brain metastases or radiation of the head, spinal cord compression, pain and edema related to pressure on nerves or bone metastases, graft-versus-host disease after bone marrow transplantation, and other disorders that occur in patients with cancer. Patients tend to feel better when taking corticosteroids, although the basic disease process may be unchanged.

Primary Central Nervous System Lymphomas Formerly considered rare tumors of older adults, central nervous system (CNS) lymphomas are being diagnosed more frequently in younger patients. They are usually associated with chronic **immunosuppression** (suppression of the immune system) caused by immunosuppressant drugs or acquired immunodeficiency syndrome (AIDS). Many of these lymphomas are very sensitive to corticosteroids, and therapy is indicated when the diagnosis is established.

Other Central Nervous System Tumors Corticosteroid therapy may be useful in both supportive and definitive treatment of brain and spinal cord tumors, and neurologic signs and symptoms often improve dramatically within 24 to 48 hours. Corticosteroids help relieve symptoms by controlling edema around the tumor, at operative sites, and at sites receiving radiation therapy. Some patients no longer require corticosteroids after surgical or radiation therapy, whereas others require continued therapy to manage neurologic symptoms. Adverse effects of long-term corticosteroid therapy may include mental changes ranging from mild agitation to psychosis and steroid myopathy (muscle weakness and atrophy) that may be confused with tumor progression. Mental symptoms usually improve if drug dosage is reduced and resolve if the drug is discontinued; steroid myopathy may persist for weeks or months.

Chemotherapy-Induced Emesis Corticosteroids have strong antiemetic effects; the mechanism is unknown. One effective regimen is a combination of an oral or intravenous (IV) dose of dexamethasone (10–20 mg) and a serotonin antagonist or metoclopramide given immediately before the chemotherapeutic drug. This regimen is the treatment of choice for chemotherapy with cisplatin, which is a strongly emetic drug.

Chronic Obstructive Pulmonary Disease

Corticosteroids are more helpful in acute exacerbations of COPD than in stable disease. However, oral corticosteroids may improve pulmonary function and symptoms in some patients. As in asthma and rhinitis, the drugs decrease mucus secretion and inflammation. For example, for a patient with inadequate relief from a bronchodilator, a trial of a corticosteroid (e.g., prednisone 20–40 mg each morning for 5–7 days)

EVIDENCE-BASED PRACTICE

Severe Hiccups During Chemotherapy: Corticosteroids are Likely Culprit

by PETER GILBAR AND IAN MCPHERSON

Journal of Oncology Pharmacy Practice
2009 December, 15, 233–236.

Corticosteroids are effective in the prevention of chemotherapy-induced nausea and vomiting. However, the administration of corticosteroids in patients receiving chemotherapy reported hiccups beginning the day after the initiation of chemotherapy. One patient suffered with severe hiccups for 30 hours. Sucking the juice of a fresh lemon provided relief. When dexamethasone was withheld before chemotherapy, the patient did not experience hiccups. He also did not suffer from the chemotherapy-related nausea and vomiting. The authors state that corticosteroids are an important protocol in the treatment of hematological malignancies and are necessary in controlling severe nausea and vomiting. However, the onset of hiccups is more likely a result of the corticosteroid and not the chemotherapy agent.

IMPLICATIONS FOR NURSING PRACTICE: It is important that the nurse instruct the patient and family regarding the onset of hiccups following the administration of corticosteroids and chemotherapy.

may be justified. Treatment should be continued only if there is significant improvement. As in other conditions, the lowest effective dose is needed to minimize adverse drug effects. Schweiger and Zdanowicz (2010) conducted a literature review to determine if data supported the current treatment guidelines in the administration of systemic corticosteroids. The authors found if patients with COPD received systemic corticosteroids during acute exacerbations, the airflow limitations improved, relapses decreased, and length of hospital stays decreased.

Inhaled corticosteroids can also be used. The inhaled corticosteroids produce minimal adverse effects, but their effectiveness in COPD has not been clearly demonstrated.

Inflammatory Bowel Disease

Patients who suffer from Crohn's disease or ulcerative colitis often require periodic corticosteroid therapy. In moderate Crohn's disease, oral prednisone, 40 mg daily, is usually given until symptoms subside. With severe disease, patients often require hospitalization, IV fluids for hydration, and parenteral corticosteroids until symptoms subside. An oral form of budesonide (Entocort EC) may be used for Crohn's disease. The capsule dissolves in the small intestine and acts locally before being absorbed into the bloodstream and transported to the liver for metabolism. It has fewer adverse effects than systemic corticosteroids but is also less effective and more expensive.

In ulcerative colitis, corticosteroids are usually used when aminosalicylates (e.g., mesalamine) are not effective or when symptoms are more severe. Initially, hydrocortisone enemas may be effective. If they are not, oral prednisone (20–60 mg daily) may be given until symptoms subside. In severe disease, oral prednisone may be required initially. After remission of symptoms is achieved, the dose can be tapered by 2.5 to 5 mg per day each week to a dose of 20 mg. Then, tapering may be slowed to 2.5 to 5 mg per day every other week. As in Crohn's disease, patients with severe ulcerative colitis often require hospitalization and parenteral corticosteroids. One regimen uses IV hydrocortisone 300 mg per day or the equivalent dose of another drug. When the patient's condition improves, oral prednisone can replace the IV corticosteroid.

Spinal Cord Injury

High-dose corticosteroid therapy to treat spinal cord injury is a common practice in clinical settings, although controversy exists regarding its use. Data suggest that methylprednisolone may be effective in acute spinal cord injury when given in high doses within 8 hours of the injury. Methylprednisolone improves neurologic recovery, although it does not improve mortality, and its use is unlikely to result in normal neurologic function. In addition, severe adverse outcomes, including wound and systemic infections, GI hemorrhage, and pneumonia, have been reported.

Prevention of Acute Adrenocortical Insufficiency

Suppression of the HPA axis may occur with corticosteroid therapy and may lead to life-threatening inability to increase cortisol secretion when needed to cope with stress. It is most likely to occur with abrupt withdrawal of systemic corticosteroid drugs. The risk of HPA suppression is high with systemic drugs given for more than a few days, although patients vary in degree and duration of suppression with comparable doses, and the minimum dose and duration of therapy that cause suppression are unknown.

When corticosteroids are given for replacement therapy, adrenal insufficiency is lifelong, and drug administration must be continued (see Chap. 43). When the drugs are given for purposes other than replacement and then discontinued, the HPA axis usually recovers within several weeks to months, but recovery may take a year. Several strategies have been developed to minimize HPA suppression and risks of acute adrenal insufficiency, including

- Administering a systemic corticosteroid during high-stress situations (e.g., moderate or severe illness, trauma, surgery) to patients who have received pharmacologic doses for 2 weeks within the previous year or who receive long-term systemic therapy (i.e., are steroid dependent)
- Giving short courses of systemic therapy for acute disorders, such as asthma attacks, then decreasing the dose or stopping the drug within a few days
- Gradually tapering the dose of any systemic corticosteroid. Although specific guidelines for tapering dosage have not been developed, higher doses and longer durations of administration in general require slower tapering, possibly over several weeks. The goal of tapering may be to stop the drug or to decrease the dosage to the lowest effective amount.
- Using local rather than systemic therapy when possible, alone or in combination with low doses of systemic drugs.

Numerous preparations are available for local application, including aerosols for oral or nasal inhalation; formulations for topical application to the skin, eyes, and ears; and drugs for intraarticular injections.

- Using alternate-day therapy (ADT), which involves titrating the daily dose to the lowest effective maintenance level, then giving a double dose every other day.

Use in Special Populations

Use in Children

Corticosteroids are used for the same conditions in children as in adults; a common indication is for treatment of asthma. With severe asthma, continual corticosteroid therapy may be required. For children with asthma, evidence indicates that with inhaled corticosteroids, starting with a moderate dose of the drug is comparable with starting with a high dose and titrating down. A concern with children is growth retardation, which can occur short term with small doses and administration by inhalation. Many children have a growth spurt when the corticosteroid is discontinued. Adult stature does not appear to be affected by inhaled corticosteroid therapy during childhood.

Parents and prescribers can monitor drug effects by recording height and weight weekly. ADT is less likely to impair normal growth and development than daily administration. In addition, for both systemic and inhaled corticosteroids, each child's dose should be titrated to the lowest effective amount.

Use in Older Adults

Corticosteroids are used for the same conditions in older adults as in younger ones. Older adults are especially likely to have conditions that are aggravated by the drugs (e.g., heart failure, hypertension, diabetes mellitus, arthritis, osteoporosis, increased susceptibility to infection, concomitant drug therapy that increases risks of GI ulceration, and bleeding). According to Cerullo (2008), adverse effects such as mania, depression, psychosis, and delirium are extremely common in older patients treated with corticosteroids. Consequently, it is important to consider risk–benefit ratios of systemic corticosteroid therapy carefully, especially for long-term therapy.

When used, lower doses are usually indicated because of decreased muscle mass, plasma volume, hepatic metabolism, and renal excretion in older adults. In addition, therapeutic and adverse responses should be monitored regularly by a health care provider (e.g., blood pressure, serum electrolytes, and blood glucose levels at least every 6 months). As in other populations, adverse effects are less likely to occur with oral or nasal inhalations than with oral drugs.

QSEN Safety Alert

When caring for a patient with COPD and a history of heart failure who takes a tapering dose of prednisone, it is necessary to instruct the patient to check his or her weight daily. The patient should also assess his or her extremities for edema. If the patient's weight increases, edema is evident, and shortness of breath develops, the patient should notify the primary health provider.

Use in Patients With Renal Impairment

It is necessary to use systemic corticosteroids with caution because of slowed excretion, with possible accumulation and signs and symptoms of hypercorticism. In renal transplantation, use of corticosteroids, along with other immunosuppressive drugs, to prevent or treat rejection reactions, is extensive. In these patients, as in others, adverse effects of systemic corticosteroids may include infections, hypertension, glucose intolerance, obesity, cosmetic changes, bone loss, growth retardation in children, cataracts, pancreatitis, peptic ulcerations, and psychiatric disturbances. Prescribers should keep doses to a minimum, and eventually withdrawal of drugs may be necessary in some patients.

Use in Patients With Hepatic Impairment

Metabolism of corticosteroids is slowed by severe hepatic disease, and corticosteroids may accumulate and cause signs and symptoms of hypercorticism. In addition, patients with liver disease should take prednisolone rather than prednisone. Liver metabolism of prednisone is required to convert it to its active form, prednisolone.

Use in Patients With Critical Illness

Use of corticosteroids in the treatment of serious illness has been extensive, with much empiric usage.

Adrenal Insufficiency Adrenal insufficiency is the most clear-cut indication for use of a corticosteroid, and even a slight impairment of the adrenal response during severe illness can be lethal if corticosteroid therapy is not instituted. Adrenal insufficiency is covered in depth in Chapter 43.

Acute Respiratory Failure in Chronic Obstructive Pulmonary Disease Some studies of patients with COPD have found that the parenteral administration of methylprednisolone may be effective for the treatment of acute respiratory failure. However, if other medications do not produce adequate bronchodilation, IV corticosteroid therapy is a reasonable treatment choice in the first 72 hours of the illness. The nurse assesses the patient for pulmonary infection because corticosteroid therapy places the patient at increased risk for pulmonary infection.

Adult Respiratory Distress Syndrome Although corticosteroids have been widely used, several well-controlled studies demonstrate that high doses of the drugs are not beneficial in early treatment or in prevention of adult respiratory distress syndrome (ARDS). Bream-Rouwenhorst, Beltz, Ross, and Moores (2008) reported that some trials have found increased complications and mortality with the use of corticosteroids in patients with ARDS. The authors found that conservative fluid management significantly reduces morbidity in these patients. Also, the use of low tidal volume ventilations has been a standard of care. Thus, the early administration of moderate doses of corticosteroids, conservative fluid volumes, and low tidal volume ventilation is beneficial in the care of patients with ARDS. Sessler and Gay (2010) found that prolonged low-to-moderate dose corticosteroids is beneficial for the treatment of ARDS. They state that drug stoppage should not be abrupt and that the patient should be monitored for infection.

Acquired Immunodeficiency Syndrome Health care providers are increasingly recognizing adrenal insufficiency in patients with AIDS, who require assessment and treatment for the condition, if indicated. Corticosteroids improve survival and decrease risks of respiratory failure with pneumocystosis, a common cause of death in patients with AIDS. The recommended regimen is prednisone 40 mg twice daily for 5 days, then 40 mg once daily for 5 days, then 20 mg daily until completion of treatment for pneumocystosis. The effect of corticosteroids on risks of other opportunistic infections or neoplasms is unknown.

Use in Patients Receiving Home Care

Corticosteroids are extensively used in the home setting, by all age groups, for a wide variety of disorders, and by most routes of administration. Because of potentially serious adverse effects, especially with oral drugs, it is extremely important that these drugs be used as prescribed. A major responsibility of home care nurses is to teach, demonstrate, supervise, monitor, or do whatever is needed to facilitate correct use. In addition, home care nurses must teach patients and caregivers interventions to minimize adverse effects of these drugs.

Clinical Application 15-2

Mrs. Thompson states, "since I have been taking this prednisone, the arthritis pain in my knees doesn't seem as bad."
- Why has her arthritic pain in her knees decreased with the administration of oral prednisone?
- What patient teaching is specific to the administration of prednisone?

NCLEX Success

6. A patient is taking fluticasone (Flovent) 440 mcg inhaled two times per day. The patient is being seen in the pulmonary clinic and says, "I have been very congested and it has been hard to breathe, so for the past 10 days I have been using my inhaler four times per day." The nurse should assess the patient for which of the following systemic adverse effects?

   A. hypoglycemia
   B. hypercalcemia
   C. anxiety
   D. hypothalamic–pituitary–adrenal (HPA) suppression

7. A liver transplant patient is receiving corticosteroids. These drugs are important to the care of this patient because they

   A. prevent thrombocytopenia
   B. increase immunity
   C. prevent tissue rejection
   D. decrease inflammation

8. A cancer patient asks the nurse why he is being given a corticosteroid before his chemotherapy. Which of the following is the nurse's best response?

   A. It will prevent the development of anemia related to the chemotherapy.
   B. It will prevent the development of hiccups, which is associated with chemotherapy.
   C. It will prevent nausea and vomiting that occurs with chemotherapy.
   D. It will boost your immune system and prevent infection.

9. When administering long-term systemic corticosteroid medications, which of the following dosing schedules is recommended?

   A. alternate-day therapy
   B. once daily at noon
   C. weekly therapy
   D. nightly therapy

Adverse Effects

Administration of more than 5 mg daily of corticosteroids results in adverse reactions. Possible adverse effects include the following:

- **Adrenocortical insufficiency:** fainting, weakness, anorexia, nausea, vomiting, hypotension, shock, and death (if untreated)
- **Adrenocortical excess**
- **Cushingoid features:** "moon face" and buffalo hump due to the redistribution of fat
- **CNS effects:** vertigo, headache, paresthesias, insomnia, and seizures
- **Cardiovascular symptoms:** hypotension, shock, hypertension, heart failure, thromboembolism, thrombophlebitis, fat embolism, and cardiac dysrhythmias
- **Diminished immunity:** increased susceptibility to infection
- **Endocrine effects:** diabetes mellitus, hyperglycemia, and hypercholesterolemia; diminished T_3 and T_4 levels, resulting in hypothyroidism; reduced growth because of altered synthesis of DNA
- **Fluid and electrolyte effects:** fluid retention, hypokalemia, hypocalcemia
- **Integumentary effects:** reddened skin, thinner skin, stretch marks, skin tears, delayed wound healing
- **Musculoskeletal effects:** hypocalcemia, which places the patient at risk for osteoporosis and fracture development; serum hypocalcemia, which increases the release parathyroid hormone, increasing the loss of calcium from bone
- **Ocular effects:** cataracts and glaucoma
- **Reproductive effects:** amenorrhea or irregular menstrual cycles

Contraindications

Corticosteroids are contraindicated in patients who experience allergic response to the medications. Patients with systemic fungal infections should not receive corticosteroids. Other contraindications include amebiasis, hepatitis B, vaccinia, varicella, and antibiotic-resistant infections. Also, patients who have been diagnosed with immunosuppression should not take corticosteroids. Patients receiving corticosteroids should not receive live virus vaccines, due to the risk of contracting the virus.

Caution is necessary when administering corticosteroids to patients with kidney disease, liver disease, hypothyroidism, recent GI surgery, peptic ulcer and inflammatory bowel disease, heart failure, thrombophlebitis, and diabetes mellitus.

Nursing Implications

Many factors have an effect on drug dosage, such as the specific drug to be given, the desired route of administration, the reason for use, expected adverse effects, and patient characteristics. In general, the patient should take the smallest effective dose for the shortest effective time. It is necessary to individualize the dosage according to the severity of the disorder being treated, whether the disease is acute or chronic, and the patient's response to drug therapy. (Calculation of dosages for children depends on severity of disease rather than weight.) If life-threatening disease is present, patients usually receive high doses until acute symptoms subside. Gradual dose reduction follows, until a maintenance dose is determined or the drug is discontinued. If life-threatening disease is not present, patients may still receive relatively high doses initially and then lower ones. Gradual reduction (tapering) over several days is necessary. With long-term corticosteroid therapy, periodic attempts to reduce dosage are desirable to decrease adverse effects. One way is to reduce the dose gradually until symptoms worsen, indicating the minimally effective dose.

Prescribers order physiologic doses (~15 to 20 mg of hydrocortisone or its equivalent daily) to replace or substitute for endogenous adrenocortical hormone. They usually order pharmacologic doses (supraphysiologic amounts) for anti-inflammatory, antiallergic, antistress, and immunosuppressive effects.

Compared with hydrocortisone, newer corticosteroids are more potent on a weight basis but are equipotent in anti-inflammatory effects when given in equivalent doses. Statements of equivalency with hydrocortisone are helpful in evaluating new drugs, comparing different drugs, and changing drugs or dosages. However, dosage equivalents apply only to drugs given orally or intravenously.

Preventing Interactions

Many medications increase or decrease the therapeutic effects of corticosteroids. Herbal interactions with corticosteroids are most often related to changes in sodium and potassium (Box 15.3). Licorice increases the effects of corticosteroids, which may potentiate its effects; cautious use of licorice with corticosteroids is necessary.

Administering the Medication

Corticosteroids can be given by several different routes to produce local or systemic effects, depending on the clinical problem. If feasible, these drugs should be given locally rather than systemically to prevent or decrease systemic toxicity. In recent years, several formulations have been developed for oral

---

> **BOX 15.3   Drug Interactions: Corticosteroids**
>
> **Drugs That Increase the Effects of Corticosteroids**
>
> ■ Estrogens, oral contraceptives, ketoconazole, macrolide antibiotics (e.g., erythromycin)
>
> *Increase the effects of corticosteroids by inhibiting the enzymes that normally metabolize corticosteroids in the liver.*
>
> ■ Diuretics (e.g., furosemide and thiazides)
>
> *Increase hypokalemia*
>
> **Drugs That Decrease the Effects of Corticosteroids**
>
> ■ Antacids and cholestyramine
>
> *Decrease the absorption of corticosteroids*
>
> ■ Carbamazepine, phenytoin, rifampin
>
> *Induce microsomal enzymes in the liver and increase the rate at which corticosteroids are metabolized or deactivated*

---

inhalation in the treatment of asthma and for nasal inhalation in the treatment of allergic rhinitis. When these drugs must be given systemically, the oral route is preferred. Parenteral administration is indicated only for patients who are seriously ill or unable to take oral medications. For intramuscular or IV injections, sodium phosphate or sodium succinate salts are used because they are most soluble in water. For intraarticular or intralesional injections, acetate salts are used because they have low solubility in water and provide prolonged local action.

Scheduling of drug administration is more important with corticosteroids than with most other drug classes. Most adverse effects occur with long-term administration of high doses. A major adverse reaction is suppression of the HPA axis and subsequent loss of adrenocortical function. Certain schedules are often recommended to prevent or minimize HPA suppression.

Corticosteroids can be given in relatively large, divided doses for approximately 48 to 72 hours in acute situations until the condition has been brought under control. After acute symptoms subside or 48 to 72 hours have passed, the dosage is tapered so that a slightly smaller dose is given each day until the drug can be discontinued completely (total period of use: ~1 week). Such a regimen may be useful in allergic reactions, contact dermatitis, exacerbations of chronic conditions (e.g., bronchial asthma), and stressful situations such as surgery.

Daily administration is required in cases of chronic adrenocortical insufficiency. The entire daily dose can be taken each morning, between 6:00 and 9:00 AM. This schedule simulates normal endogenous corticosteroid secretion.

Stress Dosage Therapy

As previously stated, long-term use of pharmacologic doses (e.g., more than 5 mg of prednisone daily) of corticosteroids produces adverse reactions. For this reason, such corticosteroid therapy should be reserved for life-threatening conditions or severe, disabling symptoms that do not respond to treatment with more benign drugs or other measures. For people receiving chronic corticosteroid therapy, dosage must be increased during periods of stress or illness. Some common sources of stress for most people include surgery and anesthesia, infections, anxiety, and extremes of temperature. Note that events that are stressful for one patient may not be stressful for another. Some guidelines for corticosteroid dosage during stress include the following:

- During minor or relatively mild illness (e.g., viral upper respiratory infection, any febrile illness, strenuous exercise, gastroenteritis with vomiting and diarrhea, minor surgery), doubling the daily maintenance dose is usually adequate. After the stress period is over, it is appropriate to reduce the dosage abruptly to the usual maintenance dose.

- During major stress or severe illness, even larger doses are necessary. For example, a patient undergoing abdominal surgery may require 300 to 400 mg of hydrocortisone on the day of surgery. Gradual dose reduction to usual maintenance doses within approximately 5 days is sufficient if postoperative recovery is uncomplicated. As a general rule, it is better to administer excessive doses temporarily than to risk inadequate doses and adrenal insufficiency. The patient also may require sodium chloride and fluid replacement, antibiotic therapy if infection is present, and supportive measures if shock occurs.

- During acute stress situations of short duration, such as traumatic injury or invasive diagnostic tests (e.g., angiography), a single dose of approximately 100 mg of hydrocortisone immediately after the injury or before the diagnostic test is usually sufficient.

- Many chronic diseases that require long-term corticosteroid therapy are characterized by exacerbations and remissions. It is usually necessary to increase the dosage of corticosteroids during acute flare-ups of disease symptoms but can then decrease the dosage gradually to maintenance levels.

Alternate-Day Therapy

ADT, in which a double dose is taken every other morning, is usually preferred for other chronic conditions. This schedule allows rest periods so that adverse effects are decreased while anti-inflammatory effects continue. ADT seems to be as effective as more frequent administration in most patients with bronchial asthma, ulcerative colitis, and other conditions for which long-term corticosteroid therapy is prescribed. ADT is used only for maintenance therapy (i.e., clinical signs and symptoms are controlled initially with more frequent drug administration). ADT can be started after symptoms have subsided and stabilized.

Intermediate-acting glucocorticoids (e.g., prednisone, prednisolone, methylprednisolone) are the drugs of choice for ADT. Long-acting drugs (e.g., betamethasone, dexamethasone) are not recommended because of their prolonged suppression of adrenocortical function.

ADT has other advantages. It probably decreases susceptibility to infection and does not retard growth in children, as do other schedules.

ADT is not usually indicated in patients who have previously received corticosteroids on a long-term basis. First, these patients already have maximal HPA suppression, so a major advantage of ADT is lost. Second, if these patients begin ADT, recurrence of symptoms and considerable discomfort may occur on days when drugs are omitted. Patients with severe disease and very painful or disabling symptoms also may experience severe discomfort with ADT.

Assessing for Therapeutic Effects

The goal of corticosteroid therapy is usually to reduce symptoms to a tolerable level. Total suppression of symptoms may require excessively large doses and produce excessive adverse effects. Because systemic corticosteroids can cause serious adverse reactions, indications for their clinical use should be as clear-cut as possible. Therapeutic effects depend largely on the reason for use.

Prescribers order hydrocortisone (Solu-Cortef) for the treatment of Addison's disease. Following the parenteral administration of the medication, the nurse monitors the patient for activity tolerance, ability to move in bed, and restoration of fluid balance. Decreases in weakness weight loss and anorexia, nausea and vomiting, hyperpigmentation, hypotension, hyponatremia, and hyperkalemia should be evident.

Prednisone is the drug of choice for nonendocrine disorders in which anti-inflammatory, antiallergic, antistress, and immunosuppressive effects are desired. The nurse assesses the patient for diminished inflammation. Inhaled corticosteroids also reduce inflammation and allergic responses and do not lead to the serious adverse effects of systemic corticosteroids.

Health care providers consider dexamethasone (parenteral or oral) the corticosteroid of choice for cerebral edema associated with brain tumors, craniotomy, or head injury, because it is thought to penetrate the blood–brain barrier more readily and achieve higher concentrations in cerebrospinal fluids and tissues. It also has minimal sodium and water-retaining properties. With brain tumors, the drug is more effective in metastatic lesions and glioblastomas than astrocytomas and meningiomas. The therapeutic response to the medication is decreased intracranial pressure.

In patients treated for rheumatoid arthritis with corticosteroid agents, the nurse assesses for decreased pain and edema in the joints, increased mobility, and increased ability to perform activities of daily living.

Organ transplant recipients administered corticosteroids to prevent rejection of the transplanted tissues should have absence of signs and symptoms of rejections.

Assessing for Adverse Effects

It is necessary to assess patients for a variety of adverse effects, which may affect every body tissue and organ. The nurse assesses patients with adrenocortical insufficiency for fainting, weakness, anorexia, nausea, vomiting, hypotension, and shock. He or she assesses patients with adrenocortical excess for "moon face," "buffalo hump," diabetes mellitus, nervousness, euphoria, anxiety, and behavioral changes. Adrenocortical excess also leads to the musculoskeletal conditions, such as osteoporosis, fractures, muscle weakness and atrophy, and growth retardation in children. Cardiovascular effects include fluid and electrolyte changes, with fluid retention, edema, hypertension, heart failure, hypernatremia, hypokalemia, and metabolic acidosis. Ocular changes include increased intraocular pressure, glaucoma, and cataracts. The nurse assesses for increased susceptibility to infection and changes to the skin, including redness, thinning, stretch marks, and tissue injury.

Women may experience menstrual irregularities, acne, and excessive facial hair.

Patient Teaching

Box 15.4 identifies patient teaching guidelines for corticosteroids.

BOX 15.4   Patient Teaching Guidelines for Long-Term Corticosteroid Therapy

General Considerations

■ Realize that in most instances, corticosteroids are used to relieve symptoms; they do not cure the underlying disease process. However, they can improve comfort and quality of life.

■ When taking an oral corticosteroid (e.g., prednisone) for longer than 2 weeks, take the drug as directed. This is extremely important. Missing a dose or two, stopping the drug, changing the amount or time of administration, taking extra drug (except as specifically directed during stress situations), or any other alterations may result in complications. Some complications are relatively minor; several are serious, even life threatening. When these drugs are being discontinued, the dosage is gradually reduced over several weeks. They must not be stopped abruptly.

■ Wear a special medical alert bracelet or tag or carry an identification card stating the drug being taken; the dosage; the prescriber's name, address, and telephone number; and instructions for emergency treatment. If an accident or emergency situation occurs, health care providers must know about corticosteroid drug therapy to give additional amounts during the stress of the emergency.

■ Report to all health care providers consulted that corticosteroid drugs are being taken or have been taken within the past year. Current or previous corticosteroid therapy can influence treatment measures, and such knowledge increases the ability to provide appropriate treatment.

■ Maintain regular medical supervision. This is extremely important so that the prescriber can detect adverse reactions, evaluate disease status, and evaluate drug response and indications for dosage change, as well as other responsibilities that can be carried out only with personal contact between the prescriber and the patient. Periodic blood tests, x-ray studies, and other tests may be performed during long-term corticosteroid therapy.

■ Take no other drugs, prescription or nonprescription, without notifying the prescriber who is supervising corticosteroid therapy. Corticosteroid drugs influence reactions to other drugs, and some other drugs interact with corticosteroids either to increase or decrease their effects. Thus, taking other drugs can decrease the expected therapeutic benefits or increase the incidence or severity of adverse effects.

■ Avoid exposure to infection when possible. Avoid crowds and people known to have an infection. Also, wash hands frequently and thoroughly. These drugs increase the likelihood of infection, so preventive measures are necessary. Also, if infection does occur, healing is likely to be slow.

■ Practice safety measures to avoid accidents (e.g., falls and possible fractures due to osteoporosis, cuts or other injuries because of delayed wound healing, soft tissue trauma because of increased tendency to bruise easily).

■ Weigh frequently when starting corticosteroid therapy and at least weekly during long-term maintenance. An initial weight gain is likely to occur and is usually attributed to increased appetite. Later weight gains may be caused by fluid retention.

■ Ask the prescriber about the amount and kind of activity or exercise needed. As a general rule, being as active as possible helps prevent or delay osteoporosis, a common adverse effect. However, increased activity may not be desirable for everyone. A patient with rheumatoid arthritis, for example, may become too active when drug therapy relieves joint pain and increases mobility.

■ Follow instructions for other measures used in treatment of the particular condition (e.g., other drugs and physical therapy for rheumatoid arthritis). Such measures may allow smaller doses of corticosteroids and decrease adverse effects.

■ Understand that the dosage may need to be temporarily increased with illness, surgery, or other stressful situations because corticosteroids impair the ability to respond to stress. Clarify with the prescriber predictable sources of stress and the amount of drug to be taken if the stress cannot be avoided.

■ In addition to stressful situations, report sore throat, fever, or other signs of infection; weight gain of 5 pounds or more in a week; or swelling in the ankles or elsewhere. These symptoms may indicate adverse drug effects and changes in corticosteroid therapy may be indicated.

■ Realize that muscle weakness and fatigue or disease symptoms may occur when drug dosage is reduced, withdrawn, or omitted (e.g., the nondrug day of alternate-day therapy). Although these symptoms may cause some discomfort, they should be tolerated if possible rather than increasing the corticosteroid dose. If severe, of course, dosage or time of administration may have to be changed.

■ Understand that dietary changes may be helpful in reducing some adverse effects of corticosteroid therapy. Decreasing salt intake (e.g., by not adding table salt to foods and avoiding obviously salty foods, such as many snack foods and prepared sandwich meats) may help decrease swelling. Eating high-potassium foods, such as citrus fruits and juices or bananas, may help prevent potassium loss. An adequate intake of calcium, protein, and vitamin D (meat and dairy products are good sources) may help to prevent or delay osteoporosis. Vitamin C (e.g., from citrus fruits) may help to prevent excessive bruising.

BOX 15.4   Patient Teaching Guidelines for Long-Term Corticosteroid Therapy (Continued)

■ Do not object when your prescriber reduces your dose of oral corticosteroid, with the goal of stopping the drug entirely or continuing with a smaller dose. Long-term therapy should be used only when necessary because of the potential for serious adverse effects, and the lowest effective dose should be given.

■ Understand that with local applications of corticosteroids, there is usually little systemic absorption and few adverse effects, compared with oral or injected drugs. When effective in relieving symptoms, it is better to use a local than a systemic corticosteroid. In some instances, combined systemic and local application allows administration of a lesser dose of the systemic drug.

   Commonly used local applications are applied topically for skin disorders; by oral inhalation for asthma; and by nasal inhalation for allergic rhinitis. Although long-term use is usually well tolerated, systemic toxicity can occur if excess corticosteroid is inhaled or if occlusive dressings are used over skin lesions. Thus, a corticosteroid for local application must be applied correctly and not overused.

■ Know that corticosteroids are not the same as the steroids often abused by athletes and body builders. Those are anabolic steroids derived from testosterone, the male sex hormone.

Self- or Caregiver Administration

■ Take an oral corticosteroid with a meal or snack to decrease GI upset.

■ If taking the medication once a day or every other day, take before 9:00 AM if taking multiple doses, take at evenly spaced intervals throughout the day.

■ Report to the prescriber if unable to take a dose orally because of vomiting or some other problem. In some circumstances, the dose may need to be given by injection.

■ If taking an oral corticosteroid in tapering doses, be sure to follow instructions exactly to avoid adverse effects.

■ When applying a corticosteroid to skin lesions, do not apply more often than ordered and do not cover with an occlusive dressing unless specifically instructed to do so.

■ With an intranasal corticosteroid, use on a regular basis (usually once or twice daily) for the best anti-inflammatory effects.

■ With an oral-inhalation corticosteroid, use on a regular schedule for anti-inflammatory effects. The drugs are *not* effective in relieving acute asthma attacks or shortness of breath and should not be used "as needed" for that purpose. Use metered-dose inhalers as follows (unless instructed otherwise by a health care provider):

1. Shake canister thoroughly.
2. Place canister between lips (both open and pursed lips have been recommended) or outside lips.
3. Exhale completely.
4. Activate canister while taking a slow, deep breath.
5. Hold breath for 10 seconds or as long as possible.
6. Wait at least 1 minute before taking additional inhalations.
7. Rinse mouth after inhalations to decrease the incidence of oral thrush (a fungal infection).
8. Rinse mouthpiece at least once per day.

Clinical Application 15-3

The home care nurse is visiting Mrs. Thompson. She says, "I am having itching in my vaginal area, and drinking citrus juices is painful." During the assessment, the nurse notices white patches in her mouth.

- What are the white patches in Mrs. Thompson's mouth?
- Why has she developed itching in the vaginal area?
- What is the cause of these symptoms?

NCLEX Success

10. A child is taking long-term systemic corticosteroids. What factor influences the child's diminished growth?

    A. hypokalemia
    B. fluid retention
    C. altered DNA synthesis
    D. increase in parathyroid hormone

11. A woman is being treated with long-term corticosteroid therapy. Her husband has just received a diagnosis of terminal cancer. How is his diagnosis likely to affect her treatment?

    A. She may need to have her dose of corticosteroid increased because of the stress.
    B. She may need a decrease in corticosteroids because of the increase in cortisol.
    C. She may need to be changed to a different corticosteroid because of the stress.
    D. She may be switched to a parenteral form of corticosteroid.

The Nursing Process

Assessment

• With the initiation of corticosteroid therapy:
   • For a patient receiving short-term corticosteroid therapy, assess the extent and severity of symptoms. This will be a baseline to evaluate the effectiveness of corticosteroid therapy.

- For a patient receiving long-term systemic corticosteroid therapy, it is necessary to make a thorough assessment. Assess for such conditions as diabetes mellitus, tuberculosis, and peptic ulcer disease, because corticosteroids may result in the development or exacerbation of these disorders. If one of these conditions is present, it is essential that corticosteroid therapy be altered and other medications given concomitantly.
- Assess for signs and symptoms of infection. If acute infection is present, treatment with appropriate antibiotics either before corticosteroid drugs are started or concomitantly with corticosteroid therapy is necessary. Continue to assess for infection-related symptoms, which should decrease.
- Assess for wound healing because corticosteroids impair healing.
- With previous or current corticosteroid therapy:
- If the patient has taken corticosteroids before, assess his or her past response to corticosteroids.
- Assess the patient for significant sources of stress, such as hospitalization, diagnostic testing, infection, illness, and psychosocial problems.
- Assess the type of systemic corticosteroid medication the patient is taking, the dosage and schedule of administration, the purpose for which the medication has been prescribed, and the length of time to be administered.
- If the patient undergoes anesthesia and surgery, expect that higher doses of corticosteroids will be given for several days. This may be done by changing the drug, the route of administration, and the dosage. Specific regimens vary according to the type of anesthesia, surgical procedure, patient condition, prescriber preference, and other variables. A patient having major abdominal surgery may be given 300 to 400 mg of hydrocortisone (or the equivalent dosage of other drugs) on the day of surgery, then tapered back to maintenance dosage within a few days.
- Expect that a patient undergoing an invasive diagnostic test may be given one extra dose of corticosteroid.
- Assess for acute adrenal insufficiency.
- Assess for signs and symptoms of adrenocortical excess and adverse drug effects.
- Assess for signs and symptoms of the disease for which long-term corticosteroid therapy is given.

Nursing Diagnoses

- Disturbed body image related to cushingoid changes in appearance
- Imbalanced nutrition: Less than body requirements related to protein and potassium losses
- Imbalanced nutrition: More than body requirements related to sodium and water retention and hyperglycemia
- Excess fluid volume related to sodium and water retention
- Risk for injury related to adverse drug effects of impaired wound healing, increased susceptibility to infection, weakening of skin and muscles, osteoporosis, GI ulceration, diabetes mellitus, hypertension, and acute adrenocortical insufficiency

- Ineffective coping related to chronic illness; long-term drug therapy and drug-induced mood changes, irritability, and insomnia
- Deficient knowledge related to disease process and corticosteroid drug therapy

Planning/Goals

The patient will

- Take the drug correctly.
- Practice measures to decrease the need for corticosteroids and minimize adverse effects.
- See a health care provider regularly to monitor for adverse drug effects.
- Keep scheduled appointments for follow-up care.
- Seek the health care provider for strategies to cope with body image changes.
- Verbalize or demonstrate essential drug information.

Nursing Interventions

For patients on long-term, systemic corticosteroid therapy, the nurse will

- Help patients set reasonable goals of drug therapy. For example, partial relief of symptoms may be better than complete relief if the latter requires larger doses or longer periods of treatment with systemic drugs.
- Instruct patients with bronchial asthma and COPD to continue with other treatment measures during corticosteroid therapy. Patients with asthma need to take corticosteroids on a regular schedule; they can usually take inhaled bronchodilators as needed.
- Instruct patients with rheumatoid arthritis to continue with rest, physical therapy, and salicylates or other nonsteroidal anti-inflammatory drugs. Systemic corticosteroid therapy is reserved for severe, acute exacerbations when possible.
- Help patients identify stressors and find ways to modify or avoid stressful situations when possible. For example, most patients probably do not think of extreme heat or cold or minor infections as significant stressors. However, they can be for people taking corticosteroids. It is necessary to individualize this assessment of potential stressors because a situation viewed as stressful by one patient may not be stressful to another.
- Encourage activity, if not contraindicated, to slow demineralization of bone (osteoporosis). This is especially important in postmenopausal women who are not taking replacement estrogens, because they are very susceptible to osteoporosis. Walking is preferred if the patient is able. Range-of-motion exercises are indicated in immobilized or bedridden people. Also, bedridden patients taking corticosteroids should have their positions changed frequently because these drugs thin the skin and increase the risk of pressure ulcers. This risk is further increased if edema also is present.
- Encourage dietary changes when they may be beneficial. Salt restriction may help prevent hypernatremia, fluid retention, and edema. Foods high in potassium may help prevent hypokalemia. A diet high in protein, calcium,

and vitamin D may help prevent osteoporosis. Increased intake of vitamin C may help decrease bleeding in the skin and soft tissues.

- Avoid exposing the patient to potential sources of infection by washing hands frequently; using aseptic technique when changing dressings; keeping health care personnel and visitors with colds or other infections away from the patient; and following other appropriate measures. Reverse or protective isolation is sometimes indicated, commonly for those patients who have had organ transplantation and are receiving corticosteroids to help prevent rejection of the transplanted organ.
- Handle tissues very gently during any procedures (e.g., bathing, assisting out of bed, venipunctures). Because long-term corticosteroid therapy weakens the skin and bones, there are risks of skin damage and fractures with even minor trauma.

Evaluation

- Interview and observe for relief of symptoms for which corticosteroids were prescribed.
- Interview and observe for accurate drug administration.
- Interview and observe for use of nondrug measures indicated for the condition being treated.
- Interview and observe for adverse drug effects on a regular basis.
- Interview regarding drug knowledge and effects to be reported to health care providers.

NCLEX Success

12. **A patient diagnosed with Addison's disease is taking exogenous corticosteroids. The nurse should assess the patient for which of the following adverse effects?**
    A. hyperglycemia
    B. hyperkalemia
    C. hypercalcemia
    D. hypermagnesemia

13. **Which of the following psychosocial changes are most likely to occur with the administration of corticosteroids?**
    A. lethargy
    B. malaise
    C. ataxia
    D. euphoria

14. **A patient is taking systemic corticosteroids. Which of the following nursing interventions is most important to implement?**
    A. Assess for signs and symptoms of adrenocortical excess.
    B. Hold the corticosteroid before surgery or diagnostic testing.
    C. Assess for fluid volume deficit.
    D. Decrease the intake of vitamin C

Key Concepts

- The most frequently desired pharmacologic effects of exogenous corticosteroids are anti-inflammatory, immunosuppressive, antiallergic, and antistress functions.
- Mineralocorticoid and androgenic effects of exogenous corticosteroids are usually considered adverse reactions.
- Daily administration of corticosteroids and mineralocorticoids is required in cases of chronic adrenocortical insufficiency (Addison's disease).
- Adrenocortical hyperfunction (Cushing's disease) may result from excessive corticotropin or a primary adrenal tumor.
- Strategies to minimize HPA suppression and risks of acute adrenal insufficiency include (1) administering a systemic corticosteroid during high-stress situations to patients who receive long-term systemic therapy (i.e., are steroid dependent); (2) giving short courses of systemic therapy for acute disorders; (3) gradually tapering the dose of any systemic corticosteroid; (4) using local rather than systemic therapy when possible, alone or in combination with low doses of systemic drugs; and (5) using ADT.
- Adverse effects of systemic corticosteroids may include infections, hypertension, glucose intolerance, obesity, cosmetic changes, bone loss, growth retardation in children, cataracts, pancreatitis, peptic ulcerations, and psychiatric disturbances.
- A **BLACK BOX WARNING** ◆ has been issued by the FDA for people who switch from a systemically active corticosteroid to a flunisolide inhaler; deaths have been reported from adrenal insufficiency.

Critical Thinking Questions

15-1. A 48-year-old patient is admitted to hospice. He has an aggressive form of brain cancer. He is having nausea and vomiting at least five times per day. He is also complaining of increasing headaches and pain on the right side of the head near the temporal lobe. The hospice physician has prescribed dexamethasone sodium phosphate (Decadron) 16 mg IM.

- Why has dexamethasone sodium phosphate been ordered for this patient?

- What is the action of dexamethasone?

15-2. A 60-year-old woman has been diagnosed with ovarian cancer. Two weeks following her total hysterectomy, she is to begin chemotherapy. She asks the nurse how to handle the chemotherapy and about the occurrence of any nausea or vomiting. The nurse informs her that antiemetic medications are very effective in treating chemotherapy-induced emesis; for example, corticosteroids can assist in preventing emesis.

- How does dexamethasone sodium phosphate (Decadron) assist in preventing chemotherapy-induced emesis?

- What other medications will assist in preventing chemotherapy-induced emesis particularly when cisplatin is administered?

References and Resources

Baptist, A. P., & Reddy, R. C. (2009). Inhaled corticosteroids for asthma: are they all the same? *Journal of Clinical Pharmacy and Therapeutics, 34,* 1–12.

Bederman, S. S., Bhandarie, M., McKee, M. D. & Schemitsch, E. H. (2009). Do corticosteroids reduce the risk of fat embolism syndrome in patients with long-bone fractures? A meta-analysis. *Canadian Journal of Surgery, 52*(5), 386–393.

Bream-Rouwenhorst, H. R., Beltz, E. A., Ross, M.B. & Moores, K. G. (2008). Recent developments in the management of acute respiratory distress syndrome in adults. *American Journal of Health-System Pharmacy, 65,* January 1, 2008, 29–36.

Cerullo, M. A. (2008). Expect Pyschiatric side effects from corticosteroid use in the elderly. *Geriatrics, 63*(1), 15–18.

Gilbar, P., & McPherson, I. (2009). Case report severe hiccups during chemotherapy: corticosteroids the likely culprit. *Journal of Oncology Pharmacy Practice, 15,* 233–236.

Karch, A. M. (2013). *2013 Lippincott's nursing drug guide.* Philadelphia, PA: Lippincott Williams & Wilkins.

Kuhn, M. A., & Winston, D. *Herbal therapy supplements a scientific and traditional approach* (2nd ed.). Philadelphia, PA: Lippincott Williams & Wilkins.

Liao, H., Ma, T., Li, Y, Chen, J., & Chang, Y. (2010). Concurrent use of corticosteroids with licorice-containing TCM preparations in Taiwan: A national health insurance database study. *The Journal of Alternative and Complementary Medicine, 16*(6), 539–544.

Porth, C. M., & Matfin, G. (2009). *Pathophysiology concepts of altered health states.* Philadelphia, PA: Lippincott Williams & Wilkins.

Schweiger, T. A., & Zdanowicz, M. Systemic corticosteroids in the treatment of acute exacerbations of chronic obstructive pulmonary disease. *American Journal of Health-System Pharmacy, 67,* July 1, 2010, 1061–1069.

Sessler, C. N., & Gay, P. C. (2010). Are corticosteroids useful in late-stage acute respiratory distress syndrome? *Respiratory Care, 55*(1), 43–55.

Smeltzer, S. C., Bare, B. G., Hinkle, J. H., & Cheever, K. H. (2008). *Brunner & Suddarth's textbook of medical-surgical nursing* (11th ed.). Philadelphia, PA: Lippincott Williams & Wilkins.

16 Drug Therapy With Beta-Lactam Antibacterial Agents

LEARNING OBJECTIVES

After studying this chapter, you should be able to:

1 Describe general characteristics of beta-lactam antibiotics.

2 Discuss the penicillins in relation to effectiveness, safety, spectrum of antibacterial activity, mechanism of action, indications for use, administration, observation of patient response, and teaching of patients.

3 Recognize the importance of questioning patients about allergies before the initial dose of all drugs, especially penicillins.

4 Describe characteristics of beta-lactamase inhibitor drugs.

5 Give the rationale for combining a penicillin and a beta-lactamase inhibitor drug.

6 Discuss the cephalosporins in relation to effectiveness, safety, spectrum of antibacterial activity, mechanism of action, indications for use, administration, observation of patient response, and teaching of patients.

7 Discuss the carbapenems in relation to effectiveness, safety, spectrum of antibacterial activity, mechanism of action, indications for use, administration, observation of patient response, and teaching of patients.

8 Discuss the one monobactam drug in relation to effectiveness, safety, spectrum of antibacterial activity, mechanism of action, indications for use, administration, observation of patient response, and teaching of patients.

9 Use the nursing process in the care of patients receiving beta-lactam antibacterials.

Clinical Application Case Study

Paul O'Brian, a 55-year-old professional musician who travels frequently, has no known drug allergies. He is being scheduled for the placement of a new cardiac pacemaker tomorrow. The physician orders that cefazolin be administered "on call" for the procedure (1 g IV).

KEY TERMS

Beta-lactamase: enzyme produced by some bacteria that attacks the beta-lactam ring, rendering the drug ineffective and leading to a resistance to beta-lactam antibiotics

Cross-allergenicity: allergy to a drug of another class with a similar chemical structure

Extended-spectrum: bactericidal activity against a wide range of bacteria

Superinfection: infection after a previous infection; typically caused by microorganisms that are resistant to the antibiotics used previously

Introduction

This chapter discusses the pharmacological care of the patient who is receiving a drug in the antibiotic class of beta-lactam antibacterials, specifically the penicillins, cephalosporins, carbapenems, and monobactams. Beta-lactam antibacterial drugs inhibit synthesis of bacterial cell walls by binding to proteins (penicillin-binding proteins; see Chap. 13) in bacterial cell membranes. This binding produces a defective cell wall that allows leakage of the intracellular contents, destroying the microorganisms. Beta-lactam antibacterial drugs are typically considered bactericidal.

Beta-lactam antibacterials derive their name from the beta-lactam ring that is part of their chemical structure. An intact beta-lactam ring is essential for the antibacterial activity of these drugs. Several gram-positive and gram-negative bacteria produce **beta-lactamases**, which are enzymes that disrupt the beta-lactam ring and inactivate the beta-lactam antibacterial drugs. This is the major mechanism by which microorganisms acquire resistance to these drugs. Penicillinase and cephalosporinase are beta-lactamase enzymes that act on penicillins and cephalosporins to render them resistant and ineffective. Patients receive beta-lactamase inhibitors concurrently with the beta-lactam antibacterial drugs to overcome this resistance.

Although a beta-lactam ring is common to all beta-lactam antibiotics, the characteristics of these drugs vary widely because of differences in their chemical structures. Because of these differences, the range of activity to particular bacteria is also different. The drugs may also differ in the routes of administration, susceptibility to beta-lactamase enzymes, and adverse effects. Table 16.1 lists the various types of beta-lactam antibiotics.

TABLE 16.1

Beta-Lactamase Antibacterials Administered for the Treatment of Infection

Drug Class	Prototype	Other Drugs in the Class
Penicillins	Ampicillin (Principen)	Amoxicillin (Amoxil, Trimox) Carbenicillin indanyl sodium (Geocillin) Penicillin G benzathine (Bicillin LA) Penicillin G procaine (Wycillin) Penicillin V (Veetids) Dicloxacillin Nafcillin Oxacillin Ampicillin–sulbactam (Unasyn) Amoxicillin–clavulanate (Augmentin)
Cephalosporins	Cefazolin (Kefzol, Ancef)	Cefadroxil (Duricef) Cefaclor (Ceclor) Cefprozil (Cefzil) Cefuroxime (Ceftin) Cefdinir (Omnicef) Cefditoren pivoxil (Spectracef) Cefixime (Suprax) Cefpodoxime (Vantin) Ceftibuten (Cedax) Cefotetan (Cefotan) Cefoxitin (Mefoxin) Cefuroxime (Kefurox, Zinacef) Cefotaxime (Claforan) Ceftazidime (Fortaz) Ceftizoxime (Cefizox) Ceftriaxone (Rocephin) Cefepime (Maxipime) Ceftaroline (Teflaro) Cephalexin (Keflex)
Carbapenems	Imipenem–cilastatin (Primaxin)	Ertapenem (Invanz) Meropenem (Merrem) Doripenem (Doribax)
Monobactam	Aztreonam (Azactam)	

Penicillins

The penicillins are effective and safe, and they are among the most commonly prescribed antibacterials. The first antibiotic developed was penicillin, which was discovered from the *Penicillium* mold. When penicillin was introduced, it was effective against many organisms. It was once necessary to give the drug parenterally because it was destroyed by gastric acid, and injections were painful. With extensive use, strains of drug-resistant staphylococci appeared. Scientists developed semisynthetic derivatives, formed by adding side chains to the penicillin nucleus, to increase gastric acid stability, beta-lactamase stability, and antimicrobial spectrum of activity, especially against gram-negative microorganisms. As a class, penicillins usually are more effective in treating infections caused by gram-positive bacteria than those caused by gram-negative bacteria. However, their clinical usefulness varies significantly according to the subgroup or individual drug and microbial patterns of resistance.

Ⓟ **Ampicillin** (Principen) is the prototype penicillin.

Pharmacokinetics

After absorption, ampicillin is widely distributed. Penetration into the cerebrospinal fluid (CSF) occurs only with inflamed meninges. The kidneys rapidly excrete ampicillin, largely as unchanged drug, and it produces high drug concentrations in the urine. It is present in breast milk, and the volume of distribution increases during pregnancy, when the half-life, generally 1 to 2 hours, is decreased.

Action

Ampicillin, like all penicillins, inhibits bacterial cell wall synthesis by binding to one or multiple penicillin-binding proteins.

Use

Clinical indications for use of ampicillin include bacterial infections caused by susceptible microorganisms. Health care providers use the drug in the treatment or prophylaxis of infective endocarditis. The drug's broad spectrum is often useful in skin, soft tissue, respiratory, gastrointestinal (GI), and genitourinary infections. The broad-spectrum coverage of ampicillin extends its activity against gram-negative bacilli. Table 16.2 provides route and dosage information for the individual penicillins.

The incidence of resistance among streptococci, staphylococci, and other microorganisms continues to increase.

TABLE 16.2

DRUGS AT A GLANCE: Penicillins

Drug	Pregnancy Category	Routes and Dosage Ranges	
		Adults	Children
Penicillins G and V			
These drugs remain effective for a limited number of uses. They are the drugs of choice for the treatment of streptococcal pharyngitis, for prevention of recurrent attacks in patients who have had previous acute rheumatic fever due to group A streptococcus and for treatment of neurosyphilis.			
Penicillin G benzathine (Bicillin LA)	B	IM 1.2–2.4 million units in a single dose Prophylaxis of recurrent rheumatic fever, IM 1.2 million units every 3–4 wk Treatment of syphilis, IM 2.4 million units (1.2 million units in each buttock) as a single dose	IM 25,000–50,000 units/kg (max 2.4 million units) Prophylaxis of recurrent rheumatic fever, 25,000–50,000 units/kg times one dose every 3–4 wk (maximum 1.2 million units)
Penicillin G procaine (Wycillin)	B	IM 600,000–4.8 million units daily in 1 or 2 doses	IM 25,000–50,000 units/kg/d in divided doses every 12–24 h
Penicillin V (Veetids)	B	PO 125–500 mg every 6–8 h	PO 125–250 mg twice daily
Penicillinase-Resistant (Antistaphylococcal) Penicillins			
Penicillinase-resistant penicillins are the drugs of choice for methicillin-susceptible *Staphylococcus aureus*. Although called "methicillin resistant," these staphylococcal microorganisms are also resistant to other antistaphylococcal penicillins.			
Dicloxacillin	B	PO 125–1000 mg every 6 h	Not recommended in newborns ≤40 kg: 12.5–100 mg/kg/d divided every 6 h ≥40 kg: 125–500 mg every 6 h

(Continued on page 294)

TABLE 16.2

DRUGS AT A GLANCE: Penicillins (Continued)

Drug	Pregnancy Category	Routes and Dosage Ranges	
		Adults	Children
Nafcillin	B	IM 500 mg every 4–6 h IV 500 mg–2 g every 4–6 h; max daily dose 18 g for serious infections	IM 25 mg/kg every 12 h IV 50–200 mg/kg/d in divided doses every 4–6 h
Oxacillin	B	IM, IV 250–2000 mg every 4–6 h	≤40 kg: IM, IV 100–200 mg/kg/d in divided doses every 6 h >40 kg: same as adults

Aminopenicillins

The aminopenicillins are drugs of choice for prevention of bacterial endocarditis due to procedures that produce transient bacteremia. Ampicillin is excreted mainly by the kidneys; thus, it is useful in some urinary tract infections (UTIs). Because some is excreted in bile, it is useful in biliary tract infections not caused by biliary obstruction. It is used in the treatment of bronchitis, sinusitis, and otitis media.

Drug	Pregnancy Category	Adults	Children
Ⓟ **Ampicillin** (Principen)	B	PO, IM, IV 250–500 mg every 6 h. In severe infections, doses up to 2 g every 4 h may be given IV.	Infants/children: PO 50–100 mg/kg/d in divided doses every 6 h (max dose 2–4 g/d) IM, IV 100–400 mg/kg/d in divided doses every 6 h (max dose 12 g/d)
Amoxicillin (Amoxil, Trimox)	B	PO 250–500 mg every 8 h or 500–875 mg every 12 h	3 mo or more: PO 20–30 mg/kg/d in divided doses every 12 h More than 3 mo: 20–50 mg/kg/d in divided doses every 8–12 h
Carbenicillin indanyl sodium (Geocillin)	B	PO 1–2 tabs 4 times daily	PO 30–50 mg/kg/d in divided doses every 6 h
Ticarcillin (Ticar)	B	IM, IV 1–4 g every 4–6 h; IM injections should not exceed 2 g/injection (max dose 24 g/d)	Infants/children: IM 50–100 mg/kg/d in divided doses every 6–8 h; IV 50–300 mg/kg/d in divided doses every 4–8 h (do not exceed adult max dose)
Piperacillin (Pipracil)	B	IM, IV 200–300 mg/kg/d in divided doses every 4–6 h. IM injections should not exceed 2 g/injection and use should be reserved for uncomplicated infections. Usual adult dosage, 3–4 g every 4–6 h; max daily dose 24 g	Infants/children/adolescents (non-FDA approved) IV 200–300 mg/kg/d in divided doses every 4–6 h; max daily dose 24 g/d

Penicillin–Beta-Lactamase Inhibitor Combinations

The beta-lactamase inhibitors display negligible antimicrobial activity but contain the beta-lactam ring. Coadministered with beta-lactam antibiotics, the inhibitors sole function is to bind with the beta-lactamases (enzymes that degrade the beta-lactam ring) to prevent inactivation of the beta-lactam antibiotics.

Drug	Pregnancy Category	Adults	Children
Ampicillin–sulbactam (Unasyn)	B	IM, IV 1.5–3 g every 6 h. Maximum dose of 4 g/d of sulbactam.	1 y or older: IV 100–400 mg/kg/d in divided doses every 6 h (max 8 g ampicillin/d; 12 g Unasyn) Doses up to 300 mg/kg/d may be given for severe infections in infants older than 1 mo of age.

TABLE 16.2
DRUGS AT A GLANCE: Penicillins (Continued)

Drug	Pregnancy Category	Routes and Dosage Ranges	
		Adults	*Children*
Amoxicillin–clavulanate (Augmentin)	B	PO 250–500 mg every 8 h; or 875 mg every 12 h	≥40 kg: same as adults <40 kg: 20–90 mg/kg/d in divided doses every 8–12 h
Piperacillin–tazobactam (Zosyn)	B	IV 2.25–4.5 g every 6–8 h	≥40 kg: same as adults IV 80–100 mg/kg/d based on piperacillin component every 8 h
Ticarcillin–clavulanate (Timentin)	B	IV 3.1 g every 4–6 h	<60 kg: IV 200–300 mg/kg/d based on ticarcillin component in divided doses every 4–6 h (max dose 18–24 g/d)

QSEN Safety Alert

Before prescribing ampicillin or other penicillins for streptococcal infections, clinicians should perform culture and susceptibility studies and be aware of local patterns of streptococcal susceptibility or resistance.

Use in Children

Ampicillin and other penicillins are widely used to treat infections in children and are generally safe. However, caution is necessary in neonates because immature kidney function slows drug elimination. Dosage should be based on age, weight, severity of the infection being treated, and renal function. Specialized pediatric dosing references provide guidance to dosing based on age and weight.

Use in Older Adults

Ampicillin and other penicillins are relatively safe in older adults. However, decreased renal function, other disease processes, and concurrent drug therapies increase the risks of adverse effects.

Use in Patients With Renal Impairment

Because ampicillin is excreted primarily by the kidneys, it is important to use caution with renal impairment.

Use in Patients With Hepatic Impairment

Ampicillin can be used in patients with hepatic impairment, as can almost all the penicillins. Caution is necessary when using amoxicillin–clavulanate (Augmentin) in patients with hepatic injury or destruction. No specific recommendations for dosage adjustment are available. Development of cholestatic jaundice and hepatic dysfunction with previous use of the drug are contraindications. Cholestatic liver impairment usually subsides when the drug is stopped.

Use in Patients With Critical Illness

Use of ampicillin in the people who are critically ill is not nearly as great as it once was, primarily because resistance to the drug has emerged and other broad-spectrum agents are available. Patients frequently take other beta-lactam agents concomitantly with other antimicrobial drugs because critically ill patients often have multiple organisms that cause infections. The **extended-spectrum** drugs (e.g., piperacillin, which is a derivative of ampicillin) and penicillin–beta-lactamase inhibitor combinations (e.g., Zosyn), which have bactericidal activity against a wide range of bacteria, are most likely to be used in critical care units for the treatment of respiratory diseases such as pneumonia, blood, or other infections. Through chemical modification, these extended-spectrum drugs affect additional types of bacteria, typically gram-negative bacteria. With cephalosporins, third- and fourth-generation drugs are commonly used and are usually given by intermittent intravenous (IV) infusions every 8 or 12 hours. Blood levels of penicillins need to be maintained above the minimum inhibitory concentration (MIC) of the microorganisms causing the infection. Thus, continuous or extended infusions may be of benefit with serious infections, especially those caused by relatively resistant organisms such as *Pseudomonas* or *Acinetobacter*. It is necessary to monitor function of the kidneys, liver, and other organs in critically ill patients and to reduce drug dosages when indicated.

Use in Patients Receiving Home Care

When using oral beta-lactam antibiotics such as ampicillin, the home care nurse mainly needs to teach patients about accurate administration of the drug and observation for therapeutic and adverse effects. With using liquid suspensions for children, shaking to resuspend the medication and measuring with a measuring spoon or calibrated device to ensure safe dosing are required. Household spoons should not be used because they vary widely in capacity and may lead to incorrect dosing.

Adverse Effects

The most common adverse effects of ampicillin are hypersensitivity reactions, including rash and/or anaphylactoid reactions. Commonly reported GI adverse effects include abdominal pain, diarrhea, gastritis, and nausea and vomiting. Nephropathy, such as interstitial nephritis, although infrequent, has occurred with all penicillins. It is most often associated with high doses of parenteral penicillins and is attributed to hypersensitivity reactions.

The U.S. Food and Drug Administration (FDA) has issued a **BLACK BOX WARNING** ◆ to alert health care providers that inadvertent IV administration of penicillin G benzathine may result in cardiopulmonary arrest and death. Long-acting repository forms have additives that decrease their solubility in tissue fluids and delay their absorption.

Contraindications

Contraindications include hypersensitivity or allergic reactions to any penicillin formulation. An allergic reaction to one penicillin means the patient is allergic to all drugs of the penicillin class. The potential for **cross-allergenicity** (allergy to a drug of another class with similar chemical structure) with cephalosporins and carbapenems exists; each has the characteristic bicyclic core structure, the chemical unit thought to be most responsible for beta-lactam hypersensitivity. Recent data suggest that the incidence is less than 1%, lower than previously thought.

Nursing Implications

Preventing Interactions

Many medications and herbs interact with ampicillin, increasing or decreasing its effects (Boxes 16.1 and 16.2). In addition, ampicillin inhibits the renal tubular secretion of methotrexate, which may lead to prolonged and higher drug concentrations of methotrexate.

Penicillins are often given concomitantly with aminoglycosides for serious infections, such as those caused by *Pseudomonas*

BOX 16.1   Drug Interactions: Ampicillin

Drugs That Increase the Effects of Ampicillin
- Allopurinol
  Increases the incidence of skin rash
- Clavulanic acid
  Overcomes resistance in bacteria that secrete beta-lactamase
- Probenecid
  Inhibits the renal tubular secretion
- Uricosuric drugs
  Block renal excretion

Drugs That Decrease the Effects of Ampicillin
- Chloroquine
  Decreases the serum concentration
- Fusidic acid
  Diminishes the therapeutic effect
- Tetracycline derivatives:
  Diminish the therapeutic effect

BOX 16.2   Herb and Dietary Interactions: Ampicillin

Herbs and Foods That Decrease the Effects of Ampicillin
- Food
  Decreases absorption
- Khat
  Decreases absorption

---

aeruginosa. These drugs should not be admixed in a syringe, given in an IV solution, or administered via Y-site, because the penicillin inactivates the aminoglycoside. If feasible, dose separation is ideal.

Administering the Medication

It is necessary to give oral ampicillin, like most oral penicillins, on an empty stomach, approximately 1 hour before or 2 hours after a meal. Patients should take the oral drug with a full glass of water, preferably to promote absorption and decrease inactivation, which may occur in an acidic environment. If need be, they may take it with food; however, the absorption rate decreases with food. Oral suspensions of the drug are stable for 7 days at room temperature and 14 days when refrigerated.

When diluted with 0.9% sodium chloride, ampicillin is stable for 8 hours for concentrations up to 30 mg/mL. It is stable for only 1 hour when diluted with dextrose-containing solutions for concentrations of 10 to 20 mg/mL. It is necessary to give IV penicillins for the full prescribed course of treatment to prevent complications such as rheumatic fever, endocarditis, and glomerulonephritis. IV concentrations should not exceed 30 mg/mL.

Assessing for Therapeutic Effects

It is not necessary to obtain drug levels when administering ampicillin or any of the antimicrobials in the penicillin class. When administering ampicillin, it is recommended that serum creatinine and blood urea nitrogen (BUN) be monitored.

Assessing for Adverse Effects

The nurse carefully assesses the characteristics of a rash, if present. It is necessary to distinguish, if possible, a hypersensitivity reaction from a nonallergic ampicillin rash.

Patient Teaching

The nurse instructs patients to take oral penicillins for the full prescribed course of treatment to prevent complications. Box 16.3 outlines patient teaching guidelines for ampicillin and other oral penicillins.

Other Drugs in the Class

Antistaphylococcal Penicillins and Aminopenicillins

Choice of a beta-lactam antibacterial depends on the organism causing the infection, severity of the infection, and other factors. Penicillin G or the aminopenicillin amoxicillin is the drug of choice in many infections. Other aminopenicillins are indicated in *Pseudomonas* infections. Antistaphylococcal penicillin is indicated in staphylococcal infections; the antistaphylococcal drugs of choice are nafcillin for IV use and dicloxacillin for oral use.

| **BOX 16.3** | **Patient Teaching Guidelines for Oral Penicillins** |

General Considerations

■ Do not take any penicillin if you have ever had an allergic reaction to penicillin in which you had difficulty breathing, swelling, or skin rash. However, some people who call a minor stomach upset an allergic reaction, which is incorrect, are not given penicillin when that is the best antibiotic in a given situation.

■ Complete the full course of drug treatment for greater effectiveness and prevention of secondary infection with drug-resistant bacteria.

■ Follow instructions carefully about the dose and how often it is taken. Drug effectiveness depends on maintaining adequate blood levels. Penicillins often need more frequent administration than some other antibiotics, because they are rapidly excreted by the kidneys.

Self- or Caregiver Administration

■ Take most penicillins on an empty stomach, 1 hour before or 2 hours after a meal. Penicillin V, amoxicillin, and Augmentin can be taken with food. (Take Augmentin with meals to increase absorption and decrease gastrointestinal upset.)

■ Take each dose with a full glass of water; do not take with orange juice or with other acidic fluids (they may destroy the drug).

■ Take at even intervals, preferably around the clock.

■ Shake liquid penicillins well, to mix thoroughly and measure the dose accurately.

■ Discard liquid penicillin after 1 week if stored at room temperature or after 2 weeks if refrigerated. Liquid forms deteriorate and should not be taken after their expiration dates.

■ Report skin rash, hives, itching, severe diarrhea, shortness of breath, fever, sore throat, black tongue, or any unusual bleeding to your health care provider. These symptoms may indicate an allergy to penicillin.

Proper administration of penicillins is important. With intramuscular (IM) penicillins, it is necessary to inject them deep into large muscle masses to decrease tissue irritation. With IV penicillins, it is necessary to usually first dilute reconstituted penicillins in 50 to 100 mL of 5% dextrose or 0.9% sodium chloride injection and infuse them over 30 to 60 minutes to minimize vascular irritation and phlebitis. It should be noted that ticarcillin may cause decreased platelet aggregation.

Penicillin–Beta-Lactamase Inhibitor Combinations

Beta-lactamase inhibitors are drugs with a beta-lactam structure but minimal antibacterial activity. They bind with and inactivate the beta-lactamase enzymes produced by many bacteria (e.g., *Escherichia coli*; *Klebsiella*, *Enterobacter*, and *Bacteroides* species; *Staphylococcus aureus*). When combined with a penicillin, the beta-lactamase inhibitor protects the penicillin from destruction by the enzymes and extends the penicillin's spectrum of antimicrobial activity. Thus, the combination drug may be effective in infections caused by bacteria that are resistant to a beta-lactam antibiotic alone.

Clavulanate, sulbactam, and tazobactam are the beta-lactamase inhibitors available in combinations with penicillins.

- Ampicillin and sulbactam is available as Unasyn, in vials with 1 g of ampicillin and 0.5 g of sulbactam, or 2 g of ampicillin and 1 g of sulbactam.
- Amoxicillin and clavulanate is marketed as Augmentin, in 250-, 500-, and 875-mg tablets, each of which contains 125 mg of clavulanate.

QSEN Safety Alert ❗

Thus, two 250-mg tablets are not equivalent to one 500-mg tablet.

- Augmentin is also available as 1000-mg extended-release tablets containing 62.5 mg of clavulanate. In addition, a chewable formulation is available as 200 mg

of amoxicillin and 28.5 mg of clavulanate, as well as 400 mg of amoxicillin and 57 mg of clavulanate.

- Ticarcillin and clavulanate is available as Timentin, an IV formulation containing 3 g of ticarcillin and 100 mg of clavulanate.
- Piperacillin and tazobactam is marketed as Zosyn, an IV formulation. Three dosage strengths are available, with 2 g piperacillin and 0.25 g tazobactam, 3 g piperacillin and 0.375 g tazobactam, or 4 g piperacillin and 0.5 g tazobactam.

NCLEX Success

1. A nurse is preparing to administer the first dose of piperacillin–tazobactam (Zosyn) to a patient in an infusion clinic. The nurse should take which of the following precautions?

   A. Ask the patient about past allergic reactions to penicillins.
   B. Ask the patient about past allergic reactions to aminoglycosides.
   C. Mix the piperacillin–tazobactam with lidocaine to reduce pain of infusion.
   D. Instruct the patient to eat a snack to decrease stomach upset from piperacillin–tazobactam.

2. A woman is to receive amoxicillin–clavulanate (Augmentin) 500 mg PO every 8 hours for bronchitis. The nurse retrieves two 250-mg tablets from the medication cart. This is incorrect for which of the following reasons?

   A. The amount of sulbactam in amoxicillin–clavulanate 250 mg is 62.5 mg per tablet, twice the intended amount.
   B. This provides twice the intended dose of clavulanate.
   C. The 250-mg tablets have less absorption than the 500-mg tablets.
   D. Administration of amoxicillin–clavulanate is only intravenous, so selecting tablets means that the wrong drug is being administered.

Cephalosporins

Cephalosporins are a widely used group of drugs derived from a fungus and closely related chemically to the penicillins. Although technically cefoxitin and cefotetan are not cephalosporins, they are categorized with the cephalosporins because of their similarities to the group. Cephalosporins are broad-spectrum agents with activity against both gram-positive and gram-negative bacteria. Compared with penicillins, these drugs are generally less active against gram-positive organisms but more active against gram-negative ones.

Classification

Cephalosporins are classified into five subgroups, or "generations," based on their pharmacology and spectrum of activity.

First-Generation Cephalosporins

The first cephalosporin, cephalothin, is no longer available for clinical use. However, it may be used to determine susceptibility to first-generation cephalosporins, which have essentially the same spectrum of antimicrobial activity. In general, first-generation cephalosporins have strong activity against gram-positive bacteria and poor activity against gram-negative bacteria. Therefore, these drugs are effective against streptococci, staphylococci (except methicillin-resistant *S. aureus* [MRSA]), *Shigella*, *E. coli*, *Proteus mirabilis*, and *Bacteroides* species (except *Bacteroides fragilis*). They are not effective against *Enterobacter*, *Pseudomonas*, and *Serratia* species.

Often, health care providers use first-generation cephalosporins for surgical prophylaxis, especially with prosthetic implants, because gram-positive organisms such as staphylococci cause most infections of surgical sites. Prescribers may also order them for treatment of infections caused by susceptible organisms in body sites where drug penetration and host defenses are adequate.

Ⓟ **Cefazolin**, the prototype cephalosporin, is the drug of choice for surgical prophylaxis in most surgical procedures. Some advantages of cefazolin over other first-generation cephalosporins include less frequent dosing, higher blood levels after parenteral administration, and increased gram-positive coverage.

Second-Generation Cephalosporins

Second-generation cephalosporins are more active against some gram-negative organisms and somewhat less active against gram-positive cocci than the first-generation agents. Thus, they may be effective in infections resistant to other antibiotics, including infections caused by *Haemophilus influenzae*, *Klebsiella* species, *E. coli*, and some strains of *Proteus*. Because each of these drugs has a different antimicrobial spectrum, susceptibility tests must be performed for each drug rather than for the entire group, as may be done with first-generation drugs. Cefoxitin (Mefoxin), for example, is active against *B. fragilis*, an anaerobic organism resistant to most drugs.

Often, other uses for second-generation cephalosporins also include surgical prophylaxis, especially for gynecologic and colorectal surgery. Prescribers also order the drugs for treatment of intra-abdominal infections such as pelvic inflammatory disease, diverticulitis, and other infections caused by organisms inhabiting pelvic and colorectal areas (perhaps caused by penetrating wounds of the abdomen).

Third-Generation Cephalosporins

Third-generation cephalosporins further extend the spectrum of activity against gram-negative organisms. In addition to activity against the usual enteric pathogens (e.g., *E. coli*, *Proteus* and *Klebsiella* species), they are also active against several strains resistant to other antibiotics and to first- and second-generation cephalosporins. Thus, they may be useful in infections caused by unusual strains of enteric organisms such as the group Enterobacteriaceae (which includes *Citrobacter*, *Serratia*, *Enterobacter*, *P. mirabilis*, and *E. coli*). Another difference is the ability of third-generation cephalosporins to penetrate inflamed meninges to reach therapeutic concentrations in CSF. Thus, they may be useful in meningeal infections caused by common pathogens, including *H. influenzae*, *Neisseria meningitidis*, and *Streptococcus pneumoniae*. Although some of the drugs are active against *Pseudomonas* organisms, drug-resistant strains may emerge when a cephalosporin is used alone for treatment of pseudomonal infection.

Overall, cephalosporins gain gram-negative activity and lose gram-positive activity as they move from the first to the third generation. The second- and third-generation drugs are more active against gram-negative organisms because they are more resistant to the beta-lactamase enzymes (cephalosporinases) produced by some bacteria to inactivate cephalosporins.

Fourth-Generation Cephalosporins

Fourth-generation cephalosporins have a greater spectrum of antimicrobial activity and greater stability against breakdown by beta-lactamase enzymes compared with third-generation drugs. Cefepime, the first fourth-generation cephalosporin to be developed, is active against both gram-positive and gram-negative organisms. With gram-positive organisms, it is active against streptococci and staphylococci (except for methicillin-resistant staphylococci). With gram-negative organisms, its activity against *P. aeruginosa* is similar to that of ceftazidime, and its activity against Enterobacteriaceae is greater than that of third-generation cephalosporins. Moreover, cefepime retains activity against strains of Enterobacteriaceae and *P. aeruginosa* that have acquired resistance to third-generation agents.

Fifth-Generation Cephalosporins

Ceftaroline (Teflaro) is an IV cephalosporin for the treatment of community-acquired pneumonia and skin infections. It is the first cephalosporin to be considered active against resistant gram-positive organisms, such as MRSA, vancomycin-resistant *S. aureus* (VRSA), vancomycin-insensitive *S. aureus* (VISA), and heteroresistant VISA.

Pharmacokinetics

After the cephalosporins are absorbed, they achieve therapeutic concentrations in most body fluids and tissues, with maximum concentrations in the liver and kidneys. However, many cephalosporins do not reach therapeutic levels in the CSF.

Most third-generation cephalosporins achieve more consistent CSF penetration in those patients with inflamed meninges.

Cefazolin is distributed into most body tissues and crosses the placenta. The onset of action is rapid with both IV and IM administration. The drug peaks at the end of IV infusion and within 1 to 2 hours with IM injection. The duration of action is 6 to 12 hours. The drug, which is largely excreted unchanged via the kidneys, concentrates in the urine. Thus, metabolism is not hepatic. Therefore, no dosage adjustments are necessary with hepatic impairment.

Action

Cefazolin inhibits the third and last step of bacterial wall synthesis by binding to one or more penicillin-binding proteins.

Use

Cefazolin is a frequently used parenteral agent. It reaches a higher serum concentration, is more protein bound, and has a slower rate of elimination than other first-generation drugs.

These factors prolong serum half-life, which means that cefazolin can be given less frequently.

Clinical indications for the use of the cephalosporins include surgical prophylaxis and treatment of infections of the respiratory tract, skin and soft tissues, bones and joints, urinary tract, brain and spinal cord, and bloodstream (septicemia). In infections caused by MRSA, cephalosporins are not clinically effective even if in vitro testing indicates susceptibility (except for the newest cephalosporin, ceftaroline). Infections caused by *Neisseria gonorrhoeae*, at one time susceptible to penicillin, are now treated with a third-generation cephalosporin such as ceftriaxone.

Tables 16.3 and 16.4 provide important information about parenteral and oral cephalosporins, respectively.

Use in Children

As with penicillins, cefazolin and other cephalosporins are extensively used to treat infections in children and are commonly safe. They should be used cautiously in neonates because immature kidney function slows their elimination. Dosage should be based on age, weight, severity of the infection, and renal function.

TABLE 16.3
DRUGS AT A GLANCE: Parenteral Cephalosporins

Drug	Pregnancy Category	Characteristics/ Indications	Routes and Dosage Ranges	
			Adults	*Children*
First Generation				
℗ **Cefazolin** (Kefzol, Ancef)	B	Active against streptococci, staphylococci, *Neisseria*, *Salmonella*, *Shigella*, *Escherichia*, *Klebsiella*, *Listeria*, *Bacillus*, *Haemophilus influenzae*, *Corynebacterium diphtheriae*, *Proteus mirabilis*, and *Bacteroides* (except *B. fragilis*)	IM, IV 250 mg–2 g every 6–12 h (max dose 12 g/d)	IM, IV 25–100 mg/kg/d in divided doses every 6–8 h (max dose 6 g/d)
Second Generation				
Cefotetan (Cefotan)	B	1. Effective against most organisms except *Pseudomonas* 2. Highly resistant to beta-lactamase enzymes	IV, IM 1–6 g/d in divided doses every 12 h Surgical prophylaxis, IV 1–2 g 30–60 min before surgery	IV, IM 20–40 mg/kg every 12 h (max 6 g/d)
Cefoxitin (Mefoxin)	B	1. The first cephamycin (derived from a different fungus than cephalosporins) 2. A major clinical use may stem from increased activity against *B. fragilis*, an organism resistant to most other antimicrobial drugs.	IV 1–2 g every 6–8 h Surgical prophylaxis, IV 1 or 2 g 30–60 min before surgery	IV 80–160 mg/kg/d in divided doses every 4–6 h. Do not exceed 12 g/d.

(*Continued on page 300*)

TABLE 16.3

DRUGS AT A GLANCE: Parenteral Cephalosporins (Continued)

Drug	Pregnancy Category	Characteristics/ Indications	Routes and Dosage Ranges	
			Adults	*Children*
Second Generation (Continued)				
Cefuroxime (Kefurox, Zinacef)	B	1. Similar to other second-generation cephalosporins 2. Penetrates cerebrospinal fluid in presence of inflamed meninges	IV, IM 500 mg–1.5 g every 6–8 h Surgical prophylaxis, IV 1.5 g 30–60 min before initial skin incision	IV, IM 50–150 mg/kg/d in divided doses every 6–8 h (max dose 6 g/d)
Cefotaxime (Claforan)	B	1. Antibacterial activity against most gram-positive and gram-negative bacteria, including several strains resistant to other antibiotics 2. Recommended for serious infections caused by susceptible microorganisms	IV, IM 1–2 g every 4–12 h; max dose, 12 g/d	>50 kg: same as adults <50 kg to 12y and age >1 mo: IV, IM 50–200 mg/kg/d, in divided doses every 6–8 h
Ceftazidime (Fortaz)	B	1. Active against gram-positive and gram-negative organisms 2. Especially effective against gram-negative organisms, including *Pseudomonas aeruginosa* and other bacterial strains resistant to aminoglycosides 3. Indicated for serious infections caused by susceptible organisms	IV, IM 500–2000 mg every 8–12 h	1 mo–12 y: IV 30–50 mg/kg every 8 h, not to exceed 6 g/d
Ceftizoxime (Cefizox)	B	1. Broader gram-negative and anaerobic activity, especially against B. fragilis 2. More active against Enterobacteriaceae than cefoperazone 3. Dosage must be reduced with even mild renal insufficiency (CrCl <80 mL/min).	IV, IM 1–4 g every 8–12 h	More than 6 mo: IV, IM 150–200 mg/kg/d in divided doses every 6–8 h (max dose 12 g/d)
Third Generation				
Ceftriaxone (Rocephin)	B	1. First third-generation cephalosporin approved for once-daily dosing 2. Antibacterial activity against most gram-positive and gram-negative bacteria, including several strains resistant to other antibiotics	IV, IM 1–2 g every 12–24 h	Infants/children IM, IV 50–100 mg/kg/d in 1–2 divided doses (max dose 4 g/d) Meningitis, IV, IM 100 mg/kg/d, not to exceed 4 g daily, in divided doses every 12 h

TABLE 16.3

DRUGS AT A GLANCE: Parenteral Cephalosporins (Continued)

Drug	Pregnancy Category	Characteristics/ Indications	Routes and Dosage Ranges	
			Adults	Children
Fourth Generation				
Cefepime (Maxipime)	B	1. Indicated for use in sepsis; in severe infections of the lower respiratory and urinary tract, skin and soft tissue, and female reproductive tract; and in febrile neutropenic patients 2. May be used as monotherapy for all infections caused by susceptible organisms except *P. aeruginosa*. A combination of drugs should be used for serious pseudomonal infections. 3. Essential to reduce dosage with renal impairment	IV 1–2 g every 8–12 h IM 0.5–1 g every 12 h	IM, IV 50 mg/kg every 8–12 h, not to exceed recommended adult dose
Fifth Generation				
Ceftaroline (Teflaro)	B	Indicated for the treatment of acute bacterial skin and skin structure infections and community-acquired bacterial pneumonia	IV 600 mg every 12 h	Safety and efficacy not yet established

TABLE 16.4

DRUGS AT A GLANCE: Oral Cephalosporins

Drug	Pregnancy Category	Characteristics/ Indications	Routes and Dosage Ranges	
			Adults	Children
First Generation				
Cefadroxil (Duricef)	B	A derivative of cephalexin that has a longer half-life and can be given less often	PO 1–2 g twice daily	30 mg/kg/d in divided doses every 12 h (max 2 g/d)
Cephalexin (Keflex)	B	First oral cephalosporin; still used extensively	PO 250–1000 mg every 6 h (max 4 g/d)	PO 25–100 mg/kg/d in divided doses every 6–8 h (max 4 g/d)
Second Generation				
Cefaclor (Ceclor)	B	More active against *Haemophilus influenzae* and *Escherichia coli* than first-generation drugs	PO 250–500 mg every 8 h	PO 20–40 mg/kg/d in divided doses every 8–12 h (max 1 g/d)

(Continued on page 302)

TABLE 16.4

DRUGS AT A GLANCE: Oral Cephalosporins (Continued)

Drug	Pregnancy Category	Characteristics/ Indications	Routes and Dosage Ranges	
			Adults	*Children*
Second Generation (Continued)				
Cefprozil (Cefzil)	B	Similar to cefaclor	PO 250–500 mg every 12–24 h	PO 7.5–15 mg/kg/d in divided doses every 12 h (max 1 g/d)
Cefuroxime (Ceftin)	B	Tablets and oral suspension are not considered bioequivalent and should not be interchanged on an mg per mg basis; can also be given parenterally.	PO 250–500 mg every 12 h; IV, IM 500 mg–1.5 g every 8 h	Under 13 y: PO Suspension 20–30 mg/kg/d in two divided doses. PO tablet 125–250 mg every 12 h. IM, IV 75–150 mg/kg/d in divided doses every 8 h (max dose 6 g/d) 13 y or older: same as adults
Third Generation				
Cefdinir (Omnicef)	B	Indicated for bronchitis, pharyngitis, and otitis media caused by streptococci or *H. influenzae*. Also indicated for uncomplicated skin structure infections	PO 300 mg every 12 h or 600 mg every 24 h for 10 d	13 y or older, PO same as adults 6 mo–12 y, PO 7 mg/kg every 12 h or 14 mg/kg every 24 h for 10 d
Cefditoren pivoxil (Spectracef)	B	Indicated for pharyngitis, bacterial exacerbations of chronic bronchitis, community-acquired pneumonia, and skin/skin structure infections	PO 400 mg twice daily (every 12 h) for 10 d Skin infections, PO 200 mg twice daily for 10 d	12 y or older, same as adults
Cefixime (Suprax)	B	First oral third-generation drug	PO 200 mg every 12 h or 400 mg every 24 h	Children ≥6 mo: 8–20 mg/kg/d in divided doses every 12–24 h (max dose 400 mg/d) PO give adult dose to children 50 kg of weight or 12 y or older
Cefpodoxime (Vantin)	B	Similar to cefixime except has some activity against staphylococci (except methicillin-resistant *Staphylococcus aureus*)	PO 100–400 mg every 12 h	PO 10 mg/kg/d divided every 12 h ≥12 y give adult dose
Ceftibuten (Cedax)	B	1. Indicated for bronchitis, otitis media, pharyngitis, or tonsillitis caused by streptococci or *H. influenzae* 2. Can be given once daily 3. Available in a capsule for oral use and an oral pediatric suspension that comes in two concentrations (90 mg/5 mL)	PO 400 mg daily for 10 d	9 mg/kg/d for 10 d (max dose 400 mg/d)

Use in Older Adults

As with penicillins, cefazolin and other cephalosporins are relatively safe, although decreased renal function, other disease processes, and concurrent drug therapies increase the risks of adverse effects in older adults.

Use in Patients With Renal Impairment

Cefazolin and all other parenteral cephalosporins, except ceftriaxone, require dosage adjustment in patients with renal impairment. Usual doses may produce high and prolonged serum drug levels, and therefore, a lower dose or an increased period between doses is necessary. Cefazolin is moderately dialyzable, and the normal dose or a supplemental dose should be administered after dialysis.

Use in Patients With Critical Illness

Some cephalosporins are used in surgical prophylaxis. The particular drug depends largely on the type of organism likely to be encountered in the operative area. First-generation cephalosporins, mainly cefazolin, are used for procedures associated with gram-positive postoperative infections because of activity against streptococci and methicillin-susceptible staphylococci. Second-generation cephalosporins, mainly cefotetan and cefoxitin, are often used for abdominal procedures, especially gynecologic and colorectal surgery, in which enteric gram-negative postoperative infections may occur. Third-generation cephalosporins should not be used for surgical prophylaxis because they are less active against staphylococci than cefazolin and the gram-negative organisms they are most useful against are rarely encountered in elective surgery. Additionally, fourth- and fifth-generation cephalosporins are not typically used for surgical prophylaxis. Widespread usage for prophylaxis promotes emergence of drug-resistant organisms.

A single dose is usually sufficient, although repeat doses are necessary in patients undergoing a surgical procedure exceeding 4 hours or procedures involving major blood loss. (Postoperative doses are rarely necessary but, if used, should generally not be given more than 24 hours after surgery.) Blood levels of cephalosporins need to be maintained above the MIC of the microorganisms causing the infection being treated. Thus, continuous infusions may be of benefit with serious infections, especially those caused by relatively resistant organisms such as *Pseudomonas* or *Acinetobacter*.

Use in Patients Receiving Home Care

With cefazolin as well as with oral agents such as cephalexin and cefprozil, the home care nurse mainly needs to teach patients about accurate administration and observation for therapeutic and adverse effects. With cefazolin or other parenteral cephalosporins, the nurse should teach the patient and family how to administer the drug and not to use the drug if (1) it is cloudy or discolored or if (2) the vial is damaged. It is important to keep needles and syringes out of the reach of children and pets and dispose of them properly.

Adverse Effects

Adverse effects to cefazolin and the other cephalosporins are similar to those of most other antibiotics: abdominal pain, diarrhea, gastritis, nausea, and vomiting. Primarily, effects of particular importance are hypersensitivity reactions and **superinfections** (infection after a previous infection, typically caused by microorganisms that are resistant to the antibiotics used earlier).

BOX 16.4 Drug Interactions: Cephalosporins

Drugs That Increase the Effects of Cephalosporins

■ Aminoglycosides
Increase the risk of nephrotoxicity

■ Entecavir
Leads to competitive inhibition of transporters in renal tubules

■ Furosemide
Increases the risk of nephrotoxicity

■ Nimodipine
Increases the risk of nephrotoxicity

■ Vancomycin
Increases the risk of nephrotoxicity

Contraindications

A contraindication to the use of a cephalosporin is a previous severe anaphylactic reaction to a penicillin. Because cephalosporins are chemically similar to penicillins, there is a risk of cross-sensitivity. However, incidence of cross-sensitivity is low, especially in patients who have had delayed reactions (e.g., skin rash) to penicillins. Another contraindication is cephalosporin allergy. Immediate allergic reactions with anaphylaxis, bronchospasm, and urticaria occur less often than delayed reactions with skin rash, drug fever, and eosinophilia.

Nursing Implications

Preventing Interactions

Cephalosporins have been associated with a decrease in prothrombin activity, which may be due to depletion of vitamin K depletion in the gut flora. It is necessary to monitor patients

previously stabilized on anticoagulants. Box 16.4 outlines drug–drug interactions. There are no identified herbal interactions. However, each gram of cefazolin has 46 mg (2 mEq) of sodium, which may have a negative effect on patients with heart failure.

Administering the Medication

To prevent complications, it is essential to administer cefazolin and other cephalosporins for the full prescribed course of treatment.

QSEN Safety Alert

It is important to avoid giving cephalosporins to people with life-threatening allergic reactions to penicillin (anaphylaxis, laryngeal swelling angioedema, or hives).

The nurse should not mix ceftriaxone and IV solutions of calcium-containing salts, or administer these drugs simultaneously, because of the potential for ceftriaxone–calcium precipitation. Adverse effects can be minimized by administering most oral cephalosporins with food or milk.

Assessing for Therapeutic Effects

Drug levels are not required when administering cefazolin or any of the cephalosporins. If the patient is experiencing renal impairment, monitoring of serum creatinine and BUN is recommended, because adjustment for renal dysfunction may be necessary.

Assessing for Adverse Effects

The nurse carefully evaluates any rash. If possible, it is necessary to distinguish a hypersensitivity reaction from a nonallergic cefazolin rash.

Patient Teaching

The nurse instructs patients that cephalosporins, like all antibiotics, should be given for the full prescribed course of treatment

BOX 16.5 Patient Teaching Guidelines for Oral Cephalosporins

General Considerations

■ Inform your physician if you have ever had a severe allergic reaction to penicillin in which you had difficulty breathing, swelling, or skin rash. A small number of people are allergic to both penicillins and cephalosporins because the drugs are somewhat similar in their chemical structures.

■ Also inform your physician if you have had a previous allergic reaction to a cephalosporin (e.g., Ceclor, Keflex). If not sure whether a new prescription is a cephalosporin, ask the pharmacist before having the prescription filled.

■ Complete the full course of drug treatment for greater effectiveness and prevention of secondary infection with drug-resistant bacteria.

■ Follow instructions about dosing frequency; effectiveness depends on maintaining adequate blood levels.

Self- or Caregiver Administration

■ Take most oral drugs with food or milk to prevent stomach upset.

■ Take cefpodoxime (Vantin) and cefuroxime (Ceftin) with food to increase absorption.

■ Do not take cefaclor, cefdinir (Omnicef), or cefpodoxime (Vantin) with antacids containing aluminum or magnesium (e.g., Maalox, Mylanta) or with Pepcid, Tagamet, or Zantac. These drugs decrease absorption of these antibiotics and make them less effective. If necessary to take one of the drugs, take it 2 hours before or 2 hours after a dose of these antibiotics.

■ Shake liquid preparations well to mix thoroughly and measure the dose accurately.

■ Report the occurrence of diarrhea, especially if it is severe or contains blood, pus, or mucus. Cephalosporins can cause antibiotic-associated colitis, and the drug may need to be stopped.

■ Inform your health care provider if you are breastfeeding. These drugs enter breast milk.

to prevent complications. Box 16.5 outlines patient teaching guidelines.

Other Drugs in the Class

As previously described, cephalosporins are grouped into generations by their antimicrobial properties. Each newer generation of cephalosporins has significantly greater gram-negative antimicrobial properties than the preceding generation, with decreased activity against gram-positive organisms. Fourth-generation cephalosporins, however, have true broad-spectrum activity acting against some gram-positive and many gram-negative organisms, including greater stability against degradation by beta-lactamase enzymes. Fifth-generation cephalosporins include anti-MRSA and anti-*Pseudomonas* activity in the spectrum of coverage.

Cefoperazone and cefotetan may cause hypoprothrombinemia (by killing intestinal bacteria that normally produce vitamin K or a chemical structure that prevents activation of prothrombin) or platelet dysfunction. Treatment of bleeding may involve giving vitamin K but does not restore normal platelet function or normal bacterial flora in the intestines.

NCLEX Success

3. A cardiac surgeon orders cefazolin 1 g IV "on call" to the operating room for a patient scheduled for a heart valve replacement. The surgery is scheduled for 7:00 AM the next morning. What is the rationale for giving the antibiotic at 6:30 AM? The last dose was administered more than 8 hours ago.

   A. The cefazolin must be given 60 minutes before the procedure for legal reasons.

   B. The cefazolin must be given within 60 minutes before the first skin incision to reach therapeutic concentrations.

   C. The cefazolin trough level will be checked at 6:00 AM, which would allow the level to come back before administration of the "on call" dose.

   D. The last dose was administered yesterday.

4. Which of the following classes of cephalosporins has the best activity against gram-positive organisms?

   A. first-generation cephalosporins

   B. second-generation cephalosporins

   C. third-generation cephalosporins

   D. fourth-generation cephalosporins

Clinical Application 16-1

The nurse asks Mr. O'Brian if he has had an allergy to penicillin or cephalosporins. He denies any known allergies to drugs.

- Why is cefazolin the drug of choice for his cardiac pacemaker procedure?

- Before administrating this medication, what factors should the nurse assess?

- Why did the nurse ask the patient about a penicillin allergy with the administration of a cephalosporin?

Carbapenems

Carbapenems are broad-spectrum, bactericidal beta-lactam antimicrobials. The group consists of four drugs. ⓟ **Imipenem–cilastatin** (Primaxin) is the prototype.

Pharmacokinetics

Imipenem–cilastatin, which is given parenterally, is distributed in most body fluids and body tissues. The drug has a rapid onset of action, peaks at the end of the infusion, and has a duration of 6 to 8 hours. An enzyme (dehydropeptidase) in renal tubules rapidly breaks down the imipenem component; therefore, the drug reaches only low concentrations in the urine. However, the cilastatin inhibits the destruction of imipenem, increasing the urinary concentration of imipenem and reducing its potential renal toxicity. Recommended doses indicate the amount of imipenem; the solution contains an equivalent amount of cilastatin. The drugs are available only in the combined form.

Action

Like other beta-lactam drugs, imipenem–cilastatin and the other carbapenems inhibit synthesis of bacterial cell walls by binding with penicillin-binding proteins.

Use

Imipenem–cilastatin is effective in infections caused by a wide range of bacteria, including penicillinase-producing staphylococci, *E. coli*, *Proteus* species, *Enterobacter–Klebsiella–Serratia* species, *P. aeruginosa*, and *Enterococcus faecalis*. Its main use is in the treatment of infections caused by organisms resistant to other drugs. Considered to be a very broad-spectrum antibiotic, imipenem–cilastatin covers a range of gram-negative and gram-positive aerobes and anaerobes. It is used to treat infections of the lower respiratory tract, urinary tract, intra-abdominal infections, bone and joints, and skin and skin structures. It can also be used to treat polymicrobial infections (caused by multiple microorganisms), bacterial septicemia, and endocarditis.

Table 16.5 gives specific dosage information for carbapenems.

Use in Children

Use of imipenem–cilastatin is appropriate in children. However, children with CNS infections should not receive the drug because of the risk of seizures. Caution with all carbapenems is warranted in neonates because immature kidney function slows their elimination. Dosages are calculated based on age, weight, severity of infection, and renal function. Specialized pediatric dosing references can provide guidance to dosing of most carbapenems based on the child's age and weight.

Use in Older Adults

Imipenem–cilastatin and other carbapenems are relatively safe, although decreased renal function, other disease processes, and concurrent drug therapies increase the risks of adverse effects in older adults. Lower doses may be necessary in the elderly, depending on renal function and severity of infection.

TABLE 16.5

DRUGS AT A GLANCE: Carbapenems

Drug	Pregnancy Category	Routes and Dosage Ranges	
		Adults	*Children*
℗ **Imipenem–cilastatin** (Primaxin)	C	IV 250–1000 mg every 6–8 h based on imipenem component (max dose 4 g/d) IM 500–750 mg every 12 h	>3 mo: non-CNS infections IV 15–25 mg/kg every 6 h (max dose 4 g/d)
Doripenem (Doribax)	B	IV 500 mg every 8 h	Safety and efficacy not yet established
Ertapenem (Invanz)	B	IV, IM 1 g once daily	3 mo–12 y: IV, IM 15 mg/kg twice daily (max dose 1 g/d)
Meropenem (Merrem)	B	IV 1.5–6 g/d in divided doses every 8 h	≥3 mo: 10–40 mg/kg in divided doses every 8 h (max dose 6 g/d)

Use in Patients With Renal Impairment

It is necessary to reduce the dosage of imipenem–cilastatin and all other carbapenems in most patients with renal impairment, and caution is warranted in patients with creatinine clearance ≤20 mL/min because of the increased risk of seizures. Patients with severe renal impairment (≤5 mL/min) should not receive imipenem–cilastatin unless hemodialysis is initiated within 48 hours.

Use in Patients With Hepatic Impairment

Imipenem–cilastatin may cause abnormalities in liver function test results (i.e., elevated alanine and aspartate aminotransferases, alkaline phosphatase), but hepatitis and jaundice rarely occur. There are no specific recommendations or guidelines for dosage adjustment in patients with hepatic impairment.

Use in Patients With Critical Illness

Imipenem–cilastatin is typically used for illnesses that are considered critical. It has a broad spectrum of activity and has less resistant patterns than the penicillins and cephalosporins. Carbapenems generally resist cleavage by most beta-lactamases. Carbapenem-resistant strains of *P. aeruginosa* are arising due to the altered permeability to this class of drugs and specific changes that occur on the protein outer membranes.

Use in Patients Receiving Home Care

The need for frequent dosing means that imipenem–cilastatin is not typically given in the home setting. However, basic principles of IV care are an important component in administering this medication at home. Potential for secondary infections is a concern.

Adverse Effects

Adverse effects, including the risk of cross-sensitivity in patients with penicillin hypersensitivity and gastric disturbances, are similar to those of other beta-lactam antibiotics. In addition, there have been reports of central nervous system toxicity, including seizures. Seizures are more likely in patients with a preexisting seizure disorder or when recommended doses are exceeded; however, they have occurred in other patients as well.

Contraindications

Contraindications to imipenem–cilastatin include a hypersensitivity to carbapenems. There is a potential for cross-reactivity with patients that have a severe penicillin allergy due to the common beta-lactam ring. Patients with severe shock or atrioventricular block should not receive the IM formulation (containing lidocaine).

Nursing Implications

Preventing Interactions

Box 16.6 outlines drug–drug interactions with imipenem–cilastatin. There are no herbal interactions. All carbapenems may decrease the serum concentrations of divalproex. The drug may cause positive Coombs test results.

Administering the Medication

It is important to avoid administering imipenem–cilastatin and the other carbapenems to people with life-threatening allergic reactions to penicillin (anaphylaxis, laryngeal swelling angioedema, or hives). In addition, IM administration of imipenem–cilastatin is not recommended for people with severe or life-threatening infections such as endocarditis, shock, or septicemia. To prepare imipenem–cilastatin for IM

BOX 16.6   Drug Interactions: Imipenem–Cilastatin

Drugs That Increase the Effects of Imipenem–cilastatin

- Cyclosporine
  May increase central nervous system effects
- Ganciclovir
  May lead to generalized seizures
- Probenecid
  Increases drug level and half-life

injection, lidocaine, a local anesthetic, is added to decrease pain. The solution is contraindicated in people allergic to this type of local anesthetic. The IM formulation is not for IV use.

Assessing for Therapeutic Effects

Drug levels are not required when administering imipenem–cilastatin or any of the carbapenems. It is recommended that serum creatinine and BUN be monitored instead.

Assessing for Adverse Effects

The nurse carefully assesses any rash. It is necessary to distinguish, if possible, a hypersensitivity reaction from a nonallergic imipenem–cilastatin rash.

Patient Teaching

Imipenem–cilastatin and the other carbapenems are typically used for illnesses that are considered critical. Therefore, patient teaching guidelines focus on instructing the patient and family about the purpose of the drug and the importance of reporting adverse effects.

Other Drugs in the Class

The overall spectrum of meropenem is similar to imipenem, although meropenem is less active against gram-positive bacteria. The drug is frequently given in the treatment of febrile neutropenia, which frequently occurs in patients with hematological malignancies and in cancer patients receiving chemotherapeutic drugs that cause bone marrow suppression.

Monobactams

Currently, the only monobactam available for use is ℗ **aztreonam** (Azactam), which serves as the prototype of this class. Aztreonam is active against aerobic gram-negative bacteria, including Enterobacteriaceae and *P. aeruginosa*, and many strains that are resistant to multiple antibiotics. The coverage is similar to that of the aminoglycosides, but the drug does not cause kidney damage or hearing loss. Because gram-positive and anaerobic bacteria are resistant to aztreonam, the drug's ability to preserve normal gram-positive and anaerobic flora may be an advantage compared with other antimicrobial agents.

Pharmacokinetics

Aztreonam, which is given parenterally, is distributed in most body fluids and tissues, including the lungs, liver, kidney, bone, uterus, intestine, sputum, bile, pleural fluid, and synovial fluids. In addition, the drug also crosses the placenta and is excreted in breast milk. It is stable in the presence of beta-lactamase enzymes. Peak action occurs in 1 hour, with a duration of 4 to 12 hours; the onset of action depends on the organism and dose. Aztreonam is metabolized in the liver to inactive metabolites, which are excreted in the urine.

Action

Like other beta-lactam drugs, aztreonam inhibits synthesis of bacterial cell walls by binding with penicillin-binding proteins. However, aztreonam, because of its monobactam structure, has limited cross-allergenicity between itself and other beta-lactam antibiotics; it is generally considered safe to administer aztreonam to patients with a penicillin allergy.

Use

Aztreonam is effective in infections caused by *N. gonorrhoeae*, *H. influenzae*, and most *Enterobacter–Klebsiella–Serratia* species, and often active against *P. aeruginosa*. Although it is often considered to have similar coverage to aminoglycosides, extended-spectrum penicillins, and third-generation cephalosporins, aztreonam lacks gram-positive coverage. Also, anaerobes are not susceptible to aztreonam. Indications for use include infections of the urinary tract, skin and skin structures, and lower respiratory tract. Other indications include intra-abdominal and gynecologic infections as well as gram-negative septicemia. The FDA considers aztreonam solution for inhalation as an orphan drug for control of gram-negative bacteria in the respiratory tracts of patients diagnosed with cystic fibrosis.

It should be noted that aztreonam may cause an elevation in hepatic enzymes; however, on discontinuation of the drug, most enzymes return to pretherapy levels. There are no specific recommendations or guidelines for dosage adjustment in patients with hepatic impairment.

Table 16.6 presents general route and dosage information for aztreonam.

TABLE 16.6

DRUGS AT A GLANCE: Aztreonam

Drug	Pregnancy Category	Routes and Dosage Ranges	
		Adults	Children
℗ **Aztreonam** (Azactam)	B	For urinary tract infection: IM, IV 0.5–1 g every 8–12 h For moderate systemic infection: IM, IV 1 g every 8–12 h or IV 2 g every 8–12 h For meningitis: IV 2 g every 6–8 h	IM, IV 30 mg/kg every 6–8 h

Use in Children

Aztreonam can be used in children older than 1 month of age. Some adverse effects occur more frequently in children. This increased incidence could result from the severity of the illness being treated or the higher doses that are typically administered in pediatrics. Dosages should be based on age, weight, severity of infection, and renal function.

Use in Older Adults

Aztreonam is relatively safe, although decreased renal function, other disease processes, and concurrent drug therapies increase the risks of adverse effects in older adults.

Use in Patients With Renal Impairment

It is necessary to reduce the dosage of aztreonam in patients with renal impairment. Aztreonam is moderately dialyzable, and patients with life-threatening infections should receive a supplemental dose after each hemodialysis session.

Use in Patients With Critical Illness

Aztreonam is used for some critical illnesses. However, use typically is reserved for those patients with a severe penicillin allergy. Monotherapy with aztreonam may lead to resistant *P. aeruginosa* infections. Often, combination therapy is recommended.

Use in Patients Receiving Home Care

The need for frequent dosing means that aztreonam is not typically given in the home setting. However, basic principles of IV care are an important component in administering this medication at home. Potential for secondary infections is a concern.

Adverse Effects

In general, adverse effects of aztreonam are similar to those of other beta-lactam antibiotics, including possible hypersensitivity reactions. The most common adverse effects include rash, diarrhea, nausea, vomiting, and localized thrombophlebitis.

Prolonged use may cause fungal or bacterial superinfections. *Clostridium difficile*–associated diarrhea and pseudomembranous colitis should be concerns with extended use.

Contraindications

Contraindications to aztreonam include a hypersensitivity to any component of aztreonam.

Nursing Implications

Preventing Interactions

Box 16.7 outlines drug–drug interactions for aztreonam. As yet, there are no identified herb or food interactions. Aztreonam and aminoglycosides, when used in combination, can demonstrate synergistic effects against some strains of organisms, specifically *P. aeruginosa* and some Enterobacteriaceae. This synergy has also been seen with other beta-lactam antibiotics. There is a potential for false-positive reactions in urine glucose tests using Benedict's solution, Clinitest, or Fehling's solution.

Administering the Medication

Aztreonam may be administered intravenously or intramuscularly.

BOX 16.7	Drug Interactions: Aztreonam

Drugs That Increase the Effects of Aztreonam
- Aminoglycosides
  Increase the risk of nephrotoxicity
- Furosemide
  May increase serum levels

Drugs That Decrease the Effects of Aztreonam
- Cefoxitin
  Induces the production of beta-lactamases
- Chloramphenicol
  May antagonize bactericidal activity

Assessing for Therapeutic Effects

Drug levels are not required when administering aztreonam. Monitoring of serum creatinine, BUN, and liver function tests is recommended in patients taking aztreonam.

Assessing for Adverse Effects

The nurse carefully assesses any rash. It is important to distinguish a hypersensitivity reaction from a nonallergic aztreonam rash, if possible.

Patient Teaching

Aztreonam is typically used for illnesses that are considered critical. Therefore, patient teaching guidelines focus on instructing the patient and family about the purpose of the drug and important of reporting adverse effects.

NCLEX Success

5. A nurse working in the neurointensive care unit is caring for a patient with a head injury who has been experiencing seizures and now has pneumonia caused by *Pseudomonas aeruginosa*. The physician has prescribed imipenem 1 g IV every 6 hours plus gentamicin for the pneumonia. Before administering the antibiotics, the nurse should do which of the following?
   A. Avoid mixing the imipenem and gentamicin in the same IV bag to prevent inactivation of the gentamicin.
   B. Remind the physician of the patient's seizures and inquire whether a different antibiotic might be safer.
   C. Suggest to the physician that imipenem is used to treat gram-positive infections and will not be effective in this patient.
   D. Set the infusion pump to deliver the imipenem over 15 minutes.

6. In acute renal failure, doses of which of the following antibiotics must be reduced? (Check all that apply.)
   A. nafcillin
   B. cefazolin
   C. meropenem
   D. aztreonam

The Nursing Process

General aspects of the nursing process in antimicrobial drug therapy apply to the patient receiving penicillins, cephalosporins, carbapenems, and the monobactam aztreonam. In this chapter, only those aspects related specifically to these drugs are included.

Assessment

- With penicillins, ask patients if they have ever taken a penicillin and, if so, whether they ever had a skin rash, hives, swelling, or difficulty breathing associated with the drug.
- With cephalosporins, ask patients if they have ever taken one of the drugs and whether they ever had a severe reaction to penicillin. Naming a few cephalosporins (e.g., Ceclor, Keflex, Rocephin, Suprax) may help the patient identify previous usage.
- With carbapenems, ask patients if they have ever taken one of the drugs and whether they ever had a severe reaction to penicillin. Assess for decreased renal function.
- With aztreonam, ask patients whether they have ever had a reaction to the drug.

Nursing Diagnoses

- Risk for injury: hypersensitivity reactions with penicillins, cephalosporins, or aztreonam
- Risk for injury: renal impairment with cephalosporins and carbapenems
- Deficient knowledge: correct home care administration and usage of oral beta-lactams

Planning/Goals

The patient will

- Take oral beta-lactam antibacterials as directed
- Receive parenteral beta-lactam drugs by appropriate techniques to minimize tissue irritation
- Receive prompt and appropriate treatment if hypersensitivity reactions occur

Nursing Interventions

The nurse will

- In any patient care setting, keep emergency equipment and supplies readily available.
- Monitor patient response to beta-lactam drugs.
- Monitor dosages of beta-lactam drugs for patients with impaired renal function.
- Provide patient teaching regarding drug therapy (see Boxes 16.3 and 16.5).

Evaluation

- Observe for improvement in signs of infection.
- Interview and observe for adverse drug effects.

Clinical Application 16-2

- Mr. O'Brian is discharged the next day, and 4 hours later, he calls the office to report a skin rash and difficulty breathing. He tells the nurse that his wife remembered that he had an allergic reaction to penicillin more than 20 years ago. What action should the nurse take?

Key Concepts

- Beta-lactam antibiotics include penicillins, cephalosporins, carbapenems, and monobactams.
- Choice of a beta-lactam antibacterial depends on the organism causing the infection, the severity of the infection, and other factors.
- Several gram-positive and gram-negative bacteria produce beta-lactamases, which are enzymes that disrupt the beta-lactam ring and inactivate these drugs. This is the major mechanism by which microorganisms acquire resistance to beta-lactam antibiotics.
- As a class, penicillins usually are more effective in infections caused by gram-positive bacteria than those caused by gram-negative bacteria.
- In the rare instance in which penicillin is considered essential, a skin test may be helpful in assessing hypersensitivity.
- Metabolic and electrolyte imbalances may occur in patients receiving penicillins who have renal impairment or congestive heart failure: hypernatremia and hypokalemic metabolic acidosis is most likely to occur with ticarcillin; hyperkalemia with large IV doses of penicillin G potassium.

- A **BLACK BOX WARNING** ◆ alerts health care providers that inadvertent IV administration of penicillin G benzathine may result in cardiopulmonary arrest and death. Long-acting repository forms have additives that decrease their solubility in tissue fluids and delay their absorption.

- Cephalosporins are classified into five subgroups, or "generations," based on their pharmacology and spectrum of activity.

- Ceftaroline (Teflaro) is the first cephalosporin to be considered active against resistant gram-positive organisms, such as MRSA, VRSA, and VISA.

- Cephalosporins and carbapenems are closely related chemically to the penicillin and cross-sensitivity should be anticipated.

- Because of its monobactam structure, aztreonam has limited cross-allergenicity between itself and other beta-lactam antibiotics and is generally considered safe to use in patients who are allergic to penicillin.

Critical Thinking Questions

16-1. Ed Beatty is a 52-year-old man with a history of chronic renal insufficiency who presents to a medical clinic complaining of a severe sore throat. He receives a diagnosis of streptococcal pharyngitis. Mr. Beatty's primary care provider informs him that he will be treated with an intramuscular injection of penicillin G.

- What information should the nurse collect from Mr. Beatty before the administration of the penicillin G occurs?

- Mr. Beatty asks why he cannot receive the medication in oral form. How should the nurse respond?

- Describe the equipment that should be available before the medication is administered to Mr. Beatty. Why is this necessary?

- After receiving the penicillin G, Mr. Beatty experiences cardiac arrest. He is successfully resuscitated. Discuss the potential causes of the cardiac arrest.

- Mr. Beatty has recovered from the cardiac arrest, and the nurse is preparing his discharge teaching. What information related to the penicillin G should the nurse include?

References and Resources

Antunez, C. (2006). Immediate allergic reactions to cephalosporins: Evaluation of cross-reactivity with a panel of penicillins and cephalosporins. *Journal of Allergy and Clinical Immunology, 117*(2), 404–410.

Corwin, E. J. (2006). *Handbook of pathophysiology* (3rd ed.). Philadelphia, PA: Lippincott Williams & Wilkins.

Cunha, B. A. (2006). Antibiotic selection in the penicillin-resistant patient. *Medical Clinics of North America, 90*(6), 1257–1264.

Drug facts and comparisons. (Updated monthly). St. Louis, MO: Facts and Comparisons.

Elston, D. M. (2007). Methicillin-sensitive and methicillin-resistant *Staphylococcus aureus*: Management principles and selection of antibiotic therapy. *Dermatology Clinics, 25*(2), 157–164, vi.

Freifeld, A. G., Bow, E. J., Sepkowitz, K. A., Boeckh, M. J., Ito, J. I., Mullen, C. A., et al. (2011). Antimicrobial agents in neutropenic patients with cancer: 2010 Update by the Infectious Diseases Society of America. *Clinical Infectious Diseases, 52*, e56–e93.

Karch, A. M. (2013). *2013 Lippincott's nursing drug guide.* Philadelphia, PA: Lippincott, Williams, and Wilkins.

Khardori, N. (2006). Antibiotics- past, present, and future. *Medical Clinics of North America, 90*(6), 1049–1076.

Lacy, C. F., Armstrong, L. L., Goldman, M. P., & Lance, L. L. (2010). *Lexi-Comp's drug information handbook* (19th ed.). Hudson, OH: American Pharmaceutical Association.

Pichichero, M. E. (2005). A review of evidence supporting the American Academy of Pediatrics recommendation for prescribing cephalosporin antibiotics for penicillin-allergic patients. *Pediatrics, 115*, 1048–1057.

Porth, C. M. (2009). *Pathophysiology: Concepts of altered health status* (8th ed.). Philadelphia, PA: Lippincott, Williams, and Wilkins.

Shoemaker, D. M., Jiang, P. P., Williamson, H., & Roland, W. E. (2007). Infectious diseases. In R. E. Rakel (Ed.), *Textbook of family medicine* (pp. 317–351), Philadelphia, PA: Elsevier.

Slama, T. G., Amin, A., Brunton, S. A., File, T. M., Milkovich, G. Rodvold, K. A., et al. (2005). A clinician's guide to the appropriate and accurate use of antibiotics: The Council for Appropriate and Rational Antibiotic Therapy (CARAT) criteria. *The American Journal of Medicine, 118* (7A), 1S–6S.

17 Drug Therapy With Aminoglycosides and Fluoroquinolones

LEARNING OBJECTIVES

After studying this chapter, you should be able to:

1. State the rationale for the increasing use of single daily doses of aminoglycosides.

2. Discuss the importance of measuring serum drug levels during aminoglycoside therapy.

3. Describe measures to decrease nephrotoxicity and ototoxicity with aminoglycosides.

4. Identify characteristics of aminoglycosides and fluoroquinolones in relation to effectiveness, safety, spectrum of antimicrobial activity, indications for use, administration, and observation of patient responses.

5. Recognize factors influencing selection and dosage of aminoglycosides and fluoroquinolones.

6. Describe characteristics, uses, adverse effects, and nursing process implications of fluoroquinolones.

7. Discuss principles of using aminoglycosides and fluoroquinolones in renal impairment and critical illness.

Clinical Application Case Study

Edward Louis, an 84-year-old man, is taking ciprofloxacin (Cipro) 500 mg PO every 12 hours for an infected leg wound. He has experienced arterial insufficiency to his lower extremities for many years, secondary to atherosclerosis. The medical plan is to clear the infection so that he can have surgery to restore circulation to his lower extremities.

KEY TERMS

Concentration-dependent bactericidal effect: relation of bactericidal ability of a drug to its concentration; the greater the concentration of the drug, the faster and the more extensive the killing of the bacteria. The goal is to maximize concentration of the drug. Once-daily dosing—single daily aminoglycoside dosing, typically using a dose of 7 mg per kg every 24 hours, or longer in patients with renal impairment.

Ototoxicity: adverse effects on the structures of the ear, especially the cochlea and auditory nerve

Postantibiotic effect: persistent effect of an antimicrobial on bacterial growth after brief exposure of the organisms to a drug

Introduction

Health care practitioners have used the aminoglycosides to treat serious aerobic gram-negative infections extensively for many years. Select aminoglycosides have shown stability in the face of the emergence of resistance. The quinolones are also older drugs originally used only for the treatment of urinary tract infections (see Chap. 18). Synthesis of the quinolones involves adding a fluorine molecule to the quinolone structure. This addition increases drug activity against gram-negative microorganisms, broadens the antimicrobial spectrum to include several other microorganisms, and allows the use of the drugs in treating systemic infections. General characteristics, mechanisms of action, indications for and contraindications to use, nursing process implications, and principles of therapy for these drugs are described in this chapter. Individual drugs and the prototype drugs, with routes of administration and dosage ranges, are presented in the Drugs at a Glance tables.

Aminoglycosides

Aminoglycosides are bactericidal agents with similar pharmacologic, antimicrobial, and toxicologic characteristics. They are used to treat infections caused by gram-negative microorganisms such as *Pseudomonas* and *Proteus* species, *Escherichia coli*, and *Klebsiella*, *Enterobacter*, and *Serratia* species. Ⓟ **Gentamicin** (Garamycin), the most widely used aminoglycoside, is the prototype. Patients often receive gentamicin for systemic infections in the clinical setting. If it is a concern, patients may receive amikacin or tobramycin because these drugs are usually less susceptible to drug-destroying enzymes.

Maintenance doses are based on serum drug concentrations. Peak serum concentrations should be determined 30 to 60 minutes after drug administration (5 to 8 mcg per mL for gentamicin and tobramycin; 20 to 30 mcg per mL for amikacin). Measurement of both peak and trough levels helps maintain therapeutic serum levels without excessive toxicity. For gentamicin and tobramycin, peak levels above 10 to 12 mcg per mL and trough levels above 2 mcg per mL for prolonged periods have been associated with nephrotoxicity. For accuracy, it is necessary to draw blood samples at the correct times and to document the timing of drug administration and blood sampling accurately, based on institutional recommendations.

Pharmacokinetics

Gentamicin is poorly absorbed from the gastrointestinal (GI) tract. Thus, when given orally, the drug exerts local effects in the GI tract. It is rapidly and completely absorbed from intramuscular (IM) injection sites and reaches peak effects in 30 to 90 minutes if circulatory status is proficient. After intravenous (IV) administration, the peak effect occurs 30 minutes after a 30-minute infusion. Plasma half-life is 2 to 4 hours in patients with normal renal function. The volume of distribution is increased by edema, ascites, and fluid overload, and it is decreased with dehydration.

After parenteral administration, gentamicin is widely distributed in extracellular fluid and reaches therapeutic levels in blood, urine, bone, inflamed joints, and pleural and ascitic fluids. Gentamicin accumulates in high concentrations in the proximal renal tubules of the kidney, potentially leading to acute tubular necrosis. This damage to the kidney is termed nephrotoxicity. Gentamicin also accumulates in high concentrations in the inner ear, damaging sensory cells in the cochlea (disrupting hearing) and the vestibular apparatus (disturbing balance). This damage to the inner ear is termed **ototoxicity**. Gentamicin is poorly distributed in the central nervous system, intraocular fluids, and respiratory tract secretions.

Action

Aminoglycosides penetrate the cell walls of susceptible bacteria and bind irreversibly to 30S and 50S ribosomal subunits, intracellular structures that synthesize proteins. As a result, the bacteria cell membrane becomes defective and cannot synthesize the proteins necessary for their function and replication.

Use

The major clinical use of gentamicin (most commonly with other antibacterial agents) is empiric therapy for serious infections caused by susceptible aerobic gram-negative organisms. Treatment of infections such as septicemia, respiratory tract infections, urinary tract infections, intra-abdominal infections, and osteomyelitis often involves gentamicin. In pseudomonal infections, patients may receive gentamicin concurrently with an antipseudomonal penicillin (e.g., piperacillin/tazobactam) for synergistic therapeutic effects. The penicillin-induced breakdown of the bacterial cell wall makes it easier for gentamicin to reach its site of action inside the bacterial cell. Researchers have demonstrated decreased mortality from combination antibiotic therapy in treatment of infections due to *Pseudomonas aeruginosa* and other multidrug-resistant gram-negative bacilli.

Table 17.1 presents dosage information for gentamicin and the other aminoglycosides.

Use in Children

Caution is necessary when using gentamicin and other aminoglycosides in children. Individualization of the dose is extremely critical because of the low therapeutic index of the drug. Larger individual doses or more frequent dosing intervals may be necessary in certain clinical situations (cystic fibrosis). Initial doses of gentamicin in neonates and children are based on age. Serum levels should be obtained to assess the pharmacokinetic parameters to establish the frequency and dose of subsequent doses. It should be noted that the risk of nephrotoxicity and ototoxicity may be increased in neonates because of their immature renal function.

Use in Older Adults

As in children, individualized dosing of gentamicin is critical in older adults because of the low therapeutic index of the drug. Decreased renal function, other disease processes, and concurrent drug therapies increase the adverse effects in older adults, specifically aminoglycoside-induced nephrotoxicity and ototoxicity. Monitoring of renal function during treatment with gentamicin, as well as other aminoglycosides, is extremely

TABLE 17.1

DRUGS AT A GLANCE: Aminoglycosides

Drug	Pregnancy Category	Characteristics	Routes and Dosage Ranges	
			Adults	*Children*
℗ **Gentamicin** (Garamycin)	D	Effective against several gram-negative organisms, although some strains have become resistant Acts synergistically with antipseudomonal penicillins against *P. aeruginosa* and with ampicillin or vancomycin against enterococci	Conventional dosing IM, IV 1–2.5 mg/kg/ dose every 8–24 h depending on renal function ODA dosing: 4–7 mg/kg/ dose once daily	<5 y: IM, IV 2.5 mg/kg/ dose every 8 h ≥5 y: IM, IV 2–2.5 mg/ kg/dose every 8 h
Amikacin (Amikin)	D	Retains a broader spectrum of antibacterial activity than other aminoglycosides because it resists degradation by most enzymes that inactivate gentamicin and tobramycin. Major clinical use is in infections caused by organisms resistant to other aminoglycosides (e.g., *Pseudomonas, Proteus, E. coli, Klebsiella, Enterobacter, Serratia*), whether community or hospital acquired.	IM, IV 15–20 mg/kg every 24 h Renal dosing: 5–7.5 mg/kg/dose every 8–24 h	*Older children:* Same as adults *Neonates:* IM, IV 10 mg/ kg initially, then 7.5 mg/kg every 12 h
Kanamycin (Kantrex)	D	Occasionally used to decrease bowel organisms before surgery, treat hepatic coma, or treat multidrug-resistant tuberculosis	IV, IM 15 mg/kg/d, in divided doses every 8–12 h	IV, IM same as adults
Neomycin	D	Given orally or topically to prepare GI tract for surgery. Although poorly absorbed from the GI tract, toxic levels may accumulate in the presence of renal failure. Used topically, often in combination with other drugs, to treat infections of the eye, ear, and skin (burns, wounds, ulcers, dermatoses). When used for wound or bladder irrigations, systemic absorption may occur if the area is large or if drug concentration exceeds 0.1%.	PO, suppression of intestinal bacteria (with erythromycin 1 g) 1 g given at 1 PM, 2 PM, and 11 PM the day before an 8 AM surgery; hepatic coma, 4–12 g daily in divided doses every 4–6 h for 5–6 d	
Streptomycin	D	May be used in a 4- to 6-drug regimen for treatment of multidrug-resistant tuberculosis	IM 15/kg/d or 1–2 g/d	IM 20–40 mg/kg/d in 2 divided doses, every 12 h (maximum dose, 1 g/d)
Tobramycin	D	Similar to gentamicin in antibacterial spectrum, but may be more active against *Pseudomonas* organisms Often used with other antibiotics for septicemia and infections of burn wounds, other soft tissues, bone, the urinary tract, and the central nervous system	Conventional dosing: IM, IV 1–2.5 mg/kg/ dose every 8–24 h depending on renal function ODA dosing: 4–7 mg/ kg/dose once daily	<5 y: IM, IV 2.5 mg/kg/ dose every 8 h ≥5 y: 2–2.5 mg/kg/dose every 8 h

GI, gastrointestinal; IM, intramuscular; IV, intravenous; ODA, once-daily aminoglycoside important. Prolonged therapy (longer than 1 week) increases the risk of toxicity and should be avoided when possible.

Use in Patients With Renal Impairment

With impaired renal function, a reduction in dosage of aminoglycosides is essential. Gentamicin may accumulate in the serum and tissues of patients being treated with higher doses and for longer periods. Methods of adjusting dosage include lengthening the time between doses or reducing doses. For specific recommendations on adjusting aminoglycoside doses for renal impairment, nurses and other health care practitioners should consult references. In urinary tract infections, smaller doses can be used than in systemic infections because the aminoglycosides reach high concentrations in the urine.

Use in Patients With Hepatic Impairment

Gentamicin is appropriate for use in patients with hepatic impairment. No adjustment in dosage or frequency is indicated. However, it is necessary to continue to monitor plasma concentrations. Gentamicin should be used with caution in severe hepatic disease, such as cirrhosis, because of the possibility of precipitating hepatorenal syndrome.

Use in Patients With Critical Illness

Primary uses for gentamicin (in combination with other antibacterial agents) include serious infections caused by aerobic gram-negative bacilli that result in septicemia, nosocomial respiratory infections, complicated urinary tract infections and intra-abdominal infections, osteomyelitis, and endocarditis. The drug also demonstrates in vitro activity against methicillin-susceptible *Staphylococcus aureus*. Patients should not take gentamicin as monotherapy. Serious infections caused by *Serratia, Pseudomonas, Citrobacter, Acinetobacter,* and *Enterobacter* species warrant its use in combination with piperacillin/tazobactam, cefepime, meropenem, or imipenem/cilastatin. However, once susceptibilities to the identified organism are determined, prescribers usually discontinue aminoglycosides if a less toxic antibiotic may be used to complete the typical course of treatment. Because patients who are critically ill are at high risk for development of nephrotoxicity and ototoxicity with aminoglycosides, it is essential to follow guidelines for safe drug usage strictly.

Use in Patients Receiving Home Care

Administration of gentamicin does not typically occur in the home setting. However, instruction about IV care is essential for caregivers who are giving this medication at home. Potential for secondary infections is of concern.

Adverse Effects

Gentamicin and other aminoglycosides result in similar adverse reactions. A **BLACK BOX WARNING** ◆ alerts health care professionals that these drugs are nephrotoxic and ototoxic and must be used very cautiously in the presence of renal impairment.

A well-known adverse reaction associated with aminoglycoside therapy, nephrotoxicity, occurs more frequently in patients with a history of renal impairment. Extended duration of treatment with gentamicin may also contribute to nephrotoxicity. In most cases, nephrotoxicity is reversible on discontinuation of the drug. Ototoxicity (auditory or vestibular) may develop after extended use and may not be reversible. Dizziness, vertigo, tinnitus, and hearing loss may be signs of ototoxicity. Peripheral nephropathy, including numbness, skin tingling, and muscle twitching, also occurs. Therefore, use of gentamicin in patients with myasthenia gravis and other neuromuscular disorders warrants caution, because increased muscle weakness may occur.

Contraindications

Contraindications include a hypersensitivity to aminoglycosides. Prescribers generally reserve aminoglycosides are for infections that have not responded to less toxic drugs.

Nursing Implications

Dosage of aminoglycosides must be carefully monitored based on serum concentrations. Two major dosing schedules are used: one involving multiple daily doses (conventional dosing) and one involving a single daily dose (**once-daily dosing**, or once-daily aminoglycosides [ODA]). The use of ODA dosing, unless contraindicated, has replaced the common multiple daily dosing in many people. The ODA method uses higher doses (e.g., 4 to 7 mg per kg) to produce high initial drug concentrations, with no repeat dosing until the serum concentration is quite low (typically 24 hours later). The rationale for this dosing approach is a potential increase in efficacy with a reduced incidence of nephrotoxicity. Most patients can be successfully treated using ODA. However, ODA is not appropriate for certain people. In general, the following circumstances contraindicate its use: age of 18 years or less, pregnancy or postpartum status, and endocarditis.

The ODA dosing practice evolved from increased knowledge about the concentration-dependent bactericidal effects and postantibiotic effects of aminoglycosides. **Concentration-dependent bactericidal effects** mean that a large dose of aminoglycosides, with high peak serum concentrations, kills more microorganisms. **Postantibiotic effects** mean that aminoglycosides continue killing microorganisms even at low serum concentrations. Monitoring of random level (12-hour) serum evaluation in a single dosing regimen replaces traditional peak and trough serum monitoring.

With the multiple-dose regimen, a patient receives an initial loading dose, based on patient weight and the desired peak serum concentration, to achieve therapeutic serum concentrations rapidly. If the patient is obese, adjusted body weight should be used because aminoglycosides are not significantly distributed in body fat. In patients with normal renal function, recommended loading doses for selected aminoglycosides are the following:

- Gentamicin: 1 to 2.5 mg per kg
- Tobramycin: 1 to 2.5 mg per kg
- Amikacin: 5 to 7.5 mg per kg

BOX 17.1 Drug Interactions: Gentamicin

Drugs That Increase the Effects of Gentamicin

■ Acyclovir, amphotericin B, carboplatin and cisplatin, cyclosporine, ganciclovir, pamidronate, salicylates, vancomycin
  Increase the risk of nephrotoxicity
■ Loop diuretics
  Increase the risk of nephrotoxicity and ototoxicity

Drugs That Decrease the Effects of Gentamicin

■ Penicillins
  Decrease serum concentrations

Prescribers adjust dosages according to serum drug levels and creatinine clearance (CrCl). With conventional dosing, it is necessary to take gentamicin peak levels 30 minutes after the end of a 30 minute IV infusion or 1 hour after IM injection. The nurse ensures that trough levels are obtained immediately before the next dose is given. With ODA dosing, it is necessary to obtain a 12-hour random gentamicin level 12 hours after the start of the infusion.

Preventing Interactions

Many medications interact with gentamicin, increasing or decreasing its effects (Box 17.1). When patients who are taking agents that may lead to nephrotoxicity receive gentamicin, careful monitoring and caution are necessary. Caution is also warranted when administering diphenhydramine and chlorpheniramine with gentamicin, because gentamicin may mask symptoms of ototoxicity. In addition, ginger may increase the effect of gentamicin by masking these effects. No herbs or foods appear to increase the effect of the drug.

The nurse should not mix penicillins and aminoglycosides in a syringe or IV solution, or administer them via a Y-site, because the penicillin inactivates the aminoglycoside. If feasible, dose separation is ideal.

Administering the Medication

The nurse uses only the IV route of administration if possible, because IM injections may be erratic. If gentamicin is used concomitantly with a penicillin-class agent, it is necessary to administer the penicillin 1 hour before or after the gentamicin infusion. Gentamicin is available in an ophthalmic preparation, and other ophthalmics should be administered 10 minutes before or after the gentamicin preparation.

QSEN Safety Alert

The nurse demonstrates consistent practice in administering antibiotics that require peak and trough levels by checking, prior to administration, for the latest values and next order for peak and trough levels. Effective standardized practices help ensure safety and quality and reduce harm to the patient.

Assessing for Therapeutic Effects

The nurse assesses for response to drug therapy and ensures that signs and symptoms of the infection are resolving. These infections may include septicemia, respiratory tract infections, urinary tract infections, intra-abdominal infections, and osteomyelitis. It is important to observe for return to baseline vital signs and normalization of white blood count. The nurse assesses for absence of local signs of infection.

Assessing for Adverse Effects

Monitoring of gentamicin serum concentrations is crucial for both effectiveness and the avoidance of toxicity. Serum concentrations should be evaluated when the patient has received three or four doses for a conventional dosing regimen. Once the desired peak and trough have been achieved, periodic monitoring is necessary.

In addition, monitoring of renal function is essential in aminoglycoside therapy. It is necessary to discontinue treatment if signs of nephrotoxicity occur. In addition, patients with vertigo or tinnitus may demonstrate signs of vestibular injury, and ototoxicity should be a consideration. It is also necessary to discontinue treatment if signs of ototoxicity occur. Other adverse effects to assess for include edema, skin itching, reddening of skin, and possible rash.

Patient Teaching

Patient teaching guidelines are outlined in Box 17.2.

Other Drugs in the Class

A few other aminoglycosides are used to treat infection and carry the same risks of ototoxicity and nephrotoxicity. The aminoglycosides are poorly absorbed from the GI tract. Thus, when given orally, they exert local effects on the GI tract. Specifically, neomycin is given orally to prepare the GI tract for surgery. It is not recommended for use in infants and children. Tobramycin, which is given intravenously, is similar to gentamicin but may be more active against *Pseudomonas* organisms. Amikacin, which is also given intravenously, retains a broader spectrum of antibacterial of activity because it resists degradation by most enzymes that inactivate gentamicin and tobramycin.

BOX 17.2 Patient Teaching Guidelines for Aminoglycosides

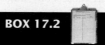

General Considerations

■ If receiving an aminoglycoside antibiotic in the home care setting, make sure to administer it at regular intervals.
■ Put all needles and syringes in a "sharps" container.

Self-Administration

■ If using a gentamicin ophthalmic preparation, do not take it by mouth. Wash hands before and after use. Administer any other ophthalmic preparations 10 minutes before or after gentamicin ophthalmic.

Fluoroquinolones

Fluoroquinolones are synthetic drugs with activity against gram-negative and gram-positive organisms. ℗ **Ciprofloxacin** (Cipro) is the prototype. When administered orally, fluoroquinolones allow ambulatory treatment of infections that previously required parenteral therapy and hospitalization.

Pharmacokinetics

Ciprofloxacin is well absorbed from the upper GI tract, like all quinolones; it achieves 70% bioavailability. Once absorbed, it achieves therapeutic concentrations in most body fluids. With immediate-release ciprofloxacin, concentrations peak in 30 minutes to 2 hours. Ciprofloxacin is partially metabolized in the liver; it forms four metabolites, which have limited activity. Hepatic conversion of ciprofloxacin to active metabolites is 10% to 20% of ciprofloxacin elimination. The kidneys are the main route of elimination, and approximately 30% to 60% of an oral dose is excreted unchanged in the urine. Additional excretion is achieved via the feces.

Action

Fluoroquinolones are bactericidal agents that cause cell death. Ciprofloxacin acts by interfering with enzymes required for synthesis of bacterial DNA and therefore necessary for bacterial growth and replication.

Use

Ciprofloxacin is the most potent fluoroquinolone against gram-negative bacteria. Like most fluoroquinolones, it is indicated for various infections caused by aerobic gram-negative and other microorganisms. Fluoroquinolones may be used to treat infections of the respiratory, genitourinary, and GI tracts, as well as infections of bones, joints, skin, and soft tissues. As of April 2007, the Centers for Disease Control and Prevention (CDC) no longer recommends the use of fluoroquinolones for gonococcal disease, unless no other option exists and susceptibility can be confirmed. Recommendations for treatment of gonorrhea change as resistance becomes more prevalent; thus, it is necessary to consult the CDC Web site on sexually transmitted diseases for the most current recommendations.

Ciprofloxacin has multiple indications and can be used for acute sinusitis, lower respiratory infections, pneumonia, skin and soft tissue infections, prostatitis, and urinary tract infections. Currently, it is recommended as first-line treatment for suspected *Bacillus anthracis* infections (anthrax) until culture and susceptibility results are available. Table 17.2 presents important information about the fluoroquinolones.

Use in Children

Ciprofloxacin, and other fluoroquinolones, should not be used routinely in children younger than 18 years of age. Some studies have demonstrated the development of an arthritic sensation with erosions of the cartilage of the weight-bearing joints. However, there is developing evidence that in some children, particularly those with cystic fibrosis, the benefit of using quinolones outweighs the small risk of joint toxicity. Ciprofloxacin has been approved for use in children with complicated urinary tract infections and pyelonephritis.

Use in Older Adults

Ciprofloxacin is relatively safe, although decreased renal function, other disease processes, and concurrent drug therapies increase the risks of adverse effects in older adults. In older adults with normal renal function, fluoroquinolones should be accompanied by an adequate fluid intake and urine output to prevent drug crystals from forming in the urinary tract. In addition, urinary alkalinizing agents should be avoided because drug crystals form more readily in alkaline urine. In older adults with impaired renal function, a common condition in this population, caution and reduced dosages are necessary.

Use in Patients With Renal Impairment

Ciprofloxacin requires a dose adjustment in renal impairment because usual doses may produce high and prolonged serum drug levels. However, even in renal failure, moxifloxacin (Avelox) does not require a dose adjustment. Reported renal effects include azotemia, crystalluria, hematuria, interstitial nephritis, nephropathy, and renal failure. Crystalluria rarely occurs in acidic urine but may occur in alkaline urine. Guidelines for reducing nephrotoxicity include using lower dosages, having longer intervals between doses, receiving adequate hydration, and avoiding substances that alkalinize the urine.

TABLE 17.2

DRUGS AT A GLANCE: Fluoroquinolones

Drug	Pregnancy Category	Characteristics	Routes and Dosage Ranges for Adults
Ⓟ **Ciprofloxacin** (Cipro)	C	Effective in respiratory tract, urinary tract, gastrointestinal tract, and skin and soft tissue infections Used as one of 4–6 drugs in treatment of multidrug-resistant tuberculosis Used to treat anthrax infections No longer recommended by CDC for treatment of gonococcal infections due to increased prevalence of resistance	PO 250–750 mg every 12 hr UTI/pyelonephritis; extended-release tablets 500 mg–1 g every 24 hr IV 200–400 mg every 12 hr
Gatifloxacin (Tequin)	C	Indicated for pneumonia, bronchitis, sinusitis, skin and soft tissue infections, urinary infections, pyelonephritis, and gonorrhea	PO, IV infusion 400 mg once daily. Give IV dose over 60 min; avoid rapid administration.
Gemifloxacin (Factive)	C	Indicated for acute bacterial exacerbation of chronic bronchitis and community-acquired pneumonia (mild to moderate severity)	PO 320 mg once daily for 5–7 d
Levofloxacin (Levaquin)	C	A broad-spectrum agent effective for treatment of bronchitis, cystitis, pneumonia, sinusitis, skin and skin structure infections, and pyelonephritis	PO, IV 250–750 mg once daily. Infuse 250–500 mg IV dose slowly over 60 min. Infuse 750 mg IV dose over 90 min.
Moxifloxacin (Avelox)	C	Indicated for community-acquired pneumonia, sinusitis, bronchitis, skin and soft tissue infections, and intra-abdominal infections	PO, IV 400 mg once daily. Infuse IV dose slowly over 60 min.
Norfloxacin (Noroxin)	C	Used only for UTI	PO 400 mg twice daily
Ofloxacin (Floxin)	C	See ciprofloxacin, above	PO 200–400 mg every 12 h for 3–10 d

CDC, Centers for Disease Control and Prevention; UTI, urinary tract infection; IV, intravenous.

Use in Patients With Hepatic Impairment

It appears that dosage adjustment is not necessary in hepatic impairment. However, ciprofloxacin should be used with caution in patients with hepatic disease such as cirrhosis.

Use in Patients With Critical Illness

Ciprofloxacin is commonly used in the critical care setting because of its broad spectrum of coverage. However, resistance is emerging because of overuse of the fluoroquinolones. The rate of resistance in *P. aeruginosa* is increasing due to the increased use of this drug class. Most activity of the fluoroquinolones is against aerobic gram-negative organisms, especially Enterobacteriaceae, *Moraxella catarrhalis*, *Haemophilus*, and *Neisseria* species. Also, fluoroquinolones have activity against *P. aeruginosa* and *Staphylococcus*. Levofloxacin and moxifloxacin have increased potency against gram-positive infections, and moxifloxacin has activity against anaerobic organisms.

Some quinolones, including ciprofloxacin, have atypical pneumonia coverage as well.

Use in Patients Receiving Home Care

Ciprofloxacin is given in the home setting as are other fluoroquinolones. The drug may be given with food to help minimize GI upset. Patients should space out ciprofloxacin administration 4 to 6 hours with any of the following: antacids, multivitamins, sucralfate, or other products containing calcium, iron, or zinc. Absorption of ciprofloxacin may be impaired when these substances are administered together with ciprofloxacin, resulting in a decreased antibiotic effect. Administration of the oral suspension of ciprofloxacin via feeding tubes should not occur, because the oil-based formulation tends to adhere to the feeding tube. The American College of Chest Physicians has issued recommendations for the range of aspects of home care for patients with pneumonia, who may be taking fluoroquinolones.

EVIDENCE-BASED PRACTICE

Home Antibiotic Therapy for Community-Acquired Pneumonia

by J. RAMSDELL, G. L. NARSAVAGE, J. B. FINK

Management of community-acquired pneumonia in the home: an American College of Chest Physicians clinical position statement

Chest
2005, 127(5), 1752–1763

An increasing number of people with community-acquired pneumonia (CAP) are being treated at home for a number of reasons, including increased availability and cost considerations of oral antibiotics. Oral drugs have demonstrated effectiveness and are the preferred route for individuals and family members, but management of people with oral drugs has widely varied. The American College of Chest Physicians position statement, cosponsored by the American Academy of Home Care Physicians, outlines recommendations for home care for patients with CAP. These include recommendations for evaluation and diagnosis in the home and the determination of the site of care and the plan of care and guidelines for monitoring and follow-up.

IMPLICATIONS FOR NURSING PRACTICE: Recommendations in the position statement take into consideration the best plan of care, incorporating the best available evidence with clinician judgment and patient preferences.

Adverse Effects

Ciprofloxacin is generally well tolerated. The most frequent adverse effects are GI side effects and include nausea, vomiting, and abdominal discomfort. Some patients experience dizziness and mild headache. Allergic and skin reactions have occurred. Photosensitivity can occur while taking ciprofloxacin with exposure to direct or indirect sunlight. Artificial light, or sunlamps, may also precipitate photosensitivity reactions. Reportedly, tendon rupture and tendinitis occur with the fluoroquinolones. The FDA has issued a **BLACK BOX WARNING** ◆ for fluoroquinolones, alerting health professionals to the increased risk of tendinitis and tendon rupture. The risk is greater for people older than 60 years of age; those with heart, kidney, and lung transplants; and those taking corticosteroid medications. Discontinuation of the fluoroquinolone is necessary. Arthropathy and cartilage erosion may be apparent in children. QT interval prolongation may occur, and the degree of severity varies by agent.

Contraindications

Contraindications include hypersensitivity and age younger than 18 years if alternatives are available. Limited data on the safety of fluoroquinolones in pregnant or lactating women are

BOX 17.3 — Drug Interactions: Ciprofloxacin

Drugs That Increase the Effects of Ciprofloxacin

- Antidysrhythmics
  Possibly prolong QT interval
- Corticosteroids
  Increase risk of tendon-related side effects
- Theophylline
  Reduces theophylline clearance
- Warfarin
  Increases international normalized ratio

Drugs That Decrease the Effects of Ciprofloxacin

- Aluminum-, calcium-, iron-, and magnesium-containing products
  Impair absorption
- Didanosine
  Decreases serum concentrations
- Sucralfate
  Impairs absorption
- Quinapril (contains magnesium)
  Impairs absorption

available; unless the benefits outweigh the potential risks, the drugs should not be used. Concurrent use of tizanidine is also a contraindication to ciprofloxacin use.

Nursing Implications

Preventing Interactions

Many medications interact with ciprofloxacin, increasing or decreasing its effects (Box 17.3). Fluoroquinolones have the potential to prolong the QT interval and may increase the risks of torsade de pointes and sudden death. Patients should not receive drugs such as the antidysrhythmic amiodarone, which prolong the QT interval, in conjunction with fluoroquinolones. Ciprofloxacin reduces theophylline clearance by 30%. Reportedly, fatal reactions have occurred after concurrent use of ciprofloxacin and theophylline.

Herbs and foods also interact with ciprofloxacin (Box 17.4). Ciprofloxacin can chelate with cations, and drugs containing

BOX 17.4 — Herb and Dietary Interactions: Ciprofloxacin

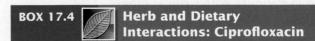

Herbs and Foods That Alter the Effects of Ciprofloxacin

- Aluminum-, magnesium-, calcium-, and iron-containing herbs and foods
- Dairy products
- Dong quai
- Enteral feedings
- St. John's wort

iron, multivitamins, calcium, magnesium, aluminum salt, and sucralfate may significantly reduce the absorption of ciprofloxacin. Therefore, patients should take oral ciprofloxacin 2 hours before or 6 hours after such agents. They should also avoid taking oral ciprofloxacin with dairy products or other calcium-containing foods. In addition, patients should not take didanosine and ciprofloxacin simultaneously.

The nurse should also watch for severe hypoglycemia, which has developed in patients receiving concomitant glyburide and fluoroquinolones, including ciprofloxacin. Although most cases have affected patients with diabetes, severe cases of hyperglycemia have occurred in patients not previously diagnosed with the disease.

Clinical Application 17-1

- Mr. Louis' wound is not responding to treatment. Because of his need for surgery, he is admitted for IV antibiotic therapy. His physician orders that gentamicin IV be administered every 24 hours. Mr. Louis receives doses for 3 days. What assessments should the nurse perform to check for toxicity?

Administering the Medication

Severe hypersensitivity reactions have occurred with the administration of fluoroquinolones. The nurse discontinues the antibiotic immediately if skin rash or other signs or symptoms occur. To reduce the risk of irritation to the veins causing burning, swelling, and pain, the nurse administers the IV formulation over 60 minutes. If administration through a nasogastric tube is necessary, the nurse crushes immediate-release tablets and mixes them with water. Enteral feedings may affect the serum concentration of ciprofloxacin, and

the nurse gives tube feedings 1 hour before and 2 hours after administering the drug. Patients should take fluoroquinolones, like all antibiotics, for the full prescribed course of treatment to prevent complications.

Assessing for Therapeutic Effects

Assessing for factors that increase the risk of adverse effects is important. For example, impaired renal function, inadequate fluid intake, concomitant use of multivitamins or antacids, or frequent exposure to sunlight in the usual activities of daily living.

It is not necessary to take drug levels when administering ciprofloxacin or any of the fluoroquinolones. Serum creatinine and blood urea nitrogen (BUN) are recommended values to monitor when administering ciprofloxacin.

Assessing for Adverse Effects

The nurse assesses adverse effects, such as nausea, diarrhea, vomiting, abdominal pain, headache, increased liver enzymes, and injection site reactions. It may be necessary to stop ciprofloxacin therapy if a harmful effect is severe enough. Any rash warrants careful evaluation, and if a hypersensitivity reaction occurs, the nurse discontinues therapy immediately.

Patient Teaching

Patient teaching guidelines are outlined in Box 17.5.

Other Drugs in the Class

Levofloxacin is a broad-spectrum agent, similar to ciprofloxacin. It is effective for bronchitis, cystitis, pneumonia, sinusitis, skin and skin structure infections, and pyelonephritis. Moxifloxacin is available for oral or IV administration, like ciprofloxacin. No dosage adjustment is necessary in renal impairment. The drug is not recommended for urinary tract infections. Other fluoroquinolones include gatifloxacin, gemifloxacin, norfloxacin, and ofloxacin.

BOX 17.5   Patient Teaching Guidelines for the Fluoroquinolones

General Considerations

- Avoid exposure to sunlight during and for several days after taking one of these drugs. Stop taking the drug and notify the prescribing physician if skin burning, redness, swelling, rash, or itching occurs. Sunscreen lotions do not prevent photosensitivity reactions.
- Be very careful if driving or doing other tasks requiring alertness or physical coordination. These drugs may cause dizziness or light-headedness.
- If receiving a fluoroquinolone antibiotic in the home care setting, make sure to administer it at regular intervals.
- Put all needles and syringes in a "sharps" container.

Self-Administration

- Take norfloxacin (Noroxin), levofloxacin (Levaquin) solution, and ofloxacin (Floxin) 1 hour before or

2 hours after meals on an empty stomach. Ciprofloxacin (Cipro) may be taken with food to decrease gastrointestinal upset. Gemifloxacin (Factive), levofloxacin tablets, and moxifloxacin (Avelox) can be taken with or without regard to meals.
- Drink 2 to 3 quarts of fluid daily if you are able. This helps prevent kidney problems.
- Do not take antacids containing magnesium or aluminum (e.g., Mylanta or Maalox); any products containing iron, magnesium, calcium (e.g., Tums), or zinc (e.g., multivitamins); or sucralfate, or buffered didanosine preparations at the same time, or for several hours before or after a dose of the fluoroquinolone. (Consult product-specific information for individual drug recommendations.)

The Nursing Process

General aspects of the nursing process in antimicrobial drug therapy apply to the patient receiving aminoglycosides and fluoroquinolones. In this chapter, only those aspects related specifically to these drugs are included.

Assessment

With aminoglycosides, assess for the presence of factors that predispose the patient to nephrotoxicity or ototoxicity.

- Check laboratory reports of renal function (e.g., serum creatinine, CrCl, BUN) for abnormal values.
- Assess for impairment of balance or hearing, including audiometry reports if available.
- Analyze current medications for drugs that interact with aminoglycosides to increase risks of nephrotoxicity or ototoxicity.
- With fluoroquinolones, assess for the presence of factors that increase risks of adverse drug effects (e.g., impaired renal function, inadequate fluid intake, concomitant use of multivitamins or antacids, frequent or prolonged exposure to sunlight in usual activities of daily living).
- Assess laboratory tests (e.g., complete blood counts, tests of renal and hepatic function) for abnormal values.

Nursing Diagnoses

- Risk for injury: hypersensitivity reactions with aminoglycosides and fluoroquinolones
- Risk for injury: renal impairment with aminoglycosides and fluoroquinolones
- Deficient knowledge: correct home care administration and usage of oral fluoroquinolones

Planning/Goals

The patent will

- Receive aminoglycoside dosages that are individualized by age, weight, renal function, and serum drug levels
- Have serum aminoglycoside levels monitored when indicated
- Have renal function tests performed regularly during aminoglycoside and fluoroquinolone therapy
- Receive adequate hydration during aminoglycoside and fluoroquinolone therapy
- Regularly monitored for adverse drug effects

Nursing Interventions

The nurse will

- With aminoglycosides, weigh patients accurately (dosage is based on total body weight for nonobese patients and adjusted body weight for obese patients) and monitor laboratory reports of BUN, serum creatinine levels, serum drug levels, and urinalysis for abnormal values.
- Force fluids to at least 2000 to 3000 mL daily if not contraindicated. Keeping the patient well hydrated reduces risks of nephrotoxicity with aminoglycosides and crystalluria with fluoroquinolones.

- Avoid concurrent use of other nephrotoxic drugs when possible
- Provide appropriate teaching (see Boxes 17.2 and 17.5)

Evaluation

- Interview and observe for improvement in the infection being treated.
- Interview and observe for adverse drug effects.

Clinical Application 17-2

- Mr. Louis says that he is experiencing a moderate amount of indigestion and asks what he should use to treat it. How does the nurse respond?

NCLEX Success

3. A patient from a nursing home arrives at the emergency department with acute pyelonephritis. The physician prescribes ciprofloxacin 500 mg PO twice daily. The patient has a history of seizures and bradycardia. The nurse should
   A. counsel the patient's caregiver to avoid administering the ciprofloxacin with the patient's anticonvulsant
   B. ask the physician to check blood levels of the patient's anticonvulsant(s) before giving the first dose of ciprofloxacin
   C. call the patient's seizure and dysrhythmia history to the physician's attention and inquire whether another type of antibiotic might be selected
   D. counsel the patient's caregiver to discontinue the ciprofloxacin after the patient's fever is gone

4. A nurse reading a patient's chart notices that the patient is scheduled to receive ciprofloxacin 500 mg PO at 9:00 AM. The medication administration record also indicates that Maalox 30 mL PO and hydrochlorothiazide 25 mg PO are due at 9:00 AM. The nurse should
   A. administer all the medications as scheduled
   B. hold the Maalox until 11:00 AM
   C. ask the physician to discontinue hydrochlorothiazide because of increased risk of ototoxicity
   D. administer the Maalox and ciprofloxacin but hold the hydrochlorothiazide

5. An outpatient has just received a prescription for ciprofloxacin 500 mg PO twice daily for acute bronchitis. The nurse should teach the patient
   A. not to take ciprofloxacin with a meal
   B. to restrict fluid intake to avoid fluid overload
   C. to take ciprofloxacin with an antacid (e.g., Tums) to decrease the chance of stomach upset
   D. to avoid prolonged exposure to sunlight

Key Concepts

- The choice of aminoglycoside depends on local susceptibility patterns and specific organisms causing an infection.

- The major clinical use of parenteral aminoglycosides is to treat serious systemic infections caused by susceptible aerobic gram-negative organisms.

- A **BLACK BOX WARNING** ◆ alerts health care professionals that aminoglycosides are nephrotoxic and ototoxic and require very cautious use in the presence of renal impairment.

- Neomycin and kanamycin may be given to suppress intestinal bacteria before bowel surgery and to treat hepatic coma.

- Multiple-dose regimens (conventional dosing) of aminoglycosides must be carefully monitored with evaluation of peak and trough serum levels. Once-daily regimens are monitored with random level (12-hour) serum evaluation.

- Drugs reach higher concentrations in the kidneys and inner ears than in other body tissues; this is a major factor in nephrotoxicity and ototoxicity.

- Fluoroquinolones are associated with hyperglycemia and hypoglycemia and older patients may be more at risk for these glucose disturbances.

- The FDA has issued a **BLACK BOX WARNING** ◆ for fluoroquinolones, alerting health professionals to the increased risk of developing tendinitis and tendon rupture.

- The CDC no longer recommends fluoroquinolones for the treatment of gonococcal infections because of increased prevalence of resistance.

Critical Thinking Questions

17-1. Mr. Roberts, a 72-year-old retired teacher, presents with difficulty breathing. A chest x-ray shows pneumonia. His white blood cell count is elevated, and he is running a fever.
Mr. Roberts is admitted to the hospital and started on IV antibiotics, gentamicin (Garamycin) and piperacillin and tazobactam for injection (Zosyn). He has a previous history of *P. aeruginosa* pneumonia.

- How would you assess the patient for nephrotoxicity or ototoxicity?

- What is the reason for giving an aminoglycoside and an antipseudomonal penicillin in the treatment of serious infections caused by P. aeruginosa?

- Why should an aminoglycoside and an antipseudomonal penicillin not be combined in a syringe or IV fluid for administration?

- Which laboratory tests need to be monitored regularly for a patient receiving a systemic aminoglycoside?

References and Resources

Centers for Disease Control and Prevention. Sexually Transmitted Diseases (STDs) Web site. Available at http://www.cdc.gov/std

Centers for Disease Control and Prevention. (2007). Update to CDC's sexually transmitted diseases treatment guidelines, 2006: Fluoroquinolones no longer recommended for treatment of gonococcal infections. *Morbidity and Mortality Weekly Report, 56*(14), 332–336.

Drug facts and comparisons. (Updated monthly). St. Louis, MO: Facts and Comparisons.

Lacy, C. F., Armstrong, L. L., Goldman, M. P., & Lance, L. L. (2010). *Lexi-Comp's drug information handbook* (19th ed.). Hudson, OH: American Pharmaceutical Association.

Karch, A. M. (2010). *2010 Lippincott's nursing drug guide.* Philadelphia, PA: Lippincott Williams & Wilkins.

Murray, T. S. (2007). Pediatric uses of fluoroquinolone antibiotics. *Pediatric Annals, 36*(6), 336–342.

Nazarian, D. J., Eddy, O. L., Lukens, T. W., Weingart, S. D., & Decker, W. W. (2009). Clinical policy: Critical issues in the management of adult patients presenting to the emergency department with community-acquired pneumonia. *Annals of Emergency Medicine, 54*(5), 704–731.

Porth, C. M. (2009). *Pathophysiology: Concepts of altered health status* (8th ed.). Philadelphia, PA: Lippincott Williams & Wilkins.

Ramsdell, J., Narsavage, G. L., & Fink, J. B. (2005). Management of community-acquired pneumonia in the home: an American College of Chest Physicians clinical position statement. *Chest, 127*(5), 1752–1763.

18 Drug Therapy With Tetracyclines, Sulfonamides, and Urinary Antiseptics

LEARNING OBJECTIVES

After studying this chapter, you should be able to:

1 Identify the prototype and describe the characteristics, action, use, adverse effects, contraindications, and nursing implications of the tetracyclines.

2 Identify the prototype and describe the characteristics, action, use, adverse effects, contraindications, and nursing implications of the sulfonamides.

3 Identify the prototype and describe the action, use, adverse effects, contraindications, and nursing implications for the adjuvant urinary antiseptic agents used in the treatment of urinary tract infections.

4 Implement the nursing process in the care of patients being treated with tetracyclines, sulfonamides, or urinary antiseptics.

Clinical Application Case Study

Sharon Dee is an 18-year-old college student. She comes to the health clinic with complaints of urinary frequency and burning on urination. Her medication history includes ongoing, long-term treatment of acne with a tetracycline. She takes 250 mg of the drug orally daily. The physician diagnoses her with a urinary tract infection and prescribes trimethoprim–sulfamethoxazole (Bactrim) 160/800 mg orally every 12 hours for 10 days.

KEY TERMS

Crystalluria: presence of crystals in the urine, indicating renal irritation

Sulfonamide: older, broad-spectrum, bacteriostatic drug (organic sulfur compounds) that is rarely used for systemic infection because of microbial resistance and the development of more effective or less toxic drugs; also known as sulfa drug

Tetracycline: antibiotic derived from chlortetracycline; used to treat a broad variety of infections

Urinary antiseptic: drug that exerts antimicrobial activity in the urine but has little or no systemic antibacterial effect; usefulness is limited to therapy and prevention of urinary tract infections

Introduction

This chapter introduces the pharmacological care of the patient experiencing an infection that is treated with tetracyclines or sulfonamides. Tetracyclines and sulfonamides are older, broad-spectrum, bacteriostatic drugs that are rarely used for systemic infections because of microbial resistance and the development of more effective or less toxic drugs. This discussion also introduces the urinary antiseptic agents administered for urinary tract infections (UTIs). The Drugs at a Glance tables present information about routes of administration and dosage ranges for both prototypes and other related drugs.

Tetracyclines

The **tetracyclines** are antibiotics, derived from chlortetracycline, that may be used to treat a broad variety of infections. The drugs in this class have similar pharmacologic properties and antimicrobial activity. Although tetracyclines are effective against both gram-negative and gram-positive microorganisms, they are usually not drugs of choice. Many gram-negative microorganisms have developed resistance to tetracyclines. However, prescribers still order them for bacterial infections caused by *Brucella* and *Vibrio cholerae*. The drugs also remain effective against rickettsiae, chlamydia, some protozoa, spirochetes, and others (see "Use" of tetracyclines). ℗ **Tetracycline hydrochloride** is the prototype of this class.

Pharmacokinetics

Administration of tetracycline is oral, and the stomach absorbs 75% of the medication. Its peak of action is 2 to 4 hours. Tetracycline is widely distributed to the tissues, with 65% of the drug protein bound. It has the ability to cross the placenta and enter the breast milk. Elimination of 50% to 60% of the drug occurs in the urine within 72 hours. Its half-life in patients with normal renal function is 8 to 11 hours.

Action

Tetracycline penetrates microbial cells by passive diffusion and an active transport system. Intracellularly, it binds to the 30S ribosomes and possibly the 50S ribosomes and inhibits microbial protein synthesis. In patients with acne, it suppresses the growth of *Propionibacterium acnes* with sebaceous follicles, reducing the free fatty acid content in the sebum.

Use

Tetracycline is effective for treating *Mycoplasma*, *Chlamydia*, and *Rickettsia*. Health care providers administer it for the treatment of acne, chronic bronchitis, gonorrhea, and syphilis in patients with a known allergy to penicillin. Combined with other drugs, it may be effective in the eradication of *Helicobacter pylori*, thus reducing the risk of duodenal ulcers. Tetracycline is also useful in treating small animal bites and Lyme disease. In addition, it may be useful as adjunctive therapy for acute intestinal amebiasis and acne vulgaris. Finally, prescribers order tetracycline when penicillin is contraindicated to treat infections caused by *Klebsiella*, *Neisseria gonorrhoeae*, *Treponema pallidum*, *Listeria monocytogenes*, *Clostridium*, *Bacillus anthracis*, *Fusobacterium fusiform*, and *Actinomyces*.

Table 18.1 provides useful information about tetracycline and related drugs.

Use in Children

Children younger than 8 years of age should not take tetracyclines because of their effects on teeth and bones. In teeth, the drugs interfere with enamel development and may cause a permanent yellow, gray, or brown discoloration. In bone, the drugs form a stable compound in bone-forming tissue and may interfere with bone growth.

Use in Older Adults

A major concern with the use of tetracyclines is renal impairment, which commonly occurs in older adults. It is also necessary to monitor hepatic function in elderly patients during the administration of these drugs.

Use in Patients With Renal Impairment

Patients with renal impairment should not take tetracyclines. High concentrations of these drugs inhibit protein synthesis in human cells. This antianabolic effect increases tissue breakdown (catabolism) and the amount of waste products to be excreted by the kidneys. Normally functioning kidneys can handle the increased workload, but when renal function is impaired, the body retains these waste products. This leads to azotemia, increased blood urea nitrogen (BUN), hyperphosphatemia, hyperkalemia, and acidosis. If a tetracycline is necessary because of an organism's sensitivity or a patient's inability to take other antimicrobial drugs, administration of doxycycline or minocycline is necessary.

Use in Patients With Hepatic Impairment

The development of hepatotoxicity is rare, but caution is warranted when the medication is administered to patients with known hepatotoxicity. Tetracycline is generally contraindicated in pregnancy because it may cause fatal hepatic necrosis in the mother (as well as interfere with bone and tooth development in the fetus). However, there are some disorders where the benefit to the mother may outweigh the risk of hepatic dysfunction; these include rickettsial infections, ehrlichiosis, inhalational anthrax, and malaria.

Adverse Effects

Several adverse effects may occur following the administration of tetracycline. These include the following:

- Hypersensitivity such as rash, urticaria, serum sickness, or anaphylaxis. Maculopapular and erythematous rashes may also occur.
- Central nervous system (CNS) conditions such as intracranial hypertension (most severe CNS effect)
- Gastrointestinal (GI) conditions such as flatulence, diarrhea, nausea, vomiting, and epigastric distress (commonly reported). Esophagitis, pancreatitis, and staphylococcal enterocolitis may also occur.

TABLE 18.1

DRUGS AT A GLANCE: Tetracyclines

Drug	Pregnancy Category	Routes and Dosage Ranges	
		Adults	*Children*
Ⓟ **Tetracycline hydro-chloride** (Sumycin)	D	250–500 mg PO every 6 h	Older than 8 y: 25–50 mg/kg/d PO in four divided doses
Demeclocycline hydrochloride (Declomycin)	D	150 mg PO every 6 h or 300 mg every 12 h	Older than 8 y: 8–12 mg/kg/d PO in two to four divided doses
Doxycycline (Vibramycin)	D	100–200 mg/d PO/IV, in one to two divided doses.	Older than 8 y: Weight <45 kg: 2–5 mg/kg/d PO/IV in one to two divided doses (max dose 200 mg/d) Weight ≥45 kg: same as adults
Minocycline hydrochloride (Minocin)	D	200 mg PO initially, then 100 mg every 12 h (max dose 400 mg/d) 200 mg IV initially, followed by 100 mg every 12 h Acne: 45–54 kg: 45 mg PO daily 55–77 kg: 65 mg PO daily 78–102 kg: 90 mg PO daily 103–125 kg: 115 mg PO daily 126–136 kg: 135 mg PO daily	Older than 8 y: 4 mg/kg PO initially, then 2 mg/kg every 12 h; 4 mg/kg IV, followed by 2 mg/kg every 12 h

EVIDENCE-BASED PRACTICE

Increase in Resistance Rates of H. pylori Isolates to Metronidazole and Tetracycline-Comparison of Three 3-Year Studies

by FARIDAEH SIAVOSHI, PhD, PARASTOO SANIEE, MSc, SAEID LATIFI-NAVID, PhD, SADEGH MASSARRATE, MD, ARGHAVAN SHEYKHOLESLAMI, MD

Archives of Iranian Medicine.
2010, 13(3): 177–187.

The aim of this 3-year study was to determine the usefulness of the treatment of *Helicobacter pylori* in dyspeptic diseases. The current trend of anti-infective agent use has contributed to the problem of resistant strains of *H. pylori*. The study included 110 *H. pylori* strains that were isolated in dyspeptic patients. The patients were tested for their susceptibility to anti-infective agents. It was found that 38.1% of the patients were resistant to tetracycline in the treatment of *H. pylori*.

IMPLICATIONS FOR NURSING PRACTICE: The resistance of anti-infective agents used in the treatment of infectious diseases is increasing. This requires that nurses carefully assess for the decrease of symptoms of the infectious disease when administering tetracycline.

- Superinfection:
  - Candidal: sore throat, white patches on the oral mucosa, or a black, furry tongue
  - GI: pseudomembranous colitis
- Other conditions such as increased pigmentation, photosensitivity reactions, azotemia, renal and hepatic toxicity, as well as retardation of bone growth. Discoloration of the teeth and enamel hypoplasia may occur in children younger than 8 years of age.

Contraindications

Contraindications to tetracycline include renal failure and known hypersensitivity to the drug. Other contraindications are young age (less than 8 years) and pregnancy; as previously stated, the drug causes permanent discoloration of teeth, defects in tooth enamel, and retardation of bone growth. Women who are breast-feeding should not take the drug because they secrete it into their breast milk. Possible hepatotoxicity may also be a problem.

Nursing Implications

Preventing Interactions

Many medications interact with tetracycline hydrochloride, increasing or decreasing its effects (Box 18.1). Tetracycline also affects the action of several drugs. Administering oral anticoagulants with tetracycline enhances the effect of vitamin K. Digoxin combined with tetracycline leads to increased digoxin absorption, resulting in digoxin toxicity. Giving penicillins with tetracycline interferes with the bactericidal effects

BOX 18.1   Drug Interactions: Tetracycline

Drugs That Increase the Effects of Tetracycline
- Methoxyflurane
  Increases the risk of nephrotoxicity

Drugs That Decrease the Effects of Tetracycline
- Aluminum, antacids, bismuth subsalicylate, didanosine, ferrous sulfate, calcium, kaolin, laxatives, magnesium, pectin, zinc
  Decrease antibiotic absorption

BOX 18.2   Patient Teaching Guidelines for Tetracycline

- Take tetracycline around the clock because it inhibits bacteria rather than kill the bacteria.
- Avoid sunlamps, tanning beds, and intense or prolonged exposure to sunlight.
- Wear sunscreen and protective clothing when in the sun.
- Report severe nausea, vomiting, diarrhea, skin rash, or perineal itching to your health care provider. These symptoms may indicate a need to change or stop the drug.
- Take the drug on an empty stomach, at least 1 hour before or 2 hours after meals.
- Do not take the drug with or within 2 hours of taking dairy products, antacids, or iron supplements.
- If you must take an antacid, take it at least 2 hours before or 4 hours after tetracycline.
- Take each dose with 8 ounces of water.
- If you are taking an oral contraceptive, use another form of birth control for the duration of therapy. The effectiveness of oral contraceptives is decreased when combined with tetracycline.
- Never take outdated tetracycline due to the risk of severe reactions.

of the penicillins. The combination of oral contraceptives and tetracycline results in diminished contraceptive effects. Some women need to use an additional form of birth control.

Foods that affect the action of tetracycline include dairy products, which decrease the absorption of the antibiotic.

Administering the Medication

It is important to obtain a culture and sensitivity prior to beginning therapy with tetracycline. Administration of the drug is oral. The medication is most effective when taken on an empty stomach. Patients should take the medication 1 hour before meals or 2 hours after meals. It is important not to take it with dairy products, antacids, or iron supplements. The combination of tetracycline with metallic ions such as aluminum, calcium, iron, or magnesium inhibits tetracycline absorption. If the patient has consumed dairy products or antacids, it is necessary to withhold tetracycline for 2 hours. Also, it is essential that tetracycline never be used after the expiration date. The administration of outdated tetracycline causes severe kidney damage.

Assessing for Therapeutic Effects

The nurse assesses for decreased signs and symptoms of the infection for which the medication is being administered. He or she checks for decreased pain and fever.

Assessing for Adverse Effects

The nurse assesses for GI irritation, nausea, epigastric distress, diarrhea, and vomiting. He or she also assesses for rash, anaphylaxis, and serum sickness. If a patient is exposed to sunlight, it is necessary to assess for sunburn or photosensitivity reactions. In addition, the nurse checks the patient's complete blood count for anemia and signs and symptoms of superinfection.

Patient Teaching

Box 18.2 identifies patient teaching guidelines for tetracycline.

Other Drugs in the Class

Demeclocycline hydrochloride (Declomycin) is useful in the treatment of bacterial infections such as acne, pertussis, and UTIs caused by gram-positive or gram-negative organisms. An unlabeled use is for the treatment of chronic syndrome of inappropriate secretion of antidiuretic hormone. When administering demeclocycline, it is important to monitor the patient's BUN. Increases in the BUN are secondary to antianabolic effects. Demeclocycline is the tetracycline most likely to cause photosensitivity.

Doxycycline (Vibramycin) is one of the drugs of choice for *B. anthracis* (anthrax); it is part of a combination drug regimen for postexposure prophylaxis and treatment. Patients who are exposed to anthrax should receive doxycycline for 60 days following exposure. The drug is also useful for infections with *Chlamydia trachomatis* and in respiratory tract infections due to *Mycoplasma pneumoniae*. In addition, people take doxycycline to prevent traveler's diarrhea due to enterotoxic strains of *Escherichia coli*. Finally, it is effective in treating gonorrhea in patients who are allergic to penicillin.

The oral form of doxycycline, which is well absorbed in the GI tract, reaches serum levels equivalent to those obtained with parenteral administration. It is highly lipid soluble, reaching therapeutic levels in the cerebrospinal fluid (CSF), eye, and prostate gland. It can be administered in smaller doses and less frequently than other tetracyclines because of its long serum half-life of 18 hours. Excretion occurs in the kidneys; however, authorities consider the drug safe for patients with impaired renal function.

Parenteral administration of doxycycline requires mixing with lactated Ringer's or dextrose 5% and lactated Ringer's. Slow infusion is necessary. The minimum infusion period is 1 hour. Complete infusion should occur in 12 hours. Doxycycline is incompatible with allopurinol, barbiturates, erythromycin lactobionate, heparin, meropenem, nafcillin, penicillin, piperacillin, sulfonamides, and riboflavin.

Minocycline hydrochloride (Minocin) is a semisynthetic tetracycline derivative. It is useful in the treatment of mucopurulent cervicitis, lower respiratory tract infections caused by *M. pneumoniae*, and rickettsial and chlamydial infections. Administration of the drug is oral. Absorption is good, and foods and fluids affect absorption of minocycline less than other tetracyclines. It readily penetrates the CSF, eye, and prostate gland. From 70% to 75% of the drug is protein bound, and metabolism occurs in the liver. Excretion takes place in the urine and feces.

Intravenous (IV) administration of minocycline requires slow infusion. Prolonged IV administration of minocycline may be associated with thrombophlebitis. The drug is stable in all IV solutions but is incompatible with calcium-containing solutions.

Clinical Application 18-1

A nurse at the college health center is interviewing Ms. Dee about her recent health history. The nurse inquires if Ms. Dee is sexually active. She replies that she has a new boyfriend with whom she has had sexual intercourse every day for the past 5 days. She says she is taking oral contraceptives. The nurse also gathers information regarding Ms. Dee's sunbathing practices (the college is on the Gulf Coast). Ms. Dee reports that she has been going to the beach daily.

- Based on the information gathered in the interview regarding the fact she is sexually active, what should the nurse instruct Ms. Dee on related to the tetracycline she is taking?

- What teaching should the nurse at the health center provide related to the administration of tetracycline?

- Based on the fact that Ms. Dee has been going to the beach daily, what is she at risk for developing?

NCLEX Success

1. A patient is admitted to the emergency department following opening an envelope containing a substance that experts have identified as anthrax. Which of the following medications is administered?

   A. tetracycline
   B. doxycycline
   C. amoxicillin–clavulanic acid combination
   D. neomycin

2. A patient receiving tetracycline should receive the following instruction regarding the medication?

   A. Take tetracycline with food.
   B. Take tetracycline in combination with antacids.
   C. Take the first dose and then obtain a test known as culture and sensitivity.
   D. Take tetracycline with a full glass of water.

3. Which of the following foods should not be taken with tetracycline?

   A. orange juice with calcium
   B. cranberry juice cocktail
   C. tomato juice
   D. lemonade

4. A man is receiving treatment for a *Mycoplasma pneumoniae* infection. He says that drinking orange juice hurts his mouth. What priority assessment should the nurse make?

   A. Assess the patient's fecal output for signs and symptoms of diarrhea.
   B. Assess the patient's mouth for signs of candidal infection.
   C. Assess the patient's lung sounds for rales or rhonchi.
   D. Assess the patient's intake and output.

5. Which laboratory value should the nurse assess in patients who are receiving demeclocycline?

   A. blood urea nitrogen
   B. aspartate aminotransferase
   C. alanine aminotransferase
   D. creatinine

Sulfonamides

Sulfonamides are bacteriostatic drugs that were once effective against a wide range of gram-positive and gram-negative bacteria. However, increasing resistance is making them less useful. It is important to document susceptibility with culture and sensitivity testing, but sulfonamides may be active against *Streptococcus pyogenes*, some staphylococcal strains, *Haemophilus influenzae*, *Nocardia*, *C. trachomatis*, and toxoplasmosis. The combination of trimethoprim and sulfamethoxazole (Bactrim, Septra) is useful in bronchitis, UTIs due to Enterobacteriaceae, and *Pneumocystis jiroveci* infection (in high doses). Individual drugs vary in extent of systemic absorption and clinical indications. Some sulfonamides are well absorbed and can be used in systemic infections; others are poorly absorbed and have more local effects. **Ⓟ Sulfisoxazole** is the prototype sulfonamide, but it is distributed in a combination form with erythromycin. The following sections discuss only sulfisoxazole. Chapter 19 discusses erythromycin. Table 18.2 summarizes key information about sulfonamides.

Pharmacokinetics

Sulfisoxazole is rapidly absorbed in the GI tract, reaching its peak in 2 to 4 hours. The half-life of the medication is 4.6 to 7.8 hours. Sulfisoxazole enters the extracellular spaces, crosses the placental and blood–brain barriers, and appears in breast milk. Metabolism occurs in the liver, and excretion takes place in the kidneys.

Action

Sulfisoxazole and other sulfonamides act as antimetabolites of para-aminobenzoic acid (PABA), which microorganisms require to produce folic acid. In turn, folic acid is necessary for the production of bacterial intracellular proteins. Sulfonamides enter into the reaction instead of PABA, compete for the enzyme involved, and cause formation of nonfunctional derivatives of folic acid. Thus, sulfonamides halt multiplication of new bacteria but do not kill mature, fully formed bacteria. With the exception of the topical sulfonamides used in burn therapy,

TABLE 18.2

DRUGS AT A GLANCE: Sulfonamides

Drug	Pregnancy Category	Routes and Dosage Ranges	
		Adults	Children
Ⓟ **Sulfisoxazole**	C D (last trimester)	2–4 g PO initially, then 4–8 g daily in four to six divided doses	Older than 2 mo: 75 mg/kg of body weight PO initially, then 120–150 mg/kg/d in four to six divided doses; max daily dose, 6 g
Mafenide acetate (Sulfamylon)	C	Topical application to burned area, once or twice daily, in a thin layer	Same as adults
Sulfadiazine (Microsulfon)	C D (last trimester)	2–8 g PO daily in divided doses every 6 h	>2 y 100–200 mg/kg/d PO in divided doses every 6 h Neonate: 50 mg/kg every 12 h for 12 mo
Silver sulfadiazine (Silvadene)	B	Cover burned area with cream one to two times daily.	Same as adults
Sulfasalazine (Azulfidine)	B	Ulcerative colitis: 3–4 g PO daily in four divided doses initially; 2 g daily in divided doses for maintenance; max dose, 4 g Rheumatoid arthritis: maintenance, 2 g PO daily in divided doses, every 12 h	30–60 mg/kg/d PO in two to six divided doses initially, followed by 30 mg/kg/d in four divided doses; max daily dose, 2 g
Trimethoprim–sulfamethoxazole (TMP-SMZ, Bactrim, Septra, others)	C	UTI: trimethoprim 160 mg and sulfamethoxazole 800 mg PO every 12 h for 10–14 d	UTI and otitis media: PO 8 mg/kg trimethoprim and 40 mg/kg sulfamethoxazole in two divided doses every 12 h for 10 d
Combination drug in which the dosage is based on trimethoprim component	D (last trimester)	Shigellosis: same dose as above for 5 d Severe UTI: IV 8–10 mg (trimethoprim component)/kg/d in two to four divided doses, up to 14 d P. jiroveci pneumonia: IV 15–20 mg (trimethoprim component)/kg/d in three or four divided doses, every 6–8 h up to 21 d; IV doses should be given over 60–90 min	Shigellosis: same dose as above for 5 d Severe UTI: IV 8–10 mg (trimethoprim component)/kg in two to four divided doses, every 6–8 h or every 12 h, up to 14 d P. jiroveci pneumonia: IV 15–20 mg (trimethoprim component)/kg/d in three or four divided doses, every 6–8 h up to 21 d

the presence of pus, serum, or necrotic tissue interferes with sulfonamide action because these materials contain PABA. Some bacteria can change their metabolic pathways to use precursors or other forms of folic acid and thereby develop resistance to the antibacterial action of sulfonamides. After resistance to one sulfonamide develops, cross-resistance to others is common.

Use

Uses for sulfisoxazole include treatment of UTIs—acute, recurrent, and chronic. The drug may also be a part of adjunctive therapy for trachoma, chloroquine-resistant malaria, acute otitis media, and meningococcal meningitis caused by

H. influenzae. Prescribers order the ophthalmic preparation for the treatment of conjunctivitis, superficial eye infections, and corneal ulcers (see Chap. 58). They may prescribe the topical vaginal preparation for *Haemophilus vaginalis* vaginitis.

Use in Children

Children younger than 2 months of age should not receive sulfisoxazole and other systemic sulfonamides. If a fetus or young infant receives a sulfonamide by placental transfer, in breast milk, or by direct administration, the drug displaces bilirubin from binding sites on albumin. As a result, bilirubin may accumulate in the bloodstream (hyperbilirubinemia) and CNS (kernicterus), resulting in life-threatening toxicity.

Use in Older Adults

When administering sulfisoxazole to older adults, it is important to assess the patient's renal function. Sulfisoxazole may cause renal impairment.

Use in Patients With Renal Impairment

Patients with renal impairment should probably avoid taking sulfisoxazole and other systemic sulfonamides, if other effective drugs are available. Acute renal failure has occurred when the drugs or their metabolites precipitated in renal tubules and caused obstruction. Preventive measures include intake of 1.5 to 3 L of fluid daily to reduce the formation of crystals and stones in the urinary tract.

Use in Patients With Hepatic Impairment

Metabolism of sulfisoxazole occurs in the liver. Thus, patients with altered liver function should avoid it.

Adverse Effects

Sulfisoxazole has several adverse effects. These include the following:

- GI effects: nausea, vomiting, diarrhea, jaundice, hepatitis, pancreatitis, and stomatitis (most common). A small percentage of patients develop cholestatic jaundice.
- Hematological effects: acute hemolytic anemia in patients with a deficiency of glucose-6-phosphate dehydrogenase (G6PD), aplastic anemia, agranulocytosis, thrombocytopenia, and leukopenia
- Dermatological effects: pruritus, urticaria, Stevens-Johnson syndrome, and exfoliative dermatitis
- Urinary effects: **crystalluria** (crystals in the urine, causing renal irritation), hematuria, anuria, and reduction in sperm count

Contraindications

Contraindications include a known hypersensitivity to sulfisoxazole or any other of the sulfonamides, salicylates, or chemically related medications used to treat group A beta-hemolytic streptococcal infections. Porphyria, G6PD deficiency, hepatic disease, and renal disease are also contraindications. Patients with intestinal or urinary obstruction should not receive the drug. Sulfonylureas combined with sulfisoxazole or any sulfonamide have the potential to produce increased hypoglycemic reactions in patients with diabetes.

Nursing Implications

When administering sulfonamides, it is important to monitor the pH of the urine. Alkalinization may be necessary; this involves giving sodium bicarbonate. Alkaline urine increases drug solubility and helps prevent crystalluria. It also increases the rate of sulfonamide excretion and the concentration of sulfonamide in the urine. However, alkalinization is not required with sulfisoxazole, because this drug is highly soluble, or sulfonamides used to treat intestinal infections or burn wounds, because there is little systemic absorption.

BOX 18.3 Drug Interactions: Sulfisoxazole

Drugs That Increase the Effects of Sulfisoxazole

- Alkalinizing agents such as sodium bicarbonate
  Increase the rate of urinary excretion, raising the levels of sulfonamides in the urinary tract and increasing effectiveness in urinary tract infections
- Methenamine compounds such as urinary acidifiers
  Increase the risk of nephrotoxicity
- Salicylates, nonsteroidal anti-inflammatory agents, oral anticoagulants, phenytoin, methotrexate
  Increase the risk of nephrotoxicity by displacing sulfonamides from plasma protein binding sites
- Sulfonylureas
  Increase hypoglycemic reactions

Preventing Interactions

Many medication and herbs interact with sulfisoxazole, increasing or decreasing its effects (Boxes 18.3 and 18.4). Sulfisoxazole and other sulfonamides are cytochrome P450 2C9 (CYP2C9) enzyme inhibitors. When combined with other medications that are CYP2C9 inhibitors, the resulting drug interaction causes pronounced effects because of the inhibition of sulfisoxazole's metabolism by the liver. Thus, in the end, there is an increased effect. The combination of sulfisoxazole or other sulfonamides with warfarin results in increased blood clotting. The combination of phenytoin with sulfisoxazole leads to increased CNS depression.

Administering the Medication

It is important to take oral sulfisoxazole before or after meals with a full glass of water. Storage in a light-resistant container at 15°C to 30°C (59–86°F) is essential.

Assessing for Therapeutic Effects

If the patient is taking sulfisoxazole for treatment of a UTI, the nurse assesses for decreased symptoms of this infection, such as the elimination of pain when voiding, cloudy urine, and fever. He or she assesses the patient with trachoma or conjunctivitis for a decrease in eye discharge, swelling, and redness. If the patient is taking sulfisoxazole for treatment of meningococcal meningitis, it is important to assess for decreased nuchal rigidity, pain, fever, jaundice, and lethargy. The level of consciousness should increase as the infection and inflammation of the meninges diminishes.

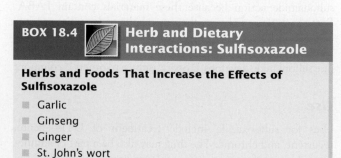

BOX 18.4 Herb and Dietary Interactions: Sulfisoxazole

Herbs and Foods That Increase the Effects of Sulfisoxazole

- Garlic
- Ginseng
- Ginger
- St. John's wort

BOX 18.5	Patient Teaching Guidelines for Sulfisoxazole

- Take sulfisoxazole with 8 ounces of water
- Take the drug before or after meals
- Drink a minimum of 2 to 3 L of fluid per day
- The effectiveness of oral contraceptives is decreased when combined with sulfisoxazole
- Avoid sunlamps, tanning beds, and intense or prolonged exposure to sunlight
- When in the sun wear sunscreen and protective clothing
- Do not take any over-the-counter medications without the prescriber's knowledge
- Inform your dentist or physician that you are taking a sulfonamide. Changes in laboratory values may occur as a result of taking the drug
- If you have diabetes, be sure to monitor your blood sugar values. Reduced blood sugar levels can occur.

Assessing for Adverse Effects

The nurse assesses the patient's intake and output. The output should be approximately 1500 mL. If the intake is greater than the output, assessment of renal function is necessary. The nurse also assesses for anemia and changes in the complete blood count that are indicative of blood dyscrasias. In addition, it is necessary to assess for signs and symptoms of superinfection or hypersensitivity reactions.

Patient Teaching

Box 18.5 identifies patient teaching guidelines for sulfisoxazole.

Other Drugs in the Class

Mafenide (Sulfamylon) is a topical anti-infective agent administered for bacteriostatic treatment of gram-negative and gram-positive organisms such as *Pseudomonas aeruginosa* and other anaerobes that may be associated with second- and third-degree burns. Topical application with sterile gloved hands follows cleansing of the burn site. The drug is absorbed rapidly, reaching its peak in 2 to 4 hours. It is inactivated in the blood to a weak carbonic anhydrase inhibitor and eliminated by the kidneys. Close monitoring of the patient's fluid and electrolyte status is necessary. Metabolic acidosis is a possibility. The nurse attempts to assess for signs and symptoms of allergic reaction; however, it is difficult to determine whether the reaction is due to allergy or severe burns.

Sulfadiazine (Microsulfon) is a short-acting sulfonamide that interferes with bacterial utilization of PABA. It inhibits folic acid biosynthesis that is required for the bacteria's growth. It is used in combination with pyrimethamine for the treatment of cerebral toxoplasmosis and chloroquine-resistant malaria. When this medication is used, it is imperative that the patient maintain a fluid intake that allows for an output of 1500 mL of urine in 24 hours. Combination with pyrimethamine decreases the development of crystalluria and stone

formation. It is important to instruct the patient to consume fluids liberally and report any symptoms of blood dyscrasias, such as pallor, fever, or sore throat.

Silver sulfadiazine (Silvadene), a silver salt, has bactericidal effects on the bacterial cell wall and cell membrane that inhibit folic acid synthesis. It has antimicrobial activity against bacteria and yeast. This medication is indicated for the treatment of second- and third-degree burns. It is effective against *Pseudomonas*, *E. coli*, *Klebsiella*, *Proteus*, *Staphylococcus*, and *Streptococcus*. Topical application with sterile gloved hands one to two times per day follows cleansing of the burn site in a whirlpool bath or spot cleansing. With large burn areas and prolonged use, patients may absorb significant amounts of silver sulfadiazine systemically. It is necessary to monitor for adverse effects of sulfonamides. Contraindications include pregnancy and age less than 1 month.

Sulfasalazine (Azulfidine) is used for ulcerative colitis and rheumatoid arthritis. The bacteriostatic action of the medication occurs in the intestine, where the intestinal flora convert the drug to two metabolites, one of which acts as an anti-inflammatory agent. It reduces *Clostridium* and *E. coli* in the stools. Sulfasalazine is contraindicated in patients who have an allergy to salicylates. The nurse instructs patients that taking this drug may make their urine yellow-orange.

Trimethoprim–sulfamethoxazole (TMP-SMZ; Bactrim, Septra) is a combination of anti-infective sulfonamide and trimethoprim. (Trimethoprim is a synthetic anti-infective agent.) The two drugs act by inhibiting bacterial synthesis of essential nucleic acids and proteins. Uses include the treatment of *P. jiroveci* pneumonitis, severe UTIs, *Shigella enteritis*, and Enterobacteriaceae. Other organisms treated with TMP-SMZ are *Streptococcus viridans*, *Staphylococcus epidermidis*, *Staphylococcus aureus*, *E. coli*, *Salmonella*, *Klebsiella*, *Nocardia*, and *Pseudomonas*.

QSEN Safety Alert

When administering TMP-SMZ parenterally, it is important that the medication is diluted in 5% dextrose and water. It is incompatible in other types of fluids.

It is essential that this drug combination not be mixed with other drugs or solutions and that IV lines be flushed to remove any residual drug. The IV medication Septra contains sodium metabisulfite, which has a potential of producing allergic reactions in some patients. The nurse assesses the patient for hives, skin redness, itching, wheezing, shortness of breath, and possible anaphylaxis.

Clinical Application 18-2

- What aspects of patient teaching should the nurse at the college health center provide to Ms. Dee regarding the administration of sulfamethoxazole and trimethoprim?

- The nurse should tell Ms. Dee about which adverse effects?

NCLEX Success

6. A woman develops a urinary tract infection following the delivery of an infant. The nurse practitioner is considering prescribing trimethoprim–sulfamethoxazole. What assessment is necessary to make?

   A. if the woman is breast-feeding
   B. if the woman has been treated with the medication in the past
   C. if anyone in her family has a known allergy to the drug
   D. if she is experiencing hematuria

7. When administering a sulfonamide, which of the following interventions is most effective in decreasing crystalluria?

   A. administering 8 ounces of cranberry juice
   B. providing a full liquid diet during the course of drug therapy
   C. inserting a Foley catheter for the measurement of an accurate intake and output
   D. providing a minimum of 2000 mL of fluid per day

8. A physician has ordered sulfisoxazole for a woman with a urinary tract infection. The nurse has asked the patient about whether she takes any over-the-counter medications. The patient reports that she regularly takes St. John's wort as a mood elevator. Which of the following patient teaching interventions is most important?

   A. Taking St. John's wort and sulfisoxazole results in no known interactions.
   B. Sulfisoxazole combined with St. John's wort leads to an increased therapeutic effect of the sulfisoxazole.
   C. Sulfisoxazole has a decreased effect when given with St. John's wort.
   D. When given in combination, sulfisoxazole and St. John's wort result in manic tendencies.

9. A nurse is applying silver sulfadiazine (Silvadene) to a child's burns. Which of the following nursing actions is most important when applying the medication?

   A. providing pain medication
   B. using sterile gloves
   C. giving the child a bath
   D. teaching the parent to apply the medication

10. A physician has ordered intravenous sulfamethoxazole with trimethoprim. How should the nurse administer the medication?

    A. in 500 mL of 0.45% normal saline
    B. in 150 mL of 10% dextrose and water
    C. in 125 mL of 5% dextrose and water
    D. in 125 mL of 5% dextrose and 0.45% normal saline

Adjuvant Medications Used to Treat Urinary Tract Infections: Urinary Antiseptics

The adjuvant medications used to treat UTIs are trimethoprim and the urinary antiseptic agents. **Urinary antiseptics** may be bactericidal for sensitive organisms in the urinary tract because these drugs are concentrated in renal tubules and reach high levels in urine. They are not used in systemic infections because they do not attain therapeutic plasma levels. The adjuvant medications include nitrofurantoin, phenazopyridine, and trimethoprim. Table 18.3 provides dosage information for the adjuvant urinary tract agents administered as adjunctive therapy for UTIs.

Nitrofurantoin

ⓟ **Nitrofurantoin** (Furadantin, Macrodantin, Macrobid) is an anti-infective agent that is administered for the treatment and prophylaxis of UTIs. The drug is effective for UTIs caused by *E. coli*, *S. aureus*, *Enterobacter*, *Enterococcus*, and *Klebsiella*. Administration of nitrofurantoin with food aids in absorption and decreases the onset of adverse effects. Older people should not take the medication due to the risk of renal, pulmonary, and hepatic toxicity. Contraindications include late pregnancy (last 5 weeks) and renal insufficiency. Significant adverse effects of nitrofurantoin included nonspecific ST- and T-wave changes and bundle branch block. CNS changes include fever, malaise, depression, headache, lethargy, vertigo, and pseudotumor cerebri. The nurse assesses for these conditions as well as hyperphosphatemia, pulmonary insufficiency, and blood dyscrasias.

Phenazopyridine

ⓟ **Phenazopyridine hydrochloride** (Pyridium, Azo-Standard) is a urinary analgesic that is administered to provide pain relief related to burning, urgency, frequency, and irritation of the lower urinary tract mucosa. The pain is a result of infection, trauma, cystoscopic examinations, surgery, or catheter insertion. Phenazopyridine, an azo dye, is a drug that acts directly on the urinary tract mucosa to provide analgesia. Metabolism occurs in the liver. It is necessary to administer the medication with food to decrease GI distress. The nurse should tell the patient that his or urine will turn reddish-orange. A **BLACK BOX WARNING** ◆ points out that if the patient's skin turns yellow, it is important to report this to the health care provider immediately. This is a sign that the drug is accumulating in the patient's system. It is also necessary to report a sore throat, fever, bruising, or bleeding. Contraindications to phenazopyridine include renal insufficiency and hepatitis.

Trimethoprim

ⓟ **Trimethoprim** (Primsol) is a folate antagonist that is a urinary tract anti-infective. Most commonly administered in combination with sulfamethoxazole or as an adjuvant

TABLE 18.3

DRUGS AT A GLANCE: Adjuvant Drugs for Urinary Tract Infections/ Urinary Antiseptics

Drug	Pregnancy Category	Routes and Dosage Ranges	
		Adults	*Children*
Ⓟ **Nitrofurantoin** (Furadantin, Macrodantin, Macrobid)	B	Macrodantin: 50–100 mg PO four times daily; Macrobid: 100 mg every 12 h for 7 d Prophylaxis of recurrent urinary tract infection (UTI) in women, Macrodantin: 50–100 mg PO at bedtime	Children older than 12 y: dual-release capsules: 100 mg every 12 h for 7 d Children 1 mo and older: macrocrystal capsules: 5–7 mg/kg/d PO in four divided doses for 7 d
Ⓟ **Phenazopyridine** hydrochloride (Azo-Standard, Pyridium)	B	100–200 mg PO three times daily after meals	6–12 y: 12 mg/kg/d PO, in three divided doses after meals for 2 d
Ⓟ **Trimethoprim** (Primsol, Proloprim)	C	100 mg PO every 12 h for 10 d or 200 mg every 24 h for 10 d	4–6 mg/kg/d in divided doses every 12 h Otitis media: Children ≥ 10 mg/kg/d PO in divided doses every 12 h for 10 d

agent with the sulfonamides (see Sulfonamides), it is also given singly. Prescribers order it for susceptible infections and UTIs. The Centers for Disease Control and Prevention has recommended that trimethoprim be used (unlabeled use) in the treatment of *P. jiroveci* pneumonia. This drug inhibits folic acid reduction to tetrahydrofolate, thus interfering with the bacterial cell growth. Contraindications include a known folate deficiency, fragile X syndrome, and a creatinine clearance less than 15 mL/min. Patient teaching should include taking the entire course of medication even if symptoms improve; having a sufficient fluid intake (2,000 to 3,000 mL/24 hours); and reporting symptoms such as sore throat, fever, bruising, or rash to the health care provider. Rash and pruritus are the most common adverse effects. There also have been occasional reports of nausea, vomiting, thrombocytopenia, and leukopenia.

NCLEX Success

11. A nurse practitioner has prescribed nitrofurantoin (Macrodantin) for a woman with a urinary tract infection. Which of the following cardiovascular adverse effects is this patient at risk for developing?

    A. inverted T wave
    B. widened QRS
    C. premature ventricular contraction (PVC)
    D. bundle branch block

12. A man has had a urinary tract infection, and a prescriber orders phenazopyridine (Pyridium). Which of the following adverse effects should he report to his health care provider?

    A. yellowing of the skin
    B. edema
    C. pain
    D. malaise

Clinical Application 18-3

In addition to the sulfamethoxazole with trimethoprim, Ms. Dee receives a prescription for phenazopyridine 200 mg three times per day.

■ What patient teaching related to the administration of phenazopyridine does the nurse provide to Ms. Dee?

■ The nurse should teach Ms. Dee that phenazopyridine will affect her urine in what way?

■ What other patient teaching should Ms. Dee receive?

The Nursing Process

General aspects of the nursing process in antimicrobial drug therapy, described in Chapter 13, apply to the patient receiving tetracyclines, sulfonamides, and urinary antiseptics. In this chapter, only those aspects related specifically to these drugs are included.

Assessment

● With tetracyclines, assess for conditions in which the drugs must be used cautiously or are contraindicated, such as impaired renal or hepatic function.

● With sulfonamides, assess for signs and symptoms of disorders for which the drugs are used:

  ● For UTIs, assess urinalysis reports for white blood cell and bacteria counts; urine culture reports for type of bacteria; and symptoms of dysuria, frequency, and urgency of urination.

  ● For burns, assess the size of the wound, amount and type of drainage, presence of edema, and amount of eschar.

- Ask patients specifically if they have ever taken a sulfonamide and, if so, whether they had an allergic reaction.
- With urinary antiseptics, assess for signs and symptoms of UTI.

Nursing Diagnoses

- Risk for injury: hypersensitivity reaction, kidney, liver, or blood disorders with sulfonamides
- Deficient knowledge: correct administration and use of tetracyclines, sulfonamides, and urinary antiseptics

Planning/Goals

The patent will

- Receive or self-administer the drugs as directed
- Receive prompt and appropriate treatment if adverse effects occur

Nursing Interventions

The nurse will

- During tetracycline therapy for systemic infections, monitor laboratory tests of renal function for abnormal values.
- During sulfonamide therapy, encourage sufficient fluids to produce a urine output of at least 1500 mL daily. A high fluid intake decreases the risk of crystalluria (precipitation of drug crystals in the urine).
- Avoid urinary catheterization when possible. If catheterization is necessary, use sterile technique. The urinary tract is normally sterile except for the lower third of the urethra. Introduction of any bacteria into the bladder may cause infection.

- A single catheterization may cause infection. With indwelling catheters, bacteria colonize the bladder and produce infection within 2 to 3 weeks, even with meticulous care.
- When indwelling catheters must be used, measures to decrease UTI include using a closed drainage system; keeping the perineal area clean; forcing fluids, if not contraindicated, to maintain a dilute urine; and removing the catheter as soon as possible. Do not disconnect the system and irrigate the catheter unless obstruction is suspected. Never raise the urinary drainage bag above bladder level.
- Force fluids in anyone with a UTI unless contraindicated. Bacteria do not multiply as rapidly in dilute urine. In addition, emptying the bladder frequently allows it to refill with uninfected urine. This decreases the bacterial population of the bladder.
- Teach women to cleanse themselves from the urethral area toward the rectum after voiding or defecating to avoid contamination of the urethral area with bacteria from the vagina and rectum. Also, voiding after sexual intercourse helps cleanse the lower urethra and prevent UTI.
- Provide appropriate teaching related to any drug therapy (see Boxes 18.2 and 18.5).

Evaluation

- Interview and observe for improvement in the infection being treated.
- Interview and observe for adverse drug effects.

Key Concepts

- Tetracyclines are effective against both gram-positive and gram-negative organisms, although they are usually not drugs of choice. Many gram-negative organisms have developed resistance to tetracyclines.
- Demeclocycline hydrochloride (Declomycin) is used to treat bacterial infections such as acne, pertussis, and urinary tract infections.
- Doxycycline (Vibramycin) is the drug of choice for *B. anthracis*, and is used to prevent traveler's diarrhea.
- Minocycline hydrochloride (Minocin) is a semisynthetic tetracycline derivative used to treat mucopurulent cervicitis, *M. pneumoniae*, *Rickettsia*, and *Chlamydia*.
- Sulfonamides are bacteriostatic against a wide range of gram-positive and gram-negative bacteria, although increasing resistance is making them less useful.
- Mafenide (Sulfamylon) is a topical anti-infective agent applied to second- and third-degree burns that when inactivated in the blood becomes a weak carbonic anhydrase inhibitor.
- Silver sulfadiazine (Silvadene) is a silver salt that provides bactericidal effects on the bacterial cell wall and cell membrane to inhibit folic acid synthesis.
- Trimethoprim–sulfamethoxazole (TMP-SMZ; Bactrim, Septra) is a combination of anti-infective sulfonamide and trimethoprim. (Trimethoprim is a synthetic anti-infective agent.)
- Sulfasalazine (Azulfidine) is contraindicated in people who are allergic to salicylates.
- Both tetracyclines (except doxycycline) and sulfonamides are contraindicated in patients with renal failure.
- Urinary antiseptics may be bactericidal for sensitive organisms in the urinary tract because these drugs are concentrated in renal tubules and reach high levels in urine but are not used in systemic infections because they do not attain therapeutic plasma levels.
- A **BLACK BOX WARNING** ◆ stipulates that the administration of phenazopyridine should be discontinued if the patient's skin turns yellow.

Critical Thinking Questions

18-1. Jake Purcell is a home care patient with an indwelling catheter. Previously, he received treatment for a urinary tract infection (UTI) with trimethoprim. Last evening he began running a fever of 102.5°F. His urine is cloudy with streaks of blood. A urine specimen is sent to the laboratory for culture and sensitivity. Following collection of the culture, a nurse practitioner prescribes trimethoprim–sulfamethoxazole (TMP-SMZ). The culture reveals that his urine is growing *Klebsiella* and *Escherichia coli*.

- Will TMP-SMZ be effective against *Klebsiella* and *E. coli*?
- What medication will be effective for the treatment of a UTI caused by *Klebsiella* and *E. coli*?

References and Resources

Harvey, R. A., & Champe, P. C. (2008). *Lippincott's illustrated reviews: Pharmacology.* Philadelphia, PA: Lippincott Williams & Wilkins.

Karch, A. M. (2011). *2011 Lippincott's nursing drug guide.* Philadelphia, PA: Lippincott Williams & Wilkins.

Kuhn, M. A. & Winston, D. *Herbal therapy supplements a scientific and traditional approach* (2nd ed.). Philadelphia, PA: Lippincott Williams, & Wilkins.

Porth, C. M. & Matfin, G. (2009). *Pathophysiology: Concepts of altered health states,* Philadelphia, PA: Lippincott Williams & Wilkins.

Siavoshi, F., Saniee, P., Fatifi-Navid, S., Massarrate, S., & Sheykholeslami, A. (2010). Increase in resistance rates of *H. pylori* isolates to metronidazole and tetracycline-comparison of three year studies. *Archives of Iranian Medicine, 13*(3), 177–187.

Smeltzer, S. C., Bare, B. G., Hinkle, J. H., & Cheever, K. H. (2008). *Brunner & Suddarth's textbook of medical-surgical nursing* (11th ed.). Philadelphia, PA: Lippincott Williams & Wilkins.

Up-To-Date. (2012). *Demeclocycline: Drug Information.* Lexi-Comp. Inc.

Up-To-Date. (2012). *Doxycycline: Drug Information.* Lexi-Comp. Inc.

Up-To-Date. (2012). *Erythromycin and Sulfisoxazole: Drug Information.* LexiComp. Inc.

Up-To-Date. (2012). *Mafenide: Drug Information.* LexiComp. Inc.

Up-To-Date. (2012). *Minocycline hydrochloride: Drug Information.* LexiComp. Inc.

Up-To-Date. (2012). *Nitrofurantoin: Drug Information.* Lexi-Comp. Inc.

Up-To-Date. (2012). *Phenazopyridine: Drug Information.* LexiComp. Inc.

Up-To-Date. (2012). *Sulfadiazine: Drug Information.* Lexi-Comp. Inc.

Up-To-Date. (2012). *Sulfasalazine: Drug Information.* Lexi-Comp. Inc.

Up-To-Date. (2012). *Sulfamethoxazole Trimethoprim: Drug Information.* LexiComp. Inc.

Up-To-Date. (2012). *Tetracycline: Drug Information.* Lexi-Comp. Inc.

Up-To-Date. (2012). *Trimethoprim: Drug Information.* Lexi-Comp. Inc.

19 Drug Therapy With Macrolides, Ketolides, and Miscellaneous Anti-Infective Agents

Clinical Application Case Study

Juro Nikki, a 65-year-old man, has had chronic obstructive pulmonary disease for a number of years. He presents to the physician's office with a respiratory tract infection. He begins taking azithromycin, 500 mg for one dose, then 250 mg orally daily for 4 days.

KEY TERMS

Glycylcyclines: class of anti-infective agents that are structurally related to the tetracyclines and share many of the same properties; used for the treatment of complicated skin and skin structure infections caused by methicillin-resistant *Staphylococcus aureus* and vancomycin-sensitive *Enterococcus faecalis*, as well as treatment of complicated intra-abdominal infections

Gray syndrome: dangerous condition that occurs in newborns who are given chloramphenicol; may lead to fatalities

Ketolides: newer class of antibiotics that belong to the macrolide group; have a more broad-spectrum effect compared to macrolides, especially *Streptococcus pneumoniae* infections

Lincosamides: similar to macrolides in their mechanism of action and antimicrobial spectrum

Lipopeptides: a new class of antibiotics that kills gram-positive bacteria by inhibiting synthesis of bacterial proteins, DNA, and RNA

Macrolides: may be bacteriostatic or bactericidal, depending on drug concentrations in infected tissues; widely used for treatment of respiratory tract and skin/soft tissue infections caused by streptococci and staphylococci

Methicillin-resistant _Staphylococcus aureus_ : microorganisms resistant to broad-spectrum antibiotics such as penicillin and erythromycin; frequently colonizes nasal passages of health care workers and is increasing as a cause of infection in health care facilities

Methicillin-resistant _Staphylococcus species non-aureus_ : other strains of antibiotic-resistant staphylococci

Methicillin-susceptible _Staphylococcus aureus_ : methicillin-susceptible strains of _Staphylococcus aureus_

Mycobacterium avium complex: caused by atypical mycobacteria; opportunistic infection that occurs mainly in people with advanced human immunodeficiency virus infection

Oxazolidinones: newer class of antibiotics; active against aerobic gram-positive bacteria by inhibiting protein synthesis

Red man syndrome: adverse reaction when vancomycin is administered too quickly; characterized by hypotension, flushing, and skin rash

Streptogramins: class of antibacterial drugs; produced by _Streptomyces graminofaciens_ bacteria

Vancomycin-resistant enterococci: pathogenic bacteria that are resistant to vancomycin

Vancomycin-resistant _Enterococcus faecium_ : _Enterococcus faecium_ that is resistant to vancomycin

Introduction

The drugs described in this chapter are heterogeneous in their antimicrobial spectra, characteristics, and clinical uses. Some are used often, and some are used only in specific circumstances. The drugs to be described in the following sections include the macrolides, ketolides, and miscellaneous anti-infective agents. The Drugs at a Glance tables present information about individual drugs and the prototype drugs, with routes of administration and dosage ranges.

Macrolides

The **macrolides**, which include erythromycin, azithromycin, and clarithromycin, have similar antibacterial spectra and mechanisms of action. Macrolides are widely distributed into body tissues and fluids and may be bacteriostatic or bactericidal, depending on drug concentration in infected tissues. They are effective against gram-positive cocci, including group A streptococci, pneumococci, and most staphylococci. They are also effective against species of _Corynebacterium_, _Treponema_, _Legionella_, _Chlamydia_, _Neisseria_, and _Mycoplasma_ and against some anaerobic species of genera such as _Bacteroides_ and _Clostridia_.

The prototype macrolide is Ⓟ **erythromycin.** This drug is now used less often because of microbial resistance, numerous drug interactions, and the development of newer macrolides. Compared with erythromycin, the newer drugs, such as azithromycin and clarithromycin, have enhanced antibacterial activity, require less frequent administration, and cause less nausea, vomiting, and diarrhea (see Other Drugs in the Class). Erythromycin is available in several preparations. Ophthalmic and topical preparations are discussed in Chapters 58 and 60, respectively.

Pharmacokinetics

The oral preparation of erythromycin is absorbed in the small intestine and has an onset of action in 1 to 2 hours. The medication reaches its peak in 1 to 4 hours. The intravenous (IV) preparation has a rapid onset of action, reaching a peak of action in less than 1 hour. Both the oral and parenteral forms cross the placenta and enter the breast milk. Erythromycin is metabolized in the liver by the cytochrome P450 3A4 (CYP3A4) isoenzymes and excreted mainly in bile; approximately 20% is excreted in urine. Depending on the specific salt formulation used, food can have a variable effect on the absorption of oral erythromycin.

Action

Erythromycin enters the microbial cells and reversibly binds to the 50S subunits of ribosomes, thereby inhibiting microbial protein synthesis and leading to cell death. The medication has bacteriostatic or bactericidal activity against susceptible bacteria.

Use

Erythromycin is useful as a penicillin substitute in patients who are allergic to penicillin; for prevention of rheumatic fever, gonorrhea, syphilis, pertussis, and chlamydial conjunctivitis in newborns (ophthalmic ointment); and to treat other infections (e.g., Legionnaire's disease, genitourinary infections caused by _Chlamydia trachomatis_, intestinal amebiasis caused by _Entamoeba histolytica_). The drug is administered for upper respiratory infections caused by group A beta-hemolytic streptococci. It is used for with sulfonamides for upper respiratory infections caused by _Haemophilus influenzae_. Prophylactically, erythromycin is administered to prevent alpha-hemolytic streptococcal endocarditis before dental or other procedures in patients who have valvular heart disease and are allergic to

TABLE 19.1

DRUGS AT A GLANCE: Macrolides

Drug	Pregnancy Category	Routes and Dosage Ranges	
		Adults	Children
Ⓟ **Erythromycin** (E-mycin)	B	250–500 mg PO every 6–12 h Severe infections: up to 4 g daily in divided doses	PO 30–50 mg/kg/d PO in divided doses every 6–12 h
Erythromycin ethylsuccinate (E.E.S.)	B	250–500 PO mg every 6–12 h Severe infections: up to 4 g daily in divided doses	30–50 mg/kg/d PO in divided doses every 6–12 h
Erythromycin lactobionate	B	15–20 mg/kg/d IV in divided doses every 6 h or 500 mg–1 g every 6 h or may be given as a continuous infusion over 24 h (max dose 4 g/d) Severe infections: up to 4 g daily in divided doses	15–50 mg/kg/d IV in divided doses every 6 h, not to exceed 4 g/d
Erythromycin stearate (Erythrocin stearate)	B	250 mg every 6 h or 500 mg every 12 h PO Severe infections: up to 4 g daily in divided doses	30–50 mg/kg/d PO in 2–4 divided doses
Azithromycin (Zithromax)	B	Respiratory and skin infections: 500 mg PO as a single dose on day 1, then 250 mg once daily for 4 d (Zpak) Nongonococcal urethritis and cervicitis caused by C. trachomatis, 1 g as a single dose MAC: prevention, 1200 mg PO once per week; treatment, 600 mg PO once daily Bacterial sinusitis: Tri-pak 500 mg PO daily for 3 d, or Zmax extended-release formula 2 g PO as a single dose CAP: IV 500 mg daily for at least 2 d followed by 500 mg PO daily for total of 7–10 d treatment	6 mo to 2 y, otitis media: 10 mg/kg PO on day 1 (not to exceed 500 mg), then 5 mg/kg once daily for 4 d (not to exceed 250 mg/d) 2 y and older, pharyngitis/tonsillitis: 12 mg/kg PO (not to exceed 500 mg) once daily for 5 d
Clarithromycin (Biaxin, Biaxin XL)	C	250–500 mg PO every 12 h for 7–14 d Prevention/treatment of MAC: 500 mg PO every 12 h or 1000 mg XL daily Bronchitis and CAP (extended-release): 1000 mg daily PO for 7 d Acute maxillary sinusitis: 1000 mg PO daily for 14 d	7.5 mg/kg PO, not to exceed 500 mg every 12 h Prevention/treatment of MAC: same as above

IV, intravenous; CAP, community-acquired pneumonia; MAC, *Mycobacterium avium* complex.

penicillin. Table 19.1 provides route and dosage information for erythromycin and other macrolides.

Use in Patients With Hepatic Impairment

Using erythromycin warrants caution, if the drug is given at all, to patients with hepatic impairment, because it is metabolized in the liver to an active metabolite that is excreted in the bile. Avoiding the drug or dosage reduction may be necessary in hepatic failure. It has also been associated with cholestatic hepatitis.

Use in Patients With Critical Illness

Erythromycin is seldom used in critical care settings, partly because broader spectrum bactericidal drugs are usually needed in critically ill patients and partly because it inhibits liver metabolism and slows elimination of several other drugs. For a critically ill patient who needs a macrolide antibiotic, one of the newer macrolides is preferred because the newer drugs have activity against several groups of microorganisms and fewer effects on the metabolism of other drugs.

Adverse Effects

Erythromycin may result in several adverse effects. Gastrointestinal (GI) effects include nausea, vomiting, diarrhea, cramping, anorexia, hepatotoxicity, and pseudomembranous colitis. If fever and jaundice occur after 1 to 2 weeks of drug administration, they subside after the drug is discontinued. Central nervous system (CNS) effects are reversible hearing loss, confusion, lability of emotions, and alterations in thought processes. Cardiac effects, with the IV form of the drug, include possible ventricular dysrhythmias. Allergic reactions include redness of the skin, rash, bronchospasm, or anaphylaxis.

Contraindications

Contraindications to erythromycin include a known hypersensitivity reaction to the drug or any macrolide. As previously stated, hepatic insufficiency requires careful use. The U.S. Food and Drug Administration (FDA) has issued a **BLACK BOX WARNING** ◆ regarding erythromycin estolate, a Canadian preparation of erythromycin; administration to patients with known liver disease warrants caution. Women who are breast-feeding should not take erythromycin because the drug is concentrated in the breast milk. This can alter the bowel flora of the infant and interfere with fever assessments. Also, people should not take erythromycin if they are concurrently using drugs highly dependent on CYP3A4 liver enzymes for metabolism.

Nursing Implications

Preventing Interactions

Many medication and herbs interact with erythromycin, increasing or decreasing its effects (Boxes 19.1 and 19.2).

In addition, as stated previously, the CYP3A4 isoenzymes in the liver metabolize erythromycin. The drug interacts with other drugs metabolized by the same isoenzyme and interferes with the elimination of several drugs. As a result, the affected drugs are eliminated more slowly, their serum

---

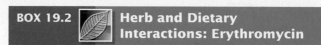

BOX 19.1 Drug Interactions: Erythromycin

Drugs That Increase the Effects of Erythromycin
- Chloramphenicol
  Increases effectiveness against strains of resistant S. aureus
- Streptomycin
  Increases effectiveness against Enterococcus in bacteremia, brain abscess, endocarditis, meningitis, and urinary tract infection

Drugs That Decrease the Effects of Erythromycin
- Antacids, calcium, magnesium, aluminum, and zinc
  Decrease antibiotic absorption
- Etravirine and lincosamide antibiotics
  Decrease serum concentration of erythromycin
- Ethanol
  Decreases the absorption of erythromycin

BOX 19.2 Herb and Dietary Interactions: Erythromycin

Herbs and Foods That Decrease the Effects of Erythromycin
- Grapefruit juice
  Decreases antibiotic absorption
- St. John's Wort
  Decreases antibiotic absorption

---

levels are increased, and they are more likely to cause adverse effects and toxicity unless the erythromycin dosage is reduced. In combination with potent inhibitors of CYP3A4 (e.g., fluconazole, diltiazem), erythromycin increases the risk of sudden cardiac death. A partial list of other interacting drugs includes carbamazepine (Tegretol), cyclosporine (Sandimmune), digoxin (Lanoxin), disopyramide (Norpace), lopinavir/ritonavir (Kaletra), lovastatin (Mevacor), nevirapine (Viramune), pimozide (Orap), quinidine, rifampin (Rifadin), ritonavir (Norvir), simvastatin (Zocor), theophylline (Theo-Dur), triazolam (Halcion), and warfarin (Coumadin). These drugs represent a variety of drug classes.

Administering the Medication

It is necessary to take oral erythromycin according to manufacturer's instructions. Drinking 6 to 8 ounces of water with the medication is important; adequate water aids absorption of the medication. It is necessary to take the drug on an empty stomach at evenly spaced intervals around the clock. Regular intervals help maintain therapeutic blood levels. People should not take erythromycin after taking antacids. Antacids decrease the absorption of both the tablet and suspension form of erythromycin.

The nurse may administer the IV administration preparation of erythromycin without regard to meals. It is important to consult the manufacturer's instructions for dissolving, diluting, and administering the parenteral form of erythromycin to achieve therapeutic effects. The IV formulation has limited stability in the solution. Also, instructions differ for intermittent and continuous infusions. The nurse infuses the medication in a peripheral or central IV site every 6 hours over 30 to 60 minutes.

Assessing Therapeutic Effects

The nurse assesses for decreased pain, fever, and malaise. Both the local and systemic signs of the infection are decreased, and the patient has decreased signs and symptoms of the specific infection for which erythromycin is being administered.

Assessing for Adverse Effects

With erythromycin, it is important to assess the patient's hearing. The loss of hearing is reversible with the discontinuation of the medication. The nurse also assesses for nausea, vomiting, and diarrhea. These symptoms may be severe and result in an alteration in acid–base balance. In addition, the nurse assesses for superinfection, as noted, with the development of pseudomembranous colitis. It is important to assess the patient's psychosocial responses that are adverse effects of erythromycin, such as crying, laughing, and altered thought processes. Finally, the nurse assesses for skin

BOX 19.3	Patient Teaching Guidelines for Erythromycin

- Erythromycin should be taken around the clock because it inhibits bacteria; it does not kill them.
- Take erythromycin on an empty stomach, 1 hour before meals or 2 to 3 hours after meals.
- Do not drink grapefruit juice while taking erythromycin.
- Complete the full course of the prescription.
- Do not take with or within 2 hours of dairy products or antacids.
- Take each dose with 8 ounces of water.
- Be aware that the effectiveness of oral contraceptives is decreased when combined with erythromycin.
- Adverse effects that you may experience include stomach cramping, gastrointestinal discomfort, labile emotions, crying, laughing, and abnormal thinking.
- Report severe or watery diarrhea, nausea, vomiting, dark urine, yellowing of the eyes or skin, loss of hearing, itching, and rash to your prescriber.

rash, urticaria, edema, dermatitis, and bronchospasm. These symptoms are indicative of an allergic reaction to erythromycin.

When administering the IV form of the drug, the nurse assesses the infusion site for phlebitis.

Patient Teaching

Box 19.3 identifies patient teaching guidelines for erythromycin.

Other Drugs in the Class

The macrolides azithromycin and clarithromycin are active against the atypical mycobacteria that cause **Mycobacterium avium complex** (MAC) disease. MAC disease (see Chap. 20) is an opportunistic infection that occurs mainly in people with advanced human immunodeficiency virus (HIV) infection. *Helicobacter pylori*, a pathogen implicated in peptic ulcer disease, is also susceptible to treatment with azithromycin or clarithromycin as part of a combination regimen (see Chap. 35).

Azithromycin (Zithromax) is useful in the treatment of lower respiratory infections, pharyngitis, and tonsillitis caused by *Haemophilus ducreyi*, *H. influenzae*, *Moraxella catarrhalis*, and *Streptococcus pneumoniae*. Prescribers order the drug for children older than 6 months of age for otitis media. It is also effective for treatment of community-acquired pneumonia (CAP) caused by *S. pneumoniae* as well as for genital ulcer disease in men and pelvic inflammatory disease in women. As previously stated, people with advanced HIV take azithromycin for MAC.

The onset of action of azithromycin is rapid, with a peak of action in 2.5 to 3.2 hours. The duration of action is 24 hours. The medication is metabolized in the liver and is distributed extensively to the tissues, skin, lungs, sputum, tonsils, and cervix. A minimal amount enters the cerebrospinal fluid (CSF). Major elimination of the drug is in the bile, with only 6% of excretion in the urine. The mechanism of action is the inhibition of RNA-dependent protein synthesis at the chain elongation step; the drug binds to the 50S ribosomal subunit to block the involved transpeptide. The parenteral form of azithromycin is stable in 5% dextrose and water,

5% dextrose and lactated Ringer's solution, lactated Ringer's solution, normal saline, and all 5% dextrose and saline IV fluids.

The adverse effects of azithromycin are similar to those of erythromycin. Caution is necessary with azithromycin in patients who have gonorrhea, syphilis, pseudomembranous colitis, and hepatic and renal impairment, as well as in lactating women. Alfuzosin, amiodarone, and artemether combined with azithromycin can enhance QT elongations. Careful assessment of the cardiac status is crucial when these medications are combined. Close monitoring of the international normalized ratio (INR) and prothrombin time is necessary when azithromycin is administered with warfarin. Patients should take the oral medication on an empty stomach, 2 hours before or after the administration of aluminum- or magnesium-containing antacids.

Clarithromycin (Biaxin, Biaxin XL) is a macrolide administered for bronchitis, sinusitis, otitis media, MAC, peptic ulcer disease, pertussis, pharyngitis, tonsillitis, and pneumonia. Prescribers also order the drug for prophylactic use in patients with underlying cardiac conditions who are undergoing invasive procedures that predispose them to infective endocarditis. It is also useful in skin infections caused by *Staphylococcus aureus* and *Streptococcus pyogenes* as well as in duodenal ulcers caused by *H. pylori*.

Absorption of clarithromycin is rapid, and the serum half-life is 3 to 7 hours. The drug is 42% to 50% protein bound, and it is widely distributed to all body tissues except the CNS. The metabolism of the medication takes place partially in the liver with CYP3A4 and is converted to the active metabolite. Metabolism occurs in the liver, and elimination takes place in the urine, with 20% to 40% of the drug unchanged. (An additional 10% to 15% remains as the metabolite.) Clarithromycin binds to the 50S ribosome to inhibit protein synthesis. One of its metabolites is two times as active as the parent compound against certain organisms.

The adverse effects of clarithromycin are headache, rash, abnormal taste, nausea, vomiting, abdominal pain, and dyspepsia. People should not take the drug with ergot derivatives, pimozide, cisapride, astemizole, colchicine, or terfenadine due to the risk of increased levels of the medications and toxicity. Generally, people may take it with or without food; however, they should take the extended-release form on an empty stomach. As with the other macrolides, use of aluminum- or magnesium-containing antacids within 2 hours of administration of clarithromycin decreases absorption of the antibiotic.

Clinical Application 19-1

The home care nurse is visiting Mr. Nikki to assess his lung status and medication regimen. Along with azithromycin, Mr. Nikki is taking omeprazole 20 mg orally daily for gastric reflux and 30 mL of Maalox at night. Since his myocardial infarction 6 months ago, he has been also taking warfarin 2 mg orally daily.

- The nurse is educating Mr. Nikki on all aspects of azithromycin. Identify all aspects of patient teaching to be provided to him.
- What instructions does the nurse provide regarding the other medications Mr. Nikki is taking?
- What laboratory tests are important to monitor during the administration of azithromycin?

NCLEX Success

1. A patient is admitted to the critical care unit with a diagnosis of Legionnaire's disease. Based on your knowledge of pharmacology, which medication is the drug of choice to treat the infection?

   A. azithromycin
   B. clarithromycin
   C. erythromycin
   D. vancomycin

2. The nurse instructs a patient on the administration of clarithromycin. Which of the following patient teaching instructions is appropriate?

   A. Take the medication on an empty stomach.
   B. Take the medication with a calcium supplement.
   C. Take the medication with a class of milk.
   D. Take the medication with cheese.

3. A teenage boy receives a prescription for erythromycin for an upper respiratory tract infection. He complains that he cannot hear the teacher, who then sends him to the school nurse's office. After assessing the patient's hearing with a tuning fork, the nurse determines that his hearing is diminished. What is the most important nursing intervention?

   A. The nurse should notify the parents to call the physician; this is an adverse effect of erythromycin.
   B. The nurse should inform the parents of a physician who specializes in ear, nose, and throat surgery.
   C. The nurse should instruct the patient to stop taking the erythromycin and his hearing will improve.
   D. The nurse should call the physician and inform the patient of a change in antibiotics.

4. A parent of a high school student calls the school nurse regarding her daughter's crying. The parent states that this behavior is unusual for her daughter. Which of the following medications contributes to changes in behavior?

   A. metronidazole
   B. naproxen sodium
   C. vitamin C
   D. erythromycin

5. A man had rheumatic fever as a child. He has an appointment for a tooth extraction. His dentist prescribes which of the following medications prior to the extraction?

   A. chloramphenicol
   B. vancomycin
   C. clarithromycin
   D. digoxin

Ketolides

The **ketolides** are related to the macrolides. ℗ **Telithromycin** (Ketek) is the prototype medication of this class. In addition to sharing the general spectrum of activity of the newer macrolides, it offers better activity against macrolide-resistant strains of *S. pneumoniae*, an increasingly common cause of infections in children and adults.

Pharmacokinetics

Telithromycin is rapidly absorbed with a peak of action in 1/2 to 4 hours. The drug is metabolized by the liver utilizing CYP3A4 and non–CYP-mediated pathways, with 60% to 70% protein bound with the majority bound to albumin. The drug's half-life is 10 hours. The urine and feces eliminate it.

Action

Telithromycin inhibits protein synthesis by binding to the 50S ribosomal unit and altering secretion of interleukin (IL)-1alpha and tumor necrosis factor (TNF)-alpha. The drug has bacteriostatic and bactericidal action on susceptible bacteria.

Use

Telithromycin is administered for the treatment of CAP caused by *S. pneumoniae*, *H. influenzae*, *Mycoplasma pneumoniae*, *M. catarrhalis*, *Bordetella pertussis*, and *Chlamydophila pneumoniae*. No adjustment in dosage is necessary for patients with hepatic impairment. Table 19.2 provides route and dosage information for telithromycin.

Use in Patients With Renal Impairment

For patients who have renal impairment, together with hepatic impairment, it is essential to reduce the dosage to 400 mg once daily. For patients with a creatinine clearance less than 30 mL per minute who are receiving dialysis, the nurse administers the medication following a dialysis session.

Adverse Effects

Cardiovascular adverse effects of telithromycin are prolonged QT interval and torsade de pointes. CNS effects include headache, dizziness, and vertigo. As for other anti-infective agents, GI-related effects include diarrhea, nausea, vomiting, alterations in taste, and pseudomembranous colitis. Superinfection, visual disturbances, and anaphylaxis may also occur.

Contraindications

Contraindications to telithromycin include a hypersensitivity reaction to macrolides or telithromycin. Concurrent administration of the drug with cisapride or pimozide should not occur due to decreased medication metabolism and possible prolonged QT wave. The FDA has issued a **BLACK BOX WARNING ◆** related to the administration of telithromycin to patients with myasthenia gravis. Life-threatening respiratory failure has occurred.

Nursing Implications

Preventing Interactions

Telithromycin is a potent CYP3A4 inhibitor. Combination of this drug with several medications results in an increased serum concentration of these other drugs. These medications are

TABLE 19.2

DRUGS AT A GLANCE: Ketolides (Telithromycin)

Drug	Pregnancy Category	Routes and Dosage Ranges	
		Adults	Children
Ⓟ **Telithromycin** (Ketek)	C	600 mg PO once daily for 7–10 d	Safety and efficacy not established

alfuzosin, alosetron, vinca alkaloids, aripiprazole, bortezomib, brentuximab, budesonide, cardiac glycosides, colchicine, conivaptan, corticosteroids, dronedarone, dutasteride, eplerenone, everolimus, fentanyl, fesoterodine, fluticasone, maraviroc, propafenone, sildenafil, tolterodine, vardenafil, vemurafenib, vilazodone, and zuclopenthixol. *Serum concentrations of digoxin are increased when combined with telithromycin.*

Many other medications interact with telithromycin, increasing or decreasing its effects (Box 19.4). St. John's wort decreases the therapeutic level of telithromycin.

Assessing for Therapeutic Effects

The nurse assesses for a decrease in the symptoms of CAP such as chest pain, fever, and productive cough. The patient has clear sputum.

Assessing for Adverse Effects

The nurse assesses the electrocardiogram for prolonged QT intervals. Also, it is important to assess for headache, dizziness, and vertigo. In addition, the nurse assesses for diarrhea, bloody diarrhea, and pseudomembranous colitis. Finally, it is essential to assess for visual changes or hypersensitivity reactions.

Patient Teaching

Box 19.5 identifies patient teaching guidelines for telithromycin.

BOX 19.4　Drug Interactions: Telithromycin

Drugs That Increase the Effects of Telithromycin

■ Atorvastatin, lovastatin, midazolam, pimozide, and simvastatin
Increase serum concentrations

■ Alfuzosin, artemether, chloroquine, ciprofloxacin, disopyramide, dronedarone, gadobutrol, indacaterol, lumefantrine, nilotinib, pimozide, quetiapine, quinine, tetrabenazine, thioridazine, toremifene, vandetanib,and ziprasidone
Produce prolonged QT

Drugs That Decrease the Effects of Telithromycin

■ Carbamazepine, phenobarbital, phenytoin, and rifampin
Decrease serum levels and lead to loss of therapeutic effectiveness

Clinical Application 19-2

Mr. Nikko develops symptoms of community-acquired pneumonia. He has a temperature of 103°F; a productive cough with yellow, thick tenacious sputum; and right-sided chest pain. His prescriber orders telithromycin 400 mg orally daily.

- The recommended dosage of telithromycin is 600 mg PO daily. What is the rationale for the diminished dose of telithromycin?
- What is the action of telithromycin?
- What patient teaching does the nurse provide to Mr. Nikko?

NCLEX Success

6. Which of the following adverse effects of telithromycin indicates a superinfection?

   A. diarrhea
   B. bloody diarrhea
   C. nausea
   D. vomiting

7. Torsade de pointes is a lengthened QT interval. Which of the following medications combined with telithromycin results in this condition?

   A. acetaminophen
   B. naproxen sodium
   C. regular insulin
   D. ciprofloxacin

8. A patient is prescribed telithromycin 800 mg orally for community-acquired pneumonia. Prior to administering the medication, the nurse reviews the patient's laboratory values. Which of the following laboratory values would recommend a reduction in dosage to 400 mg? (Select all that apply.)

   A. creatinine, 3.3 mg per dL
   B. alanine aminotransferase, 98 units per L
   C. aspartate aminotransferase, 60 units per L
   D. sodium, 145 mEq per L

| BOX 19.5 | Patient Teaching Guidelines for Telithromycin |

- Swallow the tablets whole. Do not chew or crush them.
- Take the tablets without regard to food.
- If you have gastrointestinal upset when taking the tablets, eat some food when you take them.
- Take the tablets with a full glass of water.
- Take the pills at the same time every day.
- Do not look quickly between objects in the distance if visual difficulties result.
- Complete the full course of the prescription.
- Report bloody diarrhea, rash, fainting, or yellowing of the eyes or skin to your prescriber.
- Maintain safety if headache, dizziness, or vertigo result.
- Do not drive or operate machinery if you have visual disturbances.

Miscellaneous Anti-Infective Agents

The miscellaneous anti-infective agents have properties similar to those of other drug classes, and they belong to new classes. To simplify the understanding of these medications, they are introduced in a summary format. The medications discussed in this section include chloramphenicol, clindamycin, daptomycin, tigecycline, linezolid, metronidazole, quinupristin–dalfopristin, rifaximin, spectinomycin, and vancomycin. Table 19.3 summarizes route and dosage information for these antibacterial drugs.

QSEN Safety Alert

Prior to beginning therapy with anti-infective agents, it is necessary to review the prescriber's orders and culture the suspected site of infection. The culture and sensitivity report determines the anti-infective agent that is most effective in treating the infection.

This is particularly important before starting vancomycin, quinupristin–dalfopristin, daptomycin, or linezolid. These drugs have relatively narrow spectra of activity, and it is critical to determine appropriate indications for their use to decrease the likelihood of resistance.

Chloramphenicol

Chloramphenicol (Chloromycetin) is a broad-spectrum, bacteriostatic antibiotic that is active against most gram-positive and gram-negative bacteria, rickettsiae, chlamydiae, and treponemes. It acts by interfering with microbial protein synthesis. It is well absorbed and diffuses well into body tissues and fluids, including CSF, but low drug levels are obtained in urine. It is metabolized in the liver and excreted in the urine.

Chloramphenicol is rarely used now to treat infections because of the effectiveness and low toxicity of alternative drugs. However, it is still used in serious infections for which no adequate substitute drug is available. Specific infections include meningococcal, pneumococcal, or *Haemophilus pneumoniae* type b (Hib) meningitis in penicillin-allergic patients; anaerobic brain abscess; *Bacteroides fragilis* infections; and rickettsial infections and brucellosis when tetracyclines are contraindicated. In infections due to **vancomycin-resistant enterococci (VRE)**, pathogenic bacteria that are resistant to vancomycin, chloramphenicol is effective against some enterococcal strains.

Chloramphenicol is associated with several adverse effects. The FDA has issued a **BLACK BOX WARNING** ◆ reporting the development of serious and fatal blood dyscrasias with chloramphenicol use. Irreversible bone marrow depression, which may lead to aplastic anemia, may appear weeks or months after therapy. A dose-related reversible bone marrow depression usually responds to discontinuation of the drug. Monitoring with a complete blood count, platelet count, reticulocyte count, and serum iron test every 2 days is essential. Experts recommend that patients be hospitalized to facilitate close monitoring. In addition, periodic measurements of serum drug levels are recommended when possible. Therapeutic levels are 5 to 20 μg per mL. Discontinuation of therapy should occur as soon as possible, and use of the drug for trivial infections or for prophylaxis of infections should not take place. Also, chloramphenicol concentrations may increase in patients with impaired renal function. Dose adjustments may be necessary. In addition, the patient may need an increase in dietary riboflavin, pyridoxine, and vitamin B_{12}. It is important to consult a dietician regarding dietary needs.

Neonates should not receive chloramphenicol because of the risk of **gray syndrome**, a dangerous condition that occurs in newborns. Symptoms of gray syndrome begin 3 to 4 days after the drug is administered. Infants present with abdominal distention, progressive pallid cyanosis, vasomotor collapse, irregular respirations, and death. If drug therapy is stopped within a few hours of symptom onset of gray syndrome, affected infants will recover. Infants are also at risk for gray syndrome if their mothers are receiving chloramphenicol and are breast-feeding.

When administering chloramphenicol, the nurse reconstitutes the drug in 50 to 100 mL of 5% dextrose and water and infuses it over 15 to 30 minutes. Chloramphenicol combined with rifampin or phenobarbital results in accelerated hepatic metabolism of chloramphenicol.

Clindamycin

Clindamycin hydrochloride (Cleocin), a **lincosamide**, is similar to the macrolides in its mechanism of action and antimicrobial spectrum. Bacteriostatic in usual doses, this drug is effective against gram-positive cocci, including group A streptococci, pneumococci, most staphylococci, and some anaerobes such as *Bacteroides* and *Clostridia*. Clindamycin enters microbial cells and attaches to 50S subunits of ribosomes, thereby inhibiting microbial protein synthesis.

Clindamycin is often used to treat infections caused by *B. fragilis*. Because these bacteria are usually mixed with gram-negative organisms from the gynecologic or GI tracts, prescribers usually order that clindamycin be given with another drug, such as an aminoglycoside or a fluoroquinolone, to treat mixed infections. The drug may be useful as a penicillin substitute in patients who are allergic to penicillin and who have serious streptococcal, staphylococcal, or pneumococcal infections in which

TABLE 19.3

DRUGS AT A GLANCE: Miscellaneous Anti-Infective Agents

Drug	Pregnancy Category	Routes and Dosage Ranges	
		Adults	*Children*
Chloramphenicol (Chloromycetin)	C	IV 50–100 mg/kg/d in divided doses every 6 h (max dose 4 g/d)	Meningitis (infants older than 30 d and children): 50–100 mg/kg/d in divided doses every 6 h Other infections (infants older than 30 d and children): 50–75 mg/kg/d in divided doses every 6 h (max daily dose 4 g)
Clindamycin hydrochloride (Cleocin)	B	150–450 mg PO every 6–8 h (max dose 1.8 g/d) 1.2–2.7 g/d IM or IV in 2–4 divided doses; max dose: 4.8 g/d	PO 8–16 mg/kg/d in divided doses every 6–8 h; up to 20 mg/kg/d in severe infections Neonates, 15–20 mg/kg/d in divided doses every 6–8 h 1 mo and older, IM, IV 20–40 mg/kg/d in divided doses every 6–8 h; up to 40 mg/kg/d in severe infections
Daptomycin (Cubicin)	B	Skin/soft tissue infections: 4 mg/kg IV every 24 h for 7–14 d MSSA, MRSA bacteremia or right-sided endocarditis: 6 mg/kg/d for 2–6 wk	Safety and efficacy not established
Linezolid (Zyvox)	C	400–600 mg PO or IV every 12 h for 10–28 d	Younger than 7 d, 10 mg/kg PO or IV every 12 h; 7 d–11 y, PO, IV 10 mg/kg every 8 h; 12 y and older: PO, IV 600 mg every 12 h
Metronidazole (Flagyl)	B	Anaerobic bacterial infection: 500 mg PO, IV every 6–8 h, not to exceed 4 g/d Surgical prophylaxis, colorectal surgery: 500 mg IV infused over 30–60 min 0.5–1 h before surgery C. *difficile* colitis: 250–500 mg PO every 6–8 h for 10–14 d	Anaerobic infections (older than 7 d and weight 1200–2000 g): 15 mg/kg/d PO, IV in divided doses every 12 h Anaerobic infections in children *older than* 7 d and weighing *more than* 2000 g: 30 mg/kg/d in divided doses every 12 h ≥1 mo, 15–35 mg/kg/d PO in divided doses every 8 h; 30 mg/kg/d IV in divided doses every 6 h
Quinupristin–dalfopristin (Synercid)	B	Skin and skin structure infections: 7.5 mg/kg IV over 60 min every 12 h VREF bacteremia: 7.5 mg/kg IV over 60 min every 8 h	Same as adults Shunt infection due to VRE: 7.5 mg/kg/dose every 8 h
Rifaximin (Xifaxan)	C	200 mg PO 3 times daily for 3 d	12 y and older: same as adults
Tigecycline (Tygacil)	D	100 mg IV single dose initially; maintenance dose 50 mg every 12 h for 5–14 d	Dosage and safety not established
Vancomycin (Vancocin)	B	Antibiotic-associated pseudomembranous colitis: 100–500 mg PO every 6 h (PO dose not for treating systemic infections) 20–45 mg/kg/d IV in divided doses	Antibiotic-associated pseudomembranous colitis: 40 PO mg/kg/d in divided doses every 6–8 h (PO dose not for treating systemic infections) 1 mo and older, 10–15 mg/kg IV every 6 h

IV, intravenous; MRSA, methicillin-resistant *Staphylococcus aureus*; MSSA, methicillin-susceptible *Staphylococcus aureus*; VREF, vancomycin-resistant *Enterococcus faecium*; VRE, vancomycin-resistant enterococci.

the causative organism is susceptible to clindamycin (including prevention of perinatal group B streptococcal disease). A topical solution is useful in the treatment of acne, and a vaginal cream is available. Clindamycin does not reach therapeutic concentrations in the CNS and cannot be used for treating meningitis.

Clindamycin is well absorbed with oral administration and reaches peak plasma levels within 1 hour after a dose. It is widely distributed in body tissues and fluids, except CSF, and it crosses the placenta. It is highly bound (90%) to plasma proteins. It is metabolized in the liver, and the metabolites are excreted in the bile and urine.

Adverse effects associated with clindamycin are many. It may be necessary to reduce the dosage in patients with severe hepatic failure to prevent accumulation and toxic effects. The FDA has issued a **BLACK BOX WARNING** ◆ for clindamycin regarding the potential of severe and possible fatal colitis. If diarrhea develops in a patient receiving clindamycin, discontinuation of the drug is essential. With severe and persistent diarrhea, it is critical to check the stools for white blood cells, blood, mucus, and the presence of *Clostridium difficile* toxin. It may be necessary to perform sigmoidoscopy to more definitively determine whether the patient has pseudomembranous colitis. The appearance of lesions on sigmoidoscopy means that the clindamycin should be stopped immediately. Although pseudomembranous colitis may occur with any antibiotic, it has often been associated with clindamycin therapy. Other adverse effects of clindamycin include nausea and vomiting.

Neonates and infants should receive clindamycin only if the drug is clearly indicated, and then monitoring of liver and kidney function is necessary. Diarrhea and pseudomembranous colitis may occur with topical clindamycin for treatment of acne. Clindamycin should be used cautiously in patients with liver impairment since it is excreted through the liver.

People should take oral clindamycin with a full glass of water to avoid esophageal irritation. It is important to *not* refrigerate the reconstituted oral solution. When administering clindamycin intramuscularly, the nurse gives no more than 600 mg in one injection. To avoid pain, induration, and abscess formation, it is necessary to administer the medication into the deep tissues. When administering clindamycin intravenously, the nurse dilutes 300 to 600 mg of the drug in 50 mL of IV fluid and gives it over 10 to 20 minutes, or he or she dilutes 900 mg in 50 to 100 mL and administers it over 20 minutes. The dilution of the medication in IV fluids decreases the risk of phlebitis. The patient is at risk for cardiac arrest if the medication is administered as a bolus. It is important that clindamycin not be administered with erythromycin; the combination decreases the effects of clindamycin.

Daptomycin

Daptomycin (Cubicin) belongs to the **lipopeptide** class, a new class of antibiotics. It is a bactericidal agent effective only for gram-positive infections due to *S. aureus* (including oxacillin-resistant strains), *S. pyogenes*, group B streptococci, and *Enterococcus faecalis* (vancomycin-susceptible strains only). In combination with gentamicin, daptomycin is synergistic in killing staphylococci and enterococci. Indications are limited to the treatment of complicated skin and skin structure infections caused by the above organisms.

Available only for IV administration, daptomycin reaches target concentrations by the third daily dose. The drug is excreted primarily by the kidneys. Its mechanism of action is unique. Daptomycin kills bacteria by inhibiting synthesis of bacterial proteins, DNA, and RNA.

The most common adverse effects of daptomycin are constipation, nausea, diarrhea, and vomiting. Adverse musculoskeletal effects have occurred, primarily at increased serum creatine kinase (CK) levels. These effects are usually asymptomatic, but it is necessary to discontinue the drug in patients who develop muscle pain or weakness. Unexplained increases in serum CK levels associated with symptoms of myopathy should have a prompt discontinuation of daptomycin. Also, if daptomycin is combined with "statin" cholesterol-lowering medications, the risk of musculoskeletal adverse effects is greater. If possible, concomitant use of these "statins" should be avoided. In addition, no information regarding use in children or during pregnancy and lactation is available.

When administering daptomycin intravenously, the nurse mixes the daptomycin with normal saline or lactated Ringer's solution and infuses it over 30 minutes. The drug is incompatible with dextrose-containing IV solutions.

Linezolid

Linezolid (Zyvox) is a member of the **oxazolidinone** class, a newer class of antibiotics. It is active against aerobic gram-positive bacteria. The drug exhibits bactericidal activity against most staphylococci, enterococci, and streptococci. It is indicated for pneumonia (both community-acquired and nosocomial), complicated and uncomplicated skin and skin structure infections, and **vancomycin-resistant *Enterococcus faecium*** (VREF) infections. The drug is bacteriostatic against enterococci (including *E. faecalis* and *E. faecium*) and staphylococci (including methicillin-resistant strains) and bactericidal for most streptococci.

Linezolid acts by inhibiting protein synthesis by a unique mechanism. The drug binds to the bacterial 23S ribosomal RNA of the 50S subunit, thus preventing an essential component of the bacterial translation process. It is well absorbed orally, distributes widely, and undergoes hepatic elimination.

The FDA has issued a **BLACK BOX WARNING** ◆ stating that linezolid should not be administered to patients who are currently taking selective serotonin reuptake inhibitors, serotonin–norepinephrine reuptake inhibitors, tricyclic antidepressants, or monoamine oxidase inhibitors. It is thought that linezolid inhibits the action of monoamine oxidase A, an enzyme responsible for breaking down serotonin in the brain. Thus, high levels of serotonin build up in the brain, causing toxicity. This buildup of serotonin is referred to as serotonin syndrome. The patient presents with muscle twitching, excessive sweating, shivering, shaking, fever, and diarrhea. The combination results in severe CNS reactions. It is necessary to discontinue the psychiatric agent prior to administration of the linezolid and closely monitor the patient for CNS adverse effects. The nurse assesses for mental status changes, muscle twitching, shivering, and lack of coordination.

Also, myelosuppression (bone marrow depression; e.g., anemia, leukopenia, pancytopenia, thrombocytopenia) is a serious adverse effect that may occur with prolonged linezolid therapy, longer than 2 weeks. Monitoring of the patient's complete blood count is necessary; if myelosuppression occurs, discontinuation of the drug is warranted. Myelosuppression usually improves with drug discontinuation. Pseudomembranous colitis may also occur. Mild cases usually resolve with drug discontinuation; moderate or severe cases may require fluid and electrolyte replacement and an antibacterial drug that is effective against C. *difficile* organisms. Hypertension may occur with the concomitant ingestion of linezolid and adrenergic drugs (e.g., dopamine, epinephrine).

In 2007, an alert issued by the FDA noted an increased rate of death in people treated with linezolid for catheter-related bacteremia and catheter site infections and emphasized that linezolid is not approved for site infections or bacteremia due to catheters or for gram-negative infections. In 2011, another FDA alert stated that serious CNS reactions have been reported when linezolid is combined with selective serotonin reuptake inhibitors.

The effects of linezolid in pregnant women and in children are largely unknown. Because linezolid is a weak monoamine oxidase inhibitor, patients should avoid food high in tyramine content (aged cheeses, fermented or air-dried meats, sauerkraut, soy sauce, tap beers, red wine) while taking the drug.

When administering the IV preparation of linezolid, the nurse infuses the drug over 30 to 120 minutes. It is important to infuse no other medications with linezolid sequentially and flush the line with 5% dextrose and water, normal saline, or lactated Ringer's solution.

Metronidazole

Metronidazole (Flagyl) is effective against anaerobic bacteria, including gram-negative bacilli such as *Bacteroides*, gram-positive bacilli such as *Clostridia*, and some gram-positive cocci. The drug is also effective against protozoa that cause amebiasis, giardiasis, and trichomoniasis (see Chap. 23). It achieves therapeutic concentrations in body fluids and tissues and can be used to treat anaerobic brain abscesses. Metronidazole is eliminated by the liver and kidneys.

Clinical indications for metronidazole include prevention or treatment of anaerobic bacterial infections (e.g., in colorectal surgery, intra-abdominal infections) and treatment of C. *difficile* infections associated with pseudomembranous colitis. As part of a combination regimen, the drug is also useful in treatment of infections due to H. *pylori*. It is contraindicated during the first trimester of pregnancy and must be used with caution in patients with CNS or blood disorders. The safety and efficacy of metronidazole have been established in children only for the treatment of amebiasis, although the drug is used for other infections in pediatric patients without reported unusual adverse effects.

Metronidazole has several adverse effects. Dermatological effects are skin rash, pruritus, and thrombophlebitis at the infusion site. CNS effects include seizures, peripheral paresthesias, ataxia, confusion, dizziness, and headache. The most common GI effects are nausea, vomiting, diarrhea, and metallic taste. The nurse tells the patient that consumption of alcohol when taking metronidazole will produce a disulfiram reaction. This reaction results in symptoms of flushing, headache, nausea, vomiting, and chest and abdominal pain.

Prior to administering metronidazole, it is important to review the manufacturer's instructions for administration. Metronidazole requires specific techniques for preparation and administration.

Quinupristin–Dalfopristin

Quinupristin–dalfopristin (Synercid) belongs to a class of antimicrobials referred to as **streptogramins**, produced by the bacterium *Streptomyces graminofaciens*. Both components are active antimicrobials that affect bacterial ribosomes to decrease protein synthesis. The combination is bacteriostatic against E. *faecium* (including vancomycin-resistant strains) and bactericidal against **methicillin-susceptible Staphylococcus aureus** (MSSA). It is not active against E. *faecalis*. Quinupristin–dalfopristin is indicated for skin and skin structure infections caused by S. *aureus* or group A streptococcus. It is also used for treatment of patients with serious or life-threatening infections associated with VREF bacteremia. However, a **BLACK BOX WARNING** ◆ reports that FDA approval for this use is based on the ability of quinupristin–dalfopristin to clear bacteria from the bloodstream rather than on its ability to cure the underlying infection. Further clinical studies are underway to verify the clinical benefits of the drug for curing VREF infections.

Quinupristin–dalfopristin undergoes biliary excretion and fecal elimination. The drug combination is a strong inhibitor of CYP3A4 enzymes and therefore interferes with the metabolism of drugs such as cyclosporine, antiretrovirals, carbamazepine, and many others. Toxicity may occur with the inhibited drugs.

When administering quinupristin–dalfopristin parenterally, the nurse mixes it in a minimum of 250 mL of 5% dextrose solution and infuses it over 60 minutes to decrease venous irritation. Medication toxicity may occur if it is administered in shorter infusion times. To decrease irritation, it may be necessary to use a central venous catheter for drug administration. The medication is not to be mixed with any other drug. The IV line should not be flushed with saline- or heparin-containing solutions. Quinupristin–dalfopristin is incompatible with saline- and heparin-containing solutions. The medication is compatible with anidulafungin, aztreonam, caspofungin, ciprofloxacin, fenoldopam, fluconazole, haloperidol, metoclopramide, and potassium chloride. When administering quinupristin–dalfopristin with these medications, the nurse must infuse them with 5% dextrose and water.

Rifaximin

Rifaximin (Xifaxan) is a structural analog of rifampin. It is useful in infectious (travelers') diarrhea due to *Escherichia coli* but is not effective in diarrhea due to *Campylobacter jejuni* (see Chap. 38). Whether rifaximin is effective to treat diarrhea due to *Shigella* or *Salmonella* species is not known. Because of its very limited systemic absorption (97% eliminated in feces), health care providers cannot use rifaximin to treat systemic infections, including infections due to invasive strains of E. *coli*. Therefore, diarrhea occurring with fever or bloody stools requires treatment with alternative agents. After treatment with rifaximin begins, patients reporting worsening or persistent diarrhea for longer than 24 to 48 hours, fever, or blood in the stool should receive therapy with an alternative agent. Patients may take rifaximin before or after meals.

Adverse effects of rifaximin are flatulence, headache, abdominal pain, nausea, constipation, and vomiting. Prolonged use of rifaximin may result in bacterial or fungal superinfection.

The patient may develop C. *difficile* or pseudomembranous colitis more than 2 months after the discontinuation of antibiotic therapy.

Tigecycline

Tigecycline (Tygacil) is a **glycylcycline** anti-infective agent structurally related to the tetracyclines. Health care providers use it for CAP, complicated intra-abdominal infections, and skin or skin structure infections. The drug has both bactericidal and bacteriostatic properties. It is a derivative of minocycline but is not classified as a tetracycline. Tigecycline is effective in treating **methicillin-resistant *Staphylococcus aureus* (MRSA)**. The drug is distributed extensively to the tissues and is highly protein bound. The medication is metabolized in the liver and excreted in the feces and urine. It acts by binding to the 30S ribosome of susceptible bacteria to inhibit protein synthesis.

The nurse administers tigecycline intravenously over 30 to 60 minutes in a dedicated IV line or a Y-site connection. The medication is stable in normal saline, lactated Ringer's solution, and 5% dextrose and water. It is incompatible with amphotericin B, chlorpromazine, diazepam, methylprednisolone, sodium succinate, and voriconazole.

Vancomycin

Vancomycin (Vancocin) is active only against gram-positive microorganisms. Parenteral vancomycin has been used extensively to treat infections caused by MRSA and **methicillin-resistant staphylococcal species non-aureus** (SSNA, including *Staphylococcus epidermidis*) as well as endocarditis caused by *Streptococcus viridans* (in patients allergic to or with infections resistant to penicillins and cephalosporins) or *E. faecalis* (with an aminoglycoside).

S. pneumoniae remain susceptible to vancomycin, although vancomycin-tolerant strains have been identified. Prophylactic use of the drug for gram-positive infections in patients who are at high risk of developing MRSA infections (e.g., those with diabetes, previous hospitalization, or MRSA in their nasal passages) and who require placement of long-term intravascular catheters and other invasive treatment or monitoring devices is extensive. Oral vancomycin is useful only to treat staphylococcal enterocolitis and pseudomembranous colitis caused by C. *difficile*.

Partly because of this widespread use, health care providers encounter VRE more often, especially in critical care units, and treatment options for infections caused by these organisms are limited. To decrease the spread of VRE, the Centers for Disease Control and Prevention (CDC) recommends limiting the use of vancomycin. Specific recommendations include avoiding or minimizing use in empiric treatment of febrile patients with neutropenia (unless the prevalence of MRSA or SSNA is high); in initial treatment for C. *difficile* colitis (metronidazole is preferred); and as prophylaxis for surgery, low birth weight infants, intravascular catheter colonization or infection, and peritoneal dialysis.

Vancomycin acts by inhibiting cell wall synthesis. Excretion of vancomycin occurs in the kidneys; it is necessary to reduce the dosage in the presence of renal impairment. In bacterial colitis, administration of vancomycin is oral because the drug is not absorbed from the GI tract and acts within the bowel lumen. Elimination of large amounts of vancomycin in the feces occurs after oral administration.

For systemic infections, administration of the drug is IV, and it reaches therapeutic plasma levels within 1 hour after infusion. It is very important to give IV infusions slowly, over 1 to 2 hours, to avoid an adverse reaction characterized by hypotension, flushing, and skin rash. This reaction, sometimes called **red man syndrome**, is attributed to histamine release. Close monitoring of serum drug levels of IV vancomycin is important. When administering IV vancomycin, the nurse dilutes 500-mg doses in 100 mL and 1-g doses in 200 mL of 0.9% NaCl or 5% dextrose injection and infuses it over at least 60 minutes.

EVIDENCE-BASED PRACTICE

Risk of Hepatic Events in Patients Treated With Vancomycin in Clinical Studies A Systemic Review and Meta-Analysis

by YAN CHEN, XIAO YAN YANG, MICHAEL ZECKEL, CHRIS KILLIAN, KENNETH HORNBUCKLE, ARIEREGEV, SIMON VOSS

Drug Safety
2011, 34(1), 73–82

Vancomycin is effective as a bactericidal agent against most gram-positive organisms, including penicillin-resistant S. *aureus*. The agent was discovered in 1956 but was not widely used until the 1980s. Early use of the drug revealed adverse effects of ototoxicity and nephrotoxicity. These adverse effects have decreased; the impurities of the drug have been eliminated. The Eli Lilly and Company reviewed the drug for safety from July 2007 to June 2008. During this review period, there were 14 cases of hepatic enzyme and bilirubin elevations with the administration of vancomycin. The company also conducted a systematic review of articles published several peer-reviewed medical and nursing journals from 1950 to 2010. The keywords in this search included vancomycin, clinical trial, therapeutic use, hepatocellular injury, drug-induced liver injury, hepatotoxicity, hepatic dysfunction, liver enzyme, and treatment outcome. The results revealed an increased incidence of hepatic events such as an elevation of alanine aminotransferase and aspartate aminotransferase in patients receiving vancomycin, but the majority of the events were considered mild to moderate. Thus, no evidence exists that the use of vancomycin places the patient at risk for progressive or severe drug-induced liver injury.

IMPLICATIONS FOR NURSING PRACTICE: The results of this study indicate that there is a mild to moderate risk of hepatotoxicity with vancomycin. It is important that the nurse monitor liver enzymes closely when the drug is used.

Clinical Application 19-3

Mr. Nikko develops bloody diarrhea that is positive for *C. difficile* on culture. His prescriber now orders vancomycin 500 mg orally every 6 hours.
- What is the action of vancomycin?
- Why is vancomycin administered orally?

NCLEX Success

9. A nurse practitioner sees a 19-year-old college student in the student health center for severe diarrhea. The nurse diagnoses travelers' diarrhea based on the young woman's history; she had recently returned from Mexico. She receives a prescription for rifaximin 200 mg orally three times daily for 3 days. Four days later, she calls the office and reports to the nurse that she has a fever and that the diarrhea has not resolved. Which of the following is the most appropriate information to communicate to the student?

   A. Advise the student to return to the clinic for further tests and a different antibiotic.

   B. Call the pharmacy and authorize one refill of rifaximin.

   C. Advise the student that it takes up to 48 to 72 hours after the completion of treatment for the diarrhea to completely resolve.

   D. Tell the student to continue to drink plenty of fluids and report back in 24 hours.

10. A recent nursing graduate is preparing to administer vancomycin to a man intravenously. The nurse states the patient reported that he experienced flushing with his last dose of vancomycin. The nurse should

   A. infuse the vancomycin over 30 minutes to decrease the chance of a reaction

   B. hold the vancomycin dose until the physician's rounds the following morning

   C. dilute the vancomycin in 50 mL of normal saline solution and infuse over 60 minutes

   D. contact the physician, report the reaction, and request an order for diphenhydramine pretreatment

The Nursing Process

Assessment

- Assess for infections that macrolides, ketolides, and the designated miscellaneous drugs are used to prevent or treat.

- Assess each patient for signs and symptoms of the specific current infection.
- Assess culture and susceptibility reports when available.
- Assess each patient for risk factors that increase risks of infection (e.g., immunosuppression) or risks of adverse drug reactions (e.g., impaired renal or hepatic function).

Nursing Diagnoses

- Deficient knowledge related to type of infection and appropriate use of prescribed antimicrobial drugs
- Risk for injury related to adverse drug effects
- Risk for injury related to infection with antibiotic-resistant microorganisms

Planning/Goals

The patient will

- Take or receive macrolides, ketolides, and miscellaneous antimicrobials accurately, for the prescribed length of time
- Experience decreased signs and symptoms of the infection being treated
- Be monitored regularly for therapeutic and adverse drug effects
- Verbalize and practice measures to prevent recurrent infection

Nursing Interventions

The nurse will

- Use measures to prevent and minimize the spread of infection (see Chap. 13).
- Monitor for fever and other signs and symptoms of infection.
- Monitor laboratory reports for indications of the patient's response to drug therapy (e.g., white blood cell count, tests of renal function).
- Encourage fluid intake to decrease fever and maintain good urinary tract function.
- Provide foods and fluids with adequate nutrients to maintain or improve nutritional status, especially if febrile and hypermetabolic.
- Assist patients to prevent or minimize infections with streptococci, staphylococci, and other gram-positive organisms.
- Provide appropriate patient teaching for any drug therapy (see accompanying display).

Evaluation

- Interview and observe for improvement in the infection being treated.
- Interview and observe for adverse drug effects.

Key Concepts

- Macrolides, which include erythromycin, azithromycin, and clarithromycin, inhibit microbial protein synthesis.

- The FDA has issued a **BLACK BOX WARNING** ◆ concerning erythromycin estolate, a Canadian preparation of erythromycin; administration to patients with known liver disease requires caution. The use of erythromycin concurrently with drugs highly dependent on CYP3A4 liver enzymes for metabolism is contraindicated.

- Erythromycin shares a similar antibacterial spectrum with penicillin, making it a good choice for patients with penicillin allergy.

- The ketolide telithromycin is approved only for CAP. Its mechanism of action is inhibition of microbial protein synthesis.

- The FDA has issued a **BLACK BOX WARNING** ◆ related to the administration of telithromycin to patients with myasthenia gravis. Life-threatening respiratory failure has occurred.

- Chloramphenicol, which is effective against some strains of VRE, is rarely used because of possible blood dyscrasias. The FDA has issued a **BLACK BOX WARNING** ◆ reporting serious and fatal blood dyscrasias with chloramphenicol administration.

- Clindamycin belongs to the lincosamide class of antimicrobials, similar to macrolides in its mechanism of action and antimicrobial spectrum.

- The FDA has issued a **BLACK BOX WARNING** ◆ for clindamycin regarding the potential for severe and possible fatal colitis.

- Daptomycin belongs to the lipopeptide class of antibiotics, which kills gram-positive bacteria by inhibiting synthesis of bacterial proteins, DNA, and RNA.

- Linezolid belongs to the oxazolidinone class of antibiotics. It is effective against MRSA and VRE.

- A **BLACK BOX WARNING** ◆ states that linezolid is contraindicated with selective serotonin reuptake inhibitors, serotonin–norepinephrine reuptake inhibitors, tricyclic antidepressants, and monoamine oxidase inhibitors.

- Metronidazole is effective against infections with anaerobic bacteria and some protozoa.

- Quinupristin–dalfopristin belongs to the streptogramin class of antibiotics. It is indicated for VREF and MSSA.

- A **BLACK BOX WARNING** ◆ for quinupristin–dalfopristin reports that FDA approval for use in VREF bacteremia is based on the ability of the drug to clear bacteria from the bloodstream rather than its ability to cure the underlying infection.

- Rifaximin is prescribed for travelers' diarrhea due to *E. coli* infection.

- Tigecycline is a glycylcycline anti-infective agent administered for CAP, complicated intra-abdominal infections, and skin or skin structure infections. It is distributed extensively to the tissues and is highly protein bound.

- Vancomycin is effective against gram-positive organisms only, including MRSA and SSNA.

Critical Thinking Questions

19-1. A 47-year-old woman with bipolar disorder is admitted to a hospital with a diagnosis of a vancomycin-resistant skin infection. She is taking lithium carbonate 300 mg orally three times per day. The medical intern orders linezolid 600 mg intravenously every 12 hours for 14 days.

- What is problematic about the use of linezolid and lithium carbonate?
- What is the action of linezolid (Zyvox)?
- What central nervous system adverse effects does the nurse need to assess for?
- Can the patient safely receive any other medications to treat her bipolar disorder?
- How is intravenous (IV) linezolid (Zyvox) administered?

19-2. A 38-year-old man sustained a construction-related injury 2 weeks ago. The wound site is reddened and draining. He is admitted to an infection control unit and placed on wound precautions. After obtaining a culture and sensitivity, a physician prescribes quinupristin–dalfopristin 7.5 mg per kg intravenously every 12 hours for 7 days.

- What organisms does quinupristin–dalfopristin effectively treat?
- The patient complains of severe venous irritation during the administration of the first dose. What action should the nurse take to prevent this discomfort with future infusions?
- Which IV fluid does the nurse use for quinupristin–dalfopristin administration?
- It is necessary to infuse quinupristin–dalfopristin for what length of time?
- The patient develops gastroesophageal reflux. An intern orders IV metoclopramide. What precaution does the nurse need to take in administering these two IV medications?

References and Resources

Chen, Y., Yang, X., Zeckel, M., Killian, C., Hornbuckle, K., & Regev, A. (2011). *Drug Safety, 34*(1), 73–82.

Karch, A. M. (2011). *2011 Lippincott's nursing drug guide.* Philadelphia, PA: Lippincott Williams & Wilkins.

Kuhn, M. A., & Winston, D. *Herbal therapy supplements a scientific and traditional approach.* (2nd ed.). Philadelphia, PA: Lippincott Williams & Wilkins.

Porth, C. M., & Matfin, G. (2009). *Pathophysiology: Concepts of altered health states,* Philadelphia, PA: Lippincott Williams & Wilkins.

Smeltzer, S. C., Bare, B. G., Hinkle, J. H., & Cheever, K. H. (2010). *Brunner & Suddarth's textbook of medical-surgical nursing* (11th ed.). Philadelphia, PA: Lippincott Williams & Wilkins.

Up-To-Date. (2012). *Azithromycin (systemic): Drug Information.* LexiComp. Inc.

Up-To-Date. (2012). *Chloramphenicol: Drug Information.* LexiComp. Inc.

Up-To-Date. (2012). *Clindamycin (systemic): Drug Information.* LexiComp. Inc.

Up-To-Date. (2012). *Erythromycin (systemic): Drug Information.* LexiComp. Inc.

Up-To-Date. (2012). *Linezolid: Drug Information.* LexiComp. Inc.

Up-To-Date. (2012). *Quinupristin and dalfopristin: Drug Information.* LexiComp. Inc.

Up-To-Date. (2012). *Telithromycin: Drug Information.* LexiComp. Inc.

U.S. Department of Health and Human Services. (2011). FDA Drug Safety Communication: Serious CNS reactions possible when linezolid (Zyvox) is given to patients taking certain psychiatric medications. Retrieved: February 12, 2012 http://www.fda.gov/Drugs/DrugSafety/ucm265305.htm

20 Drug Therapy for Tuberculosis and *Mycobacterium avium* Complex Disease

LEARNING OBJECTIVES

After studying this chapter, you should be able to:

1. Describe the etiology and pathophysiology of tuberculosis and *Mycobacterium avium* complex.
2. Describe the characteristics of latent, active, and drug-resistant tuberculosis.
3. Describe drug therapy for tuberculosis, including the rationale for multiple-drug therapy.
4. List the action, uses, adverse effects, and nursing implications of first-line antitubercular drugs.
5. Describe how second-line antitubercular drugs are added to drug regimens to treat multidrug-resistant tuberculosis.
6. Describe the drugs used to prevent or treat *Mycobacterium avium* complex.
7. Discuss ways to increase adherence to antitubercular drug therapy regimens.
8. Understand how to implement the nursing process in the care of patients undergoing drug therapy for tuberculosis.

Clinical Application Case Study

Ramon Diaz is a 58-year-old homeless man. He is spending the night at a shelter where one of your coworkers volunteers one evening a month. Mr. Diaz has a productive cough, and your coworker asks him how he feels; he has visibly lost weight since he was in the shelter 1 month ago. He says he sweats a lot at night and thinks he has a fever. At a free clinic, his sputum test is positive for *Mycobacterium tuberculosis*. From the clinic, Mr. Diaz is sent to the county jail, where he will stay until his sputum test is negative. He is started on a regimen, once daily, of isoniazid 300 mg for 6 months, rifampin 600 mg for 6 months, pyrazinamide 2000 mg for 2 months, and ethambutol 1200 mg for 2 months. The health department supplies his medications and is responsible for overseeing his course of therapy. You are a nurse working for the health department.

KEY TERMS

Directly observed therapy: method of medication administration where a nurse (or responsible adult) observes a patient taking a dose of antitubercular drug; highly recommended when using intermittent regimens and for high-risk patients

Extensively drug-resistant tuberculosis: relatively rare type of multidrug-resistant tuberculosis that is resistant to isoniazid and rifampin plus resistant to any fluoroquinolone and at least one of three injectable second-line drugs (i.e., amikacin, kanamycin, or capreomycin).

Hepatitis: inflammation of the liver; usually caused by an infectious agent, toxin, or drug

Jaundice: yellow discoloration of the skin and of body tissues and fluids resulting from abnormally high levels of bilirubin in the blood; common symptom when drugs cause liver damage.

Multidrug-resistant tuberculosis: tuberculosis that is resistant to isoniazid and rifampin

Introduction

Tuberculosis (TB) is an infectious disease that usually affects the lungs but may involve the lymph nodes, pleurae, bones, joints, kidneys, and the gastrointestinal (GI) tract. TB, which commonly occurs in many parts of the world, infects one third of the world's population. In 2010, a total of 8.8 million people worldwide became sick with TB. In the United States, active disease has decreased to a low level in U.S.-born people; most new cases occur in foreign-born immigrants. Large numbers of people have inactive or latent TB infection. Contributing factors include increased exposure during a resurgence of active disease between 1985 and 1992, immigration from countries where the disease commonly occurs (e.g., the Philippines, Vietnam, India, and China), and increasing numbers of people with conditions or medications that depress the immune system. TB is a leading killer of people living with human immunodeficiency virus (HIV).

Overview of Tuberculosis and *Mycobacterium avium* Complex Disease

Etiology

Mycobacterium tuberculosis, the tubercle bacillus, is the cause of TB. In general, these bacilli multiply slowly, and they may lie dormant in the body for many years. *Mycobacterium avium* and *Mycobacterium intracellulare*, which may also cause lung disease, are different types of mycobacteria that resemble each other so closely that they are usually grouped together as *Mycobacterium avium* complex (MAC). These atypical mycobacteria are found in water (including natural water sources, indoor water systems, pools, and hot tubs) and soil throughout the United States as well as in animals.

Pathophysiology

There are four phases in the initiation and progression of TB:

1. **Transmission**. This occurs when an uninfected person inhales infected airborne droplets that are exhaled by an infected person. Major factors affecting transmission are the number of bacteria expelled by the infected person and the closeness and duration of the contact between the infected and the uninfected person.

2. **Primary infection**. Authorities estimate that 30% of people who are exposed to TB bacilli become infected and develop a mild, pneumonia-like illness that is often undiagnosed. The initial infection occurs about 2 to 10 weeks after exposure. Within approximately 6 months of exposure, macrophages encapsulate the bacilli in calcified tubercles. The macrophages are unable to eliminate the bacteria completely. In the center of the calcified tubercle lies a caseous (cheesy) mass that contains small numbers of viable but dormant TB bacilli. The calcified tubercles, most commonly located in the upper lobes of the lungs, are visible on a chest radiograph.

3. **Latent tuberculosis infection**. The immune system is able to stop bacterial growth in most people who become infected with TB bacteria. The bacteria become inactive, although they remain alive in the body and can become active later. People with inactive or latent TB infection have no symptoms, do not feel sick, and do not spread TB to others. Active TB can develop years later if the latent infection is not effectively treated. In many people with latent TB, the infection remains inactive throughout their lives. In others, the TB bacteria become active and cause disease, usually when a person's immune system becomes weak as a result of disease, immunosuppressive drugs, or aging.

4. **Active tuberculosis**. About 5% to 10% of people develop active TB when they are first infected. People with latent TB develop active disease in two ways: further exposure to infected airborne droplets or reactivation of the latent TB because of weakened immune status. Although the lungs are the most common site for an active TB infection, the disease can spread to other parts of the body. Disseminated TB can infect the musculoskeletal system; the spine is the most common site, followed by the knees and hips. Other sites include the brain, liver, and kidneys.

Both new and reactivated infections of TB are more likely in people whose immune system is depressed by diseases such as HIV, diabetes mellitus, or cancer. Immunosuppression results from drugs used during cancer treatment and after organ transplantation. In people with both TB and HIV, TB progresses more rapidly, often involves extrapulmonary sites, is more severe, and is often fatal.

In addition to latent TB, a major concern among public health and infectious disease authorities is an increase in drug-resistant infections. Drug-resistant mutants of M. *tuberculosis* microorganisms may be present in any infected person. When infected people receive anti-TB drugs, the drugs do not kill or weaken the drug-resistant mutants. Instead, the resistant bacteria are able to reproduce in the presence of the drugs and to transmit the property of drug resistance to newly produced bacteria. Eventually, the majority of TB bacilli in the body are drug resistant. Once a drug-resistant strain of TB emerges, it can be transmitted to other people just like a drug-susceptible strain.

The emergence of drug-resistant TB organisms has long been attributed mainly to poor patient adherence to prescribed anti-TB drug therapy—that is, when previously infected patients do not take the drugs and doses prescribed for the length of time prescribed. However, drug-resistant strains can spread from one person to another, and there is increasing evidence that many drug-resistant infections are new infections, especially in people whose immune system is suppressed. Drug-resistant TB has been identified in many parts of the world, especially in Africa and Asia, and is a major concern in HIV-infected people. Most cases in the United States occur in foreign-born people. Factors contributing to the development of drug-resistant disease include delayed diagnosis and delayed determination of drug susceptibility (which can take several weeks). In addition, some countries lack adequate laboratory facilities or do not test TB bacteria for susceptibility to second-line anti-TB drugs. These delays in effective treatment allow rapid disease progression and rapid transmission to others, especially to those with impaired immune systems. Important risk factors for drug-resistant TB include history of previous TB treatment; contact with patients infected with drug-resistant TB; HIV co-infection; and being a member of a population group with a high prevalence of drug-resistant TB (Albanna & Menzies, 2011).

Drug-resistant TB is TB that is resistant to one first-line drug. **Multidrug-resistant tuberculosis (MDR-TB)** is TB that is resistant to isoniazid (INH) and rifampin, two of the most effective anti-TB drugs available (with or without resistance to other anti-TB drugs). MDR-TB is associated with rapid progression, with 4 to 16 weeks from diagnosis to death, and a high death rate (50% to 80%). It is also difficult and expensive to treat; most experts recommend 24 months of drug therapy. The cure rate is only about 50% or less for MDR-TB compared with a cure rate of 90% or more for drug-susceptible strains of TB. Authorities now describe some MDR-TB cases as **extensively drug-resistant TB (XDR-TB)**, an even more worrisome threat to public health. XDR-TB is resistance to the second-line drugs used to treat MDR-TB. Some cases of TB are resistant to six or seven drugs, and there are essentially no effective drugs for their treatment.

Experts believe that the organisms that cause MAC are transmitted by inhalation of droplets of contaminated water; there is no evidence of spread to humans from animals or other humans. MAC rarely causes significant disease in immunocompetent people but causes an opportunistic pulmonary infection in approximately 50% of patients with advanced HIV infection.

Clinical Manifestations

The initial symptoms of TB are a low-grade temperature, weight loss, cough, fatigue, and night sweats. The cough may be nonproductive or productive. Pulmonary and systemic symptoms may be present for weeks to months. Hemoptysis may occur. Dyspnea and orthopnea become progressively worse as TB becomes more advanced. Symptoms are less pronounced in the elderly. Disseminated TB occurs in 16% of U.S. cases; it is more prevalent in patients with HIV disease (Smeltzer, Bare, Hinkle & Cheever, 2010).

Symptoms of MAC include a productive cough, weight loss, hemoptysis, and fever. As the disease becomes disseminated through the body, chronic lung disease develops, and the bacteria are found in the blood, bone marrow, liver, lymph nodes, and other body tissues.

Box 20.1 gives information about the tuberculin skin test reactions and TB blood tests, which may be useful in diagnosis.

BOX 20.1 | **Guidelines for Interpretation of Tests for Tuberculosis**

Mantoux Skin Test
Intradermal injection of 5 tuberculin units of purified protein derived from *Mycobacterium tuberculosis*

When to Use
(general)
■ For people who are at high risk for acquiring tuberculosis (TB) because of exposure to someone with TB
■ For people who are at high risk to progression from latent to active TB because of other medical conditions

How to Interpret Results
Induration: 5 or more mm
■ Consider positive in:
  ■ HIV-infected persons
  ■ Recent contact with a person with TB
  ■ People with changes on chest radiograph consistent with prior TB

■ People with organ transplants
■ People who are immunosuppressed for other reasons (e.g., prednisone use)

Induration: 10 or more mm
■ Consider positive in:
  ■ Recent immigrants from high-prevalence countries
  ■ Injectable drug users
  ■ Residents and employees of high-risk congregate settings (e.g., long-term care facilities or prisons)
  ■ Mycobacteriology laboratory personnel
  ■ People in high-risk clinical positions
  ■ Children younger than 4 years of age
  ■ Infants, children, and adolescents exposed to high-risk adults

Induration: 15 or more mm
■ Consider positive in any person, including people with no known risk of TB

BOX 20.1	Guidelines for Interpretation of Tests for Tuberculosis (Continued)

False-Positive Reactions Possible

■ When a non-TB mycobacterial infection is present or when the patient has had previous bacillus Calmette-Guérin (BCG) vaccination (BCG, derived from *Mycobacterium bovis*, is used to vaccinate children against TB in many parts of the world.)

False-Negative Reactions Possible

■ When the patient's weakened immune system is unable to react to the skin test

■ There has been a very recent TB infection (within 8 to 10 weeks of exposure)

■ When live-virus vaccinations (e.g., measles or smallpox) have been given recently

Blood Test

Interferon-gamma release assay (IGRA) measures the concentration of a substance (interferon-gamma), which is released from white blood cells when the blood of a

person infected with *M. tuberculosis* is mixed with antigens derived from *M. tuberculosis* (e.g., QuantiFERON-TB Gold)

When to Use

■ The Centers for Disease Control and Prevention (CDC) states that this test can be used in place of tuberculin skin testing in all situations in which a tuberculin skin test is recommended.*

How to Interpret Results

■ Positive: indicates a patient has been infected with TB

■ Negative: indicates that infection with TB is unlikely

■ Indeterminate: also possible

Major Advantages

■ People need only a single visit for the test; results are available in 24 hours.

■ People who have received previous BCG vaccinations do not have false-positive results.

*The IGRA does not determine whether there is latent TB or active disease.

Clinical Application 20-1

• Identify the signs and symptoms of TB with which Mr. Diaz presents. Does he have latent TB or active TB disease?

Drug Therapy

Drugs are used to treat both latent TB and active TB. Patients with latent TB cannot spread the disease to others, but treatment of the latent disease prevents progression of the disease to an active state. It is particularly important to treat latent TB in those patients who are at high risk for progression to active TB. Treatment of active TB prevents worsening of the disease in the individual patient and prevents spread of the disease to others. *It is essential to initiate drug therapy promptly and to complete the entire course of treatment.*

Four treatment regimens have been approved for latent TB. Fewer drugs are necessary to treat latent TB because fewer mycobacterial organisms are present. The drugs used in the four treatment regimens are INH, rifampin, and rifapentine (Table 20.1).

The U.S. Food and Drug Administration (FDA) has approved 10 drugs for the treatment of active TB. However, the following discussion considers only the first-line anti-TB drugs, which are INH, rifampin, and other rifamycins, ethambutol, and pyrazinamide. (Note that more drugs are necessary to treat active TB, because more mycobacterial organisms are present.) People with active TB need to take several drugs for 6 to 9 months.

Use of multiple drugs to treat TB is necessary to prevent the development of drug-resistant TB. TB regimens are modified for use with HIV, drug resistance, and pregnancy, as well as in children. Because drug susceptibility testing results can be delayed, treatment always begins empirically; it may be necessary to adjust the regimen when results are known (Table 20.2).

Second-line anti-TB drugs are also used in combination with other drugs when there is drug resistance to one of the first-line drugs or the patient is unable to tolerate use of a first-line drug. The second-line drugs are certain aminoglycoside antibiotics (amikacin [Amikin], capreomycin sulfate [Capastat], kanamycin [Kantrex], and streptomycin); cycloserine (Seromycin); ethionamide (Trecator); aminosalicylic acid (Paser); and certain fluoroquinolones (most commonly used are moxifloxacin [Avelox], levofloxacin [Levaquin], ofloxacin [Floxin], and ciprofloxacin [Cipro]).

Adequate drug therapy of patients with active TB usually produces improvement within 2 to 3 weeks, with decreased fever and cough, weight gain, improved well-being, and improved chest radiographs. Most patients have negative sputum cultures within 3 to 6 months. If the patient is symptomatic or if the culture is positive after 3 months, nonadherence or drug resistance must be considered. Cultures that are positive after 6 months often include drug-resistant organisms.

If the initial drug regimen seems to be ineffective, the health care practitioner must suspect drug resistance. The

TABLE 20.1			
Treatment Regimens for Latent Tuberculosis			
Drugs	Duration	Interval	Minimum Dosage
Isoniazid	9 mo	Daily	270 doses
		Twice weekly	76 doses
Isoniazid	6 mo	Daily	180 doses
		Twice weekly	52 doses
Isoniazid and rifapentine	3 mo	Once weekly	12 doses
Rifampin	4 mo	Daily	120 doses

TABLE 20.2

Basic Treatment Regimens for Active Tuberculosis

	Preferred Regimen	Alternative Regimen No. 1	Alternative Regimen No. 2
Initial phase	INH, RIF, PZA, and EMB* daily for 8 wk	INH, RIF, PZA, and EMB* daily for 2 wk, then twice weekly for 6 wk	INH, RIF, PZA, and EMB* three times weekly for 8 wk
Continuation phase†	INH and RIF daily for 18 wk **OR** INH and RIF twice weekly for 18 wk	INH and RIF twice weekly for 18 wk	INH and RIF three times weekly for 18 wk

*EMB can be discontinued if drug susceptibility studies demonstrate susceptibility to first-line drugs.

†A continuation phase of weekly INH/rifapentine can be used for HIV-negative patients who do not have cavities on a chest radiograph *and* who have negative acid-fast bacilli smears at the completion of the initial phase of treatment.

INH, isoniazid; RIF, rifampin; PZA, pyrazinamide; EMB, ethambutol.

patient undergoes repeated sensitivity testing and begins to take at least three new anti-TB drugs (Albanna & Menzies, 2011). When the results of the second sensitivity testing are available, the prescriber removes drugs to which the mycobacteria are resistant and adds additional drugs. Table 20.3 lists the drugs used for MDR-TB. The regimen for treating drug-resistant TB (resistant to single first-line agent) or MDR-TB (resistant to both INH and rifampin) may include four to six drugs, including an injectable agent to which the organism is sensitive. Treatment includes second-line drugs that have many adverse effects and are more expensive and less effective than first-line drugs. A regimen for drug-resistant TB or MDR-TB

includes whichever first-line agents are effective against the organism, an injectable agent, and a fluoroquinolone; if more drugs are necessary, second-line oral anti-TB drugs are useful (see Table 20.3) (Sia & Wieland, 2011).

Albanna and Menzies (2011) describe considerations that are taken into account when designing treatment regimens for resistant TB. Administration daily, rather than at intervals, is best. Treatment lasts 24 months after repeat sputum cultures are negative. XDR-TB, along with resistance to first-line agents, is also typically resistant to an injectable agent and a fluoroquinolone. Treatment for XDR-TB is similar to that for MDR-TB but with use of even more drugs;

TABLE 20.3

Drugs Administered for the Treatment of Multidrug-Resistant Tuberculosis

Drugs	Use
First-Line Drugs *Oral agents* Isoniazid Rifamycins: rifampin, rifabutin, rifapentine, Ethambutol Pyrazinamide	These agents are used if the mycobacterial strain is susceptible to the drug
Second-Line Drugs* *Injectable agents* Aminoglycosides: amikacin, kanamycin, streptomycin, capreomycin	Amikacin and kanamycin are used first because of low cost and likely better activity These agents are used during intensive phase of treatment
Fluoroquinolones Levofloxacin, moxifloxacin, gatifloxacin, ofloxacin	New-generation fluoroquinolones (moxifloxacin, levofloxacin) are the first choice; levofloxacin is often preferred because it is available in a generic form Ciprofloxacin is not recommended
Oral bacteriostatic agents Para-aminosalicylic acid, cycloserine, ethionamide, prothionamide	Ethionamide is preferred; cycloserine is the second choice Para-aminosalicylic acid is the least preferable (least beneficial, significant adverse effects, high cost) These agents have a high rate of adverse reactions and a relatively high cost

*Agents with unclear anti-TB activity include linezolid, amoxicillin/clavulanate, imipenem/cilastatin, clarithromycin, and others; these drugs have many adverse effects. These may be used when other treatments are inadequate, but routine use is not recommended.

Adapted from Albanna, A. S. & Menzies, D. (2011). Drug-resistant tuberculosis: What are the treatment options? *Drugs, 71,* 817–818.

prescribers often include high-dose INH and new-generation fluoroquinolones. Therapy is extremely difficult, and there are no specific guidelines. Compared with treatment of MDR-TB, treatment of XDR-TB has a lower success rate and a higher mortality rate.

Clinical Application 20-2

- Mr. Diaz is taking INH, rifampin, pyrazinamide, and ethambutol for his TB. Why is he taking these four drugs? For what length of time does he take each drug?

Isoniazid

(P) **Isoniazid** (INH), the most commonly used anti-TB drug and the prototype, is bactericidal, relatively inexpensive, and nontoxic. Although use by itself for treatment of latent TB is appropriate, use with other anti-TB drugs is essential for treatment of active TB.

Pharmacokinetics

INH is well absorbed from the GI tract, with peak serum concentrations occurring 1 to 2 hours after a 300-mg dose. Food slows absorption. The drug penetrates and reaches therapeutic concentrations in essentially all body fluids and cavities, including the cerebrospinal fluid (CSF). Its half-life is 1 to 4 hours. It is acetylated in the liver to acetylisoniazid, which is excreted by the kidneys. Metabolism of INH is genetically determined; some people are "slow acetylators" and others are "rapid acetylators." A person's rate of acetylation affects

response to INH. If the rate is slow, INH is more likely to accumulate to toxic concentrations, and the development of peripheral neuropathy is more likely. However, there is no significant difference in the clinical effectiveness of INH. Liver or kidney impairment may slow elimination.

Action

INH penetrates body cells and mycobacteria, inhibiting formation of bacterial cell walls. The drug not only kills actively growing intracellular and extracellular organisms but it inhibits the growth of dormant organisms in macrophages and tuberculous lesions.

Use

It is appropriate to use INH alone or in combination with other anti-TB drugs in the treatment of latent TB. However, it is essential that it *always* be given in combination with other anti-TB drugs in the treatment of active TB. Table 20.4 gives route of administration and dosage information for INH.

For the treatment of TB in pregnant women, the initial regimen should be INH, rifampin, and ethambutol for at least 9 months (Sia & Wieland, 2011). Box 20.2 contains more information about the use of anti-TB drugs in pregnancy.

Use in Children

Changing INH therapy from daily to twice weekly may be problematic for infants and toddlers because the increased medication volume can result in medication intolerance and vomiting. Young children may need to remain on daily therapy for a longer time. INH suspension is sorbitol based and can cause GI distress or diarrhea. If a child is able to take soft foods, it may be necessary to crush INH tablets and mix them with semisolid foods (Cruz & Starke, 2010).

TABLE 20.4

DRUGS AT A GLANCE: Isoniazid

Drug	Pregnancy Category	Routes and Dosage Ranges	
		Adults	*Children*
(P) **Isoniazid** (INH)	C	PO or intramuscular (IM) Latent tuberculosis (TB): 5 mg/kg once daily (maximum 300 mg/dose) for 9 mo (6 mo if cost reduction is necessary) OR 15 mg/kg twice weekly (maximum 900 mg/dose) for 9 mo HIV disease: therapy for 9 mo Interruption in treatment: therapy for 12 mo Active TB: 5 mg/kg/d once daily (usually 300 mg/d) for 6 mo OR 15 mg/kg twice weekly (maximum 900 mg/dose) for 6 mo; when treating active TB, INH is part of a multidrug regimen HIV disease: therapy for 9 mo Extrapulmonary TB: same regimen as pulmonary TB TB meningitis: therapy for 9–12 mo	Infants and children up to age 15, PO or IM Latent TB: 10–20 mg/kg/d once daily (maximum 300 mg/dose) for 9 mo OR 20–40 mg/kg twice weekly (maximum 900 mg/dose) for 9 mo Active TB: 10–15 mg/kg/d once daily (maximum 300 mg/d) for 6 mo OR 20–30 mg/kg twice weekly (maximum 900 mg/dose) for 6 mo; when treating active TB, INH is part of a multidrug regimen HIV disease: same regimen as active TB extended for 9 mo Central nervous system or disseminated TB: therapy for 9–12 mo

HIV, human immunodeficiency virus.

BOX 20.2   Treatment of Tuberculosis in Pregnancy

Initial regimen: isoniazid (INH), rifampin, and ethambutol for at least 9 months.

> INH: good safety record in pregnancy.
>> Breastfeeding should not be discouraged during treatment with INH.
>> Pregnant and breastfeeding women who are receiving INH should take vitamin B$_6$ (pyridoxine) supplementation, and their breastfed infants should also receive pyridoxine.
> Rifampin: good safety record in pregnancy; breastfeeding should not be discouraged during treatment.
> Ethambutol: may cause ophthalmic abnormalities in infants born to women receiving ethambutol; drug should be used in pregnancy if the benefits outweigh the risks.

Pyrazinamide: not part of the initial treatment regimen for pregnant women but is probably safe for use during pregnancy.

INH therapy appears to be more effective in children than in adults, and the risk of INH-related **hepatitis** (inflammation of the liver) is minimal in infants, children, and adolescents, who generally tolerate the drug better than adults. Authorities do not recommend the routine administration of vitamin B$_6$ (pyridoxine) for children taking INH but stipulate that it be given to breastfeeding infants, children, and adolescents with vitamin B$_6$-deficient diets, as well as to children who experience paresthesias when taking INH.

Use in Older Adults

Although INH is the drug of choice for treatment of latent TB, its use is controversial in older adults. Because risks of drug-induced hepatotoxicity are higher in this population, some clinicians believe patients with positive skin tests should have additional risk factors (e.g., recent skin test conversion, immunosuppression, and previous gastrectomy) before receiving INH.

Use in Patients With Renal Impairment

In a patient with healthy kidneys, no adjustment in dosage is necessary with INH. However, because the drug is eliminated in the urine, severe renal impairment may affect elimination; caution is warranted when severe renal impairment is present.

Use in Patients With Hepatic Impairment

Damage to the liver is a serious adverse effect of INH. This risk is compounded because INH is given concurrently with other anti-TB drugs that also can cause liver damage. The risk of INH-induced hepatitis worsens if the patient consumes alcohol daily. The nurse assesses the patient monthly for symptoms of hepatitis (anorexia, nausea, fatigue, malaise, **jaundice** [yellowish discoloration of the skin and tissues]). The FDA has issued a **BLACK BOX WARNING ◆** for INH, stating that severe and sometimes fatal hepatitis may occur, usually within the first 3 months of treatment, although it may develop even after many months of therapy. Therefore, it is important that liver function tests be monitored and that the drug be discontinued if signs and symptoms of hepatotoxicity occur. Hepatitis and liver damage are more likely to occur during the first 8 weeks of INH therapy and in middle-aged and older adults. However, the risk of hepatotoxicity is possible even in children who take INH.

Use in Patients With Critical Illness

TB is a common opportunistic infection in people with advanced HIV infection. It may develop from an initial infection or reactivation of latent TB.

Use in Patients Receiving Home Care

If individual patients take INH and other anti-TB drugs for latent or active infection, the home care nurse needs to ensure that the patient takes the drugs as directed. The nurse may need to carry out **directly observed therapy** (DOT), which involves observing the patient taking the anti-TB medication. The Centers for Disease Control and Prevention (CDC) highly recommends DOT when using intermittent regimens and for high-risk patients, such as those whose treatment has been interrupted or who often do not obtain necessary medication refills (CDC, 2011).

Other specific interventions vary widely and may include teaching about the importance of taking the drugs and the possible consequences of not taking them (i.e., spreading the disease to others, more severe disease, longer treatment regimens with more toxic drugs); monitoring for adverse drug effects

---

EVIDENCE-BASED PRACTICE

Adverse Events With 4 Months of Rifampin Therapy or 9 Months of Isoniazid Therapy for Latent Tuberculosis Infection

by D. MENZIES, R. LONG, A. TRAJMAN, M. DION, J. YANG, H. AL JAHDALI, ET AL.

Annals of Internal Medicine
2008, 149, 10

The researchers compare adverse events occurring with 9 months of isoniazid (INH) therapy versus 4 months of rifampin therapy for latent tuberculosis (TB). This study, conducted in university hospital TB clinics in Canada, Brazil, and Saudi Arabia, looks at occurrence of adverse events and patient adherence to therapy and completion of the drug regimen. A 4-month regimen of rifampin led to fewer adverse events and better adherence to therapy than a 9-month regimen of INH.

IMPLICATIONS FOR NURSING PRACTICE: **Nurses have an important role to play in helping patients adhere to their anti-TB drug regimens. Expected adverse effects can be discussed with patients during initial teaching and during follow-up visits. Nurses can work with the health care provider who is managing the anti-TB therapy to modify or change drug regimens to make patient adherence easier. Nurses must counsel and support patients to ensure completion of the drug regimen.**

(especially signs and symptoms of hepatotoxicity); assisting the patient to manage adverse effects or report them to the prescriber; assisting in obtaining the drugs; and keeping follow-up appointments for blood tests and chest radiographs.

Adverse Effects

Potentially serious adverse effects of INH include hepatotoxicity and peripheral neuropathy. Manifestations of hepatotoxicity are symptoms of hepatitis or elevated liver enzymes. Indications of peripheral neuropathy may include numbness and tingling in the hands and feet. This is most likely to occur in patients who are malnourished or older or who have alcoholism, diabetes mellitus, or uremia.

Contraindications

Contraindications to INH includes a hypersensitivity to the drug, acute hepatic disease, or INH-induced liver damage. Caution is warranted in elderly patients, as well as in those people with chronic non–INH-related liver disease or chronic alcoholism, in those with seizure disorders (especially if taking phenytoin), and in those with severe renal impairment. It may be necessary to delay INH treatment of latent TB in patients with acute liver disease.

Clinical Application 20-3

- It is very important that the health department keep track of Mr. Diaz's treatment to ensure that he takes his prescribed medications. Why is it essential that Mr. Diaz take the full course of his therapy? What is directly observed therapy (DOT)? Why is DOT used with Mr. Diaz?

Nursing Implications

Preventing Interactions

Some drugs increase the effects of INH. Rifampin and pyrazinamide, frequently given in combination with INH, are hepatotoxic, and their administration with INH increases the risk of liver injury.

Alcohol increases the risk of hepatotoxicity even if alcohol use is stopped during INH therapy. INH increases the risks of toxicity associated with several drugs by inhibiting their metabolism and increasing their blood levels. These include carbamazepine, fluconazole, haloperidol, phenytoin, and vincristine. INH increases hepatotoxicity with most of these drugs; concurrent use should be avoided when possible or blood levels of the drug whose metabolism is inhibited should be monitored. With vincristine, INH may increase peripheral neuropathy. INH may enhance the adverse hepatic effects of acetaminophen. INH may decrease the metabolism of benzodiazepines, which are metabolized by oxidation. Antacids and food slow the absorption of INH.

Administering the Medication

Administration of INH is usually oral, but an intramuscular (IM) form is also available. Regardless of the route, it is necessary to take liver enzymes prior to beginning administration and then monthly thereafter. Patients should take INH on an empty stomach, 1 hour before or 2 hours after a meal, with a full glass of water. Food delays absorption. However, people may take INH with food if it causes GI upset.

Only patients who are unable to take the drug orally should receive INH parenterally. The nurse gives INH by deep injection into a large muscle mass at an approved site. It is necessary to rotate the site. Local pain and irritation may accompany the injection.

Assessing for Therapeutic Effects

If the patient is being treated with INH for latent TB, the nurse observes for signs and symptoms of active disease, such as fever, productive cough, positive sputum cultures, night sweats, fatigue, and malaise. If the patient is being treated for active TB, the nurse observes for clinical improvement, such as a decrease in the following symptoms—cough, sputum production, fever, night sweats, and fatigue; the nurse should also see an increased appetite and weight as well as an increasing feeling of well-being. Follow-up sputum smears and sputum cultures should be negative for acid-fast bacilli. It is necessary to obtain sputum cultures monthly until two consecutive cultures are negative. The appearance of the chest radiograph should also improve.

Assessing for Adverse Effects

The nurse frequently assesses for signs and symptoms of hepatotoxicity, including hepatitis (jaundice, anorexia, nausea, vomiting, and abdominal pain). The nurse reports their development to the health care provider promptly to prevent possible liver failure and death. Also, he or she must report any increase in liver enzymes or bilirubin immediately. In addition, the nurse assesses for signs and symptoms of peripheral neuropathy (tingling, numbness, and paresthesias of the extremities).

Patient Teaching

Box 20.3 presents patient teaching guidelines for INH.

Clinical Application 20-4

- The nurse has multiple opportunities to assess Mr. Diaz when he receives his medication. For what adverse effects of INH does the nurse plan to monitor him?

NCLEX Success

1. The nurse who is giving INH anticipates an order for which one of the following vitamins, which is usually given with INH?
   A. Vitamin B_3 (niacin)
   B. Vitamin B_6 (pyridoxine)
   C. Folic acid (folate)
   D. Vitamin D (calcitriol)

BOX 20.3	**Patient Teaching Guidelines for Isoniazid**

■ If you have a positive tuberculin skin test and you are taking isoniazid (INH) to treat latent tuberculosis (TB), follow the drug regimen exactly or the length of time prescribed to prevent development of active TB. Treatment may last for months or years.

■ If you are being treated for active TB, you should begin to feel better in about 2 to 3 weeks. If you do not, notify the health care provider who is managing the TB infection.

■ When you take your INH every day, take the ordered dose of vitamin B₆ (pyridoxine) at the same time, so you do not forget to take your vitamin B₆. Vitamin B₆ helps prevent the adverse effects of leg numbness and tingling.

■ Take INH on an empty stomach if possible, 1 hour before or 2 hours after a meal. If stomach upset occurs, take the drug with food.

■ Take all other anti-TB drugs prescribed along with INH.

■ Avoid alcoholic beverages while taking INH.

■ INH can cause liver damage. Watch for the following signs and symptoms of liver damage (i.e., hepatitis): loss of appetite, nausea, yellowing of skin or eyes (jaundice), light-colored stools, dark urine, fatigue, and malaise. If such symptoms occur, stop taking INH and **immediately** report the symptoms to the health care provider who is managing the TB infection.

■ If you begin to experience numbness, burning, or tingling of your arms or legs, notify the TB health care provider. These are the symptoms of another adverse effect of INH.

■ The health care provider will order blood tests to check your liver function. Be sure to keep these appointments to have blood drawn. You may also need to have sputum cultures.

---

2. The nurse should teach patients taking INH to avoid alcohol because of the increased risk of

A. central nervous system depression
B. liver damage
C. drug-resistant tuberculous organisms
D. rapid drug metabolism

3. The nurse would assess a patient taking INH for

A. elevated levels of serum aspartate aminotransferase
B. symptoms of hyperkalemia
C. decreased urine output
D. hearing loss

4. A patient is taking INH. Which one of the following adverse effects does the nurse include in discharge teaching?

A. Numbness and tingling of extremities
B. Thirst and decreased urine output
C. Loose, watery bowel movements
D. Eye pain and visual disturbances

Rifamycins

Rifamycins are a class of drugs that is bactericidal for the treatment of intracellular and extracellular TB organisms. ℗ **Rifampin** (Rifadin) is the prototype rifamycin. Rifampin and INH are synergistic in combination, eliminating TB bacilli from sputum and producing clinical improvement faster than any other drug regimen, unless the causal bacteria are resistant to one or both drugs.

Pharmacokinetics

Rifampin is well absorbed with oral administration and diffuses well into body tissues and fluids, with highest concentrations occurring in the liver, lungs, gallbladder, and kidneys.

Peak serum concentration occurs in 1 to 3 hours with oral administration and immediately with intravenous (IV) administration. The drug crosses the blood–brain barrier and enters the CSF. The drug is metabolized in the liver and excreted primarily in bile; a small amount is excreted in urine. Its elimination half-life is approximately 3 to 5 hours, depending on the dose. Because it is a strong inducer of drug-metabolizing enzymes, its half-life becomes shorter with continued use.

Action

Rifampin is bactericidal for TB organisms. It kills mycobacteria by inhibiting synthesis of RNA and thereby causing production of defective, nonfunctional proteins.

Use

Health care providers use rifampin to treat susceptible TB infections. Patients use it alone for latent TB and in combination with other anti-TB drugs for active TB. For the use of rifampin in pregnancy, see Box 20.2. Home care considerations with rifampin and the other rifamycins are the same as for INH.

Rifampin has important uses other than in the treatment of TB, including prophylaxis for people exposed to meningococcal meningitis as well as in the treatment of MAC. An unlabeled use is in the treatment of leprosy, which is caused by *Mycobacterium leprae*. The drug also has several other unlabeled uses: treatment of prosthetic valve endocarditis due to methicillin-resistant *Staphylococcus aureus* (MRSA), prophylaxis for exposure to *Haemophilus influenzae* infections and *Neisseria meningitidis*, and treatment of certain staphylococcal infections (including MRSA) when combined with another antistaphylococcal antibiotic to prevent resistance.

Table 20.5 gives route and dosage information for rifampin and the other rifamycins.

Use in Children

Children take rifampin if their TB is INH resistant.

TABLE 20.5

DRUGS AT A GLANCE: Rifamycins

Drug	Pregnancy Category	Routes and Dosage Ranges	
		Adults	Children
Ⓟ **Rifampin** (Rifadin)	C	PO or intravenous (IV) Latent tuberculosis (TB): 10 mg/kg/d (maximum 600 mg/d) for 4 mo Active TB: 10 mg/kg/d (maximum 600 mg/d) OR 10 mg/kg twice weekly (maximum 600 mg); when treating active TB, rifampin is part of a multidrug regimen	PO or IV Latent TB: 10–20 mg/kg/d once daily (maximum 600 mg/d) for 4 mos Active TB: 10–20 mg/kg/d (maximum 600 mg/dose) OR 10–20 mg/kg twice weekly (maximum dose 600 mg); when treating active TB, rifampin is part of a multidrug regimen
Rifapentine (Priftin)	C	Active TB: initial phase, 600 mg PO twice weekly with an interval of not <72 h between doses; continuation phase, 600 mg PO once weekly for 4 mo; when treating active TB, rifapentine is part of a multidrug regimen	Children younger than 2 y of age, not recommended Children ages 2–11, case by case use only Children 12 y and older, use adult dosage
Rifabutin (Mycobutin)*	B	Latent TB: 300 mg PO once daily for 4 mo Active TB: 300 mg PO once daily as part of a multidrug regimen Disseminated MAC in advanced HIV infection Prophylaxis: 300 mg PO once daily (150 mg twice daily if GI upset) Treatment: 300 mg PO once daily as second-line therapy added to first-line therapy with clarithromycin and ethambutol	Infants and children TB: 10–20 mg/kg PO once daily (maximum dose 300 mg) MAC Prophylaxis (for patients 6 y or older): 300 mg PO once daily Treatment (add-on therapy for severe infection): 10–20 mg/kg PO once daily (maximum 300 mg) Adolescents, same as adult

*Administered as alternative to rifampin.
GI, gastrointestinal; MAC, *Mycobacterium avium* complex.

Use in Patients With Hepatic Impairment

With rifampin, liver damage is most likely to occur with preexisting liver disease or concurrent use of other hepatotoxic drugs. Monitoring for symptoms of hepatotoxicity at least monthly is necessary. It is important to measure liver enzymes before starting and periodically during rifampin therapy. If signs of liver damage occur, it is essential to discontinue the drug, check the liver enzymes, and perform a medical evaluation. A dosage reduction to lower the risk of hepatotoxicity is necessary in at-risk patients.

Use in Patients With Critical Illness

Rifampin interacts with many non-nucleoside reverse transcriptase inhibitors (NNRTIs) and protease inhibitors (PIs), generally reducing the effectiveness of these antiretroviral drugs. Rifampin decreases blood levels and therapeutic effects of the anti-HIV drugs. However, this effect is much less pronounced with rifabutin, another rifamycin (see *Other Drugs in the Class*).

Adverse Effects

Adverse effects of rifampin include GI upset, skin rashes, hepatotoxicity, and acute renal failure. The drug causes a harmless red–orange discoloration of urine, tears, sweat, and other body fluids. It may stain soft contact lenses permanently. Prolonged use

may result in bacterial or fungal superinfections, including pseudomembranous colitis or *Clostridium difficile*–associated diarrhea.

Contraindications

Contraindications to rifampin include hypersensitivity to the drug (or other rifamycins). Caution is warranted in patients who have a history of liver disease, in those who are currently receiving medications known to cause harm to the liver (particularly pyrazinamide), in those with a history of alcoholism, or in those who are receiving treatment for HIV.

Nursing Implications

Preventing Interactions

Rifampin has many interactions with other drugs. It induces hepatic cytochrome P450 3A4 enzymes and accelerates the metabolism of numerous other drugs, thereby decreasing their serum concentrations, half-lives, and therapeutic effects. Use of rifampin requires careful review of the patient's drug regimen for potential interactions.

Drugs that rifampin affects include antiretroviral drugs (NNRTIs and PIs), benzodiazepines, corticosteroids, cyclosporine, estrogens, fluconazole, methadone, metoprolol, phenytoin, propranolol, oral contraceptives, oral sulfonylureas, theophylline, verapamil, and warfarin. The following examples illustrate the effects of rifampin on other drugs. Rifampin may decrease the serum concentration of the NNRTIs efavirenz and nevirapine. The anti-TB drug also decreases the serum concentration of the PI ritonavir. Rifampin interacts with warfarin; a decreased anticoagulant effect occurs approximately 5 to 8 days after rifampin is started and lasts for 5 to 7 days after rifampin is stopped. Close monitoring of the prothrombin time and INR is essential with an increase of the dosage of warfarin as necessary. In addition, rifampin decreases the effectiveness of oral contraceptives, and women who use these contraceptives and take rifampin should use another method of birth control. Finally, concurrent administration with rifampin with methadone may precipitate signs and symptoms of opiate withdrawal unless methadone dosage is increased.

Administering the Medication

Oral administration involves taking rifampin once, twice, or three times weekly, usually. Less frequent administration is more convenient, and patients are more likely follow such as treatment program. They should take the drug on an empty stomach, either 1 hour before or 2 hours after a meal. However, if patients are unable to tolerate it on an empty stomach, they may take it with a meal and a large glass of water. Food may delay or reduce the peak of action.

Rifampin is available for IV administration. The nurse reconstitutes the drug with 10 mL of sterile water to yield 60 mg/mL. He or she adds this to D_5W 100 mL and infuses it over 30 minutes or adds this to D_5W 500 mL and infuses it over 3 hours. The infusion rate should range from 30 minutes to 3 hours depending on the dose and volume of IV solution. The final concentration should not exceed 6 mg/mL.

Assessing for Therapeutic Effects

If the patient is being treated with rifampin for latent TB, the nurse observes for signs and symptoms of active disease. If the patient is being treated with the drug for active disease, the nurse observes for clinical improvement. Therapeutic effects are usually apparent with the first 2 to 3 weeks of drug therapy for active disease.

Assessing for Adverse Effects

The nurse assesses for GI adverse effects such as anorexia, epigastric distress, abdominal cramps, nausea, vomiting, and diarrhea. Even pseudomembranous colitis is possible. The nurse observes for hypersensitivity reactions such as fever, tachycardia, anorexia, and malaise; flushing, itching, and rash may also occur. Rifampin can also produce a flu-like syndrome of fever, chills, and muscle aches.

The patient taking rifampin must be observed for signs and symptoms of hepatotoxicity—increased serum liver enzymes and bilirubin, jaundice, anorexia, abdominal pain, nausea, and vomiting. Observation for these adverse effects is crucial if the patient already has liver damage, liver disease, or is taking another drug that also causes hepatotoxicity. Any symptoms of hepatotoxicity must be reported immediately to the health care provider to prevent further liver damage, liver failure, or death.

Patient Teaching

Box 20.4 presents patient teaching guidelines for rifampin and the rifamycins.

BOX 20.4　Patient Teaching Guidelines for the Rifamycins

■ If you have a positive tuberculin skin test and you are receiving rifampin or rifapentine to treat latent tuberculosis (TB), you should follow the drug regimen exactly for the length of time prescribed to prevent development of active TB. Treatment may last for months.

■ If you are being treated for active TB, you should begin to feel better in about 2 to 3 weeks. If you do not, notify the health care provider who is managing the TB infection.

■ Take rifampin on an empty stomach, 1 hour before or 2 hours after a meal. If you cannot tolerate the drug on an empty stomach, take the drug with meals and with a full glass of water.

■ If you are unable to swallow capsules, notify your prescriber and contact your pharmacists. Rifampin is available as an oral suspension.

■ Take all other anti-TB drugs prescribed along with rifampin.

■ Avoid alcoholic beverages while taking rifampin.

■ Rifampin can cause liver damage. Watch for signs and symptoms of hepatitis: fever, loss of appetite, nausea, vomiting, yellowing of skin or eyes, light-colored stools, dark urine, and malaise. If such

symptoms occur, stop taking rifampin immediately and promptly report the symptoms to the health care provider who is managing the TB infection.

■ The health care provider will order blood tests to check on liver function throughout your rifampin therapy. Keep all appointments.

■ Rifampin causes a red–orange discoloration of tears, saliva, urine, and other body secretions. Although the discoloration is harmless, it may permanently stain soft contact lenses. Consult an eye care professional; you may need to refrain from wearing your soft contact lenses.

■ Rifampin decreases the effectiveness of oral contraceptives. Use a barrier type of contraception during rifampin therapy.

■ If you are taking rifabutin, report the following symptoms of uveitis (sensitivity to light, excessive tears, or eye pain) to the health care provider as soon as possible.

■ Ask a medical professional for information about any drugs that you take that may interact with rifampin and the other rifamycins. Learn about those signs and symptoms that indicate drug ineffectiveness and that need to be reported to the health care provider.

Other Drugs in the Class

Rifapentine (Priftin) is a first-line drug used for the treatment of TB. This bactericidal drug is similar to rifampin in effectiveness, adverse effects, and enzyme induction activity. Patients must use rifapentine with at least one other drug, such as INH, to which the causative bacteria are susceptible. They may take it, in combination with INH, in a 3-month regimen for the treatment of latent TB. The major advantage of rifapentine is that it can be used in combination with INH in a once-weekly dosing regimen during the 4-month continuation phase of treatment for active TB.

When taking rifapentine, mild GI adverse effects, such as nausea and vomiting, may occur. Another common adverse effect is hyperuricemia. Like rifampin, rifapentine also produces orange discoloration of body fluids. Severe adverse effects include leukopenia, neutropenia, and thrombocytosis, as well as hepatotoxicity, which is rare. Contraindications include hyperemotivity to rifamycins. Caution is warranted in liver disease. Careful monitoring for liver damage is necessary.

Rifabutin (Mycobutin), a bactericidal rifamycin, is also a first-line drug for the treatment of TB. Other uses include treatment of MAC in people with advanced HIV disease and substituting for rifampin in patients with HIV disease. Like rifapentine, rifabutin decreases blood levels and therapeutic effects of the anti-HIV drugs (as well as many other drugs). However, this effect is much less pronounced with rifabutin. Rifabutin has no advantage over rifampin in the treatment of TB, but patients may take it concurrently with INH to patients who need prophylaxis against both M. *tuberculosis* and M. *avium*.

Like rifampin and rifapentine, rifabutin causes a harmless red–orange discoloration of body fluids and permanent staining of soft contact lenses. Adverse effects include GI upset (nausea, vomiting, and diarrhea), hepatitis, muscular aches, neutropenia, skin rash, and uveitis (an eye disorder with inflammation, pain, and impaired vision).

Clinical Application 20-5

- The nurse is teaching Mr. Diaz about his medication. What adverse effect of rifampin (Rifadin) should the nurse include in patient teaching so that the patient does not become alarmed and stop taking the medication?

NCLEX Success

5. The nurse is caring for a patient who is taking INH and rifampin (Rifadin). Which one of the following groups of symptoms is indicative of an adverse effect that is worsened by the combination of the two drugs?

   A. Numbness and tingling of the extremities
   B. Nausea, abdominal pain, and jaundice
   C. Decreased urine output and elevated blood urea nitrogen
   D. Dizziness and loss of hearing

6. A health care provider has prescribed rifampin (Rifadin) for a patient who is being discharged to home. The nurse should include which one of the following in the discharge teaching?

   A. "You will have to measure your urine output while taking rifampin."
   B. "Rifampin increases the risk of having seizures or convulsions."
   C. "Ask your eye care provider about wearing your contact lenses."
   D. "There is no necessary follow-up blood work."

7. A patient with HIV is taking rifampin (Rifadin) and a PI. The nurse should assess the patient for what condition?

   A. A worsened allergic reaction to rifampin
   B. Elevated blood urea nitrogen and serum creatinine
   C. Drowsiness, lethargy, and decreased responsiveness
   D. Increased viral load and decreased CD4 count

8. The nurse is reviewing a patient's medications and sees that the patient is receiving rifampin (Rifadin). The nurse's greatest concern about rifampin and its drug interactions is

   A. it decreases the metabolism of many other drugs
   B. it increases the metabolism of many other drugs
   C. it increases the risk for GI bleeding if given with warfarin
   D. it increases the risk of adverse effects from antiseizure drugs.

Adjuvant First-Line Antitubercular Drugs

Several other drugs are used to treat TB. Table 20.6 contains route and dosage information for these drugs.

Pyrazinamide

Pyrazinamide is part of a multidrug anti-TB regimen used with INH, rifampin, and ethambutol during the first 2 months, the initial phase, of treatment for active TB. This drug is bactericidal against actively growing mycobacteria in macrophages, but its exact mechanism of action is unknown. It is well absorbed from the GI tract and penetrates most body fluids and tissues, including macrophages containing tuberculous mycobacteria. It has a rapid onset and peaks in 2 hours. It is metabolized in the liver and excreted mainly by the kidneys. Its half-life is 9 to 10 hours.

The most common adverse effect of pyrazinamide is GI upset. Another adverse effects is gout. Pyrazinamide inhibits urate excretion, and this characteristic causes hyperuricemia in most patients and may cause acute attacks of gout. The most severe adverse effect is hepatotoxicity; a patient with preexisting liver impairment should not take the drug unless it is essential. Pyrazinamide enhances the hepatotoxic effect of rifampin. The nurse must assess patients without liver impairment for symptoms of liver dysfunction every 2 weeks during the usual 8 weeks of therapy. If such symptoms occur, measurement

TABLE 20.6

DRUGS AT A GLANCE: Adjuvant First-Line Antitubercular Drugs*

Drug	Pregnancy Category	Routes and Dosage Ranges†	
		Adults	*Children*
Pyrazinamide	C	Active TB: PO during the initial 8 wk of treatment Daily therapy (maximum dose 2000 regardless of weight) 40–55 kg: 1000 mg 56–75 kg: 1500 mg 76–90 kg: 2000 mg Twice-weekly therapy (maximum dose 4000 mg regardless of weight) 40–55 kg: 2000 mg 56–75 kg: 3000 mg 76–90 kg: 4000 mg	Active TB: PO during the initial 8 wk of treatment Daily therapy, 15–30 mg/kg/d (maximum 2 g/d) Twice weekly therapy, 50 mg/kg/dose once daily (maximum 2 g/d)
Ethambutol (Myambutol)	C	Active TB Initial dose, 15 mg/kg PO once daily (maximum 1.5 g); then suggested by lean body weight Daily therapy, 15–25 mg/kg (maximum 1.6 g) 40–55 kg: 800 mg 56–75 kg: 1200 mg 76–90 kg: 1600 mg Twice weekly therapy, 50 mg/kg (maximum 4 g) 40–55 kg: 2000 mg 56–75 kg: 2800 mg 76–90 kg: 4000 mg Disseminated MAC in advanced HIV infection: 15 mg/kg once daily; when treating MAC, ethambutol is given in combination with clarithromycin or azithromycin with/without rifabutin	Active TB Children Daily therapy, 15–20 mg/kg/d PO (maximum 1 g/d) Twice weekly, 50 mg/kg PO (maximum 2.5 g/dose) Adolescents 13 y of age or older, use adult dosage MAC, secondary prophylaxis or treatment (if HIV exposed or infected) Infants and children, 15–25 mg/kg/d once daily (maximum 2.5 g/d) with clarithromycin (or azithromycin) with or without rifabutin Adolescents 13 y old or older, use adult dosages

*When treating active TB, pyrazinamide and ethambutol are part of a multidrug regimen.
†Twice-weekly therapy should always be administered using directly observed therapy (DOT). For three times weekly therapy, consult the literature.
HIV, human immunodeficiency virus; MAC, *Mycobacterium avium* complex.

of liver enzymes is necessary. If significant liver damage is indicated, it is essential to discontinue the pyrazinamide.

Contraindications to pyrazinamide include a hypersensitivity to the drug pyrazinamide, severe preexisting hepatic damage, or acute attacks of gout. Caution is warranted in patients with a history of alcoholism.

Ethambutol

Ethambutol (Myambutol) is a tuberculostatic drug that inhibits synthesis of RNA and thus interferes with mycobacterial protein metabolism. It may be a component in a four-drug regimen for initial treatment of active TB that may be caused by drug-resistant organisms. When culture and susceptibility reports become available (usually after several weeks), it may be appropriate to stop ethambutol if the causative organisms are susceptible to INH and rifampin or continue it if the organisms

are resistant to either INH or rifampin and susceptible to ethambutol. To achieve therapeutic serum levels, patients should take the total daily dose of ethambutol at one time. Mycobacterial resistance to the drug develops slowly.

Ethambutol is well absorbed from the GI tract, even when given with food. The drug has a rapid onset, peaks in 2 to 4 hours, and lasts 20 to 24 hours. It is metabolized in the liver and excreted primarily by the kidneys. (Dosage reduction is necessary with impaired renal function.) The half-life is 3 to 4 hours.

A major adverse effect of ethambutol is optic neuritis, an inflammatory, demyelinating disorder of the optic nerve that decreases visual acuity and ability to differentiate red from green. Authorities recommend that patients have tests of visual acuity and red–green discrimination before starting therapy and periodically thereafter. If optic neuritis develops, it is necessary to discontinue the drug promptly. Recovery usually occurs when ethambutol is stopped.

9. A male patient is receiving pyrazinamide. The nurse assesses him for which of the following?

   A. Elevated liver enzymes and jaundice
   B. Elevated white blood cell count and fever
   C. Elevated cardiac troponin levels and chest pain
   D. Elevated creatine kinase and muscle weakness

10. The nurse questions an order for pyrazinamide for a patient with

   A. active TB
   B. a recent heart attack
   C. an acute attack of gout
   D. a history of smoking

11. A patient who is receiving ethambutol comes into the clinic for a follow-up visit. Which finding on the assessment indicates a serious adverse reaction to the drug?

   A. A sputum culture that is negative for acid-fast bacilli
   B. Changes in visual acuity
   C. Poor appetite and GI upset
   D. Dizziness and hearing loss

First-Line Drug Combinations Used to Treat Tuberculosis

INH/rifampin (Rifamate) and INH/rifampin/pyrazinamide (Rifater) are combination products developed to increase convenience for patients and promote adherence to the prescribed drug therapy regimen for drug-susceptible TB. A tablet of Rifamate contains 150 mg of INH and 300 mg of rifampin, and two tablets daily provide the recommended doses for a 6-month, short-course treatment regimen. A tablet of Rifater contains 150 mg of INH, 120 mg rifampin, and 300 mg pyrazinamide and is FDA approved for the first 2 months of a 6-month, short-course treatment. Dosage depends on weight, with four tablets daily for patients weighing 44 kg or less; five tablets daily for those weighing 45 to 54 kg, and six tablets daily for those weighing 55 kg or more. Rifater not only reduces the number of pills a patient has to take each day, it also prevents the patient from taking only one of the three medications, which can lead to multiple MDR-TB.

Second-Line Drugs Used to Treat Tuberculosis

The second-line anti-TB drugs are indicated for treatment of the following infections:

- Strains of M. *tuberculosis* that are resistant to first-line drugs
- TB when the patient has a hypersensitivity or inability to tolerate a first-line drug
- MDR-TB and XDR-TB

The second-line drugs are always used in combination regimens with first-line drugs. In many cases, the second-line drugs are less effective than the first-line drugs. Second-line drugs often have more frequent and severe adverse effects, and they may be more expensive as well. Little research exists on the use of the second-line drugs to treat latent TB in people exposed to MDR-TB. Health care providers have gained experience in the use of combinations of first-line and second-line drugs in the treatment of MDR-TB and XDR-TB. Table 20.3 provides a summary of the first-line drugs and the different classes of second-line drugs.

Clinical Application 20-6

- Mr. Diaz completes his course of anti-TB therapy. However, his TB does not resolve. Susceptibility tests indicate that he has drug-resistant TB. What changes does his prescriber make to his drug regimen?

Drugs Used to Treat *Mycobacterium avium* Complex Disease

The main drugs used in prevention of MAC disease in patients with HIV are the macrolides azithromycin and clarithromycin (see Chap. 19) as well as ethambutol and rifabutin (described earlier in this chapter). Treatment of MAC begins with once-daily administration of clarithromycin 500 mg and azithromycin 600 mg. Therapy may also involve ethambutol and rifabutin. Ethambutol is preferable because its use is associated with a lower relapse rate. Also, rifabutin interacts with clarithromycin, decreasing clarithromycin levels. In patients who are severely immunocompromised, amikacin or streptomycin may also be useful.

The United States Public Health Service and the Infectious Disease Society of America recommend at least 12 months of therapy. In some patients whose immune status improves with antiretroviral therapy, MAC treatment can be discontinued. However, the experts have not yet determined an exact timeline for discontinuing the anti-MAC drugs, and close follow-up is necessary to prevent relapse. For patients with HIV whose immune status does not improve with antiretroviral therapy, the recommended duration of treatment for disseminated MAC is lifelong.

Special Strategies to Increase Adherence to Antitubercular Drug Regimens

The complex drug regimens necessary to treat TB require special strategies to assist patients in adhering to their drug treatment plan. The combination of complex drug regimens administered over long periods of time and the risk of transmission of the disease to others if the patient does not adhere to the drug regimen present the nurse with unique challenges.

Strategies for successful drug treatment involve the nurse, the treating physician, the family and friends of the patient, public health departments, and the community as a whole. The nurse has a role in each of the following strategies.

- Supporting the use of short-course regimens, intermittent drug administration, and DOT. Shorter regimens and intermittent drug administration, if possible, make adherence easier for patients. Fixed-dose combinations of drugs are useful; they reduce the number of pills needed. The CDC and other experts strongly recommend DOT to ensure patient adherence. Incentives and enablers also prove useful. These include assistance with transportation to the health care provider for follow-up evaluations and tokens or food coupons given to patients each time they appear at the health care facility for treatment or follow-up.
- Educating patients, family members, and patient contacts. This may be especially important with treatment of latent TB. Most people are more motivated to take medications and schedule follow-up care when they have symptoms than when they feel well and have no symptoms. It is essential to emphasize the importance of treatment for the future health of the individual person, significant others, and the community. In addition, the patient should receive information about common and potential adverse effects of drug therapy and what to do if they occur.
- Providing support services and resources. These require substantial financial resources and may include more workers to provide DOT at the patient's location, flexible clinic hours, and reduced waiting times and to assist patients with child care, transportation, or other social service needs that encourage them to initiate and continue treatment. Lack of these services (e.g., clinics far from patients' homes, with inconvenient hours, long waiting times, and unsupportive staff) may deter patients from seeking evaluation for a positive skin test, initiating treatment, or completing the prescribed treatment and follow-up care.
- Individualizing treatment regimens. Individualized treatment is necessary whenever possible to increase patient convenience and minimize disruption of usual activities of daily living.
- Promoting communication and continuity of care. With patients for whom English is not their first language, it is desirable to have a health care provider who speaks their language or who belongs to their ethnic group. This provider may be able to teach patients more effectively, elicit cooperation with treatment, administer DOT, and be a consistent support person.

NCLEX Success

12. **The nurse taking care of a patient with TB receives an order for levofloxacin (Levaquin). This drug may be used to treat**
    A. latent TB
    B. active TB
    C. drug-resistant TB
    D. adverse effects of INH

13. **A female patient has not adhered to her drug regimen for TB. Which of the following is most effective to enhance adherence?**
    A. Explaining the importance of adherence
    B. Having the patient's family administer the medication
    C. Evaluating serum drug levels to determine adherence
    D. Having nursing staff directly watch her take her medication

The Nursing Process

Assessment

- Assess for latent or active TB infection.
- For latent TB infection, identify high-risk patients:
  - Close contacts of someone with active TB
  - Elderly or undernourished patients
  - Patients with AIDS, diabetes mellitus, silicosis, Hodgkin's disease, or leukemia
  - Alcoholics
  - Patients receiving immunosuppressive drugs
  - Immigrants from parts of the world where the disease is endemic
- For active disease, observe for fatigue, weight loss, anorexia, malaise, fever, and a productive cough. In early phases, however, there may be no symptoms. If available, check diagnostic test reports for indications of TB (chest radiograph, tuberculin skin test, or sputum smear and culture).
  - In children, initial signs and symptoms may occur within a few weeks after exposure, before skin tests become positive, and resemble those of bacterial pneumonia. In addition, indications of disease in lymph nodes, GI and urinary tracts, bone marrow, and meninges may be present.
  - In older adults, signs and symptoms of TB are often less prominent than in younger adults, or are similar to those in other respiratory disorders. Thus, an older adult is less likely to have a fever, a positive skin test, significant sputum production, hemoptysis, or night sweats. However, mental status changes and mortality are higher in older than in younger adults.
  - In patients with HIV infection, skin tests showing 5 mm of induration are considered positive. In addition, disease manifestations in patients with AIDS differ from those in people with undamaged immune systems. For example, malaise, weight loss, weakness, and fever are prominent. Other symptoms often resemble those of bacterial pneumonia, involve multiple lobes of the lungs, and involve extrapulmonary sites of infection.
- Assess candidates for anti-TB drug therapy for previous exposure and reaction to the primary drugs and for the current use of drugs that interact with the primary drugs.
- Assess for signs and symptoms of MAC disease, especially in patients with advanced HIV infection who have a CD4+ cell count of 100/mm^3 or less.

Nursing Diagnoses

- Anxiety related to health status
- Risk for injury related to adverse effect of anti-TB medications
- Deficient knowledge related to TB disease process
- Deficient knowledge related to correct use of anti-TB medications
- Deficient knowledge related to consequences of noncompliance with the drug therapy regimen
- Noncompliance related to failure to follow the drug treatment regimen

Planning/Goals

The patient will

- Take medications as prescribed.
- Keep appointments for follow-up care.
- Report adverse drug effects.
- Act to prevent the spread of TB.

Nursing Interventions

The nurse will

- Assist patients to understand the disease process and the necessity for long-term treatment and follow-up.
- Provide information about TB and its treatment through the use of written materials which are age appropriate,

appropriate to the patient's educational background, and in the patient's own language.

- Teach the patient about measures to prevent the spread of TB.
- Teach the patient how to correctly follow the multidrug regimen through correct administration of the drugs for the correct length of time.
- Teach the patient what the signs and symptoms of adverse drug reactions are and which ones need to be reported to the health care provider.
- Follow hospital policies and procedures regarding appropriate isolation techniques for hospitalized patients with TB.

Evaluation

- Observe for improvement in signs and symptoms of TB and MAC disease.
- Interview and observe for adverse drug effects and check laboratory reports of hepatic and renal function (when available).
- Question the patient regarding compliance with instructions for taking anti-TB and anti-MAC drugs.

Key Concepts

- TB is a worldwide problem. Although not as extensive in the United States as in many other countries, the public health infrastructure for diagnosing and treating TB needs to be maintained.
- MDR-TB and XDR-TB are of increasing concern.
- DOT is recommended to prevent inadequate drug therapy and development of drug-resistant TB organisms.
- INH is the treatment of choice for latent TB.
- The FDA has issued a **BLACK BOX WARNING ◆** for INH, stating that severe and sometimes fatal hepatitis may occur, usually within the first 3 months of treatment, although it may develop even after many months of therapy.
- In drug-susceptible active TB, the treatment of choice is 2 months of INH, rifampin, pyrazinamide, and ethambutol, followed by 4 months of INH and rifampin.
- In drug-resistant TB, there is no standardized treatment regimen; treatment must be individualized for each patient according to drug susceptibility reports. The second-line anti-TB drugs are used in the treatment of drug-resistant TB; typically an injectable drug and a fluoroquinolone are added to the regimen.

Critical Thinking Questions

20-1. Several of the anti-TB drugs a 42-year-old woman is taking are hepatotoxic.

- What assessments does the nurse perform before drug therapy to prevent hepatotoxicity?
- What tests does the health care provider order before therapy with these drugs to check for active liver disease?
- For what does the nurse assess at each follow-up visit?

References and Resources

Albanna, A. S. & Menzies, D. (2011). Drug-resistant tuberculosis: What are the treatment options? *Drugs, 71,* 815–822.

Aschenbrenner, D. S. & Venable, S. J. (2012). *Drug therapy in nursing* (4th ed.). Philadelphia, PA: Wolters Kluwer Health/Lippincott Williams & Wilkins.

Centers for Disease Control and Prevention. (2011). *Tuberculosis (TB).* Fact sheets. Retrieved February 1, 2012 from www.cdc.gov/tb/publications/factsheets.

Cruz, A. T. & Storke, J. R. (2010). Pediatric tuberculosis. *Pediatrics in review, 31,* 12–26.

Currier, J. S. (2010). *Mycobacterium avium* complex (MAC) infections in HIV-infected patients. *UpToDate.* Retrieved March 12, 2012 from www.uptodate.com./contents/mycobacterim-avium-complex.

Menzies, D., Long, R., Trajman, A., Dion, M., Yang, J., Al Jahdali, H., et al. (2008). Adverse events with 4 months of rifampin therapy or 9 months of isoniazid therapy for latent tuberculosis infection: A randomized trial. *Annals of Internal Medicine, 149*(10), 689–697. Retrieved March 26, 2012 from CINAHL.

Nursing 2012. (2012). *Drug handbook.* Philadelphia, PA: Wolters Kluwer Health/Lippincott Williams & Wilkins.

Porth, C. M. & Matfin, G. (2009). *Pathophysiology: Concepts of altered health states* (8th ed.). Philadelphia, PA: Wolters Kluwer Health/Lippincott Williams & Wilkins.

Smeltzer, S. C., Bare, B. G., Hinkle, J. L. & Cheever, K. H. (2010). *Brunner & Suddarth's textbook of medical-surgical nursing* (12th ed.). Philadelphia, PA: Wolters Kluwer Health/Lippincott Williams & Wilkins.

Sia, I. G. & Wieland, M. L. (2011). Current concepts in the management of tuberculosis. *Mayo Clinic Proceedings, 86*(4), 348–361.

UpToDate, Inc. (2012). Rifabutin: Drug Information. Lexi-Comp, Inc.

21 Drug Therapy for Viral Infections

LEARNING OBJECTIVES

After studying this chapter, you should be able to :

1 Identify the characteristics of viruses and common viral infections.

2 Identify the major clinical manifestations of common viral infections.

3 Identify the prototype and describe the action, use, adverse effects, contraindications, and nursing implications for antiviral agents administered for herpes simplex and varicella-zoster virus.

4 Identify the prototype and describe the action, use, adverse effects, contraindications, and nursing implications for antiviral agents administered for cytomegalovirus.

5 Identify the prototype and describe the action, use, adverse effects, contraindications, and nursing implications of drugs administered for respiratory syncytial virus.

6 Identify the prototypes and describe their action, use, adverse effects, contraindications, and nursing implications for administration in influenza.

7 Identify the prototype and describe the action, use, adverse effects, contraindications, and nursing implications for the nucleoside analog antiviral agents administered for hepatitis.

8 Identify the prototype and describe the action, use, adverse effects, contraindications, and nursing implications for the nucleoside reverse transcriptase inhibitors administered for human immunodeficiency virus (HIV).

9 Identify the prototype and describe the action, use, adverse effects, contraindications, and nursing implications for the nonnucleoside reverse transcriptase inhibitors administered for HIV.

10 Identify the prototype and describe the action, use, adverse effects, contraindications, and nursing implications for the protease inhibitors administered for HIV.

11 Identify the prototype and describe the action, use, adverse effects, contraindications, and nursing implications for the integrase strand transfer inhibitors administered for HIV.

12 Identify the prototype and describe the action, use, adverse effects, contraindications, and nursing implications for fusion protein inhibitors administered for HIV.

13 Identify the prototype and describe the action, use, adverse effects, contraindications, and nursing implications for CCR5 antagonists administered for HIV.

14 Implement the nursing process in the care of the patient undergoing drug therapy for viral infections.

Clinical Application Case Study

Ann Jackson calls her primary health care provider's office. She says that she has a cold sore under her nose on the right side. Since childhood, she has had outbreaks of this infection occasionally. Her physician orders acyclovir (Zovirax) 200 mg orally every 4 hours (5 doses daily) for 5 days.

KEY TERMS

Antiretroviral drugs: antiviral medications used in the treatment of retroviral infections such as human immunodeficiency virus (HIV)

Genital herpes: a herpesvirus that appears on the genitals

Hepatitis: liver inflammation due to a virus; five different viruses cause viral hepatitis—hepatitis A, B, C, D, and G

Herpesvirus: any virus belonging to the family of the Herpesviridae

Highly active antiretroviral therapy (HAART): several combinations of antiretroviral drugs used at one time to treat HIV/AIDS

Human immunodeficiency virus (HIV): an infection caused by a retrovirus that infects the immune system, leading to acquired immunodeficiency syndrome (AIDS). There are two types of HIV virus, HIV-1 and HIV-2; most infections in the United States are caused by HIV-1 and infections with HIV-2 occur mainly in Africa

Immunocompetent: having a normal immune response

Retrovirus: virus with an RNA genome that relies on reverse transcriptase to transform its genome from RNA to DNA (e.g., HIV)

Viral load: number of HIV RNA particles in the blood; does not measure viral levels in tissues, where viral reproduction may be continuing

Introduction

Viruses cause pneumonia, hepatitis, acquired immunodeficiency syndrome (AIDS), and other disorders that affect most body systems. Many potentially pathogenic viral strains exist, including more than 150 that infect the human respiratory tract. Viral infections vary from mild, localized diseases with few symptoms to severe systemic illnesses and death. Viruses replicate in the host with the use of metabolic processes. Antiviral agents that possess a narrow spectrum of effect on the viral process have the ability to target the invading virus. This chapter describes general characteristics of viruses and viral infections. Box 21.1 provides more specific information about selected viral infections. The text then discusses antiviral agents.

Overview of Viruses and Viral Infections

Etiology

Viruses, the infectious agents that cause viral infections, are intracellular parasites that gain entry to human host cells by binding to receptors on cell membranes. Methods of spread of viral infections include secretions from infected people, ingestion of contaminated food or water, breaks in the skin or mucous membranes, sexual contact, pregnancy, breastfeeding, and organ transplantation. All human cells do not have receptors for all viruses; cells that lack receptors for a particular virus are resistant to infection by that virus. Thus, the locations and numbers of the receptors determine which host cells can be infected by a virus. For example, the mucous membranes lining the tracheobronchial tree have receptors for the influenza A virus; helper T lymphocytes and other white blood cells have CD4 molecules, which are the receptors for the **human immunodeficiency virus (HIV)**.

Pathophysiology

Inside host cells, viruses use cellular metabolic activities for their own survival and replication. Viral replication involves dissolution of the protein coating and exposure of the genetic material (deoxyribonucleic acid [DNA] or ribonucleic acid [RNA]). With DNA viruses, the viral DNA enters the host cell's nucleus, where it becomes incorporated into the host cell's chromosomal DNA. Then, host cell genes are coded to produce new viruses. In addition, the viral DNA incorporated with host DNA is transmitted to the host's daughter cells during host cell mitosis and becomes part of the inherited genetic information of the host cell and its progeny. With RNA viruses (e.g., HIV), or **retroviruses**, viral RNA must be converted to DNA by an enzyme called reverse transcriptase before replication can occur. HIV is an infection caused by a retrovirus that infects the immune system, leading to AIDS.

After new viruses are formed, they are released from the infected cell either by budding and breaking off from the cell membrane (leaving the host cell intact) or by causing lysis of the cell. When the cell is destroyed, the viruses are released into the blood and surrounding tissues, from which they can transmit the viral infection to other host cells.

Viruses induce antibodies and immunity. Antibodies are proteins that defend against microbial or viral invasion. They are very specific (i.e., an antibody protects only against a specific virus or other antigen). For example, in a person who

BOX 21.1 Selected Viral Infections

Avian Influenza A (H5N1)

In recent years, the highly pathogenic H5N1 subtype of influenza A has been found in numerous countries. It occurs mainly in birds and poultry, but a few hundred human cases have been confirmed. Most human cases occur after exposure to infected poultry or surfaces contaminated with poultry droppings. Because human infection may cause respiratory failure and has a high mortality rate, the possibility that these viral strains might mutate so that they infect humans more easily is a major public health concern. This virus is considered the most likely cause of a future worldwide influenza epidemic.

Herpesvirus Infections

Cytomegalovirus Infection and Retinitis

Cytomegalovirus (CMV) infection is common, and most people become infected by adulthood. Infection is usually asymptomatic in healthy, immunocompetent adults. Like other herpesviruses, CMV can cause a primary infection, then remain latent in body tissues, probably for life. This means the virus can be shed in secretions of an asymptomatic host and spread to others by contact with infected saliva, blood, urine, semen, breast milk, and cervical secretions. It also means the virus may lead to an opportunistic infection when the host becomes immunosuppressed. During pregnancy, CMV is transmitted to the fetus across the placenta and may cause infection in the brain, inner ears, eyes, liver, and bone marrow. Learning disabilities and mental retardation can result from congenital CMV infection. Children spread the virus to each other in saliva or urine, whereas adolescents and adults transmit the virus mainly through sexual contact.

Major populations at risk for development of active CMV infection are patients with cancer who receive immunosuppressant drugs and organ transplant recipients, who must receive immunosuppressant drugs to prevent their body's rejection of the transplanted organ. Patients with advanced HIV infection are also at risk, but the incidence has decreased with **highly active antiretroviral therapy (HAART)**. Systemic CMV infection occurs mainly from reactivation of endogenous virus, although it may occur from an exogenous source. Active CMV infection may cause cellular necrosis and inflammation in various body tissues. Common manifestations of disease include pneumonitis, hepatitis, encephalitis, adrenal insufficiency, gastrointestinal (GI) inflammation, and gastric ulcerations.

In the eye, CMV infection produces retinitis, usually characterized by blurred vision and decreased visual acuity. Visual impairment is progressive and irreversible and, if untreated, may result in blindness. CMV retinitis may also indicate systemic CMV infection or may be entirely asymptomatic.

Genital Herpes Infection

Genital herpes infection is caused by the herpes simplex virus (HSV) and produces recurrent, painful, blister-like lesions on skin and mucous membranes. HSV is usually transmitted from person to person by direct contact with open lesions or secretions, including genital secretions. Primary infection occurs at a site of viral entry, where the virus infects epithelial cells, produces progeny viruses, and eventually causes cell death. After primary infection, latent virus may become dormant within sensory nerve cells. In response to various stimuli (e.g., intense sunlight, emotional stress, febrile illness, menstruation), latent virus may become reactivated and lead to viral reproduction and shedding.

In the fetus, HSV may be transmitted from an infected birth canal, and neonatal herpes is a serious complication of maternal genital herpes. Neonatal herpes usually becomes evident within the first week of life and may be manifested by the typical clusters of blister-like lesions on skin or mucous membranes. Irritability, lethargy, jaundice, altered blood clotting, respiratory distress, seizures, or coma may also occur. The lesions may heal in 1 to 2 weeks, but neonatal herpes carries a high mortality rate. In immunosuppressed patients, HSV infection may result in severe, systemic disease.

Herpes Zoster

Herpes zoster is caused by the VZV, which is highly contagious and present worldwide. Most children in the United States are infected by early school age. The virus produces chickenpox on first exposure and is spread from person to person by the respiratory route or by contact with secretions from skin lesions. Recovery from the primary infection leaves latent infection in nerve cells. Reactivation of the latent infection (usually later in life) causes herpes zoster (more commonly known as "shingles"), a localized cluster of painful and blister-like skin lesions. The skin lesions have the same appearance as those of chickenpox and genital herpes. Over several days, the vesicles become pustules, then rupture and heal. Because the virus remains in sensory nerve cells, pain can persist for months after the skin lesions heal. Most cases of herpes zoster infection occur among the elderly and the immunocompromised.

Human Immunodeficiency Virus Infection

HIV infection is caused by a retrovirus that infects the immune system. Two types of HIV virus have been identified, HIV-1 and HIV-2. Most infections in the United States are caused by HIV-1; HIV-2 infections occur mainly in Africa. HIV binds to receptors on the surface of CD4+ cells (especially T lymphocytes or helper T cells). HIV entry and replication eventually results in cell death. Because CD4+ cells play major roles in regulating immune function, their destruction results in serious impairment of the immune system.

The initial phase of HIV infection is characterized by influenza-like symptoms (e.g., fever, chills, muscle aches) that may last several weeks. During this time, the virus undergoes rapid replication. The next phase is characterized by a dramatic decline in the rate of viral replication, attributed to a partially effective immune response. During this phase, no visible manifestations of HIV infection may be present. However, replication of HIV continues and antibodies may be detected in the serum. During this period, the person is seropositive (HIV+) and infectious but asymptomatic. Eventually, the immune system is substantially damaged and the rate of viral reproduction accelerates. When viral load and immunodeficiency reach significant levels, the illness is termed acquired immunodeficiency syndrome (AIDS) and serious opportunistic infections occur. With effective drug therapy, viral load decreases and the CD4+ cell count increases, so that HIV-infected people may live for many years without progression to AIDS.

HIV infection occurs in all age groups and can spread to a new host during any phase of infection. The virus is commonly spread by sexual intercourse, by injection of intravenous drugs with contaminated needles, by mucous membrane contact with infected blood or body fluids,

BOX 21.1   Selected Viral Infections (Continued)

and perinatally from mother to fetus. Although the virus is found in most body fluids, infection has primarily been associated with exposure to blood, semen, or vaginal secretions. The virus is not spread through casual contact. Health care workers may be infected by needle-stick injuries. They should be aware that postexposure prophylaxis is available and may significantly reduce the risk of transmission.

Human Papilloma Virus (HPV) Infection

HPV infection, the most common sexually transmitted infection, is spread by contact with infected lesions. It affects both men and women and can cause genital warts and several types of cancer (e.g., cervical, vaginal, vulvar, anal, and penile). In women, 80% reportedly become infected within 5 years of becoming sexually active.

Respiratory Syncytial Virus Infection

Respiratory syncytial virus (RSV) is a highly contagious virus that is present worldwide and infects most children by school age. Epidemics of RSV infection often occur in nurseries, daycare centers, and pediatric hospital units during winter months. RSV infects and destroys respiratory epithelium in the bronchi, bronchioles, and alveoli. It is spread by respiratory droplets and secretions, direct contact with an infected person, and contact with fomites, including the hands of caregivers.

RSV is the most common cause of bronchiolitis and pneumonia in infants and causes severe illness in those younger than 6 months of age. These infants usually have wheezing, cough, respiratory distress, and fever. The infection is usually self-limited and resolves in 1 to 2 weeks. Antiviral therapy with ribavirin is used in some cases. The mortality rate from RSV infection is low in children who are generally healthy but increases substantially in those with congenital heart disease or immunosuppression. Recurrent infection occurs but is usually less severe than primary infection. In older children, RSV infection produces much milder disease but may be associated with acute exacerbations of asthma.

In adults, RSV infection causes colds and bronchitis, with symptoms of fever, cough, and nasal congestion. Infection occurs most often in those with household or other close contact with children, including pediatric health care workers. In older adults, RSV infection may cause pneumonia requiring hospitalization. In immunocompromised patients, RSV infection may cause severe and potentially fatal pneumonia.

Viral Hepatitis

There are several types of viral **hepatitis**, and new hepatitis viruses are still being identified. Worldwide, viral hepatitis has increased in recent years. All hepatitis viruses have similar effects on the liver, although they differ in some other characteristics. Common types of viral hepatitis are described below. Vaccines are available to prevent hepatitis A and B (see Chap. 10).

Hepatitis A virus (HAV) is transmitted mainly by the fecal–oral route and close contact with an infected person; foodborne outbreaks also occur, usually from infected food handlers or contaminated produce in the United States. The virus survives for long periods in the environment (e.g., in water and soil) and on human hands and inanimate objects. It resists freezing, detergents, and acids but can be inactivated by chlorine and temperatures above 185°F.

The HAV reproduces only in liver and GI cells, from which viral particles are released into blood and bile. The average incubation period is 25 to 30 days. The patient is infectious during the incubation period and for 7 to 10 days after symptoms develop. In infected adults, about 70% develop symptoms, including fever and jaundice, which may last as long as 2 months. Most recover without treatment and develop immunity against future HAV infections; 10% to 20% require hospitalization. In children, many are asymptomatic or develop flu-like or nonspecific symptoms without jaundice. However, even children with few or no symptoms may shed virus in their stools and be a source of community infection for as long as 6 months. The availability of hepatitis A vaccine has greatly decreased the number of reported cases. The vaccine is recommended for children and adults at increased risk of contracting the disease (e.g., travelers to certain countries, men who have sex with men, drug abusers, recipients of clotting factor replacement) and for persons with chronic liver disease.

Hepatitis B virus (HBV) can be transmitted by contact with contaminated blood and other body fluids (e.g., perinatally, during sexual contact with an infected person, by sharing needles during IV drug use, and undergoing acupuncture, hemodialysis, tattooing, or ear and body piercing). In addition, health care and public safety workers are at increased risk of developing HBV infection from injuries with contaminated equipment (e.g., contaminated needles) and from other exposures to infected body fluid. Any person exposed to infected body fluids should be evaluated for HBV infection; any person diagnosed with HBV infection should be evaluated for liver disease and for HIV infection. It is estimated that 70,000 Americans become infected with HBV every year, and approximately 5000 of them will die of the complications caused by the infection. Many Americans have chronic HBV infection; asymptomatic chronic carriers of HBV may transmit the infection to others. Hepatitis B can lead to cirrhosis, liver cancer, liver failure, and death.

The HBV can live up to 3 days on various surfaces that appear clean. The incubation period is 30 to 180 days. Increased hepatitis B surface antigens and liver enzymes (ALT, AST) occur before symptoms of HBV infection develop. After symptoms develop, antibodies to the viral antigens are produced, and the presence of antigens and viral DNA in the patient's blood indicate that the patient is infectious.

Hepatitis C virus (HCV) can be transmitted by contact with contaminated blood or other body fluids. Persons at high risk of exposure include health care and public safety workers; IV drug users; those with multiple sex partners; those undergoing hemodialysis, tattoos, or body piercings; and those who received blood transfusions before 1990, when screening blood for HCV was started. In addition, pregnant women may transmit the virus to their infants, and mothers with symptoms and high viral titers may transmit the virus to nursing infants.

The HCV incubation period is 14 to 80 days; infection is diagnosed by testing for viral DNA or antibodies. HCV infection affects people of all ages but is most often found among 20- to 39-year-olds. Infected persons can be asymptomatic for years, but most eventually develop chronic liver disease. In the United States, HCV infection is the leading cause of cirrhosis, liver cancer, and liver transplants. Effective drug therapy may cure HCV infection.

Other hepatitis viruses (e.g., D, G, and a "transfusion-transmissible" virus) have been identified; they, like HBV and HCV, are transmitted through contact with infected blood and body fluids.

has had measles, antibody protection (immunity) develops against future infection by the measles virus, but immunity does not develop against other viral infections, such as chickenpox or hepatitis. People who are **immunocompetent** have intact immune systems. Most adults possess immunity to some viral diseases because they have become infected earlier in their lives. The primary infection remains latent in the tissue and is spread by blood and body fluids. Patients who are immunocompromised have impaired or weakened immune systems and may develop the infection due to decreased immunity.

The protein coat of the virus allows the immune system of the host to recognize the virus as a "foreign invader" and to produce antibodies against it. This system works well for most viruses but does not work for the influenza A virus, which can alter its protein covering so much and so often that the immune system does not recognize it as foreign to the body. Thus, last year's antibody cannot recognize and neutralize this year's virus.

Antibodies against infecting viruses can prevent the viruses from reaching the bloodstream or, if they are already in the bloodstream, prevent their invasion of host cells. After the virus has penetrated the cell, it is protected from antibody action, and the host depends on cell-mediated immunity (lymphocytes and macrophages) to eradicate the virus along with the cell harboring it.

Clinical Manifestations

Viral infection may occur without signs and symptoms of illness. If illness does occur, the clinical course is usually short and self-limited. Recovery occurs as the virus is eliminated from the body. Some viruses (e.g., herpesvirus) can survive in host cells for many years and cause a chronic, latent infection that periodically becomes reactivated. Also, autoimmune diseases may be caused by viral alteration of host cells so that lymphocytes recognize the host's own tissues as being foreign.

Symptoms usually associated with acute viral infections include fever, headache, cough, malaise, muscle pain, nausea and vomiting, diarrhea, insomnia, and photophobia. White blood cell counts usually remain normal. Other signs and symptoms vary with the type of virus and body organs involved.

Drug Therapy

Scientists have developed several vaccines (see Chap. 10) to prevent viral infections as well as numerous drugs to treat HIV and other viral infections. Most of these antiviral drugs inhibit viral reproduction but do not eliminate viruses from tissues. In general, available drugs are expensive, relatively toxic, and effective in a limited number of infections. Some may be useful in treating an established infection if given promptly and in chemoprophylaxis if given before or soon after exposure. Protection conferred by chemoprophylaxis is immediate but lasts only while the drug is being taken. The remainder of this chapter describes the subgroups of antiviral drugs. Table 21.1 summarizes the medications used to treat viral infections.

Drugs for Herpesvirus Infections

DRUGS FOR HERPES SIMPLEX VIRUS AND VARICELLA-ZOSTER VIRUS

The **herpesviruses** include herpes simplex virus (HSV), varicella-zoster virus (VZV), and cytomegalovirus (CMV). There are two types of herpes viral infections: HSV-1 and HSV-2. HSV-1 causes fever blisters or cold sores on the lips, mouth, or face and HSV-2 causes genital warts. Ⓟ **Acyclovir** (Zovirax), the prototype antiviral agent used to combat the herpesviruses, is an oral, parenteral, and topical antiviral drug.

Pharmacokinetics

After oral administration, the body absorbs 15% to 30% of the acyclovir dosage of acyclovir, reaching a peak of action in 1.5 to 2 hours. The drug is distributed to the tissues of the lower levels distributed to the central nervous system (CNS). It is 9% to 33% protein bound and has a half-life of 3 hours. Acyclovir crosses the placenta and enters the breast milk. Excretion of unchanged drug occurs in the urine.

Action

Following uptake by infected cells, acyclovir is converted to acyclovir monophosphate by the enzyme thymidine kinase. Acyclovir triphosphate inhibits DNA polymerase, thus interrupting viral DNA replication.

Use

Immunocompromised patients take acyclovir for initial and recurrent cutaneous and mucosal HSV and VZV. Prescribers also order the drug for the treatment of **genital herpes** (a herpesvirus that appears on the genitals); it decreases viral shedding as well as the duration of skin lesions and pain. Acyclovir does not eliminate inactive virus in the body and thus does not prevent recurrence of the disease unless oral drug therapy is continued. However, prolonged or repeated courses of drug therapy may result in the emergence of acyclovir-resistant viral strains, especially in immunocompromised patients. In patients with an altered immune response, authorities recommend the intravenous (IV) form for severe genital herpes, and nonimmunocompromised patients should also receive IV preparations. Table 21.2 presents route and dosage information for acyclovir and other drugs used for HSV and VZV.

Use in Patients With Renal Impairment

There have been reports of renal failure with acyclovir use. It is necessary to reduce the dosage of acyclovir in patients with altered renal function according to the creatinine clearance (CrCl).

Adverse Effects

Acyclovir has minimal adverse effects. The most commonly reported adverse effects are malaise, headache, nausea, vomiting,

TABLE 21.1

Drugs Administered for the Treatment of Viral Infections

Drug Class/Type	Prototype	Other Drugs in the Class/Related Drugs
Drugs for Herpesvirus Infections Drugs for herpes simplex virus and varicella-zoster virus	Acyclovir (Zovirax)	Docosanol (Abreva) Famciclovir (Famvir) Penciclovir (Denavir) Valacyclovir (Valtrex)
Drugs for cytomegalovirus	Ganciclovir (Cytovene)	Cidofovir (Vistide) Foscarnet (Foscavir) Valganciclovir (Valcyte)
Drugs for Respiratory Syncytial Virus	Ribavirin (Copegus, Rebetol, Ribasphere, Virazole)	Palivizumab (Synagis)
Drugs for Influenza Adamantanes	Amantadine hydrochloride (Symmetrel)	Rimantadine (Flumadine)
Neuraminidases	Oseltamivir phosphate (Tamiflu)	Zanamivir (Relenza)
Drugs for Hepatitis: Nucleoside Analogs	Lamivudine (Epivir, Epivir-hepatitis B virus [HBV])	Adefovir dipivoxil (Hepsera) Entecavir (Baraclude) Ribavirin (Copegus, Rebetol, Ribasphere, Virazole) Telbivudine (Tyzeka) Tenofovir disoproxil fumarate (Viread)
Antiretroviral Drugs Nucleoside reverse transcriptase inhibitors	Zidovudine (AZT)	Abacavir sulfate (Ziagen) Abacavir, lamivudine, and zidovudine (Trizivir) Didanosine (Videx, Videx EC) Emtricitabine (Emtriva) Emtricitabine and tenofovir (Truvada) Emtricitabine, tenofovir, emtricitabine (Atripla) Lamivudine (Epivir) Stavudine (Zerit) Tenofovir disoproxil fumarate (Viread) Zidovudine and lamivudine (Combivir)
Non-nucleoside reverse transcriptase inhibitors	Efavirenz (Sustiva)	Delavirdine mesylate (Rescriptor) Etravirine (Intelence) Nevirapine (Viramune)
Protease inhibitors	Saquinavir mesylate (Invirase)	Atazanavir (Reyataz) Darunavir (Prezista) Fosamprenavir calcium (Lexiva) Indinavir sulfate (Crixivan) Lopinavir/ritonavir (Kaletra) Nelfinavir mesylate (Viracept) Ritonavir (Norvir) Tipranavir (Aptivus)
Integrase strand transfer inhibitor	Raltegravir (Isentress)	
Fusion protein inhibitor	Enfuvirtide (Fuzeon)	
CCR5 antagonist	Maraviroc	

TABLE 21.2

DRUGS AT A GLANCE: Drugs for Herpes Simplex Virus (HSV) and Varicella-Zoster Virus (VZV)

Drug	Pregnancy Category	Routes and Dosage Ranges	
		Adults	**Children**
Ⓟ **Acyclovir** (Zovirax)	B	Genital herpes: 200 mg PO every 4 h, 5 times daily for 10 d for initial infection; 400 mg 2 times daily to prevent recurrence of chronic infection; 200 mg every 4 h 5 times daily for 5 d to treat recurrence Herpes zoster: 800 mg PO every 4 h 5 times daily for 7–10 d Chickenpox: 20 mg/kg PO (maximum dose 800 mg) 4 times daily for 5 d Mucosal and cutaneous HSV infections in ICH: 5 mg/kg IV infused over 1 h, every 8 h for 7 d VZV in ICH: 10 mg/kg IV infused over 1 h, every 8 h for 7 d HSV encephalitis: 10 mg/kg IV infused over 1 h, every 8 h for 10 d Topically to lesions every 3 h 6 times daily for 7 d	Younger than 12 y 10 or 20 mg/kg IV every 8 h for 7 or 10 d, depending on the condition being treated—chickenpox: 2 y and older and weight 40 kg or less, 20 mg/kg PO 4 times daily for 5 d Weight above 40 kg, 800 mg PO 4 times daily for 5 d 12 y and older, topical, same as adults
Docosanol (Abreva)	C	Topically to lesions 5 times daily for up to 10 d	Older than 12 y: adult dosage
Famciclovir (Famvir)	B	Herpes zoster: 500 mg PO every 8 h for 7 d Genital herpes: 125 mg PO twice daily for 5 d	Safety and efficacy not established
Penciclovir (Denavir)	B	Topically every 2 h while awake for 4 d	Safety and efficacy not established
Valacyclovir (Valtrex)	B	Herpes labialis: 2 g PO twice daily for 1 d Herpes zoster: 1 g PO every 8 h for 7 d Recurrent genital herpes: PO 500 mg PO every 12 h daily for 5 d Reduce dosage with renal impairment	Herpes labialis: adolescents, same as adults Safety not established

ICH, immunocompromised host.

and diarrhea. The parenteral form may lead to phlebitis at the injection site, hives, itching, rash, nausea, vomiting, elevated liver enzymes, and acute renal failure. The parenteral form may result in encephalopathy, a rare but potentially serious adverse effect.

Contraindications

Contraindications to acyclovir include a known hypersensitivity to the drug, heart failure, renal disease, and lactation.

Nursing Implications

Preventing Interactions

The most significant interactions with acyclovir include increased serum concentrations with probenecid, drowsiness with zidovudine, and renal insufficiency when combined with medications that cause renal toxicity.

Administering the Medication

With the topical preparation of acyclovir, it is important to wash the hands thoroughly prior to administration and apply with a gloved hand. It is crucial that the medication be prescribed and therapy started as soon as symptoms arise. With the oral medication, patients may take the drug without respect to food intake. With the parenteral form of acyclovir, it is necessary to infuse it over 1 hour to prevent renal damage. The nurse ensures that the patient is well hydrated with 2 to 3 L of fluid per 24 hours. Acyclovir is incompatible with blood products and protein-containing solutions. In patients who are obese, it is essential to calculate acyclovir dosages according to ideal body weight.

Assess for Therapeutic Effects

The nurse assesses for the healing of lesions, decreased pain, and itching. When administering acyclovir prophylactically for genital herpes, he or she assesses for fewer recurrences.

Assessing for Adverse Effects

The nurse assesses for signs and symptoms of hypersensitivity to the acyclovir. With the topical drug, he or she assesses for burning, stinging, and pruritus. With the parenteral drug, the nurse assesses for phlebitis at the injection site. It is also necessary to assess for confusion, coma, seizures, and tremors. In addition, the nurse assesses the aspartate aminotransferase (AST) and alanine aminotransferase (ALT) for elevations as well as blood urea nitrogen (BUN) and serum creatinine for increases.

Patient Teaching

Box 21.2 identifies general patient teaching guidelines for the antiviral drugs.

Other Drugs in the Class

Docosanol (Abreva) is an over-the-counter topical antiviral agent that works in the early stages of intracellular events of viral entry into the target cells. Uses include the treatment of HSV of the face and lips. The dosage of the topical cream is five applications per day for 10 days beginning at the onset of symptoms. The patient should notify his/her primary health care provider if symptoms do not resolve in 10 days.

Famciclovir (Famvir) is an oral antiviral agent administered for herpes zoster and recurrent genital herpes. Famciclovir

is metabolized to penciclovir, its active form, and excreted mainly in the urine. Drug therapy should be started within 72 hours of the appearance of a rash or within 6 hours of the onset of genital herpes lesions. A CrCl less than 60 mL/min necessitates a dosage reduction. For patients receiving hemodialysis, dosage is calculated according to CrCl, with daily doses given after dialysis. Adverse effects of the medication include purpura, headache, nausea, vomiting, dizziness, paresthesias, and constipation. Patients on extended drug therapy should have periodic complete blood counts (CBCs) to identify blood dyscrasias.

Penciclovir (Denavir) is a topical drug used for the treatment of recurrent herpes labialis. The cold sore minimally absorbs the drug. The patient should apply the ointment every 2 hours for 4 days. If the lesion does not improve, it is important to notify the primary health care provider.

Valacyclovir (Valtrex) penetrates virus-infected cells, becomes activated by an enzyme, and inhibits viral DNA reproduction. Uses include the treatment of herpes simplex and herpes zoster infections. Metabolism occurs in the liver, and excretion takes place in the kidneys. In patients with renal impairment, the drug may accumulate, produce higher blood levels, have a longer half-life, and cause toxicity.

BOX 21.2 Patient Teaching Guidelines for Antiviral Drugs

■ Prevention is better than treatment, partly because medications used to treat viral infections may cause serious adverse effects. Thus, whenever possible, it is important to use techniques to prevent viral infections, such as limiting exposure with those infected with a viral illness.

■ Wash hands frequently and thoroughly; this helps prevent most infections.

■ Have immunizations against viral infections as indicated.

■ With genital herpes, avoid sexual intercourse when visible lesions are present and always wash hands after touching any lesion.

■ Understand that drugs may relieve symptoms but do not cure viral infections. For example, treatment of genital herpes does not prevent transmission to others, and treatment of cytomegalovirus (CMV) retinitis may not prevent disease progression.

■ Ask a health care provider for information about managing adverse drug effects.

■ If taking foscarnet or ganciclovir for CMV retinitis, have eye examinations approximately every 6 weeks.

■ If taking ganciclovir, maintain regular appointments for the assessment of the complete blood count and renal function.

■ Administer antiviral agents for recurrent genital herpes lesions as soon as signs and symptoms begin.

■ Use gloves to apply topical antiviral ointment to lesions.

NCLEX Success

1. A man with a fever, cough, and clear drainage from the nose presents to the clinic. A nurse practitioner diagnoses a viral infection. Which of the following describes the replication of the viral infection?
   A. The RNA of an infected person has invaded the man's mucous membranes.
   B. There are breaks in the cell membrane of the infected cells.
   C. Antibodies are defending against microbial cell invasion.
   D. The white blood cell count increases.

2. Why would patients with genital herpes receive acyclovir (Zovirax)?
   A. It decreases viral shedding and pain related to outbreak.
   B. It eliminates future viral outbreaks.
   C. It prevents sterility in infected patients.
   D. It prevents the development of CMV.

3. A woman is using topical acyclovir (Zovirax). Which of the following is the most important intervention to instruct the patient regarding medication administration?
   A. Administer the medication after meals to enhance absorption.
   B. Discontinue the medication when lesions are crusted over.
   C. Apply the medication to the lesions with a gloved hand.
   D. Increase oral fluids to enhance healing.

4. **A man has an elevated uric acid level, and he receives a prescription for probenecid. He also has cold sores on his mouth due to exposure to the sun, which is being treated with acyclovir. What effect will occur with the administration of these medications?**

   A. decreased serum acyclovir
   B. elevated AST and ALT
   C. increased serum uric acid
   D. increased serum acyclovir

5. **A woman experiences recurrences of herpes simplex, with an outbreak on her lips. Which medication can she apply in the early stages of the viral illness?**

   A. docosanol (Abreva)
   B. valganciclovir (Valcyte)
   C. neosporin
   D. tobramycin (Tobrex)

Clinical Application 21-1

- What is a cold sore? How does acyclovir work to decrease Ms. Jackson's symptoms and ultimately heal the cold sore?

- What patient teaching does the nurse provide to Ms. Jackson?

DRUGS FOR CYTOMEGALOVIRUS

CMV is a type of herpesvirus. The first agent developed for the treatment of CMV infection was ⓟ **ganciclovir** (Cytovene), the prototype. Prescribers use ganciclovir to treat CMV in immunocompromised patients, including those with AIDS and patients who have received transplants.

Pharmacokinetics

With oral administration, the onset of action of ganciclovir is 2 to 4 hours, and with IV administration, the onset of action is 1 hour. The drug is distributed widely to all tissues, including the cerebrospinal fluid (CSF) and eye tissue. The half-life is 1.7 to 5.8 hours, and in renal impairment, the half-life is prolonged. It is excreted unchanged in the urine.

Action

Like acyclovir, ganciclovir inhibits viral DNA synthesis. It is changed to a substrate that inhibits the binding of deoxyguanosine triphosphate to DNA polymerase.

Use

The IV form of ganciclovir is for the treatment of CMV retinitis in immunocompromised patients. Also, this preparation is for the treatment or prevention of CMV in transplant recipients. Patients take oral ganciclovir for the prevention of CMV

if they have advanced HIV infection or are at risk for disease development. In 2009, the Centers for Disease Control and Prevention (CDC) identified an unlabeled use of intravitreal ganciclovir plus systemic foscarnet for the treatment of VZV in patients with progressive outer retinal necrosis in patients with HIV. Table 21.3 summarizes route and dosage information for ganciclovir and related drugs.

Use in Older Adult Patients

Ganciclovir administration should proceed cautiously in older adults, who often have impaired organ function and concomitant diseases and use other drugs. Renal impairment is common in older adults, and risk of toxicity is greater because excretion of the drug occurs in the kidneys. Dose reduction, when indicated by decreased CrCl, may minimize these risks.

Use in Patients With Renal Impairment

It is necessary to reduce the dosage of ganciclovir according to the CrCl. Hemodialysis patients should receive ganciclovir following dialysis. The IV dosage for dialysis patients is 1.25 mg/kg every 48 to 72 hours, with maintenance dose of 0.625 mg/kg every 48 to 72 hours.

Adverse Effects

Adverse effects of ganciclovir include chills, fever, pruritus, anorexia, nausea, vomiting, anemia, leukopenia, neutropenia, thrombocytopenia, neuropathy, retinal detachment, hematuria, and sepsis. There may be increases in BUN and serum creatinine. Ganciclovir causes granulocytopenia and thrombocytopenia in 20% to 40% of recipients, often during the first 2 weeks of therapy. The U.S. Food and Drug Administration (FDA) has issued a **BLACK BOX WARNING** ◆ for ganciclovir; granulocytopenia (neutropenia), anemia, and thrombocytopenia may occur. If severe bone marrow depression occurs, it is essential that the drug be discontinued; recovery usually occurs within a week of stopping the drug. A second **BLACK BOX WARNING** ◆ advises female and male patients of childbearing age to maintain contraceptive precautions during ganciclovir therapy and for a minimum of 90 days after drug therapy.

Contraindications

Patients should not receive ganciclovir if their neutrophil count is less than 500/mm³ or platelet count is below 25,000/mm³. A known hypersensitivity to ganciclovir or any of the antiviral agents is also a contraindication. Caution is warranted in renal impairment.

Nursing Implications

Preventing Interactions

Several drugs interact with ganciclovir. Imipenem combined with ganciclovir increases the risk of seizure activity. Amphotericin B, antineoplastic agents, didanosine, dapsone, pentamidine, probenecid, trimethoprim-sulfamethoxazole, and zidovudine administered with ganciclovir

TABLE 21.3
DRUGS AT A GLANCE: Drugs for Cytomegalovirus (CMV)

Drug	Pregnancy Category	Routes and Dosage Ranges	
		Adults	Children
Ganciclovir (Cytovene)	C	CMV retinitis: induction therapy, 5 mg/kg/dose IV every 12 h for 14–21 d; maintenance therapy, 5 mg/kg/dose as a single daily dose for 7 d/wk or 6 mg/kg/d for 5 d/wk Prevention of CMV disease in transplant patients: same as induction and maintenance therapy, but the induction course is 7–14 d	CMV central nervous system (CNS) disease in human immunodeficiency virus (HIV)-exposed patients: 5 mg/kg/dose every 12 h plus foscarnet until symptoms improve followed by chronic suppression CMV retinitis: same as adult dose (slow infusion) Prevention of CMV in transplant patients: same as adult dose Neonatal congenital CMV: 6 mg/kg/dose every 12 h for 6 wk; if HIV positive a longer duration of therapy is considered
Cidofovir (Vistide) Note: Probenecid must be administered with each dose (25–40 mg/kg/dose in children)	C	Induction therapy, 5 mg/kg IV once weekly for 2 consecutive weeks; maintenance therapy, 5 mg/kg IV every 2 wk. Administer 1 L of normal saline IV before each infusion over 1–2 h and 1 L at the start of the infusion or immediately following over 1–3 h	Induction therapy, 5 mg/kg/dose IV once weekly for 2 consecutive weeks; maintenance therapy, 5 mg/kg/dose IV once every 2 wk until consecutive negative adenovirus sample. Hydrate with 20 mL/kg of normal saline for 1 h before induction therapy followed by 2 h of maintenance fluid
Foscarnet (Foscavir)	C	CMV retinitis: induction therapy, 60 mg/kg/dose IV every 8 h for 14–21 d or 90 mg/k IV every 12 h for 14–21 d; maintenance therapy, 90–120 mg every 12 h for 2 wk, followed by 120 mg/kg daily for ≥2 wk Acyclovir-resistant HSV: 40 mg/kg/dose IV every 8–12 h for 14–21 d	CMV CNS disease: 60 mg/kg/dose IV every 8 h in combination with ganciclovir followed by 90–120 mg/kg/dose daily CMV retinitis: 60 mg/kg/ dose IV every 8 h for 14–21 d with or without ganciclovir followed by 90–120 mg/kg/dose daily Acyclovir-resistant herpes simplex: 40–60 mg/kg/dose IV every 8 h until lesions heal Chickenpox not responding to acyclovir: 40–60 mg/kg/dose IV every 8 h for 7–10 d
Valganciclovir (Valcyte)	C	CMV retinitis: 900 mg PO twice daily for 21 d, then 900 mg PO once daily Prevention of CMV disease following kidney or heart transplant: 900 mg PO once daily beginning within 10 d of transplant; continue therapy until 100 d with heart or kidney transplant or 200 d for kidney transplant	1–3 mo, 16 mg/kg/dose PO every 12 h 4 mo to 16 y, dose in mg = 7 × body surface × CrCl (begin within 10 d of transplant and continue until 100 days post-transplant); doses should be rounded to the nearest 25-mg increment); maximum dose 900 mg/d

increase the risk of bone marrow suppression. Cyclosporine and ganciclovir result in nephrotoxicity. Mycophenolate, probenecid, and tenofovir increase the serum concentration of ganciclovir–valganciclovir.

Some foods and herbs interact with ganciclovir (Box 21.3).

Administering the Medication

Parenteral ganciclovir requires slow infusion, over at least 1 hour. Too rapid administration results in toxicity and excessive plasma levels. The medication is compatible with 5% dextrose

---

BOX 21.3   Herb and Dietary Interactions: Ganciclovir

■ Salt/sodium

May lead to hypernatremia when combined with certain preparations of ganciclovir

■ Echinacea

Has a potential for stimulating an autoimmune response in patients with the human immunodeficiency virus

and water, lactated Ringer's, and normal saline. Administration using intramuscular, subcutaneous, or IV push is contraindicated. Ganciclovir is a hazardous medication, and it is necessary to use appropriate precautions for handling and disposal. The nurse checks the manufacturer's guidelines and does not allow the powder or the reconstituted medication to touch the skin. The nurse does not administer the drug to patients with a platelet count less than 25,000/mm^3 or a neutrophil count less than 500/mm^3.

Assessing for Therapeutic Effects

The nurse assesses the patient for improvement in vision and visual acuity related to retinitis. It is also important to assess for improvement in symptoms related to pneumonia, hepatitis, encephalitis, adrenal insufficiency, and gastrointestinal (GI) inflammation or ulcerations.

Assessing for Adverse Effects

The nurse assesses BUN, creatinine, CrCl, CBC, and platelet count for impaired renal function and bone marrow depression. He or she assesses for signs and symptoms of hypersensitivity reactions. It is important to assess for neuropathic changes such as pain and diminished sensation.

Patient Teaching

Box 21.2 identifies general patient teaching guidelines for the antiviral drugs.

Other Drugs in the Class

Cidofovir (Vistide) is an IV drug indicated for treatment of CMV retinitis in patients with AIDS. After conversion to cidofovir diphosphate, it suppresses CMV replication by selective inhibition of viral DNA synthesis. Distribution in the CSF is limited. If the patient's serum creatinine increases by 0.3 to 0.4 mg/dL, it is necessary to reduce the dose to 3 mg/kg. If the creatinine is greater than 1.5 mg/dL, it is important to discontinue therapy. The FDA has issued three **BLACK BOX WARNINGS** ◆ for cidofovir. The drug has possible carcinogenic and teratogenic adverse effects. It may also be nephrotoxic, and prior to administration, the patient should receive 1 L of normal saline and oral probenecid. In addition, it places the patient at risk for neutropenia.

Foscarnet (Foscavir) is an IV drug administered for CMV retinitis, acyclovir-resistant HSV, and other CMV infections related to diminished immune response. The infusion rate should not exceed 1 mg/kg/min. When given by central venous access, it is possible to administer 24 mg/mL undiluted, and in abut when given through a peripheral vein, it is necessary to dilute the solution to 12 mg/mL. The nurse gives 750 to 1000 mL of normal saline or 5% dextrose and water to initiate diuresis. The patient should be well hydrated throughout the infusion of the medication. In addition to the warning related to potential renal impairment, the FDA has issued a **BLACK BOX WARNING** ◆ regarding seizures with use of foscarnet, which may occur related to impaired renal function, diminished serum calcium, and CNS conditions. It is important to use foscarnet cautiously in patients with renal disease and to assess for signs of renal impairment. Manifestations of renal impairment are most likely to occur during the second week of induction therapy but may appear any time during treatment.

To minimize renal impairment, it helps to monitor renal function (e.g., at baseline; two or three times weekly during induction; at least every 1 or 2 weeks during maintenance therapy) and reduce the dosage accordingly. If the CrCl drops below 0.4 mL/min/kg, it is necessary to discontinue the drug.

Valganciclovir is an oral drug administered for CMV retinitis and prevention of CMV infections following organ transplant. The medication inhibits viral reproduction after it is activated by a viral enzyme found in virus-infected cells. Valganciclovir has the same **BLACK BOX WARNINGS** ◆ as ganciclovir. Patients should take this drug with a high-fat diet to enhance absorption.

NCLEX Success

6. A man with HIV is on hemodialysis for renal failure. CMV retinitis develops. Which of the following is most important when administer ganciclovir?
   A. Administer the medication on an empty stomach.
   B. Assess the patient's vision following the medication administration.
   C. Administer ganciclovir after dialysis is completed.
   D. Assess the patient's sodium level following dialysis.

7. A patient receives a prescription for valganciclovir for the prevention of CMV infections following organ transplantation. Which of the following nursing interventions should be implemented?
   A. Instruct the patient to take the medication following a meal high in fat.
   B. Instruct the patient to take the meal with large amounts of fluids.
   C. Instruct the patient to report abdominal pain.
   D. Instruct the patient to report diminished sense of hearing.

Drugs for Respiratory Syncytial Virus

The Ⓟ **ribavirin** (Virazole), a synthetic nucleoside antiviral drug, is one of the few antiviral drugs that is indicated for use in children. Its main use is for the treatment of respiratory syncytial virus (RSV) infections.

Pharmacokinetics

Ribavirin, which is inhaled systemically, has a slow onset of action. It reaches its peak of action in 60 to 90 minutes. The medication is metabolized at the cellular level, with a 9.5-hour half-life. It is excreted in the feces and urine.

Action and Use

Ribavirin inhibits the replication of RNA and DNA viruses to stop the influenza virus RNA polymerase activity. This action interferes with the elongation and initiation of RNA fragments, which stops protein synthesis. Inhaled ribavirin may be effective in infants and children with severe RSV infection of

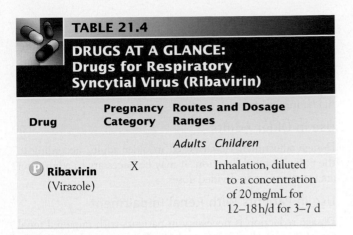

Drug	Pregnancy Category	Routes and Dosage Ranges	
		Adults	Children
Ⓟ Ribavirin (Virazole)	X		Inhalation, diluted to a concentration of 20 mg/mL for 12–18 h/d for 3–7 d

the lower respiratory tract. Table 21.4 presents route and dosage information for ribavirin.

Adverse Effects

Adverse effects experienced by patients are fatigue, insomnia, headache, anemia, nausea, and anorexia. Less than 1% of the population experiences hypotension, cardiac arrest, conjunctivitis, bronchospasm, apnea, and decline in respiratory function. Health care workers caring for children treated with RSV may report headache, conjunctivitis, nausea, rash, dizziness, chest pain, bronchospasm, pharyngitis, and rhinitis. The FDA has issued a **BLACK BOX WARNING** ◆ for ribavirin; the drug causes significant teratogenic effects, according to animal studies. Pregnant women or those who plan to become pregnant should not care for children receiving inhalation therapy or be in the room when it is being administered.

Contraindications

Contraindications to ribavirin include a known hypersensitivity to the drug or its components.

Nursing Implications

Preventing Interactions

There are no known drug or herb interactions with inhaled ribavirin. However, mixing the drug with other inhaled or aerosol medications is to be avoided.

Administering the Medication

Administration in a well-ventilated room is necessary; there should be six air exchanges per hour. Patients who are mechanically ventilated require monitoring for malfunction or obstruction of the expiratory valve, which could result in high positive end-expiratory pressures. The nurse should know that when using a SPAG-2 unit for administration, it is important to discard solutions every 24 hours and when the liquid level is low.

Assess for Therapeutic Effects

The nurse assesses respiratory status, including dyspnea, apnea, labored respirations, nasal flaring, contractions, shallow respirations, wheezing, rales, and rhonchi.

Assess for Adverse Effects

The nurse assesses level of comfort; crying, grimacing, and anxiety could indicate pain. The level of activity may indicate increased fatigue. The nurse also assesses the airway for bronchospasm or alterations in pulmonary function, including cyanosis. In addition, he or she assesses vital signs for hypotension and changes in cardiac status.

Patient Teaching

Box 21.2 identifies general patient teaching guidelines for the antiviral drugs. In addition, the nurse instructs families about the risk of exposure with pregnancy and aspects of ribavirin administration.

Clinical Application 21-2

Ms. Jackson's 1-year-old child, James, is admitted to the pediatric medical division with a diagnosis of respiratory syncytial virus (RSV). Ms. Jackson is pregnant with twins.
- What precautions does the nurse need to take with Ms. Jackson and her child?
- What patient teaching does the nurse provide to Ms. Jackson and her family?
- What assessments does the nurse implement when caring for James?

NCLEX Success

8. A 5-month-old infant is receiving ribavirin for RSV. The nurse assesses the infant visually. Which of the following indicates that the infant's pulmonary status is impaired?

   A. shallow respirations
   B. nasal flaring
   C. respiratory rate of 36 breaths/min
   D. sleeping

9. When caring for an infant receiving ribavirin, the nurse notes the fluid level is low in the SPAG-2 unit. What action should the nurse take?

   A. Discard the remaining fluid and add more fluid.
   B. Add 10 mL of normal saline to the SPAG-2 unit.
   C. Discard the SPAG-2 unit.
   D. Add sterile water to the SPAG-2 unit.

Drugs for Influenza

Two classes of drugs are used for the prophylaxis and treatment of influenza A. The first class is adamantanes, which includes Ⓟ **amantadine hydrochloride** (Symmetrel). Amantadine hydrochloride is also discussed in Chapter 47 with regard to its use in the treatment of Parkinson's disease. The second class is the neuraminidase inhibitors, which includes Ⓟ **oseltamivir phosphate** (Tamiflu).

ADAMANTANES

Amantadine hydrochloride is a synthetic antiviral agent administered for the treatment of influenza A, an RNA virus. This drug is not effective against influenza B. In the January 21, 2011 *Morbidity and Mortality Weekly Report*, the CDC recommends that amantadine (and rimantadine; see *Other Drugs in the Class*) not be administered because of the high levels of resistance of circulating influenza A virus to these drugs. However, this chapter discusses amantadine because it may be used in the event of the reemergence of adamantane-susceptible strains.

Pharmacokinetics

Amantadine is well absorbed, with an onset of action in 48 hours and a peak of action in 1 to 4 hours. It is distributed throughout the body fluids, with the highest concentrations in the lung tissues. The medication is not metabolized, and 80% to 90% of the drug is eliminated unchanged in the urine.

Action and Use

Amantadine blocks the uncoating of the virus, thus preventing penetration in the host. Its uses include prophylactic and symptomatic treatment of influenza A. Table 21.5 summarizes route and dosage information for the adamantanes and the neuraminidase inhibitors.

Use in Older Adults

Dosage adjustment is warranted in older adults, according to the patient's renal function. It may be necessary to administer amantadine in two divided doses.

Use in Patients With Renal Impairment

Dosage reduction is necessary in patients with impaired renal function according to the CrCl. Patients on hemodialysis should take amantadine 200 mg orally every 7 days.

Adverse Effects

Use of amantadine is associated with several adverse effects. CNS effects may include depression as well as dizziness,

TABLE 21.5

DRUGS AT A GLANCE: Drugs for Influenza

Drug	Pregnancy Category	Routes and Dosage Ranges	
		Adults	Children
Adamantanes			
Ⓟ **Amantadine hydro-chloride** (Symmetrel)	C	Influenza A prophylaxis: 200 mg PO daily or 100 mg PO twice daily for 10 d after exposure Uncomplicated influenza: same as above; continue 24–48 h after symptoms subside	Not recommended for age <1 y Influenza A prophylaxis: 1–9 y: 4.4–8.8 mg/kg/d PO in one or two divided doses not to exceed 150 mg/d Uncomplicated influenza: same as above; continue 24–48 h after symptoms subside
Rimantadine (Flumadine)	C	Influenza A: prophylaxis, 100 mg PO twice daily; treatment, 100 mg PO twice daily start within 48 h of symptoms for 5–7 d	1–9 y, 5 mg/kg/d PO in divided doses (maximum dose: 150 mg/d) 10 y and older, same as adults
Neuraminidase Inhibitors			
Ⓟ **Oseltamivir phos-phate** (Tamiflu)	C	Prophylaxis, 75 mg PO daily for 10 d begin within 2 d after exposure Treatment, 75 mg PO twice daily for 5 d within 2 d of exposure	Birth to 1 y, consult manufacturer's recommendations Infants <1 y, weight-based dosing; 3 mg/kg/dose twice daily for 5 d 1–12 y Prophylaxis, ≤15 kg, 30 mg/d PO; 15–23 kg, 45 mg/d PO; 23–40 kg, 60 mg/d PO; >40 kg 75 mg/d; all for 10 d Treatment, 30–75 mg PO twice daily for 5 d
Zanamivir (Relenza)	C	Prophylaxis, 2 inhalations per day for 28 d Treatment, 2 inhalations (10 mg total) every 12 h for 5 d (begin within 2 d of symptoms), first day two inhalations 2 h apart then every 12 h	Prophylaxis (5 y and older), same as adult Treatment (7 y and older), same as adult

lightheadedness, nervousness with anxiety, and inability to concentrate. Cardiovascular adverse effects include orthostatic hypotension and peripheral edema. Other adverse effects are anorexia, constipation, nausea, diarrhea, dry nose, and bluish mottling of the skin on the legs and hands.

Contraindications

Contraindications to amantadine include a known hypersensitivity to the medication.

Nursing Implications

Preventing Interactions

Anticholinergic agents administered during the course of amantadine therapy may enhance the anticholinergic effects such as urinary retention, dry mouth, narrow-angle glaucoma, and hypertension. Alcohol increases CNS depression.

Administering the Medication

Patients should take the first dose of amantadine early in the morning and the second dose in the early evening, 12 hours later. They should take the drug with a full glass of water or with food to prevent disruptive sleep patterns. It is necessary to store the medication at room temperature in a tightly closed, light-protected container. High-risk patients who have not been vaccinated previously with the influenza A vaccine can receive amantadine with the vaccine.

Assess for Therapeutic Effects

The nurse assesses for a decrease in flu-like symptoms such as decreased fever, malaise, pain, cough, and rhinitis.

Assess for Adverse Effects

The nurse assesses the patient's mental status regarding alertness and ability to cope. Also, it is necessary to assess for dizziness and lightheadedness as well as for pedal edema and signs of orthostatic hypotension with position changes.

Patient Teaching

Box 21.2 identifies general patient teaching guidelines for the antiviral drugs.

Other Drugs in the Class

Rimantadine (Flumadine) is an oral drug used to control outbreaks of influenza A. The drug can be used in combination with oseltamivir or zanamivir but is not recommended in combination with amantadine. It reaches a peak of action in 6 hours. Rimantadine is metabolized in the liver and is excreted unchanged in the urine. The serum half-life is 25.4 hours, which may be prolonged with liver or renal impairment.

NEURAMINIDASE INHIBITORS

The neuraminidase inhibitors are active against influenza A or B virus. As reported by the *Morbidity and Mortality Weekly Report* (January 21, 2011), the CDC recommends these antiviral medications be used for influenza; "on the basis of recent viral surveillance and resistance data, the greater than 99% of currently calculated

influenza virus strains are sensitive to these medications." In this class, the prototype drug is ⓟ **oseltamivir**. The CDC (2011) recommends antiviral treatment of influenza or suspected influenza begin as soon as possible with oseltamivir and zanamivir.

Pharmacokinetics

Oseltamivir is well absorbed and distributed as oseltamivir carboxylate. The half-life of the drug is 1 to 3 hours. It is metabolized in the liver, and 90% is excreted in the urine with the remainder excreted in the feces.

Action

Oseltamivir, in its active form oseltamivir carboxylate, acts to inhibit the viral enzyme neuraminidase. This enzyme helps the newly formed virus to exit the host cell. By inhibiting this viral enzyme, oseltamivir carboxylate prevents new virus from infecting other cells.

Use

Oseltamivir is an oral drug administered to adults and children 1 year or older who have contracted influenza A or B. The recipients of treatment must have been symptomatic for 2 days or less. Adults and children 1 year of age or older may also take it prophylactically. Table 21.5 gives route and dosage information for oseltamivir.

Adverse Effects and Contraindications

The adverse effects of oseltamivir are nausea, vomiting, abdominal pain, diarrhea, conjunctivitis, and epistaxis. Contraindications include a known hypersensitivity to the medication. Women who are breastfeeding should not take oseltamivir.

Nursing Implications

Preventing Interactions

Probenecid increases the serum concentration of oseltamivir. It is necessary to assess for thrombocytopenia if these drugs are administered together. People should not take oseltamivir 48 hours before receiving the influenza virus vaccine or for 2 weeks after receiving the vaccine.

Administering the Medication

According to the FDA, the manufacturer of the oral suspension of oseltamivir has changed the concentration from 12 to 6 mg/mL. The lower concentration allows for more accurate measurement because it does not become as frothy as the 12-mg concentration.

QSEN Safety Alert

It is important to read the label carefully, because the 12-mg/mL preparation is still available in some areas.

People may take oseltamivir with food to improve tolerance and prevent GI upset. If necessary, capsules can be opened and the powder mixed in a sweetened liquid to make the drug more palatable.

Assessing for Therapeutic Effects

The nurse assesses for a decrease in flu-like symptoms such as fever, malaise, pain, cough, and rhinitis.

Assessing for Adverse Effects

The nurse assesses the patient for GI upset, including nausea, vomiting, and diarrhea. It is also necessary to assess the nares for signs of bleeding and irritation as well as the conjunctiva for irritation, redness, and drainage.

Patient Teaching

Box 21.2 identifies general patient teaching guidelines for the antiviral drugs.

Other Drugs in the Class

Zanamivir (Relenza) has a similar action to oseltamivir. Patients take the medication using a Diskhaler delivery system, which should be used cautiously in patients with chronic obstructive pulmonary disease and asthma because of the risk of bronchospasm. A rapid-acting inhaled bronchodilator should be available. It is important that the nurse instruct all patients about the use of the inhaler and report worsening respiratory symptoms or the occurrence of diarrhea, nausea, and vomiting. Zanamivir has an unlabeled use in H1N1 virus infection.

NCLEX Success

10. A 55-year-old woman takes oseltamivir for the treatment of influenza A. Which viral enzyme does it inhibit in the treatment of influenza?

    A. trypsin
    B. amylase
    C. lipase
    D. neuraminidase

11. A 25-year-old man with asthma develops influenza A. Which of the following medications is contraindicated for the treatment of influenza A in this case?

    A. acetaminophen
    B. pseudoephedrine
    C. oseltamivir
    D. zanamivir

Drugs for Hepatitis: Nucleoside Analogs

Drug therapy for hepatitis B virus (HBV) includes pegylated interferon and antiviral agents, particularly lamivudine. The goal of therapy is to reduce the risk of transmission to others and prevent long-term complications such as cirrhosis or hepatocellular carcinoma. The following section discusses the nucleoside analog Ⓟ **lamivudine** (Epivir, Epivir HBV) as the prototype antiviral agent for HBV.

Pharmacokinetics

Lamivudine is rapidly absorbed in the GI tract, after which it is distributed with less than 36% of the drug bound by plasma protein. Approximately 4.2% of the drug is metabolized to a trans-sulfoxide metabolite. The half-life of the drug is 2 hours in children and 5 to 7 hours in adults. The drug is excreted unchanged in the urine.

Action

Incorporation of a monophosphate form of lamivudine into the viral DNA of HBV polymerase results in the termination of the DNA chain. The drug also inhibits the transcription of the viral RNA chain in HBV. In addition, as a cytosine analog, lamivudine inhibits HIV reverse transcriptase of the viral RNA chain.

Use

Prescribers order lamivudine for the treatment of chronic hepatitis B in patients who have evidence of hepatitis B viral replication and active inflammation of the liver. Patients with HIV may also take the drug when antiretroviral therapy with a multidrug regimen is necessary. An unlabeled use is for postexposure to HIV as part of a multidrug regimen. Table 21.6 gives route and dosage information for lamivudine and the other antiviral agents used for hepatitis.

Use in Children

Pancreatitis is prevalent in children who take lamivudine. Close monitoring is necessary. If signs and symptoms of pancreatitis such as upper abdominal pain, back pain, and vomiting develop, it is essential to discontinue the drug.

Use in Patients With Renal Impairment

The presence of renal impairment warrants a reduction in the lamivudine dosage according to the CrCl.

Adverse Effects

A main adverse effect of lamivudine is pancreatitis. Other adverse effects include nausea, vomiting, diarrhea, abdominal pain, neutropenia, myalgia, neuropathy, and musculoskeletal pain. In addition, patients have reported headache; fatigue; insomnia; cough; sinusitis; and infections of the ear, nose, and throat. The FDA has issued a **BLACK BOX WARNING** ◆ for the nucleoside analogs, stating that lactic acidosis and severe hepatomegaly with steatosis have been reported.

Contraindications

Contraindications to lamivudine include a known hypersensitivity to the drug or any of the components of the drug.

Nursing Implications

Preventing Interactions

Several drugs interact with lamivudine. Trimethoprim–sulfamethoxazole increases the serum level of lamivudine. Ganciclovir–valganciclovir may enhance the adverse effects of lamivudine. Ribavirin increases the hepatotoxic effects of lamivudine. In addition, administration of lamivudine and

TABLE 21.6

DRUGS AT A GLANCE: Drugs for Hepatitis: Nucleoside Analogs

Drug	Pregnancy Category	Routes and Dosage Ranges	
		Adults	Children
Ⓟ **Lamivudine** (Epivir, Epivir-HBV)	C	100 mg PO daily	2–17 y, 3 mg/kg PO daily up to maximum 100 mg daily
Adefovir dipivoxil (Hepsera)	C	10 mg PO daily	Younger than 12 y, safety and efficacy have not been established
Entecavir (Baraclude)	C	0.5 mg/kg PO 2 h before or 2 h after a meal History of viremia, also receiving lamivudine or with known resistance to mutations: 1 mg PO daily on empty stomach	Younger than 16 y, safety and efficacy have not been established
Ribavirin (Riba Tab)	X	75 kg or less, two 200-mg capsules PO in AM, three 200 mg capsules PO in PM with Intron A, 3 million international units Sub-Q 3 times per week; or with 180 mcg of Pegasys Sub-Q per week for 48 wk More than 75 kg, three 200-mg capsules PO in AM, three 200 mg capsules in PM with 3 million international units of Intron A subcutaneously 3 times per week; or with 180 mcg Pegasys Sub-Q per week for 48 wk	3 y and older, 15 mg/kg PO daily in divided doses (give with interferon alfa-2a, 3 million international units/m², subcutaneously 3 times per week); children 25 kg or more who cannot swallow tablets may use oral solution
Telbivudine (Tyzeka)	B	600 mg PO daily	Safety and efficacy have not been established
Tenofovir disoproxil fumarate (Viread)	B	300 mg PO daily	Safety and efficacy have not been established

zidovudine increases the serum level of zidovudine. Zalcitabine and lamivudine result in the inactivation of both drugs.

Administering the Medication

Patients may take lamivudine with or without food.

Assessing for Therapeutic Effects

The nurse assesses for decreased malaise, myalgia, loss of appetite, and abdominal pain. If the patient had jaundice, the nurse assesses for diminished yellowing of the skin and sclera. It is necessary to palpate the liver and lymph nodes for decreased size. Monitoring AST and ALT for decreasing serum levels is important. The administration of lamivudine decreases the effects of hepatitis, leading to an improvement in the serum liver enzyme levels.

Assessing for Adverse Effects

The nurse assesses for abdominal pain, particularly in pediatric patients. Such pain may be indicative of pancreatitis. Also, the nurse assesses for GI effects such as nausea, vomiting, and diarrhea, as well as for headache, myalgia, and musculoskeletal pain. It is also necessary to assess for upper respiratory effects such as sinusitis and infections.

Patient Teaching

Box 21.2 identifies general patient teaching guidelines for antiviral drugs. In addition, the nurse teaches the patient the signs of symptoms of lactic acidosis, including musculoskeletal pain.

Other Drugs in the Class

Adefovir dipivoxil (Hepsera) is a purine nucleotide analog administered for chronic hepatitis B with active viral replication producing elevation in AST/ALT. The drug requires cautious use in renal dysfunction. Experts do not recommend using adefovir for first-line therapy of chronic hepatitis B because of its weak antiviral activity, leading to viral resistance to the drug.

Entecavir (Baraclude) inhibits the HBV polymerase to reduce viral DNA levels. To aid in the absorption of the medication, administration on an empty stomach is necessary. The rapid onset of action and the peak of action occur in ½ to 1½ hours. Excretion is in the urine.

Ribavirin (Ribatab) is an oral antiviral drug administered in combination with peginterferon alfa-2a or peginterferon alfa-2b for chronic hepatitis B. People should take the drug on an empty stomach to aid in absorption and without antacids and nucleoside reverse transcriptase inhibitors (NRTIs). The FDA has issued a **BLACK BOX WARNING** ◆ for ribavirin, stating that it can produce hemolytic anemia, which could lead to myocardial infarction. Patients with unstable cardiovascular disease should not take the drug. Patients 3 years and older may take ribavirin (Copegus, Rebetol, Ribasphere, Virazole) with peginterferon alfa-2a or peginterferon alfa-2b (see Chap. 9) for the treatment of hepatitis C.

Tenofovir disoproxil (Viread) is useful for the treatment of chronic hepatitis B in patients with compensated or decompensated liver disease. It is also used in combination with other antiretrovirals for HIV infection. It is necessary to monitor frequently for demineralization that may lead to pathological fractures. The nurse teaches the patient to increase calcium intake with the use of dairy products.

Telbivudine (Tyzeka) is an oral drug used for the treatment of hepatitis B. Its metabolite inhibits the hepatitis B DNA polymerase through competition with the natural nucleoside substrate. The DNA chain is then terminated, inhibiting the replication of hepatitis B. Telbivudine has a peak of action of 1 to 4 hours, with minimal protein binding. It is widely distributed in tissues and eliminated unchanged in the urine.

NCLEX Success

12. A man is taking lamivudine. He states that he has severe upper abdominal pain. On assessment, he has guarding. What would the nurse suspect is wrong with the patient?

   A. hepatomegaly
   B. pancreatitis
   C. epiglottitis
   D. cardiomyopathy

13. A woman is taking lamivudine for chronic hepatitis B. She reports that her stools float and are clay colored. In addition, she complains of musculoskeletal pain. What would the nurse suspect has contributed to the development of these clinical manifestations?

   A. cirrhosis
   B. ascites
   C. lactic acidosis
   D. pulmonary edema

Drugs for Human Immunodeficiency Virus (Antiretroviral Drugs)

Health care providers use a variety of **antiretroviral drugs** to fight HIV, an infection that infects the immune system caused by a retrovirus. The broad classification of these drugs are the NRTIs, non-nucleoside reverse transcriptase inhibitors (NNRTIs), protease inhibitors (PIs), the integrase strand transfer inhibitors, the fusion protein inhibitors, and the CCR5 antagonists (Fig. 21.1). In general, newer drugs and drug combinations are more effective for viral suppression, cause fewer serious adverse effects, and are more convenient for patients to take. The regimen usually consists of two NRTIs with an NNRTI or a PI (Bartlett, 2012). **Highly active antiretroviral therapy** (HAART) involves the use of several combinations of antiretroviral drugs in the treatment of HIV/AIDS. Authorities do not recommend using some of the older drugs for initial treatment but may suggest them when drug-resistant infections develop with the newer drugs. Patients often undergo genotypic or phenotypic testing for drug resistance to guide antiretroviral therapy.

When administering antiretroviral agents, it is important to distinguish whether the patient has taken the antiretroviral agents in the past. Patients who have received antiretroviral agents are *treatment experienced*, whereas those who have not received them are *treatment naïve*.

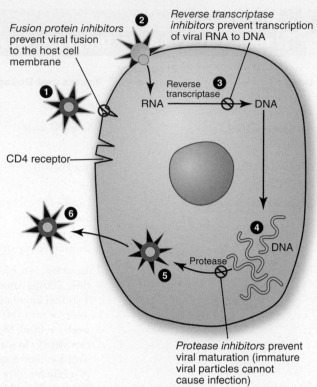

Figure 21.1 Human immunodeficiency virus (HIV) entry into cells and replication; actions of anti-HIV drugs. (1) The virus attaches to receptors (e.g., CD4 molecules) and co-receptors (CCR5 molecules) on the host cell membrane. (2) The virus becomes uncoated and releases its RNA into the host cell. (3) The enzyme reverse transcriptase converts RNA to DNA, which is necessary for viral replication. (4) The DNA codes for protein synthesis, which produces immature viral particles. (5) The enzyme protease assembles the immature viral particles into mature viruses. (6) Mature viruses are released from the host cell.

NUCLEOSIDE REVERSE TRANSCRIPTASE INHIBITORS

The NRTIs are structurally similar to DNA components (adenosine, cytosine, guanosine, and thymidine) and thus easily enter human cells and viruses in human cells. For example, ⓟ **zidovudine** (AZT, Retrovir), the prototype, is able to substitute for thymidine. The drugs are more active in slowing the progression of acute infection rather than in treating chronically infected cells. Thus, they do not cure HIV infection or prevent transmission of the virus through sexual contact or blood contamination.

Pharmacokinetics

The oral preparation of zidovudine is quickly absorbed in the GI tract, reaching a peak of action in ½ to 1½ hours. The drug, which can cross the blood–brain barrier, is readily distributed to the CSF. It also crosses the placenta. Zidovudine is metabolized in the liver. It is 25% to 38% protein bound with a half-life of 1½ to 3 hours. It is excreted in the urine; 72% to 74% is excreted as metabolites, with 14% to 18% excreted unchanged. (With the IV preparation, 45% to 60% is excreted as metabolites and 18% to 29% as unchanged drug.)

Action

Like all NRTIs, zidovudine has the ability to incorporate into the DNA chains by viral reverse transcriptase. (HIV needs this enzyme to convert RNA to DNA and replicate.) Thus, the drug blocks the addition of further nucleotides and terminates viral replication.

Use

Patients take zidovudine for the treatment of HIV infection—in combination with two or more other antiretroviral agents. Pregnant women who are infected with HIV take the drug as monotherapy to prevent the transmission of HIV to the fetus. An unlabeled use is postexposure prophylaxis for HIV exposure with a multidrug regimen. Table 21.7 presents route and dosage information for zidovudine and other NRTIs.

Use in Children

To prevent maternal–fetal HIV transmission in neonates, experts recommend that zidovudine be given as soon as possible after birth—6 to 12 hours after delivery. It is necessary to continue the dose until the neonate is 6 weeks of age. Infants born to mothers whose **viral load** (number of HIV RNA particles within the blood) is significantly below normal should receive zidovudine combined with nevirapine. If the infant develops a rash, there should be no dosage increase during the 14-day lead-in period.

Use in Patients With Renal Impairment

For patients on hemodialysis or peritoneal dialysis and a CrCl less than 15 mL/min, the oral dose should be 100 mg every 6 to 8 hours or 300 mg daily. The IV dose should be 1 mg/kg every 6 to 8 hours.

TABLE 21.7

DRUGS AT A GLANCE: Antiretroviral Drugs: Nucleoside Reverse Transcriptase Inhibitors

Drug	Pregnancy Category	Routes and Dosage Ranges	
		Adults	*Children*
(P) **Zidovudine** (AZT, Retrovir)	C	300 mg PO twice daily or 200 mg PO 3 times per day; 1 mg/kg/dose IV every 4 h Prevention of maternal–fetal human immunodeficiency virus (HIV) transmission during labor and delivery (give when labor begins): 2 mg/kg IV as loading dose followed by a continuous IV infusion of 1 mg/kg/h until umbilical cord is clamped Cesarean section: begin 3 h before surgery Prevention of HIV following needlesticks: begin 2 h after exposure, 200 mg PO 3 times per day plus lamivudine 150 mg twice daily and a PI for high-risk exposure	Neonatal HIV: use in combination with other antiretroviral agents Premature infants <35 wk gestational age, 2 mg/kg dose PO every 12 h or 1.5 mg/kg/dose IV every 12 h Infants <30 wk, increase dose to every 8 h at 4 wk of age Infants ≥30 wk, increase dose to every 8 h at 2 wk of age Full-term infants, 2 mg/kg/dose PO every 6 h or 1.5 mg/kg/dose every 6 h Prevention of maternal–fetal HIV transmission (zidovudine is used in neonates as monotherapy) 2 mg/kg/dose PO every 12 h or 1.5 mg/dose IV every 12 h; increase to every 8 h as follows: Preterm infants <30 wk, increase dose to every 8 h at 4 wk of age ≥30 wk, increase above dose to every 8 h at 2 wk of age Full-term infants 2 mg/kg PO every 6 h; alternate dosing <2.5 kg, 10 mg PO twice daily >2.5 kg, 15 mg PO twice daily 1.5 mg/kg IV every 6 h HIV: <6 wk, 2 mg/kg/dose PO every 6 h 6 wk to <12 y, 20 mg/m²/h IV continuous infusion 120 mg/m²/dose IV every 6 h ≥12 y, 1 mg/kg/dose IV intermittent infusion every 4 h around the clock

(Continued on page 384)

TABLE 21.7

DRUGS AT A GLANCE: Antiretroviral Drugs: Nucleoside Reverse Transcriptase Inhibitors (Continued)

Drug	Pregnancy Category	Routes and Dosage Ranges	
		Adults	Children
Abacavir sulfate (Ziagen)	C	300 mg PO twice daily or 600 mg daily 1 mg/kg/dose IV every 4 h Hepatic impairment: 200 mg PO 2 times per day	3 mo to 16 y, 8 mg/kg PO twice daily, not to exceed 300 mg/dose
Abacavir and lamivudine (Epzicom)	C	Abacavir 600 mg and lamivudine 300 mg PO daily	Not recommended
Abacavir, lamivudine, and zidovudine (Trizivir)	C	1 tablet PO twice daily; not recommended for patients who weigh <40 kg	Not recommended
Didanosine (Videx, Videx EC)	B	Videx <60 kg, 125 mg PO twice daily or 250 mg PO daily ≥60 kg, 200 mg PO twice daily or 400 mg PO daily Videx EC 25 to <60 kg, 250 mg PO daily ≥60 kg, 400 mg PO daily When taken with tenofovir, <60 kg and CrCl ≥60 mL/min, 200 mg once daily; ≥60 kg and CrCl ≥60 mL/min: 250 mg once daily	Videx 2 wk to 8 mo, 100 mg/m² PO twice daily >8 mo, 120 mg/m² PO twice daily (not to exceed adult dose) Videx EC ≥6 y 20 to <25 kg, 200 mg PO once daily 25 to <60 kg, 250 mg PO once daily ≥60 kg, 400 mg PO once daily
Emtricitabine (Emtriva)	D	Capsules, 200 mg PO daily Solution, 240 mg PO daily	0–3 mo, 3 mg/kg/d PO 3 mo to 17 y, >33 kg, 200 mg PO once daily Solution, 6 mg/kg per PO per day
Emtricitabine and tenofovir (Truvada)	B	Emtricitabine 200 mg and tenofovir 300 mg, one tablet PO daily	Not intended for children
Emtricitabine, tenofovir, and efavirenz (Atripla)	D	Emtricitabine 200 mg, tenofovir disoproxil 300 mg, and efavirenz 600 mg; 1 tablet PO daily	Not intended for children
Lamivudine (Epivir)	C	150 mg PO 2 times per day or 300 mg/d; PO as a single dose in combination with other antiretroviral agents	1–3 mo, 4 mg/kg PO twice daily 3 m to 16 y, 4 mg/kg PO 2 times per day; maximum dose 150 mg 2 times daily
Stavudine (Zerit)	C	<60 kg, 30 mg PO every 12 h ≥60 kg, 40 mg PO every 12 h	Birth to 13 d, 0.5 mg/kg PO every 12 h ≥14 d and <30 kg, 1 mg/kg PO every 12 h ≥30 kg, same as adults
Tenofovir disoproxil fumarate (Viread)	B	300 mg PO daily with meals	≥12 y and ≥35 kg, same as adults
Zidovudine and lamivudine (Combivir)	C	Zidovudine 300 mg and lamivudine 150 mg PO daily	Adolescents ≥30 kg, same as adults

Adverse Effects

Patients administered zidovudine has reported headache and malaise. Other significant adverse effects include nausea, vomiting, and anorexia. The FDA has issued **BLACK BOX WARNING ◆** related to the adverse effects of granulocytopenia, aplastic or hemolytic anemia, pancytopenia with bone marrow hypoplasia, leukopenia, and lymphadenopathy with zidovudine. It is necessary to adjust the dosage in patients who develop anemia or neutropenia. Two other **BLACK BOX WARNINGS ◆** for zidovudine relate to lactic acidosis and severe hepatomegaly with steatosis and symptomatic myopathy and myositis. The risk of liver disease increases in females, obese patients, and pregnant patients, and with prolonged use. If clinical or laboratory signs of lactic acidosis or hepatotoxicity develop, it is essential that the drug be discontinued.

Contraindications

Contraindications to zidovudine include a known hypersensitivity to the drug or history of lactic acidosis.

Nursing Implications

Preventing Interactions

Antiretroviral agents administered in combination with zidovudine result in an increased risk of lactic acidosis and hepatomegaly. Other drugs also have significant effects when taken with zidovudine. Clozapine increases the risk of agranulocytosis. If possible, patients should not receive clozapine and zidovudine together. Acyclovir and valacyclovir enhance CNS depression. Ribavirin enhances the development of anemia. Acetaminophen, ganciclovir, and interferon alfa enhance bone marrow suppression. Other medications interact with zidovudine, increasing or decreasing its effects (Box 21.4).

Administering the Medication

Patients may take oral preparation of zidovudine with or without food. They should take the drug around the clock to avoid variations in serum peak and trough levels. The nurse should mix the parenteral preparation in 5% dextrose and water or normal saline. Infusion should take place over ½ hour in neonates and 1 hour in children and adults. Zidovudine is incompatible with blood products and protein solutions.

Assessing for Therapeutic Effects

The nurse monitors the patient's CD4 and cell count for increase or decrease in viral load. An increase in the CD4 count indicates a decrease in viral load and the ability to fight viral infections. In addition, the nurse assesses the patient's clinical status for decrease in the development of opportunistic infections.

Assessing for Adverse Effects

The nurse assesses for malaise, CNS depression, and GI symptoms such as nausea, vomiting, and diarrhea. He or she assesses for myalgia and hepatomegaly. The development of anemia usually occurs 2 to 4 weeks after the start of therapy. Neutropenia is most likely to occur in 6 to 8 weeks. It is important to obtain the patient's CBC as a baseline measure before therapy begins and then every 2 weeks from then on. In addition, the nurse assesses the hemoglobin, hematocrit, and granulocyte count for hematologic toxicity. If the hemoglobin level is less than 7.5 g/dL or the reduction is greater than 25% of the baseline value, it may be necessary to interrupt therapy and administer transfusions. This is also the case if the granulocyte count is less than 750/mm³ or greater than 50% of the baseline measure.

Patient Teaching

Box 21.5 identifies general patient teaching guidelines for antiretroviral drugs. Because lactic acidosis may develop, the nurse teaches the patient the signs and symptoms of this condition, including musculoskeletal pain.

Other Drugs in the Class

Abacavir sulfate (Ziagen) inhibits the viral reverse transcriptase through competition with the natural DNA nucleoside and incorporation into viral DNA. It is contraindicated in moderate to severe hepatic impairment. Abacavir is administered in combination with other antiretroviral agents. The FDA has issued a **BLACK BOX WARNING** ◆ stating that patients taking abacavir may have serious and sometimes fatal hypersensitivity reactions. Patients who test positive for HLAB*5701 allele are at greatest risk for hypersensitivity reactions. Patients may also be at risk for lactic acidosis.

Didanosine (Videx, Videx EC) is an oral antiretroviral that is administered 30 minutes before meals or 2 hours after meals. The drug blocks the HIV replication in T cells and monocytes to block viral DNA synthesis and replication. Patients should not combine it with alcohol due to the increased risk of pancreatitis. It is necessary to reduce the drug dosage in renal impairment.

Emtricitabine (Emtriva) inhibits HIV-1 reverse transcriptase to inhibit HIV activity. Again, dosage reduction in renal impairment is necessary. Prior to beginning therapy, it is important to check liver function and assess it periodically throughout treatment. The nurse also assesses patients with depression for suicidal ideation. In addition, the nurse instructs patients to avoid driving or operating machinery until their response to the medication is known.

Stavudine is an NRTI that is administered in combination with other antiretroviral medications. The World Health Organization recommends 30 mg every 12 hours in all adult and adolescent patients regardless of their weight (Up-To-Date, 2012). Geriatric patients require close monitoring for peripheral neuropathy. The dosage of stavudine should be reduced in patients with renal impairment.

NCLEX Success

14. An infant is born to a mother infected with HIV. When is it appropriate to administer zidovudine?
    A. following a positive HIV test
    B. within 6 to 12 hours after birth
    C. within the first 2 days of life
    D. only is the viral load is decreased

15. The mother of an infant infected with HIV has a low viral load and gives birth to a healthy baby boy. What is the most appropriate medical intervention?
    A. Administer the adult dose of stavudine to the infant.
    B. Administer zidovudine and nevirapine.
    C. Assess the infant's viral load.
    D. Perform HIV testing on delivery.

BOX 21.4　Drug Interactions: Zidovudine

Drugs That Increase the Effect of Zidovudine
- Divalproex, doxorubicin, fluconazole, flucytosine, indomethacin, methadone, pentamidine, probenecid, vincristine, and valproic acid
  Decrease the metabolism of zidovudine, thus increasing serum levels, leading to toxicity

Drugs That Decrease the Effect of Zidovudine
- Protease inhibitors, rifamycin derivatives (excluding rifabutin)
  Decrease serum concentration

| BOX 21.5 | **Patient Teaching Guidelines for Antiretroviral Drugs** |

■ Prevention is better than treatment, partly because medications used to treat viral infections may cause serious adverse effects. Thus, whenever possible, techniques to prevent viral infections should be used.

■ Wash hands frequently and thoroughly; this helps prevent most infections.

■ Have immunizations against viral infections as indicated.

■ Always practice safe sex. Men should use a condom.

■ In cases of intravenous drug use, use and promote the use of clean needles.

■ Drugs may relieve symptoms but do not cure human immunodeficiency virus (HIV) infection, prevent transmission of the virus, or prevent other illnesses associated with advanced HIV infection.

■ Effective treatment of HIV infection requires close adherence to drug therapy regimens involving several drugs and daily doses. Missing as few as one or two doses can decrease blood levels of antiretroviral drugs and result in increased HIV replication and development of drug-resistant viral strains.

■ It is generally recommended that herbal products not be used with antiretroviral medications. St. John's wort may decrease blood levels of some anti-HIV medications and make them less effective; echinacea should be avoided because it may stimulate viral replication.

■ Request information about adverse effects associated with the specific drugs you are taking and what you should do if they occur. Adverse effects vary among the drugs; some are potentially serious.

■ Have regular blood tests, including viral load, CD4+ cell count, complete blood count, and others as indicated (e.g., tests of kidney and liver function).

■ Keep your health care providers informed about all medications being taken; do not take any other drugs (including drugs of abuse, herbal preparations, vitamin/mineral supplements, nonprescription drugs) without consulting a health care provider. These preparations may make anti-HIV medications less effective or more toxic.

■ Take the medications exactly as prescribed. Do not change doses or stop the medications without consulting a health care provider. If a dose is missed, do not double the next dose. The drugs must be taken consistently to suppress HIV infection and minimize adverse drug effects.

■ These medications vary in their interactions with food and should be taken appropriately for optimal benefit. Unless otherwise instructed, take the drugs as follows:
  ■ Abacavir, Combivir, emtricitabine, famciclovir, fosamprenavir, Kaletra tablets, lamivudine, nevirapine, tenofovir, Trizivir, valacyclovir, and zidovudine with or without food. However, do not take abacavir or efavirenz with a high-fat meal.
  ■ Atripla, efavirenz, entecavir, or indinavir on an empty stomach, 1 hour before, or 2 hours after a meal.
  ■ Atazanavir, darunavir, ganciclovir, Kaletra oral solution, nelfinavir, ritonavir, and tipranavir with food. Saquinavir within 2 hours after a meal or with a full meal.

■ To give nelfinavir to infants and young children, the oral powder can be mixed with a small amount of water, milk, or formula (if necessary). After it is mixed, give the entire amount to the child, who must take it all to obtain the full dose. Do not use acidic foods or juices (e.g., applesauce, orange juice, apple juice) because they produce a bitter taste.

NON-NUCLEOSIDE REVERSE TRANSCRIPTASE INHIBITORS

The NNRTIs inhibit viral replication in infected cells by directly binding to reverse transcriptase and preventing its function. NRTIs and NNRTIs inhibit reverse transcriptase by different mechanisms, and therefore they may have synergistic antiviral effects. The prototype NNRTI is Ⓟ **efavirenz** (Sustiva).

Pharmacokinetics

An oral drug, efavirenz, is absorbed in the GI tract. Absorption is increased after consumption of a fatty meal. Its peak of action occurs in 3 to 5 hours. Efavirenz is approximately 99% protein bound, primarily to albumin. The drug is metabolized by the hepatic enzymes cytochrome P450 (CYP) enzymes CYP3A4 and CYP2B6, which convert it to inactivated hydroxylated metabolites. The serum half-life is 52 to 76 hours after a single dose and 40 to 55 hours after multiple doses. It is eliminated as metabolites in the feces (16%–61%) and the urine (14%–34%).

Action and Use

Efavirenz binds to reverse transcriptase to block RNA-dependent and DNA-dependent polymerase activities that include HIV-1

replication. People take the medication in combination with other antiretroviral agents for HIV-1 infection. Table 21.8 presents route and dosage information for efavirenz and the other NNRTIs.

Use in Patients With Hepatic Impairment

Patients with moderate to severe hepatic impairment should not take efavirenz.

Adverse Effects

CNS adverse effects include dizziness, headache, insomnia, altered ability to concentrate, abnormal dreams, nervousness, and depression. Genitourinary adverse effects are renal calculus and hematuria. Patients may experience fever and fatigue, skin rash, erythema multiforme, Stevens-Johnson syndrome, and toxic epidermal necrolysis. In addition, patients may have increased levels of serum cholesterol, AST, and ALT.

Contraindications

Contraindications to efavirenz include a known hypersensitivity to the medication and suicidal ideation. Because the drug may cause untoward fetal effects, particularly in the first trimester, women who are pregnant should not take it. Efavirenz is also contraindicated in breastfeeding women.

TABLE 21.8

DRUGS AT A GLANCE: Antiretroviral Drugs: Non-nucleoside Reverse Transcriptase Inhibitors

Drug	Pregnancy Category	Routes and Dosage Ranges	
		Adults	*Children*
Ⓟ **Efavirenz** (Sustiva)	D	600 mg PO daily Dosage adjustments: with concomitant rifampin (if patient ≥50 kg), 800 mg PO daily; with concomitant voriconazole, efavirenz 300 mg PO daily and voriconazole 400 mg PO every 12 h	10 kg to >15 kg, 200 mg PO daily 5 kg to <20 kg, 250 mg PO daily 20 kg to <25 kg, 300 mg PO daily 25 to <32.5 kg, 350 mg PO daily 32.5 to <40 kg, 400 mg PO once daily ≥40 kg, 600 mg PO daily
Delavirdine mesylate (Rescriptor)	C	400 mg PO 3 times per day	≥16 y: same as adult dose
Etravirine (Intelence)	B	200 mg PO twice daily after meals	Not recommended
Nevirapine (Viramune)	B	Initial, 200 mg twice daily for 14 d; maintenance, 200 mg PO twice daily (immediate-release tablets) in combination with additional antiretroviral medications; 400 mg PO once daily (extended-release tablets)	Immediate-release tablets, 150 mg/m²/dose PO once daily for the first 14 d (maximum dose: 200 mg/d); increase dose to 150 mg/m²/dose PO twice daily if no rash or untoward effects (maximum 400 mg/d)

Nursing Implications

Preventing Interactions

Many medications and herbs interact with efavirenz, increasing or decreasing its effects (Boxes 21.6 and 21.7).

Administering the Medication

Patients who experience CNS adverse effects, such as CNS depression, should take efavirenz at bedtime. They may take the medication as administered on an empty stomach. After consuming a high-fat meal, patients should not take it for 2 hours. They should not discontinue efavirenz suddenly or without the consent of the prescriber.

Assessing for Therapeutic Effects

The nurse assesses the CD4 count for increased ability to fight against viral infections.

BOX 21.6 Drug Interactions: Efavirenz

Drugs That Increase the Effect of Efavirenz
■ Fluconazole, ritonavir
Increase serum levels
■ Alcohol
Increases central nervous system depression

Drugs That Decrease the Effects of Efavirenz
■ Rifampin, saquinavir
Decrease serum levels

Assessing for Adverse Effects

The nurse assesses for skin rash and onset of Stevens-Johnson syndrome as well as for lack of concentration, increased nervousness, and impaired psychiatric effects. It is also necessary to assess for alterations in GI status such as nausea, vomiting, and diarrhea, as well as urinary output for bleeding and complaints of pain related to renal calculi. In addition, the nurse assesses the serum cholesterol, AST, and ALT values for possible increases.

Patient Teaching

Box 21.5 identifies general patient teaching guidelines for antiretroviral drugs. The nurse should teach patients to use barrier contraceptives when taking efavirenz, not to drive or operate machinery until the effects of the medication are known, and to notify the prescriber in the event of pregnancy.

Other Drugs in the Class

Delavirdine mesylate (Rescriptor) is an NNRTI that is indicated for combined use with other antiretroviral agents. The potential for life-threatening adverse effects have been noted when delavirdine is combined with CYP3A4 inducers. The drugs of greatest concern are dysrhythmic agents,

BOX 21.7 Herb and Dietary Interactions: Efavirenz

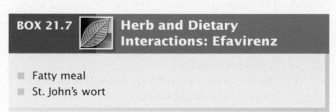

■ Fatty meal
■ St. John's wort

clarithromycin, dapsone, rifabutin, benzodiazepines, calcium channel blockers, ergot derivatives, indinavir, saquinavir, quinidine, and warfarin. In patients who have an absence of hydrochloric acid in the gastric juices, it is necessary to administer the drug with an acidic beverage. Taking delavirdine requires mixing it with a minimum of 3 ounces of water. The solution should stand for a few minutes, and then the patient should drink the solution. After rinsing the glass, the patient should drink the rinse to obtain the entire dosage of the medication. Then he or she should rinse the mouth and swallow that solution.

Etravirine (Intelence) is an NNRTI that is used in combination with a minimum of two additional antiretroviral agents to treatment-experienced HIV patients. Patients should take it with food to aid absorption. Metabolism by CYP3A4, CYP2C9, and CYP2C19 occurs in the liver; this leads to reduced serum levels of other medications metabolized by the same substrates. For example, administration of etravirine with antifungal agents increases serum levels of etravirine and decreases antifungal activity.

Nevirapine (Viramune) is an NNRTI used in combination with other antiretroviral agents. Pregnant women with HIV may also take the drug in combination with zidovudine for the prevention of transmission of HIV to the fetus. It is essential that nevirapine not be given to children exposed to the drug during prevention of transmission of HIV from the mother to the fetus. Patients may take the drug without regard to food intake. The **BLACK BOX WARNING** ◆ issued by the FDA states that the most significant adverse effect of nevirapine is the abrupt onset of flu-like symptoms, abdominal pain, fever with or without a rash, and jaundice. These adverse effects may progress to hepatic failure and encephalopathy.

NCLEX Success

16. A man infected with HIV is taking nevirapine (Viramune) and zidovudine (AZT). He develops a fever, malaise, and jaundice. He is at risk for which of the following conditions?

 A. hepatic failure
 B. heart failure
 C. pneumonia
 D. Methicillin-resistant *Staphylococcus aureus*

17. An HIV-positive man who takes etravirine (Intelence) develops a fungal infection following a trip to the Caribbean. He is admitted to the hospital, where he receives IV amphotericin B for the fungal infection. What effect will etravirine have on amphotericin B?

 A. The antifungal activity will be diminished when combined with etravirine.
 B. The serum amphotericin B level will become toxic.
 C. The patient will require a stronger antifungal agent to prevent resistance.
 D. The two drugs are synergistic and will work together to fight the fungal infection.

PROTEASE INHIBITORS

The PIs are antiretroviral drugs that exert their effects against HIV at a different phase of its life cycle than reverse transcriptase inhibitors. They inhibit the HIV enzyme protease, which is required to process viral protein precursors into mature particles capable of infecting other cells. Thus, they are active in both acutely and chronically infected cells. According to Bartlett (2012), compared with the NNRTIs and the integrase inhibitors, the PIs have a high genetic barrier to resistance. **ⓟ Saquinavir mesylate** (Invirase) is the prototype PI, but Bartlett states that lopinavir/ritonavir (Kaletra) is the preferred PI. However, other PIs are useful because lopinavir/ritonavir has significant adverse effects, including hypertriglyceridemia, myocardial infarction, and GI toxicity.

Pharmacokinetics

Absorption of saquinavir mesylate is in the GI tract. However, absorption is enhanced when the drug is taken with a high-fat meal. It is 99% protein bound, and there is no distribution in the CSF. Saquinavir is metabolized by the liver enzyme CYP3A4 with extensive first-pass effect. The half-life is 13 hours. Saquinavir is excreted primarily in the feces (only 1%–3% in the urine) within 5 days.

Action

Saquinavir binds to the site of HIV-1 protease activity to prevent the cleavage of viral gag-pol polyproteins that are required for the maturation of the HIV virus. This action produces immature noninfectious viral particles.

Use

The main purpose of using saquinavir is to reduce the viral load in HIV—in combination with other antiretroviral agents. Prescribers may also order it with colchicine for familial Mediterranean fever, gout prophylaxis, and gout flare-up and with phosphodiesterase-5 enzyme inhibitors for pulmonary hypertension or erectile dysfunction. Table 21.9 summarizes route and dosage information for saquinavir and the other PIs.

Use in Older Adults

Administration in the elderly warrants caution because of the risk of organ dysfunction.

Adverse Effects

Cardiovascular adverse effects include hypertension, hypotension, and chest pain. CNS adverse effects include back pain, fatigue, neuropathy, paresthesia, anxiety, depression, and suicidal ideation. Dermatologic adverse effects are pruritus, rash, and eczema. Hematologic adverse effects are thrombocytopenia, pancytopenia, and anemia. Elevations in creatinine kinase, AST and ALT, and bilirubin have occurred.

Contraindications

Contraindications to saquinavir include a known hypersensitivity to the drug. Other conditions that preclude its use are

TABLE 21.9

DRUGS AT A GLANCE: Antiretroviral Drugs: Protease Inhibitors

Drug	Pregnancy Category	Routes and Dosage Ranges	
		Adults	Children
℗ **Saquinavir mesylate** (Invirase)	B	1000 mg PO twice daily with ritonavir 100 mg in combination with a full meal	>16 y: same as adults
Atazanavir (Reyataz)	B	Antiretroviral-naïve, 300 mg PO once daily plus ritonavir 100 mg; patients who do not tolerate ritonavir: 400 mg PO once daily Antiretroviral-experienced, 300 mg PO once daily plus ritonavir 100 mg Pregnant patients, 300 mg PO once daily plus ritonavir 100 mg once daily	6–12 y Antiretroviral-naïve 15–24 kg, 150 mg PO once daily plus ritonavir 80 mg once daily 25–31 kg, 200 mg PO once daily plus ritonavir 100 mg PO once daily 32–38 kg, 250 mg once daily plus ritonavir 100 mg PO once daily ≥39 kg, 300 mg PO once daily plus 100 mg once daily Antiretroviral-experienced 25–31 kg, 200 mg PO once daily plus ritonavir 100 mg PO once daily 32–38 kg, 250 mg once daily plus ritonavir 100 mg PO once daily ≥39 kg, 300 mg PO once daily plus 100 mg once daily
Darunavir (Prezista)	C	Antiretroviral-naïve, 800 mg PO once daily with ritonavir 100 mg Antiretroviral-experienced, if genotypic testing is not possible, 600 mg PO with ritonavir 100 mg once daily	≥6 y ≥20 to <30 kg, 375 mg PO twice daily with ritonavir 50 mg twice daily ≥30 to <40 mg, 450 mg PO twice daily with ritonavir 60 mg twice daily ≥40 kg, 600 mg PO twice daily with ritonavir 100 mg twice daily
Fosamprenavir calcium (Lexiva)	C	Unboosted regimen: 1400 mg PO twice daily Ritonavir-boosted regimen, 1400 mg PO plus ritonavir 100–200 mg once daily (not recommended in PI-experienced patients) Or 700 mg PO plus ritonavir 100 mg twice daily	Antiretroviral-naïve 2–5 y, 30 mg/kg/dose PO twice daily ≥6 y Unboosted regimen, 30 mg/kg/dose; Ritonavir-boosted regimen, 18 mg/kg/dose plus 3 mg/kg/dose ritonavir PO twice daily (do not exceed adult dosage)
Indinavir sulfate (Crixivan)	C	Unboosted regimen, 800 mg PO every 8 h Boosted regimen, 800 mg PO twice daily with ritonavir 100–200 mg When combined with other antiretroviral agents, consult manufacturer's recommendations	Safety and efficacy not established
Lopinavir/ritonavir (Kaletra)	C	Antiretroviral-naïve or antiretroviral-experienced, lopinavir 400 mg/ritonavir 100 mg PO twice daily Antiretroviral-naïve or antiretroviral-experienced with efavirenz, fosamprenavir, nelfinavir, nevirapine, lopinavir 500 mg/ritonavir 125 mg twice daily or lopinavir 533 mg/ritonavir 133 mg solution PO twice daily Once-daily dosing, lopinavir 800 mg/ritonavir 200 mg PO once daily	14 d to 6 mo, 16 mg/kg PO twice daily 6 mo to 18 y <15 kg, 12 mg/kg PO twice dailyw 15–40 kg, 10 mg/kg PO twice daily >40 kg, lopinavir 400 mg/ritonavir 100 mg PO twice daily Combination therapy with efavirenz, fosamprenavir, nelfinavir, or nevirapine 6 mo to 18 y: <15 kg, 13 mg/kg PO twice daily 15–45 kg, 11 mg/kg PO twice daily >45 kg: same as adults
Nelfinavir mesylate (Viracept)	B	750 mg PO 3 times per day or 1250 mg PO twice daily	2–13 y: 45–55 mg/kg PO twice daily or 25–35 mg/kg PO 3 times daily not to exceed 2500 mg/d (mix oral powder in milk or water/do not mix with acidic juices)

(Continued on page 390)

TABLE 21.9

DRUGS AT A GLANCE: Antiretroviral Drugs: Protease Inhibitors (Continued)

Drug	Pregnancy Category	Routes and Dosage Ranges	
		Adults	Children
Ritonavir (Norvir)	B	600 mg PO twice daily; increase dose as follows: 300 mg twice daily for 1 d, 400 mg twice daily for 2 d, and 500 mg twice daily for 1 d. Then increase by 100 mg twice daily every 2–3 d to recommended dosage of 600 mg PO twice daily	>1 mo: 350–400 mg/m² PO twice daily; initial dose 250 mg/m² PO twice daily; titrate upward every 2–3 d by 50 mg/m² PO twice daily
Tipranavir (Aptivus)	C	500 mg PO twice daily (administer with ritonavir 200 mg PO twice daily)	≥2 y: 14 mg/kg or 375 mg/m² PO twice daily; maximum 500 mg/dose (administer with ritonavir 6 mg/kg or 150 mg/m² twice daily)

congenital or acquired prolongation of the QT interval, atrioventricular block, hepatic impairment, refractory hypokalemia, or hypomagnesemia.

Nursing Implications

Preventing Interactions

Medications as well as herbs and foods interact with saquinavir, increasing or decreasing its effects (Boxes 21.8 and 21.9). The use of ergot alkaloids with PIs increases the risk of ergot toxicity.

Administering the Medication

Patients should take saquinavir with ritonavir. To ensure maximum bioavailability, the nurse should instruct patients to take saquinavir within 2 hours of a meal or on a full stomach. Patients should have an electrocardiogram (ECG) prior to the start of therapy and 3 to 4 days after therapy is begun. It is also necessary to measure serum potassium, magnesium, triglycerides, and cholesterol before the initiation of therapy.

Assessing for Therapeutic Effects

The nurse assesses for an increase in T-helper CD4 cells. The CD4 count is a measure of the ability to fight infections.

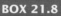

BOX 21.8 **Drug Interactions: Saquinavir**

Drugs That Increase Effects of Saquinavir
■ Delavirdine, clarithromycin, indinavir, ketoconazole, ritonavir
Increase serum levels

Drugs That Decrease the Effects of Saquinavir
■ Carbamazepine, dexamethasone, phenobarbital, phenytoin, rifabutin, rifampin
Decrease serum levels

Assessing for Adverse Effects

The nurse assesses for ECG-related changes, specifically QT prolongation. Also, he or she also assesses for signs and symptoms of peripheral neuropathy. In addition, the nurse assesses the mouth for signs of ulcerations related to increase gastric acid.

It is important to check laboratory results. The nurse assesses the CBC and bilirubin for anemia, thrombocytopenia, and pancytopenia; serum potassium and magnesium levels; and AST or ALT for elevation.

Patient Teaching

Box 21.5 presents patient teaching guidelines for antiretroviral drugs.

Other Drugs in the Class

Atazanavir (Reyataz) is a PI that is administered to treatment-naïve and treatment-experienced patients, often with ritonavir. It is necessary to take the drug with food. Monitoring of the patient's cholesterol level for increase of greater than 240 mg/dL is important. Contraindications to atazanavir include hypersensitivity to the drug—because of the risk of Stevens-Johnson syndrome.

Darunavir (Prezista) is very similar to atazanavir.

Fosamprenavir (Lexiva) is an oral PI administered with or without ritonavir. It is 63% absorbed and hydrolyzed to amprenavir by the stomach enzymes, reaching a peak of action in 2.5 hours. It is metabolized in the liver by CYP3A4 and eliminated in the urine and feces. Fosamprenavir has similar adverse effects as other drugs in the class.

Indinavir (Crixivan) is an oral PI administered with ritonavir. The medication binds to the site of HIV-1 protease

BOX 21.9 **Herb and Dietary Interactions: Saquinavir**

■ St. John's wort
■ Garlic
■ Grapefruit juice (1 quart per day)

activity to inhibit the functional proteins of infectious HIV, resulting in noninfectious viral particles. Patients should take it without food and they should drink 48 ounces of fluids per day.

Lopinavir/ritonavir (Kaletra) is an oral PI administered in treatment-naïve and treatment-experienced patients. Lopinavir, in this combination, may be part of a multidrug antiretroviral regimen. Patients should take it with food. Monitoring for signs and symptoms of pancreatitis, onset of diabetes, and triglyceride elevation is necessary. The nurse should instruct the patient about blood glucose testing and keeping regularly scheduled laboratory appointments to check amylase, triglycerides, inorganic phosphorous, thyroid function, and CBC.

Nelfinavir mesylate (Viracept) is an oral PI that patients should take with food to enhance absorption. It is distributed with 98% of the drug being protein bound. The nurse instructs the patient to take nelfinavir exactly as prescribed and not to alter the dose. The patient should report the onset of diarrhea. If necessary, the patient may mix the oral powder preparation of the drug with dietary supplements, regular or soy milk, or water but not with acidic liquids.

Ritonavir (Norvir) is an oral PI administered alone or in combination with other antiretroviral agents. Authorities do not recommend it as a primary PI. The medication is contraindicated with saquinavir in patients who have cardiac conduction insufficiency disorders. It is necessary to assess for GI distress, peripheral neuropathy, palpitations, syncope, tachycardia, and a prolonged QT interval.

Tipranavir (Aptivus) is a PI for treatment-experienced patients or patients with HIV-1 strains that are resistant to multiple PIs. Caution is warranted when administering it to patients receiving sulfonamides. It is necessary to monitor blood glucose to check for loss of glycemic control. The nurse instructs the patient to apply sunscreen because of possible photosensitivity reactions.

NCLEX Success

18. Which of the following electrocardiographic changes warrant the discontinuation of saquinavir mesylate (Invirase)?

A. prolongation of the QT interval
B. inverted T wave
C. elongated ST segment
D. premature ventricular contraction

19. A 2-year-old child is started on nelfinavir mesylate (Viracept). The nurse is instructing the mother on the proper administration of the medication. Which of the following is most appropriate to teach the mother?

A. squirt the medication in the mouth with a syringe.
B. tilt the head back and place the medicine in a nipple.
C. mix the medicine with water, milk, or formula.
D. mix the medicine in orange juice.

EVIDENCE-BASED PRACTICE

Atazanavir Plasma Concentrations are Impaired in HIV-1 Infected Adults Simultaneously Taking a Methadone Oral Solution in a Once Daily Observed Therapy Setting
by ANNETTE HABERL, MANFRED MOESCH, GABRIELE NISISU, CHRISTOPH STEPHAN, MARKUS BICKEL, PAVEL KHAYKIN, MICHAEL KUROWSKI, REINHARD BRODT, NILS VON HENTIF

European Journal of Pharmacology
2010, 66, 375–381

The objective of this study was to determine if the serum levels of atazanavir were decreased when people infected with the human immunodeficiency virus (HIV) took atazanavir oral methadone. Former opiate users often take oral methadone as a substitute. This study focused on 24 patients (12 men and 12 women) taking atazanavir/ritonavir 330/100 mg daily plus reverse transcriptase inhibitors with or without methadone. The results revealed that the patients taking methadone and atazanavir had lower serum atazanavir levels compared with the patients not taking methadone. The pharmacokinetics was similar for each group taking ritonavir.

IMPLICATIONS FOR NURSING PRACTICE: Many former intravenous (IV) drug (heroin) users receive methadone. The administration of methadone and the antiretroviral agent atazanavir protect former heroin addicts from desiring heroin, thus preventing the onset of withdrawal symptoms. Former IV drug users who are HIV positive require protease inhibitors and reverse transcriptase inhibitors to boost their CD4 counts. If they are also taking methadone, they are at risk for low CD4 counts when methadone and atazanavir are combined. It is important that the nurse assess CD4 counts when caring for patients who are receiving atazanavir and methadone.

INTEGRASE STRAND TRANSFER INHIBITORS

Integrase strand transfer inhibitors block the action of integrase, a viral enzyme of HIV-1 essential for viral replication. The only member of this drug class approved by the FDA is **raltegravir** (Isentress). This drug is comparable to efavirenz in terms of its ability to suppress HIV.

Pharmacokinetics

Raltegravir is absorbed by the GI tract. The rate of absorption is doubled if the drug is taken with a high-fat meal. It is 83% protein bound. Raltegravir is metabolized by hepatic

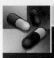

TABLE 21.10

DRUGS AT A GLANCE: Antiretroviral Drugs: Integrase Strand Transfer Inhibitors, Fusion Protein Inhibitors, and CCR5 Antagonists

Drug	Pregnancy Category	Routes and Dosage Ranges	
		Adults	Children
Integrase Strand Transfer Inhibitors			
ⓟ **Raltegravir** (Isentress)	C	400 mg PO twice daily	2 to <12 y 10 to <14 kg: 75 mg PO twice daily 14 to <20 kg: 100 mg PO twice daily 20 to <28 kg: 150 mg PO twice daily 28 to <40 kg: 200 mg PO twice daily ≥40 kg: 300 mg PO twice daily >12 y: see adults
Fusion Protein Inhibitors			
ⓟ **Enfuvirtide** (Fuzeon)	B	90 mg Sub-Q twice daily	6–16 y, 2 mg/kg Sub-Q twice daily
CCR5 Antagonists			
ⓟ **Maraviroc** (Selzentry)	C	300 mg PO twice daily	<16 y: safety and efficacy have not been established >16 y, same as adults

glucuronidation mediated by UGT1A1. The serum half-life is 9 hours. The drug is eliminated in the feces and urine.

Action

Raltegravir blocks HIV-1 integrase to prevent the formation of the HIV-1 provirus to decrease the viral load and increase the active CD4 cells. Specifically, after HIV reverse transcriptase enters CD4 T cells, the enzyme transcribes viral RNA into DNA. As the integrase combines with viral DNA and other cellular cofactors, it forms the preintegration complex. The integrase removes the nucleotide from the 3′ terminus to expose reactive hydroxyl groups. The preintegration complex enters the host cell nucleus, binding to host cell DNA. Integrase then nicks each strand of the host cell DNA, exposing 5′ phosphate groups to enable covalent bonding of host and viral DNA. When the strand transfer is complete, the host cell enzymes repair the gaps between the viral and host DNA (Hicks, 2012).

Use

Raltegravir is a first-line antiviral agent that is administered with tenofovir and emtricitabine to treatment-experienced adults. These patients must have evidence of viral replication and HIV-1 strains resistant to multiple antiretroviral drugs. Table 21.10 supplies information about the route of administration and dosage for raltegravir.

Adverse Effects and Contraindications

Few adverse effects occur with raltegravir. The most common include headache, dizziness, nausea, diarrhea, vomiting, abdominal pain, fever, and rhabdomyolysis. Sometimes serum glucose

level, hepatic enzymes, and lipase level increase. However, in a double-blind study of treatment-naïve patients over 192 weeks of follow-up, researchers found that patients showed excellent tolerance and lack of effect on lipids (Bartlett, 2012).

Contraindications include a known hypersensitivity to the medication. The drug is not suitable for treatment-naïve patients and breastfeeding women.

Nursing Implications

Preventing Interactions

Some medications interact with raltegravir, increasing or decreasing its effects (Box 21.10). St. John's wort decreases the effects of raltegravir.

Administering the Medication

Patients may take raltegravir with or without meals.

Assessing Therapeutic and Adverse Effects

The nurse assesses for an increase in T-helper CD4 cells. The CD4 count measures the ability to fight against infections.

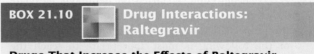

BOX 21.10   Drug Interactions: Raltegravir

Drugs That Increase the Effects of Raltegravir
- Proton pump inhibitors
  Increase the serum concentration

Drugs That Decrease the Effects of Raltegravir
- Efavirenz, fosamprenavir, rifampin, tipranavir
  Decrease the serum concentration

In addition, the nurse assesses for GI upset, headache, dizziness, fever, and rhabdomyolysis. It is necessary to monitor blood sugar, liver enzymes, and lipase levels for increases.

Patient Teaching

Box 21.5 presents patient teaching guidelines for antiretroviral drugs.

FUSION PROTEIN INHIBITORS

The drugs in this new class inhibit the HIV virus from binding to, fusing with, and entering the human cell. Ⓟ **Enfuvirtide** (Fuzeon) is the only drug in this class. This drug is for use only by patients who have previously been treated with antiretroviral agents. Antiretroviral therapy–naïve patients should not use it.

Pharmacokinetics

Following subcutaneous administration, enfuvirtide has a peak of action of 4 to 8 hours. The drug is 84% absorbed and distributed to the CSF in 2 to 18 hours. It is 92% protein bound. Enfuvirtide is metabolized by proteolytic hydrolysis in which it is catabolized into amino acids. The medication is not excreted; the amino acids are recycled.

Action and Use

Enfuvirtide inhibits the fusion of the membrane of the HIV-1 virus with that of the cell, thus preventing HIV from entering the cell. It is used in combination with other antiretrovirals in treating HIV-1. Table 21.10 gives route of administration and dosage information for enfuvirtide.

Adverse Effects and Contraindications

The most commonly reported adverse effects to enfuvirtide are fatigue, insomnia, nausea, and diarrhea. Injection site reactions such as rash, pain, discomfort, redness, hypersensitivity, rash, and nodule development may also occur. Researchers have reported bacterial pneumonia in 3% of the patients who used enfuvirtide. Less than 10% of the patients may have elevated serum creatine phosphokinase, myalgia, and limb pain.

Contraindications to enfuvirtide include a hypersensitivity to the drug and lactation.

Nursing Implications

Preventing Interactions

PIs increase serum enfuvirtide levels.

Administering the Medication

The nurse injects enfuvirtide subcutaneously into the upper arm, abdomen, or anterior thigh. Injection of the drug into blood vessels, navel, moles, scars, or other areas of skin change should never occur. Rotation of injection sites and assessment of the sites for reactions is necessary. It is important not to inject enfuvirtide into large nerves that are close to the skin near the buttocks, elbow, knee, or groin.

Assessing for Therapeutic and Adverse Effects

The nurse assesses for an increase in T-helper CD4 cells. The CD4 count measures the ability to fight against infections.

Also, the nurse assesses the injection site for signs of hypersensitivity such as rash, redness, nodules, or pain. He or she also assesses for diarrhea, nausea, or other signs of GI distress. In addition, it is necessary to assess the serum creatine phosphokinase for elevation along with myalgia or limb pain. Finally, the nurse assesses pulmonary status, looking for cough, fever, or bacterial pneumonia.

Patient Teaching

The nurse instructs the patient or family about the proper technique for the administration of the enfuvirtide. Daily administration is necessary, and if a dose is missed, it is important to notify the primary care provider. Instruct the rotation of injection sites and assessment of site for changes. Box 21.5 provides general patient teaching guidelines for antiretroviral drugs.

CCR5 ANTAGONISTS

Currently, there is only one member of this antiretroviral class, Ⓟ **maraviroc** (Selzentry). It blocks the receptor site to which the HIV needs to interact to enter the cell.

Pharmacokinetics

Maraviroc is absorbed in the GI tract. The drug has a slow onset of action, reaching a peak of action in ½ to 4 hours. Its half-life is 14 to 18 hours. Maraviroc is 76% protein bound. The drug is metabolized by the liver with the CYP3A enzyme to inactive metabolites. It is excreted in the urine (20%; 8% remains unchanged) and kidneys (76%; 25% remains unchanged).

Action and Use

Maraviroc binds to the human chemokine receptor on the cell membrane. This action prevents the interaction of HIV-1 and CCR5 that is needed for HIV to enter the cell and replicate.

People with HIV take maraviroc in combination with other antiretroviral agents for detectable CCR5-tropic HIV-1 possessing evidence of viral replication. They may have HIV-1 strains that are resistant to many other antiretroviral drugs. Those with a CrCl less than 30 mL/min or with end-stage renal disease should not take maraviroc. Table 21.10 gives route of administration and dosage information for maraviroc.

Adverse Effects

The most common adverse effects of maraviroc are fever; rash; upper respiratory infection with cough; vascular hypertension; and CNS depression with dizziness, anxiety, and depression. Other less significant adverse effects are lipodystrophy, pruritus, benign skin neoplasms, genital warts, elevated bilirubin, joint pain, conjunctivitis, and otitis media. The FDA has issued a **BLACK BOX WARNING** ◆ for maraviroc, stating that it may lead to drug-induced hepatotoxicity with allergic features following 1 month of treatment. Allergic reactions such as pruritic rash, fever, eosinophilia, fever, increased IgE, and symptoms of hepatitis that can be life threatening may precede this condition.

Contraindications

Contraindications to maraviroc include severe renal impairment and use of medications that are potent CYP3A4 inhibitors.

Nursing Implications

Preventing Interactions

Several medications interact with maraviroc, increasing or decreasing its effects (Box 21.11). St. John's wort decreases the effects of the drug.

Administering the Medication

Patients may take maraviroc before meals, with meals, or after meals. However, high-fat food enhance absorption.

Assessing for Therapeutic and Adverse Effects

The nurse assesses for an increase in T-helper CD4 cells. The CD4 count measures the ability to fight against infections.

In addition, the nurse assesses the bilirubin, AST, and ALT levels for signs of hepatotoxicity. It is also necessary to assess the temperature for fever and monitor the IgE levels, which are indicative of the onset of hepatitis. The nurse assesses for rash or other skin changes such as the development of neoplasms. He or she assesses for cough and upper respiratory infection. Finally, the nurse assesses the ear canal for otitis media or complaints of ear pain.

Patient Teaching

The nurse instructs the patient to use caution when changing positions due to possible drug-induced dizziness. He or she also tells the patient to report rash, yellow skin or eyes, muscle pain, or fatigue. In addition, the general patient teaching guidelines presented in Box 21.5 may be useful.

NCLEX Success

20. **What is the action of raltegravir?**

A. It blocks HIV integrase.
B. It increases viral load.
C. It diminishes cell membrane permeability.
D. It increases white blood cell count.

21. **A patient has been admitted to the infectious disease division. The physician has ordered enfuvirtide 90 mg twice daily. What is the recommended route of administration of enfuvirtide?**

A. intravenous
B. oral
C. intramuscular
D. subcutaneous

22. **A physician prescribes maraviroc for a man with HIV. The nurse should instruct the man to be alert for what adverse effect?**

A. edema
B. cardiac abnormality with chest pain
C. yellowing of skin
D. bronchospasm

The Nursing Process

Assessment

- Assess signs and symptoms of viral infections and resolution of signs and symptoms following the administration antiviral medications.
- Assess renal and hepatic function.
- Assess viral hepatitis risk factors, exposure, and signs and symptoms of liver dysfunction.
- Assess baseline data to assist in monitoring response to drug therapy:
  - Vital signs, weight, and nutritional status
  - Signs and symptoms of disease and opportunistic infections associated with disease and immunosuppression.
  - CBC; CD4+; lymphocyte count; plasma levels of viral RNA, BUN, AST, ALT, AST, and creatinine

Nursing Diagnoses

- Anxiety related to a medical diagnosis of serious viral infection (e.g., HIV infection and viral hepatitis)
- Altered sexuality patterns related to sexually transmitted viral infections (HIV infection and genital herpes)
- Disturbed body image related to sexually transmitted infection
- Social isolation related to a medical diagnosis of HIV infection or genital herpes
- Deficient knowledge: disease process and methods of spread; availability of vaccines and other prophylactic interventions
- Risk for injury: recurrent infection; adverse drug effects; adverse drug interactions; infections and other problems associated with a compromised immune system in HIV infection; liver damage or failure with viral hepatitis

Planning/Goals

The patient will

- Receive or take antiviral drugs as prescribed.
- Be safeguarded against new or recurrent infection.

- Act to prevent spread of viral infection to others and recurrence in self.
- Avoid preventable adverse drug effects and drug interactions.
- Receive emotional support and counseling to assist in coping with HIV infection or genital herpes.

Nursing Interventions

The nurse will

- Follow recommended policies and procedures for preventing spread of viral infections.
- Assist patients in learning ways to control spread and recurrence of viral infections.
- Assist patients to maintain immunizations against viral infections.
- For patients receiving systemic antiviral drugs, monitor serum creatinine and other tests of renal function, CBC, and fluid balance.

- For patients with HIV infection, assist to schedule their drug therapy regimen as conveniently as possible (to promote adherence), monitor for changes in baseline data during each contact, prevent opportunistic infections (e.g., herpes infections) when possible, and manage adverse effects of drug therapy to promote quality of life.

Evaluation

- Observe for improvement in signs and symptoms of the viral infection for which a drug is given.
- Interview outpatients regarding their compliance with instructions for taking antiviral drugs.
- Interview and observe for use of infection control measures.
- Interview and observe for adverse drug effects.
- Observe the extent and severity of any symptoms in patients with HIV infection or viral hepatitis.

Key Concepts

- Viral infections commonly occur in all age groups.
- Vaccinations, avoiding contact with people who have viral infections, and thorough hand hygiene are effective ways to prevent viral infections.
- Health care providers use a variety of antiviral drugs to fight viral infections.
- Because viruses are intracellular parasites, antiviral drugs are relatively toxic to human cells.
- Viral infections for which drug therapy is available include HSV, VZV, CMV, RSV, influenza, hepatitis B and C, and HIV infection.
- The FDA has issued two **BLACK BOX WARNINGS** ◆ for ganciclovir. The first states that granulocytopenia (neutropenia), anemia, and thrombocytopenia may occur. If severe bone marrow depression occurs, ganciclovir should be discontinued; recovery usually occurs within a week of stopping the drug. The second advises female and male patients of childbearing age to maintain contraceptive precautions during ganciclovir therapy and for a minimum of 90 days after drug therapy.
- The FDA has issued three **BLACK BOX WARNINGS** ◆ for cidofovir. The drug has possible carcinogenic and teratogenic adverse effects. It may also be nephrotoxic, and prior to administration, the patient should receive 1 L of normal saline and oral probenecid. In addition, it places the patient at risk for neutropenia.
- The FDA has issued a **BLACK BOX WARNING** ◆ for foscarnet. Seizures may occur related to impaired renal function, diminished serum calcium, and CNS conditions.
- Valganciclovir has the same **BLACK BOX WARNINGS** ◆ as ganciclovir.
- The FDA has issued two **BLACK BOX WARNINGS** ◆ for ribavirin. The first states that this drug causes significant teratogenic effects according to animal studies. Pregnant women or those who plan to become pregnant should not care for children receiving inhalation therapy or be in the room when it is being administered. Ribavirin is contraindicated in infants and children who have a known hypersensitivity to the drug or its components. The second states that the drug can produce hemolytic anemia, which could lead to myocardial infarction. Patients with unstable cardiovascular disease should not take the drug.
- Antiretroviral drugs are given in combination to increase effectiveness and decrease emergence of drug-resistant viruses. The antiretroviral drugs include the NRTIs, NNRTIs, PIs, the integrase strand transfer inhibitors, the fusion protein inhibitors, and the CCR5 antagonists.
- The FDA has issued a **BLACK BOX WARNING** ◆ for the nucleoside analogs, including lamivudine. There are reports of lactic acidosis and severe hepatomegaly with steatosis.

- The FDA has issued several **BLACK BOX WARNINGS** ◆ for zidovudine. One relates to the adverse effects of granulocytopenia, aplastic or hemolytic anemia, pancytopenia with bone marrow hypoplasia, leukopenia, and lymphadenopathy. Dosage adjustment is necessary in patients who develop anemia or neutropenia. Other warnings relate to lactic acidosis and severe hepatomegaly with steatosis and symptomatic myopathy and myositis.

- The FDA has issued a **BLACK BOX WARNING** ◆ for abacavir. Patients may have serious and sometimes fatal hypersensitivity reactions. Those who test positive for HLAB*5701 allele are at greatest risk for hypersensitivity reactions.

- The FDA has issued a **BLACK BOX WARNING** ◆ for nevirapine. Its most significant adverse effect is the abrupt onset of flu-like symptoms, abdominal pain, fever with or without a rash, and jaundice.

- The FDA has issued a **BLACK BOX WARNING** ◆ for maraviroc. Drug-induced hepatotoxicity with allergic features may occur following 1 month of treatment.

Critical Thinking Questions

21-1. A 17-year-old man has severe pneumonia, and he receives a diagnosis of Pneumocystis pneumonia. On further evaluation, he is tested for human immunodeficiency virus (HIV). He tests positive, and he begins taking zidovudine, saquinavir, and ritonavir.

- What is the action of zidovudine?
- What is the action of saquinavir?
- What is the rationale for the administration of ritonavir with saquinavir and zidovudine?
- What testing should the patient have prior to beginning saquinavir and ritonavir therapy?
- What patient teaching does the nurse provide about HIV and antiretroviral therapy?

References and Resources

Bartlett, J. G. (2012). Selecting antiretroviral regimens for the treatment naïve HIV-infected patient. *Up-To-Date.* Lexi Comp, Inc.

Fiore, A. E., Fry, A., Shay, D., Gubareva, L., Breesee, J. S., & Uyeki, T. M. (2011). Antiviral agents for the treatment and chemoprophylaxis of influenza, recommendations of the Advisory Committee on Immunization Practices (ACIP). *Morbidity and Mortality Weekly Reports*, 60(1), 1–26.

Hall, C. (2012). Antiviral drugs for the prevention and treatment of seasonal influenza in children. *Up-To-Date.* Lexi Comp, Inc.

Hicks, C. B. (2012). Pharmacology of integrase inhibitors. *Up-To-Date.* Lexi Comp, Inc.

Karch, A. M. (2011). *2010 Lippincott's nursing drug guide.* Philadelphia, PA: Lippincott Williams & Wilkins.

Nursing 2011 drug handbook. (2011). Philadelphia, PA: Lippincott William & Wilkins.

Porth, C. M., & Matfin, G. (2009). *Pathophysiology concepts of altered health states.* Philadelphia, PA: Lippincott Williams & Wilkins.

Rodriguez, M., & Zachary, K. C. (2012). Foscarnet: An overview. *Up-To-Date.* Lexi Comp, Inc.

Sax, P. E. (2012). Clinical trials of HIV antiretroviral therapy: CCR5 antagonists. *Up-To-Date.* Lexi-Comp. Inc.

Smeltzer, S. C., Bare, B. G., Hinkle, J. H., & Cheever, K. H. (2010). *Brunner & Suddarth's textbook of medical-surgical nursing* (12th ed.). Philadelphia, PA: Lippincott Williams & Wilkins.

Up-To-Date. (2012). *Abacavir an lamivudine: Drug information.* Lexi Comp, Inc.

Up-To-Date. (2012). *Abacavir: Drug information.* Lexi Comp, Inc.

Up-To-Date. (2012). *Abacavir, lamivudine, and zidovudine: Drug information.* Lexi Comp, Inc.

Up-To-Date. (2012). *Acyclovir (systemic): Drug information.* Lexi Comp, Inc.

Up-To-Date. (2012). *Adefovir: Drug information.* Lexi Comp, Inc.

Up-To-Date. (2012). *Amantadine: Drug information.* Lexi Comp, Inc.

Up-To-Date. (2012). *Atazanavir: Drug information.* Lexi Comp, Inc.

Up-To-Date. (2012). *Cidofovir: Drug information.* Lexi Comp, Inc.

Up-To-Date. (2012). *Darunavir: Drug information.* Lexi Comp, Inc.

Up-To-Date. (2012). *Delavirdine: Drug information.* Lexi Comp, Inc.

Up-To-Date. (2012). *Didanosine: Drug information.* Lexi Comp, Inc.

Up-To-Date. (2012). *Efavirenz: Drug information.* Lexi Comp, Inc.

Up-To-Date. (2012). *Emtricitabine: Drug information.* Lexi Comp, Inc.

Up-To-Date. (2012). *Emtricitabine and Tenofovir: Drug information.* Lexi Comp, Inc.

Up-To-Date. (2012). *Emtricitabine, tenofovir, and efavirenz: Drug information.* Lexi Comp, Inc.

Up-To-Date. (2012). *Enfuvirtide: Drug information.* Lexi Comp, Inc.

Up-To-Date. (2012). *Etravirine: Drug information.* Lexi Comp, Inc.

Up-To-Date. (2012). *Famciclovir: Drug information.* Lexi Comp, Inc.

Up-To-Date. (2012). *Fosamprenavir: Drug information.* Lexi Comp, Inc.

Up-To-Date. (2012). *Foscarnet: Drug information.* Lexi Comp, Inc.

Up-To-Date. (2012). *Foscarnet: Pediatric drug information.* Lexi Comp, Inc.

Up-To-Date. (2012). *Ganciclovir (systemic): Drug information.* Lexi Comp, Inc.

Up-To-Date. (2012). *Indinavir: Drug information.* Lexi Comp, Inc.

Up-To-Date. (2012). *Lamivudine: Drug information.* Lexi Comp, Inc.

Up-To-Date. (2012). *Lopinavir and ritonavir: Drug information.* Lexi Comp, Inc.

Up-To-Date. (2012). *Maraviroc: Drug information.* Lexi Comp, Inc.

Up-To-Date. (2012). *Nelfinavir: Drug information.* Lexi Comp, Inc.

Up-To-Date. (2012). *Nevirapine: Drug information.* Lexi Comp, Inc.

Up-To-Date. (2012). *Oseltamivir: Drug information.* Lexi Comp, Inc.

Up-To-Date. (2012). *Raltegravir: Drug information.* Lexi Comp, Inc.

Up-To-Date. (2012). *Ribavirin: Drug information.* Lexi Comp, Inc.

Up-To-Date. (2012). *Ritonavir: Drug information.* Lexi Comp, Inc.

Up-To-Date. (2012). *Saquinavir: Drug information.* Lexi Comp, Inc.

Up-To-Date. (2012). *Tenofovir: Drug information.* Lexi Comp, Inc.

Up-To-Date. (2012). *Tipranavir: Drug information.* Lexi Comp, Inc.

Up-To-Date. (2012). *Valganciclovir: Drug information.* Lexi Comp, Inc.

Up-To-Date. (2012). *Valganciclovir: Pediatric drug information.* Lexi Comp, Inc.

Zachary, K. C. (2012). Acyclovir: An overview. *Up-To-Date.* Lexi Comp, Inc.

Zachary, K. C. (2012). Ganciclovir: An overview. *Up-To-Date.* Lexi Comp, Inc.

Zachary, K. C. (2012). Treatment of seasonal influenza in adults. *Up-To-Date.* Lexi Comp, Inc.

Zachary, K. C. (2012). Valacyclovir: An overview. *Up-To-Date.* Lexi Comp, Inc.

U. S. Department of Health and Human Services. (2011). *Tamiflu (oseltamivir phosphate) for oral suspension: Label change-new concentration (6 mg/mL).* http://www.fda.gov/Safety/MedWatch/SafetyInformation/SafetyAlertsforHumanMedicalPractice Retrieved: 2/19/2012.

22 Drug Therapy for Fungal Infections

Clinical Application Case Study

Maria Angelo, age 21, is receiving antibiotic therapy for a strep throat. Following the completion of the course of antibiotics, she begins complaining of vaginal itching. She also notices a cheesy yellow vaginal discharge. Her primary care provider diagnoses *Candida albicans* vaginal infection and prescribes fluconazole (Diflucan) 150 mg PO, one dose.

KEY TERMS

Candidiasis: infection either containing or caused by *Candida* fungi

Dermatophytes: fungal parasites that grow in or on the skin

Fungi: plant-like organisms that live as parasites on living tissue or as saprophytes on decaying organic matter

Immunocompromised: having an impaired or weakened immune system

Molds: fungi that are widely dispersed in the environment and either saprophytic or parasitic; multicellular organisms composed of colonies of tangled strands

Mycoses: disease induced by a fungus or resembling such a disease

Yeasts: unicellular fungi of the genus *Saccharomyces* or *Candida*

Introduction

This chapter provides an introduction to the pharmacological care of the patient diagnosed with a fungal infection. There are three broad classifications of antifungal agents prescribed in the treatment of fungal infections. The first group discussed is the polyenes, which are administered in the treatment of severe fungal infections. The second group discussed is the azoles, which are the most commonly prescribed antifungal medications. The azoles are administered topically and vaginally. The third group of antifungal agents is the echinocandins, which have fungicidal activity against *Candida*, including azole-resistant organisms, and fungistatic activity against *Aspergillus*. This chapter also discusses antifungal agents used in the treatment of dermatophytic infections.

Overview of Fungal Infections

Etiology

Fungi are molds and yeasts that are widely dispersed in the environment and are either saprophytic (i.e., obtaining food from dead organic matter) or parasitic (i.e., obtaining nourishment from living organisms). **Molds** are multicellular organisms composed of colonies of tangled strands. They form a fuzzy coating on various surfaces (e.g., the mold that forms on spoiled food, the mildew that forms in damp environments). **Yeasts** are unicellular organisms. Some fungi, called **dermatophytes**, can grow only at the cooler temperatures of body surfaces. Other fungi, termed dimorphic, can grow as molds outside the body and as yeasts in the warm temperatures of the body. As molds, these fungi produce spores that can persist indefinitely in the environment and can be carried by the wind to distant locations. When these mold spores enter the body, most often by inhalation, they rapidly become yeasts that can invade body tissues. Dimorphic fungi include a number of human pathogens such as those that cause blastomycosis, histoplasmosis, and coccidioidomycosis.

Structurally, fungi are larger and more complex than bacteria. They have a thick, rigid cell wall, of which glucan is one of the components. Glucan is formed by the fungal enzyme, glucan synthetase. Fungi also have a cell membrane composed mainly of ergosterol, a lipid that is similar to cholesterol in human cell membranes. Within the cell membrane, structures are mostly the same as those in human cells (e.g., a nucleus, mitochondria, Golgi apparatus, ribosomes attached to endoplasmic reticulum, a cytoskeleton with microtubules, and filaments).

Fungal infections may be mild and superficial or life-threatening and systemic. Fungi that are pathogenic in humans exist in soil, decaying plants, and other environmental habitats. Some are even part of the endogenous human flora. For example, *Candida albicans* organisms are part of the normal microbial flora of the skin, mouth, gastrointestinal (GI) tract, and vagina. Growth of *Candida* organisms is normally restrained by intact immune mechanisms and bacterial competition for nutrients. When these restraining forces are altered (e.g., by suppression of the immune system and antibacterial drug therapy), fungal overgrowth and opportunistic infection can occur, leading to the fungal infection called **candidiasis**. Dermatophytes cause superficial infections of the skin, hair, and nails. They obtain nourishment from keratin, a protein in skin, hair, and nails. Dermatophytic infections include tinea pedis (athlete's foot) and tinea capitis (ringworm of the scalp) (see Chap. 60).

Systemic or invasive **mycoses** include the endemic mycoses that can cause disease (e.g., blastomycosis, coccidioidomycosis, histoplasmosis, sporotrichosis) in healthy hosts who are exposed to them in the environment and the opportunistic mycoses (e.g., aspergillosis, candidiasis, cryptococcosis) that cause serious infection mainly in immunosuppressed hosts. The fungi that cause endemic mycoses exist as molds in the environment; they grow in soil and decaying organic matter. Infection is acquired by inhalation of airborne spores from contaminated soil. Histoplasmosis, coccidioidomycosis, and blastomycosis usually occur as pulmonary disease but may be systemic. These infections often mimic common bacterial infections, and their severity is determined both by the extent of the exposure to the organism and by the immune status of the host. The fungi that cause opportunistic mycoses may be part of the normal body flora (e.g., *Candida* species) or exist in the environment (*Aspergillus*, *Cryptococcus*). Infection occurs after inhalation or inoculation of the fungus into body tissues. Fungi may have characteristics that enhance their ability to cause disease. *Cryptococcus neoformans* organisms, for example, can become encapsulated, which allows them to evade the normal immune defense mechanism of phagocytosis. *Aspergillus* organisms produce protease, an enzyme that allows them to destroy structural proteins and penetrate body tissues.

Most fungal infections occur in healthy people but are more severe and invasive in **immunocompromised** hosts. Serious infections are increasing in incidence, largely because of human immunodeficiency virus (HIV) infections, the use of immunosuppressant drugs to treat patients with cancer or organ transplants, the use of indwelling intravenous (IV) catheters for prolonged drug therapy or parenteral nutrition, implantation of prosthetic devices, and widespread use of broad-spectrum antibacterial drugs.

Pathophysiology and Clinical Manifestations

Pathophysiologic changes associated with fungal infections relate to the causal fungus and the tissue in which it has been colonized. Box 22.1 describes the characteristics of selected fungal infections and associated pathophysiologic changes. This box also identifies the clinical manifestations that result from fungal infection.

Drug Therapy

Development of drugs that are effective against fungal cells without being excessively toxic to human cells has been limited because fungal cells are similar to human cells. Most of the available drugs target the fungal cell membrane and produce potentially serious toxicities and drug interactions. In general, antifungal drugs disrupt the structure and function of fungal cell components (Fig. 22.1).

BOX 22.1 Selected Fungal Infections

Aspergillosis occurs in debilitated and immunocompromised people, including those with leukemia, lymphoma, or acquired immunodeficiency syndrome (AIDS), and those with neutropenia. Invasive aspergillosis is a serious illness characterized by inflammatory granulomatous lesions, which may develop in the bronchi, lungs, ear canal, skin, or mucous membranes of the eye, nose, or urethra. It may extend into blood vessels, which leads to infection of the brain, heart, kidneys, and other organs. It is associated with thrombosis, ischemic infarction of involved tissues, and progressive disease. It is often fatal.

Allergic bronchopulmonary aspergillosis, an allergic reaction to inhaled *Aspergillus* spores, may develop in people with asthma and cause bronchoconstriction, wheezing, dyspnea, cough, muscle aches, and fever. The condition is aggravated if the spores germinate and grow in the airways, thereby producing chronic exposure to the antigen and permanent fibrotic damage.

Aspergillus mold is widespread in the environment; spores are released into the air during soil excavations (e.g., for construction of buildings) or handling of decaying plant matter and are carried into most human environments. Spores have been found in water (e.g., hot water faucets, saunas, shower heads, swimming pools), public buildings and private homes (e.g., basements, bedding, humidifiers, ventilation ducts, potted plants, house dust), and foods (e.g., peppers and spices, pasta, peanuts, cashews, coffee beans). In hospitals, sources of infection include contaminated air from building renovations and new construction; hospital water, which may become aerosolized during activities such as patient showering; and cereals, powdered milk, tea, and soy sauce ingested by neutropenic patients. As *Aspergillus* molds grow, they produce toxins (e.g., aflatoxin, one of the strongest carcinogens known) that contaminate the food chain.

There are several species that cause invasive disease in humans, but *Aspergillus fumigatus* is the most common. *A. fumigatus* reproduces by releasing spores, which are small enough to reach the alveoli when inhaled. Most *Aspergillus* organisms enter the body through the respiratory system, and pulmonary aspergillosis is acquired by inhalation of the spores. Other potential entry sites include damaged skin (e.g., burn wounds, intravenous [IV] catheter insertion sites), operative wounds, the cornea, and the ear.

Blastomycosis occurs with inhalation of spores from a fungus that grows in soil and decaying organic matter. The organism is widespread in the United States. Sporadic cases most often occur in adult males who have extensive exposure to woods and streams with vocational or recreational activities. The infection may be asymptomatic or produce pulmonary symptoms resembling pneumonia, tuberculosis, or lung cancer. It may also be systemic and involve other organs, especially the skin and bone. Skin lesions (e.g., pustules, ulcerations, abscesses) may progress over a period of years and eventually involve large areas of the body. Bone invasion, with arthritis and bone destruction, occurs in 25% to 50% of patients.

Blastomycosis can occur in healthy people with sufficient exposure but is more severe and more likely to involve multiple organs and central nervous system (CNS) disease in immunocompromised patients.

Candidiasis occurs in patients with malignant lymphomas, diabetes mellitus, or AIDS and in patients receiving antibiotic, antineoplastic, corticosteroid, and immunosuppressant drug therapy. *Candida* organisms are found in soil, on inanimate objects, in hospital environments, and in food. In the human body, they are found on skin and in the gastrointestinal (GI) and genitourinary tracts, including the urine of patients with indwelling bladder catheters. Historically, most infections arose from the normal endogenous organisms of the GI tract and were caused by *Candida albicans*. In recent years, however, the incidence of infections caused by other candidal strains has greatly increased. Oral, intestinal, vaginal, and systemic candidiasis can occur. Early recognition and treatment of local infections may prevent systemic candidiasis.

■ Oral candidiasis (thrush) produces painless white plaques on oral and pharyngeal mucosa. It often occurs in newborn infants who become infected during passage through an infected or colonized vagina. In older children and adults, thrush may occur as a complication of diabetes mellitus, as a result of poor oral hygiene, or after taking antibiotics or corticosteroids. It may also occur as an early manifestation of AIDS.

■ GI candidiasis often occurs after broad-spectrum antibacterial therapy, which destroys a large part of the normal flora of the intestine. The main symptom is diarrhea.

■ Vaginal candidiasis occurs in women who are pregnant, have diabetes mellitus, or take oral contraceptives or antibacterial drugs. The main symptom is a yellowish vaginal discharge. The infection may produce inflammation of the perineal area and spread to the buttocks and thighs.

■ Skin candidiasis occurs in people with continuously moist skinfolds or moist surgical dressings. The organism also may cause diaper rash and perineal rashes. Skin lesions are red and macerated.

■ Systemic or invasive candidiasis occurs when the organism gets into the bloodstream and is circulated throughout the body, with the brain, heart, kidneys, and eyes as the most common sites of infection. It occurs as a nosocomial infection in patients with serious illness or who are undergoing drug therapy that suppresses the immune system and may be fatal. Invasive infections may be present in any organ and may produce such disorders as urinary tract infection, endocarditis, and meningitis. It may be diagnosed by positive cultures of blood or tissue. Signs and symptoms depend on the severity of the infection and the organs affected and are indistinguishable from those occurring with bacterial infections.

The incidence of severe candidal infections has increased in recent years, in part because of increased numbers of neutropenic and immunodeficient patients. In addition, the frequent use of broad-spectrum antibiotics leads to extensive candidal colonization in debilitated patients, and the widespread use of medical devices (e.g., intravascular catheters, monitoring equipment, endotracheal tubes, urinary catheters) allows the organisms to reach sites that are normally sterile. People who use IV drugs also develop invasive candidiasis because the injections inoculate the fungi directly into the bloodstream.

Coccidioidomycosis is caused by an organism that grows as a mold in soil and decaying organic matter and is commonly found in the southwestern United States and northern Mexico. Infection results from inhalation of spores that convert to yeasts in the warm environment of the body and

BOX 22.1 **Selected Fungal Infections** (Continued)

often cause asymptomatic or mild respiratory infection. However, the organism may cause acute pulmonary infection with fever, chest pain, cough, headache, and loss of appetite. Radiographs may show small nodules in the lung like those seen in tuberculosis. In some cases, chronic disease develops in which the organisms remain localized and cause large, organism-filled cavities in the lung. These cavities may become fibrotic and require surgical excision. In a few cases, severe, disseminated disease occurs, either soon after the primary infection or after years of chronic pulmonary disease. Disseminated coccidioidomycosis may produce acute or chronic meningitis or a generalized disease with lesions in many internal organs. Skin lesions appear as granulomas that may eventually heal or become ulcerations. Most patients with primary infection recover without treatment; patients with disseminated disease require long-term treatment.

Coccidioidomycosis may occur in healthy or immunocompromised people but is more severe and more likely to become systemic in immunocompromised patients. For example, patients with AIDS who live in endemic areas are highly susceptible to this infection. The severity of the disease also increases with intensity of exposure.

Cryptococcosis is caused by inhalation of spores of *Cryptococcus neoformans*, an organism found worldwide, especially in bird droppings. The spores have also been found in fruits, vegetables, and dairy products.

When cryptococcosis occurs in healthy people, the primary infection is localized in the lungs, is asymptomatic or produces mild symptoms, and heals without treatment. However, pneumonia may occur and lead to spread of the organisms by the bloodstream. When cryptococcosis occurs in immunocompromised people, it is likely to be more severe and to become disseminated to the CNS, skin, and other organs. People with AIDS are highly susceptible, and cryptococcosis is a frequent opportunistic infection in this population. Infection most often affects the lungs and CNS. Cryptococcal pneumonia in patients with AIDS has a high mortality rate. Cryptococcal meningitis, the most common manifestation of disseminated disease, often produces abscesses in the brain. Clinical manifestations include headache, dizziness, and neck stiffness, and the condition is often mistaken for brain tumor. Later symptoms include coma, respiratory failure, and death if the meningitis is not treated effectively.

Histoplasmosis is a common infection that occurs worldwide, especially in the central and mid-eastern United States. The causative fungus is found in soil and organic debris around chicken houses, bird roosts, and caves inhabited by bats. Exposure to spores may result from activities such as demolishing or remodeling old buildings or cleaning chicken coops. Spores can be picked up by the wind and spread over large areas. Histoplasmosis develops when the spores are inhaled into the lungs, where they rapidly develop into the tissue-invasive yeast cells that reach the bloodstream and become distributed throughout the

body. In most cases, the organisms are destroyed or encapsulated by the host's immune system. The lung lesions heal by fibrosis and calcification and resemble the lesions of tuberculosis. Some people develop histoplasmosis years after the primary infection, probably from reactivation of a latent infection.

Clinical manifestations may vary widely. In people with a normal immune response, manifestations can be correlated with the extent of exposure. Most infections are asymptomatic or produce minimal symptoms for which treatment is not sought. When symptoms occur, they usually resemble an acute, influenza-like respiratory infection and improve within a few weeks. However, people exposed to large amounts of spores may have a high fever and severe pneumonia, which usually resolves with a low mortality rate. Some people, most often adult men with emphysema or other lung diseases, develop chronic pulmonary histoplasmosis with recurrent episodes of cough, fever, and weakness. In addition, histoplasmosis occasionally infects the liver, spleen, and other organs and is rapidly fatal if not treated effectively. The severe, disseminated form usually occurs in patients whose immune system is suppressed by diseases or drugs.

Pneumocystosis is caused by *Pneumocystis jiroveci*, an organism formerly considered a protozoan but now identified as a fungus. The organism is widespread in the environment, and most people are exposed at an early age. Infections are mild or asymptomatic in immunocompetent people. However, the organism can form cysts in the lungs, persist for long periods, and become activated in immunocompromised hosts. Activation produces an acute, life-threatening pneumonia (pneumocystis pneumonia) characterized by cough, fever, dyspnea, and presence of the organism in sputum. Groups at risk include human immunodeficiency virus (HIV)-seropositive people, those receiving corticosteroids or antineoplastics and other immunosuppressive drugs, and caregivers of infected people.

Sporotrichosis occurs when contaminated soil or plant material is inoculated into the skin through small wounds (e.g., thorn pricks) on the fingers, hands, or arms. It is most likely to occur among people who handle sphagnum moss, roses, or baled hay. Thus, infection is a hazard for gardeners and greenhouse workers. It can occur in both healthy and immunocompromised people but is more severe and disseminated in immunocompromised hosts.

Initial lesions, which are usually small, painless bumps resembling insect bites, occur 1 week to 6 months after inoculation. The subcutaneous nodule develops into a necrotic ulcer, which heals slowly as new ulcers appear in adjacent areas. Local lymphatic channels and lymph nodes also develop abscesses, nodules, and ulcers that may persist for years if the disease is not treated effectively. In immunocompromised people, sporotrichosis may spread to various tissues, including the meninges.

Polyenes (e.g., amphotericin B), azoles (e.g., fluconazole), and the miscellaneous agent griseofulvin act on ergosterol to disrupt the fungal cell membrane. Amphotericin B (and nystatin) binds to ergosterol and forms holes in the membrane, causing leakage of fungal cell contents and lysis of the cell. The azole drugs bind to an enzyme that is required for synthesis of ergosterol. This action causes production of a defective cell membrane, which also allows leakage of

intracellular contents and destruction of the cell. Both types of drugs also affect cholesterol in human cell membranes, a characteristic considered mainly responsible for the drugs' adverse effects.

Echinocandins (e.g., caspofungin) disrupt fungal cell walls rather than fungal cell membranes. They inhibit glucan synthetase, an enzyme required for synthesis of glucan. Glucan is a component of the fungal cell wall; its depletion leads to leakage

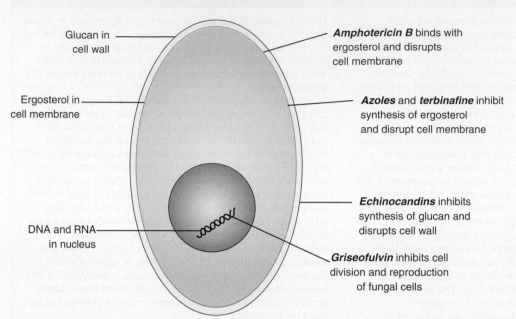

Fungal cell

Glucan in cell wall

Ergosterol in cell membrane

DNA and RNA in nucleus

Amphotericin B binds with ergosterol and disrupts cell membrane

Azoles and ***terbinafine*** inhibit synthesis of ergosterol and disrupt cell membrane

Echinocandins inhibits synthesis of glucan and disrupts cell wall

Griseofulvin inhibits cell division and reproduction of fungal cells

Figure 22.1 Actions of antifungal drugs on fungal cells.

of cellular contents and cell death. Because human cells do not contain cell walls, these drugs are less toxic than the polyene and azole antifungals.

Drugs for superficial fungal infections of skin and mucous membranes are often applied topically. Numerous preparations are available, many without a prescription. Drugs for systemic infections are given intravenously or orally. Patients with

HIV infection or severe neutropenia due to treatment with cytotoxic cancer drugs require aggressive treatment of fungal infections, because they are at high risk for developing life-threatening systemic mycoses. Selected antifungal drugs are further described in the following sections.

Table 22.1 summarizes the medications used in the treatment of fungal infections.

TABLE 22.1

Drugs Administered for Fungal Infections (Antifungal Agents)

Drug Class	Prototype	Other Drugs in the Class
Polyenes	Amphotericin B • Deoxycholate formulation (Fungizone) • Lipid formulations (Abelcet, AmBisome, Amphotec)	Nystatin (Mycostatin)
Azoles	Fluconazole (Diflucan)	Butoconazole (Femstat, Gynazole) Clotrimazole (Lotrimin, Mycelex, Gyne-Lotrimin) Econazole (Spectazole) Itraconazole (Sporanox) Ketoconazole (Nizoral) Miconazole (Monistat) Oxiconazole (Oxistat) Posaconazole (Noxafil) Sulconazole (Exelderm) Terconazole (Terazol) Tioconazole (Vagistat) Voriconazole (Vfend)
Echinocandins	Caspofungin (Cancidas)	Anidulafungin (Eraxis) Micafungin (Mycamine)
Miscellaneous antifungal agents for superficial mycoses	Griseofulvin	Ciclopirox (Penlac Nail Lacquer) Terbinafine (Lamisil)
Pyrimidine analog	Flucytosine (Ancobon)	

Clinical Application 22-1

- Ms. Angelo is told that she has a Candida infection. What does the nurse tell her about the cause of the fungal infection?

- What symptoms does Ms. Angelo experience?

NCLEX Success

1. Which of the following patients is at greatest risk for developing a life-threatening system mycoses?

    A. a patient who develops a sexually transmitted disease and is being treated with doxycycline hyclate (Vibramycin)

    B. a patient with breast cancer being treated with the chemotherapeutic agent cyclophosphamide (Cytoxan)

    C. a patient who is taking warfarin (Coumadin) for the prevention of a thromboemboli

    D. a patient with a strep throat who is being treated with cephalexin (Keflex)

2. A 32-year-old construction worker visits the occupational health clinic of the company where he is employed. The man has a high temperature, pain in the right middle and lower lobe of the lung, dyspnea, and malaise. During the admission interview, he states he has been working to restore homes in an urban area with 150-year-old houses. What does the nurse suspect is the cause of his symptoms?

    A. pneumocystosis
    B. sporotrichosis
    C. cryptococcosis
    D. histoplasmosis

Polyenes

Ⓟ **Amphotericin B**, the prototype polyene, is active against most types of pathogenic fungi and is fungicidal or fungistatic, depending on the concentration in body fluids and the susceptibility of the causative fungus. Because of its toxicity, the drug is used only for serious fungal infections. It is usually given for 4 to 12 weeks. There are three additional formulations of amphotericin B. Amphotericin B lipid-based formulations include Abelcet, AmBisome, and Amphotec.

Pharmacokinetics

Amphotericin B must be given intravenously for systemic infections. After infusion, the drug is rapidly taken up by the liver and other organs. It is then slowly released back into the bloodstream. Despite its long-term use, little is known about its distribution and metabolic pathways. Drug concentrations in most body fluids are higher in the presence of inflammation; concentrations in cerebrospinal fluid (CSF) are low with or without inflammation. The drug has an initial serum half-life of 24 hours, which represents redistribution from the bloodstream to tissues. This is followed by a second elimination phase, with a half-life of 15 days, which represents elimination from tissue storage sites. Most of the drug is thought to be metabolized in the tissues; some is excreted in the urine and can be detected for several weeks.

Lipid formulations (Abelcet, AmBisome, Amphotec) reach higher concentrations in diseased tissues than in normal tissues, so that larger doses can be given to increase therapeutic effects. At the same time, they cause less damage to normal tissues and decrease adverse effects. These products are much more expensive than the deoxycholate formulation (Fungizone). They are most likely to be used for patients with preexisting renal impairment or conditions in which other nephrotoxic drugs are routinely given (e.g., bone marrow transplant recipients) and when high doses are needed for difficult-to-treat infections. The lipid preparations differ in their characteristics and cannot be used interchangeably.

Action

Amphotericin B binds to the sterols within the fungal cell membrane, resulting in a change in the membrane permeability. This action destroys the fungal cells and prevents them from reproducing. Depending on the concentration of the medication, it has either a fungicidal or fungistatic effect.

Use

Amphotericin B is reserved for patients with progressive and potentially fatal infections resulting from cryptococcosis, North American blastomycosis, systemic candidiasis, disseminated moniliasis, coccidioidomycosis, and histoplasmosis. It is also used for mucormycosis caused by the species of *Mucor, Rhizopus, Absidia, Conidiobolus, Basidiobolus*; sporotrichosis; and aspergillosis. The drug is also given as an adjunctive agent in the treatment of American mucocutaneous leishmaniasis. A **BLACK BOX WARNING** ◆ issued by the Food and Drug Administration (FDA) states that amphotericin B should be reserved for progressive or potentially fatal infections. It is not recommended for use in noninvasive disease due to the risk of toxicity.

Abelcet is used in the treatment of aspergillosis. Likewise, Amphotec is given to treat aspergillosis if renal toxicity prevents the use of amphotericin B. AmBisome is used in the treatment of cryptococcal meningitis in HIV-infected patients. Patients who are febrile and neutropenic are given AmBisome for presumed fungal infections. Also, AmBisome is administered in the treatment of *Aspergillus, Candida,* or *Cryptococcus* when conventional amphotericin is not tolerated (Karch, 2011).

Table 22.2 presents specific information about the use of polyenes, including dosages for adults and children.

Use in Children

Children may take amphotericin B, but such use requires assessment of electrolytes due to magnesium wasting. Health care providers have used the drug successfully to treat children with serious fungal infections, without unusual or severe adverse effects.

TABLE 22.2

DRUGS AT A GLANCE: Polyenes

Drug	Pregnancy Category	Type of Infection Treated	Routes and Dosage Ranges	
			Adults	*Children*
Ⓟ **Amphotericin B deoxycholate** (Fungizone)	B	Serious, systemic fungal infections (e.g., candidiasis, histoplasmosis) Cutaneous candidiasis Oral candidiasis	Dosage is individualized according to the disease severity Initial IV dose: 0.25 mg/kg/d; gradually increase dosage to 0.5–1 mg/kg/d, infused over 2–6 h Topical: Apply 2–4 times daily for 1–4 wk Oral suspension: 100 mg/mL, 1 mL swish-and-swallow 4 times per day	Same as for adults for IV, skin preparations, and oral suspension
Amphotericin B lipid complex (Abelcet)	B	Systemic infections in patients who do not tolerate Fungizone	IV 5 mg/kg/d	Same as adults
Liposomal amphotericin B (AmBisome)	B	Systemic infections in patients who do not tolerate Fungizone Empiric treatment of presumed fungal infections in febrile, neutropenic patients	IV 3–5 mg/kg/d	Same as adults
Nystatin (Mycostatin)	C	Candidiasis of skin, mucous membrane, and intestinal tract	Oral or intestinal infection, PO tablets 1–2 (500,000–1,000,000 units) 3 times daily; oral suspension, 4–6 mL (400,000–600,000 units) 4 times daily; oral troches 1–2 (200,000–400,000 units) 4–5 times daily Topically to skin lesions, 2–3 times daily Intravaginally, 1 vaginal tablet once daily for 14 d	Oral suspension, older than 1 y:, same as adults; infants, 2 mL (200,000 units) 4 times daily Oral troches, same as adults for children old enough to suck on the lozenge until it dissolves

Use in Older Adults

Older adults, with the impaired renal and cardiovascular functions that usually accompany aging, are especially vulnerable to serious adverse effects. They require close monitoring to reduce the incidence and severity of nephrotoxicity, hypokalemia, and other adverse drug reactions. Lipid formulations of amphotericin B are less nephrotoxic than the conventional deoxycholate formulation and may be preferred.

Use in Patients With Renal Impairment

Amphotericin B deoxycholate (Fungizone) is nephrotoxic. Renal impairment occurs in most patients (up to 80%) within the first

2 weeks of therapy but usually subsides with dosage reduction or drug discontinuation. Permanent impairment occurs in a few patients. Recommendations to decrease nephrotoxicity include hydrating patients with a liter of 0.9% sodium chloride solution intravenously and monitoring serum creatinine and blood urea nitrogen (BUN) at least weekly. If the patient's BUN exceeds 40 mg/dL or serum creatinine exceeds 3 mg/dL, the drug should be stopped or dosage should be reduced until renal function recovers. Another strategy is to give a lipid formulation (e.g., Abelcet, AmBisome, Amphotec), which is less nephrotoxic. For patients who already have renal impairment or other risk factors for development of renal impairment, a lipid formulation is indicated. Renal function should still be monitored frequently.

Use in Patients With Hepatic Impairment

Although the main concern with amphotericin B is nephrotoxicity, monitoring of hepatic function during use is recommended.

Use in Patients With Critical Illness

As previously stated, amphotericin B penetrates tissues well, except for the CSF, and only small amounts are excreted in the urine. With prolonged administration, the half-life increases from 1 to 15 days. Hemodialysis does not remove the drug. Lipid formulations may be preferred in critically ill patients because of less nephrotoxicity.

Use in Patients Receiving Home Care

It is important that the home care nurse assess the patient's immune function with the administration of amphotericin B. The patient's home should be kept meticulously clean and free of mold-producing substances such as potted plants, fresh flowers, and adhesive nonslip bathtub appliques. The bathroom should be cleaned daily with bleach, and air conditioning and air-filtration systems should be kept clean.

Adverse Effects

Adverse effects of amphotericin B are often severe, with the most serious being multiple organ failure, respiratory arrest, and cardiac arrest. Other adverse affects include:

- GI: nausea, vomiting, dyspepsia, (GI) bleeding
- Genitourinary: hypokalemia, azotemia, renal failure
- Hematological: leukopenia, thrombocytopenia

Contraindications

Patients with a known allergy to amphotericin B and impairment of renal function should not receive the drug. Women who are lactating should not take it except in life-threatening situations.

Nursing Implications

Preventing Interactions

Many medications interact with amphotericin B, increasing or decreasing its effect (Box 22.2). Researchers have not reported that any herbs interact with the drug.

Administering the Drug

The pharmacy should reconstitute and prepare amphotericin B for IV administration. It is necessary to infuse the prepared solutions of amphotericin within 8 hours of reconstitution. The patient should receive a test dose to assess tolerance for the drug. Doubling maintenance doses and infusing them on alternate days is fine. However, a single daily dose of Fungizone should not exceed 1.5 mg/kg; overdoses can result in cardiorespiratory arrest. Larger doses of the lipid preparations are recommended to achieve therapeutic effects similar to those of the deoxycholate preparation. When possible, it is best to administer amphotericin B through a separate IV line. When injecting it into an existing IV line, flushing of the line with a 5% dextrose solution should occur before and after administration with both deoxycholate and

---

> **BOX 22.2** ■ **Drug Interactions: Amphotericin B**
>
> **Drugs That Increase the Effects of Amphotericin B**
> - Antibiotics *(nephrotoxic)*
>   *Increase the risk of nephrotoxicity*
> - Antineoplastic agents
>   *Increase renal toxicity, bronchospasm, and hypotension*
> - Cardiac glycosides
>   *Increase the risk of digitalis toxicity due to hypokalemia*
> - Corticosteroid, corticotropin, skeletal muscle relaxants
>   *Increase potassium depletion*
>
> **Drugs That Decrease the Effects of Amphotericin B**
> - Clotrimazole, fluconazole, ketoconazole
>   *Increase resistance to fungal infection*
> - Flucytosine
>   *Increase flucytosine toxicity*

lipid formulations. An in-line filter may be used with Fungizone and AmBisome but not with Abelcet or Amphotec.

Specific instructions for administration of the various forms of amphotericin B are

- Fungizone (IV form): give in 5% dextrose in water over 2 to 6 hours with the use of in-line filter. This drug should not be mixed with any other medications.
- Abelcet: give over 2 hours without the use of an in-line filter.
- Amphotec: give over a minimum of 2 hours without the use of an in-line filter.
- Amphotericin cream or lotion: apply liberally to skin lesions and rub in gently.

Prior to beginning treatment, it is necessary to obtain a culture of the infection. However, treatment with amphotericin B should begin prior to the culture results. The nurse monitors injection sites for signs of phlebitis. He or she gives aspirin, antihistamines, and antiemetics, which are used to manage adverse effects, prior to the administration of amphotericin B. It is essential to assess the sodium balance throughout the administration. By maintaining the serum sodium level within normal range, the patient has decreased symptoms of drug discomfort. Small doses of corticosteroids or meperidine assist in diminishing chills related to drug administration.

Assessing for Therapeutic Effects

The nurse assesses for decrease in symptoms of the fungal infection. The administration of amphotericin B is consistent with the cure of infection. When the infection is controlled, the administration of amphotericin B continues with a maintenance dose for an indefinite period (Smeltzer, Bare, Hinkle, & Cheever, 2010).

Assessing for Adverse Effects

The nurse assesses for severe chilling, headaches, malaise, nausea, vomiting, and generalized pain. (As previously stated, management of these symptoms requires aspirin, antihistamines, and antiemetics.) It is necessary to monitor the patient's electrolytes for hypokalemia and hyponatremia. When administering amphotericin topically, the nurse assesses for a hypersensitivity reaction at the site of the application. IV administration of amphotericin is irritating to the injection and requires assessment for phlebitis and thrombophlebitis.

Patient Teaching

Box 22.3 identifies patient teaching guidelines for amphotericin B.

Other Drugs in the Class

Nystatin has the same mechanism of action as amphotericin B. However, it is used only for topical therapy of oral, intestinal, and vaginal candidiasis because it is too toxic for systemic use. Although given orally for oral or intestinal infections, the drug is not absorbed systemically and is excreted in the feces. With

---

EVIDENCE-BASED PRACTICE

Topical Amphotericin B and Subconjunctival Injection of Fluconazole (Combination Therapy) Versus Topical Amphotericin B (Monotherapy) in Treatment of Keratomycosis

by RHEDA MAHDY, WALEED NADA, AND MOSTAFA WAGEH

Journal of Ocular Pharmacology and Therapeutics 2010, 26(3), 281–285

The purpose of this study was to compare (1) combination therapy of topical amphotericin B (0.5 mg/mL) eye drops together with subconjunctival injection of fluconazole (2 mg/mL) with (2) topical amphotericin B (0.5 mg/mL) eye drops in the treatment of fungal keratitis. The study involved 48 patients who presented with fungal keratitis. Predisposing factors for fungal keratitis included immunocompromise, advancing age, history of resistant corneal ulcers, corneal scarring, trauma, laser-assisted in situ keratomileusis (LASIK) corneal surgery, vernal keratoconjunctivitis, and contact lens wearing. The study revealed that treatment with combination therapy of topical amphotericin B eye drops and subconjunctival injection of fluconazole was more effective than the use of amphotericin B drops alone in the treatment of fungal keratitis.

IMPLICATIONS FOR NURSING PRACTICE: When caring for a patient with predisposing factors to the development of fungal keratitis, the nurse should consult the physician regarding the administration of amphotericin B and subconjunctival injection of fluconazole in the event that fungal keratitis develops.

BOX 22.3 Patient Teaching Guidelines for Amphotericin B

- Long-term use of amphotericin is necessary.
- You may not notice the effects of the medication for several weeks.
- Use good hygiene to prevent reinfection or spread of infection.
- You may experience side effects such as nausea and vomiting, so eat small, frequent meals.
- Be aware that topical administration of the medication may cause staining of clothes.
- Report skin irritations with the use of topical amphotericin.
- Report fever, chills, muscle aches, and headache.
- Report irritation at the injection site.

---

oral use, adverse effects include nausea, vomiting, and diarrhea; with vaginal application, adverse effects include local irritation and burning.

NCLEX Success

3. A 53-year-old man has asthma. He is admitted to the emergency department with wheezing, dyspnea, muscle aches, and a high fever. He owns and operates a swimming pool business in which he sells aboveground swimming pools and hot tubs. His business has a showroom with functioning pools and hot tubs. What fungal infection do you suspect the patient is suffering from?

   A. blastomycosis
   B. histoplasmosis
   C. aspergillosis
   D. candidiasis

4. A patient is diagnosed with cryptococcal meningitis. Which of the following medications is administered to treat cryptococcal meningitis?

   A. amphotericin B
   B. Rocephin
   C. bleomycin
   D. mupirocin

5. When administering amphotericin B, what drug is administered to prevent the development of chilling, fever, malaise, and nausea?

   A. aminophylline
   B. ibuprofen
   C. penicillin G
   D. aspirin

Azoles

The azoles are the largest group of commonly used antifungal agents. Many are used topically, and some are available without a prescription for dermatologic (see Chap. 60) or vaginal use (e.g., butoconazole, clotrimazole, miconazole, terconazole, tioconazole). It is necessary to obtain a prescription to use azoles for other indications.

Systemic azoles include ketoconazole, fluconazole, itraconazole, posaconazole, and voriconazole. Although ketoconazole was the first azole developed, Ⓟ **fluconazole** (Diflucan) is considered to be the prototype medication of the class. Fluconazole and other drugs in the class have a broader spectrum of fungal activity, are distributed more effectively, and have fewer adverse effects and drug interactions.

Pharmacokinetics

Fluconazole is administered orally or parenterally. The oral preparation has a slow onset of action with a peak of action in 1 to 2 hours and duration of action 2 to 4 days. The oral drug is well absorbed and reaches therapeutic levels in most body fluids and tissues, including the meninges. The IV preparation has a rapid onset of action, with a peak of action in 1 hour and the same duration of action 2 to 4 days. The azoles interact with cytochrome P450 (CYP) enzymes, which can potentially produce significant interactions with many other drugs (those in which there is a decrease in the metabolism and increase in the risk of toxicity with affected drugs).

Fluconazole is apparently a less potent inhibitor of CYP3A4 enzymes than ketoconazole and itraconazole. As a result, drug interactions with fluconazole are of lesser magnitude and usually occur only with dosages of 200 mg per day or more. However, fluconazole is a strong inhibitor of CYP2C9 enzymes. Fluconazole crosses the placenta and enters the breast milk. It is excreted in the urine.

Action

Fluconazole binds to sterols in the fungal cell membrane. This action changes the membrane's permeability, producing a fungicidal or fungistatic effect depending on the drug concentration and the fungal organism.

Use

Fluconazole and the other azoles discussed in this section are used systemically or both topically and systemically. Fluconazole is often the drug of choice for localized candidal infections (e.g., urinary tract infections, thrush) and is useful for systemic candidiasis. However, resistant strains of *Candida* organisms occur with extensive use of fluconazole. In vaginal candidiasis, a single oral dose of 150 mg is usually effective. Fluconazole is also used for long-term suppression of cryptococcal meningitis in patients with acquired immunodeficiency syndrome (AIDS), after initial use of amphotericin B. It is used prophylactically in the prevention of candidiasis in patients with bone marrow transplants.

Table 22.3 provides detailed information about the use of azoles, including dosages for adults and children.

Use in Children

Fluconazole is commonly used in children with *Candida* infections. However, the maximum daily dosage should not exceed 600 mg per day.

Use in Older Adults

Fluconazole is routinely administered to older patients with *Candida* infections. However, it is necessary to monitor the creatinine clearance (CrCl) and hepatic enzymes.

Use in Patients With Renal Impairment

In patients with a CrCl of 50 mL per minute or less, the patient should take 50% of the recommended dose. Patients receiving hemodialysis receive a full dose following each dialysis treatment.

TABLE 22.3

DRUGS AT A GLANCE: Azoles

Drug	Pregnancy Category	Type of Infection Treated	Routes and Dosage Ranges	
			Adults	Children
Ⓟ **Fluconazole** (Diflucan)	C	Oropharyngeal, esophageal, vaginal, and systemic candidiasis Prevention of candidiasis after bone marrow transplantation Cryptococcal meningitis	Oropharyngeal candidiasis, PO, IV 200 mg first day, then 100 mg daily for 2 wk Esophageal candidiasis, PO, IV, 200 mg first day, then 100 mg daily for at least 3 wk Vaginal candidiasis, PO 150 mg as a single dose Systemic candidiasis, PO, IV 400 mg first day, then 200 mg daily for at least 4 wk Prophylaxis, PO, IV 400 mg once daily Cryptococcal meningitis, PO, IV, 400 mg first day, then 200–400 mg/d for 10–12 wk	Oropharyngeal candidiasis, PO, IV 6 mg/kg first day, then 3 mg/kg/d for at least 2 wk Esophageal candidiasis, PO, IV, 6 mg/kg first day, then 3 mg/kg/d for at least 3 wk Systemic candidiasis, PO, IV 6–12 mg/kg/d Cryptococcal meningitis, PO, IV 12 mg/kg first day, then 6 mg/kg/d for 10–12 wk

(*Continued on page 408*)

TABLE 22.3

DRUGS AT A GLANCE: Azoles (Continued)

Drug	Pregnancy Category	Type of Infection Treated	Routes and Dosage Ranges	
			Adults	Children
Itraconazole (Sporanox)	C	Systemic fungal infections, including aspergillosis, in neutropenic and immunocompromised hosts Onychomycosis Tinea infections	Systemic infection, PO 200 mg once or twice daily for 3 mo Blastomycosis, histoplasmosis, aspergillosis, IV 200 mg twice daily for 4 doses, then 200 mg/d Onychomycosis, fingernail, PO 200 mg twice daily for 1 wk, no drug for 3 wk, then repeat dosage for 1 wk; toenail, PO 200 mg once daily for 12 consecutive weeks Oral solution, 100–200 mg daily (10–20 mL), swish and swallow 3 times daily for 3–5 d Tinea infections, PO 100–200 mg daily for 1–4 wk	Safety and efficacy not established. *3–16-y-old* patients have been treated with 100 mg daily for systemic infections and patients *6 mo to 12 y* have been treated with 5 mg/kg once daily for 2 wk without serious or unusual adverse effects
Ketoconazole (Nizoral)	C	Candidiasis, histoplasmosis, coccidioidomycosis Cutaneous candidiasis Tinea infections	PO 200 mg once daily, increased to 400 mg once daily if necessary in severe infections Topically, once daily for 2–6 wk	*2 y and older*: PO 3.3–6.6 mg/kg/d as a single dose
Posaconazole (Noxafil)	C	Treatment of oropharyngeal candidiasis Prevention of invasive fungal infection	Prevention: PO 200 mg 3 times daily Oropharyngeal candidiasis PO 100 mg twice daily initially, then 200 mg once daily for 13 d	Dosage not established
Voriconazole (Vfend)	D	Esophageal candidiasis Invasive aspergillosis Other serious fungal infections	Esophageal candidiasis, PO 200 mg every 12 h for weight of ≥40 kg; 100 mg every 12 h for weight <40 kg. Give at least 14 d or 7 d after symptoms resolve Aspergillosis and other serious infections, IV 6 mg/kg every 12 h for 2 doses (loading dose), then 4 mg/kg every 12 h (maintenance dose)	Safety and efficacy not established for children younger than 12 y

Use in Patients With Hepatic Impairment

The azoles may cause hepatotoxicity, ranging from mild elevations in alanine aminotransferase (ALT) and aspartate aminotransferase (AST) to clinical hepatitis, cholestasis, hepatic failure, and death. Fatal hepatic damage has occurred mainly in patients with serious underlying conditions, such as AIDS or malignancy, and with multiple concomitant medications. The drugs are relatively contraindicated in patients with increased liver enzymes, active liver disease, or a history of liver damage with other drugs. They should be used only if expected benefits outweigh risks of liver injury. It is necessary to check ALT, AST, and serum bilirubin before drug use, after several weeks of drug use, and every 1 to 2 months during long-term therapy. If ALT and AST increase to more than three times the normal range, the azole should be discontinued. Hepatotoxicity may be reversible if drug therapy is stopped.

Use in Patients With Critical Illness

Fluconazole penetrates tissues well, including CSF. Although IV administration may be necessary in many critically ill patients, the drug is well absorbed when administered orally (or by nasogastric tube).

Use in Patients Receiving Home Care

When administering the azoles in the home setting, it is important that the home care nurse instruct the patient and family on the management of the environment with the implementation of good hand hygiene, household cleanliness, removal of potted plants and fresh flowers, and the use of air-conditioning and air-filtration systems. The nurse should also tell the patient and family about measures to prevent the reinfection and spread of the fungal infection.

Adverse Effects

Although fluconazole is usually well tolerated, it may cause nausea, vomiting, diarrhea, abdominal pain, headache, and skin rash. In addition, elevation of liver enzymes and hepatic necrosis have reportedly occurred, and alopecia often occurs in patients receiving prolonged, high-dose treatment.

Contraindications

Fluconazole is contraindicated in patients who have experienced a hypersensitivity reaction to the azole medications. It is also contraindicated in pregnancy and lactation. It should be administered cautiously with renal or hepatic impairment.

Nursing Implications

Preventing Interactions

Azoles inhibit the metabolism of many drugs (by inhibiting CYP drug-metabolizing enzymes in the liver and small intestine, especially CYP3A4 enzymes), thus increasing the effects and possible toxicity of azoles. Many medications increase or decrease the effects of fluconazole (Box 22.4). Researchers have not identified any herbs that interact with fluconazole.

Although the main concern about azole drug interactions is increased toxicity of inhibited drugs, ketoconazole may be given with cyclosporine and tacrolimus to decrease dosages

---

BOX 22.4 **Drug Interactions: Fluconazole**

Drugs That Increase the Effects of Fluconazole
- Benzodiazepines (alprazolam, midazolam, triazolam), calcium channel blockers (felodipine, nifedipine), cyclosporine, phenytoin, statins (atorvastatin, simvastatin), sulfonylureas, tacrolimus, theophylline, warfarin, vincristine, zidovudine
  Increase serum levels and toxic effects of these drugs due to inhibition of cytochrome P450

Drugs That Decrease the Effects of Fluconazole
- Cimetidine, rifampin
  Decrease serum level of fluconazole

---

and costs of the immunosuppressant drugs. There may also be a reduced risk of fungal infections, which commonly occur in people with an impaired immune system.

The nurse should note that fluconazole is apparently a less potent inhibitor of CYP3A4 enzymes than ketoconazole and itraconazole. As a result, drug interactions with fluconazole are of lesser magnitude and usually occur only with dosages of 200 mg per day or more. However, fluconazole is a strong inhibitor of CYP2C9 enzymes, and concurrent administration of losartan, phenytoin, or warfarin results in greater risks of toxicity with the inhibited drugs.

Administering the Medication

When administering IV fluconazole, it is necessary to follow the manufacturer's recommendations. Until the nurse prepares the medication for administration, he or she should not remove the overwrap of the package. The inner bag maintains the sterility of the medication. The nurse assesses the bag for minute leaks by squeezing it firmly. If any leaks are apparent, it is necessary to discard the medication. The nurse should never mix fluconazole with any other medications. Continuous infusion of fluconazole occurs at a maximum rate of 200 mg per hour. When administering the oral suspension, it is necessary to shake the elixir vigorously prior to pouring the dose. To decrease gastric upset, the nurse administers the medication with food.

Assessing for Therapeutic Effects

When administering fluconazole, the nurse assesses the therapeutic effects of the medication. The patient who is treated for a systemic mycoses should have a decrease in fever and malaise. There is also healing of skin and mucous membrane lesions. Treatment of intestinal candidiasis results in diminished diarrhea. The female patient who has experienced discomfort from vaginal candidiasis should have decreased burning and itching along with diminished vaginal discharge.

Assessing for Adverse Effects

The nurse must assess the skin for signs of skin rash. The GI assessment should include assessing for nausea, vomiting, diarrhea, and abdominal pain. All of the azoles cause hepatotoxicity with an elevation of the AST and ALT levels. Thus, it is necessary to assess hepatic enzymes monthly during therapy. Assessment of renal function tests should occur weekly, with dosage reduction or discontinuation of the drug if renal toxicity results.

Patient Teaching

Box 22.5 identifies patient teaching guidelines for fluconazole.

Other Drugs in the Class

Although ketoconazole (Nizoral) has largely been replaced by the newer drugs, it may still be used for long-term therapy because it is less expensive than other azoles. It may also be used with cyclosporine and tacrolimus because it increases blood levels of these immunosuppressant drugs and allows smaller dosages in patients with organ transplants.

Itraconazole (Sporanox) is a drug of choice for many fungal infections. It can be given orally or intravenously. Drug absorption may be decreased in patients with achlorhydria and in those

Patient Teaching Guidelines for Fluconazole

■ Take the medication for the complete course to ensure adequate results.

■ Implement hand hygiene and maintain environmental cleanliness.

■ Have renal function tests as ordered.

■ Have hepatic function tests as ordered.

■ To avoid experiencing side effects such as nausea and vomiting, eat small, frequent meals.

■ Report any skin eruption to the prescriber.

■ Report any changes in stool or urine to the prescriber.

■ Find out about adverse effects of the drug and report any adverse effects to the prescriber.

Clinical Application 22-2

■ Before Ms. Angelo takes fluconazole, what assessments should the nurse make?

■ What is the action of fluconazole?

■ Ms. Angelo returns to the primary care provider's office 2 weeks later. She has an active *C. albicans* infection. The primary care provider prescribes fluconazole 200 mg PO for one dose, then 100 mg PO daily for 14 days. What adverse effects should the nurse tell the patient to watch for?

receiving a concurrent antacid, histamine H_2 antagonist, or proton pump inhibitor. Serum levels should be measured to ensure adequate absorption. Drug concentrations are higher in visceral organs than in serum; little drug appears in urine or CSF.

Usual doses may cause GI upset, and higher doses may cause hypokalemia, hypertension, edema, and heart failure. Itraconazole has many drug interactions. Drugs that increase the pH of gastric acid (e.g., antacids, histamine H_2 blockers, proton pump inhibitors) decrease absorption of itraconazole and should be given at least 2 hours after itraconazole. Drugs that induce drug-metabolizing enzymes (e.g., carbamazepine, phenytoin, and rifampin) decrease serum levels of itraconazole. Itraconazole increases serum levels of cyclosporine, digoxin, oral sulfonylureas, and warfarin; it decreases serum levels of carbamazepine, phenytoin, and rifampin. The FDA has issued a **BLACK BOX WARNING** ◆ about the risks of heart failure and drug interactions with itraconazole.

Posaconazole (Noxafil) is a second-generation azole with activity against *Candida* and *Aspergillus* species. It is available as an oral suspension; after administration, it reaches maximum concentration in the body in 3 to 5 hours and steady state in 7 to 10 days. It is highly protein bound and eliminated mainly in feces. Patients with severe vomiting and diarrhea or renal impairment should be monitored for breakthrough fungal infections. If given with drugs metabolized by the CYP3A4 enzymes in the liver, posaconazole increases blood levels and risks of adverse effects with the other drugs.

Voriconazole (Vfend) is a second-generation azole with activity against species of *Candida* and *Aspergillus*. It is well absorbed with oral administration and reaches peak serum levels in less than 2 hours. It is widely distributed in body tissues and metabolized in the liver by CYP2C9, CYP2C19, and CYP3A4. The metabolites are excreted renally. Transient visual disturbance is a common adverse effect, occurring in approximately 30% of recipients. Significant drug interactions include reduced voriconazole levels with enzyme inducers (e.g., rifampin, rifabutin, carbamazepine) and increased sirolimus levels with voriconazole administration, possibly to toxic levels. These drugs are contraindicated during voriconazole therapy, and concomitant administration of cyclosporine, tacrolimus, or warfarin requires vigilant monitoring. Dosage of voriconazole should be reduced with impaired liver function.

NCLEX Success

6. A patient who is being treated for a seizure disorder with phenytoin (Dilantin) receives a diagnosis of candidiasis. The prescriber orders fluconazole. What effect does fluconazole have on phenytoin?

A. The dosage of phenytoin should be increased.

B. The fluconazole will be ineffective with the phenytoin.

C. The patient should be assessed for phenytoin toxicity.

D. The fluconazole dosage will need to be increased.

7. A prescriber writes an order for fluconazole 250 mg IV per hour. Which of the following nursing actions is most appropriate?

A. Begin the IV infusion at 125 mg per hour and increase it to 250 mg per hour after 4 hours.

B. Inform the prescriber that the maximum dose is 200 mg per hour IV.

C. Administer the fluconazole at 250 mg per hour IV.

D. Administer the fluconazole at 200 mg per hour IV.

8. A patient who is undergoing hemodialysis has received a diagnosis of a systemic *Candida* infection. Which of the following interventions should be implemented when administering fluconazole?

A. Administer the full dose of fluconazole after dialysis.

B. Administer the full dose of fluconazole before dialysis.

C. Administer one-half of the dose of fluconazole after dialysis.

D. Administer one-half of the dose of fluconazole before dialysis.

9. A patient is receiving a high dose of fluconazole intravenously. Which of the following laboratory values indicate the development of hepatic necrosis?

A. CrCl of 50 mL per minute

B. BUN of 15 mg/dL

C. AST of 10 Units/L

D. ALT of 200 Units/L

10. **A prescriber has ordered oral fluconazole. Which of the following patient teaching guidelines is important to implement?**
    A. Administer the medication on an empty stomach.
    B. Administer the medication 2 hours following breakfast.
    C. Administer the medication with meals.
    D. Administer the medication with a full glass of water.

Echinocandins

The echinocandins have fungal activity against *Candida*, including azole-resistant organisms, and fungistatic activity against *Aspergillus*. The prototype for this class of antifungals is Ⓟ **caspofungin** (Cancidas).

Pharmacokinetics

Caspofungin is highly bound to plasma albumin. It is metabolized in the liver and by the plasma to inactive metabolites.

(In older adults, the use of this drug requires reduced dosage if there is hepatic insufficiency.) It is excreted in the urine and feces. Its half-life is 9 to 11 hours.

Action

Caspofungin inhibits the synthesis of the fungal cell wall, interfering with the reproduction and growth of susceptible fungi.

Use

Caspofungin is used to treat invasive aspergillosis in patients who do not tolerate other antifungal drugs. It is also used to treat *Candida* infections related to intraabdominal, pleural space, or esophageal abscesses, or peritonitis. In addition, it is given to febrile neutropenic patients who possess a suspected fungal infection.

Table 22.4 provides information about the use of echinocandins, including dosages.

Use in Children

Caspofungin is approved for use in children older than 3 months of age for the treatment of candidemia and invasive candidiasis. It is recommended that the dosage be established

TABLE 22.4
DRUGS AT A GLANCE: Echinocandins

Drug	Pregnancy Category	Type of Infection Treated	Routes and Dosage Ranges	
			Adults	*Children*
Ⓟ **Caspofungin** (Cancidas)	C	Invasive aspergillosis Candidiasis	IV infusion over 1 h, 70 mg initially, then 50 mg daily Hepatic impairment, 70 mg initially, then 35 mg daily	Safety and efficacy not established in children younger than 3 mo of age Infants and children 3 mo to 17 y are administered 70 mg/m²/dose on the first day and 50 mg/m²/dose daily. The dosage may be increased to 70 mg/m²/dose daily
Anidulafungin (Eraxis)	C	Treatment of candidemia, esophageal candidiasis, and other *Candida* infections	Candidemia, IV infusion 200 mg initially, then 100 mg daily Esophageal candidiasis, IV infusion 100 mg initially, then 50 mg daily	Dosage not established
Micafungin (Mycamine)	C	Treatment of esophageal candidiasis Prevention of *Candida* infections in patients undergoing hematopoietic stem cell transplantation	Treatment: IV infusion 150 mg daily Prevention: IV infusion 50 mg daily	Dosage not established

based on body surface area rather than weight. Patients who are receiving rifampin or phenytoin require an increased dose (Campbell & Kauffman, 2011).

Use in Patients With Renal Impairment

No dosage adjustment is necessary when using in patients with renal impairment.

Adverse Effects

Adverse effects of caspofungin include fever, headache, nausea, skin rash, vomiting, and phlebitis at the injection site.

Contraindications

Caspofungin is contraindicated in patients who have experienced a hypersensitivity reaction to the medication. It should be not administered with mannitol.

Nursing Implications

Preventing Interactions

Certain medications interact with caspofungin, increasing or decreasing its effects (Box 22.6). Researchers have not reported any interaction of herbs with caspofungin.

Administering the Medication

It is essential to administer caspofungin intravenously, and the drug is incompatible with any other IV medication, including dextrose. The medication should be at room temperature prior to administration. It is necessary to reconstitute the 50-mg or 70-mg vials of caspofungin in 10.5 mL of normal saline or sterile water. The reconstituted medication yields 5 mg/mL or 7 mg/mL, respectively. Reconstituted solutions are stable for 24 hours when stored at 25°C. Addition of the medication to 250 mL of normal saline or half normal saline follows. The nurse administers the medication slowly over 1 hour.

Prior to administering the first dose of caspofungin, the nurse assesses baseline liver and renal function along with electrolytes, complete blood count, and platelet count. During administration, the nurse assesses for hypersensitivity reactions and phlebitis at the infusion site. If it is administered concurrently with tacrolimus, it is necessary to assess serum blood levels.

BOX 22.6 **Drug Interactions: Caspofungin**

Drugs That Increase the Effects of Caspofungin

■ Cyclosporine

Increases serum effects (when cyclosporine and caspofungin are administered together)

Drugs That Decrease the Effects of Caspofungin

■ Antiseizure medications (e.g., carbamazepine, phenytoin); antiviral medications used to treat human immunodeficiency virus (HIV) (e.g., efavirenz, nelfinavir, nevirapine); dexamethasone; rifampin

Reduce blood levels and therapeutic effectiveness

Assessing for Therapeutic Effects

The therapeutic effect of caspofungin is a decrease in the growth of fungi. The patient has decreased symptoms of malaise, fever, and GI symptoms.

Assessing for Adverse Effects

When administering 50 mg daily of caspofungin, the nurse observes for nausea, vomiting, and phlebitis at the infusion site. When administering 50 to 70 mg, the nurse assesses for these adverse effects plus fever, headache, and abnormal laboratory reports (e.g., decreased white blood cells, hemoglobin and hematocrit, increased serum potassium, and liver aminotransferase enzymes). In addition, he or she assesses for a histamine reaction, including facial edema, wheezing, dyspnea, chest tightness, skin eruptions, and itching. Patients suffering from any cardiovascular disease warrant assessment for increasing weight and peripheral edema.

Patient Teaching

Caspofungin is administered in the acute care setting. The patient should receive instruction about the histamine reaction to the medication and the necessity of reporting any cardiac symptoms.

Other Drugs in the Class

Anidulafungin (Eraxis) is a semisynthetic antifungal medication that inhibits glucan synthase, an essential component in the fungal cell wall. It is used to treat esophageal candidiasis and other *Candida* infections. It produces similar adverse effects as caspofungin and warrants cautious use with hepatic impairment.

NCLEX Success

11. You are the preceptor assigned to a senior level nursing student. Which of the following nursing actions would be inappropriate for the nursing student to implement when administering caspofungin?
    A. administering the caspofungin with dextrose
    B. assessing the baseline electrolytes and liver enzymes
    C. keeping the medication at room temperature prior to administration
    D. administering the medication slowly over 1 hour

12. The nursing student has reconstituted the caspofungin. Which of the following solutions should the student use in the administration of caspofungin?
    A. 250 mL of lactated Ringer's solution
    B. 250 mL of normal saline
    C. 500 mL of 0.45% normal saline
    D. 50 mL of dextrose and normal saline

Miscellaneous Antifungal Agents for Superficial Mycoses

The miscellaneous antifungal agents are administered for dermatophyte infections of the scalp and nails. Ⓟ **Griseofulvin** is the prototype for this class.

TABLE 22.5

DRUGS AT A GLANCE: Miscellaneous Antifungal Agents for Superficial Mycoses

Drug	Pregnancy Category	Type of Infection Treated	Routes and Dosage Ranges	
			Adults	Children
Ⓟ **Griseofulvin**	C	Dermatophytosis (skin, hair, nails)	PO Microsize: 500–1000 mg/d in single or divided doses Ultramicrosize: 375 mg/d in single or divided doses; up to 750 mg/d has been used to eradicate tinea unguium, tinea pedis	Children >2 y PO Microsize: 10–20 mg/kg/d in single or divided doses; tinea capitis, 20–25 mg/ kg/d for 8–12 wk Ultramicrosize: 7.3 mg/kg/d in single dose or 2 divided doses; maximum dosage is 750 mg/d
Terbinafine (Lamisil)		Tinea infections Onychomycosis of fingernails or toenails	Tinea infections, topically to skin, once or twice daily for at least 1 wk and no longer than 4 wk Onychomycosis, fingernail, PO 250 mg daily for 6 wk; toenail, PO 250 mg daily for 12 wk	

Pharmacokinetics

Griseofulvin is absorbed in the GI tract and metabolized in the liver. The serum half-life is 9 to 22 hours. The medication is excreted in the urine, feces, and perspiration.

Action

Griseofulvin disrupts the metaphase of cell division by binding to keratin, making it resistant to fungal invasion (Up-To-Date, 2011c).

Use

Griseofulvin is used for the treatment of susceptible tinea infections of the skin, hair, and nails. Table 22.5 gives specific information about the use of miscellaneous antifungal agents, including dosages for adults and children.

Use in Children

Safety has not been established in children 2 years of age and younger.

Use in Patients With Hepatic Impairment

Patients with hepatic impairment should not take the drug.

Adverse Effects

Adverse effects of griseofulvin include

- CNS effects: dizziness, fatigue, headache, insomnia, and mental confusion
- Dermatological reactions: erythema, photosensitivity, and urticaria

- GI: sometimes gastric upset with nausea and vomiting
- Other: hepatotoxicity and proteinuria

Contraindications

Griseofulvin is contraindicated in patients with a known hypersensitivity reaction. It is also contraindicated with liver disease, porphyria, and pregnancy.

Nursing Implications

Preventing Interactions

Some medications interact with griseofulvin, increasing or decreasing its effect (Box 22.7). Substances that increase the effect of griseofulvin include alcohol and vitamin E.

Administering the Medication

It is necessary to administer griseofulvin with meals to decrease gastric upset. Greater absorption occurs when the drug is given with a high-fat meal. Storage in a tightly covered container at 15°C to 30°C is required. For treatment of tinea corporis, the duration of therapy is 2 to 4 weeks; for tinea capitis, it is 4 to

---

BOX 22.7   Drug Interactions: Griseofulvin

Drugs That Increase the Effects of Griseofulvin
■ Estrogen
Possible breakthrough bleeding

Drugs That Decrease the Effects of Griseofulvin
■ Barbiturates and rifampin
Decrease griseofulvin drug action

Patient Teaching Guidelines for Griseofulvin

- Take the entire prescription to prevent reemergence of symptoms.
- Avoid exposure to sunlight or extreme artificial light.
- Know that oral contraceptive effects are diminished.

6 weeks but may be extended for 8 to 12 weeks; for tinea pedis, it is 4 to 8 weeks; and for tinea unguium, it is 4 to 6 months.

Assessing for Therapeutic Effects

Tinea infections of skin (e.g., ringworm) improve in 3 to 8 weeks. Onychomycosis of toenails may require a year or more. The most effective therapeutic results are achieved when the patient has two to three consecutive negative cultures.

Assessing for Adverse Effects

The nurse assesses for safety related to CNS depression. He or she also assesses for dermatologic reactions such as rash, photosensitivity, or urticaria. In addition, it is necessary to assess the urine for evidence of protein and check liver enzymes for signs and symptoms of hepatotoxicity. Finally, clinicians have reported hypersensitivity reactions in patients who are allergic to penicillin.

Patient Teaching

Box 22.8 identifies patient teaching guidelines for griseofulvin.

Other Drugs in the Class

Terbinafine (Lamisil) is a broad-spectrum antifungal that inhibits an enzyme needed for synthesis of ergosterol, a structural component of fungal cell membranes. It has fungicidal activity against dermatophytes and has been used mainly for topical treatment of ringworm infections and oral treatment of onychomycosis. Therapeutic effects may not be evident until months after drug therapy is stopped, because of the time required for growth of healthy nail. The drug is metabolized to inactive metabolites and excreted in the urine.

Common adverse effects with oral terbinafine include headache, diarrhea, and abdominal discomfort, and with long-term use for onychomycosis, skin reactions and liver failure may also occur. Hepatotoxicity is uncommon but has occurred in

people with and without preexisting liver disease and has led to liver transplant or death. Terbinafine is not recommended for patients with chronic or active liver disease, and serum ALT and AST should be checked before starting the drug. The FDA has issued a **BLACK BOX WARNING** ◆ regarding the risk of hepatotoxicity.

NCLEX Success

13. **When instructing a patient on the administration of griseofulvin, which of the following is most appropriate?**

    A. Take the medication on an empty stomach.
    B. Take the medication while consuming a high-fat diet.
    C. Take the medication with a full glass of water.
    D. Take the medication 1 hour after a meal.

14. **Which of the following patients should not receive griseofulvin?**

    A. 18-year-old woman who is taking oral contraceptives
    B. 55-year-old man who is taking ibuprofen
    C. 38-year-old man who is taking phenytoin
    D. 35-year-old man who is allergic to penicillin

Pyrimidine Analog

Ⓟ **Flucytosine**, the prototype pyrimidine analog, is an antifungal agent used to treat cryptococcosis, candidiasis, and chromomycosis. This drug is similar in structure to cytosine. As the fungal agent attempts to use flucytosine in place of cytosine to construct DNA, fungal cell division is interrupted.

QSEN Safety Alert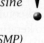

Safety alerts for the administration of flucytosine include the following:

- *The Institute for Safe Medication Practices (ISMP) states that flucytosine causes a significant risk of patient harm when used in error (Up-to-Date, 2011).*
- *Sound-alike/look-alike issues: flucytosine may be confused with fluorouracil, and Ancobon, the trade name for flucytosine, may be confused with Oncovin, the trade name for vincristine (Up-to-Date, 2011).*

TABLE 22.6

DRUGS AT A GLANCE: Flucytosine

Drug	Pregnancy Category	Type of Infection Treated	Routes and Dosage Ranges	
			Adults	**Children**
Ⓟ **Flucytosine** (Ancobon)	C	Serious infections caused by *Candida, Cryptococcus*	50–150 mg/kg PO every 6 h	Neonates: 25–100 mg/kg/d PO in divided doses every 12–24 h Infants and children: 50–150 mg/kg/d PO in divided doses every 6 h

Pharmacokinetics

Flucytosine is absorbed by the GI tract and distributed to the CSF, aqueous humor, joints, peritoneal fluid, and bronchial secretions. It is 3% to 4% protein bound and metabolized by the liver. The serum half-life with normal renal function is 2 to 5 hours. In patients with anuria, the half-life ranges from 30 to 250 hours. In patients with end-stage renal disease, the serum half-life is 75 to 200 hours. Flucytosine is excreted in the urine, greater than 90% unchanged (Up-to-Date, 2011a).

Action

Flucytosine affects the cell membrane of the fungus to cause fungal death. The exact mechanism is unknown (Karch, 2011).

Use

Flucytosine is used as an adjunctive agent with amphotericin B for the treatment of systemic fungal infections caused by *Candida* and *Cryptococcus*. Flucytosine is added to the therapy due to its anticandidal activity and ability to penetrate the CSF and brain tissue (Kauffman, 2011). It can be administered in combination with another antifungal agents for the treatment of chromomycosis and aspergillosis.

Table 22.6 presents specific information about the use of the pyrimidine analog flucytosine, including dosages for adults and children.

Use in Children

Flucytosine should be used in combination with amphotericin B in children because of the development of resistance (Up-to-Date, 2011b).

Use in Older Adults

In the presence of renal insufficiency, the dosage of flucytosine should be reduced.

Use in Patients With Renal Impairment

When administering flucytosine to patients with impaired renal function, a reduced dosage is used at the beginning. For patients with a CrCl of 20 to 40 mL per minute, an individual dose is administered every 12 hours. For those with a CrCl of 10 to 20 mL per minute, an individual dose is administered every 24 hours. For those with a CrCl of less than 10 mL per minute, an individual dose is administered every 24 to 48 hours. The FDA has issued a **BLACK BOX WARNING ◆** to use extreme caution in patients with renal impairment.

Patients receiving hemodialysis should be given 20 to 50 mg/kg following the dialysis treatment.

Use in Patients With Hepatic Impairment

Hepatotoxicity and bone marrow toxicity appear to be related. Hepatic function should be monitored closely and the dose adjusted according to the hepatic function (Semla, Belzer, & Higbee, 2010).

Adverse Effects

Adverse effects of flucytosine include

- GI: nausea, vomiting, diarrhea, duodenal ulcer, and GI bleeding
- Bone marrow depression: after 10 to 26 days of therapy. Bone marrow depression and hepatotoxicity are related to the administration of higher doses.
- Dermatologic: rash, photosensitivity, pruritus, and urticaria

Contraindications

Flucytosine is contraindicated in patients who have a known hypersensitivity to the medication or any component of the formulation. It is also contraindicated in pregnancy and lactation.

Nursing Implications

Preventing Interactions

Certain medications interact with flucytosine, increasing or decreasing its effect (Box 22.9). No documented interactions between flucytosine and herbs exist. When the drug is given with food, the rate of absorption decreases.

Administering the Medication

It is necessary to perform a culture and sensitivity before the initiation of therapy and at intervals throughout the course of treatment.

When treating endocarditis, it is necessary to give amphotericin B in combination with flucytosine. The oral dosage of amphotericin B is 25 to 37.5 mg/kg every 6 hours for at least 6 weeks after valve replacement. When treating meningoencephalitis caused by cryptococcal fungi, the oral dosage of amphotericin B is 25 mg/kg every 6 hours for 2 weeks. If the patient's clinical condition improves, the flucytosine and amphotericin B are discontinued and the patient is started on fluconazole 400 mg per day. The administration of the medication with food decreases the rate but not the extent of drug absorption.

Assessing for Therapeutic Effects

The patient has decreased symptoms of the fungal infection related to endocarditis and meningoencephalitis caused by *Candida* or *Cryptococcus*.

BOX 22.9 Drug Interactions: Flucytosine

Drugs That Increase the Effects of Flucytosine
- Amphotericin B
  Increases serum levels of flucytosine

Drugs That Decrease the Effects of Flucytosine
- *Saccharomyces boulardii* (probiotic; Florastor)
  Flucytosine decreases the levels of Saccharomyces boulardii

BOX 22.10 **Patient Teaching Guidelines for Flucytosine**

- Report any unusual bleeding such as bleeding of the gums or mouth.
- Take the entire course of treatment which could be a minimum of 4 to 6 weeks.

Assessing for Adverse Effects

The nurse assesses for dermatologic reactions such as rash, photosensitivity, pruritus, and urticaria. He or she also assesses baseline hepatic and renal function prior to beginning therapy and at frequent intervals throughout therapy due to the adverse effect of hepatotoxicity and renal toxicity. It is necessary to check leukocyte and differential counts weekly as well as platelet counts to rule out bone marrow depression. In addition, the nurse assesses intake and output to determine any change in pattern or amount of urine output.

Patient Teaching

Box 22.10 identifies patient teaching guidelines for flucytosine.

NCLEX Success

15. A patient with a fungal infection is taking flucytosine. Which of the following medications enhance the effectiveness of flucytosine in the treatment of the fungal infection?

    A. fluconazole
    B. fluorouracil
    C. Oncovin
    D. amphotericin B

The Nursing Process

Assessment

Assess for fungal infections. Specific signs and symptoms vary with location and type of infection.

- Superficial lesions of skin, hair, and nails are usually characterized by pain, burning, and itching. Some lesions are moist; others are dry and scaling. They also may appear inflamed or discolored.
- Candidiasis occurs in warm, moist areas of the body. Skin lesions are likely to occur in perineal and intertriginous areas. They are usually moist, inflamed, pruritic areas with papules, vesicles, and pustules. Oral lesions are white patches that adhere to the buccal mucosa. Vaginal infection causes a cheesy vaginal discharge, burning, and itching. Intestinal infection causes diarrhea. Systemic infection causes chills and fever, myalgia, arthralgia, and prostration.
- Blastomycosis, coccidioidomycosis, and histoplasmosis may be asymptomatic or mimic influenza, pneumonia, or tuberculosis, with cough, fever, malaise, and other pulmonary manifestations. Severe histoplasmosis may also cause

fever, anemia, enlarged spleen and liver, leukopenia, and GI tract ulcers.
- Cryptococcosis may involve the lungs, skin, and other body organs. In patients with AIDS or other immunosuppressant disorders, it often involves the CNS and produces mental status changes, headache, dizziness, and neck stiffness.
- Sporotrichosis involves the skin and lymph nodes. It usually produces small nodules that look like insect bites initially and ulcerations later. Nodules and ulcers also may develop in local lymphatic channels and nodes. The infection can spread to other parts of the body in immunocompromised patients.
- Systemic mycoses produce severe symptoms and may be life-threatening. They are confirmed by recovery of organisms from specimens of body tissues or fluids.

Nursing Diagnoses

- Risk for injury related to fungal infection
- Deficient knowledge: Prevention of fungal infection; accurate drug usage
- Noncompliance related to the need for long-term therapy
- Risk for injury: Adverse drug effects with systemic antifungal drugs

Planning/Goals

The patient will

- Take or receive systemic antifungal drugs as prescribed.
- Apply topical drugs accurately.
- Act to prevent recurrence of fungal infection.
- Avoid preventable adverse effects from systemic drugs.

Nursing Interventions

The nurse will

- Observe standard precautions while assessing or providing care to patients with skin lesions. Superficial infections (e.g., ringworm) are highly contagious and can be spread by sharing towels and hairbrushes. Systemic mycoses are not usually contagious.
- Decrease patient exposure to environmental fungi. For inpatients who are neutropenic or otherwise immunocompromised, do not allow soil-containing plants in the room and request regular cleaning and inspection of air-conditioning systems. Aspergillosis has occurred after inhalation of airborne mold spores from air-conditioning units and hospital water supplies. For outpatients, assist to identify and avoid areas of potential exposure (e.g., soil contaminated by chicken, bird, or bat droppings; areas where buildings are being razed, constructed, or renovated). If exposure is unavoidable, instruct to spray areas with water to minimize airborne spores and to wear disposable clothing and a face mask. For patients at risk for exposure to sporotrichosis (e.g., those who garden or work in plant nurseries), assist to identify risk factors and preventive measures (e.g., wearing gloves and long sleeves).
- Implement measures for obese patients with skin candidiasis. Apply dry padding to intertriginous areas to help prevent irritation and candidal growth.

- Implement measures for patients with oropharyngeal ulcerations. Provide soothing oral hygiene, nonacidic fluids, and soft, bland foods.
- Implement measures for patients with systemic fungal infections. Monitor respiratory, cardiovascular, and neurologic status at least every 8 hours. Provide comfort measures and medications (e.g., analgesics, antihistamines, antipyretics, antiemetics) for patients receiving IV amphotericin B.

Evaluation

- Observe for relief of symptoms for which an antifungal drug was prescribed.
- Interview outpatients regarding their compliance with instructions for using antifungal drugs.
- Interview and observe for adverse drug effects with systemic antifungal agents.

Key Concepts

- Serious fungal infections and infections with nonalbicans *Candida* strains are increasing.
- Patients whose immune systems are suppressed are at high risk for serious fungal infections.
- Fungal infections often require long-term drug therapy.
- Systemic antifungal drugs may cause serious adverse effects. For example, nephrotoxicity is associated with amphotericin B, and hepatotoxicity is associated with azole drugs.
- Liver function should be monitored with all systemic antifungal drugs, and both hepatic and renal function should be monitored with amphotericin B.
- A **BLACK BOX WARNING** ◆ states that amphotericin B be reserved for progressive or potentially fatal infections.
- A **BLACK BOX WARNING** ◆ points out the risks of heart failure and drug interactions associated with itraconazole.
- A **BLACK BOX WARNING** ◆ warns about the risk of hepatotoxicity with terfinadine.
- A **BLACK BOX WARNING** ◆ states that extreme caution be used when administering flucytosine to patients with renal impairment.

Critical Thinking Questions

22-1. A 48-year-old man is admitted to the infectious disease division of an urban hospital. He has been rehabilitating a home he purchased 3 months ago. It is in a revitalized area of the city's oldest residential district. The attic of the home has been a roost for pigeons and bats. The patient has developed influenza-like symptoms, including fever, malaise, cough, and pulmonary congestion. He has an IV line running of D_5 NS at 125 mL per hour. He is to receive IV amphotericin B deoxycholate (Fungizone) 0.25 mg/kg/d for the first day, then 1 mg/kg/d infused over 2 hours. The patient's weight is 70 kg.

- What fungal infection does the nurse suspect the patient has?
- How much amphotericin B does the patient receive the first day he is in the hospital?
- How much amphotericin B does the patient receive for each day of the remainder of his hospital stay?
- What is the action of amphotericin B?
- What adverse effects does the nurse need to assess for?

22-2. A 48-year-old woman has developed cryptococcal meningoencephalitis. She is to receive flucytosine 25 mg/kg per dose with amphotericin B every 6 hours for 2 weeks. She has been taking ibuprofen (Motrin) 600 mg three times per day for the last 15 years. Her CrCl is 10 to 20 mL per minute.

- What is the action of flucytosine?
- Why is it administered with amphotericin B?
- How is the dosage of flucytosine affected due to the CrCl of 10 to 20 mL per minute?

References and Resources

Ashley, E. D. & Perfect, J. R. (2009, September 13). Pharmacology of azoles. *Up-To-Date*. Retrieved February 1, 2011.

Campbell, J. R. & Kauffman, C. A. (2011, January). Treatment of candidemia in children. *Up-To-Date*. Retrieved May 9, 2011.

Karch, A. M. (2011). *2011 Lippincott's nursing drug guide*. Philadelphia, PA: Lippincott Williams & Wilkins.

Kauffman, C. A. (2011, January). Candida infections of the central nervous system. *Up-To-Date. Retrieved May 9, 2011.*

Mahdy, R. A., Nada, W. M., & Wageh, M. M. (2010). Topical amphotericin b and subconjunctival injection of fluconazole (combination therapy) versus topical amphotericin B (monotherapy) in treatment of keratomycosis. *Journal of Ocular Pharmacology and Therapeutics, 26*(10), 281–285.

Moen, M. D., Lyseng-Williamson, K. A., & Scott, L. J. (2009). Liposomal amphotericin B: a review of its use in empirical therapy in febrile neutropenia in the treatment of invasive fungal infections. *Drugs, 69*(3), 361–392.

Nursing 2011 Drug Handbook. (2011). Philadelphia, PA: Lippincott Williams & Wilkins.

Porth, C. M., & Matfin, G. (2009). *Pathophysiology concepts of altered health states*. Philadelphia, PA: Lippincott Williams & Wilkins.

Semla, T. P., Belzer, J. L., & Higbee, M. D. (2010). *Geriatric dosage handbook* (15th ed.). Hudson, OH: Lexi-Comp.

Smeltzer, S. C., Bare, B. G., Hinkle, J. H., & Cheever, K. H. (2010). *Brunner & Suddarth's textbook of medical-surgical nursing* (12th ed.). Philadelphia, PA: Lippincott Williams & Wilkins.

Up-To-Date. (2011a). Flucytosine Drug Information. *Lexi-Comp, Inc.* Retrieved February 25, 2011.

Up-To-Date. (2011b). Flucytosine Pediatric Drug Information. *Lexi-Comp, Inc.* Retrieved February 25, 2011.

Up-To-Date. (2011c). Griseofulvin Drug Information. *Lexi-Comp, Inc.* Retrieved February 25, 2011.

23 Drug Therapy for Parasitic Infections

419

LEARNING OBJECTIVES

After studying this chapter, you should be able to:

1. Describe the etiology, pathophysiology, and clinical manifestations of parasitic infections.

2. Identify the prototype and describe the action, use, adverse effects, contraindications, and nursing implications for the amebicides.

3. Identify the prototype and describe the action, use, adverse effects, contraindications, and nursing implications for the antimalarial drugs.

4. Identify the prototype and describe the action, use, adverse effects, contraindications, and nursing implications for the anthelmintic drugs.

5. Identify the prototype and describe the action, use, adverse effects, contraindications, and nursing implications for the scabicides and pediculicides.

6. Implement the nursing process in the care of the patient being treated with antiparasitic agents.

Clinical Application Case Study

Lacy Michelson, a 35-year-old woman, is a missionary. She has just returned from a 2-year stay in a developing country. She comes to the clinic with severe diarrhea, fever, chills, headache, and myalgia. Ms. Michelson receives a diagnosis of giardiasis and malaria as well as a prescription for chloroquine 500 mg daily by mouth for 3 weeks and metronidazole 250 mg three times a day by mouth for 7 days.

KEY TERMS

Amebicides: drugs that destroy amebae and are classified according to the site of action

Anthelmintics: drugs used for treatment of helminthiasis, which is an infestation of parasitic worms

Larva: developmental form of a parasite

Parasite: organism that lives in or on the host and gains nutrition from the host

Pediculicides: drugs that have the ability to destroy lice

Plasmodium: genus of ameboid parasites that causes malaria

Introduction

A **parasite** is a living organism that survives at the expense of another organism, called the host. Parasitic infestations are common human ailments worldwide. The effects of parasitic diseases on human hosts vary from minor to major and can be life-threatening. Parasitic diseases discussed in this chapter are those caused by protozoa, helminths (worms), scabies, and pediculi (lice).

Overview of Parasitic Infections

Protozoa can infect the digestive tract and other body tissues, and resulting infections include amebiasis, giardiasis, malaria, toxoplasmosis, and trichomoniasis. Helminths can also infect these sites, causing a number of infections. Scabies and pediculi affect the skin.

Etiology and Pathophysiology

Protozoal Infections

Amebiasis

Amebiasis is a common disease in Africa, Asia, and Latin America, but it can occur in any geographic region. In the United States, it is most likely to occur in residents of institutions for the mentally challenged, in men who have sex with men, and in travelers from countries with poor sanitation.

Amebiasis is caused by the pathogenic protozoan *Entamoeba histolytica*, which exists in two forms, cysts and trophozoites. Cysts are inactive; resistant to drugs, heat, cold, and drying; and can survive outside the body for long periods. Transmission occurs by ingestion of food or water contaminated with human feces containing amebic cysts. After people ingest the cysts, some cysts remain intact to be expelled in feces and continue the chain of infection, and some open in the ileum to release amebae, which produce trophozoites. Trophozoites are active amebae that feed, multiply, move about, and produce clinical manifestations of amebiasis.

Trophozoites produce an enzyme that allows them to invade body tissues. They may form erosions and ulcerations in the intestinal wall with resultant diarrhea (this form of the disease is called intestinal amebiasis or amebic dysentery), or they may penetrate blood vessels and be carried to other organs, where they form abscesses. These abscesses are usually found in the liver (hepatic amebiasis) but also may occur in the lungs or brain.

Giardiasis

Giardiasis is a protozoal disease that may affect children more than adults and may cause community outbreaks of diarrhea. It also occurs in people who camp or hike in wilderness areas or who drink untreated well water in areas where sanitation is poor.

Giardiasis is caused by *Giardia lamblia*, a common intestinal parasite. The disease spreads by ingestion of food or water contaminated with human feces containing encysted forms of the organism or by contact with infected people or animals. Infections occur 1 to 2 weeks after ingestion of the cysts. Person-to-person spread often occurs in children in day care centers, in people in institutions, and in men who have sex with men.

Malaria

Malaria is a common cause of morbidity and mortality in many parts of the world, especially in tropical regions. In the United States, malaria is rare and affects travelers or immigrants from malarious areas.

Malaria is caused by four species of protozoa of the genus *Plasmodium*. The human being is the only natural reservoir of these parasites. Only *Anopheles* mosquitoes transmit the malarial plasmodia. *Plasmodium vivax*, *Plasmodium malariae*, and *Plasmodium ovale* cause recurrent malaria by forming reservoirs in the human host. In these types of malaria, signs and symptoms may occur months or years after the initial attack. *Plasmodium falciparum* causes the most life-threatening type of malaria but does not lead to formation of a reservoir. This type of malaria may be cured and prevented from recurring.

The plasmodia protozoa have a life cycle in which one stage of development occurs within the human body. When an uninfected *Anopheles* mosquito bites a person with malaria, it ingests blood that contains gametocytes (male and female forms of the protozoan parasite). These forms produce sporozoites, which are transported to the mosquito's salivary glands. When the mosquito bites the next person, the sporozoites are injected into that person's bloodstream. From the bloodstream, the organisms lodge in the liver and other tissues, where they reproduce and form merozoites. The liver cells containing the parasite eventually rupture and release the merozoites into the bloodstream, where they invade red blood cells. After a period of growth and reproduction, merozoites rupture red blood cells, invade other erythrocytes, form gametocytes, and continue the cycle.

Trichomoniasis

Trichomoniasis is caused by *Trichomonas vaginalis*, a single-cell protozoan. The disease is usually spread by men who have no signs and symptoms of infection who engage in sexual intercourse. Women are more likely than men to become infected.

Helminthiasis

Helminthiasis, or infestation with parasitic worms, often occurs in many parts of the world. It affects about 1 billion people, making it one of the most common of all diseases. Although helminthiasis is quite frequent in topical areas, it is also found in other regions, including countries such as the United States and Canada. Box 23.1 describes the etiology and pathophysiology of some helminthic infections.

Scabies and Pediculosis

Scabies and pediculosis are parasitic infestations of the skin. Scabies is caused by the "itch mite" (*Sarcoptes scabiei*), which burrows into the skin and lays eggs that hatch in 4 to 8 days.

Pediculosis may be caused by one of three types of lice. *Pediculosis capitis* (head lice) is the most common type in the United States. It is diagnosed by finding louse eggs (nits) attached to hair shafts close to the scalp. *Pediculosis corporis* (body lice) is diagnosed by finding lice in clothing, especially in seams. *Pediculosis pubis* (pubic or crab lice) is diagnosed by the presence of nits in the pubic and genital areas. Although

| **BOX 23.1** | **Helminthic Infections** |

Hookworm infections are caused by *N. americanus*, a species found in the United States, and *A. duodenale*, a species found in Europe, the Middle East, and North Africa. Hookworm is spread by ova-containing feces from infected people. Ova develop into larvae when deposited on the soil. Larvae burrow through the skin (e.g., if the person walks on the soil with bare feet), enter blood vessels, and migrate through the lungs to the pharynx, where they are swallowed. Larvae develop into adult hookworms in the small intestine and attach themselves to the intestinal mucosa.

Pinworm infections (enterobiasis), caused by *E. vermicularis*, are the most common parasitic worm infections in the United States. They are highly communicable and often involve schoolchildren and household contacts. Infection occurs from contact with ova in food or water or on bed linens. The female pinworm migrates from the bowel to the perianal area to deposit eggs, especially at night. Touching or scratching the perianal area deposits ova on hands and any objects touched by the contaminated hands.

Roundworm infections (ascariasis), caused by *A. lumbricoides*, are the most common parasitic worm infections in the world. They occur most often in tropical regions but may occur wherever sanitation is poor. The infection is transmitted by ingesting food or water contaminated with feces from infected people. Ova are swallowed and hatch into larvae in the intestine. The larvae penetrate blood vessels and migrate through the lungs before returning to the intestines, where they develop into adult worms.

Tapeworms attach themselves to the intestinal wall and may grow as long as several yards. Segments called *proglottids*, which contain tapeworm eggs, are expelled in feces. Tapeworms are transmitted by ingestion of contaminated, raw, or improperly cooked beef, pork, or fish. Beef and fish tapeworm infections are not usually considered serious illnesses. Pork tapeworm, which is uncommon in the United States, is more serious because it produces larvae that enter the bloodstream and migrate to other body tissues (i.e., muscles, liver, lungs, and brain).

Threadworm infections (strongyloidiasis), caused by *S. stercoralis*, are potentially serious infections. This worm burrows into the mucosa of the small intestine, where the female lays eggs. The eggs hatch into larvae that can penetrate all body tissues.

Trichinosis, a parasitic worm infection caused by *Trichinella spiralis*, occurs worldwide. It is caused by ingestion of inadequately cooked meat, especially pork. Encysted larvae are ingested in infected pork. In the intestine, the larvae excyst, mature, and produce eggs that hatch into new larvae. The larvae enter blood and lymphatic vessels and are transported throughout the body. They penetrate various body tissues (e.g., muscles and brain) and evoke inflammatory reactions. Eventually, the larvae are reencysted or walled off in the tissues and may remain for 10 years or longer.

Whipworm infections (trichuriasis) are caused by *T. trichiura*. Whipworms attach themselves to the wall of the colon.

---

scabies and pediculosis are caused by different parasites, the conditions have two common characteristics:

- They are more likely to occur in areas of poverty, overcrowding, and poor sanitation. However, they may occur in people from any socioeconomic group, in any geographic area.
- They are highly communicable and transmitted by direct contact with an infected person or the person's personal effects (e.g., clothing, combs and hairbrushes, bed linens).

Clinical Manifestations

Amebiasis may be asymptomatic. Affected people may have nausea, vomiting, diarrhea, abdominal cramping, and weakness. If the disease is severe, prolonged, and untreated, these people may experience symptoms from ulcerations of the colon or abscesses of the liver (hepatic amebiasis).

Giardiasis may be asymptomatic or produce diarrhea, abdominal cramping, and distention. If the infection is untreated, it may resolve spontaneously or progress to a chronic disease with anorexia, nausea, malaise, weight loss, and continued diarrhea with large, foul-smelling stools. Deficiencies of vitamin B_{12} and fat-soluble vitamins (see Chapter 33) may occur.

Malaria initially seems to resemble influenza in terms of its symptoms (e.g., headache, myalgia). The characteristic paroxysms of chills, fever, and copious perspiration may not be present at the early stage of disease. During acute malarial attacks, the cycles occur every 36 to 72 hours. Clinical symptoms occur because of

the large parasite burden. The characteristic cycles correspond to the release of merozoites from erythrocytes. Additional manifestations include nausea and vomiting, splenomegaly, hepatomegaly, anemia, leukopenia, thrombocytopenia, and hyperbilirubinemia.

Trichomoniasis affects women and men differently. Women usually have vaginal burning, itching, and foul-smelling yellow–gray, frothy discharge. Men may be asymptomatic or have symptoms of urethritis.

Helminthiasis involves worm infestations; helminths are most often found in the gastrointestinal (GI) tract. However, several types penetrate body tissues or produce **larvae** (developmental forms of parasites) that migrate to the blood, lymph channels, lungs, liver, and other body tissues. Hookworm, roundworm, and threadworm larvae migrate through the lungs and may cause symptoms of pulmonary congestion. The hookworm may cause anemia by feeding on blood from the intestinal mucosa; the fish tapeworm may cause megaloblastic or pernicious anemia by absorbing folic acid and vitamin B_{12}. Large masses of roundworms or tapeworms may cause intestinal obstruction. The major symptom usually associated with pinworms is intense itching in the perianal area (pruritus ani).

Scabies is characterized by burrows produced by the mite that create visible skin lesions, most often between the fingers, around the nails, and on the elbows and wrists. The lesions may also involve skin that is usually covered by clothing; the buttocks, belt line, penis, and skin around the nipples are likely places for mites to burrow.

Pediculosis leads to pruritus, which is usually the major symptom of the disease. This symptom results from an allergic reaction to parasite secretions. In addition to the intense discomfort associated with pruritus, scratching is likely to cause skin excoriation with secondary bacterial infection and formation of vesicles, pustules, and crusts.

NCLEX Success

1. During the second week of July, the emergency department of a local hospital treats 45 residents of one neighborhood for diarrhea. The neighborhood has a swimming pool, and in the past 10 days, 42 of the 45 affected people swam in the pool. What should the emergency department staff consider to be the cause of this outbreak of diarrhea?

   A. *Salmonella*
   B. *Clostridium difficile*
   C. *Pseudomonas*
   D. *Giardia*

2. A woman has received a diagnosis of *Trichomonas vaginalis*. What should the nurse teach the patient?

   A. Avoid yeast-containing foods.
   B. Wear a feminine pad to absorb the drainage.
   C. Use acetic acid douches.
   D. Avoid sexual intercourse.

Clinical Application 23-1

- Ms. Michelson has received a diagnosis of a *Giardia* infection. What vitamin deficiency is she at risk for developing?
- What are the initial symptoms of giardiasis?

Drug Therapy

To combat parasitic diseases, health care professionals use antiparasitic drugs, including amebicides, antimalarials, other antiprotozoal agents, anthelmintics, scabicides, and pediculicides. Table 23.1 lists these drugs.

Amebicides

Amebicides, or drugs used to treat amebiasis, are classified according to their site of action. The prototype Ⓟ **metronidazole** (Flagyl), a synthetic compound with amebicidal and trichomonacidal activity, is effective in both intestinal and extraintestinal amebiasis. Chloroquine is a tissue or extraintestinal amebicide because it acts in the bowel wall, liver, and other tissues. Chloroquine is discussed as an antimalarial agent because it is most commonly used for the prevention and treatment of malaria.

Ⓟ **Tetracycline** and doxycycline, which are antibacterial drugs (see Chapter 18), act against amebae in the intestinal lumen by altering the bacterial flora required for amebic viability. One of these drugs may be used with other amebicides in the treatment of all forms of amebiasis except asymptomatic intestinal amebiasis.

Pharmacokinetics

Metronidazole is 80% absorbed by the GI tract, reaching a peak of action in 1 to 3 hours. The drug is widely distributed to the cerebrospinal fluid, bone, and cerebral and hepatic abscesses. Its half-life is 6 to 8 hours. Metronidazole is metabolized in the liver (30%–60%), with most excreted in the urine (77%) and some in the feces (14%). The drug readily crosses the placenta and enters the breast milk.

TABLE 23.1

Drugs Administered for Parasitic Infections

Drug Class	Prototype	Other Drugs in the Class
Amebicide	Metronidazole (Flagyl)	Iodoquinol (Yodoxin) Nitazoxanide (Alinia) Tinidazole (Tindamax)
Antibacterial	Tetracycline	Doxycycline
Antimalarial	Chloroquine phosphate (Aralen)	Artemether/lumefantrine (Coartem) Atovaquone/proguanil (Malarone) Chloroquine with primaquine Hydroxychloroquine (Plaquenil) Mefloquine (Lariam) Primaquine Quinine
Anthelmintic	Mebendazole (Vermox)	Ivermectin (Stromectol) Pyrantel (Pin-Rid)
Scabicide/pediculicide	Permethrin (Nix, Elimite)	Lindane Malathion (Ovide) Spinosad (Natroba)

TABLE 23.2
DRUGS AT A GLANCE: Amebicides

Drug	Pregnancy Category	Routes and Dosage Ranges	
		Adults	*Children*
Ⓟ **Metronidazole** (Flagyl)	B	Amebiasis: 750 mg PO for 5–10 d (in amebic dysentery combine iodoquinol 650 mg PO 3 times per day for 20 d) Giardiasis: 250 mg PO 3 times per day for 7 d Trichomoniasis: 2 g PO in 1 d or 250 mg PO 3 times per day for 7 d	Amebiasis: 35–50 mg/kg PO in three divided doses for days
Iodoquinol (Yodoxin)	C	Asymptomatic carriers: 650 mg/d PO Symptomatic intestinal amebiasis: 650 mg PO 3 times daily after meals for 20 d; repeat after 2–3 wk if necessary	40 mg/kg/d PO in three divided doses for 20 d (max 2 g/d); repeat after 2–3 wk if necessary
Nitazoxanide (Alinia)	B	*G. lamblia* or *C. parvum*: 500 mg PO every 12 h for 3 d	1–3 y: 100 mg PO every 12 h for 3 d (increase duration to 14 d in HIV-exposed or patients infected with cryptosporidia) 4–11 y: 200 mg PO every 12 h for 3 d (increase duration to 14 d in HIV-exposed or patients infected with cryptosporidia) ≥12 y: refer to adult dosing
Tinidazole (Tindamax)	C	Amebiasis: 2 g/d PO for 3 d Amebiasis, liver abscess: 2 g/d PO for 3–5 d Bacterial vaginosis: 2 g/d PO for 2 d or 1 g/d PO for 5 d Giardiasis: 2 g/d PO for 2 d or 1 g/d PO for 5 d Trichomoniasis: 2 g PO as single dose	Intestinal amebiasis or amebiasis liver abscess (age > 3 y): 50 mg/kg/d PO for 3–5 d (max 2 g/d)

Action and Use

Metronidazole diffuses across the cell membrane of anaerobic and aerobic microorganisms to cause cell death. The biochemical mechanism of action of the drug is unknown. Indications include intestinal amebiasis, amebic liver abscess, trichomoniasis, and bacterial vaginosis. The U.S. Food and Drug Administration (FDA) has not approved this drug or any other amebicide for the prophylaxis of amebiasis. Table 23.2 gives route and dosage information for metronidazole and other amebicides.

Adverse Effects and Contraindications

The adverse effects of metronidazole include headache, dizziness, ataxia, darkening of urine, diarrhea, nausea, vomiting, and an unpleasant metallic taste. Contraindications include a known hypersensitivity to the drug. Pregnancy is also a contraindication.

Nursing Implications

Preventing Interactions

Concomitant use of metronidazole with barbiturates increases the metabolism of the antiamebic drug, thus decreasing its therapeutic effect. Administration of metronidazole with anticoagulants (e.g., warfarin) increases bleeding tendencies due to decreased vitamin K metabolism. Also, disulfiram and alcohol combined with metronidazole may lead to a disulfiram-like reaction, with tachycardia, nausea, flushing, and vomiting. No herbal interactions with metronidazole reportedly occur.

Administering the Drug

Patients may take metronidazole with food to improve medication adsorption. It is important not to crush extended-release preparations. If the patient is unable to swallow regular metronidazole pills, it may be necessary to crush them.

Assessing for Therapeutic Effects

The nurse assesses patients with intestinal amebiasis for decreased abdominal pain and diarrhea. It is necessary to assess stool specimens for amebic cysts and trophozoites periodically for 6 months. Also, the nurse checks the feces for increase in form that is indicative of diminished diarrhea stools and improved hydration.

It is important to assess women with trichomoniasis for decreased vaginal drainage and odor.

Assessing for Adverse Effects

It is necessary to assess for headache; diminished muscular coordination; GI upset, including metallic taste; and hypersensitivity reactions such as rash and bronchospasm.

BOX 23.2 — Patient Teaching Guidelines for Antiparasitic Drugs

General Considerations

▪ Use measures to prevent parasitic infection or reinfection:

- ▪ Support public health measures to maintain a clean environment (i.e., sanitary sewers, clean water, regulation of food-handling establishments and food-handling personnel).
- ▪ When traveling to wilderness areas or to tropical or developing countries, check with the local health department about precautions needed to avoid parasitic infections.
- ▪ Practice good hand hygiene and other personal hygienic practices.
- ▪ When a family member or other close contact contracts a parasitic infection, be sure to complete appropriate treatment and follow-up care.
- ▪ Avoid ingesting raw fish and undercooked meat.
- ▪ With vaginal infections, avoid sexual intercourse or use a condom.

Self- or Caregiver Administration

▪ Use antiparasitic drugs as prescribed; their effectiveness depends on accurate use. Take the full course of the medication. For malaria prophylaxis, for example, take chloroquine at the same time each week, and set up a calendar with time and date of administration.

▪ Take atovaquone/proguanil, chloroquine and related drugs, iodoquinol, oral metronidazole, and tinidazole with or after meals. Food increases absorption of atovaquone and decreases gastrointestinal irritation with the other drugs.

▪ Avoid alcoholic beverages while taking metronidazole or tinidazole and for 3 days after the drugs are stopped. Flushing, headache, nausea, sweating, and vomiting may occur if alcohol is ingested.

▪ Metronidazole has an unpleasant metallic taste. Taking this drug will make your urine dark in color. Do not be alarmed.

▪ Have an ophthalmic examination at the start of chloroquine use and every 3 months during drug therapy. It is important to have complete blood count studies as ordered.

▪ Take or give most anthelmintics without regard to mealtimes or food ingestion. Mebendazole tablets should be chewed or crushed and mixed with food.

▪ Have a culture for ova and parasites 3 weeks after initial mebendazole use. Eat frequent small meals and maintain excellent hydration if diarrhea develops. Report fever and severe diarrhea.

▪ With a pinworm infection, adhere to the following instructions:

- ▪ Disinfect the toilet facilities after use.
- ▪ Launder bed linens, nightclothes, undergarments, and towels every day.
- ▪ Family members should also be treated for pinworms due to the fact they are highly contagious.
- ▪ Follow strict handwashing and excellent hygienic practices.

▪ Use pediculicides and scabicides as directed on the label or product insert. Instructions vary among preparations. Use gloves prior to applying permethrin cream rinse, cream, or lotion.

▪ With pediculosis and scabies, wash bed linens, towels, undergarments, and clothes daily.

▪ Inspect the head, genital area, and other parts of the body for lice and scabies to determine if they have been killed.

▪ With the administration of permethrin, report stinging, tingling, skin numbness, rash, itching, and rash to the prescriber.

Patient Teaching

Box 23.2 identifies patient teaching guidelines for antiparasitic drugs, including metronidazole.

Other Drugs in the Class

Iodoquinol (Yodoxin) is an iodine compound that acts against active amebae (trophozoites) in the intestinal lumen. This drug may be used alone in asymptomatic intestinal amebiasis to decrease the number of amebic cysts passed in the feces. When given for symptomatic intestinal amebiasis (e.g., amebic dysentery), it is usually given with other amebicides in concurrent or alternating courses. Iodoquinol is ineffective in amebic hepatitis and abscess formation. The drug is contraindicated in iodine allergy and liver disease.

Nitazoxanide (Alinia) is a less commonly used drug. In *Cryptosporidium parvum* infection, it inhibits the growth of sporozoites and oocysts. In G. *lamblia* infection, it inhibits the growth of trophozoites. Nitazoxanide is administered with food for the treatment of diarrhea.

Tinidazole (Tindamax), a chemical relative of metronidazole, has FDA approval for the treatment of amebiasis, giardiasis, and trichomoniasis. Cytochrome P450 3A4 enzymes in the liver metabolize the drug, and caution is warranted with use in people with impaired liver function. The most common adverse effects are a bitter metallic taste and nausea.

NCLEX Success

3. A man with intestinal amebiasis has received a prescription for metronidazole (Flagyl). He later develops a cough and takes a prescription cough syrup. What adverse effect will he experience?

   A. edema
   B. bronchospasm
   C. flushing
   D. bradycardia

4. What assessment should the nurse implement when caring for a patient who is receiving metronidazole (Flagyl) for intestinal amebiasis?

   A. diminished diarrhea
   B. hypomagnesemia
   C. increased temperature
   D. hyperkalemia

Clinical Application 23-2

- What is the action of metronidazole (Flagyl)?
- What patient teaching should the nurse provide to Ms. Michelson?

Antimalarials

Antimalarials act at different stages in the life cycle of plasmodial parasites. Some drugs such as ℗ **chloroquine phosphate** (Aralen) are effective against erythrocytic forms and are therefore useful in preventing or treating acute attacks of malaria. Although these drugs do not prevent infection with the parasite, they do prevent clinical manifestations. Other drugs such as primaquine act against exoerythrocytic or tissue forms of the parasite to prevent initial infection and recurrent attacks or to cure some types of malaria. Combination drug therapy, administered concomitantly or consecutively, is common with antimalarial drugs.

EVIDENCE-BASED PRACTICE

Disparities Exist in the Availability of Outpatient Malaria Treatment in Maryland, USA

by BEAR, K. A., HIGGINSON, A. L., AND HICKEY, P. W.

Journal of Travel Medicine
2010, 17(4), 228–232

This study examined the malaria cases in the Washington, DC, region. It determined that pharmacies in high-income postal zip codes were more likely to maintain a stock of first-line medications to prevent malaria. Pharmacies in areas with moderate-to-low income residents were less likely to stock antimalarial medications. These areas had a higher incidence of people from Western Africa who would go back to visit family and friends, thus placing them at increased risk for the development of malaria.

IMPLICATIONS FOR NURSING PRACTICE: The public health nurses of regions with an increased population from West Africa should assess the availability of antimalarial agents in the prevention of malaria cases.

Pharmacokinetics

Chloroquine is rapidly absorbed by the GI tract, and the drug is widely distributed and retained throughout the body tissues such as the central nervous system (CNS), eyes, cardiopulmonary system, liver, kidneys, and spleen. The peak of action is 1 to 2 hours with a serum half-life of 3 to 5 days. It is 55% protein bound and partially metabolized by the liver. Chloroquine is excreted by the kidneys. Small amounts of the drug are present in the urine for months following the discontinuation of drug therapy.

Action and Use

Chloroquine inhibits DNA and RNA polymerase to interfere with the metabolism and hemoglobin used by parasites. The drug also inhibits prostaglandin effects while concentrating within the parasitic acid vesicles. It raises the internal pH to inhibit parasitic growth. Uses of chloroquine include the suppression and chemoprophylaxis of malaria. Health care providers also use it for the treatment of acute malaria caused by *P. malariae*, *P. ovale*, and *P. falciparum*, as well as for extraintestinal amebiasis. Table 23.3 gives route and dosage information for chloroquine and the other antimalarial drugs.

Adverse Effects

Adverse effects of chloroquine are usually mild because small doses are used for prophylaxis; administration of the larger doses required for treatment of acute attacks occurs only for short periods. CNS changes include visual disturbances with retinal damage and difficulty to focus. Cardiovascular adverse effects include electrocardiogram changes with prolonged QRS intervals and hypotension. Other significant adverse effects are nausea, vomiting, diarrhea, loss of appetite, skin rash, pruritus, and hair loss. Reportedly, ototoxicity and muscle weakness may also occur.

Contraindications

Contraindications to chloroquine include a known hypersensitivity to 4-aminoquinolone compounds and the presence of retinal and visual field changes. Caution is necessary in porphyria, psoriasis, retinal disease, deficiency of glucose-6-phosphate dehydrogenase, alcoholism, pregnancy, and lactation.

Nursing Implications

Preventing Interactions

Some medications interact with chloroquine, increasing or decreasing its effects (Box 23.3). When the drug is combined with alcohol, the risk of GI distress increases.

Administering the Medication

For malaria prophylaxis, it is necessary to take chloroquine on the same day each week. The nurse may set up a calendar to assist with adherence. For malaria treatment, it is necessary to take the drug as prescribed (perhaps at the same time each day). It is appropriate to take chloroquine with food to reduce

TABLE 23.3

DRUGS AT A GLANCE: Antimalarials

Drug	Pregnancy Category	Routes and Dosage Ranges	
		Adults	*Children*
Ⓟ **Chloroquine phosphate** (Aralen)	C	Prophylaxis: 500 mg/wk PO on the same day each week; start 1–2 wk prior to exposure; continue while in endemic area and for 4 wk after leaving the endemic area Treatment: 1 g PO, followed by 500 mg 6, 24, and 48 h after first dose Extraintestinal amebiasis: 1 g/d PO for 2 d followed by 500 mg/d for at least 2–3 wk	Prophylaxis: 8.3 mg/kg/wk PO on the same day each week (do not exceed 500 mg/dose); begin 1–2 wk prior to exposure; continue while in the endemic area and for 4 wk after leaving endemic area Treatment: 16.6 mg/kg PO (max 1000 mg), followed by 8.3 mg/kg (max 500 mg) 6, 24, and 48 h after first dose
Artemether/ lumefantrine	C	Uncomplicated disease: 25–35 kg, 3 tablets PO at hour 0 and hour 8 the first day, then 3 tablets twice daily on day 2 and day 3 (total of 18 tablets per treatment course) ≥35 kg, 4 tablets PO at hour 0 and hour 8 the first day, then 4 tablets twice daily on day 2 and day 3 (total of 24 tablets per treatment course)	Uncomplicated disease: 5–15 kg, 1 tablet PO at hour 0 and hour 8 the first day, then 1 tablets twice daily on day 2 and day 3 (total of 6 tablets per treatment course) 15–25 kg, 2 tablets PO at hour 0 and hour 8 the first day, then 2 tablets twice daily on day 2 and day 3 (total of 12 tablets per treatment course) 25–35 kg, 3 tablets at hour 0 and hour 8 on the first day, then 3 tablets twice daily on day 2 and day 3 (total of 18 tablets per treatment course) ≥35 kg, 4 tablets PO at hour 0 and hour 8 the first day, then 4 tablets twice daily on day 2 and day 3 (total of 24 tablets per treatment course)
Atovaquone/proguanil (Malarone)	C	Prophylaxis: 250 mg/100 mg PO once daily; start 1–2 d prior to entering malaria-endemic area, continue throughout the stay and for 7 d after returning Acute treatment: 1 g/400 mg PO as a single dose, once daily for 3 consecutive days	Prophylaxis (begin 1–2 d prior to entering a malaria-endemic area; continue throughout the stay and for 7 d after returning; take as a single dose, once daily): 5–8 kg, 31–25 mg/12.5 mg 9–10 kg, 46.8 mg/18.75 mg 11–20 kg, 62.5 mg/25 mg 21–30 kg, 125 mg/50 mg 31–40 kg, 187.5 mg/75 mg >40 kg, 250 mg/100 mg PO Acute treatment: 5–8 kg, 125 mg/50 mg 9–10 kg, 187.5 mg/75 mg 11–20 kg, 250 mg/100 mg 21–30 kg, 500 mg/200 mg 31–40 kg, 750 mg/300 mg >40 kg, 1 g/400 mg PO as a single dose once daily for 3 consecutive days
Chloroquine with primaquine		Prophylaxis: 1 tablet PO weekly for 2 wk before entering and 8 wk after leaving endemic area	Prophylaxis: Same as adults for weight above 45 kg; 1/2 tablet for weight of 25–45 kg For younger children, a suspension is prepared (e.g., 40 mg of chloroquine and 6 mg of primaquine in 5 mL); given weekly for 2 wk before entering and 8 wk after leaving malarious areas; dosages are 2.5 mL for weight of 5–7 kg; 5 mL for 8–11 kg; 7.5 mL for 12–15 kg; 10 mL for 16–20 kg; and 12.5 mL for 21–24 kg

TABLE 23.3

DRUGS AT A GLANCE: Antimalarials (Continued)

Drug	Pregnancy Category	Routes and Dosage Ranges	
		Adults	*Children*
Hydroxychloroquine (Plaquenil)		Prophylaxis: 5 mg/kg PO, not to exceed 310 mg, once weekly for 2 wk before entering and 8 wk after leaving endemic area Treatment of acute disease: 620 mg PO initially, then 310 mg 6 h later, and 310 mg/d for 2 d (total of four doses)	Prophylaxis: 5 mg/kg PO once weekly for 2 wk before entering and 8 wk after leaving endemic area Treatment of acute disease: 10 mg/kg PO initially, then 5 mg/kg 6 h later, and 5 mg/kg/d PO for two doses (total of four doses)
Mefloquine (Lariam)		Prophylaxis: 250 mg PO 1 wk before travel, then 250 mg weekly during travel and for 4 wk after leaving a endemic area Treatment: 1250 mg (5 tablets) as a single dose	Prophylaxis: 1/4 tablet PO for 15–19 kg weight; 1/2 tablet for 20–30 kg; 3/4 tablet for 31–45 kg; and 1 tablet for above 45 kg, according to the schedule for adults
Primaquine		26.3 mg (15 mg of primaquine base) PO daily for 14 d, beginning immediately after leaving a malarious area, or 79 mg (45 mg of base) once weekly for 8 wk; to prevent relapse, the same dose is given with chloroquine or a related drug daily for 14 d	0.3 mg of base/kg/d PO for 14 d, according to the schedule for adults, or 0.9 mg of base/kg/wk for 8 wk
Quinine		650 mg PO every 8 h for 10–14 d	25 mg/kg/d PO in divided doses every 8 h for 10–14 d

gastric distress. When administering chloroquine to children, it is essential to double-check the dosage because young people are especially sensitive to the 4-aminoquinoline compounds that the drug contains.

Assessing for Therapeutic and Adverse Effects

The nurse assesses for a decrease in signs and symptoms of malaria. Fever and chills usually subside in 24 to 48 hours. Blood smears for plasmodia are negative in 24 to 72 hours.

Also, the nurse assesses for nausea, vomiting, diarrhea, pruritus, rash, headache, and visual changes.

Patient Teaching

Box 23.2 identifies patient teaching guidelines for antiparasitic drugs, including chloroquine phosphate.

BOX 23.3   Drug Interactions: Chloroquine

Drugs That Increase the Effects of Chloroquine
■ Cimetidine
May increase the plasma concentration

Drugs That Decrease the Effects of Chloroquine
■ Magnesium trisilicate
May reduce bioavailability
■ Vitamin C
Increases urinary excretion

Other Drugs in the Class

Artemether/lumefantrine (Coartem) is a combination product administered for the treatment of uncomplicated malaria. People may take Coartem with a full meal for optimal absorption. It may be necessary (1) to crush the tablets and mix them in 5 to 10 mL of water and (2) to rinse the container and ingest the contents. If vomiting occurs, it is important to repeat the dosage in 2 hours. People with known QT prolongation should avoid taking Coartem. If people take this combination drug with grapefruit juice, the potential for QT prolongation is enhanced.

Atovaquone/proguanil (Malarone) is a combination product with adult and pediatric formulations. The constituent drugs inhibit different pathways in plasmodial reproduction. Uses include the prevention and treatment of malaria, including chloroquine-resistant strains.

Chloroquine with primaquine is a mixture available in tablets containing chloroquine phosphate 500 mg (equivalent to 300 mg of chloroquine base) and primaquine phosphate 79 mg (equivalent to 45 mg of primaquine base). This combination is effective for prophylaxis of malaria and may be more acceptable to patients. It also may be more convenient for use in children because no pediatric formulation of primaquine is available.

Hydroxychloroquine (Plaquenil) is a derivative of chloroquine with essentially the same actions and uses with fewer adverse effects. Other uses of this drug include treatment of rheumatoid arthritis and lupus erythematosus.

Mefloquine (Lariam) is used to prevent *P. falciparum* malaria, including chloroquine-resistant strains, and to treat acute malaria caused by *P. falciparum* or *P. vivax*.

Primaquine is an antimalarial drug used to prevent the initial occurrence of malaria; to prevent recurrent attacks of malaria caused by *P. vivax, P. malariae,* and *P. ovale*; and to achieve "radical cure" (i.e., eradicating the tissue forms of the plasmodium and preventing survival of the blood forms) of these three types of malaria. It is especially effective in *P. vivax* malaria. When used to prevent initial occurrence of malaria (causal prophylaxis), people should take primaquine concurrently with a suppressive agent (e.g., chloroquine, hydroxychloroquine) after they have returned from a malarious area. Primaquine is not effective for treatment of acute attacks of malaria.

Quinine was the primary antimalarial drug for many years, but synthetic agents that cause fewer adverse reactions have largely replaced it. However, this drug may still be useful in the treatment of chloroquine-resistant *P. falciparum* malaria. Also, it relaxes skeletal muscles and may be effective in the prevention and treatment of nocturnal leg cramps.

NCLEX Success

5. **A nurse who is scheduled to work at a hospital in Haiti in 2 weeks comes to the clinic for antimalarial medication. A health care provider should prescribe which of the following drugs prior to the nurse's trip?**

   A. primaquine
   B. metronidazole (Flagyl)
   C. amitriptyline (Elavil)
   D. clindamycin

6. **Which of the following aspects of teaching is most important to provide to a patient who is taking chloroquine phosphate (Aralen)?**

   A. Take chloroquine with vitamin C.
   B. Have frequent ophthalmologic examinations.
   C. Administer antacids to reduce gastric distress.
   D. Take chloroquine on an empty stomach.

Clinical Application 23-3

- When providing patient teaching to Ms. Michelson regarding the chloroquine, what is most important that the nurse impart?

Anthelmintics

Health care providers use **anthelmintics** used for the treatment of helminthiasis. Most of these drugs act locally to kill or cause expulsion of parasitic worms from the intestines. Some of these medications act systemically against parasites that have penetrated various body tissues. The goal of anthelmintic therapy may be to eradicate the parasite completely or

to decrease the magnitude of infestation ("worm burden"). **Mebendazole** (Vermox) is the prototype of this class of medications.

Pharmacokinetics

Mebendazole is administered orally with a slow onset of action. The drug reaches peak of action in 2 to 4 hours. Approximately 2% to 10% is absorbed. It reaches its highest concentrations in the liver and muscle. Mebendazole is 95% protein bound and has an elimination half-life of 3 to 6 hours. The drug is metabolized extensively by the liver. It is excreted mostly in the feces and minimally in the urine.

Action

Mebendazole blocks glucose uptake by susceptible helminths. The drug depletes glycogen stores that the worms need for survival and reproduction, resulting in their death.

Use

Uses for mebendazole include the treatment of infections with *Enterobius vermicularis* (pinworm), *Trichuris trichiura* (whipworm), and *Ascaris lumbricoides* (roundworm), as well as *Ancylostoma duodenale* and *Necator americanus* (hookworms). Unlabeled uses of this drug are infections with *Ancylostoma caninum* (eosinophilic enterocolitis), *Capillaria philippinensis* (capillariasis), *G. lamblia* (giardiasis), *Mansonella perstans* (filariasis), and visceral larva migrans (toxocariasis). Table 23.4 presents route and dosage information for mebendazole and the other anthelmintics.

Adverse Effects

Dizziness, drowsiness, headaches, seizures, transient abdominal pain, diarrhea, nausea, and vomiting may occur with mebendazole. Hematologic effects such as agranulocytosis, anemia, leukopenia, and neutropenia sometimes take place. The hepatic enzymes alanine aminotransferase (ALT) and aspartate aminotransferase (AST) may be increased. Genitourinary effects include casts in the urine, glomerulonephritis, and hematuria. Finally, hypersensitivity reactions have reportedly occurred.

Contraindications

Contraindications to mebendazole include known hypersensitivity to the drug. It is also embryotoxic and teratogenic, particularly in the first trimester of pregnancy. Caution is necessary with lactation.

Nursing Implications
Preventing Interactions

Certain medications interact with mebendazole, increasing or decreasing its effects (Box 23.4). Serum levels of mebendazole may be increased with food.

TABLE 23.4

DRUGS AT A GLANCE: Anthelmintics

Drug	Pregnancy Category	Routes and Dosage Ranges	
		Adults	*Children*
Mebendazole (Vermox)	C	Trichuriasis, ascariasis, and hookworm: 1 tablet PO morning and evening on 3 consecutive days Enterobiasis: 1 tablet PO once; repeat treatment if not cured in 3 wk	Children 2 y of age and older, same as adults Safety and efficacy has not been established younger than 2 y of age
Ivermectin (Stromectol)	C	Strongyloidiasis: PO 200 mcg/kg as a single dose	5 y and older, 150 mcg/kg PO as a single dose
Pyrantel (Pin-Rid)	C	Ascariasis and enterobiasis: 11 mg/kg PO (max 1 g) as a single dose Hookworm: 11 mg/kg PO (max 1 g) daily for 3 consecutive days; course of therapy may be repeated in 1 mo, if necessary	Children 2 y of age and older, same as adults Safety and efficacy has not been established younger than 2 y of age

Administering the Medication

Administering mebendazole involves chewing and swallowing the tablets or crushing them and mixing them with food, whether solid or liquid. Taking the drug with food increases its serum levels.

Assessing for Adverse Effects

The nurse assesses for CNS depression, dizziness, and seizure activity. He or she also assesses for GI disorders, including nausea, vomiting, diarrhea, and alterations in fluid volume. In addition, it is important to assess the hepatic enzymes AST and ALT for elevations leading to hepatic failure. Finally, the nurse assesses for blood in the urine and glomerulonephritis. Assessing for rash and alterations in pulmonary status related to hypersensitivity to the medication is also necessary.

Assessing for Therapeutic Effects

The nurse obtains a stool sample for culture for ova and parasites after 3 weeks of drug administration. A negative stool culture is the optimum outcome of drug therapy. There is a complete eradication of the parasite, and any "worm burden" is now nonexistent.

BOX 23.4 | Drug Interactions: Mebendazole

Drugs That Increase the Effects of Mebendazole

■ Metronidazole
Enhances the toxic effect of mebendazole and the development of adverse effects

Drugs That Decrease the Effects of Mebendazole

■ Aminoquinolines (antimalarials), carbamazepine, phenytoin
Decrease the serum concentration

Patient Teaching

Box 23.2 identifies patient teaching guidelines for antiparasitic drugs, including mebendazole.

Other Drugs in the Class

Ivermectin (Stromectol), which is used for numerous parasitic infections, is most active against strongyloidiasis (caused by the roundworm *Strongyloides stercoralis*). Another use for this drug is in the oral treatment of resistant lice infestations. It has relatively few adverse effects but may cause some nausea and vomiting.

Pyrantel (Pin-Rid) is effective in infestations of roundworms, pinworms, and hookworms. The drug acts locally to paralyze worms in the intestinal tract. It is poorly absorbed from the GI tract, and most of an administered dose may be recovered in feces. Pyrantel is contraindicated in pregnancy.

NCLEX Success

7. A 4-year-old child receives a diagnosis of enterobiasis, an infection with *Enterobius vermicularis*. What is *E. vermicularis*?

   A. pinworm
   B. hookworm
   C. whipworm
   D. roundworm

8. A patient who has enterobiasis, which is caused by *Enterobius vermicularis*, is receiving treatment with mebenadazole. Which of the following agents decreases the serum concentration of mebendazole?

   A. alcohol
   B. phenytoin (Dilantin)
   C. ampicillin
   D. metronidazole (Flagyl)

TABLE 23.5

DRUGS AT A GLANCE: Scabicides and Pediculicides

Drug	Pregnancy Category	Routes and Dosage Ranges	
		Adults	*Children*
℗ **Permethrin** (Nix, Elimite)	B	Head lice: apply large volume of cream rinse to clean, damp hair to saturate hair and scalp; apply behind ears and at base of neck; leave on for 10 min before rinsing with water; repeat in 1 wk if lice and nits are present Scabies: apply cream head to toe; leave on 8–14 h before washing off with water; reapply in 1 wk if mites appear.	Same as adults
Lindane	B	Head lice: rub cream or lotion into affected area, leave in place for 12 h, then wash or shampoo (rub into the affected area for 4 min and rinse thoroughly) Scabies: apply to entire skin except the face, neck, and scalp; leave in place for 24 h; then remove by shower.	Same as adults
Malathion (Ovide)	B	Head lice: apply to hair, rub in well to wet hair, then dry hair without covering or using a hair dryer; after 8–12 h, shampoo, rinse, and comb hair with a fine-toothed comb to remove dead lice and eggs; if necessary, repeat in 7–9 d.	Same as adults
Spinosad (Natroba)	B	Apply to dry scalp and rub in gently then apply to hair; leave on for 10 min, then rinse with warm water and shampoo; repeat in 7 d if the first treatment is ineffective.	≥6 mo to <4 y: apply to dry scalp; may repeat in 7 d if needed

Scabicides and Pediculicides

Topical and oral medications are administered for the treatment scabies as well as for head or pubic lice. ℗ **Permethrin** (Nix, Elimite), a **pediculicide**, is the prototype for the treatment of lice and scabies, caused by *P. capitis* and *S. scabei*, respectively.

Pharmacokinetics and Action

After topical administration of permethrin, 2% is absorbed through the skin and metabolized in the liver by ester hydrolysis to inactive metabolites. The drug is then excreted in the urine. It inhibits the influx of sodium ions through the nerve cell membranes channels of the parasites to delay the repolarization, resulting in the paralysis or death of the lice or scabies.

Use

A single application of permethrin is useful in the treatment of infestation with *P. capitis* or *S. scabei*. Prophylactic applications are effective during epidemics of lice. Table 23.5 presents route and dosage information for permethrin and related drugs.

Adverse Effects and Contraindications

The most common adverse effects of permethrin are pruritus, rash of the scalp, erythema, burning, tingling, numbness or pain of the scalp, and edema. Contraindications include a known hypersensitivity to chrysanthemums, pyrethroid, or pyrethrin, as well as age less than 2 months.

Administering the Medication

QSEN Safety Alert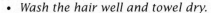

When administering permethrin for head lice, it is necessary to wear gloves and follow these directions:

- *Wash the hair well and towel dry.*
- *Apply a large amount of cream rinse to saturate the hair and scalp as well as behind the ears and at the base of the neck.*
- *Leave the medication on for 10 minutes before rinsing it with water.*

Administration should occur again in 1 week if lice and nits are present. The second time, the hair is dry and the drug stays on for 8 to 14 hours (e.g., overnight).

When administering permethrin for scabies, it is necessary to follow these directions:

- Apply the cream from head to toe.
- Leave it on for 8 to 14 hours, and then wash it off with water.

Assessing for Therapeutic and Adverse effects

The nurse assesses for lice or scabies. It is also necessary to assess the areas of application of permethrin for inflammation, pruritus, erythema, and rash. The nurse asks the patient if there is any burning, stinging, tingling, scalp numbness or pain, or edema.

Patient Teaching

Box 23.2 identifies patient teaching guidelines for antiparasitic drugs, including permethrin.

Other Drugs in the Class

Lindane is a second-line drug for scabies and pediculosis. It may be useful in people who have hypersensitivity reactions or resistance to treatment with permethrin. Administration is topical, and absorption through intact skin is substantial. CNS toxicity has been reported with excessive use, especially in infants and children. The drug is available in a 1% concentration as a cream, lotion, and shampoo.

Malathion (Ovide) is a pediculicide used in the treatment of resistant head lice infestations, and pyrethrin preparations are available over-the-counter for treatment of pediculosis. These preparations require two applications approximately 10 days apart.

Spinosad (Natroba), a pediculicidal and ovicidal drug, is useful for the treatment of head lice. It causes insect paralysis and death due to excitation of the CNS of the parasite. Topical administration results in no absorption.

NCLEX Success

9. **A prescriber has ordered permethrin for an elderly patient who has received a diagnosis of scabies. What is the action of permethrin?**

   A. It inhibits the influx of sodium through the nerve cell membranes to paralyze the parasite.
   B. It inhibits the influx of calcium through the nerve cell membranes to paralyze the parasite.
   C. It inhibits the influx of potassium through the nerve cell membranes to paralyze the parasite.
   D. It inhibits the influx of chloride through the nerve cell membranes to paralyze the parasite.

10. **When applying spinosad (Natroba) to a dry scalp for treatment of head lice, how long should it be left on?**

    A. 5 minutes
    B. 10 minutes
    C. 20 minutes
    D. 30 minutes

The Nursing Process

Assessment

- Assess for exposure to parasites. Although exposure is influenced by many variables (e.g., geographic location, personal hygiene, environmental sanitation), some useful questions may include the following:
  - Does the person live in an institution, an area of poor sanitation, an underdeveloped country, a tropical region, or an area of overcrowded housing? These conditions predispose to parasitic infestations with lice, scabies, protozoa, and worms.
  - Are parasitic diseases present in the person's environment? For example, head lice, scabies, and pinworm infestations often affect school-age children and their families.
  - Has the person recently traveled (within the previous 1–3 weeks) in malarious regions? If so, were prophylactic measures used appropriately?
  - With vaginal trichomoniasis, assess in relation to sexual activity. The disease is spread by sexual intercourse, and sexual partners need simultaneous treatment to prevent reinfection.
  - With pubic (crab) lice, assess sexual activity. Lice may be transmitted by sexual and other close contact and by contact with infested bed linens.
- Assess for signs and symptoms. These vary greatly, depending on the type and extent of parasitic infestation.
  - Amebiasis. Affected people may complain of GI symptoms such as nausea, vomiting, and diarrhea. Alternatively, if the disease is severe, prolonged, and untreated, ulceration of the colon or abscesses of the liver (amebic hepatitis) may result. Diagnosis involves identifying cysts or trophozoites of *E. histolytica* in stool specimens.
  - Malaria. Initial symptoms resemble those of influenza (e.g., headache, myalgia). During acute malarial attacks, the cycles with the characteristic chills and fever occur every 36 to 72 hours. Diagnosis involves identifying the plasmodial parasite in peripheral blood smears (by microscopic examination).
  - Trichomoniasis. Women usually have vaginal burning, itching, and yellowish discharge, and men may be asymptomatic or appear to have urethritis. Diagnosis involves finding *T. vaginalis* organisms in a wet smear of vaginal exudate, semen, prostatic fluid, or urinary sediment (by microscopic examination). Cultures may be necessary.
  - Helminthiasis. Light infestations may be asymptomatic. Heavy infestations produce symptoms according to the particular parasitic worm. Diagnosis of helminthiasis involves microscopic identification of parasites or ova in stool specimens. Diagnosis of pinworm infestation involves identifying ova on anal swabs, obtained by touching the sticky side of cellophane tape to the anal area. (Early morning swabs are best because the female pinworm deposits eggs during sleeping hours.)
  - Scabies and pediculosis. Pruritus is the primary symptom. Secondary symptoms result from scratching and often include skin excoriation and infection (i.e., vesicles, pustules, and crusts). Diagnosis of pediculosis involves visual identification of lice or ova (nits) on the patient's body or clothing.

Nursing Diagnoses

- Deficient knowledge: management of disease process and prevention of recurrence
- Deficient knowledge: accurate drug administration
- Imbalanced nutrition: less than body requirements related to parasitic disease or drug therapy
- Self-esteem disturbance related to a medical diagnosis of parasitic infestation
- Noncompliance related to need for hygienic and other measures to prevent and treat parasitic infestations

Planning/Goals

The patient will

- Experience relief of symptoms for which antiparasitic drugs were taken
- Self-administer drugs accurately
- Avoid preventable adverse effects
- Act to prevent recurrent infestation
- Keep appointments for follow-up care

Nursing Interventions

The nurse will

- Use environmental health measures to avoid exposure to or prevent transmission of parasitic diseases such as
  - Sanitary sewers to prevent deposition of feces on surface soil and the resultant exposure to helminths
  - Monitoring of community water supplies, food-handling establishments, and food-handling personnel
  - Follow-up examination and possibly treatment of household and other close contacts of people with helminthiasis, amebiasis, trichomoniasis, scabies, and pediculosis
  - Mosquito control in malarious areas and prophylactic drug therapy for travelers to malarious areas. In addition, teach travelers to decrease exposure to mosquito bites (e.g., wear long-sleeved, dark clothing; use an effective insect repellent such as DEET; sleep in well-screened rooms or under mosquito netting). These measures are especially needed at dusk and dawn, the maximal feeding times for mosquitoes.
- Use personal and other health measures to avoid exposure or prevent transmission of parasitic disease, such as
  - Maintain personal hygiene (i.e., regular bathing and shampooing, performing hand hygiene before eating or handling food and after defecation or urination).

- Avoid raw fish and undercooked meat. This is especially important for anyone with immunosuppression.
- Avoid contaminating streams or other water sources with feces.
- Control flies and avoid foods exposed to flies.
- With scabies and pediculosis infestations, drug therapy must be accompanied by measures to avoid reinfection or transmission to others. For example, close contacts should be examined carefully and treated if indicated. Clothes, bed linens, and towels should be washed and dried on hot cycles. Clothes that cannot be washed should be dry cleaned. With head lice, combs and brushes should be cleaned and disinfected; carpets and upholstered furniture should be vacuumed.
- With pinworms, clothing, bed linens, and towels should be washed daily on hot cycles. Toilet seats should be disinfected daily.
- Ensure follow-up measures, such as testing of stool specimens; vaginal examinations; anal swabs; smears; and cultures.
- With vaginal infections, avoid sexual intercourse, or have the male partner use a condom.

Evaluation

- Interview and observe for relief of symptoms.
- Interview outpatients regarding compliance with instructions for taking antiparasitic drugs and measures to prevent recurrence of infestation.
- Interview and observe for adverse drug effects.
- Interview and observe regarding food intake or changes in weight.

Key Concepts

- Parasitic infestations injure host tissues.
- Amebiasis is caused by the pathogenic protozoan E. histolytica. It is transmitted by the fecal–oral route, such as by ingesting food or water contaminated with human feces containing amebic cysts.
- Helminthiasis is an infestation of parasitic worms and is most commonly found in the GI tract.
- Scabies and pediculosis are parasitic infestations of the skin.
- Scabies is caused by S. scabiei.
- Pediculosis is caused by three types of lice.
- Amebicides are effective against the protozoans that cause amebiasis.
- Travelers to malarious regions should generally receive chloroquine to prevent malaria and take precautions to avoid or minimize exposure to the causative mosquito.
- Anthelmintics are used in the treatment of parasitic infections by hookworms, pinworms, roundworms, and whipworms.
- Scabies and pediculosis are treated with the topical agents.
- Personal and public health hygienic practices can prevent many parasitic infections and should be followed diligently.

Critical Thinking Questions

23.1. A 16-year-old female high school student has been taking ciprofloxacin for the past 10 days for the treatment of a "strep" throat. She visits the school nurse with the complaint of vaginal burning and itching along with a foul-smelling vaginal drainage. The school nurse, who is a family nurse practitioner, prescribes metronidazole (Flagyl) 500 mg every 6 to 8 hours for 7 days.

• What is the action of metronidazole?

• The nurse should provide what patient teaching to the girl?

References and Resources

Baer, K. A., Higginson, A. I., & Hickey, P. W. (2010). Disparities exist in the availability of outpatient malaria treatment in Maryland, USA. *Journal of Travel Medicine, 17*(4), 228–232.

Daily, J. (2012). Treatment of uncomplicated falciparum malaria. *Up-to-date.* LexiComp, Inc.

Goldstein, A. & Goldstein, B. Patient information: Head lice. *Up-to-date.* LexiComp, Inc.

Goldstein, A. & Goldstein, B. Scabies. *Up-to-date.* LexiComp, Inc.

Johnson, M. (2012). Metronidazole: An overview. *Up-to-date.* LexiComp, Inc.

Karch, A. M. (2011). *2011 Lippincott's nursing drug guide.* Philadelphia, PA: Lippincott Williams & Wilkins.

Kuhn, M. A. & Winston, D. *Herbal therapy supplements a scientific and traditional approach* (2nd ed.). Philadelphia, PA: Lippincott Williams & Wilkins.

Leder, K. & Weller, P. F. (2012). Treatment and prevention of cryptosporidiosis. *Up-to-date.* LexiComp, Inc.

Mitchell, C., Balkus, J., Agnew, K., Lawler, R. & Hitti, J. (2009). Changes in the vaginal microenvironment with metronidazole treatment for bacterial vaginosis in early pregnancy. *Journal of Women's Health, 18*(11), 1817–1824.

Porth, C. M. & Matfin, G. (2009). *Pathophysiology: Concepts of altered health states.* Philadelphia, PA: Lippincott Williams & Wilkins.

Smeltzer, S. C., Bare, B. G., Hinkle, J. H., & Cheever, K. H. (2008). *Brunner & Suddarth's textbook of medical-surgical nursing* (11th ed.). Philadelphia, PA: Lippincott Williams & Wilkins.

Taylor, T. E. (2012). Treatment of severe falciparum malaria. *Up-to-date.* LexiComp, Inc.

Up-To-Date (2012). *Artemether and lumefantrine: Drug information.* LexiComp, Inc.

Up-To-Date (2012). *Mebendazole: Drug information.* LexiComp, Inc.

Up-To-Date (2012). *Metronidazole (systemic): Drug information.* LexiComp, Inc.

Up-To-Date (2012). *Nitazoxanide: Drug information.* LexiComp, Inc.

Up-To-Date (2012). *Permethrin: Drug information.* LexiComp, Inc.

Up-To-Date (2012). *Tinidazole: Drug information.* LexiComp, Inc.

Weller, P. F. (2012). Antihelminthic therapies. *Up-to-date.* LexiComp, Inc.

Weller, P. F. (2012). Antiprotozoal therapies. *Up-to-date.* LexiComp, Inc.

SECTION 5

Drugs Affecting the Cardiovascular System

Drugs Affecting the Cardiovascular System

CHAPTER OUTLINE

24 Drug Therapy for Heart Failure

LEARNING OBJECTIVES

After studying this chapter, you should be able to:

1. Understand the pathophysiology of right-sided and left-sided heart failure.

2. Identify the major manifestations of heart failure.

3. Identify the prototype and describe the action, use, adverse effects, contraindications, and nursing implications for the inotrope (cardiac glycoside) drug class.

4. Identify the prototype and describe the action, use, adverse effects, contraindications, and nursing implications for the phosphodiesterase inhibitors (cardiotonic–inotropic agents).

5. Identify the prototype and describe the action, use, adverse effects, contraindications, and nursing implications for human B-type natriuretic peptide.

6. Identify the prototype and describe the action, use, adverse effects, contraindications, and nursing implications for adjuvant drugs used in the treatment of heart failure.

7. Implement the nursing process in the care of patients undergoing drug therapy for heart failure.

Clinical Application Case Study

Dr. Adams is a 59-year-old professor of history at a 4-year college. He states to the nurse practitioner at the campus health center that he has been experiencing shortness of breath and fatigue for the last 4 weeks. The nurse practitioner asks Dr. Adams questions to ascertain his past medical history. He states that he has been taking enalapril maleate, 20 mg one time per day for hypertension. Dr. Adams also states that his ankles seem to be swollen. On examination, the nurse practitioner notes that Dr. Adams has pitting edema in his feet and ankles. The nurse practitioner advises Dr. Adams to make an appointment with his physician immediately. The physician diagnoses Dr. Adams with heart failure and prescribes digoxin (Lanoxin), 0.125 mg every morning, and spironolactone (Aldactone), 25 mg every morning in addition to the enalapril maleate.

KEY TERMS

Catecholamines: active amines (e.g., epinephrine, norepinephrine, dopamine) that have an effect on the cardiovascular system

Decompensation: the inability of the heart to adequately circulate oxygenated blood to the body's vital organs

Diastolic dysfunction: impaired relaxation and filling of the ventricles during diastole

Digitalis toxicity: an accumulation of digitalis in the body that leads to nausea, vomiting, and atrial tachycardia

Digitalization: the administration of a loading dose of digoxin (Lanoxin) to achieve a therapeutic blood level of the medication more rapidly

Endothelin: a peptide that raises blood pressure, constricts blood vessels, and contributes to the onset of heart failure

Inotropic: related to or influencing the force of myocardial contractility

Renin: an enzyme produced by the kidney that divides angiotensinogen to form angiotensin I, which is then changed to angiotensin II to produce vasoconstriction

Systolic dysfunction: impaired myocardial contraction during systole

Therapeutic index: the blood level of a medication that will produce therapeutic effects

Ventricular remodeling: dilatation and hypertrophy of the ventricles in the initial phases of heart failure, causing the ventricle to assume a spherical shape

Introduction

In this chapter, you are introduced to the pharmacological care of the patient who is experiencing heart failure. Heart failure is a complex clinical condition that occurs when the heart cannot pump enough blood to meet the body tissue's needs for oxygen and nutrients. Heart failure can result from impaired myocardial contraction during systole (**systolic dysfunction**), impaired relaxation and filling of ventricles during diastole (**diastolic dysfunction**), or a combination of both systolic and diastolic dysfunction. Heart failure can result in an accumulation of fluid in the lungs and peripheral tissues.

Overview of Heart Failure

To adequately understand the pharmacologic treatment of heart failure, it is important to understand the causes, pathophysiology, and clinical manifestations of heart failure. It is also important to understand the difference between right-sided and left-sided heart failure.

Etiology

Heart failure is caused by various conditions that prevent the contractile myocardial cells and the endothelial cells that line the heart and blood vessels from functioning properly. Hypertension, cardiomyopathy, and acute myocardial infarction can affect myocardial or endothelial cell function, leading to heart failure. Heart failure can also be caused by volume overload, renal failure, or hypermetabolic states.

Endothelial dysfunction promotes processes that can lead to narrowing of the blood vessel lumen, such as the accumulation of atherosclerotic plaque, abnormal cell growth, inflammation, or platelet activation. The narrowing of the lumen can lead to blood clot formation and vasoconstriction. These are the major factors in coronary artery disease and hypertension and the most common conditions that lead to heart failure.

Hyperthyroidism is a hypermetabolic condition that is a major causative factor in the development of heart failure. Thyroid function is increased, which causes an increase in heart rate and myocardial contractility and ultimately cardiac output. The patient is prone to heart failure due to the increased cardiac output.

Fluid volume overload impairs the pumping ability of the heart, contributing to the development of heart failure. Fluid volume overload can occur in patients with renal failure. Fluid volume overload can also be caused by the excessive administration of intravenous (IV) fluids or blood transfusions, or therapy with certain medications such as corticosteroids, estrogens, and nonsteroidal anti-inflammatory agents (which promote sodium and water retention).

Pathophysiology

Heart failure results in low cardiac output and inadequate filling of the arteries. As a result, the neurohormonal system activates several feedback mechanisms. The baroreceptors in the aortic arch and carotid sinus that normally inhibit sympathetic nervous system activity are blunted in the patient who is experiencing heart failure. This results in high levels of circulating **catecholamines** (active amines, such as epinephrine, norepinephrine, and dopamine, that have an effect on the cardiovascular system). The circulating catecholamines increase the force of myocardial contractility, as does the increased activity of the sympathetic nervous system. The patient's heart rate increases, and the blood vessels constrict. Levels of endothelin, a peptide secreted by the endothelial cells, are increased in heart failure. **Endothelin** is a potent vasoconstrictor and may exert direct toxic effects on the heart.

The renin–angiotensin–aldosterone system is also activated. **Renin** is an enzyme produced in the kidneys in response to impaired blood flow and tissue perfusion. The release of renin stimulates the production of angiotensin II. Angiotensin II is a powerful vasoconstrictor. Arterial vasoconstriction impairs cardiac function by increasing the resistance (afterload) against which the ventricle ejects blood. This increases the filling pressures inside the heart, which in turn, increases the stress on the heart by stretching the walls of the heart muscle, predisposing the patient to subendocardial ischemia. Patients with severe heart failure have constriction of the arterioles in the cerebral, myocardial, renal, hepatic, and mesenteric vascular beds. This results in increased organ hypoperfusion and dysfunction.

Right-Sided Heart Failure

Right-sided heart failure results from an accumulation of blood in the systemic venous system. There are two pumps within the heart. The right-sided pump pumps unoxygenated blood from the systemic circulation into the pulmonary circulation. Failure of the right-sided pump results in an increase in the right atrial, right ventricular, end-diastolic, and systemic venous pressures.

The causes of right-sided heart failure are stenosis or regurgitation of the pulmonic or tricuspid valves, right-sided ventricular infarction, cardiomyopathy, or recurrent left-sided heart failure. In some cases severe pneumonia, pulmonary embolus, or pulmonary hypertension can result in right-sided heart failure.

Left-Sided Heart Failure

Left-sided heart failure results in a decrease in cardiac output related to an increase in left atrial and left ventricular end-diastolic pressures and congestion in the pulmonary circulation. The left side of the heart normally moves blood from the low-pressure pulmonary circulation to the higher pressure arterial side of the systemic circulation.

Left-sided heart failure is most commonly caused by a myocardial infarction or cardiomyopathy. The patient experiences pulmonary edema at night while supine in bed because the left ventricle cannot pump the blood effectively out of the ventricle into the aorta and the systemic circulation. The pressure in the left atrium increases, resulting in decreased blood flow from the pulmonary vessels. The increase in pulmonary venous pressure forces fluid from the pulmonary capillaries into the alveoli, impairing gas exchange.

Clinical Manifestations

The cardinal manifestations of heart failure are dyspnea and fatigue, which can lead to exercise intolerance and fluid retention. Fluid retention results in the development of pulmonary congestion and peripheral edema. Patients with compensated or asymptomatic heart failure usually have no symptoms at rest and no edema. In these patients, dyspnea and fatigue occur only with activities that require moderate- to high-level exertion. Patients with symptomatic heart failure have symptoms that occur with minimal exertion or at rest, ankle edema, and distention of the jugular vein. These signs and symptoms reflect **decompensation** (the inability of the heart to adequately circulate oxygenated blood to the body's vital organs). Acute, severe cardiac decompensation is manifested by pulmonary edema, a medical emergency that requires immediate treatment. Clinical manifestations of heart failure are summarized in Box 24.1.

EVIDENCE-BASED PRACTICE

Hypoxic Liver Injury
by ELLEN C. EBERT, MD

www.mayoclinicproceedings.com
September 2006, 81(9), 1232–1236
Retrieved: July 13, 2009

Hypoxic liver injury (hypoxic hepatitis) is caused by insufficient hepatic perfusion. It primarily occurs in elderly patients with right-sided heart failure. Factors that precipitate the development of hypoxic liver injury include arrhythmias or pulmonary edema. The patient will have weakness, dyspnea, and right upper quadrant pain. A massive but transient increase in serum transaminase levels in the absence of other acute causes of liver damage is seen. This increase in serum transaminase levels is related to the imbalance between hepatic oxygen supply and demand.

IMPLICATIONS FOR NURSING PRACTICE: When providing care to a geriatric patient with right-sided heart failure, it is important to assess liver enzymes due to the hepatotoxic effects of medications and the possible development of hypoxic liver injury.

BOX 24.1 Clinical Manifestations of Heart Failure

Right-Sided Heart Failure
- Edema of the lower extremities
- Weight gain
- Dyspnea
- Fatigue
- Hepatomegaly
- Ascites
- Anorexia
- Nausea or abdominal pain

Left-Sided Heart Failure
- Pulmonary congestion
- Dyspnea with possible orthopnea
- Cough
- Audible crackles in the bases of the lung
- Audible S3 or ventricular gallop

TABLE 24.1		
Medications Administered for the Treatment of Heart Failure		
Drug Class	**Prototype**	**Other Drugs in the Class**
Inotropes (cardiac glycosides)	Digoxin (Lanoxin)	
Phosphodiesterase inhibitors (cardiotonic–inotropic agents)	Milrinone lactate (Primacor)	
Human B-type natriuretic peptide (BNP)	Nesiritide (Natrecor)	
Loop diuretics	Furosemide (Lasix)	Bumetanide (Bumex) Ethacrynate sodium (Sodium Edecrin) Ethacrynic acid (Edecrin) Torsemide (Demadex)
Thiazide diuretics	Hydrochlorothiazide (HCTZ)	Chlorothiazide sodium (Diuril) Methyclothiazide (Enduron)
Angiotensin-converting enzyme (ACE) inhibitors	Enalapril maleate (Vasotec)	Benazepril hydrochloride (Lotensin) Captopril (Capoten) Fosinopril (Monopril) Lisinopril (Prinivil, Zestril) Moexipril hydrochloride (Univasc) Perindopril erbumine (Aceon) Quinapril hydrochloride (Accupril) Ramipril (Altace) Trandolapril (Mavik)
Angiotensin II–receptor blockers (ARBs)	Losartan potassium (Cozaar)	Candesartan cilexetil (Atacand) Eprosartan mesylate (Teveten) Irbesartan potassium (Avapro) Olmesartan medoxomil (Benicar) Telmisartan (Micardis) Valsartan (Diovan)
Beta-adrenergic blocking agents	Propranolol (Inderal)	Acebutolol hydrochloride (Monitan) Atenolol (Tenormin) Betaxolol hydrochloride (Kerlone) Bisoprolol fumarate (Zebeta) Carteolol hydrochloride (Cartrol, Ocupress) Carvedilol (Coreg) Esmolol hydrochloride (Brevibloc) Labetalol hydrochloride (Trandate) Metoprolol tartrate (Lopressor, Toprol XL) Nadolol (Corgard) Penbutolol (Levatol) Pindolol (Visken) Sotalol (Betapace)
Aldosterone antagonists	Spironolactone (Aldactone)	Eplerenone (Inspra)

Drug Therapy

Medications used in the treatment of heart failure are summarized in Table 24.1. Treatment guidelines are based on signs and symptoms (Table 24.2).

Clinical Application 24-1

- Does Dr. Adams have right-sided or left-sided heart failure?

NCLEX Success

1. An elderly patient is admitted to the cardiac intensive care unit with right-sided heart failure. Which of the following blood values is most important to monitor based on the patient's risk factors?

   A. complete blood count (CBC)
   B. blood glucose
   C. bleeding and clotting time
   D. liver enzymes

TABLE 24.2

Classifying Signs and Symptoms of Heart Failure and the Associated Treatment as Developed by the American College of Cardiology (ACC) and American Heart Association (AHA) Task Force

Guidelines	Recommendations
Stage A: Patient presents without signs and symptoms of heart failure but is placed at high risk for the development of heart failure. Patients at risk for developing heart failure are those with hypertension, diabetes, history of alcohol abuse, family history of cardiomyopathy, or past history of treatment with chemotherapeutic agents.	• Smoking cessation • Alcohol avoidance • Treatment of hypertension with angiotensin-converting enzyme (ACE) inhibitors or angiotensin receptor blockers (ARBs) • Control of blood glucose levels
Stage B: Patient presents without signs and symptoms of heart failure but has structural cardiac changes that place the patient at risk for heart failure. The structural changes most often associated with Stage B are past myocardial infarction, left ventricular hypertrophy, and valvular disorders of the heart.	• Smoking cessation • Alcohol avoidance • Treatment with an ARB • Treatment with an ACE inhibitor and beta blocker • Valve replacement or repair for patients with hemodynamically significant valvular stenosis or regurgitation • Implantable defibrillator if indicated
Stage C: Patient presents with symptoms of heart failure. Most common symptoms noted include dyspnea, fatigue, peripheral edema, hepatomegaly with jugular vein distention, and ascites.	• Smoking cessation • Alcohol avoidance • Sodium restriction • Treatment with an inotrope (cardiac glycoside) • Treatment with diuretics • Treatment with ACE inhibitors and beta-blockers • If ACE inhibitors are not tolerated due to cough, treatment is with ARBs such as valsartan (Diovan) or candesartan cilexetil (Atacand). • Nonsteroidal anti-inflammatory agents, antidysrhythmic agents, and calcium channel blockers should not be used.
Stage D: The patient presents with debilitating symptoms of heart failure at rest. The patient has symptoms related to advanced heart disease and requires aggressive treatment.	• All therapies for stages A, B, and C • Permanent mechanical support with implantable defibrillators • Continuous inotropic therapy • Heart transplant • Hospice/palliative care

Hunt, S. A., Abraham, W. T., Chin, M. H., Feldman, F. A., Francis, G. S., Ganiats, T. G., et al. (2005). ACC/AHA 2005 *guideline update for the diagnosis and management of chronic heart failure for the adult-summary article: A report of the American College of Cardiology/American Heart Association Task Force for Practice Guidelines (writing committee to revise the 2001 Guidelines for the Evaluation and Management of Heart Failure)*. Retrieved July 14, 2009, from http://www.guidelines.gov/summary/summary.aspx?doc_id=7664

2. **A patient is diagnosed with acute myocardial infarction. Which of the following medications will precipitate the development of left-sided heart failure in this patient?**

   A. ibuprofen (Motrin)
   B. furosemide (Lasix)
   C. gabapentin (Neurontin)
   D. fexofenadine (Allegra)

Inotropes (Cardiac Glycosides)

Inotropes (cardiac glycosides) act to influence the contractility of the heart muscle. (**Inotropic** means related to, or influencing

the force of, myocardial contractility.) ℗ **Digoxin** (Lanoxin) is the prototype drug of this class. Digoxin is derived from the digitalis plant. It is used to treat heart failure, atrial fibrillation, and atrial flutter.

Pharmacokinetics

There are various preparations of digoxin. It is primarily given orally either as a tablet or elixir. The elixir is absorbed more effectively than the tablet and is used primarily with infants and children. When digoxin is given orally, absorption varies among available preparations. With tablets, the most frequently used formulation, differences in bioavailability are important because a person who is stabilized on one formulation may be underdosed or overdosed if another formulation

TABLE 24.3

DRUGS AT A GLANCE: Digoxin

Drug	Pregnancy Category	Routes and Dosage Ranges	
		Adults	Children
℗ **Digoxin** (Lanoxin, Lanoxicaps)	C	0.75–1.5 mg PO 0.125–0.25 mg IV	Neonate: 25–35 mcg/kg PO 20–30 mcg/kg IV Child (1–24 mo): 35–60 mcg/kg PO 30–50 mcg/kg IV Child (2–5 y): 30–40 mcg/kg PO 25–35 mcg/kg IV Child (5–10 y): 20–30 mcg/kg PO 15–30 mcg/kg IV Child (older than 10 y): 10–15 mcg/kg PO 8–12 mcg/kg IV

is administered. The differences are attributed to the rate and extent of tablet dissolution rather than the amounts of digoxin. Another popular form of the medication is Lanoxicaps, which are liquid-filled capsules. Digoxin is also given by injection and is supplied as 0.25 mg/mL or 0.1 mg/mL. Digoxin dosages are summarized in Table 24.3.

When given orally, the onset of action occurs in 30 minutes to 2 hours, with the peak effect of the medication occurring in approximately 6 hours. When digoxin is given parenterally through the IV route, the onset of action occurs within 10 to 30 minutes and reaches a peak effect in 1 to 5 hours.

Digitalization is the administration of a loading dose (a dose larger than the regular prescribed daily dosage) of digoxin to reach the **therapeutic index** (the blood level of the medication that will produce therapeutic effects) rapidly. The administration of digoxin for rapid digitalization is usually done for atrial tachydysrhythmias rather than heart failure. The digitalizing dosage schedule requires the nurse to administer a total dose of 0.75 to 1.5 mg of digoxin in divided doses, 6 to 8 hours apart, over a 24-hour period. It is important to note that rapid digitalization places the patient at risk for developing digoxin toxicity. Thus, the nurse must be alert to signs and symptoms of toxicity, which include very slow or very rapid ventricular rhythm, nausea, vomiting, loss of appetite, abdominal distention, blurred vision, and mental changes. During rapid digitalization, the patient is monitored continuously on a cardiac monitor.

Another form of digitalization is slow digitalization. This can be accomplished by initiating therapy with a maintenance dose of digoxin (i.e., a dose administered daily to control symptoms). Digitalization with a maintenance dose will reach therapeutic effects in approximately 1 week. Decreased absorption of digoxin can result in **digitalis toxicity** (an accumulation of digitalis in the body that leads to nausea, vomiting, and atrial tachycardia). Factors that decrease the absorption of digoxin

include the presence of food in the gastrointestinal (GI) tract, malabsorption syndromes, and the concurrent administration of antacids or cholestyramine. The administration of digoxin should take place at least 1 hour before the administration of an antacid. It is important to note that when digoxin is discontinued, it takes approximately 1 week for the drug to be eliminated from the body.

Action

A patient with heart failure is experiencing decreased contractility of the heart, which impairs the heart's ability to pump blood adequately. Digoxin produces a cardiotonic (positive inotropic) effect that improves the contractility and pumping ability of the heart. Digoxin increases the force of myocardial contractility by inhibiting sodium, potassium, adenosine triphosphatase (Na, K-ATPase), an enzyme in cardiac cell membranes that decreases the movement of sodium out of myocardial cells after contraction. As a result, calcium enters the cell in exchange for sodium, causing additional calcium to be released from intracellular binding sites and increasing myocardial contractility.

In a patient with an atrial dysrhythmia, digoxin slows the rate of ventricular contraction (negative chronotropic effect). Negative chronotropic effects are probably caused by several factors. First, digoxin has a direct depressant effect on cardiac contraction tissues, especially at the atrioventricular (AV) node. This action decreases the number of electrical impulses allowed to reach the ventricles from supraventricular sources. Second, digoxin indirectly stimulates the vagus nerve. Third, increased efficiency of myocardial contraction and vagal stimulation decrease compensatory tachycardia that results from the sympathetic nervous system response to inadequate circulation.

EVIDENCE-BASED PRACTICE

Use of Digoxin in the Treatment of Chronic Heart Failure

by WONG, B., AND FLATTERY, M. P.

Progress in Cardiovascular Nursing
Summer 2006, 158–161
Retrieved: July 22, 2009

This review of literature revealed that digoxin improves symptoms in patients with systolic heart failure with neutral effect on mortality regardless of the presence of atrial fibrillation. Based on guidelines from the Heart Failure Society of America, patients with left ventricular systolic dysfunction and who have persistent symptoms of heart failure should be treated with digoxin, angiotensin-converting enzyme (ACE) inhibitors, beta-blockers, diuretics, and possibly aldosterone antagonists.

IMPLICATIONS FOR NURSING PRACTICE: The nurse must be aware of the effects of all these medications in the treatment of the patient with heart failure. The nurse must assess for adverse effects and the patient's response to treatment. The nurse must educate the patient and family on the need to these medications to control symptoms of heart failure.

Use

The clinical indications for use of digoxin include the management of heart failure, atrial fibrillation, and atrial flutter. Digoxin is administered to patients with acute or chronic conditions, patients who are being digitalized, or for maintenance therapy.

Use in Children

Digoxin is commonly used in children and has the same indications as in adults. When used in children, digoxin therapy should be prescribed and supervised by a pediatric cardiologist when possible. The response to a given dose varies with age and size. The child's renal and hepatic function also affect the child's response to the medication. There may be little difference between a therapeutic dose and a toxic dose. Very small amounts are often given to children. These factors increase the risk for dosage errors in children. In a hospital setting, institutional policies may require that each dose be verified with another nurse before it is administered. Liquid digoxin must be precisely measured in a syringe and the dose should never be rounded. It is imperative that the dosage administered is accurate. Electrocardiographic monitoring is desirable when digoxin therapy is initiated.

As in adults, the dosage of digoxin in children is individualized and carefully titrated. Digoxin is primarily excreted by the kidneys, and the dosage should be reduced in the presence of renal impairment. In general, divided daily doses should be given to infants and children younger than 10 years of age, and adult dosages adjusted to weight should be given to children older than 10 years of age. Larger doses are usually needed to slow a too rapid ventricular rate in children with atrial fibrillation or flutter. Differences in bioavailability of different preparations (parenterals, capsules, tablets, and elixirs) must be considered when switching from one preparation to another.

Neonates vary in tolerance of digoxin, depending on their degree of maturity. Premature infants are especially sensitive to drug effects. The dosage must be reduced, and digitalization should be even more individualized and cautiously approached than in more mature infants and children. Early signs of toxicity in newborns are undue slowing of the sinus rate, sinoatrial (SA) arrest, and prolongation of the P–R interval.

Use in Older Adults

Digoxin is a frequent cause of adverse effects in older adults. Reduced dosages are usually required because of decreased liver or kidney function, decreased lean body weight, and advanced cardiovascular disease. Impaired renal function leads to slower drug excretion and increased risk of accumulation. Dosage must be reduced by approximately 50% with renal failure or concurrent administration of amiodarone hydrochloride (Cordarone), quinidine, nifedipine (Procardia), or verapamil hydrochloride (Calan). These drugs increase the serum digoxin level and increase the risk for toxicity if the dosage is not reduced. The most commonly recommended dose is 0.125 mg daily.

Use in Patients With Renal Impairment

Digoxin must be used cautiously in patients with diminished renal function, because renal impairment delays the drug's excretion. Both loading and maintenance doses should be reduced. Patients with advanced renal impairment can achieve therapeutic serum concentrations with a dosage of 0.125 mg three to five times per week. In patients with reduced blood flow to the kidneys (e.g., as a result of fluid volume depletion or acute heart failure), digoxin may be reabsorbed in the renal tubules. As a result, less digoxin is excreted through the kidneys, and maintenance doses may need to be even less than the dosage amount calculated according to creatinine clearance.

Digoxin toxicity develops more often and lasts longer in patients with renal impairment. Patients with renal impairment who are receiving digoxin, even in small doses, must be monitored for adverse effects, and serum digoxin levels must be monitored periodically.

Digoxin can be administered with milrinone lactate (Primacor) to control acute, severe heart failure. Milrinone lactate is excreted primarily by the kidneys; thus, renal impairment significantly increases elimination half-life, drug accumulation, and adverse effects. Dosage must be reduced according to the creatinine clearance. The nurse consults the manufacturer's instructions for reduced dosages related to the creatinine clearance.

Use in Patients With Hepatic Impairment

Hepatic function has little effect on digoxin clearance. Adjustments in the dosage amount are not required for patients with hepatic impairment.

Use in Patients With Critical Illness

Critically ill patients often have multiple cardiovascular and other disorders that require drug therapy. Acute heart failure may be the patient's primary critical illness. However, that episode of heart failure may be precipitated by other illnesses and treatments that alter fluid balance, impair myocardial contractility, or increase the workload of the heart beyond its capacity to accommodate. Management of the critically ill patient is often symptomatic, with the choice of drug and dosage requiring careful titration and frequent monitoring of the patient's response. Cardiotonic, diuretic, and vasodilator drugs are often required. All of these medications should be used cautiously in critically ill patients.

Use in Patients Receiving Home Care

Most digoxin is taken at home, and the home care nurse shares the responsibility for teaching patients how to use the drug effectively and how to recognize medication responses that should be reported to the health care provider. Accurate dosing is vitally important because underuse may cause the recurrence of symptoms and overuse may cause toxicity. Either condition may be life-threatening. The nurse instructs the patient and any caregivers that if symptoms of heart failure or digoxin toxicity develop, it is necessary to seek medical intervention immediately. The home care nurse also monitors the patient's response to the drug and changes in the patient's condition or drug therapy that increase the patient's risk for toxicity.

When a patient is receiving a combination of drugs for management of heart failure, the nurse assists the patient in understanding that the different types of drugs have different actions and produce different responses. As a result, the medications work together to be more effective and maintain a more balanced state of cardiovascular function. Changing medications or dosages can upset the balance and lead to acute and severe symptoms that require hospitalization and may even cause death from heart failure. Thus, it is extremely important that the patient takes all the medications that have been prescribed. If the patient is unable to take the medications for any reason, the health care provider should be notified.

Adverse Effects

Because of digoxin's narrow therapeutic index, the patient is at greater risk for developing digoxin toxicity. Factors that contribute

---

> ### BOX 24.2   Factors That Contribute to Digoxin (Lanoxin) Toxicity
>
> ■ An accumulation of larger-than-necessary maintenance doses
> ■ Rapid loading or digitalization, whether by one or more large doses or frequent administration of small doses
> ■ Extremes in age (young and old)
> ■ Electrolyte imbalance (hypokalemia, hypomagnesemia, hypercalcemia)
> ■ Hypoxia due to heart or lung disease (hypoxia increases myocardial sensitivity to digoxin)
> ■ Hypothyroidism (slows metabolism of digoxin)
> ■ Concurrent treatment with other drugs affecting the heart, such as quinidine, verapamil (Calan), or nifedipine (Procardia)

to the development of digoxin toxicity are summarized in Box 24.2. Patients with hypokalemia can develop digoxin toxicity even when the serum digoxin level is not considered to be elevated.

The signs of toxicity include potentially life-threatening heart rhythm disturbances, ranging from slow to rapid ventricular rhythm. Premature ventricular contractions (PVCs) occur commonly with digoxin toxicity and are usually perceived as "skipped" heartbeats by patients. However, PVCs have many possible causes and therefore are not specific for digoxin toxicity. Other adverse effects include nausea, vomiting, loss of appetite, abdominal discomfort, blurred vision, and mental changes. Box 24.3 identifies medications administered to treat digoxin toxicity.

Contraindications

Digoxin is contraindicated in patients with severe myocarditis, ventricular tachycardia, or ventricular fibrillation. It should be administered cautiously in patients with acute myocardial infarction, heart block, Stokes-Adams syndrome, or Wolff-Parkinson-White syndrome, because it may place these patients at risk for fatal dysrhythmias. Patients with hypokalemia,

---

> ### BOX 24.3   Management of Digoxin (Lanoxin) Toxicity
>
> ■ Digoxin is discontinued, not just reduced in dosage. (Most patients with mild or early toxicity recover completely within a few days after the drug is stopped.)
>
> **In the Presence of Serious Cardiac Dysrhythmias:**
>
> ■ Potassium chloride, a myocardial depressant that acts to decrease myocardial excitability, is administered if the potassium level is low. The dose depends on the severity of the toxicity, the serum potassium level, and the patient's response. Potassium is contraindicated in patients with renal failure and should be used with caution in the presence of cardiac conduction defects.
> ■ Lidocaine is an antidysrhythmic local anesthetic agent used to decrease myocardial irritability.
> ■ Atropine or isoproterenol is used to manage bradycardia or conduction defects.
>
> ■ Other antidysrhythmic drugs may be used but are generally less effective in digoxin-induced dysrhythmias (as compared with dysrhythmias due to other causes).
> ■ Digoxin immune fab (Digibind) is a digoxin-binding antidote derived from antidigoxin antibodies produced in sheep. It is recommended only for serious toxicity. Digoxin immune fab combines with digoxin, pulling it out of the tissues and into the bloodstream. This causes serum digoxin levels to be high, but the drug is bound to the antibody and therefore inactive. Digoxin immune fab is given intravenously, as a bolus injection if the patient is in danger of immediate cardiac arrest, but preferably over 15 to 30 minutes. Dosage varies and is calculated according to the amount of digoxin ingested or the serum digoxin level. Dosage instructions are provided by the manufacturer and must be followed.

BOX 24.4 Drug Interactions: Digoxin

Drugs That Increase the Effects of Digoxin

■ Adrenergic agents, such as epinephrine (Adrenaline), ephedrine sulfate, and isoproterenol hydrochloride (Isuprel)

Increase the risk for cardiac dysrhythmias

■ Antidysrhythmics, such as amiodarone hydrochloride, propafenone hydrochloride, and quinidine

Decrease clearance of digoxin, thereby increasing serum digoxin levels and the risk for toxicity

■ Calcium preparations

Increase absorption of oral digoxin by slowing transit time through the gastrointestinal tract

■ Calcium channel blockers, such as diltiazem hydrochloride, felodipine (Plendil), nifedipine (Procardia), and verapamil (Calan)

Decrease clearance of digoxin, thereby increasing serum digoxin levels and the risk for toxicity.

Drugs That Decrease the Effects of Digoxin

■ Antacids, cholestyramine (Questran), colestipol hydrochloride (Colestid), oral laxatives, aminoglycosides (e.g., neomycin sulfate)

Decrease absorption of oral digoxin

hypomagnesemia, or hypercalcemia should also be administered digoxin cautiously due to the risk of dysrhythmia. Renal impairment requires an alteration in dosage and cautious administration.

Nursing Implications

Preventing Interactions

Many medications and herbs interact with digoxin, increasing or decreasing its effect (Boxes 24.4 and 24.5).

Administering the Medication

The therapeutic serum digoxin level is 0.8 to 2.0 ng/mL. The serum blood level is drawn prior to the administration of the digoxin dose. The blood sample is drawn at least 6 hours after the previous dose, because distribution of digoxin to the tissues requires about 6 hours. If the blood is drawn before 6 hours, the serum digoxin level may be elevated.

The administration of digoxin requires the nurse to thoroughly assess the patient's cardiac status. The nurse assesses the

BOX 24.5 Herb and Dietary Interactions: Digoxin

Herbs and Foods That Increase the Effects of Digoxin

■ Ginseng
■ Hawthorne
■ Licorice

Herbs and Foods That Decrease the Effects of Digoxin

■ Psyllium
■ St. John's wort

apical pulse at the point of maximal impulse (PMI) for 1 full minute. If the rate is less than 60 beats/min in adults, 70 beats/min in older children, or 100 beats/min in younger children, the dose is omitted and the health care provider is notified. The nurse also assesses the patient for a pulse deficit. The goal of therapy is to eliminate a pulse deficit in the patient with atrial fibrillation. In patients with atrial fibrillation, slowing of the heart rate and elimination of the pulse deficit are clinical indicators that digitalization has occurred.

Digoxin is administered with food or after meals. The administration of digoxin with food minimizes gastric irritation and symptoms of anorexia, nausea, and vomiting. However, these symptoms probably arise from drug stimulation of chemoreceptors in the medulla rather than as a direct irritant effect of the drug on the GI tract.

If possible, the same nurse administers each dose of digoxin to the patient. This enhances patient safety because consistency allows the nurse to recognize changes in rate and rhythm. When administering IV digoxin, the dose is administered by IV push slowly over at least 5 minutes. The same oral and IV formulation and brand is used for each dose, because digoxin formulations vary in concentration and bioavailability and cannot be used interchangeably.

QSEN Safety Alert

It is important to determine the brand of digoxin the patient was receiving at home and try to administer the same brand to the patient in the hospital. If a different brand is administered, it is important to assess the patient's response to the medication closely due to the changes in each brand's bioavailability.

Assessing for Therapeutic Effects

When administering digoxin and related medications in the treatment of heart failure, the nurse assesses the therapeutic effects of the medications. The pulmonary symptoms that develop with heart failure are a direct result of events initiated by inadequate cardiac output. The left side of the heart is unable to accommodate incoming blood flow from the lungs. The resulting back pressure in pulmonary veins and capillaries causes leakage of fluid from blood vessels into tissue spaces and alveoli. Fluid accumulation may result in severe respiratory difficulty and pulmonary edema, a life-threatening development. The improved strength of myocardial contraction resulting from cardiotonic–inotropic drugs reverses this potentially fatal chain of events. The nurse observes for signs and symptoms of pulmonary congestion, such as dyspnea, orthopnea, cyanosis, cough, hemoptysis, crackles, anxiety, and restlessness. The nurse also assesses the patient daily for edema. The absence of pitting edema, decreased size of ankles and abdominal girth, and decreased weight improves circulation and increases renal blood flow. The diminished fluid is indicative of an improved blood supply to the body tissues.

Assessing for Adverse Effects

The nurse assesses the patient for signs and symptoms of digitalis toxicity, including bradycardia and cardiac dysrhythmias such as PVCs, paroxysmal atrial tachycardia with heart block, AV tachycardia, and AV block (also known as second- or third-degree heart block). These are the most severe adverse effects associated with digoxin therapy. They are detected as abnormalities on electrocardiograms (ECGs) and in pulse rate or rhythm. PVCs are among the most common digoxin-induced dysrhythmias. Excessive slowing of the heart rate is an extension of the drug's therapeutic action of slowing conduction through the AV node and possibly depressing the SA node as well. Electrocardiography is necessary for identification of nodal rhythms and heart block.

The GI assessment is crucial in determining the onset of digoxin toxicity. The nurse assesses the patient for anorexia, nausea, and vomiting, which are common with digoxin therapy because digoxin stimulates the vomiting center of the brain. The presence of these symptoms raises the suspicion for digitalis toxicity, but is not specific because other conditions or medications (e.g., diuretics, potassium supplements) may also cause GI adverse effects. The nurse instructs the patient to report any of these symptoms immediately to the health care provider.

Other symptoms of digoxin toxicity include headache, drowsiness, and confusion. These adverse effects are more commonly seen in older adults. Visual disturbances (such as blurred vision, photophobia, altered perception of color, and flickering dots) indicate acute toxicity and must be reported to the health care provider immediately.

Patient Teaching

Box 24.6 identifies patient teaching guidelines for digoxin.

Clinical Application 24-2

- Dr. Adams' cardiologist has ordered digoxin to be administered. The cardiologist states that he is going to begin digitalization of Dr. Adams. What is meant by digitalization?

- Following digitalization, Dr. Adams is to take digoxin 0.125 mg by mouth per day. On the 2nd day of the drug administration regimen, the pharmacy delivers Lanoxicaps 0.125 mg. Is this the same as digoxin and should it be administered?

NCLEX Success

3. A patient is taking digoxin (Lanoxin) for atrial fibrillation. Which of the following assessment findings would indicate that the digoxin should be held and the health care provider should be notified?

A. respiratory rate of 20 breaths/min
B. pulse rate of 80 beats/min
C. respiratory rate of 12 breaths/min
D. pulse rate of 52 beats/min

BOX 24.6   Patient Teaching Guidelines for Digoxin (Lanoxin)

- Digoxin may be used in the treatment of heart failure or atrial fibrillation.
  - In heart failure, digoxin strengthens the heart beat to relieve symptoms such as ankle swelling, shortness of breath, and fatigue.
  - In atrial fibrillation, digoxin slows the heart beat and decreases symptoms such as fatigue.
- Digoxin is administered long-term because heart failure is a chronic condition.
- Digoxin is given daily at the same time to produce therapeutic blood levels.
- Overuse of digoxin will cause adverse effects.
- Use the same brand and type of digoxin all the time.
- Never miss a dose of digoxin. Take your prescribed dose at the same time every day and keep a written record of the date and time of administration.
- If you forget to take your daily dose and it is within 6 hours of the time you usually take the dose, take your daily dose.
- Do not take an extra dose.
- Do not take a double dose to make up for a missed dose.
- Count your pulse for a full minute prior to taking your daily dose of digoxin. If your pulse rate is less than 60 beats/min, hold the dose of digoxin and notify your health care provider.
- Take digoxin with food or after a meal. Dairy products will delay absorption.

- If needed, the tablets can be crushed. Capsules should be swallowed whole.
- Digoxin elixir must be measured accurately. A few drops more could produce overdosage, with serious adverse effects; a few drops less could produce underdosage, with a loss or decrease of therapeutic effects.
- Do not take other prescription or nonprescription drugs without consulting a health care provider.
- Have periodic physical examinations, electrocardiograms, and blood tests as ordered. These tests are used to check digoxin and electrolyte (sodium, potassium, magnesium) levels, to monitor your body's response to the digoxin, and to determine needed dosage changes.
- Digoxin is one drug in the management regimen of several drugs for heart disease. Together, the drugs in the management regimen help maintain a balance in the cardiovascular system. Never change the regimen unless you are told to do so by your health care provider.
- Limit sodium intake and get an adequate intake of potassium if you are also taking a loop diuretic. Low potassium levels can contribute to causing adverse effects of digoxin.
  - Report adverse effects such as changes in heart rate or rhythm, nausea, vomiting, or visual changes to your health care provider immediately.

4. **How does digoxin (Lanoxin) exert a negative chronotropic effect?**

   A. Digoxin has a direct depressant effect on cardiac conduction tissue.
   B. Digoxin increases electrical impulses through the ventricles.
   C. Digoxin depresses the vagal nerve to increase contractility.
   D. Digoxin prevents calcium from entering the myocardial cell.

5. **The home care nurse is visiting a patient who has a history of heart failure. The patient is taking digoxin (Lanoxin) 0.125 mg orally each day. During the assessment, the patient states he has been nauseated since the home care visit 3 days ago. The nurse suspects he has developed digoxin toxicity. Which of the following factors makes this patient more prone to the development of digoxin toxicity?**

   A. creatinine level of 2.0 mg/dL
   B. potassium level of 4.0 mEq/L
   C. calcium level of 8.5 mg/100 mL
   D. magnesium level of 2.0 mg/100 mL

6. **A patient being digitalized in the cardiac intensive care unit is noted to have frequent PVCs. What should the nurse suspect in this patient?**

   A. myocardial infarction
   B. pulmonary embolism
   C. digitalis toxicity
   D. hyperkalemia

7. **A patient is being treated for hypothyroidism. She is also taking digoxin (Lanoxin) for chronic heart failure. Which of the following factors places the patient at risk for digoxin toxicity?**

   A. impaired renal function
   B. impaired liver function
   C. tachycardia
   D. decreased metabolic rate

Phosphodiesterase Inhibitors (Cardiotonic–Inotropic Agents)

Ⓟ **Milrinone lactate** (Primacor) is the most commonly used phosphodiesterase inhibitor administered for short-term management of acute to severe heart failure in patients who do not respond to treatment with digoxin (Lanoxin), diuretics, and vasodilators. Milrinone lactate can be used alone or with other drugs such as dobutamine hydrochloride (Dobutrex) and nitroprusside sodium (Nitropress) for the treatment of heart failure.

Pharmacokinetics

Milrinone lactate is a potent inotropic agent that is given intravenously by bolus injection followed by continuous infusion. The flow rate of the drug is titrated to maintain adequate circulation. The IV administration of milrinone lactate produces an immediate effect. The half-life of this medication is approximately 80 hours, which can lead to accumulation of the medication with prolonged infusions. Dosages for milrinone lactate are given in Table 24.4.

TABLE 24.4

DRUGS AT A GLANCE: Milrinone Lactate

Drug	Pregnancy Category	Routes and Dosage Ranges	
		Adults	*Children*
Ⓟ **Milrinone lactate** (Primacor)	C	General: Loading dose 50 mcg/kg IV bolus, given over 10 min Maintenance infusion 0.375–0.75 mcg/kg/min Total dose not to exceed 1.13 mg/kg/d Older adult: Total dose not to exceed 1.13 mg/kg/d Renal impairment: Creatinine clearance (mL/min) 5 mL/min infusion rate: 0.2 mcg/kg/min 10 mL/min infusion rate: 0.23 mcg/kg/min 20 mL/min infusion rate: 0.28 mcg/kg/min 30 mL/min infusion rate: 0.33 mcg/kg/min 40 mL/min infusion rate: 0.38 mcg/kg/min 50 mL/min infusion rate: 0.43 mcg/kg/min Dilution: Dilute with 0.9% or 0.45% sodium chloride or 5% dextrose; administer the solution within 24 h	Not recommended for use in children

Action

Milrinone lactate's therapeutic action is to increase the force of contraction of the ventricles, providing a positive inotropic effect. It causes vasodilation by exerting a direct relaxant effect on the vascular smooth muscle, decreasing both preload and afterload. The drug increases the levels of cyclic adenosine monophosphate (cAMP) in myocardial cells by inhibiting phosphodiesterase, the enzyme that normally metabolizes cAMP. The effects of this drug are additive to those of digoxin and vasodilators, increasing cardiac output. Milrinone lactate may provide a synergistic effect with adrenergic drugs such as dobutamine hydrochloride (Dobutrex).

Use

Milrinone lactate is indicated for use in patients whose symptoms of heart failure are not controlled with digoxin, diuretics, and vasodilators. It is recommended for short-term IV administration in patients with acute decompensated heart failure. Milrinone lactate is not recommended for use in children. Because impairment of hepatic function has little effect on milrinone lactate clearance, dosage adjustments are not required for patients with hepatic impairment.

Use in Older Adults

Milrinone lactate must be used cautiously in the elderly because the aging process results in decreased renal function. The administration of milrinone lactate in older adults should not exceed 1.13 mg/kg/day.

Use in Patients With Renal Impairment

The creatinine clearance level is used to determine the dosage administration for patients with renal impairment (see Table 24.4).

Use in Patients With Critical Illness

Milrinone lactate should be administered only in a cardiac intensive care unit. The patient's hemodynamic and clinical response to the medication is monitored carefully.

Adverse Effects

The most serious adverse effect associated with the administration of milrinone lactate is the development of potentially fatal ventricular dysrhythmias, which reportedly occur in 12% of patients. Hypotension, supraventricular dysrhythmias, chest pain, angina, headache, thrombocytopenia, and hypokalemia may also occur. Hypotension and headache occur in 3% of patients.

Contraindications

Milrinone lactate, a category C medication, should be administered cautiously in pregnant and lactating women (Karch, 2012). It is contraindicated in patients who are allergic to milrinone lactate or bisulfites. It is also contraindicated in patients with severe aortic or pulmonic valvular disease.

Nursing Implications

Administering the Medication

Prior to administering milrinone lactate, the nurse assesses the patient for allergy to milrinone lactate or bisulfites. The nurse also obtains an accurate weight and assesses the patient for renal impairment to ensure that an accurate dosage of medication is administered. The patient's cardiac rhythm, blood pressure, and pulse are monitored continuously, and a baseline pulse and blood pressure are recorded. If a marked decline in blood pressure or pulse rate occurs, the rate of administration should be reduced. The nurse assesses for adventitious breath sounds prior to administration and periodically throughout the administration of the drug. A platelet count is drawn prior to administration and at least one time during drug therapy to rule out thrombocytopenia. Serum electrolyte levels are monitored periodically throughout the administration of the drug. The nurse also monitors and records fluid intake and output.

Milrinone lactate is not compatible with other medications and should not be mixed with any other medications during administration. Furosemide (Lasix) should not be administered through the same IV line because a precipitate may form.

Patient Teaching

Box 24.7 identifies patient teaching guidelines for milrinone lactate.

NCLEX Success

8. **Which of the following best describes the action of milrinone lactate (Primacor)?**
   A. It relaxes the smooth muscles of the blood vessels to make the vessels wider.
   B. Titration of the medication provides an inotropic effect.
   C. It produces vasoconstriction to increase both the preload and afterload.
   D. The medication decreases the levels of cyclic adenosine monophosphate (cAMP).

9. **During the administration of milrinone lactate (Primacor), the patient's blood pressure decreases from 170/96 mm Hg to 96/60 mm Hg. What is the most appropriate nursing action?**
   A. Call the physician.
   B. Administer a vasoconstrictor.
   C. Reduce the infusion rate.
   D. Reassess the blood pressure.

Human B-Type Natriuretic Peptides

Ⓟ **Nesiritide** (Natrecor) is the prototype drug in the human B-type natriuretic peptide class of drugs. Nesiritide, a vasodilator, is identical to endogenous human B-type natriuretic peptide (BNP), which is secreted primarily by the ventricles in response to fluid and pressure overload. The medication is produced by recombinant DNA technology.

BOX 24.7 — Patient Teaching Guidelines for Milrinone Lactate (Primacor)

■ While you are taking this medication, frequent monitoring of your blood pressure, pulse, and heart rhythm will be necessary.

■ You may experience increased urination while you are taking this medication. Because bed rest must be maintained, please call for assistance with toileting.

■ Report pain at the injection site to the nurse.

■ Report any numbness or tingling, shortness of breath, or chest pain.

Pharmacokinetics

Nesiritide is administered as a bolus dose followed by a continuous infusion. The onset of action of nesiritide is immediate, with peak effects attained in 15 minutes. Nesiritide (Natrecor) dosages are given in Table 24.5. Clearance of the drug is proportional to body weight.

Action

Nesiritide acts to compensate for deteriorating cardiac function by reducing cardiac preload and afterload. It produces a diuretic effect by increasing sodium secretion and suppressing the renin–angiotensin–aldosterone system. Nesiritide also decreases secretion of the neurohormones endothelin and norepinephrine, resulting in relaxation of the smooth muscle.

Use

Nesiritide is indicated for use in decompensated patients with acute heart failure (i.e., those who experience dyspnea at rest and on minimal exertion). Nesiritide is not recommended for administration to children and must be administered cautiously to patients who have impaired renal function.

Adverse Effects

Adverse effects of nesiritide include hypotension, headache, nausea, back pain, ventricular tachycardia, dizziness, anxiety, insomnia, bradycardia, and vomiting. Hypotension occurs in approximately 11% of patients receiving nesiritide. Nausea and back pain have been reported in 8% and 4% of patients, respectively. The remaining adverse effects occur in 1% to 3% of patients.

Contraindications

Nesiritide is contraindicated in patients who have a known hypersensitivity to natriuretic peptide agents. It is also contraindicated in patients in cardiogenic shock. It should not be administered if the systolic blood pressure is less than 90 mm Hg.

Nursing Implications

Nesiritide is used infrequently.

Preventing Interactions

The administration of antihypertensive agents with nesiritide will increase nesiritide's hypotensive effects.

Nesiritide administered with bayberry, black cohosh, cayenne, ephedra, ginger, kola, or licorice will increase blood pressure. Nesiritide administered with goldenseal, hawthorne, mistletoe, periwinkle, or quinine will enhance hypotension.

Administering the Medication

Nesiritide is administered through a separate IV line because it should not be mixed with other medications. In the event of severe hypotension, the administration of nesiritide should be discontinued. It is important that the patient be adequately hydrated during the administration of nesiritide. The reconstituted solution of the medication must be replaced every 24 hours. Hemodynamic monitoring of the pulmonary artery pressure is mandatory to determine drug effectiveness.

Patient Teaching

Patient teaching guidelines are found in Box 24.8.

NCLEX Success

10. A patient is admitted to the emergency department with uncontrolled shortness of breath and is diagnosed with acute heart failure. The patient is given nesiritide (Natrecor), 140 mcg by IV bolus. Which of the following symptoms would result in the discontinuation of nesiritide?

A. bradycardia
B. tachycardia
C. hypertension
D. hypotension

TABLE 24.5 — DRUGS AT A GLANCE: Nesiritide (Natrecor)

Drug	Pregnancy Category	Routes and Dosage Ranges	
		Adults	Children
Ⓟ Nesiritide (Natrecor)	C	2 mcg/kg IV bolus followed by a continuous infusion of 0.01 mcg/kg for no longer than 48 h	Not recommended for use in children

<table>
<tr><td>**BOX 24.8**</td><td>**Patient Teaching Guidelines for Nesiritide (Natrecor)**</td></tr>
</table>

- While you are taking this medication, frequent monitoring of your blood pressure, pulse, and heart rhythm will be necessary.
- Because bed rest must be maintained, please call for assistance with toileting.
- Report pain at the injection site to the nurse.
- Report any numbness or tingling, shortness of breath, or chest pain.

Adjuvant Medications Used to Treat Heart Failure

Adjuvant medications are administered for heart failure to support the treatment and resolution of symptoms. These adjuvant medications are summarized in Table 24.6.

Loop Diuretics

ⓟ **Furosemide** (Lasix) is the prototype for the loop diuretics. Furosemide is administered to patients with moderate to severe heart failure to reduce edema. Furosemide is administered with food to prevent gastric upset. When a patient is being treated with furosemide, the nurse weighs the patient daily and reports any increase in weight of greater than 2 pounds in 24 hours to the health care provider. Fluid and electrolyte levels must be assessed frequently to identify extracellular fluid overload or dehydration. The nurse assesses blood pressure, pulse, and respirations daily. A potassium-rich, low-sodium diet is recommended, and potassium supplements may be ordered. In patients with diabetes mellitus, the nurse assesses blood glucose levels frequently because furosemide therapy may cause an increase in blood glucose levels.

Thiazide Diuretics

The prototype drug for the thiazide diuretics is ⓟ **hydrochlorothiazide** (HCTZ, HydroDIURIL). Hydrochlorothiazide inhibits the reabsorption of sodium and chloride in the distal

TABLE 24.6

DRUGS AT A GLANCE: Adjuvant Drugs for the Treatment of Heart Failure

Drug	Pregnancy Category	Routes and Dosage Ranges	
		Adults	*Children*
ⓟ **Furosemide** (Lasix)	C	20–80 mg PO daily; a second dose can be administered 6–8 h after the initial daily dose 20–40 mg IV push over 1–2 min; dose can be increased in increments of 20 mg in 2 h Renal impairment: Up to 4 mg/d has been tolerated IV bolus injection should not exceed 1 g/d given over 30 min	2 mg/kg PO daily 1 mg/kg IV or IM; may increase dosage by 1 mg/kg in 2 h until desired effect is seen
ⓟ **Hydrochlorothiazide** (HCTZ, HydroDIURIL)	B	25–100 mg PO daily until adequate fluid loss is attained, then 25–100 mg PO daily Total dose not to exceed 200 mg/d	1–2 mg/kg/d PO in 1–2 doses
ⓟ **Enalapril maleate** (Vasotec)	C in first trimester D in second and third trimesters	2.5 mg PO daily or BID in conjunction with diuretic and digitalis; maintenance daily dosage is 2.5–20 mg/daily 0.625 mg IV over 5 min Renal impairment: Use smaller initial dose and adjust upward to a maximum of 40 mg/d PO	1 mon to 16 y: initial dose 0.08 mg/kg PO once daily; maximum dose is 5 mg
ⓟ **Losartan potassium** (Cozaar)	C in first trimester D in second and third trimesters	Starting dose of 50 mg PO daily	6 y and older: 0.7 mg/kg daily; not to exceed a maximum dose of 50 mg/d
ⓟ **Propranolol hydrochloride** (Inderal)	C	40 mg PO twice daily Sustained release: 80 mg PO daily Total dose not to exceed 640 mg PO daily	Not recommended for use in children
ⓟ **Spironolactone** (Aldactone)	C	100 mg/d PO initially; 25–200 mg/d when given as the sole agent; continue at least 5 d, then adjust dose or add another diuretic	Not recommended for use in children

renal tubule, increasing the excretion of sodium and water by the kidneys. It is administered for edema associated with early or mild heart failure. Decreasing the plasma volume increases cardiac output and decreases preload.

Prior to administering hydrochlorothiazide, the nurse assesses the patient for allergy to thiazides and sulfonamides. The nurse also assesses the blood pressure and pulse before administering the medication and periodically following administration. Hydrochlorothiazide is administered with food to prevent gastric upset. Throughout therapy, the nurse assesses the patient's lungs (for adventitious sounds), heart (for an S3), and extremities (for peripheral edema); the patient's fluid and electrolyte status; and the patient's weight (daily). Any increase in weight of greater than 2 pounds in 24 hours must be reported to the primary health care provider.

Angiotensin-Converting Enzyme Inhibitors

The prototype agent for the angiotensin-converting enzyme (ACE) inhibitors is Ⓟ **enalapril maleate** (Vasotec). Enalapril maleate blocks the conversion of angiotensin I to angiotensin II, which is a potent vasoconstrictor. By blocking the production of angiotensin II, enalapril maleate promotes vasodilation (decreasing blood pressure) and decreases aldosterone secretion (increasing serum potassium levels and reducing sodium and water retention). The medication also increases prostaglandin synthesis to decrease blood pressure.

Enalapril maleate is used to treat hypertension, acute and chronic heart failure, and asymptomatic left ventricular dysfunction. The ACE inhibitors are the first choice of drugs used to treat chronic heart failure. All of the ACE inhibitors have similar effects, but enalapril, captopril (Capoten), lisinopril (Prinivil, Zestril), quinapril hydrochloride (Accupril), and ramipril (Altace) are Food and Drug Administration (FDA)– approved for the treatment of heart failure.

As with the diuretic agents, the nurse assesses the patient for allergy to the drug or any drug in the class. The nurse assesses the patient's fluid volume status and withholds the medication held in the event of fluid volume depletion. The nurse assesses the patient's blood pressure and pulse prior to administration and periodically 4 to 6 hours after administration, because that is the peak of action. The nurse teaches the patient not to stop the medication without the primary health care provider's knowledge and how to recognize adverse effects that need to be reported immediately to the health care provider. The nurse instructs women of childbearing age to use contraception while taking the medication because of the risk for fetal abnormalities or death.

Angiotensin II–Receptor Blockers

Ⓟ **Losartan potassium** (Cozaar) is the prototype drug for the angiotensin II–receptor blocker (ARB) class of drugs. Losartan potassium selectively blocks the binding of angiotensin II to specific tissue receptors found in the vascular smooth muscle and adrenal glands. This, in turn, blocks the vasoconstrictive effect of the renin–angiotensin system and the release of aldosterone, leading to a decrease in the patient's blood pressure.

Losartan potassium is administered singly or in combination with other medications for the treatment of hypertension. The control of blood pressure prevents vasoconstriction, which contributes to heart failure. All of the ARBs are approved for the treatment of hypertension; however, only valsartan (Diovan) has received FDA approval for treatment of patients with moderate to severe heart failure and those unable to tolerate ACE inhibitors due to adverse effects such as cough.

Prior to administering losartan potassium, the nurse assesses the patient for pregnancy and hypersensitivity reactions to this class of medications and for the use of herbs that could interfere with drug's action. The nurse assesses the patient's blood pressure, pulse, respirations, and lung sounds prior to administering the medication. In the event of hypovolemia, the medication is held. The nurse teaches the patient to take the medication as ordered and to protect from injury related to decreases in blood pressure.

Beta-Adrenergic Blocking Agents

Beta-adrenergic blocking agents have become an adjuvant medication in the treatment of heart failure in light of increased evidence that supports their ability to decrease morbidity and mortality in patients with chronic heart failure. Beta-blockers suppress the sympathetic nervous system and the resulting catecholamine excess that eventually damages myocardial cells, reduces myocardial beta receptors, and reduces cardiac output. As a result, over time, **ventricular remodeling** (dilatation and hypertrophy of the ventricles) regresses, the heart returns toward a normal shape and function, and cardiac output increases. The prototype medication for the beta-adrenergic blocking agents is Ⓟ **propranolol hydrochloride** (Inderal).

Propranolol hydrochloride (Inderal) competitively blocks the beta-adrenergic receptors in the heart and juxtaglomerular apparatus to decrease the influence of the sympathetic nervous system on these tissues. The resultant diminished excitability of the heart reduces cardiac workload and oxygen consumption.

Prior to the administration of propranolol hydrochloride, the nurse determines if the patient has had any hypersensitivity reactions to beta-blockers or conditions that contraindicate use of the medication. Use of the herb betel palm blocks the reduction in heart rate that is produced by beta-adrenergic blocking agents. The nurse assesses the patient's weight and cardiopulmonary status and for the presence of dizziness, drowsiness, syncope, or blurred vision. The nurse instructs the patient to report shortness of breath, night cough, edema, slow pulse, confusion, depression, rash, fever, or sore throat and explains that therapy with propranolol should never be stopped abruptly.

The FDA has issued a **BLACK BOX WARNING** ◆ for beta-adrenergic blocking agents for patients with coronary artery disease: withdrawing oral forms of the class may result in exacerbation of angina, increased incidence of ventricular dysrhythmias, and the occurrence of myocardial infarctions.

Aldosterone Antagonists

Increased aldosterone is a major factor in the pathophysiology of heart failure. Increased aldosterone levels result in interstitial fibrosis, which may decrease systolic function and increase the risk for dysrhythmias. ℗ **Spironolactone** (Aldactone), the prototype drug in this class, is an aldosterone antagonist that reduces aldosterone-induced retention of sodium and water and impaired vascular function. In patients with heart failure and inadequate renal function, the addition of spironolactone allows smaller doses of loop diuretics and potassium supplements to be administered. Overall, studies indicate that the addition of spironolactone improves cardiac function and reduces symptoms, hospitalizations, and mortality in patients with heart failure.

Spironolactone is used to decrease edema in patients with heart failure. A second drug in this class, eplerenone (Inspra), is approved for use in the management of heart failure after myocardial infarction to improve survival.

The nurse assesses the patient's blood pressure and pulse prior to administering the medication. Prior to beginning therapy, a baseline ECG is obtained and electrolyte status and renal function are assessed. The nurse instructs the patient to take salicylates only if prescribed by the health care provider, because salicylates can decrease the effects of aldosterone antagonists. The nurse also advises the patient to avoid using herb licorice, which blocks the effects of aldosterone antagonists.

Clinical Application 24-3

- In addition to digoxin, the cardiologist prescribed spironolactone and enalapril maleate for Dr. Adams. How will digoxin, spironolactone, and enalapril maleate assist in decreasing Dr. Adams' symptoms?

NCLEX Success

11. **A patient is taking furosemide (Lasix), 40 mg daily, to decrease extracellular fluid related to heart failure. During patient teaching, which of the following points is most important for the nurse to convey?**

    A. Sodium intake should be increased due to fluid loss.
    B. Administration of the medication with food will decrease absorption.
    C. The skin should be protected from sun exposure using sunscreen.
    D. Foods that contain potassium should be limited to prevent hyperkalemia.

12. **A 35-year-old woman has been prescribed enalapril maleate (Vasotec). What should the nurse teach the patient?**

    A. Use effective contraception.
    B. Double the dose if one is missed.
    C. If dizziness occurs, it is not a concern.
    D. There is no change in dose with impaired renal function.

13. **What is the purpose of administering an angiotensin II–receptor blocker to a patient with heart failure?**

    A. It will increase vasoconstriction to increase myocardial contractility.
    B. It will block the influx of calcium across the sinoatrial node.
    C. It will inhibit the enzyme that catalyzes cholesterol synthesis.
    D. It will block the renin–angiotensin II system to increase vasodilation.

The Nursing Process

Assessment

- **Assess for current or potential heart failure.**
  - Identify risk factors for heart failure.
    - Cardiovascular disorders: atherosclerosis, hypertension, coronary artery disease, myocardial infarction, cardiac dysrhythmias, cardiac valvular disease
    - Noncardiovascular disorders: severe infections, hyperthyroidism, pulmonary disease (e.g., cor pulmonale)
    - Other factors: fluid volume overload related to parenteral fluids or blood transfusions, increased age, third spacing
  - Interview and observe for signs and symptoms of chronic heart failure.
    - Mild heart failure: peripheral edema (feet and ankles), dyspnea on exertion, fatigue with ordinary activity
    - Moderate to severe heart failure: more extensive edema, dyspnea at rest, orthopnea, paroxysmal nocturnal dyspnea, cough related to congestion of the respiratory tract with venous blood, confusion from cerebral hypoxia, oliguria from decreased blood flow to the kidneys, anxiety
  - Observe for signs and symptoms of acute heart failure (a medical emergency).
    - Acute pulmonary edema
- **Assess for atrial tachydysrhythmias.**
  - Record the rate and rhythm of apical and radial pulses.
  - Check the electrocardiogram (ECG) for abnormal P waves, rapid ventricular rate, and QRS complexes of normal configuration but irregular intervals.
- **Assess baseline vital signs, weight, edema, serum electrolytes (including potassium, magnesium, and calcium), and other laboratory values indicative of cardiovascular function.**
- **Assess baseline ECG before initiating digoxin therapy. ECG changes from normal could indicate digitalis toxic-**

ity. **Changes from baseline may promote early recognition of drug-induced dysrhythmias.**

Nursing Diagnoses

- Ineffective tissue perfusion related to decreased cardiac output
- Anxiety related to chronic illness and lifestyle changes
- Impaired gas exchange related to venous congestion and fluid accumulation in the lungs
- Activity intolerance related to impaired gas exchange and fatigue
- Imbalanced nutrition: less than body requirements related to digoxin-induced anorexia, nausea, and vomiting
- Noncompliance related to the need for long-term drug therapy and regular medical supervision
- Deficient knowledge: managing drug therapy regimen safely and effectively

Planning/Goals

The patient will

- Take digoxin and other medications safely and accurately
- Experience improved breathing and less fatigue and edema
- Maintain serum digoxin level within therapeutic ranges
- Be closely monitored for therapeutic and adverse effects, especially related to digitalization; changes in dosage; and when other drugs are added to or removed from the management regimen
- Maintain appointments with health care providers to monitor vital signs, serum electrolyte levels, serum digoxin levels, and renal function

Nursing Interventions

The nurse will

- Implement measures to minimize and prevent heart failure and atrial dysrhythmias
- Instruct the patient on sensible eating habits, which include a balanced diet, avoidance of excessive saturated fat and salt, and weight control
- Instruct the patient to avoid cigarette smoking
- Instruct the patient on the implementation of regular exercise
- Implement measures to treat hypertension
- Implement measures to reduce hypoxia
- Implement a low-sodium diet
- Avoid fluid overload, especially in elderly patients
- Maintain management programs for heart failure, atrial dysrhythmias, and other cardiovascular or noncardiovascular disorders
- Monitor vital signs, urine output, and serum potassium levels regularly, and compare with baseline values
- Monitor ECGs when available and compare with baseline or previous ECGs

- Implement appropriate teaching related to drug therapy
- Administer oxygen if needed to relieve dyspnea, improve oxygen delivery, reduce the work of breathing, and decrease the constriction of pulmonary blood vessels

Evaluation

- Interview and observe for relief of symptoms (weight loss, increased urine output, decreased peripheral edema, decreased or elimination of shortness of breath, improved activity tolerance, diminished heart rate, increased ability to perform self-care).
- Observe serum drug levels for normal or abnormal values.
- Interview regarding compliance with instructions for the administration of medications.
- Interview and observe for adverse drug effects.

Clinical Application 24-4

- What aspects of patient teaching are most important in the care of Dr. Adams?
- What dietary modifications are important in Dr. Adams' care?

NCLEX Success

14. **A patient is diagnosed with heart failure. Which of the following nonpharmacological interventions will be a priority in decreasing edema?**

    A. Administer a diuretic agent.
    B. Limit dietary sodium.
    C. Place the patient on bed rest.
    D. Increase dietary protein.

15. **A patient is coughing and short of breath. He has productive frothy sputum. He is diagnosed with heart failure. Which of the following nursing diagnoses is most appropriate given the assessment data?**

    A. Ineffective Tissue Perfusion
    B. Activity Intolerance
    C. Impaired Gas Exchange
    D. Anxiety

16. **Which of the following patient goals indicates that the patient will maintain adequate follow-up care related to heart failure?**

    A. maintain weight reduction
    B. experience less fatigue
    C. administer medications
    D. maintain regular medical appointments

Key Concepts

- Heart failure results from impaired myocardial contractility during systole (systolic dysfunction), impaired relaxation and filing of ventricles during diastole (diastolic dysfunction), or a combination of systolic and diastolic dysfunction.
- Right-sided heart failure results from an accumulation of blood in the systemic venous system.
- Left-sided heart failure results in a decrease in cardiac output related to an increase in left atrial and left ventricular end-diastolic pressures and congestion in the pulmonary circulation.
- Cardinal manifestations of heart failure are dyspnea and fatigue, which lead to exercise intolerance and fluid retention, resulting in pulmonary congestion and peripheral edema.
- Digoxin (Lanoxin) produces a cardiotonic or positive inotropic effect, which improves contractility and pumping ability of the heart.
- Digitalis toxicity is one of the most commonly encountered drug-related reasons for hospitalization because digitalis has a narrow therapeutic index and the end point of effective therapy is often difficult to define and measure.
- The normal digoxin level is 0.8 to 2.0 nanograms per milliliter.
- Milrinone lactate (Primacor) is administered for short-term management of acute or severe heart failure in patients who do not respond to treatment with digoxin, diuretics, and vasodilators.
- Nesiritide (Natrecor) is a vasodilator used in the management of heart failure.
- For acute heart failure, the first drugs of choice may include a loop diuretic administered intravenously, a cardiotonic–inotropic agent (e.g., digoxin, milrinone), and vasodilators.
- The FDA has issued a **BLACK BOX WARNING** ◆ for beta-adrenergic blocking agents for patients with coronary artery disease: withdrawing oral forms of the class may result in exacerbation of angina, increased incidence of ventricular dysrhythmias, and the occurrence of myocardial infarctions.

Critical Thinking Questions

24-1. A 72-year-old patient who weighs 74 kg is admitted to the cardiac intensive care unit in severe heart failure. The physician has ordered a loading dose of milrinone lactate (Primacor) of 50 mcg/kg IV bolus followed by a maintenance dose of 0.5 mcg/kg/min.

- What amount of milrinone lactate is to be administered in the IV bolus? Is the dose in an acceptable range?
- What is the amount of milrinone lactate to be administered in the maintenance dose? Is the dose in an acceptable range?
- What is the action of milrinone lactate?
- What are the adverse effects of milrinone lactate?
- What are the nursing interventions to be implemented in the administration of milrinone lactate?

24-2. A patient has a past history of heart failure and is controlled on digoxin (Lanoxin), 0.125 mg daily. The nurse in the hospital and the home care nurse provided the patient with information about the adverse effects of digoxin, including digoxin toxicity. The patient has noticed that for the past 2 days, she has not had an appetite and she is nauseated. She makes an appointment with her health care provider, who orders a serum digoxin level and serum electrolyte panel. The results of the blood tests reveal a digoxin level of 10 ng/mL and a calcium level of 12 mg/dL. The patient is administered digoxin immune fab (Digibind), 9.5 mg. Additional diagnostic studies are ordered, including a chest radiograph. The chest radiograph reveals a large mass in the right lower lobe of the lung.

- What is digoxin immune fab (Digibind)? How does digoxin immune fab (Digibind) work?
- How is the development of digoxin toxicity related to the increase in serum calcium levels?

References and Resources

American Heart Association. (2006). *AHA statistical update: Heart and stroke statistics 2006*. Retrieved July 1, 2009, from http://circ.ahajournals.org/cgi/content/short/113/6/e85

American Heart Association. (2009). *Medications commonly used to treat heart failure*. Retrieved June 29, 2009, from http://www.americanheart.org/presenter.jhtml?identifier=118

Drug facts and comparisons. (Updated monthly). St. Louis, MO: Facts and Comparisons.

Ebert, E. (2006). *Hypoxic liver injury*. Retrieved July 13, 2009, from www.mayoclinicproceedings.com. *81*(9), 1231–1236.

Hunt, S. A., Abraham, W. T., Chin, M. H., Feldman, F. A., Francis, G. S., Ganiats, T. G., et al. (2005). ACC/AHA 2005 *guideline update for the diagnosis and management of chronic heart failure for the adult-summary article: A report of the American College of Cardiology/American Heart Association Task Force for Practice Guidelines (writing committee to revise the 2001 Guidelines for the Evaluation and Management of Heart Failure)*. Retrieved July 14, 2009, from http://www.guidelines.gov/summary/summary.aspx?doc_id=7664

Karch, A. M. (2012). *2012 Lippincott's nursing drug guide*. Philadelphia, PA: Lippincott Williams & Wilkins.

Lexi-Comp. Nesiritide Drug Information. Retrieved August 1, 2009, from http://www.merck.com/mmpe/lexicomp/nesiritide.html

Porth, C. M. (2009). *Pathophysiology: Concepts of altered health status* (8th ed.). Philadelphia, PA: Lippincott Williams & Wilkins.

Rasmussen, K. D., Hall, J. A., & Renlund, D. G. (2006). Heart failure epidemic boiling to the surface. *The Nurse Practitioner, 31*(11). Retrieved July 14, 2009, from www.tnpj.com

Smeltzer, S. C., Bare, B. G., Hinkle, J. L., & Cheever, K. H. (2008). *Brunner and Suddarth's: Textbook of medical-surgical nursing* (11th ed). Philadelphia, PA: Lippincott Williams & Wilkins.

25 Drug Therapy for Dysrhythmias

LEARNING OBJECTIVES

After studying this chapter, you should be able to:

1. Give an overview of the cardiac electrophysiology and an outline of specific cardiac dysrhythmias that affect heart rhythm, heart rate, or both.

2. Describe principles of therapy in the management of dysrhythmias, including measures that do not involve antidysrhythmic drugs.

3. Identify the prototype and describe the action, use, adverse effects, contraindications, and nursing implications for class I sodium channel blockers.

4. Identify the prototype and outline the action, use, adverse effects, contraindications, and nursing implications for beta-adrenergic blockers.

5. Identify the prototype and explain the action, use, adverse effects, contraindications, and nursing implications for potassium channel blockers.

6. Identify the prototype and describe the action, use, adverse effects, contraindications, and nursing implications for calcium channel blockers.

7. Describe the nursing process implications and actions related to caring for patients using selected antidysrhythmic drugs.

Clinical Application Case Study

Bill Brown is a 74-year-old man with cardiovascular disease. He has just undergone cardiac bypass surgery for two coronary artery bypasses. During the postoperative period, he develops premature ventricular complexes followed by atrial fibrillation.

KEY TERMS

Antidysrhythmic: medication used for prevention and treatment of a cardiac dysrhythmia.

Automaticity: ability of the heart to generate an electrical impulse.

Conductivity: ability of cardiac tissue to transmit electrical impulses.

Dysrhythmia: abnormality in heart rate or rhythm.

Ectopic: when an electrical impulse arises from an abnormal focus, anywhere other than the sinoatrial node.

Excitability: ability of a cardiac muscle cell to respond to an electrical stimulus.

Prodysrhythmic effects: tendency of antidysrhythmic drugs to cause the development of new dysrhythmias.

Tachydysrhythmia: dysrhythmia of greater than 100 beats per minute.

Introduction

This chapter discusses the **antidysrhythmic** agents, the medications that are used for prevention and treatment of cardiac dysrhythmias. A **dysrhythmia** is an abnormality in heart rate or rhythm. It can become significant if it interferes with cardiac function, thereby altering the ability to adequately pump and causing inadequate perfusion of the body tissues.

Overview of Dysrhythmias

Physiology

To aid in understanding antidysrhythmic drug therapy, it is necessary to review the physiology of the cardiac electrophysiologic conduction system. The heart is an electrical pump. The "electrical" activity resides primarily in the specialized tissues that can generate and conduct an electrical impulse. The mechanical or "pump" activity resides in contractile tissue. Normally, the synchronization of these activities results in effective cardiac contraction and distribution of blood throughout the body. Each heartbeat occurs at regular intervals and consists of four events: stimulation from an electrical impulse, transmission of the electrical impulse to adjacent conductive or contractile tissue, contraction of atria and then ventricles, and then relaxation of atria and then ventricles. Certain properties are inherent in cardiac cells. Two of these properties are automaticity and conductivity.

Automaticity

Automaticity is the heart's ability to generate an electrical impulse. Any part of the conduction system can spontaneously start an impulse, but the sinoatrial (SA) node normally has the fastest rate of automaticity and therefore the faster rate of spontaneous impulse formation.

Initiation of an electrical impulse depends predominantly on the movement of sodium and calcium ions into a myocardial cell and movement of potassium ions out of the cell. Normally, the cell membrane becomes more permeable to sodium and opens certain channels to allow rapid movement of sodium into the cell. Calcium ions follow sodium ions into the cell at a slower rate and through different channels. As sodium and calcium ions move into cells, potassium ions move out of cells. The movement of the ions changes the membrane from its resting state of electrical neutrality to an activated state of electrical energy buildup. After the electrical energy is discharged (depolarization), muscle contraction occurs. The ease in which cardiac cells undergoes this series of events is call cardiac **excitability**.

Conductivity

Conductivity is the ability of cardiac tissue to transmit electrical impulses. The orderly, rhythmic transmission of impulses to all cells is needed for effective myocardial contraction. The cardiac conduction system is shown in Figure 25.1. Normally, electrical impulses originate in the SA node and are transmitted through internodal pathways to the atrioventricular (AV) node, where the impulse is delayed for a period of time. Then the impulse travels through the bundle of His, bundle branches, Purkinje fibers, and throughout the ventricular muscle.

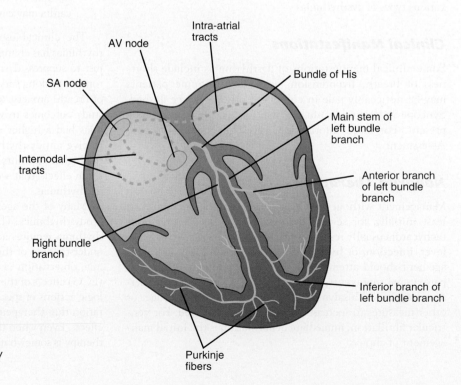

Figure 25.1 The conducting system of the heart. Impulses originating in the sinoatrial (SA) node are transmitted through the atria, into the atrioventricular (AV) node to the Bundle of His, and by way of Purkinje fibers through the ventricles.

Etiology

Cardiac dysrhythmias originate in any part of the conduction system or in atrial or ventricular muscle. They result from disturbances in electrical impulse formation (automaticity), conduction (conductivity), or both. The inherent characteristic of automaticity allows myocardial cells other than the SA node to depolarize and initiate the electrical impulse that culminates in contraction. This may occur when the SA node fails to initiate an impulse or does so too slowly. When the electrical impulse arises anywhere other than the SA node, the focus is abnormal or **ectopic**. If the ectopic focus depolarizes at a rate faster than the SA node, the ectopic focus becomes the dominant pacemaker. Conditions such as hypoxia, ischemia, or hypokalemia may activate ectopic pacemakers. Ectopic foci indicate myocardial irritability, which can increase responsiveness to stimuli, leading to potentially serious impairment of cardiac function. Atrial fibrillation is the most common dysrhythmia.

Pathophysiology

Dysrhythmias may be clinically significant if they interfere with cardiac function and thus alter the heart's ability to pump sufficient blood to body tissues. The normal heart can maintain an adequate cardiac output with ventricular rates ranging from 40 to 150 beats per minute. The diseased heart, however, may not be able to maintain an adequate cardiac output with heart rates below 60 or above 120 beats per minute. These alterations in rates are referred to as dysrhythmias, which are usually categorized by rate, location, or patterns of conduction. **Tachydysrhythmias** are heart rates greater than 100 beats per minute. Bradydysrhythmias are those less than 60 beats per minute. Atropine, which is used to treat bradydysrhythmias, is discussed in Chapter 47, and digoxin, which is used to treat atrial fibrillation, is discussed in Chapter 24. Box 25.1 describes various types of dysrhythmias.

Clinical Manifestations

Some clinical manifestations of dysrhythmias include shortness of breath, hypotension, and anxiety. Some patients may be noticeably pale in color, and others may be flushed. Syncope or mental confusion may occur. Oliguria may be present. For more information, see The Nursing Process, Assessment.

Nondrug Therapy

Management without the use of drugs may be preferable, at least initially, for several dysrhythmias. For example, sinus tachycardia usually results from such disorders as dehydration, fever, infection, or hypotension, and intervention and management should attempt to relieve the underlying cause. For paroxysmal supraventricular tachycardia with mild or moderate symptoms, Valsalva maneuver, carotid sinus massage, or other measures to increase vagal tone are preferred. For ventricular fibrillation, immediate defibrillation is the initial management of choice.

In addition to these strategies, use of other measures is increasing. The impetus for nonpharmacologic management developed mainly from studies demonstrating that antidysrhythmic drugs could worsen existing dysrhythmias, cause new dysrhythmias, and cause higher mortality rates in patients receiving the drugs than patients not receiving the drugs. Current technology allows clinicians to insert pacemakers and defibrillators (e.g., implantable cardioverter defibrillators) to control bradydysrhythmias or tachydysrhythmias and to use radio waves (radiofrequency catheter ablation) or surgery to deactivate ectopic foci.

Drug Therapy

All drugs used to combat dysrhythmias alter the electrical conduction system of the heart. The drugs used for the treatment of tachydysrhythmias are the focus of this chapter. They reduce automaticity, which is the spontaneous depolarization of myocardial cells, including ectopic pacemakers. They also slow conduction of electrical impulses through the heart and prolong the refractory period of myocardial cells so they are less likely to be prematurely activated by adjacent cells. Antidysrhythmic drug therapy is commonly indicated in the following conditions:

- Conversion of atrial fibrillation or atrial flutter to normal sinus rhythm (NSR)
- Maintaining NSR after conversion from atrial fibrillation or atrial flutter
- Suppression of a fast or irregular ventricular rate, which alters the cardiac output. Altered cardiac output leads to symptoms of decreased coronary, cerebral, and/or systemic circulation.
- Presence of dangerous dysrhythmias that may be fatal if not quickly terminated. For example, ventricular tachycardia may cause cardiac arrest.

The clinical use of antidysrhythmic drugs for tachydysrhythmias has changed over the years. Clinicians use drugs not just to suppress dysrhythmias but to prevent or relieve symptoms or prolong survival. Symptoms may manifest as shortness of breath, anxiety, or racing heart. This change resulted from study outcomes in which patients treated for some dysrhythmias had a higher mortality rate than patients who did not receive antidysrhythmic drug therapy. Researchers attributed the higher mortality rate to **prodysrhythmic effects**, which are those effects that worsen existing dysrhythmias or cause new dysrhythmias.

Many of the agents used to treat dysrhythmias are in fact prodysrhythmics. Thus, rational drug therapy for a cardiac dysrhythmia requires accurate identification of the dysrhythmia, understanding of the basic mechanisms causing the dysrhythmia, observation of the hemodynamic and electrocardiogram (ECG) effects of the dysrhythmia, knowledge of the pharmacologic actions of specific antidysrhythmic drugs, and the expectation that therapeutic effects will outweigh potential adverse effects. Even when these criteria are met, antidysrhythmic drug therapy is somewhat empiric.

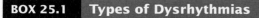

BOX 25.1   Types of Dysrhythmias

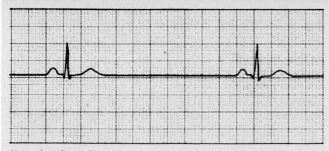

Sinus bradycardia

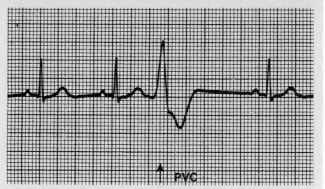

Premature ventricular contraction

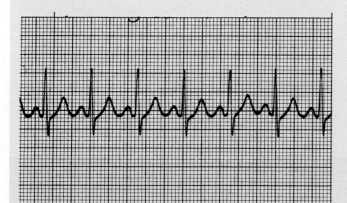

Sinus tachycardia

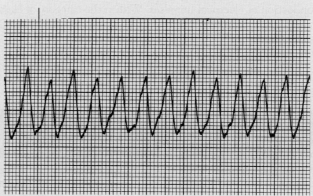

Ventricular tachycardia

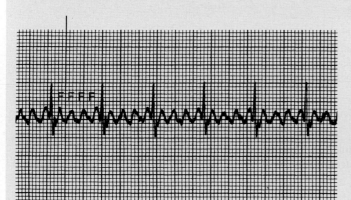

Atrial flutter

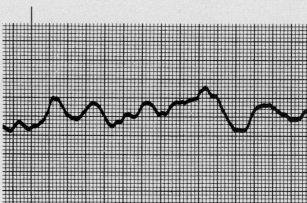

Ventricular fibrillation

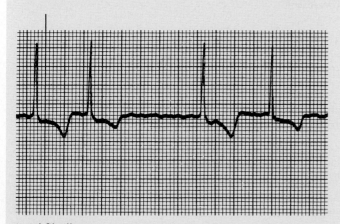

Atrial fibrillation

Several different groups of drugs function as antidysrhythmics. They are classified according to their mechanisms of action and effects on the conduction system, even though they differ in other respects. Some drugs have characteristics of more than one group. There are various types of antidysrhythmics: class I sodium channel blockers, class II beta-adrenergic blockers, class III potassium channel blockers, and class IV calcium channel blockers (Table 25.1).

Class I Sodium Channel Blockers

Class I drugs block cardiac sodium channels and slow conduction velocity, prolonging refractoriness and decreasing automaticity of sodium-dependent tissue. This results in a membrane-stabilizing effect and also decreases formation and conduction of electrical impulses. Within the category of class I drugs are subcategories, the class IA, class IB, and class IC medications.

CLASS IA

The prototype class IA drug is Ⓟ **quinidine**. Table 25.2 presents dosages for quinidine and the other class IA sodium channel blockers.

Pharmacokinetics

Quinidine is well absorbed after oral administration, with a usual onset of 1 to 3 hours. After intramuscular (IM) administration, onset occurs within 30 to 90 minutes, and after intravenous (IV) administration, onset is rapid. Therapeutic serum levels (2–6 mcg/mL) are attained within 1 hour and persist for 6 to 8 hours. (Serum levels greater than 6 mcg/mL are toxic.) Quinidine is highly bound to serum albumin and has a half-life of about 6 to 7 hours. It is metabolized by the liver (about 80%) and excreted in the urine (about 20%) as well as the feces. In alkaline urine (i.e., pH > 7), renal excretion of quinidine decreases, and serum levels may rise.

TABLE 25.1			
Drugs Administered for the Treatment of Dysrhythmias			
Class of Antidysrhythmic Drug	**Prototype**	**Other Drugs in the Class**	**Use**
Class I Sodium Channel Blockers			
Class IA	Quinidine	Procainamide (Pronestyl, Procanbid) Disopyramide (Norpace)	Maintenance of normal sinus rhythm after conversion of A-fib or atrial flutter; treatment of symptomatic PVCs, SVT, and VT; prevention of V-fib
Class IB	Lidocaine (Xylocaine)	Mexiletine (Mexitil)	Treatment of symptomatic PVCs and VT; prevention of V-fib
Class IC		Flecainide (Tambocor) Propafenone (Rythmol)	Treatment of life-threatening VT or V-fib and SVT unresponsive to other drugs
Class II Beta-Adrenergic Blockers			
	Propranolol (Inderal)	Acebutolol (Sectral) Esmolol (Brevibloc) Sotalol (Betapace)	Treatment of SVT
Class III Potassium Channel Blockers			
	Amiodarone (Cordarone)	Dofetilide (Tikosyn) Ibutilide (Corvert) Sotalol (Betapace)	Treatment of VT and V-fib; conversion of atrial flutter or A-fib to sinus rhythm; maintenance of sinus rhythm
Class IV Calcium Channel Blockers			
	Diltiazem (Cardizem)	Verapamil (Calan, Isoptin)	Treatment of SVT
Unclassified			
		Adenosine Magnesium sulfate	Treatment of tachydysrhythmias; adenosine, SVT; magnesium sulfate, torsades de pointes

A-fib, atrial fibrillation; PVC, premature ventricular contractions; SVT, supraventricular tachycardia; V-fib, ventricular fibrillation; VT, ventricular tachycardia.

TABLE 25.2

DRUGS AT A GLANCE: Class I Sodium Channel Blockers

Drug	Pregnancy Category	Routes and Dosage Ranges	
		Adults	Children
Class IA ⓟ **Quinidine**	C	PO 200–300 mg every 6–8 h, or extended-action tablets, 300–600 mg every 8–12 h	PO 300 mg/kg/24 h in five equally divided doses; 2–10 mg/kg/dose IV every 3–6 h has been used, but this route is not recommended
Procainamide (Pronestyl, Procanbid)	C	PO 50 mg/kg/d in divided doses every 3 h. Maintenance dose of 50 mg/kg/d in divided doses every 6 h, starting 2–3 h after last dose of standard oral preparation IM loading dose, 0.5–1 g every 4–8 h until oral therapy can be started IV loading dose 100 mg every 5 min at a rate not to exceed 25–50 mg/min (max dose 1 g) IV infusion following a 500–600 mg loading dose over 25–30 min, then 2–6 mg/min	PO 15–50 mg/kg/d in three to six divided doses every 3–6 h, maximum, 4 g/d IM 20–30 mg/kg/d divided every 4–6 h; maximum 4 g/d IV loading dose 3–6 mg/kg over 5 min; maintenance dose of 20–80 mcg/kg/min continuous infusion; max 100 mg/d dose or 2 g/d. 2–5 mg/kg (maximum 100 mg repeated as necessary every 5–10 min; or, 15 mg/kg given over 30–60 min, followed by maintenance infusion
Disopyramide (Norpace)	C	PO 300 mg (immediate release), if no response within 6 h, give 200 mg every 6 h; may increase to 250–300 mg every 6 h if not response in 48 h	12–18 y: PO 6–15 mg/kg/d in equal divided doses 5–12 y: PO 10–15 mg/kg/d in equal divided doses 1–4 y: PO 10–20 mg/kg/d in equal divided doses <1 y : PO 10–30 mg/kg/d in equal divided doses
Class IB ⓟ **Lidocaine** (Xylocaine)	B	IV 50–100 mg at a rate of 25–50 mg/min; give a second bolus dose after 5 min if needed, not to exceed 200–300 mg in 1 h followed by a continuous infusion of 1–4 mg/min (or 20–50 mcg/kg/min) IM only use the 10% solution 300 mg in the deltoid or thigh muscle; may repeat in 60–90 min	Safety and efficacy have not been established IV injection 0.5–1 mg/kg bolus, followed by IV infusion of 30 mcg/kg/min with caution
Mexiletine (Mexitil)	C	PO 200 mg every 8 h initially, increased in 50 to 100 mg increments every 2–3 d if necessary to a maximum of 1200 mg/d	Safety and efficacy not established
Class IC Flecainide (Tambocor)	C	PO 50 mg every 12 h initially, increased by 50 mg every 12 h every 4 d until effective; maximum dose, 300 mg/d	Safety and efficacy in patients younger than 18 y have not been established
Propafenone (Rythmol)	C	PO 150 mg every 8 h initially, increase at 3–4 d intervals to 225 mg every 8 h, then to 300 mg every 8 h; maximum dose of 900 mg/d PO (extended release) 225 mg every 12 h initially, may increase at 5-d intervals; maximum 425 mg every 12 h	Safety and efficacy not established

Action

Quinidine reduces automaticity and slows conduction throughout the cardiac system. In addition, it prolongs the refractory period of the myocardial cells.

Use

Indications for quinidine include the treatment of (1) atrial dysrhythmias and (2) paroxysmal supraventricular tachycardia or chronic ventricular tachycardia without heart block. However, the drug is usually contraindicated in patients with severe, uncompensated heart failure or with heart block because it depresses myocardial contractility and conduction through the AV node. For disopyramide, another class IA drug, the Food and Drug Administration (FDA) has issued a **BLACK BOX WARNING** ◆ because of the drug's known prodysrhythmic properties; the drug should be reserved for patients with life-threatening ventricular dysrhythmias.

Use in Children

Pediatric patients take quinidine in the oral form. Although the IV route may be used, it is not recommended.

Use in Older Adults

There are no recommendations for precautions regarding the use of quinidine in older adults. However, because of the likelihood that aging may result in renal and hepatic problems, precautions regarding the use of quinidine in older patients should be considered.

Use in Patients With Renal Impairment

Reduced dosages of quinidine are necessary, with close monitoring. Caution is necessary, especially in patients with renal tubular acidosis.

Use in Patients With Hepatic Impairment

Hepatic impairment increases the plasma half-life of several antidysrhythmic drugs, including quinidine, and patients with hepatic impairment usually receive a reduced dosage. Close monitoring is essential. In addition, caution is warranted, especially in patients with hepatic insufficiency.

Use in Patients With Critical Illness

Critically ill patients often have multiple cardiovascular disorders as well as other conditions that increase the risk of acute, serious, and potentially life-threatening dysrhythmias. Patients may also have refractory dysrhythmias that require strong, potentially toxic antidysrhythmic drugs. Thus, antidysrhythmic drugs are often given intravenously in critical care settings for rapid reversal of a fast rhythm. After reversal, transitioning from IV drugs to oral ones is often necessary to prevent recurrence of the dysrhythmia. Frequently, potentials for renal and/or hepatic involvement are greater in patients who are critically ill. It is important to monitor responses to quinidine carefully, especially when beginning therapy.

Use in Patients Receiving Home Care

Patients receiving chronic antidysrhythmic drug therapy are likely to have significant cardiovascular disease. At each visit to the home, the nurse assesses the patient's physical, mental, and functional status and evaluates pulse and blood pressure. In addition, he or she also instructs patients and caregivers to report symptoms (e.g., dizziness or fainting, chest pain) and avoid over-the-counter agents unless approved by a health care provider.

Adverse Effects

Adverse effects of quinidine include central nervous system (CNS) changes, cardiac dysrhythmias, and gastrointestinal (GI) changes, as well as hematologic and hypersensitivity alterations. Most of the CNS changes relate to vision changes, including photophobia, blurring, loss of night vision, and diplopia. Cardiac dysrhythmias include conduction disturbances, including heart block and hypotension. GI effects include nausea, vomiting, diarrhea, and liver toxicity.

Contraindications

Quinidine is contraindicated in patients with an allergy to the drug. It is also contraindicated in second- or third-degree heart block, myasthenia gravis, pregnancy, lactation, and thrombocytopenic purpura.

Nursing Implications

Prior to the start of any new therapy, it is necessary to assess for allergies, second- or third-degree heart block, myasthenia gravis, pregnancy, lactation, and thrombocytopenic purpura. Physical assessment includes inspection of skin for color and the presence of lesions, determination of orientation status, assessment of cranial nerves, determination of bilateral grip strength and reflexes, auscultation of pulse and blood pressure, interpretation of the ECG, checking for edema, and auscultation of bowel sounds. It is also necessary to evaluate hepatic and renal function as well as to perform a urinalysis and complete blood count. The findings of the physical assessment as well as results of the laboratory work and diagnostic tests help develop the nursing plan of care for the patient who is beginning sodium channel blocker therapy.

Preventing Interactions

Preventing drug-drug and drug-food interactions requires knowledge of potential effects. Several medications interact with quinidine, increasing or decreasing its effect (Box 25.2).

BOX 25.2   Drug Interactions: Quinidine

Drugs That Increase the Effects of Quinidine
■ Cimetidine, amiodarone, verapamil
   Increase the risk of possible quinidine toxicity

Drugs That Decrease the Effects of Quinidine
■ Sodium bicarbonate
   Increases cardiac depressant effects
■ Phenobarbital, hydantoins, rifampin, sucralfate
   Decrease the levels of quinidine, leading to dysrhythmias

Use of quinidine with certain other drugs has specific results. With succinylcholine, neuromuscular blocking effects may increase. With digoxin, increased digoxin level and toxicity result. With oral anticoagulants, anticoagulant effect increases, and bleeding may occur. In addition, grapefruit juice, when given with quinidine, decreases the metabolism of quinidine and increases the risk of toxic drug effects.

Administering the Medication

When administering quinidine in the IV form, preparation includes diluting 800 mg in 50 mL of 5% dextrose. With an IV infusion, it is necessary to inject the quinidine slowly at a rate of 1 mL/min. The nurse should note that if Y-site administration is needed, quinidine is not compatible with furosemide.

Assessing for Therapeutic Effects

The nurse assesses for improvement in symptoms and for return of an organized cardiac rhythm. Physical assessment includes inspection of skin for adequate color and perfusion, clear mentation, and pulse and blood pressure within the patient's normal limits. It is also necessary to evaluate the adequacy of hepatic and renal function through laboratory testing.

Assessing for Adverse Effects

The nurse monitors patients who are taking quinidine for adverse effects. Physical assessment of the body systems that are potentially affected by the action of quinidine provide this surveillance. Of particular concern are the CNS, cardiac, GI, and hematologic systems, as well as possible hypersensitivity. It is necessary to determine whether adverse effects, particularly diarrhea, are manageable and are not complicating treatment.

Patient Teaching

The nurse gives teaching points to each patient to empower the patient and encourage and foster an environment inclusive of the patient's opinion and perspective. Quinidine, like any other drug, is taken exactly as prescribed. Sustained-release tablets should not be chewed. If GI upset occurs, then the medication may be taken with food. The nurse reminds the patient that frequent cardiac monitoring and blood tests are important for follow-up; these include regular checks of heart rhythm and blood counts. The patient teaching guidelines presented in Box 25.3 are important.

CLASS IB

Class IB drugs shorten the repolarization phase. ℗ **Lidocaine** (Xylocaine), the prototype class IB drug, is the drug of choice for treating serious ventricular dysrhythmias associated with acute myocardial infarction, cardiac catheterization, cardiac surgery, and digitalis-induced ventricular dysrhythmias. It decreases myocardial irritability (automaticity) in the ventricles. Lidocaine has little effect on atrial tissue and thus is not

---

BOX 25.3 **Patient Teaching Guidelines for Antidysrhythmic Drugs**

■ A fast heartbeat normally occurs in response to exercise, fever, and other conditions so that more blood can be pumped and carried to body tissues. An irregular heartbeat occurs occasionally in most people. However, when your health care provider prescribes a long-term medication to slow or regularize your heartbeat, this means that you have a potentially serious condition. In addition, the medications can cause potentially serious adverse effects. So, it is extremely important that you take the medications exactly as prescribed. Taking extra doses is dangerous; skipping doses or waiting longer between doses may lead to loss of control of the heart problem.

■ You may be given a drug classified as an antidysrhythmic or a drug from another group that has antidysrhythmic effects (e.g., a beta blocker such as propranolol, a calcium channel blocker such as diltiazem or verapamil). Follow the instructions for the specific drug ordered.

■ Be sure you know the names (generic and brand) of the medication, why you are receiving it, and what effects you can expect (therapeutic and adverse).

■ You will need continued medical supervision, along with periodic measurements of heart rate and blood pressure, blood tests, and electrocardiograms. Be sure to keep all health care appointments.

■ Try to learn the triggers for your irregular heartbeats and avoid them when possible (e.g., excessive caffeinated beverages, strenuous or excessive exercise).

■ Avoid over-the-counter cold and asthma remedies, appetite suppressants, and antisleep preparations, which are all stimulants that can cause or aggravate irregular heartbeats.

■ Take or give medications at evenly spaced intervals to maintain adequate blood levels. Take your medications at the same time each day.

■ Take amiodarone, mexiletine, and quinidine with food to decrease gastrointestinal symptoms.

■ Do not crush or chew sustained-release tablets or capsules.

■ Do not drink grapefruit juice if you are taking quinidine.

■ Wear a medical alert tag if recommended stating the health condition you have or the medications you are taking.

■ Report dizziness or fainting spells to your health care provider. This may mean the medication is decreasing your blood pressure too much, which is more likely to occur when starting or increasing the dose of an antidysrhythmic drug. Drug dosages may need to be adjusted.

■ Report any change in vision and complaints of nausea or vomiting, sun sensitivity, tremors, or loss of coordination to your health care provider. In addition, report unusual bleeding or bruising, fever, chills, intolerance to heat or cold, shortness of breath, difficulty breathing, cough, swelling of ankles or fingers, palpitation, or difficulty with vision.

useful in treating atrial dysrhythmias. The drug differs from quinidine in that it must be given by injection, does not decrease AV conduction with usual therapeutic doses, and has a rapid onset and short duration of action. After IV administration of a bolus dose, therapeutic effects occur within 1 to 2 minutes and last approximately 10 to 20 minutes. This characteristic is advantageous in emergency management but limits the use of lidocaine to intensive care settings. Lidocaine is metabolized in the liver; thus dosage must be reduced in patients with hepatic insufficiency or right-sided heart failure to avoid drug accumulation and toxicity. Serious adverse reactions with lidocaine are uncommon.

Therapeutic serum levels of lidocaine are 1.5 to 6 mcg/mL. Toxic serum levels are greater than 6 mcg/mL. Lidocaine is contraindicated in patients allergic to related local anesthetics (e.g., procaine). Anaphylactic reactions may occur in sensitized persons. Give lidocaine parenterally only as solutions labeled "for cardiac dysrhythmias," and do not use solutions containing epinephrine. Give an IV bolus over 2 minutes. Table 25.2 provides information about the dosages of lidocaine and related drugs.

QSEN Safety Alert

Lidocaine solutions that contain epinephrine are for local anesthesia only. It is essential that epinephrine-containing lidocaine solutions never be given intravenously to patients with cardiac dysrhythmias because the epinephrine can cause or aggravate dysrhythmias. Rapid injection of lidocaine (within approximately 30 seconds) produces transient blood levels several times greater than therapeutic range limits. Therefore, there is an increased risk of toxicity without a concomitant increase in therapeutic effectiveness.

Clinical Application 25-1

Mr. Brown begins taking IV lidocaine to control premature ventricular contractions. What therapeutic level of lidocaine should be the goal for this patient?

CLASS IC

Class IC drugs have no effect on the repolarization phase but slow conduction velocity and the refractory period. Flecainide and propafenone are oral agents that greatly decrease conduction in the ventricles. These drugs may cause new dysrhythmias or aggravate pre-existing dysrhythmias, sometimes causing sustained ventricular tachycardia or ventricular fibrillation. Thus, it is necessary to begin therapy in a hospital setting in patients with continuous ECG monitoring. The new or aggravated dysrhythmias are more likely to occur with high doses and rapid dose increases. Table 25.2 presents dosage information for these drugs.

Flecainide or propafenone may be used to suppress paroxysmal atrial flutter and fibrillation in patients with minimal or no heart disease. These class IC drugs are recommended for use in life-threatening ventricular dysrhythmias. The FDA has issued two **BLACK BOX WARNINGS** ◆ for flecainide:

- Drug treatment increases the risk of nonfatal cardiac arrest and death in patients with recent myocardial infarction or chronic atrial fibrillation.
- It is necessary to monitor carefully for a risk of potentially fatal prodysrhythmic effects.

NCLEX Success

1. A nurse is monitoring a patient who has been receiving quinidine in the critical care unit. The laboratory technician calls to report that the patient's serum quinidine level is 8 mcg/mL. The patient has also developed diarrhea. The priority action is to
   A. Report the findings to the provider immediately.
   B. Administer the medication as ordered.
   C. Anticipate that the dosage of the medication will increase.
   D. Anticipate that the dosage of the medication will decrease.

2. Ms. Ferguson, age 58, is admitted to the coronary care unit for treatment of an acute anterior myocardial infarction. That evening, she experiences frequent runs of ventricular tachycardia. The provider tells the nurse to prepare an IV bolus dose of lidocaine. Why is lidocaine administered intravenously at this time—and not orally?
   A. Lidocaine absorption is too erratic when administered orally.
   B. Lidocaine is inactivated by hydrochloric acid.
   C. Most of an absorbed oral dose of lidocaine undergoes first-pass metabolism in the liver.
   D. The onset of action for oral lidocaine is greater than 8 hours.

Class II Beta-Adrenergic Blockers

Beta-adrenergic blocking agents (see Chap. 28) exert antidysrhythmic effects by slowing the stimulation of beta receptors in the heart by the sympathetic nervous system, slowing SA and AV nodal conduction. Blockage of receptors in the SA node and ectopic pacemakers decreases automaticity, and blockage of receptors in the AV node increases the refractory period. Beta-adrenergic blockers are effective for management of dysrhythmias resulting from excessive sympathetic activity. They are most often used to slow the ventricular rate of contraction in atrial flutter and atrial fibrillation.

Class II beta-adrenergic blockers are being used more extensively because of their effectiveness in reducing mortality in patients following myocardial infarction and heart failure. Reduced mortality may result from the ability of the drugs to prevent ventricular fibrillation. Ⓟ **Propranolol** (Inderal), the prototype class II drug, may be given orally for chronic therapy to prevent ventricular dysrhythmias,

TABLE 25.3

DRUGS AT A GLANCE: Class II Beta-Adrenergic Blockers

Drug	Pregnancy Category	Routes and Dosage Ranges	
		Adults	Children
℗ **Propranolol** (Inderal) Beta₁ Beta₂	C	PO 10–30 mg every 6–8 h; IV 1–3 mg with careful monitoring, not to exceed 1 mg/min; may give second dose in 2 min but then do not repeat for 4 h	Safety and efficacy not established
Acebutolol (Sectral) Beta₁	B	PO 200 mg every 12 h, increased gradually to 600–1200 mg/d in two divided doses	Safety and efficacy not established
Esmolol (Brevibloc) Beta₁	C	IV 500 mcg/kg/min initially as a loading dose for 1 min, followed by a maintenance dose of 50 mcg/kg/min over 4 min. If no response in 5 min, repeat the same loading dose, and increase maintenance doses to 100 mcg/kg/min for 4 min, continue to increase by 50 mcg/kg/min up to 200 mcg/kg/min for 4 min. Once desired response is attained, stop loading dose and increase infusion by no more than 25 mcg/kg/min. Average maintenance dose 50–200 mcg/kg/min. Infusion administered up to 24; up to 48 h may be well tolerated. Not to exceed 300 mcg/kg/min	Safety and efficacy not established
Sotalol (Betapace) Beta₁ Beta₂	B	PO 80 mg every 12 h initially, titrated to response; average dose, 240–320 mg daily	Older than 2 y with normal renal function PO 30 mg/m² 3 times daily can titrate to a maximum of 60 mg/m². Allow 36 h between increments. Pediatric patients younger than 2 y: see manufacturer's instructions

especially those precipitated by exercise. It may be administered intravenously for life-threatening dysrhythmias, including those that occur during anesthesia. Table 25.3 presents dosage information for propranolol and the other class II beta-adrenergic blockers.

Pharmacokinetics

For the oral route, the onset of action is 20 to 30 minutes, with a peak in 60 to 90 minutes and a duration of 6 to 12 hours. For the IV route, the onset of action is immediate, with a peak effect in 1 minute and a duration of more than 4 to 6 hours. The drug is metabolized in the liver, and the half-life is 3 to 5 hours (8–11 hours with the sustained release form of the medication). It is excreted in the urine.

Action

Propranolol competitively blocks beta-adrenergic receptors in the heart and juxtaglomerular apparatus. This action causes a decrease in the influence of the sympathetic nervous system on these tissues and a decrease in the excitability of the heart, cardiac workload, and oxygen consumption. This then causes a release of renin and lowers the blood pressure. In addition,

propranolol has a membrane stabilizing effect that contributes to its antidysrhythmic action.

Use

Propranolol is used in the treatment of cardiac dysrhythmias, especially supraventricular tachycardia. In addition, it has been found to be effective in the treatment of ventricular tachycardia. The safety and efficacy of this drug have not been established in pediatric patients. There are no known precautions regarding administration of propranolol in older adults or in those with renal impairment.

Use in Patients With Hepatic Impairment

As previously stated, propranolol is metabolized in the liver. Therefore, it should be used cautiously with patients with hepatic impairment.

Use in Patients With Critical Illness

Critically ill patients with cardiovascular disorders have an increased the risk of acute, serious, and potentially life-threatening dysrhythmias. Thus, as with quinidine, it is important to monitor responses to propranolol carefully, especially when beginning therapy.

Use in Patients Receiving Home Care

Patients receiving chronic antidysrhythmic drug therapy are likely to have significant cardiovascular disease. So, as with the administration of quinidine, the nurse assesses patients receiving beta-adrenergic agents both physically and mentally. It is important to assess for alterations in functional status and for changes in pulse and blood pressure.

Adverse Effects

Some of the known adverse effects to propranolol include allergic reactions, specifically laryngospasm and CNS changes. Specific cardiovascular effects are bradycardia, heart failure, cardiac dysrhythmias, SA or AV nodal block, peripheral vascular insufficiency, claudication, stroke, pulmonary edema, and hypotension. In addition, dermatologic, GI, genitourinary, musculoskeletal, and respiratory changes occur. Bronchospasm and laryngospasm are the most serious adverse respiratory effects and warrant careful monitoring.

Contraindications

Contraindications to the use of propranolol include allergy to beta-blocking agents, sinus bradycardia, and second- or third-degree heart block. In addition, other contraindications may include cardiogenic shock, heart failure, bronchial asthma, bronchospasm, chronic obstructive pulmonary disease, pregnancy, and lactation.

Nursing Implications

Preventing Interactions

The nurse monitors for important drug-drug interactions when a patient is taking propranolol as well as interference with laboratory tests. Several medications interact with propranolol, increasing or decreasing its effect (Box 25.4). Also, concomitant use of propranolol and glycerin leads to prolonged hypoglycemic effects. Additionally, propranolol interferes with glucose tolerance tests and insulin tolerance tests as well as with glaucoma screening tests.

Administering the Medication

Routes of administration of propranolol (in adults) are oral as well as parenteral. Patients take the oral form with meals. It is

---

BOX 25.4 | **Drug Interactions: Propranolol**

Drugs That Increase the Effects of Propranolol
- Verapamil
  Increases the risk of heart block effect

Drugs That Decrease the Effects of Propranolol
- Indomethacin, ibuprofen, piroxicam, sulindac, barbiturates
  Decrease the effects of blocking the beta-adrenergic receptors in the heart; have less influence on the sympathetic nervous system, excitability of the heart, cardiac workload, and oxygen consumption

---

essential that the drug not be discontinued abruptly after long-term therapy; a hypersensitivity to catecholamines may have developed, exacerbating ventricular dysrhythmias. Gradual tapering over a 2-week period, with patient monitoring, is necessary.

Assessing for Therapeutic Effects

After the nurse administers propranolol, he or she monitors the patient until determining that the dysrhythmia has resolved. If the patient has received the maximum amount of beta-adrenergic medication, it may be necessary to consider another pharmacologic agent.

Assessing for Adverse Effects

Allergic reaction, including laryngospasm, is one adverse effect. Cardiovascular effects include bradycardia, heart failure, cardiac dysrhythmias, SA or AV nodal block, peripheral vascular insufficiency, claudication, stroke, pulmonary edema, and hypotension. ECG changes to watch for include heart rates less than 60 beats per minute, abnormal heart rhythms, or heart blocks (first-, second-, or third-degree) and/or sinus exit blocks. Other adverse effects relate to the dermatologic, GI, genitourologic, and respiratory systems.

Patient Teaching

The nurse instructs patients to take propranolol with meals. It is important that patients report night cough, swelling of the extremities, slow pulse, confusion, depression, rash, fever, or sore throat to the prescriber. Patients need to realize that they should not stop taking propranolol abruptly because this action can cause the dysrhythmia to worsen. In addition, the nurse should inform patients with diabetes mellitus that propranolol may mask the normal signs of hypoglycemia (e.g., cool, clammy skin; tachycardia); it is necessary to monitor blood or urine glucose carefully. Box 25.3 presents some patient teaching considerations for all antidysthymics.

Class III Potassium Channel Blockers

Although all these drugs share a common mechanism of action, they are very different. The prototype potassium channel blocker ⓟ **amiodarone** (Cordarone) has electrophysiologic characteristics of sodium channel blockers, beta blockers, and calcium channel blockers. Thus, it has vasodilating effects and decreases systemic vascular resistance, it prolongs conduction in all cardiac tissues and decreases heart rate, and it decreases contractility of the left ventricle. Table 25.4 presents dosage information for amiodarone and the other class III potassium channel blockers.

Pharmacokinetics

The oral form of amiodarone has an onset of 2 to 3 days, with a peak in 3 to 7 hours and a duration of 6 to 8 hours. However, the action may be delayed from 3 days up to 3 weeks. The IV form has an immediate onset, with a peak in 20 minutes and a duration for as long as the infusion continues. Amiodarone is extensively metabolized in the liver and produces active

TABLE 25.4

DRUGS AT A GLANCE: Class III Potassium Channel Blockers

Drug	Pregnancy Category	Routes and Dosage Ranges	
		Adults	*Children*
Ⓟ **Amiodarone** (Cordarone)	D	Loading dose, IV 150 mg over 10 min (15 mg/min), then 360 mg over the next 6 h (1 mg/min), then 540 mg over the next 18 h (0.5 mg/min); maintenance dose, IV 720 mg/24 h (0.5 mg/min) Loading dose, PO 800–1600 mg/d for 1–3 wk, with a gradual decrease to 600–800 mg/d for 1 mo; maintenance dose, PO 400 mg/d	IV safety and efficacy have not been established
Dofetilide (Tikosyn)	C	Creatinine clearance > 60 mL/min, 500 mcg twice daily Creatinine clearance 40–60 mL/min, 250 mcg twice daily Creatinine clearance 20–<40 mL/min, 125 mcg twice daily Creatinine clearance < 20 mL/min, use is contraindicated	Not recommended
Ibutilide (Corvert)	C	Weight > 60 kg: IV infusion over 10 min, 1 mg Weight < 60 kg: IV infusion over 10 min, 0.01 mg/kg The dose can be repeated once, after 10 min, if necessary	Not recommended
Sotalol (Betapace) *Class II and class III effects*	B	PO 80 mg every 12 h initially, adjust gradually every 3 d; may require 240–320 mg daily. See manufacturer's recommendations for dosing in renal failure	Older than 2 y with normal renal function PO 30 mh/m² 3 times daily; can titrate to a maximum of 60 mg/m²; allow 38 h between increments. Younger than 2 y, see manufacturer's instructions

metabolites. The drug and its metabolites accumulate in the liver, lungs, fat, skin, and other tissues. It has a half-life of 10 days. Because of the long serum half-life of amiodarone, loading doses are usually given. These loading doses reduce the time required for therapeutic effects. However, effects may persist for several weeks after the drug is discontinued.

Action

Potassium channel blockers such as amiodarone prolong duration of the action potential, slow repolarization, and prolong the refractory period in both the atria and ventricles. To perform these actions, they block cardiac potassium channels.

Use

Amiodarone is used for various types of life-threatening tachydysrhythmias, both ventricular and atrial dysrhythmias. The IV and oral forms of amiodarone differ in their electrophysiologic effects. The oral form is given to treat recurrent ventricular tachycardia or ventricular fibrillation and to maintain a NSR after conversion of atrial fibrillation and atrial flutter. The IV form is given mainly for acute suppression of refractory, hemodynamically destabilizing ventricular tachycardia and ventricular fibrillation. The major effect is slowing conduction through the AV node and prolonging the effective refractory period.

The FDA has issued a **BLACK BOX WARNING ◆** for amiodarone, recommending use only in patients with life-threatening dysrhythmias because of the risk of the development of potentially fatal pulmonary toxicity. Low-dose amiodarone may be a pharmacologic choice for preventing recurrent atrial fibrillation after electrical or pharmacologic conversion. The low doses cause fewer adverse effects than the higher ones used for life-threatening ventricular dysrhythmias.

Use in Children

Safety and efficacy have not been established in pediatric patients.

Use in Patients With Hepatic Impairment

Amiodarone is hepatotoxic. Thus, it is necessary to evaluate the liver and monitor liver function tests closely in patients who take amiodarone.

Use in Patients With Critical Illness

Amiodarone is used only for treatment of life-threatening recurrent ventricular dysrhythmias that do not respond to adequate doses of other antidysrhythmics or when patients do not respond to alternative agents. Yet because of the potential complications of use of the medication, authorities strongly recommend adjusting to the lowest possible IV dose to limit the side effects and switching to the oral form as soon as possible.

Medical Response Team Saves Lives by Empowering Nurses to Recognize and Act on Early Warning Signs of Trouble.

by HENZE, T.

2010. *Medical Response Team Saves Lives by Empowering Nurses to Recognize and Act on Early Warning Signs of Trouble.* AHRQ Health Care Innovations Exchange. Accessed December 17, 2010. http://www.innovations.ahrq.gov/content.aspx?id=1761

The medical response team at a hospital responds to nurse and family reports of early warning signs that patients are in cardiopulmonary distress. This team then moves quickly to "rescue" the patient before the situation progresses to a medical emergency. The responsiveness of the team has reduced the number of cardiac arrests in this hospital by 26%. In addition, a number of nursing interventions have saved lives through: (1) increasing nurses' ability to recognize the early warning signs of patient distress, (2) empowering nurses to communicate with providers, and (3) permitting the initiation of effective interventions at the time of recognition of the near-event.

IMPLICATIONS FOR NURSING PRACTICE: Early identification of warning signs of a patient's deteriorating condition can improve patient outcomes and reduce medical emergencies. Health care systems that facilitate interdisciplinary collaboration at the point-of-care provide prompt intervention to reverse potential crises in individual patients and supports early communication among health care providers.

Use in Patients Receiving Home Care

Due to the close monitoring needed even with changes in the drug dosage, careful patient assessment and evaluation are necessary. Continual monitoring of cardiac response to titrate the dosage is essential.

Adverse Effects

Authorities consider most adverse effects of amiodarone to be dose dependent and reversible. However, maintenance dose selection is difficult because absorption and elimination are variable. With the use of amiodarone, CNS adverse effects, including malaise, fatigue, dizziness, tremors, and ataxia, are the most common. Other common adverse effects include cardiac dysrhythmias (which can be life-threatening), hypotension, and heart failure. GI conditions include nausea, vomiting, anorexia, and constipation.

Amiodarone is an iodine-rich drug that has been associated with thyroid dysfunction, with hypothyroidism occurring more frequently than hyperthyroidism. Respiratory adverse effects include serious, potentially fatal pulmonary toxicity (pulmonary fibrosis, pneumonitis, acute respiratory distress syndrome), which may begin with progressive dyspnea and cough with crackles, decreased breath sounds, and pleurisy. Liver function tests are abnormal. Hepatotoxicity may occur and can be life threatening.

Corneal microdeposits occur in almost all patients treated for more than 2 months and can lead to blurry vision. Photosensitivity is also an adverse effect.

Contraindications

Contraindications include hypersensitivity to amiodarone as well as sinus node dysfunction, heart block, cardiogenic shock, severe bradycardia, hypokalemia, lactation, and sensitivity to iodine. Caution is necessary when giving amiodarone to patients who are pregnant or have thyroid dysfunction.

Nursing Implications

QSEN Safety Alert

The names amrinone and amiodarone have given rise to confusion (the name amrinone has now been changed to inamrinone, but confusion may still occur). Caution is necessary.

Preventing Interactions

When oral amiodarone is used long term, it increases the effects of numerous drugs, worsening existing dysrhythmias or producing new dysrhythmias. Drugs that interact with amiodarone include beta blockers, oral anticoagulants, digoxin, and phenytoin. The effects of interactions with amiodarone may not be apparent until about 7 weeks after the initiation of therapy.

Administering the Medication

Careful patient assessment and evaluation with continual monitoring of cardiac response are necessary for titrating the dosage. Therapy should begin in the hospital with continual monitoring and emergency equipment on standby.

Assessing for Therapeutic Effects

An effect of the medication is to increase the ventricular fibrillation threshold. The nurse assesses the patient's heart rate and the cardiac rhythm; the heart rate and rhythm should be regular, with a rate between 60 and 100 beats per minute.

Assessing for Adverse Effects

If the nurse notes any change in heart rate greater than 100 beats per minute or any change in the regularity of the rhythm, increased vigilance in assessing cardiac status is warranted. In addition, the nurse assesses for ectopy and calls its attention to the physician.

Patient Teaching

Patients should understand that if drug dosages are changed in relation to response of dysrhythmias, they will need to be hospitalized during the initiation of amiodarone therapy. Additionally, the nurse should stress the importance of keeping follow-up appointments, including chest x-ray, pulmonary function tests, and ophthalmic examinations. Box 25.3 presents patient teaching information for antidysrhythmic agents.

Other Drugs in the Class

Dofetilide is indicated for the maintenance of NSR in symptomatic patients who are in atrial fibrillation for longer than 1 week. Adverse effects increase with decreasing creatinine clearance levels; thus, assessment of renal function is necessary and initial dosage is dependent on creatinine clearance levels. High dosages in patients with renal dysfunction result in accumulation of dofetilide and prodysrhythmia (torsades de pointes). The drug has an elimination half-life of approximately 8 hours, with the kidneys being the major route of elimination. It should initially be administered in a setting with personnel and equipment available for emergency use.

Ibutilide is indicated for management of recent onset of atrial fibrillation or atrial flutter, in which the goal is conversion to NSR. The drug enhances the efficacy of cardioversion. Ibutilide is structurally similar to sotalol but lacks clinically significant beta-blocking activity. Ibutilide is widely distributed and has an elimination half-life of about 6 hours. Most of a dose is metabolized, and the metabolites are excreted in urine and feces. Adverse effects include supraventricular and ventricular dysrhythmias (particularly torsades de pointes) and hypotension. Ibutilide should be administered in a setting with trained personnel and equipment available for emergency use.

Sotalol is approved for prevention or management of ventricular tachycardia and fibrillation. It has also been used, usually in smaller doses, to prevent or treat atrial fibrillation. However, it is less effective than amiodarone in the prophylaxis of atrial fibrillation. It has both beta-adrenergic–blocking and potassium channel–blocking activity. Class II effects predominate at lower doses, and class III effects predominate at higher doses. Sotalol is well absorbed after oral administration, and peak serum levels are reached in 2 to 4 hours. It has an elimination half-life of approximately 12 hours, and 80% to 90% is excreted unchanged by the kidneys.

Contraindications to the use of sotalol include asthma, sinus bradycardia, heart block, cardiogenic shock, heart failure, and previous hypersensitivity to sotalol. The dosage should be individualized, reduced with renal impairment, and increased slowly (e.g., every 2–3 days with normal renal function, at longer intervals with impaired renal function). Dysrhythmogenic effects are most likely to occur when therapy is started or when the dosage is increased. Heart failure may occur in patients with markedly depressed left ventricular systolic function. Most adverse effects are attributed to beta-blocking activity. Like amiodarone, sotalol may be preferred over a class I agent because it is more effective in reducing recurrent ventricular tachycardia, ventricular fibrillation, and death.

NCLEX Success

3. The clinical use of class III agents rather than class I agents is preferred for patients with heart disease because the class III agents are associated with

A. less ventricular fibrillation
B. increased mortality
C. more sustained effects
D. milder adverse effects

4. Mr. Conley, who is 53 years of age, is about to be discharged from the hospital after treatment for recurrent ventricular fibrillation. To prevent breakthrough ventricular ectopy, his prescriber orders amiodarone (Cordarone), 1000 mg PO daily as a loading dose for 2 weeks. What patient teaching implications are important regarding this loading dose?

A. Most of the drug is destroyed in the gastrointestinal tract, and thus a large dose needs to be given.
B. Males require large dosages because of their faster metabolic rate.
C. A history of ventricular dysrhythmia necessitates a higher dose.
D. The drug has a long serum half-life.

Clinical Application 25-2

Mr. Brown's atrial fibrillation is converted to NSR pharmacologically. The physician prescribes amiodarone at 200 mg PO daily.
- Why is he taking amiodarone?
- What therapeutic level of amiodarone should be the goal for this patient?

Class IV Calcium Channel Blockers

Ⓟ **Diltiazem** (Cardizem), the prototype class IV drug, and verapamil are the only calcium channel blockers approved for management of dysrhythmias. Table 25.5 presents dosage information for these drugs.

Pharmacokinetics

When given intravenously, diltiazem acts within 15 minutes and lasts up to 6 hours. Diltiazem and verapamil are metabolized by the liver, and metabolites are primarily excreted by the kidneys.

Action

Calcium channel blockers (see Chap. 26) obstruct the movement of calcium into conductive and contractile myocardial cells by inhibiting the influx of calcium through its channels, causing a slower conduction through the SA and AV nodes. As antidysrhythmic agents, they act primarily against tachydysrhythmias at SA and AV nodes because the cardiac cells slow channels that depend on calcium influx are found mainly at these sites. Thus, they reduce automaticity of the SA and AV nodes, slow conduction, and prolong the refractory period in the AV node.

Use

Diltiazem, as well as verapamil, is effective only in supraventricular tachycardias. The drug may be given intravenously to

TABLE 25.5

DRUGS AT A GLANCE: Class IV Calcium Channel Blockers

Drug	Pregnancy Category	Routes and Dosage Ranges	
		Adults	*Children*
ⓟ **Diltiazem** (Cardizem)	C	IV injection 0.25 mg/kg (average dose 20 mg) over 2 min. A second dose of 0.35 mg/kg (average, 20 mg) may be given in 15 min, and an IV infusion of 5–15 mg/h may be given up to 24 h, if necessary	Safety and efficacy have not been established
Verapamil (Calan, Isoptin)	C	PO 40–120 mg every 6–8 h IV 5–10 mg initially, then 10 mg 30 min later, if necessary	1–15 y: IV injection 0.1–0.3 mg/kg (usual range 2–5 mg for a single dose) over 2 min with continuous ECG monitoring; repeat in 30 min if necessary <1 y: IV injection 0.1–0.2 mg/kg over 2 min with continuous ECG monitoring

terminate acute paroxysmal supraventricular tachycardia, usually within 2 minutes, and in atrial fibrillation and atrial flutter. It is also effective in exercise-related tachycardias. One antidysrhythmic drug may not maintain an NSR, and the use of more than one agent is often necessary.

With diltiazem, the following usage information may be important:

- Safety and efficacy have not been established in pediatric patients.
- There are no recommendations regarding specific use in older adults
- Impaired renal function is a contraindication.
- Impaired hepatic function is a contraindication.

Use in Patients With Critical Illness

Cardiac function in the critically ill patient warrants carefully evaluation. Sick sinus syndrome, heart block (either second- or third-degree), severe hypertension, cardiogenic shock, and acute myocardial infarction with cardiogenic shock are all situations where use of diltiazem is contraindicated.

Use in Patients Receiving Home Care

When patients are receiving home care and are taking diltiazem, it is necessary to perform a physical assessment, including pulse and blood pressure, with each visit. The home care nurse arranges for follow-up with a 12-lead ECG if alterations in cardiac rhythm occur (e.g., irregular rate or change in baseline heart rate).

Adverse Effects

Some of the most common adverse effects associated with diltiazem are CNS conditions, including dizziness, lightheadedness, headache, and asthenia. Cardiovascular adverse effects include peripheral edema, bradycardia, and AV block. If asystole occurs, it is necessary to start cardiopulmonary resuscitation immediately. Dermatologic effects include flushing. The GI effects most often noted are complaints of nausea.

Contraindications

Contraindications to the use of diltiazem include allergy to diltiazem, impaired hepatic or renal function, sick sinus syndrome, heart block, severe hypertension, cardiogenic shock, acute myocardial infarction with cardiogenic shock, and lactation. Diltiazem, as well as verapamil, is contraindicated in digoxin toxicity because it may worsen heart block. If diltiazem is used with propranolol or digoxin, it is necessary to exercise caution to avoid further impairment of myocardial contractility. Use of IV verapamil with IV propranolol should not take place; it may result in potentially fatal bradycardia and hypotension.

Nursing Implications

Preventing Interactions

Certain drugs increase the effects of diltiazem (Box 25.5). Also, diltiazem increases the serum levels and toxicity of cyclosporine. In addition, there is a decreased metabolism and increased risk of toxic effects if diltiazem is taken with grapefruit juice.

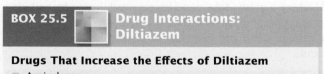

BOX 25.5 Drug Interactions: Diltiazem

Drugs That Increase the Effects of Diltiazem

- Amiodarone
  Increases the risk of sinus arrest, decreased myocardial contractility, and hypotension
- Atazanavir
  Increases the risk of conduction disturbances and atrioventricular block
- Beta-adrenergic blockers, flecainide
  Cause additive reductions in heart rate, cardiac conduction, and contractility

Administering the Medication

Careful evaluation to determine the appropriate dosing of calcium channel blockers is warranted. Ensuring that the patient swallows the extended-release or the sustained-release preparations whole rather than cutting, crushing, or chewing is a must.

Assessing for Therapeutic Effects

In determining the effects of the use of calcium channel blockers, the nurse monitors the cardiac rate and rhythm for a return to the patient's normal baseline.

Assessing for Adverse Effects

When caring for patients who are receiving diltiazem, the nurse monitors carefully for changes in blood pressure and cardiac rhythm as well as output. (Checking the blood pressure is especially important if the patient is taking nitrates concurrently.) In addition, it is necessary to monitor the cardiac rhythm regularly during dosage stabilization and periodically during long-term therapy. The nurse should also observe for safety issues associated with the development of symptoms such as dizziness and lightheadedness.

Patient Teaching

It is important to instruct the patient to report any adverse effects. Box 25.3 outlines patient teaching guidelines.

Unclassified Antidysrhythmic Drugs

Adenosine, a naturally occurring component of all body cells, differs chemically from other antidysrhythmic drugs but acts like the calcium channel blockers. It depresses conduction at the AV node and is used to restore NSR in patients with paroxysmal supraventricular tachycardia; it is ineffective in other dysrhythmias. The drug has a very short duration of action (serum half-life of less than 10 seconds) and a high degree of effectiveness. It must be given by a rapid bolus injection, preferably through a central venous line. If given slowly, it is eliminated before it can reach cardiac tissues and exert its action.

Magnesium sulfate is another of the unclassified drugs given intravenously in the management of severe tachydysrhythmias, including treatment of torsades de pointes and management of digitalis-induced dysrhythmias. Its antidysrhythmic effects may derive from imbalances of magnesium, potassium, and calcium. Hypomagnesemia increases myocardial irritability and is a risk factor for both atrial and ventricular dysrhythmias. Thus, serum magnesium levels should be monitored in patients at risk and replacement therapy instituted when indicated. However, in some instances, magnesium sulfate seems to have antidysrhythmic effects even when serum magnesium levels are normal.

Clinical Application 25-3

- While Mr. Brown is receiving his IV lidocaine, his heart rate decreases to 52 beats per minute with continued premature ventricular contractions. The nurse continues to monitor the IV line and the ECG. What should he or she then do?

The Nursing Process

Assessment

- **Assess the patient's condition in relation to cardiac dysrhythmias.**
- **Identify conditions or risk factors that may precipitate dysrhythmias. These include the following:**
  - Hypoxia
  - Electrolyte imbalances (e.g., hypokalemia, hypomagnesemia, hypocalcemia)
  - Acid–base imbalances
  - Acute coronary syndrome (angina pectoris, myocardial infarction)
  - Cardiac valvular disease
  - Febrile illness
  - Respiratory disorders (e.g., chronic lung disease)
  - Exercise
  - Emotional upset
  - Excessive ingestion of caffeine-containing beverages (e.g., coffee, tea, colas)
  - Cigarette smoking
  - Drug therapy with digoxin, antidysrhythmic drugs, CNS stimulants, anorexiants, and tricyclic antidepressants
  - Hyperthyroidism
- **Observe for clinical signs and symptoms of dysrhythmias. Mild or infrequent dysrhythmias may be perceived by the patient as palpitations or skipped heartbeats. More severe dysrhythmias may produce manifestations that reflect decreased cardiac output and other hemodynamic changes, as follows:**
  - Hypotension, bradycardia or tachycardia, and irregular rhythm
  - Shortness of breath, dyspnea, and cough from impaired respiration
  - Syncope or mental confusion from reduced cerebral blood flow
  - Chest pain from decreased coronary artery blood flow. Angina pectoris or myocardial infarction may occur.
  - Oliguria from decreased renal blood flow
- **When ECG monitoring is available (e.g., 12-lead ECG or continuous ECG monitoring), assess for indications of dysrhythmias.**

Nursing Diagnoses

- Decreased cardiac output related to ineffective rhythm of the heart
- Decreased tissue perfusion, cerebral and peripheral, related to compromised cardiac output or medication-induced hypotension
- Impaired gas exchange related to decreased tissue perfusion
- Excess fluid volume: peripheral edema and pulmonary congestion related to alteration in cardiac output
- Activity intolerance related to weakness and fatigue
- Anxiety related to potentially serious illness
- Deficient knowledge: pharmacologic and nonpharmacologic management of dysrhythmias

Planning/Goals

The patient will

- Receive or take antidysrhythmic drugs accurately
- Avoid conditions that precipitate dysrhythmias, when feasible
- Experience improved heart rate, circulation, and activity tolerance
- Be monitored for therapeutic and adverse drug effects
- Avoid preventable adverse drug effects
- Have adverse drug effects promptly recognized and treated if they occur
- Keep follow-up appointments for monitoring responses to treatment measures

Nursing Interventions

The nurse will

- Use measures to detect, prevent, and/or minimize dysrhythmias.
- Treat underlying disease processes that contribute to dysrhythmia development. These include cardiovascular (e.g., acute myocardial infarction) and noncardiovascular (e.g., chronic lung disease) disorders.
- Prevent or treat other conditions that predispose to dysrhythmias (e.g., hypoxia, electrolyte imbalance, pain, acid-base imbalance, fluid alterations).
- Help the patient understand the negative effects of cigarette smoking, overeating, excessive coffee drinking, and other habits that may cause or aggravate dysrhythmias. Encourage the patient to avoid such behaviors. Long-term supervision and counseling may be needed.
- For the patient receiving antidysrhythmic drugs, implement measures to minimize the incidence and severity of acute dysrhythmias and help the patient comply with drug therapy.
- Monitor heart rate and rhythm and blood pressure every 4 to 6 hours (or as often as is the standard for the care environment where assessing the patient).
- During IV administration of antidysrhythmic drugs, maintain continuous cardiac monitoring and check blood pressure about every 1 to 5 minutes, depending on the onset of action of the drug.

TABLE 25.6

Therapeutic Serum Drug Level Ranges of Common Antidysrhythmics

Drug	Therapeutic Range (mcg/mL)
Class IA	
Quinidine	2–6
Procainamide	4–10
Disopyramide	2–8
Class IB	
Lidocaine	1–5
Mexiletine	0.5–2
Class IC	
Flecainide	0.2–1
Propafenone	0.06–1
Class II	
Propranolol	0.05–0.1
Class III	
Amiodarone	0.5–2.5
Class IV	
Verapamil	0.08–0.3

- Check laboratory reports of serum electrolytes and serum drug levels when available. See Table 25.6 for commonly reported serum levels of antidysrhythmic agents. Report and treat abnormal values using established protocols and/or physician orders.
- Provide appropriate patient teaching related to drug therapy (see Box 25.3).

Evaluation

- Check vital signs for improved heart rate and rhythm.
- Interview and observe for relief of symptoms and improved functioning in activities of daily living.
- Interview and observe for irregular rhythms, hypotension, and other adverse drug effects.
- Interview and observe for compliance with instructions for taking antidysrhythmic drugs and other aspects of care.

Key Concepts

- Atrial fibrillation is a common dysrhythmia.
- Initiation of an electrical impulse depends predominantly on the movement of sodium and calcium ions into a myocardial cell and movement of potassium ions out of the cell.
- Quinidine, the prototype of class IA antidysrhythmics, reduces automaticity, slows conduction, and prolongs the refractory period.
- Lidocaine is the prototype of class IB antidysrhythmics used for treating serious ventricular dysrhythmias associated with acute myocardial infarction, cardiac catheterization, cardiac surgery, and digitalis-induced ventricular dysrhythmias.
- Cautions for flecainide use include the following:
  - A **BLACK BOX WARNING** ◆ states that drug treatment increases the risk of nonfatal cardiac arrest and death in patients with recent myocardial infarction or chronic atrial fibrillation.

- A **BLACK BOX WARNING** ◆ states that in patients with cardiac dysrhythmias, it is necessary to monitor carefully for a risk of potentially fatal prodysrhythmic effects.
- As class II drugs, beta-adrenergic blockers are used because of their effectiveness in reducing mortality in post–myocardial infarction and heart failure patients.
- As class IV drugs, diltiazem and verapamil are the only calcium channel blockers approved for management of dysrhythmias.
- The FDA has issued a **BLACK BOX WARNING** ◆ for disopyramide because of its known prodysrhythmic properties; the drug should be reserved for patients with life-threatening ventricular dysrhythmias.
- Amiodarone is a potassium channel blocker that prolongs conduction in all cardiac tissues and decreases heart rate, and it decreases contractility of the left ventricle.
- The FDA has issued a **BLACK BOX WARNING** ◆ for amiodarone, recommending use only in patients with life-threatening dysrhythmias because of the risk of the development of potentially fatal pulmonary toxicity.

Critical Thinking Questions

25-1. A female patient in a cardiology unit has continuous telemetry monitoring. The monitor technician pages the health care team and reports that she has become tachycardic.

- What are the priority considerations of this new finding?
- What are the possible treatment options for this patient?
- What nursing care interventions decrease the risk of dysrhythmias?
- What risk factors predispose this patient to the development of dysrhythmias?

References and Resources

Aliot, E. M., Stevenson, W. G., Almendral-Garrote, J. M., Bogun, F., Calkins, C. H., Delacretaz, E., et al. European Heart Rhythm Association (EHRA); Registered Branch of the European Society of Cardiology (ESC); Heart Rhythm Society (HRS); American College of Cardiology (ACC); American Heart Association (AHA). (2009). EHRA/HRS Expert Consensus on Catheter Ablation of Ventricular Arrhythmias: developed in a partnership with the European Heart Rhythm Association (EHRA), a Registered Branch of the European Society of Cardiology (ESC), and the Heart Rhythm Society (HRS); in collaboration with the American College of Cardiology (ACC) and the American Heart Association (AHA). *Heart Rhythm*, 6(6), 886–933.

Hazinski, M. F., Nolan, J. P., Billi, J. E., Böttiger, B. W., Bossaert, L., de Caen, A. R., et al. (2010). Part 1: Executive Summary: 2010 International Consensus on Cardiopulmonary Resuscitation and Emergency Cardiovascular Care Science With Treatment Recommendations. *Circulation, 122*, S250–S275.

Karch, A. M. (2012). *2012 Lippincott's nursing drug guide.* Philadelphia, PA: Lippincott Williams & Wilkins.

Morrison, L. J., Deakin, C. D., Morley, P. T., Callaway, C. W., Kerber, R. E., Kronick, S. L. (2010). 2010 International Consensus on Cardiopulmonary Resuscitation and Emergency Cardiovascular Care Science with Treatment Recommendations Part 8: Advanced Life Support. *Circulation, 122*, S345–S421.

Nadkarni, V. M., Nolan, J. P., Billi, J. E., Bossaert, B., Böttiger, B. W., Chamberlain, D., et al. (2010). Part 2: International Collaboration in Resuscitation Science 2010 International Consensus on Cardiopulmonary Resuscitation and Emergency Cardiovascular Care Science with Treatment Recommendations. *Circulation, 122*, S276–S282.

26 Drug Therapy for Angina

After studying this chapter, you should be able to:

1. Recognize the etiology, pathophysiology, and clinical manifestations of angina.
2. Identify the prototype and describe the action, use, contraindications, adverse effects, and nursing implications for the organic nitrates.
3. Identify the prototype and outline the actions, use, adverse effects, contraindications, and nursing implications for the beta-adrenergic blockers.
4. Identify the prototype and describe the actions, use, adverse effects, contraindications, and nursing implications for the calcium channel blockers.
5. Apply the nursing process in the care of patients with angina.

Clinical Application Case Study

Richard Gerald is a 72-year-old man with a history of hypertension and coronary artery disease. He stopped smoking and began a regular exercise program after having a myocardial infarction 3 months ago.

KEY TERMS

Acute coronary syndrome: any condition brought on by sudden, reduced blood flow to the heart

Afterload: amount of vascular resistance that must be overcome to open the aortic (or pulmonic valve on the right side of the heart) and eject the blood with systole

Cardioselectivity: ability of a beta-adrenergic blocker to selectively block $beta_1$ receptors

Intima: inner layer of an artery

Media: middle layer of a vessel

Preload: passive stretch of the ventricles just prior to systole

Introduction

The continuum of coronary artery disease (CAD) progresses from angina to myocardial infarction (MI). There are three main types of angina: stable angina, unstable angina, and variant angina; however, there are also other presentations (Box 26.1). The Canadian Cardiovascular Society classifies patients with angina according to the amount of physical activity tolerated before anginal pain occurs (Box 26.2). These categories can assist in clinical assessment and evaluation of therapy.

This chapter introduces the pharmacological care for the patient experiencing angina. Nonpharmacological treatment measures are also addressed. To understand clinical use of these drugs and nonpharmacological treatment measures, it is necessary to understand the etiology, pathophysiology, and clinical manifestations of angina.

BOX 26.1 Types of Angina Pectoris and Their Symptoms

Main Types

Stable

Stable angina (also called classic, typical, or exertional angina) occurs when atherosclerotic plaque obstructs coronary arteries and the heart requires more oxygenated blood than the blocked arteries can deliver. Anginal symptoms, such as chest pressure or pain, are usually precipitated by situations that increase the workload of the heart, such as physical exertion, exposure to cold temperatures, and emotional upset. Recurrent episodes of stable angina usually have the same pattern of onset, duration, and intensity of symptoms. Pain is usually relieved by rest, a fast-acting preparation of nitroglycerin, or both.

Variant

Variant angina (also called Prinzmetal's, or vasospastic angina) occurs at rest or with minimal exertion, often at night, and results from vasospasm of an epicardial coronary artery. It often occurs at the same time each day. This form of angina is not due to an obstructive atherosclerotic lesion; the spasms of the coronary artery decrease blood flow to the myocardium producing symptoms. Pain is usually relieved by nitroglycerin. Long-term management includes avoidance of conditions that precipitate vasospasm, when possible (e.g., exposure to cold, smoking, emotional stress), as well as antianginal drugs.

Unstable

Unstable angina (also called rest, preinfarction, and crescendo angina) is a type of acute coronary syndrome that falls between classic angina and myocardial infarction. It usually occurs in patients with advanced coronary atherosclerosis and produces increased frequency, intensity, and duration of symptoms. It often leads to myocardial infarction.

Unstable angina usually develops when a minor injury ruptures atherosclerotic plaque. The resulting injury to the endothelium causes platelets to aggregate at the site of injury, form a thrombus, and release chemical mediators that cause vasoconstriction (e.g., thromboxane, serotonin, platelet-derived growth factor). The disrupted plaque, thrombus, and vasoconstriction combine to obstruct blood flow further in the affected coronary artery. When the plaque injury is mild, blockage of the coronary artery may be intermittent and cause silent myocardial ischemia or episodes of anginal pain at rest. Thrombus formation and vasoconstriction may progress until the coronary artery is completely occluded, producing myocardial infarction. Endothelial injury, with subsequent thrombus formation and vasoconstriction, may also result from therapeutic procedures (e.g., angioplasty, atherectomy).

The Agency for Healthcare Research and Quality, in its clinical practice guidelines for the management of angina, defines unstable angina as meeting one or more of the following criteria:

- Anginal pain at rest that usually lasts longer than 20 minutes
- Recent onset (<2 months) of exertional angina of at least Canadian Cardiovascular Society Classification (CCSC) class III severity
- Recent (<2 months) increase in severity as indicated by progression to at least CCSC class III

Because unstable angina often occurs hours or days before acute myocardial infarction, early recognition and effective management are extremely important in preventing progression to infarction, heart failure, or sudden cardiac death.

Other Presentations

Refractory

Chronic stable angina is classified as refractory when it is not controllable by the maximal antianginal drugs, angioplasty, stenting, or coronary artery bypass surgery. The angina can also be classed refractory in patients where the risks of coronary interventions are unjustified.

Atypical

Patients without traditional substernal chest pain or typical relief with rest or nitroglycerin are classified as having atypical angina. This different presentation is more common in women and those with diabetes, displaying variable pain intensity or thresholds, timing, and characteristics. Palpitations and jaw or back pain are confounding complaints. Patients with atypical presentations are less likely to be diagnosed accurately and promptly, often placing them outside the therapeutic window of opportunity to receive appropriate treatment (i.e., thrombolytics and interventional therapies), resulting in poorer outcomes.

Silent Ischemia

Silent myocardial ischemia (also called anginal equivalent) may be painless or silent in a substantial number of patients, particularly in the elderly and those with diabetes. Symptoms other than chest discomfort may be present, including dyspnea, diaphoresis, nausea and vomiting, weakness, and altered sensorium. Patients with silent ischemia are less likely to be diagnosed accurately and promptly, often placing them outside the therapeutic window of opportunity to receive appropriate treatment (i.e., thrombolytics and interventional therapies), resulting in poorer outcomes. Overall, the diagnosis is usually based on chest pain history, electrocardiographic evidence of ischemia, and other signs of impaired cardiac function (e.g., heart failure).

Overview of Angina

Etiology

Angina pectoris is a common manifestation of CAD. The two main causes of angina are coronary artery spasm and atherosclerotic plaque buildup, which leads to CAD. Other causes of this condition include pulmonary embolism, aortic dissection, and pericarditis. Box 26.3 outlines the multiple risk factors associated with the development of CAD.

Pathophysiology

Coronary Artery Disease

In CAD, there is a buildup of lipids and fibrous matter within the coronary artery. Increased blood levels of low-density lipoprotein (LDL) irritate and damage the inner layer (the **intima**) of the coronary artery. Once LDL has accumulated and damaged the protective layer of the vessel, fatty streaks form, with foam cells. These fatty streaks are yellow and flat and cause no significant coronary artery obstruction. The body responds by sending smooth muscle cells from the middle layer of the vessel, the **media**. This engulfs the fatty substance and the foam cells and produces a fibrous tissue, which stimulates calcium deposition. This cycle continues, and the fatty streak and foam cell eventually transform into a fibrous plaque. This forms the fibrous cap, which is made up of smooth muscle cells, macrophages, foam cells, lymphocytes, collagen, and elastin. As the lumen of the vessel becomes smaller and blood is limited, especially during times of high oxygen demand (e.g., with physical exertion) oxygen supply cannot keep up with demand. At this point, the patient may experience stable angina.

Angina pectoris is chest pain related to a lack of blood and oxygen supply to the heart muscle, producing myocardial ischemia. Myocardial oxygen demand surpasses oxygen supply. Catecholamine release along with increased sympathetic tone as seen in tachycardia of any etiology, mental stress, or exertion can lead to ischemia. Furthermore, the development of atherosclerotic plaque, as seen in CAD, narrows the lumen of the artery, which impedes the oxygen-carrying blood flow and further results in angina.

Acute coronary syndrome (any condition brought on by sudden, reduced blood flow to the heart) may be seen when the fibrous cap raptures, exposing thrombogenic material, producing a thrombus within the lumen. At this point, the intraluminal thrombi can occlude arteries outright or will detach, move into the circulation, and eventually occlude smaller, distal branches of the coronary artery causing thromboembolism and likely an acute MI or ST-segment elevation MI.

Coronary Artery Spasm

Coronary artery spasm is a transient, sudden narrowing of one of the coronary arteries. The spasm impedes blood flow through the artery, which in turn results in ischemia, leading to angina. Causes of coronary spasm include alcohol withdrawal, emotional stress, exposure to cold, vasoconstricting medications, and stimulants, such as cocaine.

Clinical Manifestations

Clinical manifestations of angina vary with the type of angina (see Box 26.1). The classic anginal pain is usually described as substernal chest pain of a constricting, squeezing, or suffocating nature. It may radiate to the jaw, neck, or shoulder; down the left or both arms; or to the back. The discomfort is sometimes mistaken for arthritis or for indigestion, because the pain may be associated with nausea, vomiting, dizziness, diaphoresis, shortness of breath, or fear of impending doom. The discomfort is usually brief, typically lasting 5 minutes or less until the balance of oxygen supply and demand is restored. Women, elderly people, and people with diabetes are more likely to have symptoms other than chest pain, including fatigue, weakness, and shortness of breath.

Nonpharmacologic Therapy

Nonpharmacologic management of angina and MI includes risk factor modification, patient education, and revascularization procedures. For patients at any stage of CAD development, irrespective of symptoms of myocardial ischemia, optimal management involves lifestyle changes and medications, if necessary, to control or reverse risk factors for disease progression. According to *The Third Report of the National Cholesterol Education Program Expert Panel on Detection, Evaluation, and Treatment of High Blood Cholesterol in Adults* (NCEP III), metabolic syndrome is a risk factor—actually a group of several cardiovascular risk factors, which are linked with obesity—elevated waist circumference, elevated triglycerides, reduced high-density lipoprotein (HDL) cholesterol, elevated blood pressure, and elevated fasting glucose. These risk factors frequently contribute to CAD and result in significant morbidity and mortality. A growing body of evidence corroborates that risk factor management in patients with CAD improves survival, enhances quality of life, reduces recurrent events, and decreases the need for revascularization. Thus, efforts to assist patients in reducing blood pressure, weight, and serum cholesterol levels, when indicated, and developing an exercise program are necessary. For patients with diabetes mellitus, glucose and blood pressure control can reduce the microvascular changes associated with the condition.

In addition, people should avoid circumstances known to precipitate acute attacks, and those who smoke should stop. Smoking is harmful because of the following factors:

- Nicotine increases catecholamines which, in turn, increase heart rate and blood pressure.
- Carboxyhemoglobin, formed from the inhalation of carbon monoxide in smoke, decreases delivery of blood and oxygen to the heart, decreases myocardial contractility, and increases the risks of life-threatening cardiac dysrhythmias (e.g., ventricular fibrillation) during ischemic episodes.
- Both nicotine and carbon monoxide increase platelet adhesiveness and aggregation, thereby promoting thrombosis.
- Smoking increases the risks for MI, sudden cardiac death, cerebrovascular disease (e.g., stroke), peripheral vascular disease (e.g., arterial insufficiency), and hypertension. It also reduces HDL cholesterol, the "good" cholesterol.

Additional nonpharmacologic management strategies include surgical revascularization (e.g., coronary artery bypass graft) and interventional procedures that reduce blockages (e.g., percutaneous transluminal coronary angioplasty [PTCA], intracoronary stents, laser therapy, rotational atherectomy). Additionally, the use of supersaturated oxygen (SSO_2) has shown significant improvement in limiting myocardial damage in patients with anterior MIs, particularly if treatment is started within 6 hours of symptom onset. In the Acute Myocardial Infarction with Hyperoxemic Therapy II (AMIHOT II) trial, infusing SSO_2 into the previously blocked artery after performing an angioplasty procedure reduced infarct zone size by 6.5%.

Nonpharmacologic management improves patient outcomes. However, most patients still require antianginal and other cardiovascular medications to manage their disease.

NCLEX Success

1. Mr. Smith, a 52-year-old African American man, is recovering from an acute MI. His father died from an MI at age 44. He has smoked one pack of cigarettes a day for 30 years. Which of the following are unmodifiable risk factors? (Check all that apply)

A. smoking
B. genetics
C. race
D. age

2. A 63-year-old woman continues to complain of chest pain although her cardiac catheterization showed no significant cardiac disease. She notes that the chest pain occurs at the same time each night and typically during the cold weather. What kind of angina is the patient likely experiencing?

A. stable angina
B. unstable angina
C. variant angina
D. acute coronary syndrome

Drug Therapy

Table 26.1 outlines the drugs used to treat angina pectoris and myocardial ischemia, which include the organic nitrates, beta-adrenergic blockers, and the calcium channel blockers. These drugs relieve anginal pain by increasing blood supply to the myocardium as well as reducing the oxygen demand of the myocardium. This chapter also addresses pharmacologic adjuncts to the management of angina, including a metabolic modulator that increases the energy production of the heart to preserve cardiac function.

Organic Nitrates

The most widely used nitrate is the prototype ℗ **nitroglycerin** (Nitro-Bid, Nitro-Dur). Available in multiple forms, it is indicated for the management and prevention of acute chest pain caused by myocardial ischemia.

Pharmacokinetics

Nitroglycerin is 60% bound to protein, undergoes extensive first-pass metabolism in the liver, and has a half-life of 1 to 4 minutes. Excretion occurs in the urine. The onset of action, peak, and duration varies with the route of administration.

- Intravenous (IV) drip: onset, immediate; peak, immediate; duration of action, 3 to 5 minutes
- Sublingual (SL): onset, 1 to 3 minutes; peak, 4 to 8 minutes; duration of action, 30 to 60 minutes

TABLE 26.1

Drugs Administered for the Treatment of Angina

Drug Class	Prototype	Other Drugs in the Class
Organic Nitrates	Nitroglycerin (Nitro-Bid, others)	Isosorbide dinitrate (Isordil) Isosorbide mononitrate (Ismo, Imdur)
Beta-Adrenergic Blockers	Atenolol (Tenormin)	Bisoprolol (Zebeta) Carvedilol (Coreg) Esmolol (Brevibloc) Metoprolol (Lopressor, Toprol XL) Nadolol (Corgard) Propranolol (Inderal)
Calcium Channel Blockers	Nifedipine (Adalat, Procardia)	Amlodipine (Norvasc) Diltiazem (Cardizem) Felodipine (Plendil) Nicardipine (Cardene) Verapamil (Calan, Isoptin)
Adjunct Medications		
Metabolic Modulator	Ranolazine (Ranexa)	
Others		Aspirin Dyslipidemic drugs Antihypertensive drugs

- Translingual spray: onset, 2 minutes; peak, 4 to 10 minutes; duration of action, 30 to 60 minutes
- Oral (PO) tablets or capsules (sustained-release): onset, 20 to 45 minutes; peak, 45 to 120 minutes; duration of action, 4 to 8 hours
- Topical ointment: onset, 15 to 60 minutes; peak, 30 to 120 hours; duration of action, 2 to 12 hours
- Topical transdermal disk: onset, 40 to 60 minutes; peak, 60 to 180 minutes; duration of action, 18 to 24 hours

Action

Organic nitrates are converted to nitric oxide, a potent vasodilator, which relaxes smooth muscle in blood vessel walls. Anginal pain is relieved by nitrates by several mechanisms:

- Venous dilation, which reduces venous pressure and decreases venous return to the heart. This decreases blood volume and pressure within the heart (**preload**), which in turn decreases cardiac workload and oxygen demand. This is the main mechanism by which nitroglycerin relieves angina.
- Coronary artery dilation at higher doses, which can increase blood flow to ischemic areas of the myocardium.
- Arteriole dilation, which lowers peripheral vascular resistance (**afterload**). This results in lower systolic blood pressure and, consequently, reduced cardiac workload and balancing supply and demand in the heart.

Use

For relief of sudden-onset angina, fast-acting preparations of nitroglycerin include SL and chewable tablets and

transmucosal spray. Indications for these preparations include acute-onset chest pain and prophylaxis prior to activities known to provoke angina, such as walking, dancing, or mowing the lawn.

For management of recurrent, chronic angina, long-acting preparations include PO sustained-release tablets and transdermal ointment. With these longer acting forms, intolerance to their hemodynamic effects may develop, and therefore the drugs do not relieve chest pain.

QSEN Safety Alert

To avoid development of tolerance to nitroglycerin, it is essential to observe a 10- to 12-hour nitrate-free interval.

In clinical practice, patients are usually nitrate free during the night, while sleeping. The oral form of the drug undergoes rapid metabolism in the liver, and relatively small portions ultimately reach the systemic circulation. Thus, the PO form does not relieve acute chest pain and may be useful prophylactically in chronic chest pain. Nitroglycerin ointment is indicated for prevention of chronic angina. This route is convenient to use when the patient can have nothing by mouth (NPO) before surgery and cannot take the usually PO dose.

Angina that is unresponsive to SL, PO, or transdermal preparations calls for IV nitroglycerin. Prescribers may typically order the IV form for an MI. IV nitroglycerin is useful in the management of angina that is unresponsive to organic nitrates via other routes or to beta-adrenergic blockers. It also may be used to control blood pressure in perioperative or emergency situations and to reduce preload and afterload in severe heart failure.

National Clinical Guideline Centre. Management of stable angina.

by NATIONAL INSTITUTE FOR HEALTH AND CLINICAL EXCELLENCE (NICE) (CLINICAL GUIDELINE, NUMBER 126)

Retrieved from: http://www.guideline.gov/content. aspx?id=34825&search=angina

The National Institute for Health and Clinical Excellence published evidence-based clinical practice guidelines regarding management of stable angina based on expert consensus after a systematic review of the literature. Pharmacologic recommendations include the following:

• The use of a beta-blocker or a calcium channel blocker is the first-line treatment for stable angina. The choice of drug is based on contraindications, other medical conditions, and patient preference. Other drugs to treat angina should not be used routinely as first-line treatment. It may be necessary to consider the other drug class if the drug is not tolerated or if symptoms are not adequately managed.

• If a patient must take a beta-adrenergic blocker and calcium channel blocker in combination to manage symptoms, he or she should use a dihydropyridine calcium channel blocker (nifedipine, amlodipine, or felodipine).

• If either class is not tolerated or contraindicated, the health care provider should consider another drug based on contraindications, other medical conditions, contraindications, cost, and patient preference, such as a long-acting nitrate or ranolazine.

• People who have controlled stable angina with two antianginal drugs should not use a third antianginal drug. However, if symptoms are not adequately controlled, a third antianginal drug may be necessary if the person is awaiting revascularization or if revascularization is not an option.

IMPLICATIONS FOR NURSING PRACTICE: Evidence from a comprehensive review of the literature demonstrates a stepped approach to the management of stable angina. The nurse should be aware of the recommendations when caring for patients with angina.

Table 26.2 presents route and dosage information for nitroglycerin and other nitrates.

Use in Children

IV nitroglycerin is the only form of nitroglycerin approved for use in children. It may be used to treat hypertension and heart failure. Caution and close monitoring are necessary.

Use in Older Adults

Older adults may be more vulnerable to hypotension when taking nitroglycerin due to volume depletion, concurrent use of other medication, and loss of sympathetic tone.

QSEN Safety Alert

Therefore, older adults may be at greater risk of falling than younger patients at the therapeutic doses of nitroglycerin due to their risk of hypotension.

Use in Patients With Critical Illness

IV nitroglycerin is commonly used in the critical care setting. Angina related to MI may be a patient's principal issue in the intensive care unit (ICU); however, he or she may also have heart failure, hypertension, renal failure, and/or anemia and therefore could be receiving multiple drugs such as heparin, nitroglycerin, and dobutamine.

QSEN Safety Alert

The nurse must always check IV compatibility when administering drugs by that route.

Close monitoring of vital signs, along with frequent titration of IV medications, is important.

Adverse Effects

The majority of adverse effects of nitroglycerin are related to the hemodynamic changes responsible for preload reduction and vasodilation. The most common adverse effect is a severe headache, which is typically treated with acetaminophen. Other common adverse effects include dizziness, bradycardia, syncope, hypotension, and orthostatic hypotension.

Contraindications

Contraindications to nitroglycerin include hypersensitivity reactions, severe anemia, hypotension, and hypovolemia.

QSEN Safety Alert

Men who take nitroglycerin or any other nitrate should not use phosphodiesterase enzyme type 5 inhibitors, such as sildenafil (Viagra) and vardenafil (Levitra) for erectile dysfunction.

Nitrates and phosphodiesterase enzyme type 5 inhibitors decrease blood pressure, and the combined effect can produce profound, life-threatening hypotension.

Caution is necessary in the following situations:

• in the presence of head injury or cerebral hemorrhage because it may increase intracranial pressure
• with the use of other antihypertensive agents such as beta-adrenergic blockers. It is essential to observe for extreme episodes of hypotension.
• with renal impairment ■

TABLE 26.2

DRUGS AT A GLANCE: Organic Nitrates

Drug	Pregnancy Category	Routes and Dosage Ranges (Adults [unless indicated])
Ⓟ **Nitroglycerin** (Nitro-Bid, others)	C	Immediate-release tablets, 2.5–9 mg PO 2 or 3 times/d Sustained-release tablets or capsules, 2.5 mg PO 3 or 4 times/d Sublingual, 0.15–0.6 mg as needed for chest pain Translingual spray, one or two metered doses (0.4 mg/dose) sprayed onto oral mucosa at onset of anginal pain, to a maximum of three doses in 15 min Transmucosal tablet, 1 mg every 3–5 h while awake, placed between upper lip and gum or cheek and gum Topical ointment, 1/2–2 inches every 4–8 h; do not rub in Topical transdermal disc, applied once daily IV, 5–10 mcg/min initially, increased in 10–20 mcg/min increments up to 100 mcg/min or more if necessary to relieve pain
Isosorbide dinitrate (Isordil)	C	Sublingual, 2.5–10 mg as needed or every 2–4 h Regular tablets, 5–40 mg PO 4 times/d Chewable tablets, 5–10 mg PO every 2–3 h Sustained-release capsules, 40 mg PO every 6–12 h
Isosorbide mononi-trate (Ismo, Imdur)	C	5–20 mg PO twice daily, with first dose on arising and the second dose 7 h later Extended-release tablets (Imdur), 30–60 mg once daily PO in the morning, increased after several days; maximum dose 240 mg once daily

Nursing Implications

Preventing Interactions

Many drugs interact with nitroglycerin, increasing or decreasing its effects (Box 26.4). Several herbs interact with nitroglycerin and cause profound hypotension or negate the effects of nitroglycerin (Box 26.5).

Administering the Medication

It is important to take a patient's vital signs prior to administration of any form of nitroglycerin. The nurse should withhold the medication with hypotension (systolic blood pressure less than 90 or 30 mm Hg below the patient's normal blood pressure) as well as tachycardia with a heart rate greater than 100 beats per minute.

Administration of SL nitroglycerin or transdermal spray is essential as soon as chest pain develops. If a patient is hospitalized, it is necessary to call the patient's health care provider and obtain a 12-lead electrocardiogram (ECG) at the onset of chest pain. The SL nitroglycerin container should stay in a dry, cool, dark environment, and replacement every 6 months is necessary. Exposure to light deactivates the nitroglycerin.

Application of nitroglycerin ointment requires using the dose-measuring application papers supplied with ointment. It is necessary to do the following:

- Squeeze the ointment onto a measuring scale printed on paper; typically, this is 1 or 1/2 inch depending on the practitioner's order.

BOX 26.4 Drug Interactions: Nitroglycerin

Drugs That Increase the Effects of Nitroglycerin

- Adalat and other calcium channel blockers, alcohol, aripiprazole, benazepril and other angiotensin-converting enzyme inhibitors, codeine and other narcotics, diphenhydramine, tizanidine
  Increase the risk of orthostatic hypotension
- Sildenafil, tadalafil, vardenafil
  Increase the risk of life-threatening hypotension

Drugs That Decrease the Effects of Nitroglycerin

- Acetaminophen, chloral hydrate, dihydroergotamine, sulfonylureas, vasopressin
  Decrease vasodilating effects

BOX 26.5 Herb and Dietary Interactions: Nitroglycerin

Herbs and Foods That Increase the Effects of Nitroglycerin

- *N*-Acetyl cysteine
- Arginine, folate, vitamin E
- Hawthorn

Herbs and Foods That Decrease the Effects of Nitroglycerin

- Vitamin C

- Use the paper to spread ointment onto a nonhairy area of skin (chest, abdomen, thighs; avoid distal extremities) in a thin, even layer, covering a 2- to 3-inch area.
- Do not allow the ointment to come in contact with the hand. Do not massage the ointment into the patient's skin because absorption will be increased and interfere with the sustained action.

People should take PO nitrates in the morning after a nitrate-free interval (typically during the night). They should take the tablets or capsules 1 to 2 hours before meals. It is important not to break, crush, or chew sustained-release preparations.

IV nitroglycerin preparations come in a glass bottle, and nurses should use them only with special tubing provided by the manufacturer because polyvinyl chloride plastic tubing absorbs up to 80% of the nitroglycerin. They should ensure that patients receiving IV nitroglycerin are on a cardiac monitor. Many hospitals require patients to be in ICU or step-down unit while the nitroglycerin drip is actively being titrated. As previously stated, it is essential to take vital signs frequently with IV administration and recheck them with each titration.

Assessing for Therapeutic Effects

Therapeutic effects of some forms of nitroglycerin may include the relief of acute chest pain as well as a modest decrease in blood pressure. With oral preparations, a decreased frequency of chronic chest pain should occur. Overall, patients should report that they feel better and demonstrate a higher activity tolerance.

Patient Teaching

Box 26.6 reviews general patient teaching guidelines regarding drugs for the management of angina, including nitroglycerin.

Other Drugs in the Class

Isosorbide dinitrate (Isordil) is useful for reducing the frequency and severity of acute anginal episodes, not for acute relief of anginal symptoms. When given sublingually or in chewable tablets, it acts in about 2 minutes, and its effects last for 2 to 3 hours. When higher doses are given orally, more drug escapes metabolism in the liver and produces systemic effects in approximately 30 minutes. Therapeutic effects last about 4 hours after PO administration. The effective PO dose is usually determined by increasing the dose until headache occurs, indicating the maximum tolerable dose. Sustained-release capsules also are available.

Isosorbide mononitrate (Ismo, Imdur) is the metabolite and active component of isosorbide dinitrate. It is well absorbed after PO administration and almost 100% bioavailable. Unlike other PO nitrates, this drug is not subject to first-pass hepatic metabolism. Onset of action occurs within 1 hour, peak effects occur between 1 and 4 hours, and the elimination half-life is approximately 5 hours. It is used only for prophylaxis of angina; it does not act rapidly enough to relieve acute attacks.

BOX 26.6   **Patient Teaching Guidelines for Antianginal Drugs**

General Considerations

- Angina is chest pain that occurs because your heart is not getting enough blood and oxygen. The most common causes are hypertension and atherosclerosis of the coronary arteries. The chest pain usually lasts less than 5 minutes and episodes can be managed for years without causing permanent heart damage. However, if the pain is severe or prolonged, a heart attack and heart damage may develop. Seek information about your heart condition to prevent or decrease episodes of angina and prevent a heart attack.

- Several types of drugs are used in angina, and you may need a combination of drugs for the best effects. Most patients take one or more long-acting drugs to prevent anginal attacks and a fast, short-acting drug (usually nitroglycerin tablets that you dissolve under your tongue, or a nitroglycerin solution that you spray into your mouth) to relieve acute attacks. Seek emergency care immediately if rest, and three sublingual tablets or oral sprays 5 minutes apart do not relieve chest pain. The long-acting medications are not effective in relieving sudden anginal pain.

- As with any medications for serious or potentially serious conditions, it is extremely important to take antianginal medications as prescribed. Do not increase dosage or discontinue the drugs without specific instructions from your health care provider.

- With sublingual nitroglycerin tablets, keep them in the original container; carry them so that they are always within reach but not where they are exposed to body heat; and replace them approximately every 6 months because they become ineffective.

- It may be helpful to record the number and severity of anginal episodes, the number of nitroglycerin tablets required to relieve the attack, and the total number of tablets taken daily. Such a record can help your health care provider know when to change your medications or your dosages.

- Headache and dizziness may occur with nitrate antianginal drugs, especially sublingual nitroglycerin. These effects are usually temporary and dissipate with continued therapy. If dizziness occurs, avoid strenuous activity and stand up slowly for approximately an hour after taking the drugs. If headache is severe, you may take aspirin or acetaminophen with the nitrate drug. Do not reduce drug dosage or take the drug less often to avoid headache; loss of effectiveness may occur.

- Keep family members or support people informed about the location and use of antianginal medications in case help is needed.

- Avoid over-the-counter decongestants, cold remedies, and diet pills, which stimulate the heart and constrict blood vessels and thus may cause angina.

(Continued on page 482)

BOX 26.6 **Patient Teaching Guidelines for Antianginal Drugs** (Continued)

■ With nitrate antianginal drugs, avoid alcohol. Both the drugs and alcohol dilate blood vessels, and an excessive reduction in blood pressure (with dizziness and fainting) may occur with the combination.

■ With a metabolic modulator, avoid concurrent intake of grapefruit juice: grapefruit juice increases serum drug levels.

■ Several calcium channel blockers are available in both immediate-acting and long-acting (sustained-release) forms. The brand names often differ very little (e.g., Procardia is a brand name of immediate-release nifedipine; Procardia XL is a long-acting formulation). It is extremely important that the correct formulation is used consistently.

■ Keep all appointments with your health care provider.

Self- or Caregiver Administration

■ Take or give antianginal drugs as instructed; specific instructions differ with the type of drug being taken.

■ Take or give antianginal drugs on a regular schedule, at evenly spaced intervals. This increases drug effectiveness in preventing acute attacks of angina.

■ With nitroglycerin and other nitrate preparations:

■ Use according to instructions for the particular dosage form. The dosage forms were developed for specific routes of administration and are not interchangeable.

■ Take your blood pressure before administering the medication as possible and anticipate that the drug can decrease blood pressure from original reading. For sublingual nitroglycerin tablets, place them under the tongue until they dissolve. Take at the first sign of an anginal attack, before severe pain develops. If chest pain is not relieved in 5 minutes, dissolve a second tablet under the tongue. If pain is not relieved within another 5 minutes, dissolve a third tablet. If pain continues or becomes more severe, notify your health care provider immediately or report to the nearest hospital emergency room. Sit down when you take the medications. This may help relieve pain and prevent dizziness from the drug.

■ For the translingual solution of nitroglycerin, spray onto or under the tongue; do not inhale the spray.

■ For transmucosal tablets of nitroglycerin, place them under the upper lip or between the cheek and gum and allow them to dissolve slowly over 3 to 5 hours. Do not chew or swallow the tablets.

■ For nitroglycerin ointment, use the special paper to measure the dose. Place the ointment on a nonhairy part of the upper body and apply with the applicator paper. Cover the area with plastic wrap or tape. Rotate application sites (because the ointment can irritate the skin) and wipe off the previous dose before applying a new dose. Wash hands after applying the ointment.

■ Use the measured paper for accurate dosage. Use the paper to apply the ointment because the drug is readily absorbed through the skin. Avoid skin contact except on the designated area of the body. Plastic wrap or tape aids absorption and prevents removal of the drug. It also prevents soiling of clothes and linens.

■ For nitroglycerin patches, apply at the same time each day to clean, dry, hairless areas on the upper body or arms. Rotate sites. Avoid applying below the knee or elbow or in areas of skin irritation or scar tissue. Correct application is necessary to promote effective and consistent drug absorption. The drug is not as well absorbed from distal portions of the extremities because of decreased blood flow. Rotation of sites decreases skin irritation. Also, dispose of used patches properly because there is enough residual nitroglycerin to be harmful, especially to children and pets.

■ Take oral nitrates on an empty stomach with a glass of water. Oral isosorbide dinitrate is available in regular and chewable tablets; be sure each type is taken appropriately. Do not crush or chew sustained-release nitrate tablets.

■ For sublingual isosorbide dinitrate tablets, place them under the tongue until they dissolve.

■ If an oral nitrate and topical nitroglycerin are being used concurrently, stagger the times of administration. This minimizes dizziness from low blood pressure and headache, which are common adverse effects of nitrate drugs.

■ Report all new dietary supplements to the prescriber because some herbs interact with nitroglycerin.

■ With beta-adrenergic blockers:

■ Do not stop taking the drug abruptly because this can cause rebound tachycardia. If withdrawal of a beta blocker is planned by your prescriber, a gradual decrease in dose should occur and you should limit physical activity to a minimum during this period.

■ Move slowly from a sitting to a standing position to avoid orthostatic hypotension.

■ Learn how to take your own pulse and blood pressure, report heart rate less than 55 beats per minutes to your health care provider, and withhold medication as instructed. Take your pulse and blood pressure more frequently when the medication is initiated and titrated up or down.

■ Be aware of possible adverse effects, including dizziness, wheezing, and low heart rate.

■ Take atenolol at the same time each day and avoid drinking large amounts of orange juice

■ With calcium channel blockers:

■ Increase water and fiber intake as tolerated to decrease constipation.

■ Elevate your feet during the day to avoid ankle swelling.

■ With sustained-release forms, which are usually taken once daily, do not take more often than prescribed and do not crush or chew.

Clinical Application 26-1

- Mr. Gerald receives a prescription for nitroglycerin in both an SL form and as a transdermal patch. While reviewing his medication instructions with him, the nurse learns he has had a history of erectile dysfunction and has sildenafil medication in the medicine cabinet that was prescribed for him before his MI. What actions should the nurse take?

NCLEX Success

3. The nurse removes a patient's transdermal nitroglycerin disk at bedtime as ordered to minimize nitrate tolerance. The patient awakens during the night and complains of anginal symptoms. The nurse's first action is to

   A. notify the health care provider.
   B. apply a new transdermal disk.
   C. obtain further history of complaints.
   D. administer a short-acting nitrate as ordered.

4. The health care provider prescribes nitroglycerin 2% ointment, 1.5-inch dose every 4 hours. To accurately apply the ointment, the patient should be instructed to

   A. rub the ointment into the skin to enhance absorption.
   B. leave previous ointment on for 4 hours after applying a new dose.
   C. rotate application sites to decrease skin irritation.
   D. place the ointment on a distal part of the lower body to increase absorption.

5. Concurrent use of nitrates in any form or route of administration with phosphodiesterase enzyme inhibitors produces

   A. enhanced erectile potential.
   B. significant tachycardia.
   C. severe hypotensive effects.
   D. mild bronchodilation.

6. A patient taking nitroglycerin for angina reports developing a headache after taking more than one tablet. The nurse should inform him that

   A. headache is a common side effect due to the vasodilating effects of the medication.
   B. a headache indicates that a person is allergic to the nitroglycerin.
   C. the experience of headache means that the levels of nitroglycerin are toxic.
   D. the experience of a headache likely means that the tablets have passed their expiration date.

7. The nurse is educating a patient taking sublingual nitroglycerin 0.4 mg for anginal pain. Which of the following statements indicate that the patient understands the instructions? (Check all that apply)

   A. "I should take one nitroglycerin tablet every 5 minute for pain, up to a total of three tablets, as needed."
   B. "I should expect that the nitroglycerin will cause a stinging sensation when placed under my tongue."
   C. "I should store my nitroglycerin in the original dark bottle to protect the tablets from light."
   D. "I should replace my nitroglycerin tablets every month whether the bottle has been opened or not."

Beta-Adrenergic Blockers

Beta-adrenergic blockers have become the cornerstone of drug therapy regimens for people with angina, hypertension, heart failure, and dysrhythmias. They decrease cardiac workload by slowing heart rate, decreasing blood pressure, and reducing contractility. The drugs are as effective as the organic nitrates in reducing the frequency and severity of anginal symptoms during exercise and present advantages to nitrate use. People taking the drugs do not develop tolerance during therapy as occurs with the organic nitrates.

The ability of a drug in this class to selectively block $beta_1$ receptors is known as **cardioselectivity**. Cardioselective beta-adrenergic blockers include atenolol, metoprolol, bisoprolol, and esmolol. These drugs block $beta_1$ receptors. Noncardioselective beta-adrenergic blockers block $beta_1$ and $beta_2$ receptors. Examples of noncardioselective beta-adrenergic blockers include propranolol, nadolol, carvedilol, and timolol. During beta-blocker therapy, the beta receptors undergo receptor upregulation. This means that the number of receptors on the surface of target cells (the beta cells) becomes more sensitive to catecholamines.

Beta-adrenergic blockers are discussed elsewhere in the text in relation to heart failure (see Chap. 24), dysrhythmias (see Chap. 25), hypertension (see Chap. 28), and glaucoma (see Chap. 58). Propranolol (Inderal), the first beta-adrenergic blocker available, is discussed in detail in Chapter 25 and is particularly useful in preventing exercise-induced tachycardia, which can precipitate anginal attacks. This chapter discusses ℗ **atenolol** (Tenormin) and other beta-adrenergic blockers used to treat angina.

Pharmacokinetics

With PO, atenolol undergoes extensive first-pass metabolism in the liver. Absorption is rapid and consistent but incomplete. Approximately only 50% of an oral dose is absorbed from the gastrointestinal (GI) tract. The drug is modestly (5%–15%) bound to plasma, is distributed to the placenta, and is secreted in breast milk. It does not readily cross the blood–brain barrier. Peak blood levels occur between 2 and 4 hours after ingestion.

With IV atenolol, onset of action is immediate, duration of action is dose dependent (half-life 6–7 hours), and peak blood levels are reached in 5 minutes. The drug is not metabolized and is excreted in the urine and feces.

Action

Atenolol is a beta$_1$ selective (cardioselective) beta-adrenergic blocker. The cardioselectivity is diminished at higher doses, where it inhibits beta$_2$ receptors in the bronchial and vascular musculature.

Use

Atenolol is useful in the treatment of angina and hypertension as well as for the prophylaxis and treatment of MI. Health care providers use atenolol and other beta-adrenergic blockers in long-term management to decrease the frequency and severity of anginal attacks, decrease the need for sublingual nitroglycerin, and increase exercise tolerance.

QSEN Safety Alert

It is important to note that beta blockers should not be used in patients with variant angina because they are ineffective and may increase the tendency to induce coronary vasospasm.

Table 26.3 presents route and dosage information for atenolol and other beta-adrenergic blockers. The U.S. Food and Drug Administration (FDA) has issued a **BLACK BOX WARNING** ◆ for the use of beta-adrenergic blockers in patients with CAD; withdrawing oral forms may result in exacerbation of angina, increased incidence of ventricular dysrhythmias, and the occurrence of MI. Therefore, it is essential to slowly taper beta-adrenergic blockers before discontinuing them.

Use in Older Adults

The prevalence of CAD increases with age and is the major cause of disability, morbidity, and mortality in older adults. The elderly have a higher incidence of multivessel coronary disease, decreased left ventricular function, and comorbid conditions. For this reason, beta-adrenergic blockers are one of the most frequently medications prescribed in older adults. Close monitoring of the patient's heart rate is essential because the incidence of sick sinus syndrome and chronotropic intolerance increases with age and predisposes these patients to bradycardia, syncope, and falls.

Use in Patients With Renal Impairment

Atenolol is well tolerated in patients with renal impairment. New study findings indicate beta blockers slow the deterioration of renal function in chronic kidney disease.

Use in Patients With Critical Illness

Administration of atenolol in the critical care setting may occur to reduce cardiovascular mortality in the management of hemodynamically stable patients with definite or suspected acute MI. IV administration should occur in a controlled setting equipped to monitor heart rate, blood pressure, and ECG. Hypotension may also occur with use, so the patient should be closely monitored for symptoms of hypotension. Unlike nitroglycerin, IV beta-adrenergic blockers are rarely used in the ICU for control of angina.

Adverse Effects

The major cardiac adverse reactions related to beta-adrenergic blockers such as atenolol include heart failure and substantial negative chronotropy. A small number of people with chronic heart failure may have an exacerbation of heart failure when they begin taking atenolol or other beta-adrenergic blockers. In these people, sympathetic drive is maintaining cardiac output. The beta-adrenergic blockers decrease this sympathetic drive and therefore cause a low cardiac output state and heart failure.

TABLE 26.3

DRUGS AT A GLANCE: Beta-Adrenergic Blockers

Drug	Pregnancy Category	Routes and Dosage Ranges (Adults [unless indicated])
Ⓟ **Atenolol** (Tenormin)	D	50 mg PO once daily, initially, increased to 100 mg daily after 1 wk, if necessary Safety and effectiveness have not been established in children
Bisoprolol (Zebeta)	C	5 mg PO once daily, initially, increased approximately every 3 d to 10 mg daily, then 20 mg once daily, if necessary
Carvedilol (Coreg)	C	6.25 mg PO twice a day with food, initially, increased to 6.25 to 25 mg PO twice a day; maximum recommended dose 50 mg/d
Metoprolol (Lopressor, Toprol XL)	C	100–450 mg PO daily in two to three divided doses Extended-release, 100 mg PO daily in a single dose
Nadolol (Corgard)	C	40–240 mg PO daily in a single dose
Propranolol (Inderal)	C	10–80 mg PO 2 to 4 times/d 0.5–3 mg IV every 4 h until desired response is obtained

The majority of patients with heart failure do benefit from beta blockade, and symptoms of heart failure abate.

Other adverse effects include slowing of the heart rate, a negative chronotropic effect. Dosage adjustments may be necessary; the target heart should be 55 to 65 beats per minute at rest. Use of beta-adrenergic blockers can lead to serious bradydysrhythmia and depression of the atrioventricular node. Noncardiac adverse effects include bronchospasm, especially in patients with chronic obstructive pulmonary disease (COPD) receiving high dosages because of blocked beta$_2$ receptors.

Contraindications

Contraindications to atenolol include known hypersensitivity to the drug, second- or third-degree heart block, and cardiogenic shock, as well as severe bradycardia, heart failure, or hypotension. Caution is warranted with milder bradycardia, heart failure, or hypotension, and asthma.

Nursing Implications

Preventing Interactions

Many medications interact with atenolol, increasing or decreasing its effects (Box 26.7). Additionally, some herbs decrease the effects of atenolol (Box 26.8).

BOX 26.7   Drug Interactions: Atenolol

Drugs That Increase the Effects of Atenolol
- Alcohol
  Increases the risk of hypotension
- Atazanavir, dolasetron, saquinavir
  Increase the risk of heart block
- Digoxin
  Increases the risk of bradycardia
- Diltiazem, verapamil
  Increase the risk of bradycardia, heart block, and increased left ventricular end-diastolic pressure
- Reserpine
  Increases the risk of hypotension and significant bradycardia
- Sildenafil, tadalafil, vardenafil
  Increase the risk of life-threatening hypotension

Drugs That Decrease the Effects of Atenolol
- Adrenergic drugs (e.g., epinephrine, isoproterenol)
  Reverse bradycardia
- Anticholinergic drugs (e.g., diphenhydramine, ipratropium)
  Increase heart rate, offsetting slower heart rates of atenolol
- Indomethacin
  Decreases the hypotensive effects

BOX 26.8 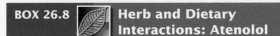 **Herb and Dietary Interactions: Atenolol**

Herbs and Foods That Decrease the Effects of Atenolol
- Betel palm
- Calcium salts
- Orange juice

Administering the Medication

Prior to giving atenolol, the nurse should check the patient's vital signs. It is important to withhold atenolol and notify the prescriber for a resting heart rate of 60 beats per minute and/or systolic blood pressure less than 90 mm Hg.

The nurse gives IV beta-adrenergic blockers over 2.5 minute. Continuous telemetry is necessary for patients receiving an IV bolus or a continuous drip. The effectiveness of beta-adrenergic blockers in relation to relieving angina is dose dependent. It is necessary to titrate the dose of the beta-adrenergic blocker for a target heart rate of 50 to 60 beats per minute with normal blood pressure. The nurse monitors the blood pressure every 5 minutes while the drip is being titrated.

Assessing for Therapeutic Effects

The nurse evaluates for three main objectives in the patient with chronic angina. One, the patient's frequency and severity of angina is reduced. Two, the patient has improved exercise capacity. Three, there is a reduction or elimination in the use of sublingual nitroglycerin. Ideally, achievement of these goals results in few adverse effects.

Assessing for Adverse Effects

The nurse closely monitors the patient's blood pressure and heart rate 2 to 4 hours after the first dose of atenolol. Signs of hypotension include dizziness and blurred vision; syncope is indicative of bradydysrhythmias. Increased shortness of breath and wheezing are adverse effects seen in patients with COPD who are taking beta-adrenergic blockers.

Patient Teaching

Box 26.6 includes patient teaching information regarding drugs for the management of angina, including atenolol.

Other Drugs in the Class

Metoprolol (Lopressor, Toprol XL) and bisoprolol (Zebeta) are other cardioselective beta-adrenergic blockers used to treat angina. These drugs block beta$_1$ receptors.

Metoprolol is used alone or in combination with other medications to treat angina and hypertension and improve survival after an MI. Extended-release tablets are used in the treatment of heart failure. The drug is lipid soluble and almost completely absorbed by the small intestine. It has a short half-life. It is eliminated by hepatic metabolism and is excreted in the urine. It has a short plasma half-life. Adverse effects include bradycardia, hypotension, dizziness, fatigue, and impotence.

Bisoprolol (Zebeta) is also used to manage hypertension (see Chap. 28) and heart failure (see Chap. 25). The drug reduces the workload of the heart and decreases myocardial oxygen demand by decreasing heart rate and the force of myocardial contractions. It is generally well tolerated, and adverse effects are mild and transient; they include nausea, diarrhea, dizziness, fatigue, impotence, bradycardia, and hypotension. At higher doses, bisoprolol can cause shortness of breath and wheezing. The drug can mask the early warning symptoms of hypoglycemia as does most of the beta-adrenergic blockers.

Noncardioselective beta-adrenergic blockers block beta$_1$ and beta$_2$ receptors. Examples of noncardioselective beta-adrenergic blockers used to treat angina include propranolol (Inderal) and nadolol (Corgard).

Propranolol (Inderal) is used to reduce the frequency and severity of acute attacks of angina. It is especially useful in preventing exercise-induced tachycardia, which can precipitate anginal attacks. Caution is warranted with hepatic impairment. Nonselective beta-adrenergic blockers such as propranolol can slow down the process of glycogenolysis. Therefore, the occurrence of hypoglycemia increases. Beta-adrenergic blockers also can mask the early symptoms of hypoglycemia such as diaphoresis and anxiety due to blocked catecholamines. Propranolol is well absorbed after oral administration. It is then metabolized extensively in the liver; a relatively small proportion of an oral dose (approximately 30%) reaches the systemic circulation. For this reason, oral doses of propranolol are much higher than IV doses. Onset of action is 30 minutes after oral administration and 1 to 2 minutes after IV injection. It is important to instruct patients to take the drug at the same time each day, preferably with or immediately following meals, because food may enhance the bioavailability of propranolol. Erectile dysfunction and wheezing are common adverse effects. Also, patients should report shortness of breath, night cough, edema, slow pulse, confusion, depression, rash, fever, or sore throat. In addition, they should understand that propranolol should never be stopped abruptly. Cimetidine may increase beta-blocking effects of propranolol by slowing its hepatic clearance and elimination.

Nadolol has the same actions, uses, and adverse effects as propranolol, but it has a long half-life and can be given once daily. The drug is excreted by the kidneys, and it is necessary to reduce the dosage in patients with renal impairment.

Clinical Application 26-2

- In addition to nitroglycerin, the nurse practitioner prescribes atenolol. Mr. Gerald understands why nitroglycerin is beneficial to his condition. He asks about the atenolol and why he needs to take this medication. How should the nurse respond?

Calcium Channel Blockers

Calcium channel blockers are used to treat an assortment of cardiovascular disorders including stable angina pectoris and variant angina. Other indications include hypertension, hypertrophic cardiomyopathy, and supraventricular dysrhythmias.

There are two main categories of calcium channel blockers: the dihydropyridines (nifedipine, amlodipine, nicardipine, nitrendipine) and the nondihydropyridines (verapamil and diltiazem). ℗ **Nifedipine** (Adalat, Procardia) is the prototype.

Pharmacokinetics

Nifedipine is well absorbed after oral administration, with an onset of action of 20 minutes or less. It reaches peak plasma levels within 1 to 2 hours (6 hours or longer for sustained-release forms). Most of the drug is more than 90% protein bound. It undergoes extensive first-pass metabolism in the liver. Excretion occurs in the feces and urine.

Action

Nifedipine inhibits the influx of calcium entering through slow channels, producing vasodilation of the peripheral blood vessels and coronary arteries (Fig. 26.1). However, the drug has a minimal effect on the sinoatrial and atrioventricular nodes. Therefore, it does not affect the heart rate.

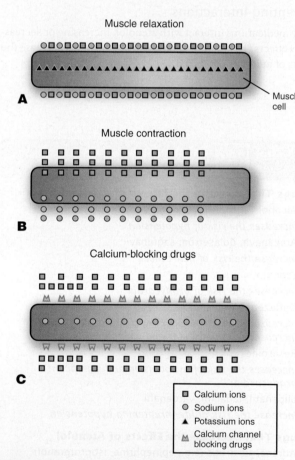

Figure 26.1 Calcium channel blockers: mechanism of action. **A.** During muscle relaxation, potassium ions are inside the muscle cell and calcium and sodium ions are outside the muscle cell. **B.** For muscle contraction to occur, potassium ions leave the cell and sodium and calcium ions enter the cell through open channels in the cell membrane. **C.** When calcium channels are blocked by drug molecules, muscle contraction is decreased because calcium ions cannot move through the cell membrane into the muscle cell.

TABLE 26.4

DRUGS AT A GLANCE: Calcium Channel Blockers

Drugs	Pregnancy Category	Routes and Dosage Ranges (Adults [unless indicated])
Ⓟ **Nifedipine** (Adalat, Procardia)	C	Angina: immediate release, 10–30 mg PO 3 times daily; sustained release, 30–60 mg PO once daily Hypertension: sustained release only, 30–60 mg once daily
Amlodipine (Norvasc)	C	5–10 mg PO once daily
Diltiazem (Cardizem)	C	Angina or hypertension (immediate release): 60–90 mg PO 4 times daily before meals and at bedtime Hypertension (sustained-release only): 120–180 mg PO twice daily Dysrhythmias (Cardizem IV only), IV injection 0.25 mg/kg (average dose 20 mg) over 2 min with a second dose of 0.35 mg/kg (average dose 25 mg) in 15 min if necessary, followed by IV infusion of 5–15 mg/h up to 24 h
Felodipine (Plendil)	C	5–10 mg PO once daily
Isradipine (DynaCirc)	C	2.5–5 mg PO twice daily
Nicardipine (Cardene)	C	Angina: immediate release only, 20–40 mg PO 3 times daily Hypertension: immediate release, same as for angina, above; sustained release, 30–60 mg PO twice daily
Verapamil (Calan, Isoptin)	C	Angina: 80–120 mg PO 3 times daily Dysrhythmias: 80–120 mg PO 3 to 4 times daily; injection, 5–10 mg IV over 2 min or longer, with continuous monitoring of electrocardiogram and blood pressure Hypertension: 80 mg PO 3 times daily or 240 mg PO (sustained release) once daily

Use

Nifedipine has been shown to be effective in the treatment for stable, variant, and unstable angina, mild-to-severe hypertension, and Raynaud's phenomenon. Table 26.4 contains route and dosage information for nifedipine and other calcium channel blockers.

Use in Children

For primary hypertension, nifedipine and other long-acting calcium channel blockers are safe. They are especially useful in children who have asthma and cannot tolerate beta-adrenergic blockers.

Use in Older Adults

Nifedipine and other calcium channel blockers are commonly used in older adults. This age group is more prone to orthostatic hypotension and is at high risk for falls while taking calcium channel blockers. Older adults may have higher plasma concentrations of nifedipine due to decreased hepatic metabolism of the drug, probably because of decreased hepatic blood flow.

Use in Patients With Renal Impairment

With nifedipine, protein binding is decreased and the elimination half-life is prolonged with renal impairment; therefore, dosage adjustment may be necessary. In a few patients, reversible elevations in blood urea nitrogen and serum creatinine have occurred.

Use in Patients With Hepatic Impairment

With nifedipine and other calcium channel blockers, impairment of liver function has profound effects on the pharmacokinetics and pharmacodynamics. Thus, use of these drugs requires caution. It is necessary to reduce dosages substantially and closely monitor patients for drug effects (including periodic measurements of liver enzymes). These recommendations stem from the following effects:

- An impaired liver produces fewer drug-binding plasma proteins such as albumin. This means that a greater proportion of a given dose is unbound and therefore active.
- In patients with cirrhosis, bioavailability of oral drugs is greatly increased and metabolism (of both oral and parenteral drugs) is greatly decreased. Both of these effects increase plasma levels of drug from a given dose (essentially an overdose). The effects result from shunting of blood around the liver so that drug molecules circulating in the bloodstream do not come in contact with drug-metabolizing enzymes and therefore are not metabolized.
- Although hepatotoxicity is uncommon, clinical symptoms of hepatitis, cholestasis, or jaundice and elevated liver enzymes (e.g., alkaline phosphatase, creatine kinase [CK],

lactate dehydrogenase [LDH], aspartate aminotransferase [AST], alanine aminotransferase [ALT]) have occurred, mainly with diltiazem, nifedipine, and verapamil. These changes resolve if the causative drug is stopped.

Use in Patients Receiving Home Care

With patients taking nifedipine, the home health nurse should check patients' blood pressure and heart rate at each visit. Also, the nurse should note adverse effects of the drug and suggest measures to minimize fall risk.

Adverse Effects

With nifedipine, cardiac adverse effects due to excessive vasodilation include hypotension, flushing, headache, dizziness, lower limb edema, and reflex tachycardia; these appear to be dose related. Noncardiac adverse effects include constipation, nausea, and gingival hyperplasia.

Contraindications

Contraindications to nifedipine include known hypersensitivity to the drug. It is important not to use nifedipine in the treatment of angina related to overdose with cocaine, amphetamines, or other alpha-adrenergic stimulants. This leads to unopposed stimulation of alpha-adrenergic receptors, causing vasoconstriction and severe, life-threatening hypertension.

Nursing Implications

Preventing Interactions

Many medications interact with nifedipine, increasing or decreasing its effect (Box 26.9). People should not take grapefruit juice with nifedipine because a two-fold increase in the effects of the drug may occur. Nifedipine may interact with quinidine, decreasing plasma levels, and digoxin, increasing levels.

BOX 26.9   **Drug Interactions: Nifedipine**

Drugs That Increase the Effects of Nifedipine

- Cisapride, dolasetron, pimozide
  Increases risk of prolongation of QT interval, second- and third-degree heart block, and ventricular dysrhythmias
- Itraconazole
  Increases dose-related negative inotropic effect
- Cimetidine
  Increases peak plasma levels
- Tizanidine
  Increases the risk of hypotension

Drugs That Decrease the Effects of Nifedipine

- Calcium-containing products
  Saturate calcium channels
- Carbamazepine, phenytoin, rifampin
  Induce hepatic enzymes and increase the rate of metabolism

Administering the Medication

People may take nifedipine with or without food. It is important not to crush or break sustained-release formulations. It is necessary to take the blood pressure prior to administering nifedipine and withhold the drug for a systolic blood pressure less than 90 mm Hg.

Assessing for Therapeutic Effects

The nurse should note a reduction of angina episodes once the patient has started taking nifedipine. Ideally, the systolic blood pressure generally should be less than 120 mm Hg.

Assessing for Adverse Effects

The nurse should assess for excessive vasodilation. Symptoms include flushing, peripheral edema, and frequent headaches. Hypotension, dizziness, lightheadedness, weakness, peripheral edema, headache, heart failure, pulmonary edema, nausea, and constipation may also occur.

Patient Teaching

QSEN Safety Alert

It is essential to teach patients to never stop taking nifedipine abruptly. This may result in rebound tachycardia.

Box 26.6 outlines patient teaching guidelines regarding drugs for the management of angina, including nifedipine.

Other Drugs in the Class

The other calcium channel blockers vary in clinical indications for use; most are used for angina or hypertension, and only diltiazem and verapamil are used to manage supraventricular tachydysrhythmias. In patients with CAD, the drugs are effective as monotherapy but are commonly prescribed in combination with beta-adrenergic blockers. In addition, nimodipine is approved for use only in subarachnoid hemorrhage, in which it decreases spasm in cerebral blood vessels and limits the extent of brain damage.

In variant angina, calcium channel blockers reduce coronary artery vasospasm. In atrial fibrillation or flutter and other supraventricular tachydysrhythmias, diltiazem and verapamil slow the rate of ventricular response. In hypertension, the drugs lower blood pressure primarily by dilating peripheral arteries.

The dihydropyridines used to treat angina besides nifedipine include amlodipine and nicardipine. Amlodipine (Norvasc) is effective in patients with exertional angina, because the drug reduces afterload decreasing myocardial oxygen demand. It is also used for the treatment of coronary spasm in variant angina. The drug is well absorbed by the PO route. Amlodipine (30–50 hours) has a long elimination half-life and therefore can be given once daily. Common adverse effects include peripheral edema, fatigue, dizziness, nausea, palpitations, and headache.

Nicardipine (Cardene) is a dihydropyridine calcium channel blocker used for the treatment of chronic stable angina (exertional), hypertension, and Raynaud's phenomenon. The drug is available in oral and intravenous forms. The most common side effects are flushing, headaches, dizziness, and peripheral edema. Nicardipine's mechanism of action and clinical effects closely resemble those of nifedipine and the other dihydropyridines,

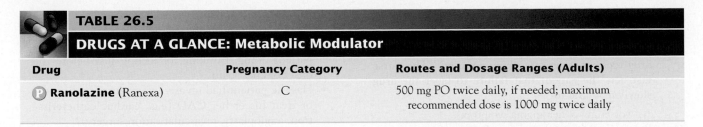

Drug	Pregnancy Category	Routes and Dosage Ranges (Adults)
Ⓟ **Ranolazine** (Ranexa)	C	500 mg PO twice daily, if needed; maximum recommended dose is 1000 mg twice daily

amlodipine and felodipine, except that nicardipine is more selective for cerebral and coronary blood vessels.

Nondihydropyridines, such as diltiazem (Cardizem) and verapamil (Calan, Isoptin), block the slow calcium channels in the heart. They also decrease the heart rate by slowing conduction through the atrioventricular node and decrease sinoatrial node automaticity. Chapter 25 describes them well. Whereas nifedipine acts mainly on vascular smooth muscle to produce vasodilation, verapamil and diltiazem have greater effects on the cardiac conduction system. For this reason, these two drugs may also be used to for supraventricular tachycardia. They are also effective in the treatment of angina, hypertension, and migraines. Diltiazem is a potent vasodilator of coronary and peripheral vessels, which decreases afterload and decreases workload on the heart. The drug has pharmacologic activity similar to verapamil, although diltiazem and verapamil differ chemically from the dihydropyridines and each other. Adverse effects include hypotension, bradycardia, dizziness, and flushing. Along with other calcium channel blockers, verapamil and diltiazem are known to induce gingival hyperplasia.

Adjuvant Medications

Metabolic Modulator: Ranolazine

The metabolic modulator Ⓟ **ranolazine** (Ranexa) is an FDA-approved first-line treatment for chronic angina. The drug increases the energy production of the heart to preserve cardiac function but does not relieve acute anginal attacks. Ranolazine performs this action without decreasing blood pressure or heart rate. Although the mechanism of action is not clearly understood, ranolazine works by preventing both calcium overload and the subsequent increase in diastolic tension. This is all related to inhibition of late inward sodium channel. Because this sodium channel frequently fails to inactivate in a number of important myocardial disease states such as ischemia and hypertrophy, excess entry of sodium ions leads to activation of the sodium–calcium exchanger, thereby raising calcium concentration. Unlike the other classes of antianginal drugs, ranolazine decreases ischemia but does not possess negative inotropic or chronotropic effects. When compared to placebo in patients with CAD, ranolazine is associated with a decreased frequency of ventricular dysrhythmias, bradycardia, and new-onset atrial fibrillation.

The FDA has recommended that ranolazine should be reserved for patients who have not had an adequate response

with other antianginal drugs due to the drug's dose-dependent ability to prolong the QT interval. Therefore, the drug is contraindicated in patients with preexisting QT-interval prolongation. It is also contraindicated in patients with hepatic disease and in patients taking other drugs that prolong the QT interval. Dose reduction of digoxin and simvastatin may be necessary with concurrent use because ranolazine affects the metabolic pathways of these drugs. Table 26.5 gives route and dosage information for ranolazine.

Other Drugs

Aspirin has become a standard in cardiac care because of its antiplatelet (i.e., antithrombotic) effects. Recommended doses vary from 81 mg daily to 325 mg daily or every other day. For tertiary prevention, such as post MI, patient should be 325 mg of aspirin a day; primary prevention dosage is 81 mg daily. Chapter 14 contains additional information regarding aspirin.

Dyslipidemic drugs (i.e., atorvastatin, cholestyramine, niacin) are useful in the management of patients with major risk factors for atherosclerosis and vascular disorders such as CAD, stroke, and peripheral arterial insufficiency when lifestyle changes alone do not reduce blood lipids. These drugs have proven efficacy, and health care providers are increasingly using them to reduce morbidity and mortality from coronary heart disease and other atherosclerosis-related cardiovascular disorders. Prescribers order dyslipidemic drugs to decrease blood lipids, prevent or delay the development of atherosclerotic plaque, promote the regression of existing atherosclerotic plaque, and reduce morbidity and mortality from cardiovascular disease. Chapter 8 discusses the dyslipidemic drugs in detail.

Besides the beta-adrenergic blockers and calcium channel blockers, antihypertensive drugs that decrease peripheral vascular resistance are useful in angina. Chapter 28 outlines antihypertensive drugs.

NCLEX Success

8. A 57-year-old man taking metoprolol (Lopressor) presents to the cardiac clinic following a myocardial infarction. He reports that he continues to smoke. Smoking may contribute to what effect on beta-blocking activity?

A. reduce the efficacy
B. potentiate an increase in intracranial pressure
C. precipitate ventricular fibrillation
D. increase the incidence of adverse effects

9. A 72-year-old woman with angina pectoris, who is being discontinued from beta-adrenergic blockers, asks the nurse, "Why can't I just stop taking the drug today if it's not working anyway?" The nurse instructs the patient that failure to taper the drug slowly may lead to

   A. worsening of her angina symptoms.
   B. significant bronchoconstriction.
   C. development of heart failure.
   D. drug fever

10. In caring for a patient with chronic angina who has been prescribed the new drug, ranolazine (Ranexa), the nurse is correct in counseling that this drug

    A. may be crushed if necessary
    B. must not be taken with beta-adrenergic blockers
    C. must not be taken with meals
    D. should not be taken with grapefruit juice

The Nursing Process

Assessment

- During the initial nursing history interview, try to answer the following questions:
  - How long has the patient been taking antianginal drugs? For what purpose are they being taken (prophylaxis, treatment of acute attacks, or both)?
  - What is the frequency and duration of acute anginal attacks? Has either increased recently? (An increase could indicate worsening coronary atherosclerosis and increased risk of MI.)
  - Do symptoms other than chest pain occur during acute attacks (e.g., shortness of breath, diaphoresis, nausea)?
  - Are there particular activities or circumstances that provoke acute attacks? Do attacks ever occur when the patient is at rest? Where does the patient fit in the Canadian Cardiovascular Society classification system?
  - What measures relieve symptoms of acute angina?
  - If the patient takes nitroglycerin, ask how often it is required, how many tablets are needed for relief of pain, how often the supply is replaced, and where the patient stores or carries the drug.
- Assess blood pressure and pulse, ECG reports, serum cholesterol, and cardiac enzymes. Elevated cholesterol is a significant risk factor for coronary atherosclerosis and angina, and the risk is directly related to the degree of elevation. Cardiac enzyme levels, such as troponin, CK, LDH, and AST, should all be normal in patients with angina.
- During an acute attack, assess the following:
  - Location and quality of the pain. Chest pain is nonspecific. It may be a symptom of numerous disorders, such as pulmonary embolism, esophageal spasm or inflammation (heartburn), costochondritis, or anxiety. Chest pain of cardiac origin is caused by myocardial ischemia and may indicate angina pectoris or MI.
  - Precipitating factors. For example, what was the patient doing, thinking, or feeling just before the onset of chest pain?
  - Has the patient had invasive procedures to diagnose or treat his or her CAD (e.g., cardiac catheterization, angioplasty, revascularization surgery)?

Nursing Diagnoses

- Decreased cardiac output related to altered stroke volume or drug therapy
- Pain, acute in chest related to inadequate perfusion of the myocardium
- Activity intolerance related to chest pain and an imbalance in cardiac supply and demand
- Knowledge, deficient related to management of disease process and drug therapy
- Ineffective individual coping related to depression, fear, anxiety, and ongoing grieving associated with the diagnosis of angina
- Sexual dysfunction related to fear of precipitating anginal symptoms

Planning/Goals

The patient will

- Receive or take antianginal drugs accurately.
- Experience relief of acute chest pain and other anginal symptoms.
- Have fewer episodes of acute chest pain and other anginal symptoms.
- Have increased activity tolerance.
- Identify and manage situations that precipitate anginal attacks.
- Be closely monitored for therapeutic and adverse effects, especially when drug therapy is started.
- Avoid preventable adverse effects.
- Verbalize essential information about the disease process, needed dietary and lifestyle changes to improve health status, and drug therapy.
- Identify available resources and support systems.
- Demonstrate appropriate coping strategies.
- Recognize signs and symptoms that necessitate professional intervention.
- Keep appointments for follow-up care and monitoring.

Nursing Interventions

The nurse will

- Use the following measures to prevent acute anginal attacks.
  - Assist in preventing, recognizing, and managing contributory disorders, such as atherosclerosis, hypertension, hyperthyroidism, hypoxia, and anemia. For example, hypertension is a common risk factor for CAD, and morbidity and mortality increase progressively with the degree of either systolic or diastolic elevation. Management of hypertension reduces morbidity and mortality rates. However, most studies indicate that the reductions stem more from

fewer strokes, less renal failure, and less heart failure than from less CAD.

- Help the patient recognize and avoid precipitating factors (e.g., heavy meals, strenuous exercise) when possible. If anxiety is a factor, relaxation techniques or psychological counseling may be helpful.
- Support the patient while identifying resources, support systems, and effective coping strategies.
- Help the patient develop a more healthful lifestyle in terms of diet and weight control, adequate rest and sleep, regular exercise, and not smoking. Ideally, these self-help interventions are practiced before illness occurs; they can help prevent or delay illness. However, most people are unmotivated until illness develops, and perhaps after it develops as well. These interventions are beneficial at any stage of CAD. For example, for a patient who already has angina, a supervised exercise program helps develop collateral circulation. Smoking has numerous ill effects on the patient with angina and decreases effectiveness of antianginal drugs.
- During an acute anginal attack in a patient known to have angina or CAD, take the following actions.
  - Assume that any chest pain may be of cardiac origin.
  - Have the patient lie down or sit down to reduce cardiac workload and provide rest.
  - Check vital signs and compare them with baseline values.
  - Record the characteristics of chest pain and the presence of other signs and symptoms.

- Have the patient take a fast-acting nitroglycerin preparation (previously prescribed), up to three SL tablets or three PO sprays, each 5 minutes apart, as necessary.
- If chest pain is not relieved with rest and nitroglycerin, assume that an MI has occurred until proven otherwise. In a health care setting, keep the patient at rest and notify the patient's prescriber immediately. Outside of a health care setting, call 911 for immediate assistance.
- Leave SL nitroglycerin at the bedside of hospitalized patients (per hospital policy). The tablets or spray should be within reach so that they can be used immediately. Record the number of tablets used daily and ensure that an adequate supply is available.
- Provide appropriate patient teaching related to drug therapy (see Box 26.6).

Evaluation

- Observe and interview for relief of acute chest pain.
- Observe and interview regarding the number of episodes of acute chest pain.
- Identify CAD lifestyle factors that are being successfully modified or require modification (e.g., diet, weight, activity, smoking cessation).
- Observe effective coping strategies and appropriate use of support system and resources.
- Interview regarding success and adherence with drug therapy.

Key Concepts

- Angina results from deficit in myocardial oxygen supply (myocardial ischemia) in relation to myocardial oxygen demand, most often caused by atherosclerotic plaque in the coronary arteries.
- The goals of antianginal drug therapy are to relieve acute anginal pain, reduce the number and severity of acute anginal attacks, improve exercise tolerance and quality of life, delay progression of CAD, prevent MI, and prevent sudden cardiac death.
- Because PO nitroglycerin is rapidly metabolized in the liver, relatively small proportions reach systemic circulation; transmucosal, transdermal, and IV preparations are more effective.
- Common drugs used for myocardial ischemia are the organic nitrates, the beta-adrenergic blockers, and the calcium channel blockers.
- Beta-adrenergic blockers are more effective than nitrates or calcium channel blockers in decreasing the likelihood of silent ischemia and improving the mortality rate after transmural MI.
- The FDA has issued a **BLACK BOX WARNING** ◆ regarding abrupt withdrawal of oral beta-adrenergic blockers, including metoprolol, in patients with angina as a severe exacerbation of angina. The occurrence of MI and ventricular dysrhythmias has been reported.
- Traditional antianginal drugs that act via hemodynamic mechanisms (e.g., beta-adrenergic blockers, calcium channel blockers, nitrates) can pose a problem in older adults because of the associated higher risk of drug interaction and greater incidence of adverse drug effects.
- Patients who take long-acting dosage forms of nitrates on a regular schedule develop tolerance to the vasodilating (antianginal) effects of the drug.
- Phosphodiesterase enzyme type 5 inhibitors for erectile dysfunction and nitrates both decrease blood pressure, and the combined effect can produce profound, life-threatening hypotension.

- In angina pectoris, calcium channel blockers improve blood supply to the myocardium by dilating coronary arteries and decrease the workload of the heart by dilating peripheral arteries; in variant angina, the drugs reduce coronary artery vasospasm.

- The metabolic modulator ranolazine increases the energy production of the heart to preserve cardiac function but does not relieve acute anginal attacks.

- Aspirin, antilipidemics, and antihypertensives are used in conjunction with antianginal drugs to prevent progression of myocardial ischemia to MI.

- Starting with relatively small doses of antianginal drugs, and increasing them at appropriate intervals as necessary should achieve optimal benefit and minimal adverse effects.

Critical Thinking Questions

26-1. Jonathan Thomas is a 58-year-old accountant who is being evaluated at the cardiology clinic for angina. He is 5 feet 9 inches tall and weighs 220 pounds, with a waist measurement of 40 inches. He has a history of hypertension, for which he has been prescribed a thiazide diuretic. He admits that he has not been taking the medication lately. His blood pressure on this visit is 154/96 mm Hg. He smokes one pack of cigarettes per day. His LDL cholesterol level is 187 mg/dL. He has no history of diabetes, and his fasting glucose level is within normal limits. He states that he "works out at the gym" 3 days per week. He admits to episodes of midsternal chest pain accompanied by dyspnea and diaphoresis and associated with activity that is usually relieved with rest. He states that these episodes have been increasing in frequency to once or twice weekly.

- The nurse is teaching Mr. Thomas about nonpharmacologic management of his angina. What measures can he take to reduce his risk?

- Mr. Thomas receives a prescription for sublingual nitroglycerin tablets to use as needed for chest pain and isosorbide mononitrate (Imdur) to take daily. He asks why he needs two prescriptions. How should the nurse respond?

- Mr. Thomas continues to experience episodes of angina despite treatment with the nitrate. He receives a prescription for ranolazine (Ranexa). He asks whether he can stop taking the nitrate now. How should the nurse answer this question?

References and Resources

Corwin, E. J. (2011). *Handbook of pathophysiology* (4th ed.). Philadelphia, PA: Lippincott Williams & Wilkins.

DiPiro, J. T., Talbert, R. L., Yee, G., Matzke, G., Wells, B., & Posey, L. M. (2011). *Pharmacotherapy: A pathophysiologic approach* (8th ed.). New York, NY: McGraw-Hill.

Facts & Comparisons. *Drug facts and comparisons.* (Updated monthly). St. Louis, MO: Facts and Comparisons.

Gerczuk, P. Z., & Kloner, R. A. (2012). An update on cardioprotection: A review of the latest adjunctive therapies to limit myocardial infarction size in clinical trials. *Journal of the American College of Cardiology, 59,* 969–978.

Guyton, A. C., & Hall, J. E. (2011). *Textbook of medical physiology* (12th ed.). Philadelphia, PA: W.B. Saunders.

Kalra, B. S., & Roy, V. (2012). Efficacy of metabolic modulators in ischemic heart disease: An overview. *The Journal of Clinical Pharmacology, 52*(3), 292–305.

Karch, A. M. (2012). *2012 Lippincott's nursing drug guide.* Philadelphia, PA: Lippincott Williams & Wilkins.

Kones, R. (2010). Recent advances in the management of chronic stable angina I: Approach to the patient, diagnosis, pathophysiology, risk stratification, and gender disparities. *Journal of Vascular Health and Risk Management, 6,* 635–656.

Lacy, C. F., Armstrong, L. L., Goldman, M. P., & Lance, L. L. (2010). *Lexi-Comp's drug information handbook* (19th ed.). Hudson, OH: American Pharmaceutical Association.

National Clinical Guideline Centre. Management of stable angina. National Institute for Health and Clinical Excellence (Clinical guideline, number 126). Retrieved May 25, 2012, from http://www.guideline.gov/content.aspx?id=34825&search=angina

National Institutes of Health Expert Panel. (2001). *Third report of the National Cholesterol Education Program (NCEP) Expert Panel on Detection, Evaluation, and Treatment of High Blood Cholesterol in Adults (Adult Treatment Panel III)* (NIH Publication No. 01-3670). Bethesda, MD: National Institutes of Health.

Porth, C. M. (2009). *Pathophysiology: Concepts of altered health status* (8th ed.). Philadelphia, PA: Lippincott Williams & Wilkins.

Smith, S. C., Benjamin, E. J., Bonow, R. O., Braun, L. T., Creager, M. A., Franklin, B. A., et al. (2011). AHA/ACCF Secondary Prevention and Risk Reduction Therapy for Patients With Coronary and Other Atherosclerotic Vascular Disease: 2011 Update: A Guideline From the American Heart Association and American College of Cardiology Foundation Endorsed by the World Heart Federation and the Preventive Cardiovascular Nurses Association. *Journal of the American College of Cardiology, 58,* 2432–2446.

Wright, R. S., Anderson, J. L., Adams, C. D., Bridges, C. R., Casey, D. E., Ettinger, S. M., et al. (2011). 2011 ACCF/AHA Focused Update of the guidelines for the management of patients with unstable angina/non-ST-elevation myocardial infarction (updating the 2007 guideline): A report of the American College of Cardiology Foundation/American Heart Association Task Force on practice guidelines developed in collaboration with the American College of Emergency Physicians, Society for Cardiovascular Angiography and Interventions, and Society of Thoracic Surgeons. *Journal of the American College of Cardiology, 57,* 1920–1959.

27 Drug Therapy to Enhance the Adrenergic Response

LEARNING OBJECTIVES

After studying this chapter, you should be able to:

1 Identify effects produced by stimulation of alpha- and beta-adrenergic receptors.

2 Discuss use of epinephrine to treat anaphylactic shock, cardiac arrest, and acute bronchospasm.

3 Identify patients at risk for the adverse effects associated with adrenergic drugs.

4 List commonly used over-the-counter preparations and herbal preparations that contain adrenergic drugs.

5 List characteristics of adrenergic drugs in terms of etiology, pathophysiology, and clinical manifestations, along with pharmacokinetics, action, use, adverse effects, contraindications, and nursing implications in use of adrenergic agents.

6 Discuss using adrenergic drugs in special patient populations.

7 Teach patients about safe, effective use of adrenergic drugs.

8 Describe signs and symptoms of toxicity due to noncatecholamine adrenergic drugs and how to treat this condition.

9 Understand the nursing process for using adrenergic drugs.

Clinical Application Case Study

Abe Sobechenko, a 71-year-old man, has chronic obstructive pulmonary disease (COPD). He has had asthma for all of his adult life and is admitted to the hospital with acute respiratory distress secondary to pneumonia. Although he has never been a smoker, he worked as a welder for 45 years. He has a very modest pension and has Medicare for health insurance, which sometimes makes it difficult for him to pay for all his medical supplies and medications.

KEY TERMS

Adrenergic drug: agent that produces effects similar to those produced by stimulation of the sympathetic nervous system and therefore has widespread effects on body tissues

Adrenergic receptor: structure that is activated by adrenaline-like compound

- **Alpha$_1$:** found on surface membranes of target tissues and organs; mainly postsynaptic
- **Alpha$_2$:** found on surface membranes of target tissues and organs; mainly presynaptic
- **Beta:** found in heart muscle, which cause increased heart rate and contractility, and in the kidney, which promote the release of renin from the kidney

Anaphylaxis: type I immunoglobulin E-mediated allergic reaction to a foreign substance (antigen) that has entered the body; occurs on second or subsequent exposure to an antigen. Symptoms develop rapidly; typical symptom onset ranges from 30 minutes to 2 hours after exposure to the antigen

Antigen: foreign substance

Decongestant: agent that reduces nasal congestion by decreasing the blood flow to the upper respiratory tract and decreasing the overproduction of secretions

Neurotransmitter: chemical substance that carries messages from one neuron to another, or from a neuron to other body tissues, such as cardiac or skeletal muscle

Postsynaptic: situated behind or occurring after a synapse

Pressor: effect that increases the blood pressure

Presynaptic: situated in front of or occurring before a synapse

Vasopressor: substance that increases the blood pressure

Introduction

Adrenergic drugs produce effects similar to those produced by stimulation of the sympathetic nervous system and therefore have widespread effects on body tissues. Major therapeutic uses and adverse effects of adrenergic medications derive from drug action on the heart, blood vessels, and lungs. Some adrenergic drugs are exogenous formulations of naturally occurring neurotransmitters and hormones, such as norepinephrine, epinephrine, and dopamine. Other adrenergic medications, such as phenylephrine, pseudoephedrine, and isoproterenol, are synthetic chemical relatives of naturally occurring neurotransmitters and hormones.

Specific effects of adrenergic medications depend mainly on the type of **adrenergic receptor** activated by the drug. Adrenergic receptors are those responses that are activated by adrenaline-like compounds. The drugs discussed in this chapter (e.g., epinephrine, pseudoephedrine, isoproterenol, phenylephrine) affect multiple adrenergic receptors and have many clinical uses. Other adrenergic drugs are more selective for specific adrenergic receptors or are given topically to produce more localized therapeutic effects and thus have fewer systemic adverse effects. These drugs have relatively restricted clinical indications and are discussed more extensively elsewhere (Chap. 29, Drug Therapy for Nasal Congestion; Chap. 31, Drugs for Asthma and Bronchoconstriction; and Chap. 57, Drug Therapy for Disorders of the Eye).

Overview of the Adrenergic Response

Physiology: Adrenergic Receptors

For the most part, adrenergic drugs interact directly with postsynaptic alpha$_1$- or beta-adrenergic receptors on the surface membrane of target organs and tissues (Fig. 27.1). **Alpha$_1$-adrenergic receptors** are receptors on surface membranes of target tissues and organs, which are mainly postsynaptic. The **beta-adrenergic receptors** reside in heart muscle, which causes increased heart rate and contractility,

and in the kidneys, which promotes the release of renin from the kidney. The drug–receptor complex then alters the permeability of the cell membrane to ions or extracellular enzymes. The influx of these molecules stimulates intracellular metabolism and production of other enzymes, structural proteins, energy, and other products required for cell function and reproduction. Epinephrine, isoproterenol, norepinephrine, and phenylephrine are examples of direct-acting adrenergic drugs.

Some adrenergic drugs exert indirect effects on postsynaptic adrenergic receptors. **Postsynaptic** means situated behind or occurring after a synapse. Indirect adrenergic effects may be produced by drugs such as amphetamines, which increase the amount of norepinephrine released into the synapse from storage sites in nerve endings (Fig. 27.2A). Norepinephrine

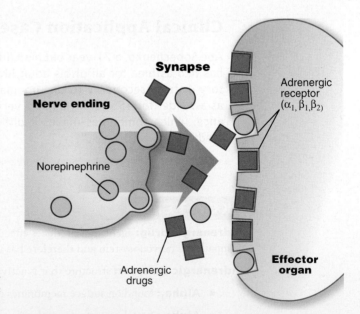

Figure 27.1 Mechanism of direct adrenergic drug action. Adrenergic drugs interact directly with postsynaptic alpha1 and beta receptors on target effector organs, activating the organ in a similar fashion as the neurotransmitter norepinephrine.

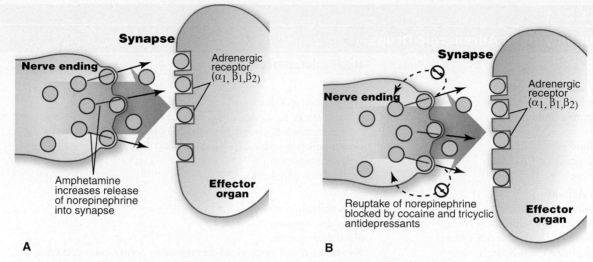

Figure 27.2 Mechanisms of indirect adrenergic drug action. Stimulation of postsynaptic alpha1, beta1, and beta2 receptors results from adrenergic medications that act indirectly, increasing the release of norepinephrine into the synapse (**A**) or inhibiting the reuptake of norepinephrine from the synapse (**B**).

then stimulates the alpha and beta receptors, producing sympathetic effects in the body. Inhibition of norepinephrine reuptake from the synapse is another mechanism that produces indirect adrenergic effects. Remember that norepinephrine reuptake is the major way that sympathetic nerve transmission is terminated. Drugs such as tricyclic antidepressants and cocaine block norepinephrine reuptake, resulting in stimulation of alpha- and beta-adrenergic receptors (Fig. 27.2B).

Other adrenergic drugs are called mixed-acting drugs. They directly stimulate adrenergic receptors by binding to them and indirectly stimulate adrenergic receptors by increasing the release of norepinephrine into synapses. Ephedrine and pseudoephedrine are examples of mixed-acting adrenergic drugs.

Because many body tissues have both alpha and beta receptors, the effect produced by an adrenergic drug depends on the type of receptor activated and the number of affected receptors in a particular body tissue. Some adrenergic drugs are nonselective, acting on both alpha and beta receptors. Other medications are more selective, acting only on certain subtypes of receptors. Table 27.1 groups commonly used adrenergic drugs by adrenergic receptor activity and gives their clinical use.

Pathophysiology of the Adrenergic Response

The effect produced by an adrenergic drug depends on the type of receptor activated and the number of affected receptors in a particular part of the body. The predominant effect in response to activation of alpha$_1$ receptors is vasoconstriction of blood vessels, which increases the blood pressure. This is sometimes referred to as a **pressor** (or **vasopressor**) effect. Alpha$_1$-activated vasoconstriction of blood vessels in nasal mucous membranes decreases nasal congestion, leading to a

decongestant effect. Other adrenergic effects resulting from alpha$_1$ activation include mydriasis, contraction of gastrointestinal (GI) and genitourinary sphincters, and elevated blood glucose.

The predominant effect in response to activation of beta$_1$ receptors in the heart is cardiac stimulation. Beta$_1$ activation causes increased force of myocardial contraction, or a positive inotropic effect; increased heart rate, or a positive chronotropic effect; and increased speed of electrical conduction in the heart, or a positive dromotropic effect. Another adrenergic effect resulting from beta$_1$ activation is increased renin secretion from the kidneys.

The predominant clinical effect in response to activation of beta$_2$ receptors is bronchodilation. Activation of beta$_2$ receptors in blood vessels causes vasodilation and increased blood flow to the heart, brain, and skeletal muscles, tissues needed for the "fight-or-flight" sympathetic response. Beta$_2$ activation also results in hepatic glycogenolysis and gluconeogenesis and decreased pancreatic insulin secretion, leading to hyperglycemia. Other adrenergic effects resulting from beta$_2$ activation include relaxation of smooth muscle in the uterus, urinary bladder, and GI tract.

Activation of beta$_3$-adrenergic receptors produces lipolysis and increased release of free fatty acids into the blood.

Drugs that activate **alpha$_2$ receptors** on presynaptic nerve fibers do not produce a sympathetic effect. Alpha$_2$ receptors are located on surface membranes of target tissues and organs and are mainly presynaptic. **Presynaptic** is defined as situated in front of or occurring before a synapse. These drugs inhibit the release of the neurotransmitter norepinephrine into synapses of the sympathetic nervous system, thus exerting an antiadrenergic response in the body. **Neurotransmitters** are chemical substances that carry messages from one neuron to another or from a neuron to other body tissues, such as cardiac or skeletal muscle.

TABLE 27.1	
Commonly Used Adrenergic Drugs	
Drug	**Major Clinical Uses**
Alpha and Beta Activity	
Dopamine	Hypotension and shock
Epinephrine (Adrenalin)	Allergic reactions, cardiac arrest, hypotension and shock, local vasoconstriction, bronchodilation, cardiac stimulation, ophthalmic conditions
Ephedrine	Bronchodilation, cardiac stimulation, nasal decongestion
Pseudoephedrine (Sudafed)	Nasal decongestion
Norepinephrine (Levophed)	Hypotension and shock
Alpha Activity	
Midodrine (ProAmatine)	Orthostatic hypotension
Naphazoline hydrochloride (Privine)	Nasal decongestion
Oxymetazoline hydrochloride (Afrin)	Nasal decongestion
Phenylephrine (Neo-Synephrine)	Hypotension and shock, nasal decongestion, ophthalmic conditions
Tetrahydrozoline hydrochloride (Tyzine, Visine)	Nasal decongestion, local vasoconstriction in the eye
Beta Activity	
Albuterol (Proventil)	Bronchodilation
Arformoterol (Brovana)	Bronchodilation
Dobutamine (Dobutrex)	Cardiac stimulation
Formoterol (Foradil)	Bronchodilation
Isoproterenol (Isuprel)	Bronchodilation, cardiac stimulation
Levalbuterol (Xopenex)	Bronchodilation
Metaproterenol (Alupent)	Bronchodilation
Pirbuterol (Maxair)	Bronchodilation
Salmeterol (Serevent)	Bronchodilation
Terbutaline (Brethine)	Bronchodilation, preterm labor inhibition

Although activation of presynaptic $alpha_2$ receptors in the periphery are not of clinical significance, activation of these receptors in the central nervous system (CNS) by medications is useful in treating hypertension (see Chap. 28).

Drug Therapy

The usefulness of adrenergic drugs stems mainly from the drugs' effects on the heart, blood vessels, and bronchi. They are often used as emergency drugs in the treatment of acute cardiovascular and respiratory collapse. In addition, adrenergic drugs are useful in the treatment of allergic reactions. Patients who benefit from these drugs include those in need of restoration of blood pressure in reversing types of hypotensive states.

Some of the pathophysiological states where adrenergic drugs are used include cardiac arrest, Stokes-Adams syndrome (sudden attacks of unconsciousness caused by heart block), and profound bradycardia. These drugs may be used as cardiac stimulants. In hypotension and shock, they may be used to increase blood pressure. In hemorrhagic or hypovolemic shock, the drugs are second-line agents that may be used if adequate fluid volume replacement does not restore sufficient blood pressure and circulation to maintain organ perfusion.

In bronchial asthma and other obstructive pulmonary diseases, adrenergic drugs are used as bronchodilators to relieve bronchoconstriction and bronchospasm. In upper respiratory infections, including the common cold and sinusitis, they may be given orally or applied topically to the nasal mucosa to reduce nasal congestion (**decongestant** effect).

Adrenergic drugs are useful in treating a variety of symptoms of allergic disorders. Severe allergic reactions are characterized by hypotension, bronchoconstriction, and laryngoedema. As vasoconstrictors, the drugs are useful in correcting the hypotension that often accompanies severe allergic reactions. The drug-induced vasoconstriction of blood vessels in mucous membranes produces a decongestant effect to relieve edema in the respiratory tract, skin, and other tissues. As bronchodilators, the drugs also help relieve the bronchospasm of severe allergic reactions. Adrenergic drugs may be used to treat allergic rhinitis, acute hypersensitivity (anaphylactic reactions to drugs, animal serums, insect stings, and other allergens), serum sickness, urticaria, and angioneurotic edema.

Other clinical uses of adrenergic drugs include relaxation of uterine musculature and inhibition of uterine contractions in preterm labor. They also may be added to local anesthetics for their vasoconstrictive effect, thus preventing unwanted systemic absorption of the anesthetic; prolonging anesthesia; and reducing bleeding. Topical uses include application to skin and mucous membranes for vasoconstriction and hemostatic effects and to the eyes for vasoconstriction and mydriasis.

Adrenergic Drugs

The adrenergic drugs have different predominant properties: alpha activity, beta activity, and alpha and beta activity. Those drugs with alpha and beta activity include dopamine, epinephrine, ephedrine, pseudoephedrine, and norepinephrine. The condition the patient has determines which adrenergic drug, with its specific effect, is necessary for treatment. Table 27.2 presents dosing recommendations for these drugs.

Ⓟ **Epinephrine** is the prototype adrenergic drug. When it is given systemically, the effects may be therapeutic or adverse, depending on the reason for use; dosage; and route of administration. Epinephrine stimulates alpha$_1$ and all beta receptors. At usual doses, beta-adrenergic effects on the heart and vascular and other smooth muscles predominate. However, at high doses, alpha$_1$-adrenergic effects (e.g., vasoconstriction) predominate.

Pharmacokinetics

Epinephrine is administered through various routes: subcutaneously, intramuscularly, intravenously, via inhalation, and even as eye drops. The subcutaneous route has an onset of 5 to 10 minutes, with a peak of 20 minutes and a duration of 20 to 30 minutes. The intramuscular route has an onset of 5 to 10 minutes, a peak in 20 minutes, and a duration of 20 to 30 minutes, the same as the subcutaneous route. The intravenous (IV) route has an instant onset, a peak of 20 minutes, and a duration of 20 to 30 minutes. The inhalation route has an onset is 3 to 5 minutes, a peak of 20 minutes, and a duration of 1 to 3 hours. Finally, administration via eye drops has an onset of less than 1 hour, a peak in 4 to 8 hours, and a duration of 24 hours. Most epinephrine is rapidly metabolized in the liver to inactive metabolites, which are then excreted in the urine. The remaining epinephrine is deactivated by reuptake at synaptic receptor sites.

The nurse should note that when given by injection, epinephrine acts rapidly but has a short duration of action. The IV form acts almost immediately to produce an increase in blood pressure; a positive inotropic and positive chronotropic effect on the myocardium; hyperglycemia; bronchodilation; and vasoconstriction of arterioles in the skin, mucosa, and most viscera. For acute asthma attacks, subcutaneous administration of epinephrine usually produces bronchodilation within 5 to 10 minutes; maximal effects may occur within 20 minutes.

Table 27.3 lists the numerous epinephrine solutions available. Solutions vary widely in the amount of drug they contain. They must be used correctly to avoid potentially serious hazards.

Action

Epinephrine is a naturally occurring neurotransmitter, the effects of which are mediated by alpha or beta receptors in specific organs. Effect on alpha receptors includes vasoconstriction, including contraction of dilator muscles of the iris. The effects on the beta receptors include positive chronotropic and inotropic effects on the heart at the beta$_1$ receptors; bronchodilation, vasodilation, and uterine relaxation of the beta$_2$ receptors; and decreased production of aqueous humor.

Use

Epinephrine is the adrenergic drug of choice for relief of anaphylactic shock, the most serious allergic reaction, as well as treatment of cardiac arrest. In addition, epinephrine is used as an additive to local anesthetics for vasoconstrictive effects, which include prolonging the action of the local anesthetic drug, preventing systemic absorption, and minimizing bleeding. Adrenergic drugs are given intravenously only for emergencies, such as anaphylactic shock, cardiac arrest, severe arterial hypotension, and circulatory shock. Because adrenergic drugs are often used in medical crises, they must be readily available in all health care settings (e.g., hospitals, long-term care facilities, physicians' offices). All health care personnel should know where emergency drugs are stored.

Use in Specific Disorders
Anaphylaxis

Anaphylactic shock or **anaphylaxis** is a type I immunoglobulin E-mediated allergic reaction to an **antigen**, a foreign substance that has entered the body. Some typical antigens include foods (e.g., shellfish, peanuts, eggs), medications (e.g., penicillin, vaccinations, enzymes, iodine-contrast media), and insect bites or stings (e.g., bees, ants). During an anaphylactic reaction, mast cells release chemical mediators such as histamine, serotonin, platelet-activating factor, prostaglandins, and leukotrienes. The resulting increased capillary permeability and smooth muscle contraction lead to edema, bronchospasm, and airway obstruction. Vasodilation results in hypotension and shock. Anaphylactic reactions occur on second or subsequent exposure to an antigen. Symptoms develop rapidly; typical symptom onset ranges from 30 minutes to 2 hours after exposure to the antigen.

IV or subcutaneous epinephrine is the drug of choice for the treatment of anaphylaxis. The drug relieves bronchospasm, laryngeal edema, and hypotension. In conjunction with its alpha (vasoconstriction) and beta (cardiac stimulation, bronchodilation) effects, it acts as a physiologic antagonist of histamine and other bronchoconstricting and vasodilating substances released during anaphylactic reactions. People susceptible to severe allergic responses should carry a syringe of epinephrine at all times. EpiPen and EpiPen Jr are prefilled, autoinjection syringes for intramuscular self-administration of epinephrine in emergency situations (Fig. 27.3). The thigh is the preferred site for autoinjection, providing more rapid absorption and higher blood levels of epinephrine than the arm in children and adults for either intramuscular or subcutaneous administration. Victims of anaphylaxis who have been taking beta-adrenergic blocking drugs (e.g., propranolol [Inderal]) do not respond as readily to epinephrine as those not taking beta blockers. Larger doses of epinephrine and large amounts of IV fluids may be required.

TABLE 27.2

DRUGS AT A GLANCE: Selected Adrenergic Drugs

Drug	Pregnancy Category	Use(s)	Routes and Dosage Ranges	
			Adults	**Children**
Ⓟ Epinephrine (Adrenalin)	C	Bronchodilation	IV: 0.1–0.25 mg (1–2.5 mL of 1:10,000 solution) injected slowly Intraspinal 0.2–0.4 mL added to anesthetic spinal fluid mixture. Concentrations of 1:100,000–1:20,000 are usually used Subcutaneous or IM for respiratory distress: 0.2–1 mL of 1:1,000 solution Metered-dose inhaler (160–250 mcg/puff): 1 puff at onset of bronchospasm. Repeat if needed after 1–5 min. Dose is individualized to patients' needs For inhalation: instill no more than 10 drops into nebulizer reservoir. Administer 1–3 inhalations not more than every 3 h	0.05 mg/kg IV and repeat every 20–30 min as needed with 1:10,000 solution For inhalation (1% solution [1:100]): instill no more than 10 drops into nebulizer reservoir. Administer 1–3 inhalations 4–6 times/d
		Profound bradycardia/ hypotension	Continuous IV infusion: 2–10 mcg/min	IV/IO injection (1:10,000 [0.1 mg/mL]): IV 0.01 mg/kg every 3–5 min PRN
		Cardiac arrest	IV injection: 0.5–1.0 mg (5–10 mL of 1:10,000) during resuscitation, 0.5 mg every 5 min. Intracardiac injection into left ventricular chamber, 0.3–0.5 mg (3–5 mL of 1:10,000 solution)	Solution (1:1,000 [1 mg/mL]): Subcutaneous /IM 0.01 mg/kg or 0.3 mL/m² (0.01 mg/kg or 0.3 mg/m²) every 4 h PRN. Maximum dose 0.5 mg
		Anaphylactic shock	Aqueous epinephrine (1:1000 [1 mg/mL]): Subcutaneous/IM 0.1–0.5 mg every 5–15 min. Maximum dose 1 mg IV injection (1:10,000 [0.1 mg/mL]): IV 0.1–0.25 mg over 5–10 min every 5–15 min PRN, *then* 1–4 mcg/min continuous infusion if severe anaphylactic shock EpiPen Autoinjector: IM 0.3 mg; may repeat	Aqueous epinephrine (1:1000 [1 mg/mL]): Subcutaneous/IM 0.01 mg/kg every 20 min–4 h PRN. Maximum dose 0.5 mg IV injection (1:100,000 [0.01 mg/mL]): IV 0.1 mg over 5–10 min once, *then* 0.1–1.5 mcg/kg/min continuous infusion EpiPen Jr Autoinjector: IM 0.15 mg; may repeat
		Ophthalmic agent	Epinephrine HCl 0.1%, 0.5%, 1%, and 2%: 1–2 drops in eyes once or twice daily	
Ephedrine (generic)	C	Asthma	PO: 12.5–25 mg every 4 h. Do not exceed 150 mg/24 h	Parenteral: 0.5 mg/kg IM or subcutaneously every 4–6 h
		Hypotension	IM, Subcutaneous: 25–50 mg IV push: 5–25 mg/dose slowly, repeated every 5–10 min as needed then every 3–4 h. Do not exceed 150 mg/24 h	Oral: Not recommended for children younger than 12 y
		Nasal congestion	PO: 25–50 mg every 4 h, 0.25% nasal spray or 1% nasal jelly	

TABLE 27.2

DRUGS AT A GLANCE: Selected Adrenergic Drugs (Continued)

Drug	Pregnancy Category	Use(s)	Routes and Dosage Ranges	
			Adults	Children
Pseudoephedrine (Sudafed)	C	Nasal congestion	60 mg PO every 4–6 h or 120 mg sustained-release formula every 12 h. Do not exceed 240 mg/24 h	6–12 y: PO 30 mg every 4–6 h; do not exceed 120 mg/24 h 2–5 y: PO 15 mg every 4–6 h; do not exceed 60 mg/24 h
Isoproterenol (Isuprel)	C	Cardiac dysrhythmia	IV 20–60 mcg (1–3 mL) bolus initially, followed by IV infusion. Can use 1:50,000 solution for IV bolus undiluted. For IV bolus using 1:5,000 solution, dilute 0.2 mg to 10 mL with sodium chloride or 5% dextrose injection and give 1–3 mL. For IV infusion, dilute 2 mg of 1:5,000 solution in 500 mL 5% dextrose injection Dosage depends on type of dysrhythmia and ranges from 0.5 to 5 mcg/min. Titrate to patient's response	No well-controlled studies in children
		Shock	IV infusion: Dilute 1 mg of 1:5,000 solution in 500 mL 5% dextrose injection. Dosage ranges from 0.5 to 5 mcg/min. Titrate to patient's response	
Phenylephrine (Neo-Synephrine, others)	C	Hypotension/ shock	IM, Subcutaneous: 2–5 mg every 1–2 h. Initial dose not to exceed 5 mg. Repeat no more often than every 10–15 min IV bolus: 0.1–0.5 mg, diluted in NaCl injection, given slowly every 10–15 min as needed. Initial dose not to exceed 0.5 mg IV infusion: 10 mg in 500 mL D5W or NS. Infuse at 100–180 mcg/min initially. When blood pressure is stable, reduce to maintenance rate of 40–60 mcg/min	
		Nasal congestion	Nasal decongestants: 0.25%, 0.5%, 1.0% solutions 2–3 drops or sprays every 3–4 h. Therapy should not exceed 3 d	Nasal solution 2–6 y: 2–3 drops of 0.125% solution in each nostril every 4 h PRN Older than 6 y: 1–2 sprays of the 0.25% solution in each nostril no more than every 4 h Oral 2–5 y: 1 dropperful of 0.25% oral drops every 4 h; do not exceed 6 doses in 24 h 6–11 y: 1 tablet every 4 h
		Ophthalmic agent/mydriatic agent	Ophthalmic preparations: 2.5% or 10% solutions. Instill one drop; may be repeated in 10–60 min	

D5W, dextrose 5% in water; NS, 0.9% sodium chloride.

TABLE 27.3

Epinephrine Concentrations and Administration Routes

Final Concentration	Route
1% (1:100)	Inhalation
0.5% (1:200)	Subcutaneous
0.1% (1:1000)	Subcutaneous
0.1% (1:1000)	Intramuscular
0.01% (1:10,000)	Intravenous
0.001% (1:100,000)	Intradermal (in combination with local anesthetics)

Clinical Application 27-1

Mr. Sobechenko receives piperacillin/tazobactam, a beta-lactam antibiotic, for treatment of his pneumonia. Within 15 minutes of the start of the antibiotic infusion, he has an anaphylactic reaction. He is agitated and flushed and complains of palpitations. He is having severe difficulty breathing due to bronchospasm. His physician then orders epinephrine.

- What are the nursing implications for this patient's reaction to the antibiotic?
- What assessment is needed relative to the adverse effects of epinephrine?

Adjunct medications that may be useful in treating severe cases of anaphylaxis include corticosteroids, norepinephrine, and aminophylline. Antihistamines are considered second-line treatment; their usefulness is limited because histamine plays a minor role in causing anaphylaxis compared with leukotrienes and other inflammatory mediators. Antihistamines should never be used alone in the treatment of anaphylaxis. Diphenhydramine is often used as a second-line adjunctive treatment; however, studies show that a combination of ranitidine and diphenhydramine is more efficacious than diphenhydramine alone.

Cardiopulmonary Resuscitation

Epinephrine is often administered during cardiopulmonary resuscitation (CPR). The most important action of epinephrine during cardiac arrest is constriction of peripheral blood vessels, which shunts blood to the central circulation and increases blood flow to the heart and brain. This beneficial effect comes at the expense of increased oxygen consumption by the myocardium, ventricular dysrhythmias, and myocardial dysfunction after resuscitation. Epinephrine is considered the drug of choice for the treatment of cardiac arrest in cases of nonventricular tachycardia/fibrillation such as asystole or pulseless electrical activity. Epinephrine is beneficial in these situations because

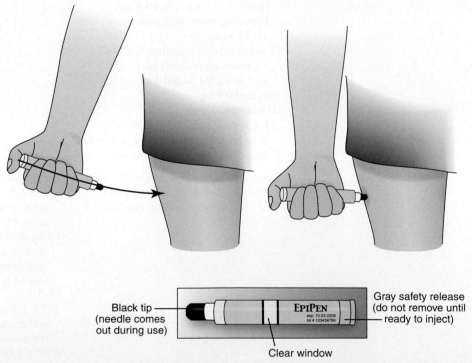

Black tip (needle comes out during use)

Clear window

Gray safety release (do not remove until ready to inject)

EPIPEN
exp: 10-23-2008
lot # 123456789

Figure 27.3 To use the EpiPen Autoinjector, grasp the unit in your fist with the black tip pointing down. When ready to inject, activate the unit by removing the gray activation cap with your other hand. Firmly thrust the device into the outer thigh at a 90-degree angle and hold in place for several seconds. After removing the autoinjector, massage the injection site to enhance absorption. (Note: The injection can be made through clothing.)

it stimulates electrical and mechanical activity and produces myocardial contraction.

The specific effects of epinephrine depend largely on the dose and route of administration. The optimal dose in CPR has not been established. Advanced Cardiovascular Life Support (ACLS) guidelines recommend administering epinephrine 1 mg intravenously every 5 minutes.

Hypotension and Shock

In hypotension and shock, initial efforts involve identifying and treating the cause when possible. Such treatments include placing the patient in the recumbent position, blood transfusions, fluid and electrolyte replacement, treatment of infection, and use of positive inotropic drugs and other medications to treat heart failure. If these measures are ineffective in raising the blood pressure enough to maintain perfusion to vital organs such as the brain, kidneys, and heart, vasopressor drugs may be used. The usual goal of vasopressor drug therapy is to maintain tissue perfusion and a mean arterial pressure of at least 80 to 100 mm Hg.

Nasal Congestion

In nasal congestion, adrenergic drugs given topically or systemically constrict blood vessels in nasal mucosa and decrease the nasal congestion associated with the common cold, allergic rhinitis, hay fever, sinusitis, or other upper respiratory allergy. The topical nasal solutions of epinephrine are for the temporary relief from nasal and nasopharyngeal mucosal congestion due to these conditions. Topical agents are effective, undergo little systemic absorption, are available over the counter (OTC), and are widely used. However, overuse leads to decreased effectiveness (tolerance), irritation and ischemic changes in the nasal mucosa, and rebound congestion. These effects can be minimized by using small doses only when necessary and for no longer than 3 to 5 days.

Oral drugs have a slower onset of action than topical ones but may last longer. They also may cause more adverse effects, which may occur with usual therapeutic doses and are especially likely with high doses. The most problematic adverse effects are cardiac and CNS stimulation; the risks of hypertension and cerebral hemorrhage are greater in people with hypertension. Commonly used oral agents are pseudoephedrine and ephedrine.

Use in Children

Clinicians use adrenergic agents to treat asthma, hypotension, shock, cardiac arrest, and anaphylaxis in children. However, guidelines for safe and effective use of adrenergic drugs in children are not well established. Children are very sensitive to drug effects, including cardiac and CNS stimulation, and recommended doses usually should not be exceeded.

Prescribers mainly order epinephrine in children for treatment of bronchospasm due to asthma or allergic reactions. Parenteral epinephrine may cause syncope when given to asthmatic children. Isoproterenol is rarely given parenterally to children. There is little reason to use the inhalation route, because in children, as in adults, selective beta₂ agonists such as albuterol are preferred for bronchodilation in asthma.

The most frequent use of phenylephrine is to relieve congestion of the upper respiratory tract and may be given topically, as nose drops. The nurse must carefully measure doses. Rebound nasal congestion occurs with overuse.

Use in Older Adults

It is necessary to use epinephrine with caution in the geriatric patient population. Clinicians use adrenergic agents to treat asthma, hypotension, shock, cardiac arrest, and anaphylaxis in older adults. These drugs stimulate the heart to increase rate and force of contraction and blood pressure. Because older adults often have chronic cardiovascular conditions (e.g., angina, dysrhythmias, heart failure, coronary artery disease, hypertension, peripheral vascular disease) that are aggravated by adrenergic drugs, careful monitoring by the nurse is required.

Prescribers often order adrenergic drugs as bronchodilators and decongestants in older adults. Therapeutic doses increase the workload of the heart and may cause symptoms of impaired cardiovascular function. Overdoses may cause severe cardiovascular dysfunction, including life-threatening dysrhythmias. The drugs also cause CNS stimulation. With therapeutic doses, anxiety, restlessness, nervousness, and insomnia often occur in older adults. Overdoses may cause hallucinations, convulsions, CNS depression, and death.

Adrenergics are ingredients in OTC asthma remedies, cold remedies, nasal decongestants, and appetite suppressants. Cautious use of these preparations is required in older adults. They should not take the drugs concurrently with prescription adrenergic drugs because of the high risk of overdose and toxicity.

Ophthalmic preparations of adrenergic drugs also require cautious use in the elderly. For example, phenylephrine acts as a vasoconstrictor and mydriatic. Applying larger-than-recommended doses to the normal eye or usual doses to the traumatized, inflamed, or diseased eye may result in sufficient systemic absorption of the drug to cause increased blood pressure and other adverse effects. The rationale for the caution in older adults is because of cardiac and CNS-stimulating effects of epinephrine.

Use in Patients With Renal Impairment

Epinephrine warrants cautious use in patients with renal failure. Adrenergic drugs exert effects on the renal system that may cause problems for patients with renal impairment. For example, adrenergic drugs with alpha₁ activity cause constriction of renal arteries, thereby diminishing renal blood flow and urine production. These drugs also constrict urinary sphincters, causing urinary retention and painful urination, especially in men with prostatic hyperplasia.

The renal system eliminates many adrenergic drugs and their metabolites. In the presence of renal disease, these compounds may accumulate and cause increased adverse effects.

Use in Patients With Hepatic Impairment

Epinephrine administration has no reported precautions for use in patients with hepatic impairment. The liver is rich in the enzymes monoamine oxidase (MAO) and catecholamine O-methyl transferase (COMT), which are responsible for metabolism of circulating epinephrine and other adrenergic drugs (e.g., norepinephrine, dopamine, isoproterenol). However, other tissues in the body also possess these enzymes and are capable of metabolizing natural and synthetic catecholamines. Any unchanged drug can be excreted in the urine. Many noncatecholamine adrenergic drugs are excreted largely unchanged in the urine. Therefore, liver disease is not usually considered a contraindication to administering adrenergic drugs.

Use in Patients With Critical Illness

Adrenergic drugs are important emergency drugs. They are essential for treating hypotension, shock, asystole and other dysrhythmias, acute bronchospasm, and anaphylaxis. Although they may save lives of critically ill patients, use of adrenergic drugs may result in secondary health problems that require monitoring and intervention. These health problems include

- Possible diminished renal perfusion and decreased urine output due to vasopressor action
- Possible decreased perfusion to the liver, with subsequent liver damage due to vasopressor action
- Possible irritable cardiac dysrhythmias due to $beta_1$ activity
- Possible increase in myocardial oxygen requirement due to $beta_1$ activity
- Hyperglycemia, hypokalemia, and hypophosphatemia due to $beta_1$ activity
- Severe hypertension and reflex bradycardia
- Tissue necrosis after extravasation
- Limb ischemia due to profound vasoconstriction

Occurrence of any of these adverse effects may complicate the already complex care of critically ill patients. Careful assessment and prompt nursing intervention are essential. The IV administration of epinephrine is used in the critical care setting in ventricular standstill to restore circulation. The injectable form of aerosols and solutions in nebulization are effective in critical ill patients who need temporary relief from acute attacks of bronchial asthma and COPD.

Use in Patients Receiving Home Care

Adrenergic drugs are often used in the home setting. Frequently prescribed drugs include bronchodilators and nasal decongestants. OTC drugs with the same effects are also commonly used to treat asthma, allergic rhinitis, cold symptoms, and appetite suppression for weight control. A major function of the home care nurse is to teach patients to use the drugs correctly (especially metered-dose inhalers), to report excessive CNS or cardiac stimulation to a health care provider, and to teach patients not to take OTC drugs or herbal preparations that have the same or similar ingredients as prescription drugs.

Excessive adverse effects are probably most likely to occur in children and older adults. Older adults often have other illnesses that may be aggravated by adrenergic drugs or they may take other drugs whose effects may be altered by concomitant

use of adrenergics. Patients who are receiving bronchodilation therapy for acute respiratory symptoms may be receiving this nebulization therapy in the home setting. In addition, routine nebulizer therapy may include an adrenergic medication.

NCLEX Success

1. **When giving a drug with beta₂ agonist activity, the nurse knows that the main therapeutic benefit is**
   A. vasoconstriction and elevation of the blood pressure
   B. relaxation of bronchial smooth muscle and bronchodilation
   C. elevated heart rate and improved force of myocardial contraction
   D. uterine contraction and induction of labor

2. **The nurse teaches the patient with diabetes using adrenergic medications to anticipate**
   A. no change in blood glucose levels
   B. a decrease in blood glucose levels
   C. an increase in blood glucose levels
   D. more fluctuation in blood glucose levels

Adverse Effects

Adverse effects occur with systemic administration, which include CNS effects and cardiovascular, GI, and genitourinary effects. The most common CNS effects include fear, anxiety, tension, restlessness, headache, lightheadedness, and dizziness. Life-threatening cardiovascular effects include hypertension, resulting in intracranial hemorrhage, cardiovascular collapse with hypotension, palpitations, tachycardia, and precordial pain in patients with ischemic heart disease. Other frequently occurring adverse effects include nausea, decreased urine formation, dysuria, vesical sphincter spasm, and pallor. Common CNS effects from ophthalmic solutions include headache, brow ache, and blurred vision, as well as transitory stinging on initial instillation at the local site.

Contraindications

Contraindications to using adrenergic drugs include cardiac dysrhythmias, angina pectoris, hypertension, hyperthyroidism, and cerebrovascular disease; stimulation of the sympathetic nervous system worsens these conditions. Narrow-angle glaucoma is a contraindication, because the drugs result in mydriasis, closure of the filtration angle of the eye, and increased intraocular pressure. Hypersensitivity to an adrenergic drug or any component is also a contraindication. For example, some adrenergic preparations contain sulfites, to which some people are allergic.

Adrenergic drugs are contraindicated with local anesthesia of distal areas with a single blood supply (e.g., fingers, toes, nose, or ears) because of potential tissue damage and sloughing from vasoconstriction. These drugs should not be given during the second stage of labor because they may delay progression. They should be used with caution in patients with anxiety, insomnia, and psychiatric disorders because of their stimulant effects on the CNS.

It is essential not to give MAO inhibitors with adrenergic drugs because the combination may cause death. Concurrent use of MAO inhibitors and adrenergic drugs may lead to a danger of cardiac dysrhythmias, respiratory depression, and acute hypertensive crisis, with possible intracranial hemorrhage, convulsions, coma, and death. Effects of an MAO inhibitor may not occur for several weeks after treatment is started and may last up to 3 weeks after the drug is stopped. The nurse should warn every patient taking an MAO inhibitor against taking any other medication without the advice of a physician or pharmacist.

Nursing Implications

Awareness and assessment of allergy or hypersensitivity to epinephrine or components of drug preparation are important issues to consider. The nurse assesses for history of narrow-angle glaucoma, shock other than anaphylactic shock, hypovolemia, general anesthesia with halogenated hydrocarbons or cyclopropane, organic brain damage, cerebral arteriosclerosis, cardiac dilation, and coronary insufficiency. In addition, assessment of history of tachyarrhythmias, ischemic heart disease, hypertension, renal impairment, COPD, diabetes mellitus, hyperthyroidism, prostatic hypertrophy, history of seizure disorders, psychoneuroses, labor and delivery, lactation, contact lens use, or being an aphakic patient is necessary.

The nurse obtains the patient's weight and assesses skin color, temperature, and turgor. Orientation status, reflexes, pulse, blood pressure, respiratory rate, and auscultation of lung sounds are also important to obtain. Required laboratory data include urinalysis, renal function, blood and urine glucose, serum electrolytes, and thyroid function. In addition, an electrocardiogram may be necessary.

Preventing Interactions

Box 27.1 lists the drugs that increase or decrease the effects of adrenergics. In addition, with the administration of epinephrine, there are excessive hypertension effects in the presence of propranolol, beta-blockers, and furazolidone.

Ephedra (ma huang) is an OTC dietary supplement used for weight control, boosting sports performance, and increasing energy levels. Ephedra is a plant source of ephedrine alkaloids, including ephedrine and pseudoephedrine, and may increase the effects of adrenergic drugs. The OTC use of ephedra has been linked to increased risk of hypertension, heart attack, stroke, and death. The Dietary Supplement Health and Education Act of 1994 granted the U.S. Food and Drug Administration (FDA) the authority to remove a dietary supplement from the market if it "presents a significant or unreasonable risk of illness or injury when used according to its labeling or under ordinary conditions of use." In 2004, using this law, the FDA prohibited the sale of any dietary supplements containing ephedrine alkaloids (i.e., ephedra).

BOX 27.1 ■ Drug Interactions: Adrenergics

Drugs That Increase the Effects of Adrenergics

- Anesthetics, general (e.g., halothane), cocaine
  Increase the risk of ventricular irritability, serious cardiac dysrhythmias, or death
- Anticholinergics (e.g., atropine)
  Increase the risk of ventricular dysrhythmias
- Tricyclic antidepressants (e.g., amitriptyline, imipramine), beta-adrenergic blocking agents (e.g., propranolol [Inderal]), doxapram (Dopram), methylphenidate (Ritalin)
  Increase the pressor response
- Antihistamines
  Increase the risk of the pressor response
- Digoxin
  Increases the risk of dysrhythmias
- Ergot alkaloids
  Increase blood pressure and ischemic response
- Monoamine oxidase (MAO) inhibitors (e.g., isocarboxazid [Marplan]); xanthines (in caffeine-containing substances, such as coffee, tea, cola drinks, and theophylline)
  Increase heart rate and blood pressure

Drugs That Decrease the Effects of Adrenergics

- Anticholinesterases (e.g., neostigmine [Prostigmin], pyridostigmine [Mestinon]) and other cholinergic drugs
  Decrease the effects of epinephrine
- Antipsychotic drugs (e.g., haloperidol [Haldol]), chlorpromazine
  Paradoxically decrease blood pressure
- Phenothiazines, phentolamine
  Inhibit or reverse the pressor effect

NCLEX Success

3. A male patient with asthma tells the nurse that he is using his metered-dose inhaler of epinephrine more frequently than prescribed to control wheezing. The nurse is concerned because this behavior may result in

   A. drug tolerance
   B. heart failure
   C. drug toxicity
   D. diabetes mellitus

4. A nurse is caring for a female patient with nasal congestion whose medical history includes depression. Which of the following medications contraindicates the use of pseudoephedrine (Sudafed) to treat her nasal congestion?

   A. fluoxetine (Prozac)
   B. amitriptyline (generic)
   C. isocarboxazid (Marplan)
   D. lithium (Lithotabs)

Administering the Medication

Administration of epinephrine is by inhalation, injection, or topical application. (Oral administration of the drug is not effective because enzymes in the GI tract and liver destroy it.) Standard doses of individual adrenergic drugs are not always effective; the dose must be individualized or titrated to the patient's response. This is especially true in emergencies but also applies in long-term use.

Assessing for Therapeutic Effects

Monitoring for the therapeutic effects of epinephrine includes assessing various parameters depending on the route of administration and the dose used. If the route has been IV for the purpose of ventricular standstill, then return of a heart rate and rhythm to normal is a positive effect. In acute asthmatic attacks, the therapeutic effect is relief of the bronchospasm or relief of the respiratory distress of the bronchial asthma. With the use of aerosols and solutions for nebulization, the expected outcome is temporary relief from acute attacks of bronchial asthma and COPD.

Assessing for Adverse Effects

Epinephrine has systemic effects that affect the CNS system. Therefore, the nurse assesses for fear, anxiety, tension, restlessness, headache, light-headedness, and dizziness. In patients who are being monitored, it is important to assess for life-threatening effects, including hypertension, which could result in intracranial hemorrhage, as well as hypotension, presence of palpitations, tachycardia, and/or precordial pain in patients with ischemic heart disease. The nurse assesses for nausea, decreased urine formation, dysuria, vesical sphincter spasm, and pallor. If a patient receives epinephrine as an ophthalmic solution, monitoring also includes assessing for presence of headache, brow ache, and blurred vision, as well as transitory stinging on initial instillation at the local site.

In addition, epinephrine is the active ingredient in many OTC inhalation products for asthma (e.g., MicroNefrin, Primatene Mist, others), producing bronchodilation. Guidelines for the optimal treatment of asthma recommend use of anti-inflammatory medications (e.g., corticosteroids) and prescription bronchodilators (e.g., beta$_2$-adrenergic agonists) (see Chap. 31). OTC epinephrine preparations have a short duration of action, which promotes frequent and excessive use. Prolonged use may cause adverse effects and result in the development of tolerance to the therapeutic effects of the drug. There is also concern by some health care professionals that reliance on OTC medications may delay the patient with asthma from seeking medical care. Another area of concern is the ozone-depleting propellants used in OTC inhalation products such as Primatene Mist. However, at this time, these medications have "essential use designation" by the FDA because they constitute the only OTC inhalation products available to people with asthma. Supporters contend that OTC bronchodilators are much less costly than prescription medications and are an affordable "rescue treatment" option for patients who do not have insurance coverage for prescription medications. People who have heart disease or are elderly should not use these OTC products on a regular basis.

Patient Teaching

Teaching tips when instructing patients about the use of epinephrine-containing medications include using the recommended dosages because adverse effects or loss of effectiveness may result. The nurse instructs patients about the side effects of epinephrine, which include dizziness, drowsiness, fatigue, apprehension, anxiety, emotional changes, nausea, vomiting, change in taste, and rapid heart rate. In addition, he or she informs patients to report chest pain, dizziness, insomnia, weakness, tremor, or irregular heartbeat, difficulty breathing, productive cough, and any failure of problems to respond to usual dosage immediately.

Nasal solutions may cause burning or stinging when first used. It is important to have patients who are to use respiratory inhalers read the instructions that come with the inhalers and ask questions if necessary. Box 27.2 presents patient teaching guidelines for epinephrine and other adrenergic drugs.

Clinical Application 27-2

Because of Mr. Sobechenko's acute reaction, his physician orders epinephrine 1:10,000 intravenously "stat." The nurse reviews the drug order. Why did the prescriber order this medication intravenously instead of orally?

Other Drugs in the Class

Pseudoephedrine (Sudafed) is a related drug, stimulating alpha$_1$ and beta receptors. It is used as a bronchodilator and nasal decongestant. Pseudoephedrine and ephedrine are ingredients used in making methamphetamine, a highly addictive and illegal drug of abuse. The Combat Methamphetamine Epidemic Act (part of the U.S. Patriot Act) requires drug stores to control OTC access to these drugs by placing these medications behind the counter and documenting each purchase by a customer.

Isoproterenol (Isuprel) is a synthetic catecholamine that acts on beta$_1$- and beta$_2$-adrenergic receptors. Its main actions are to stimulate the heart, dilate blood vessels in skeletal muscle, and relax bronchial smooth muscle. Compared with epinephrine, isoproterenol has similar cardiac stimulant effects, but it does not affect alpha receptors and therefore does not cause vasoconstriction.

Phenylephrine (e.g., Neo-Synephrine, others) is a synthetic drug that acts on alpha-adrenergic receptors to produce vasoconstriction. Vasoconstriction decreases cardiac output and renal perfusion and increases peripheral vascular resistance and blood pressure. There is little cardiac stimulation because phenylephrine does not activate beta$_1$ receptors in the heart or beta$_2$ receptors in blood vessels. The drug is excreted primarily in the urine.

Phenylephrine may be given to increase blood pressure in hypotension and shock. Compared with epinephrine, phenylephrine produces longer lasting elevation of blood pressure (20–50 minutes with injection). When given systemically, phenylephrine produces a reflex bradycardia. This effect may be

BOX 27.2   Patient Teaching Guidelines for Adrenergic Drugs

General Considerations

■ Take no other medications without the health care provider's knowledge and approval. Many over-the-counter (OTC) cold remedies and appetite suppressants contain adrenergic drugs. Use of these along with prescribed adrenergic drugs can result in overdose and serious cardiovascular or central nervous system (CNS) problems. In addition, adrenergic drugs interact with numerous other drugs to increase or decrease effects; some of these interactions may be life threatening.

■ Herbal preparations of ephedra or ma huang contain derivatives of ephedrine and should not be taken with other adrenergic medications. Excessive CNS and cardiovascular stimulation may result. (The U.S. Food and Drug Administration [FDA] banned the sale of supplements containing ephedra was in 2004.)

■ Tell your health care provider if you are pregnant, breastfeeding, taking any other prescription or OTC drugs, or allergic to sulfite preservatives.

■ Use these drugs only as directed. The potential for abuse is high, especially for the patient with asthma or other chronic lung disease who is seeking relief from labored breathing. Some of these drugs are prescribed for long-term use, but excessive use does not increase therapeutic effects. Instead, it causes tolerance and decreased benefit from usual doses and increases the incidence and severity of adverse reactions.

■ Frequent cardiac monitoring and checks of flow rate, blood pressure, and urine output are necessary if you are receiving intravenous adrenergic drugs to stimulate your heart or raise your blood pressure. These measures increase the safety and benefits of drug therapy rather than indicate the presence of a critical condition. Ask your nurse if you have concerns about your condition.

■ You may feel anxious or tense; have difficulty sleeping; and experience palpitations, blurred vision, headache, tremor, dizziness, and pallor. These are effects of the medication. Use of relaxation techniques to promote rest and decrease muscle tension may be helpful.

■ Use caution when driving or performing activities requiring alertness, dexterity, and good vision.

■ Report adverse reactions such as fast pulse, palpitations, and chest pain so that drug dosage can be reevaluated and therapy changed if needed.

Self-Administration

■ Do not use topical decongestants longer than 3 to 5 days. Long-term use may be habit forming. Burning on use and rebound congestion after the dose wears off are common side effects. Stop using the medication gradually.

■ Stinging may occur when using ophthalmic preparations. Do not let the tip of the applicator touch your eye or anything else during administration of the medication, to avoid contamination. Do not wear soft contact lenses while using ophthalmic adrenergic drugs; discoloration of the lenses may occur. Report blurred vision, headache, palpitations, and muscle tremors to your health care provider.

■ Follow guidelines for use of your inhaler. Do not increase the dosage or frequency; tolerance may occur. Report chest pain, dizziness, or failure to obtain relief of symptoms. Saliva and sputum may be discolored pink with isoproterenol.

■ Learn to self-administer an injection of epinephrine if you have severe allergies. Always carry your injection kit with you. Seek immediate medical care after self-injection of epinephrine.

■ If you have diabetes, monitor your glucose levels carefully because adrenergic medications may elevate them.

---

used therapeutically to relieve paroxysmal atrial tachycardia. However, other medications such as calcium channel blockers (Chaps. 25 and 28) are more likely to be used for this purpose. A **BLACK BOX WARNING** ◆ for parenteral use of Neo-Synephrine alerts prescribers to be familiar with complete prescribing information before use. Other uses of phenylephrine include local application for nasal decongestant and mydriatic effects. Phenylephrine is often an ingredient in prescription and nonprescription cold and allergy remedies. However, a recent systematic review and meta-analysis of oral phenylephrine demonstrated that the OTC 10-mg dose is ineffective for treatment of nasal congestion. The low bioavailability of phenylephrine (38%) may contribute to this lack of efficacy at lower doses. Dosages of 25 mg or higher did demonstrate some effectiveness in reducing nasal congestion, but this dosage exceeds the OTC recommended dose, potentially increasing the incidence of adverse effects. The reviewers recommended that OTC phenylephrine be classified as category III (data are insufficient to classify as safe and effective, and further testing is required).

Toxicity of Adrenergics: Recognition and Management

Excessive use of phenylephrine, ephedrine, and pseudoephedrine, which are ingredients in OTC products such as nasal decongestants, cold preparations, and appetite suppressants, may lead to overdose and toxicity. These drugs, unlike catecholamines, are not quickly cleared from the body. Phenylephrine and ephedrine have a narrow therapeutic index; toxic doses are only two to three times greater than the therapeutic dose. Pseudoephedrine toxicity occurs with doses four to five times greater than the normal therapeutic dose. Ephedrine and ephedra-containing herbal preparations (e.g., ma huang, herbal ecstasy) are often abused as an alternative to amphetamines. In 2004, the FDA banned the sale of these substances in the United States.

The primary clinical manifestation of this adrenergic drug toxicity is severe hypertension, which may lead to headache, confusion, seizures, and intracranial hemorrhage. Other conditions associated with phenylephrine toxicity include reflex bradycardia and atrioventricular block.

Treatment of drug toxicity involves maintaining an airway and assisting with ventilation if needed. Activated charcoal may be administered early in treatment. Aggressive use of vasodilators such as phentolamine or nitroprusside to combat the hypertension is necessary. To avoid a paradoxical increase in blood pressure, clinicians do not use beta blockers alone to treat hypertension without first administering a vasodilator. Dialysis and hemoperfusion are not effective in clearing the adrenergic drugs from the body. Urinary acidification may enhance elimination of ephedrine and pseudoephedrine; however, because of the risk of renal damage from myoglobin deposition in the kidney, use of this technique is not routine.

The Nursing Process

Assessment

Assess the patient's status in relation to the following conditions.

- Allergic disorders. It is standard procedure to question a patient about allergies on initial contact or admission to a health care agency. If the patient reports a previous allergic reaction, try to determine what caused it and what specific symptoms occurred. It may be helpful to ask if swelling, breathing difficulty, or hives (urticaria) occurred. With anaphylactic reactions, severe respiratory distress (from bronchospasm and laryngeal edema) and profound hypotension (from vasodilation) may occur.
- Asthma. If the patient is known to have asthma, assess the frequency of attacks, the specific signs and symptoms experienced, the precipitating factors, the actions taken to obtain relief, and the use of bronchodilators or other medications on a long-term basis. With acute bronchospasm, respiratory distress is clearly evidenced by loud, rapid, gasping, wheezing respirations. Acute asthma attacks may be precipitated by exposure to allergens or respiratory infections. When available, check arterial blood gas reports for the adequacy of oxygen–carbon dioxide gas exchange. Hypoxemia ($\downarrow PO_2$), hypercarbia ($\uparrow PCO_2$), and acidosis ($\downarrow pH$) may occur with acute bronchospasm.
- Chronic obstructive pulmonary disorders. Emphysema and chronic bronchitis are characterized by bronchoconstriction and dyspnea with exercise or at rest. Check arterial blood gas reports when available. Hypoxemia, hypercarbia, and acidosis are likely with chronic bronchoconstriction. Acute bronchospasm may be superimposed on the chronic bronchoconstrictive disorder, especially with a respiratory infection.
- Cardiovascular status. Assess for conditions that are caused or aggravated by adrenergic drugs (e.g., angina, hypertension, tachydysrhythmias).

Nursing Diagnoses

- Impaired gas exchange related to bronchoconstriction
- Ineffective tissue perfusion related to hypotension and shock or vasoconstriction with drug therapy

Periodic Home Visits, Specialist Visits, and Follow-up Enhances Access and Improves Outcomes for Low-Income Children With Asthma
by STANKAITIS, J.

2010, Agency for Healthcare Research and Quality (AHRQ) Innovations Exchange Accessed December 18, 2010.
http://www.innovations.ahrq.gov/content.aspx?id=1740

A medical care facility operates a pediatric asthma management program designed to improve access to and quality of care for children with asthma. Outreach workers emphasize patient education during home visits to patients with asthma, and there are periodic specialist visits. As reported, this foundation-funded pilot program led to a significant decline in the percentage of patients with moderate to severe asthma (from 51% to 26%). In addition, it improved quality of life and contributed to reductions in hospitalizations and costs.

IMPLICATIONS FOR NURSING PRACTICE: Important nursing interventions include identifying patients who are at risk for asthma; ensuring that families are contacted to schedule a visit—community-based outreach workers make initial home visits and make subsequent home visits, including follow-up visits; making certain that specialists visit; reminding patients about upcoming appointments; communicating with primary care providers; contributing to provider education and specialist consultations; promoting community-based treatment and education; and practicing self-assessment against care guidelines.

- Disturbed sleep pattern: Insomnia, nervousness
- Risk for injury related to cardiac stimulation (dysrhythmias, hypertension)
- Imbalanced nutrition: less than body requirements related to anorexia
- Noncompliance: overuse
- Deficient knowledge: drug effects and safe usage

Planning/Goals

The patient will

- Receive or self-administer drugs accurately
- Experience relief of symptoms for which adrenergic drugs are given
- Comply with instructions for safe drug use
- Demonstrate knowledge of adverse drug effects to be reported
- Avoid preventable adverse drug effects
- Avoid combinations of adrenergic drugs

Nursing Interventions

The nurse will

- Use measures to prevent or minimize conditions for which adrenergic drugs are required
- Decrease exposure to allergens. Allergens include cigarette smoke, foods, drugs, air pollutants, plant pollens, insect venoms, and animal dander. Specific allergens must be determined for each person.
- For patients with chronic lung disease, use measures to prevent respiratory infections. These include interventions to aid removal of respiratory secretions, such as adequate hydration, ambulation, deep-breathing and coughing exercises, and chest physiotherapy. Immunizations with pneumococcal pneumonia vaccine and annual influenza vaccine are also strongly recommended.
- When administering substances known to produce hypersensitivity reactions (penicillin and other antibiotics, allergy extracts, vaccines, local anesthetics), observe the recipient carefully for at least 30 minutes after administration. Have adrenergic and other emergency drugs and equipment readily available in case a reaction occurs.
- Use noninvasive interventions in addition to adrenergic medications when treating shock and hypotension. These include applying external pressure over a bleeding site to control hemorrhage and placing the patient in a recumbent position to improve venous return and blood pressure.
- Provide appropriate teaching for drug therapy (see Box 27.2)

Evaluation

- Observe for increased blood pressure and improved tissue perfusion when a drug is given for hypotension and shock or anaphylaxis.
- Interview and observe for improved breathing and arterial blood gas reports when a drug is given for bronchoconstriction or anaphylaxis.
- Interview and observe for decreased nasal congestion.

NCLEX Success

5. When the nurse responds to hypotension due to hypovolemic shock, which of the following should be administered first?

   A. epinephrine (Adrenalin)
   B. isoproterenol (Isuprel)
   C. normal saline (IV)
   D. ephedrine (generic)

6. Which of the following drugs is first administered by the nurse to treat an anaphylactic reaction to penicillin?

   A. diphenhydramine (Benadryl)
   B. epinephrine (Adrenalin)
   C. isoproterenol (Isuprel)
   D. dexamethasone (Decadron)

Key Concepts

- Adrenergic drugs produce effects similar to those produced by stimulation of the sympathetic nervous system.
- Specific effects of adrenergic medications depend mainly on the type of adrenergic receptor activated by the drug.
- Adrenergic drugs have three mechanisms of action: direct interaction with adrenergic receptors, indirect stimulation of adrenergic receptors by the neurotransmitter norepinephrine, or mixed acting, which is a combination of direct and indirect receptor stimulation.
- Because many body tissues have both alpha and beta receptors, the effect produced by an adrenergic drug depends on the type of receptor activated and the number of affected receptors in a particular body tissue.
- The predominant effect in response to activation of alpha$_1$ receptors by an adrenergic drug is vasoconstriction of blood vessels, increasing blood pressure. This is called a vasopressor or pressor effect.
- The predominant effect in response to activation of beta$_1$ receptors by an adrenergic drug is cardiac stimulation.
- The predominant effect in response to activation of beta$_2$ receptors is bronchodilation.
- The predominant effect in response to activation of beta$_3$ receptors is lipolysis and increased release of free fatty acids into the blood.
- Drugs that stimulate presynaptic alpha$_2$ receptors inhibit the release of norepinephrine into synapses of the sympathetic nervous system, thus exerting an antiadrenergic response in the body. Drugs that stimulate presynaptic alpha$_2$ receptors in the CNS are useful in treating hypertension.
- Adrenergic drugs are used as cardiac stimulants, vasopressors, bronchodilators, nasal decongestants, uterine relaxants, adjuncts to local anesthetics, and for hemostatic (topical) and mydriatic effects (topical).

- Epinephrine is the drug of choice to treat anaphylaxis.
- People who are susceptible to severe allergic reactions should carry epinephrine in the form of an autoinjector such as EpiPen or EpiPen Jr for self-administration in emergency situations. These people should also wear a Medic Alert tag or carry documentation that they have severe allergies.
- Use of beta-adrenergic blocking drugs (e.g., propranolol and others) may decrease the effectiveness of epinephrine in cases of anaphylaxis. Higher doses of epinephrine and use of IV fluids may be required to maintain a patent airway and restore blood pressure.
- Epinephrine is recommended as a vasopressor in cardiac arrest situations. A benefit of epinephrine in arrest situations due to asystole or pulseless electrical activity is the added ability to stimulate electrical and mechanical activity and produce myocardial contraction.
- Contraindications to adrenergic drugs include cardiac dysrhythmias, angina, hypertension, hyperthyroidism, cerebrovascular disease, narrow-angle glaucoma, and hypersensitivity to sulfites.
- Local anesthetics containing adrenergics should not be used in any area of the body with a single blood supply (e.g., fingers, toes, nose, ears).
- Epinephrine stimulates $alpha_1$ and beta receptors.
- Ephedrine stimulates $alpha_1$ and beta receptors.
- Pseudoephedrine stimulates $alpha_1$ and beta receptors.
- Isoproterenol stimulates $beta_1$ and $beta_2$ receptors.
- Phenylephrine stimulates $alpha_1$ receptors.
- A **BLACK BOX WARNING** ◆ for parenteral use of Neo-Synephrine alerts prescribers to be familiar with complete prescribing information before use.
- Dietary supplements containing ephedrine alkaloids (ephedra) are prohibited in the United States.

Critical Thinking Questions

27-1. A female inpatient on the postoperative surgical unit is experiencing some shortness of breath after completing physical therapy for her knee replacement. She has a cardiac history significant for nonsustained runs of ventricular tachycardia. The monitor technician alerts the staff immediately on recognition of alarms notifying that her rhythm has changed to an unstable rhythm of pulseless ventricular tachycardia.

- What adrenergic drug is the first priority for IV administration when recognizing a pulseless ventricular tachycardia?
- Administration of epinephrine stimulates which adrenergic receptors? What is the action of the stimulus?
- Why is it important to have epinephrine and other adrenergic drugs readily available in health care settings?
- If IV access in not available, by which route might a clinician give an adrenergic drug?
- What are the major adverse effects in the use of adrenergic agents?
- Why is the patient likely to experience adverse reactions to adrenergic drugs?

References and Resources

Aliot, E. M., Stevenson, W. G., Almendral-Garrote, J. M., Bogun, F., Calkins, C. H., Delacretaz, E., et al. European Heart Rhythm Association (EHRA); Registered Branch of the European Society of Cardiology (ESC); Heart Rhythm Society (HRS); American College of Cardiology (ACC); American Heart Association (AHA). (2009). EHRA/HRS Expert Consensus on Catheter Ablation of Ventricular Arrhythmias: developed in a partnership with the European Heart Rhythm Association (EHRA), a Registered Branch of the European Society of Cardiology (ESC), and the Heart Rhythm Society (HRS); in collaboration with the American College of Cardiology (ACC) and the American Heart Association (AHA). *Heart Rhythm*, 6(6), 886–933.

Hazinski, M. F., Nolan, J. P., Billi, J. E., Böttiger, B. W., Bossaert, L., de Caen, A. R., et al. (2010). Part 1: Executive Summary: 2010 International Consensus on Cardiopulmonary Resuscitation and Emergency Cardiovascular Care Science With Treatment Recommendations. *Circulation, 122*, S250–S275.

Karch, A. M. (2012). *Lippincott's nursing drug guide*. Philadelphia, PA: Lippincott Williams & Wilkins.

Montani, D., Cavailles, A., Bertoletti, L., Botelho, A., Cortot, A., Taillé, C., et al. (2010). *Revue Des Maladies Respiratoires, 27*(10), 1175–1194.

Morrison, L. J., Deakin, C. D., Morley, P. T., Callaway, C. W., Kerber, R. E., & Kronick, S. L. (2010). 2010 International Consensus on Cardiopulmonary Resuscitation and Emergency Cardiovascular Care Science With Treatment Recommendations Part 8: Advanced Life Support. *Circulation, 122*, S345–S421.

Nadkarni, V. M., Nolan, J. P., Billi, J. E., Bossaert, B., Böttiger, B. W., Chamberlain, D., et al. (2010). Part 2: International Collaboration in Resuscitation Science 2010 International Consensus on Cardiopulmonary Resuscitation and Emergency Cardiovascular Care Science With Treatment Recommendations. *Circulation, 122*, S276–S282.

Perrott, J., Henneberry, R. J., & Zed, P. J. (2010). Thrombolytics for cardiac arrest: case report and systematic review of controlled trials. *The Annals of Pharmacotherapy, 44*(12), 2007–2013.

Roberts, B. W., & Trzeciak, S. (2010). Cardiovascular effects of therapeutic hypothermia after resuscitation from cardiac arrest? *Critical Care Medicine, 38*(11), 2264–2265.

28 Drug Therapy for Hypertension

LEARNING OBJECTIVES

After studying this chapter, you should be able to:

1. Describe factors that regulate blood pressure.

2. Describe how hypertension is classified.

3. Discuss nonpharmacologic measures to control hypertension.

4. Identify the prototype and describe the action, use, contraindications, adverse effects, and nursing implications of the angiotensin-converting enzyme inhibitors.

5. Identify the prototype and describe the action, use, contraindications, adverse effects, and nursing implications of the angiotensin II receptor blockers.

6. Describe the rationale for using combination drugs in the management of hypertension.

7. Review the effects of alpha-adrenergic blockers, beta-adrenergic blockers, calcium channel blockers, and diuretics in the management of hypertension.

8. Apply the nursing process in the care of patients with hypertension.

Clinical Application Case Study

Harold Caudill, a 55-year-old African American man, is married, has four children, and works as an automobile salesman. He has a history of primary hypertension. His medical history includes type 1 diabetes mellitus, with early signs of nephropathy. After having a myocardial infarction (MI) 2 years ago, he has been treated with metoprolol, a beta blocker. In addition, he has been taking hydrochlorothiazide to treat the hypertension. His blood pressure today is 138/92 mm Hg, which is consistent with the readings on his last three visits. His physician has added captopril to his treatment regimen.

KEY TERMS

Angioedema: sudden swelling of the lips, tongue, throat, hands, or feet

Angiotensin-converting enzyme (ACE) inhibitor: drug that decreases activation of the renin–angiotensin–aldosterone system; specifically, the drug prevents inactive angiotensin I from being converted to angiotensin II

Angiotensin II receptor blocker: similar to ACE inhibitor, although the mechanism of action is blockade of the angiotensin II receptor site

Antiadrenergics: decrease or block the effects of sympathetic nerve stimulation

Autoregulation: ability of body tissues to regulate their own blood flow

Bradykinin: peptide that causes vasodilation and lowers blood pressure

Essential hypertension: high blood pressure for which no cause can be found

First-dose phenomenon: orthostatic hypotension with palpitations, dizziness, and perhaps syncope 1 to 3 hours after the first dose of a drug or an increased dose

Introduction

Antihypertensive drugs are used to treat hypertension, a common, chronic disorder affecting an estimated 50 to 60 million adults and an unknown number of children and adolescents in the United States. Hypertension increases risks of MI, heart failure, cerebral infarction and hemorrhage, and renal disease. To understand hypertension and antihypertensive drug therapy, it is necessary first to understand the physiologic mechanisms that normally control blood pressure, the characteristics of hypertension, and the characteristics of antihypertensive drugs.

Overview of Hypertension

Regulation of Blood Pressure

Arterial blood pressure reflects the force exerted on arterial walls by blood flow. Blood pressure normally remains constant because of homeostatic mechanisms that adjust blood flow to meet tissue needs. The two major determinants of arterial blood pressure are cardiac output (systolic pressure) and peripheral vascular resistance (diastolic pressure).

Cardiac output equals the product of the heart rate and stroke volume (CO = HR × SV). Stroke volume is the amount of blood ejected with each heartbeat (approximately 60–90 mL). Thus, cardiac output depends on the force of myocardial contraction, blood volume, and other factors. Peripheral vascular resistance is determined by local blood flow and the degree of constriction or dilation in arterioles and arteries (vascular tone).

Autoregulation of Blood Flow

Autoregulation is the ability of body tissues to regulate their own blood flow. This is a critical mechanism of major organs (e.g., heart, brain, kidneys) to preserve oxygenation and function. Local blood flow is regulated primarily by nutritional needs of the tissue, such as lack of oxygen or accumulation of products of cellular metabolism (e.g., carbon dioxide, lactic acid). Local tissues produce vasodilating and vasoconstricting substances to regulate local blood flow. Important tissue factors include histamine, bradykinin, serotonin, and prostaglandins.

Histamine is found mainly in mast cells surrounding blood vessels and is released when these tissues are injured. In some tissues, such as skeletal muscle, mast cell activity is mediated by the sympathetic nervous system (SNS), and histamine is released when SNS stimulation is blocked or withdrawn. In this case, vasodilation results from increased histamine release and the withdrawal of SNS vasoconstrictor activity. **Bradykinin** is released from a protein in body fluids. Kinins dilate arterioles, increase capillary permeability, and constrict venules. Serotonin is released from aggregating platelets during the blood clotting process. It causes vasoconstriction and plays a major role in control of bleeding. Prostaglandins are formed in response to tissue injury and include vasodilators (e.g., prostacyclin) and vasoconstrictors (e.g., thromboxane A_2).

An important component of regulating local blood flow is the production of several vasoactive substances by the endothelial cells that line blood vessels. Vasoconstricting substances, which increase vascular tone and blood pressure, include angiotensin II, endothelin-1, and thromboxane A_2. Vasodilating substances, which decrease vascular tone and blood pressure, include nitric oxide and prostacyclin. Excessive vasoconstrictors or deficient vasodilators may contribute to the development of atherosclerosis, hypertension, and other diseases. Injury to the endothelial lining of blood vessels by the sheer force of blood flow with hypertension or by rupture of atherosclerotic plaque leads to vasoconstriction, vasospasm, thrombus formation, and thickening of the blood vessel wall. All of these factors narrow the blood vessel lumen and increase peripheral vascular resistance.

Overall, regulation of blood pressure involves a complex, interacting, overlapping network of hormonal, neural, and vascular mechanisms, and any condition that affects heart rate, stroke volume, or peripheral vascular resistance affects arterial blood pressure. Many of these mechanisms are compensatory effects that attempt to restore balance when hypotension or hypertension occurs. Box 28.1 further describes these mechanisms.

Types of Hypertension

Hypertension is persistently high blood pressure that results from abnormalities in regulatory mechanisms. It is usually defined as a systolic pressure above 140 mm Hg or a diastolic pressure above 90 mm Hg on multiple blood pressure measurements. *The Eighth Report of the Joint National Committee on Prevention, Detection, Evaluation, and Treatment of High Blood Pressure* (JNC 8) is long awaited and expected to be released in 2012. The recommendations have been the cornerstone in the detection, evaluation, and treatment of high blood pressure. The Seventh Report, published in 2004, classifies blood pressures in adults (in mm Hg) into four categories (Box 28.2). These guidelines also recommend a goal blood pressure of less than 130/80 mm Hg for people with diabetes or renal disease.

BOX 28.1 Mechanisms That Regulate Blood Pressure

Neural

Neural regulation of blood pressure mainly involves the sympathetic nervous system (SNS). In the heart, SNS neurons control heart rate and force of contraction. In blood vessels, SNS neurons control muscle tone by maintaining a state of partial contraction, with additional constriction or dilation accomplished by altering this basal state. When hypotension and inadequate tissue perfusion occur, the SNS is activated and produces secretion of epinephrine and norepinephrine by the adrenal medulla; constriction of blood vessels in the skin, gastrointestinal tract, and kidneys; and stimulation of beta-adrenergic receptors in the heart, which increases heart rate and force of myocardial contraction. All of these mechanisms act to increase blood pressure and tissue perfusion, especially of the brain and heart.

The SNS is activated by the vasomotor center in the brain, which constantly receives messages from baroreceptors and chemoreceptors located in the circulatory system. Adequate function of these receptors is essential for rapid and short-term regulation of blood pressure. The vasomotor center interprets the messages from these receptors and modifies cardiovascular functions to maintain adequate blood flow.

More specifically, baroreceptors detect changes in pressure or stretch. For example, when a person moves from a lying to a standing position, blood pressure falls and decreases stretch in the aorta and arteries. This elicits increased heart rate and vasoconstriction to restore adequate circulation. The increased heart rate occurs rapidly and blood pressure is adjusted within 1 to 2 minutes. This quick response prevents orthostatic hypotension with dizziness and possible syncope. (Antihypertensive medications may blunt this response and cause orthostatic hypotension.)

Chemoreceptors, which are located in the aorta and carotid arteries, are in close contact with arterial blood and respond to changes in the oxygen, carbon dioxide, and hydrogen ion content of blood. Although their main function is to regulate ventilation, they also communicate with the vasomotor center and can induce vasoconstriction.

Chemoreceptors are stimulated when blood pressure drops to a certain point because oxygen is decreased and carbon dioxide and hydrogen ions are increased in arterial blood.

The central nervous system (CNS) also regulates vasomotor tone and blood pressure. Inadequate blood flow to the brain results in ischemia of the vasomotor center. When this occurs, neurons in the vasomotor center stimulate widespread vasoconstriction in an attempt to raise blood pressure and restore blood flow. This reaction, the CNS ischemic response, is an emergency measure to preserve blood flow to vital brain centers. If blood flow is not restored within 3 to 10 minutes, the neurons of the vasomotor center are unable to function, the impulses that maintain vascular muscle tone stop, and blood pressure drops to a fatal level.

Hormonal

The renin–angiotensin–aldosterone (RAA) system and vasopressin are important hormonal mechanisms in blood pressure regulation.

The RAA system is activated in response to hypotension and acts as a compensatory mechanism to restore adequate blood flow to body tissues. Renin is an enzyme that is synthesized, stored, and released from the kidneys in response to decreased blood pressure, SNS stimulation, or decreased sodium concentration in extracellular fluid. When released into the bloodstream, where its action lasts 30 to 60 minutes, renin converts angiotensinogen (a plasma protein) to angiotensin I. Angiotensin-converting enzyme (ACE) in the endothelium of pulmonary blood vessels then acts on angiotensin I to produce angiotensin II. Angiotensin II strongly constricts arterioles (and weakly constricts veins), increases peripheral resistance, and increases blood pressure by direct vasoconstriction, stimulation of the SNS, and stimulation of catecholamine release from the adrenal medulla. It also stimulates secretion of aldosterone from the adrenal cortex, which then causes the kidneys to retain sodium and water. Retention of sodium and water increases blood volume, cardiac output, and blood pressure.

Vasopressin, also called antidiuretic hormone or ADH, is a hormone secreted by the posterior pituitary gland that regulates reabsorption of water by the kidneys. It is released in response to decreased blood volume and decreased blood pressure. It causes retention of body fluids and vasoconstriction, both of which act to raise blood pressure.

Vascular

The endothelial cells that line blood vessels synthesize and secrete several substances that play important roles in regulating cardiovascular functions, including blood pressure. These substances normally maintain a balance between vasoconstriction and vasodilation. When the endothelium is damaged (e.g., by trauma, hypertension, hypercholesterolemia, or atherosclerosis), the resulting imbalance promotes production of vasoconstricting substances and also causes blood vessels to lose their ability to relax in response to dilator substances. In addition, changes in structure of endothelial and vascular smooth muscle cells (vascular remodeling) further impair vascular functions.

Vasoconstrictors increase vascular tone (i.e., constrict or narrow blood vessels so that higher blood pressure is required to pump blood to body tissues). Vasoconstricting substances produced by the endothelium include angiotensin II, endothelin-1, platelet-derived growth factor (PDGF), and thromboxane A_2. Endothelin-1 is the strongest endogenous vasoconstrictor known. Angiotensin II and thromboxane A_2 can also be produced by other types of cells, but endothelial cells can produce both. Thromboxane A_2, a product of arachidonic acid metabolism, also promotes platelet aggregation and thrombosis.

Vasodilators decrease vascular tone and blood pressure. Major vasodilating substances produced by the endothelium include nitric oxide and prostacyclin (prostaglandin I2).

Nitric oxide (NO) is a gas that can diffuse through cell membranes, trigger biochemical reactions, and then dissipate rapidly. It is formed by the action of the enzyme NO synthase on the amino acid L-arginine and continually released by normal endothelium. Its production is tightly regulated and depends on the amount of ionized calcium in the fluid portion of endothelial cells. Several substances (e.g., acetylcholine, bradykinin, catecholamines, substance P, and products of aggregating platelets such as adenosine diphosphate and serotonin) act on receptors in endothelial cell membranes to increase the cytosolic concentration of ionized calcium, activate NO synthase, and increase NO production. In addition, increased blood flow or blood pressure increases shear stress at the endothelial surface and stimulates production of NO.

BOX 28.1   Mechanisms That Regulate Blood Pressure (Continued)

Once produced, endothelium-derived NO produces vasodilation primarily by activating guanylyl cyclase in vascular smooth muscle cells and increasing intracellular cyclic 3',5'-guanosine monophosphate as a second messenger. NO also inhibits platelet aggregation and production of platelet-derived vasoconstricting substances. Because NO is released into the vessel wall (to relax smooth muscle) and into the vessel lumen (to inactivate platelets), it is thought to have protective effects against vasoconstriction and thrombosis.

NO is also produced in leukocytes, fibroblasts, and vascular smooth muscle cells and may have pathologic effects when large amounts are produced. In these tissues, NO seems to have other functions, such as modifying nerve activity in the nervous system.

Prostacyclin is synthesized and released from endothelium in response to stimulation by several factors (e.g., bradykinin, interleukin-1, serotonin, thrombin, PDGF). It produces vasodilation by activating adenylyl cyclase and increasing levels of cyclic adenosine monophosphate in smooth muscle cells. In addition, like NO, prostacyclin also inhibits platelet aggregation and production of platelet-derived vasoconstricting substances. The vasodilating effects of prostacyclin may occur independently or in conjunction with NO.

Overall, excessive vasoconstrictors or deficient vasodilators may contribute to the development of atherosclerosis, hypertension, and other diseases. Injury to the endothelial lining of blood vessels (e.g., by the sheer force of blood flow with hypertension or by rupture of atherosclerotic plaque) decreases vasodilators and leads to vasoconstriction, vasospasm, thrombus formation, and thickening of the blood vessel wall. All of these factors require the blood to flow through a narrowed lumen and increase blood pressure.

Vascular Remodeling

Vascular remodeling is similar to the left ventricular remodeling that occurs in heart failure (see Chap. 24). It results from endothelial dysfunction and produces a thickening of the blood vessel wall and a narrowing of the blood vessel lumen. Thickening of the wall makes blood vessels less flexible and less able to respond to vasodilating substances. There are also changes in endothelial cell structure (i.e., the connections between endothelial cells become looser) that lead to increased permeability. The mechanisms of these vascular changes, which promote and aggravate hypertension, are described below.

As discussed in previous chapters, normal endothelium helps maintain a balance between vasoconstriction and vasodilation, procoagulation and anticoagulation, proinflammation and anti-inflammation, and progrowth and antigrowth. In the inflammatory process, normal endothelium acts as a physical barrier against the movement of leukocytes into the subendothelial space. Endothelial products such as nitric oxide may also inhibit leukocyte activity. However, inflammatory cytokines such as tumor necrosis factor–alpha and interleukin-1 activate endothelial cells to produce adhesion molecules (which allow leukocytes to adhere to the endothelium), interleukin-8 (which attracts leukocytes to the endothelium and allows them to accumulate in subendothelial cells), and foam cells (lipid-filled monocyte/macrophages that form fatty streaks, the beginning lesions of atherosclerotic plaque). Although activation of endothelial cells may be a helpful component of the normal immune response, the resulting inflammation may contribute to disease development.

In terms of cell growth, normal endothelium limits the growth of vascular smooth muscle that underlies the endothelium and forms the vessel wall. Growth-inhibiting products of the endothelium include nitric oxide, which also inhibits platelet activation and production of growth-promoting substances. When the endothelium is damaged, endothelial cells become activated and also produce growth-promoting products. Other endothelial products (e.g., angiotensin II and endothelin-1) may also stimulate growth of vascular smooth muscle cells. Thus, damage or loss of endothelial cells stimulates growth of smooth muscle cells in the intimal layer of the blood vessel wall.

A systolic pressure of 140 mm Hg or greater, with a diastolic pressure of less than 90 mm Hg, is called isolated systolic hypertension and is more common in the elderly. Systolic–diastolic hypertension, which may also occur in older adults, involves elevations of both systolic and diastolic pressures. Both types increase cardiovascular morbidity and mortality, especially heart failure and stroke, and warrant treatment.

A hypertensive emergency or crisis is a diastolic pressure of 120 mm Hg or higher and possible target organ damage. (A hypertensive urgency is an episode of marked elevation in blood pressure without target organ damage. The goal of management is to lower blood pressure within 24 hours.)

BOX 28.2   Classification of Hypertension (all values in mm Hg)

- Normal = systolic <120 *and* diastolic <80
- Prehypertension = systolic 120–139 *or* diastolic 80–89
- Stage 1 hypertension = systolic 140–159 *or* diastolic 90–99
- Stage 2 hypertension = systolic > 160 *or* diastolic 100 or more

From U.S. Department of Health and Human Services, National Institutes of Health, National Heart, Lung, and Blood Institute, National High Blood Pressure Education Program. The Seventh Report of the Joint National Committee on Prevention, Detection, Evolution, and Treatment of High Blood Pressure (JNC 7). NIH Publication No. 04-5230, August 2004.

Etiology

Although it has frequently been indicated that the causes of primary hypertension, or **essential hypertension**, are not known, this is only partially true; genetic variations and inherited, behavioral, and environmental factors may increase blood pressure. These include obesity, high alcohol intake, insulin resistance, high salt intake in salt-sensitive people, aging, sedentary lifestyle, and stress. Furthermore, many of these factors are additive, such as obesity and alcohol intake. Primary hypertension makes up 90% to 95% of known cases. Appropriate therapy usually controls primary hypertension.

Secondary hypertension may result from renal, endocrine, or central nervous system disorders and from drugs that stimulate the SNS or cause retention of sodium and water, producing adverse effects. Secondary hypertension can sometimes be cured by managing the underlying condition or cause. Hypertensive emergencies often result from such conditions as cerebral hemorrhage, dissecting aortic aneurysm, renal disease, pheochromocytoma, or eclampsia.

Pathophysiology

Hypertension profoundly alters cardiovascular function by increasing the workload of the heart and causing thickening and sclerosis of arterial walls. The increased cardiac workload leads to myocardial hypertrophy as a compensatory mechanism, with eventual heart failure. As a result of endothelial dysfunction and arterial changes (vascular remodeling), the arterial lumen narrows, blood supply to tissues decreases, and the risk of thrombosis increases. In addition, necrotic areas may develop in arteries, and these may rupture with sustained high blood pressure. The areas of most serious damage are the heart, brain, kidneys, and eyes. These are often called target organs.

Response to Hypotension

When hypotension (and decreased tissue perfusion) occurs, the SNS is stimulated, the hormones epinephrine and norepinephrine are secreted by the adrenal medulla, angiotensin II and aldosterone are formed, and the kidneys retain fluid. These compensatory mechanisms raise the blood pressure. Specific effects include the following:

- Constriction of arterioles, which increases peripheral vascular resistance
- Constriction of veins and increased venous tone
- Stimulation of cardiac beta-adrenergic receptors, which increases heart rate and force of myocardial contraction
- Activation of the renin–angiotensin–aldosterone mechanism

Chapter 27 contains an additional discussion of the effects and management of hypotension.

Response to Hypertension

- When arterial blood pressure is elevated, the following sequence of events occurs:
- Kidneys excrete more fluid (increase urine output).
- Fluid loss reduces both extracellular fluid volume and blood volume.
- Decreased blood volume reduces venous blood flow to the heart and therefore decreases cardiac output.
- Decreased cardiac output reduces arterial blood pressure.
- The vascular endothelium produces vasodilating substances (e.g., nitric oxide, prostacyclin), which reduce blood pressure.

Clinical Manifestations

Initially, and perhaps for years, primary hypertension may produce no symptoms. If symptoms occur, they are usually vague and nonspecific. Hypertension may go undetected, or it may be incidentally discovered when blood pressure measurements are taken as part of a routine physical examination, screening test, or assessment of other disorders. Eventually, symptoms reflect target organ damage. Hypertension is often discovered after a person experiences angina pectoris, MI, heart failure, stroke, or renal disease.

Symptoms include severe headache, nausea, vomiting, visual disturbances, neurologic disturbances, disorientation, and decreased level of consciousness (drowsiness, stupor, coma). Hypertensive emergencies require immediate blood pressure reduction with parenteral antihypertensive drugs to limit damage to target organs.

Therapy

Goals of Treatment

After the diagnosis of hypertension is established, it is essential that a therapeutic regimen be designed and implemented. The goal of management for most patients is to achieve and maintain blood pressure well below 140/90 mm Hg. The target blood pressure for people with diabetes is 130/80 mm Hg. If the goal is impossible to achieve, lowering blood pressure to any extent is still considered beneficial in decreasing the incidence of coronary artery disease (CAD) and stroke. In most instances, it is better to lower blood pressure gradually and to avoid wide fluctuations in blood pressure.

Nonpharmacologic Treatment

The Joint National Committee on Prevention, Detection, Evaluation, and Treatment of High Blood Pressure (JNC 7) recommends management guidelines in which initial interventions include lifestyle modifications (i.e., reduction of weight and sodium intake, regular physical activity, moderate alcohol intake, and no smoking) to maintain normal blood pressure. If these modifications do not produce the target blood pressure or substantial progress toward the target blood pressure, it is important to initiate antihypertensive drug therapy and continue lifestyle modifications.

Dietary Management

Key behavioral determinants of blood pressure are related to dietary consumption of calories and salt; the prevalence of hypertension rises proportionally to average body mass index. The Dietary Approaches to Stop Hypertension (DASH) study demonstrated that people with prehypertension or stage 1 hypertension can reduce their blood pressures by adhering to a diet abundant in fresh fruits and vegetables and low-fat dairy products even without restricting calorie or sodium intake. The effects of the DASH diet demonstrate blood pressure–lowering effects that parallel the degree of benefit from drug monotherapy and may include dietary sodium restriction. Effects are evident in all ethnic groups, particularly African Americans.

Severe restrictions of sodium intake usually are not acceptable to people; however, moderate restrictions (4–6 g of salt a day) are beneficial and more easily implemented. Avoiding heavily salted foods (e.g., cured meats, sandwich meats, pretzels, potato chips) and not adding salt to food at the table can achieve this. Research and clinical observations indicate the following:

- Sodium restriction alone reduces blood pressure.
- Sodium restriction potentiates the antihypertensive actions of diuretics and other antihypertensive drugs. Conversely, excessive sodium intake decreases the antihypertensive actions of all antihypertensive drugs. Patients with unrestricted salt intake who are taking thiazides may lose excessive potassium and become hypokalemic.
- Sodium restriction may decrease dosage requirements of antihypertensive drugs, thereby decreasing the incidence and severity of adverse effects.

Lifestyle Management

Considerable evidence demonstrates that regular aerobic exercise by itself effectively reduces blood pressure. However, the direct benefits of exercise on blood pressure control are often difficult to isolate from those of the changes that often accompany exercise, such as improved diet, weight loss, decreased alcohol consumption, and decreased cigarette smoking. The JNC 7 recommendations include increasing exercise to at least 30 minutes per day at least 4 days per week, achieving a weight loss goal of at least 10 pounds, limiting alcohol consumption to two drinks or less per day for men and one drink or less per day for women, and ceasing smoking.

Drug Treatment

Drugs used in the management of primary hypertension belong to several different groups, including angiotensin-converting enzyme (ACE) inhibitors; **angiotensin II receptor blockers** (ARBs), also called angiotensin II receptor antagonists; antiadrenergics; calcium channel blockers; diuretics; and direct vasodilators. In general, these drugs act to decrease blood pressure by decreasing cardiac output or peripheral vascular resistance. This chapter focuses on ACE inhibitors and ARBs. Various chapters describe other drugs discussed in this chapter—for example, chapters related to heart failure (see Chap. 24), dysrhythmias (see Chap. 25), and angina (see Chap. 26).

Table 28.1 outlines the antihypertensive drugs, and Table 28.2 lists antihypertensive–diuretic combination products. Product labeling and JNC 7 recommendations are the basis for adult dosages. Product labeling and recommendations from the National High Blood Pressure Education Program Working Group on High Blood Pressure in Children and Adolescents (2004) are the basis for pediatric dosages.

The JNC 7 guidelines suggest thiazide diuretics be used as first-line therapy, either alone (monotherapy) or with a beta blocker, ACE inhibitor, ARB, or calcium channel blocker. If the initial drug (and dose) does not produce the desired blood pressure, options for further management include increasing the dose, substituting another drug, or adding a second drug from a different group. If the response is still inadequate, addition of a second or third drug, including a diuretic if not previously prescribed, is a possibility. When current management is ineffective, it is necessary to reassess the patient's adherence to lifestyle modifications and drug therapy. In addition, it is also important to review other factors that may decrease the therapeutic response, such as

the use of over-the-counter appetite suppressants, dietary or herbal supplements, or nasal decongestants, which raise blood pressure.

The guidelines of the World Health Organization and the International Society of Hypertension for management of hypertension include considering age, ethnicity, and concomitant cardiovascular disorders when choosing an antihypertensive drug; starting with a single drug, in the lowest available dose; changing to a drug from a different group, rather than increasing dosage of the first drug or adding a second drug, if the initial drug is ineffective or not well tolerated; and using long-acting drugs (i.e., a single dose effective for 24 hours). The guidelines also note that many patients require two or more drugs to achieve adequate blood pressure control. When this is the case, fixed-dose combinations or long-acting agents may be preferred, because they decrease the number of drugs and doses that are required and may increase compliance.

Variation exists in the response to drug therapy for hypertension in ethnic populations. Experts credit nearly 70% of the familial considerations related to blood pressure to shared genes rather than to shared environment. For most antihypertensive drugs, few research studies have compared effects among different genetic or ethnic groups. However, several studies indicate that beta blockers have greater effects in people of Asian heritage compared with those of Caucasian background. For hypertension, Asians in general need much smaller doses because they metabolize and excrete beta blockers slowly. Other populations known to metabolize beta blockers slowly include Arab and Egyptian Americans and possibly German Americans. In African Americans, diuretics are effective and recommended as initial drug therapy. Calcium channel blockers, alpha$_1$ receptor blockers, and the alpha–beta blocker labetalol are reportedly equally effective in African Americans and Caucasians. ACE inhibitors, some ARBs (e.g., losartan and telmisartan), and beta blockers are less effective as monotherapy in African Americans. When beta blockers are used, they are usually one component of a multidrug regimen, and higher doses may be necessary. Overall, African Americans are more likely to have severe hypertension and require multiple drugs as a result of having low circulating renin, increased salt sensitivity, and a higher incidence of obesity.

Angiotensin-Converting Enzyme Inhibitors

Authorities recommend ⓟ **captopril** (Capoten), the prototype **angiotensin-converting enzyme (ACE) inhibitor,** and other drugs in this class as first-line agents for treating hypertension in people with diabetes, particularly those with type 1 diabetes and/or diabetic nephropathy. These drugs reduce proteinuria and slow progression of renal impairment in people with this disease. (However, they may cause or aggravate proteinuria and renal damage in people who do not have diabetes.) ACE inhibitors may be used alone or in combination with other antihypertensive agents, such as thiazide diuretics.

(text continues on p.520)

TABLE 28.1

Drugs Administered for the Treatment of Hypertension

Drug Class	Prototype	Other Drugs in the Class
Angiotensin-Converting Enzyme (ACE) Inhibitors	Captopril (Capoten)	Benazepril (Lotensin) Enalapril (Vasotec) Fosinopril (Monopril) Lisinopril (Prinivil, Zestril) Moexipril (Univasc) Quinapril (Accupril) Ramipril (Altace) Trandolapril (Mavik)
Angiotensin II Receptor Blockers (ARBs)	Losartan (Cozaar)	Candesartan (Atacand) Irbesartan (Avapro) Olmesartan (Benicar) Telmisartan (Micardis) Valsartan (Diovan)
Adjuvant Medications *Direct Renin Inhibitor*	Aliskiren (Tekturna)	
Antiadrenergics *Alpha$_1$ Adrenergic Blockers*		Doxazosin (Cardura) Prazosin (Minipress) Terazosin (Hytrin)
Alpha$_2$ Agonists		Clonidine (Catapres) Guanfacine (Tenex) Methyldopa (Aldomet)
Beta-Adrenergic Blockers		Acebutolol (Sectral) Atenolol (Tenormin) Bisoprolol (Zebeta) Metoprolol (Lopressor) Nadolol (Corgard) Pindolol (Visken) Propranolol (Inderal) Timolol (Blocadren)
Alpha–Beta-Adrenergic Blockers		Carvedilol (Coreg) Labetalol (Trandate, Normodyne)
Calcium Channel Blockers		Amlodipine (Norvasc) Diltiazem (sustained release) (Cardizem SR) Felodipine (Plendil) Isradipine (DynaCirc) Nicardipine (Cardene, Cardene SR, Cardene IV) Nifedipine (Adalat, Procardia, Procardia XL) Nisoldipine (Sular) Verapamil (Calan, Calan SR, Isoptin SR)

TABLE 28.1

Drugs Administered for the Treatment of Hypertension (Continued)

Drug Class	Prototype	Other Drugs in the Class
Diuretics *Thiazide*	Hydrochlorothiazide (Esidrix, Oretic)	Chlorothiazide (Diuril) Chlorthalidone (Hygroton, Thalitone) Indapamide (Lozol) Metolazone (Zaroxolyn)
Loop	Furosemide (Lasix)	Bumetanide (Bumex) Ethacrynic acid (Edecrin) Torsemide (Demadex)
Potassium Sparing	Spironolactone (Aldactone)	Amiloride (Midamor) Triamterene (Dyrenium)
Other Vasodilators		Fenoldopam (Corlopam) Hydralazine (Apresoline) Minoxidil (Loniten) Sodium nitroprusside (Nitropress)

TABLE 28.2

DRUGS AT A GLANCE: Oral Antihypertensive Combination Products*

Trade Name	Angiotensin II Receptor Blocker	Angiotensin-Converting Enzyme Inhibitor	Beta-Adrenergic Blocker	Calcium Channel Blocker	Diuretic	Other	Dosage Ranges
Accuretic		Quinapril 10–20 mg			HCTZ 12.5–25 mg		1–2 tablets once daily
Aldactazide					HCTZ 25–50 mg; Spironolactone 25–50 mg		1–2 tablets once daily
Aldoril					HCTZ 15, 25, 30, or 50 mg	Methyldopa 250 or 500 mg	1 tablet daily
Apresazide					HCTZ 25 mg	Hydralazine 25 mg	1 tablet daily
Atacand HCT	Candesartan 16 or 32 mg				HCTZ 12.5 or 25 mg		1 tablet daily
Avalide	Irbesartan 150 or 300 mg				HCTZ 12.5 mg		1 tablet daily

(Continued on page 518)

TABLE 28.2

DRUGS AT A GLANCE: Oral Antihypertensive Combination Products* (Continued)

	Components						
Trade Name	Angiotensin II Receptor Blocker	Angiotensin-Converting Enzyme Inhibitor	Beta-Adrenergic Blocker	Calcium Channel Blocker	Diuretic	Other	Dosage Ranges
Azor	Olmesartan 20 or 40 mg			Amlodipine 5 or 10 mg			1 tablet daily
Benicar HCT	Olmesartan 20 or 40 mg				HCTZ 12.5 or 25 mg		1–2 tablets daily
Capozide		Captopril 25 or 50 mg			HCTZ 15 or 25 mg		1 tablet 2–3 times daily
Combipres					Chlorothiazide 15 mg	Clonidine 0.1–0.2 mg	1 tablet daily
Corzide			Nadolol 40 or 80 mg		Bendroflumethiazide 5 mg		1 tablet daily
Diovan HCT	Valsartan 80 or 160 mg				HCTZ 12.5 mg		1 tablet daily
Dyazide					HCTZ 25 mg; Triamterene 37.5 mg		1 tablet daily
Exforge	Valsartan 160 or 320 mg			Amlodipine 5 or 10 mg			1–2 tablets once daily
Hyzaar	Losartan 50 mg				HCTZ 12.5 mg		1 tablet daily
Inderide			Propranolol 40 or 80 mg		HCTZ 25 mg		1–2 tablets twice daily
Lexxel		Enalapril 5 mg		Felodipine 5 mg			1–2 tablets once daily
Lopressor HCT			Metoprolol 50 or 100 mg		HCTZ 25 or 50 mg		1–2 tablets daily
Lotrel		Benazepril 10 or 20 mg		Amlodipine 2.5 or 5 mg			1 capsule daily
Minizide					Polythiazide 0.5 mg	Prazosin 1, 2, or 5 mg	1 capsule 2–3 times daily

TABLE 28.2

DRUGS AT A GLANCE: Oral Antihypertensive Combination Products* (Continued)

				Components			
Trade Name	Angiotensin II Receptor Blocker	Angiotensin-Converting Enzyme Inhibitor	Beta-Adrenergic Blocker	Calcium Channel Blocker	Diuretic	Other	Dosage Ranges
Micardis HCT	Telmisartan 40 or 80 mg				HCTZ 12.5 or 25 mg		1–2 tablets daily
Moduretic					HCTZ 50 mg; Amiloride 5 mg		1 tablet daily
Prinzide		Lisinopril 20 mg			HCTZ 12.5 or 25 mg		1 tablet daily
Tarka		Trandolapril 1, 2, or 4 mg		Verapamil 180 or 240 mg		Prazosin 1, 2, or 5 mg	1 tablet daily
Tenoretic			Atenolol 100 mg		Chlorthalidone 25 mg		1 tablet daily
Teveten HCT	Eprosartan 600 mg				HCTZ 12.5 or 25 mg		1 tablet daily
Timolide			Timolol 10 mg		HCTZ 12.5		1–2 tablets daily
Twynsta	Telmisartan 40 or 80 mg			Amlodipine 5 or 10 mg			
Uniretic		Moexipril 7.5 or 15 mg daily			HCTZ 12.5 or 25 mg		1–2 tablets daily
Valturna	Valsartan 160 or 320 mg					Aliskiren 150 or 300 mg	1 tablet daily
Vaseretic		Enalapril 5 mg			HCTZ 12.5 mg		1–2 tablets daily
Zestoretic		Lisinopril 10 or 20 mg	Timolol 10 mg		HCTZ 12.5 or 25 mg		1 tablet daily
Ziac		Bisoprolol 2.5, 5, or 10 mg			HCTZ 6.25 mg		1 tablet daily

*Note that one trade-name product may be available in multiple formulations, with variable amounts of antihypertensive, diuretic, or both components.

HCTZ, hydrochlorothiazide.

EVIDENCE-BASED PRACTICE

Fixed-Dose Combinations Improve Medication Compliance: A Meta-Analysis.

by BANGALORE, S., KAMALAKKANNAN, G., PARKAR, S., MESSERLI, F. H.

American Journal of Medicine
2007, 120, 713–719

Researchers performed a meta-analysis of nine studies (11,925 patients), exploring adherence to medication administration using fixed-dose combinations compared with a regimen of drugs given individually (e.g., one pill of lisinopril plus hydrochlorothiazide versus lisinopril and hydrochlorothiazide given as two separate pills). A subgroup analysis of four retrospective studies on hypertension from this group showed that people who received fixed-dose combinations of antihypertensive medications had a reduced likelihood of nonadherence by 24% compared with people who took the same medications as separate pills. Because evidence now suggests that the majority of people with hypertension require combinations of antihypertensive medications to achieve optimal blood pressure control, simplifying the drug regimen with fixed-combination drugs can improve adherence and produce better health outcomes.

IMPLICATIONS FOR NURSING PRACTICE: The nurse should explore the level of adherence to drug therapy for patients with hypertension. The option for fixed-dose combinations can enhance adherence and lead to improved blood pressure control when patients receive prescriptions for drugs from more than one class. A thorough assessment of a patient's drug list is necessary to evaluate the option of fixed-dose combinations.

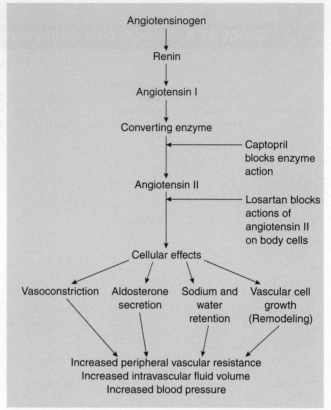

Figure 28.1 Captopril and other angiotensin-converting enzyme (ACE) inhibitors inhibit ACE and thereby prevent formation of angiotensin II. Losartan and other angiotensin II receptor blockers (ARBs) prevent angiotensin II from connecting with its receptors and thereby prevent it from acting on body tissues containing those receptors (e.g., blood vessels, adrenal cortex).

Pharmacokinetics

Captopril is well absorbed with oral administration (with absorption reduced by food), produces effects within 1 to 1½ hours, and has a prolonged serum half-life with impaired renal function. The drug is metabolized and excreted in the urine (half as unchanged drug) and is excreted in breast milk.

Action

ACE inhibitors such as captopril block the enzyme that normally converts angiotensin I to the potent vasoconstrictor angiotensin II. (ACE [also called kininase] is mainly located in the endothelial lining of blood vessels, which is the site of production of most angiotensin II. This same enzyme also metabolizes bradykinin, an endogenous substance with strong vasodilating properties.) By blocking production of angiotensin II, the ACE inhibitors decrease vasoconstriction (thus having a vasodilating effect) and decrease aldosterone production (thus reducing retention of sodium and water). Figure 28.1 describes this cascade of events. In addition to inhibiting formation of angiotensin II, ACE inhibitors also inhibit the breakdown of bradykinin, prolonging its vasodilating effects.

Use

Health care providers use captopril to prevent or reverse the remodeling of heart muscle and blood vessel walls that impairs cardiovascular function and exacerbates cardiovascular disease processes. Widely used to treat heart failure and hypertension, the drug may also decrease morbidity and mortality in other cardiovascular disorders. It may be effective as monotherapy in Caucasian patients with hypertension or in combination with a diuretic in African American hypertensive patients. Clinicians also recommend captopril and other ACE inhibitors for adults with hypertension and diabetes mellitus and kidney damage because they slow the progression of albuminuria. In addition, captopril improves post-MI survival when added to the standard therapy of aspirin, a beta blocker, and a thrombolytic.

TABLE 28.3

DRUGS AT A GLANCE: Angiotensin-Converting Enzyme Inhibitors

Drug	Pregnancy Category	Routes and Dosage Ranges	
		Adults	**Children 1–17 Y of Age (unless otherwise stated)**
Ⓟ **Captopril** (Capoten)	D	25 mg PO, 2–3 times daily initially, gradually increased to 50, 100, or 150 mg 2–3 times daily, if necessary; maximum dose 450 mg/d	1.5 mg/kg/d PO in divided doses every 8 h; maximum dose 6 mg/kg/d Neonates, 0.03–0.15 PO mg/kg/d every 8–24 h; maximum dose 2 mg/kg/d
Benazepril (Lotensin)	D	10 mg PO once daily initially, increased to 40 mg daily if necessary, in 1 or 2 doses	0.2 mg/kg PO once daily
Enalapril (Vasotec)	D	5 mg PO once daily, increased to 10–40 mg daily, in 1 or 2 doses, if necessary	0.08 mg/kg PO; maximum dose 5 mg/d
Fosinopril (Monopril)	D	10 mg PO once daily initially, increased to 40 mg daily if necessary in 1 or 2 doses	>50 kg, 5–10 mg PO once daily
Lisinopril (Prinivil, Zestril)	D	10 mg PO once daily, increased to 40 mg if necessary	≥6 y, 0.07 mg/kg PO once daily; maximum dose 5 mg/d
Moexipril (Univasc)	D	Initial dose, 7.5 mg PO (3.75 mg for those who have renal impairment or are taking a diuretic). Maintenance dose, 7.5–30 mg daily, in 1 or 2 doses, adjusted according to blood pressure control	Safety and effectiveness in children have not been established
Quinapril (Accupril)	D	10 PO mg once daily initially, increased to 20, 40, or 80 mg daily if necessary, in 1 or 2 doses; wait at least 2 wk between dose increments	5–10 PO mg once daily; maximum dose 80 mg once daily
Ramipril (Altace)	D	2.5 mg PO once daily, increased to 20 mg daily if necessary, in 1 or 2 doses	Safety and effectiveness in children have not been established
Trandolapril (Mavik)	D	Initial dose, 1 mg PO once daily (0.5 mg for those who have hepatic or renal impairment or are taking a diuretic; 2 mg for African Americans) Maintenance dose, PO 2–4 mg daily, in a single dose, adjusted according to blood pressure control	Safety and effectiveness in children have not been established

Table 28.3 presents route and dosage information for captopril and other ACE inhibitors.

Use in Children

Limited information is available on the safety and efficacy of captopril in children. Manufacturer information states that captopril should be used in children only when other measures to control blood pressure have not been successful.

Use in Patients With Renal Impairment

Captopril and other ACE inhibitors are usually effective in patients with renal impairment, but responses may vary. Careful monitoring is required, especially during the first few weeks of therapy, to prevent irreversible renal failure. For some patients, it may not be possible to normalize blood pressure and maintain adequate renal perfusion.

Use in Patients With Critical Illness

Health care providers may use captopril in patients who are critically ill. However, oral dosing may restrict use to patients who can tolerate oral medications. Urgent or emergent needs to reduce significant hypertension may require more effective management with drugs that can be administered intravenously or have a more rapid onset of action.

Adverse Effects

Captopril is well tolerated has a low incidence of serious adverse effects (e.g., neutropenia, agranulocytosis, proteinuria, glomerulonephritis, **angioedema**). However, a persistent cough develops in a significant number of patients, and this problem may lead to discontinuation of the drug. Also, acute hypotension may occur when captopril is started, especially in patients with fluid volume deficit. Starting with a low dose taken at bedtime or by stopping diuretics and reducing dosage of other antihypertensive drugs temporarily may prevent this reaction. Hyperkalemia may develop in patients with diabetes mellitus or renal impairment or who are taking nonsteroidal anti-inflammatory drugs, potassium supplements, or potassium-sparing diuretics.

Contraindications

Contraindications to captopril and other ACE inhibitors include pregnancy, and it is important to discontinue them when pregnancy is detected. The U.S. Food and Drug Administration (FDA) has issued a **BLACK BOX WARNING ◆** for use of drugs that directly affect the renin–angiotensin system, such as ACE inhibitors, during pregnancy because their use can cause injury and even death to a developing fetus. Additional contraindications to captopril include known hypersensitivity to the drug or occurrence of angioedema with previous treatment with an ACE inhibitor.

Nursing Implications

Preventing Interactions

Many medications interact with captopril, increasing or decreasing its effects (Box 28.3). Additionally, captopril may increase serum concentrations of digoxin and lithium and increase the risk of elevated serum levels and toxicity.

QSEN Safety Alert

Reportedly, salt substitutes, when taken with captopril, increase the risk of hyperkalemia.

Administering the Medication

People should take captopril 1 hour before or 2 hours after meals. If they have difficulty swallowing, they may crush the

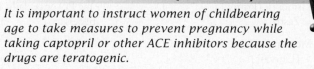

BOX 28.3 Drug Interactions: Captopril

Drugs That Increase the Effects of Captopril
- Aliskiren
  Increases the risk of hypotension, hyperkalemia, and renal impairment
- Allopurinol
  Increases the risk of severe hypersensitivity reactions, agranulocytosis, neutropenia, and serious infections
- Amiloride, cyclosporine, potassium preparations, spironolactone, tizanidine, triamterene
  Increase the risk of hyperkalemia
- Leflunomide
  Increases the risk of hepatic injury

Drugs That Decrease the Effects of Captopril
- Iron
  Decreases bioavailability

tablets. It is necessary to assess blood pressure and pulse on an ongoing basis with initial dosage adjustment and intermittently during therapy.

Assessing for Therapeutic Effects

The nurse monitors response to therapy, looking for a return of blood pressure to target limits without significant adverse effects.

Assessing for Adverse Effects

The nurse observes acute hypotension when captopril is started, to make sure the patient does not have a fluid volume deficit that would worsen the likelihood of hypotension. He or she assesses for a persistent cough. Also, it is important to check serum potassium levels to ensure a decreased risk of hyperkalemia.

Patient Teaching

QSEN Safety Alert

It is important to instruct women of childbearing age to take measures to prevent pregnancy while taking captopril or other ACE inhibitors because the drugs are teratogenic.

Box 28.4 contains additional patient education guidelines for patients taking antihypertensive drugs.

Other Drugs in the Class

Because of their effectiveness in hypertension and beneficial effects on the heart, blood vessels, and kidneys, the ACE inhibitors are increasing in importance and use. Other drugs in the class also are used in the management of hypertension and heart failure because they decrease peripheral vascular resistance, cardiac workload, and ventricular remodeling. Adverse effects for the class are similar to those outlined with captopril: specifically, there is an increased risk of cough, hyperkalemia, and angioedema, and the drugs pose a significant risk to a fetus if taken during pregnancy.

Benazepril (Lotensin) is indicated for the treatment of hypertension. Patients may take the drug alone or in combination with thiazide diuretics. Peak plasma concentrations occur within ½ to 1 hour. Once-a-day dosing means that steady-state concentrations of the drug are reached after two or three doses.

Enalapril (Vasotec) is a prodrug used in the treatment of hypertension and heart failure. Prescribers may order the drug for use alone or in combination with antihypertensive agents, particularly thiazide diuretics.

QSEN Safety Alert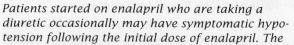

Patients started on enalapril who are taking a diuretic occasionally may have symptomatic hypotension following the initial dose of enalapril. The nurse should advocate for the patient's safety.

Fosinopril (Monopril) is indicated for the treatment of hypertension and heart failure. Patients may take the drug

BOX 28.4   Patient Teaching Guidelines for Antihypertensive Drugs

General Considerations

■ Hypertension is a major risk factor for heart attack, stroke (sometimes called brain attack), and kidney failure. Although it rarely causes symptoms unless complications occur, it can be controlled by appropriate management. Consequently, you need to learn all you can about the disease process, the factors that cause or aggravate it, and its management. In few other conditions is your knowledge and understanding about your condition as important as with hypertension.

■ For many people, lifestyle changes (i.e., a diet to avoid excessive salt and control weight and fat intake; regular exercise; and avoiding smoking) may be sufficient to control blood pressure. If drug therapy is prescribed, these measures should be continued.

■ When drug therapy is needed, your prescriber will try to choose a drug and develop a regimen that works for you. There are numerous antihypertensive drugs and many can be taken once a day, which makes their use more convenient and less disruptive of your usual activities of daily living. You may need several office visits to find the right drug or combination of drugs and the right dosage. Changes in drugs or dosages may also be needed later, especially if you develop other conditions or take other drugs that alter your response to the antihypertensive drugs.

■ Antihypertensive drug therapy is usually long term, may require more than one drug, and may produce side effects. You need to know the brand and generic names of any prescribed drugs and how to take each drug for optimal benefit and minimal adverse effects.

■ Antihypertensive drugs must be taken as prescribed for optimal benefits, even if you do not feel well when a medication is started or when dosage is increased. *No antihypertensive drug should be stopped abruptly. If problems develop, they should be discussed with the health care prescriber.* If treatment is stopped, blood pressure usually increases gradually as the medications are eliminated from the body. However, sometimes blood pressure rapidly increases to pretreatment levels or even higher. With any of these situations, you are at risk of a heart attack or stroke. In addition, stopping one drug of a multidrug regimen may lead to increased adverse effects as well as decreased antihypertensive effectiveness. To avoid these problems, antihypertensive drugs should be tapered in dosage and discontinued gradually, as directed by your health care provider.

■ Blood pressure measurements are the only way you can tell if your medication is working. Thus, you may want to monitor your blood pressure at home, especially when starting drug therapy, changing medications, or changing dosages. If so, a blood pressure machine may be purchased at a medical supply store. Follow instructions regarding use, take your blood pressure approximately the same time(s) each day (e.g., before morning and evening meals), and keep a record to show to your health care provider.

■ People sometimes feel dizzy or faint while taking antihypertensive medications. This usually means your blood pressure drops momentarily and is most likely to occur when you start a medication, increase dosage, or stand up suddenly from a sitting or lying position. This can be prevented or decreased by moving to a standing position slowly, sleeping with the head of the bed elevated, wearing elastic stockings, exercising legs, avoiding prolonged standing, and avoiding hot baths. If episodes still occur, you should sit or lie down to avoid a fall and possible injury.

■ It is very important to keep appointments for laboratory testing and follow-up care.

■ As with all drugs, keep these medications in the original container, tightly closed, and out of reach of children.

Self- or Caregiver Administration

■ Take or give antihypertensive drugs at prescribed time intervals, about the same time each day. For example, take once-daily drugs as close to every 24 hours as you can manage; twice-a-day drugs should be taken every 12 hours. If ordered four times daily, take approximately every 6 hours. Taking doses too close together can increase dizziness, weakness, and other adverse effects. Taking doses too far apart may not control blood pressure adequately and may increase risks of heart attack or stroke.

■ Take oral captopril on an empty stomach; food decreases drug absorption.

■ If you are a sexually active woman, use birth control measures when taking ACE inhibitors.

■ Take most other oral antihypertensive agents with or after food intake to decrease gastric irritation. Candesartan (Atacand), irbesartan (Avapro), losartan (Cozaar), telmisartan (Micardis), and valsartan (Diovan) may be taken with or without food.

■ When taking losartan, take the following precautions:
  ■ Avoid potassium supplements and salt substitutes containing potassium, unless directed by prescriber.
  ■ Use birth control measures if you are a woman and you are sexually active.
  ■ Contact your health care provider immediately if you suspect that you are pregnant.
  ■ Discuss with your prescriber if you are considering breastfeeding.

■ When taking aliskiren, use birth control measures if you are a woman and you are sexually active.

■ When taking ACE inhibitors, ARBs, and aliskiren, immediately report hypersensitivity reactions, especially lip or eyelid swelling, throat tightness, and difficulty breathing.

■ Avoid taking aliskiren with a high-fat meal because this significantly decreases the amount of available drug.

■ With prazosin, doxazosin, or terazosin, take the first dose and the first increased dose at bedtime to prevent dizziness and possible fainting.

■ With the clonidine skin patch, apply to a hairless area on the upper arm or torso once every 7 days. Rotate sites.

alone or in combination with thiazide diuretics. As with enalapril, symptomatic hypotension may occur following the initial dose if the patient has been taking a diuretic. A prodrug, fosinopril is absorbed very slowly after oral administration and is highly bound to protein. Time to peak concentration is about 3 hours.

Lisinopril (Prinivil, Zestril) is indicated for the treatment of hypertension and heart failure, and the drug is adjunctive therapy in the management of MI. Prescribers may order it as monotherapy or in combination with thiazide diuretics. Peak serum concentrations of lisinopril occur within about 7 hours. The drug does not undergo metabolism and is excreted unchanged entirely in the urine.

Moexipril (Univasc), which is administered orally and intravenously, is used in the treatment of hypertension. People make take the drug alone or in combination with thiazide diuretics. Peak serum concentrations occur within about ½ hours. However, absorption is significantly delayed in the presence of food, and it is important to take the drug in a fasting state. In patients who are currently taking a diuretic, symptomatic hypotension may occasionally occur following the initial dose of moexipril. The nurse should advocate for the patient's safety.

Quinapril (Accupril) may be used as monotherapy or in combination with thiazide diuretics in the treatment of hypertension or heart failure. The blood pressure–lowering effect is greater in combination than that seen with either quinapril or the thiazide diuretic alone. Following oral administration, peak concentrations are reached within 1 hour; absorption is decreased with administration with a fatty meal. The drug is highly protein bound and is primarily excreted in the urine.

Ramipril (Altace) is used alone or in combination with other medications, including thiazide diuretics, in the treatment of hypertension. It is also used to reduce the risk of heart attack and stroke in at-risk patients as well as to improve survival in patients with heart failure after a heart attack. After oral administration, peak concentration is reached in 1 hour.

Trandolapril (Mavik) is indicated for the treatment of hypertension alone or in combination with other antihypertensive agents such as hydrochlorothiazide. It is also used post-MI in patients who demonstrate left ventricular systolic dysfunction or in those who are symptomatic from heart failure immediately following an MI. The majority of drug is excreted in the stool, and the remainder is excreted in the urine. The extent of biliary excretion has not been determined.

NCLEX Success

1. In administering a newly initiated order for captopril, an ACE inhibitor, discharge instructions should indicate that which of the following adverse effects is most common?
   A. tinnitus
   B. dry, nonproductive, persistent cough
   C. muscle weakness
   D. constipation

2. Which of the following is indicated for initial drug therapy in a patient newly diagnosed with uncomplicated hypertension (stage 1)?
   A. calcium channel blocker
   B. potassium-sparing diuretic
   C. direct-acting vasodilator
   D. thiazide diuretic

3. A patient being treated with an ACE inhibitor could take which of the following drugs? (Check all that apply.)
   A. diuretics
   B. beta-adrenergic blockers
   C. calcium
   D. potassium

Angiotensin II Receptor Blockers

Scientists developed ARBs to block the strong blood pressure–raising effects of angiotensin II. These drugs resemble ACE inhibitors in their effects on blood pressure and hemodynamics and are as effective in the management of hypertension and possibly heart failure. However, they are less likely to cause hyperkalemia than ACE inhibitors, and the occurrence of a persistent cough is rare. The prototype ARB is Ⓟ **losartan** (Cozaar), the first ARB.

Pharmacokinetics

Both losartan and its metabolite are highly bound to plasma albumin, and the drug's active metabolite is 40 times more potent than losartan and largely responsible for the duration of action. The drug undergoes extensive first-pass metabolism, has an onset of 6 hours, and reaches maximum concentrations 1 to 2 hours. Absorption is good. Metabolism is rapid; the cytochrome P450 liver enzymes process losartan to an active metabolite. Excretion is through the kidneys and the liver.

Action

Instead of decreasing production of angiotensin II, like the ACE inhibitors, losartan blocks vasoconstricting and aldosterone-secreting effects of angiotensin II at various receptor sites and prevents angiotensin II from combining at various receptors sites. The drug also increases renal flow and enhances the excretion of chloride, calcium, magnesium, and phosphate.

Although multiple types of receptors have been identified, the angiotensin II receptors, type 1 (AT1) located in brain, renal, myocardial, vascular, and adrenal tissue determine most of the effects of angiotensin II on cardiovascular and renal functions. ARBs block the AT1 receptors and decrease arterial blood pressure by decreasing systemic vascular resistance (see Fig. 28.1).

Use

Prescribers primarily order losartan for use in the treatment of hypertension; the drug is effective in people with type 2 diabetes who have diabetic nephropathy. After drug therapy begins, maximal effects usually occur within 3 to 6 weeks. It is important to recognize that in African Americans, losartan and other ARBs may be ineffective when used alone. If losartan alone does not control blood pressure, a low dose of a diuretic may be added. A combination product of losartan and hydrochlorothiazide is available.

Table 28.4 presents route and dosage information for losartan and other ARBs.

Use in Older Adults

Losartan and other ARBs are metabolized by the liver and do not need dose reduction for adults with renal impairment. Use is not recommended in children who have a glomerular filtration rate less than 30 mL/min/1.73 m².

Use in Patients With Hepatic Impairment

Caution is warranted for use of all ARBs in biliary tract obstruction or hepatic impairment. Experts recommend a lower starting dose for losartan in affected patients because plasma concentrations of the drug and its active metabolite are increased and clearance is decreased approximately 50% with hepatic dysfunction.

Use in Patients With Critical Illness

Health care providers may administer losartan to critically ill patients, but monitoring is necessary to ensure that the drug produces the desired outcome without significant adverse effects. Also, it has significant drug–drug interactions and the potential to produce hyperkalemia.

Adverse Effects

Overall, losartan is generally well tolerated. Adverse effects include dizziness, muscle cramps or weakness, heartburn,

---

TABLE 28.4

DRUGS AT A GLANCE: Angiotensin II Receptor Blockers

Drug	Pregnancy Category	Routes and Dosage Ranges	
		Adults	Children 1–17 Y of Age (unless otherwise stated)
Ⓟ **Losartan** (Cozaar)	C, first trimester; D, second and third trimesters	Initial dose, 50 mg PO once daily initially (25 mg for those who have hepatic impairment or are taking a diuretic) Maintenance dose, PO 35–100 mg daily, in 1 or 2 doses, adjusted according to blood pressure control	≥6 y, 0.7 mg/kg PO once daily; maximum dose 50 mg daily
Candesartan (Atacand)	D	16 mg PO once daily initially, increased if necessary to a maximum of 32 mg daily, in 1 or 2 doses	1–<6 y, 0.05 to 0.4 mg/kg PO per day 6–<17 y of age <50 kg, 2–16 mg/d PO >50 kg, 4–32 mg/d PO
Irbesartan (Avapro)	C, first trimester; D, second and third trimesters	150 mg PO once daily initially, increased up to 300 mg, if necessary	6–16 y: 75 mg PO once daily; maximum dose 150 mg
Olmesartan (Benicar)	C, first trimester; D, second and third trimesters	20 mg PO once daily initially, increased to 40 mg after 2 wk	6–16 y 20–<35 kg, 10 mg PO once daily; maximum dose 20 mg/d >35 kg, 20 mg PO once daily; maximum dose 40 mg/d
Telmisartan (Micardis)	C, first trimester; D, second and third trimesters	40 mg PO once daily initially, increased to maximum of 80 mg daily if necessary	Safety and effectiveness in children have not been established
Valsartan (Diovan)	D	80 mg PO once daily initially, when used as monotherapy in patients who are not volume depleted; maintenance dose may be increased; however, adding a diuretic is more effective than increasing dose beyond 80 mg	6–16 y, 1.3 mg/kg PO once daily initially up to 40 mg; increase to a maximum of up to 2.7 mg/kg (up to 160 mg) once daily

diarrhea, and decreased sensitivity to touch. There are reports of angioedema, and it is important to evaluate this condition immediately.

Contraindications

Contraindications to losartan include known hypersensitivity to the drug. Additionally, the FDA has issued a **BLACK BOX WARNING** ◆ regarding the use of losartan and other ARBs, which directly affect the renin–angiotensin system, because their use can cause injury and even death to a developing fetus. Therefore, pregnancy is a contraindication to use of losartan and other ARBs, and it is essential that the drugs be discontinued as soon as pregnancy is detected.

Nursing Implications

Preventing Interactions

Many medications and herbs interact with losartan, increasing or decreasing its effects (Boxes 28.5 and 28.6).

Administering the Medication

People may take losartan without regard to meals.

Assessing for Therapeutic Effects

The nurse monitors blood pressure to evaluate drug efficacy. Also, he or she observes for the presence of lifestyle modifications that will improve baseline blood pressure readings (e.g., losing weight, stopping smoking, restricting salt intake).

BOX 28.6 **Herb and Dietary Interactions: Losartan**

Herbs and Foods That Increase the Effects of Losartan

- Alfalfa
- Aloe
- American ginseng
- Bitter melon
- Black cohosh
- California poppy
- Celery
- Coleus
- Garlic
- Ginger
- Goldenseal
- Hawthorn
- Marshmallow
- Mistletoe
- Quinine
- Shepherd's purse
- St. John's wort

Herbs and Foods That Decrease the Effects of Losartan

- American ginseng
- Bayberry
- Blue cohosh
- Grapefruit juice
- Kola
- Licorice

BOX 28.5 **Drug Interactions: Losartan**

Drugs That Increase the Effects of Losartan

- Alcohol, antihypertensive agents, diuretics
  Increase the risk of hypotension
- Aliskiren
  Increases the risk of hypotension, hyperkalemia, and renal impairment
- Fluconazole
  Increases the risk of hypotension through inhibited metabolism

Drugs That Decrease the Effects of Losartan

- CYP2C9 inducers (e.g., rifampicin, secobarbital), CYP3A4 inducers (e.g., indinavir, clarithromycin) methylphenidate, nonsteroidal anti-inflammatory drugs, peginterferon alfa-2B, yohimbine
  Decrease serum levels
- Indomethacin
  Decreases antihypertensive effects
- Phenobarbital, rifamycins
  Increase metabolism and decrease antihypertensive effects

CYP, cytochrome P450.

Assessing for Adverse Effects

The nurse assesses kidney and liver function tests, as well as serum electrolyte levels, particularly potassium. Also, he or she observes for the presence of angioedema and other hypersensitivity reactions.

Patient Teaching

Box 28.4 contains patient education guidelines for the antihypertensive drugs.

Other Drugs in the Class

Candesartan (Atacand) is used alone or in combination with other drugs to treat hypertension and heart failure. It is available in a fixed combination with hydrochlorothiazide (Avalide). The drug is highly protein bound, crosses the blood–brain barrier poorly, and is excreted in breast milk. After oral administration, the peak serum concentration is reached in about 3 to 4 hours. Food with a high fat content does not affect the bioavailability of candesartan. A portion of the drug is excreted unchanged in the urine, with the remainder excreted in stool. The adverse-effect profile is similar to losartan. Candesartan is slightly more effective in reducing blood pressure than losartan.

Irbesartan (Avapro) is used as monotherapy or in combination with other drugs to treat hypertension and is used to treat nephropathy in patients with type 2 diabetes. In patients with volume and salt depletions (e.g., those on hemodialysis), a lower initial dose is recommended. Like candesartan, irbesartan is a bit more effective in reducing blood pressure than losartan. The drug can be administered orally or intravenously. An oral preparation is available in a fixed combination with hydrochlorothiazide (Avapro HCT). Absorption of oral irbesartan is rapid, and peak concentrations occur within ½ to 2 hours after dosing. Food does not affect the drug's bioavailability. Excretion of the drug and its metabolites occurs by both the renal and biliary routes.

Olmesartan (Benicar) is used alone or in combination with other drugs to treat hypertension. It is available in a fixed combination with hydrochlorothiazide (Benicar HCT) and with Amlodipine (Azor). Absorption is good, and peak concentrations occur within 1 to 2 hours after dosing. Food does not affect the bioavailability of olmesartan. The drug is highly protein bound and crosses the blood–brain barrier poorly, but it is excreted in breast milk. The drug converts from olmesartan medoxomil to olmesartan during absorption; essentially, there is no further metabolism of olmesartan after conversion. Almost half of the absorbed drug is excreted in the urine. The remainder is excreted in the feces and via the bile.

Telmisartan (Micardis) is used as monotherapy or in combination with other drugs to treat hypertension. It is available in a fixed combination with hydrochlorothiazide (Micardis HCT) and with amlodipine (Twynsta). It is also used in patients 55 years of age or older who are at high risk for developing major cardiovascular events for the risk reduction of death from cardiovascular causes, particularly MI or stroke, and who are unable to take ACE inhibitors.

Administration of telmisartan is intravenous or oral. The drug is highly protein bound and is well absorbed, and peak concentrations occur within ½ to 1 hours after dosing. Food slightly reduces bioavailability. Telmisartan is eliminated unchanged in feces via biliary excretion, and minute amounts are found in urine.

Valsartan (Diovan) is used as monotherapy or in combination with other drugs to treat hypertension. It is available in four fixed combination: with hydrochlorothiazide (Diovan HCT), with amlodipine (Exforge), with amlodipine and hydrochlorothiazide (Exforge HCT), and with aliskiren (Valturna). The drug is available in oral (tablet and suspension) and intravenous forms. Following oral administration, peak plasma levels occur in 2 to 4 hours. With the tablet, food decreases the bioavailability and the peak plasma level. The suspension has a bioavailability about ½ times more than the tablet. The drug is excreted primarily in the feces, with a small portion in the urine. Valsartan is excreted primarily as unchanged drug, with only 1/5 of the dose recovered as metabolites.

Adjuvant Medications Used to Treat Hypertension

Prescribers may order other drugs for the treatment of hypertension. Table 28.5 presents route and dosage information for these drugs.

Direct Renin Inhibitor

Ⓟ Aliskiren (Tekturna), the only direct renin inhibitor, decreases plasma renin activity and inhibits the conversion of angiotensinogen to angiotensin I. The drug is used as monotherapy or in combination with other antihypertensive agents for the treatment of hypertension. A fixed-dose combination with valsartan (Valturna) is available. Aliskiren is poorly absorbed, and steady-state blood levels are reached in about a week. Following oral administration, peak plasma levels are reached in 1 to 3 hours. If taken with a high-fat meal, bioavailability and peak levels are decreased by about 75%. The drug is excreted in the urine. Aliskiren is contraindicated in patients with diabetes who are taking an ACE inhibitor or an ARB because of the increased risk of renal impairment, hyperkalemia, and hypotension. Angioedema may occur.

NCLEX Success

4. Which of the following drug classes are absolutely contraindicated for use in pregnant women? (Check all that apply.)
   A. ARBs
   B. calcium channel blockers
   C. direct renin inhibitors
   D. ACE inhibitors

5. Orthostatic hypotension is a potential outcome of hypertensive drugs that places the elderly at risk for injury from falls. Instructions given to the patient to decrease this effect include which of the following? (Check all that apply.)
   A. Take the dose at bedtime.
   B. Change position slowly when rising from bed or chair.
   C. Increase fluid intake by 500 mL per day.
   D. Decrease the dose until symptoms disappear.

6. Single-drug therapy with an ARB would be least effective in which of the following?
   A. children
   B. older adults
   C. hispanic people
   D. African American people

Antiadrenergics

Antiadrenergic (sympatholytic) drugs inhibit activity of the SNS. When the SNS is stimulated, the nerve impulse travels from the brain and spinal cord to the ganglia. From the ganglia, the impulse travels along postganglionic fibers to effector organs (e.g., heart, blood vessels). Although SNS stimulation produces widespread effects in the body, the effects relevant to this discussion are the increases in heart rate, force of myocardial contraction, cardiac output, and blood pressure that occur. When the nerve impulse is inhibited or blocked at any location along its pathway, the result is decreased blood pressure.

TABLE 28.5

Adjunct Medications Used for the Treatment of Hypertension

Drug	Pregnancy Category	Routes and Dosage Ranges — Adults	Routes and Dosage Ranges — Children 1–17 Y of Age (unless otherwise stated)
Direct Renin Inhibitor			
℗ **Aliskiren** (Tekturna)	D	150 mg PO once daily	Safety and effectiveness have not been established
Antiadrenergics *Alpha₁-Adrenergic Blockers*			
Doxazosin (Cardura)	C	1 mg PO once daily initially, increased to 2 mg, then to 4, 8, and 16 mg daily if necessary	Safety and effectiveness have not been established
Prazosin (Minipress)	C	1 mg PO 2–3 times daily initially, increased if necessary to 20 mg in divided doses; average maintenance dose, 6–15 mg daily	Safety and effectiveness have not been established
Terazosin (Hytrin)	C	1 mg PO at bedtime initially, may be increased gradually; usual maintenance dose, 1–5 mg once daily	Safety and effectiveness have not been established
Alpha₂ Agonists Clonidine (Catapres)	C	0.1 mg PO 2 times daily initially, gradually increased up to 2.4 mg daily, if necessary; average maintenance dose, 0.2–0.8 mg daily	5–25 mcg/kg/d PO, in divided doses, every 6 h; increase at 5–7-d intervals, if needed
Guanfacine (Tenex)	B	1 mg PO daily at bedtime, increased to 2 mg after 3–4 wk, then to 3 mg if necessary	≥12 y, 1 mg daily PO initially: maximum dose 2 mg daily
Methyldopa (Aldomet)	B	250 mg PO 2 or 3 times daily initially, increased gradually until blood pressure is controlled or a daily dose of 3 g is reached	10 mg/kg/d PO in 2–4 divided doses initially, increased or decreased according to response; maximum dose 65 mg/kg/d or 3 g daily, whichever is less
Beta-Adrenergic Blockers Acebutolol (Sectral)	B	400 mg PO once daily initially, increased to 800 mg daily if necessary	Safety and effectiveness have not been established
Atenolol (Tenormin)	D	50 mg PO once daily initially, increased in 1–2 wk to 100 mg once daily, if necessary	0.5–1 mg/kg/d PO in one or two doses; maximum dose 2 mg/kg up to 100 mg daily in one or two doses
Bisoprolol (Zebeta)	C	5 mg PO once daily, increased to a maximum of 20 mg daily if necessary	10 mg PO in a fixed combination with hydrochlorothiazide 6.25 mg daily
Metoprolol (Lopressor)	C	50 mg PO twice daily, gradually increased in weekly or longer intervals if necessary; maximum dose 450 mg daily	Immediate-release (PO), 1–2 mg/kg/d in two doses; maximum dose 6 mg/kg/d not to exceed 200 mg/d Sustained-release (PO), 1 mg/kg once daily not to exceed 50 mg/d; maximum dose not to exceed 200 mg/d

TABLE 28.5

Adjunct Medications Used for the Treatment of Hypertension (Continued)

Drug	Pregnancy Category	Routes and Dosage Ranges	
		Adults	Children 1–17 Y of Age (unless otherwise stated)
Nadolol (Corgard)	C	40 mg PO once daily initially, gradually increased if necessary; average dose, 80–320 mg daily	Safety and effectiveness have not been established
Pindolol (Visken)	B	5 mg PO 2 or 3 times daily initially, increased by 10 mg/d at 3–4-wk intervals to a maximum of 60 mg daily	Safety and effectiveness have not been established
Propranolol (Inderal)	C	40 mg PO twice daily initially, gradually increased to 160–640 mg daily	1 mg/kg/d PO initially, gradually increased to a maximum of 10 mg/kg/d
Timolol (Blocadren)	C	10 mg PO twice daily initially, increased gradually if necessary; average daily dose, 20–40 mg; maximum daily dose, 60 mg	Safety and effectiveness have not been established

Alpha–Beta-Adrenergic Blockers

Drug	Pregnancy Category	Adults	Children 1–17 Y of Age (unless otherwise stated)
Carvedilol (Coreg)	C	6.25 mg PO twice daily for 7–14 d, then increase to 12.5 mg twice daily for 7–14 d, then increase to a maximum dose of 25 mg twice daily if tolerated and needed	Not approved for children less than 18 y
Labetalol (Trandate, Normodyne)	C	100 mg PO twice daily, increased by 100 mg twice daily every 2–3 d if necessary; usual maintenance dose, 200–400 mg twice daily; severe hypertension may require 1200–2400 mg daily IV injection, 20 mg slowly over 2 min, followed by 40–80 mg every 10 min until the desired blood pressure is achieved or 300 mg has been given IV infusion, mix with IV fluids and infuse at a rate of 2 mg/min.	1–3 mg/kg PO daily initially twice daily; increase up to a maximum of 10–12 mg/kg or 1200 mg daily

Calcium Channel Blockers

Drug	Pregnancy Category	Adults	Children 1–17 Y of Age (unless otherwise stated)
Amlodipine (Norvasc)	C	5–10 mg PO once daily	≥6 y, 2.5–5 mg PO once daily
Diltiazem (sustained release) (Cardizem SR)	C	60–120 mg PO twice daily	Safety and effectiveness have not been established
Felodipine (Plendil)	C	5–10 mg PO once daily	Maximum 10 mg PO daily
Isradipine (DynaCirc)	C	2.5–5 mg PO twice daily	Immediate-release (PO), 0.25–0.2 mg/kg daily in 3–4 doses initially; maximum dose 0.8 mg/kg up to 20 mg daily Sustained-release (PO), 0.15–0.2 mg/kg daily in two divided doses initially; maximum dose 0.8 mg/kg up to 20 mg daily

(Continued on page 530)

TABLE 28.5

Adjunct Medications Used for the Treatment of Hypertension (Continued)

Drug	Pregnancy Category	Routes and Dosage Ranges	
		Adults	**Children 1–17 Y of Age (unless otherwise stated)**
Nicardipine (Cardene, Cardene SR, Cardene IV)	C	20–40 mg PO three times daily; sustained-release (PO), 30–60 mg twice daily IV infusion, 5–15 mg/h	1–3 mcg/kg/min as IV infusion for rapid reduction of blood pressure
Nifedipine (Adalat, Procardia, Procardia XL)	C	Sustained-release (PO) only, 30–60 mg once daily, increased over 1–2 wk if necessary	Sustained-release (PO), 0.25–0.5 mg/kg/d in 1–2 doses; maximum dose 3 mg/kg in 1–2 doses up to 120 mg
Nisoldipine (Sular)	C	20 mg PO once daily initially, increased by 10 mg/wk or longer intervals to a maximum of 60 mg daily; average maintenance dose, 20–40 mg daily Adults with liver impairment or >65 y, 10 mg PO once daily initially	Safety and effectiveness have not been established
Verapamil (Calan, Calan SR, Isoptin SR)	C	Immediate-release (PO), 80 mg 3 times daily Sustained-release (PO), 240 mg once daily IV, see manufacturer's instructions	IV, see manufacturer's instructions
Diuretics			
Hydrochlorothiazide (Esidrix, Oretic)	B	Hypertension: 12.5–50 mg PO 1 or 2 times daily Elderly, 12.5–25 PO mg/d	2 mg/kg/d PO in two divided doses Infants <6 mo, 2–3 mg/kg/d in 2 divided doses
Chlorothiazide (Diuril)	C	500–2000 mg/d PO divided in 1–2 times doses Elderly, 500 mg PO once daily or 1 g 3 times/wk 250–1000 mg IV once or twice daily; maximum dose 1000 mg	22 mg/kg/d PO in 2 divided doses Infants <6 mo, 20–40 mg/kg/d in 2 divided doses; maximum dose 375 mg/d IV dosing not well established
Chlorthalidone (Hygroton, Thalitone)	C	25–100 mg/d PO Elderly, 12.5–25 PO mg/d or every other day	Not approved in children
Indapamide (Lozol)	B	Hypertension: 1.25 mg PO in morning may increase to 5 mg/d	Dosage not established
Furosemide (Lasix)	C	Hypertension: 40 mg PO twice daily, gradually increased if necessary Hypertensive crisis: 40–80 mg IV injected over 1–2 min; with renal failure, much larger doses may be needed PO, IV 5–20 mg once daily	2 mg/kg PO 1 or 2 times daily initially, gradually increased by increments of 1–2 mg/kg per dose if necessary at intervals of 6–8 h; maximum daily dose 6 mg/kg 1 mg/kg IV initially; if diuretic response is not adequate, increase dosage by 1 mg/kg no sooner than 2 h after previous dose; maximum dose 6 mg/kg
Spironolactone (Aldactone)	C; D in pregnancy-induced hypertension	25–200 mg PO daily	Safety and effectiveness not established

TABLE 28.5

Adjunct Medications Used for the Treatment of Hypertension (Continued)

Drug	Pregnancy Category	Routes and Dosage Ranges Adults	Children 1–17 Y of Age (unless otherwise stated)
Amiloride (Midamor)	B	5–20 mg PO daily	Dosage not established
Triamterene (Dyrenium)	C	100–300 mg PO daily in divided doses	2–4 mg/kg/d PO in divided doses
Other Vasodilators (Direct Acting)			
Fenoldopam (Corlopam)	B	Infusion, IV, initial dose based on body weight, then flow rate titrated to achieve desired response; mix with 0.9% sodium chloride or 5% dextrose to a concentration of 40 mcg/mL (e.g., 40 mg of drug [4 mL of concentrate] in 1000 mL of IV fluid).	Infusion, IV, initial dose based on body weight (0.2 mcg/kg/min), then flow rate titrated to achieve desired response; may increase dosage every 20–30 min by up to 0.3–0.5 mcg/kg/min; maximum dose 0.8 mcg/kg/min
Hydralazine (Apresoline)	C	Chronic hypertension: 10 mg PO 4 times daily for 2–4 d, gradually increased up to 300 mg/d, if necessary Hypertensive crisis: 10–20 mg IM, IV, increased to 40 mg if necessary; repeat dose as needed	Chronic hypertension: 0.75 mg/kg/d PO initially in 4 divided doses; gradually increase over 3–4 wk to a maximum dose of 7.5 mg/kg/d if necessary Hypertensive crisis: 0.1–0.2 IM, IV mg/kg every 4–6 h as needed
Minoxidil (Loniten)	C	5 mg PO once daily initially, increased gradually until blood pressure is controlled; average daily dose, 10–40 mg; maximum daily dose, 100 mg in single or divided doses	<12 y, 0.2 mg/kg/d PO initially as a single dose, increased gradually until blood pressure is controlled; average daily dose, 0.25–1.0 mg/kg; maximum dose 50 mg/d
Sodium nitroprusside (Nitropress)	C	Infusion, IV, 0.5–10 mcg/kg/min; average dose, 3 mcg/kg/min; prepare solution by adding 50 mg of sodium nitroprusside to 250–1000 mL of 5% dextrose in water and cover promptly to protect from light	Same as adult

Alpha₁-adrenergic receptor blockers (e.g., prazosin) dilate blood vessels and decrease peripheral vascular resistance. These drugs can be used alone or in multidrug regimens. One adverse effect, called the **first-dose phenomenon**, results in orthostatic hypotension, with palpitations, dizziness, and perhaps syncope 1 to 3 hours after the first dose or an increased dose. To prevent this effect, first doses and first increased doses are taken at bedtime. Another effect, associated with long-term use or higher doses, leads to sodium and fluid retention and a need for concurrent diuretic therapy. Centrally acting sympatholytics (e.g., clonidine) stimulate presynaptic alpha₂ receptors in the brain and are classified as alpha₂ receptor agonists. Taking these drugs leads to the release of less norepinephrine and a reduction of sympathetic outflow from the vasomotor center. Stimulation of presynaptic alpha₂ receptors peripherally may also contribute

to the decreased sympathetic activity. Reduced sympathetic activity leads to decreased cardiac output, heart rate, peripheral vascular resistance, and blood pressure. Chronic use of clonidine and related drugs may result in sodium and fluid retention, especially with higher doses.

Beta-adrenergic blockers are the drugs of first choice for patients younger than 50 years of age with high-renin hypertension, tachycardia, angina pectoris, MI, or left ventricular hypertrophy. Most beta blockers have FDA approval for use in hypertension and are probably equally effective. However, the cardioselective drugs (see Chap. 26) are preferred for people with hypertension who also have asthma, peripheral vascular disease, or diabetes mellitus. Research studies demonstrate reduced morbidity and mortality with diuretics and beta blockers used in combination, especially after an MI.

Beta-adrenergic blockers (e.g., propranolol) decrease heart rate, force of myocardial contraction, cardiac output, and renin release from the kidneys. The FDA has issued a **BLACK BOX WARNING** ◆ for patients with CAD taking oral forms of atenolol, metoprolol, nadolol, propranolol, and timolol; abrupt withdrawal has resulted in exacerbation of angina, the incidence of ventricular dysrhythmias, and the occurrence of MIs. Beta blockers that normally undergo extensive first-pass hepatic metabolism (e.g., acebutolol, metoprolol, propranolol, timolol) may produce excessive blood levels in patients with cirrhosis because the blood containing the drug is shunted around the liver into the systemic circulation. It is necessary to start at a low dose and titrate the dosage carefully. Also, dosage reduction with bisoprolol and pindolol is important in patients with cirrhosis or other hepatic impairment.

Labetalol can be used as monotherapy for initial management of uncomplicated hypertension; however, thiazide diuretics are preferred by JNC 7. Administration is intravenous or oral. Occasionally following intravenous administration, orthostatic hypotension with loss of consciousness reportedly occurs; the hypotension can last for 3 hours or longer.

Other antiadrenergics include alpha blockers (phentolamine and phenoxybenzamine), which occasionally are used in hypertension resulting from catecholamine excess.

Calcium Channel Blockers

Calcium channel blockers may be used for monotherapy or in combination with other drugs. They may be especially useful for people with hypertension who also have angina pectoris or other cardiovascular disorders. The JNC 7 recommends that calcium channel blockers be considered the drug of first choice in African Americans with stage 2 hypertension. Note that sustained-release forms of nifedipine, diltiazem, verapamil, and other long-acting drugs (e.g., amlodipine, felodipine) are recommended rather than the short-acting forms because they do not cause precipitous lowering of pressure.

Calcium channel blockers (e.g., verapamil) are used for several cardiovascular disorders. Chapters 25 and 26, respectively, discuss the mechanism of action and use in the management of tachydysrhythmias and angina pectoris. In hypertension, the drugs mainly dilate peripheral arteries and decrease peripheral vascular resistance by relaxing vascular smooth muscle. As a group, the calcium channel blockers are well absorbed from the gastrointestinal tract following oral administration and are highly bound to protein. The drugs are metabolized in the liver and excreted in the urine.

Most of the available calcium channel blockers have received FDA approval for use in hypertension. Nifedipine, a short-acting calcium channel blocker, has been used to treat hypertensive emergencies or urgencies, often by puncturing the capsule and squeezing the contents under the tongue or having the patient bite and swallow the capsule.

QSEN Safety Alert ❗

Authorities no longer recommend puncturing a nifedipine capsule, because it is associated with an increased risk of adverse cardiovascular events precipitated by a rapid and severe decrease in blood pressure.

Diuretics

For mild to moderate hypertension, diuretics are often first-line drugs. In many cases of hypertension, diuretics alone may lower blood pressure. When diuretic therapy begins, blood volume and cardiac output decrease. After long-term administration, cardiac output returns to normal, but there is a persistent decrease in peripheral vascular resistance. Authorities have attributed this result to a persistent small reduction in extracellular water and plasma volume, decreased receptor sensitivity to vasopressor substances such as angiotensin, direct arteriolar vasodilation, and arteriolar vasodilation secondary to electrolyte depletion in the vessel wall. In moderate or severe hypertension that does not respond to a diuretic alone, it is necessary to continue the diuretic and add another antihypertensive drug or try monotherapy with a different type of antihypertensive drug. Health care providers prefer diuretics for initial therapy in all people with hypertension, but specifically in older adults and African American patients. They should be included in any multidrug regimen for these and other populations.

Thiazide and related diuretics are equally effective. Hydrochlorothiazide is most commonly used. Diazoxide, usually in parenteral form, is indicated for short-term treatment of malignant hypertension. The selective aldosterone blocker, eplerenone, has demonstrated efficacy in African Americans.

Loop diuretics (e.g., furosemide) or potassium-sparing diuretics (e.g., spironolactone) may be useful in some circumstances. Loop diuretics are indicated in people with renal insufficiency. Potassium-sparing diuretics may precipitate hyperkalemia. Chapter 32 discusses diuretics.

Other Vasodilators (Direct Acting)

Vasodilator antihypertensive drugs directly relax smooth muscle in blood vessels, resulting in dilation and decreased peripheral vascular resistance. As they reduce afterload, they may be used in management of heart failure. The direct-acting vasodilators are effective in managing a hypertensive emergency.

Nitroprusside (Nitropress) is a potent vasodilator that acts on arterioles and venules. Given by continuous IV infusion, the drug has a rapid onset and short duration of action, and it requires continuous blood pressure monitoring. Intraarterial blood pressure monitoring is the most effective during the infusion. Nitroprusside is metabolized to thiocyanate, and it is necessary to measure serum thiocyanate levels if the drug is given longer than 72 hours. If the serum thiocyanate level is more than 12 mg per dL, it is important to stop the infusion after 72 hours. The infusion should last no longer than 48 hours in patients with renal impairment. Hemodialysis reverses the symptoms of thiocyanate toxicity (e.g., nausea, vomiting, muscle twitching or spasm, seizures).

Fenoldopam (Plendil) is a fast-acting drug indicated only for short-term use (less than 48 hours) in hospitalized patients. Dosage is calculated according to body weight and desired effects on blood pressure. Administration is by an infusion pump, with frequent monitoring of blood pressure.

Hydralazine (Apresoline) and minoxidil act mainly on arterioles. These drugs have a limited effect on hypertension when used alone because the vasodilating action that lowers blood pressure also stimulates the SNS and triggers reflexive compensatory mechanisms (vasoconstriction, tachycardia, and increased cardiac output), which raise blood pressure. It is possible to prevent this effect during long-term therapy by also giving a drug that inhibits excessive sympathetic stimulation (e.g., propranolol, an adrenergic blocker). These drugs also cause sodium and water retention, which may be minimized by concomitant diuretic therapy. The FDA has issued a **BLACK BOX WARNING** ◆ for minoxidil because the drug can exacerbate angina and precipitate pericardial effusion (which can progress to cardiac tamponade).

Clinical Application 28-1

- Mr. Caudill states that he does not understand why he needs an additional medication considering his blood pressure is below 140 mm Hg systolic. How should the nurse respond?

NCLEX Success

7. A patient with a history of hypertension comes to the emergency department with double vision and a blood pressure of 240/120 mm Hg. The physician on call orders sodium nitroprusside (Nitropress) by continuous infusion, with continual blood pressure monitoring. This drug's immediate action is to lower blood pressure by which of the following mechanisms?

   A. increasing peripheral vascular resistance
   B. increasing cardiac output
   C. dilating venous and arterial vessels
   D. decreasing heart rate

8. A patient in the intensive care unit has been receiving sodium nitroprusside for 2 days. The nurse needs to monitor for which of the following?

   A. thiocyanate toxicity
   B. hyperglycemia
   C. hyperkalemia
   D. metabolic alkalosis

The Nursing Process

Assessment

- Identify conditions and risk factors that may lead to hypertension. These include
  - Obesity
  - Elevated serum cholesterol (total and low-density lipoprotein) and triglycerides
  - Cigarette smoking
  - Sedentary lifestyle

- Family history of hypertension or other cardiovascular disease
- African American race
- Renal disease (e.g., renal artery stenosis)
- Adrenal disease (e.g., hypersecretion of aldosterone, pheochromocytoma)
- Other cardiovascular disorders (e.g., atherosclerosis, left ventricular hypertrophy)
- Diabetes mellitus
- Use of oral contraceptives, corticosteroids, appetite suppressants, nasal decongestants, nonsteroidal anti-inflammatory agents
- Neurologic disorders (e.g., brain damage)
- Observe for signs and symptoms of hypertension.
  - Check blood pressure accurately and repeatedly. As a rule, multiple measurements in which systolic pressure is greater than 140 mm Hg, and/or diastolic pressure is greater than 90 mm Hg, are necessary to establish a diagnosis of hypertension.

    The importance of accurate blood pressure measurements cannot be overemphasized because there are many possibilities for errors. Some ways to improve accuracy and validity include using correct equipment (e.g., proper cuff size), having the patient rested and in the same position each time blood pressure is measured (e.g., sitting or supine with arm at heart level), and using the same arm for repeated measurements.
  - In most cases of early hypertension, elevated blood pressure is the only clinical manifestation. If symptoms do occur, they are usually nonspecific (e.g., headache, weakness, fatigue, tachycardia, dizziness, palpitations, epistaxis).
  - Eventually, signs and symptoms occur as target organs are damaged. Heart damage is often evidenced as angina pectoris, MI, or heart failure. Chest pain, tachycardia, dyspnea, fatigue, and edema may occur. Brain damage may be indicated by transient ischemic attacks or strokes of varying severity, with symptoms ranging from syncope to hemiparesis. Renal damage may be reflected by proteinuria, increased blood urea nitrogen, and increased serum creatinine. Ophthalmoscopic examination may reveal hemorrhages, sclerosis of arterioles, and inflammation of the optic nerve (papilledema). Because arterioles can be visualized in the retina of the eye, damage to retinal vessels may indicate damage to arterioles in the heart, brain, and kidneys.

Nursing Diagnoses

- Decreased cardiac output related to disease process or drug therapy
- Potential for ineffective self-health management related to long-term lifestyle changes and drug therapy
- Noncompliance related to lack of knowledge about hypertension and its management, costs and adverse effects of drug therapy, and psychosocial factors
- Disturbed body image related to the need for long-term management and medical supervision

- Fatigue related to antihypertensive drug therapy
- Deficient knowledge related to hypertension, antihypertensive drug therapy, and nondrug lifestyle changes
- Sexual dysfunction related to adverse drug effects

Planning/Goals

The patient will

- Receive or take antihypertensive drugs correctly
- Be monitored closely for therapeutic and adverse drug effects, especially when drug therapy is started, when changes are made in choice of drugs, and when dosages are increased or decreased
- Use nondrug measures to assist in blood pressure control
- Avoid, manage, or report adverse drug reactions
- Verbalize or demonstrate knowledge of prescribed drugs and recommended lifestyle changes
- Keep follow-up appointments

Nursing Interventions

The nurse will

- Implement measures to prevent or minimize hypertension. Preventive measures are mainly lifestyle changes to reduce risk factors. These measures should be started in childhood and continued throughout life. After hypertension is diagnosed, lifetime adherence to a therapeutic regimen may be necessary to control the disease and prevent complications. The nurse's role is important in the prevention, early detection, and management of hypertension. Some guidelines for intervention at community, family, and personal levels include the following:
  - Participate in programs to promote healthful lifestyles (e.g., improving eating habits, increasing exercise, managing stress more effectively, avoiding cigarette smoking).
  - Participate in community screening programs and make appropriate referrals when abnormal blood pressures are detected. If hypertension develops in women taking oral contraceptives, the drug should be discontinued for 3 to 6 months to see whether blood pressure decreases without antihypertensive drugs.
  - Help the patient with hypertension adhere to prescribed therapy (see Box 28.4). Nonadherence is high in patients with hypertension. Reasons given for non-

adherence include lack of symptoms; lack of motivation and self-discipline to make needed lifestyle changes (e.g., lose weight, stop smoking, restrict salt intake); perhaps experiencing more symptoms from medications than from hypertension; the cost of therapy; and the patient's failure to realize the importance of effective management, especially as related to prevention of major cardiovascular diseases (MI, stroke, and death). In addition, several studies have shown that adherence decreases as the number of drugs and number of doses increase.

The nurse can help increase adherence by teaching the patient about hypertension, helping the patient make necessary lifestyle changes, and maintaining supportive interpersonal relationships. Losing weight, stopping smoking, and other changes are most likely to be effective if attempted one at a time.

- Use recommended techniques for measuring blood pressure. Poor techniques are too often used (e.g., having the patient's arm up or down rather than at heart level; having the cuff applied over clothing, too loosely, deflated too rapidly, or reinflated before completely deflated; using a regular-sized cuff on large arms that need a large cuff; using the stethoscope diaphragm rather than the bell). It is disturbing to think that antihypertensive drugs may be prescribed and dosages changed on the basis of inaccurate blood pressures.

Evaluation

- Observe for blood pressure measurements within goal or more nearly normal ranges.
- Observe and interview regarding compliance with instructions about drug therapy and lifestyle changes.
- Observe and interview regarding adverse drug effects.

Clinical Application 28-2

- Discuss the rationale for choosing captopril in Mr. Caudill's case.
- What should the nurse include in teaching Mr. Caudill to minimize adverse effects of the captopril and metoprolol?

Key Concepts

- Hypertension is defined in adults as a systolic pressure greater than 140 mm Hg or a diastolic pressure greater than 90 mm Hg on multiple blood pressure measurements.
- Key behavioral determinants of blood pressure are related to dietary consumption of calories and salt; the prevalence of hypertension rises proportionally to average body mass index.
- African Americans are more likely to have severe hypertension and require multiple drugs as a result of having low circulating renin, increased salt sensitivity, and a higher incidence of obesity.
- ACE inhibitors and ARBs are equally effective at controlling blood pressure.
- The FDA has issued a **BLACK BOX WARNING** ◆ for ACE inhibitors and ARBs during pregnancy because their use can cause injury and even death to a developing fetus.

- Beta-adrenergic blockers are the drugs of first choice for patients younger than 50 years of age with high-renin hypertension, tachycardia, angina pectoris, MI, or left ventricular hypertrophy.

- In general, Asian Americans with hypertension require much smaller doses of beta blockers because they metabolize and excrete the drugs slowly.

- Alpha$_1$-adrenergic receptor blockers should be administered at bedtime to minimize the first-dose phenomenon.

- The FDA has issued a **BLACK BOX WARNING** ◆ for patients with CAD withdrawing from oral forms of atenolol, metoprolol, nadolol, propranolol, and timolol; abrupt withdrawal has resulted in exacerbation of angina, the incidence of ventricular dysrhythmias, and the occurrence of MIs.

- The FDA has issued a **BLACK BOX WARNING** ◆ for minoxidil because the drug can exacerbate angina and precipitate effusion (which can progress to cardiac tamponade).

Critical Thinking Questions

28-1. Mrs. Shea, a 54-year-old woman, has been admitted with hypertensive crisis and tachycardia. She received a diagnosis of hypertension 2 years ago and until now has been controlling her blood pressure with a thiazide diuretic. In taking her health history, the nurse learns that Mrs. Shea has recently started taking pseudoephedrine in oral form for sinus congestion. She tells the nurse, "I don't understand it; I have been taking my blood pressure medication regularly, as always. It has kept my blood pressure under control for 2 years. Why am I having these problems now?"

- What is the relationship between the pseudoephedrine and Mrs. Shea's hypertension?

- What should the nurse teach Mrs. Shea regarding the use of these drugs?

- What additional adverse effects related to the pseudoephedrine might the nurse expect to see in Mrs. Shea?

References and Resources

American Heart Association. (2007). Treatment of hypertension in the prevention and management of ischemic heart disease: A scientific statement from the American Heart Association. *Circulation, 115,* 2761–2788.

Bangalore, S., Kamalakkannan, G., Parkar, S., & Messerli, F. H. (2007). Fixed-dose combinations improve medication compliance: A meta-analysis. *American Journal of Medicine, 120,* 713–719.

Corwin, E. J. (2011). *Handbook of pathophysiology* (4th ed.). Philadelphia, PA: Lippincott Williams & Wilkins.

Drug facts and comparisons. (Updated monthly). St. Louis, MO: Facts and Comparisons.

Gill, V., & Edelman, M. (2012). Pediatric hypertension: A cause for concern. *Nursing, 42*(3), 54–57.

Guyton, A. C., & Hall, J. E. (2011). *Textbook of medical physiology* (12th ed.). Philadelphia, PA: W. B. Saunders.

Joint National Committee on Prevention, Detection, Evaluation, and Treatment of High Blood Pressure. (2003). *The seventh report of the Joint National Committee on Prevention, Detection, Evaluation, and Treatment of High Blood Pressure: The JNC 7 report.* Retrieved May 25, 2012, from *http://www.nhlbi.nih.gov/guidelines/hypertension*

Karch, A. M. (2012). *2012 Lippincott's nursing drug guide.* Philadelphia, PA: Lippincott Williams & Wilkins.

Lacy, C. F., Armstrong, L. L., Goldman, M. P., & Lance, L. L. (2010). *Lexi-Comp's drug information handbook* (19th ed.). Hudson, OH: American Pharmaceutical Association.

National High Blood Pressure Education Program Working Group on High Blood Pressure in Children and Adolescents (2004). *The Fourth Report on the Diagnosis, Evaluation, and Treatment of High Blood Pressure in Children and Adolescents.* Retrieved September 28, 2005, from http://www. pediatrics.org/cgi/content/full/114/2/S2/555

Porth, C. M. (2009). *Pathophysiology: Concepts of altered health status* (8th ed.). St. Louis, MO: Mosby.

U.S. Department of Health and Human Services, National Institutes of Health National Heart, Lung, and Blood Institute, National High Blood Pressure Education Program. The Seventh Report of the Joint National Committee on Prevention, Detection, Evolution, and Treatment of High Blood Pressure (JNC 7). NIH Publication No. 04-5230, August 2004.

White, W. B. (2005). Update on the drug treatment of hypertension in patients with cardiovascular disease. *American Journal of Medicine, 118,* 695–705.

World Health Organization, International Society of Hypertension (ISH) Writing Group. (2003). ISH Statement on management of hypertension. *Journal of Hypertension, 21,* 1983–1992.

Drugs Affecting the Respiratory System

Drugs Affecting the Respiratory System

CHAPTER OUTLINE

29 Drug Therapy for Nasal Congestion

LEARNING OBJECTIVES

After studying this chapter, you should be able to:

1 Describe characteristics of selected upper respiratory disorders and symptoms.

2 Identify the prototype drug for each drug class.

3 Discuss nasal decongestants in terms of their action, use, contraindications, adverse effects, and nursing implications.

4 Describe antitussive agents in terms of their action, use, contraindications, adverse effects, and nursing implications.

5 Describe expectorants in terms of their action, use, contraindications, adverse effects, and nursing implications.

6 Discuss mucolytics in terms of their action, use, contraindications, adverse effects, and nursing implications.

7 Discuss the advantages and disadvantages of using combination products to treat the common cold.

8 Understand how to use the nursing process in the care of patients receiving nasal decongestants, antitussives, expectorants, and mucolytic agents.

Clinical Application Case Study

Archie Hobbs is a 45-year-old welder at an industrial plant. The occupational nurse at the facility sees a high rate of colds. Mr. Hobbs comes to the health office complaining about his nasal congestion and cough.

KEY TERMS

Antitussive: agent used to suppress cough by depressing the cough center in the medulla oblongata or the cough receptors in the throat, trachea, or lungs

Expectorant: agent that liquefies respiratory secretions and allows for their easier removal; administered orally

Mucolytic: agent that liquefies mucus in the respiratory tract; administered by inhalation

Nasal decongestant: agent used to relieve nasal obstruction and discharge

Rhinitis: inflammation of nasal mucosa

Rhinosinusitis: inflammation of the nasal and paranasal sinus mucosa

Sinusitis: inflammation of the paranasal sinuses (air cells that connect with the nasal cavity and are lined by similar mucosa)

Introduction

This chapter introduces the pharmacological care of the patient who is receiving drugs used to treat upper respiratory disorders, such as the common cold and sinusitis, with symptoms such as nasal congestion, cough, and excessive secretions. A more extensive discussion of some of these many drugs used to treat these conditions exists in other chapters; their discussion here relates to their use in upper respiratory conditions.

Overview of Nasal Congestion and Other Respiratory Symptoms

Etiology and Pathophysiology

The Common Cold

The common cold, a viral infection of the upper respiratory tract, is the most common respiratory tract infection. Adults usually have two to four colds per year; schoolchildren may have as many as 10 colds annually. Many types of viruses, most often the rhinovirus, cause colds. Shedding of these viruses by infected people, mainly from nasal mucosa, can result in rapid spread to other people.

The viruses can enter the body through mucous membranes. Cold viruses can survive for several hours on the skin and on hard surfaces, such as wood and plastic. There may also be airborne spread from sneezing and coughing, but this source is considered secondary. After the viruses gain entry, the incubation period is generally 5 days, the most contagious period is about 3 days after symptoms begin, and the cold usually lasts near 7 days. Because of the way cold viruses spread, frequent and thorough hand hygiene (by both infected and uninfected people) is the most important protective and preventive measure. The tendency for overmedication and inappropriate use of antibiotics for the common cold is widespread and poses significant risk of complications and drug resistance.

Rhinosinusitis

Some of the most common conditions that affect the upper respiratory system are inflammatory responses. **Sinusitis** is inflammation of the mucous membranes lining the paranasal sinuses. **Rhinitis** is inflammation and congestion of nasal mucosa. Because sinusitis is almost always accompanied by inflammation of the contiguous nasal mucosa, the term **rhinosinusitis** is preferred. Sinusitis often results from a viral infection; allergic rhinitis occurs as a response to an allergen. Seasonal rhinitis, or hay fever, occurs in a specific season.

Ciliated mucous membranes help move fluid and microorganisms out of the sinuses and into the nasal cavity. (These membranes perform the same tasks in other parts of the respiratory tract.) This movement becomes impaired when sinus openings are blocked by nasal swelling, and the impairment is considered a major cause of sinus infections. Another contributing factor is decreased oxygen content in the sinuses, which aids the growth of microorganisms and impairs local defense mechanisms. In acute rhinosinusitis, the classic symptom triad is purulent nasal drainage, nasal obstruction, and facial pressure and/or pain.

Clinical Manifestations

Nasal Congestion

Nasal congestion occurs when the nasal passages become blocked as membranes lining the nose become swollen due to inflamed blood vessels. The blood vessels in the nasal mucosa become dilated, and the mucous membranes become engorged with blood. Stimulation of the nasal membranes occurs at the same time, resulting in increased mucus secretion.

Cough

Cough (a forceful expulsion of air from the lungs) is a protective reflex response to mechanical, chemical, or inflammatory irritation of the lungs mediated through neurons in the brainstem or cough center. The cough reflex involves central and peripheral mechanisms. Centrally, the cough center in the medulla oblongata receives stimuli and initiates the reflex response (deep inspiration, closed glottis, buildup of pressure within the lungs, and forceful exhalation). Peripherally, air, dryness of mucous membranes, or excessive secretions may stimulate cough receptors in the pharynx, larynx, trachea, or lungs. A cough helps remove foreign bodies, environmental irritants, or accumulated secretions from the respiratory tract. A cough is productive when secretions are expectorated; it is nonproductive when it is dry and no sputum is expectorated.

Cough is a prominent symptom of respiratory tract infections (e.g., the common cold, influenza, bronchitis, pharyngitis) as well as chronic obstructive pulmonary diseases (e.g., emphysema, chronic bronchitis). When cough is associated with the common cold, it usually stems from postnasal drainage and throat irritation.

Bronchial Secretions

Bronchial secretions can result from numerous conditions, such as the common cold, where phlegm is produced in the chest. In addition, bronchial secretions can be a symptom of pneumonia, upper respiratory infections, acute and chronic bronchitis, emphysema, and asthma. Postnasal mucus may accumulate in the chest. Alternatively, secretions may be due to nonrespiratory conditions, such as immobility, debilitation, cigarette smoking, or surgery. Surgical procedures involving the chest or abdomen are most likely to be associated with retention of secretions because pain may decrease the patient's ability to cough, breathe deeply, and ambulate.

Excessive secretions may seriously impair respiration by obstructing airways and preventing air flow to and from alveoli, where gas exchange occurs. Secretions also may cause atelectasis (a condition in which part of the lung is airless and collapses) by blocking airflow, and they may cause or aggravate infections by supporting bacterial growth.

Drug Therapy

Numerous drugs are available to treat the symptoms of respiratory disorders. Many are nonprescription drugs that can be obtained alone or in combination products on an over-the-counter (OTC) basis. Available drugs include nasal decongestants, antitussives, expectorants, and mucolytics (Table 29.1).

TABLE 29.1

Drugs Administered for the Treatment of Nasal Congestion, Cough, and Rhinosinusitis

Drug Class	Prototype	Other Drugs in the Class
Nasal Decongestants	Pseudoephedrine (Sudafed, Dimetapp)	Naphazoline (Privine) Oxymetazoline (Afrin) Phenylephrine (Neo-Synephrine)
Antitussives	Dextromethorphan (Benylin DM, others)	Benzonatate (Tessalon) Codeine Hydrocodone bitartrate (Hycodan)
Expectorants	Guaifenesin (glyceryl guaiacolate) (Robitussin, others)	
Mucolytics	Acetylcysteine (Acetadote, Mucomyst)	

Nasal Decongestants

Indications for **nasal decongestants** are the relief of nasal obstruction and discharge. Adrenergic (sympathomimetic) drugs are most often used for this purpose (see Chap. 27). These agents relieve nasal congestion and swelling by constricting arterioles and reducing blood flow to nasal mucosa. Oral and topical decongestants are available. **ⓟ Pseudoephedrine** (Sudafed) is the prototype.

Pharmacokinetics

The onset of action of oral pseudoephedrine is approximately 30 minutes and typically peaks in 1 to 2 hours. The drug has a half-life of 4 to 8 hours. Metabolism to an active metabolite occurs in the liver. Excretion is via the kidneys, and the extent of excretion, is dependent on urine pH and flow rate.

Action

Pseudoephedrine acts directly on adrenergic receptors and acts indirectly by releasing norepinephrine from its storage sites. The drug produces vasoconstriction, which shrinks nasal mucosa membranes, resulting in decreased nasal congestion. It may potentiate the drainage of sinus secretions. In addition, pseudoephedrine may increase irritability of the heart muscle, especially at high doses.

Use

Uses of pseudoephedrine include the temporary relief of symptoms associated with nasal congestion due to the common cold, allergies, and sinuses. Health care providers may also use it to reduce local blood flow before nasal surgery and to aid in visualization of the nasal mucosa during diagnostic examinations.

Table 29.2 presents dosage information about various decongestants. It is not necessary to adjust dosages for pseudoephedrine in patients with hepatic impairment. Specific guidelines for adjustment in dosage in the presence of hepatic impairment are not available.

Use in Children

Experts consider pseudoephedrine effective in children older than 4 years of age, but research studies about the drug's effectiveness in younger children are inconclusive. One issue is that the low doses found in children's preparations may be insufficient to produce therapeutic effects. As a result, some pediatricians do not recommend use of the drug, whereas others say that it may be useful in some children.

Certain organizations have expressed caution about the use of pseudoephedrine in young children.

- In 2007, the Centers for Disease Control and Prevention (CDC) warned of the risk of serious injury or fatal overdose from the administration of cough and cold products to children and infants younger than 2 years of age.
- In 2007, the U.S. Food and Drug Administration (FDA) recommended that nonprescription cough and cold products containing pseudoephedrine, dextromethorphan, chlorpheniramine, diphenhydramine, brompheniramine, phenylephrine, clemastine, or guaifenesin not be used in children younger than 6 years of age.
- In 2008, the FDA issued a Public Health Advisory recommending that OTC cough and cold products not be used in infants and children younger than 2 years of age.

Use in Older Adults

The increased risk of adverse effects from oral nasal decongestants (e.g., hypertension, cardiac dysrhythmias, nervousness, insomnia) is a major concern in older adults. Adverse effects from topical agents are less likely, but rebound nasal congestion and systemic effects may occur with overuse. Older patients with significant cardiovascular disease should avoid pseudoephedrine.

Use in Patients With Renal Impairment

Because pseudoephedrine is excreted primarily via the kidneys, caution in patients with renal impairment is important. It may be necessary to reduce the dosage to avoid potential drug accumulation and drug toxicity.

Use in Patients With Critical Illness

It is appropriate to use pseudoephedrine in patients with critical illness for relief of symptoms. However, caution is warranted

TABLE 29.2

DRUGS AT A GLANCE: Nasal Decongestants

Drug	Pregnancy Category	Routes and Dosage Ranges	
		Adults	Children
Pseudoephedrine (Sudafed, Dimetapp)	C	Regular tablets, PO 30 mg every 4 to 6 h Extended-release tablets, PO 120 mg every 12 h or 240 mg every 24 h. Maximum, 240 mg in 24 h	*12 y and older*: Same as adults for regular and extended-release tablets *6–12 y*: 30 mg every 4 to 6 h. Maximum, 120 mg/24 h *2–5 y*: PO 15 mg every 4 to 6 h. Maximum, 60 mg/24 h *under 2 y*: PO 4 mg/kg /d in divided doses every 6 h
Naphazoline (Privine) 0.05% spray or drops	C	Topically, 1–2 sprays or drops no more often than every 6 h. Maximum, 4 doses/ 24 h; not to exceed 3 continuous days	*12 y and older*: Same as adults *under 12 y*: Not recommended
Oxymetazoline (Afrin) 0.05% spray	C	Topically, 2–3 sprays in each nostril, every 10–12 h. Maximum, 2 doses/24 h	*6 y and older*: Same as adults *under 6 y*: Not recommended
Phenylephrine (Neo-Synephrine)	C	PO 10–20 mg every 4 h. Maximum, 120 mg/24 h Topically, 1–2 sprays or drops of 0.25%, 0.5%, or 1% solution in each nostril no more often than every 4 h. Maximum, 6 doses/ 24 h. not to exceed 3 continuous days	*12 y and older*: Same as adults *6–11 y*: PO 10 mg every 4 h. Maximum, 60 mg/24 h Topically, 1–2 sprays or drops of 0.25% solution in each nostril no more often than every 4 h. Maximum, 6 doses/24 h. Not to exceed 3 continuous days *2–5 y*: Topically, 1–2 sprays or drops of 0.125% solution no more often than every 4 h. Maximum, 6 doses/24 h. Not to exceed 3 continuous days

with concomitant medications and comorbid disease, such as cardiovascular disorders, glaucoma, and diabetes. In addition, pseudoephedrine may produce central nervous system (CNS) stimulation, so caution is also necessary in patients with seizure disorders.

Use in Patients Receiving Home Care

People often take pseudoephedrine in the home care setting. Household members may ask the home care nurse for advice about OTC remedies they are taking for conditions such as allergies, colds, coughs, and sinus headaches. Before recommending a particular product, the nurse needs to assess the intended recipient for conditions or other medications that contraindicate the product's use. For example, the nasal decongestant component may cause or aggravate a cardiovascular disorder (e.g., hypertension). The home care nurse also needs to evaluate other medications the patient is taking in terms of potential drug interactions with the cold remedy. In addition, the nurse must emphasize the need to read the label of any OTC medication for ingredients, precautions, contraindications, drug interactions, and administration instructions.

QSEN Safety Alert

To ensure accurate dosing in children, it is necessary to use measuring devices specifically designed for the administration of medications.

Adverse Effects

Some notable significant adverse reactions of pseudoephedrine include hypotension, dysrhythmia, impaired coordination, dizziness, excitability, headache, insomnia, restlessness, seizures, vertigo, dysuria, urinary retention, urinary difficulty, and thrombocytopenia. Some people may also experience blurred vision, tinnitus, chest tightness, dry nose, nasal congestion, and wheezing.

Contraindications

Contraindications to pseudoephedrine use include severe hypertension or coronary artery disease because of the drug's cardiac stimulating and vasoconstricting effects. Another contraindication is narrow-angle glaucoma. Caution is necessary with cardiac dysrhythmias, hyperthyroidism, diabetes mellitus, glaucoma, and prostatic hypertrophy. Patients who take tricyclic or monoamine oxidase (MAO) inhibitor antidepressants should not receive pseudoephedrine.

Nursing Implications

Preventing Interactions

Many medications interact with pseudoephedrine, increasing its effect (Box 29.1). Caffeine can enhance the adverse effects of pseudoephedrine. The herb coleus may increase the

EVIDENCE-BASED PRACTICE

Use of Over-the-Counter (OTC) Cough and Cold Medications in Children Younger Than 2 Years

by IRWIN, K.A.

Journal of Pediatric Health Care
2007, 21(4), 272–275

Reviews of the use of OTC cough and cold medicines in children younger than 2 years of age have demonstrated that the use of decongestants, antitussives, antihistamines, and expectorants as OTC cold medications in these young children should be avoided. Additionally, complementary and alternative therapies such as echinacea, vitamin C, and zinc have no beneficial effect in treating the cold symptoms in children and are not recommended for use. Investigations have demonstrated that not only are OTC cough and cold medicines no more effective than a placebo in reducing symptoms, but they may be harmful. In 2005, the Centers for Disease Control and Prevention (CDC) reviewed the deaths of three children younger than 6 months of age. The CDC discovered that the underlying cause of death was excessive levels of OTC cough and cold medicines. The main medicine prominently linked with death was pseudoephedrine.

IMPLICATIONS FOR NURSING PRACTICE: Health care providers often recommend that parents try one or more decongestants, antitussives, antihistamines, and expectorants available as OTC cold medications in treating cold symptoms in children. However, medications useful in adults may not be effective in children; the best available evidence should govern appropriate decisions regarding use of any medication in any age group.

effectiveness of the drug. Tannin-containing herbs such as green or black tea or witch hazel may decrease the absorption and effectiveness of the drug.

Administering the Medication

Patients may take the oral form of pseudoephedrine with or without food. It is important not to crush extended-release preparations.

BOX 29.1   Drug Interactions: Pseudoephedrine

Drugs That Increase the Effects of Pseudoephedrine

■ Cocaine, digoxin, general anesthetics, monoamine oxidase (MAO) inhibitors, other adrenergic drugs, thyroid preparations, xanthines
Increase the risk of cardiac dysrhythmias

■ Antihistamines, epinephrine, ergot alkaloids, MAO inhibitors, methylphenidate
Increase the risk of hypertension due to vasoconstriction

Assessing for Therapeutic Effects

The nurse assesses for decreased nasal inflammation and congestion after administration of pseudoephedrine. Laboratory monitoring is not necessary.

Assessing for Adverse Effects

The nurse must monitor for cardiac symptoms, particularly in patients with a cardiac history. If anaphylaxis, chest tightness, or throat swelling occurs, it is necessary to discontinue pseudoephedrine immediately.

Patient Teaching

Box 29.2 outlines patient teaching guidelines for nasal decongestants such as pseudoephedrine.

Other Drugs in the Class

Topical preparations (i.e., nasal solutions or sprays) are often preferred for short-term use. They are rapidly effective because they come into direct contact with nasal mucosa. Oxymetazoline (Afrin) is a commonly used nasal spray that acts directly on alpha receptors to produce vasoconstriction of the arterioles in nasal passages. If used longer than the recommended 3 days or in excessive amounts, however, rebound nasal congestion may occur. Topical decongestants are less like to produce systemic affects than oral or parenteral products, but systemic adverse effects may occur; the nurse should watch for them. For patients with cardiovascular disease, topical nasal decongestants are usually preferred. Oral agents are usually contraindicated because of cardiovascular effects (e.g., increased force of myocardial contraction, increased heart rate, increased blood pressure).

Clinical Application 29-1

■ Mr. Hobbs works in an area with many other people. What should the nurse emphasize to help prevent the further spread of infection throughout the plant?

NCLEX Success

1. In caring for a patient with nasal congestion, the nurse knows that adrenergic drugs are used as nasal decongestants to relieve symptoms by

   A. constricting arterioles and reducing blood flow to nasal mucosa
   B. stimulating air movement in the lungs
   C. stabilizing mast cells
   D. initiating the cough reflex

2. As the nurse caring for a patient with nasal congestion who is using the OTC decongestant oxymetazoline (Afrin), the nurse counsels the patient that this medication should be used only for the time recommended on the package and no longer because excessive use may produce

   A. copious lower respiratory tract secretions
   B. ringing in the ears
   C. rebound nasal congestion
   D. a suppressed cough reflex

BOX 29.2 **Patient Teaching Guidelines for Nasal Decongestants, Antitussive Medications, Expectorants, and Mucolytics**

General Considerations

■ These drugs may relieve symptoms but do not cure the disorder causing the symptoms.

■ An adequate fluid intake, humidification of the environment, and sucking on hard candy or throat lozenges can help relieve mouth dryness and cough.

■ Over-the-counter (OTC) cold remedies should not be used longer than 1 week. Do not use nose drops or sprays more often or longer than recommended. Excessive or prolonged use may damage nasal mucosa and produce chronic nasal congestion.

■ Do not increase dosage if symptoms are not relieved by recommended amounts.

■ See a health care provider if symptoms persist longer than 1 week.

■ Inform health care providers about any herbal supplements that are being taken.

■ Read the labels of OTC allergy, cold, and sinus remedies for information about ingredients; many products contain more than the active ingredient. Understand dosages, conditions, or other medications with which the drugs should not be taken and adverse effects.

■ Do not combine two drug preparations containing the same or similar active ingredients. For example, pseudoephedrine is the nasal decongestant component of most prescription and OTC sinus and multi-ingredient cold remedies. The recommended dose for immediate-release preparations is usually 30 to 60 mg of pseudoephedrine; doses in extended-release preparations are usually 120 mg. Taking more than one preparation containing pseudoephedrine (or phenylephrine, a similar drug) may increase dosage to toxic levels and cause irregular heartbeats and extreme nervousness.

■ Note that many combination products contain acetaminophen or ibuprofen as pain relievers. If you are taking another form of one of these drugs (e.g., Tylenol or Advil), there is a risk of overdosage and adverse effects. Acetaminophen can cause liver damage; ibuprofen is a relative of aspirin that can cause gastrointestinal upset and bleeding. Thus, you need to be sure your total daily dosage is not excessive (with Tylenol, above four doses of 1000 mg each; with ibuprofen, above 2400 mg).

■ People with diabetes mellitus should read OTC labels for sugar content because many decongestants and cough medicines may contain sucrose, glucose, or corn syrup as a base.

Self-Administration

■ Take medications as prescribed or as directed on the labels of OTC preparations. Taking excessive amounts or taking recommended amounts too often can lead to serious adverse effects.

■ Do not chew or crush long-acting tablets or capsules (e.g., those taken once or twice daily). Such actions can cause rapid drug absorption, high blood levels, and serious adverse effects, rather than the slow absorption and prolonged action intended with these products.

■ For OTC drugs available in different dosage strengths, start with lower recommended doses rather than "maximum strength" formulations or the highest recommended doses. It is safer to see how the drugs affect you, then increase doses if necessary.

■ With topical nasal decongestants:

■ Use only preparations labeled for intranasal use. For example, phenylephrine (Neo-Synephrine) is available in both nasal and eye formulations. The two types of solutions cannot be used interchangeably. In addition, phenylephrine preparations may contain 0.125%, 0.25%, 0.5%, or 1% of drug. Be sure the concentration is appropriate for the person to receive it (e.g., an infant, young child, older adult).

■ Blow the nose gently before instilling nasal solutions or sprays. This clears nasal passages and increases effectiveness of medications.

■ To instill nose drops, lie down or sit with the neck hyperextended and instill medication without touching the dropper to the nostrils (to avoid contamination of the dropper and medication). Rinse the medication dropper after each use.

■ For nasal sprays, sit or stand, squeeze the container once to instill medication, and rinse the spray tip after each use. Most nasal sprays are designed to deliver one dose when used correctly.

■ Report palpitations, dizziness, drowsiness, or rapid pulse. These effects may occur with nasal decongestants and cold remedies and may indicate excessive dosage.

■ Take dextromethorphan as directed; increased intake can lead to increased CNS impairment. Take cough syrups undiluted and avoid eating and drinking for approximately 30 minutes.

■ Part of the beneficial effect of cough syrups stems from soothing effects on pharyngeal mucosa. Food or fluid removes the medication from the throat.

■ If the cough has not improved after 7 days or if symptoms include high fever, skin rash, or persistent headache with cough, seek help from a health care provider.

■ If you are taking acetylcysteine, understand that increasing fluid intake as directed helps loosen and mobilize secretions. In addition:

■ The nebulization may initially cause an unpleasant odor, which soon resolves.

■ If the mask leaves a sticky residue on the face, remove it with water.

■ Clean the nebulizer equipment after use to minimize infections and prevent buildup of the drug on the equipment.

Antitussives

The goal of **antitussive** therapy is to suppress nonpurposeful coughing, not productive coughing. Locally acting agents (e.g., throat lozenges, cough drops) may suppress cough by increasing the flow of saliva and by containing demulcents or local anesthetics to decrease irritation of pharyngeal mucosa. Flavored syrups are often used as vehicles for other drugs.

The nonnarcotic drug Ⓟ **dextromethorphan** (Benylin, others) is the antitussive prototype. It is the antitussive drug of choice in most circumstances and the antitussive ingredient in almost all OTC cough remedies (often designated by "DM" on the product label). (Note that some antitussives are narcotics [e.g., codeine, hydrocodone].)

Pharmacokinetics

Following oral administration of dextromethorphan, absorption is rapid. Dextromethorphan undergoes first-pass metabolism in the liver, which results in conversion to an active metabolite, dextrorphan, by the cytochrome P450 enzyme CYP2D6. The rate of metabolism varies; about 10% of the Caucasian population has little or no CYP2D6 enzyme activity, leading to prolonged high drug levels. The duration of action is about 3 to 8 hours, with a peak cough suppressing effect in 15 to 30 minutes. The half-life of the drug is 1 to 4 hours. Food decreases the rate and extent of absorption. The majority of drug and its metabolites are excreted in urine.

Action

Antitussives suppress cough by depressing the cough center in the medulla oblongata or the cough receptors in the throat, trachea, or lungs, effectively elevating the threshold for coughing. Centrally acting antitussives include nonnarcotics and narcotics.

Use

The major clinical indication for use of dextromethorphan is a dry, hacking, nonproductive cough that interferes with rest and sleep. It is not desirable to suppress a productive cough because the secretions need to be removed. There is no information relating to the use of dextromethorphan in the elderly (compared with patients of other ages). Table 29.3 gives dosage information for various antitussives.

Recently, guidelines for treating diabetic neuropathy pain identified that moderate evidence existed for the use of dextromethorphan for this condition because it blocks pain receptors in the spinal cord. Chapter 39 discusses this use.

Use in Children

Studies have not demonstrated that antitussives, particularly dextromethorphan, are effective in children and adolescents. The American Academy of Pediatrics and several other groups advise against the use of antitussives in young people. Adverse effects of dextromethorphan in children include behavioral disturbances and respiratory depression.

TABLE 29.3

DRUGS AT A GLANCE: Antitussives

Drug	Pregnancy Category	Routes and Dosage Ranges	
		Adults	Children
Nonnarcotic			
Ⓟ **Dextromethorphan** (Benylin DM, others)	C	Liquid, lozenges, and syrup, 10–30 mg every 4–8 h. Maximum, 120 mg/24 h Sustained-action liquid (Delsym), PO 60 mg every 12 h	*12 y and older:* Same as adults 6–12 y: 5–10 mg every 4 h or 15 mg every 6–8 h; Maximum, 60 mg/24 h 2–6 y: 2.5–7.5 mg every 4–8 h. Maximum, 30 mg/24 h Sustained-action liquid, 6–12 y: 30 mg every 12 h 2–5 y: 15 mg every 12 h
Benzonatate (Tessalon)	C	PO 100–200 mg 3 times a day. Maximum, 600 mg/24 h	*10 y and older:* PO 100–200 mg 3 times a day. Maximum, 600 mg/24 h
Narcotic			
Codeine	C (D during labor)	PO 10–20 mg every 4–6 h. Maximum, 120 mg/24 h	6–12 y: PO 5–10 mg every 4–6 h. Maximum, 60 mg/24 h 2–6 y: PO 2.5–5 mg every 4–6 h. Maximum, 30 mg/24 h
Hydrocodone bitartrate (Hycodan)	C (D during labor)	PO 1 (5 mg) tablet every 4–6 h up to 6 daily	Not recommended

Use in Patients Receiving Home Care

People often take dextromethorphan and other antitussives in the home care setting, and the nurse needs to assess the effectiveness of their use. The home care nurse also must emphasize the need to read the label of any OTC medication for ingredients, precautions, contraindications, drug interactions, and administration instructions. For children, it is necessary to use measuring devices specifically designed for the administration of medications.

Adverse Effects

At normal doses, dextromethorphan is known to cause nausea, drowsiness, rash, and difficulty breathing. Doses exceeding recommendations can produce hallucinations and disassociation; dextromethorphan-containing OTC preparations have been used as recreational drugs.

Contraindications

Contraindications to dextromethorphan and other antitussives include known hypersensitivity to the drugs. Caution is necessary in atopic children due to histamine release.

Nursing Implications

Preventing Interactions

Many medications interact with dextromethorphan, increasing its effect (Box 29.3). Also, St. John's wort and tryptophan interact with the antitussive to increase the risk of serotonin syndrome. No drugs appear to decrease the effect of dextromethorphan.

Administering the Medication

It is necessary to administer dextromethorphan-containing cough syrups undiluted. The nurse instructs the patient to avoid eating and drinking for approximately 30 minutes. Some caution is warranted with lozenges, which should be dissolved in the mouth to decrease the risk of choking.

Assessing for Therapeutic Effects

The nurse observes for decreased coughing.

Assessing for Adverse Effects

The nurse observes for excessive suppression of the cough reflex (inability to cough effectively when secretions are present) or hallucinations with dosages that exceed recommendations.

BOX 29.3   Drug Interactions: Dextromethorphan

Drugs That Increase the Effects of Dextromethorphan
- Monoamine oxidase (MAO) inhibitors, serotonin reuptake inhibitors, tricyclic antidepressants, 5-HT1 receptor agonists, ergot alkaloids, lithium, phenylpiperidine opioids

  Increase the risk of serotonin syndrome
- Alcohol

  Increases central nervous system (CNS) depression

Patient Teaching

Box 29.2 outlines patient teaching guidelines for antitussives such as dextromethorphan.

Other Drugs in the Class

Benzonatate (Tessalon), another nonnarcotic antitussive agent, is a peripherally acting drug, unlike dextromethorphan. This antitussive drug acts by anesthetizing stretch receptors in the respiratory passages, thereby decreasing coughing. The nurse advises the patient to swallow the benzonatate capsules whole. Sucking or chewing them may cause numbness of the throat or mouth. Serious adverse effects include a choking feeling, chest pain or numbness, dizziness, confusion, and hallucinations.

Codeine and hydrocodone, which are both narcotics, have antitussive effects in relatively small doses. Both are centrally acting drugs, like dextromethorphan. Adverse reactions to the narcotic antitussives include nausea, vomiting, constipation, dizziness, drowsiness, pruritus, and drug dependence. Caution is necessary in asthma, head injuries and increased intracranial pressure, acute abdominal disorders, seizure disorders, renal or hepatic impairment, and prostatic hypertrophy.

Clinical Application 29-2

- Mr. Hobbs has been sick for more than 7 days. He feels that he is getting worse. When the nurse asks him what medication he is taking, he reports that he is using the oxymetazoline (Afrin) that was recommended the last time he was congested. What does the nurse tell him?

Expectorants

Expectorants are agents given orally to liquefy respiratory secretions and allow for their easier removal. The drugs act by moistening the respiratory tract to make the mucus less tenacious. ℗ **Guaifenesin** (Robitussin, others) is the prototype expectorant. It is available alone and as an ingredient in many combination cough and cold remedies.

Pharmacokinetics

Guaifenesin is well absorbed following oral administration. Onset of action is 4 to 6 hours, and the duration of action is unknown. The half-life is about 1 hour. Metabolism and excretion of guaifenesin and its metabolites occur in the urine.

Action

Guaifenesin reduces the viscosity of tenacious secretions by irritating the gastric vagal receptors stimulating respiratory tract fluid. Thus, it increases the volume and decreases the viscosity of respiratory tract secretions.

TABLE 29.4

DRUGS AT A GLANCE: Expectorants

Drug	Pregnancy Category	Routes and Dosage Ranges	
		Adults	Children
Ⓟ **Guaifenesin** (glyceryl guaiacolate) (Robitussin, Mucinex, others)	C	PO 100–400 mg every 4 h. Maximum, 2400 mg/24 h	*12 y and older*: Same as adults 6–12 y: PO 100–200 mg every 4 h. Maximum, 1200 mg/24 h 2–6 y: PO 50–100 mg every 4 h. Maximum, 600 mg/24 h

Use

Used with productive coughs, guaifenesin loosens mucus from the respiratory tract. The drug does not appear to cause unusual adverse effects or problems in older adults. There is no information identifying risk with use of guaifenesin in older patients compared with younger ones. Table 29.4 presents dosage information for the expectorants.

It is important to note that with excessive respiratory tract secretions, mechanical measures (e.g., coughing, deep breathing, ambulation, chest physiotherapy, forcing fluids) are more likely to be effective than expectorant drug therapy. Research studies do not support the drug's overall effectiveness, and many authorities do not recommend its use.

Use in Children

Guaifenesin does not appear to cause unusual problems in children. However, caution is necessary when the drug is used in children younger than 4 years of age.

Use in Patients Receiving Home Care

People use guaifenesin in the home to help liquefy mucus that is making breathing difficult. The home care nurse must emphasize the need to increase fluid intake as recommended to help facilitate mobilization of secretions. Also, the nurse must stress the importance of reading the label of any OTC medication for ingredients, precautions, contraindications, drug interactions, and administration instructions. When giving medications to children, it is necessary to use only measuring devices specifically designed for the administration of medications to young patients.

Adverse Effects

Adverse effects of guaifenesin include skin rash, headache, nausea, and vomiting.

Contraindications

Hypersensitivity to guaifenesin is the major contraindication.

Nursing Implications

Administering the Medication

It is necessary to swallow sustained-release capsules or tablets of guaifenesin whole; patients should not break, crush, or chew them. Drinking plenty of water while taking the drug may help

loosen mucus in the lungs. People can take it without regard to meals.

Assessing for Therapeutic Effects

The nurse assesses for improvement in cold symptoms, specifically reduction of cough episodes and increased ability to mobilize secretions.

Assessing for Adverse Effects

The nurse assesses for hypersensitivity to the drug and for signs of headache, nausea, and vomiting.

Patient Teaching

Box 29.2 presents patient teaching guidelines for the expectorant guaifenesin.

QSEN Safety Alert

It is important to note that guaifenesin liquefies mucus and increases the amount of mucus to be removed. Thus, suction equipment should be available (in the home, if necessary); the patient and significant others require training in proper use.

Mucolytics

Mucolytics are drugs that liquefy mucus in the respiratory tract by attacking the protein bonds of the mucus. Administration is by inhalation; solutions may be nebulized into a face mask or mouthpiece or instilled directly into the respiratory tract through a tracheostomy. Ⓟ **Acetylcysteine** (Acetadote, Mucomyst), the prototype, and sodium chloride solution are the only agents recommended for use as mucolytics.

Pharmacokinetics

Acetylcysteine is rapidly absorbed following inhalation or instillation. Onset of action is 1 minute, the maximum peak effect occurs within 5 to 10 minutes, and the duration of action is 2 to 3 hours. Metabolism occurs in the liver, with drug excretion in the urine.

Action

Acetylcysteine exerts its mucolytic action through its sulfhydryl group, which disrupts the disulfide bonds in the mucoproteins. This reduces the viscosity of mucous secretions.

TABLE 29.5

DRUGS AT A GLANCE: Mucolytics

Drug	Pregnancy Category	Routes and Dosage Ranges	
		Adults	*Children*
℗ **Acetylcysteine** (Acetadote, Mucomyst)	B	Nebulization, 1–10 mL of a 20% solution or 2–20 mL of a 10% solution every 2–6 h Instillation, 1–2 mL of a 10% or 20% solution every 1–4 h Acetaminophen overdosage, PO 140 mg/kg initially, then 70 mg/kg every 4 h for 17 doses; dilute a 10% or 20% solution to a 5% solution with cola, fruit juice, or water	Acetaminophen overdosage, see literature

Use

Acetylcysteine is used as an adjunctive agent to liquefy viscous mucous secretions. Also, the oral drug is widely used as an antidote in the treatment of acetaminophen overdosage (see Table 2.1 and Chap. 14).

Table 29.5 presents dosage information for the mucolytics. No studies of acetylcysteine focus specifically on the use of the drug in older adults.

Use in Children

Use of acetylcysteine in children does not appear to cause adverse effects. However, no specific information available compares the drug's use in children with people of other ages.

Use in Patients With Critical Illness

Although people who are critically ill may receive acetylcysteine by inhalation, they more commonly receive it by mouth as an antidote to acetaminophen poisoning. Parameters for use in critically ill patients are consistent for use in other people.

Use in Patients Receiving Home Care

People take acetylcysteine in the home in the treatment of certain lung conditions; the drug helps remove increased amounts of mucus that make breathing difficult. The home care nurse must emphasize the need to follow administration instructions, clean equipment on a scheduled basis, and increase fluid intake as recommended to help mobilize secretions. Because acetylcysteine liquefies mucus and increases the amount to be removed, suction equipment should be available. It is essential that the patient and significant others are trained in proper use.

Adverse Effects

Adverse reactions with inhalation therapy using acetylcysteine include drowsiness, nausea and vomiting, and bronchospasm.

Contraindications

Contraindications include hypersensitivity to acetylcysteine.

Nursing Implications

Administering the Medication

It is necessary to give intermittent aerosol treatments. Typically, these are on arising, before meals, and at bedtime.

Assessing for Therapeutic Effects

The nurse assesses the ability to mobilize secretions and the demonstration of improved respiratory function.

Assessing for Adverse Effects

The nurse assesses for difficulty breathing, inability to expel secretions, bronchospasm, and chest tightness. Also, he or she observes for the additional adverse effects of nausea and vomiting.

Patient Teaching

Box 29.2 outlines patient teaching guidelines for the mucolytic acetylcysteine.

Herbal Preparations

Herbal drugs have been used as cold remedies (Box 29.4).

Combination Products

Many combination products are available for treating symptoms of the common cold (Table 29.6). Many of the products contain an antihistamine, a nasal decongestant, and an analgesic. Some contain antitussives, expectorants, and other agents as well. Many cold remedies are OTC formulations. Commonly used ingredients include chlorpheniramine (antihistamine), pseudoephedrine (adrenergic nasal decongestant), acetaminophen (analgesic and antipyretic), dextromethorphan (antitussive), and guaifenesin (expectorant). Antihistamines are clearly useful in allergic conditions (e.g., allergic rhinitis; see Chap. 30), but their use to relieve cold symptoms is controversial. First-generation antihistamines (e.g., chlorpheniramine, diphenhydramine) have anticholinergic effects that may reduce sneezing, rhinorrhea, and cough. Also, their sedative effects may aid sleep. Many multi-ingredient cold remedies contain an antihistamine.

BOX 29.4   Herbal Preparations Used as Cold Remedies

■ **Echinacea** preparations differ in chemical composition depending on which of the nine species or parts of the plant (e.g., leaves, roots, whole plant) are used as well as the season of harvesting. Also, which constituents of the plants are pharmacologically active is unclear. A study concluded that there is no conclusive evidence that echinacea products effectively treat or prevent the common cold.

■ **Vitamin C** is used to reduce the incidence and severity of colds and influenza. There is no clear consensus that vitamin C shortens the duration of colds and alleviates its symptoms in adults, although clinical trials with adults have been partially positive. For those adults regularly taking vitamin C, it appears that vita-

min C plays a role in the defense mechanisms of the respiratory system. The therapeutic benefit of vitamin C in reducing cold incidence and severity in children has not been demonstrated.

■ **Zinc gluconate** lozenges are marketed as a cold remedy. However, some studies indicate beneficial effects and others do not. Most of the studies suggesting benefit are considered flawed in methodology. For example, although some studies were supposed to be blind, the lozenges' distinctive taste likely allowed the drug to be distinguished from a placebo. More recently, nasal zinc preparations (Cold-Eeze, Zicam) have been developed, and the possible risk of loss of smell with nasal zinc likely outweighs any benefit.

TABLE 29.6

Representative Multi-Ingredient Nonprescription Cold, Cough, and Sinus Remedies

Trade Name	Ingredients				
	Antihistamine	Nasal Decongestant	Analgesic	Antitussive	Expectorant
Actifed Cold & Allergy	Triprolidine 2.5 mg/ tablet	Pseudoephedrine 60 mg/tablet			
Advil Cold and Sinus Tablets		Pseudoephedrine 30 mg/tablet	Ibuprofen 200 mg/ tablet		
Cheracol D Cough Liquid				Dextromethorphan 10 mg/5 mL	Guaifenesin 100 mg/5 mL
Comtrex Cold & Sinus Tablets	Brompheniramine 2 mg/tablet	Pseudoephedrine 30 mg/tablet	Acetaminophen 500 mg/tablet		
Contac Day & Night Cold & Flu Tablets	(Night) Diphenhydramine 50 mg/tablet	Pseudoephedrine 60 mg/tablet	Acetaminophen 650 mg/tablet	(Day) Dextromethorphan 30 mg/tablet	
Coricidin D Cold, Flu & Sinus Tablets	Chlorpheniramine 2 mg/tablet	Pseudoephedrine 30 mg/tablet	Acetaminophen 325 mg/tablet		
Dimetapp Cold and Allergy Elixir	Brompheniramine 1 mg/5 mL	Pseudoephedrine 15 mg/5 mL			
Dristan Cold Formula	Chlorpheniramine 2 mg/tablet	Phenylephrine 5 mg/tablet	Acetaminophen 325 mg/tablet		
Motrin Sinus Tablets		Pseudoephedrine 30 mg/tablet	Ibuprofen 200 mg/ tablet		
Robitussin Cold and Flu Tablets		Pseudoephedrine 10 mg/tablet	Acetaminophen 325 mg/tablet	Dextromethorphan 30 mg/tablet	Guaifenesin 200 mg/tablet
Sinutab Sinus Allergy Maximum Strength Tablets	Chlorpheniramine 2 mg/tablet	Pseudoephedrine 30 mg/tablet	Acetaminophen 500 mg/tablet	Dextromethorphan 10 mg/tablet	
Theraflu Flu, Cold, and Cough Powder	Chlorpheniramine 4 mg/pack	Pseudoephedrine 60 mg/pack	Acetaminophen 650 mg/pack	Dextromethorphan 20 mg/pack	
Vicks NyQuil Cold & Flu Capsules	Doxylamine 6.25 mg/capsule	Pseudoephedrine 30 mg/capsule	Acetaminophen 250 mg/capsule	Dextromethorphan 10 mg/capsule	

The use of OTC products containing pseudoephedrine to manufacture methamphetamine has increased at an alarming rate. The Combat Methamphetamine Epidemic Act of 2005 (see Table 1.1) applies to all cough and cold products, including combination products that contain pseudoephedrine.

QSEN Safety Alert

All products, including liquids, gel caps, and pediatric formulas, are subject to law and are stored behind pharmacy counters to restrict and control sales.

Many products come in several formulations, with different ingredients, and are advertised for different purposes (e.g., allergy, sinus disorders, multisymptom cold, flu remedies). For example, allergy remedies contain an antihistamine; "nondrowsy" or "daytime" formulas contain a nasal decongestant but not an antihistamine; "PM" or "night" formulas contain a sedating antihistamine to promote sleep; pain, fever, and multisymptom formulas usually contain acetaminophen; and "maximum strength" preparations usually refer only to the amount of acetaminophen per dose, usually 1000 mg for adults. In addition, labels on OTC combination products list ingredients by generic name, without identifying the type of drug. As a result of these bewildering products, consumers, including nurses and other health care providers, may not know what medications they are taking or whether some drugs increase or block the effects of other drugs. The FDA recommends that if parents and caregivers use cough and cold products in children older than 2 years of age, it is necessary to read labels carefully, use caution when administering multiple products, and use only measuring devices specifically designed for use with medications.

It is true that single-drug formulations allow flexibility and individualization of dosage, whereas combination products may contain unneeded ingredients and are more expensive. However, many people find combination products more convenient to use.

Clinical Application 29-3

- Mr. Hobbs also complains of a productive cough. He has been taking chlorpheniramine to treat it. What advice should the nurse give to him with regard to the appropriate treatment of a productive cough?

NCLEX Success

3. A common mucolytic used to liquefy mucus in the respiratory tract is

   A. acetylcysteine (Mucomyst)
   B. ipratropium (Atrovent)
   C. dextromethorphan
   D. pseudoephedrine (Sudafed)

4. Cold remedies listed as "nondrowsy" or labeled as "daytime" formulas do not contain

   A. a nasal decongestant
   B. a first-generation antihistamine
   C. a pain reliever
   D. Any of the above

EVIDENCE-BASED PRACTICE

Cough Suppressant and Pharmacologic Protussive Therapy: ACCP Evidence-Based Clinical Practice Guidelines
by BOLSER, D. C.

Chest
2006, 129(1 Suppl), 238S–249S

The American College of Chest Physicians (ACCP) published evidence-based clinical practice guidelines regarding cough and the common cold. Pharmacologic recommendations include the following:

- Treatment of people with the common cold experiencing acute cough, postnasal drip, and throat clearing with a first-generation antihistamine/decongestant preparation (sustained-release pseudoephedrine and brompheniramine) is recommended. Naproxen can also be taken to help decrease cough in this group.
- Newer generation, nonsedating antihistamines are ineffective for reducing cough and should not be used in people with the common cold (ACCP, 2006).

IMPLICATIONS FOR NURSING PRACTICE: Not all OTC medications in a class are useful in alleviating symptoms of a cough or cold. The use of newer generation antihistamines should be discouraged in people with a cough. The nurse should be aware of the specific recommendation for drugs in a class to effectively educate patients and families.

5. Which of the following herbal preparations appears to play a role in the defense mechanisms of the respiratory system in adults?

   A. echinacea
   B. vitamin C
   C. zinc gluconate have been commonly thought to improve cold symptoms.
   D. valerian

The Nursing Process

Assessment

Assess the patient's condition in relation to disorders for which the drugs are used.

- With nasal congestion, observe for decreased ability to breathe through the nose. If nasal discharge is present, note its amount, color, and thickness. Question the patient about the duration and extent of nasal congestion and factors that precipitate or relieve it.

- With coughing, a major assessment factor is whether the cough is productive of sputum or dry and hacking. If the cough is productive, note the color, odor, viscosity, and amount of sputum. In addition, assess factors that stimulate or relieve cough and the patient's ability and willingness to cough effectively.
- Assess fluid intake and hydration status.

Nursing Diagnoses

- Risk for injury related to cardiac dysrhythmias, hypertension, and other adverse effects of nasal decongestants
- Noncompliance: overuse of nasal decongestants
- Deficient knowledge: appropriate use of single- and multi-ingredient drug formulations

Planning/Goals

The patient will

- Experience relief of symptoms
- Take drugs accurately and safely
- Avoid overuse of decongestants
- Avoid preventable adverse drug effects
- Act to avoid recurrence of symptoms

Nursing Interventions

This nurse will

- Encourage patients to use measures to prevent or minimize the incidence and severity of symptoms. Recommend to patients that they:
  - Avoid smoking cigarettes or breathing secondhand smoke, when possible. Cigarette smoke irritates respiratory tract mucosa, and this irritation causes cough, increased secretions, and decreased effectiveness of cilia in cleaning the respiratory tract.
  - Avoid or limit exposure to crowds, especially during winter when the incidence of colds and influenza is high.
  - Avoid contact with people who have colds or other respiratory infections. This is especially important for patients with chronic lung disease, because upper respiratory infections may precipitate acute attacks of asthma or bronchitis.
  - Maintain a fluid intake of 2000 to 3000 mL daily unless contraindicated by cardiovascular or renal disease.
  - Maintain nutrition, rest, activity, and other general health measures.
  - Practice good hand hygiene techniques.
  - Consider having an annual vaccination for influenza if they are elderly or have chronic respiratory, cardiovascular, or renal disorders.
- Provide appropriate teaching related to drug therapy (see Box 29.2).

Evaluation

The nurse will

- Interview and observe for relief of symptoms
- Interview and observe for tachycardia, hypertension, drowsiness, and other adverse drug effects
- Interview and observe for compliance with instructions about drug use

Key Concepts

- Most upper respiratory infections are viral in origin, and antibiotics are not generally recommended.
- Retention of secretions commonly occurs with influenza, pneumonia, upper respiratory infections, acute and chronic bronchitis, emphysema, and acute attacks of asthma.
- Nonrespiratory conditions that predispose to secretion retention include immobility, debilitation, cigarette smoking, and postoperative status.
- An adequate fluid intake, humidification of the environment, and sucking on hard candy or throat lozenges can help relieve mouth dryness and cough.
- The goal of antitussive therapy is to suppress nonpurposeful coughing, not productive coughing.
- Rebound nasal swelling can occur with excessive or extended use of nasal sprays.
- First-generation antihistamines (e.g., chlorpheniramine, diphenhydramine) have anticholinergic effects that may reduce sneezing, rhinorrhea, and cough.
- There is limited or no support for the use of dietary or herbal supplements, such as echinacea, vitamin C, and zinc, to treat symptoms of the common cold.
- Several OTC cough and cold medicines for use in infants have been recalled voluntarily due to concerns about possible misuse that could result in overdoses.
- Parents and caregivers should be educated on the importance of safe storage of OTC cough and cold medicines to prevent unintentional ingestion by children.
- For children, it is necessary to use measuring devices specifically designed for the accurate administration of medications.

Critical Thinking Questions

29-1. A 76-year-old man with a history of coronary artery disease and hypertension presents to the outpatient clinic where you work as a nurse. He is complaining of symptoms of a cold.

- What should you tell him about taking OTC nasal decongestants and cold remedies?
- He tells the nurse that his wife has been giving him echinacea and nasal preparations as a cold remedy. How does the nurse reply?

References and Resources

Bolser, D. C. (2006). Cough suppressant and pharmacologic protussive therapy: ACCP evidence-based clinical practice guidelines. *Chest, 129*(1 Suppl), 238S–249S.

Bril, V., England, J., Franklin, G.M., Backonja, M., Cohen, J., Del Toro, D., et al. (2001). Evidence-based guideline: Treatment of painful diabetic neuropathy: Report of the American Academy of Neurology, the American Association of Neuromuscular and Electrodiagnostic Medicine, and the American Academy of Physical Medicine and Rehabilitation. *Neurology, 76*, 1758–1765.

Carr, B.C. (2006). Efficacy, abuse, and toxicity of over-the-counter cough and cold medicines in the pediatric population. *Current Opinion in Pediatrics, 18*, 184–188.

Drug facts and comparisons. (Updated monthly). St. Louis, MO: Facts and Comparisons.

Guyton, A. C., & Hall, J. E. (2006). *Textbook of medical physiology* (11th ed.). Philadelphia, PA: W. B. Saunders.

Irwin, K. A. (2007). Use of over-the-counter cough and cold medications in children younger than 2 Years. *Journal of Pediatric Health Care, 21*(4), 272–275.

Karch, A. M. (2012). *2012 Lippincott's nursing drug guide.* Philadelphia, PA: Lippincott Williams & Wilkins.

Krouse, J. H. (2008). Allergic rhinitis-current pharmacotherapy. *Otolaryngologic Clinics of North America, 41*, 347–358.

Lacy, C. F., Armstrong, L. L., Goldman, M. P., & Lance, L. L. (2010). *Lexi-Comp's drug information handbook* (19th ed.). Hudson, OH: American Pharmaceutical Association.

Lazenby, R. B. (2010). *Handbook of pathophysiology* (4th ed.). Philadelphia, PA: Lippincott Williams & Wilkins.

Porth, C. M. (2009). *Pathophysiology: Concepts of altered health status.* (8th ed.). Philadelphia, PA: Lippincott Williams & Wilkins.

Pratter, M. R. (2006). Cough and the common cold: ACCP evidence-based clinical practice guidelines. *Chest, 129*(1 Suppl), 72S–74S.

Simasek, M., & Blandino, D. A. (2007). Treatment of the common cold. *American Family Physician, 75*, 515–520.

30 Drug Therapy to Decrease Histamine Effects and Allergic Response

LEARNING OBJECTIVES

After studying this chapter, you should be able to:

1. Delineate effects of histamines on selected body tissues.

2. Describe the types of hypersensitivity or allergic reactions.

3. Identify the effects of histamine that are blocked by histamine₁ (H₁) receptor antagonist drugs.

4. Discuss first-generation H₁ receptor antagonists in terms of prototype, indications and contraindications, major adverse effects, interactions, and administration.

5. Describe second-generation H₁ receptor antagonists in terms of prototype, indications and contraindications, major adverse effects, interactions, and administration.

6. Understand how to use the nursing process in the care of patients receiving antihistamines.

Clinical Application Case Study

Gene Rudolph is a 72-year-old retired mail carrier. His medical history includes hypertension, benign prostatic hypertrophy, and coronary artery disease. He is visiting a medical clinic for a routine blood pressure check. He tells the nurse that he has been having symptoms of nasal congestion, sneezing, and watering of the eyes for the past several weeks and that the symptoms started after he began working in his garden.

KEY TERMS

Anaphylactic reactions: severe, whole-body reaction after sensitization to an allergen causing a severe allergic response

Anaphylactoid reactions: anaphylaxis-like reaction to a substance without development of IgE antibody that may occur on first exposure to the causative agent

Antihistamines: drugs that antagonize the action of histamine; commonly the H₁ receptor antagonists

Histamine: first chemical mediator released in immune and inflammatory responses found mainly in mast cells surrounding blood vessels

Hypersensitivity: allergic reactions that are exaggerated responses by the immune system; produce tissue injury and may cause serious disease

Serum sickness: type III hypersensitive response is an IgG- or IgM-mediated reaction characterized by formation of antigen–antibody complexes that induce an acute inflammatory reaction in the tissues.

Introduction

The drugs that antagonize the action of histamine are commonly called **antihistamines**. There are three main types of receptors for histamine, histamine$_1$ (H$_1$), histamine$_2$ (H$_2$), and histamine$_3$ (H$_3$) receptors. This chapter focuses on those drugs that specifically prevent or reduce most of the physiologic effects that histamine normally induces at H$_1$ receptor sites. (Prescribers use some H$_2$ receptor antagonists, such as cimetidine, to treat peptic ulcers.) To understand the use of antihistamines, it is necessary to understand histamine and its effects on body tissues, the characteristics of allergic reactions, and the selected conditions for which antihistamines are used.

Overview of Histamine Release and the Allergic Response

Etiology and Pathophysiology

Histamine and Its Receptors

Histamine is the first chemical mediator to be released in immune and inflammatory responses. It is synthesized and stored in most body tissues, with high concentrations in tissues exposed to environmental substances (e.g., the skin and mucosal surfaces of the eye, nose, lungs, and gastrointestinal [GI] tract). It is also found in the central nervous system (CNS). In these tissues, histamine is located mainly in secretory granules of mast cells (tissue cells surrounding capillaries) and basophils (circulating blood cells).

Histamine is discharged from mast cells and basophils in response to certain stimuli (e.g., allergic reactions, cellular injury, extreme cold). After it is released, it diffuses rapidly into other tissues, where it interacts with H$_1$ and H$_2$ receptors on target organs. H$_1$ receptors are located mainly on smooth muscle cells in blood vessels and the respiratory and GI tracts (see Fig. 30.2). When histamine binds with these receptors and stimulates them, effects include the following:

- Contraction of smooth muscle in the bronchi and bronchioles (producing bronchoconstriction and respiratory distress)
- Stimulation of vagus nerve endings to produce reflex bronchoconstriction and cough
- Increased permeability of veins and capillaries, which allows fluid to flow into subcutaneous tissues and form edema
- Increased secretion of mucous glands. Mucosal edema and increased nasal mucus produce the nasal congestion characteristic of allergic rhinitis and the common cold.

- Stimulation of sensory peripheral nerve endings to cause pain and pruritus. Pruritus is especially prominent with allergic skin disorders.
- Dilation of capillaries in the skin, to cause flushing

When H$_2$ receptors are stimulated, the main effects are increased secretion of gastric acid and pepsin, increased rate and force of myocardial contraction, and decreased immunologic and proinflammatory reactions (e.g., decreased release of histamine from basophils, decreased movement of neutrophils and basophils into areas of injury, inhibited T- and B-lymphocyte function). Stimulation of both H$_1$ and H$_2$ receptors causes peripheral vasodilation (with hypotension, headache, and skin flushing) and increases bronchial, intestinal, and salivary secretion of mucus.

Limited information is available regarding H$_3$ receptors; they are believed to play a role in regulation of the release of histamine and other neurotransmitters from neurons. Although several drugs affecting H$_3$ receptors are currently undergoing human trials, none has a defined clinical use.

Hypersensitivity (Allergic) Reactions

In predisposed people, harmless environmental antigens that often do not cause a reaction sometimes may trigger an adaptive immune response, immunologic memory, and, on subsequent exposure to the environmental antigen, inflammation responses (see Chap. 14). **Hypersensitivity**, or allergic reactions, are exaggerated responses by the immune system that produce tissue injury and may cause serious disease. The mechanisms that eliminate pathogens in adaptive immune responses are essentially identical to those of natural immunity. Allergic reactions may result from specific antibodies, sensitized T lymphocytes, or both, formed during exposure to an antigen. Treatments and interventions are covered in other chapters.

Types of Responses to Cell-Mediated Invasion

Hypersensitivity reactions are grouped into four types according to the mechanisms by which they are produced. The substances that produce the effect for types I, II, and III hypersensitivity reactions are antibody molecules. The substances responsible for type IV reactions are antigen-specific T cells.

Type I (also called immediate hypersensitivity because it occurs within minutes of exposure to the antigen) is an immunoglobulin E (IgE)–induced response triggered by the interaction of antigen with antigen-specific IgE bound on mast cells, causing mast cell activation. Histamine and other mediators are released immediately, and cytokines, chemokines, and leukotrienes are synthesized after activation. Anaphylaxis is a type I response that may be mild (characterized mainly by urticaria, other dermatologic manifestations, or rhinitis) or severe and life threatening (characterized by respiratory distress and cardiovascular collapse). It is uncommon and does not occur on first exposure to an antigen; it occurs with a second or later exposure, after antibody formation was induced by an earlier exposure. Severe anaphylaxis (sometimes called anaphylactic shock; see Chap. 27) is characterized by cardiovascular collapse from profound vasodilation and pooling of blood in the splanchnic system so that the patient has severe hypotension and functional hypovolemia. Respiratory distress often occurs from laryngeal edema and bronchoconstriction. Urticaria often occurs because the skin has many mast cells that release histamine. Anaphylaxis is a systemic reaction that usually involves the respiratory, cardiovascular, and dermatologic systems. Severe anaphylaxis may be fatal if not treated promptly and effectively. Antihistamines are helpful in treating urticaria and pruritus but are not effective in treating bronchoconstriction and hypotension. Epinephrine, rather than an antihistamine, is the drug of choice for treating severe anaphylaxis.

Type II responses are mediated by IgG or IgM, generating direct damage to the cell surface. These cytotoxic reactions include blood transfusion reactions, hemolytic disease of newborns, autoimmune hemolytic anemia, and some drug reactions. Hemolytic anemia (caused by destruction of erythrocytes) and thrombocytopenia (caused by destruction of platelets), both type II hypersensitivity responses, are adverse effects of certain drugs (e.g., penicillin, methyldopa, heparin).

Type III is an IgG- or IgM-mediated reaction characterized by formation of antigen–antibody complexes that induce an acute inflammatory reaction in the tissues. **Serum sickness**, the prototype of these reactions, occurs when excess antigen combines with antibodies to form immune complexes. The complexes then diffuse into affected tissues, where they cause tissue damage by activating the complement system and initiating the immune response. If small amounts of immune complexes are deposited locally, the antigenic material can be phagocytized and digested by white blood cells and macrophages without tissue destruction. If large amounts are deposited locally or reach the bloodstream and become deposited in blood vessel walls, the lysosomal enzymes released during phagocytosis may cause permanent tissue destruction.

Type IV hypersensitivity (also called delayed hypersensitivity because of the lag time from exposure to antigen until the response is evident) is a cell-mediated response in which sensitized T lymphocytes react with an antigen to cause inflammation mediated by release of lymphokines, direct cytotoxicity, or both. The classic type IV hypersensitivity reaction is the tuberculin test, but similar reactions occur with contact dermatitis and some graft rejection.

Clinical Manifestations

Allergic Rhinitis

Allergic rhinitis is inflammation of nasal mucosa caused by a type I hypersensitivity reaction to inhaled allergens. It is a very common disorder characterized by nasal congestion, itching, sneezing, and watery drainage. Itching of the throat, eyes, and ears often occurs as well.

There are two types of allergic rhinitis. Seasonal disease (often called hay fever) produces acute symptoms in response to the protein components of airborne pollens from trees, grasses, and weeds, mainly in spring or fall. Perennial disease produces chronic symptoms in response to nonseasonal allergens such as dust mites, animal dander, and molds. Actually, mold spores can cause both seasonal and perennial allergies because they are present year round, with seasonal increases. Some people have both types, with chronic symptoms plus acute seasonal symptoms.

People with a personal or family history of other allergic disorders are likely to have allergic rhinitis. When mucous membranes in the nose are inflamed, symptoms can be worsened by nonallergenic irritants such as tobacco smoke, strong odors, air pollution, and climatic changes.

Allergic rhinitis is an immune response in which normal nasal breathing and filtering of air brings inhaled antigens into contact with mast cells and basophils in nasal mucosa, blood vessels, and submucosal tissues. With initial exposure, the inhaled antigens are processed by lymphocytes that produce IgE, an antigen-specific antibody that binds to mast cells. With later exposures, the IgE interacts with inhaled antigens and triggers the breakdown of the mast cell. This breakdown causes the release of histamine and other inflammatory mediators such as prostaglandins and leukotrienes (Fig. 30.1). These mediators, of which histamine may be the most important, dilate and engorge blood vessels to produce nasal congestion, stimulate secretion of mucus, and attract inflammatory cells (e.g., eosinophils, lymphocytes, monocytes, macrophages). In people with allergies, mast cells and basophils are increased in both number and reactivity. Thus, these cells may be capable of releasing large amounts of histamine and other mediators.

Allergic rhinitis that is not effectively treated may lead to chronic fatigue, impaired ability to perform usual activities of daily living, difficulty sleeping, sinus infections, postnasal drip, cough, and headache. In addition, this condition is a strong risk factor for asthma. Studies have demonstrated that although antihistamines relieve symptoms of allergic rhinitis, antihistamine are not successful or recommended for treatment of the common cold.

Chapter 31 describes the many drugs used to manage the condition besides antihistamines.

Allergic Contact Dermatitis

Allergic contact dermatitis is a type IV hypersensitivity reaction resulting from direct contact with antigens to which a person has previously become sensitized (e.g., poison ivy or poison oak, cosmetics, hair dyes, metals, drugs applied topically to the skin). This reaction, which may be acute or chronic, usually occurs more than 24 hours after reexposure to an antigen and may last from days to weeks.

Affected areas of the skin are usually inflamed, warm, edematous, intensely pruritic, and tender to touch. Skin lesions are usually erythematous macules, papules, and vesicles (blisters) that may drain, develop crusts, and become infected. Lesion location may indicate the causative antigen.

Allergic Food Reactions

Typically, food allergies are an immune response to the ingestion of a protein. Some food allergens such as shellfish, fish, corn, seeds, bananas, egg, milk, soy, peanut, and tree nuts have a higher inherent risk of triggering anaphylaxis than others. However, many other foods have been identified as allergens,

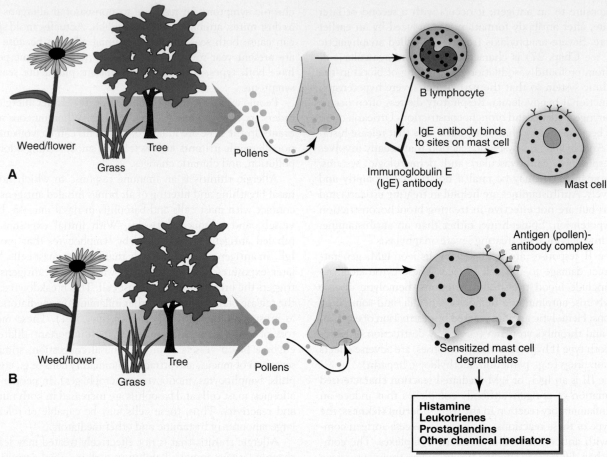

Figure 30.1 Type I hypersensitivity reaction: allergic rhinitis. **A.** The first exposure of mast cells in nasal mucosa to inhaled antigens (e.g., pollens from weeds, grasses, trees) leads to the formation of immunoglobulin E (IgE) antibody molecules. These molecules then bind to the surface membranes of mast cells. This process sensitizes mast cells to the effects of inhaled antigens (allergens). **B.** When sensitized mast cells are reexposed to inhaled pollens or other antigens, they release histamine and other chemical mediators, which then act on nasal mucosa to produce characteristic symptoms of allergic rhinitis.

including certain fruits and vegetables. Commonly, children allergic to milk, eggs, wheat, or soy outgrow their allergy. Exclusive breast-feeding has been found to be protective against the development of food allergies in early life but to increase the risk of food allergies as a person ages. There is no known preventive strategy to prevent food allergies except to delay introducing allergy-prone foods to infants until the GI tract has had time to mature. The timing for this varies from food to food and from infant to infant. The most common food allergy among adults is shellfish, often first presenting later in life.

Allergic Drug Reactions

Virtually any drug may induce an immunologic response in susceptible people, and any body tissues may be affected. Allergic drug reactions are complex and diverse and may include any of the types of hypersensitivity described previously. A single drug may induce one or more of these states and multiple symptoms. There are no specific characteristics that identify drug-related reactions, although some reactions commonly attributed to drugs (e.g., skin rashes, drug fever, hematologic

reactions, hepatic reactions) rarely occur with plant pollens and other naturally occurring antigens. Usually, however, the body responds to a drug as it does to other foreign materials (antigens). In addition, some reactions may be caused by coloring agents, preservatives, and other additives rather than the drug itself. It may be difficult to recognize in a person with atypical, resolving, or partially treated symptoms, as when skin signs such as urticaria are absent or masked by medications.

Allergic drug reactions should be considered when new signs and symptoms develop or when they differ from the usual manifestations of the illness being treated, especially if a reaction:

- Follows ingestion of a drug, especially one known to produce allergic reactions
- Is unpredictable and occurs in only a few patients when many patients receive the suspected drug
- Occurs approximately 7 to 10 days after initial exposure to the suspected drug (to allow antibody production)
- Follows a previous exposure to the same or similar drug (sensitizing exposure)
- Occurs minutes or hours after a second or subsequent exposure

Allergic Rhinitis

by UNIVERSITY OF MICHIGAN HEALTH SYSTEM

2007. Retrieved from http://www.guideline.gov/content.aspx?id=11684

Researchers completed a systematic review based on expert consensus to update the state of the science on the management of allergic rhinitis. The primary strategy to relieve the symptoms of allergic rhinitis is avoidance of the offending allergen. Should avoidance of allergens not achieve symptoms relief in patients with allergic rhinitis, indications for drug therapy suggest the following:

- Over-the-counter (OTC) second-generation antihistamines, such as loratadine, should provide symptom relief in most situations.
- Prescription drugs may be effective. These include the following:
  - Intranasal corticosteroids, such as fluticasone and flunisolide for adults, and mometasone for children (most potent drugs available to relieve symptoms except for ocular symptoms)
  - Prescription second-generation antihistamine, such as fexofenadine
  - Oral decongestants to decrease nasal swelling congestion
  - If intranasal corticosteroids are not successful or the patient is not a candidate for corticosteroids:
    ○ Leukotriene inhibitors
    ○ Intranasal OTC cromolyn (also available over-the-counter)
    ○ Intranasal antihistamines, such as azelastine (also available over-the-counter)
  - Ocular preparations for patients with allergic conjunctivitis can be considered if symptoms not adequately controlled with oral antihistamines.

IMPLICATIONS FOR NURSING PRACTICE: The use of evidence-based guidelines in the treatment of allergic rhinitis provides effective strategies for symptom relief. Appropriate drug therapy based on best practices maximizes symptom relief and reduces adverse effects, and it also decreases the cost of drug therapy. The nurse should educate patients regarding avoidance of the offending allergen and assess for effective symptom management.

- Occurs after small doses (reduces the likelihood that the reaction is due to dose-related drug toxicity)
- Occurs with other drugs that are chemically or immunologically similar to the suspected drug
- Produces signs and symptoms that differ from the usual pharmacologic actions of the suspected drug
- Produces signs and symptoms usually considered allergic in nature (e.g., anaphylaxis, urticaria, serum sickness)
- Produces similar signs and symptoms to previous allergic reactions to the same or a similar drug
- Increases eosinophils in blood or tissue
- Resolves within a few days of discontinuing the suspected drug

Virtually all drugs have been implicated in **anaphylactic reactions**. Penicillins and other antimicrobials, radiocontrast media, aspirin and other nonsteroidal anti-inflammatory drugs, and antineoplastics such as L-asparaginase and cisplatin are more common offenders. Less common causes include anesthetics (local and general), opioid analgesics, skeletal muscle relaxants used with general anesthetics, and vaccines. Approximately 10% of severe anaphylactic reactions are fatal. In many cases, it is unknown whether clinical manifestations are immunologic or nonimmunologic in origin.

Serum sickness is a delayed hypersensitivity reaction most often caused by drugs, such as antimicrobials. In addition, many drugs that produce anaphylaxis also produce serum sickness. With initial exposure to the antigen, symptoms usually develop within 7 to 10 days and include urticaria, lymphadenopathy, myalgia, arthralgia, and fever. The reaction usually resolves within a few days but may be severe or even fatal. With repeated exposure to the antigen, after prior sensitization of the host, accelerated serum sickness may develop within 2 to 4 days, with similar but often more severe signs and symptoms.

Systemic lupus erythematosus (SLE) is an autoimmune disorder that may be idiopathic from nondrug causes or induced by hydralazine, procainamide, isoniazid, and other drugs. Clinical manifestations vary greatly, depending on the location and severity of the inflammatory and immune processes, and may include skin lesions, fever, pneumonia, anemia, arthralgia, arthritis, nephritis, and others. Drug-induced lupus produces less renal and CNS involvement than idiopathic SLE.

Fever often occurs with allergic drug reactions. It may occur alone, with a skin rash and eosinophilia, or with other drug-induced allergic reactions such as serum sickness, SLE, vasculitis, and hepatitis. Dermatologic conditions (e.g., skin rash, urticaria, inflammation) commonly occur with allergic drug reactions and may be the first and most visible manifestations.

Pseudoallergic Drug Reactions

Pseudoallergic drug reactions resemble immune responses (because histamine and other chemical mediators are released), but they do not produce antibodies or sensitized T lymphocytes. **Anaphylactoid reactions** are like anaphylaxis in terms of immediate occurrence, symptoms (rash or hives, difficulty breathing, swelling of body parts), and life-threatening severity. The main difference is that they are not antigen–antibody reactions and therefore may occur on first exposure to the causative agent. The drugs bind directly to mast cells, activate the cells, and cause the release of histamine and other vasoactive chemical mediators. Contrast media for radiologic diagnostic tests are often implicated.

Drug Therapy

The H_1 receptor antagonist group contains several classes of antihistamines: alkylamines (e.g., brompheniramine),

TABLE 30.1

Drugs Administered to Decrease Histamine Release and the Allergic Response*

Drug Class	Prototype	Other Drugs in the Class
First-generation H_1 receptor antagonists	Diphenhydramine (Benadryl)	Brompheniramine (LoHist) Chlorpheniramine (Chlor-Trimeton) Clemastine (Tavist) Cyproheptadine (Periactin) Dexchlorpheniramine (Polaramine) Hydroxyzine (Vistaril) Phenindamine (Nolahist) Promethazine (Phenergan) Triprolidine (Zymine)
Second-generation H_1 receptor antagonists	Fexofenadine (Allegra)	Azelastine (Astelin) Cetirizine (Zyrtec) Desloratadine (Clarinex) Levocetirizine (Xyzal) Loratadine (Claritin) Olopatadine (Patanol)

*Table 31.1 lists inhaled drugs used to decrease the histamine response.

ethanolamines (e.g., clemastine), piperidines (e.g., cyproheptadine), piperazines (e.g., hydroxyzine), ethylenediamines (tripelennamine), phenothiazines (e.g., promethazine), and a miscellaneous group. Choosing an antihistamine is based on the desired effect, duration of action, adverse effects, and other characteristics of available drugs. For most people, a second-generation H_1 receptor antagonist is the first drug of choice. However, they are quite expensive. If costs are prohibitive for a patient, a first-generation drug may be used with minimal daytime sedation if taken at bedtime or in low initial doses, with gradual increases over a week or 2. Overall, safety should be the determining factor.

Table 30.1 lists the drugs given to block the effects of histamine. For ease of discussion in this chapter, the H_1 receptor antagonists are divided into first-generation and second-generation drugs. The division is distinguished by the level of sedative and anticholinergic effects of the drugs. The following sections and the Drugs at a Glance tables describe selected H_1 receptor and H_2 receptor antagonists. (Chap. 31 discusses inhaled drugs used to decrease the histamine response.)

The receptor activity of drugs blocking the H_2 receptor blocking agents is not related to allergic responses but is used to prevent or treat peptic ulcer disease. Chapter 35 discusses these drugs, cimetidine (Tagamet), ranitidine (Zantac), famotidine (Pepcid), and nizatidine (Axid).

First-Generation H_1 Receptor Antagonists

The oldest H_1 receptor antagonists are relatively inexpensive and widely available. They are effective in the relief of allergic symptoms but lack receptor selectivity. Their anticholinergic activity causes poor tolerability of some of these agents,

especially compared with the second-generation H_1 receptor antagonists. Patient response and occurrence of adverse drug reactions vary greatly among classes and among drugs within classes. **ⓟ Diphenhydramine** (Benadryl), the prototype first-generation antihistamine, has a high incidence of drowsiness and anticholinergic effects.

Drugs that block the H_1 receptors prevent or reduce most of the physiologic effects that histamine normally induces at H_1 receptor sites. Thus, they:

- Inhibit smooth muscle constriction in blood vessels and the respiratory and GI tracts
- Decrease capillary permeability
- Decrease salivation and tear formation

First-generation H_1 antagonists, chemically diverse antihistamines (also called nonselective or sedating agents), bind to both central and peripheral H_1 receptors and can cause CNS depression or stimulation. Many of these drugs are currently marketed with or without a prescription, both alone and in combination formulations such as cold preparations and sleep aids.

Pharmacokinetics

Diphenhydramine is well absorbed after oral administration. Immediate-release oral forms act within 15 to 60 minutes and last 4 to 6 hours. Enteric-coated or sustained-release preparations last 8 to 12 hours. For most forms, administration is oral; for a few forms, administration is parenteral. Metabolism is primarily in the liver, and excretion of metabolites and small amounts of unchanged drug occurs in the urine within 24 hours.

Action

Diphenhydramine and the other first-generation H_1 antagonists are structurally related to histamine and occupy the same

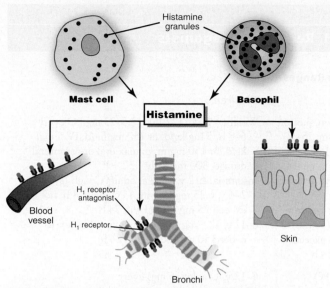

Figure 30.2 Action of antihistamine drugs. Histamine₁ (H₁) receptor antagonists bind to H₁ receptors. This prevents histamine from binding to its receptors and acting on target tissues.

receptor sites as histamine, which prevents histamine from acting on target tissues (Fig. 30.2). Thus, the drugs are effective in inhibiting vascular permeability, edema formation, bronchoconstriction, and pruritus associated with histamine release. They do not prevent histamine release or reduce the amount released.

Use

Indications for diphenhydramine include hypersensitivity reactions (allergic rhinitis, conjunctivitis, dermatitis), motion sickness, insomnia, and parkinsonism. Table 30.2 gives route and dosage information for some of the first-generation H₁ receptor antagonists.

Use in Children

Young children may experience paradoxical excitement after receiving therapeutic dosages of diphenhydramine and other first-generation H₁ receptor antagonists. After overdose, hallucinations, convulsions, and death may occur. For safe use in children, close supervision and appropriate dosages are necessary.

Diphenhydramine is not recommended for use in newborn infants (premature or full-term) or children with chickenpox or a flu-like infection. When used in young children, doses should be small because of drug effects on the brain and nervous system.

Use in Older Adults

Diphenhydramine and other first-generation H₁ receptor antagonists may cause confusion (with impaired thinking, judgment, and memory), dizziness, hypotension, sedation, syncope, unsteady gait, and paradoxical CNS stimulation in older adults. It is possible to misinterpret these effects, especially sedation, as senility or mental depression. Older men with prostatic hypertrophy may have difficulty voiding while taking these

drugs. Some of these adverse reactions derive from anticholinergic effects of the drugs and are likely to be more severe if the patient is also taking other drugs with anticholinergic effects (e.g., tricyclic antidepressants, older antipsychotic drugs, some antiparkinson drugs). However, despite the increased risk of adverse effects, diphenhydramine is sometimes prescribed as a sleep aid for occasional use in older adults. As with many other drugs, smaller-than-usual dosages are indicated.

Use in Patients With Renal Impairment

Little information is available about using first-generation H₁ receptor antagonists in patients with impaired renal function. In patients with severe renal impairment, it is necessary to give diphenhydramine at a dosing interval of 12 to 18 hours.

Use in Patients With Hepatic Impairment

In patients with hepatic impairment, single doses of diphenhydramine are probably safe, but the effects of multiple doses have not been studied.

Use in Patients With Critical Illness

The routine treatment of patients with critical illness does not often involve antihistamines. However, a patient who is having a blood transfusion or a diagnostic test may receive diphenhydramine, often by injection and usually as a single dose, to prevent allergic reactions.

Use in Patients Receiving Home Care

People often take antihistamines in the home setting, especially for allergic rhinitis and other allergic disorders. Most people are familiar with the uses and side effects of antihistamines. The home care nurse is unlikely to be involved in antihistamine drug therapy unless visiting a patient for other care and purposes.

QSEN Safety Alert

If diphenhydramine is being used, the home care nurse needs to assess for drowsiness and safety hazards in the environment (e.g., operating a car or other potentially hazardous machinery).

In most people, tolerance develops to the sedative effects within a few days if they are not taking other sedative-type drugs or alcoholic beverages. If a patient has an allergic disorder, the home care nurse may need to assist in identifying and alleviating environmental allergens (e.g., cigarette smoke, animal dander, dust mites).

Adverse Effects

Diphenhydramine and other first-generation H₁ receptor antagonists usually cause CNS depression (drowsiness, sedation) in therapeutic doses. Some studies have shown that cognitive and performance impairment occurs with the first-generation drugs even when the person does not feel drowsy or impaired. These drugs may cause CNS stimulation (anxiety, agitation) with excessive doses, especially in children. In addition, they have substantial anticholinergic effects (e.g., dry mouth, urinary retention, constipation, blurred vision).

TABLE 30.2

DRUGS AT A GLANCE: First-Generation H₁ Receptor Antagonists

Drug	Pregnancy Category	Routes and Dosage Ranges	
		Adults	*Children*
ⓟ Diphenhydramine (Benadryl)	B	Hypersensitivity reaction, motion sickness, parkinsonism: 25–50 mg PO every 4–8 h; injection 10–50 mg IV or deep IM, increased if necessary to a max daily dose of 400 mg Insomnia: PO 50 mg at bedtime Cough (syrup): 25 mg (10 mL) PO every 4 h, not to exceed 100 mg (40 mL) in 24 h	Weight >10 kg (22 lb), 12.5–25 mg PO every 6–8 h, 5 mg/kg/d, or 150 mg/m²/d; IV 5 mg/kg/d, or 150 mg/m²/d; max oral or parenteral dosage, 300 mg daily Insomnia: ≥12 y, same as adults Cough (syrup) 2–6 y, 6.25 mg (2.5 mL) PO every 4 h, not to exceed 25 mg (10 mL) in 24 h 6–12 y, 12.5 mg (5 mL) PO every 4 h, not to exceed 50 mg (20 mL) in 24 h
Brompheniramine (LoHist)	C	1–2 tablets (6–12 mg) PO every 12 h	6–12 y, 1 tablet (6 mg) every 12 h 12 y and older, same as adults
Chlorpheniramine (Chlor-Trimeton)	C	4 mg PO every 4–6 h; max dose, 24 mg in 24 h Timed-release forms, 8 mg PO every 8–12 h or 12 mg every 12 h; max dose, 24 mg in 24 h	2–6 y, 1 mg PO every 4–6 h 6–12 y, 2 mg PO every 4–6 h; max dose, 12 mg in 24 h 12 y and older, same as adults Timed-release forms, ≥12 y, 8 mg PO every 8–12 h or 12 mg every 12 h; max dose, 24 mg in 24 h
Clemastine (Tavist)	B	Allergic rhinitis: 1.34 mg PO twice daily, increased up to a max of 8.04 mg daily, if necessary Urticaria/angioedema: 2.68 mg PO one to 3 times daily	Allergic rhinitis: 6–12 y (syrup only), 0.67 mg PO twice daily, increased up to a max of 4.02 mg daily, if necessary Urticaria/angioedema: 6–12 y (syrup only), 1.34 mg PO twice daily
Cyproheptadine (Periactin)	B	4 mg PO every 8 h initially, increase if necessary; max dose 0.5 mg/kg/d	Calculate total daily dosage as 0.25 mg/kg or 8 mg/m² 2–6 y, 2 mg every 8–12 h; max dose, 12 mg/d 7–14 y, 4 mg PO every 8–12 h; max dose, 16 mg/d
Dexchlorpheniramine (Polaramine)	B	Regular tablets and syrup, PO 2 mg PO every 4–6 h Timed-release tablets, 4–6 mg PO at bedtime or every 8–12 h	2–5 y, 0.5 mg PO every 4–6 h 6–11 y, 1 mg PO every 4–6 h 12 y and older, same as adults Timed-release tablets, 12 y and older, same as adults 6–12 y, 4 mg once daily, at bedtime
Hydroxyzine (Vistaril)	C	25 mg PO every 6–8 h 25–100 mg IM as needed	Under 6 y, 50 mg PO daily in divided doses Older than 6 y, 50–100 PO mg daily in divided doses
Phenindamine (Nolahist)	B	PO 25 mg every 4–6 h; max dose 150 mg in 24 h	6–11 y, 12.5 mg every PO 4–6 h, max dose 75 mg in 24 h 12 y or older, same as adults
Promethazine (Phenergan)	C	25 mg PO, IM, rectally, every 4–6 h as needed	2 y or older, 12.5 mg every 4–6 h as needed
Triprolidine (Zymine)	C	10 mL (1.2 mg/5 mL) PO every 4–6 h, not to exceed 40 mL/24 h	4 mo–2 y, 1.25 mL every 4–6 h, not to exceed 5 mL/24 h 2–4 y, 2.5 mL every 4–6 h, not to exceed 10 mL/24 h 4–6 y, 3.75 mL every 4–6 h, not to exceed 15 mL/24 h 6–12 y, 5 mL every 4–6 h, not to exceed 20 mL/24 h 12 y or older, same as adults

BOX 30.1 — Drug–Drug Interactions With Diphenhydramine

Drugs That Increase the Effects of Diphenhydramine

- Alcohol and other central nervous system depressants (e.g., antianxiety and antipsychotic agents, opioid analgesics, sedative–hypnotics)
  Increase central nervous system depression
- Monoamine oxidase inhibitors
  Decrease metabolism, increase duration of action, and increase sedative and anticholinergic adverse effects
- Phenothiazines
  Increase the risk of dysrhythmias and excessive drowsiness
- Pramlintide
  Increases the risk of constipation
- Tricyclic antidepressants
  Increase anticholinergic adverse effects

Contraindications

Contraindications or caution is essential with diphenhydramine in pregnant women and in patients with hypersensitivity to the drugs, narrow-angle glaucoma, prostatic hypertrophy, stenosing peptic ulcer, and bladder neck obstruction.

QSEN Safety Alert

It is important not to take diphenhydramine within 14 days of taking a monoamine oxidase inhibitor (isocarboxazid, phenelzine, or tranylcypromine) because of the risk of overstimulation of the sympathetic nervous system.

Nursing Implications

Preventing Interactions

Several drugs interact with diphenhydramine, increasing its effects (Box 30.1). No drugs reportedly decrease the drug's effects, and no herbs appear to interact with it. Diphenhydramine may reduce the effectiveness of tamoxifen if used concomitantly.

Administering the Medication

People may take the oral form of diphenhydramine with or without food. Milk may help if stomach upset occurs.

QSEN Safety Alert

The nurse should give intramuscular antihistamines deeply into a large muscle mass to decrease tissue irritation; he or she injects intravenous (IV) antihistamines slowly, over a few minutes, because severe hypotension may result from rapid IV injection.

To prevent motion sickness, it is necessary to take the drug 30 to 60 minutes before travel.

Assessing for Therapeutic Effects

The nurse observes for a verbal statement of therapeutic effect (relief of symptoms):

- For decreased nasal congestion when given for hypersensitivity
- For decreased dizziness and nausea when taken for motion sickness
- For drowsiness or sleep when given for insomnia

Assessing for Adverse Effects

The nurse assesses for changes in level of consciousness; dryness of mouth, nose, and throat; blurred vision; urinary retention; and constipation. He or she also assesses for gastric effects, such as anorexia, nausea, and vomiting. In addition, particularly in children, it is necessary to observe for paradoxical excitation (restlessness, insomnia, tremors, nervousness, palpitations).

Patient Teaching

For children with allergies, family members should provide day care staff and school contacts with an emergency plan. Box 30.2 outlines patient teaching guidelines for diphenhydramine and other antihistamines.

Other Drugs in the Class

Many of the first-generation H_1 receptor antagonists are available alone and in combination with adrenergic nasal decongestants; analgesics; and allergy, cold, and sinus remedies. Several of them are available as over-the-counter (OTC) drugs, without a prescription.

Brompheniramine (LoHist) causes minimal drowsiness, with adverse effects due to the drug's anticholinergic properties. It has some antidepressant effects, inhibiting reuptake of the neurotransmitter serotonin. However, extensive clinical trials of its antidepressant properties have not been conducted.

Chlorpheniramine (Chlor-Trimeton), like brompheniramine, also causes negligible drowsiness. Chlorpheniramine, too, may have antidepressant properties. It is available in combination with hydrocodone (a narcotic) as the product Tussionex, which is indicated for treatment of cough and upper respiratory symptoms associated with allergy or cold in adults and children 6 years of age and older.

Dexchlorpheniramine (Polaramine), which also produces minimal drowsiness, is used to treat runny nose, watery eyes, hives, itching, and other symptoms of allergies and the common cold. The drug has a similar adverse effects profile as diphenhydramine. Similar interaction patterns exist with other oral H_1 receptor antagonists and diphenhydramine (see Box 30.1).

Hydroxyzine (Vistaril) or promethazine (Phenergan) may be given by injection for nausea and vomiting or to provide sedation but are not usually the first drugs of choice for these indications. Hydroxyzine and promethazine are strong CNS depressants and cause extensive drowsiness. With promethazine, cholestatic jaundice has reportedly occurred, and use of the drug warrants caution. In children, contraindications to promethazine include hepatic disease, Reye's syndrome, history of sleep apnea, or family history of sudden infant death syndrome.

BOX 30.2 **Patient Teaching Guidelines for Antihistamines**

General Considerations

■ Some antihistamines should not be taken by people with glaucoma, peptic ulcer, urinary retention, or pregnancy. Inform your physician if you have any of these conditions, or for over-the-counter (OTC) antihistamines, read the label to see if you should avoid a particular drug.

■ Antihistamines are most effective before exposure to the stimulus that causes histamine release. For instance, you may want to take these drugs during seasons of high pollen and mold counts.

■ Antihistamines may dry and thicken respiratory tract secretions and make them more difficult to remove. Thus, do not take diphenhydramine (Benadryl), which is available OTC, if you have active asthma, bronchitis, or pneumonia.

■ First-generation antihistamines cause drowsiness or dizziness and impair mental alertness, judgment, and physical coordination, especially during the first few days. Do not smoke, drive a car, operate machinery, or perform other tasks requiring alertness and physical dexterity until drowsiness has worn off, to avoid injury.

■ Avoid using sedating antihistamines with other sedative-type drugs (e.g., alcohol, medications to relieve nervousness or produce sleep), to avoid adverse effects and dangerous drug interactions. Alcohol and other drugs that depress brain function may cause excessive sedation, respiratory depression, and death.

■ Do not take more than one antihistamine at a time (e.g., two prescription drugs, two OTC drugs, or a combination of prescription and OTC drugs) because adverse effects are likely. If you do not know whether a particular medication is an antihistamine, consult a health care provider. For example, many OTC cold remedies and "nighttime" or "PM" allergy or sinus preparations contain an antihistamine. In addition, the active ingredient in OTC sleep aids is a sedating antihistamine, usually diphenhydramine (Benadryl).

■ Avoid prolonged exposure to sunlight and use sunscreens and protective clothing; some antihistamines may increase sensitivity to sunlight and risks of skin damage from sunburn.

■ Report adverse effects, such as excessive drowsiness. The health care provider may be able to change drugs or dosages to decrease adverse effects.

■ Store antihistamines out of reach of children to avoid accidental ingestion.

■ If you experience an allergic reaction to a medication, obtain information about the drug thought responsible (including its various names), acceptable alternatives for future drug therapy, and potential sources of the drug. In addition, read the list of ingredients on labels of OTC drug preparations, inform all health care providers about the drug reaction before taking any newly prescribed drug, and wear a medical alert device that lists drugs to be avoided. Note that people may be allergic to additives (e.g., dyes, binders, others) rather than the active drug.

Self-Administration

■ Take antihistamines only as prescribed or as instructed on packages of OTC preparations to increase beneficial effects and decrease adverse effects. If you miss a dose, do not take a double dose.

■ Take most antihistamines with meals to decrease stomach upset. Take loratadine (Claritin) on an empty stomach for better absorption; cetirizine (Zyrtec) and desloratadine (Clarinex) may be taken with or without food. Do not take fexofenadine and related drugs with fruit juice.

■ Do not chew or crush sustained-release tablets and do not open sustained-release capsules. Such actions can cause rapid drug absorption, high blood levels, and serious adverse effects, rather than the slow absorption and prolonged action intended with these products.

NCLEX Success

1. The nurse receives an order to administer diphenhydramine (Benadryl). This medication is recommended for use in
   A. premature or full-term infants
   B. adults to prevent allergic reactions
   C. children with chickenpox
   D. children with a flu-like infection

2. The nurse working in the emergency department anticipates an order of a severe allergic reaction with anaphylaxis, knowing that the drug of choice for severe allergic reactions with anaphylaxis is
   A. diphenhydramine (Benadryl)
   B. cimetidine (Tagamet)
   C. epinephrine
   D. loratadine (Claritin)

3. Due to the action of antihistamines on target tissues, these drugs are effective in producing which of the following actions? (Check all that apply.)
   A. inhibiting vascular permeability
   B. reducing pruritus
   C. minimizing edema formation
   D. preventing histamine release

Clinical Application 30-1

■ Mr. Rudolph tells the nurse that his wife has a prescription for diphenhydramine, which she takes intermittently at bedtime for insomnia. He says that he knows that diphenhydramine is used to treat allergies and asks if he can use it for his own symptoms. How should the nurse respond?

Second-Generation H₁ Receptor Antagonists

Unlike the first-generation H₁ receptor antagonists, the second-generation H₁ receptor antagonists do not readily enter the brain from the blood. ℗ **Fexofenadine** (Allegra), the prototype, and other drugs in this class bind preferentially to peripheral rather than central H₁ receptors. This selectivity significantly reduces the occurrence of adverse drug reactions, such as drowsiness and sedation, while still providing effective relief of allergic conditions.

The second-generation H₁ receptor antagonists are supplanting the first-generation H₁ receptor antagonists in the symptomatic treatment of allergic rhinitis and in the relief of pruritus in urticaria. In addition, these drugs have a mild beneficial effect in chronic asthma. They have not replaced the first-generation H₁ receptor antagonists for treatment of atopic dermatitis or as adjunctive treatment of pruritus and other symptoms in anaphylaxis.

Pharmacokinetics

Fexofenadine is rapidly absorbed and reaches peak serum concentrations in about 2.5 hours. It is 60% to 70% protein bound, and excretion of 95% of the unchanged drug occurs in bile and urine. Its effects last for 12 to 24 hours. The drug does not cross the blood–brain barrier, and whether the drug is excreted in breast milk is unknown.

Action

Fexofenadine competes with histamine for binding to histamine receptor sites, preventing the activation of cells by histamine. Competition for the binding sites prevents activation of the H₁ receptors by histamine, thus preventing allergy symptoms from occurring. Because the drug does not cross the blood–brain barrier, it does not cause the drowsiness associated with first-generation agents.

Use

Health care providers use fexofenadine for seasonal allergic rhinitis, other minor allergies, and urticaria (relief of pruritus). Table 30.3 presents route and dosage information for fexofenadine and the other second-generation antihistamines. A fexofenadine–pseudoephedrine combination (Allegra-D) is also available for cold and allergy relief, and it is important to review the package literature to ensure appropriate dosing.

Use in Older Adults

In general, second-generation antihistamines are much safer than first-generation agents for older adults because they do not impair consciousness, thinking, or ability to perform activities of daily living (e.g., driving a car or operating various machines).

TABLE 30.3

DRUGS AT A GLANCE: Second-Generation H₁ Receptor Antagonists

Drug	Pregnancy Category	Routes and Dosage Ranges	
		Adults	Children
℗ **Fexofenadine** (Allegra)	C	60 mg PO twice daily Renal impairment: 60 mg PO once daily	Younger than 6 y, safety and efficacy have not been established 6–11 y, 30 mg PO twice daily 12 y or older, same as adults
Azelastine (Astelin)	C	Nasal inhalation, two sprays per nostrils every 12 h	12 y or older, same as adults
Cetirizine (Zyrtec)	B	5–10 mg PO once daily Renal or hepatic impairment: 5 mg PO once daily	6 mo–5 y, PO 2.5 mg (one-half tsp) once daily 6 y or older, same as adults
Desloratadine (Clarinex)	C	5 mg PO once daily	12 y or younger, dosage not established 12 y or older, same as adults
Levocetirizine (Xyzal)	B	5 mg PO once daily	6 mo–5 y, 1.25 mg (one-half tsp) PO once daily in evening 6 y or older, same as adults
Loratadine (Claritin)	B	10 mg PO once daily Renal or hepatic impairment: 10 mg PO every other day	2–5 y, 5 mg PO daily 6 y or older, same as adults
Olopadine (Patanol)	C	Nasal inhalation, two sprays per nostrils every 12 h	12 y or older, same as adults

Use in Patients With Renal Impairment

The kidneys play a role in excretion of fexofenadine. Therefore, use of the drug in people with renal impairment warrants caution, and authorities recommend a dosage adjustment.

Use in Patients Receiving Home Care

It is common for fexofenadine to be administered in the home environment, particularly because the drug is available as an OTC preparation. As with first-generation antihistamines, the home care nurse may assess for the drug's effectiveness and provide patient teaching while visiting for other purposes. Patients likely tolerate the drug without serious adverse effects if renal function is not impaired.

Adverse Effects

Adverse effects are usually minor. These include headache, nausea, vomiting, dysmenorrhea, and fatigue.

Contraindications

Contraindications include known sensitivity to fexofenadine.

Nursing Implications

Preventing Interactions

Several drugs may interact with fexofenadine, increasing or decreasing its effects (Box 30.3). Some herbs and foods also interact with this drug (Box 30.4).

Administering the Medication

Administration should occur with water only (fruit juice may decrease absorption). It is necessary to shake oral suspensions completely before administration. Oral disintegrating tablets should remain in the blister pack until use.

BOX 30.3	**Drug Interactions: Fexofenadine**

Drugs That Increase the Effects of Fexofenadine

■ Alcohol
  Increases the potential for sedation
■ Azole antifungals (fluconazole, itraconazole, ketoconazole, miconazole)
  Increase the plasma concentration
■ Macrolide antibacterials (azithromycin, clarithromycin, erythromycin)
  Increase the plasma concentration

Drugs That Decrease the Effects of Fexofenadine

■ Antacids containing magnesium or aluminum
  Decrease the absorption
■ Rifampin
  Decreases the metabolism

BOX 30.4	**Herb and Dietary Interactions: Fexofenadine**

Herbs and Foods That Decrease the Effects of Fexofenadine

■ Fruit juice (apple, orange, grapefruit)
■ St. John's wort

QSEN Safety Alert ❗

Patients should take the tablets on an empty stomach. After placement on the tongue, the tablets dissolve in minutes, and swallowing, with or without water, may occur.

Assessing for Therapeutic Effects

The nurse assesses for relief of symptoms, including decreased nasal congestion with seasonal allergic rhinitis. In addition, he or she assesses for relief of pruritus in urticaria.

Assessing for Adverse Effects

The nurse observes for headache, nausea, vomiting, and fatigue. In women, it is also necessary to assess for dysmenorrhea.

Patient Teaching

Box 30.2 summarizes the patient teaching guidelines for antihistamines.

Other Drugs in the Class

Other second-generation H_1 receptor antagonists have similar actions and adverse effect profiles. Some have sedative properties when taken at doses that exceed the recommended dose, including loratadine and desloratadine, although cetirizine and intranasal azelastine may cause sedation at the recommended dose.

Azelastine (Astelin) and olopatadine (Patanol) are second-generation H_1 receptor antagonists that have been formulated as nasal sprays for topical use.

QSEN Safety Alert ❗

Olopatadine produces less sedation than azelastine, but patients should not perform activities that require alertness until they are sure they can engage in such activities safely.

Azelastine is available as an OTC preparation and may be used in children 5 years and older. Olopatadine is only available by prescription as a nasal spray. (However, olopatadine eye drops are available OTC.) Intranasal H_1 receptor antagonists are considered a first-line treatment for allergic rhinitis, although they are generally less effective than intranasal corticosteroids. Intranasal H_1 receptor antagonists are as effective as or superior to oral second-generation antihistamines for treating seasonal allergic rhinitis. Intranasal antihistamines have a clinically significant effect on nasal congestion. The nasal spray leaves an unpleasant taste; however, sniffing gently through the nose after each spray minimizes this taste. When applied to nasal mucosa, the drugs produce peak levels in 2 to 3 hours and last 12 to 24 hours. They are metabolized in the liver to an active metabolite and excreted mainly in feces.

Cetirizine (Zyrtec) is an active metabolite of hydroxyzine that causes less drowsiness than hydroxyzine. It reaches maximal serum concentration in 1 hour and is about 93% protein bound. About half of a dose is metabolized in the liver; the other half is excreted unchanged in the urine. The drug may be used in children 2 years of age and older. Syrup formulations are available for use in younger children. The drug can be given with food, to decrease GI upset, or without food.

Levocetirizine (Xyzal) has an onset of action of 1 hour, and a single daily dose provides antihistamine activity for 28 hours. The drug can be used with children 6 years and older. It can be given with food, to decrease GI effects, or without food.

Loratadine (Claritin) produces effects within 1 to 3 hours, which reach a maximum in 8 to 12 hours and last 24 hours or longer. The drug is metabolized in the liver, and its long duration of action is due, in part, to an active metabolite. Loratadine may be used in children 2 years of age and older. The drug should be taken on an empty stomach.

Desloratadine (Clarinex) is an active metabolite of loratadine that is marketed by same manufacturer. Desloratadine seems to offer no advantage over loratadine or other second-generation drugs. The drug may be used in children 12 years and older. It can be administered with food, to decrease GI effects, or without food.

The Nursing Process

Assessment

- Assess the patient's condition in relation to disorders for which antihistamines are used. For the patient with known allergies, try to determine the factors that precipitate or relieve allergic reactions and specific signs and symptoms experienced during a reaction.
- Assess every patient for a potential hypersensitivity reaction. For example, it is standard practice on first contact to ask a patient if he or she has any food, drug, or other allergies. The health care provider is likely to get more complete information by asking patients about allergic reactions to specific drugs (e.g., antibiotics such as penicillin, local anesthetics) rather than asking if they are allergic to or cannot take any drugs.
- If a drug allergy is identified, ask about specific signs and symptoms as well as any drugs currently being taken. With previous exposure and sensitization to the same or a similar drug, immediate allergic reactions may occur. With a new drug, antibody formation and allergic reactions usually require a week or longer. Most reactions appear within a month of starting a drug.

- When a suspected allergic reaction occurs (e.g., skin rash, fever, edema, dyspnea), interview the patient or consult medical records about the drug, dose, route, and time of administration. In addition, evaluate all the drugs a patient is taking as a potential cause of the reaction. This assessment may involve searching drug literature to see if the suspected drug is associated with allergic reactions and discussion with physicians and pharmacists.

Nursing Diagnoses

- Risk for injury related to drowsiness with first-generation antihistamines
- Deficient knowledge: safe and accurate drug use
- Deficient knowledge: strategies for minimizing exposure to allergens and irritants

Planning/Goals

The patient will

- Experience relief of symptoms
- Take antihistamines accurately
- Avoid hazardous activities if sedated from antihistamines
- Avoid preventable adverse drug effects
- Avoid taking sedative-type antihistamines with alcohol or other sedative drugs

Nursing Interventions

The nurse will

- For patients with known allergies, assist in identifying and avoiding precipitating factors when possible. If it is a drug allergy, encourage the patient to carry a medical alert device that identifies the drug.
- Monitor the patient closely for excessive drowsiness during the first few days of therapy with antihistamines known to cause sedation
- Encourage a fluid intake of 2000 to 3000 mL daily, if not contraindicated
- When indicated, obtain an order and administer an antihistamine before situations known to elicit allergic reactions (e.g., blood transfusions, diagnostic tests that involve contrast media).
- For children with allergies, provide all family members, day care staff, and school personnel with an emergency plan.

Evaluation

- Observe for relief of symptoms.
- Interview and observe for correct drug usage.
- Interview and observe for excessive drowsiness.

Clinical Application 30-2

- Mr. Rudolph informs the nurse that he thinks he is allergic to the aspirin that he has been taking for his coronary artery disease because he becomes nauseated after taking his daily dose. What questions should the nurse ask Mr. Rudolph to help determine whether he has an allergy to aspirin?

4. In explaining options for antihistamine medications to a patient, second-generation H_1 antagonists differ from first-generation H_1 antagonists in that they:

A. cause greater central nervous system sedation
B. are available only by prescription
C. are less expensive
D. do not cross the blood–brain barrier

5. A patient has asked for an antihistamine to relieve symptoms of an upper respiratory infection. The nurse explains that studies have demonstrated that for treatment of the common cold, antihistamines:

A. are effective in relieving cold symptoms
B. do not relieve symptoms and are not recommended
C. should be compounded with other products to be effective
D. relieve nonallergenic symptoms only

Key Concepts

- Virtually any drug may induce an immunologic response in susceptible people, and any body tissue may be affected.

- Allergic rhinitis is inflammation of nasal mucosa caused by a type I hypersensitivity reaction to inhaled allergens.

- Anaphylaxis is a type I hypersensitivity reaction that is uncommon and does not occur on first exposure to an antigen; it occurs with a second or later exposure, after antibody formation was induced by an earlier exposure.

- Some food allergens such as shellfish, egg, milk, peanuts, and tree nuts have a higher inherent risk for triggering anaphylaxis than others.

- Patients with drug allergies should wear a medical alert bracelet identifying the drug.

- First-generation H_1 receptor antagonists may cause drowsiness and decreased mental alertness in both children and adults.

- First-generation H_1 receptor antagonists have substantial anticholinergic effects (e.g., cause dry mouth, urinary retention, constipation, blurred vision).

- Second-generation H_1 receptor antagonists cause less CNS depression because they are selective for peripheral H_1 receptors and do not cross the blood–brain barrier.

- For children with allergies, provide all family members as well as day care and school contacts with an emergency plan.

Critical Thinking Questions

30-1. A man comes to the clinic with a red, itchy rash on both forearms. Depending on the severity of the rash, the nurse practitioner suggests treatment with topical or systemic antihistamines (or both).

- What does the nurse's assessment include?
- What does the likely plan of care include?

References and Resources

Drug facts and comparisons. (Updated monthly). St. Louis, MO: Facts and Comparisons.

Guyton, A. C., & Hall, J. E. (2006). *Textbook of medical physiology* (11th ed.). Philadelphia, PA: W. B. Saunders.

Joint Task Force on Practice Parameters, American Academy of Allergy, Asthma and Immunology, American College of Allergy, Asthma and Immunology, Joint Council of Allergy, Asthma and Immunology. (2005). The diagnosis and management of anaphylaxis: An updated practice parameter. *Journal of Allergy and Clinical Immunology, 115*(3 Suppl 2), S483–S523.

Karch, A. M. (2012). *2012 Lippincott's nursing drug guide.* Philadelphia, PA: Lippincott Williams & Wilkins.

Kobrynski, L. J. (2007). Anaphylaxis. *Clinical Pediatric Emergency Medicine, 8,* 110–116.

Lacy, C. F., Armstrong, L. L., Goldman, M. P., & Lance, L. L. (2010). *Lexi-Comp's drug information handbook* (19th ed.). Hudson, OH: American Pharmaceutical Association.

Lambert, M. (2009). Practice parameters for managing allergic rhinitis. *American Family Physician, 80*(1), 79–85.

Lazenby, R. B. (2010). *Handbook of pathophysiology* (4th ed.). Philadelphia, PA: Lippincott Williams & Wilkins.

Porth, C. M. (2009). *Pathophysiology: Concepts of altered health status.* (8th ed.). Philadelphia, PA: Lippincott Williams & Wilkins.

Simons, F. E. (2007). Risk assessment in anaphylaxis: Current and future approaches. *Journal of Allergy and Clinical Immunology, 120*(1 Suppl), S2–S24.

31 Drug Therapy for Asthma and Bronchoconstriction

Clinical Application Case Study

Terry Lee, a 38-year-old man, presents to the emergency department in severe respiratory distress, with profound dyspnea, wheezing, and circumoral cyanosis. He received a diagnosis of asthma at age 10. Mr. Lee is admitted to the intensive care unit. His treatment regimen includes albuterol via inhalation every 20 minutes for four doses and intravenous corticosteroids every 6 hours.

KEY TERMS

Airway hyperresponsiveness: exaggerated bronchoconstrictive response to stimuli

Bronchospasm (also called bronchoconstriction): constriction of the air passages of the lung (as in asthma) by spasmodic contraction of the bronchial muscles

Leukotrienes: strong chemical mediators of bronchoconstriction and inflammation, the major pathologic features of asthma

Maintenance inhalant medications: long-term control beta$_2$-agonists used to achieve and maintain prophylactic control of persistent asthma

Mast cells: cells releasing substances that produce bronchoconstriction and inflammation in response to causative stimuli

Rescue inhalant medications: quick-relief, short-acting beta$_2$-agonists used during periods of acute symptoms and exacerbations

Status asthmaticus: acute, severe asthma

Triggers: factors that initiate asthma symptoms

Work-exacerbated asthma: adverse respiratory outcome resulting from work-related conditions

TABLE 31.1

Drugs Administered for the Treatment of Asthma

Drug Class	Prototype	Other Drugs in the Class
Adrenergics	Albuterol (Proventil, Ventolin, AccuNeb)	Epinephrine (Adrenalin) Formoterol (Foradil) Levalbuterol (Xopenex [MDI], Xopenex HFA) Metaproterenol (Alupent) Pirbuterol Acetate (Maxair) Salmeterol (Serevent) Terbutaline (Brethine)
Anticholinergics	Ipratropium bromide (Atrovent)	Tiotropium (Spiriva)
Xanthines	Theophylline (aminophylline, Theochron)	
Corticosteroids	Beclomethasone (Beconase AQ, QVAR)	Budesonide (Pulmicort Turbuhaler) Ciclesonide (Omnaris) Flunisolide (AeroBid, Aerospan) Fluticasone (Flonase) Fluticasone aerosol (Flovent) Fluticasone powder (Flovent Rotadisk) Mometasone (Asmanex Twisthaler, Nasonex) Triamcinolone (Azmacort) Hydrocortisone sodium phosphate and sodium succinate Prednisone Methylprednisolone sodium succinate
Leukotriene modifiers	Montelukast (Singulair)	Zafirlukast (Accolate)
Adjuvant medications		
Mast cell stabilizer	Cromolyn (NasalCrom)	
Immunosuppressant monoclonal antibody	Omalizumab (Xolair)	

Other adrenergic drugs affect multiple adrenergic receptors and have many clinical uses; other chapters discuss these drugs more extensively (see Chaps. 29 and 58).

Administering bronchodilators by inhalation is most effective and the treatment of first choice to relieve acute asthma. Two general types of inhaled beta$_2$-adrenergic agonists are used for asthma management: **rescue inhalant medications** (quick-relief, short-acting drugs) used during periods of acute symptoms and exacerbations and **maintenance inhalant medications** (long-term control drugs used to achieve and maintain prophylactic control of persistent asthma). Box 31.3 lists the rescue and maintenance medications used in asthma therapy. ⓟ **Albuterol** (Proventil, Ventolin, AccuNeb), the prototype adrenergic bronchodilator, is a rescue medication.

Pharmacokinetics

Albuterol is rapidly absorbed following oral administration. With the oral drug, the onset of action is 15 to 30 minutes (extended release, 30 minutes), the peak is 2 to 3 hours, and the duration of action is 8 to 12 hours. With the inhaled drug (MDI), the onset of action is 5 to 15 minutes, the peak activity is 1 to 1 1/2; hours, and the duration of action is 3 to 6 hours. The drug quickly undergoes extensive metabolism in the liver. It enters breast milk.

Action

Albuterol and other drugs in the class stimulate beta$_2$-adrenergic receptors in the smooth muscle of bronchi and bronchioles. The receptors, in turn, stimulate the enzyme adenyl cyclase to increase production of cyclic AMP. The increased cyclic AMP produces bronchodilation.

BOX 31.3   Rescue and Maintenance Beta$_2$-Agonist Inhaled Medications

Short-acting rescue medications
■ Albuterol
■ Metaproterenol
■ Levalbuterol
■ Pirbuterol
■ Albuterol/ipratropium (combines a beta$_2$-agonist and an inhaled anticholinergic)

Long-acting maintenance medications
■ Formoterol
■ Salmeterol
■ Salmeterol/fluticasone (combines a beta$_2$-agonist bronchodilator and an inhaled steroid)
■ Formoterol/budesonide (combines a beta$_2$-agonist bronchodilator and an inhaled steroid)

Use

Health care providers use albuterol to treat or prevent bronchospasm in people with asthma and other reversible obstructive airway disease. They also use the drug to prevent exercise-induced bronchospasm. Table 31.2 gives route and dosage information for albuterol and other adrenergic bronchodilators. In general, children and adolescents may take antiasthmatic medications for the same indications as for adults.

Use in Older Adults

Older adults often have chronic pulmonary disorders for which albuterol and other bronchodilators are used.

QSEN Safety Alert

The main risks with adrenergic bronchodilators, particularly in older adults, are excessive cardiac and central nervous system (CNS) stimulation.

TABLE 31.2

DRUGS AT A GLANCE: Adrenergic Bronchodilators

Drug	Pregnancy Category	Routes and Dosage Ranges	
		Adults	*Children*
Ⓟ **Albuterol** (Proventil, Ventolin, AccuNeb)	C	Inhalation* aerosol (90 mcg/actuation), 1–2 oral inhalations every 4–6 h; prevention of exercise-induced bronchospasm, 2 inhalations 1 min before exercise Inhalation solution via nebulizer, 2.5 mg 3–4 times daily (in 2.5 mL sterile saline, over 5–15 min) Regular tablets, 2–4 mg PO 3–4 times daily Extended-release tablets, Proventil Repetabs 4–8 mg PO every 12 h initially; increase if necessary to a max of 32 mg/d, in divided doses, every 12 h	Inhalation aerosol, 4 y and older (12 y and older for Proventil), same as adults Nebulizer solution, 12 y and older, same as adults; 2–12 y (AccuNeb), 1.25 mg 3–4 times daily, as needed, over 5–15 min Regular tablets, 12 y and older, same as adults; 6–12 y, 2 mg 3–4 times daily Extended-release tablets: 12 y and older, same as adults 6–12 y, 4 mg PO every 12 h initially; increase if necessary to a max of 24 mg/d, in divided doses every 12 h
Epinephrine (Adrenalin)	C	Aqueous solution (epinephrine 1:1000), 0.3–0.5 mg Sub-Q; dose may be repeated after 20 min if necessary for 3 doses Inhalation by nebulizer, 1–3 inhalations of 2.25% racemic epinephrine in 2.5 mL normal saline up to every 3 h	Aqueous solution (epinephrine 1:1000), 0.01 mL/kg Sub-Q every 4 h as needed; single dose should not exceed 0.5 mL Inhalation, same as adults for nebulizer
Formoterol (Foradil)	C	Oral inhalation by special inhaler (Aerolizer), 12 mcg (contents of 1 capsule) twice daily, every 12 h	5 y and older, same as adults
Levalbuterol (Xopenex [MDI], Xopenex HFA)	C	Nebulizer, 0.63–1.25 mg 3 times daily, every 6–8 h MDI, 1–2 puffs every 4–6 h	12 y and older, same as adults 6–11 y, nebulizer, 0.31 mg 3 times daily, every 6–8 h MDI ≤4 y same as adults
Metaproterenol (Alupent)	C	Inhalation,* 2–3 inhalations (0.65 mg/dose), every 3–4 h; max dose, 12 inhalations/d	Inhalation, not recommended for use in children <12 y
Pirbuterol acetate (Maxair)	C	Inhalation by special inhaler (Autohaler),* 2 inhalations (0.20 mg/dose), every 3–4 h; max dose, 12 inhalations/d	12 y and older, same as adults
Salmeterol (Serevent)	C	Inhalation powder, 1 inhalation (50 mcg) every 12 h	<12 y, dosage not established Inhalation powder: 4 y and older, same as adults
Terbutaline (Brethine)	B	2.5–5 mg PO every 6–8 h; max dose, 15 mg/d 0.25 mg Sub-Q, repeated in 15–30 min if necessary, every 4–6 h	2.5 mg PO 3 times per day for children 12 y and older; max dose, 7.5 mg/d Sub-Q dosage not established

*Short-acting adrenergic bronchodilators are used mainly by inhalation, as needed, rather than on a regular schedule; MDI, metered-dose inhaler.

As with other populations, administering the medications by inhalation and giving the lowest effective dose decrease adverse effects.

Use in Patients With Critical Illness

People who are critically ill often use albuterol. Larger doses of bronchodilators (inhaled, systemic, or both) are usually required to relieve the symptoms of acute, severe bronchoconstriction or status asthmaticus. Then, it is necessary to reduce doses to the smallest effective amounts to attain the most therapeutic effects and produce the fewest adverse effects.

Use in Patients Receiving Home Care

Home administration of albuterol is common. Visits by a home care nurse should include assessment that the patient follows directions for administration; is not taking the drug more often than prescribed; is using the inhaler correctly; and is not manifesting signs of adverse effects, including excessive cardiac and CNS stimulation.

Adverse Effects

Administration of albuterol by MDI is associated with fewer systemic effects than administration of higher dosages orally or by nebulizer. Muscle tremor is the most frequent adverse effect. Major adverse effects are excessive cardiac and CNS stimulation. Symptoms of cardiac stimulation include angina, tachycardia, and palpitations. Symptoms of CNS stimulation consist of agitation, anxiety, insomnia, seizures, and tremors. Other reported effects may include serious dysrhythmias and cardiac arrest.

Contraindications

Contraindications to albuterol include known hypersensitivity to the drug, as well as cardiac tachydysrhythmias and severe coronary artery disease. Caution is warranted in hypertension, hyperthyroidism, diabetes mellitus, and seizure disorders.

Nursing Implications

Preventing Interactions

Some drugs interact with albuterol. Beta-blockers inhibit bronchodilation and can induce bronchospasm in patients with asthma who are taking albuterol. Thyroid hormones, theophylline, and some cold products can enhance the stimulatory adverse effects of the drug. Monoamine oxidase inhibitors should be avoided within 14 days of initiating treatment with albuterol to prevent hypertensive crisis. Caffeine-containing products, such as coffee, tea, or cola drinks, can also increase the adverse effects of cardiac and CNS stimulation.

Administering the Medication

Self-administration of albuterol and the other beta$_2$-agonists is usually by MDI. Patients should use an albuterol inhaler before they use any other inhaler. This opens the airways and allows for better absorption of the other drug. The patient should wait 5 minutes or more between using different inhalers, such as one for a corticosteroid. Although most drug references still give a regular dosing schedule (e.g., every 4–6 hours) for

beta$_2$-agonists, asthma experts recommend that the drugs be used when needed (e.g., to treat acute dyspnea or prevent dyspnea during exercise). With overuse, they lose their bronchodilating effects because the beta$_2$-adrenergic receptors become unresponsive to stimulation. (However, this tolerance does not occur with the long-acting beta$_2$-agonists.)

Assessing for Therapeutic Effects

The nurse observes for decreased dyspnea, wheezing, and respiratory secretions; relief of bronchospasm and wheezing; reduced rate and improved quality of respirations and pulmonary function; and reduced anxiety and restlessness.

Assessing for Adverse Effects

The nurse observes for tachycardia, dysrhythmias, palpitations, restlessness, agitation, and insomnia. These signs and symptoms result from cardiac and CNS stimulation.

Patient Teaching

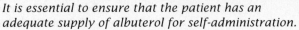

QSEN Safety Alert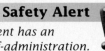

It is essential to ensure that the patient has an adequate supply of albuterol for self-administration.

In addition, the nurse helps patients recognize acute asthma attacks and have a plan to treat (or seek help for) exacerbations before respiratory distress becomes severe. Box 31.4 summarizes patient teaching guidelines for antiasthmatic drugs, including albuterol.

Other Drugs in the Class

Epinephrine (Adrenalin) is an adrenergic that may be injected subcutaneously in an acute attack of bronchoconstriction, with therapeutic rescue effects in approximately 5 minutes and lasting for approximately 4 hours. However, an inhaled selective beta$_2$-agonist is the drug of choice in this situation. Delivery by aerosol or nebulization of other selective beta$_2$-agonists is effective, even to young children and to patients on mechanical ventilation, and there is seldom a need to give epinephrine or other nonselective adrenergic drugs by injection. Cardiac stimulation is an adverse effect of bronchodilators, and in addition to beta$_2$-receptor stimulation, epinephrine also stimulates beta$_1$-adrenergic receptors in the heart to increase the rate and force of contraction.

Epinephrine is no longer available without prescription in a pressurized aerosol form (e.g., Primatene Mist); the preparation used chlorofluorocarbons (CFCs) to propel the medicine out of the inhaler. An international accord signed by the United States agreed to phase out substances that deplete the ozone layer, such as CFCs. Most prescription inhalers use hydrofluoroalkane (HFA) as a propellant.

Levalbuterol (Xopenex, Xopenex [HFA]) and pirbuterol (Maxair) are short-acting beta$_2$-adrenergic agonists used for prevention and treatment of bronchoconstriction. Pirbuterol will not be manufactured or dispensed in the United States after December 31, 2013, because it uses CFCs as a propellant; patients should be taking another drug prior to that date.

Formoterol (Foradil) and salmeterol (Serevent) are long-acting beta$_2$-adrenergic agonists used only for prophylaxis of acute bronchoconstriction. They are not effective in acute

BOX 31.4　　Patient Teaching Guidelines: Antiasthmatic Drugs

General Considerations

■ Asthma and other chronic lung diseases are characterized by constant inflammation of the airways and periodic or persistent labored breathing from constriction or narrowing of the airways. Antiasthmatic drugs are often given in combination to combat these problems. Thus, it is extremely important to know the type and purpose of each drug.

■ Except for the short-acting, inhaled bronchodilators (e.g., albuterol), antiasthmatic medications are used long term to control symptoms and prevent acute asthma attacks. This means they must be taken on a regular schedule and continued when symptom free.

■ When an asthma attack (i.e., acute bronchospasm with shortness of breath, wheezing respirations, cough) occurs, the only fast-acting, commonly used medication to relieve these symptoms is an inhaled, short-acting bronchodilator (e.g., albuterol). Other inhaled and oral drugs are not effective and should not be used.

■ Try to prevent symptoms. For example, respiratory infections can precipitate difficulty in breathing. Avoiding infections (e.g., by good hand hygiene, avoiding people with infections, annual influenza vaccinations, and other measures) can prevent acute asthma attacks. If you are allergic to tobacco smoke, perfume, or flowers, try to avoid or minimize exposure. Other substances that irritate breathing passages may include aerosol hair spray, antiperspirants, cleaning products, and automobile exhaust.

■ A common cause of acute asthma attacks is not taking medications correctly. Some studies indicate that one third to two thirds of patients with asthma do not comply with instructions for using their medications. Factors that contribute to nonadherence with drug therapy include long-term use, expense, and adverse effects. If you have difficulty taking medications as prescribed, discuss the situation with a health care provider. Cheaper medications or lower doses may be effective alternatives. Just stopping the medications may precipitate acute breathing problems.

■ If unable to prevent symptoms, early recognition and treatment may help prevent severe distress and hospitalizations. Signs of impending difficulty include increased needs for bronchodilator inhalers, activity limitations, waking at night because of asthma symptoms, and variability in the peak expiratory flow rate (PEFR), if you use a PEFR meter at home. The first treatment is to use a short-acting, inhaled bronchodilator. If this does not improve breathing, seek emergency care.

■ Keep adequate supplies of medications on hand. Missing a few doses of long-term control or "preventive" medications may precipitate an acute asthma attack; not using an inhaled bronchodilator for early breathing difficulty may lead to more severe problems and the need for emergency treatment or hospitalization.

■ Be sure you can use your metered-dose inhalers correctly. According to several research studies, many patients do not.

■ Drinking 2 to 3 quarts of fluids, as appropriate, daily helps thin secretions in the throat and lungs and makes them easier to remove.

■ Avoid excessive intake of caffeine-containing fluids such as coffee, tea, and cola drinks. These beverages may increase bronchodilation but also may increase heart rate and cause palpitations, nervousness, and insomnia with bronchodilating drugs.

■ Obtain an influenza vaccine annually and a pneumococcal vaccine at least once if you have chronic lung disease.

■ Inform all health care providers about the medications you are taking and do not take over-the-counter drugs or herbal supplements without consulting a health care provider. Some drugs can decrease beneficial effects or increase adverse effects of antiasthmatic medications. For example, over-the-counter nasal decongestants, asthma remedies, cold remedies, and antisleep medications can increase the rapid heartbeat, palpitations, and nervousness often associated with bronchodilators. With herbal remedies, none are as effective as standard antiasthmatic medication, and they may cause serious or life-threatening adverse effects.

Self-Administration

■ Follow instructions carefully. Better breathing with minimal adverse effects depends on accurate use of prescribed medications. If help is needed with metered-dose inhalers, consult a health care provider.

■ Use short-acting bronchodilator inhalers as needed, not on a regular schedule. If desired effects are not achieved or if symptoms worsen, inform the prescribing physician. Do not increase dosage or frequency of taking medication. Overuse increases adverse drug effects and decreases drug effectiveness.

■ If taking formoterol or salmeterol, which are long-acting, inhaled bronchodilators, do not use more often than every 12 hours. If constricted breathing occurs, use a short-acting bronchodilator inhaler between doses of a long-acting drug. Salmeterol does not relieve acute shortness of breath because it takes approximately 20 minutes to start acting and 1 to 4 hours to achieve maximal bronchodilating effects.

■ If taking an oral or inhaled corticosteroid, take on a regular schedule, at approximately the same time each day. The purpose of these drugs is to relieve inflammation in the airways and prevent acute respiratory distress. They are not effective unless taken regularly.

■ If taking oral theophylline, take fast-acting preparations before meals with a full glass of water, at regular intervals around the clock. If gastrointestinal upset occurs, take with food. Take long-acting preparations every 8 to 12 hours; do not chew or crush.

■ Take zafirlukast 1 hour before or 2 hours after a meal; montelukast and zileuton may be taken with or without food. Take montelukast in the evening or at bedtime. This schedule provides maximum beneficial effects during the night and early morning, when asthma symptoms often occur or worsen.

(Continued on page 576)

BOX 31.4 **Patient Teaching Guidelines: Antiasthmatic Drugs** (Continued)

■ Use inhalers correctly:

1. Shake well immediately before each use.
2. Remove the cap from the mouthpiece.
3. Exhale to the end of a normal breath.
4. With the inhaler in the upright position, place the mouthpiece just inside the mouth, and use the lips to form a tight seal or hold the mouthpiece approximately two finger-widths from the open mouth.
5. While pressing down on the inhaler, take a slow, deep breath for 3 to 5 seconds, hold the breath for approximately 10 seconds, and exhale slowly.

6. Wait 3 to 5 minutes before taking a second inhalation of the drug.
7. Rinse the mouth with water after each use.
8. Rinse the mouthpiece and store the inhaler away from heat.
9. If you have difficulty using an inhaler, ask your provider about a spacer device (a tube attached to the inhaler that makes it easier to use).

---

attacks because they have a slower onset of action than the short-acting drugs (up to 20 minutes for salmeterol). Effects last 12 hours and the drugs should not be taken more frequently. If additional bronchodilating medication is needed, a short-acting agent (e.g., albuterol) should be used. The FDA has issued a **BLACK BOX WARNING** ◆ indicating that initiating salmeterol in people with significantly worsening or acutely deteriorating asthma may be life threatening.

Metaproterenol is a relatively selective, intermediate-acting beta$_2$-adrenergic agonist that may be given orally or by MDI. It is used to treat acute bronchospasm and to prevent exercise-induced asthma. In high doses, metaproterenol loses some of its selectivity and may cause cardiac and CNS stimulation.

Terbutaline (Brethine) is a relatively selective beta$_2$-adrenergic agonist and a long-acting bronchodilator. The drug is usually well tolerated, and when symptoms occur, they are minor and require little or no treatment. Common adverse effects include shakiness, drowsiness, and headaches. When given subcutaneously, terbutaline loses its selectivity and has little advantage over epinephrine. The drug is used to treat preterm labor, although it is not approved for this use, has not been shown to be effective, and causes some safety concerns. The nurse should be aware of the FDA's recommendation that oral and injectable terbutaline should not be used for prevention or treatment of preterm labor.

Clinical Application 31-1

- Mr. Lee may experience adverse effects if albuterol is administered as ordered. For what signs and symptoms should the nurse be alert?

- Mr. Lee's wife is at his bedside. She expresses concern about his treatment with IV corticosteroids, stating that she has heard that many adverse effects are associated with these drugs. Discuss the rationale for the use of IV corticosteroids in this case.

Anticholinergics

The anticholinergic bronchodilators are most useful in the long-term management of asthma and other conditions producing bronchoconstriction, such as chronic bronchitis and emphysema. (For additional information about these drugs,

see Chap. 47.) The two drugs in the class, the prototype ⓟ **Ipratropium** (Atrovent) and tiotropium, are ineffective in relieving acute bronchospasm by themselves, and they act synergistically with other adrenergic bronchodilators. Prescribers may order them for concomitant use. The drugs improve lung function about 10% to 15% over an inhaled beta$_2$-agonist alone.

Pharmacokinetics

Ipratropium is rapidly absorbed via inhalation with an onset of action within 5 to 15 minutes, a peak effect in 1½ to 2 hours, and a duration of action of 2 to 5 hours. Absorption of the drug is negligible, with excretion in the kidneys and in the feces. Only about 15% of the drug reaches the lower airways.

Action

Ipratropium is chemically related to atropine and blocks the muscarinic acetylcholine receptors in the smooth muscles of the bronchi in the lungs, inhibiting bronchoconstriction and mucus secretion.

Use

Originally, ipratropium was formulated to be taken by inhalation for maintenance therapy of bronchoconstriction associated with asthma, chronic bronchitis, and emphysema. Improved pulmonary function usually occurs in a few minutes. Other uses include treatment of rhinorrhea associated with allergic rhinitis and the common cold. Table 31.3 presents route and dosage information for anticholinergics such as ipratropium.

Use in Patients With Critical Illness

Ipratropium can be used in the critical care setting, but it is ineffective in relieving acute bronchospasm. The drug may work synergistically with other adrenergic bronchodilators, and concomitant use may be effective. In patients who are critically ill, administering by nebulization may be necessary.

Use in Patients Receiving Home Care

Ipratropium is used in the home setting. The drug poses minimal risk of adverse effects. A major role of the home care nurse is to assist patients in using the inhaled drug safely and effectively. Several studies have indicated that many people do not use MDIs and other inhalation devices correctly. If possible, the

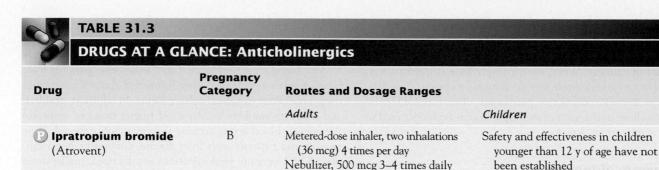

TABLE 31.3

DRUGS AT A GLANCE: Anticholinergics

Drug	Pregnancy Category	Routes and Dosage Ranges	
		Adults	Children
Ⓟ **Ipratropium bromide** (Atrovent)	B	Metered-dose inhaler, two inhalations (36 mcg) 4 times per day Nebulizer, 500 mcg 3–4 times daily every 4–6 h	Safety and effectiveness in children younger than 12 y of age have not been established
Tiotropium (Spiriva)	C	One tablet (18 mcg) in HandiHaler once daily	Dosage not established

home care nurse needs to observe a patient using an inhalation device. If the nurse detects errors in technique, further education may be necessary. With inhaled medications, a spacer device may be useful, especially for children and older adults, because less muscle coordination is required to administer a dose. Adverse effects may be minimized, as well.

Adverse Effects

Absorption of ipratropium is poor, and it produces few systemic effects. The most common adverse effects are cough, nervousness, nausea, gastrointestinal (GI) upset, headache, and dizziness.

Contraindications

Ipratropium is contraindicated with known hypersensitivity to the drug or to atropine and related substances. Caution is recommended with use in patients with narrow-angle glaucoma, prostatic hypertrophy, and bladder neck obstruction because ipratropium can worsen these conditions.

Nursing Implications

Preventing Interactions

In general, ipratropium has been shown to have limited drug–drug interactions (Box 31.5) and no herbal interactions. When given as a nasal spray, no interactions reportedly occur.

Administering the Medication

It is appropriate to mix ipratropium bromide inhalation solution in the nebulizer with albuterol or metaproterenol if the mixture is used within 1 hour.

BOX 31.5 | Drug Interactions: Ipratropium

Drugs That Increase the Effects of Ipratropium
- Atropine and other anticholinergic drugs, such as diphenhydramine, dimenhydrinate
  Increase the anticholinergic effects

Drugs That Decrease the Effects of Ipratropium
- Acetylcholinesterase inhibitors
  Decrease in therapeutic effect

QSEN Safety Alert ❗

Administering anticholinergic drugs via the respiratory route instead of the systemic route results in less thickening of respiratory secretions and therefore a reduced incidence of mucus-plugged airways.

Assessing for Therapeutic Effects

The nurse assesses for a reduced rate and improved quality of respirations and pulmonary function. The patient should report that breathing has improved and anxiety is reduced.

Assessing for Adverse Effects

The nurse observes for the presence of a cough, nervousness, nausea, GI upset, headache, and dizziness.

Patient Teaching

Box 31.4 summarizes patient teaching guidelines for antiasthmatic drugs such as ipratropium.

Other Drugs in the Class

Tiotropium (Spiriva) is a long-acting, 24-hour, anticholinergic bronchodilator taken once daily by inhalation for maintenance therapy of bronchoconstriction associated with chronic bronchitis and emphysema. A muscarinic receptor antagonist, it is closely related to ipratropium but is not used for acute bronchospasm exacerbations. The drug has different pharmacokinetic and pharmacologic properties from ipratropium, and these differences may make it superior to ipratropium as an anticholinergic agent. A patient who is taking ipratropium should not take tiotropium. The primary adverse effect of tiotropium is dry mouth. Other effects include headache, dizziness, abdominal pain, constipation, diarrhea, flu-like symptoms, and chest pain.

When taking tiotropium, the person places a capsule in a piercing chamber (HandiHaler) and then inhales the medication through the mouthpiece. It is necessary to repeat inhalations two to three times to ensure that the entire drug is inhaled. When properly administered, a distinctive flutter or rattle is audible.

Xanthines

The xanthines are a group of alkaloids commonly used for their effects as bronchodilators, mainly in treating the symptoms of asthma. ℗ **Theophylline** (aminophylline, Theochron), the prototype, is used less often than formerly and is now considered a second-line drug. It has a chemical structure similar to that of caffeine. When used, theophylline is usually given orally in an extended-release formulation for chronic disorders, such as chronic obstructive pulmonary disease (COPD). IV theophylline in the form of aminophylline is no longer used to treat acute asthma attacks.

Pharmacokinetics

Theophylline is rapidly and completely absorbed after oral administration. The onset of action occurs within 15 to 30 minutes by the oral route (extended release, 30 minutes). Peak levels occur in 1 to 2 hours, and the duration of action is 4 to 6 hours (extended release, 12 hours). Metabolism in the liver is extensive. Excretion of metabolites and some unchanged drug involves the kidneys. The drug crosses the placenta, and it enters breast milk.

Action

Theophylline works by relaxing bronchial smooth muscle promoting bronchodilation. Additionally, the drug suppresses airway responsiveness to stimuli that trigger bronchospasm.

Use

Theophylline was formerly used extensively in the prevention and treatment of bronchoconstriction associated with asthma, bronchitis, and emphysema. Now considered a second-line agent, a health care provider may add it to a regimen for severe disease that is inadequately controlled by first-line drugs.

Numerous dosage forms of theophylline are available. Theophylline ethylenediamine (aminophylline) contains approximately 85% theophylline and is the only formulation that can be given intravenously. However, authorities do not recommend IV aminophylline for emergency treatment of acute asthma; studies indicate little, if any, added benefit in adults (or children). Oral theophylline preparations may be useful in long-term treatment. Most formulations contain anhydrous theophylline (100% theophylline) as the active ingredient, and sustained-action tablets (e.g., Theochron) are more commonly used than other formulations.

To determine theophylline dosage, prescribers should measure serum theophylline levels (therapeutic range is 5–15 mcg/mL; toxic levels are 20 mcg/mL or above). It is necessary to draw blood for serum levels 1 to 2 hours after patients have taken immediate-release dosage forms and about 4 hours after they have taken sustained-release forms. In addition, children and cigarette smokers usually need higher doses to maintain therapeutic blood levels because they metabolize theophylline rapidly, and patients with liver disease, congestive heart failure, COPD, or acute viral infections usually need smaller doses because these conditions impair theophylline metabolism. For obese patients, prescribers should calculate theophylline dosage on the basis of lean or ideal body weight because theophylline is not highly distributed in fatty tissue. Table 31.4 gives the route and dosage information for long-acting and short-acting theophylline.

Use in Children

Use of theophylline necessitates close monitoring because dosage needs and rates of metabolism vary widely. In children younger than 6 months of age, especially premature infants and neonates, drug elimination may be prolonged because of immature liver function. Experts do not recommend use of theophylline preparations in such young children, except for preterm infants with apnea.

Children 6 months to 16 years of age (approximately) metabolize theophylline more rapidly than younger or older patients. Thus, they may need higher doses than adults in proportion to size and weight. Authorities do not recommend long-acting dosage forms for use in children younger than 6 years of age. Children may become hyperactive and disruptive from the CNS-stimulating effects of theophylline. Tolerance to these effects usually develops with continued use of the drug.

Use in Older Adults

It is important to monitor older patients who use theophylline carefully because effects of the drug are unpredictable. Typically, older adults require reduced doses.

Use in Patients With Renal Impairment

Patients with renal impairment can take the usual doses of theophylline, but monitoring of serum drug levels is necessary.

TABLE 31.4

DRUGS AT A GLANCE: Xanthines (Theophylline)

Drug	Pregnancy Category	Routes and Dosage Ranges	
		Adults	Children
℗ **Short-acting theophylline** (aminophylline)	C	500 mg PO, initially, then 200–300 mg every 6–8 h; Infusion, 6 mg/kg IV over 30 min, then 0.1–1.2 mg/kg/h	7.5 mg/kg PO initially, then 5–6 mg/kg every 6–8 h; Infusion, 6 mg/kg IV over 30 min, then 0.6–0.9 mg/kg/h
Long-acting theophylline (Theochron, others)	C	150–300 mg PO every 8–12 h; max dose 13 mg/kg or 900 mg daily, whichever is less	100–200 mg PO every 8–12 h; max dose 24 mg/kg/d

Use in Patients With Hepatic Impairment

Metabolism of theophylline takes place in the liver. This means that impaired liver function and decreased blood flow to the liver decrease metabolism; therefore, a dosage reduction is necessary.

Use in Patients Receiving Home Care

With theophylline, the home care nurse needs to assess the patient and the environment for substances that may affect metabolism of theophylline and decrease therapeutic effects or increase adverse effects. The nurse assesses self-administration in the home. In addition, he or she assists with periodic office or clinic visits for blood tests and other follow-up care.

Adverse Effects

The therapeutic range of theophylline is narrow, making it and other xanthines second-line asthma treatment. Signs and symptoms of theophylline overdose include anorexia, nausea, vomiting, agitation, nervousness, insomnia, tachycardia and other dysrhythmias, and tonic–clonic convulsions. Ventricular dysrhythmias or convulsions may be the first sign of toxicity. Serious adverse effects frequently occur at serum drug levels above 20 μg/mL. Overdoses with sustained-release preparations may cause a dramatic increase in serum drug concentrations much later (12 hours or longer) than the immediate-release preparations. Early treatment helps but does not prevent these delayed increases in serum drug levels. Theophylline also increases cardiac output, causes peripheral vasodilation, exerts a mild diuretic effect, and stimulates the CNS.

Contraindications

Contraindications to theophylline include acute gastritis and peptic ulcer disease. Caution is necessary in seizure disorders and cardiovascular disorders that could be aggravated by drug-induced cardiac stimulation.

Nursing Implications

Preventing Interactions

Because theophylline is metabolized by the cytochrome P450 (CYP) enzyme system, numerous drug–drug interactions using the same enzyme system exist (Box 31.6). Also, the rate of metabolism of theophylline is increased substantially in cigarette smokers (the half-life can be halved), although this metabolic increase may not be significant in those who smoke fewer than 10 cigarettes per day. In addition, caffeine reportedly produces additive cardiac and CNS stimulation. Finally, St. John's wort may decrease the effect of theophylline by increasing its metabolism.

Administering the Medication

To help regulate theophylline dosage and avoid adverse effects, it is necessary to monitor serum drug levels. Patients should take immediate-release oral theophylline before meals with a full glass of water, at regular intervals around the clock. If GI upset occurs, they may take the drug with food to promote dissolution and absorption and decrease the associated nausea and vomiting. They should take sustained-release theophylline every 8 to 12 hours, with instructions not to chew or crush. Doing so causes immediate release of potentially toxic doses.

BOX 31.6   Drug Interactions: Theophylline

Drugs That Increase the Effects of Theophylline

■ Allopurinol, propranolol, quinolones (e.g., ciprofloxacin)
   Decrease metabolism
■ Cimetidine, macrolides (e.g., erythromycin, clindamycin)
   Decrease clearance and thereby increase plasma levels

Drugs That Decrease the Effects of Theophylline

■ Carbamazepine, phenytoin, rifampicin
   Increase metabolism
■ Lithium
   Increases excretion
■ Phenobarbital
   Increases metabolism by way of enzyme induction

Assessing for Therapeutic Effects

The nurse observes for therapeutic serum levels of theophylline (5–15 mcg/mL). Chronic use of the drug results in improved arterial blood gas levels (normal values on room air: PO_2, 80–100 mm Hg; PCO_2, 35–45 mm Hg; pH, 7.35–7.45), improved exercise tolerance, and decreased incidence and severity of acute attacks of bronchospasm.

Assessing for Adverse Effects

With theophylline, the nurse monitors the serum drug level and observes for tachycardia, dysrhythmias, palpitations, restlessness, agitation, insomnia, nausea, vomiting, and convulsions. Theophylline causes cardiac and CNS stimulation. Toxic serum concentrations (>20 mcg/mL) lead to convulsions, which may occur without preceding symptoms of toxicity and may result in death. IV diazepam (Valium) may control seizures. In patients with seizures, treatment includes securing the airway, giving oxygen, injecting IV diazepam (0.1–0.3 mg/kg, up to 10 mg), monitoring vital signs, maintaining blood pressure, providing adequate hydration, and monitoring serum theophylline levels until they are between 15 and 20 μg/mL.

Theophylline also stimulates the chemoreceptor trigger zone in the medulla oblongata, causing nausea and vomiting. In patients without seizures, it may be necessary to induce vomiting, unless the level of consciousness is impaired. In these patients, precautions to prevent aspiration are necessary, especially in children. If overdose is identified within 1 hour of theophylline ingestion, gastric lavage may be helpful if health care providers are unable to induce vomiting or vomiting is contraindicated. Experts recommend administration of activated charcoal and a cathartic, especially for overdoses of sustained-release formulations—if the possible benefit exceeds the risk.

In addition, symptomatic treatment of dysrhythmias may be necessary.

Patient Teaching

With theophylline, the nurse reinforces the importance of not exceeding the prescribed dose, not crushing long-acting formulations, reporting adverse effects, and keeping appointments for follow-up care. He or she also instructs patients who smoke to notify their prescriber if they stop smoking, because the dosage of theophylline may need to be reduced. Box 31.4 presents patient teaching guidelines for antiasthmatic drugs.

NCLEX Success

1. **A woman begins using an albuterol inhaler and a beclomethasone inhaler for her asthma. She asks if it matters which inhaler she uses first. The best response by the nurse is**
   A. "You should use the albuterol inhaler first followed in 5 to 10 minutes by the beclomethasone inhaler."
   B. "You should use the beclomethasone inhaler first followed in 5 to 10 minutes by the albuterol inhaler."
   C. "The order in which you use the inhalers does not matter."
   D. "You should not use the inhalers one right after the other."

2. **The nurse notes that a patient's serum theophylline level is 25 mcg/mL and that a scheduled dose of the medication is due. The nurse should**
   A. Hold the scheduled dose, contact the health care provider, and assess the patient for signs of theophylline toxicity.
   B. Administer the dose as scheduled.
   C. Administer only half of the dose and repeat the theophylline level in 4 hours.
   D. Hold the dose until the next meal and administer at that time.

3. **A 68-year-old man who has been well controlled on theophylline for 2 years complains of insomnia, nervousness, nausea and vomiting, and tachycardia. He originally thought the nervousness was due to his recent smoking cessation. He had smoked 1 pack per day for 10 years. The nurse practitioner assesses the patient and tells him that he is likely experiencing theophylline toxicity. A serum theophylline level confirms the diagnosis. What is the best explanation for theophylline toxicity in this patient?**
   A. Because of his age, the patient is likely having renal insufficiency.
   B. The patient is not taking the medication as prescribed.
   C. A concurrent medication is altering the metabolism of theophylline.
   D. The metabolism of theophylline has decreased with the recent smoking cessation.

Corticosteroids

Chapter 15 describes corticosteroids, which are often ordered for treatment of many inflammatory conditions. The ability of the corticosteroids to suppress airway inflammation produces beneficial effects, including decreased mucus secretion, decreased edema of airway mucosa, and repair of damaged epithelium, with subsequent reduction of airway reactivity. Corticosteroids are the most consistently effective long-term control medications for asthma. The inhaled drug ℗ **beclomethasone** (Beconase AQ, QVAR) is the prototype corticosteroid in asthma.

Pharmacokinetics

Beclomethasone is rapidly absorbed from the lower respiratory tract or nasal passages. The onset of action is rapid, and the drug peaks in 1 to 2 weeks. Therapeutic effects may not occur until 4 weeks after initial use. Metabolism occurs in the lungs, GI tract, and liver, and excretion predominately occurs in the feces. The drug crosses the placenta. Whether it enters breast milk is unknown.

Action

Corticosteroids suppress the release of inflammatory mediators, block the generation of cytokines, and decrease the recruitment of airway eosinophils. The drugs increase the number and sensitivity of beta$_2$-adrenergic receptors, which restores or increases the effectiveness of beta$_2$-adrenergic bronchodilators. The number of beta$_2$ receptors increases within approximately 4 hours, and improved responsiveness to beta$_2$-agonists occurs within approximately 2 hours.

Use

Beclomethasone is effective in the prophylactic management of asthma. With inhalation, the drug controls asthma that requires corticosteroids as part of the treatment plan. In chronic asthma, patients usually take corticosteroids by inhalation, on a daily schedule. Often, they take them concomitantly with one or more bronchodilators and perhaps another anti-inflammatory drug such as a leukotriene modifier or a mast cell stabilizer. In some instances, the other drugs allow smaller doses of the corticosteroid. For acute flare-ups of symptoms during treatment of chronic asthma, a systemic corticosteroid may be needed temporarily to regain control. Intranasal administration helps relieve rhinitis that responds poorly to other treatment and minimizes the reoccurrence of nasal polyps after nasal surgery.

In early stages of progressive COPD, patients are unlikely to need corticosteroids. In later stages, however, they usually need periodic short-course therapy for episodes of respiratory distress. When corticosteroids are needed, administration is oral or parenteral because effectiveness of inhaled corticosteroids has not been established in COPD.

Table 31.5 provides route and dosage information for beclomethasone and other corticosteroid antiasthmatic drugs.

Use in Children

The effectiveness and safety of inhaled corticosteroids, including beclomethasone, in children older than 3 years of age is well established; few data are available on the use of inhaled drugs in those younger than 3 years. Major concerns about long-term use in children include decreased adrenal function, growth, and bone mass. Most corticosteroids are given by inhalation, and dosage, type of inhaler device, and characteristics of individual drugs influence the extent and severity of these systemic effects. Adrenal insufficiency is most likely to occur with systemic or high doses of inhaled corticosteroids. Although inhaled

TABLE 31.5

DRUGS AT A GLANCE: Corticosteroids

Drug	Pregnancy Category	Routes and Dosage Ranges	
		Adults	Children
P Beclomethasone (QVAR)	C	Oral inhalation, initial 40–80 mcg twice daily; max dose, 320 mcg twice daily; if on previous inhaled corticosteroids, 40–160 mcg twice daily; max dose 320 mcg twice daily	5–11 y, oral inhalation, 40 mcg twice daily; max dose 80 mcg twice daily ≥12 y, 40–80 mcg twice daily; max dose 320 mcg twice daily
P Beclomethasone (Beconase AQ)	C	Nasal inhalation, 2 sprays in each nostril twice daily (total dose 168–336 mcg/d)	≥6 y, nasal inhalation, 2 sprays in each nostril twice daily (total dose 168–336 mcg/d)
Budesonide (Pulmicort Turbuhaler)	B	Oral inhalation, 200–400 mcg twice daily	6 y, oral inhalation 200 mcg twice daily
Ciclesonide (Omnaris)	C	Oral inhalation, 80 mcg twice daily; max dose 160 mcg twice daily (if receiving bronchodilators alone); max dose 320 mcg twice daily (if receiving inhaled corticosteroids)	12 y and older, same as adults
Flunisolide (AeroBid, Aerospan*)	C	AeroBid, oral inhalation, two inhalations (0.50 mg/dose) twice daily, morning and evening; max dose four inhalations twice daily (2 mg) Aerospan, two inhalations twice daily; max dose eight inhalations daily	AeroBid, 6–15 y, oral inhalation, two inhalations twice daily; max dose eight inhalations daily Aerospan, 6–11 y, oral inhalation: one inhalation twice daily; max dose four times daily
Fluticasone (Flonase)	C	4 sprays in each nostril once daily (265 mcg/d)	12 y and older: same as adults 4–11 y: 1 spray in each nostril once daily; may increase to 2 sprays in each nostril for desired effect
Fluticasone aerosol (Flovent)	C	Aerosol, 88–440 mcg twice daily	Dosage not established
Fluticasone powder (Flovent Rotadisk)	C	Powder, 100–500 mcg twice daily	12 y and older: same as adults 4–11 y, powder, 50–100 mcg twice daily
Mometasone (Asmanex Twisthaler, Nasonex)	C	Nasal inhalation two sprays (50 mcg/spray) in each nostril once daily	12 y and older, same as adults 2–11 y, 1 spray (50 mcg) in each nostril once daily
Triamcinolone (Azmacort)	C	Oral inhalation, two (100 mcg/puff) inhalations 3 or 4 times daily or four inhalations twice daily; max dose 16 inhalations (1600 mcg)/24 h	6–12 y, one or two (100 mcg/puff) inhalations 3 or 4 times daily or two to four inhalations twice daily; max dose 12 inhalations/24 h
Hydrocortisone sodium phosphate and sodium succinate	C	100–200 mg IV every 4–6 h initially, then decreased or switched to oral form	1–5 mg/kg IV every 4–6 h
Prednisone	C	20–60 mg/d PO	2 mg/kg/d PO initially
Methylprednisolone sodium succinate	C	10–40 mg IV every 4–6 h for 48–72 h	0.5 mg/kg IV every 4–6 h

*These preparations are *not* interchangeable.

corticosteroids are the most effective anti-inflammatory medications available for asthma, high doses in children are still of concern, and monitoring of the effects is necessary. It is possible to reduce the risk by using (1) the lowest effective dose, (2) administration techniques that minimize swallowed drug, and (3) other antiasthmatic drugs to reduce corticosteroid dose. Research has not shown that nasal administration of beclomethasone affects growth. However, prolonged or high-dose use of nasal beclomethasone has the potential to influence growth.

Use in Patients With Hepatic Impairment

Because elimination of beclomethasone and most corticosteroids is hepatic, dosage reductions may be appropriate.

Use in Patients With Critical Illness

In critically ill patients, it may be necessary to replace inhaled or nasal beclomethasone by systemic corticosteroids in relatively high doses in patients whose respiratory distress is not relieved by multiple doses of inhaled beta$_2$-agonists. Administration of the systemic corticosteroid may be either IV or oral; IV administration offers no therapeutic advantage over oral administration. Relief of the symptoms of acute, severe bronchoconstriction or status asthmaticus usually requires larger doses of bronchodilators and corticosteroids (inhaled, systemic, or both). Then, dose reduction to the smallest effective amounts for long-term control is necessary.

Use in Patients Receiving Home Care

Administration of beclomethasone is common in the home setting. As with most inhaled medications, the nurse assesses the patient's ability to administer the medication as prescribed and his or her knowledge of what other medications and actions to use to treat exacerbations if symptoms occur. Also, the nurse inspects the oral cavity to monitor for the presence of fungal infection (candidiasis).

Adverse Effects

Common adverse effects of beclomethasone include headache, pharyngitis, cough, dry mouth, hoarseness, fungal infection (candidiasis), and nausea. It is possible to decrease local adverse effects of inhaled corticosteroids (oropharyngeal candidiasis, hoarseness) by reducing the dose, administering the drugs less often, rinsing the mouth and throat after use, or using a spacer device. These measures decrease the amount of drug deposited in the oral cavity.

Contraindications

Contraindications to beclomethasone include an allergy to the drug. Recent nasal surgery, injury, or ulcers preclude use of the nasal preparation; the drug can interfere with healing and increase the risk of a nasal infection.

Nursing Implications

Preventing Interactions

Little, if any, of the beclomethasone is absorbed. Therefore, no clinically significant drug–drug or herbal interactions are known to occur.

Administering the Medication

Patients should take inhaled or nasal beclomethasone on a regular schedule. After inhaling, they should rinse the mouth and throat to prevent fungal infection (candidiasis). The drug is not a rescue inhaler, and patients should not take it to resolve an acute asthma event. The recommended inhaled or nasal corticosteroid dose should be the lowest amount of drug required to control symptoms.

Assessing for Therapeutic Effects

The nurse assesses for reversal of asthma symptoms, including reduced airway inflammation, decreased mucus secretion, decreased edema of airway mucosa, and reduction of airway reactivity. With allergic rhinitis, the nurse assesses for the relief of rhinitis, including clearing of stuffy nose and postnasal drip.

Assessing for Adverse Effects

With beclomethasone and other inhaled corticosteroids, the nurse observes for the presence of headache, hoarseness, cough, throat irritation, and fungal infection (candidiasis) of mouth and throat. Inhaled corticosteroids are unlikely to produce the serious adverse effects of long-term systemic therapy (see Chap. 15).

Patient Teaching

It is important to instruct patients that oral and nasal inhalations are not interchangeable.

QSEN Safety Alert ❗

The nurse must remind patients that beclomethasone is not a fast-acting asthma treatment; the drug does not provide immediate relief from asthma-related breathing problems.

Box 31.4 outlines additional patient teaching guidelines.

Other Drugs in the Class

Budesonide (Pulmicort Turbuhaler), ciclesonide (Omnaris), flunisolide (AeroBid, Aerospan), fluticasone (Flonase), mometasone (Asmanex Twisthaler, Nasonex), and triamcinolone (Azmacort) are topical corticosteroids for inhalation. Most inhaled drugs are reformulated (indicated with HFA as the propellant being used). Topical administration minimizes systemic absorption and adverse effects; clinical effectiveness of inhaled drugs is due to direct local effects rather than systemic absorption. These preparations may substitute for or allow reduced dosage of systemic corticosteroids.

QSEN Safety Alert ❗

In people with asthma who are taking an oral corticosteroid, it is necessary to reduce the oral dosage slowly (over weeks to months) when an inhaled corticosteroid is added.

The goal is to use the lowest oral dose necessary to control symptoms.

Flunisolide and fluticasone also are available in nasal solutions for treatment of allergic rhinitis, which may play a role

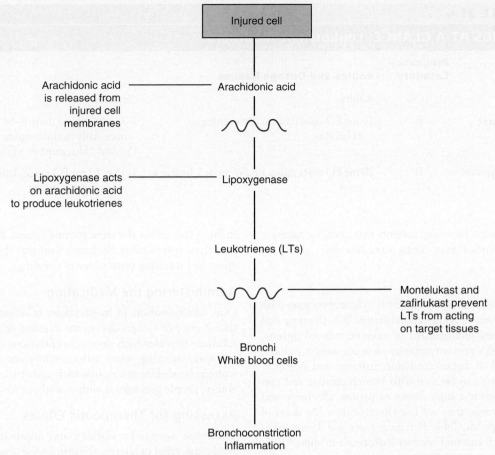

Figure 31.1 Formation of leukotrienes and actions of leukotriene-modifying drugs.

in bronchoconstriction. Ciclesonide is available only as a nasal solution. Because systemic absorption occurs in patients using inhaled corticosteroids (about 20% of a dose), high doses should be reserved for people who otherwise require oral corticosteroids.

Triamcinolone acetonide is not recommended for use in children younger than 2 years of age. Dose-related inhibition of growth has been reported in short and intermediate studies, but long-term studies have found few, if any, decreases in expected adult height. Inhaled corticosteroids have not been associated with significant decreases in bone mass, but more studies of high doses and of drug therapy in adolescents are needed.

Hydrocortisone, prednisone, and methylprednisolone are given to patients who require systemic corticosteroids. Prednisone is given orally and is highlighted as a prototype drug in Chapter 15; hydrocortisone and methylprednisolone may be given intravenously to patients who are unable to take an oral medication.

Leukotriene Modifiers

Leukotrienes are fatty compounds produced by the immune system after trauma, infection, and inflammation. They can cause sustained constriction of bronchioles and immediate hypersensitivity reactions. They also increase mucus secretion and mucosal edema in the respiratory tract. Leukotrienes are formed by the lipoxygenase pathway of arachidonic acid

metabolism (Fig. 31.1) in response to cellular injury. They are designated by LT; the letter B, C, D, or E; and the number of chemical bonds in their structure (e.g., LTB4, LTC4, and LTE4; also called slow-releasing substances of anaphylaxis, or SRS-A, because they are released more slowly than histamine).

Leukotriene modifiers are strong chemical mediators of bronchoconstriction and inflammation, the major pathologic features of asthma. The prototype leukotriene modifier, or leukotriene receptor antagonist, is Ⓟ **montelukast** (Singulair). These drugs are effective in a significant portion of patients with asthma who do not respond to other therapies.

Pharmacokinetics

Absorption from the GI tract is rapid. The CYP enzyme system is the site of metabolism, and the drug may interact with other medications metabolized by this system. Excretion of most metabolites occurs in the feces.

Action

Montelukast prevents leukotrienes from binding to its receptors reducing the bronchoconstriction and ultimate inflammation caused by leukotrienes. The drug improves symptoms and pulmonary function tests, decreases nighttime symptoms, and decreases the use of beta₂-agonist drugs. The drug is not effective in relieving

TABLE 31.6

DRUGS AT A GLANCE: Leukotriene Modifiers

Drug	Pregnancy Category	Routes and Dosage Ranges	
		Adults	Children
P **Montelukast** (Singulair)	B	10 mg PO once daily in the evening or at bedtime	2–5 y, 4 mg once daily 6–14 y, 5 mg PO once daily in the evening 15 y and older, same as adults
Zafirlukast (Accolate)	B	20 mg PO twice daily, 1 h before or 2 h after a meal	5–11 y, 10 mg PO twice daily 12 y and older, same as adults

acute asthma attacks. However, patients may continue taking it concurrently with other drugs during acute episodes.

Use

Health care providers use montelukast is indicated for long-term treatment of asthma in adults and children. It is the only oral tablet approved for management of exercise-induced asthma. The drug also helps prevent episodes of acute asthma induced by allergens, cold air, hyperventilation, irritants, and aspirin or NSAIDs. The drug can be used with bronchodilators and corticosteroids and elicit a high degree of patient adherence and satisfaction. However, they are less effective than low doses of inhaled corticosteroids. Table 31.6 gives route and dosage information for montelukast and another leukotriene modifier.

Use in Children

The FDA has approved montelukast for use in children 12 months of age and older. Film-coated tablets, chewable tablets, or granules are available.

Use in Patients With Hepatic Impairment

Montelukast produces higher blood levels in patients with hepatic impairment, and drug elimination is slower in these patients. However, no dosage adjustment is necessary for patients with mild to moderate hepatic impairment.

Use in Patients Receiving Home Care

Montelukast is self-administered at home for prevention of asthma symptoms. Prescribers often order the drug when inhaled corticosteroids and short-acting beta$_2$-agonists are unsuccessful in controlling asthma symptoms. The home health nurse assesses asthma severity and asthma control.

Adverse Effects and Contraindications

Leukotriene modifiers seem relatively devoid of serious toxicity, and adverse effects are typically mild. The most common adverse effects reported are headache, nausea, diarrhea, and infection.

Contraindications include known hypersensitivity to the drug.

Nursing Implications

Preventing Interactions

Montelukast is metabolized in the liver by the CYP enzyme system, and numerous drug–drug interactions exist, particularly

in drugs that utilize the same enzyme system. Box 31.7 summarizes these interactions. St. John's wort may decrease the drug's effect by increasing metabolism of the drug.

Administering the Medication

Oral administration of montelukast is effective. People can take it once or twice a day, in the evening or at bedtime. This schedule provides high drug concentrations during the night and early morning, when asthma symptoms tend to occur or worsen. Food does not significantly affect the drug's bioavailability; people may take it with or without food.

Assessing for Therapeutic Effects

The nurse assesses for stability and improvement of asthma symptoms, relief of allergic rhinitis, or the absence of exercise-induced respiratory symptoms. If the patient's respiratory symptoms are not stable, it is necessary to determine the current frequency and severity of acute attacks as well as factors that precipitate or relieve acute attacks.

Assessing for Adverse Effects

The nurse assesses for headache, nausea, diarrhea, or signs of an infection.

Patient Teaching

The nurse instructs the patient about recognizing signs and symptoms of infection and reporting them to his/her health care provider. Also, the nurse ensures that the patient understands appropriate use of the drug and realizes that the drug should not be used to manage acute asthma symptoms. Box 31.4 outlines additional patient teaching guidelines.

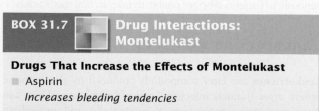

BOX 31.7   Drug Interactions: Montelukast

Drugs That Increase the Effects of Montelukast
- Aspirin
  Increases bleeding tendencies

Drugs That Decrease the Effects of Montelukast
- Carbamazepine, erythromycin, phenobarbital, phenytoin, primidone, rifamycin antibiotics, theophylline
  Decrease serum levels

Other Drugs in the Class

Montelukast has overshadowed zafirlukast (Accolate), the first leukotriene modifier. Well absorbed with oral administration, metabolism of zafirlukast by the CYP enzyme system occurs in the liver, and the drug may interact with other drugs metabolized by the hepatic system. Excretion of most metabolites occurs in the feces. Blood levels of the drug are higher and elimination is slower in older adults than in younger adults. Zafirlukast enters breast milk, and lactating women should not take it. People should take zafirlukast 1 hour before or 2 hours after a meal; food reduces the bioavailability by approximately 40%. Authorities recommend no dosage adjustments for zafirlukast in patients with renal impairment.

Adjuvant Medications Used to Treat Asthma

Mast Cell Stabilizers

Mast cell stabilizers are used as an alternative, but not preferred, medication for prophylaxis of acute asthma attacks in patients with mild, persistent asthma. They are not effective in acute bronchospasm or status asthmaticus and should not be used in these conditions. Use of one of these drugs may allow reduced dosage of bronchodilators and corticosteroids. Patients may take them prior to exercise or exposure to known allergens. **(P) Cromolyn** (NasalCrom) stabilizes mast cells and prevents the release of bronchoconstrictive and inflammatory substances when mast cells are confronted with allergens and other stimuli. Administration of mast cell stabilizers is by inhalation. Cromolyn is available in a metered-dose aerosol and a solution for use with a power-operated nebulizer. A nasal solution is also marketed for prevention and treatment of allergic rhinitis. In patients with impaired renal or hepatic function, dosage reduction is necessary.

Serious toxicity is relatively absent with mast cell stabilizers. However, the propellants in the aerosols may aggravate coronary artery disease or dysrhythmias. With cromolyn, the nurse assesses for dysrhythmias, hypotension, chest pain, restlessness, dizziness, convulsions, CNS depression, anorexia, and nausea and vomiting. Sedation and coma may occur with overdosage.

Immunosuppressant Monoclonal Antibody

Monoclonal antibodies specifically bind to target cells or proteins in the hopes of stimulating the patient's immune system to attack those cells. **(P) Omalizumab** (Xolair) combines with free immunoglobulin E (IgE)–blocking receptors on the surfaces of mast cells and basophils so that there is less IgE available to combine with allergens. This prevents IgE from attaching to the cells, thus preventing the release of substances in the body that can trigger an allergic reaction and preventing the development of inflammation. As an immunomodifier, omalizumab is indicated as adjunctive therapy in patients with moderate to severe persistent allergic asthma not well controlled by inhaled corticosteroids. Chapter 11 also discusses omalizumab.

Use of most of the drugs that have been discussed in this chapter may safely occur in the home setting. However, people must take omalizumab in the health care setting because of the risk of life-threatening anaphylaxis with administration. Due to the risk of anaphylaxis, the FDA has issued a **BLACK BOX WARNING ◆** for omalizumab. It is essential that the drug be administered to patients only in a health care setting under direct medical supervision by provider who can initiate treatment of life-threatening anaphylaxis.

Combination Regimens

Combination regimens are commonly used, and one advantage is that smaller doses of each agent can usually be given. This may decrease adverse effects and allow dosages to be increased when exacerbation of symptoms occurs. Table 31.7 summarizes information about available combination inhalation products. Advair, which was developed to treat both inflammation and bronchoconstriction, is more effective than the individual components at the same doses and as effective as concurrent use of the same drugs at the same doses. In addition, the combination reduces the corticosteroid dose by 50% and is more effective than higher doses of fluticasone alone in reducing asthma exacerbations. The combination improves symptoms within 1 week. Additional combination products are likely to be marketed and may improve patient adherence to prescribed drug therapy.

TABLE 31.7

DRUGS AT A GLANCE: Combination Regimens

Drug	Pregnancy Category	Routes and Dosage Ranges	
		Adults	Children
Fluticasone/Salmeterol (Advair)	C	Oral inhalation, one inhalation, twice daily	12 y and older, same as adults
Budesonide/Formoterol (Symbicort)	C	Oral inhalation, two inhalation, twice daily	12 y and older, same as adults
Ipratropium/Albuterol (Combivent, DuoNeb)	C	Aerosol, two inhalations 4 times daily Nebulizing solution, 1 vial 4 times daily, increased to 6 times daily if necessary	Dosage not established

Clinical Application 31-2

- Mr. Lee's symptoms subside, and he is transferred to a medical unit. Mr. Lee tells the nurse that he hopes he does not have another episode of this type again. What efforts does the nurse recommend to reduce the risk of future episodes?

NCLEX Success

4. **When teaching a patient about the proper use of metered-dose inhalers, which of the following statements should be included?**

   A. "Hold the inhaler in your mouth, take a deep breath, and then compress the inhaler."

   B. "Make sure that you puff out air repeatedly after you inhale the medication."

   C. "After you inhale the medication, hold the breath for approximately 10 seconds, and exhale slowly."

   D. "After you inhale the medication once, repeat until you obtain relief."

5. **A man who is using a steroid inhaler complains of anorexia and discomfort when he eats. The nurse reports this to the care provider, and the patient receives a diagnosis of oropharyngeal candidiasis. It is possible to decrease this adverse affect by doing which of the following? (Check all that apply.)**

   A. reducing the dose

   B. administering the drug more frequently

   C. rinsing the mouth after use

   D. using a spacer device

6. **Montelukast is effective in relieving the inflammation and bronchoconstriction associated with acute asthmatic attacks through which principal action?**

   A. stabilizing mast cells

   B. blocking leukotriene receptors

   C. binding to immunoglobulin E (IgE)

   D. decreasing prostaglandin synthesis

The Nursing Process

Assessment

- Assess the patient's pulmonary function. General assessment factors include rate and character of respiration, skin color, arterial blood gas analysis, and pulmonary function tests. Abnormal breathing patterns (e.g., rate below 12 or above 24 per minute, dyspnea, cough, orthopnea, wheezing, "noisy" respirations) may indicate respiratory distress. Severe respiratory distress is characterized by tachypnea, dyspnea, use of accessory muscles of respiration, and hypoxia. Early signs of hypoxia include mental confusion, restlessness, anxiety, and increased blood pressure and pulse rate. Late signs include cyanosis and decreased blood pressure and pulse rate. Hypoxemia is confirmed if arterial blood gas analysis shows decreased PO_2.

- In acute bronchospasm, a medical emergency, the patient is in obvious and severe respiratory distress. Assess for forceful expiration or wheezing, a characteristic feature of bronchospasm. The absence of wheezing in the presence of increased respiratory effort is an ominous sign.

- In chronic asthma, try to determine the frequency and severity of acute attacks; factors that precipitate or relieve acute attacks; antiasthmatic medications taken occasionally or regularly; allergies; and condition between acute attacks, such as restrictions in activities of daily living due to asthma.

- In chronic bronchitis or emphysema, assess for signs of respiratory distress, hypoxia, cough, amount and character of sputum, exercise tolerance (e.g., dyspnea on exertion, dyspnea at rest), medications, and nondrug treatment measures (e.g., breathing exercises, chest physiotherapy).

Nursing Diagnoses

- Impaired Gas Exchange related to bronchoconstriction and excessive mucus production
- Activity Intolerance related to impaired gas exchange and fatigue
- Risk for Injury: severe bronchospasm with asthma and adverse effects with antiasthmatic drugs
- Noncompliance: overuse of adrenergic bronchodilators
- Deficient Knowledge: factors precipitating bronchoconstriction and strategies to avoid precipitating factors
- Deficient Knowledge: accurate self-administration of drugs, including use of inhalers

Planning/Goals

The patient will

- Self-administer bronchodilating and other drugs accurately
- Experience relief of symptoms
- Avoid preventable adverse drug effects
- Avoid overusing bronchodilating drugs
- Avoid exposure to stimuli that cause bronchospasm when possible
- Avoid respiratory infections when possible

Nursing Interventions

The nurse will

- Use measures to prevent or relieve bronchoconstriction when possible. General measures include those to prevent respiratory disease or promote an adequate airway. A specific monitoring plan should be in place, whether peak flow or symptom monitoring. Some measures include the following:
  - Use mechanical measures for removing excessive respiratory tract secretions and preventing their retention. Effective measures include coughing, deep breathing, percussion, and postural drainage.
  - Help the patient identify and avoid exposure to conditions that precipitate bronchoconstriction. For example, allergens may be removed from the home, school, or work environment; cigarette smoke should be avoided when possible. When bronchospasm is precipitated by exercise, prophylaxis by prior inhalation of bronchodilating agents is better than avoiding exercise, especially in children.

- Assist patients with asthma to identify early signs of difficulty, including increased need for beta$_2$-adrenergic agonists, activity limitations, and waking at night with asthma symptoms
- Monitor the PEFR when indicated. Portable meters are available for use in clinics, physicians' offices, and patients' homes. This is an objective measure of airflow/airway obstruction and helps evaluate the patient's treatment regimen.
- Assist patients with moderate to severe asthma in obtaining meters and learning to measure PEFR. Patients with a decreased PEFR may need treatment to prevent acute, severe respiratory distress.
- Assist patients and at least one family member in developing an action plan to identify the correct action to manage acute attacks of bronchoconstriction, including when to seek emergency care
- Try to prevent or reduce anxiety, which may aggravate bronchospasm. Stay with the patient during an acute asthma attack if feasible. Patients experiencing severe and prolonged bronchospasm (status asthmaticus) should be admitted or transferred to a hospital intensive care unit.
- With any patients who smoke cigarettes, encourage cessation of smoking and provide information, resources, and assistance in doing so. Emphasize the health benefits of improved respiratory function.
- In addition, provide appropriate patient teaching related to drug therapy (see Box 31.4).

Evaluation

- Observe for relief of symptoms and improved arterial blood gas values.
- Interview and observe for correct drug administration, including use of inhalers.
- Interview and observe for tachydysrhythmias, nervousness, insomnia, and other adverse drug effects.
- Interview about and observe behaviors to avoid stimuli that cause bronchoconstriction and respiratory infections.

Key Concepts

- Management of asthma involves prevention of airway inflammation and avoidance of triggers for better symptom control.
- Guidelines for asthma care highlight the importance of four essential components: assessment and monitoring, patient education, control of factors contributing to asthma severity, and pharmacologic treatment.
- Maintenance beta$_2$-agonist inhaled medications are used to achieve and maintain control of persistent asthma, and rescue beta$_2$-agonist inhaled medications are used for quick-relief medications used during periods of acute symptoms and exacerbations.
- In an attack of acute, severe asthma, the lack of wheezing sound or coughing may indicate severe bronchoconstriction, impaired gas exchange in the lungs, and a worsening of the condition.
- Major groups of drugs used to treat asthma and other conditions causing bronchoconstriction include adrenergics, anticholinergics, xanthines, corticosteroids, leukotriene modifiers, and adjuvant medications (mast cell stabilizer and immunosuppressant monoclonal antibody).
- Because aerosol products act directly on the airways, drugs given by inhalation can usually be given in smaller doses and produce fewer adverse effects than oral or parenteral drugs.
- A selective, short-acting, inhaled beta$_2$-adrenergic agonist (e.g., albuterol) is the initial rescue drug of choice for acute bronchospasm; subcutaneous epinephrine may also be considered.
- The FDA has issued a **BLACK BOX WARNING** ◆ that initiating salmeterol in people with significantly worsening or acutely deteriorating asthma may be life threatening.
- Cigarette smoking and drugs that stimulate drug-metabolizing enzymes in the liver (e.g., phenobarbital, phenytoin) increase the rate of metabolism and therefore dosage requirements of theophylline.
- Due to the risk of anaphylaxis, the FDA has issued a **BLACK BOX WARNING** ◆ for omalizumab.

Critical Thinking Questions

31-1. An 8-year-old boy arrives at the emergency department with severe asthma. His parents have brought him there for the third time in the past month. His mother reports that they live in an old home that is full of mold and dust.

- What drug therapy should be provided to the boy in the emergency department?
- What information should the nurse share about managing the potential triggers of the boy's asthma?

References and Resources

Banasiak, N. C. (2009). Childhood asthma practice guideline part three: Update of the 2007 National Guidelines for the Diagnosis and Treatment of Asthma. The National Asthma Education and Prevention Program. *Journal of Pediatric Health Care, 23*(1), 59–61.

Blaiss, M. S. (2011). Safety update regarding intranasal corticosteroids for the treatment of allergic rhinitis. *Allergy and Asthma Proceedings, 32*(6), 413–418.

Drug facts and comparisons. (Updated monthly). St. Louis, MO: Facts and Comparisons.

Fanta, C. H. (2009). Asthma. *New England Journal of Medicine, 360*(10), 1002–1014.

Guyton, A. C., & Hall, J. E. (2006). *Textbook of medical physiology* (11th ed.). Philadelphia, PA: W. B. Saunders.

Hanania, N. A. (2007). Update on the pharmacologic therapy for chronic obstructive pulmonary disease. *Clinics in Chest Medicine, 28*, 589–607.

Henneberger, P. K., Redlich, C. A., Callahan, D. B., Harber, P., Lemière, C., Martin, J., et al.; ATS Ad Hoc Committee on Work-Exacerbated Asthma. (2011). An official American Thoracic Society statement: Work-exacerbated asthma. *American Journal of Respiratory Critical Care Medicine, 184*(3), 368–378.

Karch, A. M. (2012). *2012 Lippincott's nursing drug guide.* Philadelphia, PA: Lippincott, Williams, and Wilkins.

Lacy, C. F., Armstrong, L. L., Goldman, M. P., & Lance, L. L. (2010). *Lexi-Comp's drug information handbook* (19th ed.). Hudson, OH: American Pharmaceutical Association.

McBride, J. T. (2011). The association of acetaminophen and asthma prevalence and severity. *Pediatrics, 128*(6), 1181–1185.

National Asthma Education and Prevention Program. (2007). Expert panel report 3: Guidelines for the diagnosis and management of asthma (NIH Publication No. 08-4051). Bethesda, MD: National Institutes of Health, National Heart, Lung, and Blood Institute. Retrieved January 4, 2012, from http://www.nhlbi.nih.gov/guidelines/asthma/asthgdln.pdf

Pollart, S. M., & Elward, K. S. (2009). Overview of changes to asthma guidelines: Diagnosis and screening. *American Family Physician, 79*(9), 761–767.

Porth, C. M. (2010). *Pathophysiology: Concepts of altered health states* (8th ed.). Philadelphia, PA: Lippincott Williams & Wilkins.

Singh, S., Loke, Y. K., Enright, P. L., & Furberg, C. D. (2011). Mortality associated with tiotropium mist inhaler in patients with chronic obstructive pulmonary disease: Systematic review and meta-analysis of randomised controlled trials. *British Medical Journal, 342*, d3215.

Smeltzer, S. C., Bare, B. G., Hinkle, J. L., & Cheever, K. H. (2010). *Brunner & Suddarth's textbook of medical-surgical nursing* (12th ed.). Philadelphia, PA: Lippincott Williams & Wilkins.

Weiler, J. M. (2007). American Academy of Allergy, Asthma & Immunology Work Group report: Exercise-induced asthma. *Journal of Allergy and Clinical Immunology, 119*, 1349–1358.

Wood-Baker, R. R., Gibson, P., Hannay, M., Walters, E. H., & Walters, J. A. E. (2007). Systemic corticosteroids for acute exacerbations of chronic obstructive pulmonary disease. *The Cochrane Database of Systematic Reviews,* Issue 2.

SECTION 7

Drugs Affecting the Renal and Digestive Systems

Drugs Affecting the Renal and Digestive Systems

CHAPTER OUTLINE

32 Drug Therapy for Fluid Volume Excess

LEARNING OBJECTIVES

After studying this chapter, you should be able to:

1. Recognize normal renal physiology and the conditions requiring diuretic administration.

2. Describe the thiazide diuretics in terms of their prototype, mechanism of action, indications for use, major adverse effects, and nursing implications.

3. Describe the loop diuretics in terms of their prototype, mechanism of action, indications for use, major adverse effects, and nursing implications.

4. Describe the potassium-sparing diuretics in terms of their prototype, mechanism of action, indications for use, major adverse effects, and nursing implications.

5. Discuss the rationale for using combination products containing a potassium-losing and a potassium-sparing diuretic.

6. Discuss the rationale for concomitant use of a loop diuretic and a thiazide or related diuretic.

7. Understand how to apply the nursing process in the care of patients receiving diuretics.

Clinical Application Case Study

Agnes Bass, a 68-year-old woman, presents to the emergency department in acute heart failure complaining of an inability to "catch my breath." Her initial vital signs are temperature 99°F, pulse 108 beats per minute, respirations 28 per minute, and blood pressure 172/90 mm Hg. Her O_2 saturation is 88% on room air. Mrs. Bass has a history of uncontrolled hypertension, and her husband reports that for the past 2 months, they did not have sufficient money to buy her medications.

KEY TERMS

Anasarca: generalized massive edema

Anuria: no urine output

Ascites: accumulation of fluid in the abdominal cavity

Ceiling threshold: near-maximum response of a drug that is yielded by a certain dose

Dependent edema: localized edema occurring in the feet and ankles in people who are ambulatory

Edema: excessive accumulation of fluid in body tissues

Introduction

Drugs used to treat fluid volume excess, thereby increasing urine formation and output, are referred to as diuretics. These drugs increase renal excretion of water, sodium, and other electrolytes. They are important therapeutic agents widely used in the management of both edematous (e.g., heart failure, renal and hepatic disease) and nonedematous (e.g., hypertension, ophthalmic surgery) conditions. Diuretics are also useful in preventing renal failure by their ability to sustain urine flow. To aid understanding of diuretic drug therapy, it is necessary to understand normal renal physiology.

Renal Physiology

The primary function of the kidneys is to regulate the volume, composition, and pH of body fluids. The kidneys receive approximately 25% of the cardiac output. From this large amount of blood flow, the normally functioning kidney is efficient in retaining substances needed by the body and eliminating those not needed.

The Nephron

The nephron is the functional unit of the kidney; each kidney contains approximately 1 million nephrons. Each nephron is composed of a glomerulus and a tubule (Fig. 32.1). The glomerulus is a network of capillaries that receives blood from the renal artery. Bowman's capsule is a thin-walled structure that surrounds the glomerulus and then narrows and continues as the tubule. The tubule is a thin-walled structure of epithelial cells surrounded by peritubular capillaries. The tubule is divided into three main segments, the proximal tubule, loop of Henle, and distal tubule, which differ in structure and function.

The tubules are often called convoluted tubules because of their many twists and turns. The convolutions provide a large surface area that brings the blood flowing through the peritubular capillaries and the glomerular filtrate flowing through the tubular lumen into close proximity. Consequently, substances can be readily exchanged through the walls of the tubules.

The nephron functions by three processes: glomerular filtration, tubular reabsorption, and tubular secretion. These processes normally maintain the fluid volume, electrolyte concentration, and pH of body fluids within a relatively narrow range. They also remove waste products of cellular metabolism. A minimum daily urine output of approximately 400 mL is required to remove normal amounts of metabolic end products.

Glomerular Filtration

Arterial blood enters the glomerulus by the afferent arteriole at the relatively high pressure of approximately 70 mm Hg. This pressure pushes water, electrolytes, and other solutes out of the capillaries into Bowman's capsule and then to the proximal tubule. This fluid, called glomerular filtrate, contains the same components as blood except for blood cells, fats, and proteins that are too large to be filtered.

The glomerular filtration rate (GFR) is about 180 L/d, or 125 mL/min. Most of this fluid is reabsorbed as the glomerular filtrate travels through the tubules. The end product is about 2 L of urine daily. Because filtration is a nonselective process, the reabsorption and secretion processes determine the composition of the urine. After it is formed, urine flows into collecting tubules, which carry it to the renal pelvis, then through the ureters, bladder, and urethra for elimination from the body.

Blood that does not become part of the glomerular filtrate leaves the glomerulus through the efferent arteriole. The efferent arteriole branches into the peritubular capillaries that eventually empty into veins, which return the blood to systemic circulation.

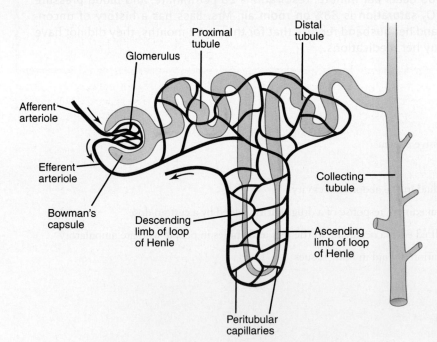

Figure 32.1 The nephron is the functional unit of the kidney.

Tubular Reabsorption

In relation to renal function, the term reabsorption indicates movement of substances from the tubule (glomerular filtrate) to the blood in the peritubular capillaries. Most reabsorption occurs in the proximal tubule. Almost all glucose and amino acids are reabsorbed; about 80% of water, sodium, potassium, chloride, and most other substances is reabsorbed. As a result, about 20% of the glomerular filtrate enters the loop of Henle. In the descending limb of the loop of Henle, water is reabsorbed; in the ascending limb, sodium is reabsorbed. A large fraction of the total amount of sodium (up to 30%) filtered by the glomeruli is reabsorbed in the loop of Henle. Additional sodium is reabsorbed in the distal tubule, primarily by the exchange of sodium ions for potassium ions secreted by epithelial cells of tubular walls. Final reabsorption of water occurs in the distal tubule and small collecting tubules. The remaining water and solutes are now appropriately called urine.

Antidiuretic hormone from the posterior pituitary gland promotes reabsorption of water from the distal tubules and the collecting ducts of the kidneys. This conserves water needed by the body and produces more concentrated urine. Aldosterone, a hormone from the adrenal cortex, promotes sodium–potassium exchange mainly in the distal tubule and collecting ducts. Thus, aldosterone promotes sodium reabsorption and potassium loss.

Tubular Secretion

The term secretion, in relation to renal function, indicates movement of substances from blood in the peritubular capillaries to glomerular filtrate flowing through the renal tubules. Secretion occurs in the proximal and distal tubules, across the epithelial cells that line the tubules. In the proximal tubule, uric acid, creatinine, hydrogen ions, and ammonia are secreted; in the distal tubule, potassium ions, hydrogen ions, and ammonia are secreted. Secretion of hydrogen ions is important in maintaining acid–base balance in body fluids.

Overview of Conditions Requiring Diuretic Agents

To adequately understand the pharmacologic treatment of fluid volume excess, it is important to understand the causes, pathophysiology, and clinical manifestations of renal disorders.

Etiology

Many clinical conditions alter renal function. In some conditions, excessive amounts of substances (e.g., sodium, water) are retained; in others, needed substances (e.g., potassium, proteins) are eliminated. Causal conditions include cardiovascular, renal, hepatic, and other disorders, which may be managed with diuretic drugs. Burns and trauma or allergic and inflammatory reactions may also lead to fluid shifts or loss.

Pathophysiology

Much of the pathophysiology related to the cause of conditions leading to the use of diuretics is discussed in other chapters. The pathophysiology of conditions producing **edema** formation (excessive accumulation of fluid in body tissues) is outlined below. Edema interferes with blood flow to tissues. Thus, it interferes with delivery of oxygen and nutrients and removal of metabolic waste products. If severe, edema may distort body features, impair movement, and interfere with activities of daily living.

Edema formation results from one or more of the following mechanisms that allow fluid to leave the bloodstream (intravascular compartment) and enter interstitial (third) spaces:

- Increased capillary permeability occurs as part of the response to tissue injury, including allergic and inflammatory reactions.
- Increased capillary hydrostatic pressure results from a sequence of events in which increased blood volume (from fluid overload or sodium and water retention) or obstruction of venous blood flow causes a high venous pressure and a high capillary pressure. This is the primary mechanism for edema formation in heart failure, pulmonary edema, and renal failure.
- Decreased plasma oncotic pressure may occur with decreased synthesis of plasma proteins (caused by liver disease or malnutrition) or increased loss of plasma proteins (caused by burn injuries or the nephrotic syndrome). Plasma proteins are important in keeping fluids within the bloodstream. When plasma proteins are lacking, fluid seeps through the capillaries and accumulates in tissues.

Clinical Manifestations

- Clinical manifestations reflect the alterations in fluid and electrolyte balance brought on by the inability of the kidneys to control the volume, composition, and pH of body fluids. Edema is a symptom of many disease processes and may occur in any part of the body. Specific manifestations of edema are determined by its location and extent. A common type of localized edema, known as **dependent edema**, occurs in the feet and ankles, especially with prolonged sitting or standing. A less common but more severe type of localized edema in the lungs is pulmonary edema, a life-threatening condition that occurs with circulatory overload (e.g., of intravenous [IV] fluids, blood transfusions) or acute heart failure. Generalized massive edema, or **anasarca**, interferes with the functions of many body organs and tissues.

Drug Therapy

Diuretic drugs act on the kidneys to decrease reabsorption of sodium, chloride, water, and other substances. Major subclasses are the thiazides and related diuretics, loop diuretics, and potassium-sparing diuretics, which act at different sites in the nephron (Fig. 32.2). The choice of diuretic drug depends primarily on the patient's condition.

Major clinical indications for diuretics are edema, heart failure, and hypertension. In edematous states, diuretics mobilize

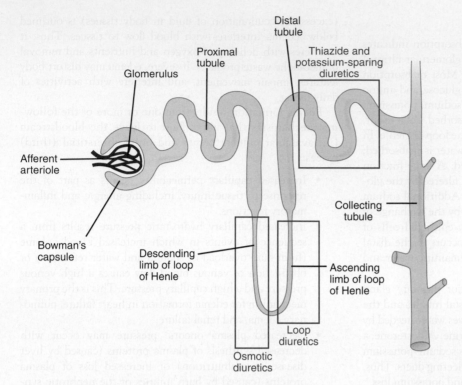

Figure 32.2 Diuretic sites of action in the nephron. Diuretics act at different sites in the nephron to decrease reabsorption of sodium and water and to increase urine output.

tissue fluids by decreasing plasma volume. In hypertension, the exact mechanism by which diuretics lower blood pressure is unknown, but antihypertensive action is usually attributed to sodium depletion. Initially, diuretics decrease blood volume and cardiac output. With chronic use, cardiac output returns to normal, but there is a persistent decrease in plasma volume and peripheral vascular resistance. Sodium depletion may have a vasodilating effect on arterioles.

Chapters 24 and 28 further discuss the use of diuretic agents in the management of heart failure and hypertension, respectively. The following section describes the types of diuretics, and Table 32.1 lists individual drugs.

Thiazide Diuretics

Thiazide diuretics are synthetic drugs that are chemically related to the sulfonamides and differ mainly in their duration of action. (P) **Hydrochlorothiazide** (Esidrix, Oretic), the most commonly used drug in the class, is the prototype. It is not a strong diuretic and works efficiently only when urine flow is adequate. Thiazide diuretics are the drugs of choice for most patients who require diuretic therapy, especially for long-term management of heart failure and hypertension. All drugs in this group have similar effects.

TABLE 32.1

Drugs Administered for the Treatment of Fluid Volume Excess

Drug Class	Prototype	Other Drugs in the Class
Thiazide Thiazide-like diuretics	Hydrochlorothiazide (Esidrix, Oretic)	Chlorothiazide (Diuril) Chlorthalidone (Hygroton, Thalitone) Indapamide (Lozol) Metolazone (Zaroxolyn)
Loop diuretics	Furosemide (Lasix)	Bumetanide (Bumex) Ethacrynic acid (Edecrin) Torsemide (Demadex)
Potassium-sparing diuretics	Spironolactone (Aldactone)	Amiloride (Midamor) Triamterene (Dyrenium)
Osmotic diuretics	Mannitol (Osmitrol)	
Combination products		Aldactazide Dyazide Maxzide Moduretic (see Table 32.6 for details)

Pharmacokinetics

Hydrochlorothiazide is administered orally and is well absorbed, widely distributed in body fluids, and highly bound to plasma proteins. The drug accumulates only in the kidneys. Diuretic effects usually occur within 2 hours, peak at 4 to 6 hours, and last 6 to 24 hours. Antihypertensive effects usually last long enough to allow use of a single daily dose. Most of the drug is excreted unchanged by the kidneys within 3 to 6 hours.

Action

Hydrochlorothiazide acts to decrease reabsorption of sodium, water, chloride, and bicarbonate in the distal convoluted tubule. Most sodium is reabsorbed before it reaches the distal convoluted tubule and only a small amount is reabsorbed at this site.

Use

Health care providers use hydrochlorothiazide to treat mild to moderate hypertension and the edema associated with heart failure and nephrotic syndrome. For most patients, this drug is effective. Table 32.2 presents route and dosage information for hydrochlorothiazide and the other thiazide diuretics.

Use in Children

Authorities have not established the safety and effectiveness of hydrochlorothiazide in children. IV chlorothiazide usually is not recommended. Thiazides do not commonly cause hyperglycemia, hyperuricemia, or hypercalcemia in children, as they do in adults.

Use in Older Adults

Prescribers often order hydrochlorothiazide and other thiazide diuretics for the management of hypertension and heart failure, which are common in older adults. Older adults are especially sensitive to adverse drug effects, such as hypotension and electrolyte imbalance. The drug may aggravate renal or hepatic impairment. With rapid or excessive diuresis, myocardial infarction, renal impairment, or cerebral thrombosis may occur from fluid volume depletion and hypotension. The smallest effective dose is recommended. Adverse effects may exceed therapeutic benefits at doses greater than 25 mg.

Use in Patients With Renal Impairment

Hydrochlorothiazide may be useful in managing edema due to renal disorders such as nephrotic syndrome and acute glomerulonephritis. However, its effectiveness decreases as the GFR decreases, and it becomes ineffective when the GFR is less than 30 mL/min. The drug may accumulate and increase

TABLE 32.2

DRUGS AT A GLANCE: Thiazide-Like Diuretics

Drug	Pregnancy Category	Routes and Dosage Ranges	
		Adults	Children
Ⓟ **Hydrochlorothiazide** (Esidrix, Oretic)	B	Edema: 25–100 mg/d PO; max dose 200 mg/d Hypertension: 12.5–50 mg PO 1 or 2 times daily Elderly, 12.5–25 mg/d PO	2 mg/kg/d PO in two divided doses Infants <6 mo, 2–3 mg/kg/d in two divided doses
Chlorothiazide (Diuril)	C	500–2000 mg/d PO divided in 1–2 times doses Elderly, 500 mg PO once daily or 1 g 3 times/wk 250–1000 mg IV once or twice daily; max dose 1000 mg	22 mg/kg/d PO in two divided doses Infants <6 mo, 20–40 mg/kg/d in two divided doses; max dose 375 mg/d IV dosing not well established
Chlorthalidone (Hygroton, Thalitone)	C	25–100 mg/d PO Elderly, 12.5–25 mg/d PO (or every other day)	Not approved in children
Indapamide (Lozol)	B	Edema: 2.5–5 mg/d PO Hypertension: 1.25 mg PO in morning; may increase to 5 mg/d	Dosage not established
Metolazone (Zaroxolyn)	B	Edema: 2.5–20 mg/d PO, depending on severity of condition and response Hypertension: 2.5 mg/d Elderly, 2.5 mg/d or every other day	Dosage not established

adverse effects in patients with impaired renal function. Thus, it is necessary to perform renal function tests periodically.

Use in Patients With Hepatic Impairment

Patients with severe hepatic impairment are at significant risk for thiazide-induced hypokalemic and hypochloremic alkalosis. Hepatic encephalopathy and death have occurred due to the electrolyte imbalances that accompany diuretic therapy. Blood ammonia levels may become increasingly elevated in people with previously elevated ammonia concentrations. Therapy with thiazide diuretics should be administered cautiously in patients with hepatic impairment and discontinued promptly if signs of impending hepatic coma (e.g., increased jaundice, tremors, confusion, and asterixis) appear.

Use in Patients With Critical Illness

Hydrochlorothiazide is ineffective when immediate diuresis is required because of its slow onset of action. The loop diuretics are more likely to be administered in a critical care setting, because more potent diuretic agents may be necessary (see later discussion).

QSEN Safety Alert ❗

It is important to note that hydrochlorothiazide should not be given the morning of surgery, because it may lead to volume depletion, causing the blood pressure to be labile and undergo frequent changes with general anesthesia.

Use in Patients Receiving Home Care

Diuretics are often taken in the home setting. The home care nurse may need to assist patients and caregivers in using the drugs safely and effectively, monitor patient responses, and provide information as indicated. With each home visit, the nurse assesses nutritional status, blood pressure, weight, and use of over-the-counter medications that may aggravate edema or hypertension.

Adverse Effects

Adverse effects of hydrochlorothiazide include hypersensitivity reactions, hypotension, weakness, dizziness, diarrhea, constipation, electrolyte imbalances (e.g., hyponatremia, hypokalemia, hypochloremia), hyperglycemia, paresthesia, and erectile dysfunction.

Contraindications

Contraindications to hydrochlorothiazide include known sensitivity to thiazides of sulfonamide-derived agents, or renal decompensation or **anuria** (no urine output).

QSEN Safety Alert ❗

It is essential to use thiazide diuretics and related drugs cautiously in patients who are allergic to sulfonamide drugs because there is a known cross-sensitivity of some sulfonamide-allergic patients to a sulfonamide nonantibiotic.

BOX 32.1   Drug Interactions: Hydrochlorothiazide

Drugs That Increase the Effects of Hydrochlorothiazide

- Alcohol, barbiturates, monoamine oxidase inhibitors, opioids, phosphodiesterase 5 inhibitors, prostacyclin analogues
  Increase hypotensive effects, possibly contributing to orthostasis
- Beta-blockers
  Increase the risk of hyperglycemia, hyperlipidemia, and hyperuricemia
- Carbamazepine
  Increases the risk of hyponatremia
- Chlorpropamide, corticosteroids, digoxin
  Increase the risk of hypokalemia

Drugs That Decrease the Effects of Hydrochlorothiazide

- Cholestyramine
  May significantly decrease absorption
- Methylphenidate, nonsteroidal anti-inflammatory drugs, yohimbine
  Decrease hypotensive effects

Also, caution is necessary during pregnancy because the drug crosses the placenta and may have adverse effects on the fetus by compromising placental perfusion. It may cause an increased risk of congenital defects.

Nursing Implications

Preventing Interactions

Several drugs and herbs increase or decrease the effects of hydrochlorothiazide (Boxes 32.1 and 32.2). The thiazide diuretic can increase the effects of angiotensin-converting enzyme inhibitors, other hypertensive agents, allopurinol, calcitriol, and lithium.

Administering the Medication

Hydrochlorothiazide, like all thiazide diuretics, has a **ceiling threshold**, which means that a certain dose yields a near-maximum diuretic response. This dose, known as the ceiling dose, is dependent on the type of diuretic and the extent of a person's disease. As the maximum effect is reached, a subsequent increase in dose does not enhance efficacy. In addition, there is a direct correlation between the dosage increase and the possible onset of adverse effects. When the diuretic dose is less than at ceiling, fluid retention remains following diuresis.

Assessing for Therapeutic Effects

The nurse assesses for the return of blood pressure to acceptable levels and improvement in the edema associated with heart failure and nephrotic syndrome.

Assessing for Adverse Effects

Monitoring for transient or irreversible hearing impairment, tinnitus, or dizziness is important. Ototoxicity is more likely to occur with high serum drug levels (e.g., high doses or in patients with severe renal impairment) or when other ototoxic drugs (e.g., aminoglycoside antibiotics) are being taken concurrently.

Patient Teaching

The nurse instructs the patient regarding the importance of taking the medication as prescribed, keeping follow-up appointments, and watching for signs and symptoms of adverse effects. Box 32.3 presents general patient teaching guidelines, which are a good reference.

Other Drugs in the Class

Chlorothiazide is the only thiazide diuretic that can be given intravenously. Related diuretics are nonthiazides whose pharmacologic actions are essentially the same as those of the thiazides; they include chlorthalidone, indapamide, and metolazone. Chlorthalidone has a longer duration of action (48–72 hours), which is attributed to slower excretion.

Indapamide, a thiazide-related drug, is the first of a new class of diuretics called the indolines. The drug is useful in the treatment of hypertension and can be given with other antihypertensive agents for an additive effect. People can take indapamide without regard to food. Its adverse effect profile is similar to that of hydrochlorothiazide.

Metolazone, another thiazide-related drug, is not generally recommended, but prescribers sometimes use it. Metolazone has some advantages over a thiazide because it is a stronger diuretic, causes less hypokalemia, and can produce diuresis in renal failure. In children, it is most often used with furosemide,

in which case it is most effective when given 30 to 60 minutes before the furosemide dose.

Loop Diuretics

Loop diuretics are the diuretics of choice when rapid effects are required (e.g., in pulmonary edema) and when renal function is impaired (creatinine clearance < 30 mL/min). Ⓟ **Furosemide** (Lasix) is the most commonly used loop diuretic and serves as the prototype for the group. Dosage can be titrated upward as needed to produce greater diuretic effects. Overall, loop diuretics are the most effective and versatile diuretics available for clinical use.

Pharmacokinetics

Furosemide is available in oral or IV forms. After oral administration, the diuretic effect of the drug occurs within 30 to 60 minutes, peaks in 1 to 2 hours, and lasts 6 to 8 hours. After IV administration, diuretic effects occur within 5 minutes, peak within 30 minutes, and last about 2 hours. Thus, furosemide produces extensive diuresis for short periods, after which the kidney tubules regain their ability to reabsorb sodium. Actually, the kidneys reabsorb more sodium than usual during this post-diuretic phase, so a high dietary intake of sodium can cause sodium retention and reduce or cancel the diuretic-induced sodium loss. Thus, dietary sodium restriction is required to achieve optimum therapeutic benefits. The drug is metabolized and excreted by the kidneys, and drug accumulation does not occur even with repeated doses.

Action

Furosemide and other loop diuretics inhibit sodium and chloride reabsorption in the ascending limb of the loop of Henle, where reabsorption of most filtered sodium occurs. Thus, these potent drugs produce significant diuresis, their sodium-losing effect being up to 10 times greater than that of thiazide diuretics.

Use

Furosemide is useful when given alone or in combination with other antihypertensive agents to treat hypertension. Uses include the management of acute pulmonary edema, heart failure, as well as hepatic and renal disease. It is feasible to titrate the dosage titrated upward as needed to produce greater diuretic effects. Table 32.3 presents route and dosage information for furosemide and the other loop diuretics.

Use in Children

Furosemide is the loop diuretic used most often in children. Oral therapy is preferred when feasible, and authorities do not recommend doses greater than 6 mg/kg of body weight per day. For maintenance therapy, it is necessary to adjust the dose to the minimum effective level. In preterm infants, furosemide stimulates production of prostaglandin E_2 in the kidneys and may increase the incidence of patent ductus arteriosus and neonatal respiratory distress syndrome. In neonates, furosemide

BOX 32.3	Patient Teaching Guidelines for Diuretics

General Considerations

■ Diuretics increase urine output and are commonly used to manage hypertension, heart failure, and edema (swelling) from heart, kidney, liver, and other disorders.

■ While taking a diuretic drug, you need to maintain regular medical supervision so drug effects can be monitored and dosages adjusted when indicated.

■ Reducing sodium intake in your diet helps diuretic drugs be more effective and allows smaller doses to be taken. Smaller doses are less likely to cause adverse effects. Thus, you need to avoid excessive table salt and obviously salty foods (e.g., ham, packaged sandwich meats, potato chips, dill pickles, most canned soups). These foods may aggravate edema or hypertension by causing sodium and water retention.

■ Diuretics may cause blood potassium imbalances, and either too little or too much damages heart function. Periodic measurements of blood potassium and other substances are one of the major reasons for regular visits to a health care provider.

   ■ Too little potassium (hypokalemia) may result from the use of potassium-losing diuretics such as hydrochlorothiazide, furosemide (Lasix), and several others. To prevent or treat hypokalemia, your physician may prescribe a potassium chloride supplement or a combination of a potassium-losing and a potassium-saving diuretic (either separately or as a combined product such as Dyazide, Maxzide, or Aldactazide). He or she may also recommend increased dietary intake of potassium-containing foods (e.g., bananas, orange juice).

   ■ Too much potassium (hyperkalemia) can result from the use of potassium-saving diuretics, the overuse of potassium supplements, or from the use of salt substitutes. Potassium-saving diuretics are not a major cause of hyperkalemia because they are usually given along with a potassium-losing diuretic. If potassium supplements are prescribed, they should be taken as directed. You should *not* use salt substitutes without consulting your primary health care provider because they contain potassium chloride instead of sodium chloride. Hyperkalemia is most likely to occur in people with decreased kidney function, which often occurs in older adults and people with diabetes.

■ With diuretic therapy, you will have increased urination, which usually lasts only a few days or weeks if you do not have edema. If you do have edema (e.g., in your ankles), you can expect weight loss and decreased swelling as well as increased urination. It is a good idea to check and record your weight two to three times per week (at same time of day with similar amount of clothing). Rapid changes in weight often indicate gain or loss of fluid.

■ Some commonly used diuretics may increase blood sugar levels and cause or aggravate diabetes. If you have diabetes, you may need larger doses of your antidiabetic medications.

■ Diuretics may cause sensitivity to sunlight. Thus, you need to avoid prolonged exposure to sunlight, use sunscreens, and wear protective clothing.

■ Do not drink alcoholic beverages or take other medications without the approval of your health care provider.

■ If you are taking a diuretic to lower your blood pressure, especially with other antihypertensive drugs, you may feel dizzy or faint when you stand up suddenly. This can be prevented or decreased by changing positions slowly. If dizziness is severe, notify your health care provider. Do not drive or operate dangerous machinery until the effects of the drug are known.

Self- or Caregiver Administration

■ Take or give a diuretic early in the day, if ordered daily, to decrease nighttime trips to the bathroom. Fewer bathroom trips mean less interference with sleep and less risk of falls. Ask someone to help you to the bathroom if you are elderly, weak, dizzy, or unsteady in walking (or use a bedside commode).

■ Take or give most diuretics with or after food to decrease stomach upset. Torsemide (Demadex) may be taken without regard to meals.

■ If you are taking digoxin, a potassium-losing diuretic, and a potassium supplement, it is very important that you take these drugs as prescribed. This is a common combination of drugs for patients with heart failure, and the drugs work together to increase beneficial effects and avoid adverse effects. Stopping or changing the dose of one of these medications while continuing the others can lead to serious illness.

---

may be given with indomethacin to prevent nonsteroidal anti-inflammatory drug–induced nephrotoxicity (toxic or damaging effects to the kidney) during therapeutic closure of a patent ductus arteriosus. In both preterm and full-term infants, the half-life of furosemide is prolonged but becomes shorter as renal and hepatic functions develop.

Use in Older Adults

In general, dose selection for the older adults requires caution, usually starting at the low end of the dosing range, reflecting the increased likelihood that older adults have decreased cardiac, renal, or hepatic function. Additionally, older adults often have concomitant disease or other drug therapy. It is necessary to monitor renal function because excessive diuresis,

particularly in older adults, may cause dehydration, blood volume reduction with circulatory collapse, and the risk of vascular thrombosis and embolism.

Use in Patients With Renal Impairment

Although furosemide and other loop diuretics are effective in patients with renal impairment, in those with chronic renal failure, the drugs have lower peak concentrations at their site of action, which decreases diuresis. Renal elimination is also prolonged. If renal dysfunction becomes more severe during treatment (e.g., oliguria, increases in blood urea nitrogen [BUN] or creatinine), it may be necessary to discontinue the drug. High doses may produce fluid volume depletion and worsen renal function.

TABLE 32.3

DRUGS AT A GLANCE: Loop Diuretics

Drug	Pregnancy Category	Routes and Dosage Ranges	
		Adults	**Children**
P **Furosemide** (Lasix)	C	Edema: 20–80 mg PO as a single dose initially; if an adequate diuretic response is not obtained, dosage may be gradually increased by 20- to 40-mg increments at intervals of 6–8 h; for maintenance, dosage range and frequency of administration vary widely and must be individualized; max daily dose, 600 mg Hypertension: 40 mg PO twice daily, gradually increased if necessary Rapid mobilization of edema: 20–40 mg IV initially, injected slowly; dose may be repeated in 2 h Acute pulmonary edema: initial dose is usually 40 mg, which may be repeated in 60–90 min Acute renal failure: 40 mg IV initially, increased if necessary; max dose, 1–2 g/24 h Hypertensive crisis: 40–80 mg IV injected over 1–2 min; with renal failure, much larger doses may be needed. 5–20 mg PO, IV once daily	2 mg/kg PO one or 2 times daily initially, gradually increased by increments of 1–2 mg/kg per dose if necessary at intervals of 6–8 h; max daily dose, 6 mg/kg 1 mg/kg IV initially; if diuretic response is not adequate, increase dosage by 1 mg/kg no sooner than 2 h after previous dose; max dose, 6 mg/kg
Bumetanide (Bumex)	C	0.5–2 mg PO daily as a single dose; may be repeated every 4–6 h to a max dose of 10 mg, if necessary; giving on alternate days or for 3–4 d with rest periods of 1–2 d is recommended for long-term control of edema 0.5–1 mg IV, IM, repeated in 2–3 h if necessary, to a max daily dose of 10 mg; give IV injections over 1–2 min	Not recommended for children <18 y
Ethacrynic acid (Edecrin)	B	Edema: 50–100 mg PO daily, increased or decreased according to severity of condition and response; max daily dose, 400 mg; rapid mobilization of edema: 50 mg IV or 0.5–1 mg/kg injected slowly to a max of 100 mg/dose	25 mg PO daily; parenteral dose not recommended in children
Torsemide (Demadex)	B	Heart failure: 10–20 mg PO, IV daily; titrate by doubling the dose to a max of 200 mg daily Hypertension: 5 mg PO daily up to 10 mg for appropriate response Chronic renal failure: 20 mg daily PO, IV; titrate by doubling the dose to a max of 200 mg daily Hepatic failure: 5–10 mg PO daily up to 40 mg for appropriate response	Safety and efficacy not established in children

EVIDENCE-BASED PRACTICE

National Collaborating Centre for Acute and Chronic Conditions (2010)

Management of chronic heart failure in adults in primary and secondary care. National Institute for Health and Clinical Excellence (NICE). (Clinical guideline; no. 108). Retrieved November 8, 2011 from http://guideline.gov/content.aspx?f=rss&id=15712

Polypharmacy for the treatment of chronic heart failure in adults is common. For the relief of congestive symptoms and fluid retention in affected patients, it is necessary to use diuretics routinely and adjust dosages according to the initiation of subsequent heart failure therapies. Patients with diagnosed heart failure with preserved ejection fraction should typically receive treatment with loop diuretics at a low to medium doses (e.g., less than 80 mg furosemide per day). Patients who do not respond to this treatment need reevaluation.

IMPLICATIONS FOR NURSING PRACTICE: Chronic health conditions, such as chronic heart failure, require balancing multiple drugs to aid symptom improvement. Diuretics are indicated to manage fluid retention. The nurse should be diligent in observing for signs of improvement in these patients and document accordingly.

Use in Patients With Hepatic Impairment

Furosemide is often used to manage edema and **ascites** (accumulation of fluid in the abdominal cavity) in patients with hepatic impairment. Caution is warranted because diuretic-induced fluid and electrolyte imbalances may precipitate or worsen hepatic encephalopathy and coma. In patients with cirrhosis, diuretic therapy should begin in a hospital setting, with small doses and careful monitoring. To prevent hypokalemia and metabolic alkalosis, supplemental potassium or spironolactone may be necessary. Potassium imbalances may occur with diuretic therapy; Box 32.4 offers prevention and management strategies for potassium imbalances.

Use in Patients With Critical Illness

Fast-acting, potent diuretics such as furosemide (and bumetanide) are the most likely diuretics to be used in critically ill patients (e.g., those with pulmonary edema). Although patients often receive IV bolus doses of the drugs, continuous IV infusions may be more effective and less likely to produce adverse effects in critically ill patients.

Use in Patients Receiving Home Care

Furosemide is commonly used in the home setting. It is critical that the drug be administered safely and effectively and that patient response is monitored. With each home visit, the nurse assesses nutritional status, blood pressure, weight, and use of over-the-counter medications that may aggravate edema or hypertension. In addition, the nurse may need to provide assistance in obtaining medications or blood for blood tests (e.g., serum potassium levels) and information as indicated.

A steady state of potassium within normal limits is necessary for cardiac function. Hypokalemia and hyperkalemia are cardiotoxic and should be prevented when possible.

Adverse Effects

Adverse effects of furosemide include fluid and electrolyte imbalances (e.g., hyponatremia, hypokalemia, fluid volume deficit) and ototoxicity. It is usually possible to avoid ototoxicity, which is associated with high plasma drug levels (greater than 50 mcg/mL), by dividing oral doses and by slow injection or continuous infusion of IV doses.

BOX 32.4   Prevention and Management of Potassium Imbalances

Hypokalemia (Serum Potassium Level < 3.5 mEq/L)
Measures to prevent or manage hypokalemia include the following:

- Giving supplemental potassium, usually potassium chloride, in an average dosage range of 20 to 60 mEq daily. Sustained-release tablets are usually better tolerated than liquid preparations.

- Increasing food intake of potassium. The minimal daily requirement of potassium is unknown; usual recommendations are 40 to 50 mEq daily for the healthy adult. Potassium loss with diuretic drugs may be several times this amount. To provide 50 mEq of potassium daily, estimated amounts of certain foods include 1000 mL of orange juice, 1600 mL of apple or grape juice, 1200 mL of pineapple juice, four to six bananas, or 30 to 40 prunes.

  - Some of these foods are high in calories and may be contraindicated, at least in large amounts, for obese patients.

- Also, the amount of carbohydrate in these foods may be a concern for patients with diabetes mellitus.

- Restricting dietary sodium intake. This reduces potassium loss by decreasing the amount of sodium available for exchange with potassium in renal tubules.

Hyperkalemia (Serum Potassium Level > 5 mEq/L)
The following measures help prevent hyperkalemia:

- Avoiding use of potassium-sparing diuretics and potassium supplements in patients with renal impairment

- Avoiding excessive amounts of potassium chloride supplements

- Avoiding salt substitutes (half of which are commonly potassium chloride)

- Maintaining urine output, the major route for eliminating potassium from the body

Contraindications

Contraindications to furosemide include known sensitivity to the drug or anuria. Patients who are allergic to sulfonamides may also be allergic to furosemide. Pregnancy is another contraindication, unless the benefits to the mother outweigh the risks to the fetus.

Nursing Implications

Preventing Interactions

Several drugs and herbs may decrease or increase the effects of furosemide (Box 32.5; see Box 32.2). Additionally, furosemide may decrease the effects of insulin or oral antidiabetic drugs; blood glucose levels may rise.

Administering the Medication

The nurse gives IV injections of furosemide over 1 to 2 minutes and administers high-dose furosemide continuous IV infusions at a rate of 4 mg/min or less. This decreases or avoids high peak serum levels, which increases the risk of adverse effects, including ototoxicity. If using high doses of furosemide, a volume-controlled IV infusion at a rate of 4 mg or less per minute may be useful. For continuous infusion, it is necessary to mix furosemide with normal saline or lactated Ringer's solution because 5% dextrose in water, or D5W, may accelerate degradation of furosemide.

Assessing for Therapeutic Effects

The nurse assesses for decreased or absent edema, increased urine output, and decreased blood pressure. In patients with heart failure or acute pulmonary edema, it is necessary to observe for decreased dyspnea, crackles, cyanosis, and cough.

Assessing for Adverse Effects

Like any effective diuretic, furosemide may cause volume depletion and electrolyte imbalance, especially in patients receiving higher doses and a restricted salt intake. Hypokalemia may develop, especially with rapid diuresis, inadequate oral electrolyte intake, or when cirrhosis is present. Digitalis therapy may exaggerate metabolic effects of hypokalemia, particularly myocardial effects. The nurse should assess the patient for diminished hearing, a sign of ototoxicity. It is necessary to monitor serum electrolytes closely in children because of the frequent changes in kidney function and fluid distribution associated with growth and development.

Patient Teaching

The reason for furosemide use should guide patient teaching. In most instances, it is necessary to initiate measures to limit sodium intake. Key considerations should include not adding salt to food during preparation or at the dinner table, reading food labels carefully to be aware of hidden sources of sodium, and avoiding processed or high-sodium foods. The nurse instructs the patient in the use of equipment needed to take routine blood pressure readings. The general teaching guidelines presented in Box 32.3 provide additional patient education information.

Other Drugs in the Class

The pharmacologic characteristics of all loop diuretics are similar; use of another loop diuretic after a lack of response to one loop diuretic at adequate doses is not indicated. Instead, it is necessary to consider combining diuretics with different sites of action if aggressive diuresis is required.

Bumetanide (Bumex) may be used to produce diuresis in some patients who are allergic to or no longer respond to furosemide. It is more potent than furosemide by drug weight, and large doses can be given in small volumes. These drugs differ mainly in potency and produce similar effects at equivalent doses (e.g., furosemide 40 mg = bumetanide 1 mg). Bumetanide should be given by IV injection over 1 to 2 minutes.

Torsemide (Demadex) is indicated for the treatment of edema associated with heart failure, renal disease, or hepatic disease. It is also used for the treatment of hypertension alone or in combination with other antihypertensive agents. This drug is highly bioavailable after oral administration. Oral and IV doses are equivalent, and it is possible to switch patients from one route to the other without changing the dosage. To decrease or avoid high peak serum levels, which increase the risk of adverse effects, including ototoxicity, it is necessary to give torsemide intravenously over 2 minutes.

BOX 32.5 | **Drug Interactions: Furosemide**

Drugs That Increase the Effects of Furosemide

- Aminoglycosides, cephalosporins
  Increase the risk of nephrotoxicity
- Corticosteroids, digoxin
  Increase the risk of hypokalemia

Drugs That Decrease the Effects of Furosemide

- Ibuprofen
  Inhibits prostaglandins
- Phenytoin
  Decreases absorption

Clinical Application 32-1

After receiving oxygen at 2 L/min on nasal cannula, placement in a high Fowlers' position, and administration of 40 mg of IV furosemide, Mrs. Bass's vital signs are temperature 99°F, pulse 102 beats per minute, respirations 26 per minute, blood pressure 172/90 mm Hg, and O_2 saturation 89%. Physical assessment findings include crackles on auscultation, productive cough, and bilateral 2+ peripheral edema to the knees. A physician makes a diagnosis of biventricular heart failure.

- What is the rationale for the use of IV furosemide to treat the heart failure?
- What is the pathophysiology of fluid overload reflected in the assessment findings?

NCLEX Success

1. A patient receives intravenous (IV) furosemide 80 mg for symptoms of severe heart failure. The nurse recognizes that administering the drug slowly by IV push reduces the likelihood of which of the following adverse effects of drug therapy?

   A. hyponatremia
   B. hypokalemia
   C. fluid volume deficit
   D. ototoxicity

2. What assessment finding in a patient with heart failure receiving furosemide (Lasix) would indicate an improvement in fluid volume status?

   A. absence of crackles on auscultation of lungs
   B. complaints of proximal nocturnal dyspnea
   C. bounding radial pulse
   D. decrease in hematocrit

3. A man who is taking an oral hypoglycemic for management of his type 2 diabetes mellitus begins taking hydrochlorothiazide. The nurse should monitor for which of the following serum laboratory changes?

   A. hypocalcemia
   B. hypercalcemia
   C. hyperglycemia
   D. hypernatremia

Potassium-Sparing Diuretics

Potassium-sparing diuretics act at the distal tubule to decrease sodium reabsorption and potassium excretion. The aldosterone antagonist and prototype is ℗ **Spironolactone** (Aldactone).

Pharmacokinetics

Given orally, the effects of spironolactone are rather slow, requiring several days before full therapeutic effect is achieved; onset, peak, and duration occur between 24 and 48 hours. The half-life of the drug is 1.3 to 2 hours. Maximal effects may not occur for 6 weeks when the drug is used as an antihypertensive. It is excreted in the feces and urine.

Action

Spironolactone competitively blocks the effects of aldosterone, a hormone secreted by the adrenal cortex, in the renal tubules. Spironolactone blocks the sodium-retaining effects of aldosterone, and aldosterone must be present for spironolactone to be effective. This effect promotes retention of sodium and water and excretion of potassium by stimulating the sodium–potassium exchange mechanism in the distal tubule. Independently, the drug is a weak diuretic because urine volume can only be slightly modified in the renal tubules; it can be combined with other diuretics to increase efficacy.

Use

Primary uses of spironolactone include treatment of heart failure, ascites (in patients with liver disease), hypokalemia, hypertension, as well as primary and secondary hyperaldosteronism. Table 32.4 gives route and dosage information for spironolactone and other potassium-sparing diuretics.

Use in Patients With Renal Impairment

Spironolactone accumulates in renal failure, and a reduction in dosage is warranted. Usually, practitioners do not use the drug in severe renal failure.

Use in Patients With Hepatic Impairment

As mentioned earlier, there is an association between hepatic encephalopathy and the administration of diuretics, including some potassium-sparing diuretics. Although diuretics are used in the management of hepatic failure, they should be used cautiously and carefully monitored in patients with significant hepatic impairment because a rapid change in fluid and electrolyte balance may lead to hepatic coma. It is important to monitor susceptible patients carefully for signs and symptoms of hepatic encephalopathy such as tremors, confusion, increased jaundice, and coma. Because spironolactone is primarily metabolized in the liver, dosage reduction may be necessary in severe hepatic impairment.

TABLE 32.4

DRUGS AT A GLANCE: Potassium-Sparing Diuretics

Drug	Pregnancy Category	Routes and Dosage Ranges	
		Adults	Children
℗ **Spironolactone** (Aldactone)	C (D in pregnancy-induced hypertension)	25–200 PO mg daily	Safety and effectiveness have not been established.
Amiloride (Midamor)	B	5–20 mg PO daily	Dosage not established
Triamterene (Dyrenium)	C	100–300 mg PO daily in divided doses	2–4 mg/kg/d PO in divided doses

Use in Patients With Critical Illness

Diuretics other than spironolactone, which is administered orally, that can be administered intravenously are more likely to be used in critically ill patients to control the volume, composition, and pH of body fluids. Additionally, because critically ill patients can develop renal insufficiency, the risk of hyperkalemia with spironolactone is potentially harmful in most critically ill patients.

Use in Patients Receiving Home Care

People may take spironolactone in the home care setting, and patients or family members may ask the home care nurse for advice about diuretic use or the clinical condition for which the drug is administered. The nurse should emphasize the need to read the labels of all over-the-counter medications as well as products, such as salt substitutes, for ingredients, adverse effects, and drug interactions that could complicate the patient's clinical condition. He or she should ensure that signs of hypotension and hyperkalemia and measures to manage these conditions are taught to the patient and the caregiver (see Box 32.4).

Adverse Effects

Common adverse effects of spironolactone include dizziness, headache, abdominal cramping, and diarrhea. Because the drug also affects androgen receptors and other steroid receptors, it can cause deepening of the voice, gynecomastia, menstrual irregularities, and testicular atrophy. Use has been known to cause an increased risk of gastric bleeding, although the mechanism is unknown.

The U.S. Food and Drug Administration (FDA) has issued a **BLACK BOX WARNING** ◆ for spironolactone. Investigations have shown that the drug is tumorigenic with chronic toxicity in rats; unnecessary use should be avoided.

Contraindications

Contraindications to spironolactone include known hypersensitivity to the drug. The presence of renal insufficiency is also a contraindication, as previously discussed, because use of spironolactone may cause hyperkalemia through the inhibition of aldosterone and the subsequent retention of potassium.

Nursing Implications

Preventing Interactions

Multiple drug and herbs interact with spironolactone, either increasing or decreasing its effects (Box 32.6; see Box 32.2). Also, spironolactone increases the half-life of digoxin, which could lead to digitalis toxicity. In addition, spironolactone may reduce renal clearance of lithium, producing a high risk of lithium toxicity.

Administering the Medication

It is necessary to administer spironolactone at the same time each day, preferably during the morning, even if the patient feels well.

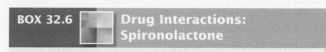

BOX 32.6   Drug Interactions: Spironolactone

Drugs That Increase the Effects of Spironolactone

- Angiotensin-converting enzyme inhibitors, angiotensin II receptor blockers, potassium-containing drugs, tacrolimus
  Increase the risk of hyperkalemia
- Beta-blockers
  Increase the risk of hyperglycemia and hypertriglyceridemia

Drugs That Decrease the Effects of Spironolactone

- Alcohol, antihypertensive drugs, in particular vasodilators and alpha-blockers
  Increase the risk of hypotension and orthostasis

Assessing for Therapeutic Effects

The nurse assesses for decrease or absence of edema, increased urine output, decreased blood pressure, or decreased ascites (in patients with liver disease). He or she measures and records weights to assist in determining the amount of mobilization of excess fluid. In patients with liver disease, it is necessary to assess abdominal girth to determine improvement in ascites.

Assessing for Adverse Effects

The nurse observes for evidence of fluid and electrolyte imbalance, including hyperkalemia, hyponatremia, hypomagnesemia, and hypochloremic alkalosis. It is necessary to perform periodic laboratory tests to measure serum electrolytes at appropriate intervals, particularly in older adults and in people with significant renal or hepatic impairment.

Patient Teaching

Routine blood pressure readings are necessary; the nurse instructs the patient in the use of equipment needed for these measurements. The nurse should instruct the patient that the drug may cause dizziness or drowsiness; the patient should curtail activities that require mental alertness (e.g., driving, operating machinery) until the effects of the drug are known. Use in pregnancy is appropriate only when the benefits to the mother outweigh the risks to the fetus. Box 32.3 contains additional patient teaching information.

Other Drugs in the Class

Amiloride (Midamor) and triamterene (Dyrenium) act directly on the distal tubules to decrease the exchange of sodium for potassium and have similar diuretic activity. Amiloride enhances renal prostaglandin production whereas triamterene decreases prostaglandin production. The choice of the specific potassium-sparing diuretic drug depends primarily on the patient's condition. Potassium-sparing diuretics are weak diuretics when used alone. Thus, they are usually given in combination with the so-called potassium-losing diuretics to increase diuretic activity and decrease potassium loss. The potassium-sparing diuretics are contraindicated in the presence of renal insufficiency because their use may cause hyperkalemia through the inhibition of aldosterone and subsequent retention of potassium. Hyperkalemia is the major adverse effect of these drugs.

QSEN Safety Alert

It is essential that patients receiving potassium-sparing diuretics do not receive potassium supplements and do not eat foods high in potassium or use salt substitutes. (Salt substitutes contain mostly potassium chloride rather than sodium chloride.)

Box 32.4 presents strategies to manage hyperkalemia.

Adjuvant Medications Used to Treat Fluid Volume Excess

Osmotic Diuretics

Osmotic diuretics produce rapid diuresis by increasing the solute load (osmotic pressure) of the glomerular filtrate. The increased osmotic pressure causes water to be pulled from extravascular sites into the bloodstream, thereby increasing blood volume and decreasing reabsorption of water and electrolytes in the renal tubules. The drug is freely filterable at the glomerular level, but it is not reabsorbed by the renal tubules. Ⓟ **Mannitol** (Osmitrol), the prototype, is useful in managing oliguria or anuria, and it may prevent acute renal failure (ARF) during prolonged surgery, trauma, or infusion of cisplatin, an antineoplastic agent. Mannitol is effective even when renal circulation and GFR are reduced (e.g., in hypovolemic shock, trauma, dehydration). When administered early in ARF, the drug tends to clear cellular debris and prevent tubular cast formation. Other important clinical uses of hyperosmolar agents include reduction of intracranial pressure before or after neurosurgery, reduction of intraocular pressure before certain types of ophthalmic surgery (see Chap. 58), and urinary excretion of toxic substances.

The onset of diuretic action of mannitol is 1 to 3 hours and reduction of intracranial pressure occurs in 15 to 30 minutes. Its half-life is approximately 1 to 1.6 hours. Excretion is primarily as unchanged drug in the urine.

Table 32.5 presents route and dosage information for mannitol.

Clinical Application 32-2

- Mrs. Bass has improved, and her vital signs are temperature 98.6°F, pulse 84 beats per minute, respirations 18 per minute, blood pressure 132/80 mm Hg, and O₂ saturation 94% on room air. Her physician orders an extra dose of 20 mg of IV furosemide, to be given now. What administration guidelines should the nurse consider?

Combination Products

Thiazide diuretics are available in numerous fixed-dose combinations with nondiuretic antihypertensive agents (see Chap. 28) and with potassium-sparing diuretics. Table 32.6 lists combination diuretic products. A major purpose of the antihypertensive combinations is to increase patient convenience and compliance with drug therapy regimens. A major purpose of the diuretic combinations is to prevent potassium imbalances.

To prevent or manage hypokalemia and to augment the diuretic effect, people may take a potassium-sparing diuretic concurrently with a potassium-losing diuretic. They may take the two drugs separately or in a fixed-dose combination product.

Alternatively, when an inadequate diuretic response occurs with one of the drugs, people sometimes take two potassium-losing diuretics concurrently. The combination of a loop and a thiazide diuretic has synergistic effects because the drugs act in different segments of the renal tubule. The synergistic effects probably result from the increased delivery of sodium to the distal tubule (where thiazides act) because a loop diuretic blocks sodium reabsorption in the loop of Henle. A commonly used combination is furosemide and hydrochlorothiazide (chlorothiazide can be given intravenously in patients who are unable to take an oral drug). Another combination is furosemide and metolazone. Generally, because a thiazide–loop diuretic combination can induce profound diuresis, with severe sodium, potassium, and volume depletion, only hospitalized patients who can be closely monitored should receive it. Ambulatory patients should take this

TABLE 32.5
DRUGS AT A GLANCE: Osmotic Diuretics (Mannitol)

Drug	Pregnancy Category	Routes and Dosage Ranges	
		Adults	*Children*
Ⓟ **Mannitol** (Osmitrol)	C	Cerebral edema: 0.25–2 g/kg IV as 15%–20% solution administered over at least 30 min, not more frequently than every 6–8 h	Cerebral edema: 1 mo to 12 y old: IV, 0.25–1.5 g/kg

TABLE 32.6

Combination Diuretic Products

Drug	Thiazide (Potassium-Losing) Diuretic	Potassium-Sparing Diuretic	Adult Dosage
Aldactazide 25/25	HCTZ 25 mg	Spironolactone 25 mg	1–8 tablets PO daily
Aldactazide 50/50	HCTZ 50 mg	Spironolactone 50 mg	1–4 tablets PO daily
Dyazide, Maxzide 25 mg/37.5 mg	HCTZ 25 mg	Triamterene 37.5 mg	Hypertension: 1 capsule PO twice daily initially, then adjusted according to response Edema: 1–2 capsules PO twice daily
Maxzide 50 mg/75 mg	HCTZ 50 mg	Triamterene 75 mg	1 tablet PO daily
Moduretic	HCTZ 50 mg	Amiloride 5 mg	1–2 tablets PO daily with meals

HCTZ, hydrochlorothiazide.

combination in very low doses or only occasionally to avoid serious adverse events.

NCLEX Success

4. Mrs. Conley, age 53, has had hypertension for 10 years and admits that she does not comply with her prescribed antihypertensive therapy. Recently, she has begun to experience shortness of breath and ankle swelling. A workup reveals the presence of chronic renal insufficiency. What classification of diuretic is the first drug of choice for the nurse practitioner to prescribe?

A. thiazide
B. loop
C. osmotic
D. potassium-sparing

5. A nurse is instructing a patient on dietary considerations while taking spironolactone (Aldactone). Which of the following statements made by the patient indicates that further teaching is necessary?

A. "I should not eat foods high in potassium while taking this medication."
B. "I should use a salt substitute instead of regular salt."
C. "I should call my nurse practitioner if I have any significant adverse effects from my medications."
D. "I should not take large amounts of potassium chloride supplements."

6. A patient reports a drug allergy to sulfonamides. Which diuretic drug class should the nurse question if ordered for the patient?

A. loop diuretics
B. thiazides
C. potassium-sparing diuretics
D. osmotic diuretics

The Nursing Process

Assessment

- Useful baseline data include serum electrolytes, creatinine, glucose, blood urea nitrogen (BUN), and uric acid, because diuretics may alter these values. Other data are blood pressure readings, weight, amount and appearance of urine output, and measurement of edematous areas such as ankles or abdomen.
- Observe for edema. Visible edema often occurs in the feet and legs of ambulatory patients. Rapid weight gain may indicate fluid retention.
  - With heart failure, numerous signs and symptoms result from edema of various organs and tissues. For example, congestion in the gastrointestinal tract may cause nausea and vomiting; liver congestion may cause abdominal pain and tenderness; and congestion in the lungs (pulmonary edema) causes rapid, labored breathing, hypoxemia, frothy sputum, and other manifestations of severe respiratory distress.
  - Cerebral edema may be manifested by confusion, headache, dizziness, convulsions, unconsciousness, bradycardia, or failure of the pupils to react to light.
  - Ascites, which occurs with hepatic cirrhosis, is an accumulation of fluid in the abdominal cavity. The abdomen appears much enlarged.
- With heart failure, fatigue and dyspnea, in addition to edema, are common symptoms.
- Hypertension (blood pressure greater than 140/90 mm Hg on several measurements) may be the only clinical manifestation present.

Nursing Diagnoses

- Excess fluid volume in edematous patients related to retention of sodium and water
- Deficient fluid volume related to increased diuresis during diuretic drug therapy

- Imbalanced nutrition: less than body requirements related to excessive loss of potassium with thiazide and loop diuretics
- Risk for injury: hypotension and dizziness as adverse drug effects
- Deficient knowledge related to the need for and correct use of diuretics
- Sexual dysfunction related to adverse drug effects

Planning/Goals

The patient will

- Take or receive diuretic drugs as prescribed
- Experience reduced edema and improved control of blood pressure
- Reduce dietary intake of sodium and increase dietary intake of potassium
- Avoid preventable adverse drug effects
- Keep appointments for follow-up monitoring of blood pressure, edema, and serum electrolytes

Nursing Interventions

The nurse will

- Promote measures to prevent or minimize conditions for which diuretic drugs are used
  - With edema, helpful measures include the following:
    - Decreasing dietary sodium intake
    - Losing weight, if obese
    - Elevating legs when sitting
    - Avoiding prolonged standing or sitting
    - Wearing support hose or elastic stockings
    - Treating the condition causing edema
  - With heart failure and in older adults, it is necessary to administer intravenous (IV) fluids or blood transfusions carefully to avoid fluid overload and pulmonary edema. Fluid overload may occur with rapid administration or excessive amounts of IV fluids.

- With hypertension, helpful measures include decreasing dietary sodium intake, exercising regularly, and losing weight, if obese.
- With edematous patients, interventions to monitor fluid losses include weighing under standardized conditions, measuring urine output, and measuring edematous sites such as the ankles or the abdomen. After the patient reaches "dry weight," these measurements stabilize and can be done less often.
- With patients who are taking digoxin, a potassium-losing diuretic, and a potassium supplement, help them understand that the drugs act together to increase therapeutic effectiveness and avoid adverse effects (e.g., hypokalemia, digoxin toxicity). Thus, stopping or changing dosage of one of these drugs can lead to serious illness.
- Provide patient teaching regarding drug therapy (see Box 32.3)

Evaluation

- Observe for reduced edema and body weight.
- Observe for reduced blood pressure.
- Observe for increased urine output.
- Monitor serum electrolytes for normal values.
- Interview regarding compliance with instructions for diet and drug therapy.
- Monitor compliance with follow-up appointments in outpatients.

Clinical Application 32-3

- Mrs. Bass says that she enjoys snacks such as potato chips and pretzels. What response should the nurse make?

Key Concepts

- Diuretic drugs act on the kidneys to decrease reabsorption of sodium, chloride, water, and other substances.
- A body weight change of 2.2 pounds (1 kg) may indicate a gain or loss of 1000 mL of fluid.
- Excessive table salt and salty foods (e.g., ham, packaged sandwich meats, potato chips, dill pickles, most canned soups) may aggravate edema or hypertension.
- Thiazide diuretics are the drugs of choice for most patients who require diuretic therapy, especially for long-term management of heart failure and hypertension.
- High-dose furosemide continuous IV infusions should be given at a rate of 4 mg/min or less to decrease or avoid risks of adverse effects, including ototoxicity.
- There is a known cross-sensitivity of some sulfonamide-allergic patients to a sulfonamide nonantibiotic, such as thiazides.
- Loop diuretics have a sodium-losing effect up to 10 times greater than that of thiazide diuretics.
- Patients with renal impairment should not take potassium-sparing diuretics because of the high risk of hyperkalemia.

- The U.S. Food and Drug Administration (FDA) has issued a **BLACK BOX WARNING** ◆ for spironolactone, which has been shown to be tumorigenic with chronic toxicity in rats; unnecessary use should be avoided.

- When digoxin and diuretics are given concomitantly, the risk of digoxin toxicity is increased due to diuretic-induced hypokalemia.

Critical Thinking Questions

32-1. Brenda Oliver, a 32-year-old executive, is diagnosed with hypertension and is starting hydrochlorothiazide. She is currently taking birth control pills and complains that she has peripheral edema in the evenings.

- What important information should be obtained from Mrs. Oliver before the discharging her from the clinic?

- What are important points to teach Mrs. Oliver about safe and effective drug usage?

- If on return to clinic, Mrs. Oliver's symptoms have not improved, what questions need answers?

References and Resources

Drug facts and comparisons. (Updated monthly). St. Louis, MO: Facts and Comparisons.

Ernst, M. E., & Gordon, J. A. (2010). Diuretic therapy: Key aspects in hypertension and renal disease. *Journal of Nephrology, 23*(5), 487–493.

Karch, A. M. (2012). *2012 Lippincott's nursing drug guide.* Philadelphia, PA: Lippincott Williams & Wilkins.

Lacy, C. F., Armstrong, L. L., Goldman, M. P., & Lance, L. L. (2010). *Lexi-Comp's drug information handbook* (19th ed.). Hudson, OH: American Pharmaceutical Association.

Munar, M. Y., & Harleen, S. (2007). Drug dosing in patients with chronic kidney disease. *American Family Physician, 75*(10), 1487–1496.

National Collaborating Centre for Acute and Chronic Conditions. (2010). Management of chronic heart failure in adults in primary and secondary care. National Institute for Health and Clinical Excellence (NICE). (Clinical guideline; no. 108). Retrieved November 8, 2011, from http://guideline.gov/content.aspx?f=rss&id=15712

Porth, C. M. (2009). *Pathophysiology: Concepts of altered health status* (8th ed.). Philadelphia, PA: Lippincott Williams & Wilkins.

Sica, D. A. (2007). Use of diuretics in the treatment of heart failure in the elderly. *Clinics in Geriatric Medicine, 23,* 107–121.

33 Nutritional Support Products, Vitamins, and Mineral Supplements

Clinical Application Case Study

Jenny Martin, an 86-year-old woman, has lived alone for 10 years since her husband died. She sometimes must limit her food purchases to pay for her medicines and utilities. Thus, her nutritional status is poor. A neighbor, who has not seen Mrs. Martin for a couple of days, finds her conscious on the kitchen floor but with slurred speech. Emergency medical personnel transport her to a hospital emergency department, where she is diagnosed with a left brain stroke with right hemiparesis, dysarthria, and dysphagia.

Mrs. Martin is unable to swallow foods safely, so the nurses insert a nasogastric tube. A dietician orders a high-calorie commercially prepared formula that contains carbohydrates, protein, fat, vitamins, and minerals.

KEY TERMS

Chelating agents: drugs used to treat metal poisoning (e.g., from iron, lead, or mercury) that bind to the toxic metal, decrease binding of the metal within the body, and promote elimination of the metal

Electrolytes: electrically charged particles found in body fluids and cells (e.g., sodium or potassium ions)

Enteral nutrition: provision of fluid and nutrients to a functional gastrointestinal tract via a feeding tube in a patient who is unable to ingest enough fluid and food

Fat-soluble vitamins: vitamins that are accumulated and stored in the body when taken in excess

Hyperkalemia: greater than normal amount of potassium in the blood

Hypokalemia: less than normal amount of potassium in the blood

Malabsorption: impaired absorption of nutrients from the gastrointestinal tract

Megaloblastic anemia: anemia characterized by the presence in the blood of megaloblasts (large, abnormal blood cells); associated with vitamin B_{12} deficiency

Megavitamins: large dose of vitamins in excess of the recommended dietary allowance

Parenteral nutrition: intravenous provision of fluid and nutrients to a patient who is unable to ingest enough fluid and food due to a nonfunctional gastrointestinal tract

Water-soluble vitamins: vitamins that are not stored in the body and are rapidly eliminated

Introduction

Water, carbohydrates, proteins, fats, vitamins, and minerals are required to promote or maintain health, to prevent illness, and to promote recovery from illness or injury. Water is necessary for cellular metabolism and excretion of metabolic waste products; people need 2000 to 3000 mL daily. Carbohydrates and fats mainly provide energy for cellular metabolism. Energy is measured in kilocalories (kcal) per gram of food oxidized in the body. Carbohydrates and proteins supply 4 kcal/g; fats supply 9 kcal/g. Proteins are structural and functional components of all body tissues; the recommended amount for adults is 50 to 60 g daily.

Vitamins are required for normal body metabolism, growth, and development. They are components of enzyme systems that release energy from ingested carbohydrates, proteins, and fats. They also are necessary for formation of genetic material, red blood cells, hormones, nerve cells, and bone and other tissues. Minerals and electrolytes are essential constituents of cell membranes, many essential enzymes, bone, teeth, and connective tissue. They function to maintain electrolyte and acid–base balance, maintain osmotic pressure, maintain nerve and muscle function, assist in transfer of compounds across cell membranes, and influence the growth process.

Patients' requirements for these nutrients vary widely, depending on age, sex, size, health or illness status, and other factors. This chapter discusses medications and products to improve nutritional status in patients with deficiency states and excess states of selected vitamins, minerals, and electrolytes.

Overview of Altered Nutritional States

Etiology

Many patients may be unable to ingest, digest, absorb, or use sufficient nutrients to improve or maintain health. Debilitating illnesses often interfere with appetite and gastrointestinal (GI) function. Drugs often cause anorexia, nausea, vomiting, or diarrhea. The lack of certain vitamins and minerals may impair the

function of body organs. Genetic disorders or traumatic injury may also affect nutritional status.

Pathophysiology

Dietary intake must provide required amino acids, fatty acids, and lipids, as well as vitamins and minerals. Both deficient and excess amounts of these nutrients adversely influence health. Nutritional status directly affects enzyme function, immune response, and wound healing.

Vitamins

Vitamins are organic compounds that help release energy from carbohydrates, fats, and proteins. They are necessary for the formation of genetic materials, red blood cells, hormones, and the nervous system, as well as for normal growth and development.

There are two types of vitamins: fat soluble and water soluble. **Fat-soluble vitamins**—vitamins A, D, E, and K—are stored in the body when taken in excess. They are absorbed from the intestine with dietary fat. Absorption requires the presence of bile salts and pancreatic lipase. (Note that vitamin D is discussed in Chap. 42 because of its major role in bone metabolism.) **Water-soluble vitamins**—B complex vitamins and vitamin C—are not stored in the body and are rapidly eliminated.

People can obtain vitamins from foods or supplements. Although experts believe foods to be the best source, studies indicate that most adults and children do not consume enough fruits, vegetables, cereal grains, dairy products, and other foods to consistently meet their vitamin requirements. In addition, some conditions increase requirements above the recommended amounts (e.g., pregnancy, lactation, and various illnesses). Historically, the major concern about vitamins concerned whether a person's intake was sufficient to promote health and prevent deficiency diseases. Hence, the Food and Nutrition Board of the National Academy of Sciences established recommendations for daily vitamin intake known as Dietary Reference Intakes (DRIs) (Box 33.1).

BOX 33.1   **Dietary Reference Intakes (DRIs)**

Dietary Reference Intakes (DRIs) are the recommended amounts of vitamins (see Table 33.1) and some minerals (see Table 33.2). The Food and Nutrition Board of the Institute of Medicine revised the current DRIs in 2006; the board intended them to replace the recommended dietary allowances (RDAs) used since 1989. DRIs consist of four subtypes of nutrient recommendations, as follows:

1. **Recommended dietary allowance (RDA)** is the amount estimated to meet the needs of approximately 98% of healthy children and adults in a specific age and gender group. The RDA is used to advise various groups about nutrient intake. It should be noted, however, that RDAs were established to prevent deficiencies and that they were extrapolated from studies of healthy adults. Thus, they may not be appropriate for all groups, such as young children and older adults.

2. **Estimated average requirement (EAR)** is the amount estimated to provide adequate intake in 50% of healthy persons in a specific group. The EAR is a median amount that takes into account the bioavailability of the nutrient and reduction of chronic disease. The EAR is used to determine the RDA.

3. **Adequate intake (AI)** is the amount thought to be sufficient when there is not enough reliable, scientific information to estimate an RDA. The AI is derived from data that show an average intake that appears to maintain health. Although an RDA is expected to meet the needs of all healthy people, an AI does not clearly indicate the percentage of people whose needs will be met.

4. **Tolerable upper intake level (UL)** is the maximum intake considered unlikely to pose a health risk in almost all healthy people in a specified group. The UL is not intended to be a recommended level of intake.

- **Vitamins.** The ULs for adults (ages 19–70 years and older) are D 50 mcg, E 1000 mg, B_3 (niacin) 35 mg, B_6 (pyridoxine) 100 mg, folate 1000 mcg, and C 2000 mg. With vitamin D, pyridoxine, and vitamin C, the UL refers to total intake from food, fortified food, and supplements. With niacin and folate, the UL applies to synthetic forms obtained from supplements, fortified food, or a combination of the two. With vitamin E, the UL applies to any form of supplemental alpha-tocopherol. *These ULs should not be exceeded.* There are inadequate data for establishing ULs for B_1 (thiamine), B_2 (riboflavin), B_5 (pantothenic acid), B_{12} (cyanocobalamin), and biotin. As a result, consuming more than the recommended amounts of these vitamins should generally be avoided.

- **Minerals.** ULs have been established for magnesium 350 mg, calcium 2.5 g, phosphorus 3 to 4 g, fluoride 10 mg, and selenium 400 mcg. *The UL should not be exceeded for any mineral–electrolyte because all minerals are toxic in overdose.* Except for magnesium, which is set for supplements only and excludes food and water sources, the stated UL amounts include those from both food and supplements.

Vitamin deficiencies occur as a result of inadequate intake or disease processes that interfere with absorption or use of vitamins. Excess states occur with excessive intake of fat-soluble vitamins because these vitamins accumulate in the body. Excess states do not occur with dietary intake of water-soluble vitamins but may occur with vitamin supplements that exceed recommended amounts.

Many authorities promote vitamin supplements as a means to improve health and prevent or treat illness. However, supplements can be harmful if overused. As a result, DRIs include tolerable upper intake levels (ULs) of some vitamins. Table 33.1 lists the function, recommended daily intake, food sources, and signs and symptoms of deficiency and excess of vitamins.

QSEN Safety Alert

No one should take more than the recommended ULs.

Although health care providers may order vitamin supplements, people mostly self-prescribe them. Because vitamins are essential nutrients, some people believe that large amounts (megadoses) promote health and provide other beneficial effects. However, excessive intake may cause harmful effects. People should never self-prescribe **megavitamins**, large doses of vitamins in excess of the recommended dietary allowance (RDA). Additional characteristics of vitamins include the following:

- Vitamins from supplements have the same physiological effects as those obtained from foods.
- Synthetic vitamins have the same structure and function as natural vitamins derived from plant and animal sources and are less expensive.
- Vitamin supplements do not require a prescription.
- Vitamin products vary widely in number, type, and amount of specific ingredients.
- Preparations should not contain more than the recommended amounts of vitamin A, vitamin D, and folic acid (a B complex vitamin).
- Multivitamin preparations often contain minerals as well. Large doses of all minerals are toxic.
- Vitamins are often marketed in combination products with each other (e.g., antioxidant vitamins) and with herbal products (e.g., B complex vitamins with ginseng). There is no reliable evidence to support the use of such products.

Some people believe that some vitamins (e.g., the vitamin A precursor beta carotene, vitamin E, and vitamin C), with their antioxidant effects, prevent heart disease, cancer, and other illnesses. Antioxidants inactivate oxygen free radicals, which are potentially toxic substances formed during normal cell metabolism, and inhibit them from damaging body cells. However, the results of most research studies with antioxidant vitamin supplements have been disappointing and inconclusive. The consensus view is that dietary vitamins

TABLE 33.1

Vitamins

Vitamin/Function	Dietary Reference Intakes	Food Sources	Signs and Symptoms of Deficiency	Signs and Symptoms of Excess
Fat-Soluble Vitamins **Vitamin A (retinol)** Required for normal vision, growth, bone development, skin, and mucous membranes	RDAs Females 14 y and older, 700 mcg Pregnancy, 750–770 mcg Lactation, 1200– 1300 mcg Males 14 y and older, 900 mcg Children 1–3 y, 300 mcg 4–8 y, 400 mcg 9–13 y, 600 mcg Infants (AIs) 0–6 mo, 400 mcg 6–12 mo, 500 mcg	Preformed vitamin A: meat, butter, fortified margarine, egg yolk, whole milk, cheese made from whole milk Carotenoids: turnip and collard greens, carrots, sweet potatoes, squash, apricots, peaches, cantaloupe	Night blindness; xerophthalmia, which may progress to corneal ulceration and blindness; changes in skin and mucous membranes that lead to skin lesions and infections; respiratory tract infections; urinary calculi	Anorexia, vomiting, irritability, skin changes (itching, desquamation, dermatitis); pain in muscles, bones, and joints; gingivitis; enlargement of spleen and liver; increased intracranial pressure; other neurological signs Congenital abnormalities in newborns whose mothers took excessive vitamin A during pregnancy Acute toxicity, with increased intracranial pressure, bulging fontanels, and vomiting, may occur in infants who are given vitamin A.
Vitamin D (see Chap. 42)				
Vitamin E Antioxidant Essential in preventing destruction of certain fats, including the lipid portion of cell membranes	RDAs* Females 14 y and older, 15 mg Pregnancy, 15 mg Lactation, 19 mg Males 14 y and older, 15 mg Children 1–3 y, 6 mg 4–8 y, 7 mg 9–13 y, 11 mg Infants (AIs) 0–6 mo, 4 mg 7–12 mo, 5 mg Older adults (UL), 1500 international unit	Cereals, green leafy vegetables, egg yolk, milk fat, butter, meat, vegetable oils	Deficiency is rare.	Fatigue, headache, blurred vision; nausea, diarrhea
Vitamin K Essential for normal blood clotting. It activates precursor proteins, found in the liver, into clotting factors II, VII, IX, and X.	RDAs Females 19 y and older, 90 mcg Pregnancy, 90 mcg If 14–18 y, 75 mcg Lactation, 90 mcg If 14–18 y, 75 mcg Males 19 y and older, 120 mcg Children 1–3 y, 30 mcg 4–8 y, 55 mcg 9–13 y, 60 mcg 14–18 y, 75 mcg	Green leafy vegetables (spinach, kale, cabbage, lettuce), cauliflower, tomatoes, wheat bran, cheese, egg yolk, liver	Abnormal bleeding (petechiae, ecchymoses, epistaxis, hematemesis, melena, hematuria, hypovolemic shock)	Clinical manifestations rare; however, when vitamin K is given to someone who is receiving warfarin (Coumadin), the patient can be made "warfarin-resistant" for 2–3 wk.

(Continued on page 612)

TABLE 33.1

Vitamins (Continued)

Vitamin/Function	Dietary Reference Intakes	Food Sources	Signs and Symptoms of Deficiency	Signs and Symptoms of Excess
Water-Soluble Vitamins *B complex Vitamins* **Vitamin B$_1$ (thiamine)** A coenzyme in carbohydrate metabolism; essential for energy production	RDAs Females 14–18 y, 1 mg 19 y and older, 1.1 mg Pregnancy, 1.4 mg Lactation, 1.4 mg Males 14 y and older, 1.2 mg Children 1–3 y, 0.5 mg 4–8 y, 0.6 mg 9–13 y, 0.9 mg Infants (AIs) 0–6 mo, 0.2 mg 7–12 mo, 0.3 mg	Meat, poultry, fish, egg yolk, dried beans, whole grain cereal products, peanuts	Mild deficiency: fatigue, anorexia; retarded growth; mental depression; irritability; apathy, lethargy Severe deficiency (beriberi): peripheral neuritis; personality disturbances; heart failure; edema Wernicke-Korsakoff syndrome in alcoholics	Not established
Vitamin B$_2$ (riboflavin) A coenzyme in metabolism; necessary for growth; may function in production of corticosteroids and red blood cells an in gluconeogenesis	RDAs Females 14–18 y, 1 mg 19 y and older, 1.1 mg Pregnancy, 1.4 mg Lactation, 1.6 mg Males 14 y and older, 1.3 mg Children 1–3 y, 0.5 mg 4–8 y, 0.6 mg 9–13 y, 0.9 mg Infants (AIs) 0–6 mo, 0.3 mg 7–12 mo, 0.4 mg	Milk, cheddar and cottage cheeses, meat, eggs, green leafy vegetables	Seborrheic dermatitis; glossitis; stomatitis; eye disorders (burning, itching, lacrimation, photophobia, vascularization of the cornea)	Not established
Biotin Part of the vitamin B$_2$ complex; essential in fat and carbohydrate metabolism	AIs Females 14–18 y, 25 mcg 19 y and older, 30 mcg Pregnancy, 30 mcg Lactation, 35 mcg Males 14–18 y, 25 mcg 19 y and older, 30 mcg Children 1–3 y, 8 mcg 4–8 y, 12 mcg 9–13 y, 20 mcg Infants 0–6 mo, 5 mcg 7–12 mo, 6 mcg	Meat, egg yolk, nuts, cereals, most vegetables	Anorexia, nausea; depression; muscle pain; dermatitis	Not established
Vitamin B$_3$ (niacin) Essential for glycolysis, fat synthesis, and tissue respiration. It functions	RDAs Females 14 y and older, 14 mg Pregnancy, 18 mg Lactation, 17 mg	Meat, poultry, fish, peanuts	Pellagra: erythematous skin lesions; GI problems (stomatitis, glossitis, enteritis, diarrhea);	Flushing, pruritus, hyperglycemia, increased liver enzymes, uricemia

TABLE 33.1

Vitamins (Continued)

Vitamin/Function	Dietary Reference Intakes	Food Sources	Signs and Symptoms of Deficiency	Signs and Symptoms of Excess
as a coenzyme in many metabolic processes (after conversion to nicotinamide, the physiologically active form).	Males 14 y and older, 16 mg Children 1–3 y, 6 mg 4–8 y, 8 mg 9–13 y, 12 mg Infants (AIs) 0–6 mo, 2 mg 7–12 mo, 4 mg		CNS problems (headache, dizziness, insomnia, depression, memory loss) Severe deficiency: delusions, hallucinations, impairment of peripheral motor and sensory nerves	
Vitamin B$_5$ (pantothenic acid) Essential for metabolism of carbohydrate, fat, and protein (e.g., release of energy from carbohydrate; fatty acid metabolism; synthesis of cholesterol, steroid hormones, and phospholipids)	AIs Females 14 y and older, 5 mg Pregnancy, 6 mg Lactation, 7 mg Males 14 y and older, 5 mg Children 1–3 y, 2 mg 4–8 y, 3 mg 9–13 y, 4 mg Infants 0–6 mo, 1.7 mg 7–12 mo, 1.8 mg	Eggs, liver, salmon, yeast, cauliflower, broccoli, lean beef, potatoes, tomatoes	No deficiency state established	Not established
Vitamin B$_6$ (pyridoxine) A coenzyme in metabolism of carbohydrate, protein, and fat; required for formation of tryptophan and conversion of tryptophan to niacin; helps release glycogen from the liver and muscle tissue; functions in metabolism of the central nervous system; helps maintain cellular immunity	DRIs Females 14–18 y, 1.2 mg 19–50 y, 1.3 mg 51–70 y and older, 1.5 mg Pregnancy, 1.9 mg Lactation, 2 mg Males 14–50 y, 1.3 mg 51–70 y and older, 1.7 mg Children 1–3 y, 0.5 mg 4–8 y, 0.6 mg 9–13 y, 1 mg Infants (AIs) 0–6 mo, 0.1 mg 7–12 mo, 0.3 mg	Yeast, wheat germ, liver and other glandular meats, whole grain cereals, potatoes, legumes	Skin and mucous membrane lesions (seborrheic dermatitis, intertrigo, stomatitis, glossitis); neurologic problems (seizures, peripheral neuritis, mental depression)	Not established
Vitamin B$_{12}$ (cyanocobalamin) Essential for normal metabolism of all body cells, normal red blood cells, normal nerve cells, growth, and metabolism of carbohydrate, protein, and fat	RDAs Females 14 y and older, 2.4 mcg Pregnancy, 2.6 mcg Lactation, 2.8 mcg Males 14 y and older, 2.4 mcg Children 1–3 y, 0.9 mcg 4–8 y, 1.2 mcg	Meat, eggs, fish, cheese	Pernicious anemia: decreased numbers of RBCs; large, immature RBCs; fatigue; dyspnea Severe deficiency: leukopenia, infection, thrombocytopenia, cardiac dysrhythmias, heart failure Neurologic signs and symptoms:	Not established

(Continued on page 614)

TABLE 33.1

Vitamins (Continued)

Vitamin/Function	Dietary Reference Intakes	Food Sources	Signs and Symptoms of Deficiency	Signs and Symptoms of Excess
	9–13 y, 1.8 mcg Infants (AIs) 0–6 mo, 0.4 mcg 7–12 mo, 0.5 mcg		paresthesias in hands and feet, unsteady gait, depressed deep tendon reflexes, loss of memory, confusion, delusions, hallucinations, psychosis Nerve damage may be irreversible.	
Folic acid (folate) A B complex vitamin; essential for normal metabolism of all body cells, normal RBCs, and growth	RDAs Females 14 y and older, 400 mcg Pregnancy, 600 mcg Lactation, 500 mcg Males 14 y and older, 400 mcg Older adults (UL), 1000 mcg Children 1–3 y, 150 mcg 4–8 y, 200 mcg 9–13 y, 300 mcg Infants (AIs) 0–6 mo, 65 mcg 7–12 mo, 80 mcg	Liver, kidney beans, fresh green vegetables (spinach, broccoli, asparagus), fortified grain products (e.g., breads, cereals, rice)	Megaloblastic anemia that cannot be distinguished from the anemia produced by vitamin B_{12} deficiency; impaired growth in children; glossitis; GI problems	Not established
Vitamin C (ascorbic acid) Essential for formation of skin, ligaments, cartilage, bone, and teeth; required for wound healing and tissue repair, metabolism of iron and folic acid, synthesis of fats and proteins, preservation of blood vessel integrity, and resistance to infection	RDAs Females 14–18 y, 65 mg 19 y and older, 75 mg Pregnancy, 80–85 mg Lactation, 115–120 mg Males 14–18 y, 75 mg 19 y and older, 90 mg Older adults (UL), 2000 mg Children 1–3 y, 15 mg 4–8 y, 25 mg 9–13 y, 45 mg Infants (AIs) 0–6 mo, 40 mg 7–12 mo: 50 mg	Fruits and vegetables, especially citrus fruits and juices	Mild deficiency: irritability, malaise, arthralgia, increased tendency to bleed Severe deficiency: scurvy and adverse effects on most body tissues (gingivitis; bleeding of gums, skin, joints, and other areas; disturbances of bone growth; anemia; and loosening of teeth); if not treated, coma and death may occur.	Renal calculi

*Vitamin E activity is expressed in milligrams of alpha-tocopherol equivalents (alpha TE).

AI, adequate intake; DRI, Dietary Reference Intake; GI, gastrointestinal; RBC, red blood cell; RDA, recommended dietary allowance.

from several daily servings of grains, fruits, and vegetables and a daily multivitamin supplement are beneficial for most children and adults, but it is not possible to make recommendations about vitamin supplements to prevent various chronic illnesses on the basis of current evidence. Because parents' desires to promote health may lead them to give children unneeded supplements or to give them more than recommended amounts, it may be necessary to give parents information about the potential hazards of vitamin overdoses.

Minerals

Minerals maintain acid–base balance and osmotic pressure. They make up part of enzymes, hormones, and vitamins. The body needs minerals for hemoglobin formation, muscle contraction, and skeletal development and maintenance. Minerals present in the body in large amounts (macrominerals) are sodium, potassium, chloride, calcium, magnesium, phosphorus, and sulfur. (Note: Calcium and phosphorus are discussed in Chapter 42 because they play major roles in bone metabolism.) Other minerals are required in small amounts (trace elements). Eight of these (chromium, cobalt, copper, fluoride, iodine, iron, selenium, and zinc) have relatively well-defined roles in human nutrition.

Minerals occur in the body and foods mainly in ionic form. When placed in solution, the components separate into **electrolytes**. Electrolytes are electrically charged particles found in body fluids and cells (e.g., sodium or potassium ions). At any given time, the body must maintain an equal number of positive and negative charges. Therefore, the ions are constantly combining and separating to maintain electrical neutrality or electrolyte balance.

Electrolytes also maintain the acid–base balance of body fluids. Acids are usually anions (e.g., bicarbonate, chloride, phosphate, or sulfate). Bases are usually cations (e.g., sodium, potassium, calcium, and magnesium). Mineral–electrolytes are obtained from foods or supplements. Although most minerals are supplied by a well-balanced diet, studies indicate that most adults and children do not ingest sufficient dietary calcium and that iron deficiency is common in some populations. In addition, some conditions increase requirements (e.g., pregnancy, lactation, and various illnesses) and some drug–drug interactions decrease absorption or use of minerals.

As with vitamins, goals for daily mineral intake have been established as DRIs. Thus far, DRIs and ULs have been established for calcium, fluoride, iron, magnesium, phosphorus, and selenium.

QSEN Safety Alert

People should not exceed the UL for any mineral–electrolyte.

Except for the stated amount for magnesium, which excludes food and water sources and considers supplements only, the ULs include those from both foods and supplements. Table 33.2 lists the function, recommended daily intake, and dietary sources of various minerals.

- Multivitamin–mineral combinations recommended for age and gender groups contain different amounts of some minerals (e.g., younger women need more iron than postmenopausal women). It is necessary to consider this when choosing a product.
- Iron supplements other than those in multivitamin–mineral combinations are usually intended for temporary use in the presence of deficiency or a period of increased need (e.g., pregnancy). People should not take them otherwise because of risks of accumulation and toxicity.
- Most adolescent and adult females probably benefit from a calcium supplement to achieve the recommended amount (1000–1300 mg daily). It is important to consider the amounts consumed in dairy products and other foods and not exceed the UL of 2500 mg daily.

Clinical Manifestations

Tables 33.1 and 33.2 list signs and symptoms associated with deficiency and excess of vitamins and minerals, respectively.

Drug Therapy

Early recognition and treatment of vitamin disorders can prevent a mild deficiency or excess from becoming severe. For deficiency states, oral vitamin preparations are preferred when possible. Multiple deficiencies are common, and a multivitamin preparation used to treat them usually contains more than the recommended daily amount. Use for limited periods is best. When fat-soluble vitamins are given to correct a deficiency, there is a risk of producing excess states. When water-soluble vitamins are given, excesses are less likely but may occur with large doses. For excess states, the usual treatment is to stop administration of the vitamin preparation. There are no specific antidotes or antagonists.

It is important to titrate the amount of mineral supplement closely to the amount needed by the body as there is a risk of producing an excess state. Oral products are preferred for replacement because they are safer, less likely to produce toxicity, more convenient to administer, and less expensive than parenteral preparations. The U.S. Food and Drug Administration (FDA) regulates content of supplements for infants and children younger than 4 years of age; however, it does not regulate the content of preparations for older children.

Children

Children need sufficient amounts of vitamins and minerals to support growth and normal body functioning. Dosages should not exceed recommended amounts. For infants (birth to 12 months), the only UL is for vitamin D. For other children, ULs vary according to age. A combined vitamin–mineral supplement every other day may be reasonable, especially for children who eat poorly.

There is a risk of overdose in children; this risk is more serious with the fat-soluble vitamins because they are stored long-term within the body. Also, all minerals and electrolytes are toxic in overdose. Because of manufacturers' marketing strategies, many supplements are available in flavors and shapes (e.g., animals, cartoon characters) designed to appeal to children.

QSEN Safety Alert

Because younger children may think of these supplements as candy and take more than recommended, it is essential that they be stored out of reach and dispensed by an adult.

Older Adults

Vitamin requirements are the same for older adults as for younger adults, but deficiencies are common, especially with the fat-soluble vitamins A and D. It is important to assess every older adult regarding vitamin intake (from food and supplements) and use of drugs that interact with dietary nutrients. For most older adults, a daily multivitamin is probably desirable, even for those who seem healthy and able to eat a well-balanced diet. In addition, requirements may be increased during illnesses, especially those affecting GI function. Overdoses, especially of the

TABLE 33.2

Minerals and Electrolytes

Mineral/Function	Dietary Reference Intakes	Food Sources	Signs and Symptoms of Deficiency	Signs and Symptoms of Excess
Macro Minerals				
Sodium Assists in regulating osmotic pressure, water balance, conduction of electrical impulses in nerves and muscles, and electrolyte and acid–base balance. Influences permeability of cell membranes and assists in movement of substances across cell membranes. Participates in many intracellular chemical reactions. Normal serum sodium = 135–145 mEq/L.	Adults (AI) 19–50 y: 1.5 g 50–70 y: 1.3 g 71 y and over: 1.2 g Adults (UL), 2.3 g	In most foods. Proteins contain large amounts; vegetables and cereals contain small to moderate amounts; fruits contain little or no sodium. Major source in the diet is table salt added to food in processing, cooking, or seasoning. One teaspoon contains 2.3 g of sodium. Water in some areas may contain significant amounts of sodium.	Serum sodium <135 mEq/L; anorexia, nausea, and vomiting; ataxia; confusion; delirium; hypotension and tachycardia; muscle tremors; oliguria and increased blood urea nitrogen; seizures; weakness	Serum sodium >145 mEq/L, disorientation, dry skin and mucous membranes, fever, hyperactive reflexes, hypotension, muscle rigidity, tremors and spasms, irritability, cerebral hemorrhage, coma, oliguria, concentrated urine, increased blood urea nitrogen
Potassium Within cells, helps maintain osmotic pressure, fluid, and electrolyte balance and acid–base balance. In extracellular fluid, is required for conduction of nerve impulses and contraction of muscle. Helps transport glucose into cells and is required for glycogen formation and storage. Required for synthesis of muscle proteins. Normal serum potassium = 3.5–5 mEq/L.	Adults (AI): 4.7 g Adults (UL), not established	Present in most foods, including meat, whole grain breads or cereals, bananas, citrus fruits, tomatoes, and broccoli	Serum potassium <3.5 mEq/L; dysrhythmias and ECG changes; cardiac arrest; confusion; delirium; hyperglycemia; postural hypotension; muscle weakness; abdominal distension, constipation, paralytic ileus; polyuria; polydipsia, nocturia. Prolonged deficiency may increase blood urea nitrogen and serum creatinine.	Serum potassium >5 mEq/L; muscle weakness; cardiotoxicity, with dysrhythmias or cardiac arrest. Cardiac effects are not usually severe until serum levels are 7 mEq/L or above.
Chloride Helps maintain osmotic pressure and electrolyte, acid–base, and water balance. Forms hydrochloric acid in gastric mucosal cells. Normal serum chloride = 95–103 mEq/L.	Adults (AI) 19–50 y: 2.3 g 50–70 y: 2 g 71 y and over: 1.8 g Adults (UL), 3.6 g	Most dietary chloride is ingested as sodium chloride, and foods high in sodium are also high in chloride.	Serum chloride <95 mEq/L; arterial blood pH >7.45; dehydration; hypotension; low respiratory rate and shallow respirations; paresthesias of face and extremities; muscle spasms and tetany, which cannot be distinguished from the tetany produced by hypocalcemia	Serum chloride >103 mEq/L; arterial blood pH <7.35; increased rate and depth of respirations; lethargy, stupor, disorientation, and coma if acidosis is not treated.

TABLE 33.2

Minerals and Electrolytes (Continued)

Mineral/Function	Dietary Reference Intakes	Food Sources	Signs and Symptoms of Deficiency	Signs and Symptoms of Excess
Magnesium Required for conduction of nerve impulses and contraction of muscle (especially important in function of cardiac and skeletal muscle). Serves as a component of many enzymes. Essential for metabolism of carbohydrate and protein. Normal serum magnesium = 1.5–2.5 mEq/L.	Adults (RDA) Females 19–30 y: 310 mg 31 y and over: 320 mg Males 19–30 y: 400 mg 31 y and over: 420 mg Adults (UL), 350 mg/d from supplements only (does not include intake from food and water)	Present in many foods; diet that is adequate in other respects contains adequate magnesium. Good food sources include nuts, cereal grains, dark green vegetables, and seafood.	Serum magnesium <1.5 mEq/L; ataxia; confusion; dizziness; irritability; muscle tremors, carpopedal spasm, nystagmus, generalized spasticity; seizures; tachycardia, hypotension, premature atrial and ventricular beats	Serum magnesium >2.5 mEq/L; skeletal muscle weakness; cardiac dysrhythmias, hypotension; respiratory insufficiency; coma
Trace Elements **Chromium** Aids glucose use by increasing effectiveness of insulin and facilitating transport of glucose across cell membranes	Adults (AI) Females 19–50 y: 25 mcg 51 y and over: 30 mcg Males 19–50 y: 35 mcg 51 y and over: 30 mcg Adults (UL), undetermined	Brewer's yeast and whole wheat products.	Impaired glucose tolerance (hyperglycemia, glucosuria); impaired growth and reproduction; decreased lifespan	Not established
Cobalt A component of vitamin B_{12} that is required for normal function of all body cells and for maturation of red blood cells	~1 mg in the form of vitamin B_{12}. There is no established RDA.	Animal foods, including liver, muscle meats, and shellfish. Fruits, vegetables, and cereals contain no cobalt as vitamin B_{12}.	Deficiency of vitamin B_{12} produces pernicious anemia.	Not established
Copper A component of many enzymes. Essential for correct functioning of the central nervous, cardiovascular, and skeletal systems. Important in formation of red blood cells, apparently by regulating storage and release of iron for hemoglobin	Adults (RDA), 900 mcg Adults (UL), 10,000 mg	Many foods, including liver, shellfish, nuts, cereals, poultry, and dried fruits.	Decreased serum levels; decreased iron absorption; anemia from impaired erythropoiesis; leukopenia. Death can occur. In infants, anemia, chronic malnutrition, and diarrhea, or Menkes syndrome (retarded growth and progressive mental deterioration), can occur.	Increased serum levels; Wilson's disease (a rare genetic disorder characterized by accumulation of copper in brain, liver, and kidneys). Signs and symptoms vary according to affected organs.
Fluoride A component of tooth enamel. Strengthens bones. Adequate intake before ages 50–60 may decrease osteoporosis and fractures during later years.	Adults (AI) Females 19–70 y and over: 3 mg Pregnancy and lactation: 5 mg Males 19–70 y and over: 4 mg	Beef, canned salmon, eggs. Very little in milk, cereal grains, fruits, and vegetables. Fluoride content of food depends on fluoride content of soil where they are grown.	Dental caries and possibly a greater incidence of osteoporosis	Mottling of teeth and osteosclerosis

(*Continued on page 618*)

TABLE 33.2

Minerals and Electrolytes (Continued)

Mineral/Function	Dietary Reference Intakes	Food Sources	Signs and Symptoms of Deficiency	Signs and Symptoms of Excess
	Children (AIs) 1–3 y: 0.7 mg 4–8 y: 1 mg 9–13 y: 2 mg 14–18 y: 3 mg Infants (AIs) 0–6 mo: 0.01 mg 7–12 mo: 0.5 mg Adults (UL), 10 mg			
Iodine Essential component of thyroid hormones	Adults (RDAs) Females 19–51 y and over: 150 mcg Pregnancy: 175 mcg Lactation: 200 mcg Males 19–51 y and over: 150 mcg Children 1–10 y: 100 mcg 11–18 y (girls): 150 mcg 11–18 y (boys): 120 mcg Infants 0–6 mo: 40 mcg 6–12 mo: 50 mcg	Iodized salt and seafood are the best sources. In vegetables, iodine content varies with the amount of iodine in soil where grown. In milk and eggs, content depends on the amount present in animal feed.	Thyroid gland enlargement; possible hypothyroidism	Iodism, with coryza, edema, fever, conjunctivitis, lymphadenopathy, stomatitis, vomiting
Iron Essential component of hemoglobin, myoglobin, and several enzymes. Hemoglobin is required for transport and use of oxygen by body cells. Myoglobin aids oxygen transport and use by muscle cells. Enzymes are important for cellular metabolism.	Adults (RDAs) Females 19–50 y: 18 mg 51 y and over: 8 mg Pregnancy: 27 mg Lactation: 9 mg Males: 8 mg Children (RDAs) 1–3 y: 7 mg 4–8 y: 10 mg 9–13 y: 8 mg 14–18 y (girls): 15 mg 14–18 y (boys): 11 mg Infants 0–6 mo: 0.27 mg (AI) 7–12 mo: 11 mg (RDA) Adults (UL), 45 mg	Liver and other organ meats, lean meat, shellfish, dried beans and vegetables, egg yolks, dried fruits, molasses, whole grain and enriched breads. Milk and milk products contain essentially no iron.	Iron deficiency anemia. With gradual development of anemia, minimal symptoms occur. With rapid development or severe anemia, dyspnea, fatigue, tachycardia, malaise, and drowsiness occur.	Acute iron intoxication: vomiting, diarrhea, melena, abdominal pain, shock, convulsions, and metabolic acidosis. Death may occur within 24 h if treatment is not prompt. Chronic iron overload (hemochromatosis): cardiac dysrhythmias, heart failure, diabetes mellitus, bronze pigmentation of skin, liver enlargement, arthropathy, and others
Selenium Important for function of myocardium and probably other muscles	Adults (RDAs) Females 19–70 y and over: 55 mcg Pregnancy: 60 mcg Lactation: 70 mcg Males 19–70 y and over: 55 mcg	Fish, meat, bread, and cereals.	Deficiency most likely with long-term IV therapy. Signs and symptoms include myocardial abnormalities and other muscle discomfort and weakness.	Highly toxic in excessive amounts. Signs and symptoms include fatigue, peripheral neuropathy, nausea, diarrhea, and alopecia.

TABLE 33.2

Minerals and Electrolytes (Continued)

Mineral/Function	Dietary Reference Intakes	Food Sources	Signs and Symptoms of Deficiency	Signs and Symptoms of Excess
	Children (RDAs) 1–3 y: 20 mcg 4–8 y: 30 mcg 9–13 y: 40 mcg 14–18 y: 55 mcg Infants (AIs) 0–6 mo: 15 mcg 7–12 mo: 20 mcg Adult UL: 400 mcg			
Zinc A component of many enzymes that is essential for normal metabolism (e.g., carbonic anhydrase, lactic dehydrogenase, alkaline phosphatase). Necessary for normal cell growth, synthesis of nucleic acids (RNA and DNA), and synthesis of carbohydrates and proteins. May be essential for use of vitamin A	Adults (RDAs) Females 19–70 y and over: 8 mg Pregnancy: 11 mg Lactation: 12 mg Males 19–70 y and over: 11 mg Children 1–3 y: 3 mg 4–8 y: 5 mg 9–13 y: 8 mg 14–18 y (girls): 9 mg 14–18 y (boys): 11 mg Infants 0–6 mo (AI): 2 mg 7–12 mo (RDA): 3 mg Adult UL: 40 mg	Animal proteins such as meat, liver, eggs, and seafood. Wheat germ is also a good source.	Most evident in growing children and includes impaired growth, hypogonadism in boys, anorexia, and sensory impairment (loss of taste and smell). Also, if the patient has had surgery, wound healing may be delayed.	Unlikely with dietary intake but may develop with excessive ingestion or inhalation of zinc. Ingestion may cause nausea, vomiting, and diarrhea; inhalation may cause vomiting, headache, and fever.

AI, adequate intake; BUN, blood urea nitrogen; DRI, Dietary Reference Intake; RDA, recommended dietary allowance.

fat-soluble vitamins A and D, may cause toxicity; it is necessary to avoid this.

Renal and Hepatic Impairment

Patients with acute renal failure who are unable to eat an adequate diet need a vitamin supplement to meet DRIs. Overall, a multivitamin with essential vitamins is recommended for daily use. Decreased renal function may promote mineral retention.

QSEN Safety Alert ❗

It is important to monitor serum electrolyte levels closely and provide supplements only with great care.

Vitamin deficiencies commonly occur in patients with chronic liver disease, because of poor intake and **malabsorption** (impaired absorption of nutrients from the GI tract). Hepatic failure results in depletion of hepatic stores of vitamin A and other vitamins.

Critical Illness

Critically ill patients often have organ failure, which alters their ability to ingest and use essential nutrients. They may be undernourished with regard to vitamins and minerals.

The Nutrition Advisory Group of the American Medical Association has established guidelines for daily intake, and parenteral multivitamin formulations are available for adults and children. Close monitoring of serum electrolytes is necessary.

Clinical Application 33-1

- Identify findings in the assessment of Mrs. Martin that would put her at risk for vitamin, mineral, and nutritional deficiency.

NCLEX Success

1. Which one of the following findings in a nursing assessment of a newly admitted patient would be most likely to result in a vitamin deficiency?

A. a history of liver disease
B. use of self-prescribed megavitamins
C. presence of a pressure ulcer
D. frequent blood transfusions

2. **A woman takes large amounts of vitamins, which she buys over the counter without a prescription. The nurse should teach the patient that excess consumption of which one of the following could result in a toxic overdose?**

   A. folic acid
   B. vitamin A
   C. vitamin B₁
   D. vitamin C

Fat-Soluble Vitamins

VITAMIN A

The following discussion concerns vitamin A, or retinol.

Pharmacokinetics and Use

After oral administration, vitamin A is absorbed from the GI tract along with dietary fat and is primarily stored in the liver. The body can store up to a year's supply of vitamin A in the liver. This vitamin, which is not soluble in the blood, is distributed by attaching to protein carriers in the blood. If a person consumes inadequate amounts of vitamin A, the body uses the vitamin stored in the liver. Vitamin A is metabolized in the liver and eliminated in the feces and urine.

The most important therapeutic use of vitamin A is for replacement in deficiency states. Table 33.3 gives route and dosage information.

Adverse Effects and Contraindications

Signs and symptoms of vitamin A toxicity include hair loss, double vision, headaches, vomiting, bone abnormalities, and liver damage. If any signs or symptoms of vitamin A excess appear, it is necessary to stop intake of any known sources of vitamin A.

Contraindications to vitamin A include a history of allergic reaction to the vitamin, hypervitaminosis A, and malabsorption syndrome (oral use only). Caution is warranted in pregnancy. Vitamin A toxicity during pregnancy can cause fetal defects (Dudek, 2010).

Nursing Implications

Preventing Interactions

Chronic use of mineral oil or bile acid sequestrants may cause vitamin A deficiency by preventing systemic absorption of vitamin A. Mineral oil combines with fat-soluble vitamins and prevents their absorption if both are taken at the same time. Bile salts increase the effects of vitamin A by increasing intestinal absorption of the vitamin. Large doses of vitamin A may increase the anticoagulant effects of warfarin. Antibiotics may cause diarrhea and subsequent malabsorption of vitamin A.

Administering the Medication

People should take vitamin A preparations before meals, on an empty stomach. However, to prevent nausea, it may be necessary to take them after food or meals. (Intramuscular [IM] administration may be necessary.) Also, people should not take oral preparations of vitamin A at the same time as mineral oil; this laxative absorbs the vitamin and thus prevents its systemic absorption.

Assessing for Therapeutic and Adverse Effects

The nurse observes for decreased signs and symptoms of deficiency, such as improved vision, especially in dim light or at night; less dryness in eyes and conjunctiva (xerophthalmia); and improvement in skin lesions. Night blindness is usually better within a few days. Skin lesions may not disappear for several weeks.

In addition, the nurse observes for signs of hypervitaminosis A, such as anorexia, vomiting, irritability, headache, skin disorders, and pain in muscles, bones, and joints. Serum levels of vitamin A greater than 1200 international unit/dL are toxic. Severity of manifestations depends largely on dose and duration of excess vitamin A intake. Very severe states produce additional clinical signs, including enlargement of the liver and spleen, altered liver function, increased intracranial pressure, and other neurologic manifestations.

Patient Teaching

Box 33.2 identifies patient teaching guidelines for vitamins, including vitamin A.

VITAMIN E

The following discussion concerns vitamin E, or alpha-tocopherol.

Pharmacokinetics and Use

Vitamin E is absorbed from the GI tract if fat absorption is normal. It is primarily stored in adipose tissue. It is metabolized in the liver and eliminated primarily in bile.

The most important therapeutic use of vitamin E is for vitamin E replacement in the narrow, specific circumstances in which vitamin E deficiency occurs. Table 33.3 gives route and dosage information for vitamin E.

Adverse Effects and Contraindications

Large amounts of vitamin E are relatively nontoxic but can interfere with vitamin K action (blood clotting) by decreasing platelet aggregation and producing a risk of bleeding. Excessive doses can also cause fatigue, headache, blurred vision, nausea, and diarrhea. If signs or symptoms of vitamin E excess appear, it is essential to stop the intake of any known source of vitamin E.

Contraindications to vitamin E include a history of allergic reaction to vitamin E or hypervitaminosis E. Patients with a history of bleeding disorders or thrombocytopenia should not take vitamin E.

Nursing Implications

Preventing Interactions

Mineral oil and cholestyramine decrease the absorption of vitamin E, which means that vitamin E should not be administered at the same time as these substances. Also, this vitamin

TABLE 33.3

DRUGS AT A GLANCE: Vitamins

Drug	Pregnancy Category	Routes and Dosage Ranges	
		Adults	*Children*
Fat-Soluble Vitamins			
Vitamin A (also called retinol)	A X if dose greater than RDA	Deficiency (severe): 100,000–500,000 international units PO or 100,000 international units IM daily for 3 d; then 50,000 international units PO or IM daily for 2 wk; then 10,000–20,000 international units PO daily for another 2 mo; follow with adequate dietary nutrition and retinol equivalent vitamin A supplements	Deficiency (severe): 1–8 y 500,000 units/kg/d PO for 5 d, then 5,000–10,000 international units daily for 2 mo or 17,000–35,000 international units IM daily for 10 d Maintenance dose to prevent return of vitamin A deficiency; follow with adequate dietary nutrition and retinol equivalent vitamin A supplements Older than 8 y: see adult dose
Vitamin E	A (if within RDA)	Deficiency: 60–75 international units PO daily Prevention of deficiency: 30 international units daily (Vitamin E may be ordered in alpha-tocopherol equivalents or ATE; 1.40 international units = 1 ATE)	Deficiency: 1 international units/kg/d PO of water miscible vitamin E Prevention of deficiency (infants): 5 international units PO per liter of formula ingested
Vitamin K or phytonadione (Mephyton)	C	Anticoagulant-induced prothrombin deficiency: 2.5–10 mg PO or subcutaneously or IM initially based on PT-INR; repeat if needed within 12–48 h of PO dose or within 6–8 h of subcutaneous or IM dose Hypoprothrombinemia due to other causes: 2.5–25 mg PO or subcutaneously or IM depending on severity; repeat and increase up to 50 mg as needed Antidote to warfarin overdose: oral dose or subcutaneous dose of 2.5–10 mg is given initially; another oral dose may be repeated in 12–48 h or another subcutaneous dose repeated in 6–8 h if needed; these dosages usually stop bleeding and return the international normalized ratio to a normal range within 24 h.	Prevention of hemorrhagic disease: 0.5–1 mg IM within 1 h after birth Treatment of hemorrhagic disease in newborns: 1 mg subcutaneously or IM daily; higher doses may be needed if mother has been receiving oral anticoagulants.
Water-Soluble Vitamins			
Vitamin B₁ (thiamine)	A If above RDA: C	Parenteral nutrition supplementation: 6 mg daily; may be increased to 25–50 mg daily with history of alcohol abuse Deficiency (beriberi): 5–30 mg IM or IV 3 times daily for 2 wk, depending on severity; then dietary correction and multivitamin supplement containing thiamine 5–30 mg PO daily for 1 mo Alcohol withdrawal syndrome: 100 mg IM or IV daily for several days, followed by 50–100 mg PO daily Wernicke's encephalopathy: initially, 100 mg IV; then, 50–100 mg IM or IV daily until patient is consuming a regular balanced diet	Deficiency (beriberi): 10–25 mg IM or IV once daily; for noncritically ill children, 10–50 mg PO daily in divided doses for several weeks with adequate diet

(Continued on page 622)

TABLE 33.3

DRUGS AT A GLANCE: Vitamins (Continued)

Drug	Pregnancy Category	Routes and Dosage Ranges	
		Adults	Children
Vitamin B$_2$ (riboflavin)	A If above RDA: C	Nutritional supplement: 5–10 mg PO daily	Nutritional supplement: 1–4 mg PO daily
Vitamin B$_3$ (niacin, nicotinic acid) Niacinamide (nicotinamide)	C	Deficiency: up to 100 mg PO daily Pellagra: initially 500 mg PO at bedtime; titrate to patient response and tolerance; max dose is 2000 mg daily Hyperlipidemia: 250 mg PO at bedtime; increase at 4–7 d intervals up to 1.5–2 g divided 2 or 3 times daily; max 6 g daily; alternatively, extended-release tablets 1–2 g PO at bedtime	Pellagra: 100–300 mg PO daily in divided doses
Vitamin B$_5$ (calcium pantothenate)	A If above RDA: C	Deficiency: 4–7 mg PO daily	
Vitamin B$_6$ (pyridoxine)	A If above RDA: C	Deficiency: 100–200 PO daily or 10–20 mg IM or IV daily for several wks; then maintenance dose of 2–5 mg PO daily for several weeks Prevention of vitamin B$_6$ deficiency during isoniazid therapy: 10–50 mg PO daily	Seizures related to vitamin B$_6$ deficiency (neonates and children): 10–100 mg IM or IV in a single dose
Vitamin B$_{12}$ (cyanocobalamin or hydroxocobalamin)	A If above RDA: C	Deficiency due to inadequate diet or causes other than pernicious anemia: as hydroxocobalamin 30 mcg IM daily for 5–10 d depending on severity; maintenance dose 100–200 mcg IM once monthly or 500 mcg gel intranasally once weekly; for subsequent prophylaxis, adequate nutrition and RDA of vitamin B$_{12}$ supplement PO Pernicious anemia or vitamin B$_{12}$ malabsorption: initially, cyanocobalamin 100 mcg subcutaneously or IM daily for 6–7 d; if response is observed, 100 mcg subcutaneously or IM every other day for 7 doses; then, 100 mcg subcutaneously or IM every 3–4 d for 2–3 wk; then, 100 mcg subcutaneously or IM once monthly	Deficiency due to inadequate diet or causes other than pernicious anemia: as hydroxocobalamin 1–5 mg in single doses of 100 mcg IM over 2 or more wks, depending on severity of deficiency; maintenance dose is 60 mcg IM monthly; for subsequent prophylaxis, adequate nutrition and RDA of vitamin B$_{12}$ supplement PO
Intranasal cyanocobalamin (Nascobal)	C	Maintenance therapy for remission of pernicious anemia after parenteral vitamin B$_{12}$ therapy: intranasal cyanocobalamin 1 spray in 1 nostril once weekly at least 1 h before or after hot liquids or foods	
Folic acid	A	Deficiency, megaloblastic anemia, hepatic disease, alcoholism: 0.4–1 mg PO, subcutaneously, or IM daily; after correction of deficiency, proper diet and RDA of folic acid supplement PO Prevention of fetal neural tube defects during pregnancy: 0.4 mg PO daily	Deficiency, megaloblastic anemia, hepatic disease Younger than 4 y: up to 0.3 mg PO, subcutaneously, or IM daily 4 y and older: same as adults
Vitamin C (ascorbic acid)	A If above RDA: C	Deficiency, depending on severity: 100–250 mg PO, subcutaneously, IM, or IV daily; then 70–150 mg PO daily for maintenance Urinary acidification; 4–12 g PO daily in divided doses	Deficiency, depending on severity: 100–300 mg PO, subcutaneously, IM, or IV daily in divided doses; then, at least 30 mg PO daily for maintenance

BOX 33.2　　Patient Teaching Guidelines for Vitamins

General Considerations

■ Certain people may need vitamin supplements. Women who are pregnant, as well as people who smoke, ingest large amounts of alcohol, have impaired immune systems, or are elderly may need to take oral vitamins.

■ Avoid taking large doses of vitamins, which do not promote health, strength, or youth.

■ Natural vitamins are advertised as being better than synthetic vitamins, but there is no evidence to support this claim. The two types are chemically identical, and the body uses them the same way. Natural vitamins are more expensive.

■ Vitamins from supplements exert the same physiological effects as those obtained from foods.

■ Multivitamin preparations often contain minerals as well, usually in smaller amounts than those recommended for daily intake. Large doses of minerals are toxic.

■ Supplementary vitamin preparations differ widely in amounts and types of vitamin content.

■ When choosing a vitamin supplement, compare ingredients and costs. Store brands are usually effective and less expensive than name brands.

Vitamin A

■ Know about dietary sources of vitamin A. Retinol occurs in liver, milk, butter, cheese, cream, egg yolk, fortified milk, margarine, and ready-to-eat cereals. Beta carotenes occur in spinach, collard greens, kale, mango, broccoli, carrots, peaches, pumpkin, red peppers, sweet potatoes, winter squash, watermelon, apricots, and cantaloupe.

■ Understand that excessive amounts of vitamin A are stored in the body and often lead to toxic effects. High doses of vitamin A can result in headaches; diarrhea; nausea; loss of appetite; dry, itching skin; and elevated blood calcium.

■ Do not take a supplementary vitamin product that contains more than recommended amounts of vitamin A because of possible adverse effects.

■ If you are pregnant or could become pregnant, know that excessive doses of vitamin A during pregnancy may cause birth defects.

Vitamin E

■ Know about dietary sources of vitamin E. This vitamin occurs in vegetable oils, margarine, salad dressing, other foods made with vegetable oil, nuts, seeds, wheat germ, dark green vegetables, whole grains, and fortified cereals.

■ Be familiar with the signs and symptoms of vitamin E overdose.

■ Do not take a supplementary vitamin product that contains more than the recommended amounts of vitamin E.

Vitamin K

■ Know about dietary sources of vitamin K. This vitamin occurs in spinach, brussels sprouts, broccoli, cabbage, cauliflower, Swiss chard, lettuce, collard greens, carrots, green beans, asparagus, and eggs.

■ Avoid excessive doses of vitamin K. Take this vitamin only as directed by a health care provider.

■ Keep intake of vitamin K–containing foods constant. Avoid sudden increases or decreases in the amounts of these foods.

■ If you are taking warfarin, report any use of vitamin K to your health care provider. During warfarin therapy, intake of vitamin K–containing foods should remain constant.

Vitamin B_1, Vitamin B_3, and Vitamin B_6

■ Know about dietary sources of vitamins B_1 (thiamine), B_3 (niacin), and B_6 (pyridoxine). Thiamine occurs in whole grain and enriched breads and cereals, liver, nuts, wheat germ, pork, and dried peas and beans. Niacin occurs in all protein foods and whole grain and enriched breads and cereals. Pyridoxine occurs in meats, fish, poultry, fruits, green leafy vegetables, whole grains, and dried peas and beans.

■ Swallow extended-release products whole; do not break, crush, or chew them. Breaking the product delivers the entire dose at once and may cause adverse effects.

■ Take oral niacin preparations, except for timed-release forms, with or after meals or at bedtime to decrease stomach irritation.

■ After taking a dose of oral niacin, sit or lie down for approximately 30 minutes after taking a dose. Niacin causes blood vessels to dilate and may cause facial flushing, dizziness, and falls. Facial flushing can be decreased by taking aspirin 325 mg orally, 30 to 60 minutes before a dose of niacin (if aspirin is not contraindicated). Itching, tingling, and headache may occur. These effects usually subside with continued use of niacin.

Vitamin B_{12} and Folic Acid

■ Know about dietary sources of vitamin B_{12}. This vitamin occurs in meat, fish, poultry, shellfish, milk, dairy products, eggs, and some fortified foods. Vitamin B_{12} does not occur in plant sources. If you are a strict vegan who consumes no animal products, you are at risk for vitamin B_{12} deficiency unless you take a supplementary source of the vitamin.

■ Know about dietary sources of folic acid. This nutrient occurs in liver, okra, spinach, asparagus, dried peas and beans, seeds, and orange juice. Breads, cereals, and other grains are fortified with folic acid.

■ Take prescribed vitamins as directed and for the appropriate time. If you have pernicious anemia, you must have vitamin B_{12} injections for the remainder of your life. Any chronic vitamin B_{12} deficiency requires lifelong treatment. If you are pregnant or breastfeeding, requirements may be greater; you usually may need additional vitamin supplements.

■ Keep appointments for follow-up visits and obtain the necessary laboratory tests.

Vitamin C

■ Know about dietary sources of vitamin C. This vitamin occurs in citrus fruits and juices, red and green peppers, broccoli, cauliflower, brussels sprouts, cantaloupe, kiwi fruit, mustard greens, strawberries, and tomatoes.

■ Be aware that vitamin C improves the absorption of iron.

■ Understand that vitamin C, which acidifies the urine, may alter the excretion of some drugs.

may increase the anticoagulant effect of warfarin. Vitamin E may increase the absorption, hepatic storage, and use of vitamin A.

Administering the Medication

People should take oral vitamin E preparations before meals on an empty stomach. However, to prevent nausea, people may also take them after food or meals.

Assessing for Therapeutic and Adverse Effects

The nurse observes for decreased signs and symptoms of vitamin E deficiency. In addition, the nurse checks for signs of hypervitaminosis E, including bleeding, fatigue, headache, blurred vision, nausea, and diarrhea.

Patient Teaching

Box 33.2 identifies patient teaching guidelines for vitamins, including vitamin E.

VITAMIN K

The following discussion concerns vitamin K, or phytonadione.

Pharmacokinetics and Use

After absorption, vitamin K is concentrated in the liver. Minimal amounts of the vitamin are stored. It crosses the placental barrier and enters breast milk. Onset of action after an oral dose is 6 to 12 hours and after a subcutaneous dose, 1 to 2 hours. Metabolism occurs rapidly in the liver, and elimination is in the bile and urine.

Vitamin K has two important therapeutic uses: (1) to correct hypoprothrombinemia caused by inadequate levels of vitamin K and (2) to reverse the effects of warfarin (Coumadin) overdose. Table 33.3 gives route and dosage information for vitamin K.

Adverse Effects and Contraindications

No symptoms have been observed from excessive intake of vitamin K. Mild adverse effects of vitamin K intake may include facial flushing, alterations in taste, or redness and pain at the injection site. The FDA has issued a **BLACK BOX WARNING** ◆ stating that IV administration of vitamin K may result in an anaphylactic type of reaction with risks of shock, cardiorespiratory arrest, and death, even with drug dilution and slow administration.

Contraindications to vitamin K include a history of allergic reaction as well as a history of allergic reaction to benzyl alcohol or castor oil.

Nursing Implications

Preventing Interactions

Mineral oil as well as cholestyramine and other bile acid sequestrants inhibit the absorption of vitamin K if taken at the same time. Increased vitamin K levels decrease the anticoagulant effect of warfarin. It is necessary to avoid the use of vitamin K as a drug when a patient is receiving warfarin, and significant increases or decreases in dietary vitamin K may necessitate adjustment of the warfarin dose.

Administering the Medication

Oral and subcutaneous routes for vitamin K administration are preferred. Both the IM route and the IV route are associated with severe hypersensitivity reactions. People may take the vitamin without regard to meals. They should avoid taking it at the same time as mineral oil or bile acid sequestrants.

It is necessary to protect all vitamin K preparations from light.

Assessing for Therapeutic and Adverse Effects

The nurse observes for decreased signs and symptoms of vitamin K deficiency. This includes decreased bleeding and more nearly normal blood coagulation tests.

Oral vitamin K rarely produces adverse reactions. Following subcutaneous injection, the nurse observes the injection site for redness and pain. Use of the IM and IV routes requires close observation for anaphylactic reaction as evidenced by chills, fever, diaphoresis, dyspnea, hypotension, bronchospasm, respiratory arrest, cardiac arrest, shock, and death. The means for emergency resuscitation must be immediately available.

Patient Teaching

Box 33.2 identifies patient teaching guidelines for vitamins, including vitamin K.

Water-Soluble Vitamins

VITAMIN B COMPLEX: VITAMIN B$_1$, VITAMIN B$_3$, AND VITAMIN B$_6$

Most vitamin B complex deficiencies are multiple, rather than single, and treatment consists of administration of a multivitamin that contains several B complex vitamins. If a single deficiency seems predominant, that vitamin may be given alone or in addition to a multivitamin preparation. Three of the vitamin B complex vitamins are presented together in this section because they have much in common and are prototypical of the B complex vitamins as a whole: vitamin B$_1$ (thiamine), vitamin B$_3$ (niacin), and vitamin B$_6$ (pyridoxine). Vitamin B$_{12}$ (cyanocobalamin) and folic acid are discussed separately below because of their common use in the treatment of anemia.

Pharmacokinetics and Use

Thiamine, niacin, and pyridoxine are absorbed from the GI tract. Thiamine is widely distributed and enters breast milk. Niacin crossed the placenta and enters breast milk. Pyridoxine is stored in the liver and crosses the placental barrier. Niacin and pyridoxine are metabolized in the liver. Thiamine, niacin, and pyridoxine are eliminated by the kidneys in the urine.

Table 33.3 gives route and dosage information for the B complex vitamins.

Use in Patients With Renal or Hepatic Impairment

Both niacin and pyridoxine warrant caution in renal impairment. People with liver disease should not take niacin because it may increase liver enzymes and bilirubin and cause further liver damage. Long-acting dosage forms may be more hepatotoxic than the fast-acting forms.

Adverse Effects and Contraindications

- Thiamine: history of an allergic reaction to the vitamin
- Niacin: hepatic impairment, active peptic ulcer disease, arterial bleeding, and lactation. Caution is necessary with a history of jaundice, hepatobiliary disease, peptic ulcers, high alcohol consumption, renal impairment, unstable angina, gout glaucoma, and diabetes mellitus. Administration causes vasodilation, which may result in dizziness, hypotension, and injury from falls.
- Pyridoxine (IV form): cardiac disease. Caution is warranted with renal impairment.

Nursing Implications

Preventing Interactions

- Thiamine: no important drug interactions
- Niacin: increases the risk of rhabdomyolysis from the statin antihyperlipidemics, increases the effectiveness of antihypertensives and vasoactive drugs, and increases the risk of bleeding from anticoagulants. Bile acid sequestrants decrease absorption.
- Pyridoxine: accelerates the peripheral conversion of levodopa into dopamine, thus decreasing the amount of levodopa that is available to cross into the central nervous system (CNS). Isoniazid decreases the effect of pyridoxine.

Administering the Medication

- Thiamine: preferred route of administration is by mouth; people may take it without regard to food. It is necessary to swallow enteric-coated tablets whole, not chewed or crushed. The IM and IV routes are for severe deficiency states only.
- Niacin: people may take oral niacin, except for timed-release forms, with or after meals, which decreases anorexia, nausea, vomiting, diarrhea, and flatulence. They should swallow timed-release forms whole, not chewed or crushed. The nurse should instruct the patient to sit or lie down for about 30 minutes after administration because niacin causes vasodilation and possible dizziness and hypotension.
- Pyridoxine: the general route of administration is oral, and people should swallow sustained-release or enteric forms of pyridoxine whole, not chewed or crushed.

Assessing for Therapeutic Effects

The nurse assesses for decreased signs and symptoms of deficiency. With B complex vitamins, it is necessary to observe for decreased or absent stomatitis, glossitis, seborrheic dermatitis, neurologic problems (neuritis, convulsions, mental deterioration, psychotic symptoms), cardiovascular problems (edema, heart failure), and eye problems (itching, burning, photophobia). Deficiencies of B complex vitamins commonly occur together and produce many similar manifestations.

Assessing for Adverse Effects

Adverse reactions are generally unlikely to occur with B complex multivitamin preparations. They are most likely to develop with large IV doses and rapid administration. The observes for the following:

- Niacin and thiamine (parenteral): hypotension and anaphylactic shock
- Niacin (oral): anorexia, nausea, vomiting, diarrhea, and postural hypotension

Patient Teaching

Box 33.2 identifies patient teaching guidelines for vitamins, including vitamins B_1, B_3, and B_6.

VITAMIN B_{12} (CYANOCOBALAMIN) AND FOLIC ACID

The following discussion concerns vitamin B_{12} (cyanocobalamin) and folic acid.

Pharmacokinetics

- Vitamin B_{12}: requires intrinsic factor, produced by the stomach, for absorption. Normally, vitamin B_{12} is widely distributed and stored principally in the liver (half-life in the liver is 400 days). Vitamin B_{12} crosses the placenta and enters breast milk. It is converted into active coenzymes in the tissues and eliminated, very slowly, in the urine.
- Folic acid: absorbed from the proximal small intestine. Folic acid is distributed to all body tissues with high concentrations in the cerebrospinal fluid. The unused portion is stored in the liver. Folic acid crosses the placenta and enters breast milk. It is metabolized in the liver to active metabolites. Elimination is in the urine, at a more rapid rate than vitamin B_{12}.

Use

Health care providers use vitamin B_{12} is used to treat vitamin B_{12} deficiency states, whether caused by dietary deficiency, malabsorption, or inadequate secretion of intrinsic factor. They use folic acid as a supplement during infancy, childhood, and pregnancy, as well as to treat folic acid deficiency caused by malabsorption (sprue) or alcoholism. Folate deficiency in alcoholism results from both poor dietary intake and interference with liver processing of folic acid. Deficiency states of both vitamin B_{12} and folic acid present similarly as **megaloblastic anemia** (characterized by abnormally large, immature red blood cells). Proper diagnosis must establish which vitamin is deficient before treatment can begin. If megaloblastic anemia is severe, treatment usually involves both vitamin B_{12} and folic acid.

In pernicious anemia (vitamin B_{12} deficiency caused by absence of intrinsic factor), vitamin B_{12} must be given by injection because oral forms are not absorbed from the GI tract. The injections must be continued for life. Vitamin B_{12} is also given to prevent pernicious anemia in patients who are strict vegetarians, who have had a gastrectomy, or who have chronic small bowel disease. Although folic acid relieves hematologic disorders of pernicious anemia, giving folic acid alone allows continued neurologic deterioration. Thus, an accurate diagnosis is required.

Table 33.3 gives route and dosage information for vitamin B_{12} and folic acid.

Adverse Effects

- Vitamin B_{12}: rare. Hypokalemia sometimes results. There is a slight risk of anaphylactic shock and sudden death.
- Folic acid: uncommon. The most serious potential adverse effect is bronchospasm.

Contraindications

- Vitamin B_{12}: history of a sensitivity to vitamin B_{12}, other cobalamins, or cobalt. Vitamin B_{12} should be used with caution when treating folic acid deficiency.
- Folic acid: undiagnosed anemia because the vitamin may mask pernicious anemia. Other contraindication includes vitamin B_{12} deficiency (the use of folic acid will improve the patient's megaloblastic anemia while doing nothing to reverse the neurological problems associated with vitamin B_{12} deficiency).

Nursing Implications

Preventing Interactions

- Vitamin B_{12}: effects decreased by omeprazole, which decreases absorption of vitamin B_{12} from food
- Folic acid: effects decreased by aspirin, chloramphenicol, nonsteroidal anti-inflammatory drugs (NSAIDs), sulfa antibiotics, sulfonylureas, triamterene, and trimethoprim. Cholestyramine, oral contraceptives, and sulfasalazine decrease absorption of folic acid. Methotrexate and phenytoin act as antagonists to folic acid. Alcohol alters liver function and leads to poor hepatic storage of folic acid. Folic acid increases phenytoin metabolism, which decreases phenytoin levels.

Administering the Medication

- Vitamin B_{12}: use of the oral form is most convenient, and administration with food increases absorption. Mixing the vitamin with fruit juice is fine, but it is important to consume the mixture quickly because ascorbic acid interferes with the stability of the vitamin. It is important to note that vitamin B_{12} is not safe for IV administration.
- Folic acid: oral administration is preferable unless severe malabsorption is present, and people may take the vitamin without regard to food. Folic acid is also available in subcutaneous, IM, or IV forms. It is necessary to protect the parenteral forms from light and heat and store them at room temperature.

Assessing for Therapeutic and Adverse Effects

With vitamin B_{12} and folic acid, the nurse observes for increased appetite, strength, and feeling of well-being; increased reticulocyte counts; and increased number of normal red blood cells, hemoglobin, and hematocrit. Therapeutic effects may be rapid and dramatic.

Patient Teaching

Box 33.2 presents patient teaching guidelines for vitamins, including vitamin B_{12} and folic acid.

VITAMIN C

The following section concerns vitamin C (ascorbic acid).

Pharmacokinetics

Vitamin C is absorbed from the GI tract and is distributed generally. It crosses the placenta and enters breast milk. The vitamin is metabolized in the liver and eliminated by the kidneys.

Use

The most important therapeutic use of vitamin C involves the prevention and treatment of scurvy. This vitamin is available alone for oral, IM, or IV administration. It is also an ingredient in most multivitamin preparations. An unlabeled use of vitamin C is to acidify the urine. There is no known benefit for taking large amounts of this vitamin, and the nurse should discourage its use.

Table 33.3 gives route and dosage information for vitamin C.

Use in Patients With Renal Impairment

Patients with acute renal failure who are unable to eat an adequate diet need a vitamin supplement to meet DRIs. However, it is imperative to avoid large doses of vitamin C because of impaired urinary excretion. Also, oxalate (a product of vitamin C catabolism) may precipitate in renal tubules or form calcium oxalate stones, obstruct urine flow, and worsen renal function. In addition, dialysis removes vitamin C, and patients receiving dialysis require vitamin C replacement.

Use in Critical Illness

Conditions that increase the need for vitamin C sometimes warrant larger doses of vitamin C. These conditions include extensive burns, delayed fracture or wound healing, delayed postoperative wound healing, or severe febrile or chronic disease states.

Adverse Effects and Contraindications

Usual doses of vitamin C are well tolerated. The most common adverse effects of oral vitamin C (especially megadoses) are abdominal cramps, nausea, vomiting, and diarrhea.

Caution is warranted in patients who are prone to kidney stones, as well as in those with glucose-6-phosphate deficiency or sickle cell anemia.

Nursing Implications

Preventing Interactions

Vitamin C, which acidifies the urine, decreases the elimination of aspirin and other salicylates, which are eliminated more rapidly in alkaline urine.

Administering the Medication

Vitamin C is available in various oral forms. Oral solutions may need mixing with food. Effervescent tablets may need dissolving in water immediately before use. Parenteral forms are also available.

Assessing for Therapeutic and Adverse Effects

Vitamin C deficiency usually begins to resolve rapidly, with improvement seen after only a few days. The nurse assesses for decreased or absent malaise, irritability, and bleeding tendencies (easy bruising of skin, bleeding gums, nosebleeds, and so forth).

Adverse reactions are rare with usual doses and methods of administration.

Patient Teaching

Box 33.2 presents patient teaching guidelines for vitamins, including vitamin C.

Clinical Application 33-2

- Mrs. Martin's physician expresses concern about her nutritional status and decides to administer a vitamin supplement. Which vitamins might he or she order?
- The physician prescribes the anticoagulant warfarin (Coumadin) for Mrs. Martin to aid in preventing another stroke. If she receives an overdose of warfarin, why does the health care prescriber order vitamin K? If she is eventually able to eat solid food, what teaching does the nurse provide concerning vitamin K in her diet and warfarin?

NCLEX Success

3. Which one of the following patients taking vitamin A supplements is of most concern to the nurse?

   A. a 21-year-old woman who is pregnant
   B. a 32-year-old man with poor night vision
   C. a 55-year-old man with hepatic cirrhosis
   D. a 79-year-old woman who is malnourished

4. The nurse administers vitamin K if a patient is bleeding from an overdose of which of the following?

   A. aspirin
   B. enoxaparin
   C. heparin
   D. warfarin

5. A nurse is planning to teach a patient about dietary sources of vitamin K. The nurse teaches that foods containing vitamin K include which of the following?

   A. spinach, brussels sprouts, and broccoli
   B. breads, cereals, and other grains
   C. citrus fruits and juices, as well as strawberries
   D. meat, fish, and poultry

6. The patient has pernicious anemia. Why does the nurse administer vitamin B_{12} by the intramuscular route?

   A. The drug cannot be administered orally.
   B. The oral form has a bitter taste.
   C. The drug is not absorbed if taken orally.
   D. The oral form causes nausea and GI upset.

EVIDENCE-BASED PRACTICE

Vitamins and Cutaneous Wound Healing

by S. SINNO, D. S. LEE, AND A. KHACHEMOUNE

Journal of Wound Care, June 2011, 20(6)

An extensive literature review reveals therapeutic uses of vitamins to enhance wound healing. The vitamin A analog tretinoin, administered topically for a short time as a pretreatment before dermatologic procedures such as dermabrasions and chemical peels, promotes skin healing following the procedure. Vitamin E (combined with vitamin C) applied topically in cosmetics and sunscreen inhibits acute ultraviolet light damage. Oral vitamin E supplements taken before and after surgery show an ability to improve the appearance of surgical scars. Vitamin K plays a role in the formation of thrombin. Sufficient vitamin K ensures that platelets are able to form a matrix with the clotting factor to develop a clot over the wound.

In general, the role of the B complex vitamins in wound healing requires further study. Only vitamin B_1 (thiamine) has an established role; thiamine supplementation has been associated with clinical improvement of human periodontal wounds. Finally, vitamin C has three major roles in wound healing: promotion of collagen synthesis, modulation of the immune function, and antioxidant action. The poor wound healing present in vitamin C deficiency (scurvy) improves rapidly when treatment with vitamin C supplements begins. Topical application of a combination of vitamin C and vitamin E provides protection against the damaging effects of light exposure and helps improve skin damaged by light exposure.

IMPLICATIONS FOR NURSING PRACTICE: Patients unfamiliar with the appropriate use of vitamins require teaching from the nurse to avoid overdosage and the risks of vitamin excess. Patients hear conflicting claims about vitamins from commercial advertising and media reports. Nurses who are familiar with the literature and the uses of vitamins in specific circumstances can offer patients clear guidance about safe use of vitamins.

Minerals

IRON

Iron deficiency is usually the result not of normal elimination but of excessive menstruation or GI bleeding. The following discussion relates to the prototype drug ℗ **ferrous sulfate** (Feosol). Ferrous sulfate is often the preparation of choice; it contains 20% elemental iron.

Pharmacokinetics and Use

The fate of iron administered in drug form is the same as that of dietary iron. Only about 10% to 15% of ingested dietary iron is absorbed; although during pregnancy or iron deficiency, this percentage increases. Iron is stored in the small intestine (and in certain other cells) as ferritin as well as in the liver. When needed, iron is released into the bloodstream, bound to transferrin, and transported to the bone marrow for incorporation into hemoglobin. Iron crosses the placenta.

Iron is not metabolized; the iron in red blood cells is reused. Small amounts of iron are eliminated daily (about 0.5–1 mg) in urine, sweat, and sloughing of intestinal mucosal cells. Excess iron is excreted in feces, which turn dark green or black.

The most important therapeutic uses of ferrous sulfate are as a supplement during periods of increased iron use and as treatment for iron deficiency. Table 33.4 gives route and dosage information for ferrous sulfate and other iron preparations. Slow-release or enteric-coated iron products decrease absorption but may cause less gastric irritation.

Adverse Effects and Contraindications

The most common adverse effects of ferrous sulfate and other oral iron preparations are GI discomfort, nausea, constipation, diarrhea, and black stools. Liquid forms of iron may temporarily stain the teeth. In iron overload, excess iron is deposited in the heart, liver, and endocrine glands resulting in organ damage and, if untreated, death.

TABLE 33.4

DRUGS AT A GLANCE: Drugs Used in Mineral–Electrolyte and Acid–Base Imbalances

Drug/Pregnancy Category	Indications for Use	Routes and Dosage Ranges	
		Adults	*Children*
Cation Exchange Resin Sodium polystyrene sulfonate (Kayexalate)/C	Treatment of hyperkalemia	15–30 g with or without sorbitol PO; may be repeated every 4–6 h as needed	
Chelating Agents (metal antagonists)			
Deferasirox (Exjade)/B	Chronic iron overload	Initially, 20 mg/kg PO daily on empty stomach 30 min before eating; adjust dose every 3–6 mo; should not exceed 40 mg/kg daily	Older than 2 y of age: same as adult
Deferoxamine (Desferal)/C	Acute iron intoxication Hemochromatosis due to blood transfusions Hemosiderosis due to hemolytic anemia	1 g IM or IV initially, then 500 mg IM or IV every 4 h for 2 doses, then 500 mg every 4–12 h if needed; max dose, 6 g/24 h; rate of IV infusion not to exceed 15 mg/kg/h.	Same as adults
Penicillamine (Cuprimine)/D NOTE: Penicillamine should always be administered with a supplement of pyridoxine 25–50 mg PO daily in both adults and children.	Wilson's disease Rheumatoid arthritis Cystinuria	Wilson's disease: 750–1000 mg PO daily in divided doses; dose based on urinary copper excretion Rheumatoid arthritis: 125–250 mg PO daily; may increase dose at 1–3 mo intervals up to 1–1.5 g PO daily (max in older adults 750 mg PO daily) Cystinuria: usually 2 g PO daily; dose titrated based on urinary cystine excretion	Wilson's disease: 20 mg/kg/d PO in 2–3 divided doses (round off to the nearest 250 mg dose); reduce dose by 25% when clinically stable; dose adjusted based on urinary copper excretion Rheumatoid arthritis: initially 3 mg/kg/d PO (≤250 mg PO daily) for 3 mo; then, 6 mg/kg/d PO (≤500 mg PO daily) in 2 divided doses for 3 mo to a max of 10 mg/kg/d PO (≤1–1.5 g PO daily) in 3–4 divided doses

TABLE 33.4

DRUGS AT A GLANCE: Drugs Used in Mineral–Electrolyte and Acid–Base Imbalances (Continued)

Drug/Pregnancy Category	Indications for Use	Routes and Dosage Ranges	
		Adults	*Children*
Succimer (Chemet)/C	Lead poisoning		10 mg/kg or 350 mg/m² PO every 8 h for 5 d, then every 12 h for 14 d (total of 19 d of drug administration); capsule comes only in 100 mg, round dose to nearest 100 mg; for young children who cannot swallow capsules, the capsule contents can be sprinkled on soft food or given with a spoon.
Iron Preparations			
Ferrous gluconate (Fergon)/A	Iron deficiency anemia	100 mg ferrous gluconate = 11.6 mg elemental iron; elemental iron doses given 60 mg 2 times daily up to 60 mg 4 times daily	Mild to moderate anemia: 3 mg/kg/d in 1–2 divided doses Severe anemia: 4–6 mg/kg/d in 3 divided doses
℗ **Ferrous sulfate** (Feosol)/A	Iron deficiency anemia	100 mg ferrous sulfate = 20 mg elemental iron; ferrous sulfate doses given 300 mg PO 2 times up to 300 mg PO 4 times daily or extended release 250 mg once daily or twice daily	Mild to moderate anemia: 3 mg/kg/d in 1–2 divided doses Severe anemia: 4–6 mg/kg/d in 3 divided doses
Iron dextran injection (INFeD)/C	Iron deficiency anemia	Dosage is calculated for individual patients according to hemoglobin and weight (see manufacturer's literature); a small test dose is required before therapeutic doses are given.	Same as adults
Magnesium Preparations Magnesium oxide/B Magnesium hydroxide/A Magnesium sulfate/A	Prevent or treat hypomagnesemia Treat hypertension or seizures associated with toxemia of pregnancy or acute nephritis in children	Hypomagnesemia: magnesium oxide 400–840 mg PO daily; magnesium sulfate 1 g IM every 6 h for 4 doses Severe hypomagnesemia: magnesium sulfate 5 g in 5% dextrose or normal saline 1000 mL infused IV over 3 h Constipation: magnesium hydroxide (milk of magnesia) 30–60 mL PO at bedtime IM Preeclampsia or eclampsia of pregnancy to prevent or control seizures: initially, magnesium sulfate 4 g in 5% dextrose or normal saline 250 mL infused IV along with magnesium sulfate 4–5 g deep IM into 2 suitable sites; then, 4–5 g deep IM every 4 h into alternate sites as needed; alternatively, magnesium sulfate in D₅W or NS 250 mL	Seizures, hypertension, and encephalopathy associated with acute nephritis in children: magnesium sulfate 20–40 mg/kg IM as needed to control seizures; dilute the 50% concentration to a 20% solution and give 0.1–0.2 mL/kg of the 20% solution; max infusion rate of magnesium sulfate given IV is 150 mg/min in children or adults

(*Continued on page 630*)

Drug/Pregnancy Category	Indications for Use	Routes and Dosage Ranges	
		Adults	*Children*
		infused IV as a loading dose; followed by 1–3 g IV hourly; total dose should not exceed 30–40 g daily	
Potassium Preparation Ⓟ **Potassium chloride** (KCl)/C NOTE: Give potassium chloride by IV infusion only, *never* IM or IV push; rapid infusion may cause fatal hyperkalemia.	Prevent or treat hypokalemia	Prevention of hypokalemia: potassium supplement 16–24 mEq PO daily in divided doses; adjust dosage based on serum potassium levels Treatment of hypokalemia: potassium supplement 40–100 mEq PO daily in 2–4 divided doses; max dose of diluted potassium chloride IV is 40 mEq infused at 10 mEq/h—*do not* exceed 200 mEq daily; further doses based on serum potassium level and blood pH; give potassium replacement IV only with monitoring of ECG and serum potassium level.	Same as adults for prevention and treatment of hypokalemia; *do not* exceed 3 mEq/kg daily
Sodium Preparation Sodium chloride (NaCl or normal saline) injection/C	Hyponatremia	1500–3000 mL of 0.22% or 0.45% solution/24 h IV depending on the patient's fluid needs; ~50 mL/h to keep IV lines open	
Zinc Preparation Zinc sulfate/C	Prevent or treat zinc deficiency	Deficiency: zinc sulfate 110–220 mg (elemental zinc 25–50 mg) PO 3 times daily	Deficiency (infants and children): elemental zinc 0.5–1 mg/kg/d once daily or in 2–3 divided doses
Multiple Mineral–Electrolyte Preparations Oral solutions (Pedialyte) IV solutions (Normosol, Plasma-Lyte 148, Ringer's solution)	Prevent or treat fluid and electrolyte deficiencies	2000–3000 mL/24 h IV, depending on individual fluid and electrolyte needs	Amount (PO, IV) individualized according to fluid and electrolyte needs based on estimated fluid loss, age, and weight (see manufacturer's literature)

Contraindications to ferrous sulfate include peptic ulceration, ulcerative colitis, regional enteritis, and repeated blood transfusions. Other contraindications are disorders that cause the accumulation of iron stores: hemosiderosis, primary hemochromatosis, and hemolytic anemia (unless iron deficiency anemia is also present).

Nursing Implications

Preventing Interactions

In general, food decreases iron absorption. Examples include cereals, cheese, coffee, eggs, milk, tea, bran and whole grain breads, and yogurt.

A few drugs increase iron absorption. Most notable is vitamin C, which increases iron absorption by acidifying gastric secretions. Vitamin C, taken at the same time as iron-containing foods or oral iron preparations, increases iron absorption. Taking ferrous sulfate with vitamin C–containing orange juice enhances iron absorption. Some oral iron preparations contain a small amount of vitamin C. Allopurinol may increase the concentration of iron in the liver.

Ferrous sulfate interferes with the absorption of the penicillamine, tetracycline, and fluoroquinolone antibiotics, possibly resulting in decreased antibiotic levels or effect. Ferrous sulfate also decreases the absorption of levodopa, methyldopa, and levothyroxine.

Administering the Medication

People should take iron tablets or capsules before meals, with 8 ounces of water or juice, if tolerated. They should not crush or chew sustained-release preparations. Oral iron preparations are better absorbed if taken on an empty stomach. However, because gastric irritation is a common adverse reaction, people more often take iron with or immediately after meals; this may decrease absorption. With liquid preparations, it is necessary to dilute them, take with a straw, and then rinse the mouth afterward to prevent temporary staining of teeth.

Certain interactions affect the timing of iron administration. Ferrous sulfate interferes with the absorption of the penicillamine, tetracycline, and fluoroquinolone antibiotics; therefore, it is necessary to take ferrous sulfate 2 to 4 hours before or after these antibiotics. Because some foods may affect iron absorption, people should take iron at least 2 hours before or after a caffeine-containing beverage or food.

Assessing for Therapeutic and Adverse Effects

The nurse observes for increased vigor and feeling of well-being, improved appetite, less fatigue, and increased red blood cells, as well as hemoglobin, hematocrit, and reticulocyte count. Therapeutic effects are usually evident within a month unless other problems are also present (e.g., vitamin deficiency, achlorhydria, infection, or malabsorption).

The nurse assesses for GI upset, which may be related to dose. GI symptoms may decrease as therapy progresses. (Enteric-coated products reduce GI upset but also reduce the amount of iron absorbed.) It is also necessary to check for stool color depending on the iron preparation. Oral iron may turn stools black. Although this unabsorbed iron is harmless, it could mask melena.

Patient Teaching

Box 33.3 presents patient teaching guidelines for minerals and electrolytes, including iron.

BOX 33.3 **Patient Teaching Guidelines for Minerals and Electrolytes**

General Considerations

- A well-balanced diet contains all the minerals needed for health in most people. Exceptions are iron and calcium, which are often needed as a dietary supplement in women and children. Note that herbal preparations of chamomile, feverfew, and St. John's wort may inhibit iron absorption. The safest action is to take mineral supplements only on a health care provider's advice, in the amounts and for length of time prescribed. All minerals are toxic when taken in excess.

- Keep all mineral or electrolyte substances out of reach of children to prevent accidental overdose. Acute iron intoxication is a common problem among young children and can be fatal. Supervise children about using fluoride supplements (e.g., remind them to spit out oral rinses and gels rather than swallow them).

- Keep appointments with health care providers for periodic blood tests and other follow-up procedures when mineral or electrolyte supplements are prescribed (e.g., potassium chloride). This helps prevent ingestion of excessive amounts.

- Minerals are often contained in multivitamin preparations, with percentages of the recommended dietary allowances supplied. These amounts differ in various preparations and should be included in estimations of daily intake.

Iron

- Know about dietary sources of iron. This mineral occurs in beef liver, red meats, fish, poultry, clams, tofu, oysters, lentils, dried peas and beans, fortified cereals, bread, and dried fruit.

- Avoid substituting one iron salt for another, because amounts of elemental iron may vary.

- Take iron preparations with or after meals, with approximately 240 mL of fluid, to prevent stomach upset. Do not take iron with coffee or other caffeine-containing beverages because caffeine decreases absorption. Take iron and caffeine preparations at least 2 hours apart.

- Do not crush or chew slow-release tablets or capsules.

- With liquid preparations, dilute with water, drink through a straw, and rinse the mouth afterward to avoid staining the teeth.

- Expect that stools will be dark green or black. Report constipation or change in color or consistency of stool to the health care provider.

Potassium

- Mix oral solutions or effervescent tablets with at least 120 mL of water or juice to improve the taste, dilute the drug, and decrease gastric irritation.

- Do not crush or chew slow-release preparations.

- Take after meals initially to decrease gastric irritation. If no nausea, vomiting, or other problems occur, the drug can be tried before meals because it is better absorbed from an empty stomach.

- *Do not stop taking the medication without notifying the health care provider who prescribed it, especially if you are also taking diuretics or digoxin.*

- Do not use salt substitutes except on the recommendation of a health care provider. Salt substitutes contain potassium chloride and may result in excessive intake.

- Serious problems may develop from either high or low levels of potassium in the blood. Know and recognize signs and symptoms of hypokalemia and hyperkalemia.

  - Signs and symptoms of hypokalemia: palpitations, confusion, dizziness, muscle weakness, abdominal distension, frequent voiding of large amounts of urine

  - Signs and symptoms of hyperkalemia: muscle weakness, palpitations, slow pulse, fatigue, shortness of breath

NCLEX Success

7. Teaching for a patient who is being started on an iron supplement should include information that the preparation:

   A. may cause diarrhea
   B. may cause stools to be dark green or black
   C. should be taken with an antacid
   D. should not be taken with fruit juice

8. When assessing a patient for therapeutic effects of iron therapy, the nurse would check the result of which laboratory study?

   A. activated partial thromboplastin time
   B. international normalized ratio
   C. reticulocyte count
   D. white blood cell count

Other Drugs Used to Treat Iron Deficiency

Iron Dextran

Iron dextran (Dexferrum, INFeD) is a parenteral form of iron useful for treating iron deficiency anemia when oral supplements cannot be used. Indications for use include peptic ulcer or inflammatory bowel disease that may be aggravated by oral iron preparations, the patient's inability or unwillingness to take oral preparations, and a shortage of time for correcting the iron deficiency (e.g., late pregnancy, preoperative status, or excessive blood loss). The FDA has issued a **BLACK BOX WARNING** ◆ for iron dextran regarding the risk of anaphylactic reactions and death. Because of this risk, administration should occur only when there is a clear indication. Contraindications include anemias not associated with iron deficiency and hypersensitivity to the drug. Caution is warranted in serious hepatic impairment, rheumatoid arthritis, or other inflammatory diseases as well as a significant history of allergies or asthma. The IV route is preferred to the IM route. It is necessary to give a small test dose before administering a therapeutic dose. The drug has a slow onset of action and peaks in 1 to 2 weeks. Dosage is calculated according to hemoglobin level and weight.

QSEN Safety Alert ❗

Equipment and drugs for emergency resuscitation must always be available whenever iron dextran IV is administered. Anaphylactic reactions may occur.

Iron Sucrose

Iron sucrose (Venofer) is a parenteral iron supplement given by IV infusion. This supplement is indicated for patients with chronic kidney disease who are not on dialysis and for those who are peritoneal dialysis-dependent or hemodialysis-dependent. It may be given alone or concurrently with erythropoietin therapy. The major advantage of iron sucrose is a lesser risk of anaphylaxis than with iron dextran; however, hypersensitivity reactions, although rare, can be fatal. Test doses are not necessary. Common adverse effects include headache, heart failure, hypotension, nausea, leg cramps, and sepsis.

POTASSIUM

The following discussion focuses on the prototype Ⓟ **potassium chloride**, or KCl. The oral form of the drug has numerous trade names.

Pharmacokinetics and Use

Potassium is absorbed from the GI tract. The potassium level is normally maintained by the kidneys.

Potassium chloride is usually the drug of choice for preventing or treating **hypokalemia** (less than normal amount of potassium in the blood) because deficiencies of potassium and chloride often occur together. Table 33.4 gives route and dosage information for this drug. Health care providers may order potassium chloride for patients who are receiving potassium-depleting diuretics (e.g., hydrochlorothiazide, furosemide), those who are receiving digoxin (hypokalemia increases the risk of digoxin toxicity), and those who are receiving IV fluids because of surgical procedures, GI disease, or other conditions. They may also use it to replace chloride in patients with hypochloremic metabolic acidosis.

Adverse Effects and Contraindications

Adverse effects of oral potassium are nausea, vomiting, abdominal pain, and diarrhea. Adverse effects of IV potassium include postinfusion phlebitis at the IV site. Overdosage with oral or IV forms or rapid infusion of IV preparations produces **hyperkalemia** (greater than normal amount of potassium in the blood), dysrhythmias, heart block, cardiac arrest, respiratory paralysis, and death. Hyperkalemia may occur with the following:

- Concurrent use of potassium chloride with angiotensin-converting enzyme inhibitors or potassium-sparing diuretics
- Salt substitutes that contain potassium instead of sodium if used with potassium supplements
- Penicillin G potassium (potassium salt of penicillin)

Contraindications to potassium supplementation include hyperkalemia, severe renal impairment, acute dehydration, heat cramps, and untreated Addison's disease. Caution is necessary in cardiac disease or renal impairment.

Nursing Implications

Administering the Medication

People should take oral preparations with or after meals; this decreases gastric irritation. They should not crush controlled-release or extended-release tablets. It is necessary to mix oral liquids, powders, and effervescent tablets in at least 120 mL of water, juice, or carbonated beverage to disguise the taste.

Intravenous (IV) potassium chloride is indicated when a patient cannot take an oral preparation or has severe hypokalemia. The nurse measures the serum potassium level and establishes that urine output is adequate before starting IV potassium therapy.

QSEN Safety Alert

It is essential to never give undiluted drug by the IV route or give it by the IV push route.

Well-diluted preparations prevent sudden hyperkalemia, cardiotoxic effects, and phlebitis at the venipuncture site. Careful administration is warranted.

Patient Teaching

Box 33.3 identifies patient teaching guidelines for minerals and electrolytes, including potassium.

Clinical Application 33-4

- Serum electrolytes reveal that Mrs. Martin is hypokalemic. The health care provider orders potassium chloride per feeding tube. What steps does the nurse take to administer this medication, and what form of potassium chloride is preferable for administration per feeding tube? What adverse effects does the nurse assess for?
- Suppose Mrs. Martin is severely hypokalemic and the health care provider orders potassium chloride to be given intravenously. What nursing interventions ensure that the ordered potassium supplement is given correctly and safely? What adverse effects may occur if IV administration of this potassium preparation occurs too rapidly?

NCLEX Success

9. Which one of the following mineral/electrolyte imbalances increases the chances of digoxin toxicity?

   A. hyperkalemia
   B. hypokalemia
   C. decreased serum iron levels
   D. elevated serum iron levels

10. A nurse should question the use of an oral potassium preparation with which one of the following drugs?

    A. ethacrynic acid (Edecrin)
    B. furosemide (Lasix)
    C. hydrochlorothiazide (HCTZ)
    D. spironolactone (Aldactone)

11. The nurse should teach a patient to avoid large amounts of potassium-containing foods or a potassium supplement if the patient is taking which one of the following drugs for control of blood pressure?

    A. an angiotensin-converting enzyme inhibitor
    B. a beta-blocker
    C. a calcium channel blocker
    D. a centrally acting alpha-agonist

ADJUVANT MINERALS

Other medications may be necessary in a variety of conditions to support the treatment and resolution of symptoms. Table 33.4 contains information about some of the agents discussed in this section.

Magnesium

Oral magnesium oxide or hydroxide may be useful for mild hypomagnesemia. Parenteral magnesium sulfate may be necessary for moderate to severe hypomagnesemia, convulsions associated with pregnancy, and prevention of hypomagnesemia in total parenteral nutrition. Therapeutic effects in these conditions are attributed to the preparations' depressant effects on the CNS as well as on smooth, skeletal, and cardiac muscle. (Discussion of the use of magnesium products as antacids and cathartics appears in Chaps. 59 and 60, respectively.)

Oral magnesium salts may cause diarrhea. Contraindications to magnesium include impaired renal function or being comatose.

Oral preparations of magnesium oxide or hydroxide act in 3 to 6 hours, are minimally absorbed systemically, and are excreted in urine. With parenteral magnesium sulfate, IM injections act in 1 hour and last 3 to 4 hours; IV administration produces immediate action that lasts 30 minutes.

Zinc

Zinc sulfate and zinc gluconate are available over the counter in various forms and strengths. Zinc is also an ingredient in several vitamin–mineral combination products. Zinc preparations are given orally as a dietary supplement to prevent or treat zinc deficiency. They have a slow onset of action and a delayed peak. They are metabolized in the liver and excreted in feces. Adverse effects of zinc sulfate are dizziness, restlessness, nausea, vomiting, gastric ulcers, and diarrhea. The FDA recommends that intranasal zinc products not be used because of reports of loss of ability to smell (anosmia) following their use. Zinc-induced anosmia is characterized by rapid onset and stinging and burning.

Multiple Mineral–Electrolyte Preparations

Oral electrolyte solutions (e.g., Pedialyte) contain several electrolytes and a small amount of dextrose. They are used to supply maintenance amounts of fluids and electrolytes when oral intake is restricted. They are especially useful in children for treatment of diarrhea and may prevent severe fluid and electrolyte depletion. The amount given must be carefully calculated, prescribed, and administered to avoid excessive intake. Oral solutions should not be used in severe circumstances in which IV fluid and electrolyte therapy is indicated, and they should not be mixed with other electrolyte-containing fluids, such as milk or fruit juices. In addition, they must be cautiously used in impaired renal function. There are numerous electrolyte solutions for IV use to maintain or replace electrolytes when the patient is unable to eat and drink.

Treatment of Mineral Excess

Penicillamine (Cuprimine)

Penicillamine (Cuprimine) is a **chelating agent**, which binds copper, lead, mercury, and zinc to form soluble complexes that are excreted in the urine. It main use is the removal of excess copper in patients with Wilson's disease, a rare condition characterized by accumulation of copper in vital organs. Prophylactic use involves giving the agent to patients in whom this hereditary condition is likely to develop, before clinical manifestations occur. Other uses for penicillamine include cystinuria, a hereditary metabolic disorder characterized by large amounts of cystine in the urine and renal calculi; lead poisoning; and severe rheumatoid arthritis that does not respond to conventional treatment measures.

Succimer (Chemet)

Succimer (Chemet) chelates lead to form water-soluble complexes that are excreted in the urine. Indications include the treatment of lead poisoning in children. After oral administration, peak blood levels are reached in 1 to 2 hours. The drug is metabolized in the liver and excreted in urine and feces, with a half-life of 2 days. The most common adverse effects are anorexia, nausea, vomiting, and diarrhea.

Deferoxamine and Deferasirox

Acute iron overdosage requires treatment with these drugs as soon as possible, even if overdosage is only suspected and the amount taken is unknown. It is unnecessary to wait until the serum iron level is measured.

Deferoxamine (Desferal) is a parenteral drug used to remove excess iron from storage sites (e.g., ferritin, hemosiderin) in the body. It combines with iron to produce a water-soluble compound that can be excreted by the kidneys. IM, IV, and subcutaneous routes may be useful in certain circumstances. The urine becomes reddish brown from the iron content. A common adverse effect is pain or induration at the injection site. The most serious adverse effect is anaphylaxis.

Deferasirox (Exjade) is an iron chelating agent used to treat chronic iron overload in children and adults who require frequent blood transfusions for severe, chronic anemia. This drug is absorbed with oral administration, with peak plasma levels in 1.5 to 4 hours. It is highly bound to serum albumin, metabolized in the liver, and excreted in bile and feces (with the iron, which binds to the drug). Oral administration should be at the same time each day, before a meal. Patients should not chew or swallow the tablets but dissolve them in water, orange juice, or apple juice. The most common adverse effects are skin rash, fever, headache, and GI problems (e.g., abdominal pain, vomiting, diarrhea, and constipation). The FDA has issued a **BLACK BOX WARNING** ◆ for deferasirox regarding the risk of hepatic and/or renal impairment and GI hemorrhage, all of which can be fatal. It is important to monitor liver and kidney function closely.

Agents Used in the Treatment of Hyperkalemia

The first step in the treatment of hyperkalemia is to eliminate any exogenous sources of potassium. It is essential to treat acidosis, if present, because potassium leaves cells and enters the serum, causing acidosis. Health care providers use measures that antagonize the effects of potassium, cause potassium to leave the serum and reenter the cells, and remove potassium from the body. Serum potassium levels and electrocardiographic (ECG) changes are the primary determinants of the treatment regimen.

Sodium Bicarbonate

Sodium bicarbonate is an agent used to control the acidosis associated with hyperkalemia. A dose of 50 mEq intravenously administered over 5 minutes causes rapid movement of potassium into cells. It may be necessary to give another dose if ECG changes persist.

Calcium Gluconate

Calcium gluconate is a mineral supplement. A 1000-mg dose is given intravenously over 5 to 7 minutes early in treatment to decrease the cardiotoxic effects of hyperkalemia. It may be necessary to give another dose if ECG changes persist or recur. Contraindications to calcium include digoxin use because hypercalcemia potentiates the cardiotoxic effects of digoxin.

Glucose and Insulin

Intravenous glucose and insulin are a treatment for hyperkalemia. Infusion causes potassium to move into cells. Glucose is given with insulin to prevent hypoglycemia. A commonly used regimen is regular insulin 10 units in 10% dextrose 500 mL infused over 1 hour. To avoid hypoglycemia, experts recommend administration of IV fluids of 10% dextrose at 50 to 75 mL/h (Mount, 2011). When glucose and insulin are used to lower serum potassium, close monitoring of blood glucose levels is necessary.

Cation Exchange: Sodium Polystyrene Sulfonate

With less severe hyperkalemia, sodium polystyrene sulfonate (Kayexalate), a cation exchange resin, administered orally, removes potassium from the body in the stool. The resin is usually mixed with water and several daily doses may be required until serum potassium is normal.

QSEN Safety Alert ❗

Although sorbitol has been given with sodium polystyrene sulfonate orally and as an enema for its laxative effect, recent studies showed an association between the combination and intestinal necrosis; in 2009, the FDA recommended that sodium polystyrene sulfonate should no longer be administered in sorbitol.

Nutritional Products

Various products are available to supplement or substitute for dietary intake. These may consist of vitamins, minerals, liquid enteral formulas, IV fluids and nutrition, and pancreatic enzymes.

Numerous liquid enteral formulas are available for oral or tube feedings, and many are nutritionally complete, except for water, when given in sufficient amounts (e.g., Ensure, Isocal, Sustacal, Resource). To meet fluid needs, it is necessary to give additional water. Most oral products come in a variety of flavors and contain 1 kcal/mL of formula. Additional products are available formulated for patients with special conditions (e.g., hepatic or renal failure, malabsorption syndromes) or needs (e.g., high protein, increased calories).

When the GI tract is functional but the patient cannot ingest sufficient food and fluid, the nurse can give high-protein, high-calorie foods (e.g., milkshakes) or nutritionally complete supplements (e.g., Ensure) with meals, between meals, and at bedtime. In patients with a feeding tube, **enteral nutrition** provides fluid and nutrients. When the GI tract is nonfunctional, the nurse often gives IV fluids, or **parenteral nutrition**. Most of these solutions are nutritionally incomplete and are used short term to supply fluids, electrolytes, and a few calories; additional nutrition may be necessary.

Use

For short-term use (e.g., 3–5 days), the goal is to provide adequate amounts of fluids and electrolytes and enough carbohydrates to minimize oxidation of body protein and fat for energy. The choice of specific solution depends on individual needs, but it should contain at least 5% dextrose. A frequently used solution is 5% dextrose in 0.45% sodium chloride, 2000 to 3000 mL per 24 hours (provides ~170 kcal/L, water, sodium, and chloride). Vitamins may be added. These solutions are nutritionally inadequate.

For long-term use (weeks to months), the goal is to provide all nutrients required for normal body functioning, including tissue repair. Basic solutions provide water, carbohydrate, protein, vitamins, and minerals. Patients usually receive fat emulsions (e.g., Intralipid) that are usually given separately to provide additional calories and essential fatty acids (500 mL of 10% emulsion provides 550 kcal).

Use in Children

For children with special needs in relation to nutrients, various enteral formulations are available. Some examples include Lofenalac for children with phenylketonuria; Nursoy and Soyalac, which contain soy protein, for children who are allergic to cow's milk; and Nutramigen and Pregestimil, which contain easily digested nutrients for children with malabsorption or other GI problems. However, parenteral nutrition may be necessary.

Use in Patients With Renal Impairment

With enteral nutrition, Amin-Aid provides amino acids, carbohydrates, and a few electrolytes for patients with renal failure. With parenteral nutrition, several amino acid solutions are available for patients with renal failure (e.g., Aminosyn-RF). Nepro is a formulation for patients receiving dialysis. Suplena, which is lower in protein and some electrolytes than Nepro, is formulated for patients who are not receiving dialysis.

Use in Patients With Hepatic Impairment

For enteral feedings (usually by GI tube) in patients with liver failure, Hepatic-Aid II is available. For parenteral feeding in patients with hepatic failure and hepatic encephalopathy, HepatAmine, a special formula of amino acids, may be useful.

Caution is warranted with the use of enteral and parenteral fat preparations in patients with hepatic impairment. Medium-chain triglycerides (e.g., MCT oil), which are used to provide calories in other malnourished patients, may lead to coma in patients with advanced cirrhosis. Patients who require parenteral nutrition may develop high serum triglyceride levels and pancreatitis if given usually amounts of IV fat emulsions.

Adverse Effects

Adverse reactions, which are usually attributed to the hypertonicity of the preparations, include tachycardia, hypotension, dehydration, nausea, vomiting, diarrhea, and increased urine output. The risk of aspiration of formula is a consideration with tube feeding.

Administering the Medication

For oral supplemental feedings, it is necessary to chill liquids or pour them over ice and give them through a straw (unless contraindicated), from a closed container, between meals. This practice may improve formula taste and decrease formula odor. A straw directs the formula toward the back of the throat and decreases contact with taste buds. A closed container also decreases odor.

For tube feedings, the nurse adheres to guidelines for safe administration (positioning, placement of tube, residual and aseptic management of formula and equipment). When medications are ordered, liquid preparations are preferable. Tablets or powders may stick in the tube lumen, which may mean the full dose of medication does not reach the stomach. Also, the obstruction of the tube is likely. It is important not to mix medications with tube feeding formula; this could interfere with drug absorption.

Assessing for Therapeutic Effects

For patients receiving nutritional formulas, the nurse observes for weight gain and increased serum albumin. For infants and children receiving milk substitutes, the nurse observes for decreased diarrhea and weight gain. Therapeutic effects depend on the reason for use (i.e., prevention or treatment of undernutrition).

Assessing for Adverse Effects

With commercial nutritional formulas (except Osmolite and Isocal), the nurse observes for tachycardia, hypotension, dehydration, nausea, vomiting, diarrhea, and increased urine output. These adverse reactions are usually attributed to the hypertonicity of the preparations. Beginning administration with small amounts of formula, given slowly, may prevent or minimize adverse effects.

Patient Teaching

Box 33.4 presents patient teaching guidelines for nutritional products.

BOX 33.4	Patient Teaching Guidelines for Nutritional Products

■ For oral supplements, take or give at the preferred time and temperature, when possible.

■ For tube feedings:

■ Use or give with the patient in a sitting position, if possible, to decrease risks of aspirating formula into the lungs.

■ Be sure the tube is placed correctly before each tube feeding. Ask a health care provider how to check placement with your type of tube.

■ Be sure the solution is room temperature. Cold formula may cause abdominal cramping.

■ Do not take or give more than 500 mL per feeding, including 60 to 90 mL of water for flushing the tube. This helps to avoid overfilling the stomach and possible vomiting.

■ Take or give slowly, over approximately 30 to 60 minutes. Rapid administration may cause nausea and vomiting.

■ With continuous feedings, change containers and tubing daily. With intermittent feedings, rinse all equipment after each use, and change at least every 24 hours. Most tube feeding formulas are milk-based and infection may occur if formulas become contaminated or equipment is not kept clean.

■ Ask a health care provider about the amount of free water. Most people receiving 1500 to 2000 mL of tube feeding daily need approximately 1000 mL or more of free water daily. However, patients' needs vary. Water can be mixed with the tube feeding formula, given after the tube feeding, or given between bolus feedings. Be sure to include the amount of water used for flushing the tube in the total daily intake.

■ For giving medications by tube:

■ Give liquid preparations when available.

■ When liquid preparations are not available, it may be necessary to crush some tablets and empty some capsules and mix them with 15 to 30 mL of water. Ask a health care provider which medications can safely be crushed or altered, because some (e.g., long-acting or enteric-coated) can be harmful if crushed.

■ Do not mix medications with the tube feeding formula because some medications may not be absorbed. If the absorption of a drug is affected by the tube feeding formula (e.g., phenytoin), discontinue the tube feeding for the recommended interval prior to drug administration; then, resume feeding at the recommended interval after drug administration.

■ Do not mix medications. Give each one separately.

■ Flush the tube with water before and after each medication to get the medication through the tube and to keep the tube open.

■ For more a more complete discussion of the care of patients with feeding tubes, administration of drugs through feeding tubes, and patient teaching guidelines for home use of feeding tubes, consult a textbook of nursing fundamentals or medical/surgical nursing.

Clinical Application 33-5

• Mrs. Martin has a percutaneous endoscopic gastrostomy tube. She is to receive a bolus tube feeding of 300 mL at 08:00, 12:00, 17:00, and 21:00 hours, with a flush of free water every 4 hours. What precautions does the nurse take to prevent aspiration of the tube feeding?

• Mrs. Martin receives several medications through the feeding tube. Explain what the nurse does if one of those medications cannot be crushed for administration through the tube. Describe the steps he or she takes to administer medications through the tube.

NCLEX Success

12. The nurse has finished administering medication through a percutaneous endoscopic gastrostomy tube. Which one of the following steps should the nurse take next?

A. Check the tube for proper placement.
B. Lower the head of the bed to a comfortable position.
C. Turn the pump on to continue the tube feeding.
D. Flush the tube with water and record the amount.

13. The patient is to receive a bolus tube feeding and a medication per tube at 08:00. When should the medication be administered?

A. prior to the feeding at 07:30
B. mixed with the feeding at 08:00
C. immediately after the feeding
D. hold the medication

The Nursing Process

Assessment

• Assess each patient for current or potential nutritional deficiencies. Some specific assessment factors include the following:

• What are usual eating patterns?

• Does the patient appear underweight? If so, assess for contributing factors (e.g., appetite or ability to obtain, cook, or chew food). Calculate or estimate the body mass index (BMI). A BMI under 18.5 kg/m^2 indicates undernutrition.

• Does the patient have symptoms, disease processes treatments, medications, or diagnostic tests that are likely to interfere with nutrition? For example, many illnesses and oral medications cause anorexia, nausea, vomiting, and diarrhea.

- With vitamins, assessment factors include the following:
  - Deficiency states are more common than excess states and people with other nutritional deficiencies are likely to have vitamin deficiencies as well.
  - Deficiencies of water-soluble vitamins (B complex and C) are more common than those of fat-soluble vitamins (A, D, E, and K).
  - Vitamin deficiencies are usually multiple and signs and symptoms often overlap, especially with B complex deficiencies.
  - Vitamin requirements are increased during infancy, pregnancy, lactation, fever, hyperthyroidism, and many illnesses. Thus, a vitamin intake that is normally adequate may be inadequate in certain circumstances.
  - Vitamin deficiencies are likely to occur in people who are poor, elderly, chronically or severely ill, or alcoholic.
  - Vitamin excess states are rarely caused by excessive dietary intake but may occur with use of vitamin drug preparations, especially if megadoses are taken.
- With mineral–electrolytes, assessment factors include the following:
  - Deficiency states are more common than excess states unless a mineral–electrolyte supplement is being taken. However, deficiencies and excesses may be equally harmful, and both must be assessed.
  - Patients with other nutritional deficiencies are likely to have mineral–electrolyte deficiencies as well. Moreover, deficiencies are likely to be multiple, with overlapping signs and symptoms.
  - Many drugs influence gains and losses of minerals and electrolytes, including diuretics and laxatives.
  - Minerals and electrolytes are lost with gastric suction, polyuria, diarrhea, excessive perspiration, and other conditions.
- Assess laboratory reports when available:
  - Check the complete blood count for decreased red blood cells, hemoglobin, and hematocrit. Reduced values may indicate iron deficiency anemia, and further assessment is needed.
  - Check serum electrolyte reports for abnormal values. All major minerals can be measured in clinical laboratories. The ones usually measured are sodium, potassium, and chloride; carbon dioxide content, a measure of bicarbonate, is also assessed.

Nursing Diagnoses

- Imbalanced nutrition: less than body requirements related to inability to absorb nutrients, inability to digest food, or inability to ingest food
- Imbalanced nutrition: more than body requirements related to excessive intake of vitamins or minerals in relation to metabolic need
- Risk for aspiration related to medication administration and tube feeding
- Risk for injury related to inadequate or excessive vitamin or mineral intake

- Deficient knowledge: nutritional needs and sources of nutrients related to unfamiliarity with information resources
- Deficient knowledge: appropriate use of vitamin/mineral supplements related to unfamiliarity with information resources
- Deficient knowledge: self-administration of vitamin/mineral drug preparations related to lack of exposure to this information

Planning/Goals

The patient will

- Improve nutritional status in relation to body needs
- Maintain fluid and electrolyte balance as measured by appropriate intake and output and serum electrolyte levels
- Ingest appropriate amounts of vitamins and mineral–electrolytes
- Avoid complications of enteral nutrition including aspiration, diarrhea, and infection
- Avoid complications of parenteral nutrition
- Avoid overdoses and adverse effects of vitamins and minerals
- Avoid mineral–electrolyte supplements unless recommended by a health care provider
- Self-administer mineral–electrolyte drugs as prescribed and have appropriate laboratory tests to monitor response

Nursing Interventions

The nurse will

- Promote a well-balanced diet for all patients. Five daily servings of fruits and vegetables provide adequate vitamins unless the patient has increased requirements or conditions that interfere with absorption or use of vitamins. An oral multivitamin may benefit most people, but it is not a substitute for and adequate diet. A diet that is adequate in protein and calories usually provides adequate minerals and electrolytes. Exceptions are calcium and iron, which are often needed as a dietary supplement in women and children.
- Provide relief for symptoms that are likely to interfere with nutrition, such as pain, nausea, vomiting, or diarrhea.
- Provide palatable supplements at appropriate times for patients who need increased protein–calorie intake and encourage patients to take them.
- Promote exercise and activity. For undernourished patients, this may increase appetite, improve digestion, and aid bowel elimination.
- Minimize the use of sedative-type drugs when appropriate. Although no one should be denied pain relief, strong analgesics and other sedatives may cause drowsiness, decreased desire or ability to eat and drink, constipation, and a feeling of fullness.
- Weigh patients at regular intervals. Calculate or estimate the BMI when indicated.
- Monitor weight, fluid intake, urine output, vital signs, blood glucose, serum electrolytes, and complete blood count for patients receiving parenteral nutrition. Obtain these values daily, weekly, or as institutional protocols dictate. Adjust monitoring based on patient status whether hospitalized or at home.

- Promote proper use of mineral supplements, which are recommended only for current or potential deficiencies and are toxic in excessive amounts.
- Follow institutional protocols in the care of patients with feeding tubes and in the administration of ordered tube feeding products. Use best practices in relation to assessing correct tube placement, maintaining patency of tubes, positioning of patients, prevention of aspiration, gravity or pump administration of feeding products, and administration of free water and flushes.
- Follow institution protocols and best practices in relation to administration of medications per feeding tubes. Included would be crushing medications only when appropriate to do so, using liquid forms when available, irrigating tubes properly to prevent occlusion, and administering drugs to minimize drug interactions with tube feeding products or other drugs.

Evaluation

- Observe undernourished patients for quantity and quality of nutrient intake, weight gain, and improvement in laboratory tests of nutritional status (e.g., serum electrolytes, glucose, and proteins).
- Observe children for quantity and quality of food intake and appropriate increases in height and weight.
- Interview and observe for signs and symptoms of complications of enteral and parenteral nutrition.
- When specific vitamins/minerals/electrolytes are being administered, therapeutically observe for improvement in deficiency or excess states as evidenced by improvement in symptoms and absence of adverse effects.

Key Concepts

- Human nutrition to maintain health requires sufficient water, carbohydrates, proteins, fats, vitamins, and minerals.
- Patients with other health problems often have nutritional deficiencies, such as protein–calorie undernutrition and vitamin deficiencies.
- All patients require assessment for nutritional status. When problems are assessed, interventions to maintain or improve nutritional status are needed.
- Fat-soluble vitamins are A, D, E, and K; water-soluble vitamins are B complex and C.
- The best source of nutrients is foods. However, it may be necessary to use oral, enteral (via GI tubes), or parenteral (IV) feedings to meet a patient's nutritional needs.
- Techniques for safe administration of oral, enteral, and parenteral feedings must be consistently followed because complications and harm to patients may occur with all methods.
- Adverse effects may occur with large doses of vitamin and mineral supplements; people should not take more than the maximum recommended amounts.
- Although most adults and children probably benefit from a daily multivitamin, large doses of single vitamins do not prevent cancer or cardiovascular disease and should be avoided.
- The FDA has issued a **BLACK BOX WARNING** ♦ for vitamin K indicating that IV administration, even with drug dilution and slow administration, may result in an anaphylactic type of reaction with risks of shock, cardiorespiratory arrest, and death.
- The FDA has issued a **BLACK BOX WARNING** ♦ for iron dextran with regard to the risk of anaphylactic reactions and death.
- The FDA has issued a **BLACK BOX WARNING** ♦ for deferasirox; there is a risk of hepatic and/or renal impairment and GI hemorrhage, all of which may be fatal.

Critical Thinking Questions

33-1. A 65-year-old man has surgery for gastric cancer and undergoes a total gastrectomy. Intrinsic factor, which is necessary for the absorption of vitamin B_{12}, is secreted by the parietal cells of the gastric mucosa. Postoperatively, the man lacks gastric mucosa and cannot secrete intrinsic factor, placing him at risk for vitamin B_{12} deficiency (pernicious anemia).

- What are the signs and symptoms of pernicious anemia? What other body system is affected by a deficiency of vitamin B_{12}?
- The health care provider orders hydroxocobalamin 30 mcg intramuscularly once daily for 5 days, then hydroxocobalamin 100 mcg intramuscularly once monthly. Why is hydroxocobalamin

ordered intramuscularly rather than orally? For what length of time will the man receive monthly injections of hydroxocobalamin?

- What teaching should the man receive in regard to self-administration of hydroxocobalamin intramuscularly?

- What adverse effects of hydroxocobalamin should the man be aware of?

- What laboratory tests are ordered to determine whether hydroxocobalamin therapy is effective?

33-2. The nurse admits a woman to the medical floor for an exacerbation of heart failure. The nurse notes she has been taking furosemide (Lasix) 80 mg orally once daily at home without a potassium supplement. Her serum potassium is 2.3 mEq/L. Her electrocardiogram is similar to one taken 3 months ago and shows no dysrhythmias.

- The health care provider orders potassium chloride 20 mEq orally three times a day. Why is the woman's serum potassium low? What factors should the nurse consider when administering this drug to this woman?

- The health care provider also orders a one-time-only dose of D5W 200 mL with potassium chloride 40 mEq to be administered intravenously at a rate of 50 mL/h per infusion pump. Is this an appropriate rate at which to administer this dose of potassium? Why is the potassium diluted in D5W and administered by IV pump instead of by IV push?

References and Resources

Dudek, S. G. (2010). *Nutrition essentials for nursing practice* (6th ed.). Philadelphia, PA: Lippincott Williams & Wilkins.

Karch, A. M. (2013). *Lippincott's nursing drug guide*. Philadelphia, PA: Lippincott Williams & Wilkins.

Mount, D. B. (2011). *Treatment and prevention of hyperkalemia*. Up-To-Date.

Nursing 2012 Drug Handbook. (2012). Philadelphia, PA: Lippincott William & Wilkins.

Porth, C. M., & Matfin, G. (2009). *Pathophysiology concepts of altered health states*. Philadelphia, PA: Lippincott Williams & Wilkins.

Sexton, D. J., & McClain, M. T. (2011). *The common cold in adults: Treatment and prevention*. Up-To-Date.

Smeltzer, S. C., Bare, B. G., Hinkle, J. H., & Cheever, K. H. (2010). *Brunner & Suddarth's textbook of medical-surgical nursing* (12th ed.). Philadelphia, PA: Lippincott Williams & Wilkins.

Taylor, C. R., Lillis, C., LeMone, P. L., & Lynn, P. (2011). *Fundamentals of nursing: The art and science of nursing care*. (7th ed.). Philadelphia PA: Lippincott Williams & Wilkins.

Up-To-Date. (2011). *Vitamin A: Pediatric drug information*. Lexi-Comp, Inc. Retrieved December 26, 2011.

Up-To-Date. (2011). *Vitamin E: Drug information*. Lexi-Comp, Inc. Retrieved December 26, 2011.

Up-To-Date. (2012). *Vitamin K₁ (phytonadione): Drug information*. Lexi-Comp, Inc. Retrieved January 1, 2012.

Up-To-Date. (2012). *Vitamin B₁ (thiamine): Drug information*. Lexi-Comp, Inc. Retrieved January 11, 2012.

Up-To-Date. (2012). *Vitamin B₅ (pantothenic acid): Drug information*. Lexi-Comp, Inc. Retrieved January 11, 2012.

Up-To-Date. (2012). *Vitamin C (ascorbic acid): Drug information*. Lexi-Comp, Inc. Retrieved January 11, 2012.

Up-To-Date. (2012). *Ferrous gluconate: Drug information*. Lexi-Comp, Inc. Retrieved January 11, 2012.

Up-To-Date. (2012). *Ferrous sulfate: Drug information*. Lexi-Comp, Inc. Retrieved January 11, 2012.

Up-To-Date. (2012). *Penicillamine: Drug information*. Lexi-Comp, Inc. Retrieved January 11, 2012.

Up-To-Date. (2012). *Zinc sulfate: Drug information*. Lexi-Comp, Inc. Retrieved January 11, 2012.

Up-To-Date. (2011). *Zinc supplements: Natural drug information*. Lexi-Comp, Inc. Retrieved December 26, 2011.

34 Drug Therapy for Weight Management

Clinical Application Case Study

Halli Vargas is a 31-year-old woman who has had a weight problem all her life. She has been on any number of diets that have a "yo-yo" effect, with weight loss followed by weight gain. She stands 5 ft 5 inches tall and weighs 265 pounds. Her nurse practitioner starts her on orlistat and prescribes a consultation with a dietitian.

KEY TERMS

Anorexiant: drug that suppresses the appetite.

Body mass index (BMI): reflection of weight in relation to height; better indicator than weight alone for determining the fitness level of a person.

Central obesity: concentration of fat in abdominal area resulting in an increase in waist size

Obesity: BMI of 30 or more kg/m^2

Overweight: BMI of 25 to 29.9 kg/m^2

Introduction

Obesity, which affects 34% of the adult population in the United States, has reached epidemic proportions. It is associated with multiple chronic diseases. Excessive amounts of any of the dietary nutrients are converted to fat and stored in the body, resulting in excess weight and obesity. Although therapeutic lifestyle changes are the cornerstone of population-based interventions to manage obesity, they are often insufficient in achieving recommended treatment targets. Once the agents are discontinued, people may regain weight. The importance of a safe and effective use of drugs coupled with therapeutic lifestyle changes has become critical. This chapter discusses obesity and weight management, specifically focusing on drugs to aid weight loss and maintain desired weight.

Overview of Weight Management

A better indicator of weight problems than weight alone, **body mass index (BMI)** reflects weight in relation to height. **Overweight** is defined as a BMI of 25 to 29.9 kg/m². **Obesity** is defined as a BMI of 30 or more kg/m². The desirable range for BMI is 18.5 to 24.9 kg/m², with any values below 18.5 indicating underweight and any values of 25 or greater indicating excessive weight (Box 34.1). A large waist circumference (greater than 35 inches for women, greater than 40 inches for men) is another risk factor for overweight and obesity. Using these definitions, it is projected that 68% of adults in America are overweight and 34% are obese.

Etiology

Carbohydrates, proteins, and fats are required for human nutrition. Either deficiencies or excesses impair health, cause illness, and interfere with recovery from illness or injury. Carbohydrates and fats serve primarily as sources of energy for cellular metabolism, and proteins are basic structural and functional components of all body cells and tissues. Energy is measured in kilocalories (kcal, commonly called calories) per gram of food oxidized in the body. Carbohydrates and proteins supply 4 kcal/g. Fats supply 9 kcal/g. Excessive amounts of any nutrient are converted to fat and stored in the body, resulting in excess weight and obesity.

The incidence of overweight and obesity has dramatically increased during the past 25 years. Obesity may occur in anyone but is more likely to occur in women, ethnic groups, and people of lower socioeconomic status. In general, more women than men are obese, whereas more men than women are overweight. African American women and Mexican American men and women have the highest rates of overweight and obesity in the United States. Women in lower socioeconomic classes are more likely to be obese than those in higher socioeconomic classes.

The etiology of excessive weight is thought to involve complex and often overlapping interactions among physiologic, genetic, environmental, psychosocial, and other factors.

BOX 34.1 Calculation of Body Mass Index (BMI) and Height and Weight Indicators for Overweight and Obese

BMI

BMI calculators are available online (http://www.nhlbisupport.com/bmi/) but can be calculated as weight in kilograms divided by height in meters, squared; or as weight in pounds divided by height in inches, squared, multiplied by a conversion factor of 704.5 (listed as 703 in some sources), as follows:

$$BMI = \frac{Weight\,(pounds)}{Height\,(inches)^2} \times 704.5$$

For example: A person who weighs 150 pounds and is 5 ft 5 inches (65 inches) tall

$$BMI = \frac{150\,pounds}{65\,in. \times 65\,in.} \times 704.5 = \frac{150}{4225} \times 704.5 = \frac{105675}{422.5} = 25$$

Weight Compared With Height as an Indicator for Being Overweight or Obese

Height (ft/in.)	Weight (Pound) Indicating Overweight (BMI 25)	Weight (Pound) Indicating Obesity (BMI 30)
5'2" (62 in.)	135	165
5'3"	140	170
5'4"	145	175
5'5"	150	180
5'6"	155	185
5'7"	160	190
5'8"	165	195
5'9"	170	200
5'10"	175	205
5'11"	180	210
6'0"	185	220
6'1"	190	225
6'2" (74 in.)	195	230

Physiologic Factors

In general, increased weight is related to an energy imbalance in which energy intake (food/calorie consumption) exceeds energy expenditure. Total energy expenditure represents the energy expended at rest (i.e., the basal or resting metabolic rate), during physical activity, and during food consumption. When a person ingests food, about 10% of the energy content of that food is expended in the digestion, absorption, and metabolism of nutrients. Foods that contain carbohydrates and proteins stimulate energy expenditure; high-fat foods have little stimulatory effect. The energy required to metabolize and to use food reaches a maximum level about 1 hour after the food is ingested. In addition, men tend to expend more energy than women because they have proportionally more muscle mass. Energy expenditure usually decreases in older men and women of all ages because these groups have less muscle tissue and more adipose tissue. Muscle is more metabolically active (i.e., has higher energy needs and burns more calories) than adipose tissue.

Excessive weight can result from eating more calories, exercising less, or a combination of the two factors. Consuming an extra 500 calories each day for a week results in 3500 excess calories or one pound of fat. Excess calories are converted to triglycerides and stored in fat cells. With continued intake of excessive calories, fat cells increase in both size and number.

Genetic Factors

Various studies indicate that a significant portion of weight variation within a given environment is genetic in origin. For example, identical twins raised in separate environments often have similar body types. Most cases of human obesity are attributed mainly to the combination of genetic susceptibility and environmental conditions.

Environmental Factors

Environmental factors contributing to the greater number of overweight and obese people include increased food consumption and decreased physical activity. The ready availability and relatively low cost of a wide variety of foods, in addition to large portion sizes and high-calorie foods, promote overeating. In addition, many social gatherings are associated with eating or overeating.

In relation to physical activity, usual activities of daily living for many people, including work-related activities, require relatively little energy expenditure. In addition, few Americans are thought to exercise in the optimal frequency, intensity, or duration to maintain health and prevent excessive weight gain. For both adults and children, increased time watching television, playing video or computer games, and working on computers contribute to less physical activity and are thought to promote weight gain and obesity. In general, however, it is still unknown whether less physical activity leads to obesity or the physical effects of obesity lead to minimal physical activity.

Psychosocial Factors

Psychosocial disorders may be either a cause or an effect of obesity. Although much is still unknown about the psychological aspects of obesity development, depression and/or abuse may play a role. Obese people often report symptoms of depression, and some people overeat and gain weight during depressive episodes. It may be that obesity and depression commonly occur together and reinforce each other. A depressed person is less likely to take the active measures in diet and exercise that are required to lose weight, even if obesity is a prominent factor in the development of depression.

Other Factors

Diseases are rarely a major cause of the development of obesity. However, numerous disease processes may limit a person's ability to engage in calorie-burning physical activity. In addition, numerous prescription medications reportedly cause weight gain in some or most of the patients who take them (Box 34.2).

Age Considerations

Overweight and Obese Children

Being overweight and obese are common and increasing among children and adolescents in epidemic proportions. It is estimated that nearly 25% of children and adolescents in the United States are overweight. Overweight is defined as a BMI above the 85th percentile for the age group and obesity as a BMI above the 95th percentile.

Childhood obesity is a major public health concern because these children have or are at risk of developing hypertension, dyslipidemias, type 2 diabetes mellitus, and other disorders that may lead to reduced quality of life, major disability, and death at younger adult ages than nonobese children. Obesity, type 2 diabetes, and other health problems are mainly attributed to poor eating habits and too little exercise. In addition, the child who is obese after 6 years of age is highly likely to be obese as an adult and develop obesity-related health problems, especially if a parent is obese. Obesity in adults that began in childhood tends to be more severe.

Under pressure from parents and advocates to prevent obesity in youth, many school districts have banned soft drinks, candy, and junk foods from school vending machines and cafeterias. The American Beverage Association agreed to a voluntary ban on the sale of all high-calorie drinks and all beverages in containers larger than 8, 10, and 12 ounces in elementary, middle, and high schools, respectively. Several additional recent initiatives to combat childhood obesity have been implemented.

In children, treatment of obesity should focus on healthy eating and increasing physical activity. In general, children should not be put on "diets." For a child who is overweight, the recommended goal is to maintain weight or slow the rate of weight gain so that weight and BMI gradually decline as the child's height increases. If the child has already reached his or her anticipated adult weight, maintenance of that weight and prevention of additional gain should be the long-term treatment goal. If the child already exceeds his or her optimal adult weight, the goal of treatment should be a slow weight loss of 10 to 12 pounds per year until this weight is reached. As with adults, increased activity is necessary for successful weight loss or management in children. It is possible to implement these measures successfully mainly within a family unit, and family support to assist the child in weight control and a more healthful lifestyle is necessary. In addition, schools should teach children the basic principles of good nutrition and why eating a balanced diet is important to health.

Overweight and Obese Older Adults

Although obesity is reported in older adults, the numbers are still significantly lower than the levels seen in the young adult population. It is speculated that socioeconomic factors may play a role in this age group when it comes to developing obesity.

Obesity does not appear to make a substantial difference to risks of death among older adults but is a major contributor to increased disability and reduced quality of life in later years. The development of type 2 diabetes mellitus remains a risk. Excess weight reduces the loss of bone mass, and overweight elderly people are less likely to suffer hip fractures, a major cause of morbidity and mortality; health risks of obesity are greater than any advantages.

BOX 34.2   Effects of Selected Medications on Weight

Antidepressants

Selective serotonin reuptake inhibitors, such as fluoxetine (Prozac, Sarafem) and related drugs, may promote weight loss with short-term use. However, with long-term use, they reportedly may cause as much weight gain as tricyclic antidepressants (TCAs) such as amitriptyline (Elavil). TCAs have long been associated with excessive appetite and weight gain. Mirtazapine (Remeron) and phenelzine (Nardil) are also associated with weight gain. The effects of bupropion (Wellbutrin and Zyban) on weight are unclear from clinical trials. Gain was reported when bupropion was used as a smoking deterrent, but both gain and loss occurred when used as an antidepressant. However, anorexia and weight loss occurred at a higher percentage rate than increased appetite and weight gain.

Antidiabetic Drugs

Although little attention is paid to the topic in most literature about diabetic drugs, weight gain apparently occurs with insulin, sulfonylureas, and the glitazones (but not with metformin, acarbose, or miglitol). Almost all patients with type 2 diabetes eventually require insulin; those who are failing on oral agents generally gain a large amount of body fat when switched to insulin therapy. Although the mechanism of weight gain is unknown, it may be related to the chronic hyperinsulinism induced by long-acting insulins and the sulfonylureas (which increase insulin secretion). Less weight is gained when oral drugs are given during the day and an intermediate- or long-acting insulin is injected at bedtime. This strategy is thought to cause less daytime hyperinsulinemia than the more traditional insulin strategies.

For near–normal-weight patients with diabetes who require drug therapy, a sulfonylurea may be given. However, for obese patients, metformin is usually the initial drug of choice because it does not promote weight gain. Metformin may also be used to treat obese diabetic children, aged 10 to 16 years, who require drug therapy.

Antiepileptic Drugs

Weight gain commonly occurs with the use of antiepileptic drugs (AEDs). This has been observed for many years with older drugs (e.g., phenytoin, valproic acid, carbamazepine) and with newer AEDs (e.g., gabapentin, lamotrigine, tiagabine). Mechanisms by which the drugs promote weight gain are unclear but may involve stimulation of appetite and/or a slowed metabolic rate. Consequences of weight gain may include increased risks of diabetes mellitus, hypertension, and other physical health problems as well as psychological distress over appearance, especially in children and adolescents.

Antihistamines

Histamine₁ (H₁) antagonists (e.g., diphenhydramine, loratadine) reportedly increase appetite and cause weight gain.

Antihypertensives

The main antihypertensive drugs reported to cause weight gain are the beta blockers. The drugs can cause fatigue and decrease exercise tolerance and metabolic rate, all of which may contribute to weight gain. Other mechanisms may also be involved. As a result, some clinicians question the use of beta blockers in overweight or obese patients with uncomplicated hypertension. Alpha blockers may also cause weight gain, but apparently at a low incidence. Angiotensin-converting enzyme (ACE) inhibitors and calcium channel blockers are not reported to promote weight gain.

Antipsychotics

Weight gain is often reported and extensively documented with antipsychotic drugs. Although the exact mechanism is unknown, weight gain has been associated with antihistaminic effects, anticholinergic effects, and blockade of serotonin receptors. In addition, dietary factors and activity levels may also play significant roles.

Clozapine and olanzapine reportedly cause significant weight gain in 40% or more of patients. Compared with clozapine and olanzapine, risperidone causes less weight gain, and quetiapine and ziprasidone cause the least weight gain. Weight gain may lead to noncompliance with drug therapy. In addition to weight gain, clozapine and olanzapine adversely affect glucose regulation and can aggravate preexisting diabetes or cause new-onset diabetes. The extent to which these effects are related to weight gain is unknown. For patients who are obese, diabetic, or at risk of developing diabetes, an antipsychotic drug that causes less weight gain would seem the better choice.

Cholesterol-Lowering Agents

Weight gain has been reported with the statin group of drugs; mechanisms and extent are unknown.

Corticosteroids

Systemic corticosteroids may cause increased appetite, weight gain, central obesity, and retention of sodium and fluid. Inhaled and intranasal corticosteroids have little effect on weight.

Gastrointestinal Drugs

Increased appetite and weight gain have been reported with the proton pump inhibitors such as omeprazole and others. The mechanisms and extent are unknown.

Hormonal Contraceptives

The weight gain associated with using hormonal contraceptives may be related more to retention of fluid and sodium than to increased body fat.

Mood-Stabilizing Agent

Weight gain has been reported with long-term use of lithium, with approximately 20% of patients gaining 10 kg (22 pounds) or more. This increased weight is attributed to fluid retention, consumption of high-calorie beverages as a result of increased thirst, or a decreased metabolic rate. Weight gain is a common reason for noncompliance with lithium therapy, and weight gain may be more common in women with lithium-induced hypothyroidism and in those who are already overweight.

Pathophysiology

Obesity results from consistent ingestion of more calories than are used for energy, and it substantially increases risks of developing numerous health problems (Box 34.3). Most obesity-related disorders are attributed mainly to the multiple metabolic abnormalities associated with obesity. Abdominal fat out of proportion to total body fat (also called visceral or **central obesity**),

which often occurs in men and postmenopausal women, is considered a greater risk factor for disease and death than lower body obesity. In addition to the many health problems associated with obesity, obesity is increasingly being considered a chronic disease in its own right. Although it has been the focus of much research in recent years, no current theory adequately explains the disorder and its resistance to treatment.

BOX 34.3   Health Risks of Obesity

Obesity is associated with serious health risks. Several disease states and chronic health problems are more prevalent in obese patients, as well as increased mortality. Studies indicate that a high body mass index (BMI) is associated with an increased risk of death from all causes, among both men and women, and in all age groups. In addition, a higher death rate occurs in people who gain weight of 10 kg or more after 18 years of age. Some of the major health risks include the disorders listed below. In general, these conditions tend to worsen as the degree of obesity increases and improve with weight loss.

Cancer

Obesity is associated with a higher prevalence of breast, colon, and endometrial cancers. With breast cancer, risks increase in postmenopausal women with increasing body weight. Women who gain more than 20 pounds from age 18 to midlife have double the risk of breast cancer compared with women who maintain a stable weight during this period of their life. In addition, central obesity apparently increases the risk of breast cancer independent of overall obesity. In women with central obesity, this additional risk factor may be related to an excess of estrogen (from conversion of androstenedione to estradiol in peripheral fatty tissue) and a deficiency of sex hormone–binding globulin to combine with the estrogen.

Colon cancer seems to be more common in obese men and women. In addition, a high BMI may be a risk factor for a higher mortality rate with colon cancer. Endometrial cancer is clearly more common in obese women, with adult weight gain again increasing risk.

Cardiovascular Disorders

Obesity is a major risk factor for cardiovascular disorders and increased mortality from cardiovascular disease. Studies have confirmed the relationship between obesity and increased risk of coronary heart disease (CHD) and stroke in both men and women. In addition, obesity during adolescence is associated with higher rates and greater severity of cardiovascular disease as adults.

Obesity increases risks by aggravating other risk factors such as hypertension, insulin resistance, low HDL cholesterol, and hypertriglyceridemia. In addition, obesity seems to be an independent risk factor for cardiovascular disorders, and central obesity may be more important than BMI as a risk factor for death from cardiovascular disease. The increased mortality rate is seen even with modest excess body weight. Hypertension, dyslipidemia, insulin resistance, and glucose intolerance are known cardiac risk factors that tend to cluster in obese people. Hypertension often occurs in obese people and is thought to play a major role in the increased incidence of cardiovascular disease and stroke observed in patients with obesity. Metabolic abnormalities that occur with obesity and type 2 diabetes mellitus (e.g., insulin resistance and the resultant hyperinsulinemia)

aggravate hypertension and increase cardiovascular risks. The combination of obesity and hypertension is associated with cardiac changes (e.g., thickening of the ventricular wall, ischemia, and increased heart volume) that lead to heart failure more rapidly. Weight loss of as little as 4.5 kg (10 pounds) can decrease blood pressure and cardiovascular risk in many people with obesity and hypertension.

Diabetes Mellitus

Obesity is strongly associated with impaired glucose tolerance, insulin resistance, and diabetes mellitus. In addition, obesity during adolescence is associated with higher rates of diabetes as adults as well as more severe complications of diabetes at younger ages.

The cellular effects by which obesity causes insulin resistance are unknown. Proposed mechanisms include down-regulation of insulin receptors, abnormal postreceptor signals, and others. Whatever the mechanism, the impaired insulin response stimulates the pancreatic beta cells to increase insulin secretion, resulting in a relative excess of insulin called hyperinsulinemia, and causes impaired lipid metabolism (increased low-density lipoprotein [LDL] cholesterol and triglycerides and decreased high-density lipoprotein [HDL] cholesterol). These metabolic changes increase hypertension and other risk factors for cardiovascular disease. As with cardiovascular disease and diabetes in general, central obesity seems to increase the likelihood of serious disease. The abdominal fat of central obesity seems to be more insulin resistant than peripheral fat deposited over the buttocks and legs. Intentional weight loss significantly reduces mortality in obese people with diabetes.

Dyslipidemias

Obesity strongly contributes to abnormal and undesirable changes in lipid metabolism (e.g., increased triglycerides and LDL cholesterol; decreased HDL cholesterol) that increase risks of cardiovascular disease and other health problems.

Gallstones

Obesity apparently increases the risk for developing gallstones by altering production and metabolism of cholesterol and bile. The risk is higher in women, especially those who have had multiple pregnancies or who are taking oral contraceptives. However, rapid weight loss with very–low-calorie diets is also associated with gallstones.

Metabolic Syndrome

Metabolic syndrome is a group of risk factors and chronic conditions that occur together and greatly increase the risks of diabetes mellitus, serious cardiovascular disease, and death. The syndrome is thought to be highly prevalent in the United States. Major characteristics include many of the health problems associated with obesity (e.g., dyslipidemias, hypertension, impaired glucose tolerance, insulin resistance,

BOX 34.3 Health Risks of Obesity (Continued)

central obesity). More specifically, metabolic syndrome includes three or more of the following abnormalities:

- Central obesity (waist circumference over 40 inches for men and over 35 inches for women)
- Serum triglycerides of 150 mg/dL or more
- HDL cholesterol below 40 mg/dL in men and below 50 mg/dL in women
- Blood pressure of 135/85 mm Hg or higher
- Serum glucose of 110 mg/dL or higher

Osteoarthritis

Obesity is associated with osteoarthritis (OA) of both weight-bearing joints, such as the hip and knee, and non–weight-bearing joints. Extra weight can stress affected bones and joints, contract muscles that normally stabilize joints, and may alter the metabolism of cartilage, collagen, and bone. In general, obese people develop OA of the knees at an earlier age and are more likely than nonobese people to require knee replacement surgery.

The important role of obesity in OA is supported by the observation that weight loss delays onset and reduces symptoms and disability. Weight reduction may also decrease infection, wound complications, and blood loss if surgery is required. Despite the benefits of weight loss, however, persons with OA have difficulty losing weight because painful joints limit exercise and activity.

Sleep Apnea

Sleep apnea commonly occurs in obese persons. A possible explanation is enlargement of soft tissue in the upper airways that leads to collapse of the upper airways with inspiration during sleep. The obstructed breathing leads to apnea with hypoxemia, hypercarbia, and a stress response. Sleep apnea is associated with increased risks of hypertension, possible right heart failure, and sudden death. Weight loss leads to improvement in sleep apnea.

Miscellaneous Effects

Obesity is associated with numerous difficulties in addition to those described above. These may include

- Nownalcoholic fatty liver disease, which is being increasingly recognized and which may lead to liver failure
- Poor wound healing
- Poor antibody response to hepatitis B vaccine
- A negative perception of people who are obese that affects their education, socioeconomic, and employment status
- High costs associated with treatment of the medical conditions caused or aggravated by obesity as well as the costs associated with weight loss efforts
- In women, obesity is associated with menstrual irregularities, difficulty in becoming pregnant, and increased complications of pregnancy (e.g., gestational diabetes, higher rates of labor induction and cesarean section, and increased risk of neural tube and other congenital defects in offspring of obese women).
- In men, obesity is associated with infertility.
- In children and adolescents, obesity increases risk of bone fractures and muscle and joint pain. Knee pain is commonly reported, and changes in the knee joint make movement and exercise more difficult.

Clinical Manifestations

Common clinical manifestations that characterize overweight and obesity are increased body weight, excess body fat, and a BMI score of 25 kg/m² or greater. Other physical findings include abnormal levels of lipids and lipoproteins, elevated serum levels of insulin, elevated blood pressure, and respiratory difficulties. These metabolic abnormalities place overweight and obese people at a significantly higher risk for hypertension, heart disease, diabetes, joint problems, and sleep apnea.

Drug Therapy

The National Heart, Lung, and Blood Institute (NHLBI) of the National Institutes of Health and most other organizations generally recommend reserving drug therapy for people with a BMI of 30 or more kg/m² and health problems (e.g., hypertension, dyslipidemia, coronary heart disease, type 2 diabetes, sleep apnea) that are likely to improve with weight loss. These organizations emphasize that drug therapy for obesity should be used as part of a weight management program that also includes a sensible diet, physical activity, and behavioral modification. The NHLBI clinical guidelines focus on the identification, evaluation, and treatment of obesity. These guidelines, outlined in Box 34.4, emphasize that drug therapy should be used to decrease medical risk and improve health rather than promote cosmetic weight loss.

Drug therapy for obesity has a problematic history, mainly because of serious adverse effects and rapid weight regain

EVIDENCE-BASED PRACTICE

Prevalence of Obesity and Trends in the Distribution of Body Mass Index Among US Adults, 1999–2010

by FLEGAL, K. M., CARROLL, M. D., KIT, B. K., & OGDEN, C. L.

Journal of the American Medical Association 2012, 307(5), 491–497.

The national obesity trends in adults from the 2009 to 2010 National Health and Nutrition Examination Survey, a nationally representative sample of the population in the United States, were examined and compared with data from 1999 to 2008. In 2009 to 2010, the age-adjusted mean body mass index was 28.7 for both women and men. No increase in the prevalence of obesity was observed from 2003 to 2008. Stabilization trends in BMI were similar to obesity trends.

IMPLICATIONS FOR NURSING PRACTICE: Although trends in obesity have stabilized, a significant number of people in the United States remain overweight or obese. These people are strong candidates for counseling regarding diet, physical activity, and behavior change.

BOX 34.4 | **National Heart, Lung, and Blood Institute (NHLBI) Report: Clinical Guidelines on the Identification, Evaluation, and Treatment of Overweight and Obesity in Adults**

■ Weight loss reduces health problems. People should decrease blood pressure if they are hypertensive; lower elevated levels of total cholesterol, low-density lipoprotein cholesterol, and triglycerides and raise low levels of high-density lipoprotein cholesterol if they are dyslipidemic; lower elevated blood glucose levels if they have type 2 diabetes.

■ Body mass index is used to assess overweight and obesity and to estimate disease risks. Measure waist circumference initially and periodically to assess abdominal fat content. Weigh regularly to monitor body weight for gain, loss, or maintenance.

■ The initial goal of weight loss therapy should be to reduce body weight by about 10% from baseline, at a rate of 1 to 2 pounds per week for a period of 6 months. Steady weight loss over a longer period reduces fat stores in the body, limits the loss of vital protein tissues, and avoids the sharp decline in metabolic rate that accompanies rapid weight loss. After weight loss, weight maintenance should be the priority goal, because weight regain is a problem with all weight loss programs. In some cases, after a period of weight maintenance, additional losses may be desirable.

■ Dietary recommendations include low-calorie diets for weight loss, mainly reducing caloric intake by 500 to 1000 cal daily. Reducing dietary fat can reduce calories. However, reducing dietary fat without reducing total caloric intake does not produce weight loss. Vitamin and mineral supplements that meet age-related requirements are usually recommended with weight loss programs that provide <1200 kcal for women or 1800 kcal for men.

■ Physical activity recommendations should be part of any weight management program because physical activity contributes to weight loss, may decrease abdominal fat, increases cardiorespiratory fitness, and

helps with weight maintenance. Initially, physical activity for 30 to 45 minutes, 3 to 5 days a week, is encouraged. On long term, adults should try to accumulate at least 30 minutes or more of moderate-intensity physical activity on most days of the week.

■ In general, weight loss and weight maintenance programs should combine reduced-calorie diets, increased physical activity, and behavior therapy. After weight loss, weight loss maintenance with dietary therapy, physical activity, and behavior therapy should be continued indefinitely. Drug therapy can also be used. However, drug safety and efficacy beyond 1 to 2 years of total treatment have not been established.

■ Behavioral modification can be helpful in a weight loss program. The goals are to help patients modify their eating, activity, and thinking habits that predispose to obesity. Techniques include identifying triggers that promote overeating and barriers that keep one from adopting a more healthful lifestyle. One strategy is keeping an accurate record of food/calorie intake and physical activity (most people tend to underestimate food intake and overestimate activity). In addition, stress management, stimulus control, and social support are helpful. Patients who eat more when stressed can learn to manage stress more healthfully. Counseling by a behavioral therapist may be needed. Stimulus control has to do with avoiding or minimizing circumstances that promote overeating (e.g., cooking calorie-dense foods; having high-calorie snacks and "junk food" readily available; eating high-fat, high-calorie foods at fast-food restaurants). Social support involves family, friends, coworkers, and fellow dieters who encourage weight loss efforts rather than sabotage them by urging one to eat high-calorie foods. In general, weight loss regimens that use several of these strategies are more effective.

---

when the drugs were stopped. The U.S. Food and Drug Administration (FDA) took some drugs (fenfluramine, dexfenfluramine, phenylpropanolamine, and sibutramine) and a component of many over-the-counter and herbal weight loss products (ephedra and ma huang) off the market because of their adverse effects. Two classes of weight loss agents, noradrenergic agents and a lipase inhibitor, are currently available by prescription. Of the adrenergic **anorexiant** drugs, only phentermine is commonly used. The lipase inhibitor orlistat is also commonly used and is the only weight loss drug approved for long-term use.

Adrenergic Anorexiants

ⓟ **Phentermine** (Adipex-P, Ionamin, Pro-Fast) is the most frequently prescribed adrenergic anorexiant and is the prototype. This Schedule IV drug is a sympathomimetic amine with pharmacologic activity similar to amphetamines.

Pharmacokinetics

Phentermine is administered orally and is primarily excreted by the kidneys. Under acidic urinary conditions, the half-life is decreased.

Action

Phentermine inhibits the reuptake of both serotonin and norepinephrine. It is an anorexiant, causing appetite suppression, which is thought to result from direct stimulation of the satiety center in the hypothalamic and limbic region.

Use

Phentermine is used to speed weight loss in people who are overweight. The drug is recommended only for short-term use (3 months or less). Combination with a healthy diet and exercise is important. Table 34.1 presents route and dosage information for phentermine.

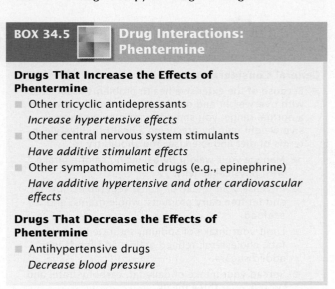

TABLE 34.1 **DRUGS AT A GLANCE: Appetite Suppressants (Phentermine)**		
Drug	**Pregnancy Category**	**Route and Dosage Ranges**
Ⓟ **Phentermine hydrochloride** (Adipex-P, Ionamin, Pro-Fast)	C	8 mg PO 3 times daily, 30 min before meals, or 15–37.5 mg daily in the morning

Limited information is available about the use of phentermine in people with hepatic impairment.

Use in Children

Although phentermine is not recommended in children, pediatric clinicians sometimes suggest treatment for children and adolescents who are overweight or obese and may have complications of obesity.

Use in Older Adults

It is important to use anorexiant drugs very cautiously, if at all in older adults. They often have cardiovascular, renal, or hepatic impairments that increase the risk of adverse drug effects.

Use in Patients With Renal Impairment

Clearance of phentermine may be decreased in patients with renal impairment, resulting in an increased risk of toxicity.

Adverse Effects

The most commonly reported adverse effects with phentermine are nervousness, hyperactivity, dry mouth, constipation, and hypertension. Impotence, insomnia, and unpleasant taste may also occur. Tolerance to the drug usually occurs within 4 to 6 weeks and is an indication for discontinuing drug administration. Continued administration or use of large doses does not maintain appetite-suppressant effects. Instead, it increases the incidence of adverse effects.

QSEN Safety Alert ❗

The nurse should emphasize to patients that phentermine may be habit-forming and should be used only as prescribed. There may be an increased risk of drowsiness, so people who take phentermine should not drive a car or operate heavy machinery until they know how the drug affects them.

Contraindications

Contraindications to phentermine use include moderate to severe hypertension, cardiovascular disease, and a history of drug abuse. Caution is warranted in anxiety or agitation because the drug may have central nervous system (CNS)-stimulating effects.

BOX 34.5   Drug Interactions: Phentermine

Drugs That Increase the Effects of Phentermine
- Other tricyclic antidepressants
  Increase hypertensive effects
- Other central nervous system stimulants
  Have additive stimulant effects
- Other sympathomimetic drugs (e.g., epinephrine)
  Have additive hypertensive and other cardiovascular effects

Drugs That Decrease the Effects of Phentermine
- Antihypertensive drugs
  Decrease blood pressure

Nursing Implications

Preventing Interactions

Several drugs interact with phentermine, increasing or decreasing its effect (Box 34.5). It is important to note that people with diabetes mellitus may require increased doses of insulin while taking phentermine because the drug produces effects similar to those caused by stimulating the sympathetic nervous system.

No herbal interactions have been identified.

Administering the Medication

It is necessary to take phentermine on an empty stomach. Recipients should take single-dose drugs in the early morning; they should take multiple-dose preparations 30 minutes before meals, with the last dose of the day about 6 hours before going to bed.

Assessing for Therapeutic Effects

The nurse assesses for the recommended rate of weight loss (1–2 pounds weekly), minimal adverse effects, and use with a healthy diet and exercise routine.

Assessing for Adverse Effects

The nurse assesses for elevated blood pressure, increased nervousness, hyperactivity, or symptoms of dry mouth or constipation.

Patient Teaching

Box 34.6 lists patient teaching guidelines for drugs used in weight management.

NCLEX Success

1. Phentermine aids weight loss by
   A. decreasing appetite
   B. increasing satiety and feelings of fullness
   C. increasing metabolism
   D. decreasing absorption of dietary fat

BOX 34.6   Patient Teaching Guidelines for Weight Management and Drugs That Aid Weight Loss

General Considerations

■ Because of the extensive health problems associated with overweight and obesity, if your weight is within a normal range, you should try to prevent excessive weight gain by practicing a healthful lifestyle in terms of diet and exercise. You should try to:

■ Manage your weight by balancing calorie intake with physical activity.

■ Increase your intake of fruits, vegetables, low-fat and fat-free dairy products, whole grains, and seafood.

■ Limit your intake of sodium, saturated and trans fats, cholesterol, refined grains, and foods with added sugars.

■ Spread your intake of daily fat, carbohydrate, and protein over three meals.

■ Further recommendations from the Dietary Guidelines for Americans 2010, published by the U.S. Department of Health and Human Services and the Department of Agriculture in January 2011 (updated every 5 years) are available online at http://www.healthierus.gov/dietaryguidelines

Self-Administration

■ Take appetite suppressants in the morning to decrease appetite during the day and avoid interference with sleep at night.

■ Do not crush or chew sustained-release products.

■ With phentermine, monitor your blood pressure. As body weight decreases, blood pressure usually decreases.

■ With orlistat (Xenical, Alli):

■ Take one capsule with each main meal or up to 1 hour after a meal, up to three capsules daily. If you miss a meal or eat a meal with no fat, you may omit a dose of orlistat.

■ Take a multivitamin containing fat-soluble vitamins (A, D, E, and K) daily, at least 2 hours before or after taking orlistat. Orlistat prevents absorption of fat-soluble vitamins from food or multivitamin preparations if taken at the same time.

■ Take the drug with a full glass of water.

2. Mr. Johnson, a 42-year-old architect, is more than 40 pounds overweight, and he has a 14-year history of type 1 diabetes mellitus. He is placed on phentermine and has been taking it for the last 8 weeks. His latest glycosylated (A_{1c}) hemoglobin concentrations have risen to 9% despite that he has maintained a healthy diet and routine exercise program. Phentermine may cause an elevation of A_{1c} levels by:

A. producing stimulant effects to the sympathetic nervous system
B. decreasing the level of fat-soluble vitamins
C. decreasing metabolism to the pancreas
D. increasing the absorption of dietary fat

Lipase Inhibitors

ⓟ **Orlistat** (Xenical, Alli) is the prototype of a new class of antiobesity agents, the lipase inhibitors. Decreased fat absorption leads to decreased caloric intake, resulting in weight loss and improved serum cholesterol values (e.g., decreased total and low-density lipoprotein [LDL] cholesterol levels). The improvement in cholesterol levels is thought to be independent of weight loss effects.

Pharmacokinetics

Orlistat is not absorbed systemically; it works in the gastrointestinal (GI) tract. The primary metabolite has a half-life of 3 hours; a second metabolite has a half-life of 13.5 hours. Nearly the entire drug is excreted in feces, 83% as unchanged drug.

Action

Orlistat binds to gastric and pancreatic lipases in the GI tract, and it can prevent the absorption of 30% of ingested fat. Triglycerides, cholesterol, and fat-soluble vitamins from fat-containing foods pass through the intestines unchanged and are not absorbed. Increasing the dose does not increase the percentage.

Use

Orlistat is intended for people who are clinically obese, not for those who want to lose a few pounds. In addition, it is still necessary to decrease consumption of high-fat foods because total caloric intake is a major determinant of weight, and adverse effects (e.g., diarrhea; fatty, malodorous stools) worsen with consumption of a large amount of fat.

The effects of long-term orlistat use are unknown. In addition to weight loss and reduced cholesterol levels, clinical trials found that orlistat results in reduced severity and improved management of other health problems associated with obesity, such as diabetes and hypertension. In general, studies have shown that the addition of orlistat therapy to diet and other lifestyle changes produces greater weight loss than addition of a placebo. In some patients with impaired glucose tolerance, weight loss with orlistat and lifestyle changes prevents or delays the occurrence of diabetes mellitus. After the medication is stopped, most patients regain weight.

Table 34.2 presents route and dosage information for orlistat.

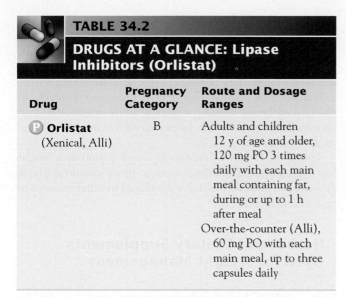

TABLE 34.2

DRUGS AT A GLANCE: Lipase Inhibitors (Orlistat)

Drug	Pregnancy Category	Route and Dosage Ranges
Ⓟ Orlistat (Xenical, Alli)	B	Adults and children 12 y of age and older, 120 mg PO 3 times daily with each main meal containing fat, during or up to 1 h after meal Over-the-counter (Alli), 60 mg PO with each main meal, up to three capsules daily

Use in Children

As previously discussed, encouraging weight control measures coupled with family involvement and support are vital to weight management in children. Methods that result in weight loss include leading a more active lifestyle, eating a low-fat diet with regular meals, avoiding high-calorie snacks, drinking water instead of calorie-containing beverages, and decreasing time spent watching television and playing computer games). Although experts do not generally recommend drug therapy for treatment of childhood obesity, the FDA has approved orlistat for use in children aged 12 and older and considers the drug to

EVIDENCE-BASED PRACTICE

Long-term Pharmacotherapy for Obesity and Overweight

by PADWAL, R., LI, S.K., & LAU, D.C.

Cochrane Database of Systematic Reviews 2007, 4, CD004094

In 11 randomized controlled trials of orlistat, overweight and obese people who took orlistat had a mean weight loss of 2.9 kg (2.9%) more than those who took placebo. In people with diabetes, in addition to improvements in total cholesterol, low-density lipoprotein cholesterol, and high-density lipoprotein cholesterol concentrations, orlistat significantly reduced the blood pressure, fasting glucose, glycosylated (A_{1c}) hemoglobin concentrations, body mass index, and waist circumference (compared with placebo).

IMPLICATIONS FOR NURSING PRACTICE: The benefits of losing weight include improvement in lipid profiles, glucose control, and blood pressure management.

be safe and effective for weight reduction in overweight adolescents (see Table 34.2).

Use in Older Adults

Little information is available about the use of orlistat in people with renal or hepatic impairment. Manufacturer recommendations advise conservative use and lower dosages, because older adults often have decreased renal, cardiac, and hepatic function.

Adverse Effects

The main adverse effects are GI symptoms: abdominal pain, oily spotting, fecal urgency and incontinence, flatulence with discharge, fatty stools, and increased defecation. These effects occur in almost all orlistat users but usually subside after a few weeks of continued drug usage with moderation of fat intake.

Contraindications

Contraindications to orlistat include known allergy to the drug and chronic malabsorption syndrome or cholestasis.

Nursing Implications

Preventing Interactions

The body does not absorb orlistat, and no reported drug interactions affecting its action have occurred. However, orlistat may slight reduce plasma concentrations of amiodarone. By partially inhibiting the absorption of dietary fat, the weight management drug may also decrease the plasma concentration of cyclosporine, which is highly lipid-soluble; patients should take orlistat and cyclosporine 2 hours apart. Concomitant use of orlistat may increase the lipid-lowering effects of pravastatin.

In addition, orlistat may reduce absorption of fat-soluble vitamins.

QSEN Safety Alert

This has implications for monitoring coagulation parameters if orlistat is use in conjunction with warfarin. The liver uses vitamin K to make blood clotting proteins; therefore, a decreased in vitamin K increases the international normalized ratio and make it more difficult to manage warfarin therapy.

Administering the Medication

It is necessary to take orlistat three times a day with meals. Because the drug prevents absorption of the fat-soluble vitamins A, D, E, and K, people who take it should also take a multivitamin daily 2 hours before or after orlistat.

Assessing for Therapeutic Effects

The nurse monitors weight loss and BMI. Most weight loss occurs in the first 6 months of therapy, but as patients continue to take orlistat, they can maintain the weight reduction. The metabolic improvements of weight loss are very beneficial for people with obesity-related health problems such as diabetes, dyslipidemia, hypertension, and metabolic syndrome.

Assessing for Adverse Effects

The nurse assesses signs of common adverse GI effects (e.g., diarrhea, flatulence) and reduced concentrations of fat-soluble vitamins. To minimize GI effects, the nurse encourages patients to distribute fat calories over the three main meals and to avoid high-fat meals.

Patient Teaching

Box 34.6 presents patient teaching guidelines for orlistat and other drugs used in weight management.

NCLEX Success

3. Orlistat (Xenical) aids weight loss by

   A. decreasing appetite
   B. increasing satiety and feelings of fullness
   C. increasing metabolism
   D. decreasing absorption of dietary fat

4. **To decrease diarrhea with orlistat (Xenical), it is important to instruct a patient to**

   A. avoid large amounts of fatty foods
   B. drink eight glasses of water daily
   C. avoid caffeine-containing beverages
   D. increase physical activity

Clinical Application 34-1

- In addition to proper administration of her medication, what strategies does the nurse review with Ms. Vargas to assist her in being successful with weight loss?
- Ms. Vargas says she needs to lose 140 pounds and would like to accomplish this by her next birthday. How does the nurse respond?

Other Drugs Used for Weight Management

Other drugs used for weight management include amphetamines and similar drugs. Experts do not recommend using amphetamines (see Chap. 56) because they are controlled substances (Schedule II), with a high potential for abuse and dependence. Amphetamines can cause a life-threatening complication in patients who take antidepressants in the form of monoamine oxidase inhibitors (i.e., isocarboxazid, phenelzine). Phentermine as well as benzphetamine, diethylpropion, and phendimetrazine are adrenergic drugs (see Chap. 27) that stimulate the release of norepinephrine and dopamine in the brain. This action in nerve terminals of the hypothalamic feeding center suppresses appetite. These anorexiants are CNS and cardiovascular stimulants and are contraindicated in

cardiovascular disease, hyperthyroidism, glaucoma, and agitated states.

Until recently, health care providers used sibutramine, a drug that suppresses appetite by inhibiting the reuptake of the neurotransmitters norepinephrine and serotonin, in the management of obesity. The drug is no longer available in the United States because a clinical study demonstrated an increased risk of cardiovascular events such as heart attack and stroke with its use.

Lastly, metformin is undergoing investigation as a weight loss drug in obese adolescents, both in those who do not have diabetes and in those who have developed insulin resistance or type 2 diabetes mellitus.

Herbal and Dietary Supplements Used for Weight Management

Many people use herbal or dietary supplements for weight loss, even though reliable evidence of safety and effectiveness is lacking. Some herbal products claim to decrease appetite and increase the rate at which the body burns calories. However, in most cases, there is no scientific evidence that they work at all. Some supplements for weight loss contain cardiovascular and CNS stimulants that may cause serious, even life-threatening, adverse effects. In general, many consumers do not seem to appreciate the benefits of proven weight management techniques (e.g., appropriate diet and exercise) or the potential risks of taking unproven weight loss products. Box 34.7 contains more information about these herbal and dietary supplements.

Clinical Application 34-2

- Ms. Vargas wants to know how orlistat will help her when nothing else in the past has been successful. How does the nurse respond?

The Nursing Process

Assessment

- Assess usual drinking and eating patterns, including healthful (e.g., whole-grain breads and cereals, fruits, vegetables, low-fat dairy products) and unhealthful (e.g., sugar-containing beverages and desserts, fried foods, saturated fat, fast foods, high-calorie snack foods) intake. The best way is to ask the patient to keep a food diary for 2 or 3 days. If food intake is not written down, people tend to underestimate the amount and caloric content. (If available, consult a nutritionist to assess a patient's diet and work with the patient to improve health and weight status.)
- Assess any obviously overweight patient for health problems caused or aggravated by excessive weight (e.g., elevated blood pressure, other cardiovascular problems, diabetes mellitus, sleep apnea, osteoarthritis, and other musculoskeletal disorders).

BOX 34.7 Selected Herbal and Dietary Supplements Used in Weight Management

■ Glucomannan expands on contact with body fluids. It is included in weight loss regimens because of its supposed ability to produce feelings of stomach fullness, thereby causing a person to eat less. It also has a laxative effect. There is little evidence to support its use as a weight loss aid. People with diabetes should not use products containing glucomannan; it may cause hypoglycemia alone and increases hypoglycemic effects of antidiabetic medications.

■ Guarana, a major source of commercial caffeine, is a component of weight loss products as well as caffeine-containing soft drinks, "energy" drinks, bodybuilding supplements, smoking-cessation products, vitamin supplements, candies, and chewing gums. Caffeine is the active ingredient; the amount varies among products, and it is not possible to determine the caffeine content of any particular product accurately. Advertisers promote guarana as a substance that decreases appetite and increases energy and mental alertness. Dysrhythmias contraindicate its use. It may aggravate gastroesophageal reflux disease and peptic ulcer disease.

Adverse effects include diuresis, cardiovascular symptoms (premature ventricular contractions, tachycardia), central nervous system (CNS) symptoms (agitation, anxiety, insomnia, seizures, tremors), and GI symptoms (nausea, vomiting, diarrhea). Such effects are more likely to occur with higher doses or concomitant use of guarana and other sources of caffeine. Adverse drug–drug interactions include additive CNS and cardiovascular stimulation with beta-adrenergic agonists (e.g., epinephrine, albuterol and related drugs, pseudoephedrine) and theophylline. In addition, concurrent use of cimetidine, fluoroquinolones, or oral contraceptives may increase or prolong serum caffeine levels and subsequent adverse effects.

■ Guar gum is a dietary fiber included in weight loss products because it is bulk forming and produces feelings of fullness. Several small studies have indicated that it is no more effective than placebo for weight loss. It may cause esophageal or intestinal obstruction if not taken with an adequate amount of water and may interfere with the absorption of other drugs if taken at the same time. Adverse effects include nausea, diarrhea, flatulence, and abdominal discomfort.

■ Hydroxycitric acid (in Citrimax and other supplements) apparently suppresses appetite in animals, but there are no reliable studies that indicate its effectiveness in humans. One 12-week study did not show weight loss.

■ Laxative and diuretic herbs (e.g., aloe, rhubarb root, buckthorn, cascara, senna, parsley, juniper, dandelion leaves) are found in several commercial products. These products cause a significant loss of body fluids and electrolytes, not fat. Adverse effects may include low serum potassium levels, with subsequent cardiac dysrhythmias and other heart problems. In addition, long-term use of laxatives may lead to loss of normal bowel function and the necessity for continued use (i.e., laxative dependency).

- Calculate the BMI (see Box 34.1) and measure waist circumference.
- Check available reports of laboratory tests. Overweight patients may have abnormally high values for total and LDL cholesterol, triglycerides, and blood sugar and low values for high-density lipoprotein (HDL) cholesterol. If no laboratory reports are available, ask patients if a health care provider has ever told them they have high cholesterol or blood sugar.
- List all prescription and nonprescription medications the patient is taking and ask about vitamins, herbals, and other dietary supplements. Review the list for drugs used to treat health problems associated with obesity, drugs that may promote weight gain, and any products that may be used to promote weight loss.
- Assess usual patterns of physical activity and exercise, including work and recreational activities.
- Assess motivation to develop and adhere to a weight management plan. Ask if there are concerns about weight; if there is interest in a weight management program to improve health; and what methods, over-the-counter products, or herbal or dietary supplements have been previously used to reduce weight, if any. The nurse must be very tactful in eliciting information and assessing whether a patient would like assistance with weight management. If the nurse–patient contact stems from a health problem caused or aggravated by excessive weight, the nurse may use this information to help motivate the patient to lose weight and improve health.

Nursing Diagnoses

- Imbalanced nutrition: more than body requirements related to excessive caloric intake
- Disturbed body image related to excessive weight
- Potential activity intolerance related to excessive weight
- Deficient knowledge: weight management

Planning/Goals

The patient will

- Reduce the impact of excessive weight on chronic health problems
- Modify lifestyle behaviors toward weight loss and weight maintenance at a more healthful level
- Avoid overuse of weight loss drugs
- Avoid unproven weight loss dietary supplements

Nursing Interventions

The nurse will

- Support programs/efforts to help promote a healthful lifestyle and prevent obesity (e.g., in families and schools).
- Serve as a role model by maintaining a healthful lifestyle and weight.
- Serve as a reliable source of information about weight loss and weight loss products and programs.
- For an obese patient who reports interest and motivation in losing weight, assist to formulate realistic goals.

Patients often expect to rapidly lose large amounts of weight with little or no effort. Most treatment programs result in a weight loss of 10% of body weight or less.

- Discuss health risks of obesity and anticipated benefits of achieving and maintaining a healthier weight. Emphasize that losing 5% to 10% of body weight is a reasonable goal and can significantly reduce the medical problems associated with being overweight.
- Assist patients to identify factors that support weight loss efforts (e.g., family and friend encouragement) and factors that sabotage weight loss efforts (e.g., having high-calorie foods readily available, frequently eating at fast-food restaurants).
- Promote exercise and activity. For overweight and obese patients, exercise may decrease appetite and distract from eating behaviors as well as increase calorie expenditure. For very sedentary, physically unfit patients, emphasize that any exercise can be beneficial and to start slowly, increasing the amount and intensity as physical condition improves.
- Encourage any efforts toward improving diet and increasing exercise to improve health.
- Weigh patients at regular intervals and measure waist circumference periodically.
- Refer patients to a dietitian or nutritionist as indicated.
- Be alert for the psychological consequences of obesity and refer patients for counseling if indicated.
- Refer overweight and obese children to pediatric obesity specialists when possible.
- Provide appropriate teaching related to drug therapy (see Box 34.6)

Evaluation

- Observe overweight or obese patients for food intake, weight loss, decreased waist circumference, and appropriate use of exercise and weight loss drugs.

NCLEX Success

5. **In counseling a patient about weight loss diets, the nurse knows that a recommended low-calorie or reduced-calorie diet**

   A. provides about 500 to 800 kcal/d
   B. reduces daily intake to about 1800 kcal/d
   C. is required for weight loss
   D. focuses on high-fat, high-carbohydrate foods

6. **Drug therapy for weight management may be prescribed for patients with which of the following?**

   A. A BMI of 22 kg/m^2 and a desire to lose 10 pounds
   B. A BMI of 24.5 kg/m^2 and physically fit
   C. A BMI of 30 kg/m^2 or more with weight-related health problems
   D. A BMI of 25 to 29 kg/m^2 and healthy

Clinical Application 34-3

- Ms. Vargas' prescription is for orlistat three times a day. She takes the dose with breakfast, lunch, and dinner. She often has a meeting that runs through lunch so she skips lunch but takes her pill on time. At her next clinic appointment, she discusses this with the nurse. How does the nurse respond?

Key Concepts

- Being overweight and obese are major concerns because of their association with numerous health problems, including diabetes, hypertension, other cardiovascular disorders, and muscle and joint disorders.
- Ingesting 500 cal more per day than those used in exercise and physical activity leads to a weight gain of 1 pound in 1 week; decreasing caloric intake or increasing caloric output of 500 cal/d for 1 week leads to a weight loss of 1 pound.
- Weight loss drugs are generally recommended only for people who are seriously overweight or have health problems associated with or aggravated by obesity.
- Many people lose weight but regain it within a few months if they do not change their lifestyle habits toward eating more healthfully and exercising more.
- Two classes of weight loss agents, noradrenergic agents (for short-term use) and a lipase inhibitor (for long-term use), are currently available by prescription.
- Orlistat prevents absorption of the fat-soluble vitamins, A, D, E, and K, so people taking the drug should also take a multivitamin containing these vitamins daily.

Critical Thinking Questions

34-1. Mrs. Williams, a 45-year-old high school teacher, is a patient in the clinic at which a nurse works. She has requested assistance in losing weight. This woman is 5 ft 7 inches tall and weighs 254 pounds. She has had a lifelong battle with her weight, and nothing she has tried has been successful.

• How does the nurse calculate Mrs. Williams' BMI?

• Given Mrs. Williams' BMI, does the nurse consider her clinically obese?

• What are some nursing interventions to assist and support Mrs. Williams to lose weight?

References and Resources

Baron, R. B. (2007). Nutrition. In: S. J. McPhee, M. A. Papadakis, & L. M. Tierney, Jr. (Eds.), *Current medical diagnosis and treatment 2007* (46th ed., pp. 1279–1310). New York: McGraw-Hill.

Daniels, J. (2006). Obesity: America's epidemic. *American Journal of Nursing, 106,* 40–49.

Dunican, K. C., Desilets, A. R., & Montalbano, J. K. (2007). Pharmacotherapeutic options for overweight adolescents. *Annals of Pharmacotherapy, 41,* 1445–1455.

Expert Panel (1998). Clinical guidelines on the identification, evaluation, and treatment of overweight and obesity in adults: Executive summary. *American Journal of Clinical Nutrition, 68,* 899–917.

Flegal, K. M., Carroll, M. D., Kit, B. K. & Ogden, C. L. (2012). Prevalence of obesity and trends in the distribution of body mass index among US adults, 1999–2010. *Journal of the American Medical Association, 307*(5), 491–497.

Kaplan, L. M. (2010). Pharmacologic therapies for obesity. *Gastroenterology Clinics of North America, 39,* 69–79.

Karch, A. M. (2012). *2012 Lippincott's nursing drug guide.* Philadelphia, PA: Lippincott Williams & Wilkins.

Lacy, C. F., Armstrong, L. L., Goldman, M. P., & Lance, L. L. (2010). *Lexi-Comp's drug information handbook* (19th ed.). Hudson, OH: American Pharmaceutical Association.

Padwal, R., Li, S. K., & Lau, D. C. (2007). Long-term pharmacotherapy for obesity and overweight. *Cochrane Database Systematic Review,* 4:CD004094.

Porth, C. M. (2009). *Pathophysiology: Concepts of altered health status* (8th ed.). Philadelphia, PA: Lippincott Williams & Wilkins.

Robinson, J. R., & Niswender, K. D. (2009). What are the risks and the benefits of current and emerging weight-loss medications? *Current Diabetes Reports, 9,* 368–375.

Rosenbaum, M. (2007). Epidemiology of pediatric obesity. *Pediatric Annals, 36,* 89–94.

Small, L., Anderson, D., & Melnyk, B. M. (2007). Prevention and early treatment of overweight and obesity in young children: A critical review and appraisal of the evidence. *Pediatric Nursing, 33,* 149–161.

Smeltzer, S. C., Bare, B. G., Hinkle, J. L., & Cheever, K. H. (2008). *Brunner & Suddarth's textbook of medical-surgical nursing* (11th ed.). Philadelphia, PA: Lippincott Williams & Wilkins.

35

Drug Therapy for Peptic Ulcer Disease and Gastroesophageal Reflux Disease

LEARNING OBJECTIVES

After studying this chapter, you should be able to:

1. Describe the main elements of peptic ulcer disease and gastroesophageal reflux disease.

2. Discuss antacids in terms of the prototype, indications and contraindications for use, routes of administration, and major adverse effects.

3. Describe histamine$_2$ receptor antagonists in terms of the prototype, indications and contraindications for use, routes of administration, and major adverse effects.

4. Discuss proton pump inhibitors in terms of the prototype, indications and contraindications for use, routes of administration, and major adverse effects.

5. Identify the adjuvant medications used to treat peptic ulcer and gastroesophageal reflux disease.

6. Understand how to use the nursing process in the care of patients receiving antacids, proton pump inhibitors, and histamine$_2$ receptor antagonists.

Clinical Application Case Study

Kathleen Daniels, a 54-year-old woman, has chronic gastroesophageal reflux disease. She takes omeprazole (Prilosec) 20 mg orally daily, as prescribed. She also takes two over-the-counter medications: famotidine (Pepcid) 10 mg twice a day as needed, to control her heartburn, and a combination antacid (Mylanta) 5 mL per dose.

KEY TERMS

Achlorhydria: low or absent production of gastric acid in the stomach

Cardia: the part of the stomach that attaches to the esophagus

Esophagitis: inflammation of the esophagus

Gastritis: acute or chronic inflammation of the gastric mucosa

Helicobacter pylori: gram-negative bacterium found in the gastric mucosa of most patients with chronic gastritis.

Hydrogen, potassium adenosine triphosphatase: enzyme system that catalyzes the production of gastric acid and acts as a gastric acid pump to move gastric acid from parietal cells in the mucosal lining of the stomach into the stomach lumen

Pepsin: proteolytic enzyme that helps digests protein foods

Pyrosis: heartburn

Stress ulcers: gastric mucosal lesions that develop in patients who are critically ill from trauma, shock, hemorrhage, sepsis, burns, acute respiratory distress syndrome, major surgical procedures, or other severe illnesses.

Introduction

Drugs to prevent or treat peptic ulcer and acid reflux disorders consist of several groups of drugs, most of which alter gastric acid and its effects on the mucosa of the upper gastrointestinal (GI) tract. To aid understanding of drug effects, this chapter presents an overview of both peptic ulcer disease and gastroesophageal reflux disease (GERD) before providing details about specific drugs. Box 35.1 gives further descriptions of selected upper GI disorders.

Overview of Peptic Ulcer Disease and Gastroesophageal Reflux Disease

Etiology and Pathophysiology

Peptic Ulcer Disease

Peptic ulcer disease is characterized by ulcer formation in the esophagus, stomach, or duodenum—areas of the GI mucosa that are exposed to gastric acid and pepsin. Gastric and duodenal ulcers are more common than esophageal ulcers. Infection with *Helicobacter pylori* and use of nonsteroidal anti-inflammatory drugs (NSAIDs) account for most cases of peptic ulcer disease. *H. pylori* is a gram-negative bacterium found in the gastric mucosa of most patients with chronic **gastritis** (inflammation of the gastric mucosa), about 75% of patients with gastric ulcers, and more than 90% of patients with duodenal ulcers. The World Health Organization reports that *H. pylori* is also present in 50% of all new cases of gastric cancer cases. This bacterium is spread mainly by the fecal–oral route. However, iatrogenic spread by contaminated endoscopes, biopsy forceps, and nasogastric tubes has also occurred.

In addition, stress (e.g., major trauma, severe medical illness) can precipitate ulcer formation. Gastric ulcers are more likely to occur in older adults, especially in the sixth and seventh decades, and to be chronic in nature. Duodenal ulcers are strongly associated with *H. pylori* infection and NSAID ingestion, may occur at any age, occur about equally in men and women, are often manifested by abdominal pain, and are usually chronic in nature. They are also associated with cigarette smoking. Compared with nonsmokers, smokers are more likely to develop duodenal ulcers, their ulcers heal more slowly with treatment, and the ulcers recur more rapidly.

Peptic ulcers seem to result from an imbalance between cell-destructive and cell-protective effects (i.e., presence of increased destructive mechanisms or presence of decreased protective mechanisms). Cell-destructive effects include those of gastric acid (hydrochloric acid), pepsin, *H. pylori* infection, and NSAID ingestion. Gastric acid, a strong acid that can digest the stomach wall, is secreted by parietal cells in the mucosa of the stomach antrum, near the pylorus. The parietal cells contain receptors for acetylcholine, gastrin, and histamine, substances that stimulate gastric acid production. Acetylcholine is released by vagus nerve endings in response to stimuli, such as thinking about or ingesting food. Gastrin is a hormone released by cells in the stomach and duodenum in response to food ingestion and stretching of the stomach wall. It is secreted into the bloodstream and eventually circulated to the parietal cells. Histamine is released from cells in the gastric mucosa and diffuses into nearby parietal cells. The enzyme system **hydrogen, potassium adenosine triphosphatase** (H^+, K^+-ATPase) catalyzes the production of gastric acid and acts as a gastric acid (proton) pump to move gastric acid from parietal cells in the mucosal lining of the stomach into the stomach lumen.

Pepsin, a proteolytic enzyme, helps digest protein foods and also can digest the stomach wall. Pepsin is derived from a precursor called pepsinogen, which is secreted by chief cells in the gastric mucosa. Pepsinogen is converted to pepsin only in a highly acidic environment (i.e., when the pH of gastric juices is 3 or less).

After *H. pylori* moves into the body, the bacterium colonizes the mucus-secreting epithelial cells of the stomach mucosa and is thought to produce gastritis and ulceration by impairing mucosal function. Eradication of the microorganism accelerates ulcer healing and significantly decreases the rate of ulcer recurrence.

Cell-protective effects (e.g., secretion of mucus and bicarbonate, dilution of gastric acid by food and secretions, prevention of diffusion of hydrochloric acid from the stomach lumen back into the gastric mucosal lining, the presence of prostaglandin E, alkalinization of gastric secretions by pancreatic juices and bile, perhaps other mechanisms) normally prevent autodigestion of stomach and duodenal tissues and ulcer formation.

A gastric or duodenal ulcer may penetrate only the mucosal surface or it may extend into the smooth muscle layers. When superficial lesions heal, no defects remain. When smooth muscle heals, however, scar tissue remains and the mucosa that regenerates to cover the scarred muscle tissue may be defective. These defects contribute to repeated episodes of ulceration.

Gastroesophageal Reflux Disease

GERD, the most common disorder of the esophagus, is a chronic digestive disease that occurs when stomach acid or, occasionally, bile refluxes into the esophagus. The backwash of acid irritates the lining of the esophagus. The main cause of GERD is thought to be an incompetent lower esophageal sphincter (LES). Normally, the LES is contracted or closed and prevents the reflux of gastric contents. It opens or relaxes on swallowing to allow passage of food or fluid, then contracts again. Several

Gastritis

Gastritis, a common disorder, is an acute or chronic inflammatory reaction of gastric mucosa. Patients with gastric or duodenal ulcers usually also have gastritis. Acute gastritis (also called gastropathy) usually results from irritation of the gastric mucosa by such substances as alcohol, aspirin or other nonsteroidal anti-inflammatory drugs (NSAIDs), and others. Chronic gastritis is usually caused by *Helicobacter pylori* infection and it persists unless the infection is treated effectively. *H. pylori* organisms may cause gastritis and ulceration by producing enzymes (e.g., urease, others) that break down mucosa; they also alter secretion of gastric acid.

Nonsteroidal Anti-Inflammatory Drug Gastropathy

NSAID gastropathy indicates damage to gastroduodenal mucosa by aspirin and other NSAIDs. The damage may range from minor superficial erosions to ulceration and bleeding. NSAID gastropathy is one of the most common causes of gastric ulcers, and it may cause duodenal ulcers as well. Many people take NSAIDs daily for pain, arthritis, and other conditions. Chronic ingestion of NSAIDs causes local irritation of gastroduodenal mucosa, inhibits the synthesis of prostaglandins (which normally protect gastric mucosa by inhibiting acid secretion, stimulating secretion of bicarbonate and mucus, and maintaining mucosal blood flow), and increases the synthesis of leukotrienes and possibly other inflammatory substances that may contribute to mucosal injury.

Stress Ulcers

Stress ulcers indicate gastric mucosal lesions that develop in patients who are critically ill from trauma, shock, hemorrhage, sepsis, burns, acute respiratory distress syndrome, major surgical procedures, or other severe illnesses. The lesions may be single or multiple ulcers or erosions. Stress ulcers are usually manifested by painless upper gastrointestinal (GI) bleeding. The frequency of occurrence has decreased, possibly because of improved management of sepsis, hypovolemia, and other disorders associated with critical illness and the prophylactic use of antiulcer drags. However, there is concern about inappropriate use of stress ulcer prophylaxis.

Although the exact mechanisms of stress ulcer formation are unknown, several factors are thought to play a role, including mucosal ischemia, reflux of bile salts into the stomach, reduced GI-tract motility, and systemic acidosis. Acidosis increases severity of lesions, and correction of acidosis decreases their formation. In addition, lesions do not form if the pH of gastric fluids is kept at about 3.5 or above and lesions apparently form only when mucosal blood flow is diminished.

Zollinger-Ellison Syndrome

Zollinger-Ellison syndrome is a rare condition characterized by excessive secretion of gastric acid and a high incidence of ulcers. It is caused by gastrin-secreting tumors in the pancreas, stomach, or duodenum. Approximately two thirds of the gastrinomas are malignant. Symptoms are those of peptic ulcer disease, and diagnosis is based on high levels of serum gastrin and gastric acid. Treatment may involve long-term use of a proton pump inhibitor to diminish gastric acid or surgical excision.

---

circumstances contribute to impaired contraction of the LES and the resulting reflux, including foods (e.g., fats, chocolate), fluids (e.g., alcohol, caffeinated beverages), medications (e.g., beta adrenergics, calcium channel blockers, nitrates), gastric distention, cigarette smoking, and recumbent posture. GERD occurs in men, women, and children but is especially common during pregnancy and after 40 years of age.

The part of the stomach that connects to the esophagus is called the **cardia**. In healthy patients, the esophagus enters the stomach at an angle, forming a valve that prevents gastric contents from traveling back into the esophagus. In patients with GERD, pathophysiologic effects and symptoms result from failure of the cardia. Additionally, *H. pylori* infection is present in nearly half of all patients with GERD.

GERD is characterized by regurgitation of duodenal bile, enzymes, and stomach acid into the esophagus and exposure of esophageal mucosa to gastric acid and pepsin. The same amount of acid–pepsin exposure may lead to different amounts of mucosal damage, possibly related to individual variations in esophageal mucosal resistance.

Clinical Manifestations

Peptic Ulcer Disease

The clinical manifestations of a gastric ulcer are almost opposite to the clinical manifestations of duodenal ulcers; the main differences are the timing and severity of the pain.

Gastric ulcers generally cause a dull aching pain, often right after eating. The intake of food does not relieve pain as is the case with a duodenal ulcer. The patient may experience bloating, indigestion, heartburn, or nausea. Gastric ulcers are often manifested by painless bleeding and take longer to heal than duodenal ulcers. Duodenal ulcers cause heartburn, bloating, severe stomach pain, and a burning sensation at the back of the throat. The symptoms may be worse when the stomach is empty and may flare at night. Typically the symptoms disappear and then return for a period of time.

Gastroesophageal Reflux Disease

Pyrosis (heartburn), which increases with a recumbent position or bending over, is the main symptom of GERD. Effortless regurgitation of acidic fluid into the mouth, especially after a meal and at night, is often indicative. Important protective mechanisms for the esophagus, including gravity, swallowing, and saliva, are effective only when people are upright. At night during sleep in a recumbent position, the effect of gravity is negated, swallowing ceases, and the secretion of saliva is decreased. Consequently, reflux that occurs at night probably results in acid staying in the esophagus longer and causing greater damage. Many people experience both pyrosis and acid reflux from time to time. When they occur regularly, they may be signs of GERD. In addition, there may also be mild to severe **esophagitis** (inflammation of the esophagus) or esophageal ulceration. Pain on swallowing usually means erosive or ulcerative esophagitis.

TABLE 35.1		
Drugs Administered for the Treatment of Peptic Ulcer Disease and Gastroesophageal Reflux Disease		
Drug Class	**Prototype(s)**	**Other Drugs in the Class**
Antacids	Mylanta Mylanta double strength	Amphojel Gelusil Maalox suspension Titralac, Tums
Histamine$_2$ Receptor Antagonists	Cimetidine (Tagamet)	Famotidine (Pepcid, Pepcid RPD) Famotidine 10 mg, calcium carbonate 800 mg, and magnesium hydroxide 165 mg (Pepcid Complete) Nizatidine (Axid) Ranitidine (Zantac)
Proton Pump Inhibitors	Omeprazole (Prilosec, Prilosec OTC)	Esomeprazole (Nexium, Nexium IV, Nexium delayed-release capsules) Lansoprazole (Prevacid, Prevacid IV) Pantoprazole (Protonix, Protonix IV) Rabeprazole (AcipHex)
Adjuvant Medications		Amoxicillin Amoxicillin, clarithromycin, and lansoprazole (Prevpac) Bismuth subsalicylate Bismuth subcitrate potassium, metronidazole, and tetracycline (Pylera) Bismuth subsalicylate, metronidazole, and tetracycline (Helidac) Clarithromycin Metronidazole Misoprostol (Cytotec) Sucralfate (Carafate) Tetracycline

Drug Therapy

Drugs used in the treatment of acid–peptic disorders promote healing of lesions and prevent recurrence of lesions by decreasing cell-destructive effects or increasing cell-protective effects. Several types of drugs are used, alone and in various combinations. Antacids neutralize gastric acid and decrease pepsin production, antimicrobials and bismuth can eliminate *H. pylori* infection, histamine$_2$ receptor antagonists (H$_2$RAs) and proton pump inhibitors (PPIs) decrease gastric acid secretion, sucralfate provides a barrier between mucosal erosions or ulcers and gastric secretions, and misoprostol restores prostaglandin activity. The following sections describe the types of drugs and individual agents. Table 35.1 lists the drugs used for peptic ulcer disease and GERD.

Available drugs are safe and effective.

QSEN Safety Alert ❗

Taking herbal supplements may delay drug treatment and have harmful consequences; therefore, it is important that nurses and other health care providers do not encourage the use of herbs for any acid–peptic disorder.

Antacids

People commonly take over-the-counter (OTC) antacids to offset the effects of GI acids. These drugs differ in their ability to neutralize gastric acid (50–80 mEq of acid is produced hourly), in onset of action, and in adverse effects. Commonly used antacids are mixtures of aluminum hydroxide and magnesium hydroxide, as well as other ingredients. The aluminum hydroxide–magnesium hydroxide–simethicone mixture Ⓟ **Mylanta** is the prototype. (In this discussion, the trade name of the drug is used to refer to this antacid.)

Some antacids contain calcium compounds. It is important to note that calcium compounds may cause hypercalcemia and hypersecretion of gastric acid ("acid rebound") due to stimulation of gastrin release, if large doses are used. Consequently, calcium compounds are rarely used in peptic ulcer disease.

Pharmacokinetics and Action

Absorption of Mylanta from the GI tract is minimal. Excretion is in the urine.

As an alkaline substance that neutralizes acids, Mylanta reacts with hydrochloric acid in the stomach to produce neutral, less acidic, or poorly absorbed salts and to raise the pH of gastric secretions. Raising the pH to approximately 3.5 neutralizes more than 90% of gastric acid and inhibits conversion of pepsinogen to pepsin. The antacid has an onset of action of 20 to 60 minutes. In general, aluminum compounds have a low neutralizing capacity (i.e., relatively large doses are required) and a slow onset of action. Magnesium-based antacids have a high neutralizing capacity and a rapid onset of action.

Simethicone, an antiflatulent drug, does not affect gastric acidity. It reportedly decreases gas bubbles, thereby reducing GI distention and abdominal discomfort.

Use

Antacids act primarily in the stomach, and people take them to prevent or treat peptic ulcer disease, GERD, esophagitis, heartburn, gastritis, GI bleeding, and stress ulcers. When pain relief is the goal of treatment, taking them on an as-needed basis is usually sufficient. However, it is important not to take them in high doses or for prolonged periods because of potential adverse effects. Table 35.2 gives route and dosage information for various antacids.

Use in Children

Ambulatory children may take Mylanta and the other antacids in doses of 5 to 15 mL every 3 to 6 hours, or after meals, and at bedtime. For prevention of GI bleeding in critically ill children, infants may receive 2 to 5 mL and children may receive 5 to 15 mL every 1 to 2 hours.

Use in Older Adults

Older adults may use all of the antiulcer, anti-heartburn drugs. With Mylanta and the other antacids, smaller doses may be effective because older adults usually secrete less gastric acid than younger adults. Also, with decreased renal function, older adults are more likely to have adverse effects, Many physicians recommend calcium carbonate antacids (e.g., Tums) as a calcium supplement in older women to prevent or treat osteoporosis.

Use in Patients With Renal Impairment

Patients with renal failure or with impaired renal function (creatinine clearance < 30 mL/min) should not take magnesium-based antacids such as Mylanta because 5% to 10% of the magnesium may be absorbed and accumulate to cause hypermagnesemia. Patients with chronic renal failure and hyperphosphatemia may take aluminum-based antacids to decrease absorption of phosphates in food. (Aluminum binds with phosphate in the GI tract, preventing phosphate absorption and hyperphosphatemia that commonly occurs in renal failure.) However, aluminum may accumulate in patients with renal failure, leading to encephalopathy, erythropoietin-resistant anemia, and osteomalacia.

Antacids containing calcium carbonate are currently recommended for the purpose of controlling phosphate levels in

TABLE 35.2

DRUGS AT A GLANCE: Representative Antacid Products

		COMPONENTS			
Drug	Pregnancy Category	Magnesium Oxide or Hydroxide	Aluminum Hydroxide	Other	Route and Dosage Ranges (Adults)
℗ Mylanta	Not classified	200 mg/tab, 200 mg/5 mL	200 mg/tab, 200 mg/5 mL	Simethicone, 25 mg/tab, 20 mg/5 mL	5–10 mL or 1–2 tablets PO every 2–4 h, between meals and at bedtime or as directed by physician
Mylanta Double strength	Not classified	400 mg/tab, 400 mg/5 mL	400 mg/tab, 400 mg/5 mL	Simethicone, 30 mg/tab, 30 mg/5 mL	Same as Mylanta
Amphojel	Not classified		300 or 600 mg/tab		600 mg PO 5 or 6 times daily
Gelusil	Not classified	200 mg/tab	200 mg/tab	Simethicone, 25 mg/tab	10 or more mL or 2 or more tablets PO after meals and at bedtime or as directed by physician to a max of 12 tablets or tsp/24 h
Maalox suspension	Not classified	200 mg/5 mL	225 mg/5 mL		30 mL PO 4 times daily, after meals and at bedtime or as directed by physician; max dose, 16 tsp/24 h
Titralac; Tums	Not classified			Calcium carbonate: 420 mg/tab, 1 g/5 mL Glycine: 180 mg/tab, 300 mg/5 mL	1 tsp or 2 tablets PO after meals or as directed by physician to max of 19 tablets or 8 tsp/24 h

patients with end-stage renal failure. Antacids with calcium carbonate can cause alkalosis and raise urine pH, and chronic use may cause renal stones and hypercalcemia.

Use in Patients With Critical Illness

To prevent **stress ulcers** (gastric mucosal lesions that occur due to physiologic stress) in critically ill patients and to treat acute GI bleeding, nearly continuous neutralization of gastric acid is desirable. Dose and frequency of administration must be sufficient to neutralize the gastric acid: a continuous intragastric drip through a nasogastric tube is effective. For patients with a nasogastric tube in place, antacid dosage may be titrated by aspirating stomach contents, determining pH, and then basing the dose on the pH. (Most gastric acid is neutralized and most pepsin activity is eliminated at a pH above 3.5.)

Use in Patients Receiving Home Care

People commonly take all of the antiulcer, anti-heartburn drugs in the home setting, usually by self-administration. The home care nurse can assist patients by providing information about taking the drugs correctly and monitoring responses.

EVIDENCE-BASED PRACTICE

Overuse of Stress Ulcer Prophylaxis in the Critical Care Setting and Beyond
by FARRELL, C. P.

Journal of Critical Care, 2010, 25(2), 214–220

A retrospective review of 210 patients indicated that 87.1% of all critical care admissions received stress ulcer prophylaxis (SUP). In patients with no risk factors, more than two thirds received SUP on critical care admission; more than three fifths continued on treatment on transfer from the area, and nearly one third were discharged home on SUP without a new indication. Although SUP in high-risk patients can decrease the incidence of gastrointestinal bleeding, inappropriate use of this regimen may increase drug reactions, needless hospital costs, and personal monetary drain on patients after discharge for over-the-counter drug purchases. The findings maintained that improvement measures to reduce overuse of SUP and to prompt discontinuation before hospital discharge were necessary.

IMPLICATIONS FOR NURSING PRACTICE: Patients admitted to the critical care units are susceptible to stress ulcers. People at high risk should receive SUP. However, increased health care costs and increased risk of adverse drug effects result with inappropriate use of SUP in the critical care area or at discharge without clear indications. Nurses should advocate for proper use of SUP in hospitalized patients.

Adverse Effects

Aluminum-containing antacids such as Mylanta can cause constipation. Hypophosphatemia and osteomalacia may develop in people who ingest large amounts of aluminum-based antacids over a long period because aluminum combines with phosphates in the GI tract and prevents phosphate absorption. Aluminum compounds are rarely used alone for acid–peptic disorders.

Mylanta also contains magnesium. Antacids with magnesium may cause diarrhea and hypermagnesemia. Older adults may experience neuromuscular effects.

Contraindications

People with any signs of appendicitis or inflamed bowel (cramping, soreness, or pain in the lower abdomen) patients with renal failure should not take Mylanta.

Nursing Implications

Preventing Interactions

Because antacids are minimally absorbed, few drugs alter their effects. Anticholinergic drugs (e.g., atropine) increase effects by delaying gastric emptying and by decreasing acid secretion themselves. Cholinergic drugs (e.g., dexpanthenol [Ilopan]) decrease effects of antacids by increasing GI motility and rate of gastric emptying. No herbs are known to alter the effects of antacids.

However, antacids may prevent absorption of most drugs taken at the same time, including benzodiazepine antianxiety drugs, corticosteroids, digoxin, H_2RAs (e.g., cimetidine), iron supplements, phenothiazine antipsychotic drugs, phenytoin, fluoroquinolone antibacterials, and tetracyclines. Antacids increase absorption of a few drugs including levodopa, quinidine, and valproic acid. To avoid or minimize these interactions, it is necessary to separate administration times by 1 to 2 hours.

Administering the Medication

Typical prescribing practices with Mylanta and other antacids used to treat active ulcers is to take them 1 hour and 3 hours after meals and at bedtime for greater acid neutralization. This schedule is effective but inconvenient for many patients. More recently, lower doses taken less often have been found effective in healing duodenal or gastric ulcers, although less acid neutralization occurs.

Authorities once thought that liquid antacid preparations were more effective. Now they consider tablets to be as effective as liquids.

QSEN Safety Alert

It is important to shake liquid antacid preparations well before measuring each dose, because these suspensions require thorough mixing.

Assessing for Therapeutic Effects

The nurse assesses for decreased epigastric pain in patients with gastric and duodenal ulcers or decreased heartburn in those with GERD. Antacids should relieve pain within a few minutes. Also, it is necessary to assess for decreased GI bleeding (e.g., absence of visible or occult blood in vomitus, gastric secretions, or feces). In addition, the nurse uses pH testing to evaluate the quantity, frequency, and duration of acid-reflux episodes, as well as to check the pH of gastric contents. The minimum acceptable pH with antacid therapy is 3.5. Healing usually occurs within 4 to 8 weeks. Finally, the nurse assesses for radiologic or endoscopic reports of ulcer healing.

Assessing for Adverse Effects

With antacids containing magnesium, such as Mylanta, the nurse assesses for diarrhea and hypermagnesemia. Combining such an antacid with one that contains aluminum or calcium may prevent this. Hypermagnesemia may occur in patients with impaired renal function. With the antacid Titralac (Tums), which contains calcium, it is important to observe for constipation. (Combining this antacid with other antacids containing magnesium may prevent this effect.)

Patient Teaching

Box 35.2 summarizes patient teaching information for antacids.

Histamine₂ Receptor Antagonists

In addition to its other effects, histamine also causes strong stimulation of gastric acid secretion. Vagal stimulation causes release of histamine from cells in the gastric mucosa. The histamine then acts on receptors located on the parietal cells to increase production of hydrochloric acid. These receptors are called the H_2 receptors. Although traditional antihistamines or H_1RAs prevent or reduce other effects of histamine, they do not block histamine effects on gastric acid production.

However, the H_2RAs inhibit both basal secretion of gastric acid and the secretion stimulated by histamine, acetylcholine, and gastrin. ⓟ **Cimetidine** (Tagamet) is the prototype of this class. OTC preparations, in relatively low doses, are available. Prescription forms are also obtainable.

Pharmacokinetics

After oral administration, absorption is good. Cimetidine is distributed in almost all body tissues. Onset varies. After a single dose, peak blood level is reached in all routes in 1 to 1.5 hours, the half-life is 2 hours, and an effective concentration is maintained for about 6 hours. Onset of the drug after intravenous (IV)

BOX 35.2 📋 **Patient Teaching Guidelines: Drugs Used for Peptic Ulcer Disease and Gastroesophageal Reflux Disease**

General Considerations

■ These drugs are commonly used to prevent and treat peptic ulcers and heartburn. Peptic ulcers usually form in the stomach or first part of the small bowel (duodenum), where tissues are exposed to stomach acid. Two common causes of peptic ulcer disease are stomach infection with a bacterium called *Helicobacter pylori* and taking nonsteroidal anti-inflammatory drugs (NSAIDs) such as ibuprofen and many others. Heartburn (also called gastroesophageal reflux disease) is caused by stomach acid splashing back onto the esophagus.

■ Peptic ulcer disease and heartburn are chronic conditions that are usually managed on an outpatient basis. Complications such as bleeding require hospitalization. Overall, these conditions can range from mild to serious, and it is important to seek information about the disease process, ways to prevent or minimize symptoms, and drug therapy.

■ With heartburn, try to minimize acid reflux by elevating the head of the bed; avoiding stomach distention by eating small meals; not lying down for 1 to 2 hours after eating; minimizing intake of fats, chocolate, citric juices, coffee, and alcohol; avoiding smoking (stimulates gastric acid production); and avoiding obesity, constipation, or other conditions that increase intra-abdominal pressure. In addition, take tablets and capsules with 8 ounce of water and do not take medications at bedtime unless instructed to do so.

■ Most medications for peptic ulcer disease and heartburn decrease stomach acid. An exception is the antibiotics used to treat ulcers caused by *H. pylori* infection.

The strongest acid reducers are omeprazole (Prilosec), esomeprazole (Nexium), lansoprazole (Prevacid), pantoprazole (Protonix), and rabeprazole (AcipHex). These are prescription drugs, except for omeprazole, which is approved for nonprescription use. Histamine-blocking drugs such as cimetidine (Tagamet), famotidine (Pepcid), and others are available as both prescription and over-the-counter (OTC) preparations. OTC products are indicated for heartburn, and smaller doses are taken than for peptic ulcer disease. These drugs usually should not be taken longer than 2 weeks without the advice of a health care provider. (A 2-week treatment with Prilosec OTC can be repeated every 4 months if needed to control heartburn.) The concern is that OTC drugs may delay diagnosis and treatment of potentially serious illness. In addition, cimetidine can increase toxic effects of numerous drugs and should be avoided if you are taking other medications.

■ Misoprostol (Cytotec) is given to prevent ulcers from NSAIDs, which are commonly used to relieve pain and inflammation with arthritis and other conditions. This drug should be taken only while taking a traditional NSAID such as ibuprofen. A related drug, celecoxib (Celebrex) is less likely to cause peptic ulcer disease. Do not take misoprostol if pregnant and do not become pregnant while taking the drug. If pregnancy occurs during misoprostol therapy, stop the drug and notify your health care provider immediately. Misoprostol can cause abdominal cramps and miscarriage.

■ Numerous antacid preparations are available, but they are not equally safe in all people and should be

BOX 35.2 | **Patient Teaching Guidelines: Drugs Used for Peptic Ulcer Disease and Gastroesophageal Reflux Disease** (Continued)

selected carefully. For example, products that contain magnesium have a laxative effect and may cause diarrhea; those that contain aluminum or calcium may cause constipation. (e.g., the antacid Titralac [Tums] contains calcium). Some commonly used antacids (e.g., Maalox, Mylanta) are a mixture of magnesium and aluminum preparations, an attempt to avoid both constipation and diarrhea. People with kidney disease should not take products that contain magnesium because magnesium can accumulate in the body and cause serious adverse effects. Thus, it is important to read product labels and, if you have a chronic illness or take other medications, ask your physician or pharmacist to help you select an antacid and an appropriate dose.

■ All H$_2$ receptor antagonists (e.g., cimetidine, famotidine) are available by prescription and OTC. When you obtain these drugs with a prescription, avoid concomitant use of OTC versions of the same or similar drugs.

Self- or Caregiver Administration

■ Take antiulcer drugs as directed. Underuse decreases therapeutic effectiveness; overuse increases adverse effects. For acute peptic ulcer disease or esophagitis, drugs are given in relatively high doses for 4 to 8 weeks to promote healing. For long-term maintenance therapy, dosage is reduced.

■ With Prilosec, AcipHex, Nexium, and Protonix, swallow the capsule whole; do not open, chew, or crush. With Prevacid, the capsule can be opened and the granules sprinkled on applesauce for patients who are unable

to swallow capsules. Also, the granules are available in a packet for preparing a liquid suspension. Follow instructions for mixing the granules exactly. The granules should not be crushed or chewed.

■ Take cimetidine with meals or at bedtime. Take famotidine, nizatidine, and ranitidine with or without food. Do not take an antacid for 1 hour before or after taking one of these drugs.

■ Take sucralfate on an empty stomach at least 1 hour before meals and at bedtime. Also, do not take an antacid for 1 hour before or after taking sucralfate.

■ Take misoprostol with food.

■ For treatment of peptic ulcer disease, take antacids 1 and 3 hours after meals and at bedtime (4–7 doses daily), 1 to 2 hours before or after other medications. Antacids decrease absorption of many medications if taken at the same time. Also, chew chewable tablets thoroughly before swallowing, then drink a glass of water; allow effervescent tablets to dissolve completely and almost stop bubbling before drinking (this increases the surface area of drug available to neutralize gastric acid); and shake liquids well before measuring the dose. A high-fiber diet, adequate fluid intake (2000–3000 mL daily), and exercise may help prevent constipation if it occurs with Mylanta therapy.

■ With Pepcid RPD orally disintegrating tablets, open the blister package with dry hands immediately before use, place the tablet on the tongue, and allow the tablet to dissolve with saliva. Taking with liquids is not necessary.

---

and intramuscular (IM) administration is rapid. Metabolism takes place in the liver. Excretion of the unchanged oral dose occurs unchanged in the urine within 24 hours; some excretion takes place in the bile, with elimination in the feces.

Action

Cimetidine inhibits the action of histamine at the H$_2$ receptors of the stomach, decreasing the amount, acidity, and pepsin content of gastric juices. A single dose can inhibit acid secretion for 6 to 12 hours, and a continuous IV infusion can inhibit secretion for prolonged periods.

Health care providers often advise taking antacids concurrently with H$_2$RAs such as cimetidine to relieve pain. The pain relief usually occurs after 1 week. Patients should not take the antacid and the H$_2$RA at the same time (except for Pepcid Complete) because the antacid reduces absorption of the H$_2$RA.

Use

Indications for use of cimetidine include prevention and treatment of peptic ulcer disease, GERD, esophagitis, GI bleeding due to acute stress ulcers, and Zollinger-Ellison syndrome. With gastric or duodenal ulcers, healing occurs within 6 to 8 weeks; with esophagitis, healing occurs in about 12 weeks. The U.S.

Food and Drug Administration (FDA) has approved the OTC preparations for the treatment of heartburn.

Table 35.3 gives route and dosage information for cimetidine and other H$_2$RAs.

Use in Older Adults

With cimetidine, older adults are more likely to experience adverse effects, especially confusion, agitation, and disorientation.

Use in Patients With Renal Impairment

Use of cimetidine in patients with impaired renal function requires caution. It is necessary to reduce the dosage of cimetidine, and other H$_2$RAs, in the presence of impaired renal function because the drugs are eliminated through the kidneys. Cimetidine may cause mental confusion in patients with renal impairment. It also blocks secretion of creatinine in renal tubules, thereby decreasing creatinine clearance and increasing serum creatinine level. Any dosage increase, if necessary, should be cautious, with close monitoring of renal function.

QSEN Safety Alert

For patients on hemodialysis, cimetidine administration should occur at the end of dialysis.

TABLE 35.3

DRUGS AT A GLANCE: Histamine₂ Receptor Antagonists

Drug	Pregnancy Category	Routes and Dosage Ranges	
		Adult	Children
Ⓟ **Cimetidine** (Tagamet)	B	Duodenal or gastric ulcer: PO 800 mg once daily at bedtime or 300 mg 4 times daily or 400 mg twice daily Maintenance: 400 mg PO at bedtime IV injection, 300 mg diluted in 20 mL of 0.9% NaCl solution every 6–8 h IV intermittent infusion: 300 mg diluted in 50 mL of dextrose or saline solution every 6 h Impaired renal function (creatinine clearance < 30 mL/min): 25 mg/h IV for prevention of GI bleeding; 300 mg PO or IV every 12 h, may increase to every 8 h if tolerated. 300 mg IM every 6–8 h GERD: 800 mg PO twice daily or 400 mg 4 times daily Prevention of upper GI bleeding: 50 mg/h continuous IV infusion Heartburn: 200 mg PO once or twice daily as needed Impaired renal function: 300 mg PO or IV every 8–12 h	Not recommended for children younger than 12 y of age
Famotidine (Pepcid, Pepcid RPD) Famotidine 10 mg, calcium 800 mg, and magnesium hydroxide 165 mg (Pepcid Complete)	B	Duodenal or gastric ulcer: 40 mg PO or IV once daily at bedtime or 20 mg twice daily for 4–8 wk; maintenance, 20 mg PO or IV once daily at bedtime Zollinger-Ellison syndrome: 20 mg PO every 6 h, increased if necessary IV injection: 20 mg every 12 h, diluted to 5 or 10 mL with 5% dextrose or 0.9% sodium chloride IV infusion: 20 mg every 12 h, diluted with 100 mL of 5% dextrose or 0.9% sodium chloride Impaired renal function (creatinine clearance <50 mL/min): 20 mg PO or IV every 24–48 h GERD: 20 mg PO twice daily for 6–12 wk Heartburn (Pepcid Complete): 1–2 tablets PO chewed, daily as needed	GERD: <3 mo, 0.5 mg/kg/dose PO daily for 8 wk 3 mo–<1 y: PO 0.5 mg/kg/dose twice daily, IV famotidine not adequately studied in patients <1 y with GERD Peptic ulcer: 1–16 y, 0.5 mg/kg/d PO at bedtime or divided twice daily up to 40 mg/d GERD with or without esophagitis: 1.0 mg/kg/d PO divided twice daily up to 40 mg twice daily
Nizatidine (Axid)	B	Duodenal or gastric ulcer: 300 mg PO once daily at bedtime or 150 mg PO twice daily; maintenance, 150 mg PO once daily at bedtime GERD: 150 mg PO twice daily Heartburn: 75 mg PO 30–60 min before meals. Impaired renal function (creatinine clearance [CrCl] 20–50 mL/min), 150 mg PO daily; CrCl <20 mL/min, 150 mg PO every 72 h	Dosing not established in children

TABLE 35.3

DRUGS AT A GLANCE: Histamine₂ Receptor Antagonists (Continued)

Drug	Pregnancy Category	Routes and Dosage Ranges	
		Adult	Children
Ranitidine (Zantac)	B	Duodenal ulcer: 300 mg PO once daily at bedtime or 150 mg PO twice daily, maintenance 150 mg PO at bedtime 50 mg IM every 6–8 h Injection, 50 mg IV diluted to 100 mL in 5% dextrose or 0.9% sodium chloride solution every 6–8 h Intermittent infusion, 50 mg IV diluted in 100 mL of 5% dextrose or 0.9% sodium chloride solution Gastric ulcer or GERD: 150 mg PO twice daily Impaired renal function (CrCl <50 mL/min): 150 mg PO every 24 h; 50 mg IV or IM every 18–24 h Heartburn: 75 mg PO as needed *H. pylori* infection: 400 mg PO twice daily for 4 wk in combination with clarithromycin	1 mo–16 y Duodenal and gastric ulcers, 2–4 mg/kg PO twice daily to a max of 300 mg/d; maintenance, 2–4 mg/kg PO once daily to a max of 150 mg/d GERD: 5–10 mg/kg/d PO, usually given as 2 divided doses

GERD, gastroesophageal reflux disease, including erosive esophagitis; GI, gastrointestinal.

Use in Patients With Hepatic Impairment

The partial metabolism of cimetidine and other H₂RAs occurs in the liver, which means that drug levels are higher than anticipated in patients with impaired liver function. Cimetidine inhibits the hepatic metabolism of many other drugs; this is a major concern.

Use in Patients With Critical Illness

H₂RAs are commonly used in critically ill patients to prevent stress-induced gastric ulceration. These are usually administered by intermittent IV infusion. Generally, information about the pharmacokinetics of these drugs in critically ill patients is limited. It appears that in patients who are critically ill, H₂RAs have a longer half-life and lower clearance rate than in people who are healthy.

Use in Patients Receiving Home Care

People take cimetidine in the home care setting. The home care nurse can assist patients by providing information about taking the drug correctly and monitoring responses. It is necessary to assess for potential drug–drug interactions with cimetidine.

Adverse Effects

Common adverse effects of cimetidine include diarrhea, dizziness, drowsiness, headache, confusion, and gynecomastia. They occur infrequently following the usual doses and standard duration of treatment. Adverse effects are more likely with prolonged use of high doses, with increasing age, and with impaired renal or hepatic function.

Contraindications

Contraindications include known hypersensitivity to cimetidine. Caution is warranted in people with renal and hepatic impairment and in women who are lactating or pregnant.

Nursing Implications

Preventing Interactions

Antacids decrease absorption of cimetidine, so the drugs should not be given at the same time. No drugs are known to increase or decrease the effects of cimetidine. Additionally, no herbs increase or decrease the effects of cimetidine.

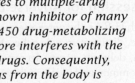

QSEN Safety Alert

However, cimetidine contributes to multiple-drug interactions, because it is a known inhibitor of many isozymes of the cytochrome P450 drug-metabolizing system in the liver and therefore interferes with the hepatic metabolism of other drugs. Consequently, the clearance of affected drugs from the body is slower; the increased serum levels means that the drugs are more likely to cause adverse effects and toxicity unless dosage is reduced.

Drugs that are affected by cimetidine include antidysrhythmics (lidocaine, propafenone, quinidine), the anticoagulant warfarin, anticonvulsants (carbamazepine, phenytoin), benzodiazepine antianxiety or hypnotic agents (alprazolam, diazepam, flurazepam, triazolam), beta-adrenergic blockers (labetalol, metoprolol, propranolol), the bronchodilator theophylline, calcium channel blocking agents (e.g., verapamil), tricyclic antidepressants (e.g., amitriptyline), and sulfonylurea antidiabetic drugs. In addition, cimetidine may increase serum levels (e.g., fluorouracil, procainamide and its active metabolite) and pharmacologic effects of other drugs (e.g., respiratory depression with opioid analgesics) by unidentified mechanisms. Cimetidine also may decrease effects of several drugs including drugs that require an acidic environment for absorption (e.g., iron salts, indomethacin, fluconazole, tetracyclines) and miscellaneous drugs (e.g., digoxin, tocainide) by unknown mechanisms. The accumulation of the antihistamines, terfenadine and astemizole, may result in a prolongation of the QT interval and could lead to the development of ventricular dysrhythmias such as torsades de pointes. Cimetidine also may decrease the effects of drugs that require an acidic environment for absorption (e.g., iron salts, indomethacin, fluconazole, tetracyclines) and miscellaneous drugs (e.g., digoxin, tocainide) by unknown mechanisms.

Administering the Medication

H₂RAs are available in a wide array of products, and it is essential to take precautions to ensure that the formulation, dosage strength, and method of administration is appropriate for the intended use.

- Oral administration of a single oral dose occurs at bedtime, and administration of multiple oral doses of cimetidine occurs with meals and at bedtime; can be taken with other drugs without regard to food intake.

QSEN Safety Alert ❗

With the oral solution, it is important to measure the liquid with a marked measuring spoon or medicine cup, not with a tablespoon.

- IV administration requires dilution and administration over at least 2 minutes. For intermittent infusion, it is necessary to dilute and infuse over 15 to 20 minutes.
- IM administration does not require dilution. Injection is given deep into a large muscle group.

Assessing for Therapeutic Effects

The nurse assesses for decreased epigastric pain with gastric and duodenal ulcers or decreased heartburn with GERD.

Assessing for Adverse Effects

With H₂RAs, the nurse assesses for diarrhea or constipation, headache, dizziness, muscle aches, fatigue, skin rashes, mental confusion, delirium, coma, depression, and fever. Adverse effects are uncommon and usually mild with recommended doses. The nurse assesses for central nervous system effects, which have been associated with high doses in patients who are elderly or in those with impaired renal function. With long-term administration of cimetidine, other observed adverse effects include decreased sperm count and gynecomastia in men and galactorrhea in women.

Patient Teaching

Box 35.2 summarizes patient teaching guidelines that apply to the H₂RAs.

Other Drugs in the Class

Unlike cimetidine, ranitidine (Zantac), famotidine (Pepcid, Pepcid RPD), and nizatidine (Axid) do not affect the cytochrome P450 drug-metabolizing system in the liver and therefore do not interfere with the metabolism of other drugs. Use of these other drugs may be preferable in patients who are critically ill because they often require numerous other drugs with which cimetidine may interact.

Ranitidine is more potent than cimetidine on a weight basis, and smaller doses can be given less frequently. Oral ranitidine reaches peak blood levels 1 to 3 hours after administration and is metabolized in the liver; approximately 30% is excreted unchanged in the urine. Parenteral ranitidine reaches peak blood levels in about 15 minutes; 65% to 80% is excreted unchanged in the urine. Famotidine and nizatidine pharmacokinetics are similar to cimetidine and ranitidine. Nizatidine is not available in a parenteral formulation. Compared with cimetidine, the other drugs cause similar effects except they are less likely to cause mental confusion and gynecomastia (antiandrogenic effects).

Ranitidine decreases absorption of diazepam if given at the same time and increases hypoglycemic effects of glipizide. Antacids probably decrease absorption of ranitidine. Nizatidine increases serum salicylate levels in people taking high doses of aspirin.

NCLEX Success

1. When taking a patient's history, the nurse notes that the patient is taking warfarin and cimetidine—a histamine₂ receptor antagonist—concurrently. The nurse should anticipate that the

   A. warfarin effects would be increased
   B. cimetidine effects would be increased
   C. warfarin effects would be decreased
   D. cimetidine effects would be decreased

2. A patient is started on Mylanta for peptic ulcer disease. It is important for the nurse to inform the patient about which of the following adverse effects?

   A. nausea
   B. vomiting
   C. diarrhea
   D. constipation

Proton Pump Inhibitors

PPIs are strong inhibitors of gastric acid secretion. PPIs are similar to the H₂RAs in terms of effects but have a different mode of action. Compared with H₂RAs, PPIs suppress gastric acid more strongly, for a longer period. This effect provides faster symptom relief and faster healing in acid-related diseases. Rates of ulcer recurrence are similar. Because PPIs are more effective than H₂RAs, certainly in the short-term, PPIs are more popular. Ⓟ **Omeprazole** (Prilosec), the first drug in the class to be developed, is still widely used.

Pharmacokinetics

Omeprazole is well absorbed after oral administration and highly bound to plasma proteins (about 95%). Metabolism occurs in the liver, and excretion takes place in the urine (about 75%) and bile or feces. The half-life of the drug is 1 to 1.5 hours. Acid-inhibiting effects occur within 2 hours and last 72 hours or longer. When the drug is discontinued, effects persist for 48 to 72 hours or longer, until the gastric parietal cells can synthesize additional H$^+$, K$^+$-ATPase.

Action

Omeprazole binds irreversibly to the gastric proton pump (e.g., the enzyme H$^+$, K$^+$-ATPase) to prevent the "pumping" or release of gastric acid from parietal cells into the stomach lumen, thereby blocking the final step of acid production. Inhibition of the proton pump suppresses gastric acid secretion in response to all primary stimuli, histamine, gastrin, and acetylcholine. Thus, omeprazole and other drugs in the class inhibit both daytime (including meal-stimulated) and nocturnal (unstimulated) acid secretion.

Use

Omeprazole and other PPIs are usually the drug class of choice for treatment of peptic ulcer disease, including duodenal and gastric ulcers; GERD with erosive esophagitis; and Zollinger-Ellison syndrome. With duodenal and gastric ulcers, healing may occur after 2 weeks compared to 4 weeks using H$_2$RAs. With GERD, PPIs usually eliminate symptoms within 1 to 2 weeks and heal esophagitis within 8 weeks. Lower doses can prevent recurrence of esophagitis, maintain symptom relief, and heal esophagitis. Higher doses or longer therapy may be needed for severe GERD.

In patients with *H. pylori*–associated ulcers, eradication of the bacterium with antimicrobial drugs is preferable to long-term maintenance therapy with antisecretory drugs. Therapy with a PPI and two antimicrobial drugs is the most effective regimen (see Medications Used to Treat *Helicobacter pylori*).

Table 35.4 presents route and dosage information for omeprazole and other PPIs.

Use in Children

Omeprazole and the other PPIs have gained widespread popularity in children and infants for the management of peptic ulcers and GERD as well as the eradication of *H. pylori*. These drugs are acid labile, and oral formulations consist of capsules that contain enteric-coated granules. A chewable form of omeprazole exists, and a pharmacist can prepare a liquid formulation.

Use in Older Adults

Older adults tolerate PPIs well. PPIs are probably the drug of choice for treating symptomatic GERD because evidence suggests that patients 60 years of age and older require stronger antisecretory effects than younger adults. However, long-term use (greater than 1 year) is associated with increased risk of hip fractures in people older than 50 years of age; the risk of fractures increases the longer the medications are taken and is greater in people who take higher dosages of PPIs. The increased risk of fractures may be due to decreased calcium absorption due to **achlorhydria** (low or absent production of gastric acid in the stomach) from PPI therapy. It is important to consider appropriate dose and duration of therapy when treating GERD in older adults.

Use in Patients With Hepatic Impairment

With omeprazole, bioavailability is increased because of decreased first-pass metabolism and plasma half-life is increased. Metabolism of PPIs occurs in the liver, and use of these drugs may cause transient elevations in liver function tests. However, dosage adjustments are not recommended.

Use in Patients With Critical Illness

The PPIs are the strongest gastric acid suppressants used in patients who are critically ill. They usually tolerate the drugs well. IV administration, if necessary, is an option.

Adverse Effects and Contraindications

Adverse effects are minimal with both short- and long-term use. Nausea, diarrhea, and headache are the most frequently reported adverse effects. High dose or long-term use of PPIs carries a possible increased risk of bone fractures. (As previously stated, this may increase in older patients.)

Contraindications include known hypersensitivity to omeprazole.

Nursing Implications

Preventing Interactions

Drug interactions with the PPIs are relatively few. Omeprazole increases blood levels of some benzodiazepines (diazepam, flurazepam, triazolam), phenytoin, and warfarin, probably by inhibiting hepatic metabolism. Coadministration of clopidogrel with PPIs may reduce the cardioprotective effects of clopidogrel. Clarithromycin increases effects of omeprazole and may increase blood levels. No herbs have been reported to increase or decrease the effects of omeprazole.

Administering the Medication

It is important that omeprazole be administered before food intake. Two 20-mg oral capsules or suspension packets are not equivalent to one 40-mg dose. The 20- and 40-mg dosages contain the same amount of sodium bicarbonate; substituting two 20-mg doses for one 40-mg dose results in the administration of too much sodium bicarbonate. The patient should swallow the tablets or capsules whole, without crushing or chewing, because the drug formulations are delayed-release and long-acting. Crushing or chewing destroys these effects.

Assessing for Therapeutic Effects

The nurse assesses for decreased epigastric pain with gastric and duodenal ulcers, and also assesses for decreased heartburn with GERDs.

Assessing for Adverse Effects

The nurse observes for the presence of headache, diarrhea, abdominal pain, nausea, and vomiting.

TABLE 35.4

DRUGS AT A GLANCE: Proton Pump Inhibitors

Drug	Pregnancy Category	Routes and Dosage Ranges	
		Adults	Children

Ⓟ **Omeprazole** (Prilosec, Prilosec OTC)	C	Gastric ulcer: 40 mg PO once daily for 4–8 wk
		Duodenal ulcer: 20 mg PO once daily for 4–8 wk
		GERD, with erosive esophagitis: 20 mg PO once daily
		Zollinger-Ellison syndrome: 60 mg PO once daily
		Heartburn: 20 mg PO for 14 d; may repeat treatment every 4 mo if needed
		H. pylori infection: 40 mg PO daily for 14 d, then 20 mg daily for 14 d, with clarithromycin
			1–16 y
			GERD:
			  5–<10 kg, 5 mg PO
			  10–<20 kg, 10 mg PO
			  ≥20 kg, 20 mg PO

Esomeprazole (Nexium, Nexium IV, Nexium delayed-release capsules)	B	GERD: 20–40 mg PO once daily for 4–8 wk; maintenance, 20 mg PO once daily, 20–40 mg IV daily up to 10 d	1 mo–<1 y, 0.5 mg/kg IV infused over 10–30 min 1–11 y, GERD: 30 mg PO once daily for up to 12 wk; >30 kg, 15 mg PO once daily for up to 12 wk 12–17 y, GERD: 10 mg PO once daily for up to 8 wk, <55 kg 10 mg IV; ≥55 kg 20 mg IV infused over 10–30 min Healing erosive esophagitis: <20 kg 10 mg PO once daily for up to 8 wk; ≥20 kg 10 or 20 mg PO once daily for up to 8 wk
Lansoprazole (Prevacid, Prevacid IV)	B	Duodenal ulcer: 15 mg PO daily for healing and maintenance Gastric ulcer: 30 mg PO once daily, up to 8 wk Erosive esophagitis: 30 mg PO daily up to 8 wk; maintenance, 15 mg PO daily; 30 mg IV daily up to 7 d *H. pylori* infection: 30 mg PO (with amoxicillin and clarithromycin) twice daily for 14 d Hypersecretory conditions: 60–90 mg PO daily	1–11 y, GERD: ≤30 kg, 30 mg PO once daily for up to 12 wk; >30 kg, 15 mg PO once daily for up to 12 wk 12–17 y GERD: 30 mg PO once daily for up to 8 wk Nonerosive GERD: 15 mg PO once daily for up to 8 wk; Healing erosive esophagitis: 15 mg PO once daily Hypersecretory conditions: 60 mg PO once daily
Pantoprazole (Protonix, Protonix IV)	B	GERD: 40 mg PO or IV once daily Zollinger-Ellison syndrome: 40–80 mg PO or IV every 12 h	5 y and more, GERD >15 kg–<40 kg, 20 mg PO once daily for up to 8 wk >40 kg, 40 mg PO once daily for up to 8 wk
Rabeprazole (AcipHex)	B	Duodenal ulcer: 20 mg PO once daily up to 4 wk GERD: 20 mg PO once daily for healing and maintenance Zollinger-Ellison syndrome: 60 mg PO once or twice daily	12 y and more, GERD 20 mg PO once daily for up to 8 wk

GERD, gastroesophageal reflux disease, including erosive esophagitis; GI, gastrointestinal; *H. pylori, Helicobacter pylori.*

Patient Teaching

Box 35.2 lists general teaching guidelines that apply to PPIs.

Other Drugs in the Class

The actions and pharmacokinetics of the other PPIs—esomeprazole (Nexium), lansoprazole (Prevacid), pantoprazole (Protonix), and rabeprazole (AcipHex)—are similar to those of omeprazole. However, the drug interactions associated of omeprazole reportedly do not occur with these other PPIs.

Esomeprazole capsules can be opened, mixed with 50 mL of water, and swallowed or administered via nasogastric tube. Flush tube with water after administration. IV esomeprazole can be injected over no less than 3 minutes or infused over 10 to 30 minutes into a dedicated IV line. Flush the IV line with 5% dextrose or lactated Ringer's solution before and after esomeprazole administration.

Lansoprazole and rabeprazole should be used cautiously and dosage should be reduced in patients with severe liver impairment. Those people with phenylketonuria should be advised that orally disintegrating tablets of lansoprazole may contain aspartame. Lansoprazole may cause drowsiness or dizziness. For patients who are unable to swallow capsules, they can have the lansoprazole (and esomeprazole) capsule opened and the granules mixed with applesauce or other acidic substances; this preserves the coating of the granules, allowing them to remain intact until they reach the small intestine. Chewing or crushing destroys the coating. For a liquid suspension, it is possible to mix the lansoprazole granules with 30 mL of water (use no other liquids), stir well, and swallow it immediately, without chewing the granules.

The nurse ensures that oral pantoprazole is taken with or without food as per the manufacturer's recommendations. The nurse may administer IV pantoprazole over 15 minutes, injecting the drug into a dedicated line or the Y-site of an IV infusion. Here are some specific directions regarding pantoprazole administration:

- Use the in-line filter provided; if injecting in a Y-site, place the filter below the Y-site closest to the patient.
- Flush the IV line with 5% dextrose, 0.9% NaCl, or lactated Ringer's solution before and after administration.

Clinical Application 35-1

In addition to taking her medication properly, the nurse should instruct Ms. Daniels to take measures to avoid gastric irritation.
- What content should the teaching plan include?

Adjuvant Medications Used to Treat Peptic Ulcer Disease and Gastroesophageal Reflux Disease

Administration of adjuvant medications may support the treatment and resolution of symptoms of acid–peptic disorders. Table 35.5 summarizes these adjuvant medications.

Miscellaneous Medications

Prostaglandin: Misoprostol

Naturally occurring prostaglandin E, which is produced in mucosal cells of the stomach and duodenum, inhibits gastric acid secretion and increases mucus and bicarbonate secretion, mucosal blood flow, and perhaps mucosal repair. It also inhibits the mucosal damage produced by gastric acid, aspirin, and NSAIDs. When synthesis of prostaglandin E is inhibited, erosion and ulceration of gastric mucosa may occur. This is the mechanism by which aspirin and other NSAIDs are thought to cause gastric and duodenal ulcers (see Chap. 14).

Misoprostol (Cytotec) (see Table 35.5) is a synthetic form of prostaglandin E approved for concurrent use with NSAIDs to protect gastric mucosa from NSAID-induced erosion and ulceration. It is indicated for patients at high risk of GI ulceration and bleeding, such as those taking high doses of NSAIDs for arthritis and older adults. The FDA has issued a **BLACK BOX WARNING ◆** to alert health care professionals that misoprostol is contraindicated in women of childbearing potential, unless effective contraceptive methods are being used, and during pregnancy, because it may induce abortion, premature birth, or birth defects. In fact, misoprostol is one of the drugs used for medical abortions in lieu of surgical evacuation.

The most common adverse effects are diarrhea (occurs in 10%–40% of recipients), which may be severe enough to lead to dosage reduction or stopping the drug, and abdominal cramping. Other adverse effects include nausea, vomiting, headache, uterine cramping, and vaginal bleeding. Older adults often take large doses of NSAIDs for arthritis and therefore are at risk for development of acute gastric ulcers and GI bleeding. Thus, they may be candidates for treatment with misoprostol. However, they may be unable to tolerate the misoprostol-induced diarrhea and abdominal discomfort. Dosage reduction to prevent severe diarrhea and abdominal cramping may be necessary.

Sucralfate

Sucralfate (Carafate) is a preparation of sulfated sucrose and aluminum hydroxide that binds to normal and ulcerated mucosa. Health care providers use it to prevent and treat peptic ulcer disease. For ulcer treatment, it requires use for 4 to 8 weeks unless healing is confirmed by radiologic or endoscopic examination. When used long term to prevent ulcer recurrence, dosage reduction is necessary.

Sucralfate is effective even though it does not inhibit secretion of gastric acid or pepsin, and it has little neutralizing effect on gastric acid. Its mechanism of action is unclear, but it is thought to act locally on the gastric and duodenal mucosa. Possible mechanisms include binding to ulcer and forming a protective barrier between the mucosa and gastric acid, pepsin, and bile salts; neutralizing pepsin; stimulating prostaglandin synthesis in the mucosa; and exerting healing effects through the aluminum component. Sucralfate is effective in healing duodenal ulcers and in maintenance therapy to prevent ulcer recurrence. In general, the rates of ulcer healing with sucralfate are similar to the rates with H₂RAs.

Adverse effects are low in incidence and severity because sucralfate is not absorbed systemically. Constipation and dry mouth are most often reported. Older adults tolerate sucralfate

TABLE 35.5

DRUGS AT A GLANCE: Adjuvant Medications Used to Treat Peptic Ulcer Disease and Gastroesophageal Reflux Disease

Drug	Pregnancy Category	Route and Dosage Ranges	
		Adults	*Children*
Misoprostol (Cytotec)	X	100–200 mg PO 4 times daily with meals and at bedtime	Safety and effectiveness not established
Sucralfate (Carafate)	B	Active ulcer: 1 g PO 4 times daily before meals and at bedtime; maintenance: 1 g PO 2 times daily	Safety and effectiveness not established
Amoxicillin	B	1 g 2–3 times daily	Dosing not established with *H. pylori* infection
Clarithromycin	C	500 mg PO 3 times daily	Dosing not established with *H. pylori* infection
Metronidazole	B	250 mg PO 4 times daily	Dosing not established with *H. pylori* infection
Tetracycline	D	500 mg PO 4 times daily	Dosing not established with *H. pylori* infection; tetracycline can discolor teeth in children 8 y of age or less.
Bismuth subsalicylate	Not rated	525 mg PO (2 tabs or 30 mL) 4 times daily	<3 y, consult physician 3–6 y, 1/3 tab or 5 mL PO 6–9 y, 2/3 tab or 10 mL PO 9–12 y, 1 tab or 15 mL PO Dosage may be repeated every 30–60 min, if needed, up to 8 doses in 24 h
Bismuth subcitrate, potassium, metronidazole, tetracycline (Pylera)	D	Bismuth subcitrate potassium 140 mg, metronidazole 125 mg, tetracycline 125 mg 3 caps PO 4 times daily with 8 ounce water after meals and at bedtime for 10 d.	Safety and effectiveness not established; tetracycline can discolor teeth in children 8 y of age or less.
Bismuth subsalicylate, metronidazole, and tetracycline (Helidac)	D	Bismuth 525 mg (2 tab), metronidazole 250 mg (1 tab), tetracycline 500 mg (1 capsule) PO 4 times daily for 14 d	Safety and effectiveness not established; tetracycline can discolor teeth in children 8 y of age or younger.
Amoxicillin, clarithromycin, and lansoprazole (Prevpac)	C	Amoxicillin 1 g, clarithromycin 500 mg, lansoprazole 30 mg PO twice daily, morning and evening, for 14 d	Safety and effectiveness not established

H. pylori, Helicobacter pylori.

well. The main disadvantages of using sucralfate are that the tablet is large; it must be given at least twice daily; it requires an acid pH for activation and should not be given with an antacid, H₂RA, or PPI; and it may bind to other drugs and prevent their absorption. Sucralfate decreases absorption of ciprofloxacin and other fluoroquinolones, digoxin, phenytoin, warfarin, as well as the PPI lansoprazole. If a person takes both sucralfate and any of these drugs, to avoid or minimize this interaction, he or she should do the following:

- Take lansoprazole about 30 minutes before sucralfate
- Take ciprofloxacin and other fluoroquinolones, digoxin, phenytoin, warfarin, or other drugs 2 hours before sucralfate, it is possible

In addition, antacids decrease the effects of sucralfate, and people should not take these within 30 minutes before or after administration of sucralfate.

Medications Used to Treat Helicobacter pylori

Combination Therapy with Antibiotics

Combination drug therapy that includes at least two antibiotics and an acid reducer (triple therapy), as well as occasionally bismuth subsalicylate, is recommended for patients with peptic ulcer disease who are known to be infected with *H. pylori*. If the selected antibiotics are not effective, the bacteria may become resistant to the action of some antibiotics. Combination regimens are the most effective way to help ensure that the bacteria do not acquire resistance to the selected antibiotics. A different combination of drug treatment may be required based on the treatment history. In situations where the first-line therapy is ineffective, rescue *H. pylori* therapy with esomeprazole, moxifloxacin, and amoxicillin has been effective and well tolerated. Data demonstrate that 14 days of treatment not only significantly improve the likelihood of eradication but also produce an increased rate of adverse events.

Over the past few years, an alternate approach to *H. pylori* treatment has demonstrated higher success rates by splitting up the antibiotics rather than taking them all at once. Sequential therapy may be more effective than standard triple therapy in light of the increasing frequency of resistant strains of *H. pylori*. Table 35.5 presents examples of drug combinations used to treat *H. pylori*. For convenience, some of the recommended drug combinations are packaged together (see Table 35.5).

Metronidazole (Flagyl), a nitroimidazole antibiotic, antiprotozoal medication, is sometimes included as part of a multidrug regimen (see Chap. 19).

QSEN Safety Alert

Consuming alcohol while using metronidazole has long been thought to have a disulfiram-like reaction with effects that can include flushing, tachycardia, diaphoresis, nausea, vomiting, or headache if alcohol ingestion occurs with use. It is important to tell patients that even a very small amount of alcohol can produce the reaction; the risk persists for up to 48 hours after completion of treatment.

Section IV of this book contains additional information about antibiotic therapy.

Bismuth Subsalicylate

Health care providers use bismuth subsalicylate to coat ulcers, protecting them from stomach acid to treat *H. pylori*. Other uses include treatment of diarrhea and nausea. Commonly known as pink bismuth, it is the active ingredient in OTC medications such as Pepto-Bismol and Kaopectate. Bismuth subsalicylate is also used in combinations with other drugs to treat *H. pylori*. As salicylate, this drug can cause serious bleeding problems when used alone in patients with ulcers.

QSEN Safety Alert

People with an allergy to aspirin or other salicylates should not take bismuth subsalicylate.

People who are taking chewable tablets should chew them and then swallow them. If they taking the liquid form of this medication, they should shake the bottle well and use a measuring device or cup. Adverse effects of bismuth subsalicylate include darkening of the stools or tongue, a harmless effect that disappears once the drug is stopped, and ringing in the ears or hearing loss. If ear-related problems occur, it is necessary to discontinue the drug and have a health care provider evaluate the patient.

NCLEX Success

3. **The nurse explains to the patient being discharged who is taking sucralfate that the medication should be administered**

   A. at the same time as an antacid
   B. after meals
   C. with meals
   D. 2 hours before other drugs

4. **A patient asks the nurse how sucralfate (Carafate) works. The nurse replies that sucralfate**

   A. inhibits gastric acid secretion
   B. increases mucus and bicarbonate secretion
   C. binds to normal and ulcerated mucosa, creating a protective barrier
   D. enhances prostaglandin synthesis

5. **One of the most common adverse effects of misoprostol that makes the drug difficult to tolerate in older adults is**

   A. headache
   B. constipation
   C. hyperphosphatemia
   D. diarrhea

The Nursing Process

Assessment

- Identify risk factors for peptic ulcer disease.
  - Cigarette smoking. Effects are thought to include stimulation of gastric acid secretion and decreased blood supply to gastric mucosa. (Nicotine constricts blood vessels.) Moreover, patients with peptic ulcers who continue to smoke heal more slowly and have more recurrent ulcers, despite usually adequate treatment, than those who stop smoking.
  - Stress, including physiologic stress (e.g., shock, sepsis, burns, surgery, head injury, severe trauma, medical illness) and psychological stress. One mechanism may be that stress activates the sympathetic nervous system, which then causes vasoconstriction in organs not needed for "fight or flight." Thus, stress may lead to ischemia in gastric mucosa, with ulceration if ischemia is severe or prolonged.
  - Drug therapy with aspirin and other NSAIDs, corticosteroids, and antineoplastics.
- Assess for signs and symptoms, which depend on the type and location of the ulcer.
  - Periodic epigastric pain, which occurs 1 to 4 hours after eating or during the night and is often described as "burning" or "gnawing," is a symptom of a chronic duodenal ulcer.
  - GI bleeding, which occurs with acute or chronic ulcers when the ulcer erodes into a blood vessel. Clinical manifestations may range from mild (e.g., occult blood

in feces, eventual anemia) to severe (e.g., hematemesis, melena, hypotension, shock).
- GERD, which produces heartburn (a substernal burning sensation).

Nursing Diagnoses

- Pain related to effects of gastric acid on peptic ulcers or inflamed esophageal tissues
- Imbalanced nutrition: less than body requirements related to anorexia and abdominal discomfort
- Constipation related to aluminum- or calcium-containing antacids and sucralfate
- Diarrhea related to magnesium-containing antacids and misoprostol
- Deficient knowledge related to drug therapy and nonpharmacologic management of GERD and peptic ulcer disease

Planning/Goals

The patient will

- Take or receive antiulcer, anti-heartburn drugs accurately.
- Experience relief of symptoms.
- Avoid situations that cause or exacerbate symptoms, when possible.
- Be observed for GI bleeding and other complications of peptic ulcer disease and GERD.
- Maintain normal patterns of bowel function.
- Avoid preventable adverse effects of drug therapy.

Nursing Interventions

The nurse will

- Use measures to prevent or minimize peptic ulcer disease and gastric acid–induced esophageal disorders.

With peptic ulcer disease, helpful interventions may include the following:

- General health measures such as a well-balanced diet, adequate rest, and regular exercise

- Avoiding cigarette smoking and gastric irritants (e.g., alcohol, aspirin and NSAIDs, caffeine)
- Reducing psychological stress (e.g., by changing environments) or learning healthful strategies of stress management (e.g., relaxation techniques, physical exercise). There is no practical way to avoid psychological stress because it is part of everyday life.
- Long-term drug therapy with small doses of H₂RAs, antacids, or sucralfate. With "active" peptic ulcer disease, help the patient follow the prescribed therapeutic regimen helps to promote healing and prevent complications (see Box 35.2).
- Diet therapy is of minor importance in prevention or treatment of peptic ulcer disease. Some physicians prescribe no dietary restrictions, whereas others suggest avoiding or minimizing highly spiced foods, gas-forming foods, and caffeine-containing beverages.
- With heartburn and esophagitis, helpful measures are those that prevent or decrease gastroesophageal reflux of gastric contents (e.g., avoiding irritant, highly spiced, or fatty foods; eating small meals; not lying down for 1 to 2 hours after eating; elevating the head of the bed; avoiding obesity, constipation, or other conditions that increase intra-abdominal pressure).

Evaluation

- Observe and interview regarding drug use.
- Observe and interview regarding relief of symptoms.
- Observe for signs and symptoms of complications.
- Observe and interview regarding adverse drug effects.

Clinical Application 35-2

- What measures should Ms. Daniels take to prevent or minimize GERD?
- What additional patient teaching regarding antacid therapy should the nurse provide Ms. Daniels?

Key Concepts

- The most common location for a peptic ulcer is the duodenum followed by the stomach and esophagus.
- Experts have attributed peptic ulcers to an imbalance between cell-destructive and cell-protective effects.
- Cell-destructive effects include gastric acid (hydrochloric acid), pepsin, *H. pylori* infection, and ingestion of NSAIDs.
- Cell-protective effects include secretion of mucus and bicarbonate, dilution of hydrochloric acid by food and secretions, prevention of diffusion of hydrochloric acid from the stomach back into the gastric mucosal lining, the presence of prostaglandin E, and alkalinization of gastric secretions by pancreatic juices and bile.
- Antacids are alkaline substances that neutralize acids.
- Aluminum antacids have low neutralizing capacity and often cause constipation.
- Magnesium antacids have high neutralizing capacity and may cause diarrhea and hypermagnesemia.

- Calcium antacids have high neutralizing capacity and rapid onset. The drugs may cause rebound acidity and hypercalcemia and so are not used for the treatment of peptic ulcer disease or GERD.

- The treatment of choice for *H. pylori* infection is multiple-drug therapy to eradicate the infection and heal the ulcer.

- The H₂RAs (e.g., cimetidine, famotidine, nizatidine, and ranitidine) inhibit secretion of gastric acid, decreasing the acidity of gastric juices. They are indicated for prevention and treatment of heartburn, peptic ulcer disease, GERD, esophagitis, GI bleeding due to stress ulcers, and hypersecretory syndromes such as Zollinger-Ellison syndrome.

- The PPIs (e.g., omeprazole, esomeprazole, lansoprazole, pantoprazole, rabeprazole) bind irreversibility to the gastric proton pump to prevent the release of gastric acid from parietal cells into the stomach lumen. They are considered drugs of choice for treatment of heartburn, gastric and duodenal ulcers, GERD, esophagitis, and hypersecretory syndromes such as Zollinger-Ellison syndrome.

- Misoprostol is a synthetic form of prostaglandin E approved for concurrent use with NSAIDs to protect the gastric mucosa from NSAID-induced erosion and ulceration.

- The FDA has issued a **BLACK BOX WARNING** ◆ to alert health care professionals that misoprostol is contraindicated in women of childbearing potential, unless effective contraceptive methods are being used, and during pregnancy, because it may induce abortion, premature birth, or birth defects.

- Sucralfate forms a protective barrier over mucosal ulcerations, protecting them from exposure to gastric juices. It requires an acid pH to be effective.

Critical Thinking Questions

35-1. Carla Sexton is a patient newly diagnosed with a duodenal ulcer associated with an *H. pylori* infection. She reports that she smokes a pack of cigarettes a day and consumes alcohol on occasion. Her physician places Ms. Sexton on lansoprazole and Helidac, a combination drug that contains bismuth, metronidazole, and tetracycline. The nurse instructs her about the importance of smoking cessation and the need to not consume alcohol with the prescribed drugs.

- Ms. Sexton asks the nurse about the Helidac. When she is informed that it contains three drugs, she responds, "Wait a minute. I don't like to take a lot of medications. Isn't this treatment excessive?" How should the nurse respond?

- How would the nurse explain that smoking cessation aids ulcer healing?

- Although the nurse told Ms. Sexton that she should not consume alcohol, she ignored the instruction and drank beer. She presents to the emergency department with tachycardia, headache, diaphoresis, and nausea and vomiting. What is the likely cause of her symptoms?

References and Resources

American Gastroenterological Association (AGA) Institute. (2008). American Gastroenterological Association medical position statement on the management of gastroesophageal reflux disease. *Gastroenterology, 135*(4), 1383–1391, 1391.e1–1391.e5.

American Society for Gastrointestinal Endoscopy (ASGE). (2007). Role of endoscopy in the management of GERD. *Gastrointestinal Endoscopy, 66*(2), 219–224.

DiPiro, J., Talbert, R. L., Yee, G., Matzke, G., Wells, B., & Posey, L. M. (Eds.). (2011). *Pharmacotherapy: A pathophysiologic approach* (8th ed.). New York: McGraw-Hill.

Drug facts and comparisons. (Updated monthly). St. Louis, MO: Facts and Comparisons.

Farrell, C. P. (2010). Overuse of stress ulcer prophylaxis in the critical care setting and beyond. *Journal of Critical Care, 25*(2), 214–220.

Marik, P. E., Vasu, T., Hirani, A., & Pachinburavan, M. (2010). Stress ulcer prophylaxis in the new millennium: A systematic review and meta-analysis. *Critical Care Medicine, 38*(11), 2222–2228.

Karch, A. M. (2012). *2012 Lippincott's nursing drug guide.* Philadelphia, PA: Lippincott Williams & Wilkins.

Lacy, C. F., Armstrong, L. L., Goldman, M. P., & Lance, L. L. (2010). *Lexi-Comp's drug information handbook* (19th ed.). Hudson, OH: American Pharmaceutical Association.

Porth, C. M. (2009). *Pathophysiology: Concepts of altered health status.* (8th ed.). Philadelphia, PA: Lippincott Williams & Wilkins.

Sacco, F., Spezzaferro, M., Amitrano, M., Grossi, L., Manzoli, L., & Marzio, L. (2009). Efficacy of four different moxifloxacin-based triple therapies for first-line *H. pylori* treatment. *Digestive and Liver Disease, 42*(2), 110–104.

Smeltzer, S. C., Bare, B. G., Hinkle J. L., & Cheever, K. H. (2009). *Brunner & Suddarth's textbook of medical-surgical nursing* (12th ed.). Philadelphia, PA: Lippincott Williams & Wilkins.

Wang, A. Y., & Peura, D. A. (2011). The prevalence and incidence of *Helicobacter Pylori*–associated peptic ulcer disease and upper gastrointestinal bleeding throughout the world. *Gastrointestinal Endoscopy Clinics of North America, 21*(4), 613–635.

36 Drug Therapy for Nausea and Vomiting

LEARNING OBJECTIVES

After studying this chapter, you should be able to:

1. Identify patients at risk for developing nausea and vomiting.

2. Discuss the phenothiazines in terms of indications and contraindications for use, routes of administration, and major adverse effects.

3. Describe selected antihistamines used to control nausea and vomiting in terms of indications and contraindications for use, routes of administration, and major adverse effects.

4. Discuss the 5-hydroxytryptamine$_3$ receptor antagonists in terms of indications and contraindications for use, routes of administration, and major adverse effects.

5. Describe the substance P/neurokinin 1 antagonist aprepitant in terms of indications and contraindications for use, routes of administration, and major adverse effects.

6. Identify the prototype drug for each drug class.

7. Identify nonpharmacologic measures to reduce nausea and vomiting.

8. Understand how to use the nursing process in the care of patients receiving drugs for the management of nausea and vomiting.

Clinical Application Case Study

Nellie Snyder is a 38-year-old woman with breast cancer who is receiving radiation and chemotherapy. She is experiencing significant nausea and vomiting.

KEY TERMS

Anticipatory nausea: conditioned response to chemotherapy or nausea in pregnancy that is triggered by fears of nausea and vomiting

Antiemetic: drug that is used to prevent or treat nausea and vomiting

Cannabinoid: derivative of marijuana

Chemoreceptor trigger zone: one of the central sites that relay stimuli to the vomiting center

Emesis: stomach contents produced with vomiting

Emetogenic: having the ability to cause vomiting

Motion sickness: action in which rapid changes in body motion stimulate receptors in the inner ear (vestibular branch of the auditory nerve, which is concerned with equilibrium), and nerve impulses are transmitted to the vomiting center.

Nausea: an unpleasant sensation of abdominal discomfort accompanied by a desire to vomit

Rescue antiemetic: antiemetic use after a prophylactic antiemetic drug regimen was unsuccessful in preventing emesis

Vomiting: expulsion of stomach contents through the mouth

Vomiting center: nucleus of cells in the medulla oblongata

Introduction

Nausea and vomiting are common symptoms experienced by virtually everyone at some time. **Nausea,** an unpleasant sensation of abdominal discomfort accompanied by a desire to vomit, may occur without vomiting, and **vomiting,** the expulsion of stomach contents through the mouth and occasionally nose, may occur without prior nausea, but the two symptoms often occur together. **Antiemetic** drugs are used to prevent or treat nausea and vomiting. They are usually contraindicated if their use may prevent or delay diagnosis or may mask signs and symptoms of drug toxicity.

Overview of Nausea and Vomiting

Etiology

Symptoms of nausea and vomiting may accompany almost any illness or stress situation. Causes of nausea and vomiting include the following:

- Gastrointestinal (GI) disorders, including infection or inflammation in the GI tract, liver, gallbladder, or pancreas; impaired GI motility and muscle tone (e.g., gastroparesis); and overeating or ingestion of foods or fluids that irritate the GI mucosa
- Cardiovascular, infectious, neurologic, or metabolic disorders
- Adverse effects of drug therapy; nausea and vomiting are the most common. Although the symptoms may occur with most drugs, they are especially associated with alcohol, aspirin, digoxin, anticancer drugs, antimicrobials, estrogen preparations, and opioid analgesics.
- Pain and other noxious stimuli, such as unpleasant sights and odors
- Emotional disturbances; physical or mental stress
- Radiation therapy
- Motion sickness
- Postoperative status, which may include pain, impaired GI motility, and receiving various medications
- Pregnancy
- Migraines

Pathophysiology

Vomiting occurs when the **vomiting center** (a nucleus of cells in the medulla oblongata) is stimulated (Fig. 36.1). Stimuli are relayed to the vomiting center by afferent signals from the **chemoreceptor trigger zone** (CTZ), as well as the cerebral cortex, the sensory organs, and the vestibular apparatus. The CTZ, composed of neurons in the fourth ventricle, can be activated by a variety of stimuli, including the presence of emetic substances (e.g., chemotherapy, opioids, ipecac) in the blood and cerebrospinal fluid and stimuli from the pharynx and GI tract. In cancer chemotherapy, **emetogenic** drugs are thought to stimulate the release of serotonin from the enterochromaffin cells of the small intestine; this released serotonin then activates 5-HT$_3$ receptors located on vagal afferent nerves in the CTZ to initiate the vomiting reflex. Activation of the CTZ is also thought to play a role in the nausea and vomiting associated with pregnancy. **Anticipatory nausea** triggered by memories and fear of nausea and vomiting is mediated by afferent signals from the higher centers of the cerebral cortex to the vomiting center. Noxious stimuli such as unpleasant odors or sights as well as pain are transmitted by afferent pathways from the sensory organs to the vomiting center. In **motion sickness**, rapid changes in body motion stimulate receptors in the inner ear (vestibular branch of the auditory nerve, which is concerned with equilibrium), and nerve impulses are transmitted to the vomiting center.

The vomiting center, CTZ, and GI tract contain benzodiazepine, cholinergic, dopamine, histamine, opiate, substance P/neurokinin, and serotonin receptors, which are stimulated by emetogenic drugs and toxins. When stimulated, the vomiting center initiates efferent impulses that stimulate the salivary center; cause closure of the glottis, contraction of abdominal muscles and the diaphragm, and relaxation of the gastroesophageal sphincter; and reverse peristalsis, which moves stomach contents toward the mouth for ejection.

Clinical Manifestations

As previously stated, nausea is an unpleasant abdominal sensation that is often, but not always, accompanied by vomiting. **Emesis** is the stomach contents produced with vomiting.

Drug Therapy

Antiemetic drugs are indicated to prevent and treat nausea and vomiting associated with surgery, pain, motion sickness, cancer chemotherapy, radiation therapy, pregnancy, and other causes. Drugs used to prevent or treat nausea and vomiting belong to several different therapeutic classifications and most have anticholinergic, antidopaminergic, antihistaminic, or antiserotonergic effects. In general, the drugs are more effective in prophylaxis than treatment. Most antiemetic agents are available in oral, parenteral, and rectal dosage forms. As a general rule, oral forms are preferred for prophylactic use, and rectal or parenteral forms are preferred for therapeutic use. When the nausea and vomiting associated with pregnancy are not controlled with lifestyle measures, some pharmacologic interventions may be appropriate. Most antiemetics prevent or relieve

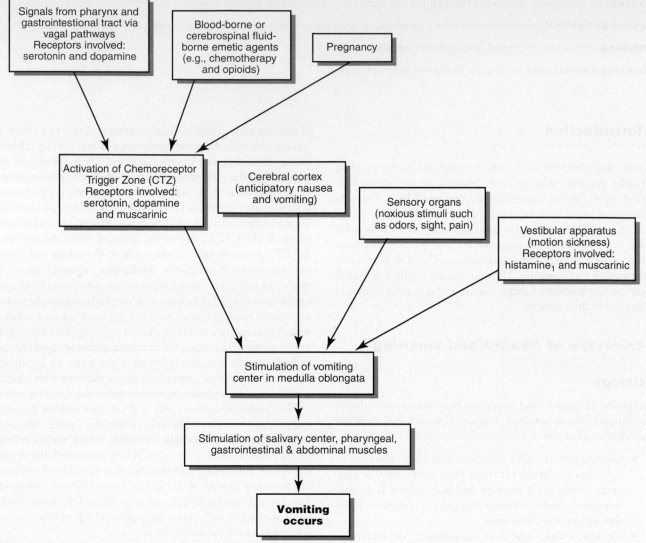

Figure 36.1 Pathophysiology of nausea and vomiting.

nausea and vomiting by acting on the vomiting center, CTZ, cerebral cortex, vestibular apparatus, or a combination of these. Table 36.1 describes major antiemetic drugs.

Phenothiazines

Phenothiazines are central nervous system (CNS) depressants that are used for a variety of reasons, including the prevention and treatment of nausea and vomiting. Dosage and route of administration depend primarily on the reason for use. Doses of phenothiazines are much smaller for antiemetic effects than for antipsychotic effects; not all phenothiazines are effective antiemetics. In this discussion, ⓟ **promethazine** (Phenergan), with its antiemetic action, serves as the prototype.

Pharmacokinetics

Promethazine is rapidly absorbed following oral administration and undergoes extensive first-pass metabolism in the

liver. Clinical effects are apparent within 20 minutes after oral, intramuscular, or rectal administration; the effects last 4 to 6 hours. Metabolism occurs in the liver, with excretion in the urine.

Action

Promethazine and other phenothiazines have widespread effects on the body. The therapeutic effects in nausea and vomiting are attributed to their ability to block dopamine from receptor sites in the brain and CTZ.

Use

Promethazine is used for the prevention and treatment of nausea and vomiting associated with surgery, anesthesia, migraines, chemotherapy, and motion sickness. Table 36.2 presents specific information about the use of promethazine and other phenothiazines, including dosages for adults and children.

EVIDENCE-BASED PRACTICE

Clinical management guidelines for obstetrician–gynecologists: Nausea and vomiting of pregnancy

by AMERICAN COLLEGE OF OBSTETRICIANS AND GYNECOLOGISTS.

2004, ACOG Practice Bulletin. Obstetrics and Gynecology, 103, 803–811

Although the cause of morning sickness remains largely unknown, effective treatments to prevent and manage the condition are available. Severe morning sickness (hyperemesis gravidarum) is the most common cause of hospitalization during early pregnancy and is the second most common reason for hospitalization during pregnancy (second only to preterm labor). Practice guidelines from the American College of Obstetricians and Gynecologists include the following evidence-based pharmacologic recommendations for treating nausea and vomiting during pregnancy:

- Taking a multivitamin at the time of conception may be effective in decreasing the severity of morning sickness.
- Taking pyridoxine (vitamin B_6) 30 to 75 mg daily in three divided doses with or without the antihistamine doxylamine 12.5 mg every 8 hours as needed is considered a first-line treatment option that is safe and effective.

IMPLICATIONS FOR NURSING PRACTICE: Nurses should be aware that pregnant women should not take any medication without the guidance of their health care provider. Some antiemetics are dangerous during pregnancy and can cause damage to the fetus. Lifestyle and dietary changes should be considered for treatment of mild cases. Prompt treatment of vomiting is more effective than managing long-term vomiting. See Chapter 6 for additional information on antiemetics used during pregnancy.

Use in Children

A **BLACK BOX WARNING** ◆ alerts nurses that promethazine is contraindicated in children younger than 2 years of age because of the risk of potentially fatal respiratory depression. Additionally, promethazine should not be used in children with hepatic disease, Reye's syndrome, a history of sleep apnea, or a family history of sudden infant death syndrome.

Use in Older Adults

Older adults may have increased concerns with the adverse anticholinergic effects (e.g., dizziness, acute confusion, delirium, dry mouth, tachycardia, blurred vision, urinary retention, constipation).

Use in Patients With Renal Impairment

A dose reduction may be necessary in patients with renal impairment to avoid the possibility of adverse effects, toxicity, or increased sensitivity to phenothiazines.

Use in Patients With Hepatic Impairment

Phenothiazines are metabolized in the liver. Therefore, the presence of liver disease (e.g., cirrhosis, hepatitis) may slow metabolism and prolong drug elimination half-life, with resultant accumulation and increased risk of adverse effects. Thus, the drugs should be used cautiously in patients with hepatic impairment. Cholestatic jaundice may occur with promethazine.

Adverse Effects

With promethazine, common side effects include blurred vision, urinary retention, dry mouth, photosensitivity, drowsiness, and confusion.

Contraindications

Contraindications to use of promethazine include known hypersensitivity to the drug. Cautious use is necessary in people with glaucoma because the drug possesses antimuscarinic activity.

Nursing Implications

Preventing Interactions

Several medications interact with promethazine, increasing its effects (Box 36.1). Herbal interactions with promethazine have been reported with kava kava, St. John's wort, and valerian; an increased risk of CNS depression is a possibility. No herbs or foods that decrease the effects of promethazine have been identified.

Administering the Medication

A **BLACK BOX WARNING** ◆ alerts nurses that promethazine is contraindicated for subcutaneous administration. The preferred route of administration is intramuscular, which reduces risk of surrounding muscle and tissue damage. However, the drug can cause pain at the injection site. The nurse avoid intravenous (IV) administration, if possible, because the drug can cause severe tissue injury.

Assessing for Therapeutic Effects

The nurse observes for prevention or resolution of nausea and vomiting.

Assessing for Adverse Effects

The nurse assesses for associated adverse anticholinergic effects (dry mouth, blurred vision, urinary retention, constipation, acute confusion, dizziness, tachycardia). It is necessary to be aware that hallucinations, convulsions, and sudden death may occur with excessive doses. The nurse also assesses tissue integrity with injection of the drug because the drug may cause severe tissue injury; burning and pain at the IV site justify immediate discontinuation of the drug.

TABLE 36.1

Drugs Administered for the Treatment of Nausea and Vomiting

Drug Class	Prototype	Other Drugs in the Class
Phenothiazines	Promethazine (Phenergan)	Chlorpromazine (Thorazine) Perphenazine (Trilafon) Prochlorperazine (Compazine)
Antihistamines	Hydroxyzine (Vistaril, Atarax)	Dimenhydrinate (Dramamine) Meclizine (Antivert, Bonine)
5-HT$_3$ (serotonin) receptor antagonists	Ondansetron (Zofran)	Dolasetron (Anzemet) Granisetron (Kytril) Palonosetron (Aloxi)
Substance P/neurokinin 1 receptor antagonist	Aprepitant (Emend)	
Miscellaneous agents		Dronabinol (Marinol) Phosphorated carbohydrate solution (Emetrol) Scopolamine (Transderm Scop)

Patient Teaching

The nurse teaches patients taking promethazine to use the lowest effective dosage and not to take other drugs with respiratory depressant effects concurrently. Box 36.2 presents additional patient teaching guidelines.

Other Drugs in the Class

Although phenothiazines are effective antiemetic agents, because of their adverse effects (e.g., sedation, cognitive impairment, extrapyramidal reactions), phenothiazines are mainly indicated if vomiting is severe and cannot be controlled by other measures or only when a few doses are needed. Prochlorperazine (Compazine), which has a side-effect profile similar to that of promethazine, is used in the treatment of severe nausea and vomiting associated with anesthesia. Chlorpromazine (Thorazine), which is more commonly used in the treatment of psychosis and psychotic symptoms in other disorders (see Chap. 55), is also used with intractable hiccups and treatment of nausea and vomiting associated with anesthesia. Perphenazine (Trilafon) is used to manage intractable hiccups and severe nausea and vomiting.

TABLE 36.2

DRUGS AT A GLANCE: Phenothiazines

Drug	Pregnancy Category	Routes and Dosage Ranges	
		Adults	*Children*
Ⓟ **Promethazine** (Phenergan)	C	PO, IM, IV, rectal suppository 12.5–25 mg every 4–6 h (max dose PO, IM, rectal 50 mg; IV 25 mg)	>2 y: PO, IM, IV rectal suppository 0.25–0.5 mg/kg every 4–6 h (max dose 25 mg); use lowest dose possible to prevent respiratory depression
Chlorpromazine (Thorazine)	C	PO 10–25 mg every 4–6 h IM, IV 25–50 mg every 4–6 h	>6 mo: PO 0.5–1 mg/kg per dose every 4–6 h; IM, IV 0.5–1 mg/kg per dose every 4–6 h <5 y: max 40 mg/d 5–12 y: max 75 mg/d
Perphenazine (Trilafon)	C	PO 8–16 mg daily in divided doses Max daily dose 24 mg if necessary IM 5 mg (deep), may repeat every 6 h	>12 y: PO 8 mg daily in divided doses. Early dose reduction is desirable. IM 5 mg (deep). May repeat every 6 h
Prochlorperazine (Compazine)	C	PO 5–10 mg 3 or 4 times daily (sustained-release capsule, 10 mg twice daily) IM 5–10 mg every 3–4 h to a maximum of 40 mg daily Rectal suppository 25 mg twice daily	>10 kg: PO 0.4 mg/kg/d, in 3 or 4 divided doses IM 0.2 mg/kg as a single dose Rectal suppository 0.4 mg/kg/d, in 3 or 4 divided doses

BOX 36.1 Drug Interactions: Promethazine

Drugs That Increase the Effects of Promethazine

- Escitalopram
  Has additive respiratory depressant effects
- Ethanol
  Increases the risk of central nervous system depression and psychomotor impairment
- Duloxetine
  Increases the plasma concentration
- Gabapentin
  Has additive respiratory depressant effects
- Zolpidem
  Has additive respiratory depressant effects

Antihistamines

Antihistamines are used primarily to prevent histamine from exerting its widespread effects on body tissues (see Chap. 30). Antihistamines used as antiemetic agents are the "classic" antihistamines or H_1 receptor blocking agents (as differentiated from cimetidine and related drugs, which are H_2 receptor blocking agents). Not all antihistamines are effective as antiemetic agents. Ⓟ **Hydroxyzine** (Vistaril, Atarax) is the prototype of the class.

Pharmacokinetics

When administered orally, hydroxyzine is rapidly absorbed from the GI tract, with its effect noticeable within 30 minutes.

The drug is metabolized in the liver, and the main metabolite is cetirizine. The half-life of hydroxyzine is, on average, 14 hours for adults, but it can be as short as 5 hours for small children and as long as 30 hours for elderly people. Hydroxyzine is excreted into the urine in the form of its metabolites.

Action

Hydroxyzine and other antihistamines are thought to relieve nausea and vomiting by blocking the action of acetylcholine in the brain.

Use

Hydroxyzine may be effective in treating nausea and vomiting and preventing and treating motion sickness. Hydroxyzine is also used as a sedative to treat anxiety. Additionally, the drug is given in combination with other medications during anesthesia. Table 36.3 presents dosage information for the antihistamines.

Use in Children

In children, the recommended dosage of hydroxyzine is based on age and weight.

Use in Older Adults

According to the Beers Criteria (see Chap. 5), hydroxyzine is considered potentially inappropriate for use in older adults. Dosage reduction may be appropriate with older adults due to an increased sedative potential.

BOX 36.2 Patient Teaching Guidelines: Antiemetic Drugs

General Considerations

- Try to identify the circumstances that cause or aggravate nausea and vomiting and avoid them when possible.
- Drugs are more effective in preventing nausea and vomiting than in stopping them. Thus, they should be taken before the causative event when possible.
- Do not eat, drink, or take oral medications during acute vomiting episodes, to avoid aggravating the stomach upset.
- Lying down may help nausea and vomiting to subside; activity tends to increase stomach upset.
- After your stomach has settled down, try to take enough fluids to prevent dehydration and potentially serious problems. Tea, broth, and gelatins are usually tolerated.
- Do not drive an automobile or operate dangerous machinery if drowsy from antiemetic drugs, to avoid injury.
- If you take antiemetic drugs regularly, do not drink alcohol or take other drugs without consulting a health care provider. Several drugs interact with antiemetic agents, to increase adverse effects.
- Dronabinol, which is derived from marijuana and recommended only for nausea and vomiting associated with cancer chemotherapy, can cause dizziness,

drowsiness, mood changes, and other mind-altering effects. You should avoid alcohol and other drugs that cause drowsiness. Also, do not drive or perform hazardous tasks requiring alertness, coordination, or physical dexterity, to decrease risks of injury.

Self- or Caregiver Administration

- Take the drugs as prescribed. Do not increase dosage, take more often, or take when drowsy, dizzy, or unsteady on your feet. Several of the drugs cause sedation and other adverse effects, which are more severe if too much is taken.
- To prevent motion sickness, take medication 30 minutes before travel and then every 4 to 6 hours, if necessary, to avoid or minimize adverse effects.
- Take or give antiemetic drugs 30 to 60 minutes before a nausea-producing event, when possible. This includes cancer chemotherapy, radiation therapy, changing of painful dressings, or other treatments.
- Take dronabinol only when you can be supervised by a responsible adult because of its sedative and mind-altering effects.
- Aprepitant (Emend) reduces the effectiveness of oral contraceptives; therefore, use an alternative form of birth control during therapy and for 1 month after therapy.

TABLE 36.3

DRUGS AT A GLANCE: Antihistamines

Drug	Pregnancy Category	Routes and Dosage Ranges	
		Adults	*Children*
Ⓟ **Hydroxyzine** (Vistaril, Atarax)	D	IM 25–100 mg every 4–6 h as needed	IM 0.5–1 mg/kg every 4–6 h
Dimenhydrinate (Dramamine)	B	PO 50–100 mg every 4–6 h as needed (max 400 mg in 24 h) IM 50 mg as needed IV 50 mg in 10 mL of sodium chloride injection, over 2 min	6–12 y: PO 25–50 mg every 4–6 h (max 150 mg in 24 h) IM 1.25 mg/kg 4 times daily (max 300 mg in 24 h)
Meclizine (Antivert, Bonine)	B	Motion sickness: PO 25–50 mg 1 h before travel Vertigo: PO 25–100 mg daily in divided doses	Motion sickness, >12 y: PO 25–50 mg/d divided into 2 or 3 doses

Use in Patients With Renal Impairment

Because hydroxyzine is excreted in the urine, dosage adjustments and more intensive monitoring of adverse effects may be required in people with renal impairment.

Use in Patients With Hepatic Impairment

Likewise, because hydroxyzine is metabolized in the liver, dosage adjustments and more intensive monitoring of adverse effects may be required in people with hepatic impairment.

Use in Patients Receiving Home Care

Antiemetics are usually given orally or by rectal suppository in the home setting. The home care nurse may need to assess patients for possible causes of nausea and vomiting and assist patients and caregivers with appropriate use of the drugs and other interventions to prevent fluid and electrolyte depletion. Excessive sedation may occur with usual doses of antiemetics and is more likely with high doses. This may be minimized by avoiding high doses and assessing the patient's level of consciousness before each dose. Teaching safety precautions with sedating drugs may also be needed.

Adverse Effects

With hydroxyzine, adverse anticholinergic effects include drowsiness, dizziness, confusion, dry mouth, thickened respiratory secretions, blurred vision, urinary retention, and tachycardia.

Contraindications

Contraindications to hydroxyzine include known sensitivity to the drug.

Nursing Implications

Preventing Interactions

Many medications interact with hydroxyzine, increasing its effects (Box 36.3). Several medications that can cause CNS depression, such as sedatives, tranquilizers, muscle relaxants, and antidepressants, can have an increased sedative effect with the concomitant use of hydroxyzine. No herbs or foods appear to decrease or increase the effects of hydroxyzine.

Administering the Medication

Oral administration of hydroxyzine is often unsuccessful with nausea and vomiting. It is important to give the medication intramuscularly deep into a large muscle, not subcutaneously. IV administration can result in a sterile abscess with damage to tissue.

Assessing for Therapeutic Effects

The nurse assesses for the absence of nausea and vomiting.

Assessing for Adverse Effects

The nurse assesses for the presence of anticholinergic effects, including blurred vision, urinary retention, constipation, thick secretions, and blurred vision. Patients with narrow-angle glaucoma, prostatic hyperplasia, and asthma are at greater risk for adverse effects.

Patient Teaching

The nurse instructs patients to take medication as directed and to enhance safety precautions due to adverse effects. Adverse effects may impair thinking or reactions, so operating a motor vehicle should be avoided. Box 36.2 outlines additional patient teaching guidelines.

BOX 36.3 | Drug Interactions: Hydroxyzine

Drugs That Increase the Effects of Hydroxyzine

■ Alcohol
  Increases the risk of respiratory depression
■ Gabapentin, levetiracetam, lamotrigine
  Increase the risk of respiratory depression
■ Seroquel
  Increases the risk of severe extrapyramidal reactions

Other Drugs in the Class

Dimenhydrinate (Dramamine) and meclizine (Antivert, Bonine) are used to prevent nausea, vomiting, dizziness, and vertigo associated with motion sickness. Meclizine is also given to manage vertigo associated with disease affecting the vestibular system. Dimenhydrinate is available over-the-counter, and meclizine is dispensed by prescription.

The initial dose should be taken 1 hour prior to travel to reduce the risk of motion sickness. Thereafter, the dose may be repeated every 24 hours for the duration of the travel. For vestibular diseases, meclizine should be taken at the onset of symptoms. As with hydroxyzine, it is necessary to instruct patients taking dimenhydrinate to use caution while driving, operating machinery, or performing other hazardous activities due to the associated drowsiness. (The addition of theophylline to the formulation is designed to counteract drowsiness.) Dimenhydrinate typically takes a minimum of 4 hours to take full effect. Meclizine becomes effective in about 1 hour. The drug is less likely to cause drowsiness, but people taking the drug should use caution when participating in hazardous activities and avoid using alcohol.

NCLEX Success

1. **The nurse knows that antiemetics are most effective when administered**

   A. before an emetogenic event occurs

   B. during an episode of nausea but before vomiting has occurred

   C. after the patient has experienced nausea and vomiting

   D. timing of administration has no impact on drug effectiveness

2. **The nurse would question an order for which of the following antiemetics for treatment of motion sickness–induced nausea?**

   A. prochlorperazine (Compazine)

   B. dimenhydrinate (Dramamine)

   C. meclizine (Antivert)

   D. scopolamine (Transderm Scop)

5-Hydroxytryptamine$_3$ (5-HT$_3$) or Serotonin Receptor Antagonists

The 5-HT$_3$ receptor antagonists are usually considered drugs of first choice for postoperative nausea and vomiting. Ⓟ **Ondansetron** (Zofran) is the prototype of the 5-HT$_3$ receptor antagonists.

Pharmacokinetics

Oral ondansetron is well absorbed from the GI tract and undergoes some first-pass metabolism. The drug's half-life is 3 to 5.5 hours in most patients and 9 to 20 hours in patients with moderate or severe liver impairment. With the oral form, action begins in 30 to 60 minutes and peaks in about 2 hours. With the IV form, onset and peak of drug action are immediate. The bioavailability is slightly increased by the presence of food but is unaffected by antacids.

Action

Ondansetron and the other 5-HT$_3$ receptor antagonists antagonize serotonin receptors, preventing their activation by the effects of emetogenic drugs and toxins.

Use

Ondansetron is used to prevent or treat moderate to severe nausea and vomiting associated with cancer chemotherapy, radiation therapy, and postoperative status. Table 36.4 presents dosage information for the 5-HT$_3$ receptor antagonists.

Use in Children

The drug is indicated for use in children, although little information is available about its use in children younger than 6 months of age. The American Society of Clinical Oncology recommends the use of a 5-HT$_3$ receptor antagonist plus a corticosteroid before administering high-dose chemotherapy or chemotherapy with high to moderate emetic risk to pediatric oncology patients.

Use in Older Adults

Dosage adjustment is not required in patients older than 65 years of age. Researchers have observed no overall differences in safety or effectiveness in older adults compared with younger patients.

Use in Patients With Hepatic Impairment

The drug's half-life is significantly increased in patients with moderate to severe hepatic impairment. This increases the risk of adverse effects.

Use in Patients Receiving Home Care

Oral administration of the drug may be given in the home setting. The home care nurse assesses for resolution of nausea and vomiting. Diarrhea is a common adverse effect; therefore, the nurse also needs to assist patients and caregivers with appropriate use of the drugs and other interventions to prevent fluid and electrolyte depletion.

Adverse Effects

Adverse effects of ondansetron are usually mild to moderate. Common ones include diarrhea, headache, dizziness, constipation, fatigue, transient elevation of liver enzymes, and pain at the injection site.

Contraindications

Contraindications to ondansetron include known hypersensitivity to the drug.

TABLE 36.4

DRUGS AT A GLANCE: 5-Hydroxytryptamine₃ (5-HT₃ or Serotonin) Receptor Antagonists

Drug	Pregnancy Category	Routes and Dosage Ranges	
		Adults	Children
Ⓟ **Ondansetron** (Zofran)	B	Chemotherapy-induced nausea and vomiting (highly emetogenic chemotherapy): PO, 24 mg, given ½ h before start of single-day chemotherapy, IV 0.15 mg/kg for 3 doses given ½ h before chemotherapy, repeat in 4 and 8 h; IV 32 mg as a single dose. Infuse over 15 min. Chemotherapy-induced nausea and vomiting (moderately emetogenic chemotherapy): PO, 8 mg for two doses, given ½ h before chemotherapy, repeat in 8 h Postoperative nausea and vomiting: PO 16 mg 1 h before anesthesia, IV 4 mg given over 2–5 min, IM 4 mg	Chemotherapy-induced nausea and vomiting: 6–18 mo: IV 0.15 mg/kg for 3 doses, given ½ h before chemotherapy, repeat in 4 and 8 h. Infuse over 15 min. 4–11 y: PO 4 mg given for 3 doses ½ h before chemotherapy, repeat in 8 and 16 h ≥12 y: PO dosage same as adults Postoperative nausea and vomiting 1 mo–12 y: ≤40 kg–IV 0.1 mg/kg ≤40 kg: IV 4 mg. Given over 2–5 min
Dolasetron (Anzemet)	C	Chemotherapy-induced nausea and vomiting: PO, 100 mg, given up to 1 h prior to chemotherapy Postoperative nausea and vomiting: IV 12.5 mg 15 min before reversal of anesthesia, PO 100 mg within 2 h prior to surgery	Chemotherapy-induced nausea and vomiting (>2 y): PO 1.8 mg/kg (max 100 mg) given up to 1 h prior to chemotherapy Postoperative nausea and vomiting (>2 y): IV 0.35 mg/kg (max 12.5 mg) 15 min before the reversal of anesthesia or with nausea or vomiting PO 1.2 mg/kg (max 100 mg) within 2 h prior to surgery
Granisetron (Kytril)	B	Chemotherapy-induced nausea and vomiting: IV, 10 µg/kg over 5 min, beginning ½ h prior to chemotherapy PO, 2 mg, given up to 1 h prior to chemotherapy, or 1 mg given up to 1 h prior to chemotherapy and repeated in 12 h Radiation-induced nausea and vomiting: PO 2 mg given up to 1 h prior to radiation Postoperative nausea and vomiting: IV 1 mg undiluted immediately before induction or reversal or after surgery	Chemotherapy-induced nausea and vomiting (2–16 y) IV 10 mcg/kg beginning ½ h prior to chemotherapy
Palonosetron (Aloxi)	B	Chemotherapy-induced nausea and vomiting: PO 0.5 mg Postoperative nausea and vomiting: IV 0.075 mg as a single dose immediately prior to induction of anesthesia	Chemotherapy-induced nausea and vomiting (>2 y): 3 mcg/kg (max 0.25 mg)

Nursing Implications

Preventing Interactions

Phenytoin, carbamazepine, rifampin, and other inducers of the cytochrome 450 (CYP) 3A4 enzymes increase the clearance of ondansetron and decrease serum concentrations. No dosage adjustment of ondansetron appears necessary for people taking these drugs based on available data. The use of ondansetron with apomorphine is contraindicated due to the potential of a significant drop of blood pressure or loss of consciousness with concurrent use. St. John's wort may decrease ondansetron levels.

Administering the Medication

It is important not to remove the tablet from the blister pack until administration. Gentle removal is essential; it is necessary to peel back the blister backing and not push the tablet through the foil.

Assessing for Therapeutic Effects

The nurse assesses for verbal reports of decreased nausea and the absence of vomiting.

Assessing for Adverse Effects

Because headache and diarrhea are the most common adverse effects, the nurse gives special attention when assessing for these effects. It is also necessary to evaluate for stamina and balance. The nurse should note that use of ondansetron may mask a progressive ileus and gastric distension following abdominal surgery or in patients with chemotherapy-induced nausea and vomiting.

Patient Teaching

The drug may impair thinking or reactions, which means that it is necessary to advise patients to use caution with driving or other tasks requiring mental alertness. The nurse teaches patients with phenylketonuria that the oral disintegrating tablets contain phenylalanine. Box 36.2 presents other patient teaching guidelines.

Other Drugs in the Class

Granisetron and dolasetron may be given intravenously or orally. The safety and efficacy of these drugs have not been established for children younger than 2 years of age.

Palonosetron is given only intravenously. The safety and efficacy of this drug has not been confirmed in patients younger than 18 years of age.

Clinical Application 36-1

- Ms. Snyder's oncologist orders ondansetron 32 mg IV to be administered 30 minutes prior to her chemotherapy and 8 to 16 mg PO every 8 hours as needed. She also receives metoclopramide 10 mg PO four times a day (30 minutes before meals and at bedtime). For what adverse effects of ondansetron does the nurse assess?

Substance P/Neurokinin 1 Antagonist: Aprepitant

Substance P is a peptide neurotransmitter in the neurokinin family. It plays a role in mediating acute chemotherapy-induced nausea and vomiting (along with serotonin) and is believed to be the primary mediator of delayed nausea and vomiting associated with chemotherapy. ℗ **Aprepitant** (Emend), the prototype of the class, is the only approved substance P/neurokinin 1 antagonist.

Pharmacokinetics

Aprepitant is orally absorbed, reaching peak levels 4 hours after administration. It is highly protein bound. The drug is metabolized in the liver and is excreted in urine and feces. Because aprepitant undergoes extensive hepatic metabolism by CYP450 enzyme systems, it has the potential for multiple drug interactions. After administration, the IV form, fosaprepitant, is rapidly converted in the body to aprepitant.

Action

Aprepitant exerts its antiemetic effect by blocking the activity of substance P at NK_1 receptors in the brain, inhibiting the signal to the brain that causes nausea. The drug has little or no effect on serotonin, dopamine, or corticosteroid receptors.

Use

Prescribers often order aprepitant as part of combination therapy along with a 5-HT_3 receptor antagonist and corticosteroids to treat both acute and delayed nausea and vomiting associated with chemotherapy. Other indications include prevention of postoperative nausea and vomiting. The U.S. Food and Drug Administration (FDA) has stipulated that the IV prodrug of the oral formulation (fosaprepitant) should no longer be used to prevent nausea and vomiting associated with cancer chemotherapy in pediatric and adult patients due to the risk of abnormal heart rhythm.

Table 36.5 contains dosage information for aprepitant. No dosage adjustment is required in patients with renal disease, including those with end-stage renal disease receiving dialysis.

Use in Children

Aprepitant appears to be well-tolerated in children receiving the drug in combination with standard antiemetics for chemotherapy-induced nausea and vomiting. Additional evidence of efficacy is necessary in this population.

Use in Patients With Hepatic Impairment

No adjustment is required in dosage for patients with mild to moderate hepatic impairment. However, no data are available regarding use in people with severe hepatic impairment, and caution is warranted in cases of serious hepatic dysfunction.

Use in Patients With Critical Illness

Aprepitant is used in patients with cancer who are receiving chemotherapy. The American Society of Clinical Oncology's antiemetic guidelines recommend the use of aprepitant in combination with a serotonin receptor antagonist and dexamethasone with chemotherapeutic drugs with high emetic risk. The drug is also recommended as part of a chemotherapy regimen in protocols including anthracycline, cyclophosphamide, and other chemotherapeutic agents known to cause moderate emetic risk.

Adverse Effects

Aprepitant is well tolerated, with the most common adverse effects being fatigue, weakness, dizziness, abnormal heart rhythm, headache, and hiccups. Infusion site pain has been reported with IV administration.

TABLE 36.5

DRUGS AT A GLANCE: Substance P/Neurokinin 1 Receptor Antagonist

Drug	Pregnancy Category	Routes and Dosage Ranges	
		Adults	Children
Ⓟ **Aprepitant** (Emend, Fosaprepitant Dimeglumine)	B	Prevention of nausea and vomiting associated with highly emetic and moderately emetic chemotherapy (administered as part of a three-drug treatment that also includes a serotonin receptor antagonist and dexamethasone): Day 1: PO 125 mg 1 h before chemotherapy or IV 115 mg ½ h over 15 min before chemotherapy Day 2, 3: PO 80 mg in the morning	Dosage not established

EVIDENCE-BASED PRACTICE

American Society of Clinical Oncology Guideline for Antiemetics in Oncology: Update 2006.

by KRIS, M. G., HESKETH, P. J., SOMERFIELD, M. R., FEYER, P., CLARK-SNOW, R., KOELLER, J. M., MORROW, G. R., CHINNERY, L. W., CHESNEY, M. J., GRALLA, R. J., & GRUNBERG, S. M

Journal of Clinical Oncology, 2006, 24, 1–16.

The American Society of Clinical Oncology has updated its 1999 guidelines regarding the use of antiemetics in oncology. The current recommendations stem from a panel's review of the literature, including randomized controlled trials, systematic reviews, and meta-analyses. The three-drug combination of a 5-HT₃ serotonin receptor antagonist, aprepitant, and dexamethasone is recommended before chemotherapy of high emetic risk. The three-drug combination is also recommended for patients receiving anthracycline and cyclophosphamide. For patients receiving other chemotherapy of moderate emetic risk, the two-drug combination of a 5-HT₃ receptor serotonin antagonist and dexamethasone continues to be recommended. Additionally, for the prevention of delayed vomiting, the group recommends that all patients receiving cisplatin and all other agents of high emetic risk receive the two-drug combination of dexamethasone and aprepitant; the combination of a 5-HT₃ serotonin receptor antagonist and dexamethasone is no longer recommended.

IMPLICATIONS FOR NURSING PRACTICE: Emetic risk categories and other characteristics guide the drug regimens used to prevent chemotherapy-induced vomiting. The recommendations serve as a framework for clinical decision making and are used along with consideration of individual variations among people.

Contraindications

Contraindications to aprepitant include known hypersensitivity to the drug or use in combination with ranolazine, pimozide, or cisapride.

Nursing Implications

Preventing Interactions

Certain drugs may increase or decrease the effects of aprepitant (Box 36.4). It is essential to reduce oral doses of dexamethasone or methylprednisolone by 50% and the IV dose of methylprednisolone by 25% when coadministered with aprepitant due to CYP3A4 inhibition.

Aprepitant also produces significant interactions that alter the effectiveness of other medications. The drug reduces the effectiveness of oral contraceptives for up to 28 days after administration; therefore, alternate contraceptive methods are recommended during treatment and for 1 month following administration of aprepitant.

QSEN Safety Alert ❗

Aprepitant induces the metabolism of warfarin. It is necessary to monitor the international normalized ratio for 2 weeks after treatment is initiated, especially for the first 7 to 10 days.

BOX 36.4 **Drug Interactions: Aprepitant**

Drugs That Increase the Effects of Aprepitant
■ CYP3A4 inhibitors, such as macrolide antibiotics, protease inhibitors, azole antifungal agents, nefazodone, cyclosporine, danazol, diltiazem, and verapamil
Alter metabolism, increasing serum levels

Drugs That Decrease the Effects of Aprepitant
■ CYP3A4 inducers, such as carbamazepine, phenytoin, rifampin, phenobarbital, and nevirapine
Alter metabolism, decreasing serum levels

Foods and herbs are also known to affect aprepitant concentrations. Grapefruit juice increases the serum levels of aprepitant. St. John's wort is known to cause a decrease in serum levels.

Administering the Medication

Patients should take aprepitant by mouth as directed with a full glass of water, with or without food. Typically, they take the first dose is taken 1 hour before chemotherapy and then daily in the morning for the next 2 days after the chemotherapy treatment. The recently approved IV form (fosaprepitant), as a dose of 115 mg, is bioequivalent to aprepitant, 125 mg, and it is appropriate to use these forms interchangeably.

Assessing for Therapeutic Effects

The nurse assesses for the absence of nausea and vomiting after chemotherapy or during the postoperative period.

Assessing for Adverse Effects

The nurse observes for the presence of adverse effects, such as fatigue, weakness, dizziness, headache, or hiccups. Additionally, it is necessary to assess for a normal heart rhythm.

Patient Teaching

The nurse instructs patients to take the medication as prescribed before the onset of nausea and vomiting. Alternate antiemetic medication (**rescue antiemetic**) may be necessary for who already have nausea and vomiting. Box 36.2 presents additional patient teaching guidelines.

Miscellaneous Antiemetics

Several miscellaneous agents are used individually or in multidrug regimens in treatment of nausea and vomiting. Table 36.6 presents the dosage information for the miscellaneous agents.

Although corticosteroids are used mainly as antiallergic, anti-inflammatory, and antistress agents (see Chap. 15), they have antiemetic effects as well. The mechanism by which the drugs exert antiemetic effects is unknown; they may block prostaglandin activity in the cerebral cortex. Dexamethasone and methylprednisolone are commonly used in the management of chemotherapy-induced emesis and postoperative nausea and vomiting, either alone or in combination with 5-HT$_3$ receptor antagonists and/or substance P/neurokinin 1 receptor antagonists. With short-term use, adverse effects associated with corticosteroids are mild (e.g., euphoria, insomnia, mild fluid retention).

Benzodiazepine antianxiety drugs (see Chap. 53) are not antiemetics, but they are often used in multidrug regimens to prevent nausea and vomiting associated with cancer chemotherapy. The drugs produce relaxation, relieve anxiety, and inhibit cerebral cortex input to the vomiting center. They are often prescribed for patients who experience anticipatory nausea and vomiting before administration of anticancer drugs. Lorazepam (Ativan) is commonly used for this purpose.

Dronabinol is a **cannabinoid** (derivative of marijuana) used in the management of nausea and vomiting associated with anticancer drugs and unrelieved by other drugs. Onset of action occurs within 12 hours, with peak intensity within 24 hours and dissipation within 96 hours. Dronabinol has the same adverse effects as marijuana, including psychiatric symptoms, and a high potential for abuse. In addition, it may cause a withdrawal syndrome when abruptly discontinued. Thus, it is a Schedule III drug under federal narcotic laws. Withdrawal symptoms (e.g., insomnia, irritability, restlessness) are most likely to occur with high doses or prolonged use, and sleep disturbances may persist for several weeks.

Marijuana cigarettes, although illegal in most states and under federal law, have been used by some people to treat chemotherapy-induced nausea and vomiting. The National Cancer Institute's Fact Sheet on Marijuana Use in Supportive Care for Cancer Patients addresses concerns surrounding lack of consistent effect due to varying potency of marijuana and points out the

TABLE 36.6

DRUGS AT A GLANCE: Miscellaneous Agents

Drug	Pregnancy Category	Routes and Dosage Ranges	
		Adults	Children
Dronabinol (Marinol)	C	PO 5 mg/m² (square meter of body surface area) 1–3 h before chemotherapy, then every 2–4 h for a total of 4–6 doses daily. Dosage can be increased by 2.5 mg/m² increments to a maximal dose of 15 mg/m² if necessary.	Same as adults for treatment of chemotherapy-induced nausea and vomiting
Phosphorated carbohydrate solution (Emetrol)	C	PO 15–30 mL repeated at 15-min intervals until vomiting ceases	PO 5–10 mL repeated at 15-min intervals until vomiting ceases
Scopolamine (Transderm Scop)	C	Motion sickness: PO, IM, subcutaneous, 0.3–0.6 mg as a single dose Transdermal disc (1.5 mg scopolamine): placed behind the ear every 3 d if needed	Motion sickness: PO, subcutaneous, 0.006 mg as a single dose

need for additional research concerning the use of marijuana for supportive care. In addition, it promotes the opinion that currently available antiemetic drugs are more effective for management of chemotherapy-induced nausea and vomiting.

Phosphorated carbohydrate solution (Emetrol) is a hyperosmolar solution with phosphoric acid. This drug is thought to reduce smooth muscle contraction in the GI tract and is available as an over-the-counter medication in syrup form.

QSEN Safety Alert

Because this solution contains fructose, patients with diabetes mellitus should consult their health care provider before using it.

Scopolamine, an anticholinergic drug (see Chap. 47), is effective in relieving nausea and vomiting associated with motion sickness and radiation therapy. It is available as a transdermal patch, which is often used to prevent motion sickness.

NCLEX Success

3. When administering 5-HT3 receptor antagonists before cancer chemotherapy, the nurse should also be prepared to administer which of the following adjunctive medications?

 A. promethazine
 B. dexamethasone
 C. dronabinol
 D. hydroxyzine

4. A woman sends her partner to the store to purchase an over-the-counter product to resolve the vomiting she has experienced during a migraine. She has a history of diabetes mellitus and hypertension. She has an appointment with her health care provider in the morning. Which of the following drugs would be the best for the partner to purchase?

 A. promethazine (Phenergan)
 B. phosphorated carbohydrate solution (Emetrol)
 C. meclizine (Antivert)
 D. dimenhydrinate (Dramamine)

Clinical Application 36-2

■ Ms. Snyder is concerned about the amount of medication she is receiving. She asks the nurse to withhold her antiemetics until she actually vomits. What is the best way to respond to Ms. Snyder?

Nonpharmacologic Management

Nonpharmacologic techniques have become an acceptable adjunct to antiemetic drug therapy. The use of herbal supplements has also received support.

Acupuncture and Acupressure

Of all the nonpharmacologic techniques, acupuncture is one of the most well-studied and accepted forms of treatment of postoperative nausea and vomiting, although the mechanism remains unclear. The use of acupressure wristbands has also been useful in the treatment of nausea and vomiting associated with motion sickness.

Herbal Supplements

The use of ginger in traditional Chinese and Indian medicine has a long history. Clinical trials indicate that the herb can effectively reduce nausea and vomiting associated with motion sickness, pregnancy, and surgery. Evidence of the herb's success against chemotherapy-induced nausea and vomiting is mixed. The herb's components are thought to interact with 5-HT$_3$ receptors, which may account for the antiemetic activity.

The Nursing Process

Assessment

- Identify risk factors for nausea and vomiting (e.g., digestive or other disorders in which nausea and vomiting are symptoms; drugs associated with nausea and vomiting).
- Interview regarding frequency, duration, and precipitating causes of nausea and vomiting. Also, question the patient about accompanying signs and symptoms, characteristics of vomitus (amount; color; odor; presence of abnormal components, such as blood), and any measures that relieve nausea and vomiting. When possible, observe and measure the vomitus.

Nursing Diagnoses

- Deficient fluid volume related to uncontrolled vomiting
- Imbalanced nutrition: less than body requirements related to impaired ability to ingest and digest food
- Altered tissue perfusion: hypotension related to fluid volume depletion or antiemetic drug effect
- Risk for injury related to adverse drug effects
- Deficient knowledge related to nondrug measures to reduce nausea and vomiting and appropriate use of antiemetic drugs

Planning/Goals

The patient will

- Receive antiemetic drugs at appropriate times, by indicated routes
- Take antiemetic drugs as prescribed for outpatient use
- Obtain relief of nausea and vomiting
- Eat and retain food and fluids
- Have increased comfort
- Maintain body weight
- Maintain normal bowel elimination patterns
- Have fewer vomiting episodes and less discomfort with cancer chemotherapy or surgical procedures

Nursing Interventions

The nurse will

- Use measures to prevent or minimize nausea and vomiting
- Assist patients to identify situations that cause or aggravate nausea and vomiting
- Avoid exposure to stimuli when feasible (e.g., unpleasant sights and odors; excessive ingestion of food, alcohol, or nonsteroidal anti-inflammatory drugs)
- Administer analgesics before painful diagnostic tests and dressing changes or other therapeutic measures may be helpful, as pain may cause nausea and vomiting
- Administer antiemetic drugs 30 to 60 minutes before a nausea-producing event, when possible (e.g., radiation therapy, cancer chemotherapy, travel)
- Adjust the timing of any oral drugs that causes gastric irritation, nausea, and vomiting by taking with or just after food. For any drug likely to cause nausea and vomiting, check reference sources to determine whether it can be given with food without altering beneficial effects.
- Assess the patient's condition and report to the health care provider if nausea and vomiting occur. In some instances, a drug (e.g., digoxin, an antibiotic) may need to be discontinued or reduced in dosage. In other instances (e.g., paralytic ileus, GI obstruction), preferred treatment is restriction of oral intake and nasogastric intubation.
- Suggest that a woman eat dry crackers before rising in the morning and ingestion of small frequent protein meals to help prevent nausea and vomiting associated with pregnancy.
- Avoid administering oral intake of food, fluids, and drugs during acute episodes of nausea and vomiting. Oral intake may increase vomiting and risks of fluid and electrolyte imbalances.
- Minimize activity during acute episodes of nausea and vomiting. Lying down and resting quietly are often helpful.

- Give supportive care during vomiting episodes
- Give replacement fluids and electrolytes. Offer small amounts of food and fluids orally when tolerated and according to patient preference.
- Record vital signs, intake and output, and body weight at regular intervals if nausea or vomiting occurs frequently
- Decrease environmental stimuli when possible (e.g., noise, odors). Allow the patient to lie quietly in bed when nauseated. Decreasing motion may decrease stimulation of the vomiting center in the brain.
- Help the patient rinse his or her mouth after vomiting. Rinsing decreases the bad taste and corrosion of tooth enamel caused by gastric acid.
- Provide requested home remedies when possible (e.g., a cool, wet washcloth to the face and neck)
- Provide appropriate education for any drug therapy (see Box 36.2)

Evaluation

- Observe and interview for decreased nausea and vomiting.
- Observe and interview regarding ability to maintain adequate intake of food and fluids.
- Compare current weight with baseline weight.
- Observe and interview regarding appropriate use of antiemetic drugs.

Clinical Application 36-3

- What nursing measures, in addition to the administration of antiemetic medication, should the nurse suggest to Ms. Snyder to reduce her nausea and vomiting?

Key Concepts

- Antiemetic drugs are used to prevent or treat nausea and vomiting associated with surgery, pain, motion sickness, cancer chemotherapy, radiation therapy, pregnancy, and other causes.
- Antiemetic drugs are most effective when given before nausea and vomiting occurs.
- The vomiting center, CTZ, and GI tract contain benzodiazepine, cholinergic (muscarinic), dopamine, histamine, opiate, substance P/neurokinin, and serotonin receptors that are stimulated by emetogenic drugs and toxins. Antiemetic drugs produce their effects by blockade of one or more of these receptors.
- The antiemetic effect of phenothiazines such as prochlorperazine and promethazine is due to blockade of dopamine receptors in the brain and CTZ. They are used to treat nausea induced by drugs, radiation therapy, surgery, and other stimuli but are considered ineffective in motion sickness.
- The FDA has issued a **BLACK BOX WARNING** ◆ stating that promethazine is contraindicated in children younger than 2 years of age because of the risk of potentially fatal respiratory depression.
- A **BLACK BOX WARNING** ◆ alerts nurses that promethazine is contraindicated for subcutaneous administration. The preferred route of administration is intramuscular, which reduces the risk of surrounding muscle and tissue damage.

- Classic H_1-blocking antihistamine drugs such as dimenhydrinate are thought to produce an antiemetic effect due to their anticholinergic properties. Antihistamines are used to prevent and treat nausea and vomiting due to motion sickness.

- The antiemetic mechanism of action of corticosteroids such as dexamethasone and methylprednisolone is unknown. These drugs are commonly used alone or in combination with 5-HT_3 serotonin receptor antagonists and/or substance P/neurokinin 1 receptor antagonists in the management of chemotherapy-induced emesis and postoperative nausea and vomiting.

- 5-HT_3 serotonin receptor antagonists such as odansetron, granisetron, dolasetron, and palonosetron antagonize serotonin receptors, preventing their activation by emetogenic drugs and toxins. They are used to prevent and treat moderate to severe nausea associated with cancer chemotherapy, radiation therapy, and postoperative conditions.

- Substance P, a peptide neurotransmitter in the neurokinin family, plays a role in acute and delayed chemotherapy-induced nausea and vomiting. Aprepitant antagonizes the neurokinin 1 receptor, preventing activation by emetogenic chemotherapeutic drugs.

- Benzodiazepines such as lorazepam produce relaxation, relieve anxiety, and inhibit cerebral cortex input to the vomiting center. They are prescribed for anticipatory nausea associated with cancer chemotherapy.

- Dronabinol is a cannabinoid used in the management of nausea and vomiting associated with chemotherapy unrelieved by other antiemetic drugs. It is a Schedule III drug under federal narcotic laws.

- Scopolamine is an anticholinergic drug effective in relieving nausea and vomiting associated with motion sickness and radiation therapy for cancer.

Critical Thinking Questions

36-1. Carol Brown, a 27-year-old teacher, is in her 10th week of pregnancy and has had mild nausea and vomiting for the past month. She presents for her second prenatal visit and asks for something to treat her morning sickness. The nurse midwife places her on vitamin B_6 25 mg three times a day plus doxylamine 12.5 mg three times a day. Ms. Brown asks if these medications are safe for her baby. She also asks if she should wait a few weeks to see if the symptoms go away on their own.

- How should the nurse respond?

References and Resources

American College of Obstetricians and Gynecologists. (2004). ACOG Practice Bulletin. Clinical management guidelines for obstetrician-gynecologists: Nausea and vomiting of pregnancy. *Obstetrics and Gynecology, 103,* 803–811.

Choi, M. R., Jiles, C., & Seibel, N. L. (2010). Aprepitant use in children, adolescents, and young adults for the control of chemotherapy-induced nausea and vomiting (CINV). *Journal of Pediatric Hematology/Oncology, 32*(7), 268–271.

DiPiro, J. T., Talbert, R. L., Yee, G. C., Matzke, G. R., Wells, B. G., & Posey, L. M. (Eds.). (2008). *Pharmacotherapy: A Pathophysiologic Approach* (7th ed.). New York: McGraw-Hill.

Drug facts and comparisons. (Updated monthly). St. Louis, MO: Facts and Comparisons.

Karch, A. M. (2012). *2012 Lippincott's nursing drug guide.* Philadelphia, PA: Lippincott Williams & Wilkins.

Kris, M. G., Hesketh, P. J., Somerfield, M. R., Feyer, P., Clark-Snow, R., Koeller, J. M., et al. (2006). American Society of Clinical Oncology: Guideline for antiemetics in oncology. *Journal of Clinical Oncology, 24,* 1–16.

Lacy, C. F., Armstrong, L. L., Goldman, M. P., & Lance, L. L. (2010). *Lexi-Comp's drug information handbook* (19th ed.). Hudson, OH: American Pharmaceutical Association.

Langford, P., & Chrisp, P. (2010). Fosaprepitant and aprepitant: An update of the evidence for their place in the prevention of chemotherapy-induced nausea and vomiting. *Core Evidence, 5,* 77–90.

Le, T. P. & Gan, T. J. (2010). Update on the management of postoperative nausea and vomiting and postdischarge nausea and vomiting in ambulatory surgery. *Anesthesiology Clinics, 28*(2), 225–249.

Lee, N. M. & Saha, S. (2011). Nausea and vomiting of pregnancy. *Gastroenterology Clinics of North America, 40*(2), 309–334.

National Cancer Institute Fact Sheet. Marijuana use in supportive care for cancer patients. Retrieved from http://www.cancer.gov/cancertopics/factsheet/Support/marijuana

Porth, C. M. (2009). *Pathophysiology: Concepts of altered health status* (8th ed.). Philadelphia, PA: Lippincott Williams & Wilkins.

Santucci, G. & Mack, J. W. (2007). Common gastrointestinal symptoms in pediatric palliative care: Nausea, vomiting, constipation, anorexia, cachexia. *Pediatric Clinics of North America, 54,* 673–689.

37 Drug Therapy for Constipation and Elimination Problems

LEARNING OBJECTIVES

After studying this chapter, you should be able to:

1. Discuss the etiology, physiology, and clinical manifestations for constipation and elimination problems.

2. Educate patients about nonpharmacologic measures to prevent or treat constipation.

3. Identify the prototype and describe the action, use, contraindications, adverse effects, and nursing implications of the laxatives.

4. Identify the prototype and describe the action, use, contraindications, adverse effects, and nursing implications of the cathartics.

5. Identify the prototype, indications, dosages, and routes for the miscellaneous agents used to treat constipation and other conditions.

6. Understand how to use the nursing process in the care of patients with constipation.

Clinical Application Case Study

Doris Campbell, an 84-year-old woman, is complaining about being constipated. Her past health history includes arthritis, osteoporosis, hemorrhoids, and peptic ulcer disease. As a home care nurse, you frequently see patients who complain of constipation.

KEY TERMS

Cathartic: drug with strong laxative effects and elimination of liquid or semiliquid stool

Constipation: infrequent and painful expulsion of hard, dry stools

Defecation: bowel elimination that is normally stimulated by movements and reflexes in the gastrointestinal tract

Flatulence: expulsion of gas through the rectum

Impaction: mass of hard, dry stool in the rectum; caused by chronic constipation

Laxative: drug with mild effects and elimination of soft, formed stool

Introduction

Constipation is a symptom, not a disease. It is the infrequent and painful expulsion of hard, dry stools. Generally, constipation is difficult to define clearly because normal frequency of stools varies as a symptom and differs from person to person. Drug therapy for constipation and elimination problems includes laxatives and cathartics, which are used to promote bowel elimination (defecation). The term **laxative** implies mild effects, with elimination of soft, formed stool. The term **cathartic** implies strong effects, with elimination of liquid or semiliquid stool. Although different effects may depend more on the dose than on the particular drug used, the names laxatives and cathartics are used in this chapter to specify the harshness of the level of response expected at normal doses of the drugs.

Overview of Constipation

Etiology

Several risk factors are associated with the development of constipation, including diet and lifestyle, particularly decreased levels of physical activity. Female sex, nonwhite status, advanced age, and low levels of education and income are related risk factors. In addition, certain drugs and disease process are associated with constipation.

Physiology and Pathophysiology

Defecation is bowel elimination that is stimulated by movements and reflexes in the gastrointestinal (GI) tract. When the stomach and duodenum are distended with food or fluids, gastrocolic and duodenocolic reflexes cause propulsive movements in the colon, which move feces into the rectum and arouse the urge to defecate. When sensory nerve fibers in the rectum are stimulated by the fecal mass, the defecation reflex causes strong peristalsis, deep breathing, closure of the glottis, contraction of abdominal muscles, contraction of the rectum, relaxation of anal sphincters, and expulsion of the fecal mass.

The cerebral cortex normally controls the defecation reflex so that defecation can occur at acceptable times and places. Voluntary control inhibits the external anal sphincter to allow defecation or contracts the sphincter to prevent defecation. When the external sphincter remains contracted, the defecation reflex dissipates, and the urge to defecate usually does not recur until additional feces enter the rectum or several hours later. In people who often inhibit the defecation reflex or fail to respond to the urge to defecate, constipation develops as the reflex weakens.

Clinical Manifestations

Constipation involves infrequent defecation. Due to variations in diet and other factors, there is no "normal" number of stools, but the traditional medical definition of constipation includes three or fewer bowel movements per week. The use of a multisymptom criterion-based checklist (Rome III criteria for functional constipation) requires two or more of six symptoms during at least one fourth of the bowel movements. Along with fewer than three stools per week, symptoms include straining, a sensation of incomplete evacuation, a sensation of anorectal blockage, hard stools, and use of manual evacuation. Normal bowel elimination should produce a soft, formed stool without pain.

Lifestyle Changes

Nonpharmacologic treatment of people with constipation has included the use of fiber, fluid supplementation, prebiotics, probiotics, and behavioral therapy. There is some evidence that fiber supplements improve the frequency and consistency of stools. No effectiveness data support increasing fluids beyond normal intake or adding behavioral interventions to reduce difficulty in passing stools.

Drug Therapy

Laxatives and cathartics are given to prevent or treat constipation and are somewhat arbitrarily classified as:

- Laxatives: bulk-forming, lubricant or emollient, and surfactant agents (stool softeners)
- Cathartics: saline and stimulant agents
- Miscellaneous agents

Table 37.1 lists the specific drugs used for the treatment of constipation by class.

Clinically, the choice of a laxative or cathartic often depends on the reason for use and the patient's condition, as shown in Table 37.2. There are several indications for use:

- To relieve constipation in pregnant women, elderly patients whose abdominal and perineal muscles have become weak and atrophied, children with megacolon, and patients receiving drugs that decrease intestinal motility (e.g., opioid analgesics, drugs with anticholinergic effects)
- To prevent straining at stool in patients with coronary artery disease (e.g., post-myocardial infarction), hypertension, cerebrovascular disease, and hemorrhoids and other rectal conditions
- To empty the bowel in preparation for bowel surgery or diagnostic procedures (e.g., colonoscopy, barium enema)
- To accelerate elimination of potentially toxic substances from the GI tract (e.g., orally ingested drugs or toxic compounds)
- To prevent absorption of intestinal ammonia in patients with hepatic encephalopathy
- To obtain a stool specimen for parasitologic examination

TABLE 37.1

Drugs Administered for the Treatment of Constipation

Drug Class	Prototype(s)	Other Drugs in the Class
Laxatives Bulk-forming	Psyllium preparations (Metamucil, Effersyllium, Serutan, Perdiem Plain)	Methylcellulose (Citrucel) Polycarbophil (FiberCon, Mitrolan)
Lubricant laxative		Mineral oil (Agoral Plain, Milkinol, Fleet Mineral Oil Enema)
Surfactant (stool softeners)		Docusate calcium (Surfak) Docusate sodium (Colace)
Cathartics Stimulant	Bisacodyl (Dulcolax)	Castor oil (Neoloid) Glycerin Senna preparations (Senokot, Black Draught)
Saline		Magnesium citrate solution Magnesium hydroxide (milk of magnesia, magnesia magma) Polyethylene glycol (PEG) solution (Miralax) Polyethylene glycol–electrolyte solution (PEG-ES) (CoLyte, GoLytely, NuLytely, OCL) Sodium phosphate and sodium biphosphate (Fleet Phosphosoda, Fleet Enema)
Miscellaneous		Lactulose (Chronulac, Cephulac) Lubiprostone (Amitiza) Sorbitol

TABLE 37.2

Use of Laxatives and Cathartics for Specific Conditions

Indication	Preferred Drug Regimen
For patients in whom straining is potentially harmful or painful such as coronary artery disease (e.g., post–myocardial infarction), hypertension, cerebrovascular disease, anal fissures, or hemorrhoids	Stool softeners (e.g., docusate sodium) are the agents of choice.
For occasional use to cleanse the bowel for endoscopic or radiologic examinations	Saline or stimulant cathartics are acceptable (e.g., magnesium citrate, polyethylene glycol–electrolyte solution, bisacodyl). These drugs should not be used more than once per week. Frequent use is likely to produce laxative abuse.
For long-term use of laxatives or cathartics in patients who are debilitated, older, or unable or unwilling to eat an adequate diet	Bulk-forming laxatives (e.g., Metamucil) usually are preferred. However, because obstruction may occur, these agents should not be given to patients with difficulty in swallowing or adhesions or strictures in the gastrointestinal (GI) tract or to those who are unable or unwilling to drink adequate fluids.
To accelerate elimination of potentially toxic substances from the GI tract (e.g., orally ingested drugs or toxic compounds)	Sorbitol may be given with activated charcoal to remove toxic substances.
To prevent absorption of intestinal ammonia in patients with hepatic encephalopathy	Lactulose acidifies the stool and traps ammonia and eliminates it with other fecal material.
For fecal impaction	A rectal suppository (e.g., bisacodyl) or an enema (e.g., oil retention or Fleet enema) is preferred. Oral laxatives are contraindicated when fecal impaction is present but may be given after the rectal mass is removed. After the impaction is relieved, measures should be taken to prevent recurrence. If dietary and other nonpharmacologic measures are ineffective or contraindicated, use of a bulk-forming agent daily or another laxative once or twice weekly may be necessary.

- To accelerate excretion of parasites after anthelmintic drugs have been administered
- To reduce serum cholesterol levels (psyllium products)

Laxatives

Bulk-forming laxatives are soluble fibers that are largely unabsorbed by the intestine. When water is added, these substances swell and become gel-like. Bulk-forming laxatives are the most physiologic laxatives because their effect is similar to that of increased intake of dietary fiber. The bulk-forming laxative ℗ **psyllium** (Metamucil, others) is the prototype laxative.

Pharmacokinetics

Psyllium usually acts within 12 to 24 hours, although it may take as long as 2 to 3 days to exert its full effects. Excretion is in the stool.

Action

Psyllium is essentially unabsorbed by the body. It works by mechanical action to absorb excess water while stimulating normal bowel elimination. The drug adds bulk and size to the fecal mass that stimulates peristalsis and defecation. It also may act by pulling water into the intestinal lumen.

Use

Uses of psyllium include treatment of occasional constipation or bowel irregularity. The drug may also help lower cholesterol when combined with a diet low in cholesterol and saturated fat. It may also be useful in the treatment of diarrhea. It should be noted that because psyllium, like most laxatives, is not absorbed or metabolized extensively, it can usually be used without difficulty in patients with hepatic impairment. Table 37.3 presents route and dosage information for the psyllium and other bulk-forming laxatives as well as surfactant and lubricant laxatives.

Use in Children

Children should obtain adequate fiber from dietary intake. Although psyllium-containing products are available without a prescription, children should take them only under the supervision of a health care provider.

Use in Older Adults

Psyllium is one of the many laxatives that is often used or overused in older adults. Nondrug measures to prevent constipation

TABLE 37.3

DRUGS AT A GLANCE: Laxatives

Drug	Pregnancy Category	Routes and Dosages Ranges	
		Adults	Children
Bulk-Forming			
℗ **Psyllium preparations** (Metamucil, Effersyllium, Serutan, Perdiem Plain)	B	PO 1 rounded tsp 1–3 times daily, stirred in at least 8 ounces water or other liquid	6–11 y: PO 1/2 the adult dosage in 8 ounces water once daily 12 y and older: PO same dosage as adults
Methylcellulose (Citrucel)	Not classified	PO 1 heaping tsp 1–3 times daily with water (8 ounces or more)	6–11 y: PO 1/2 the adult dosage in 8 ounces water once daily 12 y and older: PO same dosage as adults
Polycarbophil (FiberCon, Mitrolan)	C	PO 1 g 1–4 times daily or PRN with 8 ounces of fluid; maximum dose 4 g/24 h	2–6 y: products vary, consult labels 6–12 y: PO 500 mg 1–3 times daily or PRN; maximum dose 2 g/24 h
Surfactant (Stool Softener)			
Docusate sodium (Colace)	C	PO 50–300 mg daily	2–6 y: products vary, consult labels 6–11 y: PO 100 mg daily 12 y and older: PO same dosage as adults
Docusate calcium (Surfak)	C	PO 240 mg daily	12 y and older: PO same dosage as adults
Lubricant			
Mineral oil (Agoral Plain, Milkinol, Fleet Mineral Oil Enema)	B	PO 15–30 mL at bedtime Rectal enema, 30–60 mL	Older than 6 y: PO 5–15 mL at bedtime Rectal enema, 30–60 mL

are much preferred to laxatives in such patients. If a laxative is required on a regular basis, a bulk-forming psyllium compound (e.g., Metamucil) is best because it is most physiologic in its action.

Use in Patients with Critical Illness

Many patients with critical illness, including those with cancer, feel pain and require moderate to large amounts of opioid analgesics for pain control. The analgesics slow GI motility and cause constipation. The reduced mobility and altered bowel regimes that are often found in these patients increase the risk of constipation. Thus, they often need a bowel management program that includes routine administration of laxatives such as psyllium.

Use in Patients Receiving Home Care

Laxatives such as psyllium are commonly self-prescribed and self-administered in the home setting. When visiting patients for purposes other than providing care for patients who take laxatives, the home care nurse may become involved in their use. The functions of the home care nurse may include assessing usual patterns of bowel elimination, identifying patients at risk for constipation, promoting lifestyle interventions to prevent constipation, obtaining laxatives when indicated, and counseling about rational use of laxatives.

Adverse Effects

Psyllium or any fiber product may result in severe gas and bloating. In addition, there have been reports of abdominal cramping and esophageal or bowel obstruction.

Contraindications

Contraindications to the use of psyllium include the presence of undiagnosed abdominal pain. The danger is that the drugs may cause an inflamed organ (e.g., the appendix) to rupture and spill GI contents into the abdominal cavity with subsequent peritonitis, a life-threatening condition. Other contraindications are known allergy to the drug and intestinal obstruction and fecal **impaction**, a mass of hard, dry stool in the rectum.

QSEN Safety Alert ❗

People who have difficulty swallowing, including those with esophageal stricture or other narrowing or obstruction of the GI tract, should not take psyllium.

Nursing Implications

Preventing Interactions

With psyllium, no known drug or herbal interactions exist. However, the laxative may reduce or delay the absorption of certain medications, including carbamazepine, digoxin, lithium, tricyclic antidepressants, and warfarin. People should take psyllium at least 1 hour before or 2 to 4 hours after taking other medications. There is also a potential risk of psyllium interfering with nutrient absorption, but clear evidence is not available.

Administering the Medication

It is important to take the drug with at least 8 ounces of water or another liquid. With the psyllium-containing preparation Metamucil, there have been reports of obstruction in the GI tract when the compound was taken with insufficient fluid. People should take capsules one at a time.

Assessing for Therapeutic Effects

The nurse assesses for relief from constipation within 12 to 72 hours.

Assessing for Adverse Effects

The nurse assesses for choking or trouble swallowing, severe stomach pain or cramping, nausea or vomiting, rectal bleeding, or constipation lasting longer than 7 days.

Patient Teaching

Patients should take the medication as directed with a full glass of liquid, as soon as it is mixed. Maintaining adequate overall intake of fluids also helps improve bowel regularity.

QSEN Safety Alert ❗

Psyllium products may contain sugar, sodium, potassium, or artificial sweeteners. This may be of concern to patients who have diabetes, high blood pressure, renal disease, or phenylketonuria. It is important to teach patients to check the product label if they have these conditions.

Box 37.1 lists patient teaching guidelines for the laxatives and cathartics.

Other Drugs in the Class

Other laxatives products facilitate relief of constipation through different physiologic mechanisms. Surfactant and lubricant laxatives are briefly discussed in this section.

Lubricant Laxative

Mineral oil is the only lubricant laxative used clinically. It lubricates the fecal mass and slows colonic absorption of water from the fecal mass, but its exact mechanism of action is unknown. Effects usually occur in 6 to 8 hours. Oral mineral oil may cause several adverse effects and is not recommended for long-term use. Mineral oil is probably most useful as a retention enema to soften hard, dry feces and aid in their removal. Oral use of mineral oil may cause potentially serious adverse effects (decreased absorption of fat-soluble vitamins and some drugs; lipid pneumonia if aspirated into the lungs). Thus, mineral oil is not an oral laxative of choice in any condition, although occasional use in the alert patient is unlikely to be harmful. It should not be used regularly. With mineral oil, lipid pneumonia and decreased absorption of vitamins A, D, E, and K can occur.

BOX 37.1 Patient Teaching Guidelines for Laxatives and Cathartics

General Considerations

■ Diet, exercise, and fluid intake are important in maintaining normal bowel function and preventing or treating constipation.

■ Eat foods high in dietary fiber daily. Fiber is the portion of plant food that is not digested. It is contained in fruits, vegetables, and whole-grain cereals and breads. Bran, the outer coating of cereal grains such as wheat or oats, is an excellent source of dietary fiber and is available in numerous cereal products.

■ Drink at least 6 to 10 glasses (8 ounces each) of fluid daily if not contraindicated.

■ Exercise regularly. Walking and other activities aid movement of feces through the bowel.

■ Establish a regular time and place for bowel elimination. The defecation urge is usually strongest after eating and the defecation reflex is weakened or lost if repeatedly ignored.

■ Laxative and cathartics use should be temporary and not regular, as a general rule. Regular use may prevent normal bowel function, cause adverse drug reactions, and delay treatment for conditions that cause constipation.

■ *Never* take laxatives and cathartics when acute abdominal pain, nausea, or vomiting is present. Doing so may cause a ruptured appendix or other serious complication.

■ After taking a strong laxative or cathartic, it takes 2 to 3 days of normal eating to produce enough feces in the bowel for a bowel movement. Frequent use of a strong laxative promotes loss of normal bowel function, loss of fluids and electrolytes that your body needs, and laxative dependence.

■ If one is having chronic constipation and is unable or unwilling to eat enough fiber-containing foods in the diet, the next best action is regular use of a bulk-forming laxative (e.g., Metamucil) as a dietary supplement. These laxatives act the same way as increasing fiber in the diet and are usually best for long-term use. When taken daily, these can prevent constipation. However, these laxatives may take 2 to 3 days to work and are not effective in relieving acute constipation.

■ Urine may be discolored if one takes a laxative containing senna (e.g., Senokot). The color change is not harmful.

■ Some people use strong laxatives for weight control. This is an inappropriate use and a dangerous practice because it can lead to life-threatening fluid and electrolyte imbalances, including dehydration and cardiovascular problems.

Self- or Caregiver Administration

■ Take all laxatives and cathartics as directed and do not exceed recommended doses to avoid adverse effects.

■ With bulk-forming laxatives, mix in 8 ounces of fluid immediately before taking and follow with additional fluid, if able. *Never* take the drug dry. Adequate fluid intake is essential with these drugs.

■ With bisacodyl tablets, swallow whole (do not crush or chew), and do not take within 1 hour of an antacid or milk. This helps prevent stomach irritation, abdominal cramping, and possible vomiting.

■ Take magnesium citrate or milk of magnesia on an empty stomach with 8 ounces of fluid to increase effectiveness.

■ Refrigerate magnesium citrate before taking to improve taste and retain effectiveness.

■ Mix lactulose with fruit juice, water, or milk, if desired, to improve taste.

■ Take lubiprostone (Amitiza) with food.

■ Notify your health care provider if severe diarrhea develops while taking lubiprostone.

QSEN Safety Alert

Lipid pneumonia can be prevented by not giving mineral oil to patients with dysphagia or impaired consciousness. Decreased absorption of fat-soluble vitamins can be prevented by not giving mineral oil with or shortly after meals or for longer than 2 weeks.

Surfactant Laxatives (Stool Softeners)

Surfactant laxatives (e.g., docusate calcium or docusate sodium) decrease the surface tension of the fecal mass to allow water to penetrate into the stool. They also act as a detergent to facilitate admixing of fat and water in the stool. As a result, stools are softer and easier to expel. These agents have little, if any, laxative effect. Their main value is to prevent straining while expelling stool. They usually act within 1 to 3 days and should be taken daily.

Clinical Application 37-2

■ Based on Mrs. Campbell's past health history, what is the most likely drug of choice to relieve her constipation?

NCLEX Success

1. Which of the following points should be included when teaching patients regarding measures to promote healthy bowel function? (Select all that apply.)

A. increasing activity
B. eating a low-residue diet
C. maintaining adequate fluid intake
D. establishing regular bowel habits

EVIDENCE-BASED PRACTICE

Laxatives for the Management of Constipation in Palliative Care Patients (Cochrane Review).

by MILES, C. L., FELLOWES, D., GOODMAN, M. L., & WILKINSON, S.

Cochrane Library Database of Systematic Reviews (Online), Issue 4, 2006, CD003448

A review of research on laxatives for the management of constipation in patients receiving palliative care found insufficient data to make a recommendation on the best laxative for these patients. Bulk-forming laxatives are not usually recommended for patients with cancer because they may not be able to drink adequate amounts of fluids required with these medications. One treatment option, stimulant laxatives (e.g., bisacodyl, a senna preparation) increase intestinal motility, which is the action that opiates suppress. These drugs may cause abdominal cramping, which may be lessened by giving small doses three or four times daily.

IMPLICATIONS FOR NURSING PRACTICE: It is necessary to thoughtfully reconsider the use of laxatives and cathartics in palliative care based on the patient's clinical condition and ability to increase other measures (e.g., fluids, activity). Nurses and other health care providers need to reassess previously used measures to manage constipation given the risks posed by disease and other treatments; they may need to alter typical laxative routines.

2. Which of the following oral medications is safe to use in a 60-year-old constipated patient with dysphagia?

   A. methylcellulose (Citrucel)
   B. psyllium (Metamucil)
   C. mineral oil (Agoral Plain)
   D. docusate sodium (Colace)

3. For which of the following patients is a laxative contraindicated?

   A. a patient with cancer taking daily narcotics for pain control
   B. a patient complaining of abdominal pain and distention
   C. a patient scheduled for a colonoscopy
   D. a patient with limited mobility due to Parkinson's disease

Cathartics

The stimulant cathartics are the strongest and most abused laxative products. Two types of cathartics exist: stimulant and saline. ℗ **Bisacodyl** (Dulcolax), a stimulant cathartic, is the prototype cathartic.

Pharmacokinetics

Bisacodyl is very poorly absorbed in the small intestine following oral administration or in the large intestine following rectal administration. It has a half-life of 16 hours. The drug is metabolized in the liver. Bisacodyl is primarily excreted in the feces, and any systemically absorbed portion of the drug is excreted in the urine.

Action

Bisacodyl and other stimulant cathartics act by irritating the GI mucosa and pulling water into the bowel lumen. As a result, feces move through the bowel too rapidly to allow colonic absorption of fecal water, so there is elimination of a watery stool.

Use

Bisacodyl is prescribed for the relief of constipation and as part of bowel preparation before medical examinations and surgery. The drug is also used in the management of neurogenic bowel dysfunction. The use of bisacodyl is not restricted in patients with renal or hepatic impairment. Table 37.4 provides route and dosage information for bisacodyl as well as other stimulant and saline cathartics.

Use in Children

Stimulant laxatives are generally avoided in children younger than 6 years of age for occasional constipation, unless otherwise directed by a clinician. Bisacodyl can be used short term as rescue therapy or cautiously in children with difficult-to-treat constipation.

Use in Older Adults

There are no specific dosage recommendations for the use of bisacodyl in older adults. However, as with laxatives, cathartics are often used or overused in older adults. Measures such as maintaining adequate fluids, a high-fiber diet, and exercise are much preferred to cathartics.

Use in Patients With Critical Illness

In critically ill patients, an altered diet regime, change in bowel habits, use of medications known to cause constipation, and decreased activity with bedrest increase the risk of constipations. Often, a bowel management program that includes routine laxative administration is necessary.

Use in Patients Receiving Home Care

Bisacodyl is commonly self-prescribed and self-administered in the home setting. With all drugs used to treat constipation, it is important to identify patients at risk of developing constipation. The home care nurse assesses the usual patterns of bowel elimination, promotes lifestyle interventions to prevent constipation, and uses cathartics only as indicated.

TABLE 37.4

DRUGS AT A GLANCE: Cathartics

Drug	Pregnancy Category	Routes and Dosages Ranges	
		Adults	*Children*
Stimulants			
Ⓟ **Bisacodyl** (Dulcolax)	B	PO 10–15 mg Rectal suppository, 10 mg	6 y and older: PO 5 mg Rectal suppository, 5 mg
Castor oil (Neoloid)	X	PO 15–60 mL	Under 2 y: PO 1.25–7.5 mL depending on the strength of emulsion 5–15 y: PO 5–30 mL depending on the strength of emulsion
Glycerin	C	Rectal suppository, 3 g	Under 6 y: rectal suppository 1–1.5 g
Senna preparations (Senokot, Black Draught)	C	Granules, PO 1 level tsp once or twice daily Syrup, PO 2–3 tsp once or twice daily Tablets, PO 2 tablets once or twice daily For geriatric, obstetric, gynecologic patients, reduce all dosages by half	Weight–27 kg: PO granules, syrup, and tablets, 1/2 the adult dosage
Saline			
Magnesium citrate solution	C	PO 1/2–1 bottle at bedtime	6–11 y: PO 1/2–1/4 bottle at bedtime 12 y and older: PO same dosage as adults
Magnesium hydroxide (milk of magnesia, magnesia magma)	C	Regular liquid: PO 30–60 mL at bedtime Concentrated liquid: PO 15–30 mL at bedtime	Regular liquid: 2–5 y: PO 5–15 mL at bedtime 6–11 y: PO 15–30 mL at bedtime 12 y and older: PO same dosage as adults Concentrated liquid: 2–5 y: PO 2.5–7.5 mL at bedtime 6–11 y: PO 7.5–15 mL at bedtime 12 y and older: PO same dosage as adults
Polyethylene glycol (PEG) solution (Miralax)	C	PO 17 g in 8 ounces water	No recommended children's dose
Polyethylene glycol–electrolyte solution (PEG–ES) (CoLyte, GoLytely, NuLytely, OCL)	C	For bowel cleansing before GI examination: PO 240 mL every 10 min until 4 L is consumed	No recommended children's dose
Sodium phosphate and sodium biphosphate (Fleet Phosphosoda, Fleet Enema)	C	PO 20–40 mL in 8 ounces water Rectal enema, 60–120 mL	10 y and older: PO 10–20 mL in 8 ounces of water 5–10 y: PO 5–10 mL in 8 ounces of water Rectal enema, 60 mL

Adverse Effects

Common adverse effects of bisacodyl include abdominal pain and cramping, nausea, diarrhea, and weakness.

Contraindications

Contraindications to bisacodyl include known allergy to the drug. Additionally, the presence of undiagnosed abdominal pain or with intestinal obstruction or fecal impaction precludes its use.

Nursing Implications

Preventing Interactions

Medications interact with bisacodyl to decrease its effect (Box 37.2). Bisacodyl should not be taken within an hour after ingesting milk, because milk increases gastric pH and may reduce the resistance of the enteric coating of the tablet, resulting in earlier release of the drug.

Administering the Medication

It is necessary to take bisacodyl on an empty stomach, or at bedtime. Patients should swallow the drug whole.

People should not use bisacodyl frequently or for longer than 1 week because it may produce serum electrolyte and acid–base imbalances (e.g., hypocalcemia, hypokalemia, metabolic acidosis, or alkalosis).

The nurse inserts bisacodyl rectal suppositories to the length of the index finger, next to the rectal mucosa.

EVIDENCE-BASED PRACTICE

Evaluation and Treatment of Constipation in Infants and Children: Recommendations of the North American Society for Pediatric Gastroenterology.

by CONSTIPATION GUIDELINE COMMITTEE OF THE NORTH AMERICAN SOCIETY FOR PEDIATRIC GASTROENTEROLOGY.

Journal of Pediatric Gastroenterology and Nutrition 2006, 43, E1–E13

The North American Society for Pediatric Gastroenterology, Hepatology, and Nutrition has developed guidelines for treating constipation in infants and children. In addition to a balanced diet, containing juices that contain sorbitol, such as prune, pear, and apple juice (for infants) and whole grains, fruits, and vegetables (for children), the group recommends the following for the treatment of constipation:

- For infants:
  - Glycerin suppositories are often effective in infants and small children.
  - Lactulose or sorbitol can be used as stool softeners in infants.
  - Mineral oil or stimulant laxatives are not recommended for infants.
- For children:
  - Mineral oil, magnesium hydroxide, lactulose, and sorbitol are effective for treating constipation in children.
  - Stimulant laxatives, such as senna or bisacodyl, can be used short term as rescue therapy or in carefully selected children with difficult to treat constipation. Polyethylene glycol–electrolyte solution in low dosages may be an effective long-term treatment for difficult to treat cases.

IMPLICATIONS FOR NURSING PRACTICE: A health care provider should evaluate an infant and child to appropriately diagnose and treat ongoing constipation. It is necessary to advise parents not to give children any laxative more than once a week without consulting a health care provider and provide instruction about the best drug therapy for the age group. Evaluation of constipation involves an evaluation of dietary intake.

BOX 37.2   Drug Interactions: Bisacodyl

Drugs That Decrease the Effects of Bisacodyl

- Anticholinergic drugs (e.g., atropine)
  Slow intestinal motility, increasing constipation
- H_2 receptor blockers (e.g., ranitidine)
  Decrease stomach acid, resulting in premature tablet dissolution and gastric irritation
- Proton pump inhibitors (e.g., omeprazole)
  Decrease stomach acid, resulting in premature tablet dissolution and gastric irritation

Assessing for Therapeutic Effects

Oral formulations produce laxative effects in 6 to 12 hours, and a single bedtime dose of bisacodyl usually produces a morning bowel movement. Rectal forms of bisacodyl typically produce a bowel movement within 15 minutes to 1 hour.

Assessing for Adverse Effects

The nurse monitors for bowel elimination patterns and the presence of diarrhea. In addition, the nurse should monitor for the existence of abdominal pain and cramping, nausea, or weakness.

Patient Teaching

With bisacodyl tablets, it is important to instruct the patient to swallow the tablets without chewing and not to take them within an hour after ingesting milk or gastric antacids or while receiving H_2 receptor blocker therapy. This prevents abdominal cramping and vomiting associated with premature tablet dissolution and gastric irritation.

Box 37.1 presents additional patient teaching guidelines for the laxatives and cathartics.

Other Drugs in the Class

Stimulant Cathartics

Besides bisacodyl, other stimulant cathartics are available. In addition to irritant, stimulant effects, glycerin exerts hyperosmotic effects in the colon. It usually acts within 30 minutes. Available in the form of rectal suppositories, glycerin is not given orally for laxative effects. Oral stimulant cathartics include castor oil and senna preparations.

Saline Cathartics

Saline cathartics (e.g., magnesium citrate, milk of magnesia) are not well absorbed from the intestine. Consequently, the drugs increase osmotic pressure in the intestinal lumen and cause water to be retained. Distention of the bowel leads to increased peristalsis and decreased intestinal transit time for the fecal mass. The resultant stool is semifluid. These cathartics are used when rapid bowel evacuation is needed. With oral magnesium preparations, effects occur within ½ to 6 hours; with sodium phosphate–containing rectal enemas, effects occur within 15 minutes.

Saline cathartics are generally useful and safe for short-term treatment of constipation, cleansing the bowel before endoscopic examinations, and treating fecal impaction. However, they are not safe for frequent or prolonged usage or for certain patients because they may produce fluid and electrolyte imbalances. For example, patients with impaired renal function are at risk for hypermagnesemia with magnesium-containing laxatives because some of the magnesium is absorbed systemically. Patients with congestive heart failure are at risk for fluid retention and edema with sodium-containing cathartics. Saline cathartics containing phosphate, sodium, magnesium, or potassium salts are usually contraindicated or must be used cautiously in the presence of impaired renal function and in people who follow a sodium-restricted diet for hypertension. Ten percent or more of the magnesium in magnesium salts may be absorbed and cause hypermagnesemia; sodium phosphate and sodium biphosphate may cause hyperphosphatemia, hypernatremia, acidosis, and hypocalcemia; and potassium salts may cause hyperkalemia.

Polyethylene glycol–electrolyte solution (e.g., NuLYTELY) is formulated for rapid and effective bowel cleansing without significant changes in water or electrolyte balance. The drug is a nonabsorbable oral solution that induces diarrhea within 30 to 60 minutes and rapidly evacuates the bowel, usually within 4 hours. It is a prescription drug used for bowel cleansing before GI examination (e.g., colonoscopy) and is contraindicated in patients with GI obstruction, gastric retention, colitis, or bowel perforation. Combination products such as HalfLytely combine polyethylene glycol with a stimulant cathartic, bisacodyl, to evacuate the colon in preparation for a colonoscopy. Polyethylene glycol solution (MiraLAX) is an oral laxative that may be used to treat occasional constipation. Effects may require 2 to 4 days. It is a prescription drug, and people should not take it for longer than 2 weeks. Refrigerating magnesium citrate and polyethylene glycol electrolyte solution before giving increases the palatability and retains potency.

Miscellaneous Agents for Constipation

Several miscellaneous agents are used in the treatment of constipation. These drugs are discussed briefly below, and Table 37.5 gives dosage information.

Lactulose (Chronulac, Cephulac) is a disaccharide that is not absorbed from the GI tract. It exerts laxative effects by pulling water into the intestinal lumen. It is used to treat constipation and hepatic encephalopathy. The latter condition usually results from alcoholic liver disease in which ammonia accumulates and causes stupor or coma. Metabolism of dietary protein and intestinal bacteria produce ammonia. Lactulose decreases production of ammonia in the intestine. The goal of treatment is usually

TABLE 37.5

DRUGS AT A GLANCE: Miscellaneous Drugs Administered for the Treatment of Constipation

Drug	Pregnancy Category	Routes and Dosage Ranges	
		Adults	*Children*
Lactulose (Chronulac, Cephulac)	B	For constipation: PO 15–30 mL daily; maximum dose 60 mL daily Portal systemic encephalopathy: PO 30–45 mL 3 or 4 times daily, adjusted to produce two or three soft stools daily Rectally as retention enema, 300 mL with 700 mL water or normal saline, retained 30–60 min, every 4–6 h	Infants: PO 2.5–10 mL daily in divided doses Older children: PO 40–90 mL daily in divided doses
Lubiprostone (Amitiza)	C	For chronic idiopathic constipation: PO 24 µg twice daily with food	No recommended children's dose
Sorbitol	C	As hyperosmolar laxative PO 30–150 mL (as 70% solution) Rectal enema, 120 mL as 25% to 30% solution	2–11 y: PO 2 mg/kg (as 70% solution) Rectal enema, 30–60 mL as 25% to 30% solution 12 y and older: same as adult dose

to maintain two to three soft stools daily; effects usually occur within 24 to 48 hours. It is important to use the drug cautiously because it may produce electrolyte imbalances and dehydration.

Lubiprostone (Amitiza) is indicated for the treatment of chronic idiopathic constipation in adults. Chronic idiopathic constipation, defined as the infrequent or difficult passage of stool, is characterized by abnormal GI motility, abdominal discomfort, bloating, and straining to pass hard, lumpy stools. Lubiprostone is poorly absorbed into the circulation and exerts its effect locally, activating chloride channels in the GI tract to increase the secretion of chloride rich fluids into the intestine. Increased intestinal fluid secretion stimulates intestinal motility, improving the passage of stool. Lubiprostone is metabolized by enzymes in the stomach and excreted in the urine and feces. Adverse effects include nausea and severe diarrhea. Taking lubiprostone with food may aid in decreasing nausea.

Sorbitol is a monosaccharide that pulls water into the intestinal lumen and has laxative effects. It is often given with sodium polystyrene sulfonate (Kayexalate), a potassium-removing resin used to treat hyperkalemia, prevent constipation, and aid expulsion of the potassium–resin complex. It can also be given with activated charcoal to eliminate toxins in the body.

Clinical Application 37-3

- Mrs. Campbell is concerned about not having a bowel movement. She takes a psyllium preparation at 8 AM. She does not have a result by noon, so she takes milk of magnesia. She has not had a stool by supper, so she takes a glycerin suppository. She has diarrhea throughout the night. What patient education is appropriate?

The Nursing Process

Assessment

- Assess patients for current or potential constipation.
- Signs and symptoms, which include the following:
  - Decreased number and frequency of stools
  - Passage of dry, hard stools
  - Abdominal distention and discomfort
  - **Flatulence** (expulsion of gas through the rectum)
- Presence of risk factors
  - Diet with minimal fiber (e.g., small amounts of fruits, vegetables, and whole-grain products)
  - Low fluid intake (e.g., less than 2000 mL daily)
  - Immobility or limited activity
  - Use of drugs that reduce intestinal function and motility (e.g., opioid analgesics, antacids containing aluminum or calcium, anticholinergics, calcium channel blockers, clozapine, diuretics, iron, phenothiazines, cholestyramine, colestipol, sucralfate, tricyclic antidepressants, vincristine)
  - Overuse of antidiarrheal agents, which may also cause constipation
  - Conditions that may reduce intestinal function and motility (e.g., depression, eating disorders such as anorexia nervosa, hypothyroidism, hypercalcemia, multiple sclerosis, Parkinson's disease, spinal lesions)
  - Hemorrhoids, anal fissures, or other conditions characterized by painful bowel elimination
  - Elderly or debilitated status

Nursing Diagnoses

- Constipation related to decreased activity, inadequate dietary fiber, inadequate fluid intake, drugs, or disease processes
- Pain (abdominal cramping and distention) related to constipation or use of laxatives
- Noncompliance with recommendations for nondrug measures to prevent or treat constipation
- Risk for deficient fluid volume related to diarrhea from frequent or large doses of laxatives
- Deficient knowledge: Nondrug measures to prevent constipation and appropriate use of laxatives

Planning/Goals

The patient will

- Take laxative drugs appropriately.
- Use nondrug measures to promote normal bowel function and prevent constipation.
- Regain normal patterns of bowel elimination.
- Avoid excessive losses of fluids and electrolytes from laxative use.
- Be protected from excessive fluid loss, hypotension, and other adverse drug effects, when possible.
- Be assisted to avoid constipation when at risk (e.g., has illness or injury that prevents activity and food and fluid intake; takes medications that decrease GI function).

Nursing Interventions

The nurse will

- Assist patients with constipation and caregivers to
  - Understand the importance of diet, exercise, and fluid intake in promoting normal bowel function and preventing constipation
  - Increase activity and exercise
  - Increase intake of dietary fiber (e.g., vegetables, fruits, cereal grains)
  - Drink at least 2000 mL of fluid daily, if not contraindicated
  - Establish and maintain a routine for bowel elimination (e.g., going to the bathroom immediately after breakfast)
  - Understand and comply with drug therapy (see Box 37.1)
- Monitor patient responses.
  - Record number, amount, and type of bowel movements.
  - Record vital signs. Hypotension and weak pulse may indicate deficient fluid volume.

Evaluation

The nurse will

- Observe and interview for improved patterns of bowel elimination.
- Observe for use of nondrug measures to promote bowel function.
- Observe for appropriate use of laxatives.
- Observe and interview regarding adverse effects of laxatives.

Key Concepts

- Constipation is the infrequent and painful expulsion of hard, dry stools.

- Lifestyle modifications such as fluid and fiber intake and exercise are preferred to medications in the treatment of constipation.

- Laxatives and cathartics are drugs to promote bowel elimination.

- Common reasons for abuse of laxatives and cathartics include eating disorders, desire for strict weight control, or the belief that a daily bowel movement is necessary for health.

- Laxatives and cathartics should not be used in the presence of undiagnosed abdominal pain or other signs of intestinal obstruction due to the risks of perforation and peritonitis.

- Bulk-forming laxatives add mass to the feces, stimulating peristalsis and defecation. They must be taken with water to avoid obstruction. Generally, bulk-forming drugs are the most desirable laxative for long-term use.

- Surfactant laxatives decrease the surface tension of the fecal mass to allow water and fat to penetrate into the stool, making it softer and easier to expel. They have little true laxative effect.

- Saline laxatives increase the osmotic pressure in the intestinal lumen, resulting in the retention of water, which distends the bowel and stimulates peristalsis. They produce a semifluid stool and may lead to fluid and electrolyte imbalances.

- Polyethylene glycol–electrolyte solution is a nonabsorbable oral solution that rapidly evacuates the bowel within 4 hours. It is useful for bowel cleansing before GI procedures.

- Stimulant cathartics are the strongest and most abused laxative products. They irritate the GI mucosa, pull water into the colon, and stimulate peristalsis. They produce a watery stool and may lead to fluid, electrolyte, and acid–base imbalances.

- Lubricant laxatives lubricate the fecal mass and slow colonic absorption of water from the fecal mass. These medications may interfere with the absorption of fat-soluble vitamins and, if aspirated, may result in a lipid aspiration pneumonia.

- Lactulose exerts an osmotic effect, pulling water into the colon and stimulating peristalsis. It is also useful in treating hepatic encephalopathy by decreasing the production of the waste product ammonia.

- Sorbitol is often given with sodium polystyrene sulfonate (Kayexalate) in the treatment of hyperkalemia to aid in the expulsion of the potassium–resin complex.

- Lubiprostone (Amitiza) aids in treating chronic idiopathic constipation by increasing intestinal fluid secretion, stimulating intestinal motility and defecation.

Critical Thinking Questions

37-1. Mr. Parks is 62-year-old retired teacher who has recently been diagnosed with hepatic encephalopathy. His physician has prescribed lactulose 45 mL three or four times daily and has told Mr. Parks to adjust the amount of the medication so that he has three to four soft stools a day. A month later, Mr. Parks returns to the clinic and states that he has been taking only half of the medication once a day because he dislikes having more than one stool a day.

- What additional education regarding the lactulose and his liver disease does the nurse give to Mr. Parks?

References and Resources

Bouras, E. P., & Tangalos, E. G. (2009). Chronic constipation in the elderly. *Gastroenterology Clinics of North America, 38*(3), 463–480.

Constipation Guideline Committee of the North American Society for Pediatric Gastroenterology. (2006). Evaluation and treatment of constipation in infants and children: Recommendations of the North American Society for Pediatric Gastroenterology. *Journal of Pediatric Gastroenterology and Nutrition, 43,* E1–E13. Retrieved July 27, 2011, from http://www.guideline.gov/summary/summary.aspx?doc_id=9792&nbr=005245&string=constipation+and+infants

DiPiro, J. T., Talbert, R. L., Yee, G., Matzke, G., Wells, B., & Posey, L. M. (2011). *Pharmacotherapy: A pathophysiologic approach* (8th ed.). New York: McGraw-Hill.

Drug facts and comparisons. (Updated monthly). St. Louis, MO: Facts and Comparisons.

Karch, A. M. (2012). *2012 Lippincott's nursing drug guide.* Philadelphia, PA: Lippincott Williams & Wilkins.

Lacy, C. F., Armstrong, L. L., Goldman, M. P., & Lance, L. L. (2010). *Lexi-Comp's drug information handbook* (19th ed.). Hudson, OH: American Pharmaceutical Association.

Loening-Bauche, V. (2005). Prevalence, symptoms and outcome of constipation in infants and toddlers. *The Journal of Pediatrics, 146,* 359–363.

Miles, C. L., Fellowes, D., Goodman, M. L., & Wilkinson, S. (2006). Laxatives for the management of constipation in palliative care patients (Cochrane Review). *Cochrane database of systematic reviews (Online),* Issue 4. CD003448.

Porth, C. M. (2009). *Pathophysiology: Concepts of altered health status* (8th ed.). Philadelphia, PA: Lippincott Williams & Wilkins.

Ramkumar, D., & Rao, S. (2005). Efficacy and safety of traditional medical therapies for chronic constipation: Systematic review. *The American Journal of Gastroenterology, 100,* 936–971.

Singh, S. & Rao, S. S. C. (2010). Pharmacologic management of chronic constipation. *Gastroenterology Clinics of North America, 39*(3), 509–527.

Smeltzer, S. C., Bare, B., Hinkle, J. L., & Cheever, K. H. (2010). *Brunner & Suddarth's textbook of medical-surgical nursing* (12th ed.). Philadelphia, PA: Lippincott Williams & Wilkins.

38 Drug Therapy for Diarrhea

Clinical Application Case Study

Joseph Mendoza is a 47-year-old salesman who travels extensively as part of his job. He returned from a trip to Asia 2 days ago, and since his return, he has had abdominal cramping and bloating and an average of four watery bowel movements per day. Mr. Mendoza comes to the clinic seeking advice about how to manage his symptoms. He denies nausea and vomiting. His vital signs are temperature 99.4°F, pulse 82 beats/min, respirations 22 breaths/min, and blood pressure 124/72 mm Hg lying and 120/72 mm Hg standing.

KEY TERMS

Diarrhea: increase in the liquidity of stool or frequency of defecation to more than 3 stools per day

Inflammatory bowel disorders: disorders in which inflamed mucous membranes secrete large amounts of fluids into the intestinal lumen, along with mucus, proteins, and blood; characterized by impaired absorption of water and electrolytes

Irritable bowel syndrome: functional disorder of intestinal motility with no evidence of inflammation or tissue changes

Steatorrhea: loose, fatty stool

Travelers' diarrhea: form of diarrhea caused by the enterotoxigenic strain of *Escherichia coli*, typically from fecal contamination of food or water

Introduction

The focus of this chapter is the description of drugs used to relieve the symptoms of diarrhea, specifically the opioid-related agents. Topics of discussion include the general characteristics of these drugs, their mechanisms of action, indications for and contraindications to their use, and their nursing implications. The section on adjuvant medications briefly addresses specific drugs, including antibacterial agents, used to manage underlying disease processes that cause diarrhea.

Overview of Diarrhea

Pathophysiology

Diarrhea, an increase in the liquidity of stool or frequency of defecation to more than 3 stools per day, is a common condition experienced by virtually everyone. It is a symptom of numerous conditions and not a disease. Diarrhea is a manifestation of basic mechanisms that increase bowel motility, cause secretion or retention of fluids in the intestinal lumen (lactose intolerance or toxins such as cholera or laxatives and other drugs), or cause inflammation or irritation of the gastrointestinal (GI) tract (*Escherichia coli, Salmonella*, rotaviruses, *Giardia*). It is common for more than one of the mechanisms to be involved in the pathogenesis of a given situation. As a result, bowel contents are rapidly propelled toward the rectum, and absorption of fluids and electrolytes is limited.

Clinical Manifestations

Diarrhea may be acute or chronic and mild or severe. Most episodes of acute diarrhea are defensive mechanisms by which the body tries to rid itself of irritants, toxins, and infectious agents. These episodes of frequent liquid or semiliquid stools are usually self-limiting and subside within 24 to 48 hours without serious consequences. If severe or prolonged, acute diarrhea may lead to serious fluid and electrolyte depletion, especially in young children and older adults. Chronic diarrhea may cause malnutrition and anemia and is often characterized by remissions and exacerbations.

Fever, vomiting, and bloody stools are associated with acute diarrhea, and the presence of these symptoms may help determine the cause. Fever is common and often linked with invasive pathogens. Vomiting is frequently found in illness caused by ingestion of bacterial toxins or viruses. Invasive and cytotoxin-releasing pathogens are known to cause bloody stools, and enterotoxigenic strain *E. coli* O157:H7 infection is suspected in the absence of fecal leukocytes. Bloody stools are not associated with viral agents and enterotoxins that release bacteria.

Etiology

Some causes of diarrhea include the following:

- *Excessive use or abuse of laxatives.* Laxative abuse may accompany eating disorders such as anorexia nervosa or bulimia.

- *Undigested, coarse, or highly spiced food in the GI tract.* The food acts as an irritant and attracts fluids in a defensive attempt to dilute the irritating agent. This may result from inadequate chewing of food or lack of digestive enzymes.

- *Lack of digestive enzymes.* Deficiency of pancreatic enzymes inhibits digestion and absorption of carbohydrates, proteins, and fats. Deficiency of lactase, which breaks down lactose to simple sugars (i.e., glucose and galactose) that can be absorbed by GI mucosa, inhibits digestion of milk and milk products. Lactase deficiency commonly occurs in people of African and Asian descent.

- *Intestinal infections with viruses, bacteria, or protozoa.* A common source of infection is ingested food or fluid contaminated by a variety of organisms.

- *E. coli* O157:H7–related hemorrhagic colitis most commonly occurs with the ingestion of undercooked ground beef. A serious complication of *E. coli* O157:H7 colitis is hemolytic uremic syndrome (HUS), characterized by thrombocytopenia, microangiopathic hemolytic anemia, and renal failure. Children are especially susceptible to HUS, which is the leading cause of dialysis in pediatric patients. So-called **travelers' diarrhea** is usually caused by an enterotoxigenic strain of *E. coli* (ETEC). Fecal contamination of food or water is the most common source of ETEC-induced diarrhea.

- Consumption of improperly prepared poultry may result in diarrhea due to infection with *Campylobacter jejuni*. In the United States, this is the most common bacterial organism identified in infectious diarrhea. In addition to diarrhea, vomiting, fever, and abdominal discomfort, *Campylobacter* bacteria produce neurotoxins, which may result in paralysis.

- *Salmonella* infections may occur when contaminated poultry and other meats, eggs, and dairy products are ingested. Elderly patients are especially susceptible to *Salmonella*-associated colitis.

- Several strains of *Shigella* may produce diarrhea. Infection most often results from direct person-to-person contact but may also occur via food or water contamination. Handwashing is especially important in preventing the spread of *Shigella* from person to person.

- Other diarrhea-producing organisms associated with contamination of specific foods include *Vibrio vulnificus* and *Vibrio parahaemolyticus* contamination of raw shellfish and oysters (particularly in the Gulf Coast states), *Clostridium perfringens* contamination of inadequately heated or reheated meats, *Staphylococcus aureus* contamination of processed meats and custard-filled pastries, *Bacillus cereus* contamination of rice and bean sprouts, and *Listeria monocytogenes* contamination of hot dogs and luncheon meats. Newborns, pregnant women, and older and immunocompromised people are especially susceptible to *L. monocytogenes* infection.

- Two of the most common viral organisms responsible for gastroenteritis and diarrhea are rotavirus or Norwalk-like virus (calicivirus). Vomiting is usually a prominent symptom accompanying virus-induced diarrhea.
- **Inflammatory bowel disorders**, such as gastroenteritis, diverticulitis, ulcerative colitis, and Crohn's disease. In these disorders, inflamed mucous membranes secrete large amounts of fluids into the intestinal lumen, along with mucus, proteins, and blood, and there is impaired absorption of water and electrolytes. In addition, when the ileum is diseased or a portion is surgically excised, large amounts of bile salts reach the colon, where they act as cathartics and cause diarrhea. Bile salts are normally reabsorbed from the ileum.
- **Irritable bowel syndrome (IBS)** is a functional disorder of intestinal motility with no evidence of inflammation or tissue changes. It occurs more commonly in women than in men, affecting approximately 12% of adults in the United States. A change in bowel pattern (constipation, diarrhea, or a combination of both) accompanied by abdominal pain, bloating, and distention are the presenting symptoms. The etiology is unknown; however, activation of 5-HT$_3$ (serotonin) receptors, which affect the regulation of visceral pain, colonic motility, and GI secretions, are thought to be involved in the pathophysiology of IBS.
- *Drugs.* Many oral drugs irritate the GI tract and may cause diarrhea, including acarbose, antacids that contain magnesium, antibacterials, antineoplastic agents, colchicine, laxatives, metformin, metoclopramide, misoprostol, selective serotonin reuptake inhibitors, tacrine, and tacrolimus. Antibacterial drugs are commonly used offenders that also may cause diarrhea by altering the normal bacterial flora in the intestine.

  Antibiotic-associated colitis (also called pseudomembranous colitis) is a serious condition that results from oral or parenteral antibiotic therapy. By suppressing normal flora in the colon, antibiotics allow proliferation of other bacteria, especially gram-positive, anaerobic *Clostridium difficile* organisms. These organisms produce a toxin that causes fever, abdominal pain, inflammatory lesions of the colon, and severe diarrhea with stools containing mucus, pus, and sometimes blood. Symptoms may develop within a few days or several weeks after the causative antibiotic is discontinued. Other enteric pathogens that may overgrow in the presence of antibiotic therapy and result in colitis include *Salmonella*, *C. perfringens* type A, *S. aureus*, and *Candida albicans*. Antibiotic-associated colitis is more often associated with ampicillin, cephalosporins, and clindamycin but may occur with any antibiotic or combination of antibiotics that alters intestinal microbial flora.
- *Intestinal neoplasms.* Tumors may increase intestinal motility by occupying space and stretching the intestinal wall. Diarrhea sometimes alternates with constipation in colon cancer.
- *Functional disorders.* Diarrhea may be a symptom of stress or anxiety in some patients. No organic disease process can be found in such circumstances.

- *Hyperthyroidism.* This condition increases bowel motility.
- *Surgical excision of portions of the intestine, especially the small intestine.* Such procedures decrease the absorptive area and increase fluidity of stools.
- *Human immunodeficiency virus (HIV) infection/ acquired immunodeficiency syndrome (AIDS).* Diarrhea occurs in most patients with HIV infection, often as a chronic condition that contributes to malnutrition and weight loss. It may be caused by drug therapy, infection with a variety of microorganisms, or other factors.

Nondrug Therapy

In most cases of acute, nonspecific diarrhea in adults, fluid losses are not severe, and patients need only simple replacement of fluids and electrolytes to replace those lost in the stool. Acceptable replacement fluids during the first 24 hours include clear liquids (e.g., flat ginger ale, decaffeinated cola drinks or tea, broth, gelatin)—2 to 3 L. Also, a diet consisting of bland foods (e.g., rice, soup, bread, salted crackers, cooked cereals, baked potatoes, eggs, applesauce) is best. People may resume their regular diet after 2 or 3 days.

Drug Therapy

Antidiarrheal drugs include a variety of agents, most of which are discussed in other chapters. When used for treatment of diarrhea, health care providers may give the drugs to relieve the symptom or the underlying cause of the symptom. Overall, opiates and opiate derivatives (see Chap. 48) are the most effective agents for symptomatic treatment of diarrhea. Although morphine, codeine, and related drugs are effective in relieving diarrhea, they are rarely used for this purpose because of their adverse effects. The synthetic drugs diphenoxylate and loperamide have replaced these drugs. Uses include only treatment of diarrhea; they do not cause morphine-like adverse effects in recommended doses. Diphenoxylate requires a prescription. Table 38.1 summarizes drugs used to manage diarrhea.

Opiate-Related Antidiarrheal Agents

The oral opioid **🅟 diphenoxylate with atropine** (Lomotil) is the prototype used to treat moderate to severe diarrhea. It is a schedule IV controlled substance.

Pharmacokinetics

Diphenoxylate with atropine is well absorbed by the oral route with an onset of action of 45 to 60 minutes. The duration of action is 3 to 4 hours. The drug is metabolized in the liver to active metabolites and is excreted in bile and feces.

Action

Diphenoxylate with atropine slows peristalsis by acting on the smooth muscles in the intestine.

TABLE 38.1

Drug Therapy for Diarrhea

Drug Class	Prototype	Other Drugs in the Class
Opiate-related antidiarrheals	Diphenoxylate with atropine sulfate (Lomotil)	Loperamide (Imodium) Paregoric
Adjuvant antidiarrheal medications		Alosetron (Lotronex) Bismuth subsalicylate (Pepto-Bismol) Cholestyramine (Questran) Colestipol (Colestid) Nitazoxanide (Alinia) Octreotide (Sandostatin) Pancreatin or pancrelipase (Viokase, Pancrease, Cotazym) Polycarbophil preparations (FiberCon) Rifaximin (Xifaxan)

Use

Prescribers order diphenoxylate with atropine to treat diarrhea. Table 38.2 provides dosage information for diphenoxylate with atropine and other opiate-related drugs.

Use in Children

Signs of atropine overdose may occur with usual doses with diphenoxylate, which contains atropine. Children younger than 2 years of age should not take the drug, and those younger than 6 years of age should not take it, except with a pediatrician's supervision. Even older children should not generally use it for longer than 2 days.

Use in Older Adults

Diarrhea is less common than constipation in older adults, but it may occur from laxative abuse and bowel-cleansing procedures before GI surgery or diagnostic tests. Fluid volume deficits may

rapidly develop in older adults with diarrhea. General principles of fluid and electrolyte replacement, measures to decrease GI irritants, and drug therapy apply as for younger adults. Older people may safely take most antidiarrheal drugs, but cautious use is indicated to avoid inducing constipation.

Use in Patients With Renal and/or Hepatic Impairment

Use of diphenoxylate with atropine warrants extreme caution in patients with severe hepatorenal disease because hepatic coma may be precipitated. Care is also necessary in patients with abnormal results of liver function tests.

Use in Patients With Critical Illness

Use of diphenoxylate with atropine requires caution in critically ill patients because they may have renal or hepatic compromise.

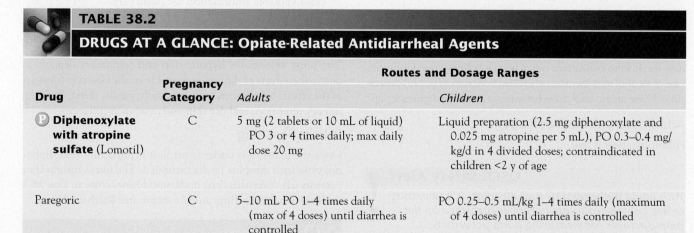

TABLE 38.2

DRUGS AT A GLANCE: Opiate-Related Antidiarrheal Agents

Drug	Pregnancy Category	Routes and Dosage Ranges	
		Adults	Children
Ⓟ **Diphenoxylate with atropine sulfate** (Lomotil)	C	5 mg (2 tablets or 10 mL of liquid) PO 3 or 4 times daily; max daily dose 20 mg	Liquid preparation (2.5 mg diphenoxylate and 0.025 mg atropine per 5 mL), PO 0.3–0.4 mg/kg/d in 4 divided doses; contraindicated in children <2 y of age
Paregoric	C	5–10 mL PO 1–4 times daily (max of 4 doses) until diarrhea is controlled	PO 0.25–0.5 mL/kg 1–4 times daily (maximum of 4 doses) until diarrhea is controlled
Loperamide (Imodium)	C	4 mg PO initially, then 2 mg after each loose stool to a maximal daily dose of 16 mg. For chronic diarrhea, dosage should be reduced to the lowest effective amount (average 4–8 mg daily)	Safety not established in for children <2 y of age 2–5 y, 13–20 kg 1 mg 3 times daily 6–8 y, 20–30 kg: PO 2 mg twice daily 8–12 y, >30 kg: PO 2 mg 3 times daily

Episodes of acute diarrhea may be defensive mechanisms by which the body tries to rid itself of irritants, toxins, and infectious agents. Antibacterial drugs administered to the critically ill may cause diarrhea by altering the normal bacterial flora in the intestine. It is important to observe for fluid and electrolyte imbalance and assess the cause of diarrhea before treating the condition. Good handwashing techniques are particularly important in preventing the spread of organisms that can cause diarrhea.

Use in Patients Receiving Home Care

People often take prescription drugs such as diphenoxylate with atropine and over-the-counter antidiarrheal aids in the home setting. The role of the home care nurse may include advising patients and caregivers about appropriate use of the drugs, trying to identify the cause and severity of the diarrhea (i.e., risk of fluid and electrolyte deficit), and teaching strategies to manage current episodes and prevent future episodes.

Adverse Effects

Adverse effects of diphenoxylate with atropine include tachycardia, dizziness, headache, flushing, nausea and vomiting, dry skin and mucous membranes, and urinary retention. Hypotension and respiratory depression have occurred, particularly with doses greater than ordered.

Contraindications

Contraindications to the use of diphenoxylate with atropine include diarrhea caused by toxic materials, microorganisms that penetrate intestinal mucosa (e.g., pathogenic *E. coli*, *Salmonella*, *Shigella*), and antibiotic-associated colitis. In these circumstances, antidiarrheal drugs that slow peristalsis may aggravate and prolong diarrhea.

Nursing Implications

Preventing Interactions

Increased levels of diphenoxylate with atropine may result with use of methotrimeprazine and pramlintide. Decreased drug levels may result from concurrent use of acetylcholinesterase inhibitors. Use of alcohol may increase central nervous system (CNS) depression. There are no known herbal interactions with diphenoxylate.

Administering the Medication

Administration is oral.

QSEN Safety Alert ❗

With liquid diphenoxylate and atropine, it is necessary to use only the calibrated dropper furnished by the manufacturer for measuring doses accurately.

Assessing for Therapeutic Effects

After drug administration, the nurse monitors the number and consistency of stools and fluid and electrolyte balance. Also, he or she assesses for the return of normal pattern of bowel movements and signs of normal fluid and electrolyte balance (adequate hydration, urine output, and skin turgor). In addition, it is important to assess for resumption of usual activities of daily living.

EVIDENCE-BASED PRACTICE

Clinical Practice Guideline: Acute Diarrhea
by WORLD GASTROENTEROLOGY ORGANISATION

2008, Retrieved November 1, 2011, from http://www.worldgastroenterology.org/assets/downloads/en/pdf/guidelines/01_acute_diarrhea.pdf

The World Gastroenterology Organisation defines acute diarrhea as an abnormally frequent discharge of semisolid or fluid bowel contents lasting less than 14 days. In people who present with acute diarrhea, it is necessary to check the history as follows:

- Evaluate history for recent intake of undercooked meat, unsanitary milk products, or ingestion of food and water from motels or other public places. Question whether others who were with the patient have a history of similar symptoms.
- Evaluate history for recent antibiotic use.

In addition, it is important to make the following physical assessments:

- Assess the pattern of loose stools regarding frequency, volume, and consistency (watery or mixed with mucus or blood). Further explore whether the stool is associated with abdominal cramps.
- Assess for the presence of fever.
- Assess hydration status.

IMPLICATIONS FOR NURSING PRACTICE: Routine administration of antidiarrheal medication without a thorough assessment of symptoms and clinical history may lead to worsening of symptoms. A review of recent history and an assessment targeting associated symptoms provides valuable information for basic care.

Assessing for Adverse Effects

The nurse assesses for hypotension and respiratory depression due to the effects of diphenoxylate. He or she observes for signs of the effects of atropine, including tachycardia, thirst, flushing, urinary retention, and dry skin and mucous membranes.

Patient Teaching

Once the diarrhea is under control, it is important that diphenoxylate with atropine be discontinued. The nurse ensures that patients who take this drug understand how to use it. Box 38.1 outlines patient teaching guidelines for antidiarrheal drugs.

NCLEX Success

1. An appropriate nursing measure when treating a 5-year-old child with a 1-day onset of mild diarrhea involves encouraging which of the following?

    A. regular diet
    B. intake of clear liquids
    C. intake of milk products
    D. no fluids for 24 hours

2. **A hospitalized patient on antibiotic therapy begins to experience fever, abdominal pain, and diarrhea containing mucus, pus, and blood. The best nursing action in this situation is to**

 A. continue the antibiotic because the patient has signs of a gastrointestinal infection

 B. monitor the patient's vital signs and notify the provider if there is further deterioration

 C. withhold the antibiotic and notify the provider of the patient's condition

 D. encourage fluid intake because fever is a sign of dehydration

Other Drugs in the Class

The choice of antidiarrheal agent depends largely on the cause, severity, and duration of diarrhea. Loperamide (Imodium) is a synthetic derivative of meperidine that decreases GI motility by its effect on intestinal muscles and is an unscheduled, nonprescription drug. Because loperamide does not penetrate the CNS well, it does not cause the CNS effects associated with opioid use and lacks potential for abuse. Although adverse effects are generally few and mild, loperamide can cause abdominal pain, constipation, drowsiness, fatigue, nausea, and vomiting. For nonprescription use, dosages for adults should not exceed 8 mg/d; with supervision by a health care provider, maximum daily dosage is 16 mg/d. In general, it is necessary to discontinue loperamide after 48 hours if clinical improvement has not occurred. With loperamide, the nurse monitors patients with hepatic impairment for signs of CNS toxicity. The drug normally undergoes extensive first-pass metabolism, which may be lessened by liver disease. As a result, a larger portion of a dose reaches the systemic circulation and may cause adverse effects. Treatment of overdose may involve naloxone, gastric lavage, and administration of activated charcoal. A dosage may be necessary.

Paregoric is a schedule III drug alone and a schedule V in the small amounts combined with other drugs; it contains 0.4 mg/mL of morphine. The main effects of paregoric are to increase the muscular tone of the intestine, to inhibit normal peristalsis, and to suppress coughing. Practitioners use it as an

---

BOX 38.1   Patient Teaching Guidelines for Antidiarrheals

General Considerations

- Taking a medication to stop diarrhea is not always needed or desirable because diarrhea may mean the body is trying to rid itself of irritants or bacteria. Treatment is indicated if diarrhea is severe, prolonged, or occurs in young children or older adults, who are highly susceptible to excessive losses of body fluids and electrolytes.
- Try to drink 2 to 3 quarts of fluid daily. This helps prevent dehydration from fluid loss in stools. Water, clear broths, and noncarbonated, caffeine-free beverages are recommended because they are unlikely to cause further diarrhea.
- Avoid highly spiced or "laxative" foods, such as fresh fruits and vegetables, until diarrhea is controlled.
- Frequent and thorough handwashing and careful food storage and preparation can help prevent diarrhea.
- Consult a health care provider if diarrhea is accompanied by severe abdominal pain or fever, lasts longer than 3 days, or if stools contain blood or mucus. These signs and symptoms may indicate more serious disorders for which other treatment measures are needed.
- Stop antidiarrheal drugs when diarrhea is controlled to avoid adverse effects such as constipation.
- Bismuth subsalicylate (Pepto-Bismol) and loperamide (Imodium A-D) are available over the counter; diphenoxylate (Lomotil) is a prescription drug.
- Diphenoxylate and loperamide may cause dizziness or drowsiness and should be used with caution if driving or performing other tasks requiring alertness, coordination, or physical dexterity. In addition, alcohol and other drugs that cause drowsiness should be avoided.
- Pepto-Bismol may temporarily discolor bowel movements a grayish-black.
- Keep antidiarrheal drugs out of reach of children.

Self- or Caregiver Administration

- Take or give antidiarrheal drugs only as prescribed or directed on nonprescription drug labels.
- Do not exceed maximal daily doses of diphenoxylate (Lomotil), loperamide, or paregoric.
- With liquid diphenoxylate, use only the calibrated dropper furnished by the manufacturer for accurate measurement of dosages.
- Use caution driving or operating heavy machinery with diphenoxylate and atropine, which may cause drowsiness or dizziness, until the effects of the medication are known.
- Diphenoxylate can cause dry mouth, so sucking on hard candy or chewing gum may alleviate the problem.
- With Pepto-Bismol liquid, shake the bottle well before measuring the dose; with tablets, chew them well or allow them to dissolve in the mouth.
- Add at least 30 mL of water to each dose of paregoric to help the drug dose reach the stomach. The mixture appears milky.
- Take cholestyramine or colestipol with at least 4 oz of water. These drugs should never be taken without fluids because they may block the gastrointestinal tract. Also, do not take within 4 hours of other drugs because they may combine with and inactivate other drugs.
- Take rifaximin with or without food for 3 days. Notify your health care prescriber if your condition worsens or does not improve after 1 to 2 days.
- Use caution driving or operating machinery if experiencing dizziness while using rifaximin.
- With Alinia, if you have diabetes, be aware that the oral suspension contains 1.48 g of sucrose per 5 mL.
- With Lotronex, if you become constipated, notice blood in your bowel movements, or experience a new worse or different pain in your stomach or abdomen, *stop* taking the drug and notify your health care prescriber.

antidiarrheal and as an antitussive. In recommended doses over the short term, paregoric does not produce euphoria, analgesia, or dependence.

QSEN Safety Alert ❗

Confusing paregoric (camphorated tincture of opium) with the much more potent drug opium tincture is a common and potentially fatal drug error. Opium tincture is much more concentrated than paregoric and contains 10 mg/mL of morphine. Labels on opium tincture packaging should identify it as a poison, giving the strength of morphine as 10 mg/mL and containing the statement, "Warning! Do not use opium tincture in place of paregoric."

Clinical Application 38-1

- What factors does the nurse practitioner include in assessment of Mr. Mendoza?
- What recommendations for management of the diarrhea does the nurse practitioner most likely make?

Adjuvant Medications Used to Treat Diarrhea

Specific drug therapy for diarrhea depends on the cause of the symptoms and may include the use of hormones, bulk-forming products, enzymatic replacement therapy, bile salt–binding drugs, antibacterial agents, and 5-HT₃ serotonin receptor antagonists. Table 38.3 presents route and dosage information for these drugs.

Bismuth Salts

Bismuth salts have antibacterial and antiviral activity. Bismuth subsalicylate (Pepto-Bismol), a commonly used over-the-counter drug, also has antisecretory and possibly anti-inflammatory effects because of its salicylate component.

QSEN Safety Alert ❗

People with an allergy to aspirin and aspirin products should not take bismuth subsalicylate.

This salt causes a temporary and harmless darkening of the tongue or stool.

Octreotide

Octreotide acetate (Sandostatin) is a synthetic form of somatostatin, a hormone produced in the anterior pituitary gland and in the pancreas. The drug may be effective in diarrhea because it decreases GI secretion and motility. Uses include diarrhea associated with carcinoid syndrome, intestinal tumors, HIV/AIDS, and diarrhea that does not respond to other antidiarrheal drugs. Commonly reported adverse effects are diarrhea, headache, cardiac dysrhythmias, and injection-site pain.

Polycarbophil

Polycarbophil (e.g., FiberCon) and psyllium are most often used as bulk-forming laxatives. They are occasionally used in diarrhea to adsorb toxins and water, decreasing the fluidity of stools. Polycarbophil is the only adsorbent drug evaluated to be effective by the U.S. Food and Drug Administration (FDA) over-the-counter review panel. Polycarbophil absorbs large amounts of water and produces stools of gelatin-like consistency. It may cause abdominal discomfort and bloating and may reduce the absorption of coadministered medications.

Enzymatic Replacement

In diarrhea caused by enzyme deficiency, pancreatic enzymes are given rather than antidiarrheal drugs. Practitioners recommend pancreatin or pancrelipase (Viokase, Pancrease, Cotazym) when a deficiency of pancreatic enzymes results in malabsorption of nutrients and **steatorrhea**, which is a loose fatty stool.

Bile-Binding Drugs

Cholestyramine (Questran) and colestipol (Colestid) are useful in treating diarrhea due to bile salt accumulation in conditions such as Crohn's disease or surgical excision of the ileum.

Antibacterial Drugs

Practitioners recommend antibacterial drugs for bacterial enteritis when diarrhea lasts longer than 48 hours, when the patient passes six or more loose stools in 24 hours, when diarrhea is associated with fever, or when blood or pus is present in the stools. In bacterial gastroenteritis or diarrhea, the choice of antibacterial drug depends on the causative microorganism and susceptibility tests. Antibacterial drugs are effective in preventing travelers' diarrhea, but authorities usually do not recommend them because their use may promote the emergence of drug-resistant microorganisms. Although effective in reducing diarrhea due to *Salmonella* and *E. coli* intestinal infections, antibiotics may induce a prolonged carrier state during which the infection can be transmitted to other people.

Rifaximin (Xifaxan) is a structural analog of the antimycobacterial drug rifampin. This nonsystemic antibiotic remains in the gut and is not absorbed into the bloodstream. Researchers developed it specifically to treat travelers' diarrhea due to noninvasive strains of *E. coli* in patients older than 12 years of age. Use for diarrhea in the presence of fever or bloody stools or due to pathogens other than *E. coli* is not warranted. As with the use of other broad-spectrum antibiotics, superinfections may occur, requiring termination of the rifaximin. Adverse effects of rifaximin may include flatulence, headache, stomach pain, urgent bowel movements, nausea, constipation, fever, vomiting, and dizziness.

Nitazoxanide (Alinia) is an antiprotozoal agent used specifically for treating diarrhea resulting from infection with *Giardia lamblia* or *Cryptosporidium parvum*. Caution is necessary when administering nitazoxanide concurrently with highly plasma protein–bound medications such as warfarin, because the active metabolite of nitazoxanide is highly plasma protein bound, and such concurrent use may result in competitive drug interactions.

TABLE 38.3

DRUGS AT A GLANCE: Adjuvant Antidiarrheal Medications

Drug	Pregnancy Category	Routes and Dosage Ranges	
		Adults	Children
Alosetron (Lotronex)	B	0.5 mg PO twice a day; may increase to 1 mg after 4 wk if needed	Not recommended
Bismuth subsalicylate (Pepto-Bismol)	C	2 tablets or 30 mL PO every 30–60 min, if needed, up to 8 doses in 24 h	Under 3 y, consult pediatrician 3–6 y, 1/3 tablet or 5 mL PO 6–9 y, 2/3 tablet or 10 mL PO 9–12 y, 1 tablet or 15 mL PO
Cholestyramine (Questran) Binds and inactivates bile salts in the intestine (see Chap. 55)	C	16–32 g/d in 120–180 mL of water PO, in 2–4 divided doses before or during meals and at bedtime	Safety and effectiveness not established
Colestipol (Colestid) Binds and inactivates bile salts in the intestine (see Chap. 55)	C	15–30 g/d in 120–180 mL of water PO, in 2–4 divided doses before or during meals and at bedtime	Safety and effectiveness not established
Nitazoxanide (Alinia) Inhibits growth of certain protozoa	B	500 mg (tablet or suspension) PO every 12 h for 3 d	12–47 mo, 5 mL (100 mg) PO every 12 h for 3 d 4–11 y, 10 mL (200 mg) PO every 12 h for 3 d ≥ 12 y, see adult dose
Octreotide (Sandostatin) Decreases secretions and motility in GI tract (see Chap. 22)	B	150–750/d Sub-Q, IV divided over 2–4 doses; start at 200–300 mcg/d divided over 2–4 doses for 2 wk, then individualize dose to response	Dosage not established
Pancreatin or pancrelipase (Viokase, Pancrease, Cotazym) Replaces pancreatic enzymes	C	1–3 tablets or capsules PO or 1–2 packets of powder with meals and snacks	1–3 tablets or capsules PO or 1–2 packets of powder with each meal
Polycarbophil preparations (FiberCon) Absorbs water and toxins and decreases fluidity of stools (see Chap. 37)	C	1 g PO, 1–4 times daily; do not exceed 4 g in 24 h; for severe diarrhea repeat dose every 30 min but do not exceed max dose	Under 6 y, products vary, so consult labels; for severe diarrhea, repeat dose every 30 min but do not exceed max dose 6–12 y, 500 mg PO 1–4 times daily; do not exceed 2 g in 24 h
Rifaximin (Xifaxan) Affects E. coli in the GI tract	C	200 mg PO 3 times a day for 3 d	Safety and effectiveness not established

AIDS, acquired immunodeficiency syndrome; GI, gastrointestinal; HIV, human immunodeficiency virus.

Selective 5-HT₃ Receptor Antagonist

Alosetron (Lotronex) is a selective 5-HT₃ receptor antagonist indicated for treating women with chronic severe diarrhea-predominant IBS that has not responded to conventional therapy. Clinical studies have not demonstrated safety and efficacy of alosetron in men. Alosetron is rapidly absorbed orally with a bioavailability of 50% to 60%. It is moderately plasma protein bound (82%). Extensively metabolized by the cytochrome 450 enzyme system (CYP2C9, CYP3A4, and CYP1A2), its multiple metabolites produced are excreted primarily in the urine. Caution is essential with concurrent administration with CYP1A2 and CYP3A4 inhibitors. Contraindications include concurrent administration with fluvoxamine and severe hepatic impairment is also a contraindication. Reduced dosages to prevent drug accumulation and toxicity may be necessary in some women older than 65 years of age.

A **BLACK BOX WARNING** ◆ alerts nurses to the serious GI adverse effects of alosetron. Severe constipation, with possible obstruction, perforation, and hemorrhage, is the most common problem. Ischemic colitis (reduced blood flow to the intestinal tract resulting in tissue damage) has also occurred. These serious conditions have resulted in hospitalizations, blood loss necessitating transfusion, surgery, and death in severe cases. It is important not to give alosetron to patients with a history of GI disorders, including chronic or severe constipation or sequelae of constipation, intestinal obstruction, stricture, toxic megacolon, GI perforation and/or adhesions, ischemic colitis, impaired intestinal circulation, thrombophlebitis or hypercoagulable state, Crohn's disease or ulcerative colitis, and diverticulitis.

To ensure safe and appropriate use of alosetron, the drug manufacturer has established a prescribing program, and only qualified health care providers enrolled in the program can prescribe this medication. Pharmacists must provide patients with a medication guide developed by the manufacturer at the time the medication is dispensed that includes the risks of taking alosetron and the situations under which the drug should be immediately discontinued. Each patient must sign a patient–physician agreement indicating that he or she (1) understands the risks of taking alosetron and agrees to take the medication, (2) will discontinue taking alosetron if constipation occurs, (3) will immediately notify the physician if constipation or signs of ischemic colitis occur, and (4) will stop taking alosetron and contact the physician after 4 weeks of therapy with alosetron if the symptoms of IBS are not controlled.

NCLEX Success

3. **A woman with diarrhea begins to complain of eye pain after administration of diphenoxylate with atropine (Lomotil). The nurse should**

   A. offer an over-the-counter analgesic such as acetaminophen
   B. discontinue the diphenoxylate with atropine and notify the provider
   C. tell the patient that this is a common side effect and will soon pass
   D. apply a cool compress to the eyes for relief of the discomfort

4. **A man tells the nurse that he has bought the over-the-counter drug bismuth subsalicylate (Pepto-Bismol) for the next episode of diarrhea. The nurse should assess for what allergy that would contraindicate use of bismuth subsalicylate?**

   A. penicillin
   B. acetaminophen
   C. aspirin
   D. sulfa

The Nursing Process

Assessment

- Try to determine the duration of diarrhea; number of stools per day; amount, consistency, color, odor, and presence of abnormal components (e.g., undigested food, blood, pus, mucus) in each stool; precipitating factors; accompanying signs and symptoms (i.e., nausea, vomiting, fever, abdominal pain, or cramping); and measures used to relieve diarrhea. When possible, look at stool specimens for possible clues to causation. Blood may indicate inflammation, infection, or neoplastic disease; pus or mucus may indicate inflammation or infection. Infections caused by *Shigella* organisms produce blood-tinged mucus. Infections caused by *Salmonella* or *E. coli* usually produce green, liquid or semiliquid stools. Inflammatory bowel disorders often produce nonbloody mucus.
- Try to determine the cause of the diarrhea. This includes questioning about such causes as chronic inflammatory diseases of the bowel, food intake, possible exposure to contaminated food, living or traveling in areas of poor sanitation, and use of laxatives or other drugs that may cause diarrhea. When available, check laboratory reports on stool specimens (e.g., culture reports).
- With severe or prolonged diarrhea, especially in young children and older adults, assess for dehydration, hypokalemia, and other fluid and electrolyte disorders.

Nursing Diagnoses

- Diarrhea related to GI infection or inflammatory disorders, other disease processes, dietary irritants, or overuse of laxatives
- Anxiety related to availability of bathroom facilities
- Deficient fluid volume related to excessive losses in liquid stools
- Pain (abdominal cramping) related to intestinal hypermotility and spasm
- Deficient knowledge: factors that cause or aggravate diarrhea and appropriate use of antidiarrheal drugs

Planning/Goals

The patient will

- Take antidiarrheal drugs appropriately
- Obtain relief from acute diarrhea (reduced number of liquid stools, reduced abdominal discomfort)
- Maintain fluid and electrolyte balance
- Maintain adequate nutritional intake
- Avoid adverse effects of antidiarrheal medications
- Reestablish normal bowel patterns after an episode of acute diarrhea
- Have fewer liquid stools with chronic diarrhea

Nursing Interventions

The nurse will

- Provide instruction about the use of measures to prevent diarrhea
  - Prepare and store food properly and avoid improperly stored foods and those prepared under unsanitary conditions. Dairy products, cream pies, and other foods may cause diarrhea (food poisoning) if not refrigerated.
  - Wash hands before handling any foods, after handling raw poultry or meat, and always before eating.
  - Chew food well.
  - Do not overuse laxatives (i.e., amount per dose or frequency of use) Many OTC products contain senna or other strong stimulant laxatives.

- Provide education about drug therapy (see Box 38.1)
- Provide supportive care, which is necessary regardless of whether antidiarrheal drugs are used
  - Replace fluids and electrolytes (2–3 quarts daily). Fluids such as weak tea; water; bouillon; clear soup; noncarbonated, caffeine-free beverages; and gelatin are usually tolerated and helpful. If the patient cannot tolerate adequate amounts of oral liquids or if diarrhea is severe or prolonged, intravenous fluids may be needed (i.e., solutions containing dextrose, sodium chloride, and potassium chloride).
  - Avoid foods and fluids that may further irritate GI mucosa (e.g., highly spiced foods; "laxative" foods, such as raw fruits and vegetables).
  - Increase frequency and length of rest periods, and decrease activity. Exercise and activity stimulate peristalsis.
  - If perianal irritation occurs because of frequent liquid stools, cleanse the area with mild soap and water after each bowel movement, then apply an emollient, such as white petrolatum (Vaseline).

Evaluation

- Observe and interview for decreased number of liquid or loose stools.
- Observe for signs of adequate food and fluid intake (e.g., good skin turgor and urine output, stable weight).
- Observe for appropriate use of antidiarrheal drugs.
- Observe and interview for return of prediarrheal patterns of bowel elimination.
- Interview regarding knowledge and use of measures to prevent or minimize diarrhea.

Clinical Application 38-2

- Mr. Mendoza's culture report identifies an enterotoxigenic strain of *E. coli* (ETEC). What is the most likely drug of choice for him?

Key Concepts

- Diarrhea is the frequent expulsion of liquid or semiliquid stools resulting from increased bowel motility, increased secretion or retention of fluids in the intestinal lumen, or inflammation/irritation of the GI tract.
- Overall, opiates and opiate derivatives are the most effective nonspecific therapy for symptomatic treatment of diarrhea.
- Use of antidiarrheal medications to treat diarrhea if it is caused by toxin-producing substances or poisoning is inappropriate.
- Specific drug therapy for diarrhea is directed at the cause of the symptoms and may include enzymatic replacement therapy, bile salt–binding drugs, antibacterial agents, and 5-HT$_3$ receptor antagonists.
- Octreotide, a synthetic form of somatostatin, decreases GI secretion and motility. Uses include diarrhea associated with carcinoid syndrome, intestinal tumors, HIV/AIDS, and diarrhea that does not respond to other antidiarrheal drugs.
- Bismuth subsalicylate has antisecretory, antimicrobial, and possibly anti-inflammatory effects. Uses include control of travelers' diarrhea and relief of abdominal cramping.
- Polycarbophil treats diarrhea by adsorbing toxins and water, decreasing the fluidity of stools.
- In bacterial gastroenteritis or diarrhea, the choice of antibacterial drug depends on the causative organism and susceptibility tests.
- Because of the risk of severe GI adverse effects, use of alosetron is subject to a mandated prescribing program. A **BLACK BOX WARNING** ◆ alerts nurses to the serious GI adverse effects of alosetron. Severe constipation, with possible obstruction, perforation, and hemorrhage, is the most common problem. Ischemic colitis (reduced blood flow to the intestinal tract resulting in tissue damage) has also occurred. These serious conditions have resulted in hospitalizations, blood loss necessitating transfusion, surgery, and death in severe cases. Only qualified health care providers enrolled in the program can prescribe this medication. Pharmacists are required to distribute educational materials when dispensing alosetron. Patients must sign a patient–physician agreement before taking this medication.

Critical Thinking Questions

38-1. Carol Rogers, a mother of an 18-month-old child, calls the health department because her son's stools have been semiliquid for the past 2 days. She has asked the nurse who has been contacted to recommend an over-the-counter antidiarrheal drug.

• Which drug does the nurse recommend, and why?

• Mrs. Rogers brings her son to the clinic for evaluation. Stool cultures are negative. What instructions does the nurse give the mother regarding the diarrhea?

References and Resources

Brye, J., Boschi-Pinto, C., Shibuya, K., Black, R. E., WHO Child Health Epidemiology Reference Group. (2005). WHO estimates of the causes of death in children. *Lancet*, 365, 1147–1152.

Centers for Disease Control and Prevention. (2006, November). *Travelers' diarrhea*. Retrieved October 31, 2011, from http://www.cdc.gov/ncidod/dbmd/diseaseinfo/travelersdiarrhea_g.htm

Drug facts and comparisons. (Updated monthly). St. Louis, MO: Facts and Comparisons.

Guerrant, R., Gilder, T., Steiner, T., Thielman, N., Slutsker, L., Tauxe, R., et al. (2001). Practice guidelines for the management of infectious diarrhea. *Clinical Infectious Diseases, 32*, 331–351.

Hatchette, T. F., & Farina, D. (2011). Infectious diarrhea: When to test and when to treat. *Canadian Medical Association Journal, 183*(3):339–344.

Institute for Safe Medication Practices. (2006, May). *Confusion between opium tinctures marks need for community high alert list*. Retrieved October 31, 2011, from http://www.ismp.org/Newsletters/ambulatory/archives/200605_1.asp

Kachrimanidou, M., & Malisiovas, N. (2011). *Clostridium difficile* infection: A comprehensive review. *Critical Reviews in Microbiology, 37*(3), 178–187.

Karch, A. M. (2012). *2012 Lippincott's nursing drug guide*. Philadelphia, PA: Lippincott Williams & Wilkins.

Li, S. T., Grossman, D. C., & Cummings, P. (2007, March). Loperamide therapy for acute diarrhea in children: Systematic review and meta-analysis. Retrieved October 24, 2011, from http://www.ncbi.nlm.nih.gov/pmc/articles/PMC1831735/

Porth, C. M. (2009). *Pathophysiology: Concepts of altered health status* (8th ed.). Philadelphia, PA: Lippincott Williams & Wilkins.

Smeltzer, S. C., Bare, B. G., Hinkle, J. L., & Cheever, K. H. (2009). *Brunner & Suddarth's textbook of medical-surgical nursing* (12th ed.). Philadelphia, PA: Lippincott Williams & Wilkins.

Spruill, W. J., & Wade, W. E. (2005). Diarrhea, constipation, and irritable bowel syndrome. In: J. T. DiPiro, R. L. Talbert, G. C. Yee, G. R. Matzke, B. G. Wells, & L. M. Posey (Eds.), *Pharmacotherapy: A pathophysiologic approach* (6th ed., pp. 677–692). New York: McGraw-Hill.

World Gastroenterology Organisation. (March 2008). *Clinical Practice Guideline: Acute Diarrhea*. Retrieved November 1, 2011, from http://www.worldgastroenterology.org/assets/downloads/en/pdf/guidelines/01_acute_diarrhea.pdf

SECTION **8**

Drugs Affecting the Endocrine System

Drugs Affecting the Endocrine System

CHAPTER OUTLINE

39 Drug Therapy for Diabetes Mellitus

Clinical Application Case Study

Alfred Smith, a 56-year-old librarian, visits his physician because he has been feeling more tired and weak than usual for the past 2 months. On questioning, the physician learns that Mr. Smith often gets up in the middle of the night to urinate and drinks a glass of water. He also has numbness and tingling in his hands and feet, as well as blurred vision, which affects his job. Laboratory results show an impaired fasting glucose of 160 mg/dL and urinalysis of 4+ glucose. His lipid panel also shows total cholesterol of 240 mg/dL, high-density lipoprotein cholesterol of 22 mg/dL, and triglycerides of 400 mg/dL. Mr. Smith receives a diagnosis of type 2 diabetes, and his physician places him on glyburide (DiaBeta) 2.5 mg by mouth with breakfast daily. He also receives information about a diet and exercise routine to help control his diabetes.

Blood glucose level: blood sugar level in the body

Blood glucose meter: device that measures how much glucose is in the blood

Diabetes mellitus: chronic disease characterized by disordered metabolism of carbohydrates, fats, and protein, and hyperglycemia, due to a deficiency in the amount on action of insulin; the three main forms of diabetes are type 1, type 2, and gestational diabetes

Glucagon: pancreatic hormone that raises blood glucose levels by stimulating the liver to convert glycogen into glucose; it opposes insulin

Gluconeogenesis: formation of glucose from noncarbohydrate sources such as fats and amino acids

Glucose: sugar in the blood; major stimulus of insulin secretion

Impaired fasting glucose: fasting blood glucose level between 100 mg/dL to 125 mg/dL; also referred to as prediabetes

Insulin: protein hormone secreted by beta cells in the pancreas; facilitates glucose utilization by cells. Absence of insulin results in diabetes mellitus

Insulin pump: wearable delivery system for continuous subcutaneous insulin infusion; the insulin dosage is programmed into the pump, and the appropriate amount of insulin is injected through a needle into the adipose tissue

Ketoacidosis: metabolic acidosis due to accumulation of ketone bodies formed by the breakdown of fatty acids and amino acids for energy in the absence of insulin

Lancet: sharp instrument used to prick the finger for a blood test

Introduction

Diabetes mellitus is characterized as a disease of insulin availability that eventually results in high blood glucose concentrations. Treatment of diabetes mellitus includes drugs to maintain blood glucose levels within the normal range and prevent complications. Insulin and oral hypoglycemic agents are two of the several types of medications used to lower blood **glucose** in diabetes mellitus. New drug therapies include amylin analogs, incretin mimetics, and dipeptidyl peptidase-4 (DPP-4) inhibitors. It is important that nurses understand the characteristic of diabetes mellitus and the clinical use of insulin, oral hypoglycemic medications, and the newer drugs. They also need to be familiar with the effects of dietary herbal supplements on blood glucose levels.

Overview of Diabetes

Metabolic problems occur early in people with diabetes mellitus and are related to changes in the metabolism of carbohydrate, fat, and protein. A major clinical manifestation of disordered metabolism is hyperglycemia, or fasting blood glucose levels exceeding 126 mg/dL. A person with a fasting blood glucose level between 100 and 125 mg/dL is said to have **impaired fasting glucose (IFG)**, or prediabetes. Indicative **blood glucose levels** for most people diagnosed with diabetes are approximately 80 to 120 mg/dL before a meal, 180 mg/dL or less after a meal, and between 100 and 140 mg/dL at bedtime.

Vascular problems include atherosclerosis throughout the body. Macrovascular (moderate and large vessels) clinical manifestations include hypertension, myocardial infarction,

stroke, and peripheral vascular disease. Changes in small blood vessels (microvasculature) especially affect the retina and kidney, resulting in retinopathy, blindness, and nephropathy.

Etiology

The two major classifications of diabetes mellitus are type 1 and type 2. Although both are characterized by hyperglycemia, they differ in onset, course, pathology, and treatment. Other types of diabetes may be induced by disease processes such as slowly progressing autoimmune disorders, certain drugs, and pregnancy (see Chap. 6).

Type 1 Diabetes

Type 1 diabetes, a common chronic disorder of childhood, results from an autoimmune disorder that destroys pancreatic beta cells. Although it may occur at any age, it usually appears after 4 years of age and peaks in incidence at 10 to 12 years for girls and 12 to 14 years for boys. A subtype of type 1 diabetes, latent autoimmune diabetes of the adult, begins in adulthood. Symptoms of traditional type 1 diabetes usually develop when 10% to 20% of functioning beta cells remain, but they may occur at any time if acute illness or stress increases the body's demand for **insulin** (a protein hormone secreted by the beta cells) beyond the capacity of the remaining beta cells to secrete insulin. Eventually, destruction of all beta cells occurs, resulting in no insulin production.

Type 1 diabetes usually has a sudden onset; produces severe symptoms; is difficult to control; produces a high incidence of complications, such as diabetic **ketoacidosis** (DKA) and renal failure; and requires administration of exogenous insulin. About 10% of people with diabetes have type 1 disease.

Type 2 Diabetes

Type 2 diabetes is characterized by hyperglycemia and insulin resistance. The hyperglycemia results from increased production of glucose by the liver and decreased uptake of glucose in liver, muscle, and fat cells. Insulin resistance means that higher-than-usual concentrations of insulin are required. Thus, insulin is present but unable to work effectively (i.e., inhibits hepatic production of glucose and causes glucose to move from the bloodstream into liver, muscle, and fat cells). Most insulin resistance is attributed to impaired insulin action at the cellular level, possibly related to postreceptor, intracellular mechanisms.

Historically, the onset of type 2 diabetes occurred after 40 years of age. More recently, however, type 2 diabetes is increasing in prevalence among children and adolescents. Compared with type 1, it usually has a gradual onset, produces less severe symptoms initially, is easier to control, causes less DKA and renal failure but more myocardial infarctions and strokes, and does not necessarily require exogenous insulin because endogenous insulin is still produced. About 90% of people with diabetes have type 2 disease; 20% to 30% of them require exogenous insulin at some point in their lives.

Type 2 is a heterogeneous disease, and etiology probably involves multiple factors such as a genetic predisposition and environmental factors. Obesity is a major cause. With obesity and chronic ingestion of excess calories, along with a sedentary lifestyle, more insulin is required. The increased need leads to prolonged stimulation and eventual "fatigue" of pancreatic beta cells. As a result, the cells become less responsive to elevated blood glucose levels and less able to produce enough insulin to meet metabolic needs. Thus, insulin is secreted but is inadequate or ineffective, especially when insulin demand is increased by obesity, pregnancy, aging, or other factors.

A risk factor for the development of type 2 diabetes is the presence of metabolic syndrome. This syndrome is characterized by a group of risk factors, including abdominal obesity (excessive fat tissue in and around the abdomen), hypertriglyceridemia, low high-density lipoprotein (HDL) cholesterol, hypertension, and/or IFG. People with metabolic syndrome have an increased risk of coronary heart disease and other diseases related to plaque buildup in artery walls (e.g., stroke and peripheral vascular disease) and type 2 diabetes. Metabolic syndrome has become increasingly common in the United States. Estimates indicate that more than 50 million Americans have it.

In the United States, African Americans, Hispanics, Native Americans, Native Alaskans, and some Asian Americans and Pacific Islanders are at high risk for type 2 diabetes. Prevalence rates are about 13.3% in African Americans and 13.9% in Hispanic Americans and 12.8% in American Indians and Alaska Natives compared with 8.7% in Caucasians. Undiagnosed diabetes is reportedly common in Mexican Americans.

Pathophysiology

Endogenous Insulin

Beta cells in the pancreas secrete insulin. The average adult pancreas secretes 40 to 60 units of insulin daily. This includes a basal amount of 1 to 2 units/h and additional amounts (4–6 units/h) after meals or when the blood glucose level exceeds 100 mg/dL. In a fasting state, serum insulin levels are low, and the body uses stored glucose and amino acids for energy needs of tissues that require glucose. After a meal, serum insulin levels increase and peak in a few minutes, then decrease to baseline levels in 2 to 3 hours.

Amylin, a pancreatic hormone secreted with insulin, delays gastric emptying, increases satiety, and suppresses **glucagon** (hormone that raises blood glucose levels by stimulating the liver to convert glycogen into glucose) secretion, thus complementing the effects of insulin on blood glucose. A synthetic form of amylin, pramlintide, has been developed to assist with glucose control in patients with diabetes (see later discussion).

Insulin is secreted into the portal circulation and transported to the liver, where about half is used or degraded. The other half reaches the systemic circulation, where it circulates mainly in an unbound form and is transported to body cells.

At the cellular level (Fig. 39.1), insulin binds with and activates receptors on the cell membranes of about 80% of body cells. Liver, muscle, and fat cells have many insulin receptors and are primary tissues for insulin action. After insulin–receptor binding occurs, cell membranes become highly permeable to glucose and allow rapid entry of glucose into the cells. The cell membranes also become more permeable to amino acids, fatty acids, and electrolytes such as potassium, magnesium, and

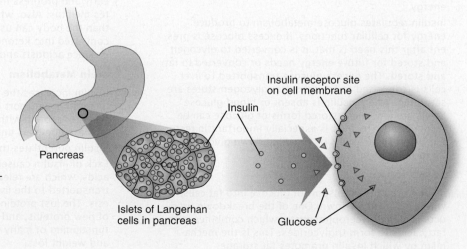

Figure 39.1 Normal glucose metabolism. After insulin binds with receptors on the cell membrane, glucose can move into the cell, promoting cellular metabolism and energy production.

Pancreas

Islets of Langerhan cells in pancreas

Insulin

Insulin receptor site on cell membrane

Glucose

phosphate ions. Cellular metabolism is altered by the movement of these substances into the cells, by activation of some enzymes and inactivation of others, by movement of proteins between intracellular compartments, by changes in the amounts of proteins produced, and perhaps by other mechanisms. Overall, the changes in cellular metabolism stimulate anabolic effects (e.g., utilization and storage of glucose, amino acids, and fatty acids) and inhibit catabolic processes (e.g., breakdown of glycogen, fat, and protein). After binding to insulin and entering the cell, receptors may be degraded or recycled back to the cell surface.

Insulin is cleared from circulating blood in 10 to 15 minutes because of rapid binding to peripheral tissues or metabolic breakdown. The insulin that does not combine with receptors is metabolized in the liver, kidneys, plasma, and muscles. In the kidneys, insulin is filtered by the glomeruli and reabsorbed by the tubules, which also degrade it. Severe renal impairment slows the clearance of insulin from the blood.

Insulin plays a major role in metabolism of carbohydrate, fat, and protein (Box 39.1). Food particles are broken down into molecules of glucose, lipids, and amino acids, respectively. The molecules enter the cells and are converted to energy for cellular activities. The energy can be used immediately or converted to storage forms for later use. When carrying out its metabolic functions, the overall effect of insulin is to lower blood glucose levels, primarily by the following mechanisms:

- In the liver, insulin acts to decrease breakdown of glycogen (glycogenolysis), form new glucose from fatty acids and amino acids (**gluconeogenesis**), and form ketone bodies (ketogenesis). At the same time, it acts to increase synthesis and storage of glycogen and fatty acids.
- In adipose tissue, insulin acts to decrease breakdown of fat (lipolysis) and to increase production of glycerol and fatty acids.

- In muscle tissue, insulin acts to decrease protein breakdown and amino acid output and to increase amino acid uptake, protein synthesis, and glycogen synthesis.

Regulation of Insulin Secretion

Insulin decreases blood sugar and regulates the amount of glucose available for cellular metabolism and energy needs, during both fasting and feeding. Insulin secretion involves coordination of various nutrients, hormones, the autonomic nervous system, and other factors.

Glucose is the major stimulus of insulin secretion; others include amino acids, fatty acids, ketone bodies (which are acidotic substances in themselves), and stimulation of beta$_2$-adrenergic receptors or vagal nerves. Oral glucose is more effective than intravenous (IV) glucose because glucose or food in the digestive tract stimulates vagal activity and induces the release of gastrointestinal (GI) hormones called incretins. Incretin hormones stimulate the release of insulin when glucose levels are normal or elevated. In addition, incretin hormones reduce glucagon production and delay gastric emptying. Two incretin hormones have been identified: glucose-dependent insulinotropic peptide and glucagon-like peptide-1 (GLP-1). GLP-1 also appears to improve insulin sensitivity and may increase the formation of new beta cells in the pancreas. The therapeutic uses of incretin hormones have recently been investigated, and this has led to the development of new drugs to treat diabetes mellitus.

Several hormones raise blood glucose levels and stimulate insulin secretion, including cortisol, glucagon, growth hormone, epinephrine, estrogen, and progesterone. Excessive, prolonged, endogenous secretion or administration of pharmacologic preparations of these hormones can exhaust the ability of pancreatic beta cells to produce insulin and thereby cause or aggravate diabetes mellitus.

BOX 39.1   Effects of Insulin on Metabolism

Carbohydrate Metabolism

- Insulin increases glucose transport into the liver, skeletal muscle, adipose tissue, the heart, and some smooth muscle organs (such as the uterus); it must be present for muscle and fat tissues to use glucose for energy.
- Insulin regulates glucose metabolism to produce energy for cellular functions. If excess glucose is present after this need is met, it is converted to glycogen and stored for future energy needs or converted to fat and stored. The excess glucose transported to liver cells is converted to fat only after glycogen stores are saturated. When insulin is absent or blood glucose levels are low, these stored forms of glucose can be reconverted. The liver is especially important in restoring blood sugar levels by breaking down glycogen or by forming new glucose.

Fat Metabolism

- Insulin promotes transport of glucose into fat cells, where it is broken down. One of the breakdown products is alpha-glycerophosphate, which combines with fatty acids to form triglycerides. This is the mechanism by which insulin promotes fat storage.

- When insulin is lacking, fat is released into the bloodstream as free fatty acids. Blood concentrations of triglycerides, cholesterol, and phospholipids are also increased. The high blood lipid concentration probably accounts for the atherosclerosis that tends to develop early and progress more rapidly in people with diabetes mellitus. Also, when more fatty acids are released than the body can use as fuel, some fatty acids are converted into ketones. Excessive amounts of ketones produce acidosis and coma.

Protein Metabolism

- Insulin increases the total amount of body protein by increasing transport of amino acids into cells and synthesis of protein within the cells. The basic mechanism of these effects is unknown.
- Insulin potentiates the effects of growth hormone.
- Lack of insulin causes protein breakdown into amino acids, which are released into the bloodstream and transported to the liver for energy or gluconeogenesis. The lost proteins are not replaced by synthesis of new proteins, and protein wasting causes abnormal functioning of many body organs, severe weakness, and weight loss.

Factors that inhibit insulin secretion include stimulation of pancreatic alpha$_2$-adrenergic receptors and stress conditions such as hypoxia, hypothermia, surgery, or severe burns.

Clinical Manifestations

Most signs and symptoms stem from a lack of effective insulin and the subsequent metabolic abnormalities. The incidence and severity depend on the amount of effective insulin, and conditions such as infection, rapid growth, pregnancy, or other factors may increase demand for insulin. Most early symptoms result from disordered carbohydrate metabolism, which causes excess glucose to accumulate in the blood (hyperglycemia). Hyperglycemia produces glucosuria, which, in turn, produces polydipsia, polyuria, dehydration, and polyphagia.

Glucosuria usually appears when the blood glucose level is approximately twice the normal value and the kidneys receive more glucose than can be reabsorbed. However, renal threshold varies, and the amount of glucose lost in the urine does not accurately reflect blood glucose. In children, glucose tends to appear in urine at much lower or even normal blood glucose levels. In older people, the kidneys may be less able to excrete excess glucose from the blood. As a result, blood glucose levels may be high with little or no glucose in the urine.

When large amounts of glucose are present, water is pulled into the renal tubule. This results in a greatly increased urine output (polyuria). The excessive loss of fluid in urine leads to increased thirst (polydipsia) and, if fluid intake is inadequate, to dehydration. Dehydration also occurs because high blood glucose levels increase osmotic pressure in the bloodstream and fluid is pulled out of the cells in the body's attempt to regain homeostasis. Polyphagia (increased appetite) occurs because the body cannot use ingested foods. People with uncontrolled diabetes lose weight because of abnormal metabolism.

Complications of diabetes mellitus are common and potentially disabling or life threatening. Diabetes is a leading cause of myocardial infarction, stroke, blindness, leg amputation, and kidney failure. These complications result from hyperglycemia and other metabolic abnormalities that accompany a lack of effective insulin. The metabolic abnormalities associated with hyperglycemia can cause early, acute complications, such as DKA or hyperosmolar hyperglycemic nonketotic coma (HHNC; Box 39.2). Eventually, metabolic abnormalities lead to damage in blood vessels and other body tissues. For example,

---

BOX 39.2   Acute Complications of Diabetes Mellitus

Diabetic Ketoacidosis (DKA)

This life-threatening complication occurs with severe insulin deficiency. In the absence of insulin, glucose cannot be used by body cells for energy, and fat is mobilized from adipose tissue to furnish a fuel source. The mobilized fat circulates in the bloodstream, from which it is extracted by the liver and broken down into glycerol and fatty acids. The fatty acids are further changed in the liver to ketones (e.g., acetoacetic acid, acetone), which then enter the bloodstream and are circulated to body cells for metabolic conversion to energy, carbon dioxide, and water.

The ketones are produced more rapidly than body cells can use them, and their accumulation produces acidemia (a drop in blood pH and an increase in blood hydrogen ions). The body attempts to buffer the acidic hydrogen ions by exchanging them for intracellular potassium ions. Hydrogen ions enter body cells, and potassium ions leave the cells to be excreted in the urine. Another attempt to remove excess acid involves the lungs. Deep, labored respirations, called *Kussmaul's respirations*, eliminate more carbon dioxide and prevent formation of carbonic acid. A third attempt to regain homeostasis involves the kidneys, which excrete some of the ketones, thereby producing acetone in the urine.

Two major causes of DKA are omission of insulin and illnesses such as infection, trauma, myocardial infarction, or stroke. DKA worsens as the compensatory mechanisms fail. Clinical signs and symptoms become progressively more severe. Early ones include blurred vision, anorexia, nausea and vomiting, thirst, and polyuria. Later ones include drowsiness, which progresses to stupor and coma; Kussmaul's respirations; dehydration and other signs of fluid and electrolyte imbalances; and decreased blood pressure, increased pulse, and other signs of shock.

Insulin therapy is a major part of any treatment for DKA. Patients with DKA have a deficiency in the total amount of insulin in the body and a resistance to the action of the insulin that is available, probably due to acidosis, hyperosmolality, infection, and other factors. To be effective, insulin therapy must be individualized according to frequent measurements of blood glucose. Low doses, given by continuous intravenous (IV) infusion, are preferred in most circumstances so that the brain has time to equilibrate and account for fluid shifts.

Additional measures include identification and treatment of conditions that precipitate DKA, administration of IV fluids to correct hyperosmolality and dehydration, administration of potassium supplements to restore and maintain normal serum potassium levels, and administration of sodium bicarbonate to correct metabolic acidosis. Infection is one of the most common causes of DKA. If no obvious source of infection is identified, cultures of blood, urine, and throat swabs are recommended. When infection is identified, antimicrobial drug therapy may be indicated.

Hyperosmolar Hyperglycemic Nonketotic Coma (HHNC)

HHNC is another type of diabetic coma that is potentially life threatening. It is relatively rare and carries a high mortality rate. The term *hyperosmolar* refers to an excessive amount of glucose, electrolytes, and other solutes in the blood in relation to the amount of water.

Like DKA, HHNC is characterized by hyperglycemia, which leads to osmotic diuresis and resultant thirst, polyuria, dehydration, and electrolyte losses, as well as neurologic signs ranging from drowsiness to stupor to coma. Additional clinical problems may include hypovolemic shock, thrombosis, renal problems, or stroke. In contrast with DKA, hyperosmolar coma occurs in people with previously unknown or mild diabetes, usually after an illness; occurs in hyperglycemic conditions other than diabetes (e.g., severe burns, corticosteroid drug therapy); and does not cause ketosis.

Treatment of HHNC is similar to that of DKA in that insulin, IV fluids, and potassium supplements are major components. Regular insulin is given by continuous IV infusion, and dosage is individualized according to frequent measurements of blood glucose levels. IV fluids are given to correct the profound dehydration and hyperosmolality, and potassium is given IV to replace the large amounts lost in urine during a hyperglycemic state.

Initiation of Intensive Diabetes Control in the First 15 Years After Diagnosis Reduces Cardiovascular Events

by AMERICAN DIABETES ASSOCIATION

Retrieved May 30, 2011, from http://www.diabetes.org/for-media/2009/factors-affecting-2009.html

Patients with diabetes mellitus are at an increased risk of developing macrovascular and microvascular complications secondary to the nature of the disease and poor glycemic control. In this study, researchers found that initiation of intensive control in the first 15 years after a diagnosis of diabetes reduced the risk of cardiovascular events, including mortality, but initiation 16 to 20 years after diagnosis yielded no such benefit. Further, initiation of intensive control 20 or more years after diagnosis actually increased the risk of cardiovascular events. Severe hypoglycemia was mentioned as a serious risk factor in tight glycemic control. Patients with severe hypoglycemic events were undoubtedly at an increased risk for cardiovascular events regardless of the degree of glycemic control.

IMPLICATIONS FOR NURSING PRACTICE: When providing care to a patient with diabetes mellitus, it is important to assess the patient's knowledge of the disease process and individual treatment plan. The nurse should teach the patient to collaborate closely with all involved members of the health care personnel directly involved in the care and management of the treatment plan. The nurse should encourage the patient to maintain a diet and exercise regimen to achieve tight glycemic control and provide education when needed.

atherosclerosis develops earlier, progresses more rapidly, and becomes more severe in people with diabetes. Microvascular changes lead to nephropathy, retinopathy, and peripheral neuropathy. Other complications include musculoskeletal disorders, increased numbers and severity of infections, and complications of pregnancy.

Drug Therapy

Medications used in the treatment of diabetes mellitus depend on the type of diabetes and degree of glycemic control. Health care providers use many medications to control diabetes (Table 39.1). Insulin is the prototype drug for treatment of type 1 diabetes. Several different classes of other drugs are also available for the treatment of type 2 diabetes (Fig. 39.2). Patients with diabetes may be using herbal supplements, and nurses should be aware that some of these substances affect blood glucose levels (Box 39.3).

Clinical Application 39-1

- ▪ What additional condition does Mr. Smith have?
- ▪ What are the complications related to this diagnosis?

NCLEX Success

1. A patient presents with a blood pressure of 162/88 mm Hg, heart rate of 100 bpm, triglycerides of 378 mg/dL, and HDL of 25 mg/dL. Which of the following are characteristics of metabolic syndrome? (Select all that apply.)

   A. blood pressure of 162/88 mm Hg
   B. heart rate of 100 bpm
   C. triglycerides of 378 mg/dL
   D. HDL of 25 mg/dL

2. A patient who has just arrived at the emergency department may be suffering from diabetic ketoacidosis. Which of the following would confirm the diagnosis?

   A. elevated serum potassium
   B. increased respiratory rate
   C. increased pH
   D. elevated blood glucose level and low plasma bicarbonate level

Insulins

Insulin in its various forms is the only effective drug treatment for type 1 diabetes, where pancreatic beta cells are unable to secrete endogenous insulin, and metabolism is severely impaired. Ⓟ **Regular insulin** (Humulin R, Novolin R) is the prototype. Insulin is also necessary in patients with type 2 diabetes who cannot control their disease with diet, weight control, and oral agents. Any person with diabetes may need insulin during times of stress, such as illness, infection, or surgery. Other uses of insulin include control of diabetes induced by chronic pancreatitis, surgical excision of pancreatic tissue, hormones and other drugs, and pregnancy (gestational diabetes). In patients who do not have diabetes, health care providers use insulin to prevent or treat hyperglycemia induced by IV parenteral nutrition and to treat hyperkalemia. In hyperkalemia, an IV infusion of insulin and dextrose solution causes potassium to move from the blood into the cells; it does not eliminate potassium from the body.

All insulin in the United States is human insulin. Pork and bovine insulins, which were more antigenic, are no longer manufactured in the United States. The name human insulin means that the synthetic product is identical to endogenous insulin (i.e., has the same number and sequence of amino acids).

Types of Insulin

Insulins differ in onset and duration of action. They are usually categorized as short, intermediate, or long acting. The synthesis of insulin analogs involves altering the type or sequence of amino acids in insulin molecules.

TABLE 39.1

Drugs Administered for the Treatment of Diabetes Mellitus

Drug Class	Prototype	Other Drugs in the Class
Insulins	Insulin (Humulin R, Novolin R)	Short-acting insulins: Insulin lispro (Humalog) Insulin aspart (NovoLog) Insulin glulisine (Apidra) Intermediate-acting insulin: Isophane insulin suspension (NPH Humulin N, Novolin N) Long-acting insulins: Insulin glargine (Lantus) Insulin levemir (Detemir)
Sulfonylureas	Glyburide (DiaBeta)	Glimepiride (Amaryl) Glipizide (Glucotrol, Glucotrol XL)
Alpha-glucosidase inhibitors	Acarbose (Precose)	Miglitol (Glyset)
Biguanide	Metformin (Fortamet, Glucophage, Glucophage XR, Glumetza, Riomet)	
Thiazolidinediones	Rosiglitazone (Avandia)	Pioglitazone (Actos)
Meglitinides	Repaglinide (Prandin)	Nateglinide (Starlix)
Dipeptidyl peptidase-4 (DPP-4) inhibitor	Sitagliptin (Januvia)	Linagliptin (Tradjenta) Saxagliptin (Onglyza)
Incretin mimetics	Exenatide (Byetta)	Liraglutide (Victoza)
Amylin	Pramlintide (Symlin)	
Angiotensin-converting enzyme inhibitor	Enalapril maleate (Vasotec)	Benazepril hydrochloride (Lotensin) Captopril (Capoten) Fosinopril (Monopril) Lisinopril (Prinivil, Zestril) Moexipril hydrochloride (Univasc) Perindopril erbumine (Aceon) Quinapril hydrochloride (Accupril) Ramipril (Altace) Trandolapril (Mavik)
HMG-CoA reductase inhibitor	Simvastatin (Zocor)	Atorvastatin calcium (Lipitor) Fluvastatin (Lescol, Lescol SL) Lovastatin (Altoprev, Mevacor) Pitavastatin calcium (Livalo) Pravastatin (Pravachol) Rosuvastatin (Crestor)

Short-acting insulins have a rapid onset (15 minutes or less) and a short duration of action (4–8 hours). Short-acting products include insulin lispro (Humalog), insulin aspart (NovoLog), and insulin glulisine (Apidra). Lispro, the first insulin analog to be marketed, is identical to human insulin except for the reversal of two amino acids (lysine and proline). It is absorbed more rapidly and has a shorter half-life after subcutaneous injection than regular (short-acting) human insulin. As a result, it is similar to physiologic insulin secretion after a meal, more effective at decreasing postprandial hyperglycemia, and less likely to cause hypoglycemia before the next meal. Injection just before a meal produces hypoglycemic effects similar to those of an injection of conventional regular insulin given 30 minutes before a meal. Aspart has an even more

rapid onset and shorter duration of action. Glulisine, the newest short-acting insulin analog, has the shortest onset of action (5–10 minutes).

Intermediate-acting insulin preparations such as isophane (NPH) suspension possess zinc insulin crystals that have been modified by protamine in a neural buffer. The addition of zinc assists in slowing the absorption and thus prolongs the duration of action.

Long-acting insulin preparations include insulin glargine and insulin detemir. Health care providers use them to provide a basal amount of insulin through 24 hours, similar to normal, endogenous insulin secretion.

Several mixtures of an intermediate- and a short-acting insulin are available and in common use. U-100, the main insulin

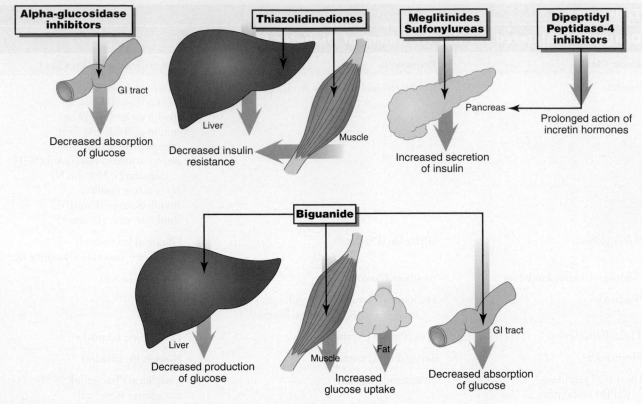

Figure 39.2 Actions of oral antidiabetic drugs. The drugs lower blood sugar by decreasing absorption or production of glucose, by increasing secretion of insulin, or by increasing the effectiveness of available insulin (decreasing insulin resistance).

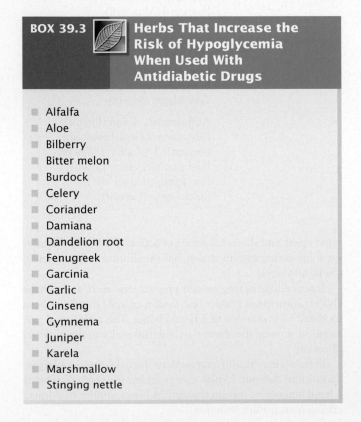

BOX 39.3   Herbs That Increase the Risk of Hypoglycemia When Used With Antidiabetic Drugs

■ Alfalfa
■ Aloe
■ Bilberry
■ Bitter melon
■ Burdock
■ Celery
■ Coriander
■ Damiana
■ Dandelion root
■ Fenugreek
■ Garcinia
■ Garlic
■ Ginseng
■ Gymnema
■ Juniper
■ Karela
■ Marshmallow
■ Stinging nettle

concentration in the United States, contains 100 units of insulin per milliliter of solution. Accurate measurement requires an orange-tipped syringe designed for use only with U-100 insulin.

After subcutaneous injection, insulin is absorbed most rapidly from the abdomen, followed by the upper arm, thigh, and buttocks. Absorption is delayed or decreased by injection into subcutaneous tissue with lipodystrophy or other lesions, by circulatory problems such as edema or hypotension, by insulin-binding antibodies (which develop after 2 or 3 months of insulin administration), and by injecting cold (i.e., refrigerated) insulin. Absorption may also be increased when administered in an extremity before the patient engages in a sport that requires use of the specific extremity (i.e., swimming, tennis, or jogging).

An inhaled insulin (Exubera) received U.S. Food and Drug Administration (FDA) approval in January 2006 for patients 18 years of age or older with type 1 or type 2 diabetes. However, by October 2007, the drug manufacturer made a decision to cease production of Exubera, citing that too few patients using inhaled insulin and the availability of other medications to lower blood sugar as reasons for discontinuing production. Currently, no FDA-approved inhaled insulins are available; however, several drug manufacturers are working to develop new forms of insulin delivery, including mouth sprays, insulin patches, and inhalers.

Table 39.2 gives information about insulins, including routes and dosages.

TABLE 39.2

DRUGS AT A GLANCE: Insulins

Drug	Characteristics*	Routes and Dosage Ranges†	Action (Hours)		
			Onset	Peak	Duration
Short-acting insulin					
Ⓟ **Insulin** (Humulin R, Novolin R)	• A clear liquid solution with the appearance of water • The hypoglycemic drug of choice for patients with diabetes in/with acute or emergency situations, diabetic ketoacidosis (DKA), hyperosmolar nonketotic coma, severe infections or other illnesses, major surgery, and pregnancy • The only insulin preparation that can be given intravenously (IV)	Sub-Q, dosage individualized according to blood glucose levels. For sliding scale dosing available as a high, medium, or low dose before meals and bedtime, depending on blood glucose levels. IV, dosage individualized. For ketoacidosis, regular insulin may be given by direct injection, intermittent infusion, or continuous infusion and is based on hourly blood and urine glucose levels.	1/2–1	2–3	5–7
Intermediate-acting insulins					
Isophane insulin suspension (NPH, Humulin N, Novolin N)	• Commonly used for long-term administration • Modified by addition of protamine (a protein) and zinc • A suspension with a cloudy appearance when correctly mixed in the drug vial • Given *only* Sub-Q • Hypoglycemic reactions are more likely to occur during mid to late afternoon • Not recommended for use in acute situations	Sub-Q, dosage individualized. Initially, 7–26 units may be given once or twice daily.	1–1 1/2	8–12	18–24
Insulin mixtures					
NPH 70%, regular 30% (Humulin 70/30, Novolin 70/30) NPH 50%, regular 50% (Humulin 50/50)	• Controls postprandial hyperglycemia • Not recommended for DKA or hyperosmolar hyperglycemic reaction				
Insulin analogs					
Insulin lispro (Humalog)	• A synthetic insulin of recombinant DNA origin, created by reversing two amino acids • Has a faster onset and a shorter duration of action than human regular insulin • Intended for use with a longer-acting insulin	Sub-Q, dosage individualized, 15 min before meals. May also be given in external insulin pumps	1/4	1–1 1/2	6–8

(Continued on page 722)

TABLE 39.2

DRUGS AT A GLANCE: Insulins (Continued)

Drug	Characteristics*	Routes and Dosage Ranges†	Action (Hours)		
			Onset	Peak	Duration
Insulin aspart (NovoLog)	Similar to lispro	Sub-Q, dosage individualized	1/4	1–3	3–5
Insulin glargine (Lantus)	• Long acting • Provides basal amount of insulin • Must *not* be diluted or mixed with any other insulin or solutions	Sub-Q, dosage individualized, once daily at bedtime	1.1	None	24
Insulin glulisine (Apidra)	• Clear, colorless solution • More rapid onset of action and shorter duration of action than regular human insulin • Should be used in regimens that include a longer-acting insulin or basal insulin analog • May be mixed with NPH insulin for injection only. Draw up Apidra first, then NPH insulin. Do NOT mix Apidra with other insulins in Sub-Q infusion pumps.	Sub-Q by injection or continuous infusion pump, dosage individualized. When used as a mealtime insulin, give up to 15 min before or within 20 min of beginning the meal.	1/12–1/6 (5–10 min)	1	4
Insulin levemir (Detemir)	• Long acting • Provides basal amount of insulin • Must not be diluted or mixed with other insulins	Sub-Q once or twice daily, dosage individualized	1	None	6–23
Analog mixtures Insulin lispro protamine 75% Insulin lispro 25% (Humalog Mix 75/25)	• Same onset, peak, and duration as individual components	Sub-Q, dosage individualized			

*All insulins are in U.S. Food and Drug Administration Pregnancy Category B.
†When mixing insulins, always draw up the clear insulin first, then add the cloudy insulin.

Choice of Insulin

When insulin therapy is indicated, the physician may choose from several preparations that vary in composition, onset, duration of action, and other characteristics. Some factors to be considered include the following:

- Regular insulin (insulin injection) has a rapid onset of action and can be given intravenously. Therefore, it is the insulin of choice during acute situations, such as DKA, severe infection or other illness, and surgical procedures.
- Isophane insulin (NPH) is often used for long-term insulin therapy. For many patients, a combination of NPH

and short-acting insulin provides more consistent control of blood glucose levels. Although several regimens are used, a common one is a mixture of regular and NPH insulins administered before the morning and evening meals. A commercial mixture is more convenient and probably more accurate than a mixture prepared by a patient or caregiver, if the proportions of insulins are appropriate for the patient.

- Insulin lispro, aspart, or glulisine may be used instead of regular subcutaneous insulin in most situations, but safe use requires both health care providers and patients to be aware of differences. Regular insulin, insulin aspart, and insulin glulisine are also approved for use in external

insulin pumps that administer a continuous subcutaneous infusion.

- Insulin glargine or insulin detemir may be used to provide a basal amount of insulin over 24 hours, with a short-acting insulin or short-acting insulin analog at meal times.

Pharmacokinetics

Regular insulin is rapidly absorbed after IV, intramuscular (IM), and subcutaneous administration. It is considered to be of short duration with a slow action. It is primarily metabolized in the liver, and a small amount is metabolized in the kidneys. Less than 2% of the drug is excreted in the urine.

Action

Insulin and its analogs (structurally similar chemicals) replace endogenous insulin, and this exogenous insulin has the same effects as the pancreatic hormone. The insulins lower blood glucose levels by increasing glucose uptake by body cells, especially skeletal muscle and fat cells, and by decreasing glucose production in the liver.

Use

Insulin is used to lower blood glucose, and the dosage must be individualized according to blood glucose levels. **Blood glucose meters** are devices that measure how much glucose is in the blood. A specially coated test strip containing a fresh sample of blood (obtained by pricking the skin, usually the finger or forearm, with a **lancet**) is inserted in the meter, which then measures the amount of glucose in the blood. The goal is to administer enough insulin to alleviate symptoms of hyperglycemia and to reestablish metabolic balance without causing hypoglycemia (Box 39.4). An initial dose of 0.5 to 1 units/ kg/d may be started and then adjusted to maintain blood glucose levels (tested before meals and at bedtime) of 90 to 130 mg/dL in adults (100–200 mg/dL in children younger than 5 years of age). However, many factors influence blood glucose response to exogenous insulin and therefore influence insulin requirements.

- Factors that increase insulin requirements include weight gain, increased caloric intake, pregnancy, decreased activity, acute infections, hyperadrenocorticism (Cushing's disease), primary hyperparathyroidism, acromegaly, hypokalemia, and drugs such as corticosteroids, epinephrine, levothyroxine, and thiazide diuretics. Patients who are obese may require 2 units/kg/d because of resistance to insulin in peripheral tissues.
- Factors that decrease insulin requirements include weight reduction; decreased caloric intake; increased physical activity; development of renal insufficiency; stopping administration of corticosteroids, epinephrine, levothyroxine, and diuretics; hypothyroidism; hypopituitarism; recovery from hyperthyroidism; recovery from acute infections; and the "honeymoon period," which may occur with type 1 diabetes.

- People who need less than 0.5 units/kg/d may produce some endogenous insulin, or their tissues may be more responsive to insulin because of exercise and good physical conditioning.
- In acute situations, dosage of regular insulin needs frequent adjustments based on measurements of blood glucose. When insulin is given intravenously in a continuous infusion, 20% to 30% binds to the IV fluid container and the infusion tubing.
- Dosage of insulin for long-term therapy is determined by blood glucose levels at various times of the day and is adjusted when indicated (e.g., because of illness or changes in physical activity). Titrating insulin dosage may be difficult and time consuming; it requires cooperation and collaboration between patients and health care providers.
- Insulin has been used successfully with all currently available types of oral agents (alpha-glucosidase inhibitors, biguanide, thiazolidinediones, meglitinides, and sulfonylureas).

Use in Children

Effective management of type 1 diabetes requires a consistent schedule of meals, snacks, blood glucose monitoring, insulin injections and dose adjustments, and exercise. Insulin is the only drug indicated for use as replacement therapy because affected children cannot produce insulin. It is essential that insulin injections be given three or four times per day. Rotation of injection sites is important in infants and young children because of the relatively small areas for injection at each anatomic site and to prevent lipodystrophy. Young children usually adjust to injections and blood glucose monitoring better when the parents express less anxiety about these vital procedures.

A healthful, varied diet, rich in whole grains, fruits, and vegetables and limited in simple sugars, is recommended. According to the American Diabetes Association (2006), medical nutrition therapy should be tailored to a person's specific health issues and personal preferences to help maintain optimum health by controlling blood glucose levels, blood pressure, cholesterol, and other risk factors.

It is essential to synchronize food intake with insulin injections, and this coordination usually involves three meals and three snacks, all at regularly scheduled times. Such a schedule is difficult to maintain in children, but it is extremely important in promoting normal growth and development. A major factor in optimal treatment is a supportive family in which at least one member is thoroughly educated about the disease and its management. Less-than-optimal treatment can lead to stunted growth, delayed puberty, and early development of complications such as retinopathy, nephropathy, or neuropathy.

Infections and other illnesses may cause wide fluctuations in blood glucose levels and interfere with metabolic control. For example, viral infections cause hypoglycemia; others, especially chronic infections, may cause hyperglycemia and insulin resistance and may precipitate ketoacidosis. As a result, insulin requirements may vary widely during illness episodes and should be based on blood glucose and urine ketone levels. Hypoglycemia often develops in young children, partly because of anorexia and smaller glycogen reserves.

BOX 39.4 Hypoglycemia: Characteristics and Management

Hypoglycemia may occur with insulin, meglitinides, oral sulfonylureas, amylin analogs (pramlintide [Symlin]), and incretin mimetics (exenatide [Byetta]). When hypoglycemia is suspected, the blood glucose level should be measured if possible, although signs and symptoms and the plasma glucose level at which they occur vary from person to person. Hypoglycemia is blood glucose below 60 to 70 mg/dL and is especially dangerous at approximately 40 mg/dL or below. Central nervous system effects may lead to accidental injury or permanent brain damage; cardiovascular effects may lead to cardiac dysrhythmias or myocardial infarction. Causes of hypoglycemia include:

■ Intensive insulin therapy (i.e., continuous subcutaneous [Sub-Q] infusion or three or more injections daily)
■ Omitting or delaying meals
■ An excessive or incorrect dose of insulin or an oral agent that causes hypoglycemia
■ Altered sensitivity to insulin
■ Decreased clearance of insulin or an oral agent (e.g., with renal insufficiency)
■ Decreased glucose intake
■ Decreased production of glucose in the liver
■ Giving an insulin injection via the intramuscular (IM) rather than the Sub-Q route
■ Drug interactions that decrease blood glucose levels
■ Increased physical exertion
■ Ethanol ingestion

Hormones That Raise Blood Sugar

Normally, when hypoglycemia occurs, several hormones (glucagon, epinephrine, growth hormone, and cortisol) work to restore and maintain blood glucose levels. Glucagon and epinephrine, the dominant counter-regulatory hormones, act rapidly because they are activated as soon as blood glucose levels start declining. Growth hormone and cortisol act more slowly, about 2 hours after hypoglycemia occurs.

People with diabetes who develop hypoglycemia may have impaired secretion of these hormones, especially those patients with type 1 diabetes. Decreased secretion of glucagon is often evident in patients who have had diabetes for 5 years or longer. Decreased secretion of epinephrine also occurs in people who have been treated with insulin for several years. Decreased epinephrine decreases tachycardia, a common sign of hypoglycemia, and may delay recognition and treatment.

The Conscious Patient

Treatment of hypoglycemic reactions consists of immediate administration of a rapidly absorbed carbohydrate. For the conscious patient who is able to swallow, the carbohydrate is given orally. Foods and fluids that provide approximately 15 g of carbohydrate include:

■ Liquids or fruit juices
■ 4 teaspoons of sugar
■ Commercial glucose products (e.g., Glutose, B-D Glucose). These products must be swallowed to be effective.
■ Symptoms usually subside within 15 to 20 minutes. If they do not subside, the patient should take another 10 to 15 g of oral carbohydrate.
■ *If acarbose or miglitol has been taken with insulin or a sulfonylurea and a hypoglycemic reaction occurs, glucose (oral or intravenous [IV]) or glucagon must be given for treatment.* Sucrose (table sugar) and other oral carbohydrates do not relieve hypoglycemia because the presence of acarbose or miglitol prevents their digestion and absorption from the gastrointestinal tract.

The Unconscious Patient

Carbohydrate cannot be given orally. Therefore, the choices are parenteral glucose or glucagon.

■ In the health care facility, administer 25% to 50% dextrose solution
■ In home or elsewhere, give Sub-Q or IM glucagon 0.5 to 1 mg if available, and there is someone to inject it.
■ Glucagon is a pancreatic hormone that increases blood sugar by converting liver glycogen to glucose. It is effective only when liver glycogen is present. Some patients cannot respond to glucagon because glycogen stores are depleted by conditions such as starvation, adrenal insufficiency, or chronic hypoglycemia. The hyperglycemic effect of glucagon occurs more slowly than that of IV glucose and is of relatively brief duration. If the patient does not respond to one or two doses of glucagon within 20 minutes, IV glucose is indicated.

Avoid Overtreatment

Caution is necessary in the treatment of hypoglycemia. Although the main goal of treatment is to relieve hypoglycemia and restore the brain's supply of glucose, a secondary goal is to avoid overtreatment and excessive hyperglycemia.

During illness, children are highly susceptible to dehydration, and an adequate fluid intake is very important. Many clinicians recommend sugar-containing liquids (e.g., regular sodas, clear juices, and regular gelatin desserts) if blood glucose values are lower than 250 mg/dL. When blood glucose values are above 250 mg/dL, children should receive diet soda, unsweetened tea, and other fluids without sugar.

Administration of insulin for infants and toddlers who weigh less than 10 kg or require less than 5 units of insulin per day can be difficult because small doses are difficult to measure in a U-100 syringe. Use of diluted insulin allows more accurate administration. The most common dilution strength is U-10 (10 units/mL), and a diluent is available from insulin manufacturers for this purpose. It is necessary to clearly label vials of diluted insulin and discard them after 1 month.

Avoiding hypoglycemia is a major goal in infants and young children because of potentially damaging effects on growth and development. There may be a delay in recognition of hypoglycemia because signs and symptoms are vague and children may be unable to communicate them to parents or caregivers. Most pediatric endocrinologists recommend maintaining blood glucose levels between 100 and 200 mg/dL to prevent hypoglycemia. It is important never to skip the bedtime snack and blood glucose measurement.

Signs and symptoms of hypoglycemia in older children are similar to those in adults (e.g., hunger, sweating, and tachycardia). In young children, hypoglycemia may be manifested by changes in behavior, including severe hunger, irritability, and lethargy. In addition, mental functioning may be impaired in all age groups, even with mild hypoglycemia. Any time, hypoglycemia is suspected; it is essential that blood glucose be tested.

Adolescents may resist adhering to their prescribed treatment regimens, and effective management may be especially difficult during this developmental period. Adolescents and young adults may delay, omit, or decrease dosage of insulin to fit in socially (e.g., by eating more, "sleeping in," drinking alcohol) or to control their weight. Omitting or decreasing insulin dosage may lead to repeated episodes of ketoacidosis. Also, adolescent females may develop eating disorders.

Health care professionals are increasingly identifying type 2 diabetes in children. This trend is attributed mainly to obesity and inadequate exercise because most children with type 2 disease are seriously overweight and have poor eating habits. In addition, most are members of high-risk ethnic groups and have relatives with diabetes. Management involves exercise; weight loss; a more healthful diet; and in some cases, drug therapy, including insulin. It is also important to attend to treating comorbid conditions such as hypertension and hyperlipidemia.

Use in Older Adults

It is estimated that at least 20% of people older than 65 years of age have diabetes. General precautions for safe and effective use of oral hypoglycemic drugs apply to older adults, including close monitoring of blood glucose levels; however, control of cardiovascular risk factors may play a greater role in reducing morbidity and mortality in this population. In addition, older adults may have impaired vision, poor manual dexterity, or other problems that decrease their ability to perform needed tasks (e.g., self-administration of insulin, monitoring blood glucose levels, managing diet, and exercise).

Use in Patients With Renal Impairment

Frequent monitoring of blood glucose levels and dosage adjustments may be necessary. It is difficult to predict dosage needs because, on the one hand, less insulin is degraded by the kidneys (normally about 25%), and this may lead to higher blood levels of insulin if dosage is not reduced. On the other hand, muscles and possibly other tissues are less sensitive to insulin, and this insulin resistance may result in an increased blood glucose level if dosage is not increased. Overall, vigilance is required to prevent dangerous hypoglycemia, especially in patients whose renal function is unstable or worsening.

Use in Patients With Hepatic Impairment

Higher blood levels of insulin may occur in patients with hepatic impairment because less insulin may be degraded. Careful monitoring of blood glucose levels and insulin dosage reductions may be needed to prevent hypoglycemia.

Use in Patients With Critical Illness

Critically ill patients, with and without diabetes mellitus, often experience hyperglycemia associated with insulin resistance. Hyperglycemia may complicate the progress of critically ill patients, resulting in increased complications such as postoperative infections, poor recovery, and increased mortality. Tight glycemic control is a key factor in preventing complications and improving mortality in the patient in an intensive care unit.

Insulin is more likely to be used in critical illness than any of the oral agents. Reasons include the greater ability to titrate dosage needs in patients who are often debilitated and unstable, with varying degrees of cardiovascular, liver, and kidney impairment. One important consideration with IV insulin therapy is that 30% or more of a dose may adsorb into containers of IV fluid or infusion sets. In addition, many critically ill patients are unable to take oral drugs. Surgery may require use of insulin. Box 39.5 provides information about perioperative insulin therapy.

Some critically ill patients are also at risk for serious hypoglycemia, especially if they are debilitated, sedated, or unable to recognize and communicate symptoms. Vigilant monitoring is essential for any patient who has diabetes and a critical illness.

Use in Patients Receiving Home Care

Most insulins are taken at home, and the home care nurse shares the responsibility for teaching patients how to use the

---

BOX 39.5 Perioperative Insulin Therapy

Patients with diabetes who undergo major surgery have increased risks of both surgical and diabetic complications. Risks associated with surgery and anesthesia are greater if diabetes is not well controlled and complications of diabetes (e.g., hypertension, nephropathy, vascular damage) are already evident. Hyperglycemia and poor metabolic control are associated with increased susceptibility to infection, poor wound healing, and fluid and electrolyte imbalances. Risks of diabetic complications are increased because the stress of surgery increases insulin requirements and may precipitate diabetic ketoacidosis. Metabolic responses to stress include increased secretion of catecholamines, cortisol, glucagon, and growth hormone, all of which increase blood glucose levels. In addition to hyperglycemia, protein breakdown, lipolysis, ketogenesis, and insulin resistance occur. The risk of hypoglycemia is also increased.

The goals of treatment are to avoid hypoglycemia, severe hyperglycemia, ketoacidosis, and fluid and electrolyte imbalances. Maintenance of blood glucose levels between 120 and 180 mg/dL during the perioperative period is desirable. In general, mild hyperglycemia (e.g., blood glucose levels between 150 and 250 mg/dL) is considered safer for the patient than hypoglycemia, which may go unrecognized during anesthesia and surgery. Because surgery is a stressful event that increases blood glucose levels and the body's need for insulin, insulin therapy is usually required.

The goal of insulin therapy is to avoid ketosis from inadequate insulin and hypoglycemia from excessive insulin. Specific actions depend largely on the severity of diabetes and the type of surgical procedure. Diabetes should be well controlled before any type of surgery. Minor procedures usually require little change in the usual treatment program; major operations usually require a different medication regimen.

drug effectively and how to recognize medication responses that should be reported to the health care provider. Accurate dosing is extremely important so that blood glucose levels can be maintained at a normal level. Hyperglycemia and hypoglycemia are both unwanted effects of poor glycemic control. The nurse instructs the patient and any caregivers that if symptoms of hypoglycemia develop, it is essential to take corrective steps immediately. The home care nurse also monitors the patient's response to insulin and changes in the patient's condition or drug therapy that increases the patient's risk for hypoglycemic episodes.

When a patient is receiving a combination of insulins for management of diabetes, the nurse assists the patient in understanding that the different types of insulins have different onsets and therapeutic ranges. As a result, the medications work together to be more effective and maintain a more stable glycemic control. Changing medications or dosages can upset the balance and lead to hyperglycemia or hypoglycemia. If the patient is unable to take the medications for any reason, it is essential to notify the health care provider.

Contraindications

The only clear-cut contraindication to the use of insulin is hypoglycemia, because of the risk of brain damage (see Box 39.4).

Nursing Implications

Preventing Interactions

Patients who take insulin may have other diseases that require therapeutic drugs. Certain medications can interfere with insulin, increasing or decreasing the effects, thus causing hypoglycemia or hyperglycemia (Box 39.6). Some herbs increase the risk of hypoglycemia (see Box 39.3).

Administering the Medication

Oral administration of insulins is not effective because the proteins are destroyed by proteolytic enzymes in the GI tract. Sub-Q administration is fine, and for regular insulin, the IV route may be appropriate.

QSEN Safety Alert

Before administering insulin, patient safety requires that two nurses always check the dosage.

Timing

Many patients who take insulin need at least two injections daily to control hyperglycemia. A common regimen is one half to two thirds of the total daily dose in the morning before breakfast and the remaining one half or one third before the evening meal or at bedtime. With regular insulin before meals, it is very important that the medication be injected 30 to 45 minutes before meals so that the insulin is available when blood sugar increases after meals. With insulin lispro, aspart, or glulisine before meals, it is important to inject the medication about 15 minutes before eating. Insulin glargine or detemir is most commonly given at bedtime. However, it may be administered in the morning or in split doses as needed.

For the patient who uses an external insulin pump, it is important for the patient to understand the pharmacokinetics

---

BOX 39.6   **Drug Interactions: Insulin**

Drugs That Increase the Effects of Insulin

■ Angiotensin-converting enzyme inhibitors (e.g., captopril)
  Increase the risk of hypoglycemia
■ Alcohol
  May promote increased hypoglycemia; inhibits gluconeogenesis (in people with or without diabetes).
■ Antidiabetic drugs, oral
  May alter blood glucose levels; increasingly being used with insulin in the treatment of type 2 diabetes. (The risks of hypoglycemia are greater with the combination.)
■ Antimicrobials (sulfonamides, tetracyclines)
  Increase the risk of hypoglycemia
■ Beta-adrenergic blocking agents (e.g., propranolol)
  Increase hypoglycemia by inhibiting the effects of catecholamines on gluconeogenesis and glycogenolysis (effects that normally raise blood glucose levels in response to hypoglycemia); may also mask signs and symptoms of hypoglycemia (e.g., tachycardia, tremors) that normally occur with a hypoglycemia-induced activation of the sympathetic nervous system

Drugs That Decrease the Effects of Insulin

■ Adrenergics (e.g., albuterol, epinephrine)
  Increase insulin requirements
■ Anabolic corticosteroids (e.g., prednisone)
  Increase insulin requirements
■ Estrogens and oral contraceptives
  Increase insulin requirements
■ Glucagon
  Raises blood glucose by converting liver glycogen to glucose
■ Levothyroxine
  Increases insulin requirements due to hyperglycemia
■ Phenytoin
  Raises blood sugar by inhibiting insulin secretion
■ Thiazide diuretics (e.g., hydrochlorothiazide)
  Increase risk of hyperglycemia due to change in glucose control

---

of the insulin used in the pump. The health care provider overseeing the patient's insulin pump sets the basal insulin settings that provide the continuous insulin needed throughout the day. However, the patient needs to have an understanding of how much and when to administer the insulin for meals. Figure 39.3 presents information concerning the insulin pump.

Selection of Subcutaneous Sites for Injections and Pumps

Several factors affect insulin absorption from injection sites, including the site location, environmental temperature, and exercise or massage. Studies indicate that insulin is absorbed fastest from the abdomen, followed by the deltoid, thigh, and hip.

Because of these differences, many clinicians recommend rotating injection sites within areas. This technique decreases

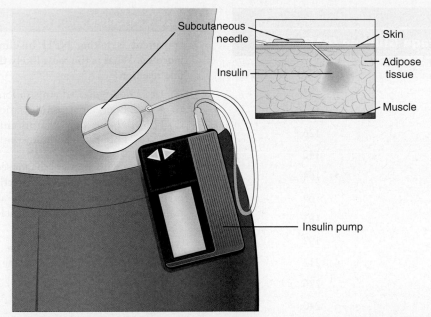

Figure 39.3 Continuous subcutaneous (Sub-Q) insulin infusion pump. The insulin dosage is programmed into the pump's computer, and the appropriate amount of insulin is injected into the adipose tissue through a needle inserted into the Sub-Q area. Insulin pumps are being increasingly used, especially by adolescents and young adults who want flexibility in diet and exercise. These devices allow continuous subcutaneous administration of regular insulin, insulin aspart, or insulin glulisine. A basal amount of insulin is injected (e.g., 1 unit/h or a calculated fraction of the dose used previously) continuously, with bolus injections before meals. This method of insulin administration maintains more normal blood glucose levels and avoids wide fluctuations. Candidates for insulin pumps include patients with diabetes that is poorly controlled with other methods and those who are able and willing to care for the devices properly.

The MiniMed Paradigm Real-Time System (Medtronic), the world's first integrated insulin pump and continuous glucose monitoring system, is now available in the United States. The Guardian RT System is an insulin pump and displays glucose readings every 5 minutes. It sounds an alarm when glucose levels reach high or low glucose limits preset by the clinical professional. The study completed on the RT System demonstrated that patients using the RT continuous glucose monitoring technology had better control of their blood glucose than patients using finger sticks only.

rotations between areas and promotes more consistent blood glucose levels. With regard to temperature, insulin is absorbed more rapidly in warmer sites and environments. In relation to exercise, people who exercise should avoid injecting insulin into subcutaneous tissue near the muscles to be used. The increased blood flow that accompanies exercise promotes rapid absorption and may lead to hypoglycemia.

For the patient with an insulin pump, the most commonly recommended sites are the abdomen and lower back so that absorption rates remain consistent (see Fig 39.3). It is extremely important that the patient rotate sites and avoid placing a site into scar tissue, which also affects insulin absorption.

Timing of Food Intake

Patients receiving insulin need food at the peak action time of the insulin and at bedtime. They usually take the food as a between-meal and a bedtime snack. These snacks help prevent hypoglycemic reactions between meals and at night. When hypoglycemia occurs during sleep, there may be a delay in recognition and treatment, which may allow the reaction to become more severe.

Assessing for Therapeutic Effects

As a general rule of thumb, it is necessary to have most patients with diabetes to check blood glucose levels at least four times a day to monitor blood glucose levels closely in response to the effects of insulin. The more often the patient can check blood glucose levels, the greater possibility of tighter glucose control. The goal of the patient taking insulin is to maintain blood glucose levels within normal range. Health care providers also look at the glycosylated hemoglobin (hemoglobin A1C) levels to assess the effectiveness of treatment. Because glucose stays attached to hemoglobin for the life of the red blood cell, which is about 120 days, the hemoglobin A1C level reflects the average blood glucose level over the past 3 months. The normal hemoglobin A1C level is less than 7% (Table 39.3).

Assessing for Adverse Effects

Assessing for signs and symptoms of hypoglycemia is essential (see Box 39.4). It is necessary to assess for tachycardia, palpitations, nervousness, weakness, confusion, hunger, and sweating. A decrease in blood glucose activates the sympathetic nervous system to produce a stress response. The nurse also assesses

TABLE 39.3

Estimated Average Glucose (eAG)

A1C (%)	eAG (mg/dL)
5	97
5.5	111
6	126
6.5	140
7	154
7.5	169
8	183
8.5	197
9	212
9.5	226
10	240
10.5	255
11	269
11.5	283
12	298

American Diabetes Association (2011). *Estimated average glucose (eAG)*. Retrieved May 29, 2011, from http://www.diabetes.org/living-with-diabetes/treatment-and-care/blood-glucose-control/estimated-average-glucose.html.

for such central nervous system effects as mental confusion, incoherent speech, visual changes, convulsions, and coma. In addition, he or she assesses the skin and subcutaneous fat for dimpling, atrophy, or hypertrophy of the injection sites. These effects are indicative of lipodystrophy that prevents proper absorption of insulin.

Patient Teaching

It is important to teach the patient and family about all aspects of diabetes care (Box 39.7). It is also essential to teach them about the insulins and their administration (Box 39.8).

Clinical Application 39-2

Mr. Smith comes back 6 months later after an increase in glyburide of up to 20 mg daily because of poor glycemic control and failure to adhere to a diet and exercise regimen. His physician orders 6 units of Humulin 70/30 once daily in the morning.

■ At what time does the nurse tell Mr. Smith to expect hypoglycemia to occur?

■ What teaching does the nurse provide to Mr. Smith about mixing insulin (if necessary) and injection technique?

NCLEX Success

3. A patient is taking NPH insulin once daily in the morning. What is the most likely time for a hypoglycemic reaction?

A. 1 to 3 hours after administration
B. 4 to 12 hours after administration
C. 12 to 18 hours after administration
D. 18 to 24 hours after administration

4. A patient with newly diagnosed type 1 diabetes is beginning daily insulin injections. The nurse is preparing to teach the patient about insulin injections. What should the nurse include in the teaching plan?

A. Understand that ketones in the urine indicate the need for a decrease in the number of units of insulin.
B. Administer the insulin at the same time every day regardless of meals.
C. Rotate the insulin injection sites.
D. Increase the insulin dosage just prior to exercise.

5. When teaching a patient who has recently received a diagnosis of diabetes how to self-administer short-acting and intermediate-acting insulin subcutaneously, which of the following instructions is correct?

A. Understand that the order of drawing up the two insulins into the syringe does not matter.
B. Draw the short-acting insulin into the syringe first, followed by the intermediate-acting insulin.
C. Draw the intermediate-acting insulin into the syringe first, followed by the short-acting insulin.
D. Give yourself two injections because mixing these insulins together is unsafe.

6. Which of the following insulins cannot be administered in a continuous subcutaneous insulin infusion pump?

A. regular insulin (Humulin R)
B. insulin aspart (NovoLog)
C. insulin glulisine (Apidra)
D. insulin glargine (Lantus)

7. A nurse is caring for a patient who is "nothing-by-mouth" (NPO) before surgery scheduled at 10:00 AM. He routinely receives 30 units of Humulin 70/30 every morning at 7:00 AM. What is the appropriate nursing action in this situation?

A. Administer 30 units of Humulin 70/30 subcutaneously.
B. Hold the insulin because the patient is NPO.
C. Give the patient a light breakfast and administer the insulin as ordered.
D. Contact the physician for a presurgery insulin order.

| BOX 39.7 | **Patient Teaching Guidelines for Antidiabetic Drugs (General)** |

■ Wear or carry diabetic identification (e.g., a Medic-Alert necklace or bracelet) at all times, to aid treatment if needed.

■ Learn as much as you can about diabetes and its management. Few other diseases require as much adaptation in activities of daily living, and you must be well informed to control the disease, minimize complications, and achieve an optimal quality of life. Although much information is available from health care providers (physicians, nurses, nurse diabetes educators, nutritionists), an additional major resource is the

American Diabetes Association
1660 Duke St.
Alexandria, VA 22314
1-800-ADA-DISC
http://www.diabetes.org

■ In general, a consistent schedule of diet, exercise, and medication produces the best control of blood sugar levels and the least risk of complications.

■ Diet, weight control, and exercise are extremely important in managing diabetes. Maintaining normal weight and avoiding excessive caloric intake decrease the need for medication and decrease the workload of the pancreas. Exercise helps body tissues use insulin better, which means that glucose moves out of the bloodstream and into muscles and other body tissues. This promotes more normal blood glucose levels and decreases long-term complications of diabetes.

■ Take antidiabetic medication as prescribed. If unable to take a medication, notify a health care provider. To control blood sugar most effectively, medications are balanced with diet and exercise. If you take insulin, you need to know what type(s) you are taking, how to obtain more, and how to store it. Unopened vials of insulin should be refrigerated. An opened vial may be stored at room temperature for 28 days. DO NOT freeze insulin. Regular and isophane (NPH) insulins and mixtures (e.g., Humulin) are available over-the-counter; Humalog, NovoLog, Lantus, Apidra, and Detemir require a prescription. Keep several days' supply of insulin and syringes on hand to allow for weather or other conditions that might prevent replacement of insulin or other supplies when needed. If you take Byetta, you should store it in the original package in the refrigerator and discard unused portion after 30 days. Alert your health care provider if you experience acute abdominal discomfort while taking Byetta. If you take Symlin, opened vials can be kept in the refrigerator or at room temperature for up to 28 days.

■ You need to know the signs and symptoms of high blood sugar (hyperglycemia): increased blood glucose and excessive thirst, hunger, and urine output. Persistent hyperglycemia may indicate a need to change some aspect of the treatment program, such as diet or medication.

■ You need to know the symptoms of low blood sugar (hypoglycemia): sweating, nervousness, hunger, weakness, tremors, and mental confusion. Hypoglycemia may indicate too much medication or exercise or too little food. Treatment is a rapidly absorbed source of sugar, which usually reverses symptoms within 10 to 20 minutes. If you are alert and able to swallow, take 4 ounces of fruit juice, 4 to 6 ounces of a sugar-containing soft drink, a piece of fruit or 1/3 cup of raisins, two to three glucose tablets (5 g each), a tube of glucose gel, 1 cup of skim milk, tea, or coffee with 2 teaspoons of sugar, or eight Lifesaver candies. Avoid taking so much sugar that hyperglycemia occurs.

■ If *you take acarbose (Precose) or miglitol (Glyset) along with insulin, glimepiride (Amaryl), glipizide (Glucotrol), or glyburide (DiaBeta, Glynase, Micronase) and a hypoglycemic reaction occurs, you must take some form of glucose (or glucagon) for treatment.* Sucrose (table sugar) and other oral carbohydrates do not relieve hypoglycemia because the presence of acarbose or miglitol prevents their digestion and absorption from the gastrointestinal (GI) tract.

■ You need to have a family member or another person who is able to recognize and manage hypoglycemia in case you are unable to obtain or swallow a source of glucose. If you take insulin, glucagon should be available in the home, and a caregiver should know how to give it.

■ The best way to prevent, delay, or decrease the severity of diabetes complications is to maintain blood sugar at a normal or near-normal level. Other measures include regular visits to health care providers, preferably a team of specialists in diabetes care; regular vision and glaucoma testing; and special foot care. In addition, if you have hypertension or elevated lipid levels, treatment can help prevent heart attacks and strokes.

■ Take only drugs prescribed by a physician who knows you have diabetes. Avoid other prescriptions and over-the-counter drugs unless these are discussed with the physician treating the diabetes because adverse reactions and interactions may occur. For example, nasal decongestants (alone or in cold remedies) and asthma medications may cause tachycardia and nervousness, which may be interpreted as hypoglycemia. In addition, liquid cold remedies and cough syrups may contain sugar and raise blood glucose levels.

■ If you wish to take any kind of herbal or dietary supplement, you should discuss this with the health care provider who is managing your diabetes. There has been little study of these preparations in relation to diabetes; many can increase or decrease blood sugar and alter diabetes control. If you start a supplement, you need to check your blood sugar frequently to see how it affects your blood glucose level.

■ Test blood regularly for glucose. A schedule individualized to your needs is best. Testing should be done more often when medication dosages are changed or when you are ill. Current blood glucose technology allows the selection of the fingertip or other location such as the forearm to obtain the blood sample. Glucose concentrations measured at different sites may vary. The fingertips are the most accurate site and should be the preferred test site if hypoglycemia is suspected.

(Continued on page 730)

BOX 39.7   **Patient Teaching Guidelines for Antidiabetic Drugs (General)** (Continued)

■ Reduce insulin dosage or eat extra food if you expect to exercise more than usual. Specific recommendations should be individualized and worked out with health care providers in relation to the type of exercise.

■ Ask for written instructions about managing "sick days" and call your physician if unsure about what you need to do. Although each person needs individualized instructions, some general guidelines include the following:

■ Continue your antidiabetic medications unless instructed otherwise. Additional insulin also may be needed, especially if ketosis develops. Ketones (acetone) in the urine indicate insulin deficiency or insulin resistance.

■ Check blood glucose levels at least four times daily; test urine for ketones when the blood glucose level exceeds 250 mg/dL or with each urination. If unable to test urine, have someone else do it.

■ Rest, keep warm, do not exercise, and keep someone with you if possible.

■ If unable to eat solid food, take easily digested liquids or semiliquid foods. About 15 g of carbohydrate every 1 to 2 hours is usually enough and can be provided by half cup of apple juice, applesauce, cola, cranberry juice, eggnog, cream of wheat

cereal, custard, vanilla ice cream, regular gelatin, or frozen yogurt.

■ Drink 2 to 3 quarts of fluids daily, especially if you have a fever. Water, tea, broths, clear soups, diet soda, or carbohydrate-containing fluids are acceptable.

■ Record the amount of fluid intake as well as the number of times you urinate, vomit, or have loose stools.

■ Seek medical attention if a premeal blood glucose level is more than 250 mg/dL, if urine acetone is present, if you have fever above 100°F, if you have several episodes of vomiting or diarrhea, or if you have difficulty in breathing, chest pain, severe abdominal pain, or severe dehydration.

■ Understand that an illness is a stress response and can increase or decrease your blood glucose. The body will have increased secretions of glucagon, epinephrine, growth hormone, cortisol, and hormones that raise blood glucose levels, and this will require an increase in medication to lower blood sugar. If you are unable to eat, hypoglycemia will result. Illnesses that lower blood sugar include viral infections, nausea, and vomiting. These conditions can result in dehydration and changes in fluids and electrolytes, leading to diabetic ketoacidosis.

Sulfonylureas

The sulfonylureas are the oldest and largest group of oral agents. Second-generation sulfonylureas have largely replaced first-generation sulfonylureas (e.g., acetohexamide, chlorpropamide, tolazamide, tolbutamide), which are not discussed further. ℗ **Glyburide** (DiaBeta) is the

prototype sulfonylurea. It is chemically related to sulfonamide antibacterial drugs.

Pharmacokinetics

After oral administration, glyburide is well absorbed, and more than 90% bound to plasma proteins. The drug is metabolized to inactive metabolites in the liver. These products are excreted

---

BOX 39.8   **Patient Teaching Guidelines for Insulin**

■ Use correct techniques for injecting insulin:

■ Follow instructions for times of administration as nearly as possible. Different types of insulin have different onsets, peaks, and durations of action. Accurate timing (e.g., in relation to meals) can increase beneficial effects and decrease risks of hypoglycemic reactions.

■ Wash hands; wash injection site, if needed.

■ Draw up insulin in a good light, being very careful to draw up the correct dose. If you have trouble seeing the syringe markers, get a magnifier or ask someone else to draw up the insulin. Prefilled syringes or cartridges for pen devices are also available.

■ Instructions may vary about cleaning the top of the insulin vial and the injection site with an alcohol swab and about pulling back on the plunger after injection to see if any blood enters the syringe. These techniques have been commonly used, but many diabetes experts do not believe they are necessary.

■ Inject straight into the fat layer under the skin, at a 90-degree angle. If very thin, pinch up a skinfold and inject at a 45-degree angle.

■ Rotate injection sites. Your health care provider may suggest a rotation plan. Many people rotate between the abdomen and the thighs. Insulin is absorbed fastest from the abdomen. Do not inject insulin within 2 inches of the "belly button" or into any skin lesions.

■ If it is necessary to mix two insulin preparations, ask for specific instructions about the technique and then follow it consistently. There is a risk of inaccurate dosage of both insulins unless measured very carefully. Commercial mixtures are also available for some combinations.

■ Change insulin dosage only if instructed to do so and the circumstances are specified.

■ Carry sugar, candy, or a commercial glucose preparation for immediate use if a hypoglycemic reaction occurs.

mainly by the kidneys; however, any whole drug is excreted about equally in urine and bile.

Action

Glyburide lowers blood glucose mainly by increasing secretion of insulin. It may also increase peripheral use of glucose, decrease production of glucose in the liver, increase the number of insulin receptors, and alter postreceptor actions to increase tissue responsiveness to insulin. Because the drug stimulates pancreatic beta cells to produce more insulin, it is effective only when functioning pancreatic beta cells are present.

Use

Health care professionals use glyburide in combination with diet to lower blood sugar in patients with type 2 diabetes mellitus. It is usually necessary to start with a low dosage and increase it gradually until the fasting blood glucose level is 110 mg/dL or less. The lowest dose that achieves normal fasting and postprandial blood sugar levels is recommended (Table 39.4).

Use in Older Adults

Older adults tend to be more sensitive to glyburide. In addition, older adults may have other disease states and may take other drugs that complicate management of diabetes. In addition, hypoglycemia is a concern. Drugs with a short duration of action and inactive metabolites are considered safer, especially in elderly people with impaired liver or kidney function. Therapy usually begins with a low dose, which is then increased or decreased according to blood glucose levels and clinical response.

Use in Patients With Renal Impairment

The kidneys are mainly responsible for excretion of metabolites, and renal impairment may lead to accumulation and hypoglycemia. Therefore, use of glyburide requires caution, with close monitoring of renal function, in patients with mild to moderate renal impairment. Use in severe renal impairment is contraindicated. Renal insufficiency may increase risks of adverse effects with oral hypoglycemic drugs, thereby increasing dosage requirements.

Use in Patients With Hepatic Impairment

Caution is warranted with use of glyburide, and monitoring of liver function is necessary. Metabolism of glyburide takes place in the liver, and hepatic impairment may result in higher serum drug levels and inadequate release of hepatic glucose in response to hypoglycemia. Glyburide may cause hypoglycemia in patients with liver disease.

Adverse Effects

The main adverse effect is hypoglycemia.

Contraindications

Contraindications include hypersensitivity to sulfa-based medications as well as sensitivity to glyburide itself. Other contraindications include severe renal or hepatic impairment. Caution is necessary with pregnancy, lactation, pituitary, or thyroid disorders.

TABLE 39.4

DRUGS AT A GLANCE: Sulfonylureas

Drug	Pregnancy Category	Routes and Dosage Ranges	
		Adults	Children
℗ **Glyburide** (DiaBeta)	C	Initial dose, 2.5–5 mg PO with breakfast Maintenance dose, 1.25–20 mg/d PO given as single or divided doses; increase in increments of no more than 2.5 mg at weekly intervals based on patient's blood glucose Older adult initial: 1.25 mg/d PO	Not recommended
Glimepiride (Amaryl)	C	Initial dose, 1–2 mg PO once daily, with breakfast or first main meal; max starting dose, 2 mg or less Maintenance dose, 1–4 mg once daily; after a dose of 2 mg is reached, increase dose in increments of 2 mg or less at 1- to 2-wk intervals, based on blood glucose levels; max recommended dose, 8 mg once daily When administered with insulin, administer glimepiride 8 mg PO once daily with insulin at the breakfast or the first main meal of the day	Safety and efficacy not established
Glipizide (Glucotrol, Glucotrol XL)	C	Initial dose, 5 mg PO daily in a single dose, 30 min before breakfast; max dose, 40 mg daily In elderly, may start with 2.5 mg daily Extended-release, once daily with breakfast	Safety and efficacy not established

Nursing Implications

In the event of high stress such as infections, surgery, or trauma, a change to insulin therapy may be warranted. In the event of severe hypoglycemia, it is necessary to administer IV glucose.

Preventing Interactions

Drugs may interact with glyburide, increasing or decreasing its effects (Box 39.9). Some herbs may increase its effects (see Box 39.3). It is extremely important that the patient inform the health care provider of all newly prescribed medications so that the patient and caregivers can be prepared to monitor for side effects related to other drugs.

Administering the Medication

Patients should take glyburide before breakfast in the morning or in divided doses before meals if the patient experiences gastric distress.

BOX 39.9 **Drug Interactions: Glyburide**

Drugs That Increase the Effects of Glyburide

■ Acarbose, miglitol, metformin, pioglitazone, rosiglitazone
  Increase risk of hypoglycemia
■ Alcohol (acute ingestion)
  Causes hypoglycemia
■ Cimetidine
  May inhibit metabolism of sulfonylureas, thereby increasing and prolonging hypoglycemic effect
■ Insulin
  May cause hypoglycemia

Drugs That Decrease the Effects of Glyburide

■ Alcohol (acute ingestion)
  Accelerates metabolism of sulfonylureas, shortening their half-lives; may produce a flushing response
■ Beta-blocking agents
  Decrease hypoglycemic effects, possibly by decreasing release of insulin in the pancreas
■ Corticosteroids, diuretics, epinephrine, estrogens, and oral contraceptives
  Have hyperglycemic effects
■ Glucagon
  Raises blood glucose levels
■ Nicotinic acid (large doses)
  Has hyperglycemic effect
■ Phenytoin
  Inhibits insulin secretion and has hyperglycemic effects
■ Rifampin
  Increases the rate of metabolism of sulfonylureas by inducing liver-metabolizing enzymes
■ Thyroid preparations
  Antagonize hypoglycemic effects of oral antidiabetic drugs

BOX 39.10 **Patient Teaching Guidelines for Oral Antidiabetic Drugs**

■ Take oral drugs as directed. Recommendations usually include the following:
  ■ Take glipizide or glyburide approximately 30 minutes before meals; take glimepiride with breakfast or the first main meal. Take Glucotrol XL with breakfast.
  ■ Take acarbose or miglitol with the first bite of each main meal. The drugs need to be in the gastrointestinal tract with food because they act by decreasing absorption of sugar in the food. Starting with a small dose and increasing it gradually helps to prevent bloating, "gas pains," and diarrhea.
  ■ Take metformin (Glucophage) with meals to decrease stomach upset.
    □ Take Glucophage XR with the evening meal.
    □ If a diagnostic test is ordered requiring a contrast media with iodine, stop metformin 48 hours before the test and do not begin taking it again until 48 hours after the test.
  ■ Take repaglinide (Prandin) or nateglinide (Starlix) about 15 to 30 minutes before meals (two, three, or four times daily). Doses may vary from 0.5 to 4.0 mg, depending on fasting blood glucose levels. Dosage changes should be at least 1 week apart. If you skip a meal, you should skip that dose of repaglinide or nateglinide; if you eat an extra meal, you should take an extra dose.
  ■ Take pioglitazone (Actos), rosiglitazone (Avandia), and sitagliptin (Januvia) without regard to meals. If you take rosiglitazone or pioglitazone, report shortness of breath, chest pain, swelling, and fatigue.
■ If you take glimepiride, glipizide, glyburide, repaglinide, or nateglinide alone or in combination with other antidiabetic drugs, be prepared to handle hypoglycemic reactions (as with insulin; see Box 39.7). Acarbose, miglitol, metformin, pioglitazone, and rosiglitazone do not cause hypoglycemia when taken alone. Do not skip meals and snacks. This increases the risk of hypoglycemic reactions.
■ If you exercise vigorously, you may need to decrease your dose of antidiabetic drug or eat more. Ask for specific instructions related to the type and frequency of the exercise. Follow the recommended diet and exercise program as ordered by the health care provider.
■ Do not stop taking your diabetic medications without consulting your health care provider.

Patient Teaching

Box 39.7 presents general patient teaching guidelines for the antidiabetic drugs. Box 39.10 presents patient teaching guidelines for the oral antidiabetic drugs, including glyburide.

Other Drugs in the Class

Other drugs in this class include glimepiride and glipizide, which resemble glyburide in terms of therapeutic and adverse effects. Glimepiride (Amaryl) stimulates the release of insulin from functioning beta cells in the pancreas and improves binding between insulin and the insulin receptors. People may take this sulfonylurea in combination with metformin or insulin for better control of glucose with diet and exercise. A reduced dosage is necessary in elderly patients as well as in patients who are malnourished or have renal or hepatic impairment. Use of glimepiride entails avoidance of alcohol.

Glipizide (Glucotrol, Glucotrol XL) also stimulates the release of insulin from functioning beta cells in the pancreas and improves binding between insulin and the insulin receptors; in addition, it may increase the number of insulin receptors. People should take the drug 30 minutes before breakfast to provide the greatest reduction in blood glucose. When beginning therapy with elderly patients, it is necessary to start with 2.5 mg/d orally, monitor them for 24 hours, and then increase the dose after several days as needed. Glipizide is associated with an increased risk of cardiovascular mortality and hematologic adverse effects such as leukopenia, thrombocytopenia, and anemia. As with the previous second-generation sulfonylureas, dosage reduction is warranted with impaired liver function.

Alpha-Glucosidase Inhibitors

Alpha-glucosidase inhibitors inhibit alpha-glucosidase enzymes (e.g., sucrase, maltase, amylase) in the GI tract, thereby delaying digestion of complex carbohydrates into glucose and other simple sugars. (P) **Acarbose** (Precose), the prototype alpha-glucosidase inhibitor, is known best for improving glycosylated hemoglobin levels. The drug is obtained through the fermentation process of microorganisms. Because acarbose does not enhance insulin, it works best when given with a sulfonylurea to control blood glucose levels.

Pharmacokinetics

Acarbose has a rapid onset of action and peaks in 1 hour. The drug is metabolized by the digestive enzymes and intestinal bacteria in the GI tract. It is minimally distributed and excreted in the urine and feces.

Action and Use

Acarbose works to delay the digestion of carbohydrates to diminish the increase in blood glucose after meals.

It may be necessary to combine acarbose with insulin or an oral agent, usually a sulfonylurea. Low initial doses and gradual increases decrease GI upset (e.g., bloating, diarrhea) and promote patient adherence. Patients taking acarbose should continue their diet, exercise, and blood glucose testing routines. Acarbose does not alter insulin secretion or cause hypoglycemia. Table 39.5 presents dosage information for acarbose and other alpha-glucosidase inhibitors.

Use in Older Adults

Some older adults have other complex diseases such as congestive heart failure, for which they may take digoxin. Acarbose can decrease digoxin levels, and patients who take both drugs need close monitoring. In addition, aging adults may have fat loss, resulting in weight reduction. In adults who weigh less than 60 kg, it is necessary to decrease the maximum dosage.

Use in Patients With Renal Impairment

Alpha-glucosidase inhibitors, which are excreted by the kidneys, accumulate in patients with renal impairment. However, dosage reduction is not helpful because the drugs act locally, within the GI tract.

Adverse Effects

There are no serious adverse effects of acarbose. However, acarbose can cause gastric upset because the drug is metabolized in the GI tract. It also has the potential to produce leukopenia, thrombocytopenia, and anemia.

Contraindications

Contraindications to acarbose include hypersensitivity, DKA, hepatic cirrhosis, inflammatory or malabsorptive intestinal disorders, and severe renal impairment.

TABLE 39.5

DRUGS AT A GLANCE: Alpha-Glucosidase Inhibitors

Drug	Pregnancy Category	Routes and Dosage Ranges	
		Adults	Children
(P) **Acarbose** (Precose)	B	Monotherapy: initially 25 mg PO 3 times/d with first bite of each meal; may start with 25 mg/d and gradually increase if gastrointestinal (GI) side effects are a problem. Patients weighing 60 kg or less, max dosage 50 mg 3 times/d PO. Patients weighing more than 60 kg, max dosage 1,000 mg 3 times/d PO	Not recommended for use in children
Miglitol (Glyset)	B	Monotherapy: initial dose 25 mg PO 3 times/d at the first bite of each meal; may start at 25 mg PO daily if severe GI effects are seen. Maintenance: 100 mg PO 3 times/d	Safety and efficacy not established

BOX 39.11
Drug Interactions: Acarbose

Drugs That Decrease the Effects of Acarbose
- Corticosteroids (systemic and inhaled)
  Result in hyperglycemia
- Luteinizing hormone, somatotropin, thiazide diuretics
  Increase risk of hyperglycemia

Drugs That Increase the Effects of Acarbose
- Corticosteroids (inhaled)
  May suppress the hypothalamic–pituitary–adrenal axis, leading to adrenal crisis, leading to hypoglycemia
- Pegvisomant
  Increased risk of hypoglycemia

Nursing Implications

Preventing Interactions

As mentioned previously, acarbose can decrease digoxin levels, and thus patients taking digoxin require close monitoring. Certain drugs may decrease the effects of acarbose (Box 39.11). The herbs that interact with acarbose are the same as those that may affect other antidiabetic agents (see Box 39.3).

Administering the Medication

People should take acarbose at the beginning of each meal so that it is present in the GI tract with food and able to delay digestion of carbohydrates.

Assessing for Therapeutic and Adverse Effects

After acarbose administration, the increase in blood glucose levels after a meal is smaller. The nurse assesses the patient's response to the medication—diminished blood glucose levels without signs and symptoms of hypoglycemia.

The nurse also assesses for GI effects such as diarrhea, abdominal pain, and flatulence. He or she should assess the complete blood (cell) count for leukopenia, thrombocytopenia, and anemia.

Patient Teaching

Box 39.7 presents general patient teaching guidelines for the antidiabetic drugs. Box 39.10 presents patient teaching guidelines for the oral antidiabetic drugs.

Other Drugs in the Class

Miglitol (Glyset) has the same action, use, adverse effects, and contraindications as acarbose.

Biguanides

The only drug available in this class is the prototype Ⓟ **metformin** (Glucophage). Experts prefer to call it an antihyperglycemic rather than a hypoglycemic because it does not cause hypoglycemia, even in large doses, when used alone.

Pharmacokinetics

Absorption of metformin occurs in the small intestine, and it circulates without binding to plasma proteins. The drug has a serum half-life of 1.3 to 4.5 hours. It is not metabolized in the liver and is excreted unchanged in the urine.

Action

Metformin reduces the production of glucose by the liver. It also decreases the intestinal absorption of glucose to increase insulin sensitivity. This action increases the uptake of glucose, thus enhancing its utilization to produce energy.

Use

People may take metformin alone or in combination with insulin or other oral agents. Prescribers widely order it as the initial drug in obese patients with newly diagnosed type 2 diabetes, mainly because it does not cause the weight gain associated with most other oral agents. Authorities consider metformin to be weight neutral and ideal for overweight people with type 2 diabetes, who have been known to lose weight on this medication, further improving insulin sensitivity. Table 39.6 presents dosage information about metformin.

Use in Older Adults

Dosage titration to the maximum amount recommended for younger adults is not appropriate for older adults. Contraindications to use of metformin in older adults often include cardiovascular disorders that increase risks of fluid retention and congestive heart failure. A **BLACK BOX WARNING** ◆ for metformin states that patients 80 years of

TABLE 39.6
DRUGS AT A GLANCE: Metformin

Drug	Pregnancy Category	Routes and Dosage Ranges	
		Adults	*Children (10 y)*
Ⓟ **Metformin** (Glucophage)	B	500 mg bid or 850 mg once daily PO; max dosage: 2,550 mg/d in divided doses	500 mg bid PO with meals; max dosage: 2,000 mg/d in divided doses 17 y and older, extended-release form may be used

age or older should not take the drug because of the risk of lactic acidosis.

Use in Patients With Renal Impairment

With metformin, periodic tests of renal function are necessary for determining dosages. Assessment of renal function should occur before starting the drug and at least annually during long-term therapy. It is essential to discontinue the metformin if renal impairment occurs or if serum lactate increases. As with other oral hypoglycemic drugs, patients taking this drug should continue their diet, exercise, and blood glucose testing regimens.

Parenteral radiographic contrast media containing iodine (e.g., Cholografin, Hypaque) may cause renal failure and have been associated with lactic acidosis in patients receiving metformin. It is important to discontinue metformin at least 48 hours before diagnostic tests are performed with these materials and resume the drug at least 48 hours after the tests are done and tests indicate that renal function is normal.

Use in Patients With Hepatic Impairment

Metformin is not recommended for use in patients with clinical or laboratory evidence of hepatic impairment because risks of lactic acidosis may be increased.

Adverse Effects

The primary adverse effect of metformin is lactic acidosis. Other adverse effects include hypersensitivity reactions, dizziness, nausea, vomiting, abdominal discomfort or cramping, malabsorption of amino acids, and diarrhea.

Contraindications

Contraindications to metformin include diabetes complicated by fever, severe infections, severe trauma, major surgery, acidosis, or pregnancy (insulin is indicated in these conditions). Patients with serious hepatic or renal impairment, cardiac or respiratory insufficiency, hypoxia, or a history of lactic acidosis should not take the drug because these conditions may increase production of lactate and the risk of potentially fatal lactic acidosis. A **BLACK BOX WARNING** ◆ alerts nurses to the dangers of lactic acidosis with metformin therapy in these patients.

Nursing Implications

Preventing Interactions

Some drugs increase the effects of metformin (Box 39.12). Use with sulfonylureas, furosemide, cationic drugs such as digoxin, and vancomycin increases the risk of hypoglycemia. Box 39.3 lists herbs that interact with metformin.

Administering the Medication

The nurse should ensure that renal function is assessed before starting metformin and at least annually during long-term therapy. Patients should take metformin with meals. They should swallow the extended-release formulation whole and take it with the evening meal. They should discontinue the drug immediately if they are diagnosed with a myocardial infarction.

BOX 39.12	Drug Interactions: Metformin

Drugs That Decrease the Effects of Metformin
- Corticosteroids (systemic and inhaled)
  Result in hyperglycemia
- Luteinizing hormone, somatotropin, thiazide diuretics
  Increase risk of hyperglycemia

Drugs That Increase the Effects of Metformin
- Alcohol
  Increases risk of hypoglycemia and lactic acidosis
- Cephalexin, cimetidine, dalfampridine, glycopyrrolate
  Interferes with metabolism and increases blood levels
- Corticosteroids (oral and inhaled)
  May suppress the hypothalamic–pituitary–adrenal axis, leading to adrenal crisis, leading to hypoglycemia
- Furosemide
  Increases blood levels
- Pegvisomant
  Increases risk of hypoglycemia
- Sulfonylurea hypoglycemic agents
  Increases risk of hypoglycemia

Assessing for Therapeutic Effects

The nurse assesses fasting, preprandial, and postprandial blood glucose for normal or near-normal levels. Also, the nurse assesses for improvement in hemoglobin A1C levels.

Assessing for Adverse Effects

The nurse assesses the skin for eczema, pruritus, erythema, and urticaria. All of these symptoms are indicative of a hypersensitivity reaction. It is also necessary to assess the GI response to the medication. In addition, the nurse assesses for abdominal pain, nausea, vomiting, and diarrhea. It is essential to check the liver function to determine the onset of lactic acidosis. Blood lactate levels are above 5 mmol/L, and blood pH is below 7.35. Symptoms and signs of lactic acidosis may include drowsiness, malaise, respiratory distress, bradycardia, and hypotension.

Patient Teaching

Box 39.7 presents general patient teaching guidelines for the antidiabetic drugs. Box 39.10 presents patient teaching guidelines for the oral antidiabetic drugs.

Thiazolidinediones

Thiazolidinediones include pioglitazone and rosiglitazone. They are sometimes called "glitazones" and are also referred to as insulin sensitizers. Thiazolidinediones decrease insulin resistance, a major factor in the pathophysiology of type 2 diabetes. Ⓟ **Rosiglitazone maleate** (Avandia) is the prototype for the thiazolidinediones.

Pharmacokinetics

Rosiglitazone has a delayed onset of action and takes up to 12 weeks to reach its maximum effects. It is 99.8% protein bound primarily by albumin. The medication is metabolized in the liver by cytochrome P450 (CYP) 2C8, and a minor portion is metabolized by CYP2C9. The serum half-life is 3 to 4 hours. The peak plasma level is reached in 1 hour, with delayed absorption when taken with food. Sixty-four percent of the medication is excreted in the urine and 23% in the feces.

Action

Rosiglitazone stimulates receptors on muscle, fat, and liver cells, thus increasing or restoring the effectiveness of circulating insulin. This change results in increased uptake of glucose by peripheral tissues and decreased production of glucose by the liver. In addition, this drug decreases insulin resistance, a major factor in the pathophysiology of type 2 diabetes.

Use

Patients may take rosiglitazone as monotherapy with diet and exercise or in combination with insulin, metformin, a sulfonylurea, an amylin analog (pramlintide), or incretin mimetic (exenatide). Table 39.7 presents dosage information for rosiglitazone.

Use in Patients With Hepatic Impairment

Rosiglitazone has been associated with hepatotoxicity and requires monitoring of liver enzymes. Liver function tests (e.g., serum aminotransferase enzymes) should be checked before starting therapy and periodically thereafter. After initiation of thiazolidinedione therapy, it is important to measure liver enzymes every 2 months for 1 year, then periodically.

Adverse Effects

GI adverse effects of thiazolidinedione include liver injury and diarrhea. The most common respiratory adverse effects are sinusitis, upper respiratory infection, rhinitis, and dyspnea.

Contraindications

Contraindications to rosiglitazone use include active liver disease or a serum alanine aminotransferase value more than 2.5 times the upper limit of normal, as well as hypersensitivity to the drug.

Caution is necessary when patients are at risk for congestive heart failure. Authorities do not recommend rosiglitazone for patients who have symptomatic congestive heart failure. Rosiglitazone increases plasma volume and may cause fluid retention. In one study, heart failure developed in 4.5% of rosiglitazone users within 10 months and in 12.4% of users within 36 months. In people who did not take a thiazolidinedione, 2.6% developed heart failure within 10 months and 8.4% within 36 months. The FDA has issued a **BLACK BOX WARNING** ◆ alerting health care professionals about the risk of congestive heart failure in patients using pioglitazone and rosiglitazone. Recent meta-analysis of several studies and clinical trials have raised concerns about increased risk of myocardial ischemic events, including angina, myocardial infarction (heart attack), and heart-related deaths, with rosiglitazone.

Nursing Implications

Preventing Interactions

Rosiglitazone serum levels may increase if the antidiabetic drug is taken with gemfibrozil, so it is essential to monitor the patient closely and make dosage adjustments if necessary. Box 39.3 lists the herbs that interact with rosiglitazone.

Administering the Medication

It is important to take rosiglitazone with meals. A patient may take a missed dose at the next meal. (However, if the patient skips a dose for an entire day, he or she should not take a double dose.)

Assessing for Therapeutic Effects

The nurse assesses fasting, preprandial, and postprandial blood glucose for normal or near-normal levels. Also, the nurse assesses for improvement in hemoglobin A1C levels.

Assessing for Adverse Effects

The nurse assesses the patient's cardiopulmonary status by auscultating the lungs for crackles or gurgles and auscultating the

TABLE 39.7
DRUGS AT A GLANCE: Thiazolidinediones

Drug	Pregnancy Category	Routes and Dosage Ranges	
		Adults	Children
(P) **Rosiglitazone** (Avandia)	C	4 mg as a single oral dose or divided into two doses; if adequate response not seen in 8–12 wk, may be increased to 8 mg PO daily	Not recommended
Pioglitazone (Actos)	C	PO 15–30 mg once daily; max dosage 45 mg Combination therapy with sulfonylurea or metformin: 15–30 mg daily PO added to the established dose of the other agent; if hypoglycemia occurs, reduce the dose of the other agent	Safety and efficacy not established

heart for an audible S_3 that indicates heart failure. Also, it is necessary to assess for signs of hepatic insufficiency and check liver enzymes. In addition, it is essential to assess for upper respiratory congestion.

Patient Teaching

The nurse teaches patients to report any signs or symptoms of congestive heart failure (e.g., dyspnea, fatigue, peripheral edema) to appropriate health care personnel. Box 39.7 presents general patient teaching guidelines for the antidiabetic drugs. Box 39.10 presents patient teaching guidelines for the oral antidiabetic drugs.

Other Drugs in the Class

Pioglitazone acts by resensitizing the tissues to insulin. This drug stimulates the insulin receptor sites, lowering blood glucose levels to improve the action of insulin. As with rosiglitazone, it has a risk of heart failure in patients. People may take pioglitazone without regard to meals. They may take a missed dose at the next scheduled time.

Meglitinides

Meglitinides are nonsulfonylureas that lower blood sugar by stimulating pancreatic secretion of insulin. ⓟ **Repaglinide** (Prandin) is the prototype meglitinide drug. The ability of repaglinide to work effectively depends on the existence of functioning beta cells left in the pancreas.

Pharmacokinetics

Absorption of repaglinide from the GI tract is good, and peak plasma level occurs within 1 hour. The drug has a plasma half-life of 1 to 1.5 hours and is highly bound (greater than 98%) to plasma proteins. Metabolism occurs in the liver. Excretion of metabolites is in urine and feces. Metabolism and removal of repaglinide from the bloodstream occurs within 3 to 4 hours after a dose. This decreases the workload of pancreatic beta cells (i.e., decreases duration of beta-cell stimulation), allows serum insulin levels to return to normal before the next meal, and decreases risks of hypoglycemic episodes.

Action

Repaglinide works by closing potassium channels in pancreatic beta cells, which causes calcium channels to open and release insulin. The ability to lower blood glucose is dependent on the amount of functioning beta cells in the pancreas.

Use

Repaglinide can be used as monotherapy with diet and exercise or in combination with metformin or thiazolidinediones. Dosage is flexible, depending on food intake, but patients should eat within a few minutes after taking a dose to avoid hypoglycemia. Table 39.8 presents dosage information for the meglitinides, including repaglinide.

Use in Patients With Renal Impairment

Assessment of renal function should occur before initiation of treatment with repaglinide and periodically during therapy. The drug requires a decrease in initial dosage in patients with renal disease as well as for those with moderate to severe renal dysfunction. It is necessary to make incremental dosage changes cautiously in patients with renal impairment or renal failure requiring hemodialysis.

Use in Patients With Hepatic Impairment

Cautious use of repaglinide is warranted in patients with moderate to severe hepatic impairment. It is necessary to make incremental dosage changes very slowly, because serum drug levels are higher for a long period.

Adverse Effects

Hypoglycemia is the most common adverse effect of repaglinide. Other adverse effects are upper respiratory congestion and gastric upset.

TABLE 39.8

DRUGS AT A GLANCE: Meglitinides

Drug	Pregnancy Category	Routes and Dosage Ranges	
		Adults	Children
ⓟ **Repaglinide** (Prandin)	C	0.5 mg–4 mg PO taken three or four times a day 15–30 min before meals; max dosage 16 mg/d PO; wait 1 wk before making dose adjustment Severe renal impairment: starting dose 0.5 mg PO	Not recommended
Nateglinide (Starlix)	C	120 mg PO 3 times daily, 1–30 min before meals; omit dose if skip a meal. 60 mg PO 3 times/d may be tried if patient is near HbA$_{1c}$ goal	Safety and efficacy not established

Contraindications

Repaglinide is contraindicated in patients with hypersensitivity. It is also contraindicated in patients with type 1 diabetes or patients with DKA.

Nursing Implications

Preventing Interactions

The risk of severe hypoglycemia is associated with the use of repaglinide with gemfibrozil and itraconazole. Therefore, such drug combinations should be avoided (Box 39.13).

Administering the Medication

Patients should take repaglinide just before or up to 30 minutes before meals. If a meal is skipped, the drug dose should be skipped; if a meal is added, a drug dose should be added.

Assessing for Adverse and Therapeutic Effects

The nurse assesses fasting, preprandial, and postprandial blood glucose for normal or near-normal levels. It is also important to assess for improvement in hemoglobin A1C levels.

The nurse assesses for dizziness, weakness, and hunger. In addition, he or she assesses for gastric upset and respiratory congestion.

BOX 39.13 **Drug Interactions: Repaglinide**

Drugs That Increase the Effects of Repaglinide

- Cimetidine, erythromycin, ketoconazole, miconazole
  Increase serum concentrations of repaglinide, leading to hypoglycemia
- Corticosteroids (oral or inhaled)
  May suppress the hypothalamic–pituitary–adrenal axis, leading to adrenal crisis, leading to hypoglycemia
- Nonsteroidal anti-inflammatory drugs and other agents that are highly bound to plasma proteins
  May displace drug from binding sites, increasing blood levels
- Pegvisomant
  Increases the risk of hypoglycemia
- Sulfonamides
  May inhibit hepatic metabolism, increasing blood levels

Drugs That Decrease the Effects of Repaglinide

- Adrenergics, corticosteroids, estrogens, niacin, oral contraceptives, and thiazide diuretics
  Increase the risk of hyperglycemia
- Corticosteroids (systemic and inhaled)
  Diminish the effect of acarbose, resulting in hyperglycemia
- Luteinizing hormone, somatotropin, thiazide diuretics
  Increase the risk of hyperglycemia
- Carbamazepine, rifampin
  Induce drug-metabolizing enzymes in the liver, which leads to faster inactivation

---

Patient Teaching

When instructing patients who have been prescribed meglitinides, it is necessary to inform them that if they skip a meal, then they should also skip the dose. If they add a meal, then they need to take a dose before the meal. Box 39.7 presents general patient teaching guidelines for the antidiabetic drugs. Box 39.10 presents patient teaching guidelines for the oral antidiabetic drugs, including repaglinide. The nurse teaches patients taking repaglinide to know and recognize the signs and symptoms of hypoglycemia and how to treat the condition immediately.

NCLEX Success

8. The nurse is assessing a patient who has just begun taking glyburide (DiaBeta). Which of the following is a therapeutic outcome for this patient? (Select all that apply.)

   A. a glycosylated hemoglobin (hemoglobin A1C) of 10%
   B. a decrease in polyuria
   C. a decrease in polyphagia
   D. a fasting blood glucose of 108 mg/dL

9. A patient with type 2 diabetes calls the nurse to report the following symptoms: blood glucose of 378 mg/dL, excessive urination, and feelings of becoming drowsier. To determine a possible diagnosis, which of the following questions is most important?

   A. "Has there been any change in diet?"
   B. "Has there been any fever?"
   C. "Have there been any ketones in the urine?"
   D. "Have you increased the amount of fluid intake?"

10. A patient with type 2 diabetes is scheduled to have a cardiac catheterization in 1 week, and the nurse makes a pre-procedure phone call. The nurse instructs the patient to stop taking which medication 2 days before the procedure?

    A. sitagliptin (Januvia)
    B. insulin
    C. glyburide (DiaBeta)
    D. metformin (Glucophage)

11. A man with type 2 diabetes mellitus has a blood glucose of more than 500 mg/dL. He is complaining of excessive urination, extreme thirst, and weakness, and he also notes recent weight loss. The nurse would expect to find which diagnosis in his chart?

    A. hypoglycemia
    B. diabetic ketoacidosis
    C. hyperglycemic hyperosmolar nonketotic syndrome
    D. hypothyroidism

12. The nurse is monitoring a patient newly diagnosed with type 2 diabetes mellitus taking repaglinide (Prandin) for complications. Which of the following, if exhibited by the patient, would indicate hypoglycemia and require immediate treatment?

    A. polyuria
    B. diaphoresis
    C. decreased heart rate
    D. hypertension

Dipeptidyl Peptidase-4 (DPP-4) Inhibitors

GLP-1 has been known for some time to have a hypoglycemic action via its ability to stimulate insulin secretion. Recent advances have overcome the problems associated with short half-life and inactivation of the incretin hormone. The DPP-4 enzyme inhibitor Ⓟ **sitagliptin phosphate** (Januvia) is a new medication that solves these problems.

Pharmacokinetics

Sitagliptin is rapidly absorbed and distributed with 3% protein bound. The drug is metabolized minimally by CYP3A4 and CYP2C8, resulting in a 12-hour circulating half-life for GLP-1. The peak of action is 1 to 4 hours. Eighty-seven percent of the medication is excreted in the urine with 79% unchanged. Approximately 13% is excreted in the feces.

Action

Sitagliptin minimizes the rate of inactivation of the incretin hormones to increase hormone levels and prolong their activity. Incretin hormones stimulate insulin release in response to a meal to normalize glucose levels. This action increases and lengthens the release of insulin and decreases hepatic glucose production to promote glycemic control.

Use

Patients with type 2 diabetes mellitus take sitagliptin in addition to following an exercise and diet regimen. They may also take it in combination with metformin and/or thiazolidinediones. Table 39.9 presents dosage information for sitagliptin and other DPP-4 enzyme inhibitors.

Use in Patients With Renal Impairment

Caution is warranted in renal insufficiency because sitagliptin is excreted by the kidneys. Patients with an elevated creatinine clearance require decreased dosages initially. Dosage adjustments are also necessary in the earlier stages of chronic kidney diseases.

Adverse Effects

Common adverse effects of sitagliptin are upper respiratory tract infection, stuffy or runny nose, sore throat, and headache.

Contraindications

Contraindications to sitagliptin use include type 1 diabetes mellitus, insulin use, or the common production of ketones in the urine. Another contraindication is end-stage renal disease. Strict avoidance of other medications known to cause hypoglycemia, such as sulfonylureas, is warranted.

Nursing Implications

Administering the Medication

Patients should take sitagliptin once daily with or without food. If they forget to take a dose, they should take it as soon as possible. However, if a dose is skipped, patients should take only one dose per day.

Assessing for Therapeutic and Adverse Effects

The nurse assesses fasting, preprandial, and postprandial blood glucose for normal or near-normal levels. It is also important to assess for improvement in hemoglobin A1C levels.

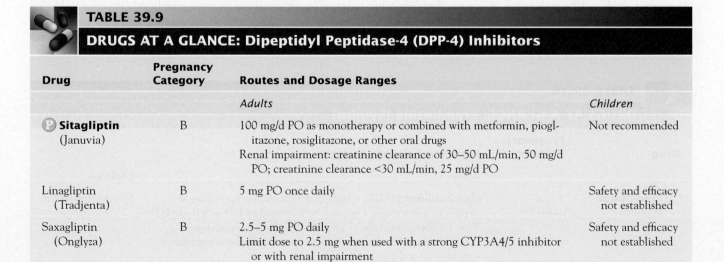

TABLE 39.9

DRUGS AT A GLANCE: Dipeptidyl Peptidase-4 (DPP-4) Inhibitors

Drug	Pregnancy Category	Routes and Dosage Ranges	
		Adults	*Children*
Ⓟ **Sitagliptin** (Januvia)	B	100 mg/d PO as monotherapy or combined with metformin, pioglitazone, rosiglitazone, or other oral drugs Renal impairment: creatinine clearance of 30–50 mL/min, 50 mg/d PO; creatinine clearance <30 mL/min, 25 mg/d PO	Not recommended
Linagliptin (Tradjenta)	B	5 mg PO once daily	Safety and efficacy not established
Saxagliptin (Onglyza)	B	2.5–5 mg PO daily Limit dose to 2.5 mg when used with a strong CYP3A4/5 inhibitor or with renal impairment	Safety and efficacy not established

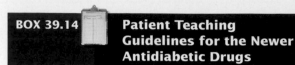

In addition, the nurse assesses the patient for signs and symptoms of upper respiratory infection.

Patient Teaching

Box 39.7 presents general patient teaching guidelines for the antidiabetic drugs. Box 39.14 gives some patient teaching guidelines for the newer antidiabetic drugs, including sitagliptin.

Amylin Analogs

Some people with type 1 or type 2 diabetes cannot achieve optimal glucose control with insulin therapy alone. Ⓟ **Pramlintide acetate** (Symlin) is a newer drug used as an adjunctive treatment with mealtime insulin that is important in the regulation of glucose control during the postprandial period. A synthetic analog of amylin, pramlintide is a peptide hormone secreted with insulin by the beta cells of the pancreas.

Pharmacokinetics

Pramlintide has a rapid onset of action, reaching its peak in 20 minutes, with a 3-hour duration of action. Sixty percent of the drug is protein bound. It is metabolized primarily in the renal system and excreted in the urine.

Action

Pramlintide slows gastric emptying, which helps regulate the postprandial rise in blood glucose. The drug also suppresses postprandial glucagon secretion, thus helping maintain better blood glucose control. It also increases the sense of satiety, possibly reducing food intake and promoting weight loss.

Use

Taken immediately before meals, pramlintide mimics the body's natural processes. Oral hypoglycemic drugs and insulin dosages are usually up to 50% lower as well, depending on the patient's response to the drug. Patients with type 2 disease may combine pramlintide and insulin therapy with metformin or sulfonylureas. Table 39.10 gives dosage information for pramlintide.

Adverse Effects

Nausea, another frequent adverse effect of pramlintide, tends to decrease with time. Careful titration of the dosage to the therapeutic level may reduce it. A **BLACK BOX WARNING** ◆ alerts nurses to the danger of severe insulin-induced hypoglycemia with pramlintide therapy, especially in type 1 diabetes.

Contraindications

The only contraindications to pramlintide are hypersensitivity and gastroparesis.

Nursing Implications

Preventing Interactions

Some drugs may increase the effects of pramlintide (Box 39.15). Pramlintide also can cause increased effects of gastric emptying if combined with anticholinergic drugs or drugs that slow gastric absorption of nutrients. It is essential to avoid pramlintide with such drugs.

Administering the Medication

Subcutaneous injection of pramlintide before meals is necessary. The patient should not use pramlintide if a meal is skipped or if a dose is forgotten. It is necessary to inject pramlintide into a site (thigh or abdomen) that is at least 2 inches away

TABLE 39.10

DRUGS AT A GLANCE: Pramlintide (Symlin)

Drug	Pregnancy Category	Routes and Dosage Ranges	
		Adults	Children
Ⓟ **Pramlintide** (Symlin)	C	Type 2 diabetes: initially 60 mcg Sub-Q injection immediately prior to major meals. Dose can be increased to 120 mcg if needed Type 1 diabetes: initially 15 mcg Sub-Q injection immediately prior to major meals; titrate 15-mcg increments to maintenance dose of 30 or 60 mcg as tolerated	Not recommended

from the insulin site injection. Opened vials of pramlintide may be stored in a refrigerator or at room temperature for up to 28 days.

It is essential not to mix pramlintide in the same injection with mealtime insulin. Patients with type 2 diabetes should take oral hypoglycemic drugs at least 1 hour before or 2 hours after injecting pramlintide.

Assessing for Therapeutic and Adverse Effects

The nurse assesses fasting, preprandial, and postprandial blood glucose for normal or near-normal levels. It is also important to assess for improvement in the hemoglobin A1C levels.

In addition, the nurse teaches the signs and symptoms of hypoglycemia, as well as its treatment. This is the only serious adverse effect.

Patient Teaching

Box 39.7 presents general patient teaching guidelines for the antidiabetic drugs. Box 39.15 gives some patient teaching guidelines for the newer antidiabetic drugs, including pramlintide.

Incretin Mimetics

Before starting a patient with type 2 diabetes on insulin, the provider should consider a new option for treatment of diabetes. With the incretin mimetic ℗ **exenatide** (Byetta), a synthetic GLP-1 analog, it is possible to improve glycemic control in patients with type 2 diabetes who are already taking an oral hypoglycemic medication but having difficulty in achieving glycemic control.

Pharmacokinetics

Exenatide has a rapid onset, and the peak effect occurs in 2 hours. The drug is metabolized minimally and has proteolytic degradation following glomerular filtration. It remains in the body for 8 to 10 hours, which means that dosages must be 6 hours apart. It has a 2.4-hour half-life and is excreted in the urine. Exenatide also crosses the placenta; thus, this drug must be used cautiously in patients who are pregnant.

Action

Exenatide acts as a natural helper hormone by stimulating the pancreas to secrete the right amount of insulin based on the food that was just eaten. This helps reduce the problem of high blood glucose after meals. The drug also halts gluconeogenesis by the liver, keeping it from making too much glucose after a meal. Exenatide slows gastric emptying, which serves to reduce the sudden rise of blood glucose after a meal, and it also quickly stimulates a feeling of satiety when eating. This fosters a sense of fullness, which causes the patient to eat less and potentially lose weight.

Use

When oral medications, diet, and exercise together have not assisted in reaching the target hemoglobin A1C goal, prescribers may now order exenatide. The FDA has approved its use with oral medications such as sulfonylureas, metformin, and/or thiazolidinediones. Major advantages of exenatide over insulin are increased satiety and weight loss. Exenatide is also now being used as monotherapy in combination with diet and exercise for newly diagnosed adults with type 2 diabetes. Table 39.11 provides route and dosage information for exenatide and other incretin mimetics.

Adverse Effects

Major adverse effects of exenatide are hypoglycemia, GI distress, and nausea. Many patients experience nausea at first, and health care providers should encourage them to continue the medication if at all possible because the nausea usually subsides and becomes a feeling of fullness. A rare but serious side effect is the development of acute pancreatitis.

TABLE 39.11

DRUGS AT A GLANCE: Incretin Mimetics

Drug	Pregnancy Category	Routes and Dosage Ranges	
		Adults	Children
℗ **Exenatide** (Byetta)	C	5 mcg by subcutaneous injection within 60 min before morning and evening meals or two main meals of day ~6 h apart; may be increased to 10 mcg twice a day after 1 mo of therapy if needed	Not recommended for use in children
Liraglutide (Victoza)	C	Initially 0.6 mg Sub-Q once daily for 1 wk; then increase dose to 1.2–1.8 mg once daily to achieve glycemic control	

Contraindications

Contraindications to exenatide include a known hypersensitivity to the drug. Patients with liver disease or elevated liver enzymes should not receive it with HMG-CoA reductase inhibitors. Lactation is also a contraindication.

Nursing Implications

Preventing Interactions

Like pramlintide, exenatide may reduce the absorption of concurrently administered oral medications due to slow gastric emptying (see Box 39.15).

Administering the Medication

Patients administer exenatide subcutaneously twice a day within 60 minutes of the morning and evening meal (at least 6 or more hours apart). No dosage adjustment is necessary based on blood glucose levels or the amount of food a patient is able to consume. If patients forget a dose, they should not inject exenatide after a meal. Injection sites include the subcutaneous tissue of the upper arm or leg and the abdomen areas.

It is essential that exenatide be stored at all times in the original packaging in a refrigerator at 36°F to 46°F, protected from light, kept dry, and discarded once opened after 30 days.

Assessing for Therapeutic Effects

The nurse assesses fasting, preprandial, and postprandial blood glucose for normal or near-normal levels. It is also important to assess for improvement in hemoglobin A1C levels.

Assessing for Adverse Effects

It is important that patients and their caregivers recognize the signs and symptoms of hypoglycemia, a possible adverse effect of exenatide, and be prepared to treat hypoglycemia with fast-acting sugar or glucagon. If patients are unable to eat or plan to skip a meal, they should not take the drug. Patients taking exenatide should report any unusual abdominal discomfort to their health care providers because acute pancreatitis is a possible adverse effect of the medication.

Patient Teaching

Box 39.7 presents general patient teaching guidelines for the antidiabetic drugs. Box 39.14 gives some patient teaching guidelines for the newer antidiabetic drugs.

NCLEX Success

13. A patient with type 2 diabetes begins taking sitagliptin (Januvia) for the management of blood glucose levels. Which statement by the patient indicates an understanding of this medication?
    A. "I will take two doses in the morning if my blood sugar is high."
    B. "By taking this medication, I am able to eat more."
    C. "Now that I am taking this medication, I don't have to exercise anymore."
    D. "I will take this medicine once a day."

14. The nurse caring for a patient with diabetes mellitus has lipodystrophy of the abdomen. What should the nurse assess?
    A. Does the patient administer the injection at a 45-degree angle?
    B. Does the patient aspirate for blood prior to giving the injection?
    C. Does the patient pinch the skin appropriately?
    D. Does the patient rotate sites for giving each injection?

15. Based on the action of pramlintide, which of the following is a primary nursing intervention?
    A. Administer glucagon during the peak of action.
    B. Assess blood sugar at 2.4 hours after medication administration.
    C. Assess respiratory status for the onset of an upper respiratory infection.
    D. Provide a meal immediately after the administration of the subcutaneous injection.

Adjuvant Medications Used to Treat Diabetes

For most patients, the goals of treatment are to maintain blood glucose at normal or near-normal levels; promote normal metabolism of carbohydrate, fat, and protein; prevent acute and long-term complications; and prevent hypoglycemic episodes. There is strong evidence that strict control of blood sugar delays the onset and slows progression of complications of diabetes. In addition to glycemic control, other measures can be used to help prevent complications of diabetes. Table 39.12 summarizes these adjuvant medications.

Angiotensin-Converting Enzyme Inhibitors

The prototype angiotensin-converting enzyme (ACE) inhibitor is ℗ **enalapril maleate** (Vasotec). Enalapril maleate blocks the conversion of angiotensin I to angiotensin II, thereby decreasing blood pressure. Enalapril maleate has protective effects on the kidneys in both type 1 and type 2 diabetes and in both normotensive and hypertensive people. Although ACE inhibitors are also used in the treatment of hypertension, their ability to delay nephropathy seems to be independent of antihypertensive effects. Additional measures to preserve renal function include effective treatment of hypertension, limited intake of dietary protein, prompt treatment of urinary tract infections, and avoidance of nephrotoxic drugs when possible.

HMG-CoA Reductase Inhibitors

The prototype HMG-CoA reductase inhibitor is ℗ **simvastatin** (Zocor). Simvastatin inhibits HMG-CoA reductase, the enzyme that catalyzes the first step in cholesterol synthesis, which ultimately reduces serum cholesterol. Current research suggests that a number of treatment strategies may be beneficial

TABLE 39.12

DRUGS AT A GLANCE: Adjuvant Drugs for the Treatment of Diabetes Mellitus

Drug	Pregnancy Category	Routes and Dosage Ranges	
		Adults	Children
Ⓟ **Enalapril maleate** (Vasotec)	D	2.5 mg PO daily or twice daily; maintenance daily dosage is 2.5–20 mg/daily Renal impairment: use smaller initial dose and adjust upward to a max of 40 mg/d PO	1 mo to 16 y, initial dose 0.08 mg/kg PO once daily; max dose 5 mg
Ⓟ **Simvastatin** (Zocor)	X	20–40 mg PO once daily in the evening Renal impairment: starting dose 5 mg/d PO and increase slowly	10–17 y: 10 mg/d PO in evening

in reducing the cardiovascular disease risk associated with type 2 diabetes mellitus. Some clinicians are recommending the routine use of statins such as simvastatin to reduce the risk of occlusive arterial disease in all patients with diabetes, regardless of cholesterol level.

Clinical Application 39-3

In addition to the addition of insulin to Mr. Smith's medication regimen, the physician also prescribes enalapril maleate (Vasotec) and simvastatin (Zocor) for Mr. Smith.

■ What is the purpose of adding these medications for Mr. Smith, and how will they assist him in his treatment of diabetes mellitus?

The Nursing Process

The best regimen for a particular patient depends on the type of diabetes, the patient's age and general condition, and the patient's ability and willingness to adhere to the prescribed therapy. In type 1 diabetes, the only effective treatment measures are insulin, diet, and exercise. In type 2, the initial treatment measures of choice are diet, exercise, and weight control. If this regimen is ineffective, the addition of oral agents or insulin may be necessary for patients with type 2 diabetes (Box 39.16). In addition, pregnant women who develop gestational diabetes also have certain regimens for care during the pregnancy to protect mother and baby (see Chap. 6).

Assessment

• Assess historic data, which include age at onset of diabetes, prescribed control measures and their effectiveness, the ease or difficulty of adhering to the prescribed treatment, occurrence of complications such as ketoacidosis, and whether other disease processes have interfered with diabetes control.

• Assess the patient's current status in relation to the following areas:
  • **Diet.** Ask about the prescribed nutritional plan, who prepares the food, what factors help in following the diet, what factors interfere with following the diet, the current weight, and whether there has been a recent weight change. Also ask if herbal or other dietary supplements are used. If so, list each one by name and frequency of use. If a nutritionist is available, ask one to assess the patient's dietary practice and needs.
  • **Activity.** Ask the patient to describe usual activities of daily living, including those related to work, home, and recreation, and whether he or she participates in a regular exercise program. If so, ask for more information about what, how often, how long, and so forth. If not, teaching is needed because exercise is extremely important in diabetes management.
  • **Medication.** If the patient takes insulin, ask what kind, how much, who administers it, usual time of administration, sites used for injections, and if a hypoglycemic reaction to insulin has ever been experienced, how it was handled. This information helps assess knowledge, usual practices, and teaching needs. If the patient takes an oral antidiabetic drug, ask the name, dosage, and time taken.
  • **Monitoring methods.** Testing the blood for glucose and the urine for ketones (e.g., when blood sugar is elevated, when ill and unable to eat) are the two main methods of self-monitoring glycemic control. Ask about the method used, the frequency of testing, and the pattern of results. If possible, observe the patient performing and interpreting an actual test to assess accuracy.
  • **Skin and mucous membranes.** Inspect for signs of infection and other lesions. Infections often occur in the axillary and groin areas because these areas have large numbers of microorganisms. Periodontal disease (pyorrhea) may be manifested by inflammation and bleeding of the gums. Women with diabetes are susceptible to monilial vaginitis and infections under the breasts. Check the sites of insulin injection for atrophy (dimpling or indentation), hypertrophy (nodules or

BOX 39.16 Combination Drug Therapy for Type 2 Diabetes

Combination drug therapy is an increasing trend in type 2 diabetes that is not controlled by diet, exercise, and single-drug therapy. Useful combinations include drugs with different mechanisms of action, and several rational combinations are currently available. Most studies have involved combinations of two drugs; some three-drug combinations are also being used. All combination therapy should be monitored with periodic measurements of fasting plasma glucose and glycosylated hemoglobin levels. If adequate glycemic control is not achieved, oral drugs may need to be discontinued and insulin therapy started. Two-drug combinations include the following:

■ **Insulin plus a sulfonylurea.** Advantages include lower fasting blood glucose levels, decreased glycosylated hemoglobin levels, increased secretion of endogenous insulin, smaller daily doses of insulin, and no significant change in body weight. The role of insulin analogs in combination therapy is not clear. One regimen, called BIDS, uses bedtime insulin, usually NPH, with a daytime sulfonylurea, usually glyburide.

■ **Insulin plus a glitazone.** Thiazolidinediones increase the effectiveness of insulin, whether endogenous or exogenous.

■ **Sulfonylurea plus acarbose or miglitol.** This combination is approved by the U.S. Food and Drug Administration (FDA) for patients who do not achieve adequate glycemic control with one of the drugs alone.

■ **Sulfonylurea plus metformin.** Glimepiride is approved by the FDA for this combination.

■ **Sulfonylurea plus a thiazolidinedione.** The sulfonylurea increases insulin, and the thiazolidinedione increases insulin effectiveness.

■ **Metformin plus a meglitinide.** If one of the drugs alone does not produce adequate glycemic control, the other one may be added. Dosage of each drug should be titrated to the minimal dose required to achieve the desired effects.

■ **Metformin plus a thiazolidinedione.** If metformin alone does not produce adequate glycemic control, a thiazolidinedione may be added. Pioglitazone is approved by the FDA for this combination.

■ **Metformin or thiazolidinedione plus sitagliptin.** Sitagliptin may be added as adjunctive therapy with metformin or a thiazolidinedione to achieve desired glycemic control.

■ **Metformin or sulfonylurea plus exenatide.** Exenatide may be added as adjunctive therapy with metformin or a sulfonylurea to achieve desired glycemic control.

■ **Mealtime insulin plus metformin, thiazolidinedione, and/or sulfonylurea plus pramlintide.** Pramlintide may be given with mealtime insulin in people with type 2 diabetes to achieve better postprandial glucose control.

---

lumps), and fibrosis (hardened areas). Check the lower leg for brown spots; these are caused by small hemorrhages into the skin and may indicate widespread changes in the blood vessels.

- Problems are especially likely to develop in the feet from infection, trauma, pressure, vascular insufficiency, and neuropathy. Therefore, inspect the feet for calluses, ulcers, and signs of infection. When such problems develop, sensory impairment from neuropathy may delay detection, and impaired circulation may delay healing. Check pedal pulses, color, and temperature in both feet to evaluate arterial blood flow. Ankle edema may indicate venous insufficiency or impaired cardiac function.

- **Eyes.** Ask about difficulties with vision and if eyes are examined regularly. Patients with diabetes are prone to development of retinopathy, cataracts, and possibly glaucoma.

- **Cardiovascular system.** Patients with diabetes have a high incidence of atherosclerosis, which makes them susceptible to hypertension, angina pectoris, myocardial infarction, peripheral vascular disease, and stroke. Therefore, check blood pressure and ask about chest pain and pain in the legs with exercise (intermittent claudication).

- **Genitourinary system.** People with diabetes often have kidney and bladder problems. Assess for signs of urinary tract infection; albumin, white blood cells, or blood in urine; edema; increased urination at night;

difficulty voiding; generalized itching; fatigue; and muscular weakness. Impotence may develop in men and is attributed to neuropathy

- **Blood glucose levels.** Assess blood sugar reports for abnormal levels. Two or more fasting blood glucose levels greater than 126 mg/dL or two random levels greater than 200 mg/dL are diagnostic of diabetes. Decreased blood sugar levels are especially dangerous at 40 mg/dL or below.

- **Glycosylated hemoglobin level.** Assess the glycosylated hemoglobin (also called glycated hemoglobin and HbA1c) level when available. This test indicates glucose bound to hemoglobin in red blood cells (RBCs) when RBCs are exposed to hyperglycemia. The binding is irreversible and lasts for the lifespan of RBCs (~120 days). The test reflects the average blood sugar during the previous 2 to 3 months. The goal is usually less than 7% (the range for people without diabetes is ~4%–6%). The test should be performed every 3 to 6 months.

- Test results are not affected by several factors that alter blood sugar levels, such as time of day, food intake, exercise, recently administered antidiabetic drugs, emotional stress, or patient cooperation. The test is especially useful in children, those whose diabetes is poorly controlled, those who do not test blood glucose regularly, and those who change their usual habits before a scheduled appointment with a health care provider so that their blood sugar control appears better than it actually is.

Nursing Diagnoses

- Ineffective tissue perfusion, peripheral, related to atherosclerosis and vascular impairment
- Disturbed sensory perception, visual and tactile, related to impaired vision or neuropathy
- Ineffective coping related to chronic illness and required treatment
- Anxiety: managing a chronic illness, finger sticks, insulin injections
- Risk for injury: trauma, infection, hypoglycemia, hyperglycemia
- Noncompliance related to inability or unwillingness to manage the disease process and required treatment
- Deficient knowledge: disease process and management; administration and effects of diabetic drugs; interrelationships among diet, exercise, and diabetic drugs; and management of hypoglycemia, "sick days," and other complications

Planning/Goals

The patient will

- Learn self-care activities
- Manage drug therapy to prevent or minimize hypoglycemia and other adverse effects
- Develop a consistent pattern of diet and exercise
- Use available resources to learn about the disease process and how to manage it
- Take diabetes medications accurately
- Self-monitor blood glucose and urine ketones appropriately
- Keep appointments for follow-up and monitoring procedures by a health care provider

Nursing Interventions

The nurse will

- Use nondrug measures to improve control of diabetes and to help prevent complications.
- Assist the patient in maintaining the prescribed diet. Specific measures vary but may include teaching the patient and family about the importance of diet, referring the patient to a dietitian, and helping the patient identify and modify factors that decrease compliance with the diet. If the patient is obese, assist in developing a program to lose weight and then maintain weight at a more nearly normal level.
- Assist the patient to develop and maintain a regular exercise program.
- Perform and interpret blood tests for glucose accurately, and assist patient and family members to do so. Self-monitoring of blood glucose levels allows the patients to see the effects of diet, exercise, and hypoglycemic medications on blood glucose levels and may promote compliance. Several products are available for home glucose monitoring. All involve obtaining a drop of capillary blood from a finger or forearm with a sterile lancet. The blood is placed on a semipermeable membrane that contains a reagent. The amount of blood glucose can be read with various machines (e.g., glucometers).
- Test urine for ketones when the patient is sick, when blood glucose levels are greater than 200 mg/dL, and when epi-

sodes of nocturnal hypoglycemia are suspected. Also teach patients and family members to test urine when indicated.
- Promote early recognition and treatment of problems by observing for signs and symptoms of urinary tract infection, peripheral vascular disease, vision changes, ketoacidosis, hypoglycemia, and others. Teach patients and families to observe for these conditions and report their occurrence.
- Discuss the importance of regular visits to health care facilities for blood sugar measurements, weights, blood pressure measurements, and eye examinations.
- Perform and teach correct foot care. Have the patient observe the following safeguards: avoid going barefoot, to prevent trauma to the feet; wear correctly fitted shoes; wash the feet daily with warm water, dry well, inspect for any lesions or pressure areas, and apply lanolin if the skin is dry; wear cotton or wool socks because they are more absorbent than synthetic materials; and cut toenails straight across and only after the feet have been soaked in warm water and washed thoroughly. Teach the patient to avoid use of hot water bottles or electric heating pads; cutting toenails if vision is impaired; use of strong antiseptics on the feet; and cutting corns or calluses. Also teach the patient to report any lesions on the feet to the physician.
- Help patients keep up with newer developments in diabetes care by providing information, sources of information, consultations with specialists, and other resources. However, do not overwhelm a patient who has just received a diagnosis of diabetes with excessive information or assume that a patient with long-term diabetes does not need information.
- Provide appropriate patient teaching for any drug therapy and combination drug therapy for patients with type 2 diabetes mellitus. (Boxes 39.7, 39.10, 39.14, and 39.16).

Evaluation

- Check blood sugar reports regularly for normal or abnormal values.
- Check glycosylated hemoglobin reports when available.
- Interview and observe for therapeutic and adverse responses to diabetic drugs.
- Interview and observe for compliance with prescribed treatment.
- Interview patients and family members about the frequency and length of hospitalizations for diabetes mellitus.

Clinical Application 39-4

The goal of care for Mr. Smith is to increase his ability to achieve good glycemic control and prevent complications related to diabetes mellitus.

- In addition to his primary physician, what other types of health care providers should be involved in his care to allow him to achieve this goal?
- What additional teaching could the nurse provide to Mr. Smith to help prevent physical and emotional complications?

40 Drug Therapy for Hyperthyroidism and Hypothyroidism

Clinical Application Case Study

Brenda Zalewski, a 45-year-old woman, had a goiter as a child and a thyroidectomy at age 12. She has been taking a synthetic thyroid preparation since that time. Ms. Zalewski takes a maintenance dose of levothyroxine (Synthroid) 0.1 mg orally daily. She is 5 feet 8 inches tall and weighs 215 pounds.

KEY TERMS

Cretinism: congenital hypothyroidism that occurs when a child is born with a poorly functioning or absent thyroid gland

Euthyroid: normal thyroid gland functioning

Goiter: visible enlargement of the thyroid gland

Graves' disease: antibody-mediated autoimmune disease resulting in hyperthyroidism; most common cause of hyperthyroidism

Hyperthyroidism: excessive secretion of thyroid hormone; usually involves an enlarged thyroid gland that has an increased number of cells and an increased rate of secretion

Hypothyroidism: diminished secretion of thyroid hormone; occurs when disease or destruction of thyroid gland tissue causes inadequate production of thyroid hormones

Myxedema: adult hypothyroidism that occurs more often in women than men

Thyroid storm: rare but severe complication characterized by extreme symptoms of hyperthyroidism; most likely to occur in patients with hyperthyroidism that has been inadequately treated, especially when stressful situations occur; also known as thyrotoxic crisis

Thyroiditis: common cause of primary hypothyroidism; an autoimmune disorder characterized by inflammation of the thyroid gland

Thyroxine: known as T_4; one of three hormones produced by the thyroid gland

Introduction

This chapter introduces the pharmacological care of the patient experiencing increased or decreased function of the thyroid gland. The two types of thyroid disorders requiring drug therapy are hyperthyroidism and hypothyroidism.

Overview of the Thyroid Gland

Physiology

Normal serum levels of thyroid hormones and a **euthyroid** physiologic state (normal thyroid function) require a functioning thyroid gland and feedback mechanism. The thyroid gland produces three hormones: thyroxine, triiodothyronine, and calcitonin. **Thyroxine** (also called T_4) contains four atoms of iodine and triiodothyronine (also called T_3) contains three atoms of iodine. T_3 is more potent than T_4 and has a more rapid onset but a shorter duration of action. Despite these minor differences, the two hormones produce the same physiologic effects and have the same actions and uses. Chapter 42 discusses calcitonin functions in calcium metabolism.

Production of T_3 and T_4 depends on the presence of iodine and tyrosine in the thyroid gland. In a series of chemical reactions, iodine atoms become attached to tyrosine, an amino acid derived from dietary protein, to form the thyroid hormones T_3 and T_4. After they are formed, the hormones are stored within the chemically inactive thyroglobulin molecule. Tyrosine forms the basic structure of thyroglobulin.

Thyroid hormones are released into the circulation when the thyroid gland is stimulated by thyroid-stimulating hormone (thyrotropin; TSH) from the anterior pituitary gland (Fig. 40.1). The hormones become largely bound to plasma proteins, with only the small unbound ones remaining biologically active. The bound thyroid hormones are released to tissue cells very slowly. In tissue cells, the hormones combine with intracellular proteins so they are again stored. They are released slowly within the cell and used over a period of days or weeks. When they are used by the cells, the thyroid hormones release iodine atoms. Most of the iodine is reabsorbed and used to produce new thyroid hormones; the remainder is excreted in the urine.

Thyroid hormones control the rate of cellular metabolism and thus influence the functioning of virtually every cell in the body. The heart, skeletal muscle, liver, and kidneys are especially responsive to the stimulating effects of thyroid hormones. The brain, spleen, and gonads are less responsive. Thyroid hormones are required for normal growth and development and are considered especially critical for brain and skeletal development and maturation. These hormones are thought to act mainly by controlling intracellular protein synthesis.

Thyroid hormones also influence linear growth; brain function, including intelligence and memory; neural development; dentition; and bone development. These hormones are thought to act mainly by controlling intracellular protein synthesis. Some specific physiologic effects include:

- Increased rate of cellular metabolism and oxygen consumption with a resultant increase in heat production
- Increased heart rate, force of contraction, and cardiac output (increased cardiac workload)
- Increased carbohydrate metabolism
- Increased fat metabolism, including increased lipolytic effects of other hormones and metabolism of cholesterol to bile acids
- Inhibition of pituitary secretion of TSH

Etiology and Pathophysiology

Hyperthyroidism

Hyperthyroidism is characterized by excessive secretion of thyroid hormone and usually involves an enlarged thyroid gland that has an increased number of cells and an increased rate of secretion. It may be associated with **Graves' disease**, nodular goiter, thyroiditis, overtreatment with thyroid drugs, functioning thyroid carcinoma, and pituitary adenoma that secretes excessive amounts of TSH.

The hyperplastic thyroid gland may secrete 5 to 15 times the normal amount of thyroid hormone. As a result, body metabolism is greatly increased. Specific physiologic effects vary (see *Clinical Manifestations*), depending on the amount of circulating thyroid hormone, and they usually increase in incidence and severity with time if hyperthyroidism is not treated.

Subclinical hyperthyroidism is defined as a reduced TSH (less than 0.1 microunit/L) and normal T_3 and T_4 levels. The most common cause is excess thyroid hormone therapy. Subclinical hyperthyroidism is a risk factor for osteoporosis in postmenopausal women who do not take estrogen replacement therapy, because it leads to reduced bone mineral density. It also greatly increases the risk of atrial fibrillation in patients older than 60 years of age.

Hypothyroidism

Hypothyroidism is characterized by diminished secretion of thyroid hormone. Primary hypothyroidism occurs when disease or destruction of thyroid gland tissue causes inadequate production of thyroid hormones. Common causes of primary

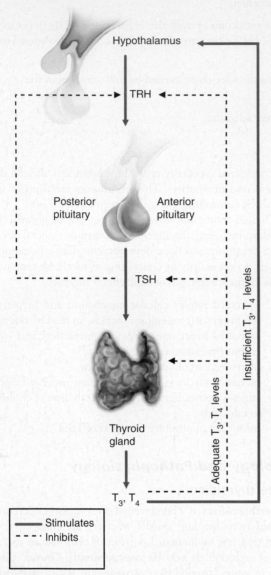

Figure 40.1 Thyroid-releasing hormone (TRH) from the hypothalamus stimulates the anterior pituitary to release thyroid-stimulating hormone (TSH). It also inhibits the hypothalamus from releasing TRH. TSH stimulates the thyroid gland to release T_3 and T_4. It also inhibits the hypothalamus from releasing TRH and the anterior pituitary from releasing more TSH. The release of T_3 and T_4 from the thyroid gland inhibits TRH release from the hypothalamus, TSH release from the pituitary, and further T_3 and T_4 release from the thyroid gland. Falling T_3 and T_4 levels stimulate the hypothalamus to release TRH, and the process repeatedly continues to maintain effective hormone levels. ACTH, adrenocorticotropic hormone; CRH, corticotropin-releasing hormone; FSH, follicle-stimulating hormone; GH, growth hormone; GHRH, growth hormone–releasing hormone; GnRH, gonadotropin-releasing hormone; LH, luteinizing hormone; PIF, prolactin-inhibiting factor; PRL, prolactin; PRF, prolactin-releasing factor; SRIF, somatotropin release–inhibiting factor.

hypothyroidism include chronic (Hashimoto's) **thyroiditis**, an autoimmune disorder characterized by inflammation of the thyroid gland, and treatment of hyperthyroidism with antithyroid drugs, radiation therapy, or surgery. Other causes include

previous radiation to the thyroid area of the neck and treatment with amiodarone, lithium, or iodine preparations. Secondary hypothyroidism occurs when there is decreased TSH from the anterior pituitary gland or decreased thyrotropin-releasing hormone (TRH) secreted from the hypothalamus.

Clinical Manifestations

Table 40.1 lists specific effects of hyperthyroidism and hypothyroidism.

Hyperthyroidism

Thyroid storm or thyrotoxic crisis is a rare but severe complication characterized by extreme symptoms of hyperthyroidism, such as severe tachycardia, fever, dehydration, heart failure, and coma. It is most likely to occur in patients with hyperthyroidism that has been inadequately treated, especially when stressful situations occur (e.g., trauma, infection, surgery, emotional upset).

It should be noted that iodine is present in foods (especially seafood and kelp) and in radiographic contrast dyes. Reports of iodine-induced hyperthyroidism have been reported after ingestion of dietary sources of iodine.

Hypothyroidism

Congenital hypothyroidism, or **cretinism**, occurs when a child is born with a poorly functioning or absent thyroid gland. Cretinism is uncommon in the United States but may occur with a lack of iodine in the mother's diet. Symptoms are rarely present at birth but develop gradually during infancy and early childhood, and they include poor growth and development, lethargy and inactivity, feeding problems, slow pulse, subnormal temperature, and constipation. If cretinism is untreated until the child is several months old, permanent mental retardation is likely to result.

Adult hypothyroidism, or **myxedema**, may be subclinical or clinical and occurs much more often in women than in men. Subclinical hypothyroidism, the most common thyroid disorder, involves a mildly elevated serum TSH and normal serum thyroxine levels. It is usually asymptomatic. If the thyroid gland cannot secrete enough hormones despite excessive release of TSH, hypothyroidism occurs, and a **goiter** (visible enlargement of the thyroid gland) may occur from the overstimulation. Clinical hypothyroidism produces variable signs and symptoms, depending on the amount of circulating thyroid hormone. Initially, manifestations (see Table 40.1) are mild and vague. They usually increase in incidence and severity over time as the thyroid gland gradually atrophies and functioning glandular tissue is replaced by nonfunctioning fibrous connective tissue.

Myxedema coma is severe, life-threatening hypothyroidism characterized by coma, hypothermia, cardiovascular collapse, hypoventilation, and severe metabolic disorders such as hyponatremia, hypoglycemia, and lactic acidosis. Predisposing factors include exposure to cold, infection, trauma, respiratory disease, and administration of central nervous system (CNS) depressants (e.g., anesthetics, analgesics, sedatives).

QSEN Safety Alert

A person with severe hypothyroidism cannot metabolize and excrete the drugs. It is necessary to assess the patient for signs of adverse drug effects.

TABLE 40.1

Thyroid Disorders and Their Effects on Body Systems

Hypothyroidism	Hyperthyroidism
Cardiovascular Effects	
Increased capillary fragility	Tachycardia
Decreased cardiac output	Increased cardiac output
Decreased blood pressure	Increased blood volume
Decreased heart rate	Increased systolic blood pressure
Cardiac enlargement	Decreased diastolic blood pressure
Congestive heart failure	Cardiac dysrhythmias
Anemia	Congestive heart failure
More rapid development of atherosclerosis and its complications (e.g., coronary artery and peripheral vascular disease)	
Central Nervous System Effects	
Apathy and lethargy	Nervousness
Emotional dullness	Emotional instability
Slow speech, perhaps slurring and hoarseness as well	Restlessness
Hypoactive reflexes	Anxiety
Forgetfulness and mental sluggishness	Insomnia
Excessive drowsiness and sleeping	Hyperactive reflexes
Metabolic Effects	
Intolerance of cold	Intolerance of heat
Subnormal temperature	Low-grade fever
Increased serum cholesterol	Weight loss despite increased appetite
Weight gain	
Gastrointestinal Effects	
Decreased appetite	Increased appetite
Constipation	Abdominal cramps
	Diarrhea
	Nausea and vomiting
Muscular Effects	
Weakness	Weakness
Fatigue	Fatigue
Vague aches and pains	Muscle atrophy
	Tremors
Integumentary Effects	
Dry, coarse, and thickened skin	Moist, warm, flushed skin due to vasodilation and increased sweating
Puffy appearance of face and eyelids	
Dry and thinned hair	Hair and nails soft
Thick and hard nails	
Reproductive Effects	
Prolonged menstrual periods	Amenorrhea or oligomenorrhea
Infertility or sterility	
Decreased libido	

(Continued on page 752)

TABLE 40.1

Thyroid Disorders and Their Effects on Body Systems (Continued)

Hypothyroidism	Hyperthyroidism
Miscellaneous Effects	
Increased susceptibility to infection	Dyspnea
Increased sensitivity to narcotics, barbiturates, and anesthetics due to slowed metabolism of these drugs	Polyuria
	Hoarse, rapid speech
	Increased susceptibility to infection
	Excessive perspiration
	Localized edema around the eyeballs, which produces characteristic eye changes, including exophthalmos

NCLEX Success

1. A 62-year-old woman has a reduced TSH level of 0.07 microunit/L and a normal T_3 and T_4. Which of the following symptoms is she at risk for developing?

   A. sinus bradycardia
   B. premature ventricular contractions
   C. atrial fibrillation
   D. prolong QT interval

2. An infant has diminished growth and development with a very slow pulse and below-normal temperature. Based on the symptoms, what disorder is suspected?

   A. cretinism
   B. Cushing's disease
   C. Addison's disease
   D. thyroid storm

3. A patient has been treated for ventricular dysrhythmias with amiodarone. What is the patient at risk for developing?

   A. Graves' disease
   B. thyroiditis
   C. thyroid storm
   D. cretinism

Drug Therapy

The goal of treatment is to restore the euthyroid state and normal metabolism. In hyperthyroidism, the goals are to reduce thyroid hormone production to relieve symptoms, return serum TSH and thyroid hormone levels to normal, and avoid complete destruction of the thyroid gland. Antithyroid drugs act by decreasing the production or release of thyroid hormones. The thioamide drugs inhibit synthesis thyroid hormones. Iodine preparations inhibit the release of thyroid hormones and cause them to be stored within the thyroid gland. Radioactive iodine emits rays that destroy the thyroid gland tissue.

In hypothyroidism, the goal (of thyroid-replacement therapy) is to administer a dosage in sufficient amounts to compensate for the thyroid deficit—to resolve symptoms and restore serum TSH and thyroid hormone to normal.

Table 40.2 summarizes the drugs administered for thyroid disease.

Antithyroid Drugs

PROPYLTHIOURACIL AND RELATED DRUGS

Ⓟ **Propylthiouracil** (PTU) is the prototype of the thioamide antithyroid drugs. The U.S. Food and Drug Administration (FDA) approved it for the treatment of hyperthyroidism more than 60 years ago.

Pharmacokinetics

PTU is well absorbed with oral administration, and peak plasma levels occur within 30 minutes. The drug's plasma half-life is 1 to 2 hours. However, its duration of action depends on the

TABLE 40.2

Drugs Administered for the Treatment of Hyperthyroidism and Hypothyroidism

Drug Class	Prototype	Other Drugs in the Class
Antithyroid drug	Propylthiouracil (PTU)	Methimazole (Tapazole) Strong iodine solution (Lugol's Solution) Saturated solution of potassium iodide (SSKI) Sodium iodide ^{131}I (Iodotope)
Beta-adrenergic–blocking agent	Propranolol hydrochloride (Inderal)	
Thyroid drug	Levothyroxine (Synthroid, Levothroid)	

half-life within the thyroid gland rather than the plasma half-life. Because this time is relatively short, PTU must be given every 8 hours. It is metabolized in the liver and excreted in urine.

Action

PTU acts by inhibiting production of thyroid hormones and peripheral conversion of T_4 to the more active T_3. The drug does not interfere with release of thyroid hormones previously produced and stored. Thus, therapeutic effects do not occur for several days or weeks until the stored hormones have been used.

Use

Health care providers may use PTU alone to treat hyperthyroidism, as part of the preoperative preparation for thyroidectomy, before or after radioactive iodine therapy, and in the treatment of thyroid storm. Treatment of hyperthyroidism changes the rate of body metabolism, including the rate of metabolism of many drugs. In the hyperthyroid state, drug metabolism may be very rapid, and higher doses of most drugs may be necessary to achieve therapeutic results. When the patient becomes euthyroid, the rate of drug metabolism decreases. Consequently, it is necessary to evaluate and to reduce doses of all medications (probably); this avoids severe adverse effects. Table 40.3 contains standard route and dosage information for PTU and the other antithyroid drugs.

Use in Children

PTU (or methimazole) is useful. Potential risks for adverse effects are similar to those in adults. Radioactive iodine may cause cancer and chromosome damage in children; therefore,

it is essential that this agent be used only for hyperthyroidism that cannot be controlled by other antithyroid drugs or surgery.

Use in Older Adults

PTU (or methimazole) may be useful. However, radioactive iodine is often preferable because it is associated with fewer adverse effects than other antithyroid drugs or surgery. It is necessary that patients be monitored closely for hypothyroidism, which usually develops within 1 year after receiving treatment for hyperthyroidism.

Use in Patients With Hepatic Impairment

The FDA has issued a **BLACK BOX WARNING ◆** for PTU stating that severe liver injury resulting in death or acute liver failure may occur within 6 months of treatment. All patients should receive instructions about the signs and symptoms of acute liver failure. Routine liver function testing to assess for liver failure is important.

Adverse Effects

Administration of PTU may have several adverse effects, including the following:

- Signs and symptoms of hypothyroidism: bradycardia, heart failure, anemia, coronary artery disease, peripheral vascular disease, slow speech and body movements, emotional and mental dullness, excessive sleeping, increased weight, constipation, and skin changes
- Hematologic effects: leukopenia, agranulocytosis (puts patient at risk for sepsis; rare but severe; earliest symptoms likely to be sore throat and fever), and hypoprothrombinemia

TABLE 40.3

DRUGS AT A GLANCE: Drugs for Hyperthyroidism (Antithyroid Drugs)

Drug	Pregnancy Category	Routes and Dosage Ranges	
		Adults	*Children*
Ⓟ **Propylthiouracil** (PTU)	D	300–400 mg/d PO in divided doses every 8 h, until the patient is euthyroid; then 100–150 mg/d in 3 divided doses, for maintenance	6–10 y, 50–150 mg/d PO in divided doses every 8 h Older than 10 y, 150–300 mg/d PO in divided doses every 8 h; usual maintenance dose, 100–300 mg/d PO in 2 divided doses, every 12 h
Methimazole (Tapazole)	D	15–60 mg/d PO initially, in divided doses every 8 hours until the patient is euthyroid; maintenance, 5–15 mg/d PO in 2 or 3 doses	0.4 mg/kg/d PO initially, in divided doses every 8 h; maintenance dose, one half initial dose
Strong iodine solution (Lugol's solution)	D	2–6 drops PO 3 times per day for 10 d before thyroidectomy	2–6 drops PO 3 times per day for 10 d before thyroidectomy
Saturated solution of potassium iodide (SSKI)	D	5 drops PO 3 times per day for 10 d before thyroidectomy	5 drops PO 3 times per day for 10 d before thyroidectomy
Sodium iodide I[131] (Iodotope)	D	Dosage (PO, IV) as calculated by a radiologist trained in nuclear medicine	Dosage (PO, IV) as calculated by a radiologist trained in nuclear medicine

- Dermatologic effects: rash, pruritus, and alopecia
- CNS effects: headache, dizziness, loss of taste, drowsiness, and paresthesias
- Gastrointestinal (GI) effects: nausea, vomiting, abdominal discomfort, gastric irritation, and cholestatic hepatitis
- Other reported effects: lymphadenopathy, edema, joint pain, and drug fever

Contraindications

The only contraindication to PTU is a known hypersensitivity reaction to the medication.

Nursing Implications

Preventing Interactions

PTU may increase the effect of anticoagulants, which may put patients at risk for bleeding. Also, use with amiodarone, potassium iodide, and sodium iodide reverses thyroid hormone efficacy. Lithium acts synergistically with PTU to produce hypothyroidism.

Administering the Drug

Patients should take PTU around the clock in evenly divided doses. If they choose to take one dose of the medication without food, they should take all doses without food. (The same is true if they take it with food.)

Assessing for Therapeutic Effects

The nurse assesses for a slower pulse rate, slow speech, normal level of activity without the signs of hyperactivity, decreased nervousness and tremors, increased sleep patterns, and weight gain. The therapeutic effects should be apparent in 1 to 2 weeks, but euthyroidism may not occur for 6 to 8 weeks.

Assessing for Adverse Effects

The nurse assesses the patient's heart rate and peripheral pulses for increases, the lung sounds for crackles, and the heart sounds for an audible S_3; these are all indicative of heart failure. It is also necessary to assess for slow speech and emotional status (dullness). In addition, the nurse checks for increased periods of

EVIDENCE-BASED PRACTICE

Amiodarone-Induced Thyroid Dysfunction: Brand-Name Versus Generic Formulations

by MEYTAL TSADOK, CYNTHIA JACKEVICIUS, ELHAM RAHME,

Canadian Medical Association Journal, 2011, 183(12), E817–E823

The administration of amiodarone in the treatment of atrial fibrillation can result in the dysfunction of the patient's thyroid gland. The researchers evaluated and compared the risk of thyroid dysfunction between patients treated with brand-name or generic amiodarone. In the study, 4.7% of the patients received brand-name formulations and 10.4% were administered the generic formulation. There was no difference between brand-name and generic amiodarone.

IMPLICATIONS FOR NURSING PRACTICE: When administering brand-name or generic amiodarone, the patient is at risk for the development of thyroiditis.

rest, increased weight, constipation, and skin changes. Finally, he or she assesses for CNS depression and gastric irritation, as well as for fever or sore throat, the first signs of agranulocytosis. It is important to assess the white blood count for leukopenia.

Patient Teaching

Box 40.1 identifies patient teaching guidelines for PTU.

Other Drugs in the Class

Methimazole (Tapazole) is similar to PTU in terms of action, use, and adverse effects. It is also well absorbed with oral administration and rapidly reaches peak plasma levels.

BOX 40.1   Patient Teaching Guidelines for Propylthiouracil

- To decrease the production of thyroid hormone by an overactive thyroid gland, it is necessary to take antithyroid drugs for 1 year or longer to return thyroid hormone levels to normal.
- Have periodic tests of thyroid function. Dosage adjustments may be necessary.
- Have periodic tests of liver function tests during the first 6 months of treatment.
- Ask the prescriber if it is necessary to avoid or restrict amounts of seafood or iodized salt. It may be necessary to reduce or omit these sources of iodide during antithyroid drug therapy.
- Take this drug at regular intervals around the clock, usually every 8 hours.

- Report fever, sore throat, unusual bleeding or bruising, headache, skin rash, yellowing of the skin, or vomiting to the prescriber. If these adverse effects occur, he or she may reduce the drug dosage or have you stop taking the drug.
- Consult a health care provider before taking over-the-counter drugs. Some drugs contain iodide, which can increase the likelihood of goiter and the risk of adverse effects from excessive doses of iodide. For example, some cough syrups, asthma medications, and multivitamins may contain iodide.
- Take your pulse daily and report rates above 100 and below 60 beats per minute to the prescriber.
- Check your weight two to three times per week, and if it increases suddenly, call your health care provider.

Strong iodine solution (Lugol's solution) and saturated solution of potassium iodide (SSKI) are iodine preparations sometimes used in short-term treatment of hyperthyroidism. These drugs inhibit release of thyroid hormones, causing them to accumulate in the thyroid gland. Lugol's solution is usually used to treat thyrotoxic crisis and to decrease the size and vascularity of the thyroid gland before thyroidectomy. SSKI is more often used as an expectorant but may be given as preparation for thyroidectomy. Iodine preparations should not be followed by PTU, methimazole, or radioactive iodine because the latter drugs cause release of stored thyroid hormone and may precipitate acute hyperthyroidism.

Sodium iodide ^{131}I (Iodotope) is a radioactive isotope of iodine. The thyroid gland cannot differentiate between regular iodide and radioactive iodide, so it picks up the radioactive iodide from the circulating blood. As a result, small amounts of radioactive iodide can be used as a diagnostic test of thyroid function, and larger doses are used therapeutically to treat hyperthyroidism. Therapeutic doses act by emitting beta and gamma rays, which destroy thyroid tissue and thereby decrease production of thyroid hormones. The drug is also used to treat thyroid cancer. It is safe, effective, inexpensive, and convenient. One disadvantage is hypothyroidism, which usually develops within a few months and requires lifelong thyroid hormone-replacement therapy. Another disadvantage is the delay in therapeutic benefits. Results may not be apparent for 3 months or longer, during which time it is necessary to bring severe hyperthyroidism under control with one of the thioamide antithyroid drugs.

ADJUVANT MEDICATION USED TO TREAT HYPERTHYROIDISM

The drug ⓟ **propranolol** (Inderal) is a beta-adrenergic blocking agent that is sometimes administered to help control the symptoms of hyperthyroidism. Most often, uses include treatment of cardiovascular conditions, such as dysrhythmias, angina pectoris, and hypertension. When given to patients with hyperthyroidism, propranolol blocks beta-adrenergic receptors in various organs and thereby controls symptoms of hyperthyroidism resulting from excessive stimulation of the sympathetic nervous system. These symptoms include tachycardia, palpitations, excessive sweating, tremors, and nervousness. Propranolol is useful for controlling symptoms during the

delayed response to thioamide drugs and radioactive iodine, before thyroidectomy, and in treating thyrotoxic crisis. When patients become euthyroid and definitive treatment has controlled hyperthyroid symptoms, it is necessary to taper propranolol and discontinue it. Table 40.4 gives route and dosage information for propranolol.

NCLEX Success

4. A patient with a diagnosis of hyperthyroidism has a blood pressure of 170/98 mm Hg. Which of the following medications might a physician prescribe to treat hypertension?
   A. PTU
   B. propranolol (Inderal)
   C. furosemide (Lasix)
   D. hydrochlorothiazide with triamterene (Maxzide)

5. How does propranolol (Inderal) control symptoms of hyperthyroidism?
   A. Propranolol blocks the alpha-adrenergic receptor sites.
   B. Propranolol stimulates the thyroid gland to decrease thyroid production.
   C. Propranolol blocks the beta-adrenergic receptors in various organs.
   D. Propranolol lowers blood pressure to decrease metabolism.

6. A woman is taking PTU and develops a sore throat and fever. What does the nurse suspect is wrong with this woman?
   A. She has developed a goiter.
   B. She has an elevated liver function.
   C. She has developed a hypersensitivity reaction.
   D. She has agranulocytosis.

Thyroid Drugs

ⓟ **Levothyroxine** (Synthroid, Levothroid), a synthetic preparation of thyroxine, serves as the prototype thyroid drug. It is the drug of choice for long-term treatment of hypothyroidism. This potent form of T_4 contains a uniform amount of hormone and can be administered parenterally.

TABLE 40.4

DRUGS AT A GLANCE: Adjuvant Drugs for the Treatment of Hyperthyroidism (Propranolol)

Drug	Pregnancy Category	Routes and Dosage Ranges	
		Adults	*Children*
ⓟ **Propranolol hydrochloride** (Inderal)	C	40–160 mg/d PO in divided doses	

Pharmacokinetics

Absorption of levothyroxine varies after oral administration from 48% to 79%. Taking the drug on an empty stomach increases absorption. In malabsorption syndromes this results in excessive loss of the drug in the feces. Most (99%) of the circulating drug is bound to serum proteins, including thyroid-binding globulin as well as thyroid-binding prealbumin and albumin. Levothyroxine has a long half-life, about 6 to 7 days in euthyroidism (normal thyroid function), but it is prolonged to 9 to 10 days in hypothyroidism and shortened to 3 to 4 days in hyperthyroidism. The drug is metabolized in the liver and excreted in the urine.

Action

Levothyroxine increases the metabolic rate in the body's tissues, increasing oxygen consumption, respiratory rate, and heart rate. It also increases the metabolism of fats, carbohydrates, and proteins and enhances the growth process.

Use

Health care providers use levothyroxine as replacement therapy for people with hypothyroidism. Other uses include the following:

- Treatment and prevention of euthyroid goiters in patients with pituitary suppression of TSH
- Management of thyroid cancer
- Prevention of goitrogenesis, hypothyroidism, and thyrotoxicosis during pregnancy (in combination with antithyroid medications)
- Treatment of myxedema coma

Table 40.5 provides route and dosage information for levothyroxine. It is important to note that the FDA has issued a **BLACK BOX WARNING** ◆ cautioning prescribers not to order thyroid hormones, either alone or with other therapeutic agents, for the treatment of obesity or for weight loss.

Significant and serious complications may develop in euthyroid people who take thyroid hormones.

Use in Children

Replacement therapy is necessary because thyroid hormone is essential for normal growth and development. As in adults, levothyroxine is the drug of choice in children, and dosage needs may change with growth. After thyroid drugs are started, determination of the maintenance dosage requires periodic radioimmunoassay of serum thyroxine levels and periodic radiographs to follow bone development. To monitor drug effects on growth in children, it is important to record height and weight and compare them with growth charts at regular intervals. Close monitoring for adverse drug effects is necessary.

Use in Older Adults

Thyroid hormone replacement with levothyroxine increases the workload of the heart and may cause serious adverse effects in older adults, especially those with cardiovascular disease. In such patients, cautious treatment is necessary because of a high risk of adverse effects on the cardiovascular system. Thus, use of smaller initial dosages and smaller drug increments at longer intervals than younger adults is essential. It is important to have periodic measurements of serum TSH levels to monitor drug therapy and to adjust doses when indicated. Also, regular monitoring of blood pressure and pulse is essential. As a general rule, levothyroxine should not be given if the resting heart rate is more than 100 beats per minute.

Use in Patients With Hepatic Impairment

QSEN Safety Alert

Hepatic metabolism in patients with hypothyroidism is slow, so drug metabolism may be delayed. Many drugs given to these patients have a prolonged effect. It is therefore important to assess drug reactions in patients with hepatic impairment.

TABLE 40.5

DRUGS AT A GLANCE: Levothyroxine

Drug	Pregnancy Category	Routes and Dosage Ranges	
		Adults	Children
℗ **Levothyroxine** (Synthroid, Levothroid)	A	0.05 mg/d PO initially, increased by 0.025 mg every 2–3 wk until desired response obtained; usual maintenance dose, 0.1–0.2 mg/d (100–200 mcg/d) Myxedema coma, IV 0.4 mg in a single dose; then 0.1–0.2 mg daily Thyroid-stimulating hormone (TSH) suppression in thyroid cancer, nodules, and euthyroid goiters, 2.6 mcg/kg/d PO for 7–10 d Older adults, patients with cardiac disorders, and patients with hypothyroidism of long duration, 0.0125–0.025 mg/d PO for 6 wk, then dose is doubled every 6–8 wk until the desired response is obtained	Congenital hypothyroidism, PO Birth–6 mo, 25–50 mcg/d (or 8–10 mcg/kg/d) 6–12 mo, 50–75 mcg/d (or 6–8 mcg/kg/d) 1–5 y, 75–100 mcg/d (or 5–6 mcg/kg/d) 6–12 y, 100–150 mcg/d (or 4–5 mcg/kg/d) Older than 12 y, >150 mcg/d (or 2–3 mcg/kg/d)

Use in Patients With Critical Illness

Management of patients in thyroid storm or thyrotoxic crisis is common in the critical care unit. Increased rate of cellular metabolism and oxygen consumption occur with a resultant increase in heat production. The hypermetabolic state increases the metabolism of medications, so increased or more frequent dosing may be necessary.

Adverse Effects

Adverse effects of levothyroxine include signs and symptoms of hyperthyroidism. Other more serious adverse effects are tachycardia, cardiac dysrhythmias, angina pectoris, myocardial infarction, and heart failure. Nervousness, hyperactivity, insomnia, diarrhea, abdominal cramps, nausea, vomiting, weight loss, fever, and an intolerance to heat have also been reported.

Most adverse reactions stem from excessive doses, and signs and symptoms produced are the same as those occurring with hyperthyroidism. Excessive thyroid hormones make the heart work very hard and fast in attempting to meet tissue demands for oxygenated blood and nutrients. Symptoms of myocardial ischemia occur when the increased cardiac workload is prolonged. Cardiovascular problems are more likely to occur in patients who are elderly or who already have heart disease.

Contraindications

Contraindications to levothyroxine include a known hypersensitivity to active or extraneous constituents of the drug, thyrotoxicosis, and acute myocardial infarction related to hypothyroidism. Caution is warranted in Addison's disease. Affected patients require corticosteroids prior to administration of levothyroxine. Thyroid hormones increase tissue metabolism and tissue demands for adrenocortical hormones. If adrenal insufficiency is not treated first, administration of thyroid hormone may cause acute adrenocortical insufficiency, a life-threatening condition. Also, caution is necessary during lactation and with coronary artery disease or angina.

Nursing Implications

Preventing Interactions

Many medications interact with levothyroxine, increasing and decreasing its effects (Box 40.2).

Administering the Medication

Several factors affect the dosage of levothyroxine: the choice of drug, age and general condition, severity and duration of hypothyroidism, and clinical response to drug therapy. It is essential to individualize the dosage to approximate the amount of thyroid hormone needed to make up the deficit in endogenous hormone production. As a general rule, the initial dosage is relatively small, and gradual increases at approximately 2-week intervals are appropriate until symptoms are relieved and a normal serum TSH level (0.5–4.2 microunits/L) is reestablished. Determination of the maintenance dosage for long-term

---

> **BOX 40.2   Drug Interactions: Levothyroxine**
>
> **Drugs That Increase the Effects of Levothyroxine**
> - Activating antidepressants (bupropion, venlafaxine), adrenergic asthmatic agents (albuterol, epinephrine), nasal decongestants
>   *Increase the effects of thyroid hormones*
>
> **Drugs That Decrease the Effects of Levothyroxine**
> - Antacids, cholestyramine, iron, sucralfate
>   *Decrease absorption of levothyroxine*
> - Antihypertensives, propranolol
>   *Decrease cardiac-stimulating effects*
> - Estrogens, oral contraceptives
>   *Increase thyroxine-binding globulin, thereby increasing the amount of bound, inactive levothyroxine in patients with hypothyroidism*
> - Phenytoin, rifampin
>   *Induce enzymes, leading to more rapid metabolism*

therapy depends on the patient's clinical status and periodic measurement of serum TSH.

People should take levothyroxine in the morning on an empty stomach. If the pulse rate prior to administering the drug is more than 100 beats per minute, it is important to notify the prescriber.

When giving levothyroxine to an infant or young child, it may be necessary to crush the tablet and add a small amount of formula or water. The child should take the solution with the medication soon after it is mixed; storing the liquid for long periods is a practice to avoid. It is also appropriate to sprinkle the crushed tablet on a small amount of food and then administer it.

Assessing for Therapeutic Effects

In hypothyroidism, thyroid-replacement therapy is lifelong. Medical supervision is necessary frequently during early treatment and at least annually after the patient's condition has stabilized and maintenance dosage has been determined. The brand of medication should be consistent; patients should not change brands. The nurse assesses for the following conditions:

- Increasing energy and diminished sleep
- Level of alertness and interest in the environment and surroundings
- Increased pulse rate and blood pressure
- Bowel regularity and decreased symptoms of constipation
- Reversal of coarseness of skin and hair
- Laboratory values (should decrease as the thyroid hormone is replaced): serum cholesterol, creatinine phosphokinase, lactate dehydrogenase, and aspartate aminotransferase

In patients with cretinism, the nurse records the patient's height periodically to determine an increased in linear growth.

In patients with myxedema, the nurse assesses for decreased edema and loss of weight.

BOX 40.3 Patient Teaching Guidelines for Levothyroxine

■ Thyroid hormone is required for normal body functioning and for life. When your thyroid gland is unable to produce enough thyroid hormone, levothyroxine is used as a synthetic substitute. Thus, levothyroxine therapy for hypothyroidism is lifelong; stopping it may lead to life-threatening illness.

■ Have periodic tests of thyroid function.

■ Understand that dosage adjustments may occur according to clinical response and results of thyroid function tests.

■ Do not switch from one drug brand to another; effects may be different.

■ Consult a health care provider before taking over-the-counter drugs that stimulate the heart or cause nervousness (e.g., asthma remedies, cold remedies, decongestants). Levothyroxine stimulates the central nervous system and the heart; excessive stimulation may occur if it is taken with other stimulating

drugs. In addition, you should probably limit your intake of caffeine-containing beverages to 2 to 3 servings daily.

■ Take the drug every morning, on an empty stomach, for best absorption. Also, do not take the drug with an antacid (e.g., Tums, Maalox), an iron preparation, or sucralfate (Carafate). These drugs decrease absorption of levothyroxine. If it is necessary to take one of these drugs, take levothyroxine 2 hours before or 4 to 6 hours after the other drug.

■ Take the drug at about the same time each day for more consistent blood levels and more normal body metabolism.

■ Report chest pain, heart palpitations, nervousness, or insomnia to the prescriber. These adverse effects result from excessive stimulation and may indicate that drug dosage or intake of other stimulants needs to be reduced.

Assessing for Adverse Effects

The nurse assesses for tachycardia and any cardiac dysrhythmias. Excessive thyroid hormones make the heart work very hard and fast in an attempt to meet the tissue demands for oxygenated blood and nutrients. It is necessary to assess for chest pain, edema, and signs of heart failure. Symptoms of myocardial infarction occur when the myocardium does not have an adequate supply of oxygenated blood. Symptoms of heart failure occur when the increased cardiac workload is prolonged.

Patient Teaching

Box 40.3 provides patient teaching guidelines for levothyroxine.

Clinical Application 40-1

■ While Ms. Zalewski is in the hospital, the nurse is administering her medications. Hospital routine is to administer all once-daily medications at 9:00 AM. When reviewing the medication administration orders, the nurse notes that Ms. Zalewski is to receive levothyroxine (Synthroid) at 9:00 AM. Patients usually receive their breakfast trays between 8:00 and 8:30 AM. What action should the nurse take with regard to the administration of levothyroxine?

NCLEX Success

7. A man asks the nurse when he should take his daily dose of levothyroxine (Synthroid). Which of the following instructions is most appropriate to teach him?

A. Take it before breakfast on an empty stomach.
B. Take it with meals every 8 hours in divided doses.
C. Take it every night at bedtime with a snack.
D. Take it every day at the same without regard to meals.

8. What assessment should the nurse implement prior to the administration of levothyroxine?

A. blood glucose
B. heart rate
C. lung sounds
D. urine output

9. The home care nurse is visiting with a patient who has a diagnosis of hypothyroidism. The patient is being treated with levothyroxine. The assessment of the patient reveals the following findings: an audible S_3, crackles in the lower lobes, edema of the lower extremities, and a heart rate of 120 beats per minute. What does the nurse suspect the patient has developed?

A. myocardial infarction
B. thrombophlebitis
C. pulmonary embolism
D. heart failure

10. A 21-year-old woman is taking levothyroxine for hypothyroidism. She has recently become sexually active and would like to take an oral contraceptive. Which of the following aspects of patient teaching is most accurate?

A. A low-dose oral contraceptive agent is permissible with levothyroxine.
B. Oral contraceptive agents increase the amount of thyroid hormone.
C. For protection from pregnancy, it is necessary to use an oral contraceptive and an alternative form of birth control.
D. Oral contraceptive agents result in diminished levothyroxine levels due to inactivation.

Clinical Application 40-2

Ms. Zalewski has been discharged from the hospital and is being seen by the home care nurse. During the visit, the nurse reviews all of Ms. Zalewski's medications. Ms. Zalewski states she is taking aluminum hydroxide gel (Amphojel) every morning when she arises to prevent gastric distress after breakfast.

- How will the administration of Amphojel affect her levothyroxine?
- What patient teaching should the home care nurse provide to Ms. Zalewski?

The Nursing Process

Assessment

- Assess for signs and symptoms of thyroid disorders (see Table 40.1). During the course of treatment with thyroid or antithyroid drugs, the patient's blood level of thyroid hormone may range from low to normal to high. At either end of the continuum, signs and symptoms may be dramatic and obvious. As blood levels change toward normal as a result of treatment, signs and symptoms become less obvious. If presenting signs and symptoms are treated too aggressively, they may change toward the opposite end of the continuum and indicate adverse drug effects. Thus, each patient receiving a drug that alters thyroid function must be assessed for indicators of hypothyroidism, euthyroidism, and hyperthyroidism.
- Check laboratory reports for serum TSH (normal = 0.5–4.2 microunits/mL) when available. An elevated serum TSH is the first indication of primary hypothyroidism and commonly occurs in middle-aged women, even in the absence of other signs and symptoms. Serum TSH is used to monitor response to drugs that alter thyroid function.

Nursing Diagnoses

- Decreased cardiac output related to disease- or drug-induced thyroid disorders
- Imbalanced nutrition: less than body requirements with hyperthyroidism
- Imbalanced nutrition: more than body requirements with hypothyroidism
- Ineffective thermoregulation related to changes in metabolism rate and body heat production
- Deficient knowledge: disease process and drug therapy

Planning/Goals

The patient will

- Achieve normal blood levels of thyroid hormone
- Receive or take drugs accurately
- Experience relief of symptoms of hypothyroidism or hyperthyroidism

- Be assisted to cope with symptoms until therapy becomes effective
- Avoid preventable adverse drug effects
- Maintain the therapeutic and avoid the adverse effects of drug therapy

Nursing Interventions

The nurse will

- Use nondrug measures to control symptoms, increase effectiveness of drug therapy, and decrease adverse reactions. Some areas for intervention include the following:
  - Environmental temperature. Regulate for the patient's comfort, when possible. Patients with hypothyroidism are very intolerant of cold, due to their slow metabolism rate. Chilling and shivering should be prevented because of added strain on the heart. Please provide blankets and warm clothes as needed. Patients with hyperthyroidism are very intolerant of heat and perspire excessively, due to their rapid metabolism rate. Provide cooling baths and lightweight clothing as needed.
  - Diet. Despite a poor appetite, hypothyroid patients are often overweight because of a slow metabolism rate. Thus, a low-calorie, weight-reduction diet may be indicated. In addition, an increased intake of high-fiber foods is usually needed to prevent constipation as a result of decreased GI secretions and motility. Despite a good appetite, hyperthyroid patients are often underweight because of a rapid metabolism rate. They often need extra calories and nutrients to prevent tissue breakdown. These can be provided by extra meals and snacks. The patient may wish to avoid highly seasoned and high-fiber foods because they may increase diarrhea.
  - Fluids. With hypothyroidism, patients need an adequate intake of low-calorie fluids to prevent constipation. With hyperthyroidism, patients need large amounts of fluids (3000–4000 mL/d) unless contraindicated by cardiac or renal disease. The fluids are needed to eliminate heat and waste products produced by the hypermetabolic state. Much of the patient's fluid loss is visible as excessive perspiration and urine output.
  - Activity. With hypothyroidism, encourage activity to maintain cardiovascular, respiratory, GI, and musculoskeletal function. With hyperthyroidism, encourage rest and quiet, nonstrenuous activity. Because patients differ in what they find restful, this must be determined with each patient. A quiet room, reading, and soft music may be helpful. Mild sedatives are often given. The patient is caught in the dilemma of needing rest because of the high metabolic rate but being unable to rest because of nervousness and excitement.
  - Skin care. Hypothyroid patients are likely to have edema and dry skin. When edema is present, inspect pressure points, turn often, and avoid trauma when possible. Edema increases risks of skin breakdown and decubitus ulcer formation. Also, increased capillary fragility increases the likelihood of bruising from seemingly minor trauma. When skin is dry, use soap sparingly and lotions and other lubricants freely.

41 Drug Therapy for Pituitary and Hypothalamic Dysfunction

Clinical Application Case Study

Jose Rojas is a 24-year-old man who has suffered a head injury while riding his motorcycle without a helmet. He has been admitted for observation, with multiple abrasions and a blow to the head. He begins to produce massive amounts of clear, pale-yellow urine. The physician diagnoses diabetes insipidus and orders desmopressin 0.2 mL intranasally in two divided doses.

KEY TERMS

Acromegaly: a chronic disease, resulting from excessive secretion of growth hormone (GH); characterized by an abnormal pattern of bone and connective tissue growth associated with an increased incidence of diabetes mellitus and hypertension

Antidiuretic hormone: functions to regulate water balance; also known as vasopressin. This hormone is secreted when body fluids become concentrated and when blood volume is low

Corticotropin: anterior pituitary hormone obtained from animal pituitary glands; also referred to as adrenocorticotropic hormone. This hormone may be used as a diagnostic test to differentiate primary adrenal insufficiency from secondary adrenal insufficiency caused by inadequate pituitary secretion of corticotropin

Corticotropin-releasing hormone or factor: causes release of corticotropin in response to stress and threatening stimuli; most often secreted during sleep

Dwarfism: a condition marked by severely decreased linear growth and frequently severely delayed mental, emotional, dental, and sexual growth; caused by a lack of GH

Gonadotropin-releasing hormone: causes release of follicle-stimulating hormone and luteinizing hormone

Growth hormone (GH): stimulates the growth of body tissues; regulates cell division and protein synthesis required for normal growth and promotes an increase in cell size and number, including growth of muscle cells and lengthening of bone

Inhibiting hormone: produced by the hypothalamus; decreases hormone secretion that corresponds to each of the major hormones of the anterior pituitary gland

Releasing hormone: produced by the hypothalamus; accelerates the secretion of the anterior pituitary hormone

Thyroid-stimulating hormone (thyrotropin): regulates secretion of thyroid hormones

Introduction

This chapter introduces the pharmacological care of the patient experiencing increased or decreased function of the hormones secreted by the hypothalamus and pituitary gland. It focuses on drug therapy for chronic precocious puberty, acromegaly, growth hormone deficiency in children, and diabetes insipidus.

The hypothalamus of the brain and the pituitary gland interact to control most metabolic functions of the body and to maintain homeostasis (Fig. 41.1). They are anatomically connected by a funnel-shaped hypophyseal stalk. The hypothalamus controls secretions of the pituitary gland. The pituitary gland, in turn, regulates secretions or functions of other body tissues called target tissues. The pituitary gland is actually two glands, each with different structures and functions. The anterior pituitary is composed of different types of glandular cells that synthesize and secrete different hormones. The posterior pituitary is anatomically an extension of the hypothalamus and is composed mainly of nerve fibers. Although it does not manufacture any hormones itself, it stores and releases hormones synthesized in the hypothalamus. Hormones are chemical messengers with specific regulatory effect on the cells that control various bodily functions.

Overview of Pituitary and Hypothalamic Dysfunction

Physiology

Anterior Pituitary Hormones

The anterior pituitary gland produces seven hormones. Two of these, growth hormone and prolactin, act directly on their target tissues; the other five act indirectly by stimulating target tissues to produce other hormones.

Corticotropin, also called adrenocorticotropic hormone (ACTH), stimulates the adrenal cortex to produce corticosteroids (see Chap. 15). The hypothalamus and plasma levels of cortisol, the major corticosteroid, control secretion of corticotropin.

A negative feedback mechanism inhibits the release of cortisol when plasma levels are adequate for body needs. After corticotropin administration, there is a greater release of corticotropin by way of negative feedback. Thus, the therapeutic effects are greater with corticotropin than with glucocorticoids, leading to a decrease in ACTH and changing the structure of the pituitary.

Growth hormone, or GH (also called somatotropin), stimulates growth of body tissues. It regulates cell division and protein synthesis required for normal growth and promotes an increase in cell size and number, including growth of muscle cells and lengthening of bone. These effects occur mainly via altered metabolism of carbohydrate, protein, and fat by direct and indirect effects. Authorities often consider GH an insulin antagonist because it suppresses the abilities of insulin to stimulate uptake of glucose in peripheral tissues and enhance glucose synthesis in the liver. Paradoxically, administration of GH produces hyperinsulinemia by stimulating insulin secretion. In addition, GH stimulates protein anabolism in many tissues. The hormone also enhances fat utilization by stimulating triglyceride breakdown and oxidation in fat-storing cells.

Levels of GH rise rapidly during adolescence, peak in the 20s, and then start to decline. In children, deficient GH produces **dwarfism,** a condition marked by severely decreased linear growth and, frequently, severely delayed mental, emotional, dental, and sexual growth. If untreated, excessive GH in preadolescents produces gigantism, resulting in heights of 8 or 9 feet.

In adults, deficient GH (less than expected for age) can cause increased fat, reduced skeletal and heart muscle mass, reduced strength, reduced ability to exercise, and worsened cholesterol levels (i.e., increased low-density lipoprotein cholesterol and decreased high-density lipoprotein cholesterol), which increases the risk of cardiovascular disease. Excessive GH in adults produces **acromegaly,** a chronic disease characterized by an abnormal pattern of bone and connective tissue growth associated with an increased incidence of diabetes mellitus and hypertension.

Thyroid-stimulating hormone (TSH) (also called thyrotropin) regulates secretion of thyroid hormones. Thyrotropin secretion is controlled by a negative feedback mechanism in proportion to

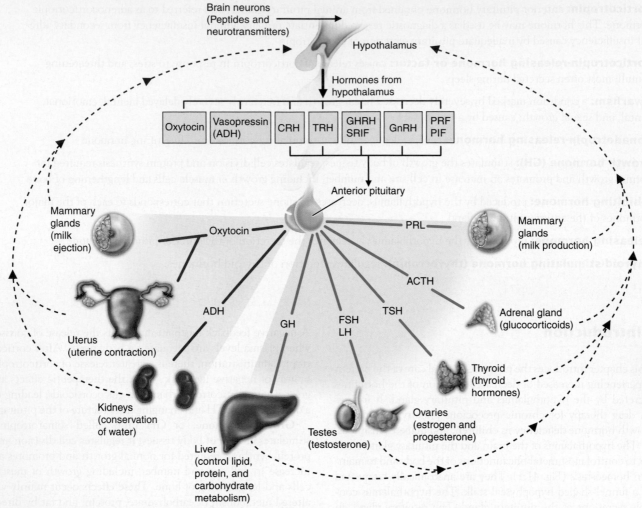

Figure 41.1 Hypothalamic and pituitary hormones and their target organs. The hypothalamus produces hormones that act on the anterior pituitary or are stored in the posterior pituitary. The anterior pituitary produces hormones that act on various body tissues and stimulate production of other hormones. T₃, triiodothyronine; T₄, thyroxine; TRH, thyrotropin-releasing hormone; TSH, thyroid-stimulating hormone.

metabolic needs. Thus, increased thyroid hormones in body fluids inhibit secretion of thyrotropin by the anterior pituitary and of thyroid-releasing hormone (TRH) by the hypothalamus.

Follicle-stimulating hormone (FSH), one of the gonadotropins, stimulates functions of sex glands. In people of both sexes, the anterior pituitary produces FSH, beginning at puberty. It acts on the ovaries in a cyclical fashion during the reproductive years, stimulating growth of ovarian follicles. These follicles then produce estrogen, which prepares the endometrium for implantation of a fertilized ovum. FSH acts on the testes to stimulate the production and growth of sperm (spermatogenesis), but it does not stimulate secretion of male sex hormones.

Luteinizing hormone (LH) (also called interstitial cell-stimulating hormone), another gonadotropin, stimulates hormone production by the gonads of both sexes. In women, LH is important in the maturation and rupture of the ovarian follicle (ovulation). After ovulation, LH acts on the cells of the collapsed follicular sac to produce the corpus luteum, which then produces progesterone during the last half of the menstrual cycle. When blood progesterone levels rise, a negative feedback effect

acts on hypothalamic and anterior pituitary secretion of gonadotropins. Decreased pituitary secretion of LH causes the corpus luteum to die and stop producing progesterone. Lack of progesterone causes slough and discharge of the endometrial lining as menstrual flow. (Of course, if the ovum has been fertilized and attached to the endometrium, menstruation does not occur.) In men, LH stimulates the Leydig cells in the spaces between the seminiferous tubules to secrete androgens, mainly testosterone.

Prolactin plays a part in milk production by nursing mothers. It is not usually secreted in nonpregnant women because of the hypothalamic hormone prolactin-inhibiting factor (PIF). During late pregnancy and lactation, various stimuli, including suckling, inhibit the production of PIF, which thus allows prolactin to best synthesized and released.

Melanocyte-stimulating hormone (MSH) plays a role in skin pigmentation, and investigators have found that it also plays important roles in feeding and energy metabolism as well as in inflammation. Recently, they have explored links between MSH, particularly gamma-MSH, and cardiovascular regulation and sodium metabolism.

Posterior Pituitary Hormones

The posterior pituitary gland stores and releases two hormones that are synthesized by nerve cells in the hypothalamus.

Antidiuretic hormone (ADH), also called vasopressin, functions to regulate water balance. ADH makes renal tubules more permeable to water. This allows water in renal tubules to be reabsorbed into the plasma and thus conserves body water. In the absence of ADH, little water is reabsorbed, and large amounts are lost in the urine.

Secretion of ADH occurs when body fluids become concentrated (high amounts of electrolytes in proportion to the amount of water) and when blood volume is low. In the first instance, ADH causes reabsorption of water, dilution of extracellular fluids, and restoration of normal osmotic pressure. In the second instance, ADH raises blood volume and arterial blood pressure toward homeostatic levels.

Oxytocin functions in childbirth and lactation. It initiates uterine contractions at the end of gestation to induce childbirth, and it causes milk to move from breast glands to nipples so the infant can obtain the milk by suckling.

Hypothalamic Hormones

The hypothalamus produces **releasing hormones** to accelerate the secretion of a given hormone or **inhibiting hormones** that decreases hormone secretion that corresponds to each of the major hormones of the anterior pituitary gland.

Corticotropin-releasing hormone or factor (CRH or CRF) causes release of corticotropin in response to stress and threatening stimuli. Secretion of CRH most often occurs during sleep; it is under the influence of several neurotransmitters. Acetylcholine and serotonin stimulate its secretion, and gamma-aminobutyric acid (GABA) and norepinephrine inhibit its secretion. ADH increases the ability of CRH to stimulate corticotropin secretion, and somatostatin and elevated levels of glucocorticoids decrease or prevent this ability. Health care providers use CRH in the diagnosis of Cushing's disease, a disorder characterized by excess cortisol.

Growth hormone–releasing hormone (GHRH) causes release of GH in response to low blood levels of GH. The neurotransmitters dopamine, norepinephrine, epinephrine, GABA, acetylcholine, and serotonin stimulate the secretion of hypothalamic GHRH. Somatostatin blocks the stimulatory effect of GHRH on secretion of GH. Uses of GHRH include testing pituitary function and stimulating growth in children with GHRH deficiency.

As previously mentioned, somatostatin (growth hormone release–inhibiting hormone) inhibits release of GH and is distributed throughout the brain and spinal cord, where it functions as a neurotransmitter. It is also found in the intestines and the pancreas, where it regulates secretion of insulin and glucagon. Several neurotransmitters, including acetylcholine, dopamine, epinephrine, GABA, and norepinephrine, increase somatostatin secretion.

Somatostatin also inhibits other functions, including secretion of corticotropin, **thyroid-stimulating hormone (TSH or thyrotropin)**, prolactin, pancreatic secretions (e.g., insulin, glucagon), and gastrointestinal (GI) secretions (gastrin, cholecystokinin, secretin, vasoactive intestinal peptide) as well as GI motility, bile flow, and mesenteric blood flow. Hypothalamic somatostatin blocks the action of GHRH and decreases thyrotropin-releasing hormone (TRH)–induced release of TSH. GH stimulates secretion of somatostatin, and the effects of somatostatin on TSH may contribute to TSH deficiency in children being treated with GH.

TRH causes release of TSH in response to stress, such as exposure to cold. TRH is useful in diagnostic tests of pituitary function and hyperthyroidism (see Chap. 40).

Gonadotropin-releasing hormone (GnRH) causes release of FSH and LH. Several synthetic equivalents of GnRH are clinically useful.

Prolactin-releasing factor is active during lactation after childbirth. PIF is active at times other than during lactation.

NCLEX Success

1. **A young woman, a graduate nurse, is scheduled to take the NCLEX examination in the morning. Which of the following hormones is released while she is asleep?**
   A. glucagon
   B. insulin
   C. corticotropin
   D. antidiuretic hormone

2. **A man has sustained burns over 80% of his body in a boating accident. Which of the following hormones is released to raise the arterial blood pressure?**
   A. antidiuretic hormone
   B. oxytocin
   C. melanocyte-stimulating hormone
   D. luteinizing hormone

3. **An adult has decreased growth hormone. Which of the following signs or symptoms is the patient likely to develop?**
   A. increased cholesterol
   B. increased muscle strength
   C. increased mental alertness
   D. increased blood glucose

Pathophysiology and Clinical Manifestations

Precocious Puberty

Children diagnosed with precocious puberty develop secondary sexual characteristics prior to the age of 9 (boys) and 8 (girls). The Lawson Wilkins Pediatric Endocrine Society recommends that African American girls who develop breast and/or pubic hair prior to age 6 and Caucasian girls who develop these characteristics prior to the age of 7 be evaluated for precocious puberty. The three types of precocious puberty involve different pathological processes.

The first type, gonadotropin-dependent precocious puberty, is also known as central precocious puberty. The cause of this disorder is early maturation of the hypothalamic–pituitary–gonadal axis. Breast enlargement and pubic hair development occur in girls, and testicular enlargement and pubic hair development occur in boys. Other signs of this disorder include accelerated linear bone growth, increased bone age, and pubertal levels of some gonadal hormones (FSH and LH in girls; testosterone in boys).

The second type, gonadotropin-independent precocious puberty, is a result of excess secretion of the estrogen and androgen sex hormones from the gonads or adrenal glands. In girls, pituitary tumors are rare but do cause this type of precocious puberty. Exposure to estrogen creams used by menopausal care providers of girls may also lead to precocious puberty. In boys, Leydig cell tumors may be the cause. These tumors, which result in an asymmetric enlargement of the testes, are benign; surgical removal is appropriate.

The third type, incomplete precocious puberty, is isolated breast development in girls or hormone-mediated characteristics (e.g., acne or axillary or pubic hair) in boys. It is necessary to confirm the diagnosis using radiographic examination of the bone age—determining when the epiphyseal maturation is marginally advanced.

Acromegaly

Acromegaly results from persistent hypersecretion of GH due to the presence of a somatotroph adenoma of the anterior pituitary or a hypothalamic tumor that releases GHRH. The hypersecretion of growth hormone then results in the liver secretion of insulin-like growth factor-1 (IGF-1). This activity produces the clinical manifestations of acromegaly. The onset of these clinical manifestations is slow, as is its progression. Patients may complain of headaches with visual changes. Women have menstrual abnormalities, hot flashes, and vaginal atrophy from decreased estrogen levels. Men have erectile dysfunction, diminished libido, and decreased testicular size. Other signs and symptoms are thickening of the skin, linear bone growth, and enlargement of the liver, lungs, kidney, thyroid, and heart. High serum levels of GH and IGF-1 result in impaired glucose tolerance, hyperinsulinism, and insulin resistance.

Growth Hormone Deficiency in Children

The definition of growth deficiency in children is growth below the third percentile of the established normal values. There are several causes of GH deficiency. Mutation of a transcription factor (POUF1; also known as PIT-1) leads to variable recessive peptide hormone deficiencies that may be associated with anterior pituitary hypoplasia. Also, mutation of a transcription factor (PROP1), which causes a failure to activate POUF1/PIT-1 gene expression, results in pituitary hypoplasia and/or familial multiple pituitary hormone deficiency. In addition, mutations in the anterior pituitary cells are sources of GH deficiency.

Idiopathic short stature is present when a child's stature falls below 2 standard deviations of the mean for age. The child has no endocrine, metabolic, or condition to account for the GH deficiency.

Diabetes Insipidus

Diabetes insipidus is a condition that results from a dysfunction in the posterior pituitary lobe. Excretion of large quantities of dilute urine results due to a deficiency in the production of ADH. With the absence of ADH, the kidneys filter the water but do not reabsorb it. When this occurs, the circulating fluid volume decreases, producing increased thirst and large amounts of urine production.

Diabetes insipidus may be idiopathic, hereditary, or acquired. Causes include lesions in the posterior pituitary, hypothalamus, or infundibular stem that interfere with ADH synthesis, transport, and release. These lesions in the central nervous system (CNS) can be the result of a tumor, aneurysm, or thrombus. Other causes are the removal of the pituitary gland, immunological disorders, or infections.

Characteristic features include polyuria, with excretion of dilute urine ranging from 4 to as much as 30 L; extreme polydipsia, with the consumption of copious amounts of water or other fluids; and hypernatremia, with increased serum osmolality. The dehydration produces dizziness, weakness, and weight loss. Children present with enuresis, irritability, diminished sleep, and decreased weight gain along with diminished linear growth. If diabetes insipidus goes untreated, it may produce circulatory collapse and CNS depression or damage in both adults and children.

Clinical Application 41-1

- How has Mr. Rojas' head injury contributed to the development of diabetes insipidus?
- Why is he producing large amounts of dilute urine?

NCLEX Success

4. A nurse is educating grandparents about child safety. Which of the following prevents precocious puberty?

   A. keeping Tylenol out of a child's reach
   B. keeping estrogen cream out of a child's reach
   C. keeping Nitro-Bid paste out of a child's reach
   D. keeping hydrocortisone out of a child's reach

5. Two weeks ago, a 4-year-old girl fell from a backyard swing and hit her head. Her mother states her potty-trained daughter has been wetting the bed for the past 3 nights. What do you suspect the bedwetting is related to?

   A. regression in development due to changes in the home
   B. drinking juices prior to bedtime
   C. a urinary tract infection
   D. possible diabetes insipidus

6. A man has received a diagnosis of acromegaly. Which of the following symptoms can cause alterations in the man's psychosocial integrity?

   A. increased libido
   B. tachycardia
   C. increased linear growth
   D. erectile dysfunction

Drug Therapy

Although pituitary and hypothalamic hormones has few therapeutic uses, they have important functions when used in certain circumstances. Hypothalamic hormones are synthesized into drug formulations that are administered to treat endometriosis, metastatic breast cancer, advanced prostate cancer, uterine fibroid tumors, vasoactive intestinal tumors, and diarrhea, as well as central precocious puberty. Manufacturers have synthesized more drug formulations. Tables 41.1 and 41.2 list the exogenous hormones used in the treatment of hormonal dysfunction.

Anterior Pituitary Hormone Drugs for Growth Deficiency in Children

The prototype anterior pituitary hormone is GH. Administered therapeutically, GH is not natural but rather synthesized from bacteria using recombinant DNA technology. Ⓟ **Somatropin**

TABLE 41.1

Drugs Administered for the Treatment of Hypothalamic Hormonal Changes

Drug Class	Prototypes	Other Drugs in the Class

Hypothalamic hormones	Leuprolide acetate (Lupron)
	Octreotide acetate
	  (Sandostatin, LAR
	  Depot)
		Goserelin (Zoladex)
		Histrelin (Vantas, Supprelin LA)
		Nafarelin (Synarel)
		Triptorelin (Trelstar)

(Humatrope, others) is therapeutically equivalent to endogenous GH produced by the anterior pituitary gland.

Pharmacokinetics

Somatropin is well absorbed. Most of the drug is metabolized in the liver and kidneys. A small amount is excreted unchanged by the kidneys.

Action

Somatropin has the same sequence of amino acids as endogenous GH; it stimulates skeletal, linear, muscle, and organ growth. Stimulation of cartilage growth at the epiphyseal plate promotes linear growth. Lean body mass and bone mass increase, and fat mass decreases. Stimulation of erythropoietin results in an increase of red blood cells. The drug increases protein synthesis and hepatic glucose output. Absorption of nutrients from the GI tract improves.

Use

The main clinical use of somatropin is for children whose growth is impaired by a deficiency of endogenous GH. The drug is ineffective when impaired growth results from other causes or after puberty, when epiphyses of the long bones have closed. Also, it is useful in the treatment of growth failure associated with chronic kidney disease as well as short stature associated with Turner syndrome, being born small for gestational age, Prader-Willi syndrome, idiopathic short stature, certain genetic mutations, and Noonan syndrome. In addition, somatropin is useful in adults with GH deficiency. Table 41.3 gives route and dosage information for somatropin and other anterior pituitary hormone drugs.

Use in Older Adults

Reduced dosages may be necessary to minimize adverse effects. Patients who are 65 years of age or older may be more sensitive to the action of GH. Clinicians should avoid using GH in the

TABLE 41.2

Drugs Administered for the Treatment of Pituitary Hormonal Changes

Hormone	Hormonal Action
Anterior Pituitary Hormones	
Corticotropin (Acthrel; HP Acthar Gel)	Stimulates the synthesis of hormones by the adrenal cortex
Cosyntropin (Cortrosyn)	Stimulates the adrenal cortex to synthesize and secrete adrenocortical hormones
Human chorionic gonadotropin (Chorex, Choron, Pregnyl); recombinant chorionic gonadotropin alpha (Ovidrel)	Induces ovulation
Follitropin alfa (Gonal-F, Gonal-F RFF pen)	Stimulates ovulation
Follitropin beta (Follistim)	Stimulates ovulation
Menotropins (Pergonal)	Induces ovulation
Pegvisomant (Somavert)	Growth hormone receptor antagonist
Somatropin (Genotropin, Humatrope, Norditropin, Nutropin, Serostim); somatrem (Protropin)	Promotion of growth in children
Thyrotropin alfa (Thyrogen)	Stimulates the secretion of thyroglobulin
Urofollitropin (Bravelle)	Stimulates ovulation
Posterior Pituitary Hormones	
Desmopressin (DDAVP, Stimate)	Increases cyclic adenosine monophosphate (cAMP)
Vasopressin (Pitressin)	Increases cAMP
Oxytocin (Pitocin)	Increases uterine contractility

TABLE 41.3

DRUGS AT A GLANCE: Anterior Pituitary Hormone Drugs

Drug	Pregnancy Category	Routes and Dosage Ranges	
		Adults	*Children*
ⓟ **Somatropin** (Genotropin, Humatrope, Norditropin, Nutropin, Serostim) Somatrem (Protropin)	C		Somatropin, up to 0.06 mg/kg IM 3 times per week Somatrem, up to 0.1 mg/kg IM 3 times per week
Corticotropin (Acthrel; HP Acthar Gel)	C	Diagnostic use, up to 80 units IM, subcutaneous as a single injection HP Acthar Gel, 40–80 units IM, subcutaneous every 24–72 h 80–120 units IM daily for 2–3 wk	
Cosyntropin (Cortrosyn)	C	0.25 mg IM, IV (equivalent to 25 units adrenocorticotropic hormone)	Older than 2 y, same as adult dose Younger than 2 y, 0.125 mg IM, IV
Human chorionic gonadotropin (hCG) (Chorex, Choron, Pregnyl)	X	Cryptorchidism and male hypogonadism: 500–4000 units IM 2–3 times per week for several weeks	Preadolescent boys, cryptorchidism and hypogonadism: see adult dose
Recombinant chorionic gonadotropin alpha (Ovidrel)	X	250 mcg subcutaneous in 1 dose, 1 d after treatment with menotropins	
Follitropin alfa (Gonal-F, Gonal-F RFF pen)	X	75 international units subcutaneous of follicle-stimulating hormone (FSH) to maximum daily dose of 300 units Prefilled pen, 300–900 international units IV of FSH as individualized dosage	
Follitropin beta (Follistim)	X	75 international units subcutaneous of FSH to maximum daily dose of 300 international units	
Menotropins (Pergonal)	X	1 ampule (75 units FSH and 75 units luteinizing hormone) IM daily for 9–12 d, followed by hCG to induce ovulation	
Pegvisomant (Somavert)	B	Load, 40 mg subcutaneous Maintenance, 10 mg subcutaneous, titrate by 5-mg increments every 4–6 wk according to insulin-like growth factor-1 levels to maximum of 30 mg/d	
Thyrotropin alfa (Thyrogen)	C	0.9 mg IM every 24 h for 2 doses or every 72 h for 3 doses	Younger than 16 y, dosage not established
Urofollitropin (Bravelle)	X	150 international units subcutaneous of FSH daily for the first 5 d to maximum daily dose of 450 units	

elderly except as hormone replacement following pituitary gland removal. Treatment should begin at the low end of the dosage range.

Use in Patients With Renal or Hepatic Impairment

Although chronic renal impairment or severe hepatic disease decreases renal or hepatic metabolism, respectively, there are no recommended dosing changes in patients with renal or hepatic dysfunction. Children treated with somatropin for chronic renal insufficiency receive the drug until renal transplantation.

Use in Patients With Critical Illness

It is important not to initiate somatropin in patients with acute critical illness due to complications following open heart or abdominal surgery, trauma, or acute respiratory failure. Increased mortality may occur.

Adverse Effects

Adverse effects are not common and are fewer in children than in adults. Mild edema, headache, localized muscle pain, weakness, and hyperglycemia may occur. Patients with diabetes are more likely to develop hyperglycemia; they require close monitoring, and diabetic medications may require adjustment. Antibodies to the drug may develop, but this does not interfere with its growth-stimulating effects. Otitis media may occur in children. Hypersensitivity reactions are possible.

Patients with chronic renal failure, Turner syndrome, and Prader-Willi syndrome are at increased risk for intracranial hypertension; symptoms include headache, papilledema, visual changes, nausea, and vomiting. When intracranial hypertension occurs, it is important to stop treatment, but it is appropriate to start the drugs again after symptoms resolve.

A special set of warnings accompanies the use of somatropin in treating short stature in patients with Prader-Willi syndrome. Fatalities have been reported following the use of somatropin in these patients. Risk factors associated with these fatalities are severe obesity, sleep apnea, respiratory impairment, respiratory infection, and male sex. It is essential to discontinue use of somatropin if any signs of upper airway obstruction occur or if snoring develops or increases.

Contraindications

Contraindications to somatropin include closed epiphyses, preproliferative or severe nonproliferative diabetic retinopathy, active malignancy, or active underlying intracranial lesions. Patients with Prader-Willi syndrome who have severe obesity or severe respiratory impairment should not take the drug.

Caution is necessary in hypothyroidism, GH deficiency caused by intracranial lesions, and diabetes.

Nursing Implications

Preventing Interactions

Long-term use of corticotropin or corticosteroids inhibits the growth response to somatropin. Patients require monitoring to determine this lack of effect. Somatropin decreases insulin sensitivity, resulting in hyperglycemia. Patients most at risk for increased insulin sensitivity are those with obesity, Turner syndrome, or a family history of diabetes mellitus. Antihyperglycemic drugs may require dosage adjustments.

Administering the Medication

Administration may be subcutaneous or intramuscular (IM). The subcutaneous route is preferred; here are guidelines for its use:

- To prepare the solution, inject the supplied diluent into the vial containing the drug by aiming the stream of liquid against the glass wall of the vial.
- Rotate injection sites.
- Then swirl the vial gently. Do not shake it.
- After reconstitution, make sure the solution is clear. Do not inject a cloudy solution.
- Store the reconstituted drug in the refrigerator; use within 14 days.
- If the patient develops sensitivity to the diluent, reconstitute the drug with sterile water for injection. When

administering the drug to infants, use only sterile water as the diluent. With sterile water, administer only one dose per vial and use the reconstituted drug within 24 hours; discard any unused portion.
- There is a preservative-free form of somatropin. Not all forms are approved for IM injection.
- Administer the correct dosage daily.

QSEN Safety Alert ❗

When administering somatropin, it is essential that after one nurse calculates the dosage, another nurse rechecks the calculation.

Assessing for Therapeutic Effects

The nurse observes for increased skeletal growth and development. Appropriate increases in height and weight should occur. It is necessary to measure the child's height frequently. The child should take somatropin until a satisfactory height has been achieved, epiphyseal closure occurs, or until no further stimulation of growth occurs. Periodic tests of growth curve and bone age are also important.

Assessing for Adverse Effects

It is important to have periodic tests of serum glucose levels and thyroid function as well as frequent eye examinations. Monitoring of serum and urine calcium should occur. Patients who fail to respond to somatropin should receive testing for GH antibodies. Children who have GH deficiency may develop slipped capital femoral epiphyses more frequently, and those with scoliosis may see a progression of the condition. The nurse assesses the patient for severe hip or knee pain or the development of a limp.

The nurse carefully assesses patients with malignancies or GH deficiency secondary to an intracranial lesion to ensure that enlargement or recurrence of the lesion is not occurring. Reportedly, there is an increased risk of a second neoplasm in adults who had cancer as children and who have been treated with somatropin. It is necessary to monitor patients with Prader-Willi syndrome carefully for signs of respiratory infection.

Patient Teaching

Box 41.1 presents patient teaching information for somatropin.

BOX 41.1   Patient Teaching Guidelines for Somatropin

Parent or Caregiver Information

- Keep appointments for all follow-up visits and diagnostic tests.
- Report any lack of growth to the health care practitioner.
- Report any new-onset limping or hip or knee pain.
- Monitor the glucose level as ordered by the health care practitioner.
- Administer the medication subcutaneously or intramuscularly and rotate sites to prevent tissue damage.

Other Anterior Pituitary Hormone Drugs

Corticotropin (ACTH, Acthar Gel), which is obtained from animal pituitary glands, is mainly of historical interest. For therapeutic purposes, adrenal corticosteroids have replaced it. It may be used occasionally as a diagnostic test to differentiate primary adrenal insufficiency (Addison's disease, which is associated with atrophy of the adrenal gland) from secondary adrenal insufficiency caused by inadequate pituitary secretion of corticotropin. However, cosyntropin (Cortrosyn), a synthetic formulation, is more commonly used to test for suspected adrenal insufficiency (see Chap. 43).

Human chorionic gonadotropin (hCG; Chorex) produces physiologic effects similar to those of naturally occurring LH. In males, it is used to evaluate the ability of Leydig cells to produce testosterone, to treat hypogonadism due to pituitary deficiency, and to treat cryptorchidism (undescended testicle) in preadolescent boys. In females, recombinant hCG choriogonadotropin alpha (Ovidrel) is used in combination with menotropins to induce ovulation in the treatment of infertility. Excessive doses or prolonged administration can lead to sexual precocity, edema, and breast enlargement caused by oversecretion of testosterone and estrogen (see Chap. 6).

Menotropins (Pergonal), a gonadotropin preparation obtained from the urine of postmenopausal women, contains both FSH and LH. It is usually combined with hCG to induce ovulation in the treatment of infertility caused by lack of pituitary gonadotropins (see Chap. 6).

Pegvisomant (Somavert) is a GH receptor antagonist used in the treatment of acromegaly in adults who are unable to tolerate or are resistant to other management strategies. The drug selectively binds to GH receptors, blocking the binding of endogenous GH. In general, it is necessary to individualize the dosage according to response. Dosage reduction of hypoglycemic agents may be required because the drug may increase glucose tolerance. Increased dosages of pegvisomant may be necessary when administered with narcotics. Caution is warranted in the elderly and in renal or hepatic disease.

Thyrotropin alfa (Thyrogen) is a synthetic formulation of TSH used as a diagnostic adjunct for serum thyroglobulin testing in people with well-differentiated thyroid cancer. The test may or may not involve radioiodine imaging. Because there is a risk of missing the diagnosis of thyroid cancer. Thyroid hormone withdrawal Tg testing radioactive imaging is the standard test for evaluating the presence, extent, and location of thyroid cancer. Thyrotropin alfa requires caution in patients with coronary artery disease and with a large amount of residual thyroid tissue; the drug produces a temporary rise of thyroid hormone concentration in the blood.

Urofollitropin (Bravelle), follitropin alfa (Gonal-F), and follitropin beta (Follistim) are drug preparations of FSH. The purpose of these drugs is to stimulate ovarian function in the treatment of infertility, and women may take sequentially with hCG. Urofollitropin, which is extracted from the urine of postmenopausal women, acts directly on the ovaries to stimulate follicular ovulation. Follitropin alfa and follitropin beta are recombinant products that appear to be well tolerated and have similar efficacy. A new liquid formulation of follitropin alfa (Gonal-F RFF Pen) is available in a prefilled and ready-to-use multidose FSH injection (see Chap. 6).

Posterior Pituitary Hormone Drugs for Diabetes Insipidus

ⓟ Desmopressin acetate (DDAVP, Stimate) is the prototype posterior pituitary hormone medication. It is a synthetic analog of ADH.

Pharmacokinetics

For the intranasal form, the onset of action is 15 to 30 minutes and the peak of action of 30 minutes. For the intravenous (IV) and subcutaneous forms, the onset of action is 1 hour and peak of action is 1.5 to 2 hours. For the oral form, the onset of action is 60 minutes and the peak of action is 60 to 90 minutes. For all forms, the duration of action is approximately 6 to 14 hours. The half-life of the intranasal, IV and subcutaneous, and oral preparations is approximately 3.5 hours, 3 hours, and 2 to 3 hours, respectively. Elimination of all forms of the medication takes place in the urine.

Action

Desmopressin increases cyclic adenosine monophosphate in the cells of the renal tubule to increase the water permeability, decreasing urine volume and increasing its osmolality. The drug increases the plasma level of von Willebrand factor, clotting factor VIII, and tissue plasminogen activator (a protein involved in the breakdown of blood clots) to shorten the activated partial thromboplastin and bleeding times.

Use

The main clinical use for desmopressin is for the treatment of neurogenic diabetes insipidus. However, synthetic hormones are useful for other purposes. Table 41.4 contains route and dosage information for desmopressin and other posterior pituitary hormones.

TABLE 41.4

DRUGS AT A GLANCE: Posterior Pituitary Hormone Drugs

Drug	Pregnancy Category	Routes and Dosage Ranges	
		Adults	*Children*
Ⓟ **Desmopressin** (DDAVP, Stimate)	C	Diabetes insipidus: intranasally 0.1–0.4 mL/d, usually in 2 divided doses Hemophilia A, von Willebrand's disease: IV 0.3 mcg/kg in 50 mL sterile saline, infused over 15–30 min	Diabetes insipidus: 3 mo–2 y: 0.05–0.3 mL/d in 1–2 doses intranasally Hemophilia A, von Willebrand's disease: weight more than 10 kg, same as adult dosage Weight 10 kg or less, 0.3 mcg/kg IV in 10 mL of sterile saline
Vasopressin (Pitressin)	C	0.25–0.5 mL (5–10 units) IM, Sub-Q, intranasally on cotton pledgets 2–3 times daily	0.125–0.5 mL (2.5–10 units) IM, Sub-Q, intranasally on cotton pledgets 3–4 times daily
Oxytocin (Pitocin)	C	See Chapter 6	

Use in Patients With Renal Impairment

A creatinine clearance less than 50 mL/min contraindicates the use of desmopressin.

Adverse Effects and Contraindications

Adverse effects of desmopressin reportedly occur in less than 5% of cases. The most common effects are erythema, swelling, and burning of the parenteral injection site. The U.S.

Food and Drug Administration (FDA) has issued a **BLACK BOX WARNING** ◆ stating that hyponatremia may develop as a result of the medication, leading to seizures. Another **BLACK BOX WARNING** ◆ stipulates that changes in fluid volume status may result in cardiac arrest in patients with known cardiovascular disease.

Contraindications include hypersensitivity to the drug or any component of its formulation.

Nursing Implications

Preventing Interactions

Several medications interact with desmopressin, increasing or decreasing its effects (Box 41.2).

Administering the Medication

Guidelines for administration are as follows:

- Use the IM, IV, and subcutaneous preparations for central diabetes insipidus. Withdraw the dosage from the ampule and administer it using a small-gauge needle and syringe (e.g., an insulin syringe).
- For hemophilia A, von Willebrand disease (type 1), and prevention of surgical bleeding in patients with uremia, infuse the IV preparation over 10 minutes.

EVIDENCE-BASED PRACTICE

Desmopressin Versus Behavioral Modifications as Initial Treatment of Primary Nocturnal Enuresis

by PATRICIA, FERA, MARIE ALICE DOS SANTOS LELIS, REGIANE DE QUADROS GLASHAN, SHEILA GONZALES PEREIRA, AND HOMERO BRUSCHINI

The purpose of this study was to investigate the effectiveness of desmopressin as compared with behavioral modifications as the initial treatment for primary monosymptomatic nocturnal enuresis. The most common type of pediatric urinary incontinence is nocturnal enuresis. This study involved 30 children age 7 to 12 years. Of these, 15 received desmopressin and 15 received treatment with behavioral modifications. The researchers determined that either intervention was effective.

IMPLICATIONS FOR NURSING PRACTICE: The authors of this article acknowledge the administration of desmopressin provides adequate results in the treatment of nocturnal enuresis. However, they state that when the desmopressin therapy stopped, some children experienced enuresis. Thus, it is important to use behavior modification in addition to desmopressin therapy.

BOX 41.2 | Drug Interactions: Desmopressin

Drugs That Increase the Effects of Desmopressin
- Carbamazepine, chlorpropamide
  Increase the risk of antidiuretic effects
- Selective serotonin reuptake inhibitors, tricyclic antidepressants
  Increase the risk of hyponatremia

Drugs That Decrease the Effects of Desmopressin
- Alcohol
  Decreases the diuretic effect

- For intranasal administration, use a rhinal tube. (The DDAVP nasal spray pump delivers 0.1 mL [10 mcg]; administer 10 mcg per nostril. Discard any solution that remains after 50 doses.)
  - Insert the top of the dropper into the tube in a downward position. Then squeeze the dropper until the solution reaches the desired calibrated dose and disconnect the dropper.
  - Hold the tube 3/4 inches from the end and insert one end into the nostril until the fingertips reach the nostril. Place the opposite end into the patient's mouth while the patient holds his or her breath.
  - Have the patient tilt the head back and blow into the tube, and into the nostril, with a strong, short puff. (In children, the nurse or an adult needs to blow into the tube.)

Assessing for Therapeutic Effects

The desired therapeutic effects are decreased urine output, increased urine specific gravity, decreased signs of dehydration, and decreased thirst. It is important to assess the serum electrolytes, particularly the sodium and potassium levels. The sodium level should be 135 to 145 mEq/L. The nurse assesses serum osmolality; it should be in the normal range of 285 to 295 mOsm/kg H_2O. It is necessary to interview the patient to determine if he or she is thirsty. The nurse assesses skin turgor, mucous membranes, and production of tears for signs of rehydration. In patients with von Willebrand disease, it is important to determine the factor VIII coagulant effect; the normal factor VIII is 55% to 145%.

Assessing for Adverse Effects

The nurse assesses for hyponatremia, which can lead to diminished mental status and seizures. Serum osmolality may be less than 285 mOsm/kg H_2O. It is also necessary to assess fluid volume status for signs of dehydration, as well as urine output and urine specific gravity. Also, the nurse assesses the parenteral injection site for rash or erythema.

Patient Teaching

Box 41.3 presents patient teaching information for desmopressin.

Other Posterior Pituitary Hormone Drugs

Vasopressin (Pitressin) is used for the treatment of central diabetes insipidus and the differential diagnosis of diabetes

---

BOX 41.3 **Patient Teaching Guidelines for Desmopressin**

- Report drowsiness, headache, dizziness, lethargy, shortness of breath, gastric irritation with heartburn, abdominal cramping, vulval pain, nasal congestion, and nasal irritation to the health care provider.
- When using the DDAVP nasal spray pump, insert the top of the dropper into the tube in a downward position. Squeeze the dropper until the solution reaches the desired calibrated dose and disconnect the dropper. Then hold the tube 3/4 inches from the end and insert it into the nostril until the fingertips reach the nostril. Place the opposite end of the tube in the mouth while holding your breath. Tilt the head back and blow into the tube with a strong, short puff into the nostril.

---

insipidus. The drug is administered intravenously, intranasally, or by endotracheal tube.

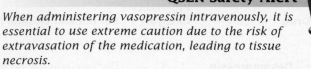

QSEN Safety Alert

When administering vasopressin intravenously, it is essential to use extreme caution due to the risk of extravasation of the medication, leading to tissue necrosis.

The drug is stable in 5% dextrose in water (D_5W).

Oxytocin (Pitocin) is a synthetic drug that exerts the same physiologic effects as the posterior pituitary hormone. Thus, it promotes uterine contractility and is used clinically to induce labor and in the postpartum period to control bleeding. It is essential that oxytocin be used only when clearly indicated and when the patient can be supervised by well-trained personnel, as in a hospital (see Chap. 6).

Clinical Application 41-2

- What are the signs and symptoms of diabetes insipidus?
- What is the action of desmopressin?
- What is the therapeutic effect of desmopressin?
- How does the nurse administer desmopressin intranasally using a rhinal tube?

NCLEX Success

9. The nurse is administering intranasal desmopressin to a child. What does he or she need to do differently from administering this drug to an adult?

   A. The nurse should question the order, because intranasal desmopressin is contraindicated in children.
   B. The nurse should encourage the mother to administer the medication in the hospital.
   C. The nurse needs to blow in the tube to administer the medication.
   D. The nurse should use parenteral administration in the child.

10. A patient has just received desmopressin. Which electrolyte is most important to assess?

   A. sodium
   B. chloride
   C. potassium
   D. calcium

Hypothalamic Hormone Drugs

DRUGS FOR CENTRAL PRECOCIOUS PUBERTY

Ⓟ **Leuprolide acetate** (Lupron) is equivalent to GnRH. The drug is more potent than the natural hormone.

Pharmacokinetics

Leuprolide has a transient onset of action. The drug is 43% to 49% protein bound. It is metabolized to pentapeptide in the hypothalamus and anterior pituitary and is excreted in the urine.

Action

An LH-releasing hormone agonist, leuprolide acts as a potent inhibitor of gonadotropin secretion, thus suppressing production of ovarian and testicular steroids. This action decreases LH and FSH to decrease testosterone in males and estrogen in females. (Testosterone levels are below levels required for reproduction.)

Use

Leuprolide is useful for the treatment of central precocious puberty in children. Experts recommended that the drug be administered to girls until age 11 and boys to age 12. Other uses include treatment of advanced prostate cancer, infertility, and endometriosis and uterine fibroids. Table 41.5 gives route and dosage information for the hypothalamic hormones.

Adverse Effects and Contraindications

The most common adverse effect of leuprolide is pain at the injection site. Less than 2% of the people who receive the drug have reported vasodilation, labile emotions, rash, acne, and allergic reaction.

Contraindications include known hypersensitivity to the medication's formulation, GnRH, or GnRH antagonists.

Nursing Implications

Preventing Interactions

Leuprolide may decrease the therapeutic effect of antidiabetic drugs, resulting in hyperglycemia.

Administering the Medication

Administration of Lupron Depot should occur as a single injection. The depot suspension is stable for 24 hours after reconstitution. It is important to rotate the injection sites and not to use areas of the body that are compressed or rubbed.

Assessing for Therapeutic Effects

The nurse assesses for a decrease in mature sexual characteristics. Gonadotropins (testosterone in males; estrogen in females) should decrease to prepubertal levels. These effects occur within 2 to 4 weeks after therapy has begun.

TABLE 41.5

DRUGS AT A GLANCE: Hypothalamic Hormones

Drug	Pregnancy Category	Routes and Dosage Ranges	
		Adults	Children
Ⓟ **Leuprolide acetate** (Lupron)	X		Central precocious puberty: 50 mcg/kg/d Sub-Q (may be titrated up to 10 mcg/kg/d) Depot-Ped, IM 5 kg or less, 7.5 mg 25–37.5 kg, 11.25 mg More than 37.5 kg, 15 mg every month
Ⓟ **Octreotide acetate** (Sandostatin; LAR Depot [long-acting])	B	Acromegaly: 50–100 mcg Sub-Q 3 times daily; long-acting: 100–200 mcg 3 times daily, may be adjusted up to 500 mcg 3 times daily	Dosage not established but 1–10 mcg/kg reportedly well tolerated in young patients
Goserelin (Zoladex)	X Pregnancy category D: with the treatment of breast cancer	Implant into upper abdominal wall, 3.6 mg Sub-Q every 28 d or 10.8 mg Sub-Q every 3 mo	
Histrelin (Vantas; Supprelin LA)	X	Implant, 1 Sub-Q every 12 mo	Central precocious puberty: Supprelin LA, Implant Sub-Q every 12 mo
Nafarelin (Synarel)	X	1 spray (200 mcg) in one nostril in the morning and 1 spray in the other nostril in the evening (400 mcg/d), starting between the 2nd and 4th days of the menstrual cycle	Central precocious puberty: 2 sprays (400 mcg) in each nostril morning and evening (1600 mcg/d), until resumption of puberty is desired
Triptorelin (Trelstar)	X	3.75 mg IM depot injection	

BOX 41.4

BOX 41.4 | **Patient Teaching Guidelines for Leuprolide**

■ Administer the medication subcutaneously or intramuscularly.

■ Use a calendar to mark the dates of future injections.

■ Report any pain, burning, itching, or tingling of the injection site to the health care provider.

■ Be aware, if you are a parent, that a female is fertile and if she is sexually active she should receive a prescription for a form of birth control.

Assessing for Adverse Effects

The nurse assesses for pain at the injection sites. It is also necessary to assess for signs of a hypersensitivity reaction to the medication such as a rash or erythema.

Patient Teaching

Box 41.4 presents patient teaching information for leuprolide.

Other Hypothalamic Hormone Drugs

Goserelin (Zoladex), histrelin (Vantas), nafarelin (Synarel), and triptorelin (Trelstar) are equivalent to GnRH. After initial stimulation of LH and FSH secretion, chronic administration of therapeutic doses inhibits gonadotropin secretion. This action results in decreased production of testosterone and estrogen, which is reversible when administration is stopped. In children with central precocious puberty, gonadotropins decline to prepubertal levels. As with leuprolide, these effects occur within 2 to 4 weeks of beginning drug treatment.

Oral administration of these GnRH equivalents is ineffective, because enzymes in the GI tract destroy the medication. Administration of most of these drugs is by injection; they are available in depot preparations that nurses can give once a month (or less often). Adverse effects are basically those of testosterone or estrogen deficiency. The drugs may also cause or aggravate depression.

DRUGS FOR ACROMEGALY

ⓟ **Octreotide acetate** (Sandostatin; Sandostatin LAR Depot) has pharmacological actions similar to the anterior pituitary hormone somatostatin. Scientists first synthesized this hormone-like drug in 1979.

Pharmacokinetics

Octreotide is rapidly and completely absorbed. It is released slowly in the microsphere of the muscle. The drug reaches a peak of action in 1 hour, with a duration of action of 6 to 12 hours. Its half-life is 1.5 hours. Octreotide is metabolized in the liver and excreted by the kidneys.

Action

Octreotide mimics the natural hormone somatostatin by inhibiting serotonin release. The drug also inhibits gastrin, vasoactive intestinal peptide, insulin, glucagon, secretin, motilin, and pancreatic polypeptide. In acromegaly, it suppresses GH and IGF-1. In fact, octreotide inhibits GH, glucagon, and insulin more than endogenous somatostatin. The drug also suppresses LH response to GnRH and the secretion of TSH.

Use

Prescribers order octreotide for patients with acromegaly to reduce levels of GH. Table 41.5 presents route and dosage information for this drug.

Use in Older Adults

In older adults, the elimination half-life of octreotide is 46% greater, and the drug's clearance is decreased by 26% less. Thus, it is necessary to reduce the dosage of the medication to the lower recommended range.

Use in Patients With Renal and Hepatic Impairment

For patients on renal dialysis, it is essential to reduce the dosage of the drug by 50%. For those with cirrhosis of the liver, the initial dosage should be 10 mg intramuscularly over 4 weeks. It is necessary to titrate the dosage weekly based on the patient's response.

Adverse Effects

Octreotide may cause CNS effects such as headache, dizziness, lightheadedness, and fatigue. Cardiac effects such as bradycardia and heart failure may also occur. Other effects include hyperglycemia, pruritus, abdominal pain, loose stools, nausea, and cholelithiasis. Reportedly, approximately 20% of patients report back pain, myalgia, upper respiratory infections, and shortness of breath.

Contraindications

Contraindications to octreotide include a known hypersensitivity to the drug or any component of the formulation.

Nursing Implications

Preventing Interactions

The combination of octreotide with alfuzosin, artemether, chloroquine, ciprofloxacin, dronedarone, indacaterol, lumefantrine, pimozide, propafenone, quetiapine, quinine, tetrabenazine, thioridazine, toremifene, vandetanib, vemurafenib, and ziprasidone results in a prolonged QTc with an increased risk of ventricular dysrhythmia and cardiac arrest. The combination of octreotide and codeine increases the metabolism of codeine, and the combination of cyclosporine and octreotide decreases the serum concentration of cyclosporine. The administration of octreotide with food may alter the absorption of dietary fats. Many herbs increase the effects of octreotide (Box 41.5).

Administering the Medication

Administration is subcutaneous or IM. It is important to administer the medication between meals to prevent fat malabsorption. Storage of the ampules requires refrigeration.

With a depot injection, administration should occur immediately after the medication is mixed. The nurse administers the depot injections intramuscularly, deep in the intragluteal

---

BOX 41.5   Herb and Dietary Interactions: Octreotide

Herbs and Foods That Increase the Effects of Octreotide

- Alfalfa
- Aloe
- Bilberry
- Bitter melon
- Burdock
- Celery
- Damiana
- Fenugreek
- Garcinia
- Garlic
- Ginger
- Ginseng
- Gymnema
- Marshmallow
- Stinging nettle

---

site—never in the deltoid. With a subcutaneous injection, he or she rotates the sites of administration.

It is necessary to withdraw the drug for 4 weeks once per year.

Assessing for Therapeutic Effects

The nurse assesses for diminished bone growth. He or she must interview the patient to determine if headaches and visual changes have subsided. Also, it is necessary to assess women for a decrease in hot flashes and regulation of the menstrual cycle.

Assessing for Adverse Effects

The nurse assesses for alertness (e.g., is there any fatigue?). It is necessary to interview the patient and ask about headache or lightheadedness. The nurse checks the blood glucose for glucose tolerance. Approximately 2% to 27% of the patients develop hyperglycemia. Also, the nurse assesses the heart rate for bradycardia and an audible S_3, indicating the onset of heart

BOX 41.6 Patient Teaching Guidelines for Octreotide

- Administer the medication subcutaneously or intramuscularly.
- Contact the health care provider to determine the time for withdrawal of the medication. It should be withdrawn for 4 weeks one time per year.
- Have follow-up diagnostic tests and keep the schedule of those tests.
- Monitor blood glucose.
- Notify the health care provider if abdominal pain or pain between the shoulder blades develops.
- Have follow-up gallbladder ultrasounds to detect cholelithiasis.

---

failure. In addition, he or she assesses for abdominal pain, nausea, or pain between the shoulder blades, indicating the onset of cholelithiasis. Finally, it is important to check for musculoskeletal pain, fever, cough, and congestion, including the respiratory rate and effort that indicates the onset of shortness of breath.

Patient Teaching

Box 41.6 presents patient teaching information for octreotide.

NCLEX Success

11. **A 30-year-old woman is receiving treatment for acromegaly. Her physician has prescribed octreotide for subcutaneous administration three times per day. What is the most important information to teach the patient?**

    A. to rotate the sites of the injections and use the sites infrequently
    B. to administer all injections in the dorsogluteal muscle
    C. to administer the injections with food
    D. to take an antacid if you experience gastric upset

12. **A man with acromegaly is planning a mission trip to Haiti to assist with rebuilding houses damaged in a recent earthquake. He is taking chloroquine to prevent malaria and octreotide for acromegaly. What is he at risk for developing?**

    A. diarrhea
    B. ventricular dysrhythmia
    C. hepatotoxicity
    D. urinary retention

The Nursing Process

Assessment

- Assess for disorders for which hypothalamic and pituitary hormones are given.
- Assess for the following:
  - For children with impaired growth, height and weight (actual and compared with growth charts) and diagnostic radiographic reports of bone age
  - For patients with diabetes insipidus, baseline blood pressure, weight, ratio of fluid intake to urine output, urine specific gravity, and laboratory reports of serum electrolytes

Nursing Diagnoses

- Deficient knowledge: drug administration and effects
- Altered growth and development
- Anxiety related to multiple injections
- Risk for injury: adverse drug effects

Planning/Goals

The patient will

- Experience relief of symptoms without serious adverse effects
- Take or receive the drug accurately
- Adhere to procedures for monitoring and follow-up

42 Drug Therapy to Regulate Calcium and Bone Metabolism

LEARNING OBJECTIVES

After studying this chapter, you should be able to:

1 Examine the roles of parathyroid hormone, calcitonin, and vitamin D in regulating calcium metabolism.

2 Evaluate the use of calcium and vitamin D supplements, as well as calcitonin, in the treatment of osteoporosis.

3 Identify the prototype and describe the action, use, adverse effects, contraindications, and nursing implications of the bisphosphonates used in the treatment of osteoporosis.

4 Outline appropriate management strategies of hypercalcemia as a medical emergency.

5 Implement the nursing process in the care of the patient receiving drug therapy to regulate calcium and bone metabolism.

Clinical Application Case Study

Carolyn Taylor, a 68-year-old retired teacher, has chronic venous insufficiency and osteoporosis. She has suffered two fractures from falls in recent years. Mrs. Taylor has been menopausal for 16 years and has not been on estrogen replacement therapy due to her vascular disease. Her health care provider prescribes alendronate once weekly.

KEY TERMS

Bisphosphonates: class of drugs that binds to bone and inhibits calcium resorption from bone

Calcitonin: hormone from the thyroid gland whose secretion is controlled by the concentration of ionized calcium in the blood flowing through the thyroid gland; lowers serum calcium in the presence of hypercalcemia

Hypercalcemia: abnormally high blood calcium level (greater than 10.5 mg/dL)

Hypocalcemia: abnormally low blood calcium level (less than 8.5 mg/dL)

Hyperparathyroidism: excessive production of parathyroid hormone (PTH)

Hypoparathyroidism: insufficient production of PTH

Osteoporosis: decreased bone density and weak, fragile bones that often lead to fractures, pain, and disability

Paget's disease: inflammatory skeletal disease that affects older people

Parathyroid hormone (PTH): hormone secreted by the parathyroid glands; secretion is stimulated by low serum calcium levels and inhibited by normal or high levels

Tetany: neuromuscular irritability characterized by numbness and tingling of the lips, fingers, and toes; twitching of facial muscles; spasms of skeletal muscle; carpopedal spasm; laryngospasm; and convulsions

Vitamin D (calciferol): fat-soluble vitamin that includes both ergocalciferol (obtained from foods) and cholecalciferol (formed by exposure of skin to sunlight); functions as a hormone and plays an important role in calcium and bone metabolism

Introduction

Three hormones regulate calcium and bone metabolism—parathyroid hormone, calcitonin, and vitamin D—and act to maintain normal serum levels of calcium. When serum calcium levels are decreased, hormonal mechanisms raise them; when they are elevated, hormonal mechanisms lower them (Fig. 42.1). Overall, the hormones alter absorption of dietary calcium from the gastrointestinal (GI) tract, movement of calcium from bone to serum, and excretion of calcium through the kidneys.

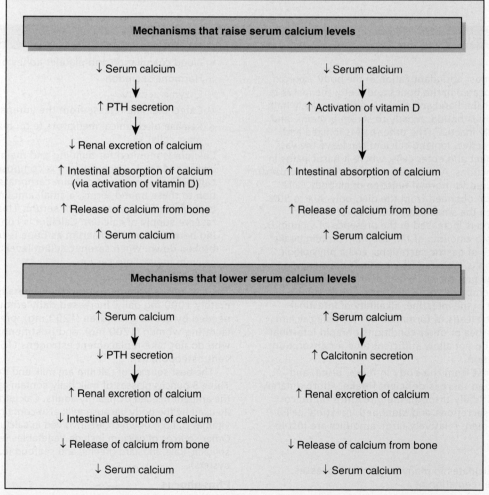

Figure 42.1 Hormonal regulation of serum calcium levels. When serum calcium levels are low (hypocalcemia), there is increased secretion of parathyroid hormone (PTH) and increased activation of vitamin D. These mechanisms lead to decreased loss of calcium in the urine, increased absorption of calcium from the intestine, and increased resorption of calcium from bone. These mechanisms work together to raise calcium levels to normal.

When serum calcium levels are high (hypercalcemia), there is decreased secretion of PTH and increased secretion of calcitonin. These mechanisms lead to increased loss of calcium from the intestine and decreased resorption of calcium from bone. These mechanisms lower serum calcium levels to normal.

Disorders of calcium and bone metabolism include hypocalcemia, hypercalcemia, osteoporosis, Paget's disease, and bone breakdown associated with breast cancer and multiple myeloma. Drugs used to treat these disorders mainly alter serum calcium levels or strengthen bone. This chapter describes the characteristics of the hormones, calcium, phosphorus, and some associated disorders.

Overview of Calcium and Bone Metabolism

Etiology and Pathophysiology

Hypocalcemia, a low serum calcium level, stimulates **parathyroid hormone (PTH)** secretion, and **hypercalcemia**, a high serum calcium level, inhibits it (a negative feedback system). Because phosphate is closely related to calcium in body functions, PTH also regulates phosphate metabolism. In general, when serum calcium levels increase, serum phosphate levels decrease, and vice versa. Thus, an inverse relationship exists between calcium and phosphate.

When the serum calcium level falls below the normal range, PTH raises the level by acting on bone, intestines, and kidneys. In bone, breakdown is increased, so that calcium moves from bone into the serum. In the intestines, there is increased absorption of calcium ingested in food (PTH activates vitamin D, which increases intestinal absorption). In the kidneys, there is increased reabsorption of calcium in the renal tubules and less urinary excretion. The opposite effects occur with phosphate (PTH decreases serum phosphate and increases urinary phosphate excretion).

Calcium and phosphorus are discussed together because they are closely related physiologically. These mineral nutrients occur in many of the same foods, from which they are absorbed together. Calcium and phosphorous both play critical roles in cellular structure and function and, as calcium phosphate, in formation and maintenance of bones and teeth. Box 42.1 summarizes their characteristics and functions.

BOX 42.1 Characteristics and Functions of Calcium and Phosphorus

Calcium

Calcium is the most abundant cation in the body. Approximately 99% is located in the bones and teeth; the rest is in the extracellular fluid and soft tissues. Approximately half of serum calcium is bound, mostly to serum proteins, and is physiologically inactive. The other half is ionized and physiologically active. Ionized calcium can leave the vascular compartment and enter cells, where it participates in intracellular functions. An adequate amount of free (ionized) calcium is required for normal function of all body cells.

Of the calcium obtained from the diet, only 30% to 50% is absorbed from the small intestine; the rest is lost in feces. Absorption is increased in the presence of vitamin D, lactose, moderate amounts of fat, and high protein intake; increased acidity of gastric secretions; and a physiologic need. Absorption is inhibited by vitamin D deficiency; a high-fat diet; the presence of oxalic acid (from beet greens, chard), which combines with calcium to form insoluble calcium oxalate in the intestine; alkalinity of intestinal secretions, which leads to formation of insoluble calcium phosphate; diarrhea or other conditions of rapid intestinal motility, which do not allow sufficient time for absorption; and immobilization.

Calcium is lost from the body in feces, urine, and sweat. Even when there is deficient intake, approximately 150 mg are lost daily through the intestines (in mucosal and biliary secretions and sloughed intestinal cells). In lactating women, relatively large amounts are lost in breast milk.

Functions

■ Calcium participates in many metabolic processes, including the regulation of
  ■ Cell membrane permeability and function
  ■ Nerve cell excitability and transmission of impulses (e.g., it is required for release of neurotransmitters at synapses)
  ■ Contraction of cardiac, skeletal, and smooth muscle
  ■ Conduction of electrical impulses in the heart

  ■ Blood coagulation and platelet adhesion processes
  ■ Hormone secretion
  ■ Enzyme activity
  ■ Catecholamine release from the adrenal medulla
  ■ Release of chemical mediators (e.g., histamine from mast cells)

■ Calcium is required for building and maintaining bones and teeth. Bone calcium is composed mainly of calcium phosphate and calcium carbonate. In addition to these bound forms, a small amount of calcium is available for exchange with serum. This acts as a reserve supply of calcium. Calcium is constantly shifting between bone and serum as bone is formed and broken down. When serum calcium levels become low, calcium moves into serum.

Requirements and Sources

The calcium requirement of normal adults is approximately 1000 mg daily. Increased daily amounts are needed by growing children (1200 mg), pregnant or lactating women (1200 mg), and postmenopausal women who do not take replacement estrogens (1500 mg to prevent osteoporosis).

The best sources of calcium are milk and milk products. Three 8-ounces glasses of milk daily contain approximately the amount needed by healthy adults. Calcium in milk is readily used by the body because milk also contains lactose and vitamin D, both of which are involved in calcium absorption. Other sources of calcium include vegetables (e.g., broccoli, spinach, kale, mustard greens) and seafood (e.g., clams, oysters).

Phosphorus

Phosphorus is one of the most important elements in normal body function. Most phosphorus is combined with calcium in bones and teeth as calcium phosphate (~ 80%). The remainder is distributed in every body cell and in extracellular fluid. It is combined with carbohydrates, lipids, proteins, and various other compounds.

Phosphorus is obtained from the diet, and approximately 70% of dietary phosphorus is absorbed from the gastrointestinal (GI) tract. The most efficient absorption occurs when calcium and phosphorus are ingested in approximately equal amounts. Because this equal ratio is present in milk, milk is probably the best source of phosphorus. In general, factors that increase or decrease calcium absorption act the same way on phosphorus absorption. Vitamin D enhances, but is not essential for, phosphorus absorption. Large amounts of calcium or aluminum in the GI tract may combine with phosphate to form insoluble compounds and thereby decrease absorption of phosphorus.

Phosphorus is lost from the body primarily in urine. In people with acute or chronic renal failure, phosphorus intake is restricted because excretion is impaired.

Functions
Phosphorus, most of which is located intracellularly as the phosphate ion, performs many metabolic functions:

- It is an essential component of deoxyribonucleic acid, ribonucleic acid, and other nucleic acids in body cells. Thus, it is required for cell reproduction and body growth.
- It combines with fatty acids to form phospholipids, which are components of all cell membranes in the body. This reaction also prevents buildup of excessive amounts of free fatty acids.

- It forms a phosphate buffer system, which helps to maintain acid–base balance. When excess hydrogen ions are present in kidney tubules, phosphate combines with them and allows their excretion in urine. At the same time, bicarbonate is retained by the kidneys and contributes to alkalinity of body fluids. Although there are other buffering systems in the body, failure of the phosphate system leads to metabolic acidosis (retained hydrogen ions or acid and lost bicarbonate ions or base).
- It is necessary for cellular use of glucose and production of energy.
- It is necessary for proper function of several B vitamins (i.e., the vitamins function as coenzymes in various chemical reactions only when combined with phosphate).

Requirements and Sources
Daily requirements for phosphorus are approximately 800 mg for normal adults and 1200 mg for growing children and pregnant or lactating women. Phosphorus is widely available in foods. Good sources are milk and other dairy products, meat, poultry, fish, eggs, and nuts. There is little risk of phosphorus deficiency with an adequate intake of calcium and protein.

Disorders of parathyroid function are related to **hypoparathyroidism** (insufficient production of PTH) or **hyperparathyroidism** (excessive production of PTH). Most often, the cause of hypoparathyroidism is removal of or damage to the parathyroid glands during neck surgery. Most often, the cause of hyperparathyroidism is a tumor or hyperplasia of a parathyroid gland. It also may result from ectopic secretion of PTH by malignant tumors (carcinomas of the lung, pancreas, kidney, ovary, prostate gland, or bladder). Clinical manifestations and treatment of hypoparathyroidism are the same as those of hypocalcemia. Clinical manifestations and treatment of hyperparathyroidism are the same as those of hypercalcemia.

Calcitonin is a hormone from the thyroid gland whose secretion is controlled by the concentration of ionized calcium in the blood flowing through the thyroid gland. When the serum level of ionized calcium increases, secretion of calcitonin increases. The function of calcitonin is to lower serum calcium in the presence of hypercalcemia, which it does by decreasing movement of calcium from bone to serum and increasing urinary excretion of calcium. The action of calcitonin is rapid but of short duration. Thus, this hormone has little effect on long-term calcium metabolism.

Vitamin D (calciferol) is a fat-soluble vitamin that includes both ergocalciferol (obtained from foods) and cholecalciferol (formed by exposure of skin to sunlight). It functions as a hormone and plays an important role in calcium and bone metabolism. The main action of vitamin D is to raise serum calcium levels by increasing intestinal absorption of calcium and mobilizing calcium from bone. It also promotes bone formation by providing adequate serum concentrations of minerals.

Vitamin D is not physiologically active in the body. It must be converted to an intermediate metabolite in the liver, then to an active metabolite (1, 25-dihydroxyvitamin D or calcitriol) in the kidneys. PTH and adequate hepatic and renal function are required to produce the active metabolite.

Deficiency of vitamin D causes inadequate absorption of calcium and phosphorus. This, in turn, leads to low levels of serum calcium and stimulation of PTH secretion. In children, this sequence of events produces inadequate mineralization of bone (rickets), a rare condition in the United States. In adults, vitamin D deficiency causes osteomalacia, a condition characterized by decreased bone density and strength.

Bone is mineralized connective tissue that functions as structural support and a reservoir for calcium, phosphorus, magnesium, sodium, and carbonate. The role of bone in maintaining serum calcium levels takes precedence over its structural function (bone may be weakened or destroyed as calcium leaves bone and enters serum). Bone tissue is constantly being formed and broken down in a process called remodeling. Bone tissue removal is referred to as resorption. During childhood, adolescence, and early adulthood, formation usually exceeds breakdown (resorption) as the person attains adult height and peak bone mass. After approximately 35 years of age, resorption is greater than formation. **Osteoporosis** occurs when bone strength (bone density and bone quality) is impaired, leading to increased porousness and vulnerability to fracture. Hormonal deficiencies, some diseases, and some medications (e.g., glucocorticoids) can also increase resorption, resulting in loss of bone mass and osteoporosis. Table 42.1 presents an overview of the prevention and treatment of osteoporosis.

TABLE 42.1

Prevention and Treatment of Osteoporosis

Prevention/Treatment	Rationale
Adequate dietary intake of calcium at all ages Calcium supplementation if needed	Promotes normal bone development and maintenance Promotes peak bone mass Allows for more bone loss before osteoporosis develops
Adequate dietary intake of vitamin D Vitamin D supplementation if at risk (older adults and patients on chronic corticosteroid therapy)	Ensures adequate stores of vitamin D to maintain normal serum and bony calcium
Lifestyle changes Adequate exercise Smoking cessation	Vigorous, weight-bearing exercise promotes and maintains strong bone. Smoking decreases amount of active estrogen which accelerates bone loss.
Use of bisphosphonates (e.g., alendronate)	Used for prevention and treatment Reduces bone resorption and increases bone mass and strength
Preventive measures for patients on chronic corticosteroid therapy (prednisone >7.5 mg daily) Calcium and vitamin D supplements Lifestyle changes Use of bisphosphonates Use of low doses of corticosteroids or nonsystemic route, if possible	Corticosteroids decrease calcium absorption, increasing risk of osteoporosis. Lower doses or nonsystemic routes decrease corticosteroid effect on calcium absorption.
Preventive measures for patients taking phenytoin Calcium and vitamin D supplements Drug treatment if bone density is low	Phenytoin increases hepatic metabolism of vitamin D.
Treatment in women (if actual bone loss is present) Calcium/vitamin D supplements Alendronate 10 mg daily or 70 mg weekly OR Risedronate 5 mg daily Estrogen supplements Dose reduction if on corticosteroids	Bisphosphonates decrease the rate of bone breakdown, slow the rate of bone loss, increase bone mineral density, reduce the risk of vertebral fractures, and slow the progression of vertebral deformities and loss of height. Estrogen protects against bone loss and fracture, but only short-term use is recommended due to the cancer risks of estrogen therapy.
Treatment in men Calcium/vitamin D supplements Use of bisphosphonates Testosterone supplements Dose reduction if on corticosteroids	Low testosterone levels may contribute to osteoporosis in men.

Clinical Manifestations

The calcium disorders are hypocalcemia and hypercalcemia, either of which can be life-threatening. Hypocalcemic emergencies, for example, may result in **tetany** (neuromuscular irritability). The bone disorders discussed in this chapter are those characterized by increased resorption of calcium and loss of bone mass. These disorders weaken bone, and possibly leading to osteoporosis, with fractures, pain, and disability. Box 42.2 describes selected calcium and bone disorders.

Drug Therapy

Health care providers use a variety of drugs to regulate calcium and bone metabolism.

- Treatment of hypocalcemia and prevention and treatment of osteoporosis: calcium and vitamin D supplements

- Treatment of hypercalcemia: bisphosphonates, calcitonin, corticosteroids, 0.9% sodium chloride intravenous (IV) infusion, and other agents
- Treatment of osteoporosis: bisphosphonates, calcitonin, estrogens, and antiestrogens

Clinical Application 42-1

- Mrs. Taylor, who has osteoporosis, should take preventive measures in addition to taking her prescribed medication. One important measure is to increase the intake of foods that contain high levels of calcium. What dietary recommendations should the nurse make?

Optimal Management of Cancer Treatment-Induced Bone Loss: Considerations for Elderly Patients

by TIPPLES, K., & ROBINSON, A.

Drugs & Aging, November 11, 2011, 867–883

The researchers conducted an extensive literature review, including abstracts from oncology and bone health conferences with a special focus on cancer treatment-induced bone loss. The treatment of many types of cancer has involved decreasing hormone levels and use of corticosteroids. Treatment of breast cancer often has concerned therapies that decrease estrogen levels, and treatment of prostate cancer has involved therapies that decrease androgen levels. Treatment of multiple myeloma uses corticosteroids. These therapies increase the risk of osteoporosis, especially in the elderly.

IMPLICATIONS FOR NURSING PRACTICE: The authors' recommendations should guide nursing practice in oncology, community health, and geriatric settings. Careful screening of at-risk patients is necessary. Bone protection therapy with a bisphosphonate is recommended, and denosumab also shows promise. Nurses can encourage the recommended lifestyle changes, including weight-bearing exercise, smoking cessation, reduction in alcohol use, increase in dietary intake of calcium, and use of calcium and vitamin D supplementation when needed. Teaching and encouragement from nurses helps ensure adherence of elderly patients to necessary drug and dietary regimens.

Calcium Preparations

Calcium is available in many different forms. These preparations differ mainly in the amounts of calcium they contain and their routes of administration. It is important to note that even if people have normal serum levels of calcium, their diets may not contain enough calcium; they may need calcium supplements. Experts believe that the diets of most people of all ages, but especially of young women and older adults, are deficient in calcium.

Pharmacokinetics and Action

Absorption of calcium occurs in the small intestine, where approximately one third of the amount consumed is actually absorbed. PTH and vitamin D increase the absorption of calcium. Excretion primarily occurs in the feces, with the remainder excreted by the kidneys. PTH decreases renal excretion of calcium.

Oral and IV calcium preparations replace lost calcium and help maintain normal calcium levels.

Use

Oral calcium (e.g., calcium carbonate or calcium citrate) provides supplemental calcium when diet alone is insufficient to meet body requirements. Also, it is useful for treatment of chronic, nonemergent hypocalcemia, regardless of cause. In addition, it provides relief from symptoms of acid indigestion and heartburn. Finally, it can decrease bone loss and fractures, especially in women. Calcium citrate is reportedly better absorbed than calcium carbonate.

IV calcium is essential for the treatment of acute, severe hypocalcemia, which is a medical emergency. It may be necessary to give repeated doses, to give a continuous infusion, or to use oral supplements to avoid symptoms of hypocalcemia and maintain normal serum calcium levels (measured every 4–6 hours). In

---

BOX 42.2 **Calcium and Bone Disorders**

Hypocalcemia

Hypocalcemia is an abnormally low blood calcium level (i.e., less than 8.5 mg/dL). Causes may include inadequate intake of calcium and vitamin D, numerous disorders (e.g., diarrhea or malabsorption syndromes that cause inadequate absorption of calcium and vitamin D, hypoparathyroidism, renal failure, severe hypomagnesemia, hypermagnesemia, acute pancreatitis, rhabdomyolysis, tumor lysis syndrome, vitamin D deficiency), and several drugs (e.g., cisplatin, cytosine arabinoside, foscarnet, ketoconazole, pentamidine, agents used to treat hypercalcemia). Calcium deficits caused by inadequate dietary intake affect bone tissue rather than serum calcium levels. Two mechanisms result in hypocalcemia associated with renal failure. First, inability to excrete phosphate in urine leads to accumulation of phosphate in the blood (hyperphosphatemia). Because phosphate levels are inversely related to calcium levels, hyperphosphatemia induces hypocalcemia. Second, when kidney function is impaired, vitamin D conversion to its active metabolite is impaired. This results in decreased intestinal absorption of calcium.

Clinical manifestations are characterized by increased neuromuscular irritability, which may progress to tetany. Tetany is characterized by numbness and tingling of the lips, fingers, and toes; twitching of facial muscles; spasms of skeletal muscle; carpopedal spasm; laryngospasm; and convulsions. In young children, hypocalcemia may be manifested by convulsions rather than tetany and erroneously diagnosed as epilepsy. This may be a serious error because anticonvulsant drugs used for epilepsy may further decrease serum calcium levels. Severe hypocalcemia may cause lethargy or confusion.

Hypercalcemia

Hypercalcemia is an abnormally high blood calcium level (i.e., greater than 10.5 mg/dL). It may be caused by hyperparathyroidism, hyperthyroidism, malignant neoplasms, vitamin D or vitamin A intoxication, aluminum intoxication, prolonged immobilization, adrenocortical insufficiency, and ingestion of thiazide diuretics, estrogens, and lithium. Cancer is a common cause, especially carcinomas (of the breast,

(Continued on page 784)

BOX 42.2 Calcium and Bone Disorders (Continued)

lung, head and neck, or kidney) and multiple myeloma. Cancer stimulates bone breakdown, which increases serum calcium levels. Increased urine output leads to fluid volume deficit. This leads, in turn, to increased reabsorption of calcium in renal tubules and decreased renal excretion of calcium. Decreased renal excretion potentiates hypercalcemia. Patients at risk for hypercalcemia should be monitored for early signs and symptoms, so treatment can be started before severe hypercalcemia develops.

Clinical manifestations are caused by the decreased ability of nerves to respond to stimuli and the decreased ability of muscles to contract and relax. Hypercalcemia has a depressant effect on nerve and muscle function. Gastrointestinal problems with hypercalcemia include anorexia, nausea, vomiting, constipation, and abdominal pain. Central nervous system problems include apathy, depression, poor memory, headache, and drowsiness. Severe hypercalcemia may produce lethargy, syncope, disorientation, hallucinations, coma, and death. Other signs and symptoms include weakness and decreased tone in skeletal and smooth muscle, dysphagia, polyuria, polyphagia, and cardiac dysrhythmias. In addition, calcium may be deposited in various tissues, such as the conjunctiva, cornea, and kidneys. Calcium deposits in the kidneys (renal calculi) may lead to irreversible damage and impairment of function.

Osteoporosis

Osteoporosis is characterized by decreased bone density (osteopenia) and weak, fragile bones that often lead to fractures, pain, and disability. Although any bones may be affected, common fracture sites are the vertebrae of the lower dorsal and lumbar spines, wrists, and hips. Risk factors include female sex, advanced age, small stature, lean body mass, white or Asian race, positive family history, low calcium intake, menopause, sedentary lifestyle, nulliparity, smoking, excessive ingestion of alcohol or caffeine, high protein intake, high phosphate intake, hyperthyroidism, and chronic use of certain medications (e.g., corticosteroids, phenytoin). Postmenopausal women who do not take estrogen replacement therapy are at high risk because of estrogen deficiency, age-related bone loss, and a low peak bone mass. Osteoporosis occurs in men but less often than in women. Both men and women who take high doses of corticosteroids are at high risk because the drugs demineralize bone. In addition, renal transplant recipients can acquire osteoporosis from corticosteroid therapy, decreased renal function, increased parathyroid hormone secretion, and cyclosporine immunosuppressant therapy.

Osteopenia or early osteoporosis may be present and undetected unless radiography or a bone density measurement is done. If detected, treatment is needed to slow bone loss. If undetected or untreated, clinical manifestations of osteoporosis include shortened stature (a measurable loss of height), back pain, spinal deformity, or a fracture. Fractures often occur with common bending or lifting movements or falling.

Paget's Disease

Paget's disease is an inflammatory skeletal disease that affects older people. Its etiology is unknown. It is characterized by a high rate of bone turnover and results in bone deformity and pain. It is treated with nonnarcotic analgesics and drugs that decrease bone resorption (e.g., bisphosphonates, calcitonin).

---

calcium blocker overdose, calcium gluconate is given by IV infusion to help reverse the vasodilation and decreased myocardial contractility caused by the calcium channel blocker.

Table 42.2 gives route and dosage information for several calcium supplements.

Use in Older Adults

Hypocalcemia is uncommon in older adults because calcium moves from bone to blood to maintain normal serum levels. However, calcium deficiency commonly occurs because of long-term dietary deficiencies of calcium and impaired absorption of calcium from the intestine. As previously stated, osteoporosis is a concern in some women. Although osteoporosis develops in older men, it occurs less often, at a later age, and to a lesser extent than in older women. Both men and women who take corticosteroids are at risk for osteoporosis. The risk is higher with systemic corticosteroids but may also occur with oral or inhaled drugs, especially at higher doses.

Use in Patients With Renal Impairment

Patients with renal impairment or failure often have disturbances in calcium and bone metabolism. Calcium acetate may be used to prevent or treat hyperphosphatemia. The calcium reduces blood levels of phosphate by reducing its absorption from foods. It binds with dietary phosphate to produce calcium phosphate, which is insoluble and excreted in feces.

Adverse Effects

Hypercalcemia produces adverse effects in several body systems. GI effects include anorexia, nausea, vomiting, abdominal pain, and constipation. Central nervous system effects are apathy, poor memory, depression, drowsiness, and disorientation. Cardiac effects include dysrhythmias, and an electrocardiogram (ECG) shows a prolonged QT interval and an inverted T wave. Weakness and decreased tone in skeletal and smooth muscles, dysphagia, polyuria, and polydipsia may also occur.

Contraindications

Contraindications to calcium preparations include cancer with bone metastases, as well as ventricular fibrillation, hypercalcemia, hypophosphatemia, and renal calculi.

Nursing Implications

Preventing Interactions

Several medications and foods interact with calcium supplements, increasing or decreasing their effects (Boxes 42.3 and 42.4).

Also, it is important to note that oral calcium preparations interfere with the absorption of numerous drugs, including

TABLE 42.2

DRUGS AT A GLANCE: Calcium and Vitamin D preparations

Drug	Pregnancy Category	Routes and Dosage Ranges	
		Adults	Children
Oral Calcium Products			
Calcium acetate (PhosLo) 25% calcium	C	1,334 mg PO with each meal; increase gradually to 2001–2,668 mg with each meal	Dosage not established
Calcium carbonate precipitated (Os-Cal, Tums) 40% calcium	C	500–2,000 mg PO 2–4 times per day	45–65 mg/kg/d PO in four divided doses
Calcium citrate (Citracal) 21% calcium	Not rated	1–2 g PO or more per day in 3–4 divided doses	45–65 mg/kg/d PO in four divided doses
Calcium gluconate 9% calcium	Not rated	2 g 2–4 PO times per day	200–500 mg/kg/d PO divided every 6 h.
Parenteral Calcium Products			
Calcium chloride 10 mL of 10% solution contains 273 mg (13.6 mEq) of calcium	A C in high doses	500 mg–1 g IV every 6 h	10–20 mg/kg/dose IV every 4–6 h
Calcium gluconate (10 mL of 10% solution contains 93 mg (4.65 mEq) of calcium	A C in high doses	2–15 g/24 h IV as a continuous infusion or in divided doses	200–500 mg/kg/d as a continuous IV infusion or in four divided doses (max 2–3 g per dose)
Vitamin D Preparations			
Calcitriol (Rocaltrol, Calcijex)	C	0.25 mcg PO daily initially; then adjusted according to serum calcium levels (usual daily maintenance dose 0.5–1 mcg)	1–5 y, 0.25–0.75 mcg PO daily 6 y or older, refer to adult dose
Cholecalciferol (Delta-D)	C	DRI (19–70 y), 600 international units PO daily	DRI Birth–12 mo AI, 400 PO international units/d 1–18 y RDA, 600 PO international units/d
Ergocalciferol (Calciferol, Drisdol)	C	19–70 y, 600 international units/d PO	Same as cholecalciferol
Paricalcitol (Zemplar)	C	Secondary hyperparathyroidism associated with chronic renal failure: 0.04–0.1 mcg/kg IV every other day initially; increase by 2–4 mcg at 2–4 wk intervals if necessary; reduce dosage or stop therapy if hypercalcemia occurs	Secondary hyperparathyroidism associated with chronic renal failure: 5 y and older, same as adults (small studies only)

AI, adequate intake; DRI, dietary reference intake; RDA, recommended dietary allowance.

atenolol and fluoroquinolones, when the calcium is taken at the same time. In the case of oral tetracyclines, the calcium combines with the antibiotic, preventing its absorption.

In addition, calcium preparations and digoxin have similar effects on the myocardium. Therefore, if a patient taking digoxin receives calcium, the risks of digoxin toxicity and cardiac dysrhythmias increase. It is essential to use this combination very cautiously. Use of calcium with phenytoin decreases absorption of both drugs. IV calcium antagonizes the effects of verapamil.

Administering the Medication

Calcium is available in many different forms; the nurse ensures that the form being given is the correct one. The nurse also makes sure to

BOX 42.3	**Drug Interactions: Calcium Preparations**

Drugs That Increase the Effects of Calcium
- Thiazide diuretics
  Reduce calcium losses in the urine
- Vitamin D
  Increases absorption of calcium

Drugs That Decrease the Effects of Calcium
- Calcitonin
  Interferes with absorption of calcium
- Corticosteroids (prednisone and others)
  Lower calcium levels by various mechanisms
- Phosphates
  Lower calcium levels by various mechanisms

- Administer oral preparations with or after meals to increase absorption. If used as an antacid, administer after a meal.
- Administer oral preparations separately from atenolol and fluoroquinolones and more than 2 to 3 hours before or after giving oral tetracycline.
- Dilute IV preparations in a compatible fluid and administer slowly as a continuous infusion or in divided doses; check pulse and blood pressure closely; monitor the ECG if possible. IV solutions may cause dysrhythmias and hypotension if administered too rapidly.
  - Carefully observe the IV site during administration because IV calcium is irritating to tissues.
  - Do not administer parenteral forms intramuscularly.

Assessing for Therapeutic Effects

The nurse observes for relief of symptoms of neuromuscular irritability and tetany, such as decreased muscle spasms, decreased paresthesias, absence of Chvostek's sign, and absence of Trousseau's sign. He or she also assesses laboratory results for return of serum calcium levels to the normal range of 8.5 to 10.5 mg/dL.

Once the hypocalcemia is stabilized, the aim of treatment is management of the underlying cause or prevention of recurrence. If diarrhea or malabsorption is the cause, treatment of the underlying condition decreases loss of calcium from the body and increases absorption. It is also necessary to measure serum magnesium levels; treatment of hypomagnesemia is essential before treatment of hypocalcemia can be effective.

BOX 42.4	**Herb and Dietary Interactions: Calcium Preparations**

Herbs and Foods That Decrease the Effects of Calcium
- Bran
- Rhubarb
- Spinach
- Whole-grain cereals

BOX 42.5	**Patient Teaching Guidelines for Calcium Preparations**

- Consult with your health care provider before taking calcium supplements.
- If you need a calcium supplement, your health care provider may recommend calcium carbonate 500 mg twice daily. This calcium supplement contains the most elemental calcium by weight (40%). It is inexpensive and available in a nonprescription form as the antacid Tums, which contains 200 mg of calcium per tablet.
- Consume good sources of dietary calcium that include milk, yogurt, hard natural cheese, bok choy, broccoli, Chinese/Napa cabbage, collards, kale, okra, turnip greens, fortified breakfast cereals, fortified orange juice, and dried peas and beans.
- Do not take a calcium supplement with an iron preparation, tetracycline, ciprofloxacin, or phenytoin. Instead, take the drugs at least 2 hours apart to avoid calcium interference with drug absorption.
- Avoid rhubarb, spinach, bran, and whole grain cereals in the meal before taking calcium because these foods interfere with calcium absorption.
- Take oral calcium 1 to 1.5 hours after meals if gastrointestinal upset occurs.
- Take oral calcium with a full glass of water.
- Report anorexia, nausea, vomiting, abdominal pain, dry mouth, thirst, or polyuria.

Assessing for Adverse Effects

The nurse assesses for increased thirst, inability to eat, and increased urination, as well as for constipation and abdominal pain. It is necessary to assess for diminished memory, disorientation, and drowsiness. The nurse checks the ECG for a prolonged QT interval and inverted T wave that results from hypercalcemia.

Patient Teaching

Box 42.5 presents patient teaching guidelines for calcium preparations.

Clinical Application 42-2

- What instructions should the nurse give Mrs. Taylor about taking oral calcium supplements?

NCLEX Success

1. The nurse must administer a tetracycline antibiotic to a patient who takes an oral calcium supplement with each meal. When should the nurse administer the tetracycline?
   A. 2 hours before meals
   B. 30 minutes before meals
   C. with meals
   D. 1 hour after meals

2. The nurse is administering a continuous IV infusion of calcium properly diluted in a compatible IV fluid. Which one of the following would it be most important for the nurse to monitor?

   A. cardiac rhythm

   B. urine output

   C. hearing changes

   D. musculoskeletal pain

Vitamin D

Vitamin D is a fat-soluble vitamin used in chronic hypocalcemia if calcium supplements alone cannot maintain serum calcium levels within a normal range. It is also used to prevent deficiency states and treat hypoparathyroidism and osteoporosis. Although authorities agree that dietary intake is better than supplements, some suggest a vitamin D supplement for people who ingest less than the recommended amount. The recommended dietary allowance, or RDA, for vitamin D is 600 international units for people 1 to 70 years of age and 800 international units daily for adults 71 years and older to prevent and treat osteoporosis. Adequate intake for infants 0 to 12 months is 400 international units daily.

Pharmacokinetics and Action

As a drug, vitamin D is absorbed from the GI tract. It is stored in the liver, skin, and other tissues for months. It is metabolized into its active form in the liver and kidneys. Half of an oral dose is eliminated in the bile.

Vitamin D increases calcium and phosphorus absorption from the GI tract. It also promotes movement of calcium and phosphorus from the bones to maintain normal serum calcium levels. In the kidneys, vitamin D decreases elimination of calcium and phosphorus.

Use

Vitamin D is useful for the treatment of rickets, other vitamin D deficiency diseases, and hypoparathyroidism. It is important to take vitamin D supplements cautiously and not overuse them; excessive amounts can cause serious problems, including hypercalcemia.

Vitamin D is also useful if a calcium preparation alone cannot maintain serum calcium levels within a normal range. When vitamin D is given to treat hypocalcemia, frequent measurements of serum calcium levels determine dosage. Usually people take higher doses initially, and lower doses are appropriate for maintenance therapy. Calcium salts and vitamin D are available over-the-counter in many combined preparations promoted as dietary supplements (Table 42.3). These mixtures are not indicated for maintenance therapy in chronic hypocalcemia.

Use in Children

Authorities recommend vitamin D supplementation for infants who are partially or completely breast-fed because breast milk contains only small quantities of vitamin D.

TABLE 42.3

Selected Calcium/Vitamin D Combination Products*

Drug	Calcium (mg of Elemental Calcium)/Tablet or Capsule	Vitamin D International Units/Tablet
Caltrate 600 + D and Caltrate Plus	600	200
Citracal caplets + D	315	200
Dical-D tablets	117	133
Dical-D wafers	233	200
Os-Cal 250 + D	250	125
Os-Cal 500 + D	500	125
Posture-D	600	125

*In general, intake of calcium should not exceed 2500 mg daily, from all sources, and intake of vitamin D should not exceed 400 international units daily.

Use in Patients With Renal Impairment

Renal disease interferes with metabolism of vitamin D precursors to the active form of vitamin D in the kidneys. If vitamin D therapy is necessary for the treatment of osteomalacia associated with renal impairment, calcitriol (Rocaltrol) is preferable. Calcitriol is the active form of vitamin D and thus undergoes no metabolism.

Adverse Effects

The principal adverse effects of excessive vitamin D use are hypervitaminosis D and hypercalcemia. This is most likely to occur with chronic ingestion of high doses daily. In children, accidental ingestion may lead to acute toxicity. Of particular significance with vitamin D excess are kidney stones, irreversible kidney damage, and muscle and bone weakness. Box 42.2 discusses symptoms of hypercalcemia, such as tetany.

Contraindications

Contraindications to vitamin D include hypercalcemia and vitamin D toxicity. It is necessary to withhold all preparations containing vitamin D.

Nursing Implications

Preventing Interactions

Several medications interact with vitamin D, increasing or decreasing its effects (Box 42.6).

Administering the Medication

People may take vitamin D without regard to food. It is important not to take both the vitamin and magnesium-containing antacids or mineral oil.

Assessing for Therapeutic Effects

The nurse observes for a decrease in symptoms of hypocalcemia and symptoms of rickets or osteomalacia. It is necessary to check that the following laboratory results are normal: serum calcium level, blood urea nitrogen and serum creatinine, and serum phosphate. Improved bone health, as documented by radiograph, should be evident.

Assessing for Adverse Effects

It is important to monitor serum calcium. If hypercalcemia occurs, the nurse must stop the drug and notify the health care provider. It is necessary to observe for signs and symptoms of vitamin D excess, including headache, somnolence, weakness, irritability, hypertension, cardiac dysrhythmias, kidney stones, polydipsia, polyuria, and bone and muscle pain.

Patient Teaching

Box 42.7 presents patient teaching guidelines for vitamin D.

Clinical Application 42-3

■ Mrs. Taylor has developed end-stage renal disease and receives hemodialysis three times per week. She requires a vitamin D supplement. Why would she receive the active form of vitamin D, calcitriol (Rocaltrol)?

Bisphosphonates

Bisphosphonates are drugs that bind to bone and inhibit calcium resorption from bone. Although indications vary, the drugs are used mainly in the treatment of hypercalcemia and osteoporosis. Ⓟ **Alendronate** (Fosamax) is the prototype bisphosphonate.

Pharmacokinetics and Action

Alendronate is poorly absorbed from the intestinal tract. It is not metabolized. The drug bound to bone is slowly released into the bloodstream. Most of the drug that is not bound to bone is excreted in the urine.

Alendronate suppresses osteoclast activity on newly formed resorption surfaces, which reduces bone turnover. This means that bone formation exceeds resorption at remodeling sites, leading to progressive gains in bone mass.

Use

Although the main use of alendronate is to prevent and treat osteoporosis in postmenopausal women, it is also used to treat osteoporosis in men. Other uses include the treatment of **Paget's disease**, an inflammatory bone disease that affects older people, and glucocorticoid-induced osteoporosis in both sexes. The drug is not useful in children. Table 42.4 gives route and dosage information for alendronate and other bisphosphonates.

Use in Patients With Renal Impairment

Experts do not recommend using alendronate in severe renal impairment (creatinine clearance < 35 mL/min).

Adverse Effects

Adverse effects of alendronate are usually minor if the doses taken for prevention or treatment of osteoporosis are used and the drug is taken as directed. Patients who do not follow the dosing instructions are at greater risk for esophagitis, dysphagia, and esophageal ulcers/erosions. Other effects include headache, musculoskeletal pain (sometimes severe), and decreased serum calcium. More severe effects may occur with the higher doses taken for Paget's disease.

Rare adverse effects include atypical femur fracture and osteonecrosis of the jaw. Patients on long-term therapy are at greater risk for femur fracture.

TABLE 42.4

DRUGS AT A GLANCE: Bisphosphonates

Drug	Pregnancy Category	Routes and Dosage Ranges	
		Adults	Children
Alendronate (Fosamax)	C	Osteoporosis: Women (postmenopausal), Prevention, 5 mg once daily PO or 35 mg PO once weekly Treatment, 10 mg once daily PO or 70 mg PO once weekly Men, 10 mg PO once daily Glucocorticoid-induced disease: 5 mg PO once daily Paget's disease: 40 mg PO daily for 6 mo; repeated if necessary	No use established
Ibandronate (Boniva)	C	Osteoporosis (postmenopausal women): prevention/treatment, 2.5 mg PO once daily, 150 mg PO every month, or 3 mg IV every 3 mo	No use established
Pamidronate (Aredia)	D	Hypercalcemia of malignancy: 60–90 mg IV as a single dose over 2–24 h Breast cancer: 90 mg IV over 2 h every 3–4 wk Multiple myeloma: 90 mg IV over 4 h once monthly Paget's disease: 30 mg IV over 4 h daily for 3 consecutive days	No use established
Risedronate (Actonel)	C	Osteoporosis (postmenopausal or glucocorticoid-induced): prevention/treatment, 5 mg PO once daily, 35 mg PO once weekly, or 150 mg PO once monthly Paget's disease: 30 mg PO (immediate-release) once daily for 2 mo	No use established
Zoledronate (Reclast, Zometa)	D	Hypercalcemia of malignancy: 4 mg IV; max given as a single dose	No use established

Contraindications

Contraindications to alendronate include hypersensitivity to the drug, abnormalities of the esophagus that delay esophageal emptying, and inability to stand or sit upright for at least 30 minutes. People with hypocalcemia require correction of the low serum calcium levels before beginning therapy with alendronate.

Caution is warranted with active upper GI conditions.

Nursing Implications

Preventing Interactions

Several medications interact with alendronate, increasing or decreasing its effects (Box 42.8). Any food interferes with absorption of alendronate.

BOX 42.8	Drug Interactions: Alendronate

Drugs That Increase the Effects of Alendronate

■ Aspirin and nonsteroidal anti-inflammatory drugs
Increase the risk of gastrointestinal effects when combined with alendronate

Drugs That Decrease the Effects of Alendronate

■ Antacids and calcium supplements
Interfere with alendronate absorption if they are taken within 2 hours of the drug

Administering the Medication

The nurse ensures proper administration of alendronate. It is always necessary to take the drug with a full glass of water, not juice or coffee, at least 30 minutes before breakfast and before taking other drugs. The person must remain upright (either with head elevated 90 degrees if in bed, sitting upright in a chair, or standing) for at least 30 minutes after administration. These interventions promote absorption and decrease esophageal and gastric irritation.

Assessing for Therapeutic and Adverse Effects

The nurse observes for improved bone density and absence of fractures. Early osteopenia and osteoporosis are asymptomatic. Measurement of bone density is the only way to quantify bone loss.

It is also necessary to observe for GI adverse effects, including abdominal distension, acid regurgitation, dysphagia, esophagitis, and flatulence.

Patient Teaching

Box 42.9 gives patient teaching guidelines for alendronate.

Other Drugs in the Class

Other bisphosphonates include ibandronate (Boniva), pamidronate (Aredia), risedronate (Actonel), and zoledronate (Reclast, Zometa). Ibandronate, risedronate, and zoledronate

BOX 42.9 **Patient Teaching Guidelines for Alendronate**

■ Take tablets on waking only with 6–8 ounces of water or more at least 30 minutes before eating or drinking anything else, including food, beverages, or other drugs. Waiting longer than 30 minutes improves absorption.

■ Do not lie down for at least 30 minutes after taking alendronate to reduce the risk of esophageal irritation and aid movement of the drug to the stomach.

■ Report adverse effects to the health care provider immediately, especially esophageal pain, irritation, or burning; heartburn; dyspepsia, nausea, vomiting; or difficulty swallowing.

(Reclast), like alendronate, are used to prevent and treat osteoporosis. Both ibandronate and risedronate are available in oral preparations to be taken once monthly. Zoledronate, as Reclast, is administered IV once a year. Pamidronate is not U.S. Food and Drug Administration (FDA) approved for osteoporosis but may be useful for various bone-related conditions such as Paget's disease and bone lesions.

Common adverse effects of bisphosphonates include nausea and vomiting. Serious adverse effects may include anemia, jaw osteonecrosis, neutropenia, infections, and renal damage.

Clinical Application 42-4

- The nurse is giving instructions to Mrs. Taylor on the proper administration method for taking alendronate. What important instructions must the nurse include?

NCLEX Success

3. **A man has a serum calcium level of 6.8 mg/dL. The health care provider orders a vitamin D supplement. Which one of the following laboratory values for serum calcium indicates that the vitamin D is effective?**

   A. 5.5 mg/dL
   B. 6.8 mg/dL
   C. 7.5 mg/dL
   D. 8.5 mg/dL

4. **The nurse is caring for a patient who takes alendronate (Fosamax). Which adverse effects should the nurse observe for?**

   A. numbness and tingling of the extremities
   B. irregular pulse rate and angina
   C. acid reflux and difficulty swallowing
   D. rash and skin lesions

5. **The health care provider has prescribed alendronate (Fosamax) for the patient. Which one of the following should the nurse include in discharge teaching?**

   A. "Take alendronate first thing in the morning with orange juice."
   B. "Take alendronate at bedtime with a glass of milk."
   C. "Take alendronate first thing in the morning with water."
   D. "Take alendronate on a full stomach after breakfast."

Other Medications Used to Treat Bone Disorders and Hypercalcemia

Other drugs are used to treat bone disorders and hypercalcemia. Table 42.5 presents route and dosage information for these drugs.

Calcitonin-salmon (Calcimar, Miacalcin) is used in the treatment of hypercalcemia, Paget's disease, and osteoporosis. In hypercalcemia, calcitonin lowers serum calcium levels by inhibiting bone resorption. Calcitonin is most likely to be effective in hypercalcemia caused by hyperparathyroidism, prolonged immobilization, or certain malignant neoplasms. In acute hypercalcemia, health care providers may use calcitonin along with other measures to lower serum calcium rapidly. A single injection of calcitonin decreases serum calcium levels in approximately 2 hours, and its effects last approximately 6 to 8 hours. In Paget's disease, calcitonin slows the rate of bone turnover, improves bone lesions on radiologic examination, and relieves bone pain. In osteoporosis, calcitonin prevents further bone loss in the presence of adequate calcium and vitamin D. In addition, calcitonin helps control pain in patients with osteoporosis or metastatic bone disease. Both subcutaneous and intranasal administrations relieve pain within 1 to 12 weeks. Initially people take the drug daily, then two to three times a week. The mechanism by which pain is reduced is unknown.

Denosumab (Prolia, Xgeva) is an antiresorptive drug. Prolia is used to treat osteoporosis in postmenopausal women at high risk of fracture. Xgeva is used to prevent skeletal-related events in bone metastases from solid tumors. Denosumab decreases bone resorption and increases bone mass and strength. The drug is administered subcutaneously at 6-month intervals. Adverse effects include fatigue, weakness, back pain, extremity pain, hypocalcemia, hypophosphatemia, nausea, and diarrhea.

Glucocorticoids (e.g., prednisone, hydrocortisone) are useful in the treatment of hypercalcemia due to malignancies or vitamin D intoxication. These drugs lower serum calcium levels by inhibiting cytokine release, by direct cytolytic effects on some tumor cells, by inhibiting calcium absorption from the intestine, and by increasing calcium excretion in the urine. The serum calcium level decreases in approximately 5 to 10 days, and after it stabilizes, gradual dosage reduction to the minimum needed to control symptoms of hypercalcemia is necessary. High dosage or prolonged administration leads to serious adverse effects.

Phosphate salts (Neutra-Phos) inhibit intestinal absorption of calcium and increase deposition of calcium in bone. (Neutra-Phos is an oral combination of sodium phosphate and

TABLE 42.5

DRUGS AT A GLANCE: Drugs Used to Treat Other Bone Disorders and Hypercalcemia

Drug	Pregnancy Category	Routes and Dosage Ranges	
		Adults	Children
Calcitonin-salmon (Calcimar, Miacalcin)	C	Hypercalcemia: 4 international units/kg subcutaneously or IM every 12 h; can be increased after 1–2 d to 8 international units/kg every 12 h; max dose 8 international units/kg every 6 h Paget's disease: 50–100 international units/d subcutaneously or IM, Postmenopausal osteoporosis: nasal spray (Miacalcin), 200 international units/d; 100 international units subcutaneously or IM every other day, 1 spray in 1 nostril	No use established
Denosumab (Prolia, Xgeva)	C	Osteoporosis, bone loss in breast and prostate cancer treatment (Prolia): 60 mg subcutaneously every 6 mo Prevention of skeletal-related events with solid tumor bone metastases (Xgeva): 120 mg subcutaneously every 4 wk	No use established
Phosphate salts (Neutra-Phos)	C	Hypercalcemia: elemental phosphorus 250–500 mg PO 4 times per day	Hypercalcemia: 4 y of age or older, elemental phosphorus 250 mg PO 4 times per day
Prednisone or hydrocortisone	C	Hypercalcemia: prednisone, 20–40 mg PO daily (or equivalent dose of another glucocorticoid) for 5–10 d, then tapered to the minimum dose required to prevent hypercalcemia; hydrocortisone, 100–500 mg/d IM or IV	Consult pediatric literature
Raloxifene (Evista)	X	Osteoporosis (postmenopausal women): prevention/treatment, 60 mg PO once daily	No use established
Teriparatide (Forteo)	C	Osteoporosis: 20 mcg subcutaneous daily	No use established

potassium phosphate.) Oral salts are effective in the treatment of hypercalcemia due to any cause. A potential adverse effect of phosphates is calcification of soft tissues due to deposition of calcium phosphate, which can lead to severe impairment of function in the kidneys and other organs. It is important to give phosphates only when hypercalcemia is accompanied by hypophosphatemia (serum phosphate < 3 mg/dL) and renal function is normal to minimize the risk of soft tissue calcification. Frequent monitoring of serum calcium, phosphate, and creatinine levels is necessary, and the dose reduction should occur if serum phosphate exceeds 4.5 mg/dL or the product of serum calcium and phosphate exceeds 60 mg/dL.

Raloxifene (Evista) is a selective estrogen receptor modulator that is used to prevent or treat postmenopausal osteoporosis. It acts like estrogen in some body tissues and prevents the action of estrogen in other body tissues. It has estrogenic effects in bone tissue, thereby decreasing bone breakdown and increasing bone mass density. It has antiestrogen effects in breast and uterine tissue. Raloxifene increases the risk of deep

vein thrombosis or pulmonary emboli; the risk of death due to stroke may be increased in women with coronary heart disease or in women at risk for coronary events.

Teriparatide (Forteo) is a recombinant DNA version of PTH that is approved for the treatment of osteoporosis in women. This drug increases bone formation by increasing the number of bone-building cells (osteoblasts). It also increases serum levels of calcium and the active form of vitamin D. In clinical trials, teriparatide increased vertebral bone mineral density and decreased vertebral fractures. Experts recommend the drug for use in patients with severe osteoporosis or those who have not responded adequately to other treatments. Patients with an increased risk of osteosarcoma, such as those with Paget's disease, prior radiation, unexplained elevation of alkaline phosphatase, and open epiphyses, should avoid using teriparatide. Adverse effects include nausea, headache, back pain, dizziness, syncope, and leg cramps. It is necessary to administer the drug with the patient sitting or lying down to prevent orthostatic hypotension.

Teriparatide is rapidly and well absorbed after subcutaneous injection. Bioavailability is 95%, and peak serum levels occur in 30 minutes. The drug is metabolized and excreted through the liver, kidneys, and bone. It is not expected to accumulate in bone or other tissues, to interact significantly with other drugs, or to require dosage adjustment with renal or hepatic impairment.

Emergency Treatment of Hypercalcemia

Acute hypercalcemia (severe symptoms or a serum calcium level > 12 mg/dL) is a medical emergency, and rehydration is a priority. It is essential to administer an IV saline solution (0.9% sodium chloride) at an initial rate of 200 to 300 mL/h and then adjust it to maintain a urine output of 100 to 150 mL/h. Authorities no long recommend the routine use of loop diuretics, such as furosemide, in the absence of heart failure or renal insufficiency. Because sodium, potassium, and water are also lost in the urine, replacement with IV fluids is necessary.

The Nursing Process

Assessment

- Assess for risk factors and manifestations of hypocalcemia and calcium deficiency:
  - Assess dietary intake of dairy products, other calcium-containing foods, and vitamin D.
  - Check serum calcium reports for abnormal values. The normal total serum calcium level is approximately 8.5 to 10.5 mg/dL (SI units 2.2–2.6 mmol/L). Approximately half of the total serum calcium (4–5 mg/dL) should be free ionized calcium, the physiologically active form. To interpret serum calcium levels accurately, serum albumin levels and acid–base status must be considered. Low serum albumin decreases the total serum level of calcium by decreasing the amount of calcium that is bound to protein; however, the ionized concentration is unaffected by serum albumin levels. Metabolic and respiratory alkalosis increase the binding of calcium to serum proteins, thereby maintaining normal serum calcium but decreasing the ionized values. Conversely, metabolic and respiratory acidosis decrease binding and therefore increase the concentration of ionized calcium.
  - Check for Chvostek's sign: Tap the facial nerve just below the temple, in front of the ear. If facial muscles twitch, hyperirritability of the nerve is present, and tetany may occur.
  - Check for Trousseau's sign: Constrict blood circulation in an arm (usually with a blood pressure cuff) for 3 to 5 minutes. This produces ischemia and increased irritability of peripheral nerves, which causes spasms of the lower arm and hand muscles (carpopedal spasm) if tetany is present.
- Assess for conditions in which hypercalcemia is likely to occur: cancer, prolonged immobilization, or vitamin D overdose.

- Observe for signs and symptoms of hypercalcemia in patients at risk. ECG changes indicative of hypercalcemia include a shortened QT interval and an inverted T wave.
- Assess for risk factors and manifestations of osteoporosis, especially in postmenopausal women and men and women on chronic corticosteroid therapy.
  - If risk factors are identified, ask if preventive measures are being used (e.g., increasing calcium intake, exercise, medications).
  - If the patient is known to have osteoporosis, ask about duration and severity of symptoms, age at onset, location, whether fractures have occurred, what treatments have been performed, and response to treatments.
- If Paget's disease is suspected, assess for an elevated serum alkaline phosphatase level and abnormal bone scan reports.

Nursing Diagnoses

- Deficient knowledge related to recommended daily amounts and dietary sources of calcium and vitamin D
- Deficient knowledge related to disease process and drug therapy for osteoporosis
- Risk for injury (risk factors: tetany, sedation, and seizures due to hypocalcemia)
- Risk for injury (risk factor: hypercalcemia due to overuse of supplements)
- Risk for injury (risk factor: hypocalcemia due to aggressive treatment of hypercalcemia)

Planning/Goals

The patient will

- Achieve and maintain normal serum levels of calcium
- Increase dietary intake of calcium-containing foods to prevent or treat osteoporosis
- Use calcium or vitamin D supplements in recommended amounts
- Adhere to instructions for safe drug use
- Be monitored closely for therapeutic and adverse effects of drugs used to treat hypercalcemia
- Adhere to procedures for follow-up treatment of hypocalcemia, hypercalcemia, or osteoporosis
- Avoid preventable adverse effects of treatment for acute hypocalcemia or hypercalcemia

Nursing Interventions

The nurse will

- Assist all patients in meeting the recommended daily requirements of calcium and vitamin D. With an adequate protein and calcium intake, patients also obtain sufficient phosphate.
- Instruct the patient that the best dietary source is milk and other dairy products, including yogurt.
- Recommend that adults drink at least two 8 ounces glasses of milk daily (unless contraindicated by the patient's condition). This furnishes approximately half the daily calcium requirement; the remainder will probably be obtained from other foods.

- Instruct parents that children need approximately four glasses of milk or an equivalent amount of calcium in milk and other foods to support normal growth and development.
- Teach pregnant and lactating women to take approximately four glasses of milk or the equivalent to meet increased needs. Vitamin and mineral supplements are often prescribed during these periods.
- Instruct postmenopausal women who take estrogens to consume at least 1000 mg of calcium daily. Those who do not take estrogen need at least 1500 mg. The dosage is adjusted to dietary calcium intake.
- Assist patients who must avoid or minimize their intake of dairy products because of calories to identify low-calorie sources such as skim milk and low-fat yogurt.
- Teach patients in need of additional vitamin D that milk that has been fortified with vitamin D is the best food source. Exposure of skin to sunlight is also needed to supply adequate amounts of vitamin D.

- Teach patients who are unable or unwilling to ingest sufficient calcium that a supplement may be needed to prevent osteoporosis.
- Instruct patients with hypercalcemia to decrease formation of renal calculi and prevent urinary tract infections by taking 3000 to 4000 mL of fluid daily (if not contraindicated).

Evaluation

- Check laboratory reports of serum calcium levels for normal values.
- Interview and observe for relief of symptoms of hypocalcemia, hypercalcemia, or osteoporosis.
- Interview and observe intake of calcium-containing foods.
- Question about normal calcium requirements and how to meet them.
- Interview and observe for accurate drug usage and adherence to follow-up procedures.
- Interview and observe for therapeutic and adverse drug effects.

Key Concepts

- Hypoparathyroidism is most often caused by removal of or damage to the parathyroid glands during neck surgery.
- Hyperparathyroidism is most often caused by a tumor or hyperplasia of a parathyroid gland.
- Deficiency of vitamin D causes inadequate absorption of calcium and phosphorus.
- In general, intake of calcium should not exceed 2500 mg from all sources, and intake of vitamin D should not exceed 400 international units daily. (The upper intake level for vitamin D is 2000 international units daily.)
- Calcium deficiency commonly occurs in the elderly because of long-term dietary deficiencies of calcium and vitamin D, impaired absorption of calcium from the intestine, lack of exposure to sunlight, and impaired liver or kidney metabolism of vitamin D to its active form.
- Postmenopausal women are at high risk for osteoporosis.
- Both men and women who take corticosteroids are at risk for osteoporosis.

Critical Thinking Questions

42-1. An 80-year-old man with bruising from the top of his left hip extending to the ankle sees his health care provider. The man's alkaline phosphatase level is extremely elevated at 220 units/L. The patient is diagnosed with Paget's disease.

- What receives a diagnosis of Paget's disease?
- The health care provider prescribes alendronate. What is this drug?
- What patient teaching related to the administration of alendronate does the nurse provide?

References and Resources

Nursing 2012. (2012). *Drug handbook*. Philadelphia, PA: Wolters Kluwer Health/Lippincott Williams & Wilkins.

Smeltzer, S. C., Bare, B. G., Hinkle, J. L., & Cheever, K. H. (2010). *Brunner & Suddarth's textbook of medical-surgical nursing* (12th ed.). Philadelphia, PA: Wolters Kluwer Health/Lippincott Williams & Wilkins.

Tipples, K., & Robinson, A. (2011). Optimal management of cancer treatment-induced bone loss: Considerations for elderly patients. *Drugs & Aging, 28*(11), 867–883. Retrieved May 25, 2012, from CINAHL.

Up-To-Date, Inc. (2012). Up-To-Date from uptodate.com.

43 Drug Therapy for Addison's Disease and Cushing's Disease

LEARNING OBJECTIVES

After studying this chapter, you should be able to:

1 Understand the etiology and pathophysiology of adrenal cortex disorders.

2 Identify the major manifestations of Addison's disease and Cushing's disease.

3 Explain how corticotropin (ACTH) is used in the diagnosis of adrenocortical insufficiency.

4 Explain how cosyntropin (Cortrosyn) is used in the diagnosis of adrenocortical insufficiency.

5 Identify the prototypes and describe the action, use, adverse effects, contraindications, and nursing implications for the drugs used in the treatment of Addison's disease.

6 Identify the prototypes and describe the action, use, adverse effects, contraindications, and nursing implications for the drugs used in the treatment of Cushing's disease.

7 Implement the nursing process in the care of the patient with Addison's disease or Cushing's disease.

Clinical Application Case Study

Rosa James is a 68-year-old woman who is being seen by her physician with symptoms of muscle weakness and fatigue. She states that she has felt depressed. Physical assessment reveals dark pigmentation of the mucous membranes and skin on the knuckles, knees, and elbows. She appears dehydrated with poor skin turgor. Her blood pressure is extremely low—84/50 mm Hg. Blood chemistry reveals of sodium level of 132 mEq/L and a potassium level of 5.5 mEq/L. Mrs. James is admitted to the hospital with suspected Addison's disease.

KEY TERMS

Addisonian crisis: acute adrenocortical insufficiency

Adrenocortical excess: increase in adrenocortical function

Adrenocortical insufficiency: decrease in adrenocortical function

Introduction

Chapter 15 discussed corticosteroids, and Chapter 41 addressed the types of hormones secreted by the hypothalamus, including corticotropin-releasing hormone (CRH). This chapter introduces the pharmacological care of the patient with adrenocortical insufficiency and the patient with adrenocortical excess. The adrenal glands are attached to the upper portion of each kidney. The adrenal cortex of each adrenal gland secretes steroid hormones. The hypothalamic–pituitary–adrenal (HPA) axis regulates hormone secretion. The hypothalamus secretes CRH, which in turn stimulates the pituitary gland to secrete adrenocorticotropic

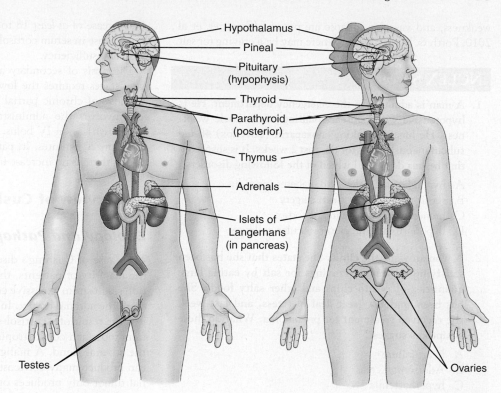

Hypothalamus
Pineal
Pituitary
(hypophysis)
Thyroid
Parathyroid
(posterior)
Thymus
Adrenals
Islets of
Langerhans
(in pancreas)
Testes
Ovaries

Figure 43.1 The adrenal glands are located on the top of each kidney. Adrenocorticotropic hormone is secreted by the pituitary gland.

hormone (ACTH) (Fig. 43.1). The ACTH then stimulates the adrenal cortex to secrete glucocorticoid hormone (cortisol). As the levels of adrenal or steroid hormones increase, the levels of CRH and ACTH decrease; this is a negative feedback mechanism (Smeltzer, Bare, Hinkle, & Cheever, 2010).

Overview of Addison's Disease

Etiology and Pathophysiology

There are two forms of **adrenocortical insufficiency**. Primary adrenal insufficiency, or Addison's disease, occurs when adrenal cortical hormones are deficient. ACTH levels are elevated because the feedback mechanism is not working. Secondary adrenal insufficiency occurs when there is a disorder in the HPA system.

Primary adrenal insufficiency most commonly results from an autoimmune disorder that has destroyed the layers of the adrenal cortex. Other causes of adrenal cortex destruction include metastatic carcinoma, fungal infections such as histoplasmosis, cytomegalovirus, amyloid disease, and hemochromatosis. Hemorrhage of the adrenal cortex related to anticoagulant therapy, open heart surgery, giving birth, or trauma also leads to primary adrenal insufficiency.

Secondary adrenal cortical insufficiency results from hypopituitarism or surgical removal of pituitary gland (Porth & Matfin, 2009). The abrupt withdrawal of oral glucocorticoids also causes secondary adrenal insufficiency. Patients who have endogenous steroid production from a nonendocrine tumor have adrenocortical insufficiency.

Primary adrenocortical insufficiency is associated with the destruction of the adrenal cortex. The resulting deficiency in the mineralocorticoids causes an increase in the loss of urinary sodium, chloride, and water. The patient becomes hyponatremic, and the cardiac output decreases. This progression of the

disease is known as **Addisonian crisis**. The loss of sodium leads to retention of potassium, resulting in symptoms of hyperkalemia.

Clinical Application 43-1

- Mrs. James is hyponatremic. When assessing her cardiac status, what findings would the nurse expect?
- On the 2nd day of Mrs. James' hospital admission, her sodium level is 125 mEq/L. What condition does the nurse suspect?

Clinical Manifestations

Clinical manifestations of adrenocortical insufficiency are evident when approximately 90% of the adrenal cortex has been destroyed. These signs and symptoms reflect loss of sodium, water, and chloride. Findings include decreased cardiac output, dehydration, weakness, and fatigue. Excessive sodium loss results in cardiovascular collapse and shock. Other symptoms include lethargy, weakness, fever, anorexia, nausea, vomiting, and weight loss. Hyperkalemia and hypoglycemia are present. (Any patient with unexplained severe hypoglycemia requires assessment for adrenal insufficiency (Nieman, 2011).) Hyperpigmentation of the gums and mucous membranes is also present; they may be bluish black. Women have diminished axillary and pubic hair, but men have few effects from the lack of androgens due to the production of hormones by the testes (Porth & Matfin, 2009).

Acute adrenal crisis, or Addisonian crisis, is a life-threatening condition that occurs when Addison's disease is the underlying problem and the patient is exposed to minor illness or increased stress. Nausea, vomiting, hypotension, muscle weakness, and vascular collapse are present (Smeltzer, et al., 2010; Porth & Matfin, 2009). There may be a craving for salt.

Diagnosis

According to Smeltzer et al. (2010), patients commonly present to their primary health care provider with vague symptoms of adrenocortical insufficiency. However, as the adrenocortical insufficiency progresses, acute hypotension results and Addisonian crisis may develop. Making the diagnosis of adrenocortical insufficiency involves laboratory work. This includes early morning serum cortisol and plasma ACTH levels. A serum cortisol level less than 3 mcg/dL, or 80 nmol/L, is indicative of adrenocortical insufficiency. (The normal morning level of serum cortisol is greater—10 to 20 mcg/dL, or 275 to 555 nmol/L.) An ACTH level greater than 22.0 nmol/L is indicative of (primary) adrenocortical insufficiency. (The normal morning level of ACTH is less than 18 nmol/L.)

Confirming the diagnosis of adrenocortical insufficiency requires a short plasma corticotropin stimulation test. The examiner administers corticotropin in the morning, and a subnormal blood cortisol level in the morning and afternoon confirms the diagnosis. A higher cortisol level in the morning is a sign that a person does not have adrenal insufficiency. In a patient with adrenal insufficiency, the response to the corticotropin, or ACTH, is the same both morning and afternoon.

Another test that confirms the diagnosis of adrenocortical insufficiency is the standard high-dose test. It is a three-step process:

1. Measurement of baseline serum cortisol
2. Intravenous (IV) administration of 250 mcg of ACTH 30 minutes later
3. Measurement of serum cortisol 30 to 60 minutes later

An increase of *at least* 18 to 20 mcg/dL is considered normal. No increase in serum cortisol indicates the presence of adrenocortical insufficiency.

Diagnosis of secondary adrenocortical insufficiency in its early stages requires the low-dose test. It is also used for the diagnosis of chronic partial pituitary ACTH deficiency. This test involves the administration of 1 mcg of cosyntropin (Cortrosyn) as an IV bolus. Normally, an increase in cortisol occurs in 20 minutes. In patients with adrenocortical insufficiency, there is no increase in the serum cortisol level.

Overview of Cushing's Disease

Etiology and Pathophysiology

The cause of Cushing's disease is **adrenocortical excess**. In the majority of patients, the increased adrenocortical function results from excessive corticotropin, leading to hyperplasia of the adrenal cortex. In a smaller percentage of patients, it is the result of a cortisol-secreting adrenal tumor, whether from too much corticotropin (ACTH) or a primary tumor of the adrenal gland. A malignant tumor of the adrenal gland can produce many corticosteroids, whereas the benign adrenal tumor only produces one corticosteroid that is secreted by the adrenal gland. Other, much less common causes are hyperplasia of the adrenal gland or ectopic production of ACTH by malignancies such as bronchogenic carcinoma (Smeltzer et al., 2010). Long-term treatment with pharmacological glucocorticoids leads to iatrogenic Cushing's syndrome.

Clinical Manifestations

Patients with Cushing's disease often present with classic signs and symptoms. These include obesity, with a heavy trunk and thin extremities; a fatty "buffalo hump" at the neck and supraclavicular region; and a moon-faced appearance. The skin becomes fragile and tears easily, and broad purple striae and bruises may develop. Wound healing may be impaired. The hair is thin. Women have virilization with the appearance of masculine traits such as increased facial hair, breast atrophy, enlarged clitoris, disrupted menses, and voice deepening. Libido is diminished or absent in men and women. Depression, weakness, and lassitude may also occur.

The excessive secretion of corticotropin leads to osteoporosis and fractures, which are caused by the increase in calcium reabsorption from the bone. Blood glucose levels are also increased, and glucose intolerance may occur as a result of increased hepatic gluconeogenesis and resistance to insulin. Peptic ulcers may develop because of increased secretion of gastric acid and pepsin.

Diagnosis

The diagnosis of Cushing's disease requires an overnight dexamethasone suppression test. The patient takes dexamethasone, a synthetic glucocorticoid, 1 mg orally at 11 PM. He or she then has a serum cortisol level drawn at 8 AM. A cortisol level of

TABLE 43.1

Drugs Administered for Addison's Disease

Drug Class	Prototypes	Other Drugs in the Class
Adrenocorticoid/ mineralocorticoids	Hydrocortisone cypionate (Cortef) Hydrocortisone sodium succinate (Solu-Cortef)	
Mineralocorticoids	Fludrocortisone acetate (Florinef Acetate)	

less than 5 mcg/dL indicates that the HPA axis is functioning normally. Cortisol levels are higher in patients with adrenal or ectopic tumors.

NCLEX Success

3. **A women receives a diagnosis of Cushing's disease. She has an excess of which of the following hormones?**

   A. luteinizing hormone
   B. glucose
   C. insulin
   D. corticotropin

4. **A man has a low level of adrenocorticotropic hormone and a high level of cortisol. What disease does he have?**

   A. Cushing's disease
   B. Addison's disease
   C. adrenal cortex hemorrhage
   D. myocardial infarction

Drugs Used to Treat Addison's Disease

The goal of treatment for Addison's disease is to replace the adrenocorticoids to correct adrenal insufficiency. It is important to replace both the mineralocorticoid and adrenocorticoid. Lifetime hormone replacement is necessary. Table 43.1 summarizes the adrenocorticoid and mineralocorticoids administered for the treatment of adrenocortical insufficiency.

ADRENOCORTICOIDS/ MINERALOCORTICOIDS

Ⓟ Hydrocortisone cypionate (Cortef) or **Ⓟ hydrocortisone sodium succinate** (Solu-Cortef) is a combination of a mineralocorticoid and adrenocorticoid. Both of these drugs are useful in acute and chronic adrenal insufficiency.

Pharmacokinetics and Action

The oral preparation of hydrocortisone has a 1- to 2-hour onset of action, a peak of action in 1 to 2 hours, and a duration of action of 1 to 1.5 days. The parenteral preparation of the drug has an immediate onset of action, an unknown peak of action, and a duration of action of 1 to 1.5 days. Metabolism occurs in the liver. Excretion is in the kidneys.

Action

Hydrocortisone enters the cells and binds to the receptors in the cytoplasm to decrease inflammation; it suppresses the migration of polymorphonuclear lymphocytes and decreases capillary permeability. The mineralocorticoid in the drug increases the retention of sodium.

Use

Health care providers used hydrocortisone to replace adrenocorticoids and mineralocorticoids in patients with Addison's disease. The drug is also useful in congenital adrenal hyperplasia. Table 43.2 gives route and dosage information for adrenocorticoids and mineralocorticoids.

TABLE 43.2

DRUGS AT A GLANCE: Adrenocorticoids/Mineralocorticoids and Mineralocorticoids

Drug	Pregnancy Category	Routes and Dosage Ranges	
		Adults	Children
Ⓟ **Hydrocortisone cypionate** (Cortef)	C	20–30 mg PO daily	Doses must be individualized by monitoring growth, bone age, and hormonal levels
Ⓟ **Hydrocortisone sodium succinate** (Solu-Cortef)	C	100–500 mg IV and every 2, 4, or 6 h based on condition and response	Doses must be individualized by monitoring growth, bone age, and hormonal levels
Ⓟ **Fludrocortisone acetate** (Florinef Acetate)	C	0.05–0.2 mg/d PO with ranges of 0.1 mg 3 times per week	0.05–0.1 mg/d

Use in Children

It is necessary to individualize the dose depending on the severity of the adrenal insufficiency and the response to the medication. The drug may affect growth velocity, and it is important to carefully assess growth and development with infants and children. Also, the nurse assesses neonate's respiratory status closely after the administration of parenteral hydrocortisone. Some preparations contain benzyl alcohol, which may cause gasping syndrome in neonates.

Use in Older Adults

Elderly people should receive the lowest possible dosage because of the increased risk of adverse effects with systemic corticosteroids.

Adverse Effects

Hydrocortisone has significant adverse effects, including the following:

- Cardiac effects: fluctuations in blood pressure, shock, dysrhythmias, myocardial infarction, embolism, circulatory collapse, heart failure, and cardiac arrest
- Central nervous system (CNS) effects: vertigo, headache, and depression
- Dermatologic effects: fragile skin that tears easily, petechiae, ecchymoses
- Gastrointestinal (GI) effects: peptic or esophageal ulcers, pancreatitis, increased appetite, and weight gain
- Hematologic effects: sodium and fluid retention
- Metabolic effects: hyperglycemia and Cushing's syndrome
- Musculoskeletal effects: osteoporosis and spontaneous fractures (long-term administration)
- Reproductive (female) effects: amenorrhea and irregular menses
- Other effects: immunosuppression, muscle weakness, impaired wound healing, and anaphylaxis

Contraindications

Contraindications to hydrocortisone include a known hypersensitivity to the drug or any component of the formulation as well as a serious infection. A **BLACK BOX WARNING** ◆ states that patients who are being treated with hydrocortisone should not receive live virus vaccines.

Nursing Implications

Preventing Interactions

Several medications and herbal supplements interact with hydrocortisone, increasing or decreasing its effects (Boxes 43.1 and 43.2). Hydrocortisone has numerous other interactions. Combination of hydrocortisone with certain drugs may result in the following effects:

- Salicylates: increased serum salicylate levels
- Acetylcholinesterase drugs: diminished therapeutic effect
- Anticoagulants: increased bleeding; it is necessary to monitor the ProTime and the International Normalized Ratio closely
- Food: interference with calcium absorption
- Alcohol: increased risk of gastric mucosal irritation and development of gastric ulcers

---

EVIDENCE-BASED PRACTICE

Cortisone Replacement Therapy in Endocrine Disorders—Quality of Self-Care

by IGOR A. HARSCH, ANDREA SCULLER, ECKHART G. HAHN, & JOHANNES HENSEN

Journal of Evaluation in Clinical Practice, International Journal of Public Health Policy and Health Services Research
2010, 16, 492–498

The authors of this study developed a questionnaire to determine patients' knowledge of Addison's disease and the treatment of the disease with cortisone replacement therapy. The first part of the questionnaire obtained some demographic information about the patient as well as his or her disease, including the length of time since diagnosis and the number of episodes of Addisonian crisis. The second part of the questionnaire focused on the instructions the patient initially received about the disease and other sources he or she used to obtain information about the disease. The third part of the questionnaire assessed the knowledge the patient now has about the disease; it asked eight multiple choice questions about the disease and its treatment. The questionnaire also asked about the ideal manner in which they learned about the disease and its treatment. The participants reported that physicians were the main source of knowledge and that the media contributed to their knowledge base. Only half of the answers to the questions about the disease and its treatment were correct. The authors concluded that improving patients' knowledge about the disease and its treatment is important.

IMPLICATIONS FOR NURSING PRACTICE: Educating all patients about Addison's disease and related treatment is a primary task that nurses should undertake. Without the proper knowledge of any disease and its treatment, patients are at risk for the development of adverse effects of medications or medications being ineffective. Proper patient teaching helps provide safe and effective care.

BOX 43.1 Drug Interactions: Hydrocortisone

Drugs That Increase the Effects of Hydrocortisone

■ Estrogen, hormonal contraceptives, ketoconazole, troleandomycin

Increase steroid blood levels

Drugs That Decrease the Effects of Hydrocortisone

■ Cholestyramine, phenobarbital, phenytoin, rifampin

Decrease steroid blood levels

BOX 43.2 Herb and Dietary Interactions: Hydrocortisone

Herbs and Foods That Increase the Effects of Hydrocortisone

- Cat's claw
- Echinacea

Herbs and Foods That Decrease the Effects of Hydrocortisone

- St. John's wort

Administering the Medication

People should take the oral preparation with food to decrease gastric irritation.

QSEN Safety Alert

Administration of hydrocortisone should take place every morning before 9 AM. This minimizes HPA suppression.

It is necessary to dilute hydrocortisone sodium succinate to 50 mg/mL and administer the drug as an IV bolus over 30 seconds or over 10 minutes for doses *greater than or equal to* 500 mg. For intermittent IV infusion, dilution to 1 mg/mL and administration over 20 to 30 minutes is appropriate.

Assessing for Therapeutic Effects

The nurse assesses the patient's blood pressure, pulse, and respirations for improved cardiac function. He or she also assesses the sodium level and fluid volume status for return to normal range with retention of sodium and water. It is important to assess for increased strength and energy as well as for improved mood and ability to cope with stress.

Assessing for Adverse Effects

The nurse assesses for hypertension, heart failure, or alterations in cardiac output. It is important to assess for normal menses and diminished virilization in women. Also, the nurse checks the patient's ability to fight infection (e.g., is the white blood cell count normal?). In addition, he or she assesses the serum blood sugar to rule out hypoglycemia or hyperglycemia.

Patient Teaching

Box 43.3 presents patient teaching guidelines for hydrocortisone.

Clinical Application 43-2

- Mrs. James' endocrinologist orders hydrocortisone sodium succinate 200 mg intravenously every 4 hours. How does the nurse dilute the drug and over what period does he or she administer it?

BOX 43.3 Patient Teaching Guidelines for Hydrocortisone

- Take the oral preparation of hydrocortisone every day at 9:00 AM.
- Space other doses of hydrocortisone evenly throughout the day.
- Do not stop the medication abruptly or without notifying the prescriber.
- Inform the health care provider of increased stress. The dosage of the medication may need to be increased.
- Increase calcium intake if hydrocortisone is administered for a prolonged period.
- Administer antacids between doses of hydrocortisone to prevent gastric irritation.
- Monitor blood sugar daily.
- Wear a medic alert bracelet.
- Report swelling, weight gain, muscle weakness, tarry stools, moon face, fever, infection, inability of wounds to heal, and fatigue.

- One hour following the administration of the medication, the endocrinologist orders blood glucose testing. What is the rationale for blood glucose testing?
- What is the action of hydrocortisone sodium succinate?

MINERALOCORTICOIDS

If a patient with Addison's disease requires additional mineralocorticoid supplementation, then Ⓟ **fludrocortisone acetate** (Florinef Acetate), a synthetic steroid, is useful. A patient usually takes it in combination with a glucocorticoid.

It is important to note that fludrocortisone has proved effective for the treatment of orthostatic hypotension in older adults.

Pharmacokinetics and Action

Fludrocortisone is absorbed rapidly and completely and is 42% protein bound. The drug reaches a peak serum level in approximately 1.7 hours, and it has a 3.5-hour serum half-life. Metabolism occurs in the liver. The site of excretion is unknown.

Fludrocortisone has strong mineralocorticoid action. This drug produces sodium retention and potassium excretion to increase blood pressure.

Use

Health care providers use fludrocortisone for partial replacement of mineralocorticoids in the treatment of primary and secondary adrenocortical insufficiency resulting from Addison's disease.

Use in Children

In young children who have taken high doses of fludrocortisone for long periods, the drug may cause hypercortisism or suppression of the HPA axis. This suppression can lead to adrenal crisis.

Use in Older Adults

Use of fludrocortisone warrants caution in older adults because they are at risk for adverse effects of the drug. It is essential that the lowest possible dose is used for the shortest possible period.

Use in Patients With Hepatic Impairment

Patients with hepatic impairment or cirrhosis who take fludrocortisone for long periods require close monitoring for fluid retention.

Adverse Effects and Contraindications

The endocrine and metabolic effects of fludrocortisone are HPA axis suppression, growth suppression, hyperglycemia, and hypokalemia alkalosis. The most commonly reported cardiopulmonary adverse effects include heart failure, edema, and hypertension. Other adverse effects include peptic ulcer, acne, bruising, rash, cataracts, muscle weakness, and diaphoresis.

Contraindications include known hypersensitivity to the medication or any component of its formulation as well as a systemic fungal infection.

Nursing Implications

Preventing Interactions

Many medications interact with fludrocortisone, increasing or decreasing its effects (Box 43.4). Amphotericin B, indacaterol, loop diuretics, and thiazide diuretics in combination with fludrocortisone enhance the hypokalemic effect of

fludrocortisone. Warfarin in combination with fludrocortisone enhances the anticoagulant effect, placing the patient at risk for hemorrhage.

Administering the Medication

People should take fludrocortisone concomitantly with a glucocorticoid to enhance effectiveness and produce a more normal adrenal response. It is necessary to store the drug in an airtight, light-protected container at 59°F to 86°F.

Assessing for Therapeutic Effects

The nurse assesses sodium levels for increased values and potassium levels for decreased values. It is also important to assess intake, output, and blood pressure. The nurse monitors the patient's weight and assesses fluid volume status. If the weight increases by 5 pounds in 1 week, it is necessary to notify the prescriber.

Assessing for Adverse Effects

In children, it is essential to assess growth patterns. In all patients, the nurse assesses the patient's fluid and electrolyte status for hypokalemia and alkalosis. He or she assesses for pedal edema, hypertension, crackles in the lungs, and an audible S_3 that is indicative of heart failure. It is important to assess the GI system for burning, epigastric pain, and bleeding, which are signs of peptic ulcer disease. The nurse assesses the skin for bruising and rash. He or she also assesses for muscle weakness.

Patient Teaching

Box 43.5 contains patient teaching guidelines for fludrocortisone.

BOX 43.4 | Drug Interactions: Fludrocortisone

Drugs That Decrease the Effects of Fludrocortisone

■ Acetylcholinesterase inhibitors, neuromuscular agents
  Increase muscle weakness
■ Aminoglutethimide
  Increases metabolism of fludrocortisone
■ Antacids
  Decrease bioavailability of fludrocortisone
■ Barbiturates, primidone
  Decrease serum concentration of fludrocortisone

Drugs That Increase the Effects of Fludrocortisone

■ Antifungal agents, calcium channel blockers, macrolide antibiotics
  Decrease the metabolism of corticosteroids
■ Aprepitant, estrogens, fosaprepitant, mifepristone, mitotane, telaprevir
  Increase serum concentration of fludrocortisone

BOX 43.5 | Patient Teaching Guidelines for Fludrocortisone

■ Eat foods high in potassium such as bananas, potatoes, and orange juice.
■ Consume foods high in calcium and vitamins A and D such as dairy products.
■ Take supplements containing vitamins B6 and C, folate, zinc, and phosphorous.
■ Decrease sodium in the diet and limit salt intake.
■ Report muscle weakness, numbness, fatigue, depression, increased urination, changes in heart rhythm, epigastric pain, and tarry stools.
■ Monitor weight and report an increase of 5 pounds to the primary health care provider.
■ See an ophthalmologist every 6 months to determine if cataracts have formed.
■ Have periodic laboratory tests as ordered by the prescriber.
■ Report swelling of feet, hands, and shortness of breath to the primary health care provider.
■ Report any infections or injuries to the primary health care provider.
■ Wear medical alert identification.

5. A patient is taking fludrocortisone acetate (Florinef Acetate) for adrenal insufficiency. Which of the following symptoms indicates that the patient is hypokalemic?

   A. tetany
   B. irregular pulse rate
   C. decreased pulse rate
   D. muscle weakness

6. The administration of fludrocortisone acetate (Florinef Acetate) is necessary in which of the following conditions?

   A. hypoglycemia
   B. hypernatremia
   C. hypercalcemia
   D. hyperphosphatemia

7. A woman receives a prescription of hydrocortisone for adrenal insufficiency. It is necessary to report which of the following conditions to the primary health care provider?

   A. fever
   B. headache
   C. insomnia
   D. neuropathic pain

Drugs Used to Treat Cushing's Disease

The treatment of Cushing's disease depends on the cause of the medical condition. The most common treatment of hypercortisolism is surgical (Nieman, 2011). Drug therapy is indicated in several situations: when surgery is contraindicated, in preparation for surgery, in occult ectopic ACTH syndrome, with a recurrence of hypercortisolism following surgery, and with treatment using radiation therapy to the pituitary (Nieman, 2011).

11-DEOXYCORTISOL INHIBITORS

In Cushing's disease, the goal of drug therapy is to inhibit one or more enzymes contained in cortisol synthesis. The antifungal drug (see Chapter 22) ℗ **ketoconazole** (Nizoral) has the ability to inhibit these enzymes. It also prevents the conversion of 11-deoxycortisol to cortisol. Table 43.3 names the drugs administered for the treatment of Cushing's disease.

Pharmacokinetics and Action

Ketoconazole is absorbed rapidly in the GI tract. The drug is protein bound. It is metabolized in the liver and excreted by the kidneys.

Ketoconazole acts by inhibiting the first step in cortisol biosynthesis and the conversion of deoxycortisol to cortisol.

Use

Health care providers use ketoconazole to control cortisol secretion in Cushing's disease. Table 43.4 presents route and dosage information for the drugs used in Cushing's disease.

Adverse Effects and Contraindications

The most commonly reported adverse effects associate with ketoconazole include pruritus, headache, sedation, nausea, vomiting, and abdominal pain. Gynecomastia, impotence, and decreased libido may occur and are related to the decrease in testosterone production. The U.S. Food and Drug Administration (FDA) has issued a **BLACK BOX WARNING** ◆ stating that ketoconazole can cause hepatotoxicity. Therefore, caution is warranted in patients with hepatic impairment.

Contraindications include a known hypersensitivity to the medication. It is essential that the drug not be administered with ergotamine agents, cisapride, or triazolam because of the risk of cardiac dysrhythmias.

Nursing Implications

Preventing Interactions

Some medications interact with ketoconazole, decreasing its effects (Box 43.6). Ketoconazole combined with echinacea puts the patient at risk for hepatotoxicity.

Administering the Medication

People should take ketoconazole with water, coffee, tea, or fruit juice. The presence of stomach acid enhances absorption.

Assessing for Therapeutic Effects and Adverse Effects

The nurse assesses for a decrease in blood pressure. He or she checks the blood glucose for normal levels. It is also important to assess for increased muscle strength and cardiopulmonary status without edema or crackles in the lower lobes and audible S_3.

Assessing for adverse effects is also necessary. The nurse assesses for skin irritation and pruritus; nausea, vomiting, and headache; and diminished libido, gynecomastia, and impotence.

TABLE 43.3

Drugs Administered for Cushing's Disease

Drug Class	Prototype	Other Drugs in the Class
11-deoxycortisol inhibitors	Ketoconazole	Metyrapone (Metopirone) Etomidate (Amidate)
Antineoplastics	Mitotane (Lysodren)	

TABLE 43.4

DRUGS AT A GLANCE: 11-Deoxycortisol Inhibitors and Antineoplastics

Drug	Pregnancy Category	Routes and Dosage Ranges	
		Adults	Children
11-Deoxycortisol Inhibitors			
℗ **Ketoconazole**	C	200–400 mg PO 2–3 times per day	Not administered to children
Metyrapone (Metopirone)	C	250 mg PO 4 times daily (max dose 6000 mg)	Diagnostic test for hypothalamic–pituitary adrenocorticotropic hormone (ACTH) function: single dose, 30 mg/kg at midnight; multiple dose, 15 mg/kg every 4 h for 6 doses
Etomidate		0.3 mg/kg IV per hour	Same as adults
Antineoplastics			
℗ **Mitotane** (Lysodren)		Adrenocortical carcinoma: 2–6 g/d in 3–4 divided doses, then increase incrementally to 9–10 g/d in 3–4 divided doses; max tolerated range is 2–16 g/d, usually 9–10 g/d; max studied dose is 18–19 g/d Cushing's syndrome: 500 mg PO 3 times per day; max dose 3000 mg 3 times per day	Safety and efficacy not established

Patient Teaching

Box 43.7 presents patient teaching guidelines for ketoconazole.

Other Drugs in the Class

Metyrapone and etomidate are also administered for their inhibition of 11-deoxycortisol. Metyrapone (Metopirone) blocks the final step in cortisol biosynthesis and increases adrenal androgen production. The drug also decreases cortisol production. It is administered as an adjunctive agent to prevent further release of ACTH in patients with mild Cushing's disease or following radiation therapy of the pituitary gland.

Etomidate (Amidate) also blocks the production of cortisol. Normally administered to produce sedation, it is a local anesthetic and is discussed in Chapter 50. Prescribers order it for patients with ectopic secretion of ACTH. Etomidate lowers serum cortisol to normal in approximately 10 hours.

ANTINEOPLASTICS

Health care providers use the antineoplastic drug ℗ **mitotane** (Lysodren) for the treatment of adrenocortical carcinoma. The drug may also be useful for therapy of Cushing's disease caused by such carcinoma.

Pharmacokinetics and Action

Mitotane is absorbed rapidly, with approximately 40% of the drug absorbed in the GI tract. The onset of action is 2 to 4 weeks. The half-life of mitotane is 18 to 159 days. The drug is metabolized in the liver and deposited in the adipose tissues. It is eliminated in the urine and feces.

Mitotane is an adrenolytic agent that causes the adrenal cortex to atrophy. The drug affects the mitochondrial adrenal

---

BOX 43.6 | **Drug Interactions: Ketoconazole**

Drugs That Decrease the Effects of Ketoconazole
- Antacids, anticholinergics
  Decrease absorption, thus decreasing serum levels
- Isoniazid, rifampin
  Increase metabolism

BOX 43.7 | **Patient Teaching Guidelines for Ketoconazole**

- Take the medication with water, coffee, tea, or fruit juice. Acidic drinks enhance absorption.
- Take the drug with food to prevent gastrointestinal upset.
- Do not take antacids.
- Maintain serum liver enzyme laboratory tests as ordered by the prescriber.
- Report clay-colored stools, extreme thirst, yellowing of skin or eyes. These signs and symptoms indicate elevated liver enzymes.

cortical cells, resulting in decreased production of cortisol. It also alters the peripheral metabolism of steroids.

Use

Mitotane is used for the treatment of an inoperable adrenocortical carcinoma. Its unlabeled use is for treatment of Cushing's syndrome. Table 43.4 gives route and dosing information for mitotane.

Adverse Effects and Contraindications

The CNS effects of mitotane include depression, lethargy, and dizziness. GI effects are anorexia, nausea, vomiting, and diarrhea. Neuromuscular effects include weakness and muscle tremors.

Contraindications include known hypersensitivity to the drug.

Nursing Implications

Preventing Interactions

Mitotane increases the metabolism of phenytoin, phenobarbital, and warfarin. The antineoplastic drug decreases the effect of potassium-sparing diuretics. Alcohol increases the CNS depression associated with mitotane.

Administering the Medication

The FDA has issued a **BLACK BOX WARNING** ◆ stating that it is necessary to withhold mitotane in the event the patient develops shock or with trauma, because the primary action of the drug is adrenal suppression. The onset of shock or trauma should lead to a temporary discontinuation of mitotane followed by the administration of steroids.

QSEN Safety Alert ▼

The Institute for Safe Medication Practices considers mitotane to be a drug that has a heightened risk of causing significant patient harm when used in error.

Assessing for Therapeutic Effects

The nurse assesses for a decrease in blood pressure. It is necessary to check the blood glucose for normal levels. The nurse also assesses for increased muscle strength and cardiopulmonary status without edema or crackles in the lower lobes and audible S_3.

Assessing for Adverse Effects

The nurse assesses for CNS depression. Such depression may place the patient at risk for injury. It is also important to assess the gait for safety with walking. The nurse assesses for decreased weight related to anorexia or fluid and electrolyte balance related to nausea and vomiting, as well as for muscle weakness and tremors.

Patient Teaching

Box 43.8 presents patient teaching guidelines for mitotane.

BOX 43.8   Patient Teaching Guidelines for Mitotane

- Understand that this drug will decrease the tumor mass but will not cure the disease.
- Report signs and symptoms of adrenal insufficiency, including weakness, fatigue, orthostatic hypotension, nausea, anorexia, vomiting, increase skin pigmentation, and weight loss.
- Do not operate machinery due to diminished alertness and central nervous system depression.

NCLEX Success

8. A woman has received a diagnosis of Cushing's disease and is taking ketoconazole. Which of the following conditions affects the treatment plan?

   A. hypertension with administration of hydrochlorothiazide
   B. type 2 diabetes with the administration of metformin
   C. migraine headaches with the administration of ergotamine
   D. heart failure with the administration of digoxin

9. A man is receiving mitotane for an inoperable adrenocortical carcinoma. He is admitted to the emergency department following an automobile accident. He is diaphoretic and unresponsive. He has a blood pressure of 80/0 mm Hg. What medication should a nurse administer?

   A. a steroid
   B. an anticoagulant
   C. a beta blocker
   D. a sulfonylurea

10. A patient is taking ketoconazole for the treatment of Cushing's disease. When providing patient teaching, which of the following is most important?

    A. Take antibiotics at the first sign of a sore throat.
    B. Have prothrombin times drawn monthly.
    C. Salt cravings mean that it is fine to increase salt intake.
    D. Take the medication with juice or an acidic beverage.

The Nursing Process

Assessment

- For the patient with Addison's disease, the major focus of the assessment should be on the severity of symptoms and the effectiveness of drug therapy for the treatment of the disease. Assess for the following:
  - Dehydration and hypovolemia
  - Nutritional status, blood glucose, and muscle weakness
  - Skin pigmentation for darkened areas
  - Mental status for depression

Drugs Affecting Women's and Men's Health

44 Drug Therapy for Women's Health

Clinical Application Case Study

Paula Bigelow, a 52-year-old woman, has been complaining of vaginal dryness, hot flashes, and night sweats for the past 6 months. She reports that her last normal menstrual period was over 1 year ago.

KEY TERMS

Estrogen: hormone produced primarily by the ovaries and secondarily by the adrenal cortex; promotes growth of specific body cells and development of most female secondary sexual characteristics

Menopause: permanent end of menstrual periods, which usually occurs in women 48 to 55 years of age

Progesterone: hormone produced in the ovaries and adrenal cortex; prepares the lining of the uterus for pregnancy

Progestin: synthetic form of progesterone that is similar to the hormone produced naturally by the body; most often used in combination with an estrogen in contraceptive products

Introduction

This chapter focuses on drug therapy in women's health care. **Estrogen** and **progesterone** are female sex hormones produced primarily by the ovaries and secondarily by the adrenal cortex in nonpregnant women. Small amounts of estrogens are also synthesized in the liver, kidney, brain, skeletal muscle, testes, and adipose tissue. In normal premenopausal women, estrogen synthesis in adipose tissue may be a significant source of the hormone. Some evidence indicates that a minimum body weight (about 105 lb) and fat content (16%–24%) are required for initiation and maintenance of the menstrual cycle. The observation that women with anorexia nervosa, chronic disease, or malnutrition, as well as women who engage in long-distance running, usually have amenorrhea supports this view. With anorexia nervosa, regaining weight and body mass usually reestablishes normal menstrual patterns.

As with other steroid hormones, estrogen and progesterone are synthesized from cholesterol. The ovaries and adrenal glands can manufacture cholesterol or extract it from the blood. Through a series of chemical reactions, cholesterol is converted to progesterone and then to androgens, testosterone, and androstenedione. The ovaries use these male sex hormones to produce estrogens. After formation, the hormones are secreted into the bloodstream in response to stimulation by the anterior pituitary gonadotropic hormones, follicle-stimulating hormone (FSH), and luteinizing hormone (LH). In the bloodstream, the hormones combine with serum proteins and are transported to target tissues, where they enter body cells. They cross cell membranes easily because of their steroid structure and lipid solubility. Inside the cells, the hormones bind to estrogen or progesterone receptors and regulate intracellular protein synthesis. Estrogen can enhance target-tissue responses to progesterone by increasing progesterone receptors. Progesterone seems to inhibit tissue responses to estrogen by decreasing estrogen receptors.

Overview of Reproduction in Women

To adequately understand the pharmacologic effects of estrogens and **progestins** (synthetic progesterone), it is important to understand the physiology of female reproductive hormones and the menstrual cycle.

Physiology

Estrogens

The main function of the estrogens is to promote growth in tissues related to reproduction and sexual characteristics in women. Estrogens also have specific effects on other body tissues (Box 44.1). Three ovarian estrogens (estradiol, estrone, and estriol, known as endogenous estrogens) are secreted in significant amounts. Estradiol is the major estrogen because it exerts more estrogenic activity than the other two estrogens combined.

In nonpregnant women, between puberty and **menopause** (permanent end of menstrual periods), estrogens are secreted in a monthly cycle called the menstrual cycle. During the first half of the cycle, before ovulation, estrogens are secreted in progressively larger amounts. During the second half of the cycle, estrogens and progesterone are secreted in increasing amounts until 2 to 3 days before the onset of menstruation. At that time, secretion of both hormones decreases abruptly. When the endometrial lining of the uterus loses its hormonal stimulation, it is discharged vaginally as menstrual flow.

During pregnancy, the placenta in conjunction with the fetus produces large amounts of estrogen causing enlargement of the uterus and breasts, growth of glandular tissue in the breasts, and relaxation of ligaments and joints in the pelvis. All these changes are necessary for the growth and birth of the fetus.

Finally, estrogens are deactivated in the liver and readily excreted through the kidneys. Metabolites are also formed in the gastrointestinal (GI) tract, brain, skin, and other steroid target tissues. Most of the conjugates are excreted in urine, and some are excreted in bile and recirculated to the liver or excreted in feces.

Progesterone

In general, progesterone has different effects on lipid metabolism compared with estrogen. That is, progesterones decrease high-density lipoprotein (HDL) cholesterol and increase low-density lipoprotein (LDL) cholesterol, both of which increase the risk of cardiovascular disease. Physiologic progesterone increases insulin levels but does not usually impair glucose tolerance. However, long-term administration of potent synthetic exogenous progestins, such as norgestrel, may decrease glucose tolerance and make diabetes mellitus more difficult to control. Like estrogen, progesterone is metabolized in the liver.

In nonpregnant women, progesterone is secreted by the corpus luteum during the last half of the menstrual cycle, which occurs after ovulation. This hormone continues the changes in the endometrial lining of the uterus begun by estrogens during the first half of the menstrual cycle. These changes provide for implantation and nourishment of a fertilized ovum. When fertilization does not take place, the estrogen and progesterone levels decrease and menstruation occurs.

If the ovum is fertilized, progesterone acts to maintain the pregnancy. The corpus luteum produces progesterone during the first few weeks of gestation. Then, the placenta produces the progesterone needed to maintain the endometrial lining of the uterus. In addition to its effects on the uterus, progesterone prepares the breasts for lactation by promoting development of milk-producing cells. Milk is not secreted, however, until the cells are further stimulated by prolactin from the anterior pituitary gland. Progesterone also may help maintain pregnancy by decreasing uterine contractility. This, in turn, decreases the risk of spontaneous abortion.

Menstrual Cycle

The menstrual cycle consists of the follicular phase (days 1–14) and the luteal phase (days 15–28). Hormones in the

BOX 44.1	Effects of Endogenous Estrogens

Breasts

■ Stimulate growth at puberty by causing deposition of fat, formation of connective tissue, and construction of ducts. These ducts become part of the milk-producing apparatus after additional stimulation by progesterone.

Sexual Organs

■ Enlarge the fallopian tubes, uterus, vagina, and external genitalia at puberty, when estrogen secretion increases greatly

■ Cause the endometrial lining of the uterus to proliferate and develop glands that later nourish the implanted ovum when pregnancy occurs

■ Increase resistance of the epithelial lining of the vagina to trauma and infection

Skeleton

■ Stimulate skeletal growth so that, beginning at puberty, height increases rapidly for several years. Estrogen then causes the epiphyses to unite with the shafts of the long bones, and linear growth is halted. This effect of estrogen is stronger than the similar effect of testosterone in the male. Consequently, women stop growing in height several years earlier than men and on the average are shorter than men.

■ Conserve calcium and phosphorus for healthy bones and teeth. This action promotes bone formation and decreases bone loss.

■ Broaden the pelvis in preparation for childbirth

Skin and Subcutaneous Tissue

■ Increase vascularity in the skin. This leads to greater skin warmth and likelihood of bleeding in women.

■ Cause deposition of fat in subcutaneous tissue, especially in the breasts, thighs, and buttocks, which produces the characteristic female figure

Anterior Pituitary Gland

■ Decrease pituitary secretion of follicle-stimulating hormone and increase secretion of luteinizing hormone when blood levels are sufficiently high (negative feedback mechanism)

Metabolism

■ Affect metabolism of both reproductive and nonreproductive tissues. Estrogen receptors are found in female reproductive organs, breast tissue, bone, the brain, liver, heart, and blood vessels. They are also found in various tissues in men.

■ Increase protein anabolism, bone growth, and epiphyseal closure in young girls

■ Decrease bone resorption

■ Increase sodium and water retention, serum triglycerides, and high-density lipoproteins (HDL or "good" cholesterol)

■ Decrease low-density lipoproteins (LDLs or "bad" cholesterol)

■ Increase the amount of cholesterol in bile and thereby increase gallstone formation

Blood Coagulation

■ Enhance coagulation by increasing blood levels of several clotting factors, including prothrombin and factors VII, IX, and X, and probably increase platelet aggregation

hypothalamus, pituitary gland, and ovary regulate this cycle. The usual length of a complete menstrual cycle is 28 days, and the first day of menstrual bleeding is day 1.

Figure 44.1 shows how the hormones interact in this cycle. Initially, the hypothalamus releases gonadotropin-releasing hormone (GnRH), which causes the anterior pituitary gland to produce FSH in the follicular phase of the cycle. FSH results in the maturing of ovarian follicles, which in turn produce estrogens. Increasing estrogen levels result in the continued maturation of the ovarian follicle and increasing growth of the endometrium. A negative feedback system responds to the increasing amounts of estrogen by decreasing the amount FSH. At midcycle (typically day 14 of a 28-day menstrual cycle), the anterior pituitary gland releases LH, resulting in the rupture of the ovarian follicle and the development of the corpus luteum. This process is ovulation. The corpus luteum releases progesterone and estrogen, which causes the endometrial lining to continue to increase in thickness and vascularity. If fertilization of the ovum does not occur, the corpus luteum atrophies, resulting in the reduced production of estrogen and progesterone. As estrogen and progesterone levels continue to decrease, the endometrium begins to

regress, causing menstruation, and the beginning of another menstrual cycle.

Drug Therapy

Women may take exogenous estrogens and progestins at various stages in the reproductive cycle. When exogenous estrogens and progestins are administered for therapeutic purposes, they produce the same effects as endogenous hormones. Multiple preparations of estrogens and progestins are available for various purposes and in several forms. Clinical indications, routes of administration, and dosages are presented in the Drugs at a Glance tables.

Clinical Application 44-1

■ Mrs. Bigelow has her FSH level measured, as ordered by her physician. Assuming Mrs. Bigelow has completed menopause, would the nurse expect the FSH levels to be high or low? Why?

TABLE 44.1

DRUGS AT A GLANCE: Estrogens

Drug	Pregnancy Category	Menopausal Symptoms	Female Hypogonadism	Prevention of Osteoporosis	Other
P **Conjugated estrogens, equine** (Premarin)	X	PO 0.3 mg–1.25 mg daily for 21 d followed by 7 d without the drug	PO 2.5–7.5 mg daily in divided doses, cyclically, 20 d on, 10 d off the drug	PO 0.625 mg daily for 21 d, then 7 d without the drug	Dysfunctional uterine bleeding: IM or IV for emergency use, 25 mg, repeated in 6–12 h if necessary. Atrophic vaginitis: topical, 2.4 g of vaginal cream inserted daily
Conjugated estrogens A, (synthetic) (Cenestin)	X	PO 0.3–1.25 mg daily			
Conjugated estrogens B, (synthetic) (Enjuvia)	X	PO 0.3–1.25 daily			
Esterified estrogens (Menest)	X	PO 0.3–1.25 mg daily	PO 2.5–7.5 mg daily in divided doses, cyclically, 20 d on, 10 d off the drug		Breast cancer (inoperable, progressing): PO 10 mg three times a day for at least 3 months in selected postmenopausal women
Estradiol acetate (Femtrace)	X	PO 0.45–1.8 mg daily or daily for 3 wk, then 1 wk off			
Estradiol cypionate (Depo-Estradiol)	X	IM 1–5 mg every 3–4 wk	IM 1.5–2 mg at monthly intervals		
Estradiol hemihydrate (Vagifem)	X				Atrophic vaginitis: 10 mcg/tablet, inserted into vagina, daily for 2 wk, then twice weekly
Estradiol, micronized (Estrace, oral or vaginal cream; Estring, vaginal ring)	X	PO 0.5–2 mg daily for 3 wk, then 1 wk off or daily Monday through Friday, none on Saturday or Sunday as prescribed		PO 0.5 mg daily for 23 d and no drug for 5 d each month	Atrophic vaginitis: Cream, 2–4 g daily for 2 wk, then 1–2 g daily for 2 wk, then 1 g 1–3 times weekly; vaginal ring (Estring), 1 every 3 mo

TABLE 44.1

DRUGS AT A GLANCE: Estrogens (Continued)

Drug	Pregnancy Category	Menopausal Symptoms	Female Hypogonadism	Prevention of Osteoporosis	Other
Estradiol transdermal system (Climara, Estraderm, Menostar, Vivelle, Vivelle-Dot, Estrasorb, Estrogel, Evamist)	X	Climara: 0.025–0.1 mg/d topically to skin every week; Estraderm: 0.05–0.1mg/d topically to skin, one patch 2 times per week; Menostar: 0.014 mg/d applied topically each week; Vivelle: 0.05–0.1 mg/d topically to skin 2 times per week; Vivelle-Dot: 0.025–0.1 mg/d topically to skin two times per week; Estrasorb (topical lotion; 1.74 g/ pouch): 2 pouches applied topically to legs every day; Estrogel (topical gel; 1.25 g per pump): One pump applied topically everyday; Evamist (topical spray; 1.53 mg per spray): One spray applied topically everyday		Climara: 0.025–0.1 mg/d topically to skin every week; Estraderm: 0.05–0.1 mg/d topically to skin, one patch 2 times per week Menostar: 0.014 mg/d applied topically each week; Vivelle: 0.05–0.1 mg/d applied topically; Vivelle-Dot: 0.025–0.1 mg/d topically to skin 2 times per week	
Estradiol valerate (Delestrogen)	X	IM 10–20 mg every 4 wk	IM 10–20 mg every 4 wk		
Estrone	X	IM 0.1–0.5 mg weekly in single or divided doses	IM 0.1–2 mg weekly		Dysfunctional uterine bleeding: IM 2–4 mg daily for several days until bleeding is controlled, followed by progestin for 1 wk
Estropipate (Ogen)	X	PO 0.625–5 mg daily, cyclically	PO 1.25–7.5 mg daily for 3 wk, followed by a rest period of 8–10 d. Repeat as needed	PO 0.625 mg daily for 25 d and no drug for 6 d each month	Ovarian failure: same dosage as for female hypogonadism Atrophic vaginitis: topical, 1–2 g vaginal cream daily

hyperplasia and may cause endometrial cancer. Women with an intact uterus should also be given a progestin, which opposes the effects of estrogen on the endometrium. Opinions differ regarding estrogens as a cause of breast cancer. Most studies indicate little risk; a few indicate some risk, especially with high doses for prolonged periods (i.e., 10 years or longer). However, estrogens do stimulate growth in breast cancers that have estrogen receptors.

The U.S. Food and Drug Administration (FDA) has issued a **BLACK BOX WARNING** ◆ regarding estrogen use; supervised use at the lowest dose for the shortest duration should be prescribed. Estrogens are associated with the following:

- An increased risk of endometrial cancer. Estrogens should not be used alone in women with an intact uterus.
- An increased risk of thromboembolic events such as myocardial infarction, stroke, deep vein thrombosis, and pulmonary embolism. Estrogens (with or without progestins) should not be used for the prevention of cardiovascular disease.
- An increased risk of dementia in postmenopausal women. Estrogens should not be used for the prevention of dementia.
- An increased risk of breast cancer development in women taking estrogen–progestin combinations.

Box 44.2 provides information about the studies on which these warnings are based.

Contraindications

Estrogens have a wide variety of effects on body tissues and a number of reported adverse reactions. Therefore, the list of contraindications is long. It is important to avoid using estrogens in the following situations:

- Known or suspected pregnancy, because teratogenic effects capable of interfering with the normal development of the fetus may result
- Thromboembolic disorders, such as thrombophlebitis, deep vein thrombosis, or pulmonary embolism
- Known or suspected cancers of breast or genital tissues, because the drugs may stimulate tumor growth. An exception is the use of estrogens for treatment of metastatic breast cancer in women at least 5 years postmenopause.
- Undiagnosed vaginal or uterine bleeding
- Fibroid tumors of the uterus
- Active liver disease, including liver cancer, impaired liver function
- History of cerebrovascular disease, coronary artery disease, thrombophlebitis, hypertension, or conditions predisposing to these disease processes
- Tobacco use. Women who smoke cigarettes have a greater risk of thromboembolic disorders if they take estrogen supplements, possibly because of increased platelet aggregation with estrogen ingestion and cigarette smoking. In addition, estrogen increases hepatic production of blood-clotting factors.
- Family history of breast or reproductive system cancer

BOX 44.2 Hormone Replacement Therapy in Postmenopausal Women

From the 1980s until mid-2002, long-term postmenopausal estrogen replacement therapy was frequently recommended for women, with the expectation that it would manage menopausal symptoms, exert cardioprotective effects, prevent osteoporosis, and prolong life. Two large-scale randomized controlled trials, the Heart and Estrogen/Progestin Replacement Study (HERS) and the Women's Health Initiative (WHI), disputed this prevailing observational data and expert opinion.

- The HERS and HERS II studies involved postmenopausal women with an intact uterus who already had coronary heart disease (CHD). Results indicated that in women who had preexisting heart disease, the hormones in hormone replacement therapy (HRT) provided no benefit in relation to preventing serious cardiovascular events; this increased interest in the NIH-funded WHI trials that were designed to evaluate primary prevention.
- The WHI study was conducted in healthy women to determine if an estrogen–progestin combination (in women with an intact uterus) or estrogen alone (in postmenopausal women who have had a hysterectomy) would prevent the development of CHD.
- Both arms of the WHI study were stopped in the interest of safety. The consensus was that with estrogen-only therapy in posthysterectomy women, the hormone increased the risk of stroke and offered no protection against heart disease. As with healthy women, the conclusion of the WHI was that the

hormones should not be started or continued for preventive purposes in women with CHD because risks were greater than benefits.

- In the arm of the study looking at postmenopausal women who have had a hysterectomy and thus do not need a progestin, estrogen-only therapy significantly increased the hazard of deep vein thrombosis and had no significant effect on the risk of colorectal or breast cancer. A reduced risk of hip and other fractures was reported. A related study also found that the hormone might also increase the risk of dementia and mild cognitive impairment in older women.
- A WHI substudy determined that there is an increased risk of invasive breast cancer in women taking estrogen–progestin combination.
- In summary, studies have demonstrated no evidence for HRT in secondary prevention of heart disease and showed increased rates of CHD, thromboembolic stroke, venous thromboembolism, dementia, and breast cancer, which outweigh the benefits of decreased risk of fracture and colon cancer. Thromboembolic disorders are most likely to occur during the first year of use, and the risk of developing breast cancer increases with the duration of drug use. FDA recommended that HRT only be used for women with symptoms severe enough to warrant its use, at the lowest dose and for the shortest duration possible, to ease the menopausal transition.

Nursing Implications

An important nursing implication associated with estrogen use is the identification of those factors that result in the contraindication of estrogen use in high-risk women. Identification of these at-risk women can be accomplished through the completion of a thorough medical and social history. This history should assess for menopausal symptoms, cardiovascular disease (hypertension, hyperlipidemia, and cerebrovascular risk), gynecological history (menstrual history, last menstrual period, and age at menopause), cancer history, and history of smoking. It is also necessary to obtain a family history relating to menopause, osteoporosis, cardiovascular disease, cerebral vascular disease, and cognitive disease, as well as allergy status. In the careful screening of any high-risk woman, the nurse assesses the blood pressure, weight, height, and pregnancy status. He or she also ensures that a lipid panel is taken. A clinical breast examination with a mammogram and pelvic examination are essential.

Preventing Interactions

Several drugs interact with estrogens, decreasing their effect (Box 44.3). With corticosteroids and estrogen, increased therapeutic effects and a risk of toxicity of the corticosteroids occur. Use of ropinirole with estrogen may require a dosage adjustment of the estrogen. Estrogens have a decreased effect on tamoxifen, sulfonylurea antidiabetic drugs, and anticoagulants, especially warfarin. St. John's wort increases the breakdown of estrogen, which may decrease the effectiveness of birth control pills.

Administering the Medication

Choice of preparation depends on the reason for use, desired route of administration, and duration of action. Although dosage needs vary with women and the health conditions for which the drugs are prescribed, a general rule is to use the smallest effective dose for the shortest effective time. Estrogens are often given cyclically. In one regimen, the drug is taken for 3 weeks and then omitted for 1 week; in another, it is omitted the first 5 days of the month. These regimens more closely resemble normal secretion of estrogen and avoid prolonged stimulation of body tissues. It is necessary to give naturally occurring, nonconjugated estrogens (estradiol, estrone) intramuscularly because they are rapidly metabolized if administered orally. Administration of nonsteroidal synthetic preparations is usually oral or topical. Women may take estrogen with food or at bedtime to decrease nausea, a common adverse reaction.

Transdermal estradiol (e.g., Climara, Estraderm, Vivelle) allows for absorption of estrogen through the skin to the bloodstream. Depending on the preparation, patients apply the patches weekly or biweekly. The total amount of drug absorbed and the resulting plasma drug concentrations from transdermal estrogen can increase during exposure to heat. The nurse should ensure that patients are advised to avoid prolonged sun exposure in the area of the patch.

Assessing for Therapeutic Effects

The therapeutic effects of estrogen vary depending on the reason of use. When treatment of menopausal symptoms is the goal, it is essential to assess for the decrease in hot flashes, vaginal dryness, and night sweats. When amenorrhea is the target, the occurrence of menstruation indicates that the hormone is working. When female hypogonadism is the treatment goal, the occurrence of menstruation and the presence of breast enlargement, axillary and pubic hair, and other secondary sexual characteristics indicate proper actions of the medication. When prevention of osteoporosis is the objective, the therapeutic effect includes the absence of bone fractures.

Assessing for Adverse Effects

The nurse should assess for the adverse effects of estrogen through the use of a history and physical examination. A careful assessment with each visit regarding the new onset of abdominal pain, chest pain, headache, vision change, and leg pain is essential in the early recognition of a potential blood clot. The nurse should ensure that blood pressure, glucose, lipid panel, pelvic examination (with Papanicolaou [Pap] smear), and mammography are monitored routinely based on the age of the patient.

Patient Teaching

Box 44.4 presents patient teaching guidelines for estrogens.

BOX 44.4

Patient Teaching Guidelines for Estrogens, Progestins, and Estrogen–Progestin Combinations

- Take your weight weekly, and report sudden weight gain to your health care provider. (Such weight gain may be due to fluid retention and edema.)
- Report any unusual vaginal bleeding immediately to your health care provider.
- Discuss the increased thromboembolic risk associated with smoking while using estrogens or progestins.
- Know the warning signs that may occur if a thromboembolism should develop—think ACHES (severe) abdominal pain, chest pain, headache, eye changes, severe leg pain. Seek medical attention immediately if such symptoms occur.
- If taking estrogen for long periods, have a physical examination at least annually. Have your blood pressure checked, as well as a breast and pelvic examination. Adverse conditions may occur when these drugs are taken for long periods. Your health care provider needs to monitor for adverse drug effects such as high blood pressure, gallbladder disease, and blood-clotting disorders.

BOX 44.3

Drug Interactions: Estrogens

Drugs That Decrease the Effects of Estrogen

- Anticonvulsants, such as carbamazepine, oxcarbazepine, phenytoin, and topiramate
  Induce enzymes that accelerate the metabolism of estrogens
- Barbiturates and rifampin
  Induce enzymes that accelerate inactivation of estrogens

Clinical Application 44-2

- Mrs. Bigelow receives a diagnosis of menopause. She inquires about hormone replacement therapy. What additional information does the nurse need to provide the best information?
- Mrs. Bigelow has no absolute contraindications to hormone replacement therapy, and her physician prescribes Prempro 0.625/2.5 mg every day. What instructions would the nurse provide to Mrs. Bigelow to ensure that she completely understands the risks, benefits, and adverse effects of the hormone replacement therapy?

NCLEX Success

3. A nurse practitioner prescribes estrogen replacement therapy to relieve severe menopausal symptoms of hot flashes or flushes, which are the result of

   A. insufficient gonadotropin secretion
   B. vasomotor instability
   C. high levels of estrogen
   D. decreased progesterone

4. Hormone therapy is indicated for

   A. treatment of osteoporosis
   B. relief of vasomotor symptoms
   C. cardiovascular disease prevention
   D. endometrial cancer treatment

Progestins

Health care providers use progestins to prevent hyperplasia of the endometrial lining of the uterus in women taking endogenous estrogen. Ⓟ **Medroxyprogesterone acetate** (Provera), a synthetic progestin and a progesterone derivative, is the prototype progestin.

Pharmacokinetics

Oral administration of medroxyprogesterone acetate and other progestins results in rapid absorption, and the drug can reach a maximum concentration in 1 to 2 hours. During the first 6 hours, half-life is about 2 to 3 hours; thereafter, half-life extends to 8 to 9 hours. Prompt degradation occurs in the liver, and metabolites are excreted primarily in the urine. Rapid absorption is also characteristic of intramuscular progestins, which have a half-life of just a few minutes. Long-acting forms can maintain effective concentrations for 3 to 6 months; maximum concentrations can be achieved in 24 hours with a half-life of about 10 weeks. Gel preparations have sustained-release properties, and absorption is prolonged with half-lives of 1 to 2 days.

Action

Medroxyprogesterone acetate and other progestins diffuse freely into cells, where they bind to progesterone receptors. The progestins act primarily on the endometrial lining of the uterus by changing it from a proliferative endometrium into a secretory endometrium. They also suppress the release of pituitary hormones, which inhibit ovulation. Finally, they inhibit spontaneous uterine contractions.

Use

Progestins have both noncontraceptive and contraceptive uses, as part of estrogen–progestin combinations or as progestin-only preparations (mini-pills). Health care providers use progestins to suppress ovarian function in dysmenorrhea, endometriosis, endometrial cancer, and uterine bleeding. These uses of progestins are extensions of the physiologic actions of progesterone on the neuroendocrine control of ovarian function and on the endometrium. Table 44.2 presents dosage information for the progestins.

For approximately 20 to 25 years, postmenopausal women with an intact uterus took progestins in combination with estrogen for long-term HRT. In HRT, the purpose of a progestin is to prevent endometrial cancer, which can occur with unopposed estrogenic stimulation. Currently, however, as previously stated, this combination is not recommended for long-term use because evidence has indicated that the adverse effects outweigh the beneficial effects. Two large-scale randomized controlled trials, the Heart and Estrogen/Progestin Replacement Study (HERS) and the Women's Health Initiative (WHI), have disputed the cardioprotective effects of postmenopausal estrogen use (see Box 44.2).

Use in Children

Progestins are not intended for use in children.

Use in Patients With Renal Impairment

Progestin metabolites are predominately excreted in urine. Therefore, patients with renal impairment require close evaluation and management, and advanced renal impairment may contraindicate progestin use.

Use in Patients With Hepatic Impairment

Metabolism of progestins occurs primarily in the liver. Therefore, impaired liver function or liver disease prohibits use.

Use in Patients With Critical Illness

Due to the increased risk of thromboembolic disorders, such as thrombophlebitis, deep vein thrombosis, and pulmonary embolism associated with the use of progestins, critical illness resulting in extended bed rest may increase the risk of using the drug. It may be less beneficial.

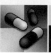

TABLE 44.2

DRUGS AT A GLANCE: Progestins

Drug	Pregnancy Category	Routes and Dosage Ranges for Various Indications			
		Menstrual Disorders	Endometriosis	Endometrial Cancer	Other
Ⓟ **Medroxyprogesterone acetate** (Provera, Depo-Provera, Depo-SubQ Provera 104)	X	Dysfunctional uterine bleeding: PO 2.5–10 mg daily for 5–10 d, beginning on 16th or 21st day of cycle	SubQ 104 mg/ 0.65 mL every 3 months	IM 400–1000 mg weekly until improvement, then 400 mg monthly	
Megestrol acetate (Megace, Megace ES)	X			PO 40–320 mg daily in four divided doses for at least 2 mo	Breast cancer: PO 160 mg daily in four divided doses for at least 2 mo Cachexia with HIV: PO initially 800 mg/d; normal range, 400–800 mg/d (suspension only) or 625 mg/d ES suspension
Norethindrone acetate (Aygestin)	X	Amenorrhea, dysfunctional uterine bleeding: PO 2.5–10 mg daily, starting on 5th day of menstrual cycle and ending on 25th day	PO 5 mg daily for 2 wk, increased by 2.5 mg daily every 2 wk to dose of 15 mg. Then give 10–15 mg daily for maintenance		
Progesterone (Crinone, Prochieve [vaginal gel], Prometrium)	X	Amenorrhea, dysfunctional uterine bleeding: IM 5–10 mg for 6–8 consecutive day			Secondary amenorrhea: 4% gel, 45 mg every other day; Infertility: 90 mg vaginally daily in women requiring progesterone supplementation

Adverse Effects

The most significant risk associated with progestins is an increased risk of cardiovascular complications, such as stroke, heart attack, hypertension, thromboembolic and thrombotic disease, thrombophlebitis, retinal thrombosis, and pulmonary embolism. Other adverse effects include the following:

- Irregular vaginal bleeding (common; decreases during the first year of use). Amenorrhea may occur.
- Weight gain and fluid retention (common)

- Ophthalmic disorders, such as sudden, partial, or complete loss of vision
- An increased risk of migraines and mental depression
- Possible skin conditions, such as rash, acne, alopecia, and hirsutism
- GI upset, with nausea and vomiting
- Bone loss. A **BLACK BOX WARNING** ◆ stipulates that some forms of medroxyprogesterone acetate cause calcium loss in bones, leading to weak bones and possible bone breakage.

Nurses should be aware that the FDA has recognized some of these problems and issued a **BLACK BOX WARNING** ◆ for the progestins, stating that the drugs:

- Should not be used in pregnancy
- Should not be used in combination with estrogen for the prevention of cardiovascular disease or dementia
- Are associated with an increased risk of thromboembolic events, such as myocardial infarction, stroke, deep vein thrombosis, and pulmonary embolism in women taking estrogen–progestin combination therapy
- Are associated with an increased risk of dementia in postmenopausal women

Contraindications

Contraindications to progestins include allergies to the drugs, pregnancy or suspected pregnancy, and breast-feeding. Other contraindications are history of active cardiovascular disease; thrombophlebitis; thromboembolic disorders; cerebral hemorrhage; renal disease; hepatic disease; and carcinoma of the breast, ovaries, or endometrium. A final contraindication is undiagnosed vaginal bleeding. A history of depression warrants caution.

Nursing Implications

Nursing implications associated with progestins are very similar to those associated with estrogens. The following information is essential in the identification of those women for whom progestin therapy is contraindicated:

- Assessment of medical and social history. The nurse assesses for menopausal symptoms, cardiovascular disease (hypertension, hyperlipidemia, and cerebral vascular risk), gynecological history (menstrual history, last menstrual period, and age at menopause), cancer history, and history of smoking.
- Assessment of family history of menopause, osteoporosis, cardiovascular disease, cerebrovascular disease, cognitive disease, including allergy status
- Assessment of blood pressure, weight, height, lipid panel, clinical breast examination with age-appropriate mammogram, pelvic examination, and Pap smear

Preventing Interactions

Progestin use often results in inaccurate liver function and endocrine function tests. It is essential that health care providers be aware that progestins are being used when laboratory testing is indicated. No reports of drug–drug, drug–food, or drug–herb interactions concerning progestin have appeared.

Administering the Medication

Progestins can be administered through a variety of routes. Oral, intramuscular, subcutaneous, intravaginal, intrauterine, and transdermal preparations of the drug are available. To reduce the GI effects of the drugs, it is necessary to take them with food or at bedtime. For treatment of dysfunctional uterine bleeding and amenorrhea, cyclic administration of the drug is often warranted.

Assessing for Therapeutic Effects

When given for menstrual disorders, such as abnormal uterine bleeding, amenorrhea, dysmenorrhea, premenstrual discomforts, and endometriosis, the nurse observes for relief of symptoms.

Assessing for Adverse Effects

The nurse observes for breakthrough bleeding and provides reassurance to affected women. He or she assesses for irregular vaginal bleeding, which is a major reason that some women do not want to take progestin-only contraceptives. The nurse ensures that lipid panels are assessed, due to the decreased HDL and increased LDL cholesterol that may occur with progestin use. These changes in LDL and HDL levels increase the risk of cardiovascular disease and may lead to discontinuation of the progestin. In women with a history of depression, discontinuation of the drug is essential at the first sign or indication of recurring depression.

Patient Teaching

Box 44.4 presents patient teaching guidelines for progestins. Women who have an intact uterus should take both estrogen and progestin; the progestin component (e.g., Provera) prevents endometrial cancer, an adverse effect of estrogen-only therapy. Posthysterectomy, women should take estrogen-only medications. Combined estrogen–progestin therapy may increase blood sugar levels in women with diabetes. This effect is attributed to progestin and is unlikely to occur with estrogen-only therapy. Women with diabetes should report increased blood glucose levels. Take progestins with food or at bedtime to decrease nausea, a common adverse reaction. Patients should take their weight weekly and report sudden weight gain, which may result from fluid retention and edema. Patients should report any unusual vaginal bleeding.

Clinical Application 44-3

- Mrs. Bigelow has been taking Prempro 0.625/ 2.5 mg every day for 1 month. She calls the office when you are on duty. She is complaining of left leg pain and swelling that has been occurring off and on for 4 days. What is the nursing intervention?

Estrogen–Progestin Combinations

The most effective and widely used contraceptives are estrogen–progestin combinations. For contraception, the prototype hormonal combination is ethinyl estradiol–norethindrone (Ortho-Novum). For HRT, the prototype drug is Ⓟ **conjugated estrogen–medroxyprogesterone** (Prempro).

Several varieties of progestins are part of combined oral contraceptives. The progestin component may determine the choice of a combination contraceptive product. Progestins have progestational, estrogenic, and androgenic qualities. These qualities vary depending on the type of the progestin and are important in the management of the adverse effects associated with hormonal contraceptives. Progestational qualities have an influence on the suppression of ovulation and reduction in menstrual bleeding. Estrogenic qualities may be associated with headache, breast tenderness, or fluid retention. Androgenic qualities are often associated with acne or hirsutism (unwanted female hair growth). Progestins with minimal androgenic activity are desogestrel and norgestimate, those with intermediate activity include norethindrone and ethynodiol, and those with high androgenic effects include norgestrel.

Pharmacokinetics

Absorption of ethinyl estradiol is good with oral administration, and it reaches peak plasma levels within 2 hours. It is 98% bound to plasma proteins, and its half-life varies from 6 to 20 hours. The estrogen undergoes extensive first-pass metabolism, additional metabolism, and conjugation in the liver; the conjugates are then excreted in bile and urine.

Action

The estrogen component of combined oral contraceptives prevents pregnancy by inhibiting ovulation; it prevents the formation of the follicle by suppressing FSH and LH and stabilizing the endometrium. The progestin component thins the endometrium, slows sperm transport, thickens cervical mucus, and suppresses the LH surge.

Use

The primary use of estrogen–progestin contraceptives is to prevent pregnancy. Three different types of hormonal contraceptives are common: monophasic contraceptives, which contain fixed amounts of both estrogen and progestin components; biphasics, which contain either fixed amounts of estrogen and varied amounts of progestin; and triphasics, which contain three different doses of estrogen and progestin (Table 44.3). Biphasic and triphasic preparations mimic normal variations of hormone secretion, decrease the total dosage of hormones, and may decrease adverse effects. These contraceptives are dispensed in containers with color-coded tablets that must be taken in the correct sequence. Dispensers with 28 tablets contain 7 inactive or placebo tablets of a third color. Several combination products and alternative dosage forms are available to help individualize treatment and promote adherence.

Health care providers also use oral contraceptive preparations to treat menstrual disorders (e.g., amenorrhea, dysmenorrhea). The FDA has approved some oral contraceptives for the treatment of acne, such as Ortho Tri-Cyclen, Estrostep, and Yaz. Prescribers order Yaz for treatment of premenstrual dysphoric disorder. Continuous-dosing oral contraceptives, which include Lybrel, Seasonale, and Seasonique, are useful in the treatment of menorrhagia, metrorrhagia, endometriosis, and premenstrual syndrome. Such continuous-dosing oral contraceptives provide birth control protection for three consecutive months while suppressing ovarian function and reducing uterine bleeding; withdrawal bleeding occurs only four times per year.

Table 44.4 presents dosage information for noncontraceptive estrogen–progestin combinations.

Use in Patients With Renal Impairment

Oral contraceptives are associated with fluid retention and dilated kidneys as a result of increased renin–angiotensin–aldosterone system activity. This alteration in the renal system occurs especially when the contraceptives are used in higher doses; therefore, patients with renal impairment require close evaluation and management. Severe renal impairment may be a contraindication to oral contraceptive use.

Use in Patients With Hepatic Impairment

Due to the metabolism of combined oral contraceptives in the liver, hepatic impairment is an absolute contraindication for use. In addition, women who have had jaundice during pregnancy have an increased risk of recurrence if they take estrogen-containing contraceptives. Any patient in whom jaundice develops when taking estrogen should stop taking the drug. Because jaundice may indicate liver damage, the cause warrants investigation.

Use in Patients With Critical Illness

Oral contraceptive use during a critical illness that results in limited mobility is contraindicated. There is an increased risk

TABLE 44.3

Estrogen–Progestin Combinations Used as Contraceptives

	Pregnancy Category	Estrogen	Progestin
Monophasics Alesse Aviane Lessina Lutera Sronyx	X	Ethinyl estradiol 20 mcg	Levonorgestrel 0.1 mg
Jolessa Levora 0.15/30 Nordette Portia	X	Ethinyl estradiol 30 mcg	Levonorgestrel 0.15 mg
Junel 21 1/20 Junel Fe 1/20 Loestrin 1/20 Loestrin Fe 1/20 Microgestin Fe 1/20	X	Ethinyl estradiol 20 mcg	Norethindrone 1.0 mg
Junel Fe 1.5/30 Junel 21 1.5/30 Loestrin 21 1.5/30 Loestrin Fe 1.5/30 Microgestin Fe 1.5/30	X	Ethinyl estradiol 30 mcg	Norethindrone 1.5 mg
Necon 1/35 Norinyl 1+35 Ortho-Novum 1/35 Ⓟ	X	Ethinyl estradiol 35 mcg	Norethindrone 1.0 mg
Balziva Femcon Fe chewable Ovcon 35 Fe Zenchent	X	Ethinyl estradiol 35 mcg	Norethindrone 0.4 mg
Brevicon Modicon Necon 0.5/35	X	Ethinyl estradiol 35 mcg	Norethindrone 0.5 mg
Ortho-Novum 1/50 Ovcon 50	X	Ethinyl estradiol 50 mcg	Norethindrone 1.0 mg
Cryselle Lo-Ovral Low-Ogestrel	X	Ethinyl estradiol 30 mcg	Norgestrel 0.3 mg
Ogestrel Ovral	X	Ethinyl estradiol 50 mcg	Norgestrel 0.5 mg
Kelnor 1/35 Zovia 1/35E	X	Ethinyl estradiol 35 mcg	Ethynodiol diacetate 1.0 mg
Zovia 1/50E	X	Ethinyl estradiol 50 mcg	Ethynodiol diacetate 1.0 mg
Apri Desogen Ortho-Cept Reclipsen	X	Ethinyl estradiol 30 mcg	Desogestrel 0.15 mg
Kariva Mircette	X	Ethinyl estradiol 20/10 mcg	Desogestrel 0.15 mg
Yasmin	X	Ethinyl estradiol 30 mcg	Drospirenone 3.0 mg
Yaz	X	Ethinyl estradiol 20 mcg	Drospirenone 3.0 mg
Mononessa Ortho-Cyclen Sprintec	X	Ethinyl estradiol 35 mcg	Norgestimate 0.25 mg

TABLE 44.3

Estrogen–Progestin Combinations Used as Contraceptives (Continued)

	Pregnancy Category	Estrogen	Progestin
Norinyl 1+50 Ortho-Novum 1/50	X	Mestranol 50 mcg	Norethindrone 1.0 mg
Extended-Cycle Monophasics Lybrel	X	Ethinyl estradiol 20 mcg	Levonorgestrel 0.09 mg
Quasense Seasonale Seasonique	X	Ethinyl estradiol 30 mcg	Levonorgestrel 0.15 mg
Lo-Seasonique	X	Ethinyl estradiol 20/10 mcg	Levonorgestrel 0.10 mg
Biphasics Necon 10/11 Ortho-Novum 10/11	X	Ethinyl estradiol 35 mcg	Norethindrone 0.5/1.0 mg
Triphasics Cesia Cyclessa Velivet	X	Ethinyl estradiol 25 mcg	Desogestrel 0.1/0.125/0.15 mg
Necon 7/7/7 Ortho-Novum 7/7/7	X	Ethinyl estradiol 35 mcg	Norethindrone 0.5/0.75/1.0 mg
Aranelle Leena/Tri-Norinyl	X	Ethinyl estradiol 35 mcg	Norethindrone 0.5/1.0/0.5 mg
Estrostep Fe	X	Ethinyl estradiol 20/30/35 mcg	Norethindrone 1.0 mg
Ortho Tri-Cyclen TriNessa Tri-Previfem Tri-Sprintec	X	Ethinyl estradiol 35 mcg	Norgestimate 0.18/0.215/0.25 mg
Ortho Tri-Cyclen Lo	X	Ethinyl estradiol 25 mcg	Norgestimate 0.18/0.215/0.25 mg
Enpresse Triphasil Trivora-28	X	Ethinyl estradiol 30/40/30 mcg	Levonorgestrel 0.05/0.075/0.125 mg
Ortho Evra transdermal patch	X	Ethinyl estradiol 750 mcg	Norelgestromin 6 mg
NuvaRing vaginal insert	X	Ethinyl estradiol 2.7 mg	Etonogestrel 11.7 mg
Progestin-Only Products Ovrette	X		Norgestrel 0.075 mg
Camila Errin Jolivette Nora-BE Nor-Q.D. Ortho Micronor	X		Norethindrone 0.35 mg
Depo-Provera	X		Depot medroxyprogesterone acetate IM
Depo-SubQ Provera	X		Depot medroxyprogesterone acetate SubQ
Mirena intrauterine device	X		Levonorgestrel-releasing intrauterine device (provides contraception for 5 years)
Implanon subdermal implant	X		Etonogestrel 68 mg subdermal (provides contraception for 3 years)

TABLE 44.4

DRUGS AT A GLANCE: Estrogen–Progestin Combinations Used for Noncontraceptive Purposes

Drug	Pregnancy Category	Routes and Dosage Ranges for Various Indications		
		Menopausal Symptoms	Female Hypogonadism	Prevention of Osteoporosis
Ⓟ **Conjugated estrogens/medroxyprogesterone acetate** (Prempro, Premphase)	X	PO 0.3/1.5 mg–0.625/2.5 mg daily		PO 0.3/1.5 mg–0.625/ 2.5 mg daily
Conjugated estrogens/ medroxyprogesterone acetate (Premphase)	X	PO 0.625/5.0 mg daily		PO 0.625/5.0 mg daily
Estradiol/norgestimate (Prefest)	X	PO 1 mg estradiol everyday for 3 d; 0.09 mg norgestimate every day for 3 d in repeating cycle		PO 1 mg estradiol everyday for 3 d; 0.09 mg norgesti- mate every day for 3 d in repeating cycle
Estradiol/norethindrone (Activella)	X	PO 0.05 mg/0.1 everyday; PO 1 mg/0.5 mg every day		PO 0.05 mg/0.1 everyday; 1 mg/0.5 mg every day
Ethinyl estradiol/norethin- drone acetate (femHRT)	X	PO 2.5 mcg/0.5 mg every day; PO 5 mcg/1 mg every day		PO 2.5 mcg/0.5 mg every day; PO 5 mcg/1 mg every day
Estradiol/drospirenone (Angeliq)	X	PO 5 mcg/1 mg every day		PO 5 mcg/1 mg every day
Estradiol/norethindrone (CombiPatch)	X	Transdermal 0.05 mg/0.14 mg twice a week; Transdermal 0.05 mg/0.25 mg twice a week		

of thromboembolic disorders, such as thrombophlebitis, deep vein thrombosis, and pulmonary embolism.

Use in Patients Receiving Home Care

Patients usually self-administer oral contraceptives. Home care nurses may encounter patients or family members taking one of the drugs when visiting the home for another reason. It may be necessary to teach or assist patients to take the drugs as prescribed. In addition, patients may need encouragement to keep appointments for follow-up supervision and blood pressure monitoring. When visiting families that include adolescent girls or young women, home care nurses may need to teach about birth control measures, adverse reactions, and adverse effects.

Adverse Effects

Adverse effects of oral contraceptives may include the GI effects of nausea and vomiting. Taking the drugs with food or at bedtime minimizes nausea. Cardiovascular effects of thromboembolism, myocardial infarction, stroke, and hypertension may also occur. Earlier oral contraceptives, which contained larger amounts of estrogen than those currently used, did cause these problems, and they are much less common in most

people who take low-dose preparations. However, for women 35 years of age and older who smoke, there is an increased risk of myocardial infarction and other cardiovascular disorders, even with low-dose pills. Also, gallbladder disease is more likely in women who use oral contraceptives or estrogen–progestin HRT than in those who do not take hormones. Researchers attribute this to increased concentration of cholesterol in bile acids, which leads to decreased solubility and increased precipitation of stones. Finally, edema, weight gain, and headache are other adverse effects that may be associated with combined oral contraceptives.

The FDA has issued the following **BLACK BOX WARNINGS ◆** regarding the use of oral contraceptives:

- Cigarette smoking increases the risk of cardiovascular adverse effects, especially in women older than 35 years of age.
- Concern about the use of Depo-Provera and Depo-SubQ Provera relates to its associated with the loss of stored calcium from bones, which increases the risk of broken bones and osteoporosis, especially after menopause. There is a greater risk of bone loss with long-term use.
- Risks of thromboembolic events increase with use of the Ortho Evra transdermal patch due to the higher levels of estrogen that are circulated into the blood.

EVIDENCE-BASED PRACTICE

Contraceptive Hormone Use and Cardiovascular Disease

by SHUFELT, C.L. AND BAIREY MERZ, C.N.

Journal of the American College of Cardiology 2009,
53(3), 221–231

Findings from the Women's Health Initiative have prompted the review of hormone therapy in women across the lifespan. Young women often receive prescriptions for hormonal contraceptives. Therefore, the purpose of this article was to review observational clinical studies for the risk of cardiovascular events in women using hormonal contraception. Observational data findings reveal that first- and second-generation oral contraceptives have been consistently associated with small but statistically significant increases in the risks of myocardial infarction and venous thromboembolism, especially in higher hormone doses and in smokers. Findings reveal that there is no cardiovascular data available for third-generation oral contraceptives or nonoral routes (transdermal and vaginal) but an increase in the risk of venous thromboembolism persists. Additional studies are warranted. Finally, the study findings recommend fasting lipid profiles for women with dyslipidemia before initiating oral contraceptives. In those women with low-density lipoprotein (LDL) cholesterol of 160 mg/dL or above, nonhormonal contraception is recommended.

IMPLICATIONS FOR NURSING PRACTICE: Appropriate health education regarding the adverse thromboembolic effects that may be associated with hormonal contraception is warranted. In women 35 years of age or older, a careful health history is essential to assess for cardiovascular risk factors. Women with LDL cholesterol of 160 mg/dL or above require nonhormonal contraception. Careful assessment and monitoring of blood pressure is essential, and elevations warrant discontinuation of hormonal contraception. Finally, hormonal contraception is contraindicated in women 35 years of age or older who are smokers.

Contraindications

Despite the decreased estrogen dosage, combined oral contraceptives are associated with several contraindications. These include cigarette smoking, age of 35 years and older, a history of thromboembolic problems, and concurrent cirrhosis or active viral hepatitis, diabetes mellitus, hypertension, or migraine with aura. When estrogen is contraindicated, it is permissible to use a progestin-only contraceptive.

Yasmin and Yaz contain the progestin drospirenone, which increases serum potassium. Therefore, contraindications to these oral contraceptives include renal, liver, or adrenal insufficiency; use of potassium-sparing diuretics; potassium supplements; angiotensin-converting enzyme inhibitors; angiotensin-II receptor agonists; heparin; and continuous, long-term use of nonsteroidal anti-inflammatory drugs.

Nursing Implications

It is necessary to assess each patient's need and desire for contraception, as well as her willingness to comply with the prescribed regimen. Assessment includes determining a patient's knowledge about birth control, both pharmacologic and nonpharmacologic, and identifying patients in whom hormonal contraceptives are contraindicated or who are at increased risk for adverse drug effects. Adherence involves the willingness to take the drugs as prescribed and to have breast and pelvic examinations and blood pressure measurements every 6 to 12 months. The goal of effective oral contraceptive use is the prevention of pregnancy with the lowest effective dose of hormones.

Preventing Interactions

Several medications may reduce the effectiveness of oral contraceptives (i.e., increase the likelihood of pregnancy; Box 44.5). These include several antibiotics and antiseizure medications. (Box 44.3 lists specific drug–drug interactions that decrease the effectiveness of estrogen.) Patients should notify all health care providers who prescribe medications that they are taking a birth control pill. Use of an additional

---

BOX 44.5 Drug Interactions: Oral Contraceptives

Drugs That Decrease the Effects of Oral Contraceptives

■ Antibiotics, such as amoxicillin, ampicillin, doxycycline, metronidazole, minocycline, neomycin, nitrofurantoin, penicillin, tetracycline
   Decrease absorption and effectiveness

■ Anticonvulsants, such as carbamazepine, hydantoins (ethotoin, mephenytoin, phenytoin), succinimides
   Induce hepatic cytochrome P450, resulting in increased metabolism

■ Barbiturates such as phenobarbital, primidone
   Increase metabolism

■ Benzodiazepines
   Activate the hepatic enzyme cytochrome P450, resulting in increased metabolism

■ Griseofulvin
   Increases metabolism

■ Rifampin
   Activates the hepatic enzyme cytochrome P450, resulting in increased metabolism

■ Topiramate
   Decreases contraceptive efficacy and increases breakthrough bleeding

or alternative method of birth control is necessary (1) if a dose is missed or (2) if the oral contraceptive cannot be taken because of illness or infection (e.g., an antibiotic is prescribed).

QSEN Safety Alert

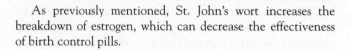

It is essential to add a different method of birth control while taking certain antibiotics (see Box 45.5) for the remainder of that reproductive cycle.

As previously mentioned, St. John's wort increases the breakdown of estrogen, which can decrease the effectiveness of birth control pills.

Administering the Medication

Numerous preparations are available, with different components and different doses of components, so that a preparation can be chosen to meet individual needs. Most oral contraceptives contain an estrogen and a progestin. The estrogen dose is usually 30 to 35 mcg. Smaller amounts (e.g., 20 mcg) may be adequate for small or underweight women; larger amounts (e.g., 50 mcg) may be needed for large or overweight women. Effects of estrogen components are similar when prescribed in equipotent doses, but progestins differ in progestogenic, estrogenic, antiestrogenic, and androgenic activity. Consequently, adverse effects may differ to some extent, and a patient may be able to tolerate one contraceptive better than another.

Assessing for Therapeutic Effects

When taken correctly, estrogen–progestin contraceptive preparations are nearly 100% effective in preventing pregnancy. Therapeutic effects of oral contraceptives include the prevention of pregnancy with regulation of menses with shorter, lighter flow and reduction in ovarian cyst formation. Improvements in hemoglobin may occur due to decreased menstrual flow or if women are taking oral contraceptives with added iron.

Assessing for Adverse Effects

It is very important to monitor for adverse drug effects such as high blood pressure, gallbladder disease, and blood-clotting disorders, which may be associated with oral contraceptive use. The assessment of weight, blood pressure, regularity of menses (occurring only on the withdrawal pills), absence of chest pain, abdominal pain, headache, vision changes, and leg pain indicates an absence of adverse effects of the oral contraceptives.

Patient Teaching

It is essential that women seek information about the use of oral contraceptives. The nurse should be sure that women understand that oral contraceptives are very effective at preventing pregnancy but *do not* prevent transmission of sexually transmitted diseases (e.g., human immunodeficiency virus [HIV], chlamydia, gonorrhea). Box 44.4 presents teaching guidelines for patients taking contraceptives.

EVIDENCE-BASED PRACTICE

Does Hormone Replacement Therapy Cause Breast Cancer? An Application of Causal Principles to Three Studies: Part 2. The Women's Health Initiative: Estrogen Plus Progestogen.
by SHAPIRO, S, FARMER, R.D., MUECK, A.O., SEAMAN, H., AND STEVENSON, J.C.

Journal of Family Planning and Reproductive Health
2011, 37(3), 165–172

Research has suggested that there is an increased risk of breast cancer in women taking combined hormone placement therapy (HRT). The findings from the Collaborative Reanalysis (CR), the Women's Health Initiative (WHI), and the Million Women Study (MWS) have established this finding. However, there has been conflicting evidence in these studies regarding the risk of breast cancer in women taking unopposed estrogen therapy. Two studies (the CR and MWS) have reported increased risks of breast cancer in women taking estrogen alone, whereas the WHI did not support this finding. The purpose of this article was to evaluate the findings of the WHI study, and they were inconclusive. Findings from the study report that HRT with estrogen and progestin may or may not increase the risk of breast cancer in women. However, the authors report that data from the WHI study do not establish a risk of increased breast cancer in women taking HRT with estrogen and progestin.

IMPLICATIONS FOR NURSING PRACTICE: Evidence-based practice is constantly evolving, and the nurse is responsible for maintaining a current knowledge base. Many patients are confused regarding medical information found in media. Nurses with up-to-date knowledge can help patients understand often complicated information.

Clinical Application 44-4

- Mrs. Bigelow has her FSH level measured, as ordered by her physician, and the levels are within normal range. After completion of her history, physical examination, and diagnostic tests, her physician begins her on hormonal contraceptives for menstrual regulation. She is on the second cycle of pills when she calls complaining of irregular bleeding on the pills and requests a new pill. What is the nurse's best response?

NCLEX Success

7. Patient teaching for a woman who will be using the transdermal patch Ortho Evra should include information about applying the patch to
   A. the skin daily
   B. clean and dry skin
   C. the same area for consistency
   D. the skin every 2 weeks

8. The nurse is preparing a presentation of the risk factors of oral contraceptives. What would factor is an absolute contraindication?
   A. bulimia
   B. cigarette smoking at age 33
   C. body mass index (BMI) of 23
   D. history of thromboembolism

9. When oral contraceptives are contraindicated in women with liver disease, what other birth control option would be safe?
   A. Ortho Evra (contraceptive patch)
   B. Depo-Provera (injectable progestin)
   C. barrier method (condoms)
   D. Implanon (subdermal implant)

10. After patient teaching of the warning signs associated with combination hormonal contraception, what statement would result in the nurse providing additional education?
    A. "Breakthrough bleeding is a sign of a uterine abnormality."
    B. "I should immediately go to the emergency department if I get a sudden, severe headache that is not relieved with rest or analgesic."
    C. "Severe leg pain and swelling should immediately be reported."
    D. "Cardiovascular problems are the most severe adverse effect associated with oral contraceptives."

The Nursing Process

Assessment

- Obtain a thorough patient history relating to general and gynecological health, social particulars, and family health.
- Obtain a history of drug and food allergies.
- Obtain baseline height, weight, BMI, and blood pressure.
- Document the last menstrual period (rule out pregnancy).

Nursing Diagnoses

- Deficient knowledge related to contraceptive method
- Risk for ineffective health maintenance related to not being familiar with the various contraceptive methods

- Fear related to
  - Unintended pregnancy if method not used correctly
  - Long-term side effects and adverse effects of contraceptive method
- Disturbed sleep pattern related to body temperature fluctuations
- Ineffective sexuality patterns related to pain during intercourse
- Deficient knowledge related to the hormonal effects on cardiovascular status
- Risk for injury related to loss of bone mass

Planning/Goals

The patient will

- Choose the birth control method with minimal risks and most benefit
- Report an understanding of the dosing schedule, risks, benefits, and warning signs of the method selected
- Self-administer oral, transdermal, topical, or vaginal medications as prescribed
- Report adverse effects of the birth control method
- Report an understanding of the risks, benefits, and warning signs associated with hormonal replacement therapy
- Report an understanding of the nonpharmacologic and pharmacologic choices of HRT
- Choose the method of HRT with minimal risks and most benefits
- Report adverse effects of the HRT

Nursing Interventions

The nurse will

- Provide health teaching regarding various birth control methods with the risks and benefits
- Identify and discuss any contraindications to birth control options
- Encourage the patient to participate in choosing the birth control method
- Provide instruction regarding the use of method chosen
- Obtain written informed consents, which imply that the patient is making an informed decision regarding the birth control method and is aware of the risks and benefits
- Review typical menopausal changes
- Identify and discuss any contraindications to HRT
- Provide health teaching regarding the nonpharmacologic and pharmacologic methods available for menopause, include risks, benefits, and warning signs

Evaluation

- Provide a follow-up visit to assess the effectiveness of the hormone therapy.
- Assess for side effects, adverse effects, and changes in the patient's health status.

Key Concepts

- When exogenous estrogens and progestins are administered for therapeutic purposes, they produce the same effects as endogenous hormones.
- Oral contraceptives are very effective at preventing pregnancy, but they do not prevent transmission of sexually transmitted diseases.
- Cigarette smoking in women who use oral contraceptives increases risks of blood clots in the legs, lungs, heart, or brain.
- Because estrogens cause epiphyseal closure, caution is necessary when used in children before completion of bone growth and attainment of adult height.
- When estrogens are used alone in postmenopausal women, they cause endometrial hyperplasia and may cause endometrial cancer. Women with an intact uterus should also be given a progestin, which opposes the effects of estrogen on the endometrium.
- Most interactions with antimicrobials have been reported with oral contraceptives. To prevent pregnancy from occurring during antimicrobial therapy, a larger dose of oral contraceptive or an additional or alternative form of birth control is probably advisable.
- The FDA has issued a **BLACK BOX WARNING** ◆ that estrogens increase the risk of developing cancer of the uterus. The warning instructs women who take estrogens with or without progestins that there is an increased risk of dementia, myocardial infarctions, strokes, breast cancer, and blood clots. In addition, a **BLACK BOX WARNING** ◆ warns that estrogens and progestins should not be used in pregnancy.
- A **BLACK BOX WARNING** ◆ outlines the concern of the use of Depo-Provera and Depo-SubQ Provera being associated with the loss of stored calcium from bones, which increases the risk of broken bones and osteoporosis, especially after menopause. There is a greater risk of bone loss with long-term use.

Critical Thinking Questions

44-1. Julie Campbell is a 35-year-old college student. She presents to student health services requesting oral contraceptives to prevent unwanted pregnancy. Julie's medical history reveals that she is taking hydrochlorothiazide 25 mg orally every day for "fluid retention." She is a cigarette smoker (a half a pack per day).

- What is the best nursing intervention regarding contraception in this case?
- Julie tells the nurse practitioner that other options for birth control are not desirable and taking the pill is her preferred method. What information can the nurse provide to have her reconsider?

References and Resources

Binder, B., Lackner, H. K., Salmhofer, W., & Hofmann-Wellenhof, R. (2009). Risk factors for deep vein thrombosis in women aged 18–50: A retrospective analysis. *Dermatologic Surgery, 35*(3), 451–456.

Buist, D. S., Anderson, M. L, Reed, S. D., Aiello Bowles, E. J., Fitzgibbons, E. D., Gandara, J. C., et al. (2009). Short-term hormone therapy suspension and mammography recall: A randomized trial. *Annals of Internal Medicine, 150*(11), 752–765.

Chlebowski, R. T., Anderson, G. L., Gass, M., Lane, D. S., Aragaki, A. K., Kuller, L. H., et al. (2010). Estrogen plus progestin and breast cancer incidence and mortality in postmenopausal women. *The Journal of the American Medical Association, 304*(15), 1684–1692.

Karch, A. (2012). *2012 Lippincott's nursing drug guide.* Philadelphia, PA: Lippincott Williams & Wilkins.

Neuhouser, M. L., Wassertheil-Smoller, S., Thomson, C., Aragaki, A., Anderson, G. L., Manson, J. E., et al. (2009). Multivitamin use and risk of cancer and cardiovascular disease in the Women's Health Initiative Cohorts. *Archives of Internal Medicine, 169*(3), 294–304.

Orshan, S. A. (2008). *Maternity, newborn, and women's health nursing: Comprehensive care across the life span.* Philadelphia, PA: Lippincott Williams & Wilkins.

Ricci, S. S. (2009). *Essentials of maternity, newborn, and women's health nursing.* Philadelphia, PA: Lippincott Williams & Wilkins.

Sarna, M. A., Hollenberg, N. K, Seely, E. W., & Ahmed, S. B. (2009). Oral contraceptive progestins and angiotensin-dependent control of the renal circulation in humans. *Journal of Human Hypertension, 23*(6), 407–414.

Sengwee, T., Hernandez-Diaz, S., Logan, R., Rossouw, J. E., Hernan, M. A. (2010). Coronary heart disease in postmenopausal recipients of estrogen plus progestin therapy: Does the increased risk ever disappear? *Annals of Internal Medicine, 152*(4), 211–217.

Shufelt, C. L., & Bairey Merz, C. N. (2009). Contraceptive hormone use and cardiovascular disease. *Journal of the American College of Cardiology, 53*(3), 221–231.

45 Drug Therapy for Men's Health

Clinical Application Case Study

Phillip Johnson, a 52-year-old veterinarian, is seen in the clinic for hypertension control. He has a one-pack per day history of cigarette smoking and has begun walking to reduce his weight. For 5 years, he has been taking hydrochlorothiazide and atenolol to lower his blood pressure, which is well controlled. He has no other chronic health problems.

However, Mr. Johnson reports significant erectile dysfunction that has progressed over the past 9 months. This has significantly distressed him and his wife and has caused considerable marital discord.

KEY TERMS

Anabolic steroids: synthetic drugs with increased anabolic activity and decreased androgenic activity compared with testosterone

Androgens: male sex hormones, primarily testosterone, secreted by the testes in men, the ovaries in women, and the adrenal cortex in both men and women

Benign prostatic hypertrophy: benign enlargement of the prostate gland; also known as benign prostatic hyperplasia

Corpora cavernosa: major erectile tissue of the penis

Erectile dysfunction: difficulty in initiating or maintaining penile erection that is satisfactory for sexual relations

Erectogenic: capable of causing an erection

Ergogenic: increase in muscular work capacity caused by drugs that enhance athletic performance

Leydig cells: cells in the testes that control androgen secretion

Testosterone: male sex hormone; secreted by the Leydig cells in the testes

Introduction

This chapter explores the drugs used to manage disorders and conditions that affect men's reproductive health. To understand the drugs discussed in this chapter, it is necessary to understand the regulation of male reproductive function as well as recognize the main disorders of male reproduction.

Overview of Reproductive Health Problems in Men

Androgens are male sex hormones secreted by the testes in men, the ovaries in women, and the adrenal cortex in both men and women. Like the female sex hormones, the naturally occurring male sex hormones are steroids synthesized from cholesterol, which is why they are called anabolic steroids. The sex organs and adrenal glands can produce cholesterol or remove it from the blood. Cholesterol then undergoes a series of conversions to progesterone, androgenic prehormones, and testosterone. The androgens produced by the ovaries have little androgenic activity and are used mainly as precursor substances for the production of naturally occurring estrogens. The adrenal glands produce several androgens, including androstenedione and dehydroepiandrosterone (DHEA). Androstenedione and DHEA are weak androgens with little masculinizing effect that are mainly converted to estrogens.

Testosterone is normally the only important androgen. This male sex hormone has several effects on body tissues (Box 45.1). Certain cells in the testes, called **Leydig cells**, secrete testosterone in response to stimulation by luteinizing hormone (LH) from the anterior pituitary gland. The increased production of testosterone results in the changes associated with puberty in the adolescent male. The main functions of testosterone concern the development of male sexual characteristics, reproduction, and metabolism. Testosterone is necessary for normal sperm development.

About 97% of the testosterone secreted by the testes binds to plasma albumin or to sex hormone–binding globulin and circulates in the blood for 30 minutes to several hours. The bound testosterone is either transferred to the tissues or broken down into inactive products that are excreted. Much of the testosterone that transfers to tissues undergoes intracellular conversion to dihydrotestosterone (DHT), which combines with receptor proteins in the cytoplasm. A series of actions stimulates production of proteins. Almost all effects of testosterone result from the increased formation of proteins throughout the body, especially in the cells of target organs and tissues responsible for development of male sexual characteristics.

The portion of testosterone that does not become attached to tissues is converted into androsterone and DHEA by the liver. These are conjugated with glucuronic or sulfuric acid and excreted in the bile or urine.

Etiology

Androgen Deficiency

Lack of sufficient testosterone can result in congenital or acquired hypogonadism in the male. Causes include genetic diseases, head or testicular trauma, alkylating agents, tumors, and radiation injury.

- Primary hypogonadism results from a testicular disorder. Common diseases that can cause primary hypogonadism are mumps, testicular inflammation, and trauma.
- Secondary hypogonadism results from a problem in the hypothalamus or the pituitary gland, areas of the brain that signal the testicles to produce testosterone. A lack of production of gonadotropin-releasing hormone from the hypothalamus or a deficiency of follicle-stimulating hormone (FSH) and LH from the anterior pituitary may result from thyroid disorders, Cushing's syndrome, or estrogen-secreting tumors. Chronic diseases (e.g., metabolic syndrome, diabetes) can lead to secondary hypogonadism.

Erectile Dysfunction

Erectile dysfunction (ED) is defined as difficulty initiating or maintaining penile erection that is satisfactory for sexual relations. The condition affects more than 50% of men between 40 and 70 years of age. Incidence increases with age. Causes may include drugs (antidepressants, antihypertensive agents, histamine receptor antagonists), lifestyle factors (alcohol, tobacco, or cocaine use), diseases (diabetes, thyroid conditions, prostate cancer, cardiovascular conditions, obesity), and spinal cord injuries. Psychological factors may also play a role. Low testosterone levels rarely lead to ED but may reduce a man's sex drive. ED and cardiovascular disease share many risk factors; the pathophysiology of both conditions is mediated through endothelial dysfunction. Cardiovascular disease enhances the risk of developing ED; conversely, ED is thought to be a powerful predictor of coronary artery disease, especially in men older than 60 years of age.

Benign Prostatic Hypertrophy

Benign prostatic hypertrophy (BPH), also known as benign prostatic hyperplasia, is benign enlargement of the prostate gland. More than 50% of men in their 60s and as many as 90% in their 70s and 80s have some symptoms of BPH. Part of the

BOX 45.1	Effects of Testosterone on Body Tissues

Fetal Development

Large amounts of chorionic gonadotropin are produced by the placenta during pregnancy. Chorionic gonadotropin is similar to luteinizing hormone (LH) from the anterior pituitary gland. It promotes development of the interstitial or Leydig cells in fetal testes, which then secrete testosterone. Testosterone production begins in the second month of fetal life. When present, testosterone promotes development of male sexual characteristics (e.g., penis, scrotum, prostate gland, seminal vesicles, and seminiferous tubules), and suppresses development of female sexual characteristics. In the absence of testosterone, the fetus develops female sexual characteristics.

Testosterone also provides the stimulus for the descent of the testes into the scrotum. This normally occurs after the seventh month of pregnancy, when the fetal testes are secreting relatively large amounts of testosterone. If the testes do not descend before birth, administration of testosterone or gonadotropic hormone, which stimulates testosterone secretion, produces descent in most cases.

Adult Development

Little testosterone is secreted in boys until 11 to 13 years of age. At the onset of puberty, testosterone secretion increases rapidly and remains at a relatively high level until about 50 years of age, after which it gradually declines.

The testosterone secreted at puberty acts as a growth hormone to produce enlargement of the penis, testes, and scrotum until approximately 20 years of age. The prostate gland, seminal vesicles, seminiferous tubules, and vas deferens also increase in size and functional ability. Under the combined influence of testosterone and follicle-stimulating hormone (FSH) from the anterior pituitary gland, sperm production is initiated and maintained throughout the man's reproductive life. It affects various parts of the body.

■ **Skin.** Testosterone increases skin thickness and activity of the sebaceous glands. Acne in the male adolescent is attributed to the increased production of testosterone.

■ **Voice.** The larynx enlarges and deepens the voice of the adult man.

■ **Hair.** Testosterone produces the distribution of hair growth on the face, limbs, and trunk typical of the adult man. In men with a genetic trait toward baldness, large amounts of testosterone cause alopecia (baldness) of the scalp.

■ **Skeletal muscles.** Testosterone is largely responsible for the larger, more powerful muscles of men. This characteristic is caused by the effects of testosterone on protein metabolism. Testosterone helps the body retain nitrogen, form new amino acids, and build new muscle protein. At the same time, it slows the loss of nitrogen and amino acids formed by the constant breakdown of body tissues. Overall, testosterone increases protein anabolism (buildup) and decreases protein catabolism (breakdown).

■ **Bone.** Testosterone makes bones thicker and longer. After puberty, more protein and calcium are deposited and retained in bone matrix. This causes a rapid rate of bone growth. The height of a male adolescent increases rapidly for a time, then stops as epiphyseal closure occurs. This happens when the cartilage at the end of the long bones in the arms and legs becomes bone. Further lengthening of the bones is then prevented.

Anterior Pituitary Function

■ High blood levels of testosterone decrease secretion of FSH and LH from the anterior pituitary gland. This, in turn, decreases testosterone production.

---

male reproductive system, the prostate is a walnut-sized gland composed of two lobes enclosed by an outer layer of tissue. This gland produces part of the seminal fluid that nourishes and transports sperm. The prostate is located in front of the rectum and below the bladder, where urine is stored, and it surrounds the urethra, the canal through which urine passes out of the body.

It is thought that BPH is a normal element of the male aging process. Causes include changes in hormone balance and cell growth. Testosterone undergoes reduction to form the more potent androgen DHT, which has greater affinity for androgen receptors than testosterone. During the formation and growth of an embryo, DHT plays a critical role in the formation of the male external genitalia, whereas in the adult, DHT acts as the primary androgen in the prostate and in hair follicles.

Pathophysiology

Androgen Deficiency

- Hypogonadism results from dysfunction of the hypothalamus, the anterior pituitary, or the gonads. Chapter 41 describes the role of the hypothalamic–pituitary–adrenal axis. Primary hypogonadism involves pathology of either

Leydig cells or the seminiferous tubules, or both. Injury to Leydig cells results in decreased testosterone production, whereas seminiferous tubule dysfunction results in decreased or absent spermatogenesis. The majority of the conditions causing testicular injury predominantly involve tubules. Gonadotropins are elevated due to loss of negative feedback.

- Secondary hypogonadism involves decreased or incorrectly normal gonadotropin levels, leading to decreased testicular stimulation, spermatogenesis, and androgen production and if prolonged, testicular atrophy.

Erectile Dysfunction

The process of achieving penile erection involves the integration of psychological, neurological, and vascular processes, which combine to initiate a physiologic response within the penile vasculature. Stimulation of penile shaft results in the secretion of nitric oxide, which causes the relaxation of the smooth muscles of the **corpora cavernosa** (the main erectile tissue of penis). This results in increased blood flow into the sinusoids of the corpora cavernosa with subsequent filling, which obstructs venous outflow from the penis by compression of the veins against the tunica albuginea, resulting in penile erection. Additionally, adequate levels of testosterone and an intact pituitary gland are required.

Benign Prostatic Hypertrophy

The prostate contains stromal and epithelial tissue. Stromal tissue is smooth muscle tissue that contracts around the urethra when activated and is regulated by alpha$_1$-adrenergic receptors. Epithelial tissue is the glandular portion of the prostate and is under the control of androgens, primarily testosterone. The enzyme 5-alpha reductase converts testosterone to DHT, its active metabolite, in epithelial tissue.

The prostate undergoes two main growth periods, first in puberty, when the prostate doubles in size, and second in early adulthood, at about 25 years of age, when the gland begins another growth phase that often results years later in BPH. A surrounding layer of tissue limits overgrowth of the epithelial or glandular tissue of the prostate, causing the gland to put pressure against the urethra. In addition, the bladder wall becomes thicker and more easily irritated; it contracts even when it contains small amounts of urine, leading to more frequent urination. At some point, the bladder weakens and loses the capacity to empty, and urine is retained in the bladder. The narrowing of the urethra and partial emptying of the bladder cause many of the problems associated with BPH.

Clinical Manifestations

Androgen Deficiency

Signs and symptoms of androgen deficiency in adult males include ED, infertility, decreased beard and body hair growth, decreased muscle mass, breast tissue (gynecomastia), and loss of bone mass (osteoporosis). Hypogonadism can also cause mental and emotional changes. As testosterone decreases, some men may experience symptoms similar to those of menopause in women, including fatigue, decreased sex drive, difficulty concentrating, and hot flashes.

To confirm a diagnosis of hypogonadism, it is necessary to perform laboratory tests. Serum testosterone is decreased. To determine the cause, it is also necessary to measure hormone levels in the serum: FSH, LH, prolactin, thyroid hormone, and estradiol. If normal or elevated FSH and LH serum levels are present with a low testosterone level and the testes are nonresponsive to hormonal stimulation, a primary hypogonadism is present. If FSH and LH are low along with the testosterone level, a secondary hypogonadism is present.

Erectile Dysfunction

The main clinical manifestation of ED is the consistent inability to attain or maintain an erection satisfactory for sexual activity. An associated symptom may be reduced sexual desire.

Benign Prostatic Hypertrophy

Clinical manifestations of BPH result from the obstruction of the urethra from the enlargement of the prostate gland, causing reduction in outflow of urine. Rarely do symptoms occur in men younger than 40 years of age. Men may experience urinary frequency, hesitancy, urgency, dribbling, and decrease force of the urinary stream. Nocturia, postvoid leakage, urinary stones, or infection can also occur.

On physical examination, a midline mass above the symphysis pubis, which likely represents an incompletely emptied bladder, may be visible. On digital rectal examination, rubbery enlargement of the prostate is present. Excretory urography may indicate emptying and filling defects in the bladder, urinary tract obstruction, calculi or tumors, and hydronephrosis.

Drug Therapy

Table 45.1 outlines the drugs used to maintain male reproductive health, which include the androgens and anabolic steroids, the phosphodiesterase type 5 (PDE5) inhibitors and prostaglandins, and the 5-alpha reductase inhibitors and the alpha$_1$-adrenergic inhibitors.

TABLE 45.1

Drugs Administered for Maintenance of Male Reproductive Health

Drug Class	Prototype	Other Drugs in the Class
Androgens	Testosterone	Testolactone (Teslac) Fluoxymesterone (Halotestin) Methyltestosterone (Android, Testred) Danazol*
Phosphodiesterase type 5 inhibitors	Sildenafil (Viagra, Revatio)	Avanafil (Stendra) Tadalafil (Cialis) Vardenafil (Levitra)
Prostaglandins		Alprostadil (Caverject aqueous, Caverject powder, Edex powder, Muse)
5-alpha reductase inhibitors	Finasteride (Proscar)	Dutasteride (Avodart)
Alpha$_1$-adrenergic blockers	Tamsulosin (Flomax)	Alfuzosin (Uroxatral) Doxazosin (Cardura) Silodosin (Rapaflo) Terazosin (Hytrin)

*Used in women

Androgens and Anabolic Steroids

When clinicians use male sex hormones or androgens from exogenous sources for therapeutic purposes, the effects are the same as those of naturally occurring hormones. These effects include inhibition of endogenous sex hormones and sperm formation through negative feedback of pituitary LH and FSH. **Anabolic steroids** are synthetic drugs with increased anabolic activity and decreased androgenic activity compared with endogenous testosterone. They were developed during attempts to modify testosterone so that its tissue-building and growth-stimulating effects could be retained while the drug's masculinizing effects could be eliminated or reduced.

Prescribers may order male sex hormones for women to antagonize or reduce the effects of female sex hormones. Thus, administration of androgenic or anabolic steroids to women causes suppression of menstruation and atrophy of the endometrial lining of the uterus.

Several dosage forms of androgens are available. They differ mainly in route of administration and pharmacokinetics. Ⓟ **Testosterone** is the prototype.

Pharmacokinetics

Like endogenous testosterone, the drug molecules are highly bound (98%) to plasma proteins and serum half-life varies (e.g., 8 days for IM testosterone cypionate, 9 hours for oral fluoxymesterone). Testosterone is extensively metabolized in its first pass through the liver, so that nearly half of a dose is lost before it reaches the systemic circulation. About 90% of a dose is excreted in urine as conjugates of testosterone and its metabolites; the remainder is excreted in feces.

Action

Like other steroid drugs, testosterone penetrates the cell membrane and binds to receptor proteins in the cell cytoplasm. The steroid–receptor complex is then transported to the nucleus, where it activates ribonucleic acid (RNA) and deoxyribonucleic acid (DNA) production and stimulates cellular synthesis of protein.

Use

With testosterone, the most clear-cut indication for use is to treat androgen deficiency states (e.g., hypogonadism, cryptorchidism, impotence, oligospermia) in boys and men. In postpubertal men who become androgen deficient, the hormone reestablishes and maintains masculine characteristics and functions. Table 45.2 gives route and dosage information for testosterone and other androgens and anabolic steroids.

TABLE 45.2

DRUGS AT A GLANCE: Androgens

Drug	Pregnancy Category	Routes and Dosage Ranges	
		Hypogonadism	*Other*
Ⓟ **Testosterone cypionate** (Depo-Testosterone)	X	50–200 mg IM every 2–4 wk	
Ⓟ **Testosterone enanthate** (Delatestryl)	X	50–200 mg IM every 2–4 wk	
Ⓟ **Testosterone gel** (AndroGel 1%)	X	Apply 5 g (50 mg of drug) once daily to skin of shoulders and upper arms or abdomen	
Ⓟ **Testosterone pellets**	X	150–450 mg Sub-Q every 3–6 mo	Delayed puberty: lower dosage range Sub-Q, for a limited duration (e.g., every 3 mo for 2–3 doses)
Ⓟ **Testosterone transdermal systems** (Androderm)		Apply two systems (dose of 5 mg) nightly to back, abdomen, upper arm, or thigh	
Testolactone (Teslac)	C		Breast cancer: 250 PO mg 4 times daily
Fluoxymesterone (Halotestin)	X	5–20 mg PO daily	
Methyltestosterone (Android, Testred)	X		Cryptorchidism: 30 mg PO daily; buccal tablets, 15 mg PO daily
Danazol	X		Endometriosis: 800 mg PO daily in two divided doses for 3–9 mo
Fibrocystic breast disease: 100–400 mg PO daily in two divided doses for 3–6 mo

Use in Children

The main indication for use of testosterone in children is for boys with established sex hormone deficiencies; the hormone stimulates the development of masculine characteristics.

QSEN Safety Alert

Because testosterone can cause epiphyseal closure, it is essential to examine a child's hands and wrists using radiography every 6 months to detect bone maturation and to check that there is no loss of height if receiving testosterone therapy.

Stimulation of skeletal growth should continue for approximately 6 months after testosterone therapy stops. If premature puberty occurs (e.g., precocious sexual development, enlarged penis), it is necessary to stop the drug. Testosterones may cause or aggravate acne. Scrupulous skin care and other antiacne treatment may be necessary, especially in adolescent boys.

Use in Older Adults

In older adults with hypertension and other cardiovascular disorders, the sodium and water retention associated with testosterone may aggravate these conditions. Also, in men, the drugs may increase prostate size and interfere with urination, increase risk of prostatic cancer, and cause excessive sexual stimulation and priapism.

Adverse Effects

Common adverse effects from testosterone include acne, change in sex drive, hair loss, headache, bitter taste or mouth irritation, or gum tenderness. Additionally, hypercalcemia, jaundice, and edema may occur. Virilizing or masculinizing effects may vary. In adult men with adequate secretion of testosterone, adverse effects include priapism, increased sexual desire, reduced sperm count, and prostate enlargement. In prepubertal boys, adverse effects may involve premature development of sex organs and secondary sexual characteristics, such as enlargement of the penis and pubic hair. Priapism may occur. In women, adverse effects include hirsutism, deepening of the voice, and menstrual irregularities.

Contraindications

Contraindications to testosterone include pregnancy (because of possible masculinizing effects on a female fetus), preexisting liver disease, and disorders of the prostate. (Men with an enlarged prostate may have additional enlargement, and men with prostate cancer may experience tumor growth.)

Nursing Implications

Preventing Interactions

Some medications and herbs interact with testosterone, decreasing its effects (Box 45.2). Androgens may increase effects of cyclosporine and warfarin, apparently by slowing their metabolism and increasing their concentrations in the blood. If possible, people should avoid using these combinations. If

---

| BOX 45.2 | Drug Interactions: Testosterone |

Drugs That Decrease the Effects of Testosterone
- Barbiturates
  Increase enzyme induction and rate of metabolism
- Calcitonin
  Decreases calcium retention, thus antagonizing the calcium-retaining effects of androgens

---

they are necessary, the nurse monitors serum creatinine and cyclosporine levels (for cyclosporine) and prothrombin time or international normalized ratio (INR) (for warfarin). Androgens also increase the effects of sulfonylureas. If possible, people should avoid using sulfonylureas concurrently.

Administering the Medication

Naturally occurring androgens are given by injection because they are metabolized rapidly by the liver if given orally. Some esters of testosterone have been modified to slow the rate of metabolism and thus prolong action. For example, intramuscular (IM) testosterone cypionate and testosterone enanthate have slow onsets of action and last 2 to 4 weeks. As a result of first-pass metabolism, doses as high as 400 mg/d may be needed to produce adequate blood levels for full replacement therapy.

Several transdermal formulations of testosterone are available. They have a rapid onset of action and last approximately 24 hours. A topical gel (a 10g dose delivers 100 mg) produces normal serum testosterone levels within 4 hours after application, and absorption of testosterone into the blood continues for 24 hours. Steady-state serum concentrations occur by the second or third day of use. When the gel is discontinued, serum testosterone levels remain in the normal range for 24 to 48 hours but decrease to pretreatment levels within about 5 days.

Assessing for Therapeutic and Adverse Effects

The nurse assesses for return of sex hormone levels, development of masculine characteristics in boys, and return of libido in adult males.

The nurse should assess for adverse effects, including hypersensitivity reaction, changes in sexual drive or masculinization, hair loss, changes in taste, oral irritation, and/or gum tenderness. The nurse also monitors serum calcium and observes for signs of hypercalcemia (e.g., kidney stones, polyuria, abdominal pain, nausea, vomiting, depression).

Patient Teaching

Box 45.3 presents patient teaching information for androgens.

Other Drugs in the Class

Danazol is a synthetic testosterone with weak androgenic activity. Clinicians may use the drug in women to prevent or treat endometriosis or fibrocystic breast disease. Danazol is seldom prescribed continuously beyond six months because it produces the same androgenic adverse effects as other androgens, which are particularly of concern in females. Although some drug

BOX 45.3   Patient Teaching Guidelines for Androgens

General Considerations

■ Take the drugs only if prescribed and as prescribed. Use by athletes for body building is inappropriate and, if not prescribed by a licensed prescriber, is illegal.

■ Continue medical supervision as long as the drugs are being taken.

■ Weigh self once or twice weekly and record the amount. An increase may indicate fluid retention and edema.

■ Practice frequent and thorough skin cleansing to decrease acne, which is most likely to occur in women and children.

■ Keep all appointments for laboratory testing and follow-up care.

■ As with all drugs, keep these medications in the original container, tightly closed, and out of reach of children.

Self-Administration

■ Take oral preparations before or with meals, in divided doses.

■ For buccal preparations, adhere to the following guidelines:
  ■ Take in divided doses.
  ■ Place the tablet between the cheek and gum and allow to dissolve (do not swallow).
  ■ Avoid eating, drinking, or smoking while the tablet is in place.

■ For transdermal systems, adhere to the following guidelines:
  ■ Apply two Androderm systems nightly to clean, dry skin on back, abdomen, upper arm, or thigh. Do not apply to scrotum. Rotate sites, with 7 days between applications to a site. Press firmly into place for adherence.
  ■ Apply the prescribed amount of gel to clean, dry, intact skin of the shoulders and upper arms or the abdomen (do not apply to the genital area), once daily, preferably in the morning. Wash hands after application and allow sites to dry before dressing. After application, wait at least 1 hour and preferably 4 to 6 hours before showering or swimming.

---

literature still lists metastatic breast cancer and some types of anemia as indications for use of androgens, newer drugs have largely replace them for these purposes. In breast cancer, androgens are second-line hormonal agents, after antiestrogens (e.g., tamoxifen). In anemia associated with renal failure, synthetic erythropoietin is more effective and more likely to be used. Administration of danazol is oral, and metabolism occurs in the liver. The route of excretion is unknown.

Fluoxymesterone is an anabolic steroid with strong androgenic properties used in the treatment of hypogonadism, delayed male puberty, and breast cancers in women. This drug is often abused to increase athletic performance.

Methyltestosterone is a synthetic formulation of testosterone that can be used in adolescent males with delayed puberty to produce puberty. The drug is less extensively metabolized by the liver and more suitable for oral administration.

Testolactone, a derivative of progesterone, is an antineoplastic agent used to treat advanced breast cancer. The drug blocks the production of estrogen, which reduces the growth of breast cancers that are activated by estrogen. It does not seem to have the masculinizing effects of testosterone.

Abuse of Androgens and Anabolic Steroids

Drugs used to enhance athletic performance are termed **ergogenic** (causing an increase in muscular work capacity). Androgens and anabolic steroids are widely abused in attempts to enhance muscle development, muscle strength, and athletic performance.

QSEN Safety Alert

Because of their abuse potential, the drugs are Schedule III controlled substances.

Although nonprescription sales of the drugs are illegal, they apparently are easily obtained.

Athletes are considered a high-risk group because some start taking the drugs as early as middle school and continue for years. The use of performance-enhancing drugs in nonathletes is also on the rise to improve performance outside of sports. The number of teens taking anabolic steroids is thought to be small in comparison with the number using marijuana, amphetamines, and other illegal drugs. However, the number is increasing, and long-term effects may be as serious as the effects that occur with use of other illegal drugs. Although steroids have a reputation for being dangerous to adult athletes, such as body builders and football players, they are considered even more dangerous for teens because teens are still growing.

QSEN Safety Alert

Anabolic steroids can stop bone growth and damage the heart, kidneys, and liver of adolescents.

In addition to those who take steroids to enhance athletic performance, some males take the drugs to produce a more muscular appearance and impress females. Steroid abusers usually take massive doses and often take several drugs or combine injectable and oral drugs for maximum effects. The large doses produce potentially serious adverse effects in several body tissues:

- Cardiovascular disorders include hypertension, decreased high-density blood lipoproteins, and increased low-density lipoproteins, all of which promote heart attacks and strokes.
- Liver disorders include benign and malignant neoplasms, cholestatic hepatitis and jaundice, and peliosis hepatis, a disorder in which blood-filled cysts develop in the liver and may lead to hemorrhage or liver failure.

- Central nervous system disorders include aggression, hostility, combativeness, and dependence characterized by preoccupation with drug use, inability to stop taking the drugs, and withdrawal symptoms similar to those that occur with alcohol, cocaine, and narcotics. In some cases, psychosis may develop.
- Reproductive system disorders include decreased testicular function (e.g., decreased secretion of endogenous testosterone, decreased formation of sperm), testicular atrophy, and impotence in men. They include amenorrhea in women.
- Metabolic disorders include atherosclerosis-promoting changes in cholesterol metabolism and retention of fluids, with edema and other imbalances. Fluid and electrolyte retention contribute to the increased weight associated with drug use.
- Dermatologic disorders include moderate to severe acne in both sexes, depending on drug dosage.

Many of these adverse effects persist several months after the drugs are stopped and may be irreversible.

Androstenedione and DHEA, androgens produced by the adrenal cortex, are also available as over-the-counter (OTC) dietary supplements. They are marketed as safe, natural, alternative androgens for building muscles. These products, which have weak androgenic activity, act mainly as precursors for the production of sex hormones. Androstenedione, for example, may be converted to testosterone by way of an enzyme found in most body tissues. However, it may also be converted to estrogens, and the testosterone that is produced may be further converted to estrogen (estradiol).

DHEA is available alone as oral capsules or tablets and in a topical cream with vitamins and herbs. Contraindications to DHEA include prostate cancer or BPH as well as estrogen-responsive breast or uterine cancer, because DHEA may stimulate growth of the cancerous tissues. It is important that patients older than 40 years of age be aggressively screened for hormonally sensitive cancers before taking DHEA.

Adverse effects of DHEA include aggressiveness, hirsutism, insomnia, and irritability. Whether large doses of the OTC products can produce some of the serious adverse effects associated with standard anabolic steroids is unknown.

NCLEX Success

1. **The most clear-cut therapeutic indication for use of male sex hormones is which of the following?**

   A. to treat androgen deficiency states in boys and men
   B. for body-building purposes
   C. to treat metastatic breast cancer
   D. to treat anemia associated with renal failure

2. **Four patients in an endocrine clinic are ordered to begin androgen therapy. The nurse reviews each patient's current medications and identifies which patient as able to begin androgen therapy without the risk of a known drug interaction?**

   A. patient 1, taking cyclosporine
   B. patient 2, taking warfarin
   C. patient 3, taking sulfonylureas
   D. patient 4, taking heparin

3. **A 19-year-old female athlete presents for her first prenatal visit and tells the nurse she has been on androgen therapy to improve her distance running. She asks the nurse if she can continue taking the androgens to maintain her "competitive edge." The nurse should instruct her that she:**

   A. can continue taking androgens, because the drugs pose no risk to the fetus
   B. can continue taking androgens, but a higher dose will be required due to increased drug metabolism during pregnancy
   C. can continue taking androgens until the third trimester, when they must be discontinued because androgens cause an increased risk of premature rupture of membranes
   D. must stop taking androgens immediately, because they pose a risk to the fetus; she should discuss this with her health care provider at today's visit

4. **Which of the following statements by a male patient taking transdermal androgens indicates that teaching has been adequate? (Choose all that apply.)**

   A. "I need to weigh myself once or twice weekly and record the amount."
   B. "I should wash my face and body thoroughly to decrease the risk of acne."
   C. "The patch systems should be applied nightly to skin on my back, abdomen, upper arm, or thigh."
   D. "I should apply the patch systems in the morning to the same site each and every day."

Clinical Application 45-1

- Mr. Johnson asks a nurse if he can take the "little blue pill that will improve his love making" (sildenafil). How should the nurse respond?

Phosphodiesterase Type 5 Inhibitors

Prescribers commonly order PDE5 inhibitors to treat ED. These drugs do not cause an erection but enhance the erection resulting from sexual stimuli by increasing blood flow to the penis. The prototype PDE5 inhibitor is ℗ **sildenafil** (Viagra).

Pharmacokinetics

Sildenafil is significantly protein bound and is rapidly absorbed by the oral route. The drug is metabolized in the liver and is primarily excreted in the feces and to a lesser extent by the kidneys. The onset of action is 20 to 60 minutes, with a duration of up to 4 hours.

Action

Sildenafil improves erectile function by inhibiting the enzyme responsible for the breakdown of cyclic guanosine monophosphate (cGMP), a vasodilatory neurotransmitter in corporal tissues of the penis. This causes a vasodilatory effect in the smooth muscle of the corpus cavernosum that allows for a harder and longer-lasting erection.

Use

Sildenafil is used for the treatment of ED in men healthy enough for sexual activity. The U.S. Food and Drug Administration (FDA) has also approved the drug for the treatment of pulmonary arterial hypertension. Women and children should not use it. Table 45.3 gives route and dosage information for sildenafil and other PDE5 inhibitors.

Use in Patients With Hepatic Impairment

Caution is warranted with the use of sildenafil with hepatic impairment. Patients with cirrhosis or other significant liver dysfunction should start with a lower dose to minimize worsening of the hepatic impairment.

Adverse Effects

Adverse reactions to sildenafil commonly include headache, facial flushing, dyspepsia, nasal congestion, and dizziness. Rarely, clinicians have reported nonarteritic ischemic optic neuropathy (NAION) due to obstruction of blood flow to the optic nerve, resulting in irreversible loss of vision in one or both eyes, as well as sudden permanent hearing loss accompanied by dizziness and tinnitus. Priapism is rare and usually associated with excessive dosing or concurrent use with another **erectogenic** drug (capable of causing an erection).

Contraindications

Contraindications to sildenafil include a known hypersensitivity to the drug.

QSEN Safety Alert

Prescribers should not order it for men who also take organic nitrates, commonly used to treat angina, because the sildenafil–nitrate combination can cause severe hypotension resulting in dizziness, syncope, heart attack, or stroke.

Also, men who are not healthy enough to engage in sexual activity should not take it.

Nursing Implications

Preventing Interactions

Sildenafil, like other PDE5 inhibitors, is primarily metabolized by the cytochrome P450 (CYP) enzyme CYP3A4. Many medications and herbs interact with sildenafil, increasing or decreasing its effects (Boxes 45.4 and 45.5).

Administering the Medication

Administration is generally oral. It is important not to take sildenafil more than once in a 24-hour period. A recent high-fat meal may delay drug action.

EVIDENCE-BASED PRACTICE

Oral Phosphodiesterase-5 Inhibitors and Hormonal Treatments for Erectile Dysfunction: A Systematic Review and Meta-Analysis

by TSERTSVADZE, A., FINK, H. A., YAZDI, F., MACDONALD, R., BELLA, A. J., ANSARI, M. T., GARRITTY, C., SOARES-WEISER, K., DANIEL, R., SAMPSON, M., FOX, S., MOHER, D., & WILT, T. J.

Annals of Internal Medicine
2009, 151(9), 650–661

Erectile dysfunction (ED) is a significant health issue reported to affect 50% of men from 40 to 70 years of age. According to the National Health and Nutrition Examination Survey, if all affected men sought care for the condition, annual treatment costs could reach $15 billion. Researchers performed a systematic review and meta-analysis of 191 distinctive studies from 10882 publications exploring the current success of treatment of ED. The review had two aims:

- To determine the relative benefits and harms of oral PDE5 inhibitors and hormonal treatments of ED
- To determine the value of hormone blood testing for identification and management of the causes of ED

Unless contraindicated, oral phosphodiesterase type 5 (PDE5) inhibitors are the first-line treatment for the management of ED. Adverse-effect profiles are similar for the products.

The review studied 15 randomized control trials that evaluated the efficacy of hormone therapy in hypogonadal men with ED. The findings were inconsistent regarding the effects of testosterone, with most indicating that testosterone was no more effective than placebo. (The study included oral, intramuscular, gel, cream, and patch testosterone.)

IMPLICATIONS FOR NURSING PRACTICE: ED is a significant problem in older men, and an assessment of the condition should occur when taking a patient's history. The introduction of the PDE5 inhibitors has changed the likelihood of successful treatment, but the drugs do have adverse effects. The nurse should be aware that there is little evidence for use of testosterone for ED despite growing popularity of androgen supplementation for various indications in aging men.

Assessing for Therapeutic and Adverse Effects

The nurse should assess that the patient reports the ability to initiate or maintain a penile erection for satisfactory sexual relations. Additionally, the nurse assesses for signs of adverse effects, including headache, facial flushing, dyspepsia, nasal congestion, and dizziness. Patients with symptoms of NAION or sudden decrease or loss of hearing should discontinue

TABLE 45.3

Drugs for Erectile Dysfunction: Phosphodiesterase Type 5 Inhibitors

Drug	Pregnancy Category	Routes and Dosage Ranges (Adult Males)
Ⓟ **Sildenafil** (Viagra, Revatio)	B	Erectile dysfunction (Viagra): 25–100 mg PO 1 h before sexual activity; reduce dose with age older than 65 years, concurrent use of CYP3A4 inhibitors*, and renal or hepatic impairment Pulmonary arterial hypertension (Revatio): 20 mg PO 3 times per day, taken 4–6 h apart; 10 mg IV 3 times per day
Avanafil (Stendra)	C	100–200 mg PO 30 min before anticipated sexual activity, reduced dose with age older than 65 years, hepatic impairment, and concurrent use of CYP3A4 inhibitors*
Tadalafil (Cialis)	B	2.5–20 mg PO 2 h or more before anticipated sexual activity, 2.5–5 mg PO once daily, reduced dose with age older than 65 years, renal or hepatic impairment, and concurrent use of CYP3A4 inhibitors*
Vardenafil (Levitra)	B	5–20 mg PO 1 h before sexual activity, reduced dose with age older than 65 years, hepatic impairment, and concurrent use of CYP3A4 inhibitors*

*CYP3A4 inhibitors include azole antifungals, erythromycin, and saquinavir.

sildenafil and seek immediate medical care. Although rare, persistent priapism requires prompt medical treatment to avoid permanent penile damage.

Patient Teaching

Box 45.6 contains patient teaching guidelines for sildenafil and other drugs for ED.

Other Drugs in the Class

Avanafil (Stendra), the newest PDE5 inhibitor, is a fast-acting and highly selective member of the class. The drug reaches its peak in 30 minutes, with a duration of 6 hours. Meals do not affect absorption rate or peak levels. Absorption and metabolism of the drug occurs in the liver through the CYP450 system. Excretion takes place in the feces through the bile. Adverse effects, common to other PDE5 inhibitors, include headache, flushing of the face, nasal congestion, and back pain.

Tadalafil (Cialis) reaches its peak in 2 hours, with a duration of 24 to 36 hours. Meals do not affect absorption rate or peak levels. Adverse effects may include back and muscle pain.

Vardenafil (Levitra) has a time to peak effect of 1 hour and a duration of action of 4 hours. As with sildenafil, a high-fat meal delays absorption and reduces peak levels.

QSEN Safety Alert

Vardenafil is the only PDE5 inhibitor that prolongs the QT interval and should not be used with other drugs with similar effect, particularly class I and II antidysrhythmics (see Chap. 25).

Like sildenafil, vardenafil reduces blood pressure and to a lesser degree increases the risk of light sensitivity, blurred vision, and loss of blue-green color discrimination.

Adjuvant Medications Used to Treat Erectile Dysfunction

Clinicians consider adjuvant drugs second-line therapy in the management of ED and generally reserve them for patients who manifest insufficient response to or adverse effects from

---

BOX 45.4   **Drug Interactions: Sildenafil**

Drugs That Increase the Effects of Sildenafil

■ Alcohol
  Increases the risk of orthostatic hypotension, tachycardia, dizziness, and headache
■ Alpha-adrenergic blockers, antihypertensive drugs, cytochrome P450 3A4 inhibitors (e.g., azole antifungals, erythromycin, saquinavir, and protease inhibitors)
  Increase risk of hypotension

BOX 45.5   **Herb and Dietary Interactions: Sildenafil**

Herbs and Foods That Increase the Effects of Sildenafil

■ Grapefruit juice
■ Saw palmetto
■ Yohimbine

Herbs and Foods That Decrease the Effects of Sildenafil

■ Fatty food

BOX 45.6	Patient Teaching Guidelines for Sildenafil and Other Drugs Used to Treat Erectile Dysfunction

General Considerations

■ Take the drugs only as prescribed.

■ Keep appointments for laboratory testing and follow-up care.

■ As with all drugs, keep these medications in the original container, tightly closed, and out of reach of children.

Self-Administration

■ Do not take any phosphodiesterase type 5 (PDE5) inhibitor with nitrates because a serious and potentially life-threatening drop in blood pressure may occur.

■ Do not take sildenafil more than once a day.

■ Avoid consuming a high-fat meal before taking sildenafil or vardenafil.

■ Seek immediate medical attention for an erection lasting 4 hours or longer.

■ Do not use intraurethral alprostadil without using a condom if your partner is pregnant.

■ If symptoms of nonarteritic ischemic optic neuropathy or a sudden decrease or loss of hearing occurs while taking PDE5 inhibitors, discontinue the drug and seek medical attention.

BOX 45.7	Adjuvant Medications Used to Treat Erectile Dysfunction: Alprostadil

Intracavernosal Injection (Caverject Aqueous, Caverject Powder, Edex Powder)

■ Injection may occur along the dorsolateral aspect of the proximal third of the penis, avoiding visible veins.

■ It is necessary to rotate injection sites from one side of the penis to the other and change injection site with each dose.

■ Self-injection may occur no more than 3 times per week and only once in 24 hours.

■ To determine dose adequate for achieving satisfactory erection without causing priapism, it is important to have an initial injection in provider's office.

Intraurethral Administration (Muse)

■ Prior to introducing pellet into urethra, it is important to void; residual urine in urethra aids in dispersing the medication.

■ Intraurethral administration may occur no more than 2 times in 24 hours.

■ To determine dose adequate for achieving satisfactory erection without causing priapism, the patient should visit the provider.

PDE5 inhibitors. Alprostadil is a synthetic enzyme that causes relaxation of cavernosal smooth muscle and dilation of cavernosal arterioles leading to increased penile blood flow. It is a prostaglandin, specifically a prostaglandin E_1.

Administration of alprostadil occurs in two ways: either as an injection into the penis or as a pellet inserted into it (via the urethral opening at the end of the penis). Box 45.7 presents notes about administering the drug. Intracavernosal alprostadil (Caverject) relaxes trabecular smooth muscle and dilates cavernosal arteries, resulting in penile engorgement and reduced venous outflow. Intraurethral alprostadil (Muse) is less efficacious than the intracavernosal drug (60% or less). Administration by either route can produce dose–response improvements in frequency of an erection sufficient for intercourse. The onset of action is immediate following injection, and erection should not last longer than 1 hour with proper dosing (determined in a provider's office).

Intracavernosal injection of alprostadil is associated with a burning sensation, prolonged erection, and priapism, and long-term use is associated with penile fibrosis. Caution is warranted in patients concurrently receiving anticoagulants due to risk of bleeding and in patients at risk for priapism (e.g., sickle cell anemia or trait, multiple myeloma, leukemia). Intraurethral use of the drug is associated with penile pain and minor urethral bleeding. Experts do not recommend alprostadil for concurrent use with other vasoactive agents.

Drugs for Benign Prostatic Hypertrophy

The 5-alpha reductase inhibitors and the alpha$_1$-adrenergic blockers are the two major drug classes used to treat BPH. Use of drugs from both classes in combination has demonstrated to be more effective than either drug class alone and is the gold standard for treatment of the symptoms associated with BPH.

5-ALPHA REDUCTASE INHIBITORS

Ⓟ **Finasteride** (Proscar), the prototype 5-alpha reductase inhibitor, represents this drug class and is used to treat BPH.

Pharmacokinetics

Finasteride is well absorbed as an oral drug. It is 90% bound to plasma proteins. The onset of action is rapid, with a duration of 5 to 7 days. The half-life is 5 to 7 hours. Finasteride may take 3 to 6 months to reach maximum effects. The drug crosses the blood–brain barrier and has been found in semen.

Action

Finasteride acts by inhibiting 5-alpha reductase, the enzyme responsible for converting testosterone to 5-alpha DHT, one of its active metabolites. This inhibits the metabolism of testosterone, causing decreased proliferation of prostatic cells, which

TABLE 45.4
DRUGS AT A GLANCE: 5-Alpha Reductase Inhibitors

Drug	Pregnancy Category	Routes and Dosage Ranges (Adult Males)
Ⓟ **Finasteride** (Proscar)	X	5 mg/d PO to max of 5 mg/d
Dutasteride (Avodart)	X	5 mg/d PO

reduces the enlargement of the prostate gland and mechanical obstruction to the urethra.

Use

Prescribers order finasteride mainly to treat BPH. However, the drug is also available in smaller doses as Propecia, which is indicated for the prevention of male pattern baldness. Table 45.4 gives route and dosage information for finasteride.

Use in Older Adults

Older adults are prone to the hypotensive and hypothermic adverse effects from the vasodilation produced by finasteride.

Use in Renal or Hepatic Impairment

Caution is necessary when administering finasteride to patients with renal or hepatic impairment.

Adverse Effects and Contraindications

Adverse effects of finasteride include various sexual dysfunctions, such as impotence, gynecomastia, reduced libido, and ejaculatory disorders. Dysfunction is usually transient. The drug may decrease sperm production, adversely affecting fertility.

Contraindications include known sensitivity to finasteride. Children and in women, particularly those who are pregnant or lactating, should not take the drug.

Nursing Implications

Preventing Interactions

Concurrent use of finasteride has led to few drug and herb interactions. Use of the drug with testosterone reduces the effects of both finasteride and testosterone. Anticholinergics may decrease the effects of finasteride. The herb saw palmetto may increase the effects of the drug.

Administering the Medication

People may take finasteride once a day around the same time each day, without regard to food.

QSEN Safety Alert ❗

Pregnant caregivers, nurses, or pharmacists should not handle the crushed drug, which can be absorbed and harmful to a male fetus.

Assessing for Therapeutic Effects

The nurse assesses for improved urinary function with patient voiding in sufficient amounts with no palpable bladder distention. Patients should report less urinary frequency, hesitancy, urgency, dribbling, nocturia, and an improved force of the urinary stream.

Assessing for Adverse Effects

The nurse should take a thorough sexual history in patients taking finasteride, including information regarding the presence of impotence, infertility, gynecomastia, reduced libido, and ejaculatory disorders, such as decreased volume of ejaculate. The effect of the drug on sexual dysfunction may be difficult to assess in older males who report these disorders with increasing age and other health conditions.

Patient Teaching

Box 45.8 presents patient teaching guidelines for finasteride and other drugs used to treat BPH.

Other Drugs in the Class

Dutasteride (Avodart) is the only other 5-alpha reductase inhibitor and has a stronger ability than finasteride to reduce the levels of DHT, causing the prostate to decrease in size. Symptoms may improve after 3 months of therapy. However, it may take 6 months or longer to determine the full benefit of the drug. Women who are pregnant or may become pregnant should not handle dutasteride capsules for fear of harming the fetus. A combination of the dutasteride and tamsulosin is available under the trade name of Jalyn. Women should not use Jalyn.

Clinical Application 45-2

- After an evaluation, the nurse practitioner suspects that Mr. Johnson's erectile dysfunction may result from the combination of obesity and antihypertensive medications. He receives a prescription for lisinopril, an angiotensin-converting enzyme inhibitor, which he will take along with hydrochlorothiazide. What patient teaching guidelines should the nurse discuss with Mr. Johnson and his wife?

ALPHA$_1$-ADRENERGIC BLOCKERS

The alpha$_1$-adrenergic blockers are the other drug class used to treat BPH. Ⓟ **Tamsulosin** (Flomax) is the prototype of the anti-BPH drugs and one of the drugs of choice in the treatment of BPH. Other drugs in the class are used to treat hypertension (see Chap. 28), nasal congestion (see Chap. 29), and ophthalmic hyperemia (see Chap. 58).

Pharmacokinetics

Tamsulosin is well absorbed and is highly protein bound. The drug is extensively metabolized by the cytochrome P450 enzyme system, mainly by CYP3A4 and CYP2D6. It is excreted by the kidneys.

BOX 45.8 Patient Teaching Guidelines for Treatment of Benign Prostatic Hypertrophy

General Considerations

■ Take finasteride as prescribed, and note that maximum benefit from the medication is achieved in 6 to 12 months.

QSEN Safety Alert

If you are pregnant, do not handle broken or crushed finasteride or dutasteride medication because the drug could have negative effects on a male fetus.

QSEN Safety Alert

While taking a 5-alpha reductase inhibitor, avoid donating blood because the blood could be given to a pregnant woman.

■ Make sure to keep appointments for laboratory testing and follow-up care.

■ Keep these medications in the original container, tightly closed, protected from light, and out of reach of children.

■ Report a sulfa allergy before beginning tamsulosin therapy; a cross-allergic reaction has been reported.

■ Seek medical care immediately if you are unable to void, if you pass bloody urine, or develop a fever.

Self-Administration

■ Take oral preparations without regard to meals.

■ Do not take other prescription or OTC medications without consulting your health care provider.

■ Be careful when changing positions because dizziness may occur when standing up.

■ If you are a woman of childbearing age and are sexually active, use a barrier contraceptive to prevent pregnancy.

■ Take terazosin at bedtime to reduce the adverse effects.

■ Note that a decrease in libido and volume of ejaculate may occur; this is usually reversible when the drug is stopped.

■ If you are having surgery, including dental surgery, tell the surgeon or dentist that you are taking tamsulosin. If you need to have eye surgery at any time during or after your treatment, be sure to tell your surgeon that you are taking or have taken tamsulosin.

■ Do not drive a car, operate machinery, or perform dangerous tasks until you know how tamsulosin affects you. This medication may make you drowsy or dizzy.

Action

Tamsulosin works by relaxing the muscles in the prostate and bladder neck, enhancing the ability to urinate. Blockage of alpha$_1$-adrenergic receptors decreases vascular smooth muscle contraction, influencing the activity of genitourinary smooth muscle.

Use

Prescribers order tamsulosin to improve urination and reduce complications in men with BPH. Table 45.5 contains route and dosage information for tamsulosin and other alpha$_1$-adrenergic receptor blockers.

Adverse Effects

Tamsulosin may cause adverse effects, including postural hypotension, weakness, sleepiness, difficulty falling or staying asleep, stuffy or runny nose, sore throat, and blurred vision. The drug may also lead to abnormal ejaculation due to inhibition of alpha$_1$A-adrenergic receptors on the vas deferens.

Contraindications

Contraindications to tamsulosin include a known hypersensitivity to the drug.

TABLE 45.5

DRUGS AT A GLANCE: Alpha$_1$ Adrenergic Blockers

Drug	Pregnancy Category	Routes and Dosage Ranges (Adult Males)
Ⓟ **Tamsulosin** (Flomax)	B	0.4 mg PO 30 min after a mean to max of 0.8 mg/d
Alfuzosin (Uroxatral)	B	10 mg/d PO to max of 10 mg/d
Doxazosin (Cardura) Doxazosin XL (Cardura XL)	C	1–8 mg/d PO to max of 8 mg/d extended release: 4–8 mg/d PO to max of 8 mg/d
Silodosin (Rapaflo)	B	8 mg/d PO
Terazosin (Hytrin)	C	Start with 1 mg PO at bedtime to 1–5 mg/d to max of 20 mg/d

Drugs That Increase the Effects of Tamsulosin
- Cimetidine
  Decreases clearance
- Other alpha blocker medications (e.g., alfuzosin, doxazosin, prazosin, terazosin); anticoagulants (e.g., warfarin); and phosphodiesterase type 5 inhibitors (e.g., avanafil, sildenafil, tadalafil, vardenafil)
  Increase the risk of orthostatic hypotension

Nursing Implications

Preventing Interactions

Some medications interact with tamsulosin, increasing its effects (Box 45.9).

Administering the Medication

People take tamsulosin 30 minutes after the same meal daily. They should swallow capsules intact; it is essential not to open, crush, or chew the capsules.

Assessing for Therapeutic Effects

The nurse assesses for improved urinary function demonstrated by decreased urinary frequency, hesitancy, urgency, dribbling, nocturia, and improved force of the urinary stream. The patient should report a decrease in the pain associated with BPH as tamsulosin relaxes the smooth muscle in the bladder neck and the prostate, decreasing the resistance to urinary flow.

Assessing for Adverse Effects

The nurse assesses for difficulty with sleep, blurred vision, nasal congestion, sore throat, weakness, sleepiness, difficulty falling or staying asleep, stuffy or runny nose, sore throat, and blurred vision. Tamsulosin may cause abnormal ejaculation due to inhibition of $alpha_1A$-adrenergic receptors on the vas deferens.

Patient Teaching

Box 45.8 contains patient education guidelines for tamsulosin and other drugs used to treat BPH.

Other Drugs in the Class

Alfuzosin (Uroxatral) is classed as a nonreceptor subtype selective $alpha_1$-adrenergic blocker also used to treat BPH. The drug is able to be uroselective due to accumulation of drug in prostatic tissue. It has a strong safety profile and is well tolerated.

Doxazosin (Cardura) is effective and widely used as a treatment for symptoms associated with BPH. The drug has a rapid onset of action (1–2 weeks). Maximal plasma concentrations are achieved within 1 to 4 hours. With the longer 22-hour half-life of doxazosin, the drug can be taken in the morning or evening, with no difference in the incidence of adverse effects. Major adverse effects include dizziness, headache, and fatigue. Sexual dysfunction is not commonly associated with drug use.

Silodosin (Rapaflo) is a selective $alpha_1A$-adrenergic receptor blocker and a drug of choice to treat BPH because of its mild adverse effects profile with fewer systemic vascular actions. Patients should take it with meals.

Terazosin (Hytrin) has an efficacy profile similar to doxazosin, as well as a similar adverse-effect profile. The drug's main variation is a shorter 12-hour half-life, which may be attributed to the increased incidence of headache, dizziness, and fatigue if the drug is administered in the morning. Consequently, experts recommend that terazosin be given at bedtime.

NCLEX Success

5. **In which of the following men would the use of sildenafil be contraindicated?**

   A. a 52-year-old with type 1 diabetes
   B. a 58-year-old with unstable angina
   C. a 69-year-old with asthma
   D. a 74-year-old with cirrhosis

6. **A 63-year-old man begins to take dutasteride for benign prostatic hypertrophy. He asks the nurse how long he will need to take the medication. The man needs to take drug for how long?**

   A. for 2 years
   B. indefinitely
   C. for two weeks
   D. until his prostate is normal

7. **Finasteride is most effective:**

   A. if started early in the development of prostatic hypertrophy
   B. for improvement of erectile dysfunction
   C. when prostatic hypertrophy is advanced
   D. to decrease the risk of prostate cancer

The Nursing Process

Assessment

- Before drug therapy begins, patients need a thorough history and physical examination. Periodic monitoring of the patient's condition is needed throughout drug therapy.
  - Assess for conditions in which the drugs are used (e.g., deficiency states, erectile dysfunction, BPH).
  - Assess the patient's attitude toward taking male sex hormones or drugs to improve sexual function or urinary flow.
  - Assess the patient's willingness to adhere to instructions for taking the drugs and follow-up procedures.
  - Assess for conditions that increase risks of adverse effects or are contraindications (e.g., pregnancy, liver disease, prostatic hypertrophy).
- With androgens, it is necessary to check several findings regularly.
  - Check laboratory reports of liver function tests (the drugs may cause cholestatic jaundice and liver damage), serum electrolyte levels (the drugs may cause sodium and water retention), and serum lipid levels (the drugs may increase levels and aggravate atherosclerosis).
  - Assess weight and blood pressure regularly. These may be elevated by retention of sodium and water with resultant edema, especially in patients with congestive heart failure.
  - For children, check radiograph examination reports of bone growth status initially and approximately every 6 months while androgens are being taken.

- With ED, assess risk factors for the development of the condition (e.g., drugs therapy, lifestyle, diseases, and injuries).
- With BPH, assess urinary function, urine stream caliber and force, any symptoms of urinary hesitancy, and difficulty starting urination.

Nursing Diagnoses

- **General**
  - Deficient knowledge: physiologic and psychological consequences of overuse and abuse of the drugs to enhance athletic performance or erectile dysfunction
  - Risk for injury: liver disease and other serious adverse drug effects
- **Androgen deficiency**
  - Disturbed body image related to masculinizing effects and menstrual irregularities (with androgens)
  - Noncompliance: overuse of drugs or dietary supplements for enhanced athletic performance or physical appearance
- **Erectile dysfunction**
  - Sexual dysfunction
  - Ineffective sexuality patterns
  - Nonadherence
- **Benign prostatic hypertrophy**
  - Urinary retention (acute or chronic) related to bladder obstruction
  - Risk for infection
  - Deficient knowledge regarding condition, prognosis, treatment, self-care, and discharge needs

Planning/Goals

The patient will

- Use the drugs only as directed
- Avoid preventable adverse drug effects

- Adhere to monitoring and follow-up procedures
- Develop prevention and self-care measures to avoid ED (e.g., limitation or avoidance of alcohol and other drugs, smoking cessation, regular exercise and rest, stress reduction)
- Report healthy sexual functioning or improved urinary patterns of elimination based on cause of drug therapy

Nursing Interventions

The nurse will

- Assist patients to use the drugs correctly (see Boxes 45.3, 45.6, and 45.8)
- Assist patient to reduce sodium intake if edema develops, with androgen use
- Record weight and blood pressure at regular intervals, with androgen use
- Participate in school or community programs to inform children, parents, coaches, athletic trainers, and others of the risks of inappropriate use of androgens, anabolic steroids, and related dietary supplements
- Consider psychological counseling and therapy, as indicated
- Demonstrate problem-solving skills regarding solutions to problems that occur

Evaluation

- Interview and observe for adherence with instructions for taking prescribed drugs.
- Interview and observe for therapeutic and adverse drug effects.
- Observe athletes for increased weight and behavioral changes that may indicate drug abuse with androgens.
- Interview and seek verbalization for satisfactory sexual performance.
- Observe for adequate urinary elimination with BPH.

Key Concepts

- The main functions of testosterone are related to the development of male sexual characteristics, reproduction, and metabolism.

- Androgens and anabolic steroids are used to enhance athletic performance and are termed ergogenic (causing an increase in muscular work capacity); they are widely abused in attempts to enhance muscle development, muscle strength, and athletic performance.

- Because of their abuse potential, androgens and anabolic steroids are classified as Schedule III controlled substances.

- Because androgens cause premature epiphyseal closure, boys with established deficiency states receiving androgens should undergo radiographic examination every 6 months to detect bone maturation and prevent loss of adult height.

- PDE5 inhibitors are successful in the treatment of ED.

- PDE5 inhibitors should not be prescribed for men who also take organic nitrates because the drug combination can cause severe hypotension resulting in dizziness, syncope, heart attack, or stroke.

- BPH is an enlargement of the prostate that occurs with increasing frequency with age.

- The combination of a 5-alpha reductase inhibitors and an alpha$_1$-adrenergic blockers is more effective than with either drug class alone and is the gold standard for treatment of the symptoms associated with BPH.

Critical Thinking Questions

45-1. Karen Watson is a 35-year-old woman with endometriosis. She is taking danazol 800 mg daily in two divided doses. The nurse is counseling her about use of danazol.

* What teaching points should the nurse discuss?

* The nurse is assessing Ms. Watson for adverse effects of danazol. For what signs and symptoms should the nurse observe?

45-2. Warren Watson, a brother of the patient in question 1, is a 27-year-old body builder with an 11-year history of abusing a variety of anabolic steroids. She is worried about him and convinces him to come to the clinic for a checkup. At the clinic, Mr. Watson states that he takes no medications. His blood pressure is 180/94 mm Hg. He says he has "white-coat syndrome" and that his blood pressure is never elevated except at the office. When the nurse practitioner mentions possible treatment for his high blood pressure, he refuses to discuss the possibility.

* What is the nurse's responsibility?

References and Resources

Carpenter, P. C. (2007). Performance-enhancing drugs in sport. *Endocrinology and Metabolism Clinics of North America*, *36*, 481–495.

Dimitrakakis, C. (2011). Androgens and breast cancer in men and women. *Endocrinology and Metabolism Clinics of North America*, *40*(3), 522–547.

Drug facts and comparisons. (Updated monthly). St. Louis, MO: Facts and Comparisons.

Erdemir, F., Harbin, A., & Hellstrom, W. J. (2008). 5-alpha reductase inhibitors and erectile dysfunction: The connection. *The Journal of Sexual Medicine*, *5*(12), 2917–2924.

Goldstein, I. (2007). A clinical paradigm for the combined management of androgen insufficiency and erectile dysfunction. *Endocrinology and Metabolism Clinics*, *36*, 435–452.

Guyton, A. C., & Hall, J. E. (2011). *Textbook of medical physiology* (12th ed.). Philadelphia, PA: W. B. Saunders.

Lacy, C. F., Armstrong, L. L., Goldman, M. P., & Lance, L. L. (2010). *Lexi-Comp's drug information handbook* (19th ed.). Hudson, OH: American Pharmaceutical Association.

Lasker, G. F., Maley, J. H., & Kadowitz, P. J. (2010). A review of the pathophysiology and novel treatments for erectile

dysfunction. *Advances in Pharmacological Sciences*, 2010, Article ID 730861, doi:10.1155/2010/730861.

McVary, K. T. (2007). Clinical practice. Erectile dysfunction. *The New England Journal of Medicine*, *357*(24), 2472–2481.

Porth, C. M., & Matfin, G. (2009). *Pathophysiology: Concepts of altered health states* (8th ed.). Philadelphia, PA: Lippincott Williams & Wilkins.

Schwartz, B. G. & Kloner, R. A. (2011). Clinical cardiology: Physician update: Erectile dysfunction and cardiovascular disease. *Circulation*, *123*, 98–101.

Tsertsvadze, A., Fink, H. A., Yazdi, F., MacDonald, R., Bella, A. J., Ansari, M. T., et al. (2009). Oral phosphodiesterase-5 inhibitors and hormonal treatments for erectile dysfunction: A systematic review and meta-analysis. *Annals of Internal Medicine*, *151*(9), 650–661.

Wei, J. T., Miner, M. M., Steers, W. D., Rosen, R. C., Seftel, A. D., Pasta, D. J., et al. (2011). Benign prostatic hyperplasia evaluation and management by urologists and primary care physicians: Practice patterns from the observational BPH registry. *The Journal of Urology*, *186*(3), 971–976.

CHAPTER OUTLINE (Continued)

46 Drug Therapy for Myasthenia Gravis and Alzheimer's Disease

LEARNING OBJECTIVES

After studying this chapter, you should be able to:

1. Understand the pathophysiology and major manifestations of myasthenia gravis.

2. Identify the prototype and describe the action, use, adverse effects, contraindications, and nursing implications for indirect-acting cholinergic drugs used in myasthenia gravis.

3. Understand the pathophysiology and major manifestations of Alzheimer's disease.

4. Identify the prototype and describe the action, use, adverse effects, contraindications, and nursing implications for reversible indirect-acting cholinergic drugs used in Alzheimer's disease.

5. Understand the etiology, pathophysiology, and clinical manifestations of urinary retention.

6. Identify the prototype and describe the action, use, adverse effects, contraindications, and nursing implications for direct-acting cholinergic drugs.

7. Describe the pharmacologic care of the patient with toxicity of irreversible anticholinesterase agents.

8. Be able to implement the nursing process in the care of patients undergoing cholinergic drug therapy for myasthenia gravis, Alzheimer's disease, and urinary retention.

Clinical Application Case Study

Mary Collins, a 35-year-old woman, who has recently been diagnosed with myasthenia gravis, arrives in the clinic. She has been quite upset about her diagnosis and has lost interest in everyday life. On assessment, the nurse notes that Ms. Collins has shortness of breath, difficulty swallowing, and a drooping eyelid on the left side. Her physician has ordered sertraline and neostigmine 50-mg extended-release tablets to control her symptoms.

KEY TERMS

Acetylcholine: neurotransmitter in the cholinergic system located in many areas of the brain, with high concentrations in the motor cortex and basal ganglia (also a neurotransmitter in the autonomic nervous system and at peripheral neuromuscular junctions); exerts excitatory effects at synapses and at the nerve–muscle junction and inhibitory effects at some peripheral sites, such as organs supplied by the vagus nerve

Acetylcholinesterase: enzyme that acts on the neurotransmitter acetylcholine, breaking it into choline and an acetate group; found mainly at neuromuscular junctions, its activity serves to terminate synaptic transmission

Alzheimer's disease: most common type of dementia; characterized by a significant loss of neurons in addition to shrinkage of large cortical neurons, with plaques and neurofibrillary tangles

Anticholinesterase drugs: indirect-acting cholinergic agents that decrease the inactivation of acetylcholine in the synapse by the enzyme acetylcholinesterase

Cholinergic drugs: agents that stimulate the parasympathetic nervous system in the same manner as acetylcholine

Myasthenia gravis: chronic autoimmune neuromuscular disease characterized by varying degrees of weakness of the skeletal (voluntary) muscles of the body

Introduction

The neuromuscular conditions myasthenia gravis and Alzheimer's disease are characterized by disruptions in neurological and autoimmune processes. This chapter discusses the anticholinesterase medications used for the treatment of myasthenia gravis as well as the medications used to improve memory related to Alzheimer's disease. It also covers selected drugs used to treat atony of the gastrointestinal (GI) and urinary smooth muscle, which may result in paralytic ileus and urinary retention.

Overview of Myasthenia Gravis

Myasthenia gravis is a chronic autoimmune neuromuscular disease characterized by varying degrees of painless weakness of the skeletal (voluntary) muscles of the body. The hallmark of the disorder is muscle weakness that increases during periods of activity and improves after periods of rest. The name myasthenia gravis, which is Latin and Greek in origin, literally means "grave muscle weakness." With the therapies currently available, however, most cases of myasthenia gravis are not as "grave" as the name implies. In fact, most people who have myasthenia gravis have a normal life expectancy.

Myasthenia gravis occurs in all ethnic groups and both genders. It most commonly affects young adult women (younger than 40 years of age) and older men (older than 60 years of age), but it can occur at any age.

Etiology

Myasthenia gravis results from a defect in the transmission of nerve impulses to muscles. Normally, when impulses travel down the nerve, the nerve endings release a neurotransmitter called **acetylcholine**. Acetylcholine travels from the neuromuscular junction and binds to acetylcholine receptors, which are activated and generate a muscle contraction.

Pathophysiology

Myasthenia gravis occurs when normal communication between the nerve and muscle is interrupted at the neuromuscular junction—the place where nerve cells connect with the muscles they control. Antibodies produced by the body's own immune system block, alter, or destroy the receptors for acetylcholine at the neuromuscular junction, which prevents muscle contraction from occurring. Because the immune system, which normally protects the body from foreign organisms, mistakenly attacks itself, myasthenia gravis is known as an autoimmune disease.

Clinical Manifestations

Although myasthenia gravis may affect any voluntary muscle, muscles that control eye and eyelid movement, facial expression, and swallowing are most frequently affected. The onset of the disorder may be sudden, and symptoms often are not immediately recognized as myasthenia gravis. In most cases, the first noticeable symptom is weakness of the eye muscles. In others, difficulty in swallowing and slurred speech may be the first signs. The degree of muscle weakness involved in myasthenia gravis varies greatly among people, ranging from a localized form limited to eye muscles (ocular myasthenia) to a severe or generalized form in which many muscles—sometimes including those that control breathing—are affected.

Symptoms, which vary in type and severity, may include a drooping of one or both eyelids (ptosis), blurred or double vision (diplopia) due to weakness of the muscles that control eye movements, unstable or waddling gait, a change in facial expression, difficulty in swallowing, shortness of breath, impaired speech (dysarthria), and weakness in the arms, hands, fingers, legs, and neck.

Drug Therapy

Cholinergic drugs stimulate the parasympathetic nervous system in the same manner as acetylcholine. The cholinergic drugs described in this chapter act indirectly by inhibiting the enzyme **acetylcholinesterase**, thereby slowing acetylcholine metabolism at autonomic nerve synapses. Other drugs act directly to stimulate cholinergic receptors (Fig. 46.1).

Anticholinesterase drugs are classified as either reversible or irreversible inhibitors of acetylcholinesterase. The reversible inhibitors exhibit a moderate duration of action and have several therapeutic uses—in myasthenia gravis and, as described later in this chapter, in Alzheimer's disease. Table 46.1 lists medications used to treat myasthenia gravis.

Clinical Application 46-1

- What does the nurse teach Ms. Collins about the pathophysiology of myasthenia gravis?

- What information does the nurse provide to Ms. Collins about the signs and symptoms she is experiencing?

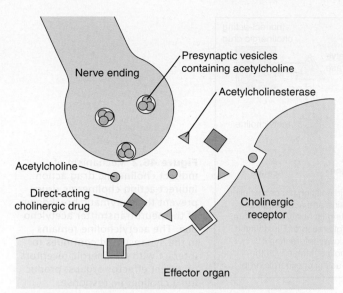

Figure 46.1 Mechanism of direct cholinergic drug action. Direct-acting cholinergic drugs interact with postsynaptic cholinergic receptors on target effector organs, activating the organ in a similar fashion as the neurotransmitter acetylcholine.

Indirect-Acting Cholinergics

The anticholinesterase drug Ⓟ **neostigmine** (Prostigmin) is the prototype drug in this class. Health care providers use this drug for the long-term treatment of myasthenia gravis and as an antidote for tubocurarine and other nondepolarizing skeletal muscle relaxants used in surgery.

Pharmacokinetics

Neostigmine is available in an oral preparation, and absorption in the GI tract is poor. An intravenous (IV) form is available (for muscle spasms). The onset of action is 20 to 30 minutes for the oral form and 15 minutes for the IV form. The half-life is 50 to 90 minutes. Metabolism occurs in the liver, and the drug does not appear to cross the placenta easily. Excretion occurs in the kidneys.

Action

Neostigmine decreases the inactivation of acetylcholine in the synapse by the enzyme acetylcholinesterase. Thus, acetylcholine accumulates in the synapse and enhances the activation of postsynaptic muscarinic as well as nicotinic receptors (Fig. 46.2). In addition to the cholinergic drug effects described above, the added effect of indirect-acting cholinergic drugs on nicotinic receptors in skeletal muscles results in improved skeletal muscle tone and strength.

In a patient with myasthenia gravis, specific effects of neostigmine include decreasing the heart rate, increasing the tone of GI smooth muscle, and stimulating the salivary glands to increase secretions. In addition, this drug increases tone and contractility of smooth muscle (detrusor) in the urinary bladder and relaxes the sphincter and bronchial smooth muscles (see Fig. 46.2).

Use

The major use of neostigmine is in the diagnosis and treatment of myasthenia gravis. In addition, prescribers order it to reverse the action of nondepolarizing neuromuscular blocking agents, such as tubocurarine, which is used in surgery. Neostigmine does not reverse the neuromuscular blockade produced by depolarizing neuromuscular blocking agents such as succinylcholine.

Table 46.2 presents dosage information for neostigmine and related drugs.

Use in Older Adults

Older adults are more likely to experience adverse drug effects because of age-related physiologic changes and superimposed pathologic conditions.

Use in Patients With Renal Impairment

Neostigmine undergoes tubular excretion in the kidneys. Therefore, renal impairment may result in accumulation and increased adverse effects, especially with chronic use. It is necessary to monitor patients with renal impairment and urinary obstruction carefully and give the drug at the lowest possible loading dose.

Use in Patients With Hepatic Impairment

Neostigmine undergoes metabolism in the liver, and hepatic disease may interfere with this, resulting in increased adverse effects. However, no dosage adjustments are necessary in patients with hepatic impairment.

TABLE 46.1		
Drugs Administered for the Treatment of Myasthenia Gravis, Alzheimer's Disease, and Urinary Retention		
Drug Class	**Prototype**	**Other Drugs in the Class**
Indirect-acting cholinergics	Neostigmine (Prostigmin)	Edrophonium (Tensilon) Physostigmine (Antilirium) Pyridostigmine (Mestinon)
Reversible indirect-acting cholinergics	Donepezil (Aricept)	Galantamine (Razadyne, Razadyne ER) Rivastigmine (Exelon), (Exelon Patch)
Direct-acting cholinergic	Bethanechol (Urecholine)	

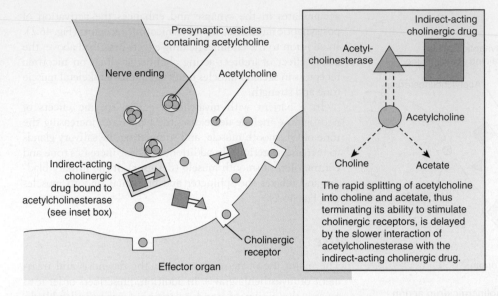

Figure 46.2 Mechanism of indirect cholinergic drug action. Indirect-acting cholinergic drugs prevent the enzymatic breakdown of the neurotransmitter acetylcholine. The acetylcholine remains in the synapse and continues to interact with cholinergic receptors on target effector organs, producing a cholinergic response.

(Inset box text:) The rapid splitting of acetylcholine into choline and acetate, thus terminating its ability to stimulate cholinergic receptors, is delayed by the slower interaction of acetylcholinesterase with the indirect-acting cholinergic drug.

TABLE 46.2

DRUGS AT A GLANCE: Indirect-Acting Cholinergics Used for the Treatment of Myasthenia Gravis

Drug	Pregnancy Category	Routes and Dosage Ranges	
		Adults	*Children*
Ⓟ **Neostigmine** (Prostigmin)	C	Diagnosis of myasthenia gravis: 0.022 mg/kg IM. Treatment of myasthenia gravis: Dosage individualized to patient needs. PO 15–375 mg/d in 3 or 4 divided doses. Subcutaneous, IV, or IM 0.5 mg initially. Individualize subsequent doses. Prevention/treatment of postoperative distention and urinary retention: 0.25–0.5 mg IM or sub-Q every 4–6 h for 2–3 d. Antidote for nondepolarizing neuromuscular blockers: Give atropine sulfate 0.6–1.2 mg IV several minutes before slow IV injection of neostigmine 0.5–2 mg. Repeat as needed; total dose not to exceed 5 mg	Diagnosis of myasthenia gravis: 0.04 mg/kg IM. Treatment of myasthenia gravis: PO 0.3–0.6 mg/kg every 3–4 h. Subcutaneous, IV, IM 0.01–0.04 mg/kg/dose every 2–3 h as needed. Prevention/treatment of postoperative distention and urinary retention: safety and efficacy not established. Antidote for nondepolarizing neuromuscular blockers: give atropine sulfate 0.008–0.025 mg/kg IV several minutes before slow IV injection of neostigmine 0.07–0.08 mg/kg
Edrophonium (Tensilon)	C	Diagnosis of myasthenia gravis: IV route preferred: 2 mg IV over 15–30 s; 8 mg IV given 45 s later if no response. Test dose may be repeated in 30 min. IM route: 10 mg; may follow up with an additional 2 mg 30 min later if no response. Differentiation of myasthenic crisis from cholinergic crisis: 2 mg IV, observe response for 60 s; may repeat with subsequent doses of 3 mg and 5 mg if no response to initial dose. *Be prepared* to intubate	Diagnosis of myasthenia gravis: Infants: 0.5 mg IV. <34 kg: 1 mg IV; may titrate up to 5 mg if no response. >34 kg: 2 mg IV; may titrate up to 10 mg if no response. Children <34 kg: 2 mg IM. Children >34 kg: 5 mg, IM
Physostigmine (Antilirium)	C	IM, IV 0.5–2 mg. Give IV slowly, no faster than 1 mg/min to avoid adverse effects of bradycardia, respiratory distress, and seizures.	Dosage not established
Pyridostigmine (Mestinon)	C	PO 60 mg 3 times daily initially; individualize dose to control symptoms. Average dose in 24 h: 600 mg. Range in 24 h: 60–1500 mg. IM, IV slowly: 1/30th the oral dose	Neonates of mothers with myasthenia gravis who have difficulty with sucking/breathing/swallowing: 0.05–0.15 mg/kg IM. Change to syrup as soon as possible

Use in Patients With Critical Illness

Neostigmine has specific uses in critical illness. These include reversal of skeletal muscle paralysis caused by nondepolarizing muscle relaxants, improvement of muscle strength, and use as an antidote to anticholinergic poisoning. In this last case, drugs such as atropine or tricyclic antidepressants are also required.

Use in Patients Receiving Home Care

Use of neostigmine in the home involves the treatment of long-term conditions such as myasthenia gravis. Self-administration may be a problem for the patient, who may have diplopia or diminished muscle strength. Strict adherence to timely medication administration promotes optimal blood levels of drugs and optimal symptom control. In the event the patient develops muscle weakness, it is essential that the primary care provider be notified immediately.

Adverse Effects

Specific Effects

Neostigmine has several adverse effects. Cardiovascular adverse effects of neostigmine are cardiac dysrhythmias, diminished cardiac output, hypotension, syncope, and cardiac arrest. Development of respiratory depression indicates cholinergic crisis. Other respiratory adverse effects include increased pharyngeal and tracheobronchial secretions, laryngospasm, bronchospasm, bronchiolar constriction, shortness of breath, and respiratory paralysis. (IV atropine sulfate is the specific antidote for cholinergic agents.) Conditions such as excessive salivation, nausea, emesis, frequent urination, or diarrhea require a reduction in dosage.

Toxicity of Neostigmine and Other Indirect-Acting Anticholinergics

Cholinergic crisis is a drug-induced overstimulation of the parasympathetic nervous system, requiring discontinuation of any anticholinesterase drug that the patient has been receiving. Atropine sulfate should be readily available whenever cholinergic drugs are given. It is important to note that atropine reverses only the muscarinic effects of cholinergic drugs, primarily in the heart, smooth muscle, and glands. Atropine does not interact with nicotinic receptors and therefore cannot reverse the nicotinic effects of skeletal muscle weakness due to overdose of indirect anticholinergic drugs.

Atropine sulfate is also administered for the management of mushroom poisoning. Muscarine, an alkaloid that is found in small quantities in the *Amanita muscaria* mushroom, is the source of the name for the muscarinic receptors in the parasympathetic nervous system; muscarine can stimulate these receptors. Some mushrooms found in North America, such as *Clitocybe* and *Inocybe* mushrooms, however, contain much larger quantities of muscarine. Accidental or intentional ingestion of these mushrooms results in cholinergic crisis and is potentially fatal.

Contraindications

Contraindications to neostigmine include known hypersensitivity. Patients with lung disease, such as bronchial asthma, or heart disease, such as sick sinus syndrome, should not take the drug. In addition, it is necessary to use caution with patients with benign prostatic hypertrophy and other urinary retention problems.

Nursing Implications

Preventing Interactions

Several drugs interact with neostigmine (Box 46.1), increasing or decreasing its effects.

Administering the Medication

When administering neostigmine, it is necessary to give the drug with food or fluid and not to crush extended-release forms. It is important to administer IV neostigmine slowly and have atropine available as an antidote in the event of a cholinergic crisis or hypersensitivity to neostigmine.

QSEN Safety Alert

When administering neostigmine to older patients, it is essential to observe for signs of cholinergic reactions, particularly when the drug is given IV. Treatment for myasthenic crisis includes administration of additional anticholinesterase medications and measures to maintain respirations until the medications are effective in improving muscle strength.

Assessing for Therapeutic Effects

The nurse assesses the patient's response to the medication. When neostigmine is given to patients with myasthenia gravis, it is necessary to observe for increased muscle strength; decreased difficulty with chewing, swallowing, and speech; and decreased or absent ptosis of eyelids.

Assessing for Adverse Effects

The nurse assesses for increased central nervous system (CNS) effects such as convulsions, dizziness, and drowsiness. He or she assesses for increased secretions, bronchospasm, laryngospasm, and respiratory failure. It is necessary to assess for nausea and vomiting, which are common GI effects. In addition, the nurse

BOX 46.2 — Patient Teaching Guidelines for Neostigmine

■ Wear a medical alert identification device if you are taking long-term cholinergic drug therapy for myasthenia gravis.

■ Record symptoms of myasthenia gravis and effects of drug therapy, especially when drug therapy is initiated and medication doses are being titrated. The amount of medication required to control symptoms of myasthenia gravis varies greatly, and the physician needs this information to adjust the dosage correctly.

■ Do not overexert yourself if you have myasthenia gravis. Rest between activities. Although the dose of medication may be increased during periods of increased activity, it is desirable to space activities to obtain optimal benefit from the drug, at the lowest possible dose, with the fewest adverse effects.

■ Report increased muscle weakness, difficulty breathing, or recurrent of myasthenic symptoms to your physician. These are signs of drug underdosage (myasthenic crisis) and indicate a need to increase or change drug therapy.

■ Report adverse reactions, including abdominal cramps, diarrhea, excessive oral secretions, difficulty in breathing, and muscle weakness. These are signs of drug overdosage (cholinergic crisis) and require immediate discontinuation of drugs and treatment by a physician. Respiratory failure can result if this condition is not recognized and treated properly. Atropine may be administered for overdose of cholinergic drugs.

observes neonates of mothers with myasthenia gravis who have received neostigmine for difficulty breathing, swallowing, or sucking.

Patient Teaching

Box 46.2 identifies patient teaching guidelines for neostigmine.

Clinical Application 46-2

■ Ms. Collins takes her neostigmine 50-mg extended-release tablet one morning. At 2:00 PM, she develops nausea and becomes diaphoretic. She calls the home care nurse about her symptoms. What does the nurse suspect has contributed to the development of these symptoms?

■ Ms. Collins continues to take the 50-mg extended-release tablets. One week later, the home care nurse visits and finds that her respirations are very shallow at a rate of 8 breaths per minute. Based on this assessment, what does the nurse suspect is wrong with the patient?

■ The home care nurse calls 9-1-1. She informs the paramedics of Ms. Collins diagnosis of myasthenia gravis and the medications she is taking. What medication do the paramedics administer?

NCLEX Success

1. A patient has received neostigmine 50 mg. Which of the following is a serious adverse effect of neostigmine (Prostigmin)?

   A. bronchospasm
   B. headache
   C. nausea
   D. sweating

2. The nursing supervisor of a skilled nursing facility observes an aide crushing an extended-release tablet of neostigmine and mixing it in applesauce. What instruction should the nurse provide to the aide?

   A. Inform the aide that it is appropriate to crush the pill.
   B. Inform the aide to order a liquid form of neostigmine.
   C. Inform the aide that this will result in too large a dose.
   D. Inform the aide that neostigmine causes respiratory depression.

3. A man receives a diagnosis of myasthenia gravis. His physician prescribes neostigmine (Prostigmin) 60 mg by mouth every 3 hours. Before administering this anticholinesterase agent, the nurse reviews the patient's history. Which preexisting condition contraindicates the use of neostigmine?

   A. ulcerative colitis
   B. blood dyscrasia
   C. intestinal obstruction
   D. urinary obstruction

Other Drugs in the Class

Edrophonium (Tensilon) is a short-acting cholinergic drug used to diagnose myasthenia gravis, to differentiate between myasthenia crisis and cholinergic crisis, and to reverse the neuromuscular blockade produced by nondepolarizing skeletal muscle relaxants. A physician administers this drug intramuscularly or IV and remains in attendance. The ideal test dose of edrophonium has not been determined. An incremental dosing schedule begins with 2 mg, followed by a 60-second period of time during which the response of the patient is observed. Subsequent doses of 3 and 5 mg may be necessary if indicated by a lack of response. If the edrophonium test causes a dramatic improvement in breathing, it is considered positive and the diagnosis is myasthenic crisis. If the edrophonium test makes the patient even weaker, the diagnosis is cholinergic crisis. Atropine, an antidote, and life-support equipment, such as ventilators and endotracheal tubes, must be available when the drug is given.

Physostigmine salicylate (Antilirium) is the only anticholinesterase drug capable of crossing the blood–brain barrier. Unlike other drugs in this group, physostigmine is not a quaternary amine, does not carry a positive charge, and therefore is more lipid soluble. It is sometimes used as an antidote for overdosage of anticholinergic drugs, including atropine, antihistamines, tricyclic antidepressants, and phenothiazine antipsychotics. However, its potential for causing serious adverse effects limits its usefulness.

Pyridostigmine (Mestinon) is similar to neostigmine in actions, uses, and in adverse effects. It may have a longer duration of action and lower incidence of adverse effects, and it is the maintenance drug of choice for patients with myasthenia gravis. An added advantage is the availability of a slow-release form, which is effective for 8 to 12 hours. When this form is taken at bedtime, the patient does not have to take other medications during the night and does not awaken too weak to swallow.

Overview of Alzheimer's Disease

Etiology

Alzheimer's disease is the most common form of dementia, a general term for memory loss and other intellectual abilities serious enough to interfere with daily life. Alzheimer's disease accounts for 50% to 80% of dementia cases. As many as 5% of people with the disease have early-onset Alzheimer's disease (also known as younger-onset), which often develops when a person is in their 40s or 50s.

Pathophysiology

Alzheimer's disease results in a significant loss of neurons, in addition to shrinkage of large cortical neurons. The neuropathologic hallmarks of Alzheimer's disease are neuritic plaques and neurofibrillary tangles, although these lesions are not unique to Alzheimer's disease and can be found in other neurodegenerative disorders and in clinically normal people as well. The number and distribution of the plaques and tangles appear to contribute to the development of dementia.

Classic neuritic plaques are spherical structures consisting of a central core of fibrous protein known as amyloid that is surrounded by degenerating or dystrophic nerve endings (neurites). Two other types of amyloid-related plaques are recognized in the brains of patients with Alzheimer's disease: diffuse plaques, which contain poorly defined amyloid but no well-circumscribed amyloid core, and "burnt-out" plaques, which consist of an isolated dense amyloid core.

Neurofibrillary tangles, found in the cytoplasm of abnormal neurons, consist of fibrous proteins that are wound around each other. These tangles are resistant to breakdown and persist in brain tissue.

Clinical Manifestations

The most common early symptom of Alzheimer's disease is difficulty remembering newly learned information because the neurologic changes typically begin in the part of the brain that affects learning. As Alzheimer's disease advances through the brain, it leads to increasingly severe symptoms, including disorientation and mood and behavior changes; deepening confusion about events, time, and place; unfounded suspicions about family, friends, and professional caregivers; more serious memory loss and behavior changes; and difficulty speaking, swallowing, and walking.

Drug Therapy

The goal of drug therapy for Alzheimer's disease is to slow the loss of memory and cognition, thus preserving the independence of the individual person for as long as possible. Studies have shown that vitamin E, estrogen, and anti-inflammatory agents lower the risk of Alzheimer's disease. Practice guidelines developed by the American Academy of Neurology (2011) recommend early diagnosis and treatment of Alzheimer's disease with cholinesterase inhibitors for all patients with mild to moderate symptoms. Although these drugs do not cure Alzheimer's disease, they do delay the onset of the disease somewhat and bring about a slight improvement in cognition and function. The reversible indirect-acting cholinergic (anticholinesterase) drugs improve memory by elevating acetylcholine in the cerebral cortex of the brain. Tacrine (available as Cognex) was the first U.S. Food and Drug Administration–approved drug for use in the treatment of Alzheimer's disease. Now it is no longer marketed in the United States, and other related drugs have taken its place.

Reversible Indirect-Acting Cholinergics

Ⓟ **Donepezil** (Aricept) is the prototype drug in this class. Treatment of Alzheimer's disease is the primary use for this centrally acting reversible cholinesterase inhibitor. Table 46.1 lists the indirect-acting cholinergics used in the management of Alzheimer's disease.

Pharmacokinetics

Absorption of donepezil after oral administration is good, and it is unaffected by food. The drug is highly bound (96%) to plasma proteins. The peak of action occurs in 3 to 4 hours. Metabolism takes place in the liver, producing several metabolites, some of which are pharmacologically active. Excretion of these metabolites and some unchanged drug occurs mainly in urine.

Action

Donepezil increases acetylcholine in the brain by inhibiting its metabolism, leading to elevated acetylcholine levels in the cortex. This slows the neuronal degradation that occurs in Alzheimer's disease.

Use

As previously stated, health care providers use donepezil to treat mild, moderate, or severe Alzheimer's disease. Long-term studies have shown that the drug delays the progression of the disease for up to 55 weeks. Other uses include enhancing memory in other neurological conditions such as multiple sclerosis, treating myasthenia gravis, or treating overdoses of atropine and centrally acting anticholinergic drugs (e.g., those used for parkinsonism). Table 46.3 presents dosage information for donepezil and related drugs.

TABLE 46.3

DRUGS AT A GLANCE: Indirect-Acting Cholinergics Used for the Treatment of Alzheimer's Disease

Drug	Pregnancy Category	Routes and Dosage Ranges	
		Adults	Children
ⓟ **Donepezil** (Aricept)	C	5 mg PO daily at bedtime for 4–6 wk, then increase to 10 mg daily if needed	Dosage not established
Galantamine (Razadyne, Razadyne ER)	C	8 mg PO daily initially, with food; increase to 16 mg/d after 4 wk if needed. May continue to increase every 4 wk up to max dose of 24 mg/d	Dosage not established
Memantine (Namenda)	B	5 mg PO daily, increase dose by 5 mg/wk over a 3-wk period; target dose: 10 mg PO 2 times/d. Severe renal impairment: 5 mg PO 2 times/d	Dosage not established
Rivastigmine (Exelon), (Exelon Patch)	C	1.5 mg PO twice daily with food initially. May titrate to higher doses at 1.5 mg intervals every 2 wk to a maximum dose of 12 mg/d. TDS initially 4–6 mg/24 h patch. Increase to 9.5 mg/24 h patch after 4 wk. Max dose 9.5 mg/24 h patch	Dosage not established

TDS, transdermal delivery system

Use in Older Adults

Older adults are more likely to experience adverse drug effects because of age-related physiologic changes and superimposed pathologic conditions.

Use in Patients With Hepatic Impairment

Liver disease may impair the hepatic metabolism of donepezil, resulting in increased adverse effects. It is important to monitor a patient's liver function and clinical response to the medication carefully.

Use in Patients With Critical Illness

Donepezil has several specific uses in critical illness, which include reducing cognitive dysfunction. Commonly, critically ill patients may have delirium, a form of acute cognitive dysfunction that manifests as a fluctuating change in mental status, with inattention and altered level of consciousness. As many as 80% of mechanically ventilated patients are in the intensive care unit; this makes donepezil is an important management drug.

Use in Patients Receiving Home Care

Patients with Alzheimer's disease may have problems with remembering to take medications and may easily underdose or overdose themselves. It is important for the home care nurse to work with responsible family members in such cases to ensure accurate drug administration.

Adverse Effects

The most common adverse effects of donepezil are headache, dizziness, depression, vertigo, and insomnia. Possible drug-related GI conditions include nausea, vomiting, diarrhea, abdominal muscle cramps, anorexia, and GI bleeding. The most serious

adverse effects are breathing problems (e.g., asthma, chronic obstructive pulmonary disease), fainting, and heart disease (e.g., sick sinus syndrome, other heart conduction disorder). Dyspnea has been reported and is more common in patients who have previous lung disease. In addition, fatigue and anorexia may occur. Other adverse effects include seizures and trouble urinating.

Contraindications

Contraindications to donepezil include known hypersensitivity to the drug. Patients with lung disease or heart disease such as sick sinus syndrome should not take this medication.

Nursing Implications

Preventing Interactions

Many medications interact with donepezil, increasing or decreasing its effects (Box 46.3).

Administering the Medication

Before administering donepezil, the nurse assesses the patient for allergy, orientation, and contraindications. Administration should occur at bedtime each day. If the patient is taking an oral disintegrating tablet, the nurse ensures that the medication is dissolved on the tongue.

QSEN Safety Alert

The brand names for donepezil (Aricept) and rabeprazole (AcipHex) are a source of confusion. It is essential to use caution when administering either of these drugs.

BOX 46.3 Drug Interactions: Donepezil

Drugs That Increase the Effects of Donepezil

■ Theophylline
 Increases the risk of toxicity

■ Cholinesterase inhibitors
 Increase the risk of toxicity

Drugs That Decrease the Effects of Donepezil

■ Anticholinergics
 Decrease the efficacy

■ Nonsteroidal anti-inflammatory drugs
 Increase the risk of gastrointestinal bleeding

Assessing for Therapeutic Effects

The nurse assesses for improved memory and reduction of dementia. This involves assessing daily for memory changes, forgetfulness, and mood.

Assessing for Adverse Effects

The nurse assesses for signs and symptoms of GI upset such as nausea, diarrhea, insomnia, and vomiting. If GI bleeding is suspected, it is important to obtain an order for laboratory tests such as complete blood count and bleeding time.

Patient Teaching

Box 46.4 identifies patient teaching guidelines for donepezil.

Other Drugs in the Class

Galantamine hydrobromide (Razadyne) is similar to donepezil in its action. Indications include mild to moderate dementia and vascular dementia (unlabeled use). Contraindications

BOX 46.4 Patient Teaching Guidelines for Donepezil

■ Take this drug exactly as prescribed, at bedtime.

■ Place orally disintegrating tablet on your tongue; allow it to dissolve and then drink water.

■ Know that this drug does not cure the disease but is thought to slow down the degeneration associated with the disease.

■ Continue taking this drug if no change in symptoms is noted.

■ Arrange for regular blood tests and follow-up visits while adjusting to this drug.

■ Note that the following side effects may occur: nausea, vomiting (eat frequent small meals), insomnia, fatigue, and confusion (use caution if driving or performing tasks that require alertness).

■ Report severe nausea, vomiting, changes in stool or urine color, diarrhea, changes in neurologic functioning, and yellowing of the eyes or skin to your health care provider.

include severe hepatic or renal impairment. The most common adverse effects are insomnia, tremor, dizziness, somnolence, headache, bradycardia, and syncope. Patients and families should receive instructions about reporting any changes in mental status. To decrease gastric upset, it is necessary to take the medication with food.

Memantine hydrochloride (Namenda) is widely administered for moderate to severe Alzheimer's disease. The drug blocks the *N*-methyl-*D*-aspartate receptors sites and slows calcium accumulation without interfering with glutamate that is required for memory. Absorption in the GI tract is complete, and excretion of unchanged drug occurs in the urine. It is necessary to monitor patients with diabetes who are taking memantine for hyperglycemia. Patients and families should receive instructions about reporting any changes in mental status or hypersensitivity to the drug. Patients should not take sodium bicarbonate because it increases serum levels of the memantine.

Rivastigmine (Exelon) is a long-acting central anticholinesterase agent approved for the treatment of mild to moderate dementia due to Alzheimer's disease as well as Parkinson's

EVIDENCE-BASED PRACTICE

A Review Comparing the Safety and Tolerability of Memantine With the Acetylcholinesterase Inhibitors
by JONES, R. W.

International Journal of Geriatric Psychiatry
2010, 24, 547–553
Retrieved January 3, 2012

The rate of Alzheimer's disease and dementia is on the rise worldwide. The treatment focuses on the alleviation of symptoms. The elderly patient is at risk for multiple adverse effects due to the fact the patient may have multiple comorbidities, which require multiple medications. Another factor that leads to an increase risk of adverse effects is the fact the Alzheimer's patient may not maintain adequate compliance with the medication regime.

In this study, the author reviewed recent safety and tolerability data for memantine and acetylcholinesterase inhibitors. The study revealed that Alzheimer's patients are vulnerable to adverse effects of medications due to polypharmacy and comorbid disease processes. However, memantine and acetylcholinesterase inhibitors are safe and well tolerated.

IMPLICATION FOR NURSING PRACTICE: When caring for patients with Alzheimer's disease, it is important that the nurse understand the effects of polypharmacy in relation to the development of adverse drug effects. It is also the nurse's responsibility to provide teaching to the patient and family about safety and the prevention of injury related to central nervous system depression.

disease. Oral rivastigmine lasts 12 hours, making twice-a-day dosing possible. Rivastigmine transdermal is applied as a patch once a day. Like other drugs in this class, it is not a cure for Alzheimer's disease but does slow the progression of symptoms. Metabolism occurs in the liver, and excretion takes place in the feces. The side-effect profile of rivastigmine is similar to that of donepezil. To minimize certain adverse effects (e.g., nausea, vomiting, loss of appetite), it is typically necessary to increase dosages slowly until the therapeutic dosage is reached. Patients may take the drug with food to decrease GI distress.

NCLEX Success

4. A nurse is teaching family members how to administer donepezil (Aricept) for Alzheimer's disease. The instructions should include which of the following?

   A. Take the medication with food.
   B. Take the medication on an empty stomach.
   C. Take the medication at bedtime.
   D. Take the medication at the start of each day.

5. A 74-year-old man has Alzheimer's disease. Which nursing diagnosis takes highest priority for this patient?

   A. Imbalanced Nutrition: Less Than Body Requirements
   B. Ineffective Airway Clearance
   C. Impaired Urinary Elimination
   D. Risk for Injury

6. A woman diagnosed with Alzheimer's disease has used donepezil (Aricept) for four years. Her daughter notices her memory is worsening. Which of the following medications might be more successful for enhancing her memory?

   A. tacrine (Cognex)
   B. rivastigmine (Exelon)
   C. memantine (Namenda)
   D. galantamine (Razadyne)

Overview of Urinary Retention

Etiology and Pathophysiology

Urinary retention may be due to several factors. The most common cause is a lack of nerve innervation; this condition is also known as neurogenic bladder. Other causes include diabetes, prostate enlargement, pregnancy, neurological disorders such as multiple sclerosis or Parkinson's disease, as well as surgery with general anesthesia. Surgery with general anesthesia that involves perineal or anal regions results in a reflex spasm of the sphincters (Smeltzer, Bare, Hinkle, & Cheever, 2010). There may be a reduction of bladder muscle innervation in the postoperative period.

The two most common neurogenic bladder disorders are the failure to store urine, known as the spastic bladder, or the failure to empty urine from the bladder, known as the flaccid bladder. The spastic bladder results from neurologic lesions above the level of the sacral micturition reflexes. The flaccid bladder results from lesions at the sacral micturition reflex.

Clinical Manifestations and Drug Therapy

A neurogenic bladder results in urinary retention or leakage. The patient may describe a sensation of bladder fullness or incomplete bladder emptying.

The pharmacological treatment of urinary retention is administration of bethanechol chloride (Urecholine) (see Table 46.1).

Direct-Acting Cholinergics

Ⓟ **Bethanechol chloride** (Urecholine) is the prototype direct-acting cholinergic agent used to increase the contraction of the detrusor muscle to relieve urinary retention.

Pharmacokinetics

Bethanechol is well absorbed in the GI tract. The onset of action is 30 minutes, and the medication reaches its peak in 60 to 90 minutes. The duration of action is 1 to 6 hours. The site of metabolism and elimination is not known. The drug does not cross the blood–brain barrier but does cross the placenta, and it enters breast milk.

Action

Bethanechol is a sympathomimetic agent that acts at the cholinergic receptors in the urinary and GI tracts to increase muscle tone. The increased tone of the detrusor muscle in the urinary bladder allows for bladder emptying.

Use

Bethanechol is administered during the acute postoperative and postpartum periods for the treatment of nonobstructed urinary retention and neurogenic atony of the bladder muscle. Table 46.4 gives dosage information for this drug.

Adverse Effects

Cardiovascular adverse effects to bethanechol include transient heart block, orthostatic hypotension with large doses, and cardiac arrest. Reported GI adverse effects are abdominal discomfort, increased salivation, nausea, vomiting, and fecal incontinence. Genitourinary effects include urinary urgency. Other adverse effects are flushing, sweating, malaise, and dyspnea.

Contraindications

Contraindications to bethanechol include known hypersensitivity to the drug or other cholinergic agent as well as hyperthyroidism, peptic ulcer disease, intestinal obstruction, asthma, bradycardia, coronary artery disease, epilepsy, and parkinsonism. Patients should not take bethanechol in the postoperative phase of bladder neck or GI surgery.

TABLE 46.4

DRUGS AT A GLANCE: Direct-Acting Cholinergic Used for the Treatment of Urinary Retention

Drug	Pregnancy Category	Routes and Dosage Ranges	
		Adults	Children
ⓟ **Bethanechol hydrochloride** (Urecholine)	C	10–50 mg PO 3–4 times/d; initial dose of 5–10 mg with gradual increases hourly until desired effect is seen; or until 50 mg is given	Safety and efficacy not established

Nursing Implications

Preventing Interactions

Several drugs, including cholinergic agents, atropine, procainamide, epinephrine, and ganglionic blockers, increase the effects of bethanechol. This causes a significant drop in blood pressure.

Administering the Medication

Administration of bethanechol should occur 1 hour before meals or 2 hours after meals to prevent nausea and vomiting. Therapy should begin using the lowest possible dosage, which is then increased as tolerated.

Assessing for Therapeutic Effects

The nurse assesses the patient's ability to void 1 hour following the administration of the medication. He or she interviews the patient regarding the relief of symptoms of bladder fullness.

Assessing for Adverse Effects

The nurse assesses the patient's blood pressure lying, sitting, and standing. It is also necessary to assess an electrocardiogram for signs of heart block or impending cardiac arrest. In addition, the nurse assesses for cholinergic crisis with sweating and flushing. Finally, he or she assesses for GI effects such as abdominal pain, nausea, and vomiting.

Patient Teaching

Box 46.5 identifies patient teaching guidelines for bethanechol.

BOX 46.5 Patient Teaching Guidelines for Bethanechol Chloride

- Take the medication on an empty stomach.
- Take the medication only as prescribed.
- Report difficulty urinating to your health care provider.
- Report diarrhea, headache, belching, substernal pressure, or pain to your health care provider.

NCLEX Success

7. The nurse should be prepared to administer which of the following drugs as an antidote to cholinergic drug overdose?
   A. epinephrine (Adrenaline)
   B. diphenhydramine (Benadryl)
   C. atropine (AtroPen)
   D. propranolol (Inderal)

8. The nurse who is working in the genitourinary surgical division of the health center has an order to administer bethanechol (Urecholine) to a patient. Which of the following statements by the patient would require the nurse to hold the medication and notify the prescriber?
   A. "I was diagnosed with hyperthyroidism this year."
   B. "I have not eaten any breakfast."
   C. "I have not urinated for 6 hours."
   D. "My mother was allergic to bethanechol."

9. The nurse has administered bethanechol (Urecholine) to a patient who has not voided in 8 hours. What is the priority assessment following the administration of bethanechol?
   A. Assess the patient's blood pressure in 2 hours.
   B. Assess the cardiac status every 15 minutes.
   C. Assess the patient's urinary output in 1 hour.
   D. Assess the patient's fluid intake for 24 hours.

10. A 40-year-old patient is taking bethanechol (Urecholine) for urinary retention. The physician increases the dosage from 30 to 40 mg. For which of the following adverse effects should the nurse assess?
    A. pulmonary edema
    B. bronchospasm
    C. orthostatic hypotension
    D. pulse deficit

Irreversible Anticholinesterase Toxicity

Most irreversible anticholinesterase agents are highly lipid soluble and can enter the body by a variety of routes, including the eye, skin, respiratory system, and GI tract. Because they readily cross the blood–brain barrier, their effects are seen peripherally as well as centrally.

Some of the agents used by terrorists are irreversible anticholinesterases. In 1995, a terrorist group released sarin gas on a number of subway trains in Tokyo, Japan. Sarin is a toxic nerve gas that produces a cholinergic crisis characterized by excessive cholinergic (muscarinic) stimulation and neuromuscular blockade. This cholinergic crisis occurs because the irreversible anticholinesterase poison binds to the enzyme anticholinesterase and inactivates it. Consequently, acetylcholine remains in cholinergic synapses and causes excessive stimulation of muscarinic and nicotinic receptors. Other nerve gases that produce these effects include tabun and soman. In addition, the organophosphate insecticides malathion and parathion have the same cholinergic effects.

Emergency treatment includes decontamination procedures such as removing contaminated clothing, flushing the poison from skin and eyes, and using activated charcoal and lavage to remove ingested poison from the GI tract. Pharmacologic treatment includes administering atropine to counteract the muscarinic effects of the poison (e.g., salivation, urination, defecation, bronchial secretions, laryngospasm, bronchospasm). Atropine acts by blocking the acetylcholine at the parasympathetic sites of the smooth muscle, salivary glands, and the CNS to dry secretions and increase cardiac output. The severity of the poisoning dictates the dosage of atropine. The U.S. Department of Defense uses atropine in the form of AtroPen for the initial treatment of muscarinic symptoms.

In addition, a second drug is necessary to relieve the neuromuscular blockade produced by nicotinic effects of the poison. This drug, pralidoxime (Protopam), a cholinesterase reactivator, is a specific antidote for overdose with irreversible anticholinesterase agents. (Other indications for pralidoxime include control of overdose by anticholinesterase drugs used to treat myasthenia gravis.) It treats toxicity by causing the anticholinesterase poison to release the enzyme acetylcholinesterase. The reactivated acetylcholinesterase can then degrade excess acetylcholine at the cholinergic synapses, including the neuromuscular junction. It is important to note that pralidoxime cannot cross the blood–brain barrier; thus, it is effective only in the peripheral areas of the body. It is essential that pralidoxime is given as soon after the poisoning as possible. If too much time passes, the bond between the irreversible anticholinesterase agent and acetylcholinesterase becomes stronger, and pralidoxime is unable to release the enzyme from the poison.

Dosage reduction is necessary in the presence of renal impairment. During the administration of the medication, continuous monitoring of the patient is essential due to the risk of tachycardia and cardiac arrest. The peak onset of action is 5 to 15 minutes. The half-life is 74 to 77 minutes. Excretion of unchanged drug occurs in the urine.

Treatment of anticholinesterase overdose may also require diazepam or lorazepam to control seizures. The mechanism of action of diazepam is not understood, but the drug is thought to act in the limbic system. It potentiates gamma-aminobutyric acid, an inhibitory neurotransmitter. Close monitoring of the patient's electrocardiogram during drug administration is necessary. Mechanical ventilation may be necessary to treat respiratory paralysis.

Table 46.5 summarizes the miscellaneous medications used for the treatment of irreversible anticholinesterase toxicity.

The Nursing Process

Assessment
- Myasthenia gravis
  - Assess for muscle weakness mild to moderate disease: ptosis (drooping) of the upper eyelid and diplopia (double vision) caused by weakness of the eye muscles.
  - In severe disease, assess for difficulty in chewing, swallowing, and speaking; accumulation of oral secretions, which the patient may be unable to expectorate or swallow; decreased skeletal muscle activity, including impaired chest expansion; and eventual respiratory failure.
- Alzheimer's disease
  - Assess for abilities and limitations in relation to memory, cognitive functioning, and self-care activities.
  - Assess for preexisting conditions that may be aggravated by a cholinergic drug.
- Urinary retention
  - Assess for bladder distention.
  - Assess for time and amount of previous urination and fluid intake.

Nursing Diagnoses
- Impaired gas exchange related to increased respiratory secretions, bronchospasm, and/or respiratory paralysis
- Ineffective breathing pattern related to bronchoconstriction
- Ineffective airway clearance related to increased respiratory secretions
- Self-care deficit related to muscle weakness, cognitive impairment, or diplopia
- Deficient knowledge: drug administration and effects
- Altered elimination pattern: decreased smooth muscle control

Planning/Goals
The patient will
- Verbalize or demonstrate correct drug administration
- Improve in self-care abilities
- Regain usual patterns of urinary and bowel elimination
- Maintain effective oxygenation of tissues
- Report adverse drug effects
- For patients with myasthenia gravis, at least one family member will verbalize or demonstrate correct drug administration, symptoms of too much or too little drug, and emergency care procedures.
- For patients with dementia, a caregiver will verbalize or demonstrate correct drug administration and knowledge of adverse effects to be reported to a health care provider.

Nursing Interventions
The nurse will
- Use measures to prevent or decrease the need for cholinergic drugs. Ambulation, adequate fluid intake, and judicious use of opioid analgesics or other sedative-type drugs help prevent postoperative urinary retention.

TABLE 46.5

DRUGS AT A GLANCE: Miscellaneous Drugs Used for Treatment of Irreversible Anticholinesterase Toxicity

Drug	Pregnancy Category	Routes and Dosage Ranges	
		Adults	*Children*
Atropine sulfate	B	Nerve agent toxicity: Mild to moderate symptoms: 0.05 mg/kg IM Severe symptoms: 0.1 mg/kg IM Repeat atropine IM at 5–10 min intervals until secretions have diminished Organophosphate poisoning: 0.02–0.05 mg/kg IV every 10–20 min until atropine effect	Nerve agent toxicity: 1 mo–2 y: Mild to moderate symptoms: 0.05 mg/kg IM or 0.02 IV Severe symptoms: 0.1 mg IM or 0.02 mg/kg IV 2–10 y: Mild to moderate symptoms: 1 mg Severe symptoms 4 mg >10 y: Mild to moderate symptoms: 2 mg Severe symptoms: 4 mg Organophosphate poisoning: 1 to ≤ 6 mo: 0.25 mg AtroPen 6 mo–4 y: 0.5 mg AtroPen 4–10 y 1 mg AtroPen >10 y: 2 mg AtroPen Mild symptoms: 1 injection Severe symptoms: Two additional injections Unconscious: Three injections in rapid succession
Pralidoxime (Protopam)	C	Use in conjunction with atropine 1–2 g IV or IM; repeat in 1–2 h if muscle weakness has not been relieved, then at 10–12 h intervals if cholinergic signs recur Organophosphate poisoning: loading dose 1000–2000 mg IV, repeat bolus of 1000–2000 mg after 1 h and repeat 10–12 h thereafter Mild symptoms: 600 mg IM, repeat every 15 min (maximum dose 1800 mg) Severe symptoms: 600 mg; repeat twice in rapid succession to deliver 1800 mg Persistent symptoms: repeat entire series beginning 1 h after last injection	Use in conjunction with atropine 20–50 mg/kg/dose; repeat in 1–2 h if muscle weakness is not improved, then 10–12 h intervals if cholinergic signs recur Organophosphate poisoning (<16 y): 20–50 mg/kg IV (max dose 2000 mg/dose); maintenance infusion 10–20 mg/kg/h Mild symptoms: 15 mg/kg repeat every 15 min for persistent symptoms (max dose: 45 mg/kg; may administer in rapid succession) Severe symptoms: 15 mg/kg; repeat twice in rapid succession 45 mg/kg total dose Persistent symptoms: may repeat entire series (45 mg/kg) beginning 1 h after last dose
Diazepam (Valium)	D	5–10 mg IV slowly; may repeat in 5–10 min; max dose: 30 mg	1 mo–5 y: 0.2–0.5 mg slowly IV every 2–5 min; max dose: 10 mg >5 y: 1 mg every 2–5 min; max dose: 10 mg

- In myasthenia gravis:
  - Schedule activities to avoid excessive fatigue and to allow adequate rest periods. This may be beneficial, because muscle weakness is aggravated by exercise and improved by rest.
  - Recommend that one or more family members be trained in cardiopulmonary resuscitation.
- In Alzheimer's disease, assist and teach caregivers to
  - Maintain a quiet, stable environment and daily routines to decrease confusion (e.g., verbal or written reminders, simple directions, adequate lighting, calendars, personal objects within view and reach).
  - Avoid altering dosage or stopping the drug without consulting the prescribing physician.

- Be sure that the patient keeps appointments for supervision and blood tests.
- Report signs and symptoms (i.e., skin rash, jaundice, light-colored stools) that may indicate hepatotoxicity for patients taking tacrine.
- Notify surgeons about tacrine therapy. Exaggerated muscle relaxation may occur if succinylcholine-type drugs are given.
- With long-term drug use, assist patients and families to establish a schedule of drug administration that best meets the patient's needs.
- Do not give cholinergic drugs for bladder atony and urinary retention or for paralytic ileus in the presence of an obstruction.

Evaluation

- Observe and interview about the adequacy of urinary elimination.
- Observe abilities and limitations in self-care.
- Question the patient and at least one family member of the patient with myasthenia gravis about correct drug

usage, symptoms of underdosage and overdosage, and emergency care procedures.
- Question caregivers of patients with dementia about the patient's level of functioning and response to medication.

Key Concepts

- Cholinergic drugs stimulate the parasympathetic nervous system directly by stimulating cholinergic receptors or indirectly by inhibiting the enzymatic metabolism of acetylcholine in synapses.

- Both direct-acting cholinergic drugs and indirect-acting cholinergic drugs (or anticholinesterase drugs) have widespread parasympathetic effects when they activate muscarinic receptors in cardiac muscle, smooth muscle, exocrine glands, and the eye.

- Indirect-acting cholinergic drugs also stimulate nicotinic receptors in skeletal muscles, resulting in improved skeletal muscle tone and strength.

- Indirect-acting cholinergic or anticholinesterase drugs are indicated to treat myasthenia gravis and Alzheimer's disease.

- Neostigmine (Prostigmin), the prototype drug used to treat myasthenia gravis, decreases the inactivation of acetylcholine in the synapse by the enzyme acetylcholinesterase.

- Edrophonium is used to differentiate between myasthenic crisis (too little cholinergic medication) and cholinergic crisis (too much cholinergic medication).

- Donepezil (Aricept) is a reversible indirect-acting cholinergic drug used in the treatment of Alzheimer's disease. It increases acetylcholine in the brain by inhibiting its metabolism leading to increased levels of acetylcholine in the cerebral cortex.

- Bethanechol chloride (Urecholine) is a direct-acting cholinergic agent administered to increase the contraction of the detrusor muscle to relieve urinary retention.

- Atropine reverses muscarinic effects due to overdose of cholinergic drugs but does not reverse the nicotinic effects of skeletal muscle weakness or paralysis due to overdose of indirect cholinergic drugs.

- Pralidoxime, a cholinesterase reactivator, is the specific treatment for neuromuscular blockade due to overdose with irreversible cholinergic drugs.

Critical Thinking Questions

46-1. A family, who just returned from a camping trip, has finished eating dinner containing wild mushrooms they picked while hiking. The 8-year-old boy begins to have trouble breathing, and he develops a high-pitched noise that is audible on inspiration. His mother notices that he is producing large amounts of saliva. Because of the child's increasing weakness and difficulty breathing, the father calls 9-1-1.

- When the emergency transport team arrives, what assessments should they make?
- What is the high-pitched audible sound on inspiration?
- What is the cause of the symptoms and what additional symptoms would the nurse expect to see?
- What is the drug of choice to relieve the symptoms?
- What is the dosage for the 8-year-old?

46-2. An 89-year-old woman has moved in with her son and daughter-in-law. She has been taking Donepezil (Aricept) for moderate Alzheimer's disease. In the past few weeks, her family states that she is increasingly more forgetful and has had episodes where she roams the house at night. She also has increased anxiety. The geriatrician has prescribed memantine (Namenda) 5 mg orally once daily.

- What is the rationale for prescribing memantine in addition to donepezil?
- What patient teaching does the nurse provide to the family?

References and Resources

Alzheimer's Association (2011). *What is Alzheimer's disease?* Retrieved August 22, 2011, from www.alz.org

American Academy of Neurology. Retrieved August 22, 2011 from http://www.aan.com.

Craig, M. C., & Murphy, D. G. (2010). Estrogen therapy and Alzheimer's dementia. *Annals of the New York Academy of Sciences, 1205,* 245–253.

Correia, S. C., Santos, R. X., Cardosa, S., Carvalho, C. Santos, M. S., Oliveria, C. R., et al. (2010). Effects of estrogen in the brain: Is it a neuroprotective agent in alzheimer's disease? *Current Aging Science, 3*(2), 113–126.

Cortese, I., Chaudhry, V., So, Y. T., Cantor, F., Comblath, D. R., & Rae-Grant, A. (2011). Evidence-based guideline update: Plasmapheresis in neurologic disorders. Report of the Therapeutics and Technology Assessment Subcommittee of the American Academy of Neurology, *Neurology, 76,* 294–300.

Ferreri, F., Määttä, S., Vecchio, F., Curcio, G., & Ferrarelli, F. (2011). Clinical neurophysiology in Alzheimer's disease. *International Journal of Alzheimer's Disease, 2011,* 134–157.

Jones, R. W. (2010). A review comparing the safety and tolerability of memantine with the anticholinesterase inhibitors. *International Journal of Geriatric Psychiatry, 24,* 547–553.

Karch, A. M. (2012). *2012 Lippincott's nursing drug guide.* Philadelphia, PA: Lippincott Williams & Wilkins.

McDade, E. M., & Petersen, R. C. (2011). *Mild cognitive impairment: Prognosis and treatment.* Up-to-Date. Lexi Comp, Inc.

National Institutes of Neurological Disease (NINDS). (2010). *Myasthenia Gravis Fact Sheet.* Retrieved August 20, 2011. NIH Publication No. 10-768.

Nursing 2011 Drug Handbook. (2011). Philadelphia, PA: Lippincott William & Wilkins.

Porth, C. M., & Matfin, G. (2009). *Pathophysiology concepts of altered health states.* Philadelphia, PA: Lippincott Williams & Wilkins.

Sathasivam, S. (2011). Current and emerging treatments for the management of myasthenia gravis. *Therapeutics and Clinical Risk Management, 7,* 313–323.

Smeltzer, S. C., Bare, B. G., Hinkle, J. H., & Cheever, K. H. (2010). *Brunner & Suddarth's textbook of medical-surgical nursing* (12th ed.). Philadelphia, PA: Lippincott Williams & Wilkins.

Up-To-Date. (2011). *Atropine: Pediatric Drug Information.* Lexi-Comp, Inc.

Up-to-Date. (2012). *Pralidoxime: Drug Information.* Lexi-Comp, Inc.

Up-to-Date. (2011). *Pralidoxime: Pediatric Drug Information.* Lexi-Comp, Inc.

Up-To-Date. (2011). *Treatment of Myasthenia Gravis.* Lexi-Comp, Inc.

47 Drug Therapy for Parkinson's Disease and Anticholinergics

LEARNING OBJECTIVES

After studying this chapter, you should be able to:

1. Describe major characteristics and manifestations of Parkinson's disease.

2. Understand the pathophysiology of Parkinson's disease.

3. Describe the types of commonly used antiparkinson drugs.

4. Identify the prototype and describe the action, use, adverse effects, contraindications, and nursing implications for the dopamine receptor agonists.

5. Identify the prototype and describe the action, use, adverse effects, contraindications, and nursing implications for the catechol-*O*-methyltransferase (COMT) inhibitors.

6. Identify the prototype and describe the action, use, adverse effects, contraindications, and nursing implications for a COMT inhibitor and decarboxylase inhibitor/dopamine precursor.

7. Implement the nursing process in the care of patients undergoing drug therapy for Parkinson's disease.

8. Describe the general characteristics of anticholinergic drugs.

9. Identify the prototype and describe the action, use, adverse effects, contraindications, and nursing implications for belladonna alkaloids and derivatives.

10. Identify the prototype and describe the action, use, adverse effects, contraindications, and nursing implications for centrally acting anticholinergic drugs.

11. Identify the prototype and describe the action, use, adverse effects, contraindications, and nursing implications for anticholinergic medications used for gastrointestinal and urinary disorders.

12. Implement the nursing process in the administration of anticholinergic agents.

Clinical Application Case Study

Lee Stokes is a 61-year-old man who visits his primary health care provider. He is experiencing pill-rolling movement of the right hand and fingers; slow, stooped movement; a shuffling gait with absence of arm movement; and excessive salivation. His physician diagnoses Mr. Stokes with Parkinson's disease and starts him on levodopa/carbidopa (Sinemet) 25 mg carbidopa/100 mg levodopa four times a day and benztropine mesylate at bedtime.

KEY TERMS

Akinesia: rigid limbs

Anticholinergic drug: drug that inhibits the actions of acetylcholine in the brain

Antimuscarinic drug: drug that interacts with muscarinic cholinergic receptors in the brain, secretory glands, heart, and smooth muscle to produce an anticholinergic response

Basal ganglia: area in the midbrain that controls smooth voluntary movement

Bradykinesia: inability to move

Catechol-*O*-methyltransferase inhibitor: medication that inhibits the metabolism of levodopa in the periphery

Cycloplegia: Paralysis in the ciliary muscle of the eye

Dopamine receptor agonist: drug that corrects the neurotransmitter imbalance by increasing levels of dopamine

Extrapyramidal reactions: movement disorders such as tardive dyskinesia (inability to initiate movement), akathisia (inability to remain motionless), dystonia, and drug-induced parkinsonism that may occur with use of antiparkinsonism and antipsychotic drugs

Hypertensive crisis: severe increase in blood pressure that can lead to a stroke

Muscarinic receptors: located in the most internal organs, including the cardiovascular, respiratory, gastrointestinal (GI), and genitourinary systems. When activated by acetylcholine, the affected cells may be excited or inhibited in their functions

Mydriasis: pupil dilation

Nicotinic receptors: located in motor nerves and skeletal muscle; when activated by acetylcholine, the cell membrane depolarizes and produces muscle contraction

"Off time": periods of the day when the medication is not working well, causing worsening of parkinsonian symptoms

Parkinson's disease: chronic, progressive, degenerative disorder of the central nervous system characterized by resting tremor, bradykinesia, rigidity, and postural instability

Parkinsonism: often defined as a parkinsonian syndrome that is idiopathic (having no known cause), although some atypical cases have a genetic origin

Quaternary amines: anticholinergic drugs that carry a positive charge and are lipid insoluble; they do not readily cross the cell membranes, are poorly absorbed from the GI tract, and do not cross the blood–brain barrier

Substantia nigra: region of the midbrain with dopamine cells

Tertiary amines: anticholinergic drugs that are unchanged lipid-soluble molecules, able to cross cell membranes readily, and are well absorbed from the GI tract and conjunctiva, and they cross the blood–brain barrier

---

The first part of this chapter discusses Parkinson's disease and the medications administered to decrease the symptoms of the disease. The second part discusses anticholinergic drugs administered to decrease secretions and prevent urinary urgency.

Overview of Parkinson's Disease

Parkinson's disease (also called **parkinsonism**) is a chronic, progressive, degenerative disorder of the central nervous system (CNS) characterized by resting tremor, bradykinesia, rigidity, and postural instability. Manifestations of Parkinson's disease also may occur with other CNS diseases, brain tumors, and head injuries. Drugs that deplete dopamine stores or block dopamine receptors, including the older antipsychotic drugs (phenothiazines and haloperidol), reserpine, and metoclopramide, can produce movement disorders such as secondary parkinsonism (which also involves **extrapyramidal reactions**; see Chap. 55). Treatment can be pharmacologic, nonpharmacologic, and/or surgical.

The Parkinson's Disease Foundation estimates that approximately 1 million people in the United States are living with Parkinson's disease (2010a). This value includes about 60,000 people who are diagnosed each year with the disease, with 96% older than 50 years of age. Parkinson's disease occurs slightly more often in men than in women and in Caucasian and Hispanic/Latino people than in African Americans.

Etiology

The cause of the nerve cell damage is unknown; age-related degeneration, genetics, and exposure to environmental toxins

TABLE 47.1

Drugs Administered for the Treatment of Parkinson's Disease

Drug Class	Prototype	Other Drugs in the Class
Dopamine receptor agonist	Levodopa/carbidopa	Amantadine (Symmetrel) Apomorphine hydrochloride (Apokyn) Bromocriptine mesylate (Parlodel, Cycloset) Cabergoline (Dostinex) Pramipexole dihydrochloride (Mirapex, Mirapex ER) Rasagiline (Azilect) Ropinirole (Requip) Rotigotine-transdermal (Neupro) Selegiline hydrochloride (Eldepryl)
Catechol-O-methyltransferase (COMT) inhibitors	Tolcapone	Entacapone
COMT inhibitor and decarboxylase inhibitor/dopamine precursor	Levodopa, carbidopa, and entacapone (Stalevo)	

are possible etiologic factors. A total of nine genetic linkages and four genes have been associated with Parkinson's disease, including mutations of alpha-synuclein and parkin genes. A high incidence of mutations in the parkin-2 gene has been associated with early-onset parkinsonism.

Pathophysiology

Idiopathic parkinsonism results from progressive destruction of or degenerative changes in dopamine-producing nerve cells in the **substantia nigra** in the **basal ganglia**, the area in the midbrain that controls smooth voluntary movement. The basal ganglia in the brain normally contain substantial amounts of the neurotransmitters dopamine and acetylcholine. The correct balance of dopamine and acetylcholine is important in regulating posture, muscle tone, and voluntary movement. People with Parkinson's disease have an imbalance in these neurotransmitters, resulting in a decrease in inhibitory brain dopamine and a relative increase in excitatory acetylcholine.

Clinical Manifestations

The first symptom of Parkinson's disease is often a resting tremor that begins in the fingers and thumb of one hand ("pill-rolling" movements), eventually spreading over one side of the body and progressing to the contralateral limbs. Other common symptoms include inability to move (**bradykinesia**), rigid limbs (**akinesia**), shuffling gait, stooped posture, mask-like facial expression, and a soft speaking voice. Less common manifestations may include depression, personality changes, loss of appetite, sleep disturbances, speech impairment, or sexual difficulty. Approximately 15% to 20% of people with Parkinson's disease develop dementia. The severity of disease manifestations usually worsen over time. However, disease progression is often quite gradual,

and patients may retain near-normal functional abilities for several years.

Drug Therapy

Drugs used in Parkinson's disease include **dopamine receptor agonists**, which help correct the neurotransmitter imbalance by increasing levels of dopamine, and **catechol-O-methyltransferase (COMT) inhibitors**, which inhibit the metabolism of levodopa in the periphery. See Table 47.1. (The older belladonna alkaloids and the newer centrally acting anticholinergic agents inhibit the actions of acetylcholine in the brain. As previously stated, these medications are discussed later in this chapter.)

Clinical Application 47-1

■ A nurse is providing patient teaching to Mr. Stokes and his family. The family inquires about the progression of Parkinson's disease. What does the nurse tell the patient and the family with regard to disease progression?

Dopamine Receptor Agonists

Levodopa (L-dopa), the original prototype dopamine receptor antagonist, was developed in the 1960s. It is routinely administered with the drug carbidopa; therefore, the combination medication is discussed as the prototype. ℗ **Levodopa/carbidopa** (Sinemet, Sinemet CR, Parcopa) is well established as the most effective drug for the symptomatic treatment of idiopathic Parkinson's disease. (Carbidopa is used only in conjunction with levodopa.) The combination is particularly effective for the management of akinetic symptoms.

Pharmacokinetics

In peripheral tissues (e.g., gastrointestinal [GI] tract, liver), levodopa is metabolized extensively by the enzyme aromatic amino acid decarboxylase (AADC) and to a lesser extent by catechol-O-methyltransferase (COMT). Because most levodopa is metabolized in peripheral tissues, large doses are required to obtain therapeutic levels of dopamine in the brain. These large amounts increase adverse drug effects. To reduce levodopa dosage and decrease adverse effects, carbidopa, an AADC inhibitor, is given to decrease the peripheral metabolism of levodopa. The combination of levodopa and carbidopa greatly increases the amount of available levodopa, so that levodopa dosage can be reduced by approximately 70%. When carbidopa inhibits the decarboxylase pathway of levodopa metabolism, the COMT pathway becomes more important (see Catechol-O-Methyltransferase Inhibitors for a discussion of entacapone and tolcapone).

Levodopa is well absorbed from the small intestine after oral administration, reaches peak serum levels within 30 to 90 minutes, and has a short serum half-life (1–3 hours). Absorption is decreased by delayed gastric emptying, hyperacidity of gastric secretions, and competition with amino acids (from digestion of protein foods) for sites of absorption in the small intestine. Pyridoxine (vitamin B_6) promotes the breakdown of levodopa, reducing its effectiveness. Levodopa is metabolized to 30 or more metabolites, some of which are pharmacologically active and probably contribute to drug toxicity; the metabolites are excreted primarily in the urine, usually within 24 hours.

Action

Dopaminergic drugs increase the amount of dopamine in the brain by various mechanisms (Fig. 47.1). If levodopa is administered alone, large doses must be taken to produce therapeutic

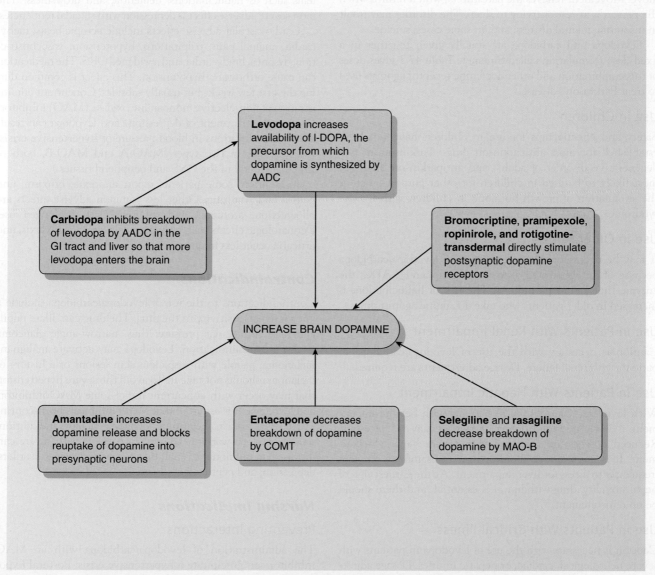

Figure 47.1 Mechanisms by which dopaminergic drugs increase dopamine in the brain. AADC, amino acid decarboxylase; COMT, catechol-O-methyltransferase; MAO-B, monoamine oxidase B.

effects. Carbidopa combined with levodopa prevents the decarboxylation of the levodopa, which makes levodopa more available for transportation to the brain. Levodopa is the metabolic precursor of dopamine, and after levodopa crosses the blood–brain barrier, it converts to dopamine in the brain. This is thought to be the mechanism whereby the drug relieves symptoms of Parkinson's disease. Carbidopa does not cross the blood–brain barrier and does not affect levodopa metabolism.

Use

Levodopa/carbidopa is a treatment of idiopathic Parkinson's disease, postencephalitic and arteriosclerotic parkinsonism, and parkinsonism related to carbon dioxide and manganese intoxication. Prescribers may also order levodopa to reduce the symptoms of restless leg syndrome (RLS). People with RLS, also known as Ekbom's syndrome, experience paresthesias of the muscles, particularly in the calf and thighs, creating the urge to move. Movement relieves the paresthesia, which returns when the person is at rest or trying to sleep. The disorder may result in insomnia; mental distress; and, in some cases, suicide.

Levodopa and carbidopa are usually given together in a fixed-dose formulation called Sinemet. Table 47.2 gives doses of this combination and other dopamine receptor agonists used to treat Parkinson's disease.

Use in Children

Safety and effectiveness for use in children have not been established for most antiparkinson drugs. Parkinsonism is a degenerative disorder of adults, and antiparkinson drugs are most likely to be used in children for other purposes such as the stimulation of growth hormone in children with Down's syndrome.

Use in Older Adults

It may be necessary to reduce dosages of levodopa/carbidopa because of an age-related decrease in peripheral AADC, the enzyme that carbidopa inhibits. The risk of hallucinations is increased in older patients who take dopamine agonist drugs.

Use in Patients With Renal Impairment

Caution is necessary with the use of levodopa/carbidopa in patients with renal failure. Dosage adjustments are required.

Use in Patients With Hepatic Impairment

With levodopa, cautious use in patients with hepatic impairment is warranted, and dosage reduction may be necessary. Reduced dosages are indicated with severe hepatic impairment. It is important to monitor liver transaminase enzymes frequently to assess for liver impairment. At the earliest sign of hepatotoxicity, drug withdrawal is essential, and there should be no reinstatement.

Use in Patients With Critical Illness

Caution is necessary with the use of levodopa in patients with severe neurological, cardiac, or hepatic injuries. Dosage adjustment to the lowest level required for therapeutic effects is essential.

Use in Patients Receiving Home Care

The home care nurse can help patients and caregivers understand that the purpose of drug therapy is to control symptoms and that noticeable improvement may not occur for several weeks. Also, the nurse can encourage patients to consult physical therapists, speech therapists, and dietitians to help maintain their ability to perform activities of daily living. In addition, teaching about preventing or managing adverse drug effects may be necessary. Caregivers may need to be informed that most activities (e.g., eating, dressing) take longer and require considerable effort by patients with parkinsonism.

Adverse Effects

Because of the adverse effects and recurrence of parkinsonism symptoms after a few years of levodopa therapy, levodopa is usually reserved for patients with significant symptoms and functional disabilities. The most common CNS adverse effects are headache and anxiety. Older patients may experience problems such as hallucinations, dementia, and drowsiness. The most severe adverse effect is depression with suicidal tendencies.

Cardiovascular adverse effects include ectopic beats, tachycardia, anginal pain, palpitations, hypotension, vasoconstriction, dyspnea, bradycardia, and a widened QRS. The medication can cause orthostatic hypotension. This effect is common during the first few weeks but usually subsides. Concurrent administration of nonselective monoamine oxidase (MAO) inhibitors (used in the treatment of depression) and levodopa can result in extreme elevations in blood pressure or **hypertensive crisis**. (MAO exists in two types, MAO-A and MAO-B, both of which are found in the CNS and peripheral tissues.)

In addition, some patients report anorexia, bruxism, and nausea and vomiting. Other less common adverse effects are piloerection, azotemia, and gangrene with prolonged use. Dermatologic effects such as hypersensitivity, anaphylaxis, and urticaria occur less frequently.

Contraindications

Contraindications to the use of levodopa/carbidopa include a known hypersensitivity to the drug. The drug can dilate pupils and raise intraocular pressure; thus, narrow-angle glaucoma is also a contraindication. Levodopa may activate malignant melanoma; people with suspicious skin lesions or a history of melanoma should not take it. To avoid the severe hypertension that may occur with concurrent use of some MAO inhibitors and levodopa, it is essential that MAO inhibitors be discontinued 14 days prior to beginning levodopa therapy. In addition, use of levodopa warrants caution in patients with severe cardiovascular, pulmonary, renal, hepatic, or endocrine disorders; depression; and peptic ulcer disease.

Nursing Implications

Preventing Interactions

The administration of levodopa/carbidopa with an MAO inhibitor can precipitate a hypertensive crisis. Postural hypotension occurs with the administration of tricyclic antidepressants and levodopa/carbidopa. Methyldopa combined

TABLE 47.2

DRUGS AT A GLANCE: Dopamine Receptor Agonists

Drug	Pregnancy Category	Routes and Dosage Ranges	
		Adults	**Children**
Ⓟ **Levodopa/ carbidopa** (Sinemet, Sinemet CR, Parcopa)	C	1 tablet containing 10 mg carbidopa and 100 mg levodopa or 25 mg carbidopa and 100 mg levodopa PO 3 times per day; increased by 1 tablet daily or every other day up to 6 tablets/d Patients who are switched from levodopa alone to levodopa/carbidopa: 1 tablet containing 25 mg carbidopa and 250 mg levodopa PO 3–4 times per day; the dosage is adjusted by 1/2–1 tablet per day (initial dose should be 20%–25% of initial dose of levodopa)	Safety and efficacy not established
Amantadine hydrochloride (Endantadine, Symmetrel)	C	*Antiparkinson:* 100 mg PO 2 times per day (maximum dosage 400 mg/d) *Antiviral:* 200 mg/d or 100 mg 2 times per day PO for 10 d after exposure, for the duration of known influenza A	Safety and efficacy have not been established in children under the age of 1 y 1–9 y: 4.4–8.8 mg/kg/d PO in one or two divided doses not to exceed 150 mg/d 9–12 y: 100 mg PO 2 times per day
Apomorphine hydrochloride (Apokyn)	C	"Off time": Monitor blood pressure with administration: 0.2 mL or 2 mg subcutaneous; if no response, administer 0.4 mL or 4 mg if well tolerated administer 0.3 mL or 30 mg; may increase by 1 mg every day Max dose: 0.6 mL as a single injection; max of 5 injections/d	Safety and efficacy not established
Bromocriptine mesylate (Parlodel, Cycloset)	C	1.25–2.5 mg PO daily (max dosage: 100 mg/d in divided doses)	Safety and efficacy not established
Cabergoline (Dostinex)	B	0.5 mg PO daily; may increase up to 2.5 mg daily (max dosage 5 mg/d)	Safety and efficacy not established
Pramipexole dihydrochloride (Mirapex, Mirapex ER)	C	0.125 mg PO 3 times per day gradually increase every 5–7 d to a max dose of 1.5 mg 3 times per day Extended release: 0.375 mg PO daily, may increase after 5 d up to a max dose of 4.5 mg/d Restless leg syndrome: 0.125 mg taken 2–3 h before bed, dose can be increased every 4–7 d Renal impairment: CrCl 35–60 mL/min: same titration schedule dosed 2 times/d (max dose: 1.5 mg 2 times per day) CrCl 15–35 mL/min (max dosage 1.5 mg/d)	Safety and efficacy not established
Rasagiline (Azilect)	C	1 mg PO daily as monotherapy; 0.5–1 mg/d PO Hepatic impairment: 0.5 mg PO daily	Safety and efficacy not established
Ropinirole hydrochloride (Requip, Requip XL)	C	0.25 mg PO 3 times per day; titrate up by 0.25 mg/dose 3 times per day every week to a target dose of 1 mg 3 times per day; may be increased by 1.5 mg/d every week (max dosage: 9 mg/d) and then 3 mg/d to a max dosage of 24 mg/d Extended release: 2 mg/d for 1–2 wk then increase by 2 mg/d at 1 wk intervals; max dosage 24 mg/d Restless leg syndrome: 0.25 mg 1–3 h before bedtime for 2 d, increase or 0.5 mg for the first week, then increase by 0.5 mg every week to a max dosage of 4 mg	Safety and efficacy not established
Selegiline hydrochloride (Eldepryl)	C	5 mg PO 2 times per day with breakfast and lunch; dosages >10 mg/d are associated with increased risk of toxicity due to MAO inhibition Geriatric dosage: Start with 5 mg in the morning	Safety and efficacy not established

BOX 47.1 Drug Interactions: Levodopa/Carbidopa

Drugs That Increase the Effects of Levodopa/Carbidopa

■ Monoamine oxidase inhibitors
Increase the risk of hypertensive crisis

Drugs That Decrease the Effect of Levodopa/Carbidopa

■ Anticholinergics
Increase anticholinergic effects by delaying gastric emptying

■ Pyridoxine (vitamin B₆)
Stimulates decarboxylase, the enzyme that converts levodopa to dopamine, causing metabolism in the peripheral tissues and decreasing medication distribution to the central nervous system

■ Phenytoin, papaverine, tricyclic antidepressants, benzodiazepines
Decrease drug efficacy

with levodopa increases CNS effects. Dysrhythmic effects are increased when combined with halogenated general anesthetics. Several drugs interact with levodopa/carbidopa, increasing or decreasing its effects (Box 47.1). A high-protein meal increases the effects of levodopa/carbidopa, and kava decreases the effects of the drug.

Administering the Medication

The nurse ensures that:

- Levodopa/carbidopa is administered with or just after food or following a meal to reduce nausea and vomiting.
- Sinemet CR is not crushed.
- Levodopa is not given with iron preparations or multivitamin–mineral preparations that contain iron.
- Levodopa/carbidopa is not administered with a high-protein diet. Adequate hydration is also necessary.

In addition, the nurse should ensure a temperature-controlled environment; this prevents hyperpyrexia.

QSEN Safety Alert

When administering levodopa, carbidopa, and other medications for Parkinson's disease, it is important that medications be given to the patient on time. Timing of medication administration is critical for optimal therapeutic effect.

Assessing for Therapeutic Effects

With levodopa and other dopaminergic agents, the nurse observes for improvement in mobility, balance, posture, gait, speech, handwriting, and self-care ability. Elimination of drooling and seborrhea may occur. Mood elevation may result. After 2 to 5 years, the medication may lose its overall effectiveness, and the dosage may need to be increased. The nurse needs to be aware of symptoms such as ataxic gait, tremors of the hands and fingers, drooling, and mask-like facial expressions.

Assessing for Adverse Effects

The nurse assesses for anorexia, nausea, and vomiting. These symptoms usually disappear after a few months of levodopa/carbidopa therapy. As previously stated, giving the drug with food minimizes these effects. The nurse also assesses the patient's blood pressure in the sitting and standing positions to identify signs of orthostatic hypotension. This effect, too, commonly dissipates a few weeks after beginning therapy. Levodopa and its metabolites stimulate beta-adrenergic receptors in the heart. Patients with preexisting coronary artery disease may take propranolol (Inderal) to counteract cardiac dysrhythmia effects. It is necessary to assess the patient for dyskinesia. The involuntary movements of the tongue, mouth, and face are common adverse effects. Decreasing the dose of the medication decreases dyskinesia.

Patient Teaching

Box 47.2 identifies patient teaching guidelines for levodopa/carbidopa.

Other Drugs in the Class

Amantadine hydrochloride (Endantadine, Symmetrel) is an antiparkinson and antiviral agent (see Chap. 21). It increases the dopamine release in the nigrostriatal pathway of patients with Parkinson's disease. It is absorbed in the GI tract with an onset of action of 36 to 48 hours, a peak of action of 1.5 to 8 hours, and a half-life of 10 to 25 hours. It crosses the placenta and enters the breast milk. It is excreted unchanged in the urine. The most common adverse effects of amantadine are dizziness, light-headedness, and insomnia. The nurse instructs the patient to report swelling of the fingers or ankles, difficulty walking, urinary retention, tremors, slurred speech, or thoughts of suicide to the health care provider. It is important not to discontinue this drug abruptly.

BOX 47.2 Patient Teaching Guidelines for Levodopa/Carbidopa

- Take the medication as prescribed.
- Do not crush the sustained-release preparation.
- Do not take multivitamin preparations containing pyridoxine.
- Understand that there are adverse effects of medication such as drowsiness, dizziness, and orthostatic hypotension.
- Change positions slowly to prevent drop in blood pressure.
- Avoid alcohol.
- Take the medication with food to prevent nausea and vomiting.
- Do not take the medication with a high-protein meal.
- Report fainting, light-headedness, irregular heart rate, uncontrolled facial movements, urinary retention, nausea, and vomiting to the prescriber.
- Notify the prescriber of any increase in symptoms such as static gait, altered mobility, and "pill rolling."

Apomorphine hydrochloride (Apokyn) is an antiparkinson agent administered for **"off time,"** or "off" episodes, of Parkinson's disease—to assist in diminishing the symptoms of hypomobility. "Off time" is the period when the medication is not adequately controlling the patient's symptoms. Patients who suffer from "off time" episodes have advanced Parkinson's disease. Administration is subcutaneous. Doses are incremental, generally ranging from 20 to 40 mg. The most common dosage is 30 mg, or 0.3 mL, and the maximum dosage is 60 mg. The patient's blood pressure must be monitored for hypertensive crisis during the administration. When apomorphine is administered to patients with a known cardiac history, periodic electrocardiogram results should be monitored as well as serum electrolytes.

Bromocriptine mesylate (Parlodel, Cycloset) is an ergot derivative that directly stimulates dopamine receptors in the brain. It is used in the treatment of idiopathic Parkinson's disease, with levodopa/carbidopa, to prolong effectiveness and to allow reduced dosage of levodopa. Administration to patients with a history of myocardial infarction with residual dysrhythmia requires caution.

Cabergoline, a synthetic ergot, is a long-acting dopamine agonist approved by the U.S. Food and Drug Administration (FDA) for use in hyperprolactinemia. This medication has an unlabeled use: to improve motor symptoms of parkinsonism. However, the higher dosage required to treat parkinsonism is associated with the development of serious heart valve damage due to fibrosis.

Pramipexole (Mirapex) and ropinirole (Requip) stimulate dopamine receptors in the brain. The FDA has approved their use in both early and late stages of Parkinson's disease. In early stages, one of these drugs can be used alone to improve motor performance, improve ability to participate in usual activities of daily living, and delay levodopa therapy. In advanced stages, one of these drugs can be used with levodopa and perhaps other antiparkinson drugs to provide more consistent relief of symptoms between doses of levodopa and allow reduced dosage of levodopa. These drugs, which are not ergot derivatives, may not cause some adverse effects associated with bromocriptine (e.g., pulmonary and peritoneal fibrosis, constriction of coronary arteries).

Pramipexole is rapidly absorbed with oral administration. Peak serum levels are reached in 1 to 3 hours after a dose and steady-state concentrations in about 2 days. The drug is less than 20% bound to plasma proteins and has an elimination half-life of 8 to 12 hours. Most of the drug is excreted unchanged in the urine; only 10% is metabolized. As a result, renal failure may cause higher-than-usual plasma levels and possible toxicity. However, hepatic disease is unlikely to alter drug effects.

Ropinirole is also well absorbed with oral administration. It reaches peak serum levels in 1 to 2 hours and steady-state concentrations within 2 days. It is 40% bound to plasma proteins and has an elimination half-life of 6 hours. It is metabolized by the cytochrome P450 enzymes in the liver to inactive metabolites, which are excreted through the kidneys. Less than 10% of ropinirole is excreted unchanged in the urine. Thus, hepatic failure may decrease metabolism, allow drug accumulation, and

increase adverse effects. Renal failure does not appear to alter drug effects.

Rasagiline (Azilect) is an irreversible MAO inhibitor. It is indicated for initial treatment for idiopathic parkinsonism and as an adjunct therapy with levodopa to reduce "off time" when movements are poorly controlled. Because it has not been determined to be selective for MAO-B in humans, care must be taken to avoid tyramine-containing foods as well as sympathomimetic medications to prevent hypertensive crisis. In addition, rasagiline has the potential to increase serotonin neurotransmission. When given with other drugs that enhance stimulation of serotonergic receptors (e.g., antidepressants, St. John's wort, dextromethorphan, and meperidine), serotonin syndrome, a potential fatal CNS toxicity reaction characterized by hyperpyrexia and death, can occur. Rasagiline should be discontinued at least 14 days before beginning treatment with most antidepressants or other MAO inhibitors. Fluoxetine should be discontinued at least 5 weeks before initiating rasagiline, due to its long half-life. Rasagiline is well absorbed orally, metabolized in the liver, and excreted primarily by the kidney. It is contraindicated with foods containing tyramine or sympathomimetic amine–containing medications (e.g., nonprescription cold preparations and anesthetics) because of the risk of hypertensive crisis and with antidepressants (e.g., tricyclic antidepressants, selective serotonin reuptake inhibitors, serotonin–norepinephrine reuptake inhibitors, mirtazapine), meperidine, and dextromethorphan because of the potential for inducing serotonin syndrome.

Selegiline (Eldepryl) inhibits metabolism of dopamine by MAO, which exists in two types (as previously stated). These types are differentiated by their relative specificities for individual catecholamines. MAO-A acts more specifically on tyramine, norepinephrine, epinephrine, and serotonin. This enzyme is the main subtype in GI mucosa and in the liver and is responsible for metabolizing dietary tyramine. If MAO-A is inhibited in the intestine, tyramine in various foods is absorbed systemically rather than deactivated. As a result, there is excessive stimulation of the sympathetic nervous system, and severe hypertension and stroke can occur. This is sometimes called the "cheese reaction" because aged cheeses are high in tyramine. This life-threatening reaction can also occur with some medications (e.g., sympathomimetics) that are normally metabolized by MAO. MAO-B metabolizes dopamine; in the brain, most MAO activity is due to type B. At oral dosages of 10 mg/d or less, selegiline inhibits MAO-B *selectively* and is unlikely to cause severe hypertension and stroke. However, at dosages greater than 10 mg/d, selectivity is lost and metabolism of both MAO-A and MAO-B is inhibited. Dosages greater than 10 mg/d should be avoided in patients with Parkinson's disease. Selegiline inhibition of MAO-B is irreversible, and drug effects persist until more MAO is synthesized in the brain, which may take several months.

In early Parkinson's disease, selegiline may be effective as monotherapy (level A). In advanced disease, prescribers order the drug to enhance the effects of levodopa. Its addition aids symptom control and allows the dosage of levodopa/carbidopa to be reduced. Once proposed to have neuroprotective properties, authorities now believe that there is insufficient evidence to recommend the use of selegiline to confer neuroprotection in patients with Parkinson's disease (level U).

NCLEX Success

1. The daughter of a 75-year-old woman states to the parish nurse that she has noticed her mother rolling her fingers together on her right hand. The nurse observes the patient and determines she is "pill rolling," which is characteristic of Parkinson's disease. Which of the following factors contributes to the development of central nervous system symptom of "pill rolling"?
   A. decrease firing of the sinoatrial node
   B. conversion of angiotensin I to angiotensin II
   C. increase in excitatory acetylcholine
   D. influx of potassium through the cell membrane

2. A 65-year-old woman has been taking levodopa for several weeks for symptoms of Parkinson's disease. Which of the following symptoms indicates that she is not receiving an adequate dose for the treatment of her symptoms?
   A. edema of the feet and ankles
   B. widened QRS complex
   C. static gait
   D. increased intraocular pressure

3. The 56-year-old man is taking levodopa/carbidopa for Parkinson's disease. During the therapy, he becomes light-headed and dizzy. Which of the following is a potentially serious adverse effect of the drug treatment?
   A. orthostatic hypotension
   B. diminished fluid volume
   C. hematuria
   D. jaundice

4. A 52-year-old man is taking selegiline for the treatment of Parkinson's disease. He consumes port wine cheese and crackers at a party. Which of the following symptoms does he develop?
   A. ataxic gait
   B. melena
   C. cardiac dysrhythmia
   D. hypertension

5. A 48-year-old man with severe akinesia develops severe symptoms of parkinsonism following the administration of his antiparkinson medications. This condition occurs only one to two times per month. Which of the following medications is the man's prescriber most likely to order?
   A. bromocriptine mesylate (Parlodel)
   B. apomorphine hydrochloride (Apokyn)
   C. cabergoline (Dostinex)
   D. pramipexole dihydrochloride (Mirapex, Mirapex ER)

Clinical Application 47-2

- Mr. Stokes has been having "off time" symptom development. His neurologist orders rasagiline (Azilect). He develops an upper respiratory viral infection with a cough. He begins to take dextromethorphan hydrobromide (Robitussin) every 4 hours. What is Mr. Stokes at risk for developing?
- What symptom does the nurse assess Mr. Stokes for when combining rasagiline and dextromethorphan hydrobromide?

Catechol-*O*-Methyltransferase Inhibitors

Ⓟ **Tolcapone** (Tasmar) is the prototype COMT inhibitor. COMT plays a role in brain metabolism of dopamine and metabolizes approximately 10% of peripheral levodopa. By inhibiting COMT, tolcapone increases levels of dopamine in the brain and relieves symptoms more effectively and consistently.

Pharmacokinetics

Tolcapone is absorbed rapidly and is highly protein bound. It is metabolized in the liver and possesses a 2 to 3 hour half-life. It crosses the placenta and enters the breast milk. It is excreted in the feces and urine.

Action

The main mechanism of action of tolcapone seems to be inhibiting the metabolism of levodopa in the bloodstream, thus increasing the plasma concentration and duration of action of the drug. It may also inhibit COMT in the brain and prolong the activity of dopamine at the synapse.

Use

Tolcapone is useful for the treatment of signs and symptoms of idiopathic Parkinson's disease. Administration is only in conjunction with levodopa/carbidopa, and a reduction in levodopa dosage is required. If a patient does not show a clinical benefit within 3 weeks of starting treatment, discontinuation of tolcapone is necessary.

Table 47.3 presents dosage information for tolcapone and other drugs in its class.

Use in Older Adults

When administering tolcapone to geriatric patients, it is important to reduce the dosage and adjust it slowly to prevent adverse effects.

Use in Patients With Renal Impairment

Caution is warranted in administration of tolcapone to patients with renal impairment because it is excreted in the urine.

TABLE 47.3
DRUGS AT A GLANCE: Catechol-O-Methyltransferase (COMT) Inhibitors

Drug	Pregnancy Category	Routes and Dosage Ranges	
		Adults	Children
Tolcapone (Tasmar)	C	100 mg PO 3 times per day (max dose: 200 mg 3 times per day)	Safety and efficacy not established
Entacapone (Comtan)	C	200 mg PO administered with each dose of levodopa/carbidopa up to 8 times per day	Safety and efficacy not established

Use in Patients With Hepatic Impairment

If liver values are greater than two times the upper limit of normal, discontinuation of tolcapone is necessary. Patients with moderate to severe hepatic impairment should not take tolcapone at doses exceeding 100 mg three times per day. The FDA has issued a **BLACK BOX WARNING** ◆ stating that patients who take tolcapone risk potentially fatal acute fulminant liver failure. It is important to monitor liver function tests before therapy begins and every 2 weeks thereafter.

Adverse Effects

Tolcapone produces adverse effects in several major body systems, including the CNS, cardiovascular system, dermatological system, GI system, and respiratory system. The most severe adverse effect is fulminant liver failure, which may be fatal. CNS adverse effects include disorientation, confusion, hallucinations, and psychosis. Dizziness and orthostatic hypotension may also occur.

Contraindications

Contraindications to tolcapone include a hypersensitivity to the drug. Other contraindications are liver disease, nontraumatic rhabdomyolysis, hyperpyrexia, and confusion. Caution is warranted with hypertension, hypotension, and renal impairment.

Nursing Implications

Preventing Interactions

It is essential that tolcapone and other COMT medications not be administered with MAO inhibitors due to the risk of hypertensive crisis.

Administering the Medication

It is necessary to administer tolcapone in conjunction with levodopa/carbidopa and to monitor the patient's response to the medication. The addition of the drug may require a decrease in the levodopa dosage. Abrupt withdrawal of tolcapone can lead to serious complications. Tapering over 2 weeks is necessary to prevent adverse effects.

Assessing for Therapeutic Effects

The decrease or absence of symptoms of Parkinson's disease such as improved gait and mobility, diminished tremors, and rigidity is indicative of tolcapone's therapeutic effectiveness.

Assessing for Adverse Effects

The nurse assesses for disorientation and confusion, lightheadedness, and orthostatic hypotension. It is necessary to take blood pressure lying down, sitting, and standing up. Frequent monitoring of liver enzymes is essential.

Patient Teaching

Box 47.3 presents patient teaching guidelines for tolcapone.

Other Drugs in the Class

Entacapone is well tolerated and safer than tolcapone, and thus, prescribers more commonly order entacapone. This COMT inhibitor is well absorbed after oral administration and reaches a peak plasma level in 1 hour. It is highly protein bound (98%), has a half-life of about 2.5 hours, and is metabolized in the liver to an inactive metabolite. Dosage must be reduced by 50% in the presence of impaired liver function. The parent drug and metabolite are 90% excreted through the biliary tract and feces, and 10% of excretion occurs in the urine. Adverse effects include confusion, dizziness, drowsiness, hallucinations, nausea, and vomiting, which can be reduced by lowering the dose of either levodopa or entacapone. Although clinical trials report few instances of liver enzyme elevation or hemoglobin decreases, it is recommended that liver enzymes and red blood cell counts be measured periodically.

BOX 47.3   Patient Teaching Guidelines for Tolcapone

- Take the medication exactly as prescribed.
- Do not stop the medication abruptly; taper it over 2 weeks.
- Take the medication in conjunction with levodopa/carbidopa.
- Use barrier contraceptives while using this medication.
- Do not breast-feed while taking the medication.
- Use caution when operating machinery due to central nervous system depression.
- Use hard candy to decrease dry mouth.
- Have liver function tests as scheduled.

6. An elderly woman is taking tolcapone. She has noticed that her skin is yellow. The nurse assesses which of the following?

   A. intake of carrots
   B. temperature related to infection
   C. sclera
   D. amount of urine output

7. A 35-year-old woman has begun to take tolcapone in addition to levodopa/carbidopa for Parkinson's disease. Which of the following is the priority nursing intervention?

   A. arrange to assess the patient for hypertension early in the morning
   B. evaluate the patient's ability care for herself
   C. have the patient take levodopa/carbidopa 2 hours after tolcapone
   D. instruct the patient to report tea-colored urine to the prescriber

Catechol-O-Methyltransferase Inhibitor and Decarboxylase Inhibitor/Dopamine Precursor

One antiparkinson drug is a combination of **ⓟ levodopa, carbidopa, and entacapone** (Stalevo). This chapter discusses this medication in a separate class because it combines medications from two separate classes. Administration of Stalevo allows for greater convenience and improved Parkinson symptom management. Use of the drug combination provides the patient with the convenience of one medication.

Pharmacokinetics

The combination drug Stalevo has the same pharmacokinetics as those of levodopa/carbidopa and entacapone.

Action

Levodopa is the metabolic precursor of dopamine. Depleted in Parkinson's disease, levodopa is circulated in the plasma and crosses the blood–brain barrier, where it is converted to dopamine by the striatal enzymes. Carbidopa inhibits the peripheral plasma breakdown of levodopa by inhibiting decarboxylation, thus increasing levodopa. Entacapone is a reversible and selective inhibitor of COMT. It alters the pharmacokinetics of levodopa, allowing for more sustained levodopa serum levels and increased concentrations for absorption across the blood–brain barrier.

Use

Stalevo is used for the treatment of idiopathic Parkinson's disease. Table 47.4 presents dosage information for Stalevo.

EVIDENCE-BASED PRACTICE

Comparison of Pharmacokinetic Profile of Levodopa Throughout the Day Between Levodopa/Carbidopa/Entacapone and Levodopa/Carbidopa When Administered Four or Five Times Daily

by KUOPPMANKI, M., KORPELA, K., MARTTILA, R., VI KAASINEN, HARTIKAINEN, P., LYYTINEN, J., KAAKKOLA, S., HANNINEN, J., LOYTTYNIEMI, E., KAILAJARVI, M., RUOKONIEMI, P., ELLMEN, J.

Eur J Clin Pharmacol 2009, 65(5),443–455
Epub 2009 Feb 20

This study compared the plasma levodopa concentrations after repeated doses of levodopa/carbidopa/entacapone and levodopa/carbidopa. The results of the study revealed that 100 to 150 mg of levodopa/carbidopa/entacapone administered four to five times per day provided a better pharmacokinetic profile than levodopa/carbidopa.

IMPLICATIONS FOR NURSING PRACTICE: Based on this study, symptom control was better than with levodopa/carbidopa and entacapone than levodopa/carbidopa alone. Thus, the administration of levodopa/carbidopa, entacapone provides better symptom control in Parkinson's patients due to the fact the trough values of levodopa were higher with the combination medication.

Use in Patients With Renal Impairment

It is necessary to administer Stalevo with caution in patients with severe renal impairment. Dosage reduction to prevent further renal insufficiency may be warranted.

Use in Patients With Hepatic Impairment

Cautious administration of Stalevo is also necessary in patients with hepatic impairment because the medication is metabolized in the liver.

Adverse Effects

Stalevo may affect the GI, dermatologic, respiratory, and cardiovascular systems. GI adverse effects include diarrhea as well as nausea, vomiting, bruxism, dry mouth, and excess salivation. The development of diarrhea is indicative of drug-induced colitis, and it is necessary to discontinue Stalevo if diarrhea occurs. Also, the risk of melanoma may increase. As with other antiparkinson medications, hypotension is a risk, along with heart attack, stroke, and cardiovascular death. The FDA is conducting an ongoing review of data to assess whether patients are at risk for cardiovascular events when taking this drug (U.S. FDA, Stalevo [carbidopa/levodopa and entacapone], 2010). Also, there is an increased risk of cardiovascular events in patients who received Stalevo versus those who received Sinemet. However, the study

TABLE 47.4

DRUGS AT A GLANCE: Catechol-*O*-Methyltransferase Inhibitor and Decarboxylase Inhibitor/Dopamine Precursor

Drug	Pregnancy Category	Routes and Dosage Range	
		Adults	Children
ⓟ **Levodopa/carbidopa/ entacapone** (Stalevo)	C	Dosing forms: Levodopa 50 mg/carbidopa 12.5 mg/ entacapone 200 mg PO daily	Safety and efficacy not established
		Levodopa 75 mg/carbidopa 18.75 mg/entacapone 200 mg	
		Levodopa 100 mg/carbidopa 25 mg/entacapone 200 mg	
		Levodopa 125 mg/carbidopa 31.25 mg/entacapone 200 mg	
		Levodopa 150 mg/carbidopa 37.5 mg/entacapone 200 mg	
		Levodopa 200 mg/carbidopa 50 mg/entacapone 200 mg	

shows that the risk of cardiovascular events is not statistically significant, but studies of the drug are continuing. The FDA is evaluating clinical data that the administration of Stalevo may increase the male patient's risk of developing prostate cancer. One trial has compared Stalevo with carbidopa and levodopa. Unexpectedly, the study has revealed that a greater number of patients taking Stalevo have prostate cancer (U. S. Food and Drug Administration. FDA Drug Safety Communication, 2010).

Contraindications

Contraindications to the use of Stalevo include a known sensitivity to the levodopa, carbidopa, or entacapone. The concurrent use of MAO inhibitors, or use within 14 days, is also a contraindication. Levodopa may trigger melanoma; therefore, patients with a history of melanoma should not receive Stalevo. Also, it is important to note that ergot-derived dopamine agonists administered with Stalevo have been associated with fibrotic complications such as pleural effusion, pleural thickening, and pulmonary infiltrates.

Nursing Implications

Preventing Interactions

The administration of catecholamines such as epinephrine, dopamine, and methyldopa enhances the action of entacapone, one of the components of Stalevo.

Administering the Medication

Patients whose medication regime is being changed to Stalevo should be administered levodopa and the adjunctive entacapone. The levodopa dose should be adjusted prior to the conversion to Stalevo therapy. The dose should be individualized based on the therapeutic response. The presence of dyskinesia necessitates a dosage adjustment. The dose may be adjusted by changing the strength or adjusting the dosing intervals.

Fractionated doses are not recommended, and only one tablet should be administered at each dosing interval. The maximum daily dose is eight 50-, 75-, 100-, 125-, and 150-mg tablets and only six 200-mg tablets. (Patients who take more than 600 mg/d of levodopa should not switch directly to Stalevo.) Patients should swallow the tablets whole—not crushed, broken, or chewed. Stalevo can be administered without regard to meals. To prevent fluctuation in levodopa absorption, it is necessary to distribute protein intake throughout the day. People should take iron, iron supplements, and multivitamins that contain minerals separately from Stalevo.

Assessing for Therapeutic Effects

The decrease or absence of Parkinson's symptoms such as muscle rigidity, excessive salivation, "pill rolling," and tremors is indicative of Stalevo's therapeutic effectiveness.

Assessing for Adverse Effects

The nurse assesses the patient's cardiovascular status, including heart rate and blood pressure, to determine alterations in cardiovascular symptoms. It is also necessary to assess for chest pain, confusion, and weakness of extremities related to cerebrovascular accident or myocardial infarction. In addition, the nurse assesses the patient's skin for unusual skin lesions and checks the patient's fecal elimination for drug-induced colitis.

Patient Teaching

Patient education for Stalevo is the same as the patient education for the drug's individual components: levodopa, carbidopa, and entacapone (see Box 47.2). With entacapone, the nurse instructs the patient to report hallucinations and diarrhea. It is also necessary to tell the patient that his or her urine may become brownish-orange. This is a normal reaction to the medication and is not harmful. In addition, the nurse tells the patient to protect against falls due to orthostatic hypotension; patients can stand up slowly.

Clinical Application 47-3

▪ Mr. Stokes' prescriber switches him from levodopa/carbidopa to levodopa/carbidopa/entacapone. He asks his nurse what the difference is between the medication he once took and what he is now taking. What patient education does the nurse provide?

NCLEX Success

8. A 76-year-old woman is taking levodopa/carbidopa/entacapone (Stalevo). Which of the following is the priority nursing intervention?

    A. administering with a high-protein meal
    B. administering with meals only
    C. assessing for diarrhea
    D. assessing for constipation

9. An elderly man begins taking levodopa/carbidopa/entacapone (Stalevo). Which of the following symptoms warrants a change in the dosage?

    A. dilated pupils
    B. static gait
    C. edema
    D. nausea

The Nursing Process

Assessment

- Assess for signs and symptoms of Parkinson's disease and drug-induced extrapyramidal reactions, such as the following, depending on the severity and stage of progression:
    - Slow movements (bradykinesia) and difficulty in changing positions, assuming an upright position, eating, dressing, and other self-care activities
    - Stooped posture
    - Accelerating gait with short steps
    - Tremor at rest (e.g., "pill-rolling" movements of fingers)
    - Rigidity of arms, legs, and neck
    - Mask-like, immobile facial expression
    - Speech problems (e.g., low volume, monotonous tone, rapid, difficult to understand)
    - Excessive salivation and drooling
    - Dysphagia
    - Excessive sweating
    - Constipation from decreased intestinal motility
    - Mental depression from self-consciousness and embarrassment over physical appearance and activity limitations. The intellect is usually intact until the late stages of the disease process.

Nursing Diagnoses

- Bathing/grooming self-care deficit related to tremors and impaired motor function
- Impaired physical mobility related to alterations in balance and coordination

- Deficient knowledge: safe usage and effects of antiparkinsonism drugs
- Imbalanced nutrition: less than body requirements related to difficulty in chewing and swallowing food
- Risk for falls: related to altered gait

Planning/Goals

The patient will

- Experience relief of excessive salivation, muscle rigidity, spasticity, and tremors
- Experience improved motor function, mobility, and self-care abilities
- Increase knowledge of the disease process and drug therapy
- Take medications as instructed
- Avoid falls and other injuries from the disease process or drug therapy

Nursing Interventions

The nurse will

- Use measures to assist the patient and family in coping with symptoms and maintaining function. These include the following:
    - Arrange for physical therapy for heel-to-toe gait training, widening stance to increase balance and base of support, and other exercises
    - Encourage ambulation and frequent changes of position, assisted if necessary
    - Help with active and passive range-of-motion exercises
    - Encourage self-care as much as possible
- It may help to cut meat; open cartons; give frequent, small meals; and allow privacy during mealtime.
- If the patient has difficulty chewing or swallowing, chopped or soft foods may be necessary.
- Hook-and-loop-type fasteners or zippers are easier to handle than buttons.
- Slip-on shoes are easier to manage than laced ones.
    - Spend time with the patient and encourage socialization with other people. Victims of Parkinson's disease tend to become withdrawn, isolated, and depressed.
    - Schedule rest periods. Tremor and rigidity are aggravated by fatigue and emotional stress.
    - Provide facial tissues if drooling is a problem.
    - Provide appropriate patient teaching related to drug therapy (see Boxes 47.2 and 47.3).

Evaluation

- Interview and observe for relief of symptoms.
- Interview and observe for increased mobility and participation in activities of daily living.
- Interview and observe regarding correct usage of medications.

Overview of Anticholinergic Drugs

Anticholinergic drugs inhibit the actions of acetylcholine in the brain and affect the parasympathetic nervous system. Most anticholinergic drugs interact with muscarinic cholinergic receptors in the brain, secretory glands, heart, and smooth muscle and are sometimes called **antimuscarinic**

TABLE 47.5

Common Tertiary Amine and Quaternary Amine Anticholinergic Drugs

Tertiary Amines	Quaternary Amines
Atropine	Glycopyrrolate (Robinul)
Benztropine mesylate (Cogentin)	Ipratropium bromide (Atrovent)
Darifenacin hydrobromide (Enablex)	Methscopolamine bromide (Pamine)
Dicyclomine hydrochloride (Bentyl)	Tiotropium bromide (Spiriva)
Flavoxate hydrochloride (Urispas)	Trospium chloride (Sanctura)
L-Hyoscyamine (Anaspaz)	
Oxybutynin chloride (Ditropan)	
Scopolamine hydrobromide	
Solifenacin succinate (Vesicare)	
Tolterodine tartrate (Detrol, Detrol LA, and Oxytrol)	
Trihexyphenidyl hydrochloride (Trihexy)	

drugs. When given at high doses, a few anticholinergic drugs are also able to block **nicotinic receptors** in autonomic ganglia and skeletal muscles. Glycopyrrolate is an example of such a medication. This drug class includes belladonna alkaloids and their derivatives, such as atropine, and many synthetic substitutes.

Most anticholinergic medications are either **tertiary amines** or **quaternary amines** (Table 47.5). Tertiary amines are uncharged lipid-soluble molecules. Atropine and scopolamine are tertiary amines and therefore are able to cross cell membranes readily. They are well absorbed from the GI tract and conjunctiva, and they cross the blood–brain barrier. Tertiary amines are excreted in the urine.

Quaternary amines carry a positive charge and are lipid insoluble. Some belladonna derivatives and synthetic anticholinergics are quaternary amines. Consequently, they do not readily cross cell membranes. They are poorly absorbed from the GI tract and do not cross the blood–brain barrier. Quaternary amines are excreted largely in the feces.

Clinical Use

The widespread effects of anticholinergic drugs limit their clinical usefulness. Consequently, several synthetic drugs have been developed in an effort to increase selectivity of action on particular body tissues, especially to retain the antispasmodic and antisecretory effects of atropine while eliminating its adverse effects. This effort has been less than successful—all the synthetic drugs produce atropine-like adverse effects when doses are sufficient.

Some synthetic drugs are used for antispasmodic effects in GI disorders and overactive urinary bladder. Another group of synthetic drugs includes centrally active anticholinergics used in the treatment of Parkinson's disease; these drugs balance the relative cholinergic dominance that causes the movement

disorders associated with parkinsonism. Specific body systems and conditions in which anticholinergic medications are administered are listed in Table 47.6.

Drug Therapy

Anticholinergic drugs act by occupying receptor sites on target organs innervated by the parasympathetic nervous system, thereby leaving fewer receptor sites free to respond to acetylcholine (Fig. 47.2). Parasympathetic response is absent or decreased, depending on the number of receptors blocked by anticholinergic drugs and the underlying degree of parasympathetic activity. Because cholinergic **muscarinic receptors** are widely distributed in the body, anticholinergic drugs produce effects in a variety of locations, including the CNS, heart, smooth muscle, glands, and the eye.

Specific effects on body tissues and organs include the following:

- CNS stimulation followed by depression, which may result in coma and death. This is most likely to occur with large doses of anticholinergic drugs that cross the blood–brain barrier (atropine, scopolamine, and antiparkinson agents).
- Decreased cardiovascular response to parasympathetic (vagal) stimulation that slows heart rate. Atropine is the anticholinergic drug most often used for its cardiovascular effects. According to Advanced Cardiac Life Support (ACLS) protocol, atropine is the drug of choice to treat symptomatic sinus bradycardia. Low doses (less than 0.5 mg) may produce a slight and temporary decrease in heart rate; however, moderate to large doses (0.5–1 mg) increase heart rate by blocking parasympathetic vagal stimulation. Although the increase in heart rate may be therapeutic in bradycardia, it can be an adverse effect in patients with other types of heart disease because

TABLE 47.6	
Body System and Indication of Anticholinergic Use	
Body System	**Indication for Anticholinergic Use**
Cardiac	Bradycardia, heart block with hypotension and shock: increases heart rate and prevent vagal stimulation
Gastrointestinal	Peptic ulcer disease, gastritis, pylorospasm, and diverticulitis: relieves pain and relaxes gastrointestinal smooth muscle Irritable bowel, colitis: reduces frequent bowel movements and abdominal discomfort
Genitourinary	Urinary incontinence and frequency: reduces urinary muscle spasm Cystitis, urethritis, and prostatitis: decreases pain and frequency Enuresis, paraplegia, and neurogenic bladder: increases bladder capacity
Otolaryngology	Head and neck surgery and bronchoscopy: reduces respiratory tract secretions
Ophthalmology	Mydriatic and cycloplegic effects: dilate pupils
Respiratory	Asthma, chronic bronchitis: produces bronchodilation
Metabolic	Mushroom poisoning and organophosphate pesticide poisoning: reduces cholinergic stimulation; salivation, urination, defecation, bronchial secretions, laryngospasm, and bronchospasm

atropine increases the myocardial oxygen demand. Atropine usually has little or no effect on blood pressure. Large doses cause facial flushing because of dilation of blood vessels in the neck.

- Bronchodilation and decreased respiratory tract secretions. Anticholinergics block the action of acetylcholine in bronchial smooth muscle when given by inhalation. This action reduces intracellular guanosine monophosphate (GMP), a bronchoconstrictive substance. When anticholinergic drugs are given systemically, respiratory secretions decrease and may become viscous, resulting in mucous plugging of small respiratory passages. Administering the medications by inhalation decreases this effect while preserving the beneficial bronchodilation effect.

- Antispasmodic effects in the GI tract due to decreased muscle tone and motility. The drugs have little inhibitory effect on gastric acid secretion with usual doses and insignificant effects on pancreatic and intestinal secretions.

- **Mydriasis** and **cycloplegia** in the eye. Normally, anticholinergics do not change intraocular pressure, but with narrow-angle glaucoma, they may increase intraocular pressure and precipitate an episode of acute glaucoma. When the pupil is fully dilated, photophobia may be uncomfortable, and reflexes to light and accommodation may disappear.

- Miscellaneous effects. These include decreased secretions from salivary and sweat glands; relaxation of ureters, urinary bladder, and the detrusor muscle; and relaxation of smooth muscle in the gallbladder and bile ducts.

Table 47.7 lists the various anticholinergic medications.

Belladonna Alkaloid and Derivatives

Ⓟ **Atropine sulfate,** the prototype of the anticholinergic drugs, is a naturally occurring belladonna alkaloid that can be extracted from the belladonna plant or prepared synthetically. It is usually prepared as atropine sulfate, a salt that is very soluble in water. Atropine sulfate is also classified as a muscarinic antagonist.

Pharmacokinetics

Atropine is well absorbed from the GI tract and distributed throughout the body. It crosses the blood–brain barrier to enter the CNS, where large doses produce stimulant effects and toxic doses produce depressant effects. The drug is also absorbed

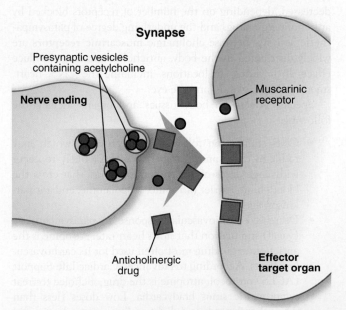

Figure 47.2 Mechanism of action of anticholinergic drugs. Anticholinergic (antimuscarinic) drugs prevent acetylcholine from interacting with muscarinic receptors on target effector organs, thus blocking or decreasing a parasympathetic response in these organs.

TABLE 47.7

Anticholinergic Medications

Drug Class	Prototype	Other Drugs in the Class
Belladonna alkaloids and derivatives	Atropine sulfate	Homatropine bromide (Isopto Homatropine) Hyoscyamine sulfate (Anaspaz) Ipratropium bromide (Atrovent) Scopolamine hydrobromide Tiotropium bromide (Spiriva)
Centrally acting anticholinergic agents	Benztropine mesylate (Cogentin)	Trihexyphenidyl hydrochloride (Trihexy)
Gastrointestinal antisecretory/antispasmodic	Dicyclomine hydrochloride (Bentyl)	Glycopyrrolate (Robinul)
Urinary antispasmodic	Oxybutynin chloride (Ditropan, Ditropan XL, Oxytrol)	Darifenacin hydrobromide (Enablex) Flavoxate hydrochloride (Urispas) Solifenacin succinate (Vesicare) Tolterodine tartrate (Detrol and Detrol LA) Trospium chloride (Sanctura)

systemically when applied locally to mucous membranes. It is metabolized in the liver. The pharmacologic effects last for about 4 hours, except for ocular effects, which may last for 7 to 14 days. Atropine is rapidly excreted in the urine.

Action

Atropine competitively blocks the effects of acetylcholine at muscarinic cholinergic receptors that mediate the effects of parasympathetic postganglionic impulses. It also prevents the action of acetylcholine in the CNS. Atropine depresses the salivary and bronchial secretions, dilates the bronchi, inhibits vagal influences on the heart, relaxes the GI and genitourinary tracts, and inhibits gastric acid secretion. In addition, it relaxes the pupil of the eye and prevents the accommodation for near vision.

Use

In the past, atropine was used to control the symptoms of Parkinson's disease—to relieve tremors and decrease rigidity. The development of the centrally acting anticholinergic agents has replaced the use of atropine for Parkinson's disease. Impaired renal or hepatic function is a contraindication to the use of atropine.

The most common use of atropine is the restoration of cardiac rate and arterial pressure during anesthesia when vagal stimulation produced by intraabdominal traction causes a decrease in pulse rate, lessening the degree of atrioventricular block when increased vagal tone is a factor. Atropine also relieves bradycardia and syncope due to hyperactive carotid sinus reflex. It also serves as an antidote for cardiac collapse with an overdose of parasympathomimetic drugs also know was cholinergic agents and cholinesterase inhibitors such as physostigmine.

Also, practitioners administer atropine in the preanesthesia stage to reduce respiratory tract secretions.

In addition, atropine is an antidote for mushroom poisoning (*Amanita muscaria*). Symptoms of muscarinic poisoning include salivation, lacrimation, visual disturbances, bronchospasm, diarrhea, bradycardia, and hypotension. Atropine prevents

the poison from interacting with muscarinic receptors, thus reversing the toxic effects. Muscarinic poisoning can also occur from cholinergic agonist drugs, cholinesterase inhibitor drugs, and insecticides that contain organophosphates.

Table 47.8 presents dosage information for atropine sulfate and the other belladonna alkaloids.

Use in Children

Systemic anticholinergics, including atropine, have essentially the same indications in children of all ages as in adults. Anticholinergic drugs cause the same adverse effects in children as in adults. However, the effects may be more severe in children, who are especially sensitive to these drugs. Facial flushing is common, and skin rashes may occur. In addition, the administration of atropine sulfate to children can cause hyperpyrexia or atropine fever.

Use in Older Adults

It is necessary to administer atropine cautiously in the geriatric population. In older adults, CNS reactions are more likely to occur.

Use in Patients With Critical Illness

When atropine is administered for cardiovascular symptoms, it is necessary to monitor the patient's cardiac status with an electrocardiogram.

Adverse Effects

Atropine sulfate may adversely affect several body systems. Cardiovascular adverse effects include bradycardia (low doses) and with tachycardia (high doses). CNS adverse effects include blurred vision, mydriasis, cycloplegia, photophobia, and increased intraocular pressure. In the geriatric population, nervousness, weakness, confusion, or excitement are common. The most severe GI adverse effect is paralytic ileus. Genitourinary effects are urinary hesitancy and retention. The patient may also complain of decreased sweating, which leads to heat prostration.

TABLE 47.8

DRUGS AT A GLANCE: Belladonna Alkaloids and Derivatives

Drug	Pregnancy Category	Routes and Dosage Ranges	
		Adults	*Children*
ⓟ **Atropine sulfate** (AtroPen, Sal-Tropine) **Ophthalmic atropine** (Isopto Atropine)	C	PO, IM, Sub-Q, IV 0.4–0.6 mg IM, Sub-Q, or IV 0.4–0.6 mg prior to induction. Use 0.4-mg dose with cyclopropane anesthesia. IV 0.5 mg (up to 3 mg) every 3–5 min PRN IV titrate large doses of 2–3 mg as needed until signs of atropine toxicity appear and cholinergic crisis is controlled. For refraction: Instill 1 or 2 drops of 1% solution into eye(s) 1 h before refraction	PO, IM, Sub-Q, IV: 7–16 lb: 0.1 mg 16–24 lb: 0.15 mg 24–40 lb: 0.2 mg 40–65 lb: 0.3 mg 65–90 lb: 0.4 mg under 90 lb: 0.4–0.6 mg 0.1 mg (newborn) to 0.6 mg (12 y) given Sub-Q 30 min prior to surgery For refraction: Instill 1–2 drops of 0.5% solution twice daily for 1–3 d before procedure.
Homatropine bromide (Isopto Homatropine)	C	For refraction: Instill 1–2 drops of 2% solution or 1 drop of 5% solution into eye before procedure. May repeat at 5–10 min intervals as needed. For uveitis: Instill 1 or 2 drops of 2% or 5% solution 2–4 times daily or every 3–4 h as needed.	For refraction: Instill 1 drop of 2% solution into eye before procedure. May repeat every 10 min as needed For uveitis: Instill 1 drop of 2% solution 2–4 times daily.
Hyoscyamine sulfate (Anaspaz)	C	PO, SL 0.125–0.25 mg 3 or 4 times daily before meals and at bedtime. PO (timed- release formula): 0.375– 0.75 mg every 12 h; IM, IV, Sub-Q: 0.25–0.5 mg every 6 h	Children under 2 y: half of the previous dose Children 2–10 y: PO 0.062– 0.125 mg every 6–8 h
Ipratropium bromide (Atrovent, Atrovent HFA)	B	Bronchodilation: 2 puffs (36 mcg) of aerosol 4 times daily. Additional inhalations may be needed. Do not exceed 12 puffs/24 h. Solution for inhalation: 500 mcg, 3 or 4 times daily. 2 sprays/nostril of 0.03% spray 2 or 3 times daily Rhinorrhea: 2 sprays/nostril of 0.06% spray 3–4 times daily	Rhinorrhea: 2 sprays/nostril of 0.03% spray 3–4 times per day
Scopolamine	C	0.4–0.8 mg daily. PO 0.32–0.65 mg Sub-Q, IM 0.32–0.65 mg IV diluted in sterile water for injection Transdermal: Apply disk 4 h before antiemetic effect is needed. Replace every 3 d. For refraction: Instill 1 or 2 drops into eye 1 h before refracting. For uveitis: Instill 1 or 2 drops into eye(s) up to 3 times daily.	Preoperative and antiemetic: 6 mcg/ kg/dose Sub-Q, IM, or IV (max dose: 0.3 mg/dose) every 6–8 h Motion sickness: Children >12 y: 1–2 tablets PO 1 h prior to exposure Apply 1 transdermal disk behind ear at least 4 h prior to exposure every 3 d as needed For refraction and iridocyclitis: Instill 1 drop of 0.25% to eye twice daily for 2 d before procedure
Tiotropium bromide (Spiriva)	C	Bronchodilation: Inhalation of con- tents of one capsule (18 mcg) daily using the HandiHaler inhalation device	Safety and efficacy have not been established.

Overdose of atropine or other anticholinergic drugs produces the usual pharmacologic effect such as decreased secretions, increased heart rate, relaxation of the bronchial smooth muscle, and decreased GI and genitourinary tone in severe and exaggerated forms. The anticholinergic overdose syndrome is characterized by hyperthermia; hot, dry, flushed skin; dry mouth; mydriasis; delirium; tachycardia; paralytic ileus; and urinary retention. Myoclonic movements and choreoathetosis may be evident. Seizures, coma, and respiratory arrest may also occur. Treatment involves use of activated charcoal to absorb the ingested drug. Hemodialysis, hemoperfusion, peritoneal dialysis, and repeated doses of charcoal are not effective.

Physostigmine salicylate (Antilirium), an acetylcholinesterase inhibitor, is a specific antidote for overdose of anticholinergics. It is usually given intravenously at a slow rate of injection, because rapid administration may cause bradycardia, hypersalivation (with subsequent respiratory distress), and seizures. The adult dose is 2 mg (no more than 1 mg/min), and the pediatric dose is 0.5 to 1 mg (no more than 0.5 mg/min). Repeated doses may be given if life-threatening dysrhythmias, convulsions, or coma occurs with anticholinergic overdose. However, the benefit of repeat dosing must be balanced against the risk of physostigmine overdose. Excessive administration of physostigmine can precipitate a cholinergic crisis, leading to seizures and dysrhythmias. Atropine is the antidote for physostigmine overdose.

Diazepam or a similar drug may be given for excessive CNS stimulation (e.g., delirium, excitement) that accompanies anticholinergic toxicity. Ice bags, cooling blankets, and tepid sponge baths may help reduce fever. Artificial ventilation and cardiopulmonary resuscitative measures are used if excessive depression of the CNS causes coma and respiratory failure. Infants, children, and the elderly are especially susceptible to the toxic effects of anticholinergic drugs.

Contraindications

Contraindications to the use of atropine include a known hypersensitivity to anticholinergic agents. Other contraindications include glaucoma, stenosing peptic ulcer, pyloroduodenal obstruction, bronchial asthma, and bladder neck obstruction, as well as hepatic or renal disease.

Nursing Implications

Preventing Interactions

Drugs that increase the anticholinergic effects of atropine include amantadine, antihistamines, tricyclic antidepressants, quinidine, disopyramide, and procainamide. Some herbs also increase the effectiveness of atropine (Box 47.4).

BOX 47.4   Herb and Dietary Interactions: Atropine Sulfate

Herbs and Foods That Increase the Effects of Atropine Sulfate

- Aloe
- Cascara
- Senna

Administering the Medication

Prior to administering atropine, the nurse assesses for hypersensitivity to anticholinergic agents, glaucoma, stenosing peptic ulcer, paralytic ileus, bronchial asthma, bladder neck obstruction, and cardiac dysrhythmias. The patient should be well hydrated and the environment should be cool to protect from hyperpyrexia. If the patient has a history of urinary retention, the patient should void before administration of the drug.

Assessing for Therapeutic Effects

The nurse assesses the heart rate if atropine is administered for bradycardia. In preoperative patients, the nurse assesses for diminished secretions, particularly when the drug is administered for head and neck surgery. Patients with Parkinson's disease or Parkinson-like syndromes require assessment for decreased spasticity and tremors.

Assessing for Adverse Effects

The nurse assesses for the following conditions, which may indicate a severe anticholinergic reaction:

- Changes in rate, quality, and rhythm of the heart that indicates ventricular tachycardia
- Urinary retention
- Bowel sounds for signs of paralytic ileus
- Photophobia, mydriasis, blurred vision, and increased intraocular pressure
- Dry mouth
- Increased temperature. Elderly people and children are prone to hyperpyrexia due to suppression of perspiration and heat loss.

Patient Teaching

Box 47.5 identifies patient teaching guidelines for atropine sulfate.

Other Drugs in the Class

Homatropine hydrobromide is a semisynthetic derivative of atropine used as eye drops to produce mydriasis and cycloplegia.

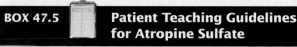

BOX 47.5   Patient Teaching Guidelines for Atropine Sulfate

- Avoid excessive high temperatures.
- Drink water frequently.
- Rinse the mouth frequently.
- Maintain good dental hygiene.
- Use hard candy to decrease dry mouth.
- Void before taking the medication.
- Visit the ophthalmologist regularly.
- Notify your prescriber is fluid intake is greater or less than urine output.
- Notify your prescriber if you develop a fever.
- Notify your prescriber if weakness becomes severe.
- Avoid the use of machinery if visual acuity or alertness is impaired.

Compared with atropine, homatropine may be preferable, because its ocular effects do not last as long.

Hyoscyamine (Anaspaz) is a belladonna alkaloid used in GI and genitourinary disorders characterized by spasm, increased secretion, and increased motility. It has the same effects as other atropine-like drugs.

Ipratropium (Atrovent) is an anticholinergic drug chemically related to atropine. When given as a nasal spray, it is useful in treating rhinorrhea due to allergy or the common cold. When given in inhaled or aerosol form to patients with chronic obstructive pulmonary disease (COPD), it is beneficial as a bronchodilator. Using the respiratory route instead of the systemic route to administer anticholinergic drugs results in less thickening of respiratory secretions and therefore a reduced incidence of mucus-plugged airways.

Scopolamine has similar uses, adverse effects, and peripheral effects when compared with atropine but is different with regard to its central effects. When scopolamine is given parenterally, it depresses the CNS and causes amnesia, drowsiness, euphoria, relaxation, and sleep. Effects of the drug appear more quickly and disappear more readily than those of atropine. Scopolamine also is used in motion sickness. It is available as oral tablets and as a transdermal adhesive disk that is placed behind the ear. The disk (Transderm-V) protects against motion sickness for 72 hours.

Tiotropium bromide (Spiriva HandiHaler) is a dry powder in capsule form intended for oral inhalation with the HandiHaler inhalation device. This long-acting, antimuscarinic, anticholinergic, quaternary ammonium compound inhibits M_3 receptors in smooth muscle, resulting in bronchodilation. Tiotropium is indicated for daily maintenance treatment of bronchospasm associated with COPD. It is not indicated for acute episodes of bronchospasm (i.e., rescue therapy). Tiotropium is eliminated via the renal system, and patients with moderate to severe renal dysfunction should be carefully monitored for drug toxicity. No dosage adjustments are required for older patients or patients with hepatic impairment or mild renal impairment.

NCLEX Success

10. A 62-year-old man is admitted to the cardiac intensive care unit. He is in sinus bradycardia with a rate of 48 beats per minute. What is the drug of choice for sinus bradycardia?

   A. atropine sulfate
   B. epinephrine (Adrenalin)
   C. isoproterenol (Isuprel)
   D. dopamine (Intropin)

11. A hospice patient has loud gurgling respirations that are audible without a stethoscope. Which of the following medications is the drug of choice to decrease the secretions?

   A. trihexyphenidyl (Trihexy)
   B. tolterodine (Detrol LA)
   C. tiotropium bromide (Spiriva HandiHaler)
   D. scopolamine

12. After a man takes atropine sulfate, he becomes nonresponsive and his respiratory rate drops. Based on these symptoms, what medication is administered?

   A. dicyclomine (Bentyl)
   B. dopamine (Intropin)
   C. physostigmine salicylate (Antilirium)
   D. diazepam (Valium)

Centrally Acting Anticholinergics

Older anticholinergic drugs such as atropine are rarely used to treat Parkinson's disease because of their undesirable peripheral effects (e.g., dry mouth, blurred vision, photophobia, constipation, urinary retention, tachycardia). Newer, centrally acting synthetic anticholinergic drugs are more selective for muscarinic receptors in the CNS and are designed to produce fewer adverse effects. The prototype centrally acting anticholinergic agent is ⓟ **benztropine mesylate** (Cogentin).

Pharmacokinetics

Benztropine is administered orally and parenterally. The oral form has an onset of action of 60 minutes and a 6- to 10-hour duration of action. The parenteral form has an onset of action in 15 minutes and a similar duration of action. The drug is absorbed from the GI tract and metabolized in the liver. It crosses the blood–brain barrier and the placenta. It is unknown how the drug is excreted.

Action

The anticholinergic activity of benztropine takes place in the CNS. Experts believe that the drug helps normalize the imbalance of cholinergic and dominergic neurotransmission in the basal ganglia of the brain to reduce rigidity, akinesia, and tremor. It suppresses the secondary symptoms of parkinsonism such as excessive salivary secretions and drooling.

Use

Benztropine mesylate is used for adjunctive therapy of all forms of parkinsonism: arteriosclerotic, idiopathic, and postencephalitic. It is also administered to control extrapyramidal disorders such as tardive dyskinesia due to neuroleptic drugs (phenothiazines). In addition, it is commonly used as a supplement with trihexyphenidyl, carbidopa, or levodopa. Table 47.9 lists the dosages of the centrally acting anticholinergic agents.

Use in Older Adults

Use of benztropine in older adults requires caution. Prescribers and nurses must adhere strictly to dosing regulations. Patients older than 60 years of age can develop increased sensitivity to the CNS effects of all anticholinergic medications.

Adverse Effects

CNS adverse effects of benztropine include disorientation, confusion, hallucinations, memory loss, psychoses, agitation, euphoria, light-headedness, depression, giddiness, and

TABLE 47.9

DRUGS AT A GLANCE: Centrally Acting Anticholinergics

Drug	Pregnancy Category	Routes and Dosages	
		Adults	Children
Ⓟ **Benztropine mesylate** (Cogentin)	C	0.5–1 mg PO, IM, IV at bedtime; may increase up to 6 mg given at bedtime or in 2–4 divided doses. For acute dystonia: IM, IV 1–2 mg; may repeat if needed. For prevention: PO 1–2 mg	Safety and efficacy have not been established.
Trihexyphenidyl (Trihexy)	C	1–2 mg PO; increase by 2-mg increments at 3- to 5-d intervals until a total of 6–10 mg is given daily in divided doses 3–4 times daily at mealtimes and bedtimes. PO 1 mg initially. Increase as needed to control symptoms.	Safety and efficacy have not been established.

heaviness of the limbs. With the administration of high doses, an inability to move certain muscle groups may occur. Peripheral anticholinergic effects include tachycardia, palpitation, hypotension, orthostatic hypotension, blurred vision, dry mouth, urinary retention, decreased sweating, and elevated temperature.

Contraindications

There are several contraindications to the use of benztropine mesylate. Glaucoma is a problem because the drug can increase intraocular pressure. GI obstruction, prostatic hypertrophy, and urinary bladder neck obstruction are other complications because of the drug's effect on smooth muscle and sphincter tone. Also, myasthenia gravis is a contraindication, because blockade of acetylcholine receptor sites at neuromuscular synapses exacerbates muscle weakness.

Caution is necessary in patients with cardiovascular disorders (e.g., tachycardia, dysrhythmias, and hypertension) because parasympathetic blockade may allow a harmful increase in sympathetic dominance. Also, caution is warranted in elderly patients with preexisting cognitive impairments because acetylcholine is an important neurotransmitter in memory function.

Nursing Implications

Preventing Interactions

Benztropine has the same interactions as atropine. Phenothiazines and tricyclic antidepressants combined with benztropine mesylate can cause confusion, hallucinations, and paralytic ileus.

Administering the Medication

If the patient is experiencing GI upset, it is necessary to administer benztropine with food. The drug may be taken before meals in the presence of a dry mouth and after meals if drooling or nausea occurs. The use of ice chips or lozenges to counteract symptoms of dry mouth may help. The patient should void prior to the administration of the medication. Dosage reduction during the summer months may be necessary.

Assessing for Therapeutic Effects

The nurse assesses for decreased rigidity and tremor. Also, he or she assesses for a decrease in oral secretions and an absence of drooling.

Assessing for Adverse Effects

The nurse monitors the patient's intake and output. If difficulty with urination results, a dosage reduction may be necessary. The nurse assesses for signs and symptoms of paralytic ileus such as intermittent constipation, abdominal pain, diminished bowel sounds on auscultation, and distention. It is also necessary to assess the heart rate for tachycardia. In addition, the nurse assesses the inability to move certain muscle groups. Checking the patient's ambulation for signs of muscle weakness and unsteady gait helps.

Patient Teaching

Box 47.6 identifies patient teaching guidelines for benztropine.

BOX 47.6   Patient Teaching Guidelines for Benztropine Mesylate

- Take the medication as prescribed.
- Avoid excessive high temperatures.
- Avoid alcohol, sedatives, and over-the-counter medications, including cough and cold remedies.
- Drink water frequently.
- Rinse the mouth frequently.
- Maintain good dental hygiene.
- Use hard candy to decrease dry mouth.
- Void before taking the medication.
- Visit the ophthalmologist regularly.
- Notify your prescriber if fluid intake is greater or less than urine output.
- Notify your prescriber of if you develop a fever.
- Notify your prescriber if weakness becomes severe.
- Avoid the use of machinery if visual acuity or alertness is impaired.

Other Drugs in the Class

Trihexyphenidyl (Trihexy) is used in the treatment of parkinsonism and extrapyramidal reactions caused by some antipsychotic drugs. This drug relieves smooth muscle spasm by a direct action on the muscle and by inhibiting the parasympathetic nervous system. It supposedly has fewer adverse effects than atropine, but approximately half of the recipients report mouth dryness, blurring of vision, and other adverse effects common to anticholinergic drugs. Trihexyphenidyl requires the same precautions as other anticholinergic drugs and is contraindicated in glaucoma.

Clinical Application 47-4

Mr. Stokes has been prescribed benztropine mesylate (Cogentin) 3 mg PO at bedtime. He resides in Wisconsin and lives there for much of the year, but he spends the winter months in Corpus Christi, Texas.

- The nurse should educate Mr. Stokes regarding the administration of benztropine mesylate (Cogentin). What specific guidelines are important to mention?
- What adverse effect is Mr. Stokes at risk for during the time he spends in Corpus Christi?

NCLEX Success

13. A 46-year-old woman is taking benztropine mesylate (Cogentin). The nurse teaches her which of the following?

   A. avoid overheating and stay well hydrated
   B. double the dose with excess secretions
   C. report diarrhea to the prescriber
   D. administer benztropine with phenothiazines

14. A patient is taking benztropine mesylate (Cogentin) and reports gastrointestinal upset following administration of the medication. The nurse teaches the patient to do what?

   A. take the medication prior to eating
   B. take the medication before bed
   C. take the medication with food
   D. take the medication with Maalox

Gastrointestinal Anticholinergics (Antisecretory/Antispasmodic)

Dicyclomine hydrochloride (Bentyl) and glycopyrrolate (Robinul) are older medications previously administered for the treatment of peptic ulcer disease. The use of these medications has declined with the advent of the proton pump inhibitors. However, they are still prescribed for irritable bowel syndrome. Ⓟ **Dicyclomine hydrochloride** (Bentyl) is the prototype GI anticholinergic medication.

Pharmacokinetics

Dicyclomine is available for oral and parenteral administration. Its onset of action in 1 to 2 hours, and its duration of action is 4 hours. It is metabolized in the liver and excreted by the kidneys. The drug crosses the placenta and enters the breast milk.

Action

Dicyclomine is a GI smooth muscle relaxant. It competitively blocks the effects of acetylcholine at muscarinic cholinergic receptors that mediate the effects of the parasympathetic postganglionic impulses.

Use

Prescribers order dicyclomine for the treatment of irritable bowel syndrome. Table 47.10 gives the dosage information for this drug and related agents.

Use in Older Adults

The onset of adverse effects is increased in elderly people. Use of dicyclomine in older patients requires caution.

Adverse Effects

Adverse effects of dicyclomine are blurred vision, dry mouth, altered taste perception, nausea, vomiting, dysphagia, urinary hesitancy, urinary retention, and irritation at the injection site.

Contraindications

Dicyclomine possesses the same contraindications as the belladonna derivatives and the centrally acting anticholinergics. Contraindications to the belladonna derivatives include hypersensitivity, glaucoma, some ulcers, bronchial asthma, urinary bladder neck obstruction, and hepatic or renal disease. Contraindications to the use of centrally acting anticholinergics also include glaucoma, GI obstruction, and urinary bladder neck obstruction, as well as prostatic hypertrophy and myasthenia gravis.

Nursing Implications

Preventing Interactions

Dicyclomine has interactions similar to those of the previous anticholinergics. The combination of antipsychotic agents with dicyclomine results in decreased effectiveness of the antipsychotic medications. Tricyclic antidepressants and amantadine combined with dicyclomine produces increased anticholinergic effects. If dicyclomine is administered with digoxin or atenolol, there is a greater reduction in the heart rate or blood pressure then if the medications are administered alone.

Administering the Medication

As with the other anticholinergic medications, it is necessary to have the patient void before taking dicyclomine. With the intramuscular preparation, it is important that the patient is switched to the oral form as soon as possible because of the increased anticholinergic effects of the parenteral formulation.

TABLE 48.10

DRUGS AT A GLANCE: Gastrointestinal Anticholinergics (Antisecretory/Antispasmodic)

Drug	Pregnancy Category	Routes and Dosage Ranges	
		Adults	Children
ⓟ **Dicyclomine hydrochloride** (Bentyl)	B	20–40 mg PO before meals and at bedtime 20 mg IM before meals and at bedtime	Safety and efficacy have not been established.
Glycopyrrolate (Robinul)	B	1–2 mg PO 2 or 3 times daily 0.1–0.2 mg IM, IV 0.004 mg/kg IM 30–60 min before anesthesia	Not recommended in children under the age of 12 y for antisecretory use Younger than 2 y: 0.004 mg/lb IM 30–60 min before anesthesia 2–12 y: 0.002–0.004 mg/lb IM 30–60 min before anesthesia

Assessing for Therapeutic Effects

If dicyclomine is working, the patient reports a decrease in abdominal pain.

Assessing for Adverse Effects

The nurse assesses for altered taste perception, dry mouth, nausea, and vomiting, as well as for urinary retention. Administering the parenteral preparation requires assessment for injection site irritation.

Patient Teaching

Patient teaching for dicyclomine is the same as for atropine and benztropine (see Boxes 47.5 and 47.6).

Urinary Antispasmodics

Anticholinergic drugs are the drugs of choice for their antispasmodic effects on smooth muscle to relieve the symptoms of urinary incontinence and frequency that accompany an overactive bladder. In infections such as cystitis, urethritis, and prostatitis, the drugs decrease the frequency and pain of urination. The drugs are also given to increase bladder capacity in enuresis, paraplegia, and neurogenic bladder. ⓟ **Oxybutynin** (Ditropan, Ditropan XL, Oxytrol), the prototype, is a urinary antispasmodic that is available in oral and transdermal forms.

Pharmacokinetics

The oral preparation of oxybutynin has an onset of action 30 to 60 minute, a peak of 3 to 6 hours, and a duration of action of 6 to 10 hours. The transdermal preparation has an onset of action of 24 to 48 hour, a variable peak, and a duration of action of 96 hours. The medication is metabolized in the liver and is excreted in the urine. It crosses the placenta and may enter the breast milk.

Action

Oxybutynin acts directly to relax the smooth muscle and inhibits the effects of acetylcholine at muscarinic receptors. A less potent anticholinergic than atropine, oxybutynin is more potent as an antispasmodic and devoid of antinicotinic activity at the skeletal neuromuscular junctions or autonomic ganglia.

Use

Oxybutynin is administered for the relief of bladder instability associated with voiding in patients with uninhibited neurogenic and reflex neurogenic bladder. The extended-release tablets decrease the symptoms of overactive bladder, incontinence, urgency, and frequency. Table 47.11 gives dosage information for oxybutynin and other urinary antispasmodics.

Use in Children

The FDA has approved the use of the extended-release formulation of oxybutynin for the treatment of symptoms of detrusor muscle overactivity associated with neurological conditions such as spina bifida in children 6 years and older.

Use in Older Adults

In older adults, the dosage of oxybutynin should not exceed 2.5 mg PO two to three times per day.

Use in Patients With Renal Impairment

The use of oxybutynin in the presence of renal impairment requires caution because of its elimination in the urine.

Use in Patients With Hepatic Impairment

The use of oxybutynin in the presence of hepatic impairment requires caution because it is metabolized by the liver.

TABLE 48.11

DRUGS AT A GLANCE: Urinary Antispasmodics

Drug	Pregnancy Category	Routes and Dosages	
		Adults	*Children*
Oxybutynin (Ditropan, Ditropan XL, Oxytrol)	B	5 mg PO 2 or 3 times daily; max dose 5 mg 4 times daily. Extended release: 5 mg PO daily up to 30 mg/daily TDS: Apply TDS every 3–4 d. Geriatric Patient: 2.5 mg PO 2–3 times per day	Children >5 y: 5 mg PO daily (max dosage 5 mg 3 times per day) >6 y: extended release 5 mg PO daily; dosage may be adjusted in 5 mg increments up to a max dose of 20 mg/d
Darifenacin hydrobromide (Enablex)	C	7.5 mg PO once daily. May increase to 15 mg if needed to control symptoms.	Safety and efficacy have not been established.
Flavoxate hydrochloride (Urispas)	B	100–200 mg PO 3 or 4 times daily. Reduce when symptoms improve.	Safety and efficacy have not been established.
Solifenacin succinate (Vesicare)	C	5 mg once PO daily. May increase to 10 mg once daily if needed to control symptoms.	Safety and efficacy have not been established.
Tolterodine tartrate (Detrol, Detrol LA)	C	2 mg PO twice daily. May decrease to 1 mg when symptoms improve. Reduce doses to 1 mg PO twice daily in presence of hepatic impairment.	Safety and efficacy have not been established.
Trospium chloride (Sanctura, Sanctura XR)	C	20 mg PO twice daily at least 1 h before meals or on an empty stomach	Safety and efficacy have not been established.

Adverse Effects

The adverse effects of oxybutynin are consistent with the previous anticholinergic agents discussed in this chapter. The most commonly reported CNS adverse effects include drowsiness, dizziness, and blurred vision. Other adverse effects are dry mouth, nausea, urinary hesitancy, and decreased sweating.

Contraindications

Contraindications to oxybutynin are hypersensitivity to the medication, pyloric or duodenal ulcer, obstructive intestinal lesions, intestinal atony, megacolon, colitis, obstructive uropathies, glaucoma, myasthenia gravis, cardiovascular instability, and urinary retention.

Nursing Implications

Preventing Interactions

Use of oxybutynin in combination with phenothiazines results in increased anticholinergic effects. The phenothiazines inhibit the cytochrome 450 enzyme CYP3A4 in the liver. This enzyme

is required in the metabolism of oxybutynin. The inhibition of the enzyme results in a greater amount of oxybutynin that has not undergone first-pass metabolism contributing to oxybutynin toxicity. This same effect occurs if haloperidol is administered with oxybutynin. Also, use of oxybutynin together with haloperidol reduces the effect of the haloperidol and results in the development of tardive dyskinesia. Administration of oxybutynin with amantadine or nitrofurantoin leads to increased toxicity of oxybutynin.

Administering the Medication

It is important that the extended-release medication is not cut, crushed, or chewed.

Assessing for Therapeutic Effects

The nurse assesses for patient reports of decreased urinary incontinence, urgency, and frequency.

Assess for Adverse Effects

The nurse assesses for CNS depression. He or she also assesses for urinary hesitancy and retention as well as for impotence. In addition, it is necessary to assess for allergic reactions to the medication such as urticarial reactions.

BOX 47.7 Patient Teaching Guidelines for Oxybutynin Chloride

- Take the medication as prescribed; do not cut, crush, or chew extended-release tablets.
- Apply the transdermal patch to dry intact skin over the abdomen, hip, or buttock every 3 to 4 days (twice weekly). Remove the old system before applying a new one. Select a new site when applying a new system.
- Have periodic bladder examinations to evaluate the therapeutic response.
- Drink water frequently.
- Rinse the mouth frequently.
- Maintain good dental hygiene.
- Use hard candy to decrease dry mouth.
- Avoid excessive high temperatures.
- Notify your prescriber if fluid intake is greater or less than urine output.
- Notify your prescriber if you develop a fever.

Patient Teaching

Box 47.7 identifies the patient teaching guidelines for oxybutynin.

Other Drugs in the Class

Darifenacin (Enablex) is a competitive, antimuscarinic, anticholinergic agent with selective affinity for M_3 receptors involved in contraction of the urinary bladder. Darifenacin is indicated for the treatment of overactive bladder, reducing symptoms of urge incontinence, urgency, and frequency. After oral administration, darifenacin is 98% protein bound and extensively metabolized in the liver by enzymes CYP3A4 and CYP2D6. A small group of people (~7% Caucasian and 2% African American) are poor metabolizers of the drug and may require reduced dosages to avoid adverse effects. Dosage should also be reduced in people with moderate hepatic dysfunction and avoided in those with severe hepatic impairment.

Flavoxate (Urispas) was developed specifically to counteract spasm in smooth muscle tissue of the urinary tract. It has anticholinergic, local anesthetic, and analgesic effects. Thus, the drug relieves dysuria, urgency, frequency, and pain with genitourinary infections, such as cystitis and prostatitis.

Solifenacin (Vesicare) is a competitive, antimuscarinic, anticholinergic agent indicated for the treatment of overactive bladder with symptoms of urgency, urge incontinence, and frequency. Solifenacin is well absorbed after oral administration, 98% bound to plasma proteins, and extensively metabolized in the liver by CYP3A4 enzymes. Dosages should be reduced in people with moderate renal or hepatic impairment, and solifenacin is not recommended for those with severe hepatic impairment. Solifenacin may prolong QT intervals, especially at higher dosages, potentially resulting in dysrhythmias.

Tolterodine (Detrol and Detrol LA) is a competitive antimuscarinic, anticholinergic agent that inhibits bladder contraction, decreases detrusor muscle pressure, and delays the urge to void. It is used to treat urinary frequency, urgency, and urge incontinence. Tolterodine is more selective

for muscarinic receptors in the urinary bladder than in other areas of the body, such as the salivary glands, and therefore, anticholinergic adverse effects are less marked. Reduced doses (1 mg) are recommended for patients with hepatic dysfunction. Tolterodine is also available in an extended-release form.

Trospium chloride (Sanctura) is an antimuscarinic, anticholinergic drug for treatment of urgency, urge incontinence, and urinary frequency associated with overactive bladder. Trospium reduces the tone of smooth muscle in the bladder, exerting an antispasmodic effect. Because of its quaternary structure, less than 10% of an orally administered dose is absorbed, and food further delays absorption. Therefore, it is recommended that the medication be taken at least 1 hour before meals or on an empty stomach. Absorbed trospium is eliminated by a combination of glomerular filtration and active tubular secretion. Trospium has the potential for interaction with other drugs that are eliminated by active tubular secretion (e.g., digoxin, procainamide, pancuronium, morphine, vancomycin, metformin, tenofovir), resulting in increased serum concentration of either trospium or the coadministered drug because of competition for the urinary tubular pump. Reduced dosages of trospium are recommended for patients with renal insufficiency and those older than 75 years of age who may be less able to tolerate the adverse effects of anticholinergic drugs.

The Nursing Process

Assessment

- Assess the patient's condition in relation to disorders for which anticholinergic drugs are used (i.e., check for bradycardia or heart block, diarrhea, dysuria, abdominal pain, and other disorders). If the patient reports or medical records indicate a specific disorder, assess for signs and symptoms of that disorder (e.g., Parkinson's disease).
- Assess for disorders in which anticholinergic drugs are contraindicated (e.g., glaucoma, prostatic hypertrophy, reflux esophagitis, myasthenia gravis, hyperthyroidism).
- Assess use of other drugs with anticholinergic effects, such as antihistamines (histamine$_1$ receptor antagonists), antipsychotic agents, and tricyclic antidepressants.

Nursing Diagnoses

- Impaired urinary elimination: decreased bladder tone and urine retention
- Constipation related to slowed gastrointestinal function
- Disturbed thought processes: confusion, disorientation, especially in older adults
- Deficient knowledge: drug effects and accurate usage
- Risk for injury related to drug-induced blurred vision and photophobia
- Risk for noncompliance related to adverse drug effects
- Risk for altered body temperature: hyperthermia

Planning/Goals

The patient will

- Receive or self-administer the drugs correctly
- Experience relief of symptoms for which anticholinergic drugs are given

- Avoid or cope with adverse drug effects on vision, thought processes, bowel and bladder elimination, and heat dissipation (with assistance, if necessary)

Nursing Interventions

The nurse will

- Instruct the patient regarding all aspects of medication administration
- Provide anticholinergic medications with meals to prevent GI upset
- Protect the patient from heat-related adverse effects

- Assess the patient's therapeutic response to the anticholinergic medication administration
- Administer anticholinergic medications at same time every day

Evaluation

- Interview and observe in relation to safe, accurate drug administration.
- Interview and observe for relief of symptoms for which the drugs are given.
- Interview and observe for adverse drug effects.

Key Concepts

- Parkinsonism is a progressive neurodegenerative disorder characterized by a deficit of dopamine and a relative excess of acetylcholine.
- Classic symptoms of Parkinson's disease include resting tremor, bradykinesia, rigidity, and postural instability.
- Dopaminergic drugs increase dopamine concentrations in the brain, exerting dopaminergic activity, directly or indirectly.
- Dopamine activity can be increased by increasing dopamine release and reducing neuronal reuptake (amantadine), directly stimulating dopamine receptors (apomorphine, bromocriptine, pramipexole, ropinirole, rotigotine-transdermal), replacement of dopamine or its precursor (levodopa,), or inhibition of metabolism of dopamine by MAO or COMT enzymes (rasagiline, selegiline, entacapone, tolcapone).
- Carbidopa prevents levodopa breakdown in the periphery, resulting in higher brain concentrations with lower levodopa dosages.
- The FDA has issued **a BLACK BOX WARNING** ◆ stating that patients who take tolcapone risk potentially fatal acute fulminant liver failure.
- Anticholinergic drugs (e.g., benztropine, trihexyphenidyl, and diphenhydramine) decrease the effect of acetylcholine in the brain.
- Combinations of antiparkinson drugs are often given to reduce dosages and achieve better control of symptoms.
- Care must be taken to avoid serious food or drug interactions that may diminish treatment effectiveness (levodopa) or be potentially fatal (selegiline and rasagiline).
- Anticholinergic drugs block the action of acetylcholine on the parasympathetic nervous system.
- Most anticholinergic drugs interact with muscarinic cholinergic receptors in the brain, secretory glands, heart, and smooth muscle and are sometimes called antimuscarinic drugs.
- Cholinergic (muscarinic) receptors are widespread throughout the body, producing effects in a variety of locations including the central nervous system, heart, smooth muscle, glands, and the eye.
- Synthetic anticholinergics were developed to exert more selective effects on particular body tissues.
- Anticholinergic drugs (e.g., dicyclomine or glycopyrrolate) are indicated for antispasmodic effects in GI disorders. Historically, they have also been used to treat peptic ulcer disease; however, they are weak inhibitors of gastric acid secretion and have been largely replaced other more effective medications (e.g., proton pump inhibitors)
- Urinary antispasmodic anticholinergic drugs are the drugs of choice for treatment of symptoms of overactive bladder.
- Ophthalmic anticholinergic preparations are indicated for mydriatic and cycloplegic effects to aid in eye examination and surgery.
- Ipratropium and tiotropium are anticholinergic medications given by inhalation for bronchodilation effects in the treatment of asthma and chronic bronchitis.

- Atropine is the drug of choice to treat bradycardia.

- Anticholinergic medications are indicated in the relief of central nervous system symptoms of Parkinson's disease or extrapyramidal symptoms associated with some antipsychotic drugs.

- Anticholinergic drugs are given preoperatively to prevent anesthesia-associated complications such as bradycardia, excessive respiratory secretions, and hypotension.

- Anticholinergic drugs are contraindicated for patients with benign prostatic hypertrophy, myasthenia gravis, hyperthyroidism, narrow-angle glaucoma, tachydysrhythmias, myocardial infarction, heart failure, or conditions associated with esophageal reflux.

- Anticholinergic overdose is characterized by hyperthermia; hot, dry, flushed skin; dry mouth; mydriasis; delirium; tachycardia; paralytic ileus; urinary retention; myoclonic movements; seizures; coma; and respiratory arrest. Physostigmine is the specific antidote for anticholinergic overdose.

- Atropine is the antidote for muscarinic agonist poisoning.

Critical Thinking Questions

47-1. An 85-year-old woman is being discharged from the hospital following a fall at her home. On admission, a fine hand tremor is apparent. She receives a diagnosis of Parkinson's disease.

- During the patient teaching session, her daughter asks the following question, "How did they figure out my mother had Parkinson's disease?"
- What are the adverse effects of levodopa/carbidopa?
- What are teaching strategies for a patient taking levodopa?

47-2. A 62-year-old postmenopausal woman is having urinary urgency and frequency. Her physician prescribes the transdermal oxybutynin (Ditropan). The nurse is instructing her about this medication.

- What is the action of oxybutynin?
- What patient teaching does the nurse provide?

References and Resources

Caslake, R., Macleod, A., Ives, N., et al. (2009). Monoamine oxidase B inhibitors versus other dopaminergic agents in early Parkinson's disease. *Cochrane Database System Review*, CD006661.

Cranwell-Bruce, L. A. (2010). Drugs for Parkinson's disease. *Medsurg Nursing*, 19(6), 347–355.

Feign, A. (2011). Gene therapy for Parkinson disease. *Science Daily*. Retrieved August 16, 2011.

Karch, A. M. (2012). *2012 Lippincott's nursing drug guide*. Philadelphia, PA: Lippincott Williams & Wilkins.

Lavsa, S. M., Fabian, T. J., Saul, M. I., Corman, S. L., & Coley, K. C. (2010). Influence of medications and diagnoses on fall risk in psychiatric patients. *American Journal of Health System Pharmacology*, 67, 1274–1280.

Lexicomp Online. (2010). *Levodopa, carbidopa, and entacapone (Stalevo): FDA evaluating trial suggesting a possible increased cardiovascular risk*. Retrieved October 3, 2011.

Kuoppamaki, M., Korpela, K., Marttila, R., Kaasinen, V., Hartikainen, P., Lyytinen, J., et al. (2009). Comparison of pharmacokinetic profile of levodopa throughout the day between levodopa/carbidopa/entacapone and levodopa/carbidopa when administered four or five times daily. *European Journal of Phamacology*, (65), 443–455.

Parkinson Disease Foundation (2010a). *Statistics on Parkinson's*. Retrieved from http://www.pdf.org/en/parkinson_statistics

Porth, C. M., & Matfin, G. (2009). *Pathophysiology concepts of altered health states*. Philadelphia, PA: Lippincott Williams & Wilkins.

Rabinak, C. A., & Nirenberg, M. J. (2010). Dopamine agonist withdrawal syndrome in Parkinson disease. *Archives of Neurology*, 67, 58.

Smeltzer, S. C., Bare, B. G., Hinkle, J. H., & Cheever, K. H. (2010). *Brunner & Suddarth's textbook of medical-surgical nursing* (12th ed.). Philadelphia, PA: Lippincott Williams & Wilkins.

Tarsey, D. (2011). *Pharmacological treatment of Parkinson disease*. Up-To-Date.

U. S. Food and Drug Administration. Stalevo (carbidopa/levodopa and entacapone): ongoing safety review: possible increased cardiovascular risk. Retrieved from http://www.fda.gov/Safety/MedWatch/SafetyInformation/SafetyAlertsforHumanMedicalProducts/ucm223423.htm. Updated August 20, 2010.

U. S. Food and Drug Administration. FDA Drug Safety Communication: ongoing safety review of Stalevo (entacapone/carbidopa/levodopa) and possible development of prostate cancer. Retrieved from http://www.fda.gov/Drugs/DrugSafety/PostmarketDrugSafetyInformationforPatientsandProviders/ucm206363.htm. Updated March 31, 2010.

48 Drug Therapy With Opioids

Clinical Application Case Study

Darlene Hoffman, a 50-year-old woman, is receiving treatment for ovarian cancer. After surgery, she arrives on the unit from the postanesthesia care unit (PACU) complaining of lower back pain of 2 out of 10 on a 10-point pain scale. She received a total of 10 mg of morphine sulfate in the PACU. Her vital signs are temperature 98.2°F, pulse 82 beats/min, respirations 22 breaths/min, and blood pressure 124/72 mm Hg, with an O_2 saturation of 94% on 2 L/min nasal cannula.

KEY TERMS

Analgesics: drugs that relieve pain without loss of consciousness

Breakthrough pain: episodic bursts of intense pain that "breaks through" the pain control of the medication regime

Ceiling effect: a phenomenon of certain drugs that limits the ability to produce a further effect above a particular dosage level

Endogenous analgesia system: nerve signals that relieve pain by suppressing the transmission of pain signals from peripheral nerves; can be activated by nerve signals entering the brain or by morphine-like drugs

Endorphins: peptides (i.e., endorphins, enkephalins, and dynorphins) that interact with receptors to inhibit perception and transmission of pain signals

Nociceptors: nerve endings that selectively respond to painful stimuli and send pain signals to the brain and spinal cord

Pain: unpleasant, sensory, emotional sensation that is associated with actual or potential tissue damage

Patient-controlled analgesia: any method used by patients to administer their own pain medication, typically used to indicate administration through a controlled intravenous pump

Preemptive analgesia: a strategy to reduce postsurgical pain by administering medications prior to the occurrence of the noxious stimuli or pain

Introduction

Pain is an unpleasant, sensory, emotional sensation associated with actual or potential tissue injury. The perception of pain is part of the clinical presentation in many acute and chronic disorders and is one of the most difficult sensations for patients to cope with during the course of a disease. It impels a person to remove the cause of the damage or seek relief from the pain. This chapter aids in the understanding of drug actions by discussing pain and pain-relieving opioid drugs.

Overview of Pain

Pain is the most common symptom prompting people to seek health care. When not managed effectively, pain may greatly impair quality of life and ability to perform activities of daily living. The Joint Commission includes assessment and management of pain for all patients (the fifth vital sign) in the standards by which it evaluates health care organizations. Opioid **analgesics** are drugs that provide pain relief by affecting people's perception and tolerance of moderate to severe pain.

Etiology

The causes of pain include nerve damage, actual tissue injury, cancer, or surgery. Pain may be classified according to its origin in body structures (e.g., somatic, visceral, neuropathic), duration (e.g., acute, chronic), or cause (e.g., cancer). Box 48.1 describes these types of pain.

Pathophysiology

Pain occurs when tissue damage activates the free nerve endings (pain receptors) of peripheral nerves. **Nociceptors**, nerve endings that selectively respond to painful stimuli, are abundant in arterial walls, joint surfaces, muscle fascia, periosteum,

---

BOX 48.1   Types of Pain

Acute pain may result from injury, trauma, spasm, disease processes, and treatment or diagnostic procedures that damage body tissues. Patients often describe it as sharp or cutting. The intensity of the pain is usually proportional to the amount of tissue damage and the pain serves as a warning system by demanding the sufferer's attention and compelling behavior to withdraw from or avoid the pain-producing stimulus.

Acute pain is called fast pain because it is felt quickly after a pain stimulus is applied. It is aroused by mechanical and thermal stimuli and conducted to the spinal cord by A-delta fibers in the peripheral nerves. Glutamate is the neurotransmitter secreted in the spinal cord at the A-delta nerve fiber endings.

Acute pain is often accompanied by anxiety and objective signs of discomfort (e.g., facial expressions of distress; moaning or crying; positioning to protect the affected part; tenderness, edema, and skin color or temperature changes in the affected part; and either restlessness and excessive movement or limited movement, if movement increases pain). It usually responds to treatment with analgesic drugs and resolves as tissue repair mechanisms heal the damaged area.

Chronic (noncancer) pain (i.e., lasting 3 months or longer) demands attention less urgently, may not be characterized by visible signs, and is often accompanied by emotional stress, increased irritability, depression, social withdrawal, financial distress, loss of libido, disturbed sleep patterns, diminished appetite, weight loss, and decreased ability to perform usual activities of daily living. It may occur with or without evidence of tissue

damage and may include acute pain that persists beyond the typical recovery time for the precipitating tissue injury, pain related to a chronic disease, pain without an identifiable cause, and pain associated with cancer. It may arise from essentially any part of the body. It may be continuous or episodic or a combination of both.

Chronic (noncancer) pain may also be called slow pain. It can be elicited by mechanical, thermal, and chemical stimuli and is described as burning, aching, or throbbing. Slow, chronic pain is transmitted by C nerve fibers to the spinal cord and brain. Substance P is the neurotransmitter at C nerve fiber endings; it is released slowly and accumulates over seconds or minutes.

Cancer pain has characteristics of both acute and chronic pain, and it may be constant or intermittent. Chronic cancer pain is often caused by tumor spread into pain-sensitive tissues and the resulting tissue destruction. It usually progresses as the disease advances and can be severe and debilitating. Acute pain is often associated with diagnostic procedures or treatment measures (e.g., surgery, chemotherapy). It may also occur with disease progression, with activity, or with the development of drug tolerance.

Somatic pain results from stimulation of nociceptors in skin, bone, muscle, and soft tissue. It is usually well localized and described as sharp, burning, gnawing, throbbing, or cramping. It may be intermittent or constant and acute or chronic. Sprains and other traumatic injuries are examples of acute somatic pain; the bone and joint pain of arthritis is an example of chronic somatic pain, although acute exacerbations may also occur.

BOX 48.1   Types of Pain (Continued)

Somatic pain of low to moderate intensity may stimulate the sympathetic nervous system and produce increased blood pressure, pulse, and respiration; dilated pupils; and increased skeletal muscle tension, such as rigid posture or clenched fists.

Visceral pain, which is diffuse and not well localized, results when nociceptors are stimulated in abdominal or thoracic organs and their surrounding tissues. It includes pain associated with cholecystitis, pancreatitis, uterine disorders, and liver disease and is often described as deep, dull, aching, or cramping. It may be referred to a different part of the body (e.g., pain from the liver can be referred to the right shoulder area; ischemic pain from the heart can be referred to the left arm or neck area). Severe visceral pain stimulates the parasympathetic nervous system and produces decreased blood pressure and pulse, nausea and vomiting, weakness, syncope, and possibly loss of consciousness.

Neuropathic pain is caused by lesions or physiologic changes that injure peripheral pain receptors, nerves, or the central nervous system. It is characterized by excessive excitability in the damaged area or surrounding normal tissues, so that nerve cells discharge more easily. As a result, pain may arise spontaneously or from a normally nonpainful stimulus such as a light touch. It is a relatively common cause of chronic pain and is usually described as severe, shooting, burning, or stabbing. It occurs with peripheral neuropathies associated with diabetes mellitus (diabetic neuropathy), herpes zoster infections (postherpetic neuralgia), traumatic nerve injuries, and some types of cancer or cancer treatments. It is difficult to treat because standard analgesics (e.g., nonsteroidal anti-inflammatory drugs and opioids) are less effective in neuropathic pain than in other types of pain. Antidepressants and anticonvulsants are often used along with analgesics.

skin, and soft tissues; they are scarce in most internal organs. Causes of tissue damage may be physical (e.g., heat, cold, pressure, stretch, spasm, and ischemia) or chemical (e.g., pain-producing substances are released into the extracellular fluid surrounding the nerve fibers that carry the pain signal). These pain-producing substances activate pain receptors, increase the sensitivity of pain receptors, or stimulate the release of inflammatory substances.

For a person to feel pain, the signal from the nociceptors in peripheral tissues must be transmitted to the spinal cord, then to the hypothalamus and cerebral cortex in the brain. The signal is carried to the spinal cord by two types of nerve cells, A-delta fibers and C fibers. A-delta fibers, which are myelinated and found mainly in skin and muscle, transmit fast, sharp, well-localized pain signals. These fibers release glutamate and aspartate (excitatory amino acid neurotransmitters) at synapses in the spinal cord. C fibers, which are unmyelinated and found in muscle, abdominal viscera, and periosteum, conduct the pain signal slowly and produce a poorly localized, dull, or burning type of pain. Tissue damage resulting from an acute injury often produces an initial sharp pain transmitted by A-delta fibers followed by a dull ache or burning sensation transmitted by C fibers. C fibers release somatostatin and substance P at synapses in the spinal cord. Glutamate, aspartate, substance P, and perhaps other chemical mediators enhance transmission of the pain signal.

The dorsal horn of the spinal cord is the control center or relay station for information from the A-delta and C nerve fibers, for local modulation of the pain impulse, and for descending influences from higher centers in the central nervous system (CNS) (e.g., attention, emotion, memory). Here, nociceptive nerve fibers synapse with nonnociceptive nerve fibers (neurons that carry information other than pain signals). The brain also contains descending pathways that inhibit nociceptive input. Some brain nuclei are serotonergic and project to the dorsal horn of the spinal cord, where they suppress nociceptive transmission. Another inhibitory pathway is noradrenergic and originates in the pons. Thus, increasing the

concentration of norepinephrine and serotonin in the synapse inhibits transmission of nerve impulses that carry pain signals to the brain and spinal cord.

In the brain, the thalamus is a relay station for incoming sensory stimuli, including pain. Perception of pain is a primitive awareness in the thalamus, and sensation is not well localized. From the thalamus, pain messages are relayed to the cerebral cortex, where they are perceived more specifically and analyzed to determine actions needed.

The CNS has its own system, the **endogenous analgesia system**, for relieving pain by suppressing the transmission of pain signals from peripheral nerves. Nerve signals entering the brain or morphine-like drugs can activate the system. Important elements include receptors and endogenous peptides with actions similar to those of morphine. Receptors are highly concentrated in some regions of the CNS, including the ascending and descending pain pathways and portions of the brain essential to the endogenous analgesia system. The peptides (i.e., **endorphins**, enkephalins, and dynorphins) interact with receptors to inhibit perception and transmission of pain signals. Endorphin release can be triggered by excitement, stress, or aerobic exercise. Enkephalins are believed to interrupt the transmission of pain signals at the spinal cord level by inhibiting the release of substance P from C nerve fibers. The endogenous analgesia system may also inhibit pain signals at other points in the pain pathway.

Clinical Manifestations

Pain is a subjective experience, and patients' self-reporting of pain is considered the gold standard of pain assessment measurements because it offers the most valid measurement of pain. However, numerous factors, including mood, sleep disturbances, fatigue, and medications, may influence self-reporting. Cultural, gender, age, and other psychosocial factors can play a role in manifestations of pain.

A variety of pain measurement tools exists, including visual analogue scales, verbal or numerical rating scales, or picture scales. The pain measurement tool chosen should be appropriate to the individual patient, considering developmental, cognitive, emotional, language, and cultural factors. A mnemonic device (SOCRATES) can be used to assess the clinical manifestations of pain. Its meaning appears below:

- Site
- Onset
- Character
- Radiation
- Associations with other symptoms
- Time course (pattern)
- Exacerbating/relieving factors
- Severity

Nurses can use observational tools for patients who cannot communicate their pain for various reasons (e.g., unconsciousness, cognitive impairment). These tools involve facial expressions, limb movements, vocalization, restlessness, and guarding as indicators of pain. In patients with pain, vital signs may demonstrate tachycardia, tachypnea, and hypertension.

EVIDENCE-BASED PRACTICE

Clinical Guidelines for the Use of Chronic Opioid Therapy in Chronic Noncancer Pain

by CHOU, R., FANCIULLO, G. J., FINE, P. G., ADLER, J. A., BALLANTYNE, J. C., DAVIES, P., DONOVAN, M. I., FISHBAIN, D. A., FOLEY, K. M., FUDIN, J., GILSON, A. M., KELTER, A., MIASKOWSKI, C., MAUSKOP, A., O'CONNOR, P. G., PASSIK, S. D., PASTERNAK, G. W., PORTENOY, R. K., RICH, B. A., ROBERTS, R. G., TODD, K. H.

The Journal of Pain
2009,10(2), 113–130

The use of long-term opioid therapy for chronic noncancer pain has escalated. A systematic review of the evidence regarding chronic opioid use for chronic cancer pain demonstrates that chronic opioid therapy can be effectively and safely administered in carefully selected and monitored patients. Clinical practice guidelines by the American Pain Society and the American Academy of Pain Medicine present recommendations to minimize adverse effects and the potential for abuse of opioids. The comprehensive recommendations provide guidance on the myriad of issues that must be considered to ensure patient safety while providing effective pain control.

IMPLICATIONS FOR NURSING PRACTICE: The safe and effective use of opioids in chronic noncancer pain involves knowledge and clinical skills. Recommendations from the clinical guidelines take into consideration the most effective plan of care, incorporating the best available evidence with clinician judgment and patient preferences to assess and manage adverse effects, abuse, and addiction.

Drug Therapy

Opioid analgesics relieve moderate to severe pain by inhibiting the transmission of pain signals from peripheral tissues to the brain, reducing the perception of pain sensation in the brain, producing sedation, and decreasing the emotional upsets often associated with pain. They also inhibit the production of pain and inflammation by prostaglandins and leukotrienes in peripheral tissues. Most of these drugs are Schedule II drugs under federal narcotics laws and may lead to drug abuse and dependence (see Chap. 1).

Table 48.1 outlines the subgroups of opioid analgesics: the opioid agonists, agonists/antagonists, and antagonists. The larger group of agonists includes morphine and morphine-like drugs. These agents have activity at mu and kappa receptors and thus produce prototypical effects. As their name indicates, the agonists/antagonists have both agonist and antagonist activity. Antagonists are antidote drugs that reverse the effects of agonists. In addition, numerous combinations of opioid and nonopioid analgesics (see Chap. 14) are available and commonly used in most health care settings. In addition, **preemptive analgesia** is used to reduce postsurgical pain by simultaneously administering medications from different drug classes to suppress pain by blocking multiple pain pathways (Box 48.2).

Opioid Agonists

Ⓟ **Morphine sulfate**, the prototype, is an opium alkaloid used mainly to relieve moderate to severe pain. A Schedule II–controlled drug, administration is most often oral or parenteral. Patient response depends on route of administration and dosage.

Pharmacokinetics

Morphine is well absorbed after oral (PO), intramuscular (IM), subcutaneous, and intravenous (IV) administration. PO formulations undergo significant first-pass metabolism in the liver, which means that PO doses must be larger than injected doses to have equivalent therapeutic effects. After PO administration of fast-acting (e.g., immediate-release) formulations, peak activity occurs in about 60 minutes. After IV injection, maximal analgesia and respiratory depression usually occur within 10 to 20 minutes. After IM injection, these effects occur in about 30 minutes. After subcutaneous injection, morphine effects may be delayed up to 60 to 90 minutes. Morphine is extensively metabolized in the liver, and metabolites are excreted in urine. Morphine is about 30% bound to plasma proteins, and its half-life is 2 to 4 hours. The duration of action is 5 to 7 hours.

Action

Morphine relieves pain by binding to receptors in the brain, spinal cord, and peripheral tissues. When bound to the drug, receptors function like gates that close and thereby block or decrease transmission of pain impulses from one nerve cell to the next. The receptors also activate the endogenous analgesia system. The major types of receptors are mu, kappa, and delta.

TABLE 48.1

Drugs (Opioids) Administered for the Treatment of Pain

Drug Class	Prototype	Other Drugs in the Class
Agonists	Morphine sulfate (MS Contin, Roxanol, others)	Codeine fentanyl (Actiq, Duragesic, and others) Hydrocodone (Lortab, Vicodin) Hydromorphone (Dilaudid) Meperidine (Demerol) Methadone (Dolophine) Oxycodone (OxyContin) Oxymorphone (Numorphan, Opana) Tramadol (Ultram)
Agonists/antagonists	Pentazocine (Talwin)	Butorphanol (Stadol) Nalbuphine (Nubain)
Antagonists	Naloxone (Narcan)	Naltrexone (Depade, ReVia)

Most of the effects of morphine (analgesia; CNS depression, with respiratory depression and sedation; euphoria; decreased gastrointestinal [GI] motility; and physical dependence) are attributed to activation of the mu receptors. Analgesia, sedation, and decreased GI motility occur with activation of kappa receptors. The endogenous analgesia system involves the delta receptors, which may not bind with opioid drugs.

Use

The main indication for morphine is to prevent or relieve acute or chronic pain. Specific conditions for morphine include acute myocardial infarction, biliary colic, renal colic, burns and other traumatic injuries, postoperative states, and cancer. Health care providers usually give morphine for chronic pain, such as that associated with terminal cancer, only when other measures and milder drugs are ineffective. Other clinical uses of morphine include the following:

- Before and during surgery to promote sedation, decrease anxiety, facilitate induction of anesthesia, and decrease the amount of anesthesia required
- During labor and delivery (obstetric analgesia)
- Treatment of GI disorders, such as abdominal cramping and diarrhea
- Treatment of acute pulmonary edema
- Treatment of severe, unproductive cough (codeine may be used)
- Unlabeled use: relief of dyspnea associated with acute left ventricular failure and pulmonary edema

Table 48.2 gives dosages of morphine sulfate and other opioid agonists.

BOX 48.2 | **Preemptive Analgesia**

To lessen postsurgical pain, simultaneous administration of medications from different drug classes creates a multi-modal approach to suppress pain by blocking multiple pain pathways. The drugs are commonly given before the start of surgery and continue through the maintenance phase. Many of these are considered opioid sparing, which allows a clinically significant reduction in dose of opioid during and after surgery. This reduces opioid adverse effects without sacrificing the control of pain. Rather than treating pain after it has occurred, the goal is to significantly suppress both short- and long-term pain. In addition, properly managed pain reduces health care costs and improves postoperative outcome. This therapeutic intervention is called preemptive analgesia.

Drugs that can be used in preemptive analgesia include

- Ketamine, primarily used for the induction and maintenance of general anesthesia, usually in combination with a sedative
- Parenteral drugs include
- Dexmedetomidine (Precedex) that has sedative and hypnotic effects similar to natural sleep without respiratory depression

- Intravenous (IV) nonsteroidal anti-inflammatory drugs (NSAIDs) such as ketorolac tromethamine (Toradol), ibuprofen (Caldolor), and the IV form of acetaminophen (Ofirmev) for short-term management of moderate to severe pain. Caution must be exercised when administering NSAIDs (see Chap. 14) as there is an elevated risk of postoperative bleeding.
- Oral medications include
  - Gabapentin (Neurontin) and pregabalin (Lyrica), both GABA analogues and anticonvulsants (Chap. 52)
  - Celecoxib (Celebrex), an NSAID and selective COX-2 inhibitor
  - Clonidine (Catapres), a direct acting alpha-2 adrenergic receptor agonist
- Neuroaxial blocks such as epidural and spinal anesthesia, peripheral regional anesthetic techniques, and local wound infiltration using long-acting local anesthetics to provide superior analgesia. Regional techniques can be combined with general anesthesia or sedation.

TABLE 48.2

DRUGS AT A GLANCE: Opioid Agonists

Drug	Pregnancy Category	Routes and Dosage Ranges	
		Adults	Children
P **Morphine sulfate** (MS Contin, Roxanol, others)	C	PO immediate release, 5–30 mg every 4 h PRN PO controlled release, 30 mg or more every 8–12 h IM, subcutaneously 5–20 mg/70 kg every 4 h PRN IV injection, 2–10 mg/70 kg, diluted in 5 mL water for injection and injected slowly, over 5 min IV continuous infusion, 0.1–1 mg/mL in 5% dextrose in water solution, by controlled infusion pump Epidurally, 2–5 mg/24 h; intrathecally, 0.2–1 mg/24 h Rectal, 10–20 mg every 4 h PCA dosing based on institutional protocols; standard parameters: 2 mg bolus, 1 mg dose, lockout interval 10 min, 4-h maximum limit 30 mg, basal rate not recommended for starting PCA Older adult, PCA dosing per institutional protocols typically 25% of adult dose and requires more intense monitoring and dose individualization	IM, Sub-Q 0.05–0.2 mg/kg (up to 15 mg) every 4 h
Codeine	C	Pain: PO, subcutaneous, IM 15–60 mg every 4–6 h PRN; usual dose 30 mg; max, 360 mg/24 h Cough: PO 10–20 mg every 4 h PRN; max, 120 mg/24 h	1 y or older, pain: PO, subcutaneous, IM 0.5 mg/kg every 4–6 h PRN 2–6 y, cough: PO 2.5–5 mg every 4–6 h; max, 30 mg/24 h 6–12 y, cough: PO 5–10 mg every 4–6 h; max, 60 mg/24 h
Fentanyl (Actiq, Duragesic, Fentora, Ionsys, Sublimaze)*	C	Preanesthetic sedation: IM 0.05–0.1 mg 30–60 min before surgery Analgesic adjunct to general anesthesia: IV total dose of 0.002–0.05 mg/kg, depending on surgical procedure Adjunct to regional anesthesia: IM or slow IV (over 1–2 min) 0.05–0.1 mg PRN Postoperative analgesia: IM 0.05–0.1 mg, repeat in 1–2 h if needed General anesthesia: IV 0.05–0.1 mg/kg with oxygen and a muscle relaxant (max dose 0.15 mg/kg with open heart surgery, other major surgeries, and complicated neurologic or orthopedic procedures) Chronic pain (Duragesic transdermal system): 2.5–10 mg every 72 h	Children weighing at least 10 kg: conscious sedation or preanesthetic sedation, 5–15 mcg/kg of body weight (100–400 mcg), depending on weight, type of procedure, and other factors; max dose, 400 mcg, regardless of age and weight. 2–12 y: general anesthesia induction and maintenance, IV 2–3 mcg/kg
Hydrocodone (with acetaminophen: Lortab, Vicodin) (with ibuprofen: Ibudone, Vicoprofen)	With acetaminophen: C; D, prolonged use or high doses near term With ibuprofen: C; D, third trimester	With acetaminophen: 1–2 tablets every 4–6 h as needed for pain, not to exceed 8 tablets daily. With ibuprofen: 1 tablet every 4–6 h as needed for pain, not to exceed 5 tablets daily; consider reducing dosing in elderly	2–13 y or <50 kg: hydrocodone 0.1–0.2 mg/kg/dose, not to exceed 6 doses a day or the max recommended dose of acetaminophen. Dosing not established for hydrocodone with ibuprofen. Extended-release products containing hydrocodone should not

TABLE 48.2

DRUGS AT A GLANCE: Opioid Agonists (Continued)

Drug	Pregnancy Category	Routes and Dosage Ranges	
		Adults	*Children*
			be given to children younger than 6 years of age and should be used with caution in children 6–12 y of age.
Hydromorphone (Dilaudid)	C	PO 2–4 mg every 4–6 h PRN IM, subcutaneous, IV 1–2 mg every 4–6 h PRN (may be increased to 4 mg for severe pain) Rectal suppository 3 mg every 6–8 h	Dosage not established
Meperidine (Demerol)	C	IM, IV, subcutaneous, PO 50–100 mg every 2–4 h Obstetric analgesia: IM, Sub-Q 50–100 mg every 2–4 h for three or four doses	IM, subcutaneous, PO 1.1–1.75 mg/kg, up to adult dose, every 3–4 h
Methadone (Dolophine)	C	IM, subcutaneous, PO 2.5–10 mg every 3–4 h PRN	Not recommended
Oxycodone (OxyContin, Roxicodone, others)	C	PO, immediate release, 5 mg every 6 h PRN (OxyIR, Oxydose, OxyFAST); 10–30 mg every 4 h PRN for other formulations PO, controlled release, 10 mg every 12 h, increased if necessary	Not recommended for children younger than 12 y of age
Oxymorphone (Numorphan, Opana)	C	PO (Opana), 10–20 mg every 4–6 h PO, extended release (Opana ER), 5 mg every 12 h, increased by 5–10 mg every 12 h every 3–7 d until pain relieved IM, subcutaneous 1–1.5 mg every 4–6 h PRN IV 0.5 mg every 4–6 h PRN Rectal, 5 mg every 4–6 h PRN Obstetric analgesia: IM 0.5–1 mg	Dosage not established
Tramadol (Ultram)	C	PO 50–100 mg every 4–6 h PRN (max, 400 mg/d) Renal impairment (CrCl < 30 mL/min): PO 50–100 mg every 12 h (max dose, 200 mg/d) Hepatic impairment (cirrhosis): PO 50 mg every 12 h Older adults (65–75 y): same as adults, unless they also have renal or hepatic impairment Older adults (>75 y): <300 mg daily, in divided doses	Dosage not established

*Actiq, Fentora, and Ionsys are special preparations for specific uses. (Check manufacturers' instructions for dosage and administration instructions.)

Use in Children

In general, experts do not completely understand the physiology, pathology, assessment, and management of pain in children. Many authorities indicate that in children pain is often ignored or undertreated, including children having surgical and other painful procedures for which adults routinely receive an anesthetic, a strong analgesic, or both. This is especially true in preterm and full-term neonates. In the past, one reason for inadequate prevention and management of pain in newborns was a common belief that they did not experience pain because of immature nervous systems. However, research indicates that neonates have abundant C fibers and that A-delta fibers are developing during the first few months of life. These nerve fibers carry pain signals from peripheral tissues to the spinal cord. In addition, brain pain centers and the endogenous analgesia system are developed and functional.

Older infants and children may experience pain even when analgesics are readily available. For example, children may be unable to communicate their discomfort, or they may fear injections. Health care providers or parents may fear adverse effects of morphine, including excessive sedation, respiratory depression, and addiction.

To make the situation more complex, formulations of morphine and other opioids for children are not generally available. Rectal suppositories, which are used more often in children than in adults, are useful when PO or parenteral routes are not indicated.

QSEN Safety Alert

When children's doses are calculated based on adult doses, fractions and decimals often result, which greatly increases the risk of a dosage error. It is advisable to have two people do the calculations independently and compare results.

With all forms of opioids, it is important to note that the effects of the drugs in children may differ from those expected in adults because of physiologic and pharmacokinetic differences. Even with suppositories, the dose of medication received by the child is unknown because drug absorption is erratic and because adult suppositories are sometimes cut in half or otherwise altered. The nurse assesses children regularly and is alert for unusual signs and symptoms.

Use in Older Adults

It is necessary to use morphine cautiously in older adults, especially if they are debilitated; have hepatic, renal, or respiratory impairment; or are receiving other drugs that depress the CNS. Older adults are especially sensitive to respiratory depression, excessive sedation, confusion, and other adverse effects. However, they should receive adequate analgesia, along with vigilant monitoring. Specific recommendations for use in older adults include the following:

- Start with low doses and increase doses gradually, if necessary.
- Give morphine less frequency than for younger adults because the duration of action may be longer.
- Monitor carefully for sedation or confusion. In addition, monitor voiding and urine output because acute urinary retention is more likely to occur in older adults.

Use in Patients With Renal Impairment

Patients with renal impairment should take minimal doses of morphine for the shortest effective time because usual doses may produce profound sedation and a prolonged duration of action. Morphine produces an active metabolite that may accumulate in patients with renal impairment.

Use in Patients With Hepatic Impairment

Morphine is extensively metabolized by the liver; therefore, morphine may accumulate and cause increased adverse effects in the presence of hepatic impairment. Drug accumulation and increased adverse effects may occur if dosage is not reduced, especially with chronic use.

Use in Patients With Critical Illness

Morphine is commonly used to manage pain associated with disease processes and invasive diagnostic and therapeutic procedures. In intensive care units, morphine and other opioid agonists are also used concurrently with sedatives and neuromuscular blocking agents, which increase the risks of adverse drug reactions and interactions. In patients with critical illness, morphine is usually given by IV bolus injection or continuous infusion. Guidelines include the following:

- Assume that all critically ill patients are in pain or at high risk for development of pain.
- When pain is thought to be present, identify and treat the underlying cause when possible.
- Prevent pain when possible. Some specific interventions include being very gentle when performing nursing care to avoid tissue trauma and positioning patients to prevent ischemia, edema, and misalignment. In addition, give analgesics before painful procedures, when indicated.
- Consider **patient-controlled analgesia** (PCA), which is any method that allows a person in pain to administer his or her own pain relief. Commonly, an IV device regulated by programmable settings delivers morphine at a preset bolus dosage when the patient presses a button. It is possible to program a lockout period into the pump so that the frequency of administration is controlled, as well as the basal amount of drug to be delivered. When starting a continuous IV infusion of pain medication, a health care professional gives a loading dose to attain therapeutic blood levels quickly. The nurse assesses pain scores after initiation, after any change in pump setting, and periodically using a standardized pain rating scale to assess pain relief response to the PCA medication based on hospital protocol. Box 48.3 outlines specific assessment considerations prior to and throughout the administration of opioids using PCA.
- Manage pain to provide relief and prevent its recurrence. In general, morphine should be given continuously or on a regular schedule of intermittent doses, with supplemental or bolus doses when needed for **breakthrough pain**, episodic bursts of intense pain that "break through" the pain control provided by the pain medication.

Use in Patients Receiving Home Care

The use of morphine is often restricted to a short period, and patients self-administer their medication. The need for strong pain medication recedes as healing occurs. The home care nurse may teach patients and caregivers safe usage of morphine (e.g., that the drugs decrease mental alertness and physical agility, so potentially hazardous activities should be avoided). It is important to consider nonpharmacologic methods of managing pain and ways to prevent adverse effects of opioids, although these do not serve

---

BOX 48.3 **Assessment for Appropriateness of Patient-Controlled Analgesia**

- Preprocedure cognitive assessment (patient must be cognitively competent to actively participate in pain management)
  - Assess mental status, level of consciousness, and developmental status.
  - Assess patient's (and family's) ability to comprehend teaching regarding his or her role in managing pain, specific information on pump operation, safety measures, and when to alert a nurse.
- Is the patient opioid-tolerant or opioid naive?
  - Opioid-tolerant: patient has been taking at least 60 mg of morphine or an equianalgesic dose of another opioid for a week or longer.
  - Opioid naive: patients who do not meet opioid-tolerant criteria and have not had narcotics in the amounts given above for a week or more.

- Pain assessment: use a consistent standard pain assessment tool, such as the 0 to 10 pain scale or the 0 to 10 Faces Pain Scale for children.
- Sedation assessment
  - Assess sedation using a consistent tool (e.g., Pasero, Ramsay, or Richmond Agitation and Sedation Scale [RASS] sedation scales).
  - This is a critical component; sedation precedes respiratory depression because less opioid is required to produce it.
- Respiratory assessment
  - Assess rate, quality, and sounds of respirations.
  - Assess oxygen saturation using pulse oximetry.

---

as a substitute for adequate pharmacologic pain relief. Physical dependence is uncommon with short-term use of morphine for acute pain.

With some types of chronic pain, such as those occurring with low back pain or osteoarthritis, morphine is not indicated for long-term use. Treatment involves nonopioid medications, physical therapy, and other measures. The home care nurse may need to explain the reasons for not using opioids on a long-term basis and help patients and caregivers learn alternative methods of relieving discomfort.

With cancer pain, the goal of treatment is to prevent or relieve pain and keep patients comfortable, without concern about addiction. Thus, the home care nurse must assist patients and caregivers in understanding the appropriate use of morphine in cancer care, including administration on a regular schedule, storing the drugs to avoid use by people other than the patient, and avoiding theft and diversion to street use. The nurse also must be proficient in using and teaching various routes of drug administration and in arranging regimens with potentially very large doses and various combinations of drugs. In addition, the nurse must make an active effort to prevent or manage adverse effects, such as a bowel program to prevent constipation.

Additional guidelines include the following:

- Morphine should be given on a regular schedule, around the clock. Patients should be awakened, if necessary, to prevent pain recurrence.
- PO, rectal, and transdermal routes of administration are generally preferred over injections.
- When long-acting forms of morphine are given on a regular schedule, fast-acting forms also need to be available for breakthrough pain (acute pain that occurs spontaneously or with activity). If supplemental or "rescue" doses are needed frequently, the baseline dose of long-acting medication may need to be increased.
- In addition to morphine, other drugs may be used to increase patient comfort (see Other Drugs in the Class). In addition, some antidepressants and anticonvulsants decrease neuropathic pain.

Adverse Effects

Morphine has widespread pharmacologic effects, especially in the CNS and the GI system. These effects occur with usual doses and may be therapeutic or adverse, depending on the reason for use. CNS effects include analgesia; CNS depression, ranging from drowsiness to sleep to unconsciousness; decreased mental and physical activity; respiratory depression; nausea and vomiting; and pupil constriction. Sedation and respiratory depression are major adverse effects and potentially life-threatening. In the GI tract, morphine slows motility, and it may cause constipation and smooth muscle spasms in the bowel and biliary tract.

Contraindications

Contraindications and cautions are respiratory depression, acute or chronic lung disease, liver or kidney disease, prostatic hypertrophy, pregnancy, increased intracranial pressure and head injury, seizure disorders, or hypersensitivity reactions to morphine. Lactation is a consideration (it may be safer to wait 4–6 hours after administration to nurse an infant). Additional contraindications may include Addison's disease, severe alcoholism, and toxic psychosis.

Nursing Implications

Preventing Interactions

Drugs that increase the effects of morphine are found in Box 48.4. Naloxone is known to reverse the effects of morphine. Herbs such as kava, valerian, and St. John's wort may increase the sedative effect of morphine.

Administering the Medication

Although the dose of morphine can be titrated upward for adequate analgesia, unacceptable adverse effects (e.g., excessive sedation, respiratory depression, nausea, and vomiting) may limit the dose. With PO administration, patients may take the drug without regard to food. However, if GI upset occurs, food is acceptable. It is essential that PO forms are not broken

BOX 48.4 Drug Interactions: Morphine Sulfate

Drugs That Increase the Effects of Morphine Sulfate

- Alcohol
  Increases sedation
- Antihistamines
  Increase sedation and the risk of constipation and urinary retention
- Antidepressants
  Increase the risk of drowsiness, confusion, memory loss, or respiratory distress
- Antipsychotics
  Increase the risk of drowsiness, confusion, memory loss, or respiratory distress
- Barbiturates
  Increase the risk of drowsiness, confusion, memory loss, or respiratory distress
- Benzodiazepines
  Increase the risk of drowsiness, confusion, memory loss, or respiratory distress
- Monoamine oxidase (MAO) inhibitors
  Increase the risk of hypotension, respiratory depression, or coma; patients should not take morphine and an MAO inhibitor within 14 days of each other.
- Other narcotics or opiates
  Increase the risk of hypotension, respiratory depression, or coma
- Sedatives
  Increase sedation

BOX 48.5 Recognition and Management of Toxicity With Opioid Use

- Acute toxicity or overdose can occur from therapeutic use or from abuse by drug-dependent people.
- Overdose may produce severe respiratory depression and coma.
- The main goal of treatment is to restore and maintain adequate respiratory function.
- Managed by inserting an endotracheal tube and starting mechanical ventilation or by giving an antagonist, such as naloxone
- Emergency supplies should be readily available in any setting where opioids are used.

Assessing for Therapeutic Effects

The nurse assesses for decreased pain (patient reports) and general feeling of well-being. The nurse ensures that the patient is free from adverse effects. Tolerance (the initial dose of a substance loses its effectiveness over time) occurs with morphine and other opioids (see Chap. 2).

Assessing for Adverse Effects

The nurse should assess for increases in respiratory distress, cardiac rhythm disturbances, and increasing somnolence. The U.S. Food and Drug Administration (FDA) has issued **BLACK BOX WARNINGS** ◆ for all opioid analgesics because of the potentially fatal adverse effects of respiratory depression, coma, and death, as well as the risks of drug abuse and dependence. Assessing for pruritus and urticaria, which may indicate an allergic reaction, is also important. Sweating may be a sign of tolerance and dependence in some patients taking morphine. Box 48.5 presents measures to recognize and manage toxicity. Additionally, Box 48.6 measures to recognize and manage withdrawal from opioids.

Patient Teaching

Box 48.7 presents patient teaching guidelines for morphine sulfate and other opioids.

or crushed. The nurse dilutes and administers IV doses slowly to minimize likelihood of adverse effects.

It is necessary to monitor respiration closely in neonates. The antagonist naloxone should be readily available (see "Opioid Antagonists"). Other guidelines for morphine administration include

- Assess for pain on a regular schedule around the clock (e.g., every 1–2 hours). It is important to use a consistent method for assessing severity, such as a visual analog or numeric scale. If the patient is able to communicate, the nurse asks about the location, severity, and so forth. If the patient is unable to communicate needs for pain relief, as is often the case during critical illnesses, the nurse must evaluate posture, body language, risk factors, and other possible indicators of pain.
- In patients with trauma and other critical illnesses, administer morphine by IV infusion over a prolonged period. Health care providers may also give the drug by transdermal patch or by epidural infusion, depending on the patient's condition. For information about the use of PCA, see Box 48.3.
- As previously stated, the nurse administers morphine by the recommended routes (e.g., PO, IV, epidural) rather than IM injections, because IM injections are painful and frightening for children. For any child receiving parenteral medications, it is essential to assess vital signs and level of consciousness regularly.

Clinical Application 48-1

- Mrs. Hoffman complains of pain in her lower back with an intensity of 7 out of 10. Her vital signs remain stable. To manage her pain, her prescriber has ordered morphine 4 to 8 mg intravenously, every 2 to 4 hours as needed, to be given over 5 minutes, as well as oxycodone 5 mg with acetaminophen 500 mg orally (after 24 hours), every 4 to 6 hours, as needed, not to exceed six doses in 24 hours. When assessing pain in Mrs. Hoffman, what are the major considerations?
- Mrs. Hoffman tells the nurse that she does not want to take morphine because she is afraid that she will become addicted. What is the best response regarding addiction to narcotics?
- What major adverse effects of analgesics should the nurse observe for in Mrs. Hoffman once the morphine is administered?

■ Abstinence from opioids after chronic use produces a withdrawal syndrome characterized by anxiety; restlessness; insomnia; perspiration; pupil dilation; piloerection (goose flesh); anorexia, nausea, and vomiting; diarrhea; elevation of body temperature, respiratory rate, and systolic blood pressure; muscle cramps; and dehydration.

■ Signs and symptoms in neonates include tremor, restlessness, increased muscle tone, screaming, fever, sweating, tachycardia, vomiting, diarrhea, respiratory distress, and possibly seizures.

■ Although all opioids produce similar withdrawal syndromes, the onset, severity, and duration vary.

■ With morphine, symptoms begin within a few hours of the last dose, reach peak intensity in 36 to 72 hours, and subside over 8 to 10 days.

■ With methadone, symptoms begin in 1 to 2 days, peak in about 3 days, and subside over several weeks.

■ Heroin, meperidine, methadone, morphine, oxycodone, and oxymorphone are associated with more severe withdrawal symptoms than other opioids.

■ If an antagonist such as naloxone (Narcan) is given, withdrawal symptoms occur rapidly and are more intense but of shorter duration.

■ Recognition and treatment of early, mild symptoms of withdrawal can prevent progression to severe symptoms.

■ One technique is to give the opioid from which the person is withdrawing, which immediately reverses the signs and symptoms of withdrawal. Then, dosage is gradually reduced over several days.

■ Another technique is to substitute a long-acting opioid (e.g., methadone) for a short acting. Methadone is usually given in an adequate dose to control symptoms, once or twice daily, and then is gradually tapered over 5 to 10 days.

■ In neonates undergoing withdrawal, methadone or paregoric may be used.

NCLEX Success

1. When caring for a patient who is receiving morphine, it is most important that the nurse regularly assess for which of the following?

   A. respiratory depression
   B. hyperactive bowel sounds
   C. frequent urination
   D. insomnia

2. A man has an order for morphine sulfate 2 mg intravenously every 2 hours following a cholecystectomy. The patient has a history of IV drug abuse. He reports that his pain is 7 out of 10 (with 10 being the worst) and requests the morphine every hour. What is the nurse's appropriate response?

   A. to instruct him about possible adverse effects
   B. to tell him that you can administer the drug only every 2 hours
   C. to use distraction techniques to help him forget his pain
   D. to notify the surgeon of his request

Other Drugs in the Class

Several other opioid agonists aside from morphine are available (see Table 48.2). Factors such as patient variability, the type of pain (i.e., acute vs. chronic), length of administration of the previous drug, and drug tolerance may be influential. To calculate the dose of a specific opioid agonist, a prescriber may consult an equianalgesic chart, a conversion table that lists equivalent doses of these pain-relieving drugs. Table 48.3 outlines the equianalgesic dosing of common opioids.

Codeine is an opium alkaloid used for analgesic and antitussive effects. This Schedule II drug produces weaker analgesic and antitussive effects and milder adverse effects than morphine. Compared with other opioid analgesics, codeine is more effective when given orally and is less likely to lead to abuse and dependence. The injected drug is more effective than the oral drug in relieving pain, but onset (15–30 minutes), peak (30–60 minutes), and duration of action (4–6 hours) are about the same. Half-life is about 3 hours. Larger doses are required for analgesic than for antitussive effects. Codeine is often given with acetaminophen for additive analgesic effects.

The cytochrome P450 2D6 (CYP2D6) family of enzymes metabolizes the opioid to morphine, which is responsible for codeine's analgesic effects. As many as 10% of Caucasians, Asians, and African Americans have inadequate amounts or activity of the CYP2D6 enzymes and may therefore receive less pain relief with usual therapeutic doses. Prescribers sometimes order codeine for moderate pain, often with a nonopioid analgesic. A combination of opioid and nonopioid drugs produces additive analgesic effects and may allow smaller doses.

Fentanyl (Duragesic, Sublimaze, others) is a potent opioid agonist that is widely used for preanesthetic medication, postoperative analgesia, and chronic pain that requires an opioid analgesic. Fentanyl is commonly given intravenously and may also be given intramuscularly. In addition, other formulations are suitable for other routes of administration. These formulations are not interchangeable—each must be used appropriately.

Two transdermal formulations of fentanyl are available.

- Ionsys is for short-term treatment of acute postoperative pain in hospitalized adults who require opioid analgesics. An adhesive skin patch, it uses a tiny electric current to deliver a dose of fentanyl through intact skin and into the bloodstream. The patch, which is placed on the patient's upper arm or chest, has a button the patient can press for a preset dose of 40 mcg. *Only* the patient should activate the patch (to avoid overdosing). After removal of the Ionsys patch, serum drug levels decline gradually.

BOX 48.7	**Patient Teaching Guidelines for Opioid Analgesics**

General Considerations

■ For acute episodes of pain that occur at irregular intervals, most opioids may be taken as needed; for acute pain that occurs daily and for chronic pain, the drugs should be taken on a regular schedule, around the clock.

■ When a choice of pain-relieving medication is available, use the least amount of the mildest drug that is likely to be effective in a particular situation.

■ Take only as prescribed. If desired effects are not achieved, report to your health care provider. Do not increase the dose and do not take medication more often than prescribed. Although these principles apply to all medications, they are especially important with opioid analgesics because of potentially serious adverse effects and because analgesics may mask pain for which medical attention is needed.

■ Do not drink alcohol or take other drugs that cause drowsiness (e.g., some antihistamines, sedative-type drugs for nervousness or anxiety, sleeping pills) while taking opioids for pain. Combining drugs with similar effects may lead to excessive sedation and difficulty in breathing.

■ Do not smoke, cook, drive a car, or operate machinery when drowsy or dizzy or when vision is blurred from medication.

■ Sit or lie down at least 30 to 60 minutes after receiving an opioid by injection. Injected drugs may cause dizziness, drowsiness, and falls when walking around. If it is necessary to stand up, ask someone for assistance.

■ If hospitalized, ask a health care provider about methods of pain management. For example, if anticipating surgery, ask how postoperative pain will be managed, how you need to report pain and request pain medication, and so on. It is better to take adequate medication and be able to cough, deep breathe, and walk around than to avoid or minimize pain medication and be unable to perform activities that promote recovery and healing. Do not object to having bed rails up or asking for assistance when receiving a strong narcotic analgesic. These are safety measures to prevent falls or other injuries because these drugs may cause drowsiness, weakness, unsteady gait, and blurred vision.

■ Avoid constipation, a common adverse effect of opioid analgesics. It may be prevented or managed by eating high-fiber foods, such as whole-grain cereals, fruits, and vegetables; drinking 2 to 3 quarts of fluid daily; and being as active as tolerated. If you take these medicines for more than a few days, or if you are the caregiver for someone who takes them, ask a health care provider about a bowel program to prevent constipation. A possible regimen is a daily stool softener (e.g., docusate) and a daily or every other day laxative (e.g., bisacodyl), preferably started at the same time as the narcotic. Docusate and bisacodyl are available over the counter.

Self-Administration

■ Take oral opioid analgesics with 6 to 8 ounces of water, with or after food to reduce nausea.

■ Do not crush or chew long-acting tablets (e.g., MS Contin, OxyContin). The tablets are formulated to release the active drug slowly, over several hours. Crushing or chewing causes immediate release of the drug, with a high risk of overdose and adverse effects, and shortens the duration of pain-relieving effects.

■ You may experience these side effects: nausea, loss of appetite (take the drug with food and lie quietly), constipation (notify your health care provider if this is severe; a laxative may help), dizziness, sedation, drowsiness, and impaired visual acuity (avoid driving or performing other tasks requiring alertness, visual acuity).

■ Omit one or more doses if severe adverse effects occur, and report to a health care provider. Also, report a skin rash.

■ Take these drugs exactly as prescribed. Avoid alcohol, antihistamines, sedatives, tranquilizers, and over-the-counter drugs.

■ Do not take any leftover medication for other disorders, and do not let anyone else take your prescription.

TABLE 48.3

Equianalgesic Dosing of Common Opioids

Drug	Intravenous (IV) to Oral	Dose Equianalgesic to 1 mg IV Morphine	Comments
Morphine	1:3	—	Route: IV, subcutaneous, intramuscular, oral, rectal, intrathecal
Oxycodone	—	—	No IV form available in the United States. Oxycodone: morphine 1:1 to 1:1.5
Fentanyl patch (Duragesic)	—	25 mcg	Also available in buccal and oral formulations
Hydromorphone	1:4	0.2 mg	Sustained-release preparation available
Methadone	1:2	Ratio increases as daily morphine dose increases	Use only by experienced prescriber is suggested.

- Duragesic is for treatment of chronic and severe malignant pain. After deposition of active drug in the skin, systemic absorption slowly occurs. Duragesic has a slow onset of action (12–24 hours), but it lasts about 72 hours. When a Duragesic patch is removed, the drug continues to be absorbed from the skin deposits for 24 hours or longer.

With both transdermal formulations, a fast-acting formulation should be available for acute pain. An oral lozenge on a stick (Actiq) and a buccal tablet (Fentora) are approved to treat acute (breakthrough) pain in people who have been receiving opioids and have become opioid-tolerant. Because of a risk of respiratory depression, recommended dosages must not be exceeded with any formulation.

Hydrocodone (Lortab, Vicodin), a Schedule III drug, is similar to codeine in its analgesic and antitussive effects. It is available only in oral combination products for cough and with acetaminophen or ibuprofen for pain. Its half-life is about 4 hours, and its duration of action is 4 to 6 hours. Hydrocodone is metabolized to hydromorphone by the CYP2D6 enzymes.

Hydromorphone (Dilaudid) is a semisynthetic derivative of morphine that has the same actions, uses, contraindications, and adverse effects as morphine. It is more potent on a milligram basis and more effective orally than morphine. Effects occur in 15 to 30 minutes, peak in 30 to 90 minutes, and last 4 to 5 hours. Hydromorphone is metabolized in the liver to inactive metabolites that are excreted through the kidneys.

Meperidine (Demerol) is a synthetic drug similar to morphine in action and adverse effects. After injection, analgesia occurs in 10 to 20 minutes, peaks in 1 hour, and lasts 2 to 4 hours. After an oral dose, about half is metabolized in the liver and never reaches the systemic circulation. Prescribers order meperidine infrequently for therapeutic purposes, mainly because it produces a neurotoxic metabolite (normeperidine). Normeperidine accumulates with chronic use, large doses, or renal failure and produces CNS stimulation characterized by agitation, hallucinations, and seizures. The half-life of normeperidine is 15 to 30 hours, depending on renal function, and the effects of normeperidine are not reversible with opioid antagonist drugs. Meperidine is not recommended for use in older adults.

Methadone (Dolophine) is a synthetic drug similar to morphine but with a longer duration of action. It is usually given orally, and onset and peak of action occur in 30 to 60 minutes. Effects last 4 to 6 hours initially and longer with repeated use. Half-life is 15 to 30 hours, and this also lengthens with repeated use. Prescribers order methadone for severe pain and in the detoxification and maintenance treatment of opiate addicts. In 2006, the FDA issued an alert about serious adverse effects (e.g., death, overdose, and serious cardiac dysrhythmias) reported in patients taking methadone. The FDA recommended that methadone dosage for pain should be carefully selected and titrated and that patients should be taught not to exceed prescribed dosage or frequency of administration.

Oxycodone (Roxicodone, others) is a derivative of codeine used to relieve moderate pain; its pharmacologic actions are similar to those of other opioid analgesics. It is a Schedule II drug of abuse. With oral administration, action starts in 15 to 30 minutes, peaks in 60 minutes, and lasts 4 to 6 hours. Its half-life is unknown. It is metabolized by the CYP2D6 enzymes and excreted through the kidneys.

Oxycodone is an agonist narcotic that is used, alone or in combination with acetaminophen, for the treatment of moderate to severe pain. Several years ago, controlled-release tablets (OxyContin) in 10-, 20-, 40-, and 80-mg sizes became available for extended treatment of such pain (only patients who have developed drug tolerance through long-term use of smaller doses should take the 80-mg tablets). When given every 12 hours, the tablets relieve pain around the clock. These effects are advantageous to patients with terminal cancer or other chronic pain conditions. However, OxyContin soon became a popular drug of abuse, leading to many deaths and much criminal activity. Most deaths have resulted from inappropriate use (i.e., not legally prescribed for the user) by chewing, crushing, and snorting through the nose, or crushing and injecting the drug. Chewing or crushing destroys the long-acting feature and constitutes an overdose. Subsequently, the manufacturer and the FDA have issued precautions for prescribing OxyContin and warnings not to crush the product. In addition, the FDA has approved a new formula that is designed to prevent the tables from being chewed or crushed; it is hoped that this will help prevent abuse of the drug.

Oxymorphone (Numorphan, Opana) is a derivative of morphine with actions, uses, and adverse effects similar to those of morphine. Formerly available as a solution for injection and as a rectal suppository, prescribers ordered it infrequently. In 2006, the FDA approved oral tablets (immediate-release and extended-release Opana).

Tramadol (Ultram) is an oral, synthetic, centrally active analgesic for moderate to severe pain. It is effective and well tolerated in older adults and in people with acute or chronic pain, back pain, fibromyalgia, osteoarthritis, and neuropathic pain. Because it has a low potential for producing tolerance and abuse, it may be used long term for the management of chronic pain. It is not chemically related to opioids and is not a controlled drug. Its mechanism of action includes binding to mu opioid receptors and inhibiting reuptake of norepinephrine and serotonin in the brain, actions that interfere with transmission of pain signals. Analgesia occurs within 1 hour of administration and peaks in 2 to 3 hours with immediate-release tablets. Tramadol causes significantly less respiratory depression than morphine but may cause other morphine-like adverse effects (e.g., drowsiness, nausea, constipation, orthostatic hypotension).

Tramadol is well absorbed after oral administration, even if taken with food. It is minimally bound to plasma proteins, and its half-life is 6 to 7 hours. The CYP3A4 and CYP2D6 enzymes metabolize the drug, and it forms an active metabolite. About 30% of a dose is excreted unchanged in the urine, and 60% is excreted as metabolites. Dosage reduction in people with renal or hepatic impairment is necessary. Tramadol is available in oral immediate-release tablets alone and in combination with acetaminophen (Ultracet) as well as an extended-release tablet (Ultram ER) that can be given once daily.

Opioid Agonists/Antagonists

Opioid agonists/antagonists act on the same pain receptors in the CNS as morphine and other opiates, resulting in interference with pain transmission and/or pain sensation. These agents have agonist activity at some receptors and antagonist activity at others. Because of their agonist activity, they are potent analgesics

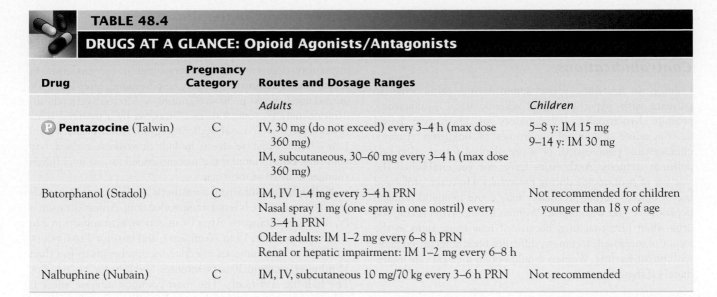

TABLE 48.4
DRUGS AT A GLANCE: Opioid Agonists/Antagonists

Drug	Pregnancy Category	Routes and Dosage Ranges	
		Adults	Children
℗ **Pentazocine** (Talwin)	C	IV, 30 mg (do not exceed) every 3–4 h (max dose 360 mg) IM, subcutaneous, 30–60 mg every 3–4 h (max dose 360 mg)	5–8 y: IM 15 mg 9–14 y: IM 30 mg
Butorphanol (Stadol)	C	IM, IV 1–4 mg every 3–4 h PRN Nasal spray 1 mg (one spray in one nostril) every 3–4 h PRN Older adults: IM 1–2 mg every 6–8 h PRN Renal or hepatic impairment: IM 1–2 mg every 6–8 h	Not recommended for children younger than 18 y of age
Nalbuphine (Nubain)	C	IM, IV, subcutaneous 10 mg/70 kg every 3–6 h PRN	Not recommended

with a lower abuse potential than pure agonists. However, they are considered second-line drugs for treatment of moderate to severe pain. Because of their antagonist activity, they should not be given to people who have been receiving analgesics, and they may produce withdrawal symptoms in people with dependence. ℗ **Pentazocine** (Talwin) is the prototype drug of this class.

Pharmacokinetics

Pentazocine is well absorbed from the GI tract. After oral administration, onset of significant analgesia usually occurs in 15 to 30 minutes, and the duration of action is usually 3 hours or longer. Concentrations in plasma coincide closely with the onset, duration, and intensity of analgesia. One study found that the time to mean peak concentration in 24 normal subjects was 1.7 hours (range, 0.5–4 hours) after oral administration and that the mean plasma elimination half-life was 3.6 hours (range, 1.5–10 hours). Pentazocine is metabolized in the liver and excreted primarily in the urine. The products of the oxidation of the terminal methyl groups and glucuronide conjugates are excreted by the kidney. Elimination of approximately 60% of the total dose occurs within 24 hours. Pentazocine crosses the placenta, and it also enters the breast milk.

Action

Pentazocine, like morphine, has sedative effect. It is a synthetic analgesic with potency that is one third of morphine. Large doses increase blood pressure and heart rate. It weakly antagonizes the analgesic effects of morphine and meperidine. In addition, it produces incomplete reversal of cardiovascular, respiratory, and behavioral depression induced by morphine and meperidine.

Use

Pentazocine (Talwin) is used to treat moderate to severe pain. Pentazocine (Talwin NX; a Talwin and naloxone combination) has been shown to be beneficial in managing chronic pain. It is also used before, during, and after surgery

for short-term sedating effects. (For more information on naloxone, see "Opioid Antagonists.") Table 48.4 presents dosage information for pentazocine and the other opioid agonists/antagonists.

Use in Children

The safety of pentazocine has not been established in children younger than 12 years of age. When used in children, pentazocine should be prescribed by weight and in lower dosage.

Use in Older Adults

Cautious use of pentazocine is warranted in older adults because it may lead to increased sedation, respiratory depression, and hepatic failure. It is necessary to begin with low doses.

Use in Patients With Hepatic Impairment

Extensive liver disease, with decreased metabolism, may predispose the patient to accentuated adverse effects. Although laboratory tests have not indicated that pentazocine causes or increases renal or hepatic impairment, caution is important when administering pentazocine to patients with such impairment.

Use in Patients With Renal Impairment

Similarly, caution is necessary in patients with renal impairment. It is important to use the lowest dose possible.

Adverse Effects

The adverse effects of pentazocine are similar to those of morphine (confusion, respiratory depression, and risk of dependence), but pentazocine may be more likely to cause hallucinations. The cardiovascular effects it may produce, which include increased blood pressure and systemic vascular resistance, make it unsuitable for use in myocardial infarction.

Unlike morphine, the respiratory depressant action of pentazocine is subject to a **ceiling effect**; this causes no further effect (in this case respiratory depression) above a particular dosage level. The drug can be used as an analgesic for dental extractions except in patients dependent on opioid agonists.

Contraindications

Caution is necessary when administering pentazocine to patients with hypothyroidism, adrenocortical insufficiency, prostate hypertrophy, inflammatory or obstructive bowel disease, acute abdominal syndromes of unknown etiology, cholecystitis, pancreatitis, or acute alcohol intoxication and delirium tremens. Authorities have not yet established the safe use of pentazocine during pregnancy. However, prolonged use of opioids during pregnancy may cause neonatal physical dependence and withdrawal. Women should avoid taking the drug when breast-feeding, because it may cause signs in the infant of increased sleepiness, difficulty breathing, or problems with breast-feeding. Women should obtain medical care immediately if these symptoms arise.

Nursing Implications

Preventing Interactions

The nurse should be aware that alcohol and other CNS depressants add to the sedative effect of pentazocine. Concomitant use with the phenothiazines increases the risk of respiratory depression, hypotension, profound sedation, or coma. Smoking tobacco could increase the metabolic clearance rate of pentazocine, decreasing the clinical effectiveness of a standard dose of pentazocine. Anticholinergics when used concurrently with opioid analgesics may result in increased risk of urinary retention and/or severe constipation, which may lead to paralytic ileus.

Administering the Medication

Administration of pentazocine is by IM and IV injection. Rarely, administration is by subcutaneous injection (lactate). It is essential to give the drug at regular intervals exactly as directed.

Assessing for Therapeutic Effects

The nurse assesses for pain relief. However, tolerance can be a problem, and it may be necessary to adjust the dosage of pentazocine.

Assessing for Adverse Effects

The nurse assesses for respiratory depression, CNS depression, and possible signs of withdrawal in opioid-tolerant patients. The signs of withdrawal from pentazocine include tremors and anxiety. The **BLACK BOX WARNING** ◆ issued for morphine also applies to pentazocine because of its potentially fatal adverse effects of respiratory depression, coma, and death, as well as risks of drug abuse and dependence.

Patient Teaching

The nurse ensures that patients are instructed to notify the prescriber if the pain does not disappear, becomes worse, or changes in location or type. Patients should not stop taking pentazocine abruptly, and they should take care when changing positions quickly or operating equipment that requires mental alertness. Box 48.7 outlines additional patient teaching guidelines.

Other Drugs in the Class

Butorphanol (Stadol) is a synthetic, Schedule IV agonist similar to morphine in analgesic effects and ability to cause respiratory depression. Prescribers order it for moderate to severe pain. Administration may be parenteral; after IM or IV use, analgesia peaks in 30 to 60 minutes. Alternatively, administration may be topical to nasal mucosa by a metered spray (Stadol NS); after nasal application, analgesia peaks within 1 to 2 hours. Adverse effects include drowsiness, nausea, and vomiting. Butorphanol is not recommended for use in children younger than 18 years of age.

Nalbuphine (Nubain) is a synthetic analgesic used for moderate to severe pain. It is not a controlled drug. Administration is IV, IM, or subcutaneous. After IV injection, action starts in 2 to 3 minutes, peaks in 15 to 20 minutes, and lasts for 3 to 6 hours. After IM or subcutaneous injection, action begins in less than 15 minutes, peaks in 30 to 60 minutes, and lasts for 3 to 6 hours. The half-life is 5 hours. The most common adverse effect is sedation; at recommended doses, other effects are minimal.

Opioid Antagonists

An antagonist (antidote) reverses analgesia and the CNS and respiratory depression caused by agonists. However, an opioid antagonist does not relieve the depressant effects of other drugs, such as sedative–hypnotic, antianxiety, and antipsychotic agents. The chief clinical use of an antagonist is to relieve opioid-induced CNS and respiratory depression. The prototype of this class is Ⓟ **naloxone** (Narcan). It is essential that this drug be readily available in all health care settings in which opioids are given.

Pharmacokinetics

Therapeutic effects occur within minutes after IV, IM, or subcutaneous injection and last 1 to 2 hours. Naloxone has a shorter duration of action than opioids, and repeated injections are usually necessary. To combat the effects of a long-acting drug such as methadone, patients may need injections for 2 to 3 days.

Action

Naloxone (antidote) reverses analgesia and the CNS and respiratory depression caused by agonists. It competes with opioids for receptor sites in the brain and thereby prevents binding with receptors or displaces opioids already occupying receptor sites. When opioids cannot bind to receptor sites, they are "neutralized" and cannot exert their effects on body cells.

Use

Naloxone has long been the drug of choice to treat respiratory depression caused by an overdose of opioids. Given intravenously, naloxone begins to reverse CNS and respiratory depression induced by opioids in minutes. Table 48.5 gives dosage information for naloxone.

Use in Children

Cautious use of naloxone is necessary in neonates and children. As usual, the dose is smaller and given according to kilogram weight. The child's renal and hepatic function also affect the response to the medication. The recommended route is IV only, to control absorption.

Use in Patients With Renal Impairment

Use of naloxone in renal impairment requires caution. If it is advised, it is necessary to give small dose. Impaired renal function leads to slower drug excretion and increased risk of accumulation.

Use in Patients With Hepatic Impairment

Similarly, use of naloxone in hepatic impairment requires caution. It is necessary to monitor the patient's liver function closely to prevent toxicity.

Use in Patients With Critical Illness

Critically ill patients who have increased intracranial pressure, seizure disorders, head trauma, or respiratory depression should not receive naloxone. However, people with coma of unknown origin may receive the drug to determine if the cause of the mental status change could result from opioids.

Adverse Effects

Adverse effects of naloxone include tremors, drowsiness, sweating, decreased respirations, hypertension, and nausea and vomiting. Naloxone itself has minimal toxicity.

Contraindications

Contraindications to naloxone include known hypersensitivity to the drug, presence of narcotic abuse, and pregnancy. The drug may precipitate withdrawal, producing tachycardia, hypertension, and violent behavior.

Nursing Implications

Assessing for Therapeutic Effects

The nurse assesses for reversal of opioid effects, including improved respiratory function and decreased sedation.

Assessing for Adverse Effects

The nurse assesses for decreased reparations and elevated blood pressure. With the use of naloxone, the nurse is prepared to repeat the dose. The return of pain is a factor to be considered.

TABLE 48.5
DRUGS AT A GLANCE: Opioid Antagonists

Drug	Pregnancy Category	Routes and Dosage Ranges Adults	Children
Ⓟ **Naloxone** (Narcan)	C	Overdose: IV 0.4–2 mg, repeat every 2–3 min if needed. Give IM or subcutaneous if unable to give IV; also may give same dose via endotracheal tube Postoperative reversal: IV 0.1–0.2 mg every 2–3 min until desired level of reversal is attained	Birth to 5 y or weight <20 kg: 0.1 mg/kg; may repeat every 2–3 min if needed Age over 5 y or weight 20 kg or more: 2 mg/dose; may repeat every 2–3 min if needed
Naltrexone (Depade, ReVia)	C	50 mg every 24 h; alternate dosing can be used with supervised administration.	Not approved by FDA for administration in children

FDA, U.S. Food and Drug Administration.

Other Drugs in the Class

Naltrexone (Depade, ReVia) is an opiate antagonist that acts in the brain to prevent opiate effects (e.g., pain relief, feelings of well-being), making it effective in decreasing the desire to take opiates and in treating alcohol abuse. Professionals commonly use naltrexone as part of a complete treatment program for substance abuse (e.g., compliance monitoring, counseling, support, behavioral contract, lifestyle modification); health care providers administer the medication. The drug decreases the desire to drink alcohol, and the dose is based on the patient's medical condition and response to treatment.

Contraindications to naltrexone include concurrent use of opiates, including methadone. Such use can cause sudden withdrawal symptoms (see Box 48.6). After discontinuing opiates, at least 7 days should pass before a person starts taking naltrexone. To confirm absence of opioids, health care providers should verify self-reporting of opioid abstinence in addicted patients using urine analysis. If opioids are positive or there are signs of opiate withdrawal, a naloxone challenge test (administering small doses of naltrexone and observing for signs of withdrawal) is typically necessary. It is important to assess liver function in patients taking naltrexone, because liver problems may occur.

NCLEX Success

5. **A man is difficult to arouse after IV administration of morphine sulfate. He has a respiratory rate of 7 breaths/min. Which of the following is the priority nursing diagnosis?**

   A. Ineffective tissue perfusion
   B. Activity intolerance
   C. Impaired gas exchange
   D. Chronic pain

6. **For an overdose of morphine sulfate, which drug should the nurse have on hand to counteract an overdose?**

   A. phenytoin (Dilantin)
   B. tramadol (Ultram)
   C. naloxone (Narcan)
   D. atropine sulfate (Atropine)

The Nursing Process

Assessment

- The nurse must assess every patient with regard to pain, initially to determine appropriate interventions and later to determine whether the interventions were effective in preventing or relieving pain. Although the patient is usually the best source of data, other people may be questioned about his or her words and behaviors that indicate pain. This is especially important with young children. During assessment, keep in mind that acute pain may coexist with or be superimposed on chronic pain. Specific assessment data include
  - Location. Determining the location may assist in relieving the pain or identifying its underlying cause.

Ask the patient to indicate where it hurts, if possible, and whether the pain stays in one place or radiates to other parts of the body.
  - Intensity or severity. Because pain is a subjective experience and cannot be objectively measured, assessment of severity is based on the patient's description and the nurse's observations. Various scales have been developed to measure and quantify pain. These include verbal descriptor scales in which the patient is asked to rate pain as mild, moderate, or severe; numeric scales, with 0 representing no pain and 10 representing severe pain; and visual analog scales, in which the patient chooses the location indicating the level of pain on a continuum.
  - Assess pain in relation to time, activities, and other signs and symptoms. Mnemonic devices, such as SOCRATES, may be helpful.
  - Assess for pain on a regular schedule around the clock (e.g., every 1–2 hours). Use a consistent method for assessing severity, such as a pain scale. If the patient is able to communicate, ask about the location, severity, and so forth. If the patient is unable to communicate needs for pain relief, as is often the case during critical illnesses, evaluate posture, body language, risk factors, and other possible indicators of pain.
- Prevent pain when possible. Interventions include being very gentle when performing nursing care to avoid tissue trauma and positioning patients to prevent ischemia, edema, and misalignment. In addition, give analgesics before painful procedures, when indicated.
- When pain occurs, manage it to provide relief and prevent its recurrence. In general, morphine should be given continuously or on a regular schedule of intermittent doses, with supplemental or bolus doses when needed for breakthrough pain. When starting a continuous intravenous (IV) infusion of pain medication, a loading dose should be given to attain therapeutic blood levels quickly.
- For uncontrolled or unexpected pain, reassess and consider alternative causes for the pain.

Nursing Diagnosis

- Acute pain related to tissue damage
- Chronic pain related to potential tissue damage
- Impaired gas exchange related to sedation and decreased mobility
- Risk for injury related to sedation and decreased mobility
- Constipation related to slowed peristalsis
- Deficient knowledge: effects and appropriate use of opioid analgesics
- Noncompliance: drug dependence related to overuse

Planning/Goals

The patient will

- Avoid or be relieved of pain
- Use opioid analgesics appropriately
- Avoid preventable adverse effects
- Be monitored for excessive sedation and respiratory depression
- Be able to communicate and perform other activities of daily living when feasible

Nursing Interventions

Use measures to prevent, relieve, or decrease pain when possible. General measures include those that promote optimal body functioning and those that prevent trauma, inflammation, infection, and other sources of painful stimuli. Specific interventions include the following:

- Encourage pulmonary hygiene techniques (e.g., coughing, deep breathing, ambulation) to promote respiration and prevent pulmonary complications, such as pneumonia and atelectasis.
- Use sterile technique when caring for wounds, urinary catheters, or IV lines.
- Use exercises, ambulation, and position changes to promote circulation and musculoskeletal function.
- Rub or massage the painful area (e.g., knee pain with osteoarthritis) if feasible and helpful. This intervention is thought to stimulate other nerve fibers that block the nerve fibers carrying pain signals from entering the spinal cord.
- Handle any injured tissue gently, to avoid further trauma.
- Prevent bowel or bladder distention.
- Apply heat or cold.
- Use relaxation or distraction techniques.
- Consider using special nursing concerns for children in pain, including the following:
  - Recognize that expressions of pain may differ according to age and developmental level. Infants may cry and have muscular rigidity and thrashing behavior. Preschoolers may behave aggressively or complain verbally of discomfort. Young school-aged children may express pain verbally or behaviorally, often with regression to behaviors used at younger ages.
  - Understand that adolescents may be reluctant to admit they are uncomfortable or need help. With chronic pain, children of all ages tend to withdraw and regress to an earlier stage of development.
  - Acknowledge that like adults, children seem more able to cope with pain when they are informed about what is happening to them and are assisted in developing coping strategies. Age-appropriate doll play, a favorite videotape/DVD, diversionary activities, and other techniques can be used effectively. However, such techniques should be used in conjunction with adequate analgesia, not as a substitute for pain medication.
- Attempt to relieve the pain as soon as possible if a patient is in pain on initial contact. After pain is controlled, plan with the patient to avoid or manage future episodes. If a patient is not in pain initially but anticipates surgery or an uncomfortable diagnostic procedure, plan with the patient ways to minimize and manage discomfort.

Evaluation

- Ask patients about their levels of comfort or relief from pain.
- Observe behaviors that indicate the presence or absence of pain.
- Observe participation and ability to function in usual activities of daily living.
- Observe for presence or absence of sedation and respiratory depression.
- Observe for inappropriate drug-seeking behavior (possibly indicating dependence).

Key Concepts

- Pain is a subjective experience, and patients' self-reporting of pain is considered the gold standard for assessment because as it is the most valid measure of pain.
- It is important to assess all patients for pain. If present, effective pain management, often with a combination of strategies that may include nonpharmacologic treatments, nonanalgesics, analgesics, and adjuvant drugs, is essential.
- Acute pain may be manifested verbally or by behavior that indicates discomfort. Chronic pain may not be manifested by visible signs and is often accompanied by anxiety and depression.
- Failure to properly manage pain is a significant contributor to elevated health care costs and poor postoperative outcome.
- Analgesics react with receptors in the CNS and peripheral tissues to inhibit transmission of pain signals, to reduce the perception of pain, and to reduce the emotional upsets often associated with pain.
- Most opioid analgesics are Schedule II–controlled drugs and may cause serious adverse effects (e.g., respiratory depression, sedation) and physical dependence. As a result, they all have **BLACK BOX WARNINGS ◆** regarding safe and appropriate use.
- Agonist drugs stimulate receptors; agonists/antagonists have agonist activity at some receptors and antagonist activity at others; antagonists reverse or block the effects of agonists.
- Selection, dosage, and route of administration should be individualized according to the patient's condition.

- For most acute and chronic pain, analgesics are more effective if given on a regular schedule, on an around-the-clock basis. When acute pain has subsided or occurs at irregular intervals and when breakthrough pain occurs in patients receiving long-term analgesic therapy for chronic pain, administration of analgesics may occur as needed.

- For patients who require large doses of opioids to relieve their pain, it is often necessary to use additional medications and interventions to manage adverse effects (e.g., nausea, constipation).

- Assess pain using a visual analogue scale, verbal or numerical rating scale, or picture scale. Mnemonic devices may be helpful, such as SOCRATES (Site, Onset, Character, Radiation, Associations, Time course, Exacerbating/Relieving factors, and Severity).

- It is essential that pain-relieving interventions are documented in patients' records.

- The **BLACK BOX WARNING** ◆ issued for morphine also applies to the opioid agonist/antagonist pentazocine because of its potentially fatal adverse effects of respiratory depression, coma, and death, as well as risks of drug abuse and dependence.

Critical Thinking Questions

48-1. Mr. Thompson, an 80-year-old man, is hospitalized and receiving controlled-release morphine sulfate (MS Contin) 30 mg every 8 hours for management of the pain associated with colon cancer. He is receiving an intravenous D_5NS infusion of 100 mL/h. The nurse assessing him one evening assessment has difficulty arousing him. His vital signs are temperature 98.4°F, pulse 104 beats/min, respirations 7 breaths/min, and blood pressure 92/52 mm Hg, with O_2 saturation 89% on room air.

- As the nurse caring for Mr. Thompson, what are the priority interventions at this time?

- Mr. Thompson arouses and is oriented to person, place, and time. He begins complaining of his usual left upper quadrant abdominal pain. His vital signs are temperature 98.4°F, pulse 90 beats/min, respirations 16 breaths/min, blood pressure 114/62 mm Hg, with an O_2 saturation of 96% on 2 L/min nasal cannula. His nurse practitioner is at the bedside and has called the pain management team to reassess his pain control. What additional assessment should be made over the next few hours?

References and Resources

Chou, R., Fanciullo, G. J., Fine, P. G., Adler, J. A., Ballantyne, J. C., Davies, P., et al. (2009). Clinical guidelines for the use of chronic opioid therapy in chronic noncancer pain. *The Journal of Pain, 10*(2), 113–130.

Gottschalk, A., & Smith, D. S. (2001). New concepts in acute pain therapy: Preemptive analgesia. *American Family Physician, 15*(6), 1979–1985.

Induru, R. A., & Lagman, R. L. (2011). Managing cancer pain: Frequently asked questions. *Cleveland Clinic Journal of Medicine, 78*(7), 449–464.

International Association for the Study of Pain (IASP). (2011). Pain: Clinical updates. The classification and treatment of neuropathic pain. Retrieved August 18, 2011, from http://www.iasp-pain.org/AM/AMTemplate. cfm?Section=Home&TEMPLATE=/CM/ContentDisplay. cfm&CONTENTID=11541&SECTION=Home

Karch, A. M. (2012). *2012 Lippincott's nursing drug guide.* Philadelphia, PA: Lippincott Williams & Wilkins.

Nalamachu, S. R., Narayana, A., & Janka, L. (2011). Long-term dosing, safety, and tolerability of fentanyl buccal tablet in the management of non-cancer-related breakthrough pain in opioid-tolerant patients. *Current Medical Research and Opinion, 27*(4), 751–760.

Nursing 2011 Drug Handbook. (2011). Philadelphia, PA: Lippincott William & Wilkins.

Porth, C. M. (2009). *Pathophysiology: Concepts of altered health status* (8th ed.). Philadelphia, PA: Lippincott Williams & Wilkins.

Up-To-Date. (2011). *Cancer pain management with opioids: Optimizing analgesia.* Lexi-Comp, Inc.

49 Drug Therapy With Local Anesthetics

Clinical Application Case Study

Lexi Scruggs, a 7-year-old girl, was swinging from the monkey bars on the school playground. She lost her grip and fell, cutting her left knee on a piece of glass. At the emergency department, she requires 10 sutures to close the jagged cut. She receives lidocaine (Xylocaine) prior to cleaning and suturing the wound.

KEY TERMS

Bier block anesthesia: regional limb anesthesia provided by local anesthesia and an extremity tourniquet

Epidural anesthesia: injection of an anesthetic into the epidural space

Local anesthetics: agents that produce loss of sensation and motor activity

Local anesthetic systemic toxicity (LAST): systemic absorption of a local anesthetic agent that results in excitation of the CNS

Spinal anesthesia: injection of anesthetic into the cerebrospinal fluid, usually in the lumbar spine

Topical anesthesia: application of a local anesthetic on the skin or mucous membranes

Introduction

This chapter introduces the fundamentals of local anesthesia and the implementation of nursing care during the administration of local anesthesia. The local anesthetic agents are classified as amides and esters. The molecular structure of the amides possess an amide linkage and the esters contains an ester linkage.

Overview of Local Anesthesia

Local anesthetics, given to produce loss of sensation and motor activity, are injected into localized areas of the body. These agents decrease the permeability of the nerve cell membrane to ions, especially sodium. This action reduces the excitability of cell membranes. When the excitability falls, the nerve impulses can no longer be initiated or conducted by the anesthetized nerves. These drugs prevent the cells from responding to pain impulses and sensory stimulation.

Local anesthetic effects diminish as the drug molecules diffuse out of the neurons into the bloodstream. The drugs are then transported to the liver for metabolism to inactive metabolites and eventual excretion in the urine.

There are three common types of local anesthesia.

- **Spinal anesthesia** involves injecting the anesthetic agent into the cerebrospinal fluid, usually in the lumbar spine. The anesthetic blocks sensory impulses at the root of peripheral nerves as they enter the spinal cord. Spinal anesthesia is especially useful for surgery involving the lower abdomen and legs.
- **Epidural anesthesia** involves injecting the anesthetic into the epidural space. It is used most often in obstetrics during labor and delivery. The epidural route is also used to provide analgesia (often with a combination of a local anesthetic and an opioid) for patients with postoperative or other pain. When the combination is used, it is essential to reduce the dosage of the anesthetic and the opioid to avoid respiratory depression and other adverse effects.
- **Topical anesthesia** involves application of a local anesthetic to skin and mucous membranes. The anesthetic is usually an ingredient in ointments, solutions, or lotions designed for use at particular sites. For example, preparations are available for use on eyes, ears, nose, oral mucosa, perineum, hemorrhoids, and skin. These preparations are used to relieve pain and itching of dermatoses, sunburn,

minor skin wounds, hemorrhoids, sore throat, and other conditions. The main adverse effect is allergic reactions.

Table 49.1 lists the drugs administered for local anesthesia. The use of topical anesthetics is especially important in children, who are administered local anesthesia before suturing, insertion of an intravenous (IV) line, or vaccination administration. Box 49.1 summarizes the use of topical anesthesia in children.

Amides

Ⓟ **Lidocaine** (Anestacon, Dilocaine, L-Caine, Lidoderm, Lidoject-1, LidoPen, Xylocaine) is the prototype amide local anesthetic. It has a rapid effect, and, when combined with epinephrine, this effect is prolonged.

Pharmacokinetics and Action

The pharmacokinetics of lidocaine depend on the route of administration. The onset of action may be almost immediate, with a peak of 2 to 5 minutes and a duration of 30 to 120 minutes. The anesthetic has an elimination half-life of 96 minutes, and therefore, a single dose should not be repeated during this time frame. It is metabolized in the liver into two active metabolites, and most is excreted in the urine.

Lidocaine diminishes pain by blocking nerve conduction. It decreases the neuronal membrane's permeability to sodium

TABLE 49.1

Drugs Administered for Local Anesthesia

Drug Class	Prototype	Other Drugs in the Class
Amides	Lidocaine (Anestacon, Dilocaine, L-Caine, Lidoderm, Lidoject-1, LidoPen, Xylocaine)	Bupivacaine (Marcaine, Sensorcaine), dibucaine (Nupercainal), mepivacaine (Carbocaine, Polocaine), prilocaine (Citanest), ropivacaine
Esters	Procaine hydrochloride (Novocaine)	Benzocaine (Americaine, Anbesol, Dermoplast, Orajel, Solarcaine), cocaine hydrochloride, tetracaine hydrochloride

BOX 49.1	Topical Anesthesia Used in Children

■ Eutectic mixture of local anesthetics (EMLA): This cream-based mixture of lidocaine and prilocaine is applied to intact skin. The cream penetrates intact skin to provide local anesthesia and decrease pain of vaccinations and venipuncture. The cream is applied at the injection site with an occlusive dressing at least 60 minutes before the vaccination or venipuncture. EMLA should never be applied to abraded skin or mucous membranes.

■ Lidocaine, epinephrine, and tetracaine (LET): This combination of lidocaine (4%), epinephrine (0.1%), and tetracaine (0.5%) is an aqueous solution or gel that blocks the sensory and motor nerves. It inhibits axonal sodium channels, thus blocking conduction of action potential. Epinephrine causes local vasoconstriction, whereas lidocaine and tetracaine produce numbness and weakness. It is used for laceration repair.

■ Needle-free lidocaine delivery: Lidocaine is administered by compressed gas. It reduces pain at the site of venipunctures or intravenous line insertion.

■ Liposomal lidocaine (LMX 4 or LMX 5): This solution contains lidocaine encapsulated in liposomes. It is applied to intact skin with the use of an occlusive dressing.

- 4% solution: administered through a nebulizer and inhaled into the lungs to produce anesthesia for a diagnostic procedure, such as a bronchoscopy.

Table 49.2 gives route and dosage information for lidocaine and other amide local anesthetics.

Adverse Effects

Local anesthetic systemic toxicity (LAST) is the most severe and life-threatening effect associated with the use of lidocaine or any local anesthetic. LAST occurs when the local anesthetic is absorbed systemically, resulting in extreme central nervous system (CNS) excitation followed by cardiovascular excitation and cardiovascular collapse. Initial symptoms may include analgesia, circumoral numbness, metallic taste, tinnitus or auditory changes, and agitation. These may progress to seizure activity and then lead to symptoms of CNS depression, including coma, respiratory arrest, and cardiovascular depression.

Contraindications

A known hypersensitivity or allergic reaction to an amide local anesthetic rules out the use of lidocaine in any form. Any patient may experience hypersensitivity reactions to any local anesthetic. If lidocaine is combined with sulfites, the patient may develop a

ions. This action then inhibits the depolarization and blocks nerve conduction.

Use

Clinicians use lidocaine in its various forms to obtain local anesthesia. Specific uses include

- Topical preparation: used to relieve pain associated with postherpetic neuralgia
- Injectable solution: used for infiltration of the skin or subcutaneous administration prior to the insertion of an IV or central venous catheter, spinal, epidural or a minor emergency procedure such as suturing or a minor surgical procedure.
  - 2% solution: administered intravenously preceding administration of a painful IV medication such as propofol (Diprivan) in the surgical arena. Lidocaine 2% is also used in conjunction with other local anesthetics to achieve epidural anesthesia, appropriate for surgical procedures, treatment of postoperative pain, or management of labor pain. In addition, it can be administered as surface anesthesia for a diagnostic procedure of the upper respiratory tract, such as a medical thoracoscopy.
  - 0.5% to 2% solution: administered for IV regional anesthesia. **Bier block anesthesia** is regional limb anesthesia produced by a local anesthetic such as lidocaine and a pneumatic extremity tourniquet. The tourniquet prevents lidocaine and blood flow from the extremity to enter the general circulation.

EVIDENCE-BASED PRACTICE

Successful Resuscitation From Bupivacaine-Induced Cardiovascular Collapse With Intravenous Lipid Emulsion Following Femoral Nerve Block in an Emergency Department

by HARVEY, M., CAVE, G., CHANWAI, G., & NICHOLSON, T.

Emergency Medicine Australia, 2011, 23, 209–214

This article is a case report concerning a 60-year-old woman who sustained an intertrochanteric fracture of the left proximal femur. In the emergency room, she underwent a femoral nerve block. She received a combination of anesthetic agents that primarily contained bupivacaine and epinephrine. Thirty seconds after the clinician removed the needle, she became unresponsive with tonic–clonic seizure activity. She received intravenous (IV) atropine and epinephrine. Eight minutes into the resuscitation, she received metaraminol and one bolus of intralipid over a 2-minute period. The woman's blood pressure rose, and she subsequently stabilized.

IMPLICATIONS FOR NURSING PRACTICE: When administering amide anesthetic agents in the emergency department, it is essential that IV lipid preparations are readily available for the treatment of local anesthetic systemic toxicity (LAST).

TABLE 49.2

DRUGS AT A GLANCE: Amides

Drug	Pregnancy Category	Routes and Dosage Ranges	
		Adults	*Children*
Ⓟ **Lidocaine** (Anestacon, Dilocaine, L-Caine, Lidoderm, Lidoject-1, LidoPen, Xylocaine)	B	Infiltration: 0.5%–1% solution Nerve block: 1%–2% solution Epidural: 1%–2% solution Caudal: 1%–1.5% solution Saddle block: 1.5% with dextrose Topical: 2.5–5 jelly, ointment, cream, solution Max dosage is 4.5 mg/kg/dose, not to exceed 300 mg, do not repeat for 2 h	Same as adults: administer lowest concentrations
Bupivacaine (Marcaine, Sensorcaine)	C	Local anesthesia: 0.25% locally (max dose 175 mg) Caudal block: 15–30 mL of 0.25% or 0.5% Epidural block: 3–5-mL increments, allowing time to detect toxic manifestations Epidural with maximum muscle relaxation: 10–20 mL of 0.75% Peripheral nerve block: 5 mL of 0.025% or 0.5% (max dose 400 mg/d)	Children >12 y: same as adults
Dibucaine (Nupercainal)	Safe during pregnancy	Apply cream or ointment to skin of affected area as needed (max application 1 ounce or 28 g/24 h) Rectal cream, apply in the morning, at night, and after bowel movements	Apply cream or ointment to skin of affected area as needed (max application 1/4 ounce or 7 g/24 h)
Mepivacaine (Carbocaine, Polocaine)	C	Local anesthesia: max dose 400 mg, do not exceed 1000 mg/24 h Infiltration: up to 40 mL of 1% solution (max 400 mg) Therapeutic block pain management: 1–5 mL of 1% solution (max dose 50 mg) Epidural block: 15–30 mL of 1% solution (max 300 mg) or 10–25 mL solution (max 375 mg) or 10–20 mL of 2% solution (max 100 mg)	Max dose 5–6 mg/kg; concentration <2% should be used in children <3 y or <14 kg
Prilocaine (Citanest)	B	Dental anesthesia: 40–80 mg as a 4% solution (max 400 mg)	<10 y, >40 mg as a 4% solution >10 y, same as adult
Ropivacaine	B	Lumbar epidural: 20–30 mL dose of 5% solution or 15–20 mL of 0.75% solution Labor pain management: lumbar epidural initial dose of 10–20 mL of 0.2% solution; continuous infusion dose of 6–14 mL/h of 0.2% solution with incremental injections of 10–15 mL/h of 0.2% solution Postoperative pain management: peripheral nerve block 5–10 mL/h of 0.2% solution Lumbar or thoracic nerve block: 6–14 mL/h of 0.2% solution	

laryngospasm. Other contraindications include severe trauma, sepsis, blood dyscrasias, and cardiac abnormalities, including heart block.

Nursing Implications

Preventing Interactions

Some medications interact with lidocaine, increasing or decreasing its effects (Box 49.2). St. John's wort decreases the serum concentration of the anesthetic.

Administering the Medication

The nurse ensures that the appropriate preparation of lidocaine is administered properly. For topical anesthesia, it is necessary to

- Apply the gel formulation to the skin of the affected area, approximately 1/8 inch thick. The area becomes numb in 20 to 60 minutes.

BOX 49.2   Drug Interactions: Lidocaine

Drugs That Increase the Effects of Lidocaine

■ Antidysrhythmic drugs (amiodarone and dronedarone, beta blockers, mexiletine), barbiturates, darunavir
Increase serum concentration
■ Procainamide
Increases the neurologic and cardiac effects

BOX 49.3   Patient Teaching Guidelines for Lidocaine

■ Report pain.
■ Report tachycardia and anxiety.
■ Do not drink fluids or eat after gargling with viscous lidocaine for at least 60 minutes due to risk of aspiration.
■ Prior to applying lido patch, remove the old patch, cleanse the skin, and apply the new patch to the most painful site.

- Swish the oral solution in the mouth and then spit it out. When pharyngeal anesthesia is needed, the patient gargles and then swallows the medication.
- Apply Lidoderm to the most painful area of the skin. Patients should not expose this preparation to an external heat source such as a heating pad.
- Apply the lido patch (lidocaine and menthol) to the most painful area of the skin after removing the protective film. First remove the old patch and cleanse the skin.
- Use a nebulizer following dilution in normal saline or sterile water.

QSEN Safety Alert

A physician or nurse anesthetist administers the injectable form of lidocaine. It is essential that it not be administered into blood vessels.

Assessing for Therapeutic Effects

The therapeutic effect of lidocaine is dependent on the route of administration, concentration of the medication, vascularization of the site, and the patient's physical condition. The nurse assesses the patient's sense of touch at 2 to 5 minutes after the application of lidocaine to determine if the patient is experiencing numbness at the site. It is also important to ask the patient if he or she senses any pain, pressure, or discomfort. The nurse should ask the patient questions throughout the procedure to determine if feeling is returning to the site.

Assessing for Adverse Effects

The nurse assesses the skin for redness, hives, or rash, indicating a hypersensitivity reaction. It is necessary to assess the respiratory status and lung sounds for signs of bronchospasm related to hypersensitivity. (Respiratory adverse effects are more common when lidocaine is administered by nebulizer.) The nurse assesses the CNS for excitability such as anxiety, tremors, and seizures. Also, he or she assesses the cardiovascular status for tachycardia and hypertension, leading to cardiovascular collapse.

Patient Teaching

Box 49.3 identifies patient teaching guidelines for lidocaine.

Other Drugs in the Class

Bupivacaine (Marcaine, Sensorcaine) is used for local, regional, and spinal anesthesia for diagnostic and therapeutic procedures. Obstetric patients receive the lowest concentrations, and elderly, debilitated, and acutely ill patients receive reduced concentrations. It is important to administer a test dose before the full dosage and ensure that resuscitative equipment is available. Adverse effects include hypersensitivity and LAST. In obstetrics, a clinician infuses bupivacaine epidurally with the opioid analgesic fentanyl. It is important to reduce the dosage of both agents to decrease the risk of respiratory arrest.

Dibucaine (Nupercainal) is local anesthetic administered topically to the affected area to induce pain relief. It is not absorbed systemically; therefore, it is considered safe during pregnancy. It is necessary to assess the area of application for edema, redness, and contact dermatitis.

Mepivacaine (Carbocaine, Polocaine) is used to produce local or regional analgesia. It is also used for local infiltration, peripheral neural, and central neural with epidural and caudal anesthesia. Adverse effects include hypersensitivity and LAST.

NCLEX Success

3. Which of the following medications increases the effectiveness of local anesthetics?
   A. norepinephrine
   B. epinephrine
   C. calcium
   D. phosphorous

4. A patient has been administered lidocaine hydrochloride epidural. Which of the following symptoms indicates the patient is having a serious reaction to the anesthesia?
   A. blood pressure of 130/86 mm Hg
   B. pulse rate of 76 beats/min
   C. crackles in the right lower lobe of the lung
   D. anxiety

Clinical Application 49-1

- How does lidocaine produce numbness in Lexi's knee?
- What assessments does the nurse make to determine whether Lexi is anesthetized so that the wound can be cleaned?

Esters

ⓟ **Procaine hydrochloride** (Novocaine) is the prototype ester local anesthetic. Researchers first synthesized it more than 100 years ago.

Pharmacokinetics

Procaine is absorbed rapidly at the injection site. The onset of action is 2 to 5 minutes, with a duration of 1 hour. The serum half-life is 7 minutes. It is hydrolyzed by plasma pseudocholinesterase in the liver, and 80% of the metabolites are excreted in the urine.

Action and Use

The action of procaine is similar to that of lidocaine. Procaine decreases the influx of sodium into the nerve cell and depresses depolarization to prevent conduction of the nerve impulse. Table 49.3 gives route and dosage information for procaine and other ester local anesthetics.

Adverse Effects and Contraindications

The adverse effects of procaine, as with lidocaine, include LAST and hypersensitivity reactions.

Contraindications include known hypersensitivity to procaine or similar drugs that contain parabens. Other contraindications are sepsis or inflammation, meningitis, syphilis, increased abdominal pressure, and impaired cardiac function.

Nursing Implications

Preventing Interactions

Sulfonamides and antihypertensive drugs may cause hypotension. Also, St. John's wort decreases the serum concentration of procaine.

Assessing for Therapeutic and Adverse Effects

Assessing for the therapeutic and adverse effects of procaine is the same as for lidocaine. The therapeutic effect of procaine is dependent on the route of administration, concentration of the medication, vascularization of the site, and the patient's physical condition. It is necessary to assess the sense of touch and to ask the patient if he or she senses any pain, pressure, or discomfort.

Also, the nurse assesses the skin for redness, hives, or rash, indicating a hypersensitivity reaction. It is necessary to assess the respiratory status and lung sounds for signs of bronchospasm related to hypersensitivity. The nurse assesses the CNS for excitability and the cardiovascular status for tachycardia and hypertension, leading to cardiovascular collapse.

Patient Teaching

Box 49.4 identifies patient teaching guidelines for procaine.

Other Drugs in the Class

Benzocaine (Americaine, Anbesol, Dermoplast, Orajel, Solarcaine) is an ester local anesthetic applied for skin irritation related to minor burns, sunburns, and insect bites. Application of the 5% to 20% topical solution relieves hemorrhoid pain.

TABLE 49.3

DRUGS AT A GLANCE: Esters

Drug	Pregnancy Category	Routes and Dosage Ranges	
		Adults	Children
ⓟ **Procaine hydrochloride** (Novocaine)	C	Spinal anesthesia: 10% solution diluted with normal saline at 1 mL/5 s Infiltration anesthesia/peripheral nerve block: 0.25%–0.5% solution	Check product insert for pediatric dosage
Benzocaine (Americaine, Anbesol, Dermoplast, Orajel, Solarcaine)	C	Topical anesthesia: 1–2 drops of 0.5% solution or 1.25–2.5 cm of ointment in the lower conjunctival fornix or 0.5% solution or ointment to the nose or throat Spinal anesthesia: 1% solution diluted with equal volume of 10% dextrose injected in the subarachnoid space	Check product insert for pediatric dosage
Cocaine hydrochloride	C	1%–10% solution (max single dose 1 mg/kg)	Check product insert for pediatric dosage
Tetracaine hydrochloride	C	Topical anesthesia: 1–2 drops of 0.5% solution or 1/25–2.5 cm of ointment in lower conjunctival fornix or 0.5% solution or ointment to nose or throat Spinal anesthesia: 1% solution diluted with equal amount of 10% dextrose injected in the subarachnoid space	Check product insert for pediatric dosage

<table>
<tr><td>

BOX 49.4   **Patient Teaching Guidelines for Procaine**

■ Following dental procedures, do not eat or drink until numbness disappears.

■ When numbness dissipates following spinal anesthesia, do not ambulate without assistance.

■ Report anxiety, rash, hives, or redness.

</td></tr>
</table>

Use of oral solutions relieves mouth and gum irritation, such as teething pain in infants ≥4 months of age.

Topical cocaine is an anesthetic administered to the ear, nose, or throat to produce adequate anesthesia and vasoconstriction of the mucous membranes. The drug has a rapid onset of action and reaches a peak in 5 minutes. It is metabolized by the liver and excreted in the urine.

Tetracaine is a topical, ophthalmic, and spinal anesthetic that is metabolized in the liver and excreted in the urine. The topical preparation is applied to the nose and throat prior to diagnostic procedures such as rhinolaryngology. Ophthalmic drops are instilled in the eye for ocular procedures. When administering the drops, care is necessary so the eye is not touched with the applicator. Spinal anesthesia is accomplished by the injection of tetracaine in the subarachnoid space. The patient is at risk for cardiac arrest if the medication is administered too rapidly. It is important to have resuscitation equipment available.

NCLEX Success

5. **A child returns to school after a dental procedure requiring anesthesia. He visits the school nurse's office to take his pain medication. What is the most important assessment the nurse should make prior to the administration of the pain medication?**

   A. Assess the prescription for an expiration date.
   B. Assess the child's blood pressure and pulse.
   C. Assess the child's mouth for bleeding.
   D. Assess the child's mouth for numbness.

6. **What is the rationale for withholding food or fluids following the application of a local anesthetic to the mouth or throat?**

   A. It prevents aspiration.
   B. It prevents infection.
   C. It prevents a hypersensitivity reaction.
   D. It enhances pain control.

The Nursing Process

Assessment

* Assess the patient's status in relation to the application and response of the local anesthetic.

* Assess his or her understanding of the administration of the topical, spinal, and epidural anesthesia.
* Interview him or her regarding any past experience with anesthesia, particularly the development of LAST.
* Identify what medications, both prescription and over-the-counter or complementary and alternative therapies, he or she is taking.
* Assess his or her skin integrity.
* If the patient is to receive local anesthesia for treatment of an injury, assess his or her psychosocial response to the injury and administration of local anesthesia.
* If the patient is to receive local anesthesia for a procedure, assess his or her vital signs preprocedure, immediately following the administration of the local anesthetic, throughout the procedure, and postprocedure.

Nursing Diagnoses

* Acute pain related to preoperative illness or surgery
* Anxiety related to anesthesia, surgery, or diagnostic procedure
* Deficient knowledge related to anesthesia and surgery
* Disturbed sensory perception related to anesthesia medications
* Risk for falls related to diminished sensation of the lower extremities
* Risk of aspiration related to consumption of food or fluids with facial and mouth numbness
* Risk for impaired tissue perfusion related to the onset of LAST

Planning/Goals

The patient will

* Experience a reduced level of anxiety in the preprocedure and postprocedure phases
* Understand the benefits and risks of local anesthesia
* Have no adverse effects from local anesthesia
* Understand the expected outcome or limitations of local anesthesia, including the following
  * Postprocedure pain
  * Limited mobility
  * Recovery

Nursing Interventions

The nurse will

* Instruct the patient to report symptoms of redness, hives, or rash
* Instruct the patient to report anxiety
* Provide accurate information to the patient regarding surgery, emergency care, the diagnostic procedure, or during the obstetrical delivery
* Assess the patient's psychosocial status
* Monitor vital signs before, during, and after the local anesthetic has been administered
* Instruct the patient about postanesthesia care

Evaluation

- Be familiar with your institution's practice guidelines and benchmark goals to help direct therapy and evaluate recovery from anesthesia.
- Observe that patient planning/goals are met.
- Assess the effectiveness of perioperative nursing interventions and medication therapy.

Clinical Application 49-2

- What does the nurse teach Lexi's mother about the anesthetic?

Key Concepts

- Local anesthetics are given to produced loss of sensation and motor activity.
- Local anesthetic agents may be topical, spinal, or epidural.
- Lidocaine is classified as an amide local anesthetic.
- Procaine is classified as an ester local anesthetic.
- Local anesthetic systemic toxicity (LAST) is the most severe and life-threatening effect with the administration of any local anesthetic.

Critical Thinking Questions

49-1. The staff nurse in the emergency department is the preceptor of a nursing student. The nursing student has never used eutectic mixture of local anesthetics (EMLA).

- What is EMLA?
- When is EMLA administered?
- What precautions should the nurse take when applying EMLA?

References and Resources

Baldor, R., & Mathies, B. M. (2012). Digital nerve block. *Up-To-Date*. Lexi-Comp, Inc.

Carpenito, L. J. (2013). *Nursing diagnosis application to clinical practice* (14th ed.). Philadelphia, PA: Lippincott Williams & Wilkins.

Donnelly, A. J., Baughman, V. L., Gonzales, J. P., Golembiewski, J., Tomsik, E. A. (2006). *Anesthesiology & critical care drug handbook*. Hudson, OH: Lexi-Comp, Inc.

Halm, M. A. (2008). Effects of local anesthetics on pain with intravenous catheter insertion. *American Journal of Critical Care, 17*, 265–268.

Harvey, M., Cave, G., Chanwai, G., & Nicholson, T. (2011). Successful resuscitation from bupivacaine-induced cardiovascular collapse with intravenous lipid emulsion following femoral nerve block in an emergency department. *Emergency Medicine Australia, 23*, 209–214.

Hsu, D. C. (2012). Topical anesthetics in children. *Up-To-Date*, Lexi-Comp Inc.

Hsu, D. C. (2012). Infiltration of local anesthetics. *Up-To-Date*, Lexi-Comp Inc.

Neal, J. M., Bernards, C. M., Butterworth, J. F., Gregorio, G. D., Drasner, K., Hejtmanek, M. R., et al. (2010). ASRA Practice Advisory on local anesthetic systemic toxicity. *Regional Anesthesia and Pain Medicine, 35*, 152–161.

Ouellette, R., & Joyce, J. A. (2011). *Pharmacology for nurse anesthesiology*. Sudbury, MA: Jones & Bartlett Learning, LLC.

Schatz, M. (2012). Allergic reactions to local anesthetics. *Up-To-Date*. Waltham, MA: Lexi-Comp, Inc.

Stoelting, R. K., & Hillier, S. C. (2006). *Pharmacology & physiology in anesthetic practice* (4th ed.). Philadelphia, PA: Lippincott Williams & Wilkins.

Up-To-Date. (2012). *Bupivacaine: Drug information*. Lexi-Comp Inc.

Up-To-Date. (2012). *Cocaine: Drug information*. Lexi-Comp Inc.

Up-To-Date. (2012). *Chloroprocaine: Pediatric drug information*. Lexi-Comp Inc.

Up-To-Date. (2012). *Dibucaine: Drug information*. Lexi-Comp Inc.

Up-To-Date. (2012). *Lidocaine (systemic): Drug information*. Lexi-Comp Inc.

Up-To-Date. (2012). *Lidocaine (topical): Drug information*. Lexi-Comp Inc.

Up-To-Date. (2012). *Mepivacaine: Drug information*. Lexi-Comp Inc.

Up-To-Date. (2012). *Prilocaine: Drug information*. Lexi-Comp Inc.

Up-To-Date. (2012). *Ropivacaine: Drug information*. Lexi-Comp Inc.

Up-To-Date. (2012). *Tetracaine: Drug information*. Lexi-Comp Inc.

50 Drug Therapy With General Anesthetics

LEARNING OBJECTIVES

After studying this chapter, you should be able to:

1. Define general anesthesia.

2. Describe the three phases of general anesthesia.

3. Describe the fundamental principles of balanced anesthesia.

4. Describe how inhalation anesthetics are delivered and describe how this process is different from intravenous anesthetics.

5. Identify the prototype and describe the action, use, adverse effects, contraindications, and nursing implications for the inhalation and intravenous general anesthetic agents.

6. Identify the prototype and describe the action, use, adverse effects, contraindications, and nursing implications for the neuromuscular blocking agents.

7. Identify the prototype and describe the action, use, adverse effects, contraindications, and nursing implications for the adjuvant medications administered to patients receiving general anesthesia.

8. Implement the nursing process in the care of patients receiving general anesthesia.

Clinical Application Case Study

Harriet Wilberson is a mildly obese 60-year-old woman with chronic cholecystitis and a history of allergic asthma. Despite dietary modification, she continues to have right abdomen pain, nausea, and bloating sensation. Ms. Wilberson believes that her numerous food allergies are the cause of these symptoms. She is scheduled for a laparoscopic cholecystectomy in an ambulatory surgical facility. Because Ms. Wilberson has an anaphylactic penicillin allergy, the surgeon has ordered preoperative intravenous gentamicin and clindamycin. The anesthesia provider has completed a preanesthetic evaluation and plans to administer a general endotracheal anesthetic. You are the nurse assigned to her care.

KEY TERMS

Amnesia: memory loss (of limited duration in anesthesia)

Balanced anesthesia: four elements of general anesthesia (amnesia, analgesia, hypnosis, and muscle relaxation) achieved by a combination of medications to produce a state of physiologic and pharmacologic equilibrium

Emergence: return to consciousness from general anesthesia

Fasciculation: transitory muscle contractions that occur after the administration of a depolarizing muscle relaxant

General anesthesia: medication-induced reversible unconsciousness with loss of protective reflexes

Hypnosis: unconsciousness

Induction: rendering the patient unconscious by using inhalation anesthetics, intravenous anesthetics, or both

Maintenance anesthesia: administering a continuous level of inhalation and/or intravenous anesthetic to sustain general anesthesia until the procedure is complete

Malignant hyperthermia: potentially fatal hypermetabolic response after exposure to volatile inhalation anesthetics or the drug succinylcholine

Minimum alveolar concentration: quantitative measure of the potency of inhalation anesthetics

Monitored anesthesia care: sedation administered by an anesthesia provider

Recurarization: residual weakness after assumed recovery from the effects of nondepolarizing muscle relaxants

Total intravenous anesthesia: a method of general anesthesia that replaces the inhalation agent with an intravenous anesthetic for the induction and maintenance of anesthesia

Introduction

In this chapter, you are introduced to the fundamentals of general anesthesia and the implementation of nursing care during the administration of general anesthesia. The administration of general anesthesia is a complex task that requires the expertise of a certified registered nurse anesthetist (CRNA), anesthesiologist (physician), or both. The CRNA and anesthesiologist may practice independently or as a team. They are physically present and actively providing care during the entire anesthetic process.

The goal of this chapter is to learn the basic aspects of anesthesia and anesthetic medications. With knowledge of anesthesia drug classes and their actions, the nurse is able to recognize adverse consequences and intervene to avoid detrimental outcomes. In some circumstances, complications arising from anesthesia can be immediately life threatening. For this reason, the operating room and postanesthesia care unit (PACU) must be a controlled environment to promote patient safety. The nurse must have an organized differential approach to clinical problems. It is necessary to provide life-saving interventions and then seek the cause of the difficulty. Airway, breathing, circulation, and supplemental oxygen, or ABC+O, is an important approach to all clinical problems. Fortunately, present-day anesthetic medications are generally safe with rapid onset and recovery. Because this chapter is not about medication therapy for a disease process, the content focuses on understanding the medications, adverse effects (or after effects), and nursing care.

Overview of General Anesthesia

General anesthesia is defined as a medication-induced reversible unconsciousness with loss of protective reflexes. There is the misconception that general anesthesia is a deep sleep. It is much deeper and more like a drug-induced coma. Arousal, even to painful stimuli, cannot occur. Therefore, it is possible to perform surgery or other unpleasant therapeutic or diagnostic procedures such as endoscopy or interventional radiology that would be unreasonable or impossible to accomplish in a conscious person.

Clinical Manifestations

The concept of using several drugs to achieve a state of physiologic and pharmacologic equilibrium under general anesthesia is called **balanced anesthesia**. Balanced anesthesia refers to the following four elements of general anesthesia designed to work collectively to produce a superior outcome:

1. **Amnesia**, or memory loss (of limited duration in anesthesia)
2. **Analgesia**, or a reduction or absence of pain
3. **Hypnosis**, or unconsciousness
4. Muscle relaxation, or immobility

Depending on the procedure, the anesthesia provider combines one or more of these elements by selecting appropriate medications. Generally, a major surgical procedure that requires tracheal intubation requires all of these elements to some degree.

Drug Therapy

Selection of anesthesia and adjuvant medications depends on a variety of conditions. This includes the requirements of the procedure, the patient's age and health status, medical conditions, weight, drug allergies, the results of laboratory or diagnostic tests, and the patient's preferences (if relevant). Using this information, the anesthesia provider develops a plan of care that maintains the patients; health and physiologic homeostasis.

The administration of a general anesthetic can be divided into three phases. The first phase is **induction**, which is rendering the patient unconscious by using inhalation anesthetics, intravenous anesthetics, or both. Adult patients usually receive a rapid-acting intravenous anesthetic medication. Pediatric patients more often breathe an inhalation anesthetic through a face mask. Called a mask induction, this allows an anesthesia provider or a nurse to perform the venipuncture for intravenous solutions after the patient is under general anesthesia. Before induction, the patient, whether adult or child, may receive a benzodiazepine that provides rapid anxiolytic and amnestic effects. The induction phase also includes securing and maintaining a patent airway.

The next phase is **maintenance** or **maintenance anesthesia**, which is administering a continuous level of inhalation and/or intravenous anesthetics until the procedure is complete. Adjunctive medications may be used at this time, such as antiemetics (see Chap. 36), opioids (see Chap. 48), and neuromuscular blocking agents.

The concluding phase is **emergence**. As the procedure ends, the general anesthetic medications are stopped, and the patient is permitted to wake up. As the patient emerges from the anesthetic, the anesthesia provider may use medications to reverse the effects of neuromuscular blocking agents. The patient is then transported to the PACU or perhaps the intensive care unit (ICU) for close observation, monitoring of vital signs and neurological status, and additional nursing or medical care.

Five drug classes are used to achieve balanced anesthesia: benzodiazepines, analgesics, inhalation anesthetics, intravenous anesthetics, and neuromuscular blocking agents. Benzodiazepines or inhalation anesthetics are used to achieve amnesia. Opioid or nonopioid medications are used to achieve analgesia. Inhalation or intravenous anesthetics are used to achieve hypnosis. Neuromuscular blocking agents and, to some extent, inhalation anesthetics are used to achieve muscle relaxation. Within each class, every medication has unique properties that determine onset, duration, elimination, and other characteristics. The anesthesia provider can select from several medications in each class to achieve balanced anesthesia. Knowledge of the synergistic, additive, or antagonistic effects of anesthetic medications helps decide the appropriate dose and combination.

Table 50.1 lists the general anesthetics and neuromuscular blocking agents discussed in this chapter.

Inhalation Anesthetics

Inhalation anesthetics are volatile organic liquids administered by inhalation for induction and maintenance of general anesthesia. Volatile means having the ability to evaporate

TABLE 50.1
General Anesthetics and Neuromuscular Blocking Agents

Drug Class	Prototype	Other Drugs in the Class
Inhalation anesthetics	Isoflurane (Forane)	Desflurane (Suprane) Enflurane (Ethrane) Nitrous oxide Sevoflurane (Ultane)
Intravenous anesthetics	Propofol (Diprivan)	Etomidate (Amidate) Fospropofol (Lusedra) Ketamine (Ketalar) Methohexital (Brevital)
Neuromuscular blocking agents	Vecuronium (Norcuron)	Atracurium (Tracrium) Cisatracurium (Nimbex) Pancuronium (Pavulon) Rocuronium (Zemuron) Succinylcholine (Anectine, Quelicin)

readily and release a gas. Today's volatile inhalation anesthetics are halogenated ethers, which contain fluorine. The stability of the fluorine carbon bond helps reduce solubility, decreasing metabolism and organ toxicity. **Ⓟ Isoflurane** (Forane), an extremely physically stable methyl ethyl ether, is the prototype inhalation anesthetic. Although not the first inhalation anesthetic introduced for clinical use, it deserves recognition for its wide acceptance. Its improved potency, low tissue solubility and metabolism, and chemical stability earned isoflurane the gold standard. Currently, it is the most potent inhalation anesthetic available. Isoflurane has a mild pungent or ethereal odor and can irritate the airways when concentration increases. Therefore, it does not lend itself to inhalation mask inductions. However, it makes an excellent maintenance anesthetic after using an intravenous induction medication.

Pharmacokinetics

Inhalation of isoflurane results in its delivery as a gas to the lungs. From there it diffuses rapidly into the arterial vascular system, travels throughout the vascular system, and crosses the blood–brain barrier. As the inhaled concentration of the anesthetic increases or decreases, the depth of anesthesia also changes. Several factors determine the speed of onset, but the desired level of anesthesia can be obtained in just a few minutes. The characteristics of intermediate solubility and high potency of isoflurane allow for easy regulation of the depth of anesthesia, and it is possible to sustain its effect on the brain without significant absorption into blood or body tissues. This means that induction and emergence are rapid.

Metabolism of isoflurane principally occurs in the liver, although some metabolism takes place in the kidney. Approximately 0.2% of the anesthetic undergoes complete metabolism. Therefore, absorption (uptake) and excretion are primarily through the alveoli and involve ventilation of the lungs. At the conclusion of the anesthesia, the patient receives 100% oxygen. This creates a reverse gradient, and the lungs eliminate the anesthetic. Awakening usually takes place within 10 minutes, and the patient is coherent within 15 to 30 minutes.

Action

Isoflurane produces amnesia, skeletal muscle relaxation, and hypnosis. It therefore blocks the perception of pain. Its ability to provide analgesia is unclear. The exact mechanism of action of inhalation anesthetics has not been established. However, the drug may amplify the effect of inhibitory neurotransmitter targets such as the gamma-aminobutyric acid (GABA) and glycine receptors. Activation of brain GABA receptors results in a loss of consciousness and amnesia, and the spinal cord glycine receptors cause immobility or absence of response to noxious stimuli. The action of inhalation anesthetics also involves the antagonism of excitatory N-methyl-D-aspartate (NMDA) receptors and possibly other unidentified molecular sites.

Isoflurane produces a dose-dependent change in several organ systems. As the isoflurane concentration increases, the blood pressure decreases and the heart rate may increase.

TABLE 50.2
DRUGS AT A GLANCE: Inhalation Anesthetics

Drug	Pregnancy Category	Routes and Dosage Ranges	
		Adults	Children
℗ Isoflurane (Forane)	C	MAC in 100% O₂, 30–55 years old: 1.15% (range 0.7%–2.5%)	MAC values are generally lower in newborns but higher in infants, and then progressively decreasing with age.
Desflurane (Suprane)	B	MAC in 100% O₂, 30–55 years old: 6% (range 3%–7%)	
Enflurane (Ethrane)	B	MAC in 100% O₂, 30–55 years old: 1.63% (range 1%–3%)	Agents are titrated according to patient response and depth of anesthesia
Nitrous oxide	D or X	MAC in 100% O₂, 30–55 years old: 104% (range up to 70%)	
Sevoflurane (Ultane)	B	MAC in 100% O₂, 30–55 years old: 1.85% (range 1%–3%)	

MAC, minimum alveolar concentration.

The respiratory rate increases, but the tidal volume diminishes. If necessary, this is reversed by the anesthesia provider with assisted ventilation. There is minimal bronchodilation. Once the patient emerges from general anesthesia, the depressant effects normally resolve within 30 minutes. Therefore, residual effects may be observed in the PACU. In addition, as concentration increases, there is progressive skeletal muscle relaxation likely due to the effect on spinal cord glycine receptors. This enhances the action of neuromuscular blocking agents.

Use

Isoflurane is indicated for the induction and maintenance of general anesthesia in people of all ages, in those who are healthy, and in those who are critically ill. It can be used alone to maintain general anesthesia or more commonly in combination with other agents to produce balanced anesthesia. Table 50.2 summarizes the use of the inhalation anesthetic agents.

Use in Patients With Renal Impairment

Isoflurane reduces renal blood flow and urine output. Adequate hydration during the perioperative period maintains normal renal function. Therefore, administration of isoflurane to patients with renal impairment or insufficiency is considered safe.

Use in Patients With Hepatic Impairment

Isoflurane is associated with very mild and brief postoperative hepatic dysfunction. Any disease that impairs liver function such as hepatic cirrhosis may place the patient at risk. The incidence of hepatotoxicity is rare. Therefore, isoflurane can be administered to patients with hepatic disease.

Adverse Effects

Inhalation anesthetics such as isoflurane are associated with cardiovascular and respiratory depression. They can also cause airway irritation and progress to coughing, laryngospasm, or bronchospasm in susceptible patients such as smokers or asthmatics. In addition, inhalation anesthetics are known to cause vomiting, especially after 2 or more hours of exposure.

There is also a very rare possibility of immune-mediated hepatotoxicity that can result in death. Although all halogenated inhalation anesthetics can produce hepatic injury, this phenomenon was usually associated with halothane, which has been discontinued. In the obstetrical patient, all volatile inhalation anesthetics, including isoflurane, decrease the tone of uterine smooth muscle, making it susceptible to bleeding during surgery such as caesarean section. Additionally, an alteration in the thermoregulatory system with or without hypothermia may cause shivering after emergence.

Malignant hyperthermia, a genetic disorder, is a potentially fatal hypermetabolic response after exposure to volatile inhalation anesthetics or to the neuromuscular blocking agent succinylcholine. Several myopathies such as muscular dystrophy have a predisposition to malignant hyperthermia. The presentation of malignant hyperthermia may be highly variable, and the response time may be immediate or delayed. The signs include tachycardia, elevated temperature, body rigidity, mixed metabolic and respiratory acidosis, mottling and sweating, masseter spasm (rigid jaw), hyperkalemia, elevated creatine kinase (CK), myoglobinuria, and renal failure. The treatment consists of intravenous dantrolene sodium (Dantrium) (see Chap. 52), oxygenation and hyperventilation, hydration, and body cooling. Additional medications are necessary to treat the acidosis, hyperkalemia, and dysrhythmias and to prevent renal failure. After recognition, therapy must begin immediately to avoid poor outcome.

Contraindications

If there is an actual or suggestive family history of malignant hyperthermia, or disease processes associated with this serious disease, the anesthesia provider will not use a volatile anesthetic. Patients with a history of hepatic dysfunction after exposure to halogenated inhalation anesthetics or those at risk for developing a sensitivity reaction should not receive isoflurane. If a patient reports that he or she is allergic to general anesthesia, the anesthesia provider will attempt to determine the specific reaction. The avoidance of inhalation anesthetics may be necessary. In patients who have history of severe postoperative nausea and vomiting, the anesthetist may substitute the inhalation anesthetic with a technique called **total intravenous anesthesia** (TIVA). TIVA replaces the inhalation agent with a less emetic and nonmalignant hyperthermia triggering intravenous anesthetic for the induction and maintenance of anesthesia.

QSEN Safety Alert

With the exception of cesarean section, surgery while pregnant would be performed to save life, limb, or eyesight. The benefits of surgery (e.g., to save life, limb, or sight) must outweigh the risks. Therefore, a preoperative pregnancy test is routinely ordered in women of childbearing age. The anesthesia provider designs effective strategies and tailors the anesthetic to avoid the possibility of patient harm and fetal teratogenicity.

The more advanced the pregnancy, the smaller the chance that the medications and inhalation anesthetics affect the unborn child. Authorities generally agree that anesthesia and surgery after the first trimester can be conducted in a safe manner and that the risk of fetal teratogenicity is minimal to nonexistent. Both the nurse and anesthesia provider serve as an advocate and minimize the possibility of harm to the patient and unborn child.

Nursing Implications

Anesthesia providers use inhalation anesthetics widely in their daily practice. The choice of inhalation anesthetic is based on several factors such as the pharmacokinetic profile, preexisting medical conditions, and history of previous reactions.

Preventing Interactions

Isoflurane combined with dopamine, ephedrine, epinephrine, isoproterenol, or norepinephrine may be capable of producing cardiac dysrhythmias. Alcohol and some herbs may increase the effect of isoflurane (Box 50.1).

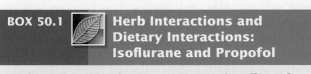

BOX 50.1	Herb Interactions and Dietary Interactions: Isoflurane and Propofol

Herbs and Foods That May Increase the Effect of Isoflurane and Propofol

- Alcohol
- Kava
- St. John's Wort
- Valerian Root

Administering the Medication

The administration of inhalation anesthetics requires the use of an anesthesia machine. These devices vary in features and sophistication. It only takes a very small amount of anesthetic (1%–3%) to produce general anesthesia. The mixture of agents is delivered to the patient's lungs through a plastic breathing circuit that connects to a mask, endotracheal tube, or supraglottic airway device such as the laryngeal mask airway.

The term **minimum alveolar concentration** (MAC) is a quantitative measure of the potency of an anesthetic. It is the concentration of anesthetic necessary to suppress a response to pain in 50% of patients who receive a noxious stimulus such as a surgical incision. The MAC values vary with the age of the patient. Furthermore, MAC values are additive. With the addition of other medications such as opioids, intravenous anesthetics, or nitrous oxide, the MAC values decrease. For example, the MAC of isoflurane is 1.15% in adults when it is administered alone. However, when in combination with 70% nitrous oxide, the MAC of isoflurane decreases to 0.5%.

Assessing for Therapeutic Effects

Assessing the patient for the therapeutic effects of inhalation anesthetics is the responsibility of the anesthesia provider.

Assessing for Adverse Effects

Because inhalation anesthetics may lead to low blood pressure and respiratory depression, it is prudent to provide oxygen and frequently assess the blood pressure and quality of breathing or ventilation early in the postoperative period. Monitoring oxygen saturation as measured by pulse oximetry helps guide therapy. The nurse may treat postoperative shivering with warm blankets or forced-air warming devices. Nausea and vomiting may occur after surgery using isoflurane. Treatment involves antiemetics (see Chap. 36). If there are symptoms suspicious of malignant hyperthermia, it is imperative that the nurse notify the anesthesia provider immediately.

Patient Teaching

Box 50.2 identifies patient teaching guidelines for the inhalation anesthetics, including isoflurane.

Other Drugs in the Class

Several other inhaled anesthetic agents are available. The introduction of desflurane (Suprane) in 1992 and sevoflurane (Ultane) in 1994 represented a new era of completely fluorinated ethers. These inhalation anesthetics further reduce body tissue solubility and allow rapid induction and emergence from anesthesia. They are valuable adjuncts in today's extensive practice of ambulatory surgery.

Desflurane (Suprane) is a completely fluorinated methyl ethyl ether. Of the currently available inhalation anesthetics, it is the least soluble and least potent. These characteristics favor rapid induction and emergence, return of protective airway reflexes, and negligible metabolism. Patients benefit from faster recovery and return of normal cognition. However, desflurane is very pungent, making mask inhalation induction impractical. Moreover, desflurane produces airway irritation and increases the incidence of coughing, breath holding, or

BOX 50.2 **Patient Teaching Guidelines for General Anesthetics**

- Ask your health care provider for information about the administration and effects of the general anesthetic agent(s) you may receive. Feel free to ask questions. Learn about the postoperative/postprocedural recovery phase.
- If you will be receiving an intravenous anesthetics such as propofol, be aware that there may be pain, burning, or stinging when the medication is injected into the intravenous catheter and flows into the vein. (Preinduction narcotics and simultaneous administration of intravenous lidocaine also help relieve the discomfort.)
- Refrain from smoking prior to surgery.
- Discontinue complementary and alternative medicine products, including herbal supplements, for 2 weeks prior to surgery.
- Do not ingest alcohol for 24 hours prior to their scheduled surgery or procedure.
- Ask your health care provider about diagnostic testing to screen for malignant hyperthermia or atypical plasma cholinesterase if you have a family history.

laryngospasm. Unlike other inhalation anesthetics, desflurane may cause mild bronchoconstriction.

Enflurane (Ethrane) is a potent methyl ethyl ether that has a profile similar to isoflurane. It is slightly more soluble, and therefore the induction and emergence is somewhat slower. Unfortunately, enflurane has two limitations. First, it may promote seizures at high concentrations. Second, its metabolism to fluoride carries a risk of nephrotoxicity. Therefore, it is contraindicated in patients with epilepsy or diminished renal function.

Sevoflurane (Ultane) is a completely fluorinated methyl isopropyl ether that has about half the potency of isoflurane. Its solubility is extremely low. Therefore, induction, emergence, and recovery are fast. In addition, sevoflurane is nonpungent and results in the least amount of airway irritation. It provides a pleasant inhalation mask induction in both adults and children without the need of an initial intravenous anesthetic. Furthermore, it produces bronchodilation similar or perhaps greater than isoflurane. These properties make sevoflurane a popular choice for patients with reactive airway disease or chronic obstructive pulmonary disease. In young children, sevoflurane is associated with emergence or postoperative agitation but does not seem to have long-term implications.

In addition to the volatile anesthetics, the inorganic inhalation agent nitrous oxide is commonly used in combination with other anesthetic medications. Also known as laughing gas, it is not a volatile agent like isoflurane because it is a gas at room temperature. Unfortunately, the potency of nitrous oxide is low, and it cannot produce general anesthesia by itself. However, its additive effect will permit a lower concentration or dose of the volatile or intravenous anesthetics. Nitrous oxide produces amnesia, analgesia, and euphoria. Because it has a greater solubility in blood than nitrogen, it diffuses into closed body cavities and expands. This can place undue pressure in the bowels, middle ear, and other spaces created by surgery or disease. As a

result, it is contraindicated in many types of surgeries and preexisting medical conditions. Nitrous oxide is also implicated in exacerbating postoperative nausea and vomiting, possibly due to gas expansion in the bowel.

NCLEX Success

1. The nurse is circulating in the operating room when the anesthesia provider declares a malignant hyperthermia emergency. Which of the following symptoms are indicative of malignant hyperthermia?

   A. muscle rigidity
   B. bradycardia
   C. hypokalemia
   D. increased serum creatinine

2. A 32-year-old woman is admitted to the hospital with right lower quadrant abdominal pain. She has a history of absence seizures. Which of the following inhalation anesthetic agents is contraindicated?

   A. isoflurane
   B. sevoflurane
   C. desflurane
   D. enflurane

Clinical Application 50-1

- The anesthesia provider has decided to use sevoflurane, an inhalation anesthetic, for Ms. Wilberson's cholecystectomy. Why is this anesthetic an appropriate choice?

Intravenous Anesthetics

Intravenous anesthetics render a patient unconscious in a fast and safe manner. Introduced in 1934, the fast-acting barbiturates revolutionized the often slow and difficult procedure of inducing the surgical patient using only an inhalation anesthetic. Ⓟ **Propofol** (Diprivan) is the prototype intravenous anesthetic because of its wide acceptance in the United States since 1986. Propofol is formulated in an oil-in-water emulsion derived from soybean oil, glycerol, and egg lecithin. For that reason, it has the appearance of milk or intravenous lipids. Unlike barbiturates, awakening from propofol is associated with negligible after affects such as lingering sedation, confusion, and nausea. Therefore, propofol is the most widely administered intravenous anesthetic and is used extensively for ambulatory surgery and diagnostic procedures. Fortunately, no intravenous anesthetic triggers malignant hyperthermia.

Pharmacokinetics

Following intravenous administration, propofol provides smooth hypnosis in the time it takes the drug to travel from the injection site to the brain. This occurs in about 30 to 45 seconds. It is chiefly metabolized in the liver to water-soluble inactive metabolites, which are then excreted by the kidney. Elimination of the anesthetic is not altered by chronic hepatic or renal impairment. Propofol, which is very lipid soluble, easily crosses the blood–brain barrier. The cessation of the effect of propofol is dependent on its redistribution away from the central nervous system (CNS). Therefore, because of both extensive redistribution and high metabolic clearance, recovery from anesthesia is rapid, usually within 10 minutes. However, very long administration times, with large dosages, can result in delayed emergence from anesthesia.

Action

Propofol produces amnesia, euphoria, and hypnosis. It therefore blocks the perception of pain. It does not provide analgesia. Propofol causes depression of the CNS by amplifying the inhibitory neurotransmitter GABA. The action of propofol may also involve modulation of excitatory NMDA receptors, glycine receptors, and the endocannabinoid system. Furthermore, propofol has anticonvulsant properties.

Propofol produces a dose-dependent change in several organ systems. This effect is exacerbated in hypovolemia, critically ill, significant cardiac disease, or elderly patients. There are reductions in blood pressure and cardiac output. The tidal volume and respiratory rate decrease and may necessitate assisted ventilation. Unlike inhalation anesthetics, propofol does not alter the actions of neuromuscular blocking agents.

Use

Propofol is indicated for the induction and maintenance of general anesthesia in all people of all ages, including those who are healthy as well as those who are critically ill. It can be used alone to maintain general anesthesia (TIVA) or more commonly combined with other medications to produce a balanced anesthesia. Because of propofol's antiemetic properties, it is frequently used for the induction and maintenance of general anesthesia with patients at high risk for postoperative nausea and vomiting. Propofol can produce bronchodilation, which is therapeutic for patients with asthma and chronic obstructive pulmonary disease. Moreover, propofol suppresses laryngeal reflexes, making it a suitable choice when inserting a supraglottic airway device.

Propofol can be titrated and used in lesser amounts to provide sedation, which is a much less deep state of "sleep" than general anesthesia. When an anesthesia provider administers propofol or similar medications for sedation, it is called **monitored anesthesia care**. During conscious or moderate sedation, the patient can be aroused with stimulation and maintains protective airway reflexes. However, anesthesia providers may provide deep sedation in particularly uncomfortable procedures or minor surgery. Deeply sedated patients are not easily aroused and may partially or entirely lose protective airway reflexes. The level of deep sedation can rapidly change into general anesthesia, necessitating a clinician educated in airway management and the recognition and treatment of anesthetic related complications.

Table 50.3 summarizes the use of the intravenous anesthetics.

Use in Children

Propofol is used for general anesthesia and short-term sedation in infants and children.

Use in Patients With Critical Illness

Propofol infusion syndrome is a rare but sometimes fatal side effect of long-term infusion with high doses usually observed

TABLE 50.3

DRUGS AT A GLANCE: Intravenous Anesthetics

Drug	Pregnancy Category	Routes and Dosage Ranges	
		Adults	*Children*
Ⓟ **Propofol** (Diprivan)	B	Induction: Healthy: 2–2.5 mg/kg IV or 40 mg every 10 s until hypnosis Elderly or debilitated: 1–1.5 mg/kg IV or 20 mg every 10 s until hypnosis Maintenance: 50–200 mcg/kg/min IV Sedation: 10 mg IV PRN titrated to effect or 25–75 mcg/kg/min IV	Induction: Healthy: 2.5–3.5 mg/kg Debilitated: lower dose Maintenance: 125–300 mcg/kg/min IV
Etomidate (Amidate)	C	Induction: 0.2–0.6 mg/kg IV, average dose 0.3 mg/kg IV	Induction: 0.2–0.4 mg/kg IV (>10 y of age)
Fospropofol (Lusedra)	B	Initial dose 6.5 mg/kg IV, supplemental dose 1.6 mg/kg every 4 or more minutes PRN	Not recommended in children
Ketamine (Ketalar)	C	Induction: 1–2 mg/kg IV Maintenance Infusion: 10–30 mcg/kg/min Sedation and analgesia: 0.2–0.5 mg/kg IV PRN	Induction: 0.5–3 mg/kg IV; 5–10 mg/kg IM Maintenance infusion: 0.5–1 mg/kg IV every 15–30 min PRN
Methohexital (Brevital)	B	Induction: 1–2 mg/kg IV Sedation: 5–30 mg IV PRN titrated to effect	Induction: 1–2.5 mg/kg IV

in critically ill ICU patients. Propofol is used to sedate patients on mechanical ventilation. The syndrome affects both children and adults and is characterized by metabolic acidosis, rhabdomyolysis, dysrhythmias, and multiorgan failure. Along with other indicators, monitoring for elevations in lactic acidosis, CK levels, and triglyceride levels help avoid this situation.

Adverse Effects

The rapid intravenous administration of propofol can be unpleasant because of the emulsion formula. On injection, pain, burning, or stinging at the intravenous site may occur. Occasionally, hiccups and myoclonic movements are observed during induction with propofol.

Contraindications

The anesthesia provider should exercise caution in patients with disorders of lipid metabolism and pancreatitis. Patients who are allergic to soybean or soy products, or eggs or egg products, should not receive propofol. Generic formulations of propofol may contain the preservative sodium metabisulfite or benzyl alcohol, whereas the trade preparation Diprivan contains disodium edetate. Metabisulfite can cause bronchoconstriction and wheezing in susceptible patients. Therefore, the anesthetic provider must exercise discretion in choice of propofol formulation in patients with a history of reactive airway disease or an allergy to sulfites.

Nursing Implications

Similar to inhalation anesthetics, propofol is widely used in daily practice. The choice of propofol is based on several factors such as the pharmacokinetic profile, preexisting medical conditions, and allergies.

Preventing Interactions

The same foods and herbs that interact with isoflurane may also increase the effect of propofol (see Box 50.1).

Administering the Medication

An anesthesia provider administers anesthesia or sedation with propofol. It may be administered in the ICU, where the nurse managing the patient must be skilled in the care of critically ill patients and educated in advanced life support to include airway management. Propofol is an intravenous drug that is either injected manually or attached to an electronic syringe pump to provide a precisely controlled administration. Electronic pumps are especially useful for maintenance anesthesia or sedation.

The administration of propofol should be individualized according to concomitant anesthetic medications and comorbidities. It should be titrated to the desired effect while maintaining cardiovascular stability. Age-appropriate doses are necessary. The handling of propofol requires aseptic technique because the emulsion-based formulation favors the growth of pathogens.

Assessing for Adverse Effects

When caring for a patient who received propofol, the hypnosis or sedation dissipates quickly. Adverse effects are few.

Patient Teaching

Box 50.2 identifies patient teaching guidelines for intravenous anesthetics, including propofol.

Other Drugs in the Class

Other intravenous anesthetics are useful. Etomidate (Amidate) is a short-acting anesthetic that appears to promote cardiovascular stability, even in critically ill patients. As an imidazole-containing compound, it is structurally dissimilar to the other intravenous anesthetics. Like propofol, etomidate amplifies the inhibitory neurotransmitter GABA and results in quick patient recovery because of its redistribution to other tissues. However, etomidate suppresses steroid synthesis, leading to short-term adrenocortical suppression. Symptoms may include weakness and hypotension. Also, when compared with other intravenous anesthetics, etomidate causes more postoperative nausea and vomiting.

Fospropofol (Lusedra) is a water-soluble prodrug of propofol that received U.S. Food and Drug Administration (FDA) approval in 2008. An intravenous sedative-hypnotic agent, it is used for procedures such as endoscopy or interventional radiology. After injection, fospropofol is metabolized in the liver by the enzyme alkaline phosphatase to the active drug propofol. Because this prodrug is soluble in water, there is no pain on injection. However, the onset of fospropofol is delayed by approximately 8 minutes because of the liver metabolism. Many patients report a transient burning or tingling sensation in the perineal region after the initial injection.

Ketamine is a dissociative anesthetic, which means that it produces a trance-like state or detached feeling. It causes hypnosis, amnesia, and potent analgesia. Opioid-sparing, it does not rely on opioid receptors. Because of these unique properties, ketamine can be used as a sedative or total anesthetic. Ketamine has sympathomimetic effects and is commonly used in the care of critically ill patients because it maintains blood pressure and heart rate as long as catecholamine reserves are present. The anesthetic has a versatile profile, and its administration may be intravenous, intramuscular, oral, or nasal. When carefully titrated, ketamine preserves airway reflexes and adequate ventilation. It is also an excellent bronchodilator. Because ketamine increases salivation, prior administration of glycopyrrolate is recommended.

The FDA has issued a **BLACK BOX WARNING** ◆ for ketamine. A phencyclidine derivative, it can produce emergence delirium, hallucinations, and unpleasant dreams. Symptoms of this effect may include confusion, agitation, and nystagmus. Psychological effects can last up to 24 hours. Reducing adverse effects involves using the lowest necessary doses and premedicating with benzodiazepines. With the exception of required nursing care and vital signs, the nurse minimizes stimulation and permits the patient to recover in a calm, quiet environment with gentle reorientation. Monitoring to ensure a complete recovery from anesthesia is essential. The anesthesia provider may have to treat severe reactions. A responsible adult should accompany the patient home.

Methohexital sodium (Brevital) and sodium thiopental (Pentothal) are both ultrashort-acting barbiturates. Although they were predominantly used to induce anesthesia before the introduction of propofol, they may be used to induce rapid anesthesia, which is then maintained with an inhaled anesthetic. Both anesthetics depress the cardiovascular and respiratory system. Methohexital is more potent and has a faster recovery period than thiopental. Patients with porphyria should not receive barbiturates. Barbiturates are highly alkaline and cause venous irritation. Venous infiltration results in local tissue damage. Incompatibility with other medications results in precipitation, so it is necessary to flush the intravenous line before and after injecting barbiturates. Methohexital does not raise the seizure threshold. Therefore, it is the drug of choice when providing short-term anesthesia prior to electroconvulsive therapy.

The FDA has issued a **BLACK BOX WARNING ◆** for methohexital. Appropriately educated clinicians should be available to continuously monitor the patient and provide age-specific resuscitative measures if necessary. The use of deep sedation requires that clinician be dedicated to patient monitoring and care and not be participating in the surgery or procedure.

Clinical Application 50-2

- Ms. Wilberson stated in the nursing interview that she has a history of food allergies. Before administration of the anesthetic, the nurse and anesthesia provider need to assess for which food allergies.

NCLEX Success

3. A patient is admitted to the diagnostic procedure center for a routine colonoscopy. Propofol is the drug of choice for sedation. Which of the following food allergies should the nurse report to the anesthesia provider?

   A. eggs
   B. peanuts
   C. shrimp
   D. strawberries

4. What is the rationale for the administration of propofol?

   A. It has fewer lingering sedative effects.
   B. It can be administered without risk.
   C. It slowly crosses the blood–brain barrier.
   D. There is less infusion pain with administration.

5. A seriously ill pediatric patient has been admitted to the ICU. The patient is intubated, and propofol is used for long-term sedation so the patient does not "fight" the ventilator. Which of the following laboratory values should be monitored?

   A. complete blood count
   B. alkaline phosphatase
   C. creatine kinase
   D. luteinizing hormone

6. A 30-year-old woman suffering from postpartum depression is scheduled to receive electroconvulsant therapy. Which of the following anesthetic agents will most likely be administered?

   A. methotrexate sodium
   B. methohexital sodium
   C. methocarbamol (Robaxin)
   D. methimazole (Tapazole)

Neuromuscular Blocking Agents

Modern neuromuscular blocking agents, or muscle relaxants, are divided into two classes, the depolarizing and nondepolarizing muscle relaxants. ℗ **Vecuronium** (Norcuron), a nondepolarizing aminosteroid compound, is the prototype. This widely accepted agent has been in extensive use since the early 1980s. There are several nondepolarizing muscle relaxants. Succinylcholine is the only depolarizing agent used in the United States. Each agent has unique characteristics (see Other Drugs in the Class), and the anesthesia provider makes the appropriate choice based on the health history of the patient as well as the length and type of procedure.

Pharmacokinetics

Maximum neuromuscular blockade with vecuronium occurs within 3 to 5 minutes, and the duration of action is 25 to 40 minutes. The onset and duration are dose dependent. For example, larger doses result in faster onset and longer duration. The cessation of effect is dependent on the redistribution of the medication away from the neuromuscular junction. Vecuronium has an extensive hepatic uptake and metabolism, which accounts for a rapid decline in plasma concentration. Because of its lipid solubility, about 40% of the vecuronium is excreted in the bile. Hepatic metabolites and unchanged vecuronium are excreted in the urine. Because of the distribution to peripheral compartments, large and repeated dosing can result in accumulation of vecuronium and active metabolites.

Action

Vecuronium acts by temporarily suspending nerve impulses at the neuromuscular junction. It can be titrated to produce weakness through complete paralysis. The inhibition of nerve transmission occurs at the postsynaptic nicotinic acetylcholine (ACh) receptors. Because vecuronium is structurally similar to ACh, it binds to the receptors on the muscle and prevents normal function of ACh, producing skeletal muscle paralysis. As vecuronium redistributes and metabolizes, ACh effectively takes over, and normal functioning of skeletal muscle resumes. Vecuronium has no abnormal effects on the cardiovascular system.

Use

The use of vecuronium and other neuromuscular blocking agents is often necessary because inhalation or intravenous anesthetics alone may not produce the skeletal muscle

TABLE 50.4
DRUGS AT A GLANCE: Neuromuscular Blocking Agents

Drug	Pregnancy Category	Routes and Dosage Ranges	
		Adults	*Children*
Ⓟ **Vecuronium** (Norcuron)	C	Intubation: 0.08–0.12 mg/kg IV Rapid sequence induction: 0.2–0.4 mg/kg IV Maintenance: 0.015–0.05 mg/kg IV PRN	Intubation: 0.07–0.1 mg/kg IV Rapid sequence induction: 0.2 mg/kg IV Maintenance: 0.02–0.03 mg/kg IV PRN
Atracurium (Tracrium)	C	Intubation: 0.4–0.6 mg/kg IV Rapid sequence induction: 0.75–1.5 mg/kg IV Maintenance: 0.15–0.25 mg/kg IV PRN	Intubation: 0.3–0.5 mg/kg IV Maintenance: 0.1–0.2 mg/kg IV PRN
Cisatracurium (Nimbex)	B	Intubation: 0.15–0.2 mg/kg IV Rapid sequence induction: 0.4 mg/kg IV Maintenance: 0.03–0.05 mg/kg IV PRN	Intubation; 0.1–0.2 mg/kg IV Maintenance: 0.02–0.04 mg/kg IV PRN
Pancuronium (Pavulon)	C	Intubation: 0.08–0.10 mg/kg IV Rapid sequence induction 0.15–0.2 mg/kg IV Maintenance 0.015–0.06 mg/kg IV PRN	Intubation: 0.1–0.15 mg/kg IV Maintenance 0.02–0.1 mg/kg IV PRN
Rocuronium (Zemuron)	C	Intubation: 0.45–0.8 mg/kg IV Rapid sequence induction: 1–1.2 mg/kg IV Maintenance: 0.1–0.3 mg/kg IV PRN	Intubation: 0.6–1 mg/kg IV Rapid sequence induction: 1.2 mg/kg IV Maintenance: 0.075–0.3 mg/kg IV PRN
Succinylcholine (Anectine, Quelicin)	C	Intubation: 1–1.5 mg/kg IV 2.5–4 mg/kg deep IM (150 mg max)	Intubation: Neonate 2 mg/kg IV Infant 2–3 mg/kg IV Child 1–1.5 mg/kg IV Child 4 mg/kg IM

relaxation a surgeon needs when performing an operation. Muscles may need to be relaxed, so that proper exposure occurs. Also, absolutely no movement is essential for delicate repairs. In addition, neuromuscular blocking agents facilitate easy tracheal intubation and mechanical ventilation by relaxing the vocal cords, jaw, and associated respiratory muscles.

Table 50.4 summarizes the use of the neuromuscular blocking agents.

Clinical Application 50-3

- During laparoscopic procedures such as Ms. Wilberson's cholecystectomy, the surgeon has long metal instruments inside the body, perhaps next to major blood vessels. The anesthesia provider administers vecuronium during the procedure, in addition to the sevoflurane. What is the purpose of using vecuronium?

Use in Children

Children have a larger volume of distribution than adults. In addition, they have a high clearance rate. Therefore, children younger than 10 years of age may require higher initial doses and more frequent supplementation to maintain sedation. However, infants between the age of 7 weeks and 1 year are more sensitive to vecuronium and take longer to recover.

Use in Older Adults

Cautious use of vecuronium is necessary in elderly patients. An age-related reduction in organ clearance prolongs the effect of the anesthetic.

Use in Patients With Renal Impairment

Some vecuronium is excreted unchanged in the urine. Therefore, when larger doses of vecuronium are administered and the patient has significant renal dysfunction, the clearance is inhibited. This can result in drug accumulation and prolonged muscle paralysis.

Use in Patients With Hepatic Impairment

Because of the extensive hepatic metabolism and biliary excretion of vecuronium, patients with significant hepatic impairment such as cirrhosis or cholestasis can experience slow elimination and prolonged muscle paralysis.

Use in Patients With Critical Illness

Vecuronium or other nondepolarizing neuromuscular blocking agents are administered in critical care situations to enhance the therapeutic effects of mechanical ventilation.

Adverse Effects

Nondepolarizing neuromuscular blocking agents can result in allergic reactions during anesthesia such as anaphylaxis or mild dermatological conditions such as urticaria or erythema.

Contraindications

In the case of a patient who reports a known hypersensitivity or allergy to vecuronium or nondepolarizing neuromuscular blocking agents, the anesthesia provider modifies the anesthetic plan.

Nursing Implications

The maintenance of the patient's airway and respiratory function following the administration of neuromuscular blocking agents such as vecuronium is the most important nursing implication. The anesthetist ensures respiratory function during the period of anesthesia.

Preventing Interactions

Numerous medications interact with vecuronium (Box 50.3).

Administering the Medication

Neuromuscular blocking agents are intravenous drugs that may be injected manually. Or, like propofol, they may be attached to an electronic syringe pump to provide controlled administration.

After administration of vecuronium is complete, it may be necessary to reverse its effects so that the patient can regain baseline skeletal muscle function. The anesthetist uses neostigmine, edrophonium, or pyridostigmine, which inhibit acetylcholinesterase, the enzyme responsible for degrading ACh. This allows an increase in synaptic ACh, which displaces the neuromuscular blocking agent, thus resulting in a regaining muscle movement.

Assessing for Therapeutic Effects

Most often, anesthesia providers use a device called a peripheral nerve stimulator to monitor the level of paralysis. Using this as a guide, the anesthesia provider is better able to select the correct dosing regimen. When administered in the ICU, the

---

BOX 50.3 | **Drug Interactions: Vecuronium**

Drugs That Increase the Effects of Vecuronium

■ Abobotulinumtoxin A, aminoglycosides, calcium channel blockers, cyclosporine, inhalation anesthetics, lincosamide antibiotics, lithium, local anesthetics, magnesium salts, polymyxins, quinidine, spironolactone, vancomycin

Act in a complex way

Drugs That Decrease the Effects of Vecuronium

■ Acetylcholinesterase inhibitors; calcium; chronic use of carbamazepine, fosphenytoin, or phenytoin

Act in a complex way

Drugs That May Increase or Decrease the Effects of Vecuronium Depending on Dose and Comorbidities

■ Corticosteroids, loop diuretics

Act in a complex way

EVIDENCE-BASED PRACTICE

Sugammadex, a Selective Reversal Medication for Preventing Postoperative Residual Neuromuscular Blockade

by ABRISHAMI A, HO J, WONG J, YIN L, & CHUNG F.

Cochrane Database of Systematic Reviews
October 2009, (4), CD007362

Sugammadex is a new medication that specifically reverses the action of rocuronium and vecuronium. A cyclodextrin with a unique mechanism of action, sugammadex encapsulates the steroidal nondepolarizing muscle relaxant that effectively reverses the neuromuscular paralysis. To further explore the efficacy and safety of sugammadex, the investigators conducted a meta-analysis of 18 randomized controlled trials (n = 1321 patients). They concluded that sugammadex is effective and there is no difference in the incidence of side effects when compared with placebo or the acetylcholinesterase inhibitor neostigmine.

IMPLICATIONS FOR NURSING PRACTICE: The acetylcholinesterase inhibitors used for reversal of neuromuscular paralysis have limitations and unpleasant side effects. A major limitation is ineffective reversal and recurarization after admission to the postanesthesia care unit (PACU). Adverse effects include postoperative nausea and vomiting and alternations in hemodynamics. Recurarization can lead to generalized weakness, respiratory compromise, aspiration, and hypoxia, all of which can cause serious harm and delayed recovery. When appropriately dosed at the conclusion of surgery, sugammadex has a rapid onset and is not associated with recurarization or the side effects of traditional acetylcholinesterase inhibitors. Therefore, sugammadex improves patient safety and alleviates the concern of residual paralysis and reversal induced side effects in the PACU. In addition, differential diagnosis is simplified when untoward situations arise. Without the worry of recurarization, the nurse can redirect attention to other aspects of perianesthesia nursing care.

---

nurse may be responsible for monitoring the level of paralysis. Because nondepolarizing neuromuscular blocking agents have no anesthetic or analgesic properties, medication induced hypnosis and amnesia must be provided to ensure patient comfort.

Assessing for Adverse Effects

The actions of nondepolarizing neuromuscular blocking agents such as vecuronium may persist after emergence from anesthesia and manifest in the PACU. This may occur after improper reversal or no reversal. This persistent or return of weakness after assumed recovery from the effects of nonpolarizing neuromuscular blocking agents is known as **recurarization**. Patients at risk include those with liver and kidney disease, acid–base or electrolyte imbalance, hypothermia, critical illness, myopathic disorders, and neuromuscular diseases such as myasthenia gravis or myasthenic (Eaton-Lambert) syndrome. Also, elderly patients or those taking medications that may intensify or prolong the actions of neuromuscular blocking agents are at risk. Recurarization can elevate the risk of upper airway obstruction, aspiration, and hypoventilation with respiratory acidosis and hypoxia. Therefore, it is essential to assess airway, breathing, and circulation. The nurse assesses the quality of respirations by observing the rate and depth. Subtle signs such as difficulty swallowing or double vision may be present, and patients may have a weak and ineffective cough. Difficulties with vocalization and taking a deep breath are possible. The nurse assesses the patient's ability to sustain a head lift for 5 seconds and assesses the strength of the patient's hand grip. If the patient shows any signs or symptoms of respiratory distress, the nurse immediately begins supplemental high-flow oxygen by mask and notifies the anesthesia provider. Reversal medications or supported ventilation are necessary.

Patient Teaching

Box 50.2 identifies patient teaching guidelines for vecuronium.

Clinical Application 50-4

- On admission to the PACU, Ms. Wilberson complains of difficulty breathing in a weak voice. She has trouble lifting her head. What would be the initial nursing actions?
- What aspect of Ms. Wilberson's care and anesthetic provide clues as to the cause of her symptoms?

Other Drugs in the Class

Nondepolarizing Neuromuscular Blocking Agents

Other aminosteroids in addition to vecuronium include the long acting (greater than 60 minutes) pancuronium and the intermediate acting (less than 60 minutes) rocuronium. Pancuronium is useful when prolonged paralysis is indicated. In addition, it has the ability to stimulate the vagus nerve and accelerate the heart rate. However, patients with hepatic and renal insufficiency or significant disease may experience prolonged paralysis. Rocuronium has a rapid onset in high doses and is the drug of choice when succinylcholine is contraindicated.

The isoquinoline derivative intermediate-acting nondepolarizing neuromuscular blocking agents are cisatracurium and atracurium. Cisatracurium, an isomer of atracurium, is three times as potent. Both drugs are useful when anesthetizing patients with compromised renal or hepatic function, because elimination is not dependent on enzymatic, liver, or kidney pathways. Cisatracurium has a longer duration than atracurium. At higher doses, atracurium releases histamine, whereas cisatracurium does not. Histamine can produce hypotension, bronchospasm, tachycardia, and skin flushing.

Depolarizing Neuromuscular Blocking Agent

Succinylcholine (Anectine, Quelicin) is a rapid onset and short duration muscle relaxant administered by intravenous or intramuscular injection. The depolarization caused by succinylcholine results momentary contractions of the muscles called **fasciculation**; the patient's entire body may twitch and move for about 5 to 10 seconds. After the fasciculation, the succinylcholine remains attached to the receptor, and there is muscle paralysis for approximately 5 to 10 minutes. Succinylcholine is metabolized by plasma cholinesterase. There are no reversal medications for succinylcholine.

The primary use for succinylcholine is paralysis for tracheal intubation, especially when it is necessary to quickly protect the airway. When tracheal intubation is combined with cricoid pressure to occlude the esophagus, it is referred to as rapid sequence induction. This type of induction is indicated in emergency procedures when an empty stomach cannot be guaranteed. Succinylcholine is also used to relax the vocal cords and terminate a laryngospasm.

The adverse effects of succinylcholine include bradycardia, hyperkalemia, and postoperative myalgia. Because there is a risk of abrupt hyperkalemia and cardiac arrest, it is important to avoid using succinylcholine in patients with preexisting hyperkalemia, major burns or extensive tissue damage, denervation conditions such as paraplegia, prolonged illness with immobility, stroke, or motor neuron disease. In patients at risk, serum electrolytes with potassium levels help guide therapy. Malignant hyperthermia is also possible with succinylcholine, so it is contraindicated with confirmed or suspicious history of this condition. In addition, it is avoided in disease processes associated with malignant hyperthermia. Finally, two scenarios cause prolonged paralysis after administration of succinylcholine. The first is decreased plasma cholinesterase, which can result from severe illness that may include liver disease and interactions with other medications. The prolonged effect is usually small. The other scenario is the genetic condition called atypical plasma cholinesterase. Paralysis can last from approximately 30 minutes to many hours. Patients remain intubated and are observed in the ICU until the paralysis spontaneously resolves. During this time, they receive a drug to induce hypnosis.

The FDA has issued a **BLACK BOX WARNING ◆** for succinylcholine because of the risk of sudden cardiac arrest from rapid onset rhabdomyolysis and hyperkalemia. (This condition most likely occurs in boys younger than 8 years of age with Duchenne muscular dystrophy.) Because of the possibility of undiagnosed myopathy in children, the use of succinylcholine in this population is reserved for emergency airway control and intubation to prevent aspiration.

NCLEX Success

7. **An anesthesia provider administers vecuronium. What is the expected effect of this drug?**

   A. decrease in anxiety
   B. induction of paralysis
   C. decrease in spasticity
   D. reduction in tachycardia

8. **A surgical patient with which of the following conditions may experience recurarization following the administration of vecuronium?**

   A. hypertension
   B. hyperthyroidism
   C. myasthenia gravis
   D. patient with the diagnosis of Parkinson's disease

9. **A man is admitted to the PACU following surgery, where he received vecuronium. He is unable to raise his head and develops shortness of breath. What is the priority nursing intervention?**

   A. Notify the anesthesia provider.
   B. Administer furosemide.
   C. Apply high flow oxygen.
   D. Intubate the patient.

Adjuvant Medications Used in General Anesthesia

The adjuvant medications are administered during the preoperative, intraoperative, and postoperative phase in support of balanced anesthesia. Table 50.5 summarizes the chief adjuvant medications administered to support balanced anesthesia.

Benzodiazepines

Benzodiazepines are a valuable adjunct to all types of anesthesia. This includes sedation, regional techniques such peripheral nerve blocks, spinal anesthetics, epidural anesthetics, and general anesthesia. Benzodiazepines produce amnesia, anxiolysis, sedation, and have anticonvulsant properties (see Chap. 52). At high doses, benzodiazepines can induce hypnosis. Ⓟ **Midazolam** (Versed), the prototype drug in this class, is a short-acting intravenous medication. Midazolam is the most common medication administered prior to surgery or procedures. Furthermore, when given for procedures that only require sedation, midazolam can be continuously administered to maintain sedation. Because midazolam can be administered in flavored syrup by mouth or intramuscularly, it is a valuable adjunct in pediatric anesthesia.

The FDA has issued a **BLACK BOX WARNING** ◆ for midazolam because of profound respiratory depression that may result in hypoxia, brain damage, or death. Rapid intravenous administration to neonates has resulted in hypotension and seizures. It is essential to titrate midazolam carefully according to age and medical conditions. Following administration of midazolam, continuous monitoring for respiratory depression is required, and if necessary, age specific resuscitative measures should be implemented. Flumazenil (Romazicon) is a benzodiazepine antagonist that reverses the effects of midazolam.

Opioid Analgesics

When pain is anticipated, opioid analgesics are a component of the anesthetic technique. Opioids (see Chap. 48) bind to several classes of opioid receptors in the nervous system and tissues. The prototype intravenous opioid analgesic is Ⓟ **fentanyl** (Sublimaze). A synthetic opioid that is about 100 times more potent than morphine sulfate, fentanyl can be used to supplement sedation, regional techniques, and general anesthesia. Common adverse effects of all opioids are respiratory depression, nausea and vomiting, altered mentation, urinary retention, and itching. Naloxone (Narcan) (see Chap. 48) is an antagonist that reverses the effects of opioids.

The Nursing Process

Assessment

A systematic preoperative interview is conducted prior to the surgery or diagnostic procedure to determine the physical and psychological preparation of the patient. This helps predict the possible implications or interactions with anesthesia. Although the anesthesia provider is responsible for the assessment and treatment of the patient, the care of the patient is a team process. The nurse is a patient advocate and must be cognizant of perianesthesia process and the needs of the anesthesia provider. The assessment must be completed before the administration of any anesthetic medications.

TABLE 50.5

DRUGS AT A GLANCE: Adjuvant Drugs Used in General Anesthesia

		Routes and Dosage Ranges	
Drug	Pregnancy Category	Adults	Children
Ⓟ **Midazolam** (Versed)	D	0.015–0.07 mg/kg IV PRN titrated to effect; usually given in 0.5–1 mg increments	0.25–1 mg/kg PO (15 mg max) 0.08–0.2 mg/kg IM 0.02–0.1 mg/kg IV divided doses
Ⓟ **Fentanyl** (Sublimaze)	C	Balanced anesthesia: 2–8 mcg/kg with 50%–75% of total dose at induction Higher doses may be used for complex surgeries Sedation/analgesia; 25–50 mcg IV PRN titrated to effect	Balanced anesthesia: 1–3 mcg/kg standard range 4–10 mcg/kg higher range for complex surgeries

- **Assess the patient's status in relation to the anesthesia administration and his or her surgical experience preoperatively.**
  - Assess the patient's understanding of the perioperative process.
  - Assess the patient for comorbid conditions that increase the patient's risk related to anesthesia administration.
  - Assess the patient's health and surgical history, including allergies to medications, eggs or soy products, latex, or anesthesia related products.
  - Interview the patient about the surgical experience and administration of anesthetics, including a family or patient history of malignant hyperthermia or atypical plasma cholinesterase.
  - Assess medications, both prescription and over-the-counter or complementary and alternative therapies taken in the last 2 weeks.
  - Assess the time of the last fluid intake prior to surgery.
  - Assess the time of the last meal and its contents.
  - Assess medications taken the day of surgery
- **Implement preoperative assessments.**
  - Assess blood count, chemistry panel, coagulation profile, fasting blood sugar, glycated hemoglobin or HbA1c, electrocardiogram, chest radiation, and pregnancy test (obtained depending on age, sex, and comorbidities)
  - Assess baseline vital signs, level of consciousness, and orientation.
  - Assess psychosocial status.
  - Assess for pain using a pain scale.
- **Assess the patient's response to general anesthesia.**
  - Assess vital signs continuously.
  - Assess physiological response to anesthesia.
- **Implement postanesthesia/postoperative assessment.**
  - Assess airway and respiratory function.
  - Assess vital signs continuously.
  - Assess level of consciousness.
  - Assess pain using a pain scale.
  - Assess for postoperative nausea and vomiting.

Nursing Diagnoses

- Acute pain related to preoperative illness or surgery
- Anxiety related to anesthesia, surgery, or diagnostic procedure
- Deficient knowledge related to anesthesia and surgery
- Disturbed sensory perception related to anesthesia medications
- Decreased cardiac output related to hypovolemia, heart rate and rhythm, or effects of anesthetic medications
- Ineffective breathing pattern related to general anesthesia
- Nausea related to general anesthesia
- Risk for aspiration related to a full stomach
- Risk for bleeding related to surgical intervention
- Risk for unstable blood glucose level related to surgical intervention
- Risk for electrolyte imbalance related to surgery and comorbidity
- Risk for imbalanced body temperature related to hypothermia

Planning/Goals

The patient will

- Understand the benefits and risks of the planned anesthesia, surgery, or diagnostic procedure
- Understand the expected outcome or limitations of the anesthesia, including the following:
  - Predicted postoperative level of pain
  - Predicted severity of postoperative nausea and vomiting
  - Expectations during the surgery or procedure and recovery period
- Adhere to preoperative instructions (a coherent patient may be necessary for selected surgical or diagnostic procedures):
  - Cessation of alcohol, complementary and alternative therapies, and smoking
  - Age-appropriate fasting
  - Essential medications day of surgery
- Experience reduced level of stress and anxiety prior to the surgery or procedure
- Experience partial or complete amnesia while in the surgical suite
- Return to acceptable or baseline physiologic status postoperatively appropriate for extent and complexity of anesthesia and surgery
- Experience control of pain to acceptable level
- Experience control of postoperative nausea and vomiting so as not to cause excessive pain, dehydration, or disrupt the surgical repair
- Have no adverse effects from the anesthesia

Nursing Interventions

The nurse will

- Provide accurate information to the patient about the surgical or diagnostic procedure, the planned anesthetic, and the expected outcomes
- Instruct the patient to report symptoms such as pain, nausea, difficult breathing, weakness, lightheadedness, itching, and chest pain
- Assess the patient's preoperative psychological status
  - Collaborate with family or significant others
  - Use age appropriate teaching, answer questions, and reassurance, which helps reduce stress, anxiety, and fear
    - Simple and truthful conversation reduces the fear of parental separation and the unknown.
    - Behavioral preparation programs, parental presence during the anesthesia induction, or the use of premedication such as midazolam reduce stress.
- Keep the operating room quiet during induction and emergence. Do not manipulate or move the patient during this process
- Be available to assist the anesthesia provider during tracheal intubation and extubation
- Secure the patient to the operating room table and pad to prevent injury
- Monitor vital signs, fluid intake or output, or other responsibilities in coordination with the anesthesia provider
- Do not move or reposition an intubated patient without prior coordination with the anesthesia provider

- Know the location of emergency equipment such as a difficult airway cart, malignant hyperthermia cart, or code cart
- Refrain from inappropriate discussion during surgery. Even during general anesthesia or sedation, a patient may have recall of conversation or events
- Be cognizant that anesthetics have the potential for rapid and profound changes in physiologic stability and that the nurse may be required to assist the anesthesia provider at any time
- Assist the anesthesia provider with the transport from the operating room to the PACU or ICU
  - Continue to evaluate airway patency, breathing, and circulation during transport and on arrival to the PACU or ICU. Supplemental oxygen may be necessary, especially for pediatric and elderly patients.
    - Assess for shortness of breath or hypoventilation
    - Assess for diminished mental status
    - High-risk patients may require additional monitoring during transport
      - Pulse oximetry oxygen saturation
      - Assess for symptomatic changes in blood pressure or pulse
- If you are the accepting perianesthesia nurse, be prepared to receive the detailed report provided by the anesthesia provider. Information includes the anesthetic technique and medications used, time of last narcotic, intake and output, pertinent events during the surgery or procedure, length of anesthetic, stability during procedure, and whether neuromuscular blocking agents were reversed and at what time.

- Provide the accepting perianesthesia nurse with pertinent information obtained in the preoperative interview.
- Develop a customized plan of patient care with the anesthesia provider.
- Ensure a smooth transition of care from the operating room to the PACU or ICU. Ensure that the patient is continually monitored in the PACU or ICU. The patient's medical condition dictates the appropriate methods and acuity of observation and monitoring. During the assessment, the nurse is cognizant of adverse anesthesia medication effects.
  - Pulse oximetry oxygen saturation
  - Ventilation: patent airway, unimpaired breathing pattern
  - Circulation (blood pressure, electrocardiograph, peripheral pulses, skin color)
  - Level of consciousness and motor function
  - Temperature
  - Pain
  - Postoperative nausea and vomiting
  - Emotional comfort
  - Intake and output

Evaluation

- Be familiar with your institution's practice guidelines and benchmark goals to help direct therapy and evaluate recovery from anesthesia.
- Observe that patient planning/goals are met.
- Assess the effectiveness of perioperative nursing interventions and medication therapy.

Key Concepts

- General anesthesia is defined as a medication-induced reversible unconsciousness with loss of protective reflexes, much like a drug-induced coma.
- The administration of anesthesia and monitored anesthesia care requires a CRNA or anesthesiologist educated in advanced airway control and the recognition and treatment of anesthetic-related complications.
- The nurse solves clinical problems in an organized differential approach and temporize life-threatening situations by maintaining airway, breathing, circulation, and providing supplemental oxygen.
- Three phases of general anesthesia are induction or rendering the patient unconscious, maintenance or administering a continuous level of anesthetic, and emergence or stopping general anesthetic medications and allowing the patient to wake up.
- Balanced anesthesia combines several medications to produce amnesia, analgesia, hypnosis, and muscle relaxation, which achieves a state of physiologic and pharmacologic equilibrium while under general anesthesia.
- Volatile inhalation anesthetics are liquid halogenated hydrocarbons whose inhaled vapors produce hypnosis, amnesia, and skeletal muscle relaxation.
- Nitrous oxide is an inorganic inhalation agent in the form of a gas that produces amnesia, analgesia, and euphoria but cannot produce general anesthesia.
- Malignant hyperthermia is a genetic disorder that may trigger a potentially fatal hypermetabolic response after exposure to volatile inhalation anesthetics or succinylcholine.

- Intravenous anesthetics are used to induce hypnosis or sedation in a fasting-acting manner.
- The mishandling of the propofol syringe, vial, or ampoule can result in inadvertent bacterial contamination and elevate the risk of systemic sepsis.
- The FDA has issued a **BLACK BOX WARNING** ◆ for the intravenous anesthetic ketamine. It can produce emergence delirium, hallucinations, and unpleasant dreams. Therefore, special attention is necessary during the administration of the drug in addition to providing a safe and quiet environment during recovery.
- The FDA has also issued a **BLACK BOX WARNING** ◆ for methohexital, another intravenous anesthetic. Appropriately educated clinicians should be available to continuously monitor the patient and provide age-specific resuscitative measures if necessary.
- Neuromuscular blocking agents are divided into two classes according to their mechanism of action: depolarizing and nondepolarizing.
- Neuromuscular blocking agents are used to facilitate endotracheal intubation and mechanical ventilation, relax skeletal muscle to facilitate surgical exposure or repair, and maintain a motion-less surgical field.
- Recurarization is defined as postoperative weakness caused by residual nondepolarizing muscles relaxants which requires prompt recognition and treatment.
- Succinylcholine is a rapid onset and short duration depolarizing neuromuscular blocker that is usually given intravenously for tracheal intubation, especially when it is necessary to quickly protect the airway in rapid sequence induction.
- The FDA has released a **BLACK BOX WARNING** ◆ for succinylcholine because of the risk of sudden cardiac arrest from rapid onset rhabdomyolysis and hyperkalemia.
- The benzodiazepine midazolam produces amnesia, anxiolysis, and sedation, and it is fre-quently administered prior to surgery or a procedure. The FDA has issued a **BLACK BOX WARNING** ◆ for midazolam because of profound respiratory depression that may result in hypoxia, brain damage, or death. Rapid intravenous administration to neonates has resulted in hypotension and seizures.
- Opioids are used to reduce pain during and after surgery or procedures and are selected according to their pharmacokinetic and pharmacodynamic properties.

Critical Thinking Questions

50-1. A 45-year-old woman is having a spinal cord nerve stimulator surgically implanted under monitored anesthesia care. She has a history of complex regional pain syndrome in the lower extremities and takes several opioid analgesics at home to treat the chronic pain. In addition to propofol for hypnosis, the anesthesia provider plans to administer ketamine for analgesia and amnesia.

- Why is ketamine indicated in this procedure?
- What adverse effects may be expected during the procedure?
- What intraoperative nursing interventions can help alleviate the adverse effects?
- What other class of medication would be beneficial?

50-2. An 8-year-old boy with acute appendicitis has been admitted to the surgical suite for emergency appendectomy. Although he was not very hungry, he tried to eat about 4 hours ago; he subsequently vomited. He has no other medical history or allergies. The anesthesia provider has asked the nurse to assist in rapid sequence induction and plans to use succinylcholine to facilitate prompt tracheal intubation.

- What questions about patient and family history are important?
- Is blood laboratory analysis necessary?
- How do health care professionals prevent patient injury during the induction of anesthesia?
- What is a rapid sequence induction?
- How does the nurse assist the anesthesia provider in performing the rapid sequence induction?

References and Resources

American Association of Nurse Anesthetists (AANA). (2011). *Herbal products and your anesthetic: Information you will want to share.* Retrieved from http://www.aana.com/herbalproducts.aspx

Allain, R. M., Alston, T. A., Dunn, P. F., Kwo, J., Levine, W. C., & Rosow, C. E. (Eds.). (2010). *Handbook of clinical anesthesia procedures of the Massachusetts general hospital* (8th ed.). Philadelphia, PA: Lippincott Williams & Wilkins.

American Society of PeriAnesthesia Nurses. (2010). *2010-2012 Perianesthesia nursing standards and practice recommendations.* Cherry Hill, NJ: American Society of PeriAnesthesia Nurses.

Barash, P. G., Cahalan, M. K., Cullen, B. F., Stock, M. C., & Stoelting, R. K. (Eds.). (2009). *Clinical anesthesia* (6th ed.). Philadelphia, PA: Lippincott Williams & Wilkins.

Chaplin, R. L., Jedynak, J., Johonson, D., Heiter, D., Shovelton, L. & Garret, N. (2007). The effects of valerian on the time course of emergence from general anesthesia in Sprague-Dawley rats. *AANA Journal, 75*(6), 431–435.

Fintelmann, V., & Weiss, R. F. (2000). *Herbal medicine* (2nd ed.). New York: Thieme.

Hillier, S. C., & Stoelting, R. K. (2006). *Pharmacology and physiology in anesthesia practice* (4th ed.). Philadelphia, PA: Lippincott Williams & Wilkins.

Karch, A. M. (2012). *2012 Lippincott's nursing drug guide.* Philadelphia, PA: Lippincott Williams & Wilkins.

MHAUS. (2011). *For medical professionals.* Retrieved from http://www.mhaus.org/

Nettina, S. M. (Ed.). (2010). *Lippincott manual of nursing practice* (9th ed.). Philadelphia, PA: Lippincott Williams & Wilkins.

Tietze, K. J. (2010). *Use of neuromuscular blocking medications in critically ill patients.* Up-To-Date. Lexi-Comp, Inc.

Up-To-Date. (2011). *Acetaminophen, aspirin, and caffeine: Drug Information.* Lexi-Comp, Inc.

Up-To-Date. (2011). *Isoflurane: Drug Information.* Lexi-Comp, Inc.

Up-To-Date. (2011). *Methohexital: Drug Information.* Lexi-Comp, Inc.

Up-To-Date. (2011). *Propofol: Drug Information.* Lexi-Comp, Inc.

Up-To-Date. (2011). *Vecuronium: Drug Information.* Lexi-Comp, Inc.

Up-To-Date. (2011). *Vecuronium: Pediatric Drug Information.* Lexi-Comp, Inc.

Zaccheo, M. M., & Bucher, D. H. (2008). *Propofol infusion syndrome: A rare complication with potentially fatal results.* Critical Care Nurse, 28(3), 18–27.

51 Drug Therapy for Migraines and Other Headaches

After studying this chapter, you should be able to:

1. Understand the pathophysiology of migraine headaches.

2. Identify the major manifestations of tension headaches, cluster headaches, migraine headaches, and menstrual migraine headaches.

3. Identify the prototype and describe the action, use, adverse effects, contraindications, and nursing implications for nonsteroidal anti-inflammatory drugs administered as abortive therapy for migraines.

4. Describe the action, use, adverse effects, contraindications, and nursing implications for acetaminophen–aspirin–caffeine combinations administered as abortive therapy for headaches.

5. Identify the prototypes and describe the action, use, adverse effects, contraindications, and nursing implications for ergot alkaloids administered as abortive therapy.

6. Identify the prototypes and describe the action, adverse effects, contraindications, and nursing implications for triptans administered as abortive therapy.

7. Identify the prototype and describe the action, use, adverse effects, contraindications, and nursing implications for estrogen administered for menstrual migraines.

8. Identify the medications used for the prevention of migraine headaches.

9. Describe the action, use, adverse effects, contraindications, and nursing implications for antiemetic drugs used in the treatment of migraine headache.

10. Implement the nursing process of care of patients of all ages who suffer from migraine headaches.

Clinical Application Case Study

Tanya Van Art, an 18-year-old young woman, has experienced headaches since she was 13 years old. She has been experiencing headaches with increased severity in the past year. While at work this past week, she developed a severe headache with nausea and vomiting. She was admitted to the emergency department. On admission, her blood pressure was 180/90 mm Hg and her pain was 10 on a 10-point scale. In the emergency department, she received ketorolac tromethamine 30 mg intravenous (IV). The diagnosis was acute migraine headache.

Introduction

This chapter discusses the various types of headaches, all of which produce pain. However, the pain experienced by patients is different with each type of headache. This chapter also considers the pharmacological treatment of each of these headaches.

Different types of headaches have different symptoms. **Cluster headaches** are recurrent, severe, unilateral orbitotemporal headaches that are associated with histamine reactions. **Tension headaches** are the result of chronic contraction of the scalp muscles and are associated with nervous tension or anxiety. **Migraine headaches** are unilateral pain in the head that may or may not be accompanied by an **aura**. An aura is a subjective sensation that immediately precedes the migraine headache consisting a breeze, odor, or light. **Menstrual migraine headaches** are associated with a drop in circulating estrogen 2 to 3 days prior to the onset of menses.

Overview of Migraine Headaches

Migraine headaches are common disorders. Annually, they affect approximately 20% of women and 8% of men. Migraines demonstrate a familial pattern, and authorities believe that they are inherited as autosomal dominant traits with incomplete penetrance. Migraine headaches with an aura are more common with the genetic inheritance. During childhood, migraine headaches are evenly distributed between boys and girls; however, in adulthood, migraines affect women three times more often than men. Food that precipitate migraine effects include aged cheeses, fermented foods, aspartame, monosodium glutamate, and chocolate (Solomon & Jamieson, 2009).

Pathophysiology

Cluster Headaches

The pathophysiology of cluster headaches is not completely understood. One theory, the major one, states that primary cluster headaches are characterized by hypothalamic activation with secondary activations of the trigeminal autonomic reflex. Another theory states that neurogenic inflammation of the walls of the cavernous sinus obliterates venous outflow, injuring the transverse sympathetic fibers of the intracranial internal carotid artery and its branches (May, 2010).

Tension Headaches

The pathophysiology of tension headaches is multifactorial. A wide variation exists in the experiences of people who suffer from tension headaches, but the current theory of chronic tension headache asserts that a person experiences a sensitization of the dorsal horn neurons related to increased nociceptive inputs from pericranial myofascial tissues. Experts believe that this heightened sensitivity of pain pathways in the central nervous system (CNS) plays a critical role in the pathogenesis. With a decreased pain threshold, the person misinterprets incoming signals as pain. Decreased pain, thermal, and electrical thresholds reported in patients with chronic tension headaches probably represent a central misinterpretation of incoming signals (Taylor, 2008).

Migraine Headaches

Authorities have proposed two theories related to the pathophysiology of migraine headaches. First, at the onset of a migraine, the trigeminal nerve is stimulated, resulting in the release of neuropeptides. This leads to painful neurogenic inflammation in the meningeal vasculature characterized by plasma protein extravasation, vasodilation, and mast cell degranulation. Second, neurogenic vasodilation of the meningeal blood vessels occurs, producing inflammation. The activations of trigeminal sensory fibers cause neurogenic dural vasodilation mediated by the calcitonin gene-related peptide. The calcitonin gene-related peptide is elevated during a migraine (Porth & Matfin, 2009).

Clinical Manifestations

Cluster Headaches

Cluster headaches usually occur up to eight times per day, with severe orbital, supraorbital, or temporal pain accompanied by autonomic symptoms such as ptosis, miosis, lacrimation, conjunctival injection, rhinorrhea, and nasal congestion (May, 2010).

Tension Headaches

Characteristic signs and symptoms of tension headaches include bilateral, nonthrobbing head pain of mild to moderate intensity. Patients may describe pressure, head fullness, or a band-like sensation around the head, or they may report a feeling like a heavy weight is on their head or shoulders (Taylor, 2008).

Migraine Headaches

Migraine headaches with an aura have four phases: prodrome, aura, headache, and recovery. The prodrome phase occurs hours or days before the onset of a migraine headache. Symptoms include depression, irritability, feeling cold, cravings, loss of appetite, alterations in activity, polyuria, diarrhea, and constipation. The aura phase, which occurs only in some patients, involves an aura lasting 1 hour with focal neurologic symptoms, visual disturbances, or vision in only half of the visual field. The headache phase is characterized by vasodilation and a decline in serotonin levels. A throbbing headache becomes more intense, lasting for several hours. The headache can become incapacitating, with photophobia, nausea, and vomiting. The recovery phase involves slow subsiding of the pain. There may be muscle contractions in the neck and scalp, with localized tenderness, tiredness, and alterations in mood. The patient may sleep for hours after the recovery phase (Smeltzer, Bare, Hinkle, & Cheever, 2010).

Chronic migraine headaches may be a problem. The chronic migraine is diagnosed by the presence of a migraine headache without an aura for 8 days or more per month for 3 months. The headache is unilateral, pulsating, with moderate to severe intensity, and aggravated by activity (Garza & Schwedt, 2011).

Drug Therapy

Cluster Headaches

Treatment of cluster headaches involves subcutaneous sumatriptan and oxygen. It is important to note that although oxygen may be effective in some patients, repeated or frequent use in a short period of time should be avoided. Evidence has shown that the frequency of cluster headaches may increase in some patients with overuse of oxygen. Ergot derivatives, lidocaine, and octreotide are also effective in the treatment of acute cluster headaches.

Tension Headaches

Acute therapy for tension headaches entails the use of nonpharmacological methods such as rest, relaxation techniques, or stress-reduction strategies as well as medication. Pharmacological treatment of tension headaches includes acetaminophen, aspirin, and nonsteroidal anti-inflammatory agents (see Chap. 14).

Migraine Headaches

There are two specific courses of treatment for migraine headaches: abortive and preventive therapy. **Abortive therapy** is the administration of medications to treat the symptoms of migraine headache. **Preventive therapy** is the administration of medications to prevent the development of a migraine headache. Medications used in the treatment of migraine headaches are listed in Table 51.1.

The abortive agents administered for the treatment of migraine headaches include nonsteroidal anti-inflammatory agents, aspirin–acetaminophen with caffeine medication, the ergot alkaloids, and the triptans. According to the American Academy of Neurology, the pharmacological and nonpharmacological treatment of long-term migraine is to reduce the frequency, severity,

TABLE 51.1

Drugs Administered for the Treatment of Migraine Headache

Drug Class	Prototype	Other Drugs in the Class
Nonsteroidal anti-inflammatory drugs	Ibuprofen (Motrin, Advil)*	Naproxen* Naproxen sodium (Aleve)* Ketorolac tromethamine (Toradol)
Analgesic	Aspirin–acetaminophen–caffeine (several products)	
Ergot alkaloids	Ergotamine tartrate	Dihydroergotamine
Triptans	Sumatriptan	Almotriptan (Axert) Eletriptan (Relpax) Frovatriptan (Frova) Naratriptan (Amerge) Rizatriptan (Maxalt) Zolmitriptan (Zomig)
Estrogen	Estradiol	

*See Chap. 14 for more information. Naproxen is commonly prescribed for the treatment of migraine headaches.

and disability. The initial pharmacotherapy for acute treatment of migraine is the administration of triptans (serotonin receptor [5-HT$_{1B}$ and 5-HT$_{1D}$] agonists). Patients who experience nausea and vomiting may receive intranasal or subcutaneous sumatriptan.

Women who experience menstrual migraines take estrogen preparations. People who suffer from migraines take preventive medications, which are discussed later in this chapter.

Clinical Application 51-1

- What does the nurse teach Ms. Van Art about the pathophysiology of acute migraine?

NCLEX Success

1. A patient is admitted to the emergency department with a severe headache with nausea and vomiting. She receives a diagnosis of an acute migraine headache. Which of the following medications assists in decreasing the nausea and vomiting related to the acute migraine episode?

    A. intravenous ketorolac
    B. intranasal sumatriptan
    C. inhaled albuterol
    D. oral diclofenac

2. Which of the following medications are administered for preventive therapy in the treatment of migraine?

    A. beta blockers
    B. nonsteroidal anti-inflammatory agents
    C. ergot alkaloids
    D. analgesics

Nonsteroidal Anti-Inflammatory Agents

Ibuprofen is the prototype of the nonsteroidal anti-inflammatory agents (see Chap. 14). However, naproxen sodium is more commonly prescribed for the treatment of migraine headaches.

Thus, ℗ **naproxen** or **naproxen sodium** (Aleve) is the prototype described in detail in this chapter.

Pharmacokinetics

There are two types of naproxen: naproxen and naproxen sodium. Naproxen has an onset of action of 1 hour, a peak of action of 2 to 4 hours, and duration of action of 7 hours or less. Naproxen sodium has an onset of action of 1 hour, a peak of action of 1 to 2 hours, and the same duration of action as naproxen. Metabolism of both agents occurs in the liver, and they have a half-life of 12 to 15 hours. Excretion is in the urine. Naproxen and naproxen sodium cross the placental barrier and enter the breast milk.

Action

Naproxen is a nonselective inhibitor of cyclo-oxygenase resulting in the inhibition of prostaglandin synthesis of COX-1 and COX-2. Naproxen sodium improves the solubility of naproxen through faster absorption and rapid onset of action (Suthisisang, Poolsup, Suksomboon, Lertpipopmetha, & Tepwitukgid, 2010).

Use

Prescribers order naproxen sodium to reduce the pain resulting from an acute migraine headache. Table 51.2 presents dosage information for naproxen and related drugs.

Use in Older Adults

Older people should not take more than 200 mg of naproxen sodium every 12 hours.

Use in Patients With Renal Impairment

Caution is necessary with the administration of naproxen sodium in patients with renal disease because the renal system excretes the drug.

Use in Patients With Hepatic Impairment

Caution is warranted with the administration of naproxen sodium in patients with hepatic impairment because the site of metabolism is the liver.

TABLE 51.2

DRUGS AT A GLANCE: Nonsteroidal Anti-Inflammatory Drugs*

Drug	Pregnancy Category	Routes and Dosages	
		Adults	*Children*
℗ **Naproxen**	C	375–500 mg PO 2 times per day	10 mg/kg PO in two divided doses
℗ **Naproxen sodium** (Aleve)	C	275–550 mg PO 2 times per day May increase to 1.65 g/d for a limited period	Safety has not been established
Ketorolac tromethamine (Acular LS, Acular PF)	C (second and third trimester) D (third trimester)	30 mg IV every 6 h to a maximum of 120 mg/d	2–16 y: 0.5 mg/kg IV up to a maximum of 15 mg

*Drugs used in headache treatment.

Adverse Effects

The most severe adverse effects of naproxen sodium include bronchospasm and anaphylaxis. Gastrointestinal (GI) adverse effects include GI bleeding, nausea, dyspepsia, and GI pain. U.S. Food and Drug Administration (FDA) has issued a **BLACK BOX WARNING** ◆ stating that naproxen sodium may put patients at increased risk for cardiovascular events and GI bleeding.

Contraindications

Contraindications to naproxen or naproxen sodium include a known allergy to aspirin or other nonsteroidal anti-inflammatory drugs as well as pregnancy and lactation. It is important to administer the medication cautiously to patients with asthma, cardiovascular dysfunction, hypertension, GI bleeding, and peptic ulcer.

Nursing Implications

Preventing Interactions

The administration of naproxen sodium with lithium results in increased lithium levels and the risk of lithium toxicity.

Assessing for Therapeutic Effects

Following the administration of naproxen or naproxen sodium, the patient should exhibit diminished pain. The nurse assesses the patient's pain level using a pain scale.

Assessing for Adverse Effects

The nurse assesses the patient for GI upset, dyspepsia, or bleeding. He or she also assesses pulmonary function and lung sounds for bronchospasm or anaphylactic reaction.

Patient Teaching

Box 51.1 identifies patient teaching guidelines for naproxen sodium.

Other Drugs in the Class

Migraine sufferers often seek treatment in the emergency department when the more commonly used abortive therapies are ineffective. In the emergency setting, ketorolac tromethamine is the most frequently administered intravenous

---

BOX 51.1 **Patient Teaching Guidelines for Naproxen Sodium**

- Take the medication with meals to prevent gastrointestinal upset.
- Take medication as prescribed.
- Do not cut, crush, or chew tablets.
- Do not operate machinery if dizziness or drowsiness occurs.
- Report sore throat, fever, rash, itching, edema, visual changes, and black, tarry stools to your health care provider.

---

medication for migraine sufferers who have not responded to oral abortive therapy.

Clinical Application 51-2

- What is the rationale for administering ketorolac to Ms. Van Art?

Acetaminophen, Aspirin, and Caffeine

The combination of ⓟ **acetaminophen, aspirin,** and **caffeine** may be effective for the treatment of headaches. In the United States, brand names include Anacin Advanced Headache Formula, Excedrin Extra Strength, Excedrin Migraine, Goody's Extra Strength, and Vanquish Extra Strength Pain Reliever.

Pharmacokinetics

To understand the pharmacokinetics of acetaminophen, aspirin, and caffeine, it is important to review each medication individually. Acetaminophen reaches a peak of action in 0.5 to 2 hours and possesses a 1- to 3-hour half-life. It crosses the placental barrier and enter the breast milk. The drug is metabolized in the liver and excreted in the urine. Aspirin has an onset of action of 5 to 30 minutes, reaches a peak of action in 15 to 120 minutes, and has a duration of action of 3 to 6 hours. The half-life of aspirin is 15 minutes to 12 hours. The drug is absorbed in the stomach and metabolized in the liver. Caffeine has an onset of action of 15 minutes and reaches a peak of action in 15 to 45 minutes. It readily crosses the placental barrier and enters breast milk. Like acetaminophen and aspirin, metabolism of caffeine takes place in the liver and elimination occurs in the kidneys.

Action

Acetaminophen may act as an analgesic, and its mechanism of action is unknown. Aspirin has the ability to inhibit the synthesis of prostaglandins, which are a mediator of inflammation. Caffeine increases calcium permeability in the sarcoplasmic reticulum to promote the accumulation of cyclic adenosine monophosphate (cAMP) and block the adenosine receptors, stimulating the CNS, cardiac activity, gastric acid secretion, and diuresis. It causes constriction of the blood vessels, which is known as **vascular constriction**. Migraine headaches result from the vasodilation of blood vessels. In addition, caffeine increases the effectiveness of acetaminophen and aspirin by approximately 40%.

Use

Acetaminophen–aspirin–caffeine products are administered to reduce pain related to migraine or tension headache. Table 51.3 presents oral dosage of information for these combination products.

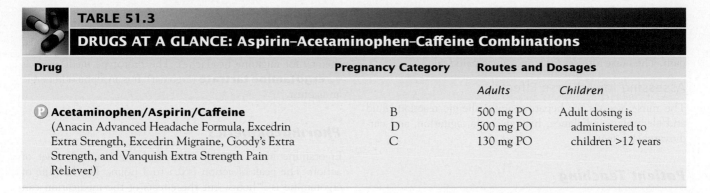

TABLE 51.3

DRUGS AT A GLANCE: Aspirin–Acetaminophen–Caffeine Combinations

Drug	Pregnancy Category	Routes and Dosages	
		Adults	Children
℗ **Acetaminophen/Aspirin/Caffeine**	B	500 mg PO	Adult dosing is
(Anacin Advanced Headache Formula, Excedrin	D	500 mg PO	administered to
Extra Strength, Excedrin Migraine, Goody's Extra	C	130 mg PO	children >12 years
Strength, and Vanquish Extra Strength Pain			
Reliever)			

Use in Children

Children older than 12 years of age may receive the adult dose of the combination agent.

Use in Patients With Hepatic Impairment

People with hepatic impairment should not receive this combination agent on an ongoing basis. They may not metabolize acetaminophen in this combined medication effectively, leading to hepatotoxicity.

Adverse Effects

Each component of the combination medication has adverse effects, which will be addressed individually. Acetaminophen may result in headache, chest pain, dyspnea, myocardial damage with doses of 5 to 8 g/day, and hepatic impairment. Aspirin may lead to GI effects such as dyspepsia, heartburn, and epigastric discomfort as well as hematologic effects such as occult blood loss and hemostatic defects. Aspirin toxicity involves respiratory alkalosis, tachypnea, hemorrhage, excitement, confusion, seizures, tetany, cardiovascular collapse, and metabolic acidosis. Caffeine may result in excitement, insomnia, restlessness, tremors, headaches, and lightheadedness, as well as cardiovascular effects such as tachycardia, hypertension, extrasystole, and palpitations.

Contraindications

Contraindications to acetaminophen include a known allergy to the drug. Caution is necessary in impaired hepatic function, chronic alcoholism, pregnancy, and lactation. Contraindications to aspirin includes a known hypersensitivity to the drug or other anti-inflammatory agents. Vigilance is warranted with renal impairment. Contraindications to caffeine include duodenal ulcers, diabetes, and lactation. Caution is essential in pregnancy, renal and hepatic impairment, and cardiovascular disease.

Nursing Implications

People most commonly take the acetaminophen–aspirin–caffeine in the home setting. It is important to be familiar with all aspects of each medication to maintain medication safety.

Preventing Interactions

Several drug–drug interactions may occur with acetaminophen–aspirin–caffeine combinations. Box 51.2 names the specific medications that increase or decrease the effects of each of the medications in the combined drug. Other drug–drug interactions include the following:

- Oral anticoagulants combined with acetaminophen increase hypothrombinemic effects.
- Aspirin combined with sulfonylureas and insulin results in greater glucose-lowering effects.
- Valproic acid combined with aspirin puts patients at risk for seizure activity secondary to protein receptor site displacement.
- Spironolactone or furosemide combined with aspirin leads to decreased diuretic effects.
- Theophylline or clozapine combined with caffeine increases the serum levels of theophylline or clozapine.

The concomitant administration of caffeine and guarana, ma huang, and ephedra with caffeine is not recommended.

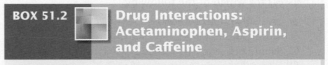

BOX 51.2 **Drug Interactions: Acetaminophen, Aspirin, and Caffeine**

Drugs That Increase the Effects of Acetaminophen
- Alcohol, barbiturates, carbamazepine, hydantoins, rifampin, sulfinpyrazone
  Increase the risk of hepatotoxicity

Drugs That Increase the Effects of Aspirin
- Alcohol, anticoagulants, nonsteroidal anti-inflammatory agents
  Increase the bleeding risk
- Carbonic anhydrase inhibitors
  Increase the risk of salicylate toxicity

Drugs That Increase the Effects of Caffeine
- Cimetidine, hormonal contraceptive, disulfiram, ciprofloxacin, mexiletine
  Increase the central nervous system effects

Drugs That Decrease the Effects of Aspirin
- Acetazolamide, methazolamide, antacids, alkalinizers
  Decrease the salicylate levels

Drugs That Decrease the Effects of Caffeine
- Nicotine
  Produces vasoconstriction

Assessing for Therapeutic Effects

Following the administration of the acetaminophen–aspirin–caffeine combination, the patient should exhibit diminished pain. The nurse assesses for pain using a pain scale.

Assessing for Adverse Effects

The nurse assesses for hepatotoxicity, allergic reaction, fluid and electrolyte imbalance, hypoglycemia, agitation, and cardiovascular effects.

Patient Teaching

Box 51.3 identifies patient teaching guidelines for acetaminophen–aspirin–caffeine combinations.

NCLEX Success

3. A patient is taking naproxen sodium for headache and lithium for manic depression. Which of the following effects occurs when the naproxen is administered in combination with lithium?

   A. increased risk of lithium toxicity
   B. increase in creatinine clearance
   C. hepatotoxicity
   D. potential GI effects

4. A teenage girl is suffering from migraine headaches. Her health care provider orders a combination of acetaminophen, aspirin, and caffeine. Prior to the administration of the medication, it is necessary to assess for which of the following?

   A. anxiety and depression
   B. history of smoking
   C. family history of migraines
   D. antacid use

BOX 51.3   Patient Teaching Guidelines for Acetaminophen–Aspirin–Caffeine Combinations

- Never exceed the recommended dosage of acetaminophen–aspirin–caffeine combinations.
- Avoid the use of over-the-counter and prescription forms of medications that contain acetaminophen.
- Keep the medication out of the reach of children.
- Take the drug with food or after meals if possible.
- Do not stop caffeine abruptly.
- Do not consume foods high in caffeine.
- Report the following conditions to your health care provider:
  - Any signs and symptoms of bleeding
  - Ringing in the ears, dizziness, confusion, abdominal pain, dyspnea, nausea, and vomiting
  - Abnormal heart rate and palpitations.

Ergot Alkaloids

The ergotamine preparations are administered for abortive therapy for migraine headaches. The prototype medication is **Ⓟ ergotamine tartrate** (Ergomar). It is an alpha-adrenergic antagonist.

Pharmacokinetics

Ergotamine has a variable rate of absorption and onset of action. The peak of action is 0.5 to 3 hours. The half-life of ergotamine is 2 hours, but the effects of the medication can continue for 24 hours. The medication is metabolized by the cytochrome P450 enzyme CYP3A4 in the liver and excreted in the bile. Ergotamine is excreted in the breast milk and may cause vomiting, diarrhea, and changes in heart rate and blood pressure in the nursing infant. It has caused fetal growth retardation in animal studies.

Action

Ergotamine produces stimulation of the cranial and peripheral vascular smooth muscles while depressing the effects of the central vasomotor centers. It is a partial agonist and antagonist that acts against tryptaminergic, dopaminergic, and alpha-adrenergic receptors to constrict the cranial and peripheral blood vessels.

Use

Prescribers order ergotamine individually or in combination with caffeine to prevent or stop migraine, cluster, or vascular headaches. Children as well as people with renal or hepatic impairment should not take ergotamine. Table 51.4 gives dosage information for the ergot alkaloids.

Use in Older Adults

It is necessary to administer ergotamine cautiously in older adults because of the drug's vasoconstrictive properties and cardiovascular adverse effects.

Adverse Effects

The cardiovascular adverse effects of ergotamine include absence of pulse, bradycardia, cardiac valvular fibrosis, cyanosis, edema, heart rhythm changes, gangrene, hypertension, ischemia, precordial distress, chest pain, tachycardia, and vasospasm. Musculoskeletal adverse effects include muscle pain, numbness, paresthesia, and weakness. Other side effects may include vertigo, nausea, vomiting, itching, pulmonary fibrosis, and genitourinary retroperitoneal fibrosis.

Contraindications

Contraindications of ergotamine include a known hypersensitivity reaction to the drug or its components. Additional contraindications are the existence of peripheral vascular disease, hepatic

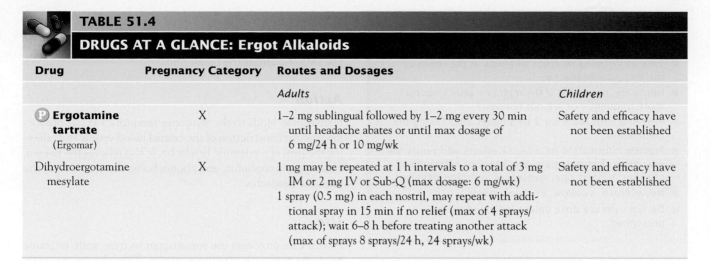

TABLE 51.4

DRUGS AT A GLANCE: Ergot Alkaloids

Drug	Pregnancy Category	Routes and Dosages	
		Adults	Children
Ⓟ Ergotamine tartrate (Ergomar)	X	1–2 mg sublingual followed by 1–2 mg every 30 min until headache abates or until max dosage of 6 mg/24 h or 10 mg/wk	Safety and efficacy have not been established
Dihydroergotamine mesylate	X	1 mg may be repeated at 1 h intervals to a total of 3 mg IM or 2 mg IV or Sub-Q (max dosage: 6 mg/wk) 1 spray (0.5 mg) in each nostril, may repeat with additional spray in 15 min if no relief (max of 4 sprays/attack); wait 6–8 h before treating another attack (max of sprays 8 sprays/24 h, 24 sprays/wk)	Safety and efficacy have not been established

and renal disease, coronary artery disease, hypertension, and sepsis. The FDA has issued a **BLACK BOX WARNING** ◆ stating that ergotamine is contraindicated with potent inhibitors of CYP3A4 medications. These medications include the protease inhibitors, azole antifungals, and some macrolide antibiotics. Concomitant use of these medications results in ergot toxicity. Pregnancy and lactation are also contraindications to the use of ergotamine.

Nursing Implications

Preventing Interactions

Many medications and foods interact with ergotamine, increasing its effect (Boxes 51.4 and 51.5).

Administering the Medication

Administration of ergotamine is sublingual, and the tablet should be dissolved under the tongue. It is important that

tablets not be crushed, chewed, or swallowed whole. Patients should not drink, eat, or smoke while the medication is in place.

Assessing for Therapeutic Effects

The nurse assesses for a decrease in headache pain.

Assessing for Adverse Effects

Following administration of ergotamine, the nurse assesses for cardiovascular adverse effects. Measurement of the pulse and blood pressure is essential. The nurse also assesses for vertigo, muscle pain, numbness, paresthesia, and weakness, as well as for signs and symptoms of a hypersensitivity reaction to ergotamine. It is important to assess the patient's fluid and electrolyte status if the patient is suffering from nausea and vomiting. In addition, the nurse assesses the patient's urinary elimination due to the adverse effect of retroperitoneal fibrosis in which the patient develops an obstruction of the ureters.

Patient Teaching

Box 51.6 identifies patient teaching guidelines for ergotamine.

Other Drugs in the Class

Dihydroergotamine mesylate reduces the rate of serotonin-induced platelet aggregation and has a weaker vasoconstrictive action than ergotamine. It has a greater adrenergic blocking activity to relieve migraine headaches.

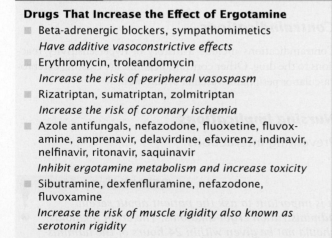

BOX 51.4 Drug Interactions: Ergotamine

Drugs That Increase the Effect of Ergotamine

- Beta-adrenergic blockers, sympathomimetics
  Have additive vasoconstrictive effects
- Erythromycin, troleandomycin
  Increase the risk of peripheral vasospasm
- Rizatriptan, sumatriptan, zolmitriptan
  Increase the risk of coronary ischemia
- Azole antifungals, nefazodone, fluoxetine, fluvoxamine, amprenavir, delavirdine, efavirenz, indinavir, nelfinavir, ritonavir, saquinavir
  Inhibit ergotamine metabolism and increase toxicity
- Sibutramine, dexfenfluramine, nefazodone, fluvoxamine
  Increase the risk of muscle rigidity also known as serotonin rigidity

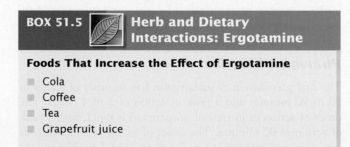

BOX 51.5 Herb and Dietary Interactions: Ergotamine

Foods That Increase the Effect of Ergotamine

- Cola
- Coffee
- Tea
- Grapefruit juice

BOX 51.6 — Patient Teaching Guidelines for Ergotamine

- Take ergotamine or ergot alkaloids at the onset of the migraine headache.
- Notify the prescriber if the migraine attacks occur more frequently or are not relieved.
- Rest in a dark room for 2 to 3 hours after taking the medication.
- Provide information on adverse effects and notify the prescriber if muscle pain, weakness of extremities, changes in heart rate, nausea, or vomiting develops.
- Never crush, swallow, or chew tablets.
- Do not increase dose unless indicated by the prescriber.

NCLEX Success

5. A patient with migraine headaches receives a prescription for an ergot alkaloid as abortive therapy. Which of the following is a priority intervention for patient education?

   A. Notify the prescriber if an aura precedes the migraine headache.
   B. Administer the medication with food.
   C. Seek emergency help if cardiac changes occur.
   D. Administer the medication with caffeinated beverages.

6. A 32-year-old woman has been taking ergotamine tartrate as abortive therapy for migraine headache for many years. For which of the following adverse effects does the nurse assess?

   A. hypotension
   B. muscle weakness
   C. hypoventilation
   D. valvular fibrosis

Triptans

Triptans are serotonin 5-HT$_{1B}$ and 5-HT$_{1D}$ agonists that affect the pathophysiologic mechanism of migraine or cluster headaches, thus relieving the associated symptoms. The advantage of the administration of triptans over the ergot alkaloids is that these medications can be easily taken by patients during their daily lives. The prototype triptan is Ⓟ **sumatriptan** (Imitrex).

Pharmacokinetics

The oral preparation of sumatriptan has an onset of action of 60 to 90 minutes and a peak of action of 2 to 4 hours. The onset of action of intranasal sumatriptan is rapid, with a peak of action of 90 minutes. The onset of action of subcutaneous sumatriptan varies, with a peak of action of 5 to 20 minutes. Sumatriptan is widely distributed and is 10% to 20% protein bound. Its therapeutic half-life is 115 minutes. Metabolism occurs in the liver. Excretion is in the urine, with excretion of the oral preparation in the feces. Sumatriptan crosses the placenta and enters the breast milk.

Action

Sumatriptan binds to the serotonin receptors 5-HT$_{1D}$, producing vascular constriction of the cranial blood vessels and relieving the pain of a migraine headache. It also relieves the nausea, vomiting, photophobia, and phonophobia that accompany the migraine headache.

Use

Health care providers use sumatriptan to treat acute migraine headache pain with or without an aura. They also use it to treat cluster headaches. Older adults should not take sumatriptan and other triptans. Table 51.5 gives dosage information for the triptans.

Use in Patients With Renal Impairment

Caution is necessary when administering sumatriptan to patients with impaired renal function because elimination takes place in the renal system.

Use in Patients With Hepatic Impairment

Caution is also warranted when administering sumatriptan to patients with impaired hepatic function because metabolism takes place in the liver.

Adverse Effects

CNS adverse effects of all sumatriptan preparations are dizziness, vertigo, headache, anxiety, malaise, myalgia, and fatigue. Cardiovascular adverse effects include alterations in blood pressure and chest pain as well as the most severe cardiovascular adverse effect, shock. The nasal administration of sumatriptan produces nausea, nasal and throat irritation, and a bad taste in the mouth. The injectable form of the drug may cause injection site discomfort.

Contraindications

Contraindications include a history of hypersensitivity reactions to the drug. Other contraindications are existing cerebrovascular or peripheral vascular syndromes.

Nursing Implications

Preventing Interactions

QSEN Safety Alert

It is important to ask the patient about recent administration ergot alkaloids. The ergot alkaloids should not be given within 24 hours of the administration of triptans.

TABLE 51.5

DRUGS AT A GLANCE: Triptans

Drug	Pregnancy Category	Routes and Dosages	
		Adults	Children
Ⓟ **Sumatriptan** (Imitrex)	C	25, 50, or 100 mg PO additional doses may be repeated in 2 h or more (max dosage 200 mg/d) 6 mg Sub-Q may be repeated in 1 h; (max dosage 12 mg/24 h) 5, 10, or 20 mg intranasal into one nostril or 10 mg divided doses of 5 mg one in each nostril, may be repeated after 2 h (max dosage 40 mg/24 h)	Safety and efficacy have not been established
Almotriptan (Axert)	C	6.25–12.5 mg PO repeat after 2 h if necessary (max, 2 doses/24 h)	Safety and efficacy have not been established
Eletriptan (Relpax)	C	20–40 mg PO as a single dose, repeat after 2 h if necessary (max dose, 80 mg/d)	Safety and efficacy have not been established
Frovatriptan (Frova)	C	2.5 mg PO; repeat after 2 h if necessary (max dose, 7.5 mg)	Safety and efficacy have not been established
Naratriptan (Amerge)	C	1–2.5 mg PO as a single dose; repeat in 4 h if necessary (max dose, 5 mg/d)	Safety and efficacy have not been established
Rizatriptan (Maxalt)	C	5–10 mg PO as a single dose; repeat after 2 h if necessary (max dose, 30 mg/d)	Safety and efficacy have not been established
Zolmitriptan (Zomig)	C	1.25–2.5 mg PO as a single dose; may repeat after 2 h if necessary (max dose, 10 mg/d) 0.5, 1, 2.5, or 5 mg intranasal by unit-dose spray device (max dose, 10 mg/d) Orally disintegrating tablets (Zomig-ZMT) 2.5–5 mg as a single dose; may repeat after 2 h if necessary (max dose, 10 mg/d)	Safety and efficacy have not been established
Sumatriptan and naproxen (Treximet)	C	1 tablet (sumatriptan 85 mg and naproxen 500 mg) PO; if migraine is not relieved in 2 h, a second dose may be administered (max dose, 2 tablets/24 h)	Safety and efficacy have not been established

The combination of ergot-containing drugs and the triptans results in cardiac ischemia. Also, administration of monoamine oxidase (MAO) inhibitors leads to increased serum levels of sumatriptan and sumatriptan toxicity. Two weeks after an MAO inhibitor has been discontinued, it is permissible to give sumatriptan in combination with the MAO inhibitor. In addition, administration of the herb St. John's wort with triptans results in triptan toxicity.

Administering the Medication

It is important to administer sumatriptan at the onset of migraine symptoms. Administration of a second dose of the oral preparation when symptoms return is acceptable but not earlier than 2 hours after the first tablet. Dosages should not exceed 100 mg in a single dose or 200 mg/d. It is necessary to administer the oral preparation with fluids and the intranasal preparation as a single dose of one spray in each nostril. With the subcutaneous preparation, administration just below the skin as soon as

symptoms develop is best. If relief does not occur or if symptoms reappear, a second injection may follow 1 hour or longer after the first one. A person may have two injections in 24 hours. With the administration of all sumatriptan preparations, it is necessary to monitor the blood pressure for hypertension.

Assessing Therapeutic Effects

The nurse assesses for diminished pain and ultimate relief of migraine headaches.

Assessing for Adverse Effects

The nurse assesses for increased blood pressure, as well as chest pain, shock, dizziness, and vertigo. With subcutaneous administration, the nurse also assesses for irritation at the injection site.

Patient Teaching

Box 51.7 identifies patient teaching guidelines for sumatriptan.

BOX 51.7 **Patient Teaching Guidelines for Sumatriptan**

■ Provide instruction about the administration of sub-cutaneous sumatriptan or use of the autoinjector.

■ Do not administer more than two injections in 24 hours.

■ Inject just below the skin as soon as symptoms are noted.

■ Properly dispose of the autoinjector, syringes, and needles.

■ Administer nasal spray as a single dose; repeat if necessary in 2 hours.

■ Do not administer the medication if you are pregnant.

■ Do not operate machinery after the administration of sumatriptan.

■ Report symptoms of hypersensitivity such as heat, flushing, tiredness, and feeling sick to your health care provider.

Other Drugs in the Class

Almotriptan (Axert) is similar in action to other triptans; however, it can be administered with MAO inhibitors. After oral administration, it has a variable onset of action and a peak of action of 1 to 3 hours. Prior to administering almotriptan, it is necessary to determine whether the patient has received any ergot alkaloids in the past 24 hours.

Eletriptan (Relpax) has a rapid onset of action with a 1.5 to 2 hour peak of action. It is administered orally in 20- or 40-mg doses. It is important to ensure the patient has not taken an ergot-containing compound within 24 hours and to control the environment for light and sound. The drug is usually well tolerated and causes no major harm; however, any elevation in blood pressure or chest pain requires discontinuation of the medication.

Frovatriptan (Frova) has a variable onset of action and reaches the peak of action in 2 to 4 hours. It interacts unfavorably with selective serotonin reuptake inhibitors such as fluoxetine, fluvoxamine, paroxetine, and sertraline, producing weakness, hyperreflexia, and diminished CNS effects such as alertness. Frovatriptan may lead to serotonin syndrome, and is a potentially life-threatening reaction that may occur when two drugs that affect serotonin levels in the body are taken concurrently. Other symptoms of serotonin syndrome include restlessness, hallucinations, fever, loss of consciousness, tachycardia, and a rapid change in blood pressure.

Naratriptan (Amerge) has a slow onset of action. Contraindications include a creatinine clearance less than 15 mL/min or severe hepatic impairment. Women of childbearing age should use barrier contraceptives due to the risk of serious birth defects.

Rizatriptan (Maxalt) is an oral preparation that can be swallowed or administered in a "melt-away" (orally disintegrating) formulation. It is effective in the treatment of acute migraine. Studies have shown that the 10-mg dosage is more effective

than the 5-mg dose. The most common adverse effects are dizziness, fatigue, nausea, and somnolence.

Zolmitriptan (Zomig) is a triptan that may be administered orally or intranasally. The onset of action of the oral drug is variable, whereas that of the intranasal preparation is 15 minutes. Two large studies have found that zolmitriptan is effective for acute migraine therapy, with an optimal starting dose of 2.5 mg. The most commonly reported adverse effects were dizziness, nausea, somnolence, paresthesia, fatigue, and tightness of the throat or chest.

Sumatriptan–naproxen sodium (Treximet) is a combination drug that is administered orally. Patients should not divide, chew, or crush the tablets. This combination is effective in treating acute migraine and decreasing photophobia. The FDA has issued two **BLACK BOX WARNINGS ◆** : (1) cardiovascular risk from sumatriptan, with an increased risk of adverse thrombotic events, including myocardial infarction and stroke, and (2) GI risk due to naproxen sodium, with an increased risk of GI irritation, inflammation, ulceration, bleeding, and perforation.

NCLEX Success

7. A 50-year-old woman has a subarachnoid bleed. She has received treatment for migraine headaches in the past. Which of the following patient teaching guidelines is a priority on her discharge from the rehabilitation facility?

   A. Take estrogen to prevent a menstrual migraine.
   B. Take gabapentin (Neurontin) for neuropathic pain.
   C. Do not take sumatriptan (Imitrex) for migraine headache.
   D. Take zolmitriptan (Zomig) because it has a more rapid onset of action.

8. A patient has taken sumatriptan–naproxen sodium (Treximet) for an acute migraine. She has also taken over-the-counter ibuprofen (Motrin) for menstrual cramps. Which of the following adverse effects is she at risk for developing?

   A. bronchospasm
   B. urinary retention
   C. edema
   D. GI bleed

Clinical Application 51-3

Ms. Van Art is discharged from the emergency department following an acute migraine headache. Her prescriber orders sumatriptan (Imitrex), to be administered subcutaneously at the onset of an acute migraine headache.

■ What education should Ms. Van Art receive prior to discharge?

■ What medications are contraindicated with the administration of sumatriptan?

Estrogen

Estrogen in the form of ⓟ **estradiol** is a treatment for menstrual migraines, which are most likely 2 days prior to menses through the third day of bleeding (Calhoun, 2011). Perimenstrual estrogen supplementation is based on evidence that the natural decline in estrogen in the late luteal phase of the menstrual cycle, prior to menstruation, is associated with the increased risk of migraine (MacGregor, 2010).

Pharmacokinetics

Metabolism of estradiol occurs in the liver. Excretion takes place in the urine. The drug crosses the placenta and enters the breast milk.

Action

Estradiol binds to intracellular receptors to form a complex that stimulates synthesis of proteins responsible for estrogenic effects. Prophylactic administration minimizes the premenstrual decline in estrogen that precipitates the development of the migraine headache (Calhoun, 2011).

Use

Transcutaneous administration of estradiol increases the estrogen levels in the late luteal phase of the menstrual cycle that contribute to the development of menstrual migraine headaches. Table 51.6 gives dosage information for estradiol.

Adverse Effects

The major adverse effect associated with the administration of estrogen preparations is thromboembolic disorders. Menstrual irregularity can occur because of the suppression of endogenous estrogen during treatment.

Contraindications

Contraindications include incomplete bone growth, which occurs in adolescents. Other contraindications are the presence of neoplasms, breast cancer, thromboembolic disorders, fibroids, endometriosis, thyroid disease, and pregnancy.

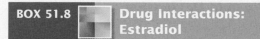

BOX 51.8   Drug Interactions: Estradiol

Drugs That Increase the Effects of Estradiol
■ Cyclosporine, theophylline, tricyclic antidepressants
  Increase serum levels

Drugs That Decrease the Effects of Estradiol
■ Phenytoin and rifampin
  Decrease serum levels
■ Nicotine
  Reduces or cancels efficacy

Nursing Implications

Preventing Interactions

Some drugs interact with estradiol, increasing or decreasing its effects (Box 51.8). In addition, the combination of estradiol and bromocriptine interferes with the effects of bromocriptine.

Administering the Medication

Prior to applying the transcutaneous preparation, it is necessary to clean and dry the skin area. It is important to apply the preparation to the trunk.

Assessing for Therapeutic Effects

The nurse assesses for the development of migraine headache in the later luteal phase of the menstrual cycle. If a headache does not develop, the dose is adequate.

Assessing for Adverse Effects

The nurse assesses for the development of leg pain or chest pain indicative of the development of thromboembolism. He or she also assesses for breakthrough bleeding.

Patient Teaching

Box 51.9 identifies patient teaching guidelines for estradiol.

Preventive Therapy for Migraine Headaches

Many medications are administered for the prevention of migraine headaches. These medications are primarily administered for the treatment of other conditions and are thoroughly covered in other chapters. Their use in the prevention of migraines medications is discussed briefly. For complete information about these drugs, one may review the information in the chapters indicated.

BOX 51.9   Patient Teaching Guidelines for Estradiol

■ Take estradiol transdermal as ordered by the prescriber.
■ Notify your health care provider of intermittent breakthrough bleeding, spotting, or unexplained pain, especially calf or chest pain.

	TABLE 51.6		
	DRUGS AT A GLANCE: Estradiol		
Drug	**Pregnancy Category**	**Routes and Dosages**	
		Adults	*Children*
ⓟ **Estradiol**	X	100-mcg patch or 1.5-mg gel	Safety and efficacy have not been established

Carboxylic Acid Derivative

Valproic acid (see Chap. 52) is a carboxylic acid derivative that is most commonly administered to control seizures. However, it has proved effective in the prevention of migraine headaches. Valproic acid is available in two forms. The dosage for valproic acid tablets is 250 mg orally two times per day, with a maximum dosage of 1000 mg. The dosage of the extended-release preparation is 500 mg orally once per day. Researchers have found that valproic acid is safe for children younger than 18 years of age. According to a study by Apostol et al. (2008), the administration of extended-release valproic acid was associated with a 75% decrease in median 4-week headache days between the first and fourth months of the study. The most common adverse effects with the administration of valproic acid were nausea, vomiting, weight gain, nasopharyngitis, migraine, and upper respiratory infection. Ten percent of subjects stated that the migraine headache worsened. According to this study, extended-release valproic acid is well tolerated by adolescents with migraine headaches.

Gamma-Aminobutyric Acid

Gabapentin (Neurontin) (see Chap. 52) is a gamma-aminobutyric acid medication commonly administered to control neuropathic pain and as an adjunctive agent for control of seizures. Studies have shown that gabapentin is effective in reducing the frequency of migraines. At the end of 12 weeks, 46% of patients who received 2400 mg/d had a 50% reduction in the 4-week rate of migraine. The most commonly reported adverse effects were dizziness and somnolence.

Sulfamate-Substituted Monosaccharide

Topiramate (Topamax) is a sulfamate-substituted monosaccharide agent used most commonly as an antiepileptic agent (see Chap. 52). It has been approved for the prevention of migraine with an initial dose of 25 mg PO in the evening during week 1, then 25 mg PO two times per day during week 2, then 25 mg PO in the morning and 50 mg PO in the evening during week 3, and 50 mg in the morning and evening during week 4. The most commonly reported adverse effects include paresthesia, fatigue, anorexia, diarrhea, weight loss, altered memory, difficulty concentrating, and nausea.

Beta-Adrenergic Blocking Agents

The most common administered beta-adrenergic blocking agent administered prophylactically for migraine headaches is propranolol (Inderal) (see Chap. 28). The recommended dosage is 80 mg/d, either in (1) sustained-release capsules, (2) extended-release tablets, or (3) divided doses. The maintenance dosage may be increased to 160 to 240 mg/d. Studies have shown that propranolol is effective in reducing migraine frequency.

Other beta blockers used for migraine prophylaxis include timolol, metoprolol, nadolol, and atenolol. It takes several weeks for the beta blockers to become effective, and it is necessary to titrate the dose for at least 3 months to ascertain effectiveness. A concern related to the use of beta blockers is the increased risk of stroke and other cardiovascular events.

Calcium Channel Blockers

Verapamil is the calcium channel blocker of choice for migraine prophylaxis. It takes several weeks for benefits of the medication to be noted. It seems to be the most effective calcium channel blocker for migraine prevention. It is necessary to take 120 mg in three divided doses.

Studies have also noted that tolerance may develop with calcium channel blockers. Tolerance to the medication can be overcome by increasing the dosage or switching to a different calcium channel blocker. Calcium channel blocking agents such as nifedipine (Procardia) (see Chap. 26) have been used for prevention of migraine headache. However, studies have shown that this class is not as effective as other agents.

Angiotensin-Converting Enzyme Inhibitors

As Chap. 28 points out, enalapril maleate is the prototype angiotensin-converting enzyme (ACE) inhibitor, but studies have shown that lisinopril seems to be more effective in the prevention of migraine headaches. A study has shown that a dose of 10 mg/d for 1 week and then 20 mg/d reduced the number of hours and days with headache and headache severity compared to a placebo. An adverse effect is the development of the ACE cough. (The cough is a result of an interference with bradykinin, substance P, or tachykinin metabolism.)

Angiotensin II Receptor Blockers

Angiotensin II receptor blockers (see Chap. 28) can be effective in the prevention of migraine headache. Studies on the effectiveness of candesartan have revealed that it produces favorable results in the prevention of migraine headaches. It is necessary to inform women of childbearing age that barrier contraceptives are required with this medication. The FDA has issued a **BLACK BOX WARNING** ◆ stating that fetal injury and death have been reported with candesartan.

Olmesartan is effective and well tolerated as a migraine prophylactic agent for patients with comorbid hypertension and prehypertension. Researchers have studied patients with hypertension and prehypertension to determine the effectiveness of this medication (Charles, Jotkowitz, & Byrd, 2006).

Tricyclic Antidepressants

Imipramine (Tofranil) and other tricyclic antidepressants (see Chap. 53) are effective in the prevention of migraine and tension headaches. Amitriptyline (Elavil) 10 to 50 mg at bedtime is also effective for migraine prophylaxis. Tricyclic antidepressants have a sedative effect, and to minimize this, it helps to administer the drugs at bedtime. Other side effects of tricyclic antidepressants include dry mouth, constipation, tachycardia, palpitations, orthostatic hypotension, weight gain, and urinary retention.

EVIDENCE-BASED PRACTICE

Antidepressants in Long-term Migraine Prevention

by HORST J. KOCH, TIM P. JÜRGENS

Drugs
2009, 69(1), 1–19

The rate of depression and migraine headache is 20% to 30%. Clinical studies have identified tricyclic antidepressants to be beneficial in the prophylactic treatment of migraine. Amitriptyline is considered the antidepressant of choice for the prophylactic treatment of migraine. In a study of 279 children with a mean age of 12 years, amitriptyline showed a reduction in the number of migraine attacks per month by 62%. Current data have shown that fluoxetine, a selective serotonin reuptake inhibitor, is also beneficial in the treatment of migraine, but the number of patients in the study was small in number, requiring further research. The authors also identified various herbal remedies such as St. John's wort, used in treatment of depression, and butterbur root and feverfew, used in treatment of migraine. St. John's wort can increase the risk of adverse effects if taken together with an antidepressant. Butterbur root has been associated with hepatotoxicity.

IMPLICATIONS FOR NURSING PRACTICE: It is imperative that the nurse interviews the patient and discovers any complementary or alternative therapies taken by the patient. This knowledge reduces the potential adverse effects that can result from the combination with antidepressants.

Herbal Supplements

People with migraines may use herbal supplements to treat these headaches (Box 51.10).

NCLEX Success

9. A 14-year-old girl is diagnosed with menstrual migraines. Which of the following factors prevents the use of estradiol for the treatment of menstrual migraines?

   A. breakthrough bleeding
   B. leg pain
   C. incomplete long bone growth
   D. anxiety

10. A 16-year-old girl develops migraine headaches. Which of the following medications is safe and effective for the treatment of migraine headaches?

    A. antiepileptic agents
    B. triptans
    C. ergot alkaloids
    D. opioids

BOX 51.10   **Herbal Supplements Used in the Treatment of Headaches**

Feverfew is an herbal medicine with some evidence of effectiveness in treatment of migraines, especially in reducing incidence and severity. Authorities think that the main active ingredient of feverfew is parthenolide. Some people believe that this agent inhibits platelet aggregation, prostaglandin synthesis, and the release of inflammatory mediators such as histamine, but its exact mechanism in migraine prophylaxis is unknown. Contraindications include pregnancy and lactation.

In general, it is necessary to encourage patients to try standard methods of preventing and treating migraine before taking products with uncertain benefits and risks. For example, commercial preparations of feverfew are not standardized and may contain different amounts of parthenolide. The usual recommended dose is 25 to 50 mg daily with food, but more studies are needed.

Adverse effects include hypersensitivity reactions in people with allergies to ragweed, asters, chrysanthemums, or daisies. Stopping the preparation abruptly can result in withdrawal symptoms of pain and stiffness. No reported interactions with over-the-counter or prescription drugs have occurred, but there is a potential for increased risks of bleeding in patients taking an antiplatelet drug (e.g., aspirin) or an anticoagulant (e.g., warfarin).

Adjuvant Medications for Migraine Headaches

Adjuvant medications administered for severe migraine headaches include antiemetics and opioids. Antiemetic agents are adjuvant medications administered to control the symptoms of nausea and vomiting related to migraine, tension, and cluster headaches. Table 51.7 gives dosage information for the antiemetics. Opioid use is controversial because these agents can contribute to the development of chronic daily headache and interference with preventive therapy (Bajwa & Sabahat, 2010). They are not discussed in this section.

Antiemetic agents may be useful for treatment of symptoms related to migraine headache. ⓟ **Chlorpromazine hydrochloride** (Thorazine) (see Chap. 55) is a phenothiazine that has been shown to be effective in treating both the headache itself and the associated nausea and vomiting. Investigators have also shown that antiemetic drugs decrease the photophobia and phonophobia that may accompany the migraine headache. The mechanism of action involved in the decrease of nausea and vomiting is related to the suppression of the chemoreceptor zone. Besides chlorpromazine, related antiemetics include metoclopramide and prochlorperazine. Parenteral preparations of these drugs appear more effective than oral preparations. When administering the antiemetic agents, it is necessary to assess the patient for relief of headache, nausea, and vomiting. Chlorpromazine also depresses the CNS, so it is important to assess the patient's level of consciousness.

TABLE 51.7
DRUGS AT A GLANCE: Antiemetics Used for the Treatment of Headaches

Drug	Pregnancy Category	Routes and Dosages	
		Adults	Children
℗ **Chlorproma-zinve hydro-chloride** (Thorazine)	C	10–25 mg PO every 4–6 h; 50- to 100-mg suppository rectally every 6–8 h; 25–50 mg IM/IV every 4–6 h	>6 mo: 0.55 mg/kg PO every 4–6 h PRN up to 500 mg/d >6 mo: 0.55 mg/kg IM/IV every 6–8 h
Metoclopramide (Reglan)	B	10–20 mg IM/IV	2 mg/kg IM/IV
Prochlorperazine (Compazine)	C	5–10 mg PO 3–4 2/d sustained release; 10–15 mg every 12 h; 5–10 mg IM every 3–4 h (max dose, 40 mg); 2.5–10 mg IV every 3–4 h (max dose, 40 mg); 25 mg per rectum 2 times per day	2.5 mg PO or per rectum 1–3 times per day or 5 mg 2 times per day (max dose, 15 mg/d; 0.13 mg/kg IM every 3–4 h)

Metoclopramide (Reglan) is a GI stimulant that is effective in reducing headache, nausea, and vomiting. It is less effective than chlorpromazine in reducing symptoms. Metoclopramide is a potent central dopamine receptor antagonist that increases esophageal sphincter tone and elevates the chemoreceptor zone threshold.

Prochlorperazine (Compazine) has the same antiemetic action as chlorpromazine and metoclopramide. When taking prochlorperazine orally, it is important to swallow it whole and not chew or crush the tablets. When administering the medication parenterally, it is necessary to give it intramuscularly (deep) and never subcutaneously. When administering metoclopramide and prochlorperazine, it is necessary to assess the patient for signs and symptoms of dystonia, which is indicative of a hypersensitivity reaction. If the patient develops dystonia, it is necessary to administer diphenhydramine (Benadryl) to counteract this reaction. With all of these medications, the patient should be assessed for urinary retention due to the anticholinergic effects.

The Nursing Process

Assessment
* Assess the severity, patterns, and occurrences of cluster, tension, or migraine headaches.

Nursing Diagnosis
* Acute pain
* Fluid volume deficit
* Activity intolerance related to pain
* Deficient knowledge: therapeutic and adverse effects of commonly administered medications

Planning/Goals
The patient will
* Take medications routinely to prevent headache
* Take medications to treat acute migraine with the onset of symptoms or aura
* Avoid trigger factors that contribute to headache symptoms
* Experience fewer and less severe attacks of migraine, tension, or cluster headaches

Nursing Interventions
The nurse will
* Implement measures to minimize and prevent the symptoms of headache
* Instruct the patient on medications to treat acute migraine headache pain
* Instruct the patient on the trigger points related to migraine and strategies to decrease trigger points
* Instruct the patient on medications to prevent migraine headaches
* Administer medications to treat acute migraine headaches
* Administer medications to prevent migraine headaches
* Administer antiemetic agents to reduce nausea and vomiting during acute episodes

Evaluation
* Interview and observe patient for relief of symptoms.
* Interview and observe patient's ability to provide self-care.
* Interview and observe patient regarding safe, effective use of the medications for the acute and preventive treatment.
* Interview and assess patient for medication compliance.

Key Concepts

- Cluster headaches are characterized by recurrent, severe, unilateral orbitotemporal headache that are associated with a histamine reaction.

- Tension headaches are associated with nervous tension or anxiety and involve the chronic contraction of the scalp muscles.

- Migraine headache are unilateral pain in the head that may or may not be accompanied by an aura, which is a subjective sensation that immediately precedes the migraine headache.

- Menstrual migraines are associated with a drop in circulating estrogen 2 to 3 days prior to the onset of menses.

- Naproxen sodium is administered for the reduction pain related to an acute migraine headache.

- The combination of acetaminophen, aspirin, and caffeine has been used for the treatment of headaches.

- Ergotamine produces stimulation of the cranial and peripheral vascular smooth muscles while depressing the effects of the central vasomotor centers. It is a partial agonist and antagonist against tryptaminergic, dopaminergic, and alpha-adrenergic receptors.

- A **BLACK BOX WARNING** ◆ stresses that ergotamine is contraindicated with potent inhibitors of CYP3A4 medications. These medications include the protease inhibitors, azole antifungals, and some macrolide antibiotics. Concomitant use of these medications results in ergot toxicity.

- Triptans are serotonin 1B/1D agonists that act on the pathophysiologic mechanism of the headache. The advantage of the administration of triptans over the ergot alkaloids is that these medications are easily administered by the patient throughout their daily lives.

- For the sumatriptan/naproxen sodium combination (Treximet), the FDA has issued two **BLACK BOX WARNINGS** ◆ : (1) cardiovascular risk from sumatriptan, which has an increased risk of adverse thrombotic events, and (2) GI effects due to naproxen sodium, which has an increased risk of GI irritation, inflammation, ulceration, bleeding, and perforation.

- Estrogen supplementation in the form of estradiol in the late luteal phase decreases symptoms of menstrual migraines.

- Abortive agents administered for the symptomatic treatment of migraine headaches include nonsteroidal anti-inflammatory agents, aspirin–acetaminophen with caffeine medication, the ergot alkaloids, and the triptans.

- Preventive agents administered to prevent development of migraine headaches include antiepileptic agents, beta blockers, calcium channel blockers, and the angiotensin II receptor blockers. Antidepressants have been identified as beneficial in long-term treatment of migraine headache.

- The FDA has issued a **BLACK BOX WARNING** ◆ stating that fetal injury and death have been reported with candesartan, an angiotensin II receptor blocker.

- The adjuvant medications administered for severe migraine headaches include antiemetics and opioids.

Critical Thinking Questions

51-1. A 20-year-old woman is diagnosed with acute migraines and is prescribed sumatriptan 6 mg to be administered with the onset of migraine symptoms. She experiences an aura prior to the onset of pain.

- What is the action of sumatriptan?
- What are the adverse effects of sumatriptan?
- When should sumatriptan be administered?
- What patient teaching does the nurse implement?

51-2. An 18-year-old woman has been suffering from migraine headaches for the past 2 years. She has been taking Excedrin Migraine (aspirin, acetaminophen, and caffeine) without relief. Her health care provider has prescribed ergotamine 2 mg sublingual every 30 minutes until headache subsides with a maximum dose of 6 mg/24 h.

- What is the action of ergotamine?
- What are the adverse effects of ergotamine?
- What patient teaching does the nurse implement?
- What medications are contraindicated with ergotamine?

References and Resources

Apostol, G., Lewis, D. W., Laforet, G. A., Robieson, W. Z., Fugate, J. M., Abi-Saab, W. M., et al. (2008). Divalproex sodium extended-release for the prophylaxis of migraine headache in adolescents: Results of a stand-alone, long-term open-label safety study. *Headache: The Journal of Head and Face Pain, 49*(1), 45–53.

Bajwa, Z. H., & Sabahat, A. (2010). *Acute treatment of migraine in adults.* Up-To-Date. Retrieved June 25, 2011.

Bajwa, Z. H., & Sabahat, A. (2011). *Preventive treatment of migraine in adults.* Up-To-Date. Retrieved June 25, 2011.

Calhoun, A. H. (2011). *Estrogen-associated migraine.* Up-To-Date. Retrieved December 13, 2011.

Charles, J. A., Jotkowitz, S., & Byrd, L. H. (2006). Prevention of migraine with olmesartan in patients with hypertension/prehypertension. *Headache: The Journal of Head and Face Pain, 46*(3), 503–507.

Garza, I., & Schwedt, T. J. (2011). *Chronic migraine.* Up-To-Date. Retrieved June 25, 2011.

Haydon, S. (2009). Pharmacological options for treatment of migraine. *Nurse Prescribing, 7*(7), 300–308.

Karch, A. M. (2012). *2012 Lippincott's nursing drug guide.* Philadelphia, PA: Lippincott Williams & Wilkins.

Koch, H. J., & Jurgens, T. P. (2009). Antidepressants in long-term migraine prevention. *Drugs, 69*(1), 1–19.

Kuhn, M. A., & Winston, D. *Herbal therapy supplements a scientific and traditional approach* (2nd ed.). Philadelphia, PA: Lippincott Williams & Wilkins.

Martin, V. T., & Lipton, R. B. (2008). Epidemiology and biology of menstrual migraine. *Headache: The Journal of Head and Face Pain, 48*(Suppl 3), S124–S130.

MacGregor, E. A. (2010). Prevention and treatment of menstrual migraine. *Drugs, 70*(14), 1799–1818.

May, A. (2011). *Cluster headache: Acute and preventive treatment.* Up-To-Date. Retrieved July 2, 2011.

May, A. (2011). *Cluster headache. Epidemiology, clinical features, and diagnosis.* Up-To-Date. Retrieved July 2, 2011.

Porth, C. & Matfin, G. (2009). *Pathophysiology: Concepts of Altered Health Status.* (8th ed.). Philadelphia, PA: Lippincott Williams & Wilkins.

Sahai-Srivastava, S., Desai, P., & Zheng, L. (2008). Analysis of headache management in a busy emergency room in the United States. *Headache: The Journal of Head and Face Pain,* June, 931–938.

Silberstein, S.; American Academy of Neurology (2000). Neurology practice parameter: Evidence-based guidelines for migraine headache (an evidence-based review): Report of the Quality Standards Subcommittee of the American Academy of Neurology. *Neurology, 55*(6), 754. Information current retrieved June 25, 2011.

Smeltzer, S. C., Bare, B. G., Hinkle, J. H., & Cheever, K. H. (2010). *Brunner and Suddarth's textbook of medical-surgical nursing* (12th ed.). Philadelphia, PA: Lippincott Williams & Wilkins.

Solomon, G. D. & Jamieson, D. G. (2009). Common Headache Disorders: Diagnosis and Management Part I. 15(11), 125–132.

Solomon, G. D. & Jamieson, D. G. (2009). Common Headache Disorders: Diagnosis and Management Part II. 15(12), 133–144.

Suthisisang, C. C., Poolsup, N., Suksomboon, N., Lertpipopmetha, V., & Tepwitukgid, B. (2010). Meta-analysis of the efficacy and safety of naproxen sodium in the acute treatment of migraine. *Headache: The Journal of Head and Face Pain, 50*(5), 808–818.

Taylor, F. R. *Tension-type headache in adults: Acute treatment.* Up-To-Date. Retrieved July 2, 2011.

Taylor, F. R. *Tension-type headache in adults: Pathophysiology, clinical features, and diagnosis.* Up-To-Date. Retrieved July 2, 2012.

Up-To-Date. (2011) *Abortive treatment of migraine: Oral and inhalation medications.* Retrieved October 15, 2011.

Up-To-Date. (2011). *Acetaminophen, aspirin, and caffeine: Drug information.* Retrieved July 2, 2011.

Up-To-Date. (2011). *Ergotamine: Drug information.* Retrieved September 6, 2011.

Up-To-Date. (2011). *Sumatriptan and naproxen: Drug information.* Retrieved October 17, 2011.

Whyte, C., Tepper, S. J., & Evans, R. W. (2010). Rescue me: Medication for migraine. *Headache: The Journal of Head and Face Pain,* February, 307–313.

Wolter's Kluwer Health (2012). *Stedman's medical dictionary for the health professions and nursing* (7th ed.). Philadelphia, PA: Lippincott Williams & Wilkins.

52 Drug Therapy for Seizure Disorders and Spasticity

Clinical Application Case Study

Two days ago, Andrew Cummings, a 7-year-old boy, was at home playing and experienced a tonic–clonic seizure, which was witnessed by his mother. On questioning the mother, a pediatric neurologist at the hospital where the boy was admitted determined that the seizure was unprovoked and had a generalized onset. The mother stated that it lasted approximately 3 minutes. The neurologist diagnoses a seizure disorder. Andrew is now taking carbamazepine (Tegretol) 50 mg orally four times per day and sodium valproate (Depakene Syrup) 20 mg/kg/d.

KEY TERMS

Antiepileptic drugs: drugs used to control seizures or convulsions; also referred to as antiseizure medications or anticonvulsants

Clonic: spasms that alternate between contraction and relaxation

Convulsion: tonic–clonic type of seizure characterized by spasmodic contractions of involuntary muscles

Epilepsy: disease where the patient has repetitive seizures

Gingival hyperplasia: overgrowth of the gums related to long-term administration of phenytoin

Malignant hyperthermia: rare but life-threatening complication of anesthesia characterized by hypercarbia, metabolic acidosis, skeletal muscle rigidity, fever, and cyanosis

Monotherapy: use of a single drug in drug therapy; advantages include fewer drug–drug interactions, lower cost, and usually greater patient adherence

Muscle spasm: sudden, involuntary, painful muscle contraction that occurs with musculoskeletal trauma or inflammation

Seizure: brief episode of abnormal electrical activity in nerve cells of the brain that may or may not be accompanied by visible changes in appearance or behavior

Spasticity: caused by nerve damage in the brain and spinal cord, it is a permanent condition that may be painful and disabling; involves increased muscle tone or contraction and stiff, awkward movements

Status epilepticus: repeated seizures or a seizure that lasts at least 30 minutes; may be convulsive, nonconvulsive, or partial

Tonic: muscle spasms with sustained contraction

Tonic–clonic: most common type of seizure; often referred to as a major motor seizure

- **Tonic phase:** sustained contraction of skeletal muscles; abnormal postures, such as opisthotonos; and absence of respirations, during which the person becomes cyanotic

- **Clonic phase:** rapid rhythmic and symmetric jerking movements of the body

Introduction

The first part of this chapter introduces the condition known as **epilepsy**, which is characterized by recurrent seizures, and discusses the pharmacological care of the patient who is experiencing a seizure. Although the terms seizure and convulsion may be used interchangeably, they have different meanings. A **seizure** involves a brief episode of abnormal electrical activity in nerve cells of the brain that may or may not be accompanied by visible changes in appearance or behavior. It refers to all types of epileptic occurrences. A **convulsion** is a tonic–clonic type of seizure characterized by spasmodic contractions of involuntary muscles.

The second part of this chapter describes the role skeletal muscle relaxants play in decreasing seizures and reducing muscle spasms and spasticity associated with neurological and musculoskeletal injuries. A **muscle spasm** is a sudden, involuntary, painful muscle contraction that occurs with musculoskeletal trauma (e.g., overuse or injury of skeletal muscle, twisting a joint, or tearing a ligament as with a sprain) or inflammation (e.g., bursitis, arthritis). Muscle spasm also occurs with acute and chronic low back pain. Spasms may be clonic (alternating contraction and relaxation) to tonic (sustained contraction). Muscle spasms commonly occur, sometimes causing significant disability with inflammation, edema, and poor coordination and mobility.

Spasticity involves increased muscle tone or contraction and stiff, awkward movements. It occurs in neurologic disorders such as multiple sclerosis, spinal cord injury, traumatic brain injury, cerebral palsy, and poststroke syndrome. Because spasticity is caused by nerve damage in the brain and spinal cord, it is a permanent condition that may be painful and disabling.

In patients with spinal cord injury, spasticity requires treatment when it impairs safety, mobility, and the ability to perform activities of daily living (e.g., self-care in hygiene, eating, dressing, and work or recreational activities). Stimuli that precipitate

spasms vary from one individual to another and may include muscle stretching, bladder infections or stones, constipation and bowel distention, or infections. It is necessary to assess each person for personal precipitating factors, so that these factors can be avoided if possible. Treatment measures include passive range-of-motion and muscle-stretching exercises and antispasmodic medications (e.g., baclofen, dantrolene).

Overview of Epilepsy

Sudden, abnormal, hypersynchronous firing of neurons is characteristic of epilepsy. Signs and symptoms of seizure activity lead to the diagnosis. On the electroencephalogram (EEG), abnormal brain wave patterns are present.

Etiology

Seizures may occur as single events in response to hypoglycemia, fever, electrolyte imbalances, overdoses of numerous medications (e.g., amphetamine, cocaine, isoniazid, lidocaine, lithium, methylphenidate, antispasmodics, theophylline), and withdrawal from alcohol or sedative–hypnotic drugs. Alternatively, seizures may be idiopathic (having no discernible cause) or attributable to a secondary cause. Authorities also classify seizures as unprovoked (idiopathic) or provoked (secondary). Secondary causes in infancy include developmental defects, metabolic disease, or birth injury. Fever is a common secondary cause in late infancy and early childhood. Inherited forms of epilepsy usually begin in childhood or adolescence. When epilepsy begins in adulthood, it is often caused by an acquired neurologic disorder (e.g., head injury, stroke, brain tumor) or alcohol and other drug effects. Toxemia is a secondary cause of seizures in pregnancy.

Some of the identified specific causes of seizures include alterations in cell membrane permeability or the distribution of ions across the neuronal cell membranes. Genetic mutations have also been linked to epilepsy. In addition, a decrease in the inhibition of thalamic or cortical neuronal activity is a cause. Finally, imbalances in the neurotransmitters gamma-aminobutyric acid (GABA) or acetylcholine excess result in seizure disorders (Porth & Matfin, 2009).

Pathophysiology

Experts broadly classify seizures as partial or generalized. Partial seizures begin in a specific area of the brain and often indicate a localized brain lesion such as birth injury, trauma, stroke, or tumor. They produce symptoms ranging from simple motor and sensory manifestations to more complex abnormal movements and bizarre behavior. Movements are usually automatic, repetitive, and inappropriate to the situation, such as chewing, swallowing, or aversive movements (automatisms). In simple partial seizures, consciousness is not impaired; in complex partial seizures, the level of consciousness is decreased.

Clinical Manifestations

Generalized seizures are bilateral and symmetric and have no discernible point of origin in the brain. The most common type is the **tonic–clonic** or major motor seizure. The **tonic phase** involves sustained contraction of skeletal muscles; abnormal postures, such as **opisthotonos**; and absence of respiration, during which the person becomes cyanotic. The **clonic phase** is characterized by rapid rhythmic and symmetric jerking movements of the body. Tonic–clonic seizures are sometimes preceded by an aura—a brief warning, such as a flash of light or a specific sound or smell. In children, febrile seizures (i.e., tonic–clonic seizures that occur with fever in the absence of other identifiable causes) are the most common form of epilepsy.

The absence seizure, which is characterized by abrupt alterations in consciousness that last only a few seconds, is a kind of generalized seizure. Other types of generalized seizures include the myoclonic type (contraction of a muscle or group of muscles) and the akinetic type (absence of movement). Some people are subject to mixed seizures.

Status epilepticus is a life-threatening emergency characterized by generalized tonic–clonic convulsions lasting for several minutes or occurring at close intervals. During this time, the patient does not regain consciousness. Hypotension, hypoxia, and cardiac dysrhythmias may also occur. There is a high risk of permanent brain damage and death unless prompt, appropriate treatment is instituted. In a person taking medications for a diagnosed seizure disorder, the most common cause of status epilepticus is abruptly stopping **antiepileptic drugs** (AEDs). In other patients, regardless of whether they have a diagnosed seizure disorder, causes of status epilepticus include brain trauma or tumors, systemic or central nervous system (CNS) infections, alcohol withdrawal, and overdoses of drugs (e.g., cocaine, theophylline).

Drug Therapy

Treatment of the underlying cause or use of an AED may relieve seizures. AEDs can usually control seizure activity but do not cure the underlying disorder. Numerous difficulties, for both clinicians and patients, have been associated with AED therapy,

including trials of different drugs; consideration of **monotherapy** (using a single drug) versus combination therapy (using two or more drugs); the need to titrate dosage over time; lack of seizure control while drugs are being selected and dosages adjusted; social stigma and adverse drug effects, often leading to poor patient adherence; and undesirable drug interactions among AEDs and between AEDs and other medications.

The AEDs used in the prevention and treatment of seizures has evolved over the years. In recent years, the U.S. Food and Drug Administration (FDA) has approved newer medications in the treatment of seizure disorders. The FDA most often classifies these medications as newer or miscellaneous drugs. The medication tables identify the newer drugs primarily as derivatives. Table 52.1 summarizes the drug classes. For specific drugs, other tables identify the AEDs administered, the dosage, pregnancy category, the type of seizure they are used to treat, and the therapeutic serum drug levels. The therapeutic serum drug level is very important because of the risk of drug toxicity.

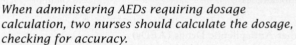

QSEN Safety Alert

When administering AEDs requiring dosage calculation, two nurses should calculate the dosage, checking for accuracy.

Clinical Application 52-1

- According to Andrew's chart, he should receive carbamazepine (Tegretol) 50 mg four times per day. The elixir is 100 mg/5 mL. The boy weighs 56 pounds. How much carbamazepine does the nurse administer?
- The physician has ordered sodium valproate (Depakene) 20 mg/kg/d for Andrew. The elixir is 250 mg/5 mL. How much sodium valproate does the nurse administer?

NCLEX Success

1. A male infant is admitted to the emergency department. His parents report that he had a seizure. The infant's aural temperature is 104.3°F. What is the most likely cause of the seizure?

   A. head injury
   B. developmental delay
   C. sepsis
   D. fever

2. A woman is admitted to the labor and delivery unit with a blood pressure of 200/90 mm Hg. The admitting diagnosis is preeclampsia. The intravenous (IV) magnesium sulfate ordered for this patient prevents?

   A. seizures
   B. myocardial damage
   C. tetany
   D. hypothermia

TABLE 52.1

Drugs Administered for Seizures (Antiepileptic Drugs)

Drug Class	Prototype	Other Drugs in the Class
Drugs Used to Treat Seizure Disorders		
Barbiturates	Phenobarbital (Luminal)	Mephobarbital (Mebaral) Pentobarbital (Nembutal) Primidone (Mysoline) Secobarbital (Seconal Sodium)
Benzodiazepines	Diazepam (Valium)	Clonazepam (Klonopin) Clorazepate (Tranxene) Lorazepam (Ativan)
Gamma-aminobutyric acid (GABA) structural analogs	Gabapentin (Neurontin)	Pregabalin (Lyrica) Tiagabine hydrochloride (Gabitril Filmtabs)
Hydantoins	Phenytoin (Dilantin)	Ethotoin (Peganone) Fosphenytoin (Cerebyx)
Iminostilbenes	Carbamazepine (Tegretol)	Oxcarbazepine (Trileptal)
Sulfonamides	Acetazolamide (Diamox)	Ethosuximide (Zarontin) Zonisamide (Zonegran)
Other Antiepileptic Drugs (AEDs)		
Carboxylic acid derivatives	Valproic acid (Depakene, Depakene Syrup)	
Functionalized amino acids	Lacosamide (Vimpat)	
Mineral electrolytes	Magnesium sulfate	
Phenyltriazine derivatives	Lamotrigine (Lamictal)	
Pyrrolidine derivatives	Levetiracetam (Keppra)	
Sulfamate-substituted monosaccharides	Topiramate (Topamax)	
Triazole derivatives	Rufinamide (Banzel)	

3. A patient is having a seizure that lasts longer than 30 minutes. What type of generalized seizure is the patient experiencing?

A. tonic–clonic
B. absence seizure
C. atonic seizure
D. status epilepticus

4. A patient is admitted to the emergency department with repeated tonic–clonic seizures. Tonic–clonic seizures may be attributed to which of following drugs?

A. ciprofloxacin hydrochloride (Cipro)
B. cimetidine (Tagamet)
C. cocaine
D. morphine sulfate

Drugs Used to Treat Seizure Disorders

BARBITURATES

ⓟ Phenobarbital (Luminal) is the prototype AED of the barbiturate class. Since its development in 1912, it has been used as an antiepileptic or sedative.

Pharmacokinetics

Phenobarbital, like all barbiturates, is absorbed rapidly through the gastrointestinal (GI) tract, usually within 1 hour. The oral drug has an onset of action of 30 to 60 minutes and a duration of 10 to 16 hours. The IV form begins to act in 5 minutes and lasts for 4 to 6 hours. Phenobarbital has a half-life of 50 to 140 hours. The drug takes approximately 2 to 3 weeks to reach therapeutic serum levels and 3 weeks to reach a steady-state concentration. It is also lipid bound, which means that it crosses the placenta and is present in breast milk. Phenobarbital is metabolized in the liver and excreted by the renal system.

Action

Phenobarbital depresses the CNS by inhibiting the conduction of impulses in the ascending reticular activating system, thus depressing the cerebral cortex and cerebellar function. Figure 52.1 indicates the site of action of barbiturates, along with other antiepileptic drugs.

Use

Prescribers order oral phenobarbital as a sedative and antiepileptic agent in the treatment of generalized tonic–clonic and partial seizures. Clinicians use the parenteral form to control acute seizures. Table 52.2 gives route and dosage information for phenobarbital and other barbiturates.

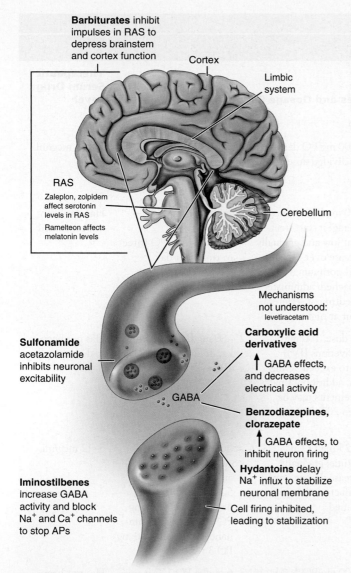

Barbiturates inhibit impulses in RAS to depress brainstem and cortex function

Cortex

Limbic system

RAS
Zaleplon, zolpidem affect serotonin levels in RAS
Ramelteon affects melatonin levels

Cerebellum

Mechanisms not understood:
levetiracetam

Sulfonamide
acetazolamide inhibits neuronal excitability

Carboxylic acid derivatives
↑ GABA effects, and decreases electrical activity

GABA

Benzodiazepines, clorazepate
↑ GABA effects, to inhibit neuron firing

Hydantoins delay Na⁺ influx to stabilize neuronal membrane

Iminostilbenes
increase GABA activity and block Na⁺ and Ca⁺ channels to stop APs

Cell firing inhibited, leading to stabilization

Figure 52.1 Sites of action of antiepileptic drugs. AP, action potential; GABA, gamma-aminobutyric acid; RAS, reticular activating system. (Adapted from Karch, A.M. (2013). *Focus on nursing pharmacology.* (5th ed.). Philadelphia, PA: Wolters Kluwer Health | Lippincott Williams & Wilkins.)

Use in Older Adults

Older adults may experience greater sedation, due to decreased absorption and altered renal excretion of phenobarbital, placing them at risk for injury. These patients may also be at risk for adverse drug reactions related to altered metabolism and excretion.

Use in Patients With Renal or Hepatic Impairment

Patients who have decreased creatinine clearance (CrCl) may not be able to excrete phenobarbital adequately. Patients with hepatic impairment require a lower dose to prevent adverse effects associated with the drug.

Use in Patients With Critical Illness

When administering phenobarbital parenterally, it is best to do so in a critical care unit. This allows for constant monitoring of drug effects and early resuscitation in the event of respiratory arrest.

Adverse Effects

As with all AEDs, CNS depression, possibly cognitive impairment with sedation, is the most common adverse effect. Other reported conditions include somnolence, agitation, confusion, vertigo, and nightmares. The most severe adverse effect is Stevens-Johnson syndrome, a hypersensitivity reaction. Respiratory problems may occur, particularly with parenteral phenobarbital. Sudden withdrawal of the medication places the patient at risk for status epilepticus. The FDA has issued a **BLACK BOX WARNING** ◆ for phenobarbital. Patients who take phenobarbital are at risk for suicidal ideation. It is important to monitor the patient for statements that indicate depression and suicide.

Contraindications

Contraindications to phenobarbital include a known hypersensitivity to barbiturates. Other contraindications include liver failure, nephritis, porphyria, respiratory depression, pregnancy, or addiction to barbiturates. Caution is necessary in acute or chronic pain, lactation, fever, hyperthyroidism, diabetes, decreased liver renal function, and pulmonary and cardiac disease.

Nursing Implications

Preventing Interactions

Several drugs interact with phenobarbital, increasing its effects (Box 52.1). Opioid analgesics combined with phenobarbital result in enhanced CNS depression. When administered with phenobarbital, corticosteroids, doxycycline, estrogens, hormonal contraceptives, oral anticoagulants, and tricyclic antidepressants have an increased metabolism and a decreased effect. Oil of primrose increases the effects of phenobarbital.

Administering the Medication

Oral administration of phenobarbital may occur without regard to food. Parenteral administration may involve combining the medication with dextrose, lactated Ringer's, or normal saline. However, if a precipitate forms, administration should not take place. Also, the drug is incompatible with acidic solutions, amphotericin B, chlorpromazine, diphenhydramine, insulin, and vancomycin. The nurse always injects IV phenobarbital into large veins at an infusion rate no faster than 60 mg/min. Inadvertent intra-arterial injection can cause spasm of the artery and gangrene. When administering the intramuscular (IM) drug, the nurse uses a large needle and injects into deep muscle.

Assessing for Therapeutic Effects

The ultimate goal of therapy with phenobarbital is to decrease seizure effects. The patient's EEG reveals decreased brain waves consistent with seizure activity.

Assessing for Adverse Effects

The nurse assesses for increases in CNS activity consistent with paradoxical excitation, as noted most often in the elderly. It is essential to assess respiratory problems such as hypoventilation, apnea, respiratory depression, laryngospasm, bronchospasm, and circulatory collapse, particularly in patients receiving parenteral phenobarbital. In addition, it is necessary to

TABLE 52.2

DRUGS AT A GLANCE: Barbiturates

Drug	Pregnancy Category	Type of Seizure Treated	Routes and Dosage Ranges		Therapeutic Serum Drug Level
			Adults	Children	
Phenobarbital (Luminal)	D	Generalized tonic–clonic and partial seizures	100–300 mg PO daily in 2–3 divided doses	5 mg/kg PO per day in 2–3 divided doses Neonates, intramuscular (IM)	10–25 mcg/mL
Mephobarbital (Mebaral)	D	Partial and generalized tonic–clonic and cortical focal seizures	32–100 mg PO 3 times/d (average); start treatment low and gradually increase over 4–5 d until optimum dosage is reached; administer at bedtime if seizures occur at night	<5 y, 16–32 mg PO 3–4 times/d >5 y, 32–64 mg PO three to times per day	Has not been determined
Pentobarbital (Nembutal)	D	Acute seizure episodes associated with anesthesia, eclampsia, meningitis, tetanus, and status epilepticus	Initial dose, 100 mg intravenous (IV), not to exceed 50 mg/min; additional small increments may be given 200–500 mg	25–80 mg IM or 206 mg/kg; do not exceed 100 mg	Has not been determined
Primidone (Mysoline)	D	Tonic–clonic, psychomotor, and focal seizures	100–125 mg PO at bedtime; gradually increase dosage until satisfactory dosage is attained	>8 y, adult dosage <8 y, day 1–3, 50 mg PO at bedtime; day 4–6, 50 mg PO 2 times/d; day 7–9, 100–125 mg PO 2 times/d; maintenance dose, 125–250 mg PO 3 times/d	5–12 mcg/mL
Secobarbital sodium (Seconal Sodium)	D	Preanesthesia prevention of seizures	200–300 mg PO 1–2 h before surgery	2–6 mg/kg PO 1–2 h before surgery; maximum dose 100 mg	Has not been determined

- Assess for bradycardia, hypotension, and syncope
- Assess the serum drug level for signs of toxicity or inadequate seizure treatment
- Assess for changes in the integumentary system indicative of the onset of Stevens-Johnson syndrome

---

BOX 52.1 — Drug Interactions: Phenobarbital

Drugs That Increase the Effects of Phenobarbital

■ Alcohol, chloramphenicol, diazepam, monoamine oxidase inhibitors
  May increase central nervous system (CNS) and respiratory depression
■ Gabapentin, valproic acid
  Increase serum level
■ Mephobarbital, primidone
  May increase serum level

Patient Teaching

Box 52.2 identifies patient teaching guidelines for phenobarbital.

BENZODIAZEPINES

Drugs belonging to this class have a broad range of uses; they may act as antidepressants, antiepileptics, or skeletal muscle relaxants. The benzodiazepines potentiate the effects of GABA by increasing the attraction to the receptor sites. The prototype of this class is **(P) diazepam** (Valium). See Figure 52.1 for the increased effects of GABA by benzodiazepines.

Pharmacokinetics

This varies with the preparation of diazepam. For the IV drug, the onset of action is 1 to 5 minutes, with a peak of 30 minutes and a duration of 15 to 60 minutes. For the oral drug, the onset of action of 30 to 60 minutes, with a peak of 1 to 2 hours and a

BOX 52.2   Patient Teaching Guidelines for Phenobarbital

- Understand that this drug is administered long term for the treatment of seizure activity.
- Take the medication as prescribed, and do not stop the medication abruptly.
- Have regular tests to determine serum levels of the drug.
- Change positions slowly. This drug may cause drowsiness or syncope.
- Do not drive or operate machinery with central nervous system (CNS) depression.
- If you are of childbearing age, use two forms of contraception.
- Notify your prescriber about the development of rashes or skin eruptions.
- Wear a medical alert bracelet or necklace stating that you have a seizure disorder and naming the medications you take.

duration of 3 hours. For the IM drug, the onset of action is generally within 15 to 30 minutes, with a peak of 30 to 45 minutes and a duration of 3 hours. For the rectal drug, the onset is rapid, with a peak of 1.5 hours and a duration of 3 hours. Its half-life, which is longer in newborns and the elderly, is 20 to 80 hours.

Diazepam crosses the placenta and enters the breast milk. It is metabolized by the liver and excreted by the kidneys.

Action

The exact mechanism of action of diazepam is unknown. However, authorities believe that the drug acts primarily on the limbic system and reticular formation to produce skeletal muscle relaxation. It potentiates the effect of GABA by increasing the attraction of the medication to the receptor sites.

Use

IV diazepam is an adjunctive skeletal muscle relaxant administered for the treatment of severe recurrent convulsive seizures and status epilepticus. Oral diazepam is an adjunctive agent used for seizure disorders. Clinicians also order benzodiazepines such as diazepam for treatment of Lennox-Gastaut syndrome, a mixed seizure disorder that presents at approximately 2 years of age. Table 52.3 gives route and dosage information for diazepam and other benzodiazepines.

Use in Children

IV diazepam is recommended for use in children age 1 month or older. Newborns require a lower dose. Oral diazepam is recommended for children older than 6 months of age. Rectal administration is not recommended in children younger than 2 years of age.

Use in Older Adults

It is necessary to reduce the dosage of diazepam administered to older adults because the drug has an extended half-life in this population.

Use in Patients With Renal or Hepatic Impairment

Diazepam is excreted by the kidneys after being metabolized in the liver. Thus, patients with renal or hepatic impairment should take reduced dosages of diazepam.

Use in Patients With Critical Illness

Patients with critical illness or those in debilitated states should take reduce dosages of diazepam. During IV administration, patients should receive oxygen.

Adverse Effects

CNS adverse effects of diazepam include depression, disorientation, restlessness, and confusion. In the first 2 weeks of treatment, paradoxical excitatory reactions may occur. The most serious cardiovascular adverse effect is cardiovascular collapse with bradycardia and hypotension. Also, potentially life-threatening tachycardia may occur. Other reported problems include constipation, diarrhea, incontinence, urinary retention, and changes in libido.

Contraindications

Patients with known hypersensitivity to benzodiazepines should not receive diazepam. Contraindications also include acute narrow-angle glaucoma, shock, coma, acute alcohol intoxication, and pregnancy.

Nursing Implications

Preventing Interactions

Many medications and herbs interact with diazepam, decreasing or increasing its effects (Boxes 52.3 and 52.4).

Administering the Medication

When preparing diazepam, the nurse does not mix the drug in plastic bags or tubing or combine it with other solutions. During administration, it is important to monitor pulse, blood pressure, and respiration. During parenteral administration, it is necessary to administer oxygen as well as to put the patient on bedrest for 3 hours. The nurse injects the IV form of the drug slowly into a large vein at 1 mL/min—over at least 3 minutes in children—never intra-arterially or into small veins. Intra-arterial administration results in arterial spasm.

Assessing for Therapeutic Effects

When administering diazepam for a seizure disorder, the goal of therapy is to control seizure activity. When administering drug for status epilepticus, the goal is to eliminate the seizure activity.

Assessing for Adverse Effects

The nurse assesses for changes in cardiovascular status that could indicate hypotension, bradycardia, or tachycardia. He or she closely monitors the CNS response. In addition, the nurse assesses for alterations in elimination patterns.

TABLE 52.3

DRUGS AT A GLANCE: Benzodiazepines

Drug	Pregnancy Category	Type of Seizure Treated	Routes and Dosage Ranges		Therapeutic Serum Drug Level
			Adults	Children	
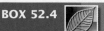 **Diazepam** (Valium)	D	Status epilepticus	Seizure control: 2–10 mg PO 3–4 times/d Status epilepticus: 5–10 mg intravenous (IV) slowly administered; may repeat every 5–10 min; maximum dose of 30 mg	Status epilepticus: older than 1 mo and younger than 5 y, 0.2–0.5 mg slowly IV every 2–5 min up to a maximum dose of 5 mg 5 y and older, 1 mg IV every 2–5 min up to a maximum dose of 10 mg	Has not been determined
Clonazepam (Klonopin)	D	Myoclonic or akinetic seizures, alone or with other antiepileptic drugs (AEDs); possibly effective in generalized tonic, clonic, and psychomotor seizures	1.5 mg PO daily increased by 0.5 mg/d every 3–7 d if necessary; maximum dose, 20 mg/d	0.01–0.03 mg/kg/d PO, increased by 0.25–0.5 mg/d every 3–7 ds if necessary; maximum dose, 0.2 mg/kg/d	20–80 ng/mL
Clorazepate (Tranxene)	D	Partial seizures, with other AEDs	7.5 mg PO 3 times daily maximum initial dose; increased by 7.5 mg every week, if necessary; maximum dose 90 mg/d	>12 y, same as adults 9–12 y, 7.5 mg PO 2 times daily maximum initial dose; increased by 7.5 mg every week, if necessary; maximum dose 60 mg/d	Has not been determined
Lorazepam (Ativan)	D	Status epilepticus	18 y and older, 4 mg IV slowly at 2 mg/min; may give another 4 mg after 10–15 min if needed	Not recommended in children younger than 12 y	Has not been determined

AED, antiepileptic drug.

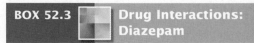

BOX 52.3 — Drug Interactions: Diazepam

Drugs That Increases the Effect of Diazepam
- Alcohol, omeprazole
  Increase central nervous system (CNS) depression
- Cimetidine, disulfiram, and hormonal contraceptives
  Increase pharmacological effects

Drugs That Decrease the Effects Diazepam
- Theophylline, ranitidine
  Decrease pharmacological effects

BOX 52.4 — Herb and Dietary Interactions: Diazepam

Herbs and Foods That Increase the Effect of Diazepam
- Kava
- Valerian
- Grapefruit juice

BOX 52.5	Patient Teaching Guidelines for Diazepam

- Take the medication as prescribed and do not skip doses or stop therapy.
- Do not use alcohol or smoke. Alcohol is more potent when combined with diazepam. Smoking may constrict blood vessels, resulting in reduced elimination of the drug.
- Obtain instructions about the administration of rectal diazepam.
- Use two types of contraceptives if you are a woman of childbearing age and are sexually active.
- Ask your prescriber about safety and central nervous system (CNS) depression. Protect yourself from falls. Do not drive or operate machinery if you have CNS depression.
- Wear a medical alert bracelet or necklace stating that you have a seizure disorder and naming the medications you take.

Patient Teaching

Box 52.5 identifies patient teaching guidelines for diazepam.

Clinical Application 52-2

- During a hospitalization, Andrew has an episode of status epilepticus. His neurologist orders diazepam (Valium) 1 mg IV every 2 to 5 minutes, with a maximum dosage of 10 mg. How does the nurse administer the medication?
- What assessments and interventions are necessary to implement before, during, and after the administration of diazepam?

NCLEX Success

5. Which of the following medications is administered for status epilepticus?

A. phenytoin (Dilantin)
B. diazepam (Valium)
C. levetiracetam (Keppra)
D. mephobarbital (Mebaral)

6. A patient is taking phenobarbital (Luminal) for a seizure disorder. Which of the following statements indicates that the patient should be seen by a health care provider immediately?

A. "I have a rash that started on my trunk, and now it is on my arms and legs."
B. "I rest if I feel tired."
C. "I take my medication routinely and do not skip doses."
D. "I have my blood levels checked if my breathing decreases."

7. A patient stops taking clonazepam (Klonopin). What adverse effect will occur?

A. status epilepticus
B. bone marrow depression
C. cerebral edema
D. lethargy

GAMMA-AMINOBUTYRIC ACID STRUCTURAL ANALOGS

In 1993, the FDA approved **Ⓟ gabapentin** (Neurontin) for treatment of partial seizures. In May of 2002, the FDA approved it for treatment of postherpetic neuralgia pain.

Pharmacokinetics and Action

Gabapentin reaches its peak in 1 hour. Metabolism occurs in the liver and elimination takes place in the urine. The drug crosses the placenta and may enter the breast milk.

Its antiepileptic action is related to its ability to inhibit postsynaptic responses and block post-tetanic potentiation.

Use

Prescribers order gabapentin as an adjunctive treatment for partial seizures. Table 52.4 gives route and dosage information for gabapentin and other GABA structural analogs.

Use in Patients With Renal Impairment

Patients with impaired renal function may require dosage adjustment depending on their CrCl.

Use in Patients With Hepatic Impairment

Patients with impaired liver function require monitoring for elevated liver enzymes.

Adverse Effects

The most common adverse effects of gabapentin are associated with CNS depression and include dizziness, somnolence, insomnia, and ataxia. Other reported adverse effects are pruritus, dry mouth, dyspepsia, nausea, vomiting, and suicidal ideation.

Contraindications

Contraindications to gabapentin include a known hypersensitivity to the medication.

Nursing Implications

Preventing Interactions

Antacids do not affect the serum level but they decrease absorption of gabapentin when administered at the same time. The herb *Ginkgo biloba* decreases the effect of the drug.

Administering the Medication

The nurse ensures that gabapentin is taken orally. People may take the drug with food to prevent GI upset.

TABLE 52.4

DRUGS AT A GLANCE: Gamma-Aminobutyric Acid Structural Analogs

Drug	Pregnancy Category	Type of Seizure Treated	Routes and Dosage Ranges		Therapeutic Serum Drug Level
			Adults	Children	
Ⓟ **Gabapentin** (Neurontin)	C	Partial seizures	Epilepsy: 300 mg PO 3 times/d initially Maintenance: 900–1800 mg/d PO in divided doses 3 times/d; maximum interval between doses should not exceed 12 h; up to 2400–3600 mg/d has been used Postherpetic neuralgia: 300 mg/d PO initially; 300 mg PO 2 times/d on day 2, 300 mg PO 3 times/d on day 3 Renal impairment: creatinine clearance (CrCl) >60 mL/min, 400 mg 3 times daily (1200 mg/d); CrCl 30–60 mL/min, 300 mg 2 times daily (600 mg/d); CrCl 15–30 mL/min, 300 mg once daily; CrCl <15 mL/min, 300 mg every other day. Patients on hemodialysis: 200–300 mg after each 4 h of hemodialysis	3–12 y, initially 10–15 mg/kg/d PO in three divided doses; 3–4 y, up to 40 mg/kg/d in three divided doses; 5 y and older, adjust upward over about 3 d to 25–35 mg/kg daily in three divided doses	Clinical trial data indicate that monitoring serum levels is not necessary for safe use
Pregabalin (Lyrica)	C	Partial-onset seizures with other antiepileptic drugs (AEDs)	Epilepsy: 150–600 mg/d PO 2–3 times/d Fibromyalgia: 75–150 mg PO 2 times/d; maximum dose, 450 mg/d Postherpetic pain: 75–150 mg PO 2 times/d; maximum dose, 600 mg/d	Safety and efficacy not established	Has not been determined
Tiagabine (Gabitril)	C	Partial seizures, with other AEDs	4 mg PO daily for 1 wk; increased by 4–8 mg/wk until desired effect; maximum dose 56 mg/d in 2–4 divided doses	<12 y, not recommended 12–18 y, 4 mg PO daily for 1 wk; increased to 8 mg/d in 2 divided doses for 1 wk; then increased by 4–8 mg/wk up to a maximum of 32 mg/d in 2 to 4 divided doses	Has not been determined

AED, antiepileptic drug.

Assessing for Therapeutic and Adverse Effects

The nurses assesses for the absence of partial seizures, the most important therapeutic effect.

It is also necessary to assess changes in mood and personality in patients receiving gabapentin, as with all antiepileptic medications, because suicidal ideation is the result of CNS depression. The nurse assesses for CNS depression that could affect patient safety.

Patient Teaching

Box 52.6 identifies patient teaching guidelines for gabapentin.

- Take the medication as prescribed and do not stop taking it abruptly.
- Take the medication with food to decrease gastrointestinal (GI) discomfort.
- Do not cut, crush, or chew extended-release capsules. If swallowing is difficult, sprinkle the contents of the capsule over soft food.
- Notify your prescriber if seizure activity occurs.
- You may experience nausea, vomiting, insomnia, fatigue, and confusion.
- Do not drive or operate machinery with central nervous system (CNS) depression.
- Report severe nausea and vomiting, changes in stool or urine color, diarrhea, or changes in neurologic function to the prescriber.

HYDANTOINS

The prototype antiepileptic of the hydantoin class is **℗ phenytoin** (Dilantin). The oldest and most widely used AED, it is often the initial drug of choice, especially in adults. In addition to using it to treat seizure disorders, prescribers sometimes order it for cardiac dysrhythmias.

Pharmacokinetics

Phenytoin is highly bound (90%) to plasma proteins, and only the free drug (the fraction not bound to plasma albumin) is therapeutically active. The oral preparation, absorbed by the GI tract, has a slow onset of action, with a peak of 2 to 12 hours and a duration of 6 to 12 hours. The IV preparation has an onset of action of 1 to 2 hours with a rapid peak and a duration of 12 to 24 hours. The drug is metabolized by the liver and excreted in the urine.

Action

Phenytoin stabilizes the neuronal membrane by delaying the influx of sodium ions into the neurons and preventing the excitability caused by excessive stimulation. See Figure 52.1 for the site of action of hydantoins.

Use

Clinicians use phenytoin to control tonic–clonic seizures, psychomotor seizures, and nonepileptic seizures. They also use it to prevent seizure activity in patients during and following neurosurgery and brain injury. Table 52.5 gives route and dosage information for phenytoin and the other hydantoins.

Phenytoin is available in several forms: a capsule (generic, Dilantin), chewable tablet, oral suspension, and injectable solution. Patients should not switch between generic and trade

TABLE 52.5

DRUGS AT A GLANCE: Hydantoins

Drug	Pregnancy Category	Type of Seizure Treated	Routes and Dosage Ranges Adults	Children	Therapeutic Serum Drug Level
℗ **Phenytoin** (Dilantin)	D	Generalized tonic–clonic and some partial seizures Prevention and treatment of seizures occurring during or after neurosurgery	100 mg PO 3 times daily initially; 300 mg (long-acting) once daily as maintenance Intravenous (IV) 100 mg every 6–8 h; maximum 50 mg/min	Neonates, 15–20 mg/ kg in divided doses of 5–10 mg/kg Older infants and children, 4–7 mg/ kg/d PO in divided doses; dosing is highly variable; dosage adjustment based on serum concentrations	5–20 mcg/mL (40–80 micromol/L)
Ethotoin (Peganone)	D	Tonic–clonic, psychomotor seizures, used with other antiepileptic drugs (AEDs)	1 g/d PO; increase gradually over several days; usual maintenance dose 2–3 g/d in 4–6 divided doses; <2 g/d is ineffective in most adults	750 mg/d PO initially in 4–6 divided doses; maintenance doses range from 500 to 1000 mg/d PO	15–50 mcg/mL
Fosphenytoin (Cerebyx)	D	Status epilepticus	Status epilepticus: 15–20 mg PE/kg administered at 100–150 PE/min	Not recommended	

PE, phenytoin equivalent.

name formulations because of differences in absorption and bioavailability. If a patient becomes stable on a generic drug and then switches to Dilantin, there is a risk of higher serum phenytoin levels and toxicity. If a patient becomes stable on Dilantin and then switches to a generic drug, there is a risk of lower serum phenytoin levels, loss of therapeutic effectiveness, and seizures. (There may also be differences in bioavailability among generic formulations manufactured by different companies.)

Use in Children

When used for status epilepticus, the IV phenytoin dose is determined according to the weight of the child. The recommended dosage is 10 to 15 mg/kg.

Use in Older Adults

It is necessary to administer phenytoin cautiously to older adults. Elderly patients may have altered albumin levels, decreasing the affinity of phenytoin for albumin and causing displacement of the drug.

Use in Patients With Renal Impairment

Renal impairment or failure also causes displacement of the drug, placing the patient at risk for toxicity.

Use in Patients With Hepatic Impairment

Hepatic impairment results in altered albumin levels, decreasing the affinity of phenytoin for albumin and causing displacement of the drug.

Use in Patients With Critical Illness

The IV administration of phenytoin can result in cardiovascular collapse. It is important to assess blood pressure, pulse, and respirations. Monitoring the patient's cardiovascular status is necessary with the use of telemetry.

Adverse Effects

The most common adverse effects of phenytoin affect the CNS (e.g., ataxia, drowsiness, lethargy) and GI tract (e.g., nausea, vomiting). **Gingival hyperplasia,** an overgrowth of gum tissue, is also common, especially in children. Long-term use may lead to an increased risk of osteoporosis because of its effect on vitamin D metabolism. Serious reactions are uncommon but may include allergic reactions, hepatitis, nephritis, bone marrow depression, and mental confusion.

Contraindications

Contraindications to phenytoin include a known hypersensitivity to the hydantoins. Other conditions that require caution are seizures related to hypoglycemia, sinus bradycardia, heart block, and Stokes-Adams syndrome. In patients exhibiting seizures related to hypoglycemia, the primary treatment involves interventions to increase blood glucose (not the use of AEDs). Given the sedative effects associated with phenytoin, the patient is at risk for decreased heart rate; thus, frequent assessment of cardiac output is required if phenytoin is administered to these patients. Caution is also required when administering

---

BOX 52.7 **Drug Interactions: Phenytoin***

Drugs That Increase the Effects of Phenytoin
- Alcohol, amiodarone, chloramphenicol, omeprazole, ticlopidine
  Increase phenytoin levels

Drugs That Decrease the Effects of Phenytoin
- Enteral feedings
  Decrease phenytoin absorption

*Complex interactions and effects may occur when phenytoin and valproic acid are taken together. Phenytoin toxicity may result with apparently normal serum phenytoin levels.

---

phenytoin to pregnant women. The risk of birth defects is a significant adverse effect.

Nursing Implications

Preventing Interactions

Several medications interact with phenytoin, increasing or decreasing its effects (Box 52.7). The effectiveness of corticosteroids, oral contraceptives, and nisoldipine is reduced when combined with phenytoin. Absorption of folic acid, calcium, and vitamin D is decreased with the administration of phenytoin. The herb *Ginkgo biloba* decreases the effect of the drug.

Administering the Medication

The injectable solution is highly irritating to tissues. Therefore, when giving the drug intravenously, it is necessary to use special techniques.

Assessing for Therapeutic and Adverse Effects

The nurse assess for the absence of tonic–clonic and psychomotor seizures.

The nurse assesses for the presence of a rash or skin eruption indicative of a hypersensitivity reaction; the presence of a skin eruption could be indicative of Stevens-Johnson syndrome. In addition, the nurse assesses for cardiovascular collapse with IV administration.

Patient Teaching

Box 52.8 identifies patient teaching guidelines for phenytoin.

IMINOSTILBENES

The AEDs classified as the iminostilbenes include the prototype Ⓟ **carbamazepine** (Tegretol).

Pharmacokinetics

Carbamazepine is administered orally and absorbed by the GI tract. The onset of action is slow in both the oral and oral extended-release preparations. The regular oral preparation peaks in 4 to 5 hours, whereas the extended-release preparation

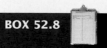

BOX 52.8 Patient Teaching Guidelines for Phenytoin

- Take the drug as prescribed and do not stop taking it abruptly.
- Take the medication with food to prevent gastric upset.
- Have serum drug levels checked as ordered by your prescriber.
- Maintain good oral hygiene (regular brushing and flossing) to prevent gum disease.
- Have regular dental check-ups.
- Use contraception if you are of childbearing age and are sexually active.
- Wear a medical alert bracelet or necklace, stating that you have a seizure disorder and naming the medications you take.

peaks in 3 to 12 hours. The half-life of the drug is 12 to 17 hours. It is metabolized by the liver and excreted in the feces and urine. Carbamazepine crosses the placenta and enters breast milk.

Action

The mechanism of action of carbamazepine is not understood, but its antiepileptic activity may be related to inhibition of polysynaptic responses that block post-tetanic potentiation.

Like the tricyclic antidepressants, the drug affects sodium channels within the cortical neurons. It has the ability to decrease action potential of the cell by inhibiting the influx of sodium into the cell. See Figure 52.1 for the site of action of the iminostilbenes.

Use

Clinicians use carbamazepine to prevent partial seizures with complex symptoms, as in patients with psychomotor and temporal lobe epilepsy. Prescribers order the drug for generalized tonic–clonic and mixed seizures, either partial or generalized. Patients who have uncontrolled seizures or CNS depression on other AEDs use it commonly. Table 52.6 presents route and dosage information for carbamazepine and another iminostilbene.

Use in Older Adults

Carbamazepine may result in increased sedation and confusion. It is necessary to assess patient safety when using this medication in older adults.

Use in Patients With Renal or Hepatic Impairment

Caution is necessary with carbamazepine in patients with renal or hepatic impairment. The drug may cause hepatic cellular necrosis.

TABLE 52.6

DRUGS AT A GLANCE: Iminostilbenes

Drug	Pregnancy Category	Type of Seizure Treated	Routes and Dosage Ranges		Therapeutic Serum Drug Level
			Adults	*Children*	
℗ **Carbamazepine** (Tegretol)	D	Partial Generalized tonic–clonic Mixed seizures	Epilepsy: 200 mg PO twice daily, increased gradually to 600–1200 mg daily if needed, in 3 or 4 divided doses Trigeminal neuralgia: 200 mg PO daily, increased gradually Bipolar disorder: 400 mg PO in divided doses, increased gradually to 1600 mg if necessary	Epilepsy: 6–12 y, 100 mg PO twice daily (tablet) or 50 mg 4 times daily (suspension), increase to 1000 mg daily if necessary in 3–4 divided doses; >12 y, 200 mg PO twice daily, increase to 1000 mg daily for children 12–15 y and 1200 mg for children older than 15 y	4–12 mcg/mL
Oxcarbazepine (Trileptal)	C	Partial seizures, as monotherapy or with other antiepileptic drugs (AEDs) in adults, with other AEDs in children 4–16 y old	600 mg PO twice daily (1200 mg/d); maximum dose, 2400 mg/d Severe renal impairment creatinine clearance (CrCl <30 mL/min): 300 mg PO twice daily (600 mg/d) and increased slowly until response achieved	With other AEDs, 8–10 mg/kg/d PO, not to exceed 600 mg twice daily; titrate to reach target dose over 2 wk	Monitor serum sodium levels prior to beginning therapy and periodically during drug therapy

AED, antiepileptic drug.

Adverse Effects

Carbamazepine may have serious adverse effects. The FDA has issued a **BLACK BOX WARNING** ◆ for carbamazepine concerning aplastic anemia and agranulocytosis. Other adverse effects include heart block, Stevens-Johnson syndrome, respiratory depression, hepatitis, massive hepatic cellular necrosis with total loss of intact liver tissue, and suicidal ideation.

Contraindications

Contraindications include a hypersensitivity reaction to carbamazepine or tricyclic antidepressants as well as administration of monoamine oxidase inhibitors. Caution is warranted in patients with a history of increased intraocular pressure; adverse hematologic reaction to other medications; cardiac, hepatic, or renal damage; and latent psychosis.

Nursing Implications

Preventing Interactions

Some medications interact with carbamazepine, increasing or decreasing its effects (Box 52.9). Warfarin combined with carbamazepine produces greater anticoagulant effects. The herb *Ginkgo biloba* decreases the effect of the drug.

Administering the Medication

It is essential that carbamazepine not be administered within 14 days of use of a monoamine oxidase inhibitor. The nurse should tell patients never to crush or chew extended-release tablets. When the nurse administers carbamazepine suspension, he or she never mixes the preparation with other liquid medications because a precipitate may develop. The nurse ensures that the medication is taken with food to prevent GI upset.

Assessing for Therapeutic Effects

The nurse assesses the patient for absence of partial, tonic–clonic, and mixed seizures.

Assessing for Adverse Effects

There is a risk of aplastic anemia with the administration of carbamazepine, and hematologic assessments are most important. The nurse also assesses the integumentary system for Stevens-Johnson syndrome. It is also important that he or she assess hepatic function to check for hepatic adverse effects, including hepatic failure.

In addition, to prevent toxicity, the nurse assesses serum levels as ordered.

Patient Teaching

Box 52.10 identifies patient teaching guidelines for carbamazepine.

Clinical Application 52-3

- If Andrew receives a carbamazepine suspension at 9:00 AM, when will the peak serum level be reached?
- At 10 years of age, Andrew develops petechiae on his face and bruising on his arms and legs. His mother calls the pediatric nurse practitioner. What does this nurse suspect is the cause of the bruising?

SULFONAMIDES

The sulfonamide diuretic ℗ **acetazolamide** (Diamox) controls fluid secretion in the CNS. It is an adjuvant medication useful in the treatment of seizures.

Pharmacokinetics and Action

Acetazolamide is absorbed by the GI tract. For regular tablets, the onset of action is 1 hour, the peak is 2 to 4 hours, and the duration of action is 6 to 12 hours. For sustained-release tablets, the onset of action is 2 hours, the peak is 3 to 6 hours, and the duration of action is 6 to 12 hours. The half-life of

---

BOX 52.9 | Drug Interactions: Carbamazepine

Drugs That Increase the Effects of Carbamazepine
- Erythromycin, troleandomycin, cimetidine, danazol, isoniazid, propoxyphene, verapamil
  Increase serum levels and manifestations of toxicity
- Lithium
  Increases central nervous system (CNS) toxicity
- Isoniazid
  Increases the risk of hepatotoxicity

Drugs That Decrease the Effects of Carbamazepine
- Barbiturates
  Decrease serum levels
- Phenytoin, primidone
  Increase drug metabolism without changing seizure control

BOX 52.10 | Patient Teaching Guidelines for Carbamazepine

- Take the medication with food.
- Do not chew or crush extended-release tablets.
- Do not stop taking the medication abruptly.
- Avoid alcohol, sleep agents, or over-the-counter medications.
- Have hematological testing as ordered by your prescriber.
- Use contraceptives if you are of childbearing age and are sexually active.
- Wear medical alert bracelet or necklace stating that you have a seizure disorder and naming the medications you take.
- Report symptoms of bruising or bleeding immediately to your prescriber.

TABLE 52.7

DRUGS AT A GLANCE: Sulfonamides

Drug	Pregnancy Category	Type of Seizure Treated	Routes and Dosage Ranges		Therapeutic Serum Drug Level
			Adults	Children	
Ⓟ **Acetazolamide** (Diamox)	C	Absence and tonic–clonic seizures	8–30 mg/kg/d PO in divided doses given in combination with other antiepileptics; starting dose 250 mg	8–30 mg/kg/d PO in divided doses given in combination with other antiepileptic drugs (AEDs); starting dose 250 mg	Has not been determined
Ethosuximide (Zarontin)	C	Absence seizures, myoclonic, and akinetic epilepsy	500 mg/d PO initially, increased by 250 mg weekly until seizures are controlled or toxicity occurs; maximum dose, 1500 mg/d	250 mg/d PO initially, increased at weekly intervals until seizures are controlled or toxicity occurs; maximum dose, ~750–1000 mg/d	40–100 mcg/mL
Zonisamide (Zonegran)	D	Partial seizures, with other antiepileptic drugs	100–200 mg PO daily as a single dose or as 2–3 divided doses; increase by 100 mg/d every 1–2 wk if necessary; maximum dose, 600 mg daily	<16 y, 1–2 mg/kg PO given once daily or in divided doses twice daily; increase by 1–2 mg/kg/d only every 1–2 wk; target range is 4–8 mg/kg/d	Has not been determined

the drug is 5 to 6 hours. Acetazolamide is concentrated in the red blood cells, plasma, and kidneys. The drug is excreted by the kidneys and eliminated in the urine. It crosses the placenta.

The antiepileptic action of acetazolamide is unclear, but it is thought to inhibit CNS carbonic anhydrase to decrease neuronal excitability.

Use

Clinicians use acetazolamide to control absence and tonic–clonic seizures. Table 52.7 presents route and dosage information for acetazolamide and other sulfonamides.

Use in Older Adults

It is necessary to use acetazolamide cautiously in older adults because of an increased risk of diuresis.

Use in Patients With Renal Impairment

In patients with a glomerular filtration rate greater than 50 mL/min, administration of acetazolamide should occur every 6 hours. If the glomerular filtration rate is 10 to 50 mL/min, administration should occur every 12 hours. With a glomerular filtration rate of less than 10 mL/min, the drug is not effective, and the patient should not receive it.

Use in Patients With Hepatic Impairment

Patients with hepatic impairment should not take acetazolamide.

Adverse Effects

The adverse effects of acetazolamide include excessive diuresis, Stevens-Johnson's syndrome, CNS depression, aplastic anemia, leukopenia, thrombocytopenia, hypokalemia, asymptomatic hyperuricemia, and hyperchloremic acidosis.

Contraindications

Contraindications to acetazolamide include hypersensitivity to the drug, hyponatremia, hypokalemia, renal or hepatic insufficiency, and chronic noncongestive angle-closure glaucoma. Administration with thiazide diuretics or antibacterial sulfonamides should not occur.

Nursing Implications

Preventing Interactions

Several medications interact with acetazolamide. There is decreased renal excretion of quinidine, amphetamine, procainamide, and tricyclic antidepressants with acetazolamide. Salicylates and lithium administered with acetazolamide result in diminished renal excretion of these drugs. There is also a risk of salicylate toxicity related to metabolic acidosis with acetazolamide

Administering the Medication

To prevent GI upset, the nurse ensures that the drug is taken with food. Crushing or chewing of regular tablets is permissible, but patients must swallow sustained-release tablets whole. It is

BOX 52.11 **Patient Teaching Guidelines for Acetazolamide**

- Take the medication with food to prevent gastric upset.
- Have annual eye examinations to assess intraocular pressure.
- Report any changes in weight, unusual bruising or bleeding, pain, or rash to your prescriber.

necessary to store the oral preparation in a container with a tight-fitting lid at 59°F to 86°F.

Assessing for Therapeutic and Adverse Effects

The patient should be without symptoms of absence or tonic–clonic seizures.

The nurse assesses the integumentary system for any sign of skin rash or eruption and fluid and electrolyte levels for metabolic acidosis. The patient should have annual eye examinations to determine if there has been an increase in intraocular pressure.

Patient Teaching

Box 52.11 identifies patient teaching guidelines for acetazolamide.

Other Antiepileptic Drugs

CARBOXYLIC ACID DERIVATIVES

Ⓟ **Valproic acid** (Depakene, Depakene Syrup), a carboxylic acid derivative, has been in use for approximately 40 years. A researcher identified its antiseizure ability while studying laboratory rats. The drug is synthesized from valeric acid found in the herb valerian.

Pharmacokinetics

The onset of action for oral valproic acid varies, and it reaches its peak in serum in 1 to 4 hours. Parenteral valproic acid has a rapid onset of action, reaching a peak in 1 hour. The drug is metabolized by the liver and excreted by the kidneys. It crosses the placenta and enters breast milk. See Figure 52.1 for the site of action of the carboxylic acid derivatives.

Action

The action of valproic acid is not understood, but it is thought to produce antiepileptic activity by increasing GABA effects, thus decreasing electrical activity.

Use

Clinicians use valproic acid alone or in combination with other AEDs for the treatment of simple and complex absence seizures, and prescribers also order the drug for the treatment of seizures related to Lennox-Gastaut syndrome. Table 52.8 presents route and dosage information for valproic acid.

Use in Children

Children aged 10 years and older may receive extended-release forms (Depakote ER) for the treatment of epilepsy. Use in children younger than age 10 requires extreme caution; fatal hepatotoxicity has occurred. The nurse must monitor the patient's liver function closely. In addition, caution is warranted in children younger than 18 months of age and those younger than 2 years of age with congenital abnormalities and severe mental disability.

Use in Older Adults

When administering valproic acid to the elderly, it is necessary to adjust the dosage slowly.

Use in Patients With Renal or Hepatic Impairment

Caution is necessary in renal or hepatic impairment.

Adverse Effects

The most life-threatening adverse effects associated with valproic acid are pancreatitis and hepatic failure. Other significant adverse effects include altered bleeding time, thrombocytopenia, bruising, and hemorrhage. The most common GI adverse effects are nausea, vomiting, indigestion, diarrhea, and abdominal cramps. CNS adverse effects include sedation, tremor, emotional upset, weakness, and suicidal ideation.

The FDA has issued several **BLACK BOX WARNINGS ◆** for valproic acid. The first instructs patients to discontinue valproic acid at any sign of pancreatitis. The development of this condition is life threatening. The second points out that valproic acid is a teratogenic medication. Women of childbearing age should not take the drug without using two forms of birth control. The third instructs the patient to check for signs of bleeding or bruising. Altered bleeding times may occur. The nurse should tell the patient to have platelet counts, bleeding time determination, and clotting times according to the prescriber's orders.

Contraindications

Contraindications to valproic acid include significant hepatic impairment as well as a hypersensitivity reaction to the drug.

Nursing Implications

Preventing Interactions

Certain medications interact with valproic acid, decreasing or increasing its effects (Box 52.12). Serum levels of phenobarbital, primidone, ethosuximide, diazepam, lamotrigine, and zidovudine may increase when these drugs are combined with valproic acid. The herb *Ginkgo biloba* decreases the effect of the drug.

Administering the Medication

The nurse dilutes the vial in 5% dextrose, 0.9% sodium chloride, or lactated Ringer's solution for IV administration. The reconstituted medication is stable for 24 hours and does not need to be refrigerated. Infusion should occur over 1 hour, no faster than 20 mg/min. IV administration is permissible only for 14 days, and a switch to an oral preparation is necessary.

TABLE 52.8

DRUGS AT A GLANCE: Other Antiepileptic Drugs

Drug	Pregnancy Category	Type of Seizure Treated	Routes and Dosage Ranges		Therapeutic Serum Drug Level
			Adults	Children	
Ⓟ Valproic acid (Depakene capsules); Sodium valproate (Depakene syrup, Depacon injection); Divalproex sodium (Depakote enteric-coated tablets)	D	Absence, mixed, and complex partial seizures	PO: 10–15 mg/kg/d, increase weekly by 5–10 mg/kg/d, until seizures controlled, adverse effects occur, or maximum dose (60 mg/kg/d) is reached; give amounts >250 mg/d in divided doses; usual daily dose, 1000–1600 mg, in divided doses IV: usual dose, diluted in 5% dextrose or 0.9% sodium chloride injection	15–30 mg/kg/d PO	50–100 mcg/mL (350–700 μmol/L)
Ⓟ Lacosamide (Vimpat)	C	Adjunctive therapy for partial seizures	17 y and older, initially 50 mg PO twice daily; increase at weekly intervals to a maximum daily dosage of 100–200 mg twice daily; intravenous (IV) administration when oral is not feasible Hepatic impairment: 300 mg maximum dosage	Safety and efficacy not established	Not available
Ⓟ Magnesium sulfate	A	Preeclampsia and eclampsia paroxysms	Eclampsia, severe preeclampsia: total initial 10–14 g; may infuse 4–5 g in 250 mL of 5% dextrose while giving intramuscular (IM) doses up to 10 g or may give initial dose of 4 g IV over 3–4 min; then inject 405 g IM into alternate buttocks every 4 h as needed depending on patellar reflex and respiratory function OR, after initial IV dose, 1–2 g/h by constant IV infusion; continue until paroxysms stop; do not exceed 30–40 g in 24 h		6 mg/100 mL

(Continued on page 966)

TABLE 52.8

DRUGS AT A GLANCE: Other Antiepileptic Drugs (Continued)

Drug	Pregnancy Category	Type of Seizure Treated	Routes and Dosage Ranges		Therapeutic Serum Drug Level
			Adults	*Children*	
Ⓟ **Lamotrigine** (Lamictal)	C	Partial seizures, with other antie-pileptic drugs (AEDs) Lennox-Gastaut syndrome, with other AEDs	With AEDs, other than valproic acid: 50 mg PO once daily for 2 wk, then 50 mg twice daily (100 mg/d) for 2 wk, then increase by 100 mg/d at weekly intervals to a main-tenance dose; usual maintenance dose, 300–500 mg/d in 2 divided doses With AEDs, including valproic acid: 25 mg PO every other day for 2 wk, then 25 mg once daily for 2 wk, then increase by 25 to 50 mg/d every 1–2 wk to a maintenance dose; usual maintenance dose: 100–150 mg/d in 2 divided doses	2–12 y, with enzyme-inducing AEDs, initially, PO 0.15 mg/kg/d in 1 or 2 doses for 2 wk; if calcu-lated dose is 2.5–5 mg, give 5 mg on alternate days for 2 wk, then 0.3 mg/kg/d in 1 or 2 doses, rounded to nearest 5 mg, for 2 wk; mainte-nance dose, PO 5–15 mg/kg/d in 2 divided doses >12 y, with enzyme-inducing AEDs, initially, PO 25 mg every other day for 2 wk, then 25 mg daily for 2 wk; maintenance dose, PO 100–400 mg daily in 1 or 2 divided doses; with val-proic acid, PO 50 mg daily for 2 wk, then 100 mg daily in 2 divided doses for 2 wk; maintenance dose, PO 300–500 mg daily in 1 or 2 doses	Has not been determined
Ⓟ **Levetiracetam** (Keppra)	C	Partial seizures, with other AEDs	500 mg PO twice daily initially, increased by 1000 mg/d every 2 wk, if necessary; maximum dose, 3000 mg daily Renal impairment: creati-nine clearance (CrCl >80 mL/min), 500–1500 mg; CrCl 50–80 mL/min, 500–1000 mg; CrCl 30–50 mL/min, 250–750 mg; CrCl <30 mL/min, 250–500 mg End-stage renal disease, on hemodialysis: 500–1000 mg, with a supplemental dose of half the total daily dose (250–500 mg)	Partial seizures or refractory seizures (adjunctive treat-ment): 4–5 y, 10 mg/kg PO twice daily; can increase the daily dose every 2 wk by incre-ments of 20 mg/kg to recommended dose of 30 mg/kg twice daily (60 mg/kg/d)	Has not been determined
Ⓟ **Topiramate** (Topamax)	C	Initial monotherapy for partial seizures or generalized tonic-clonic seizures; partial seizures,	25–50 mg PO daily, increased by 25–50 mg/wk until response; usual dose, 400 mg daily in 2 divided doses	2–16 y, week 1, 25 mg PO every PM, increase by 1–3 mg/kg/d at 1- or 2-wk intervals until response; usual dose 5–9 mg/kg/d, in 2 divided doses Monotherapy: 10 y and older, 25 mg PO twice	Has not been determined

TABLE 52.8

DRUGS AT A GLANCE: Other Antiepileptic Drugs (Continued)

Drug	Pregnancy Category	Type of Seizure Treated	Routes and Dosage Ranges		Therapeutic Serum Drug Level
			Adults	Children	
		generalized tonic clonic, and Lennox-Gastaut syndrome with other AEDs		daily, titrating to mainte- nance dose of 200 mg PO twice daily over 6 wk Week 1: 25 mg twice daily Week 2: 50 mg twice daily Week 3: 75 mg twice daily Week 4: 100 mg twice daily Week 5: 150 mg twice daily Week 6: 200 mg twice daily	
Ⓟ **Rufinamide** (Banzel)	D	Adjunctive treatment of seizures caused by Lennox-Gastaut syndrome	400–800 mg PO in 2 divided doses; maximum dosage 3200 mg/d	4 y and older, 4 mg/kg/d in 2 equally divided doses; target dose, 45 mg/kg/d in 2 equally divided doses	Not available

AED, antiepileptic drug.

When administering Depakote to children, the nurse may open the tablets and sprinkle the contents on applesauce or pudding.

Assessing for Therapeutic Effects

The absence of simple and complex absent seizures is indicative that the therapeutic effects of the valproic acid have been attained.

Assessing for Adverse Effects

The nurse assesses the patient for signs and symptoms of pancreatitis, which include severe abdominal pain and back pain (Smeltzer, Bare, Hinkle, & Cheever, 2010). The nurse should also assess for bleeding and bruising. It is essential that the patient's liver function tests be assessed routinely.

BOX 52.12 Drug Interactions: Valproic Acid*

Drugs That Increase the Effects of Valproic Acid
- Alcohol, central nervous system (CNS) depressants
  Increase sedation
- Chlorpromazine, cimetidine, erythromycin, felbamate, salicylates
  Increase serum levels and toxicity

Drugs That Decrease the Effects of Valproic Acid
- Carbamazepine, charcoal, rifampin
  Decrease drug levels
- Phenytoin

*Phenytoin may increase effects. There are complex interactions between phenytoin and valproic acid; breakthrough seizures have occurred.

Patient Teaching

Box 52.13 identifies patient teaching guidelines for valproic acid.

FUNCTIONALIZED AMINO ACIDS

Ⓟ **Lacosamide** (Vimpat) is a new AED. It is available in oral and IV preparations.

BOX 52.13 Patient Teaching Guidelines for Valproic Acid

- Take medication at regular intervals, do not skip a dose, and do not stop abruptly.
- Do not chew or crush extended-release tablets.
- Avoid alcohol and over-the-counter sleep aids.
- Keep follow-up appointments with your prescriber.
- Keep follow-up appointments for serum blood levels, platelet counts, bleeding and clotting times, liver function, and renal function.
- Use two types of birth control if you are a woman of childbearing age and are sexually active. Notify your prescriber if you become pregnant.
- Do not operate machinery with central nervous system (CNS) depression. You may have sedation, tremors, emotional upset, weakness, or suicidal ideation.
- Know the signs and symptoms of pancreatitis, such as upper abdominal pain and nausea and vomiting, which often begins or worsens after eating.
- If you have diabetes, be aware that this medication interferes with ketones.
- Report any unusual bleeding or bruising.
- Wear a medical alert bracelet or necklace stating that you have a seizure disorder and naming the medications you take.

Pharmacokinetics

Lacosamide is rapidly absorbed. The oral preparation reaches its peak in 1 to 4 hours, and the IV preparation reaches its peak at the end of the infusion. The half-life of the medication is 13 hours. The drug is metabolized by the liver and excreted in the urine. It crosses the placenta and may enter the breast milk.

Action

The mechanism of action of lacosamide is not fully understood. The drug inhibits the voltage-sensitive sodium channels, producing stabilization of the neuronal membrane and inhibition of the repetitive firing of the neuron.

Use

Indications for oral lacosamide include the treatment of partial-onset seizures. Clinicians use the IV drug on a short-term basis when oral administration is prohibited. Table 52.8 gives route and dosage information for lacosamide.

Use in Older Adults

A reduction in dosage in the elderly is not necessary unless renal impairment is apparent (Cross and Curran, 2009). It is important to determine the dosage based on the patient's hepatic and renal function.

Use in Patients With Renal Impairment

Renal function regulates dosage, because the drug is eliminated in the urine. Patients with a CrCl of 30 mL/min or less should receive 300 mg/d as the maximum dosage.

Use in Patients With Hepatic Impairment

It is necessary to titrate the dosage in patients with mild to moderate hepatic impairment. Experts do not recommend use of the drug in patients with severe hepatic impairment, because the drug possesses hepatotoxic adverse effects.

Use in Patients With Critical Illness

Critically ill patients should receive lacosamide intravenously when oral preparation is prohibited. Caution is necessary in the presence of cardiac conduction abnormalities, myocardial ischemia, and heart failure.

Adverse Effects and Contraindications

The adverse effects of lacosamide include a prolonged PR interval, dizziness, ataxia, diplopia, somnolence, suicidal ideation, headache, nausea, and vomiting.

Contraindications include a known hypersensitivity to the drug.

Nursing Implications

Preventing Interactions

It is important that lacosamide not be combined with any medication that prolongs the PR interval. Patients should not take this drug in combination with alcohol.

> **BOX 52.14** 📋 **Patient Teaching Guidelines for Lacosamide**
>
> ■ Take the medication as prescribed.
> ■ Do not discontinue the drug abruptly. If you need to stop taking it, taper the dosage.
> ■ Report any mood changes to the prescriber.
> ■ Keep follow-up appointments to monitor drug response and assessment of adverse effects.
> ■ Do not drink alcohol because of the increased risk of central nervous system (CNS) depression.
> ■ If you are a woman of childbearing age and are sexually active, use contraceptives.

Administering the Medication

The nurse may give IV lacosamide in 0.9% sodium chloride, 5% dextrose, or lactated Ringer's solution. The period of infusion is 30 to 60 minutes. Administration of lacosamide should not occur in the same IV line with other medications. The preparation is stable at room temperature for 24 hours.

Assessing for Therapeutic and Adverse Effects

The nurse assesses the patient for CNS depression and diminished partial-onset seizure activity.

The greatest risks associated with lacosamide are suicidal ideation and cardiac conduction abnormalities. The nurse assesses the patient for sudden personality changes, signs of aggression, and severe nausea and vomiting. During parenteral administration, the nurse assesses for signs of a prolonged PR interval.

Patient Teaching

Box 52.14 identifies patient teaching guidelines for lacosamide.

MINERAL ELECTROLYTES: MAGNESIUM SULFATE

It is important to understand the use and administration of the mineral electrolyte Ⓟ **magnesium sulfate** due to the fetal neuroprotection it can prove to pregnant women. This medication provides the opportunity to improve neurodevelopmental outcomes in infants by delaying preterm birth and decreasing maternal seizure risk. Table 52.8 contains some dosage information about this agent. Chapter 6 discusses the use of magnesium sulfate more fully.

PHENYLTRIAZINE DERIVATIVES

Ⓟ **Lamotrigine** (Lamictal) is used for adjunctive therapy in the treatment of partial seizures.

Pharmacokinetics

Lamotrigine is administered orally. It is absorbed by the GI tract with a rapid onset of action. Lamotrigine is metabolized by the liver and excreted in the urine. It crosses the placenta and enters the breast milk. The medication is 55% protein bound and has a 25- to 30-hour half-life.

Action

The action of lamotrigine is not well understood. It is thought to reduce the release of glutamate, an excitatory neurotransmitter, in the brain. The neurotransmitter is sensitive to sodium channels, thus decreasing seizure activity.

Use

Clinicians use lamotrigine for partial seizures as well as for generalized tonic–clonic, absence, or myoclonic seizures. Other uses include bipolar disorder. Table 52.8 gives route and dosage information for lamotrigine.

Use in Children

Children should receive lamotrigine in combination with valproic acid and other AEDs.

Use in Patients With Renal or Hepatic Impairment

It may be necessary to reduce the dosage in patients with renal or hepatic impairment.

Adverse Effects

Adverse effects of lamotrigine include dizziness, drowsiness, headache, ataxia, blurred or double vision, nausea and vomiting, and weakness. The FDA has issued a **BLACK BOX WARNING** ◆ related to the potential development of serious dermatologic reactions. Because a serious skin rash may occur, especially in children, lamotrigine should be administered cautiously to children younger than 16 years of age and should be discontinued at the first sign of skin rash in an adult. Skin rash is more likely to occur with concomitant valproic acid therapy, high lamotrigine starting dose, and rapid titration rate. It may resolve if lamotrigine is discontinued, but it progresses in some patients to more severe forms, such as Stevens-Johnson syndrome or toxic epidermal necrosis.

Contraindications

Contraindications to lamotrigine includes any hypersensitivity to the drug. Patients who have signs and symptoms of suicide, as well as in those who are pregnant or lactating, should not take it.

Nursing Implications

Preventing Interactions

Several medications and herbs interact with lamotrigine, increasing or decreasing its effects (Boxes 52.15 and 52.16).

Administering the Medication

The nurse should ensure that chewable tablets are chewed or crushed, not swallowed. If the drug is discontinued, it is essential to taper the medication over a 2-week period.

BOX 52.15	Drug Interactions: Lamotrigine

Drugs That Increase the Effects of Lamotrigine
- Valproic acid
  Significantly increases plasma concentration

Drugs That Decrease the Effects of Lamotrigine
- Carbamazepine, fosphenytoin, oral contraceptives, phenobarbital, primidone, phenytoin
  Decrease serum concentration

Assessing for Therapeutic and Adverse Effects

The nurse should assess for the lack of generalized, myoclonic, and absence seizures.

The nurse assesses the integumentary system daily for the onset of skin eruptions. He or she also questions the patient about ophthalmological changes.

Patient Teaching

Box 52.17 identifies patient teaching guidelines for lamotrigine.

NCLEX Success

8. A 12-year-old boy comes to the school nurse's office after falling during gym class. The nurse assesses the child and notes that he has bruising and petechiae over most of his legs, arms, and torso. The child has a history of absence seizures that are treated with valproic acid (Depakene). Based on the child's history, what would the nurse suspect?

   A. abuse
   B. leukemia
   C. adverse effect
   D. anemia

9. Which of the following places the patient at risk for toxicity following the administration of phenytoin (Dilantin)?

   A. The patient skips a dose of phenytoin.
   B. The patient takes a different brand of phenytoin.
   C. The patient switches to a different antiepileptic agent.
   D. The patient receives phenytoin in an enteral feeding.

10. Which of the following is most important to teach a patient who is being administered lamotrigine (Lamictal)?

    A. to report the development of edema
    B. to report anxiety
    C. to report the development of a skin rash
    D. to report anorexia

PYRROLIDINE DERIVATIVES

Ⓟ **Levetiracetam** (Keppra) is an AED that is effective in the treatment of a wide variety of seizure disorders. In a retrospective study, Gamez-Leyva, Aristin, Fernandex, and Pascual (2009) found that IV levetiracetam was effective in patients with status epilepticus. Of note, these patients had not responded well to benzodiazepines.

Pharmacokinetics

Levetiracetam is administered orally or intravenously and is rapidly absorbed, reaching its peak in 1 hour. It is 10% protein bound with minimal hepatic metabolism. It is excreted in the urine and has a 7.1-hour half-life. The half-life in older adults is 9.6 hours.

Action

Levetiracetam is chemically unrelated to other AEDs, and its mechanism of action is unknown. It inhibits abnormal neuronal firing but does not affect normal neuronal excitability or function.

Use

Clinicians use levetiracetam as adjunctive therapy for partial-onset and generalized tonic–clonic seizures. Table 52.8 presents route and dosage information for levetiracetam.

Use in Patients With Renal Impairment

It is essential to reduce the dose in patients with impaired renal function, because the kidneys eliminate the majority of a dose (66%).

Adverse Effects and Contraindications

Common adverse effects of levetiracetam include drowsiness, dizziness, and fatigue. Others include decreases in red and white blood cell counts, double vision, amnesia, anxiety, ataxia, emotional lability, hostility, nervousness, paresthesia, pharyngitis, and rhinitis.

Contraindications include a known hypersensitivity to the medication, pregnancy, lactation, and suicidal ideation.

Nursing Implications

Preventing Interactions

CNS depressants combined with levetiracetam may increase symptoms of sedation.

Administering the Medication

It is essential that the IV preparation of levetiracetam be administered only on a short-term basis. The nurse tells patients not to crush extended-release forms of the drug. To prevent GI upset, the nurse administers the oral preparation with food. He or she monitors patients for psychosis and depression.

Assessing for Therapeutic and Adverse Effects

The nurse assesses the patient for symptoms of partial-onset and generalized tonic–clonic seizures, which should be absent.

The nurse assesses the patient for ocular changes, CNS depression, and hematological changes.

Patient Teaching

Box 52.18 identifies patient teaching guidelines for levetiracetam.

SULFAMATE-SUBSTITUTED MONOSACCHARIDES

Ⓟ **Topiramate** (Topamax) is a sulfamate-substituted monosaccharide that was identified during a research project to develop a new antidiabetic agent. One study found that topiramate provides neurostabilizing effects by attenuating the excitability of brain neuronal pathways (Maryanoff, 2009).

Pharmacokinetics

Topiramate is absorbed in the GI tract and produces peak plasma levels about 2 hours after oral administration. The average half-life is about 21 hours, and steady-state concentrations are reached in about 4 days with normal renal function. The drug is 20% bound to plasma proteins. Topiramate is not extensively metabolized and is primarily eliminated via the kidneys.

Action

The mechanism of action of topiramate is not understood, but the antiepileptic action may be related to the blockage of sodium channels in neurons with sustained depolarization. This action increases GABA activity at the receptors, potentiating the inhibition of the neurotransmitters blocking excitatory neurotransmitters at the neuron receptor sites.

Use

Clinicians use topiramate as monotherapy in partial-onset or primary generalized tonic–clonic seizures as well as in adjunctive therapy for partial-onset or primary generalized seizures. Lennox-Gastaut syndrome is also an indication. In addition, prescribers order the medication as a preventive for migraine headaches. Table 52.8 gives route and dosage information for topiramate.

Use in Patients With Renal Impairment

Patients with a CrCl less than 70 mL/min should receive one-half the usual dose.

EVIDENCE-BASED PRACTICE

Novel Medications for Neonatal Seizures: Bumetanide and Topiramate
by JANET SOUL

Journal of Pediatric Neurology
2009, 85–93.
Retrieved: October 10, 2010

This review of evidence-based practice studies revealed that the diuretic bumetanide and antiepileptic topiramate suppress seizures in newborn infants. These agents have neuroprotective effects when used to treat refractory seizures resulting from acute insults to the neonatal brain. The use of antiepileptic drugs (AEDs) has not been studied in the neonatal population, who are particularly at risk for adverse effects of antiepileptic agents due to differences in pharmacokinetics and safety compared with children and adults. The main antiepileptic agents administered to neonates are phenobarbital, phenytoin, and fosphenytoin. Bumetanide and topiramate have the ability to suppress seizures in the newborn brain. Animal studies on bumetanide revealed the combination or phenobarbital with bumetanide was more effective then the administration of phenobarbital alone. Topiramate has been studied in animals and possesses neuroprotective properties in neonate animal studies.

IMPLICATIONS FOR NURSING PRACTICE: Current literature does not identify bumetanide use in seizure control in newborns. However, with further research and approval by the U.S. Food and Drug Administration (FDA), this medication could be added to the current list of antiepileptic agents.

Use in Patients With Hepatic Impairment

Patients with elevated liver enzymes should receive reduced doses of topiramate, with the dosage increased slowly over time. It is necessary to monitor patients closely for increased hepatic effects.

Adverse Effects and Contraindications

Adverse effects of topiramate include CNS effects such as ataxia, somnolence, dizziness, and nystagmus as well as GI adverse effects such as nausea and dyspepsia. Renal stones may develop. Other adverse effects are increased intraocular pressure, weight loss, and fatigue.

Contraindications include hypersensitivity to the drug and metabolic acidosis.

Nursing Implications

Preventing Interactions

Several medications interact with topiramate, increasing or decreasing its effects (Box 52.19). The drug decreases the effectiveness of oral contraceptives. The herb *Ginkgo biloba* decreases the effect of topiramate.

Administering the Medication

Topiramate has a very bitter taste. To prevent patients from tasting the bitterness, the nurse instructs them never to chew the medication. In addition, the nurse notes that it is necessary to store topiramate in a tightly closed container at 59°F to 86°F.

Assessing for Therapeutic and Adverse Effects

Patients are without symptoms of partial or generalized seizures. Those with Lennox-Gastaut syndrome have no seizure activity.

The nurse assesses the patient for pain or discomfort related to kidney stones. The patient should have an annual eye examination to determine the onset of increased intraocular pressure.

Patient Teaching

Box 52.20 identifies patient teaching guidelines for topiramate.

TRIAZOLE DERIVATIVES

Ⓟ **Rufinamide** (Banzel) is structurally unrelated to other AEDs. It produced antiepileptic effects in several animal studies including seizures induced by maximal electroshock (Perucca, Cloyd, Critchley, & Fuseau, 2008).

BOX 52.19 — Drug Interactions: Topiramate

Drugs That Increase the Effects of Topiramate
- Alcohol
  Increases central nervous system (CNS) depression
- Carbonic anhydrase inhibitors
  Increase the risk of renal stone development

Drugs That Decrease the Effects of Topiramate
- Carbamazepine, phenytoin, valproic acid
  Decrease serum levels

- Take the medication as prescribed.
- Do not stop taking the medication abruptly.
- Use two types of contraceptives if you are of child-bearing age and are sexually active.
- Do not operate machinery with central nervous system (CNS) depression.
- Drink six to eight 8-ounce glasses of water per day to decrease risk of renal stone development.

Pharmacokinetics and Action

Rufinamide is absorbed slowly by the GI tract. Peak plasma concentrations occur between 4 and 6 hours. The drug is metabolized extensively without active metabolites. It is excreted by the kidneys.

Rufinamide decreases seizure activity by prolonging the inactive sodium channels in the cortical neurons.

Use

Clinicians use rufinamide in the treatment of seizures in patients with Lennox-Gastaut syndrome. Table 52.8 gives route and dosage information for rufinamide.

Use in Patients With Hepatic Impairment

It is necessary to administer rufinamide cautiously to patients with moderate hepatic impairment. Patients with severe hepatic impairment should not take the drug.

Adverse Effects and Contraindications

The most common adverse effects of rufinamide include fatigue, headache, somnolence, vomiting, and flu-like symptoms.

Contraindications include short QT syndrome, severe hepatic impairment, pregnancy, and lactation.

Nursing Implications

Preventing Interactions

Several drugs interact with rufinamide, increasing or decreasing its effects (Box 52.21).

BOX 52.21 **Drug Interactions: Rufinamide**

Drugs That Increase the Effect of Rufinamide
- Valproic acid
  Increases plasma concentration

Drugs That Decrease the Effect of Rufinamide
- Primidone
- Carbamazepine, ethinyl estradiol, and norethindrone
  Decrease the effect of both drugs
- Phenobarbital, phenytoin
  May increase levels of these drugs as well as decrease rufinamide level

- Take the medication with food.
- Take the medication as prescribed.
- Do not stop taking the medication abruptly.
- Use two types of contraceptives if you are of child-bearing age and are sexually active.

Administering the Medication

To increase drug absorption, the nurse ensures that rufinamide is taken with food. It is acceptable to crush or split the medication for ease of administration.

Assessing for Therapeutic and Adverse Effects

The patient is without seizure activity related to Lennox-Gastaut syndrome.

It is important to assess the patient's CNS response to the medication. The nurse also assesses the patient for GI upset and flu-like symptoms.

Patient Teaching

Box 52.22 identifies patient teaching guidelines for rufinamide.

The Nursing Process

Assessment

- Assess the patient status in relation to seizure activity and other factors.
  - Interview the patient about the seizure disorder and AEDs.
    - How long has the patient had the seizure disorder?
    - How long has it been since the seizure activity occurred?
    - What is the frequency of the seizures?
    - Does any particular situation precipitate the seizure?
    - How does the seizure affect the patient (loss of consciousness, body part or parts affected, drowsiness after the seizure)?
    - What AEDs are prescribed?
    - What affect do the AEDs have on the patient?
    - Does the patient take the AEDs as prescribed?
    - What is the patient's attitude toward the seizure disorder?
    - What other medications does the patient take?
  - Assess serum levels of AEDs.
  - Identify risk factors for seizure disorders (previous seizure activity, brain surgery, head injury, hypoxia, hypoglycemia, drug overdosage, withdrawal of AEDs or CNS depressants)
  - Observe and document seizure activity accurately; location (localized or general); and specific characteristics of abnormal movements or behavior, duration, and concomitant events (loss of consciousness, incontinence, and postseizure behavior).

- Assess for risk of status epilepticus (recent changes in AED therapy, chronic alcohol ingestion, use of drugs known to cause seizures, and infection).

Nursing Diagnoses

- Ineffective coping related to denial of disease process and need for long-term drug therapy
- Deficient knowledge: disease process
- Deficient knowledge: drug effects
- Risk for injury: trauma related to ataxia, dizziness, confusion
- Risk for injury: seizure activity or drug toxicity
- Risk for seizure complications
- Ineffective management of therapeutic regimen: individual underuse of medications

Planning/Goals

The patient will

- Take the medication as prescribed
- Experience control of seizures
- Avoid serious adverse effects
- Verbalize knowledge of the disease process and treatment regimen
- Avoid discontinuing AEDs abruptly
- Keep follow-up appointments with the primary care provider

Nursing Interventions

The nurse will

- Assist the patient in the identification of conditions under which seizures are likely to occur. These precipitating factors, which are to be avoided or decreased when possible, may include ingestion of alcoholic beverages or stimulant drugs; fever; severe physical or emotional stress; and sensory stimuli, such as flashing lights and loud noises. Identification of precipitating factors is important because lifestyle changes (e.g., reducing stress, reducing alcohol and caffeine intake, increasing exercise, improving sleep, and diet) and treatment of existing disorders can reduce the frequency of seizures.
- Assist the patient in planning how to obtain adequate rest and exercise and consume a balanced diet.
- Discuss the seizure disorder, the plan of treatment, and the importance of adhering to prescribed drug therapy with the patient and family members.
- Involve the patient in decision making when possible.
- Inform the patient and family that seizure control is not gained immediately when drug therapy is started. The goal is to avoid unrealistic expectations and excessive frustration while AEDs and dosages are being changed in an effort to determine the best regimen for the patient.
- Discuss social and economic factors that promote or prevent compliance.
- Protect the patient experiencing a generalized tonic–clonic seizure by
  - Placing a small pillow or piece of clothing under the head to prevent injury from the ground or floor
  - Never restraining the patient's movements; fractures may result

- Loosening tight clothing, especially around the neck and chest, to promote respirations
- Turning the patient to one side so that accumulating secretions can drain from the mouth and throat when paroxysms stop. The cyanosis, abnormal movements, and loss of consciousness that characterize a generalized tonic–clonic seizure can be quite alarming to witnesses. Most of these seizures subside within 3 to 4 minutes, and the patient starts responding and regaining normal skin color. If the patient has one seizure after another (status epilepticus), has trouble breathing or continued cyanosis, or has sustained an injury, further care is needed, and a physician should be notified immediately.
- When risk factors for seizures, especially status epilepticus, are identified, try to prevent or minimize their occurrence.
- If an aura or smell is noted prior to the onset of seizure, be sure the patient notifies a nurse.

Evaluation

- Interview and observe for decrease in or absence of seizure activity.
- Interview and observe for avoidance of adverse drug effects, especially those that impair safety.
- When available, check laboratory reports of serum drug levels for the therapeutic ranges or evidence of underdosing or overdosing.

Overview of Spinal Cord Injury

Spinal cord injuries are classified by the spinal level at which the injury occurs. Tetraplegia, or quadriplegia, is the impairment of motor and sensory function in the arms, trunk, legs, and pelvic organs. Paraplegia is the impairment of motor and sensory function in the thoracic, lumbar, and sacral segments of the spinal cord. Upper motor neuron injuries result in spastic paralysis with hyperreflexia, preventing purposeful movement. Lower motor neuron injuries result in the flaccidity of muscles and muscle atrophy (Porth & Matfin, 2009).

Etiology

Spinal cord injury is a result of damage to the cord by trauma. The damage to the cord is related to indirect injury from vertebral fractures or contusions. The direct cause of spinal cord injury is from a penetrating wound. The indirect cause of spinal cord injury is the result of a vertebral fracture, fracture dislocations, or spinal subluxation (Porth & Matfin, 2009; Smeltzer, Bare, Hinkle, & Cheever, 2010).

Pathophysiology

Primary spinal cord injury produces hemorrhage in the gray matter of the cord with edema of the white matter and ultimate necrosis of the neural tissue. The injury is from compression, stretch, and shearing associated with spinal fracture or dislocation. An injury to the cord producing penetration of the cord is from laceration or a tear of the cord. The secondary spinal cord injury follows the primary injury with further tissue destruction and progressive damage of neurologic tissue (Porth & Matfin, 2009).

Clinical Manifestations

The clinical manifestations of a spinal cord injury are the result of the type and level of the injury. The level of the spinal cord injury produces greater loss of function and sensation. Clinical manifestations of complete spinal cord injury are irreversible with loss of autonomic, neural, and motor function. Incomplete spinal cord injuries vary in the severity of neurological loss according the severity of the damage. Changes in the autonomic nervous system affect temperature regulation, bowel and bladder function, and hypotension (Bare et al., 2009).

Drug Therapy

All skeletal muscle relaxants except dantrolene are centrally acting drugs. Pharmacologic action is usually attributed to general depression of the CNS but may involve blockage of nerve impulses that cause increased muscle tone and contraction. It is unclear whether relief of pain results from muscle relaxation or sedative effects. In addition, although parenteral administration of some drugs (e.g., diazepam, methocarbamol) relieves pain associated with acute musculoskeletal trauma or inflammation, it is uncertain whether oral administration of usual doses exerts a beneficial effect in acute or chronic disorders.

Baclofen and diazepam increase the effects of GABA, an inhibitory neurotransmitter. Tizanidine inhibits motor neurons in the brain. Dantrolene is the only skeletal muscle relaxant that acts peripherally on the muscle itself; it inhibits the release of calcium in skeletal muscle cells, thereby decreasing the strength of muscle contraction.

Table 52.9 summarizes the drug classes of skeletal muscle reactants, naming the prototype drug.

TABLE 52.9

Drugs Administered for the Treatment of Spasticity and to Relax Skeletal Muscles

Drug Class	Prototype*
Carbamate derivatives	Carisoprodol (Soma)
Gamma-aminobutyric acid (GABA) derivatives	Baclofen (Lioresal)
Hydantoin derivatives	Dantrolene sodium (Dantrium)
Tricyclic antidepressant derivatives	Cyclobenzaprine hydrochloride (Flexeril)
Imidazole derivatives	Tizanidine hydrochloride (Zanaflex)

*There are no drugs other than the prototypes in any of the classes.

Clinical Application 52-4

- Andrew is now a 20-year-old college student. While living in the dorm, he has not been consistently taking his antiepileptic medications. On his trip home for the holidays, he suffers a seizure and has an automobile accident that leaves him paralyzed. The site of the spinal cord injury is T12. This injury results in muscle spasticity. Why is muscle spasticity so severe with spinal cord injuries?

Drugs Used to Treat Muscle Spasms and Spasticity

CARBAMATE DERIVATIVES

Ⓟ **Carisoprodol** (Soma) is a centrally acting skeletal muscle relaxant. It is chemically related to meprobamate, which inhibits multineuronal spinal reflexes.

Pharmacokinetics

The onset of action of carisoprodol is 30 minutes, with a peak in 1 to 2 hours and a duration of 4 to 6 hours. The half-life is 8 hours. The drug is metabolized in the liver by the enzyme CYP2C19 and excreted in the urine. It crosses the placenta and is present in breast milk.

Action

The action of carisoprodol is not known, but animal studies have shown that the drug inhibits interneuronal activity in the descending reticular formation and spinal cord. It does not act directly to relax the skeletal muscles.

Use

Clinicians use carisoprodol in the relief of discomfort associated with acute painful musculoskeletal conditions in which relief was not attained by rest, physical therapy, or alternative measures. Table 52.10 gives route and dosage information for carisoprodol.

Adverse Effects

CNS adverse effects of carisoprodol include dizziness, drowsiness, vertigo, ataxia, tremor, agitation, and irritability. Initially, after the first, second, third, or fourth dose, patients may exhibit an allergic or idiosyncratic reaction with rash, erythema multiforme, pruritus, eosinophilia, hypotension, bronchospasm, vision and speech alterations, and the most severe adverse effect, anaphylactoid shock.

Contraindications

Contraindications to carisoprodol includes an allergic response to the drug or acute intermittent porphyria. Other contraindications are pregnancy and lactation.

TABLE 52.10

DRUGS AT A GLANCE: Drugs Used to Relax Skeletal Muscles

Drug	Pregnancy Category	Routes and Dosage Ranges	
		Adult	*Children*
Ⓟ Carisoprodol (Soma)	C	12 y and older, 350 mg PO 3–4 times daily for maximum of 2–3 wk, with last dose at bedtime Geriatric patients, patients with renal or hepatic impairment: reduce dose and monitor closely	Not recommended for children younger than 12 y
Ⓟ Baclofen (Lioresal)	C	Start at a low dosage and increase gradually until optimum effect is achieved (40–80 mg/d); 5 mg PO for 3 d; 10 mg 3 times daily for 3 d; 15 mg 3 times daily for 3 d; 20 mg 3 times daily for 3 d; may increase to a maximum of 80 mg/d (20 mg 4 times daily) Intrathecal, refer to manufacturer's instructions; testing is usually done with 50 mcg/mL injected into intrathecal space over 1 min; patient is observed for 4–8 h, then a dose of 75 mcg/ 1.5 mL is given and patient is observed for another 4–8 h; a final screening bolus of 100 mcg/2 mL is given 24 h later if response is still not adequate. Patients who do not respond to this dose are not candidates for the implant Maintenance dose: 22–1400 mcg/d (smallest dose to achieve muscle tone without adverse effects)	Safety in children younger than 12 y of age has not been established; orphan drug use to decrease spasticity in children with cerebral palsy is being studied
Ⓟ Dantrolene sodium (Dantrium)	C	Chronic spasticity: establish therapeutic goal before initiating therapy; titrate and individual- ize dosage, increasing until maximum perfor- mance is compatible to relieve dysfunction; initially 25 mg daily; increase to 25 mg 3 times daily for 7 d; then to 50 mg 3 times daily, and if necessary to 100 mg 3 times daily; most patients respond to 400 mg/d or less; maintain each dosage level for 4–7 d to evaluate response; discontinue after 45 d if benefits are not evident Preoperative prophylaxis of malignant hyperther- mia: 4–8 mg/kg/d PO in 3–4 divided doses for 1–2 d prior to surgery; give the last dose 3–4 h before scheduled surgery with minimum amount of water; adjust dose to prevent incapacitation due to drowsiness and excessive gastrointestinal (GI) irritation Postcrisis follow-up: 4–8 mg/kg/d PO in 4 divided doses for 1–3 d to prevent recurrence Parenteral administration for malignant hyperther- mia: discontinue all anesthetics as soon as prob- lem is recognized; give dantrolene by continuous rapid intravenous (IV) push beginning at minimum dose of 1 mg/kg and continuing until symptoms subside or maximum cumulative dose of 10 mg/kg has been given; if physiological and metabolic abnormalities reappear, repeat regi- men; give continuously until symptoms subside Preoperative prophylaxis of malignant hyperther- mia: 2.5 mg/kg IV 1 h before surgery infused over 1 h	Safety for children <5 y has not been established Chronic spasticity: initially 0.5 mg/ kg once daily for 7 d, followed by 0.5 mg/kg 3 times daily for 7 d; then 1 mg/kg 3 times daily for 7 d; then 2 mg/kg 3 times daily if necessary; do not exceed 100 mg 4 times daily

(Continued on page 976)

TABLE 52.10

DRUGS AT A GLANCE: Drugs Used to Relax Skeletal Muscles (Continued)

Drug	Pregnancy Category	Routes and Dosage Ranges	
		Adult	Children
Cyclobenzaprine hydrochloride (Flexeril)	B	5 mg PO 3 times daily up to 10 mg PO 3 times daily, not to exceed 60 mg/d; do not use longer than 2–3 wk; extended-release capsules: 15 mg daily; some patients may require 30 mg/d	Safety and efficacy not established in children younger than 15 y
Tizanidine hydrochloride (Zanaflex)	C	4 mg PO daily, increased in 2–4-mg increments as needed over 2–4 wk; usual maintenance dose, 8 mg PO every 6–8 h; maximum dose, 36 mg/d in divided doses; reduce dose in patients with renal impairment	Safety and efficacy not established

Nursing Implications

Preventing Interactions

CNS system depressants and alcohol combined with carisoprodol increase CNS depression.

Administering the Medication

The nurse administers carisoprodol with food to prevent GI upset, giving the last dose of medication at bedtime. It is necessary to store the mediation in a container with a tight-fitting lid.

Assessing for Therapeutic Effects

The nurse assesses the musculoskeletal area for relief of pain and spasms associated with the musculoskeletal injury.

Assessing for Adverse Effects

The nurse assesses the integumentary system for signs and symptoms of an idiosyncratic reaction after the fourth to fifth doses of carisoprodol. It is also important to observe for visual changes, speech difficulties, bronchospasm, hypotension, and anaphylaxis. Carisoprodol is habit forming and should not be stopped abruptly. Abrupt withdrawal results in headache, nausea, insomnia, and abdominal cramping.

Patient Teaching

Box 52.23 identifies patient teaching guidelines for carisoprodol.

GAMMA-AMINOBUTYRIC ACID DERIVATIVES

The GABA derivative **baclofen** (Lioresal) is an agonist-specific inhibitor to $GABA_B$ receptors located in the spinal cord. It restricts the influx of calcium to reduce the presynaptic neurotransmitter release in the excitatory spinal pathways (Gorgey, Chiodo, & Gater, 2010).

Pharmacokinetics

Oral baclofen begins to act in 1 hour, peaks in 2 hours, and lasts 4 to 8 hours. It is metabolized in the liver and excreted in urine; its half-life is 3 to 4 hours. Intrathecal baclofen has an

onset of action of 30 to 60 minutes, peaks in 4 hours, and like oral baclofen, has a duration of action 4 to 8 hours. The drug crosses the placenta and enters the breast milk.

Action

The exact mechanism of action of baclofen is unknown. It appears to reduce impulse transmissions from the spinal cord to the skeletal muscle, thus decreasing muscle spasms.

Use

Clinicians use baclofen to alleviate signs and symptoms of spasticity in patients with multiple sclerosis. It is particularly effective against flexor spasms, concomitant pain, and muscular rigidity. Other indications include the treatment of spinal cord injuries and other diseases of the spinal cord. Table 52.10 gives route and dosage information for baclofen.

Use in Older Adults

Older adults who take baclofen require close monitoring. Dosage reduction to prevent excessive CNS depression may be necessary.

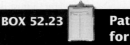

BOX 52.23   Patient Teaching Guidelines for Carisoprodol

- Do not operate machinery with central nervous system (CNS) depression.
- Do not combine with other CNS depressants or alcohol.
- Take the medication with food.
- Do not combine with over-the-counter cold remedies without approval from the prescriber.
- Do not stop the medication abruptly.
- Know the idiosyncratic effects of the drug and how to maintain safety when CNS effects are evident.
- Report signs and symptoms of idiosyncratic adverse effects.

Use in Patients With Renal Impairment

Dosage reduction is necessary in patients with renal impairment.

Adverse Effects and Contraindications

The most common adverse effects of baclofen are transient drowsiness, dizziness, weakness, fatigue, confusion, headache, insomnia, hypotension, and urinary frequency. Elevated blood sugar may occur, requiring the administration of an oral hypoglycemic agent.

Contraindications include known hypersensitivity to the drug and skeletal muscle spasms resulting from rheumatic disorders.

Nursing Implications

Preventing Interactions

When baclofen is combined with alcohol or other CNS depressants, patients experience increased CNS depression.

Administering the Medication

Administration of baclofen is oral or intrathecal. The nurse starts with a low dose that he or she increases slowly, using the smallest dose possible to achieve muscle tone without adverse effects. If the benefits of the medication are not evident during a trial period, then the medication is withdrawn gradually.

Intrathecal administration involves an implantable pump. It is best to consult the manufacturer's literature concerning the pump instructions and initiation of long-term infusions.

Assessing for Therapeutic Effects

The nurse assesses the affected musculoskeletal region for decrease in symptoms of spasticity.

Assessing for Adverse Effects

It is important to assess the degree of CNS depression. The nurse assesses the patient's blood pressure for hypotension, particularly with position changes. Genitourinary assessments include the patient's level of urinary frequency and dysuria. Other adverse effects noted are weight gain, increased aspartate aminotransferase, blood sugar, and alkaline phosphatase.

Patient Teaching

Box 52.24 identifies patient teaching guidelines for baclofen.

BOX 52.24   Patient Teaching Guidelines for Baclofen

- Do not stop taking the drug abruptly; Abrupt discontinuation may cause hallucinations or other serious side effects.
- Avoid alcohol and other central nervous system (CNS) depressants.
- Do not take if you are pregnant or breast feeding.
- Do not operate machinery.
- Report painful or frequent urination, constipation, headache, insomnia, or confusion.

Clinical Application 52-5

- Andrew is receiving baclofen (Lioresal) to treat the spasticity. He and his parents are to receive instruction about the administration of intrathecal baclofen. What aspects of the medication administration does the nurse teach?
- His parents ask the nurse why he is taking baclofen (Lioresal) and not diazepam (Valium), which he has taken in the past. What is the best response to this question?

NCLEX Success

11. A nurse administers a peripherally acting muscle relaxant to a patient with a spinal cord injury. Which of the following drugs does the nurse administer?

    A. dantrolene (Dantrium)
    B. baclofen (Lioresal)
    C. methocarbamol (Robaxin)
    D. diazepam (Valium)

12. A patient is taking carisoprodol (Soma) for back spasms related to an occupational injury. Which of the following is most important to teach the patient?

    A. to take the medication at 8:00 AM, 2:00 PM, and 8:00 PM
    B. to know the signs and symptoms of an idiosyncratic reaction
    C. to take the medication between meals
    D. to stop the medication with the first sign of abdominal cramping

13. A nurse administers baclofen (Lioresal) to a young man for a back injury. Which of the following interventions is most important related to the administration of baclofen?

    A. Assess heart rate.
    B. Assess for edema.
    C. Assess blood sugar.
    D. Assess for increased spasticity.

HYDANTOIN DERIVATIVES

Ⓟ **Dantrolene sodium** (Dantrium intravenous) is a drug administered for spasticity related to multiple sclerosis, cerebral palsy, spinal cord injury, and stroke.

Pharmacokinetics

Oral dantrolene is absorbed by the GI tract, reaching a peak in 4 to 6 hours. The duration of action is 8 to 10 hours, and the half-life is 9 hours. IV dantrolene has a rapid onset of action with a peak in 5 hours, a duration of action of 6 to 8 hours, and a half-life of 4 to 8 hours. The drug is metabolized by the liver and excreted in the urine. Dantrolene crosses the placenta and enters the breast milk.

Action

Dantrolene interferes with the release of calcium from the sarcoplasmic reticulum to relax skeletal muscle. It does not interfere with neuromuscular transmission or affect the surface membrane of the skeletal muscle.

Use

Dantrolene controls spasticity caused by upper motor neuron disorders, such as spinal cord injury, cerebrovascular accident, cerebral palsy, and multiple sclerosis. Clinicians may use it to prevent and manage **malignant hyperthermia,** a rare but life-threatening complication of anesthesia characterized by hypercarbia, metabolic acidosis, skeletal muscle rigidity, fever, and cyanosis. Table 52.10 gives route and dosage information for dantrolene.

Use in Older Adults

Aging increases the risk of liver damage as a result of the administration of dantrolene. Administration of dantrolene necessitates the close monitoring of liver enzyme levels.

Use in Patients With Hepatic Impairment

It is important not to administer dantrolene to patients with active liver disease. The development of hepatocellular damage can be fatal. As in the elderly, close monitoring of liver enzymes is necessary.

Adverse Effects

Common adverse effects of dantrolene include drowsiness, dizziness, diarrhea, and fatigue. The most serious adverse effect is potentially fatal hepatitis, with jaundice and other symptoms that usually occur within 1 month of starting drug therapy. Liver function tests should be monitored periodically in all patients receiving dantrolene. These adverse effects do not occur with short-term use of IV drug for malignant hyperthermia. The FDA has issued a **BLACK BOX WARNING ◆** stating that the patient should have liver function tests and that dantrolene be discontinued at the first indication of hepatic impairment.

Contraindications

Contraindications to dantrolene include active liver disease. Other contraindications include spasticity used to maintain an upright position and balance with locomotion as well as spasticity from rheumatic conditions.

Nursing Implications

Preventing Interactions

The patient is at risk for hyperkalemia and myocardial depression if dantrolene is combined with verapamil.

Administering the Medication

When administering dantrolene intravenously, the nurse monitors the injection sites and ensures that extravasation does not occur. Dantrolene is an alkaline agent that is irritating to the tissues.

When administering dantrolene orally, the nurse consults with other health care professionals to determine interventions that enhance mobility. Withdrawal of the oral medication should occur over 2 to 4 days. If diarrhea occurs, discontinuance of dantrolene is necessary.

If malignant hyperthermia develops, it is essential to discontinue all triggering drugs. In addition, the nurse assesses for metabolic acidosis and electrolyte imbalances. It may be necessary to use a cooling blanket.

Assessing for Therapeutic Effects

The nurse assesses the patient's response to dantrolene. The patient should have a decrease in muscle spasticity that does not affect the ability to perform activities of daily living. The IV administration for the treatment of malignant hyperthermia results in a reverse of symptoms, including decreased temperature and fluid and electrolyte balance without signs and symptoms of metabolic acidosis.

Assessing for Adverse Effects

It is necessary to check the patient's liver enzymes with the administration of oral dantrolene. The nurse assesses the patient for diarrhea, dizziness, and fatigue. Headache, anorexia, and nervousness are potentially serious adverse effects in people older than 35 years of age who have taken the drug for 60 days or longer. Women in this age group who take estrogens have the highest risk of developing these adverse effects. Hepatotoxicity can be prevented or minimized by administering the lowest effective dose, monitoring liver enzymes during therapy, and discontinuing the drug if no beneficial effects occur in 45 days.

Patient Teaching

Box 52.25 identifies the patient teaching guidelines for dantrolene.

TRICYCLIC ANTIDEPRESSANT DERIVATIVES

Ⓟ **Cyclobenzaprine hydrochloride** (Flexeril) is a centrally acting skeletal muscle relaxant administered on a short-term basis for the relief of muscle spasm.

Pharmacokinetics

Cyclobenzaprine is administered orally and is well absorbed by the GI tract. The onset of action is 1 hour, with a peak in 3 to 8 hours, and the duration of action is 12 to 24 hours. The half-life

---

| BOX 52.25 | **Patient Teaching Guidelines for Dantrolene** |

- Do not alter positions when experiencing dizziness.
- Report gastrointestinal (GI) upset and eat small frequent meals.
- Avoid alcohol and other central nervous system (CNS) depressants.
- Report severe diarrhea, headache, and anorexia.

is 1 to 3 days. The drug is highly protein bound. It is metabolized in the liver to inactive metabolites and is excreted in the urine, with some eliminated in the feces. Cyclobenzaprine crosses the placenta and is excreted in the breast milk.

Action

The mechanism of action of cyclobenzaprine is not known, but it appears to produce relaxation by acting at the brainstem and spinal cord to depress motor activity.

Use

Clinicians use cyclobenzaprine as an adjunctive to other measures such as physical therapy to relieve muscle spasm. Table 52.10 gives route and dosage information for cyclobenzaprine.

Use in Older Adults

Conventional 5-mg tablets are used in older adults, with the dosage adjusted slowly upward. Use of extended-release capsules is not recommended.

Use in Patients With Hepatic Impairment

The same recommendations for older adults apply to patients with hepatic impairment.

Adverse Effects and Contraindications

Common adverse effects of cyclobenzaprine are drowsiness, dizziness, and anticholinergic effects (e.g., dry mouth, constipation, urinary retention, tachycardia).

Contraindications include known hypersensitivity to the drug. Other contraindications include acute myocardial infarction, dysrhythmia, heart block, conduction disturbances, heart failure, and hyperthyroidism. Caution is necessary with urinary retention, increased intraocular pressure, and mild hepatic impairment.

Nursing Implications

Preventing Interactions

Increased CNS depression occurs when cyclobenzaprine is combined with alcohol or other CNS depressants.

Administering the Medication

Because of the risk of inconsistent doses, the nurse does not split the generic 10-mg tablets when administering cyclobenzaprine. He or she administers extended-release capsules whole.

Assessing for Therapeutic and Adverse Effects

The nurse assesses the patient's response to the medication, which should indicate relief of the skeletal muscle spasm, decreased pain, and increased activity.

The nurse assesses for increased CNS depression, which will place the patient at risk for falls and injury. It is necessary to assess the patient's cardiovascular status, including pulse and

blood pressure. The medication places the patient at risk for hypotension. Anticholinergic effects occur. The nurse assesses the patient for urinary retention.

Patient Teaching

Box 52.26 identifies patient teaching guidelines for cyclobenzaprine.

NCLEX Success

14. An 18-year-old man is having an open reduction external fixation of a hip following a football injury. During surgery, he develops a fever of 105°F. Which of the following medications is administered?

    A. cyclobenzaprine hydrochloride (Flexeril)
    B. dexamethasone sodium phosphate (Decadron)
    C. phenytoin (Dilantin)
    D. dantrolene sodium (Dantrium)

15. Which of the following interventions assists the patient in decreasing the anticholinergic effects of cyclobenzaprine (Flexeril)?

    A. Have the patient void before the administration of cyclobenzaprine.
    B. Give the patient lemon juice mixed with warm water to prevent constipation.
    C. Give the patient hard candy to suck on.
    D. Assess the patient's pulse and blood pressure.

IMIDAZOLINE DERIVATIVES

Ⓟ **Tizanidine hydrochloride** (Zanaflex) is a centrally acting alpha₂-adrenergic agonist administered for acute and intermittent management of increased muscle tone with spasticity.

Pharmacokinetics

Tizanidine is absorbed rapidly in the GI tract. The medication has on onset of action in 30 to 60 minutes, peak in 1 to 2 hours, and duration of action in 3 to 6 hours. It is metabolized by the liver with a 2.7- to 4.2-hour half-life, and the drug is excreted in the urine. Tizanidine crosses the placenta and enters the breast milk.

Action

Tizanidine is a centrally acting alpha$_2$-adrenergic agonist that produces antispasmodic effect as a result of indirect depression of postsynaptic reflexes by blocking the excitatory actions of spinal interneurons.

Use

Clinicians use tizanidine as indicated for use in patients who have acute and intermittent management of increased muscle tone associated with spasticity. Table 52.10 gives route and dosage information for tizanidine.

Adverse Effects and Contraindications

Common adverse effects of tizanidine include drowsiness, dizziness, constipation, dry mouth, and hypotension. Hypotension may be significant and occur at usual doses. The drug may also cause psychotic symptoms, including hallucinations.

Contraindications include hypersensitivity to the medication. Other contraindications include use of fluvoxamine and ciprofloxacin.

Nursing Implications

Preventing Interactions

The administration of alcohol, baclofen, or CNS depressants with tizanidine can increase the patient's susceptibility to symptoms of depression. Hormonal contraceptives may increase the plasma concentration of tizanidine. Administration with other alpha$_2$-agonists may have hypotensive effects. Kava and valerian may decrease the effect of the drug.

Administering the Medication

Patients may take tizanidine with or without food. However, consistent administration of the drug assists in absorption of the drug and its effect.

Assessing for Therapeutic and Adverse Effects

The nurse assesses the patient for a reduction of skeletal muscle spasms and decreased muscle tone.

The nurse assesses patients for somnolence, sedation, dizziness, and hallucinations. He or she also assesses the cardiovascular patient's status for bradycardia and hypotension. In addition, it is necessary to assess the patient's liver and renal function.

Patient Teaching

Box 52.27 identifies patient teaching guidelines for tizanidine.

BOX 52.27   Patient Teaching Guidelines for Tizanidine

■ Do not alter positions when experiencing dizziness.
■ Do not operate machinery.
■ Report unusual sensory effects such as hallucinations or delusions.

The Nursing Process

Assessment

- For muscle spasms, assess for
  - Pain: This prominent symptom of muscle spasm is usually aggravated by movement. Determine the location of the spasm, as well as the intensity, duration, and precipitating factors (e.g., traumatic injury, strenuous exercise).
  - Accompanying signs and symptoms: bruises (ecchymoses), edema, or signs of inflammation (redness, heat, edema, tenderness to the touch)
- With spasticity, assess for:
  - Pain
  - Impaired functional ability in self-care (e.g., eating, dressing, bathing)
  - Ambulation and other exercise (joint and muscle mobility)

Nursing Diagnoses

- Pain related to muscle spasm
- Impaired physical mobility related to spasm and pain
- Bathing/hygiene self-care deficit related to spasm and pain
- Deficit knowledge: nondrug measures to relieve muscle spasm, pain, spasticity and safe usage of skeletal muscle relaxants
- Risk for injury: dizziness, sedation related to CNS depression

Planning/Goals

The patient will

- Experience relief of pain and spasm
- Experience improved motor function
- Increase self-care abilities in activities of daily living
- Take medications as instructed
- Use nondrug measures appropriately
- Be safeguarded when sedated from drug therapy

Nursing Interventions

The nurse will

- Use adjunctive measures to help treat muscle spasm and spasticity
  - Physical therapy (massage, moist heat, exercises)
  - Relaxation techniques
  - Correct posture and lifting techniques (e.g., stooping rather than bending to lift objects, holding heavy objects close to the body, *not lifting excessive amounts of weight*)
  - Regular exercise and use of warm-up exercises (Strenuous exercise performed on an occasional basis [e.g., weekly or monthly] is more likely to cause acute muscle spasm.)

Evaluation

- Interview and observe for relief of symptoms.
- Interview and observe correct usage of medications and nondrug therapeutic measures.

Key Concepts

- Seizures are idiopathic or secondary (caused by tumors, metabolic disorders, overdoses of numerous drugs, or withdrawal of alcohol or sedative–hypnotic drugs).

- When seizures occur in a chronic, recurrent pattern, they characterize a disorder known as epilepsy, which usually requires long-term drug therapy.

- Types of seizures include generalized (generalized tonic–clonic seizures) and partial (simple or complex, depending on whether consciousness is altered).

- Status epilepticus is a life-threatening emergency that may result in hypotension, hypoxia, cardiac dysrhythmias, permanent brain damage, and death unless prompt, appropriate treatment is instituted.

- The FDA has issued a **BLACK BOX WARNING** ◆ for phenobarbital. Patients who take phenobarbital are at risk for suicidal ideation. It is important to monitor the patient for statements that indicate depression and suicide.

- Adverse-effect profiles vary with individual AEDs; potential teratogenic adverse effects, drug interactions, hypersensitivity reactions, and blood dyscrasias have been reported.

- The FDA has issued several **BLACK BOX WARNINGS** ◆ for valproic acid. The first instructs patients to discontinue valproic acid at any sign of pancreatitis; the development of this condition is life threatening. The second points out that valproic acid is a teratogenic medication. The third instructs the patient to check for signs of bleeding or bruising. Altered bleeding times may occur.

- The FDA has issued a **BLACK BOX WARNING** ◆ for carbamazepine concerning aplastic anemia and agranulocytosis.

- Newer AEDs have better adverse-effect profiles with enhanced seizure control and are classified as derivatives.

- The FDA has issued a **BLACK BOX WARNING** ◆ related to the potential development of serious dermatologic reactions with lamotrigine. Because a serious skin rash may occur, especially in children, lamotrigine should be administered cautiously to children younger than 16 years of age and should be discontinued at the first sign of skin rash in an adult.

- Monotherapy should guide initial management of seizure disorders.

- When an AED is being discontinued, its dosage should always be tapered gradually, usually over 1 to 3 months. Abruptly stopping an AED may exacerbate seizures or cause status epilepticus.

- Monitoring of serum drug levels is useful for most AEDs and must be interpreted in relation to clinical responses.

- Muscle spasms usually result from trauma to the affected skeletal muscle.

- Spasticity results from damage to nerves in the brain and spinal cord.

- Both muscle spasms and spasticity can cause pain and disability.

- Physical therapy and other nonpharmacologic treatments are useful in treating muscle spasm and spasticity.

- Most muscle relaxant drugs are CNS depressants; only dantrolene acts on the muscle.

- The FDA has issued a **BLACK BOX WARNING** ◆ stating that the patient should have liver function tests and that dantrolene be discontinued at the first indication of hepatic impairment.

Critical Thinking Questions

52-1. An 18-year-old man is diagnosed with generalized and partial seizures. He has experienced three tonic clonic seizures in the past 6 months and was started on phenytoin (Dilantin) 1 month ago. The phenytoin has decreased the number of seizures but has not been successful in controlling the seizures to the degree the patient would like. The prescriber has added carbamazepine (Tegretol) to the antiepileptic regimen.

- What is the action of phenytoin and carbamazepine?
- What patient teaching is most important with each of these medications?

52-2. A 57-year-old man is status postcraniotomy for brain cancer. He has a seizure disorder as a result of the brain tumor. He takes lamotrigine (Lamictal). When giving his history, he states that he smells a scent similar to ammonia prior to experiencing a seizure.

- In caring for this patient, which nursing action is most important in his care?
- What are the nursing implications regarding the administration of lamotrigine?

References and Resources

Cross, S. A., & Curran, M. P. (2009). Lacosamide in partial-onset seizures. *Drugs, 69*(4), 449–459.

Eisai Incorporated Medical Services (2010). *Banzel (Rufinamide) Drug Insert.*

Eisai Incorporated Medical Services (2010). *Banzel Therapeutic Blood Levels.* 1–4.

Gamez-Levya, G., Aristin, J. L., Fernandez, E., & Pascual, J. (2009). Experience with intravenous levetiracetam in status epilepticus. *CNS Drugs, 23*(11), 983–987.

Gorgey, A. S., Chiodo, A. D., & Gater, D. R. (2009). Oral baclofen administration in persons with chronic spinal cord injury does not prevent the protective effects of spasticity on body composition and glucose homeostasis. *Spinal Cord, 48,* 160–165.

Karch, A. M. (2013). *2013 Lippincott's nursing drug guide.* Philadelphia, PA: Lippincott Williams & Wilkins.

Kuhn, M. A., & Winston, D. (2008). *Herbal therapy supplements a scientific and traditional approach.* (2nd ed.). Philadelphia, PA: Lippincott Williams & Wilkins.

Maryanoff, B. E. (2009). Pharmaceutical "Gold" from neurostabilizing agents: Topiramate and successor molecules. ChemInform (abstract) 40(37)

Nursing 2011 drug handbook. (2011). Philadelphia, PA: Lippincott William & Wilkins.

Perucca, E., Cloyd, J., Critchley, D., & Fuseau, E. (2008). Rufinamide: Clinical pharmacokinetics and concentration–response relationships in patients with epilepsy. *Epilepsia, 47*(7), 1123–1141.

Porth, C. M., & Matfin, G. (2009). *Pathophysiology concepts of altered health states.* Philadelphia, PA: Lippincott Williams & Wilkins.

Rouse, D. J. (2011). Using magnesium sulfate for fetal neuroprotection. *Contemporary OB/GYN,* April.

Scheinfeld, N. (2003). The role of gabapentin in treating diseases with cutaneous manifestations of pain. *International Journal of Dermatology, 42,* 491–495.

Smeltzer, S. C., Bare, B. G., Hinkle, J. H., & Cheever, K. H. (2010). *Brunner & Suddarth's textbook of medical-surgical nursing* (12th ed.). Philadelphia, PA: Lippincott Williams & Wilkins.

Soul, J. (2009). Novel medications for neonatal seizures: Bumetanide and topiramate. *Journal of Pediatric Neurology,* (7), 85–93.

Up-To-Date. (2011). *Lamotrigine: Drug Information.* Lexi-Comp, Inc.

Waterhouse, C., & Hale, H. (2010). Clinical standards for phenytoin administration: The application of evidence to practice. *British Journal of Neuroscience Nursing, 6*(3), 116–122.

53 Drug Therapy to Reduce Anxiety and Produce Hypnosis

Clinical Application Case Study

Lorraine Terrence, an 83-year-old widow who lives alone, is in the early stages of Alzheimer's disease. She has a history of cardiovascular disease and hypertension and has been admitted to the local hospital for observation after complaints of chest pain. At present, she is very anxious and agitated. The admitting nurse received a telephone call from Mrs. Terrence's daughter, who lives out of town. The daughter states that her mother has experienced anxiety and depression for many years and her symptoms have worsened since her father died 6 months ago. The daughter does not know what medications her mother currently takes, and she is concerned that her mother lives alone and wants her to move to a nursing home. The physician orders the following medications: alprazolam (Xanax) for anxiety, citalopram (Celexa) for depression, and zolpidem (Ambien) for sleep.

KEY TERMS

Anterograde amnesia: short-term memory loss

Anxiety: common disorder that may be referred to as nervousness, tension, worry, or other terms that denote an unpleasant feeling

Anxiety disorder: severe anxiety that is prolonged and impairs the ability to function in usual activities of daily living

Anxiolytics: antianxiety drugs

Hypnotics: drugs that produce sleep

Insomnia: prolongs difficulty in going to sleep or staying asleep long enough to feel rested

Sedatives: drugs that produce central nervous system depression

Introduction

This chapter introduces the pharmacological care of the patient who is experiencing anxiety and/or insomnia. Antianxiety and sedative–hypnotic drugs are central nervous system (CNS) depressants that have similar effects. **Anxiolytics** are antianxiety drugs, **sedatives** promote relaxation, and **hypnotics** produce sleep. The difference between the effects depends largely on dosage. Large doses of antianxiety and sedative drugs produce sleep, and small doses of hypnotics have anxiolytic or sedative effects. Also, therapeutic doses of hypnotics taken at bedtime may have residual sedative effects ("morning hangover") the following day. Because these drugs produce varying degrees of CNS depression, some are also used as anticonvulsants and anesthetics.

Overview of Anxiety

To promote understanding of the uses and effects of both benzodiazepines and nonbenzodiazepines, anxiety and insomnia are described in the following sections. The clinical manifestations of these disorders are similar and overlapping; that is, daytime anxiety may be manifested as nighttime difficulty in sleeping because the person cannot "turn off" worries, and difficulty in sleeping may be manifested as anxiety, fatigue, and decreased ability to function during usual waking hours.

Etiology

Anxiety is a common disorder that may be referred to as nervousness, tension, worry, or other terms that denote an unpleasant feeling. It occurs when a person perceives a situation as threatening to physical, emotional, social, or economic well-being. Anxiety may occur in association with everyday events related to home, work, school, social activities, and chronic illness, or it may occur episodically, in association with acute illness, death, divorce, losing a job, starting a new job, or taking a test. Situational anxiety is a normal response to a stressful situation. It may be beneficial when it motivates the person toward constructive, problem-solving, coping activities. Symptoms may be quite severe, but they usually last only 2 to 3 weeks.

Although there is no clear boundary between normal and abnormal anxiety, when anxiety is severe or prolonged and impairs the ability to function in usual activities of daily living, it is called an **anxiety disorder**. The American Psychiatric Association delineates anxiety disorders as medical diagnoses in the *Diagnostic and Statistical Manual of Mental Disorders, 4th edition, Text Revision* (*DSM-IV-TR*). This classification includes several types of anxiety disorders, as described in Box 53.1. Generalized anxiety disorder (GAD) is emphasized in this chapter.

Pathophysiology

The pathophysiology of anxiety disorders is unknown, but there is evidence of a biologic basis and possible imbalances among several neurotransmission systems. A simplistic view involves an excess of excitatory neurotransmitters (e.g., norepinephrine) or a deficiency of inhibitory neurotransmitters (e.g., gamma-aminobutyric acid [GABA]).

The noradrenergic system is associated with the hyperarousal state experienced by patients with anxiety (i.e., feelings of panic, restlessness, tremulousness, palpitations, hyperventilation), which is attributed to excessive norepinephrine. Norepinephrine is released from the locus coeruleus (LC) in response to an actual or a perceived threat. The LC is a brainstem nucleus that contains many noradrenergic neurons and has extensive projections to the limbic system, cerebral cortex, and cerebellum. Certain observations lend support to the role of the noradrenergic system in anxiety. Drugs that stimulate activity in the LC (e.g., caffeine) may cause symptoms of anxiety, and drugs used to treat anxiety (e.g., benzodiazepines) decrease neuronal firing and norepinephrine release in the LC.

Neuroendocrine factors also play a role in anxiety disorders. Perceived threat or stress activates the hypothalamic–pituitary–adrenal axis and corticotropin-releasing factor (CRF), one of its components. CRF activates the LC, which then releases norepinephrine and generates anxiety. Overall, authorities consider CRF important in integrating the endocrine, autonomic, and behavioral responses to stress.

GABA is the major inhibitory neurotransmitter in the brain and spinal cord. Gamma-aminobutyric acid$_A$ (GABA$_A$) receptors are attached to chloride channels in nerve cell membranes. When GABA interacts with GABA$_A$ receptors, chloride channels open, chloride ions move into the neuron, and the nerve cell is less able to be excited (i.e., generate an electrical impulse).

The serotonin system, although not as well understood, also may play a role in anxiety. Both serotonin reuptake inhibitors and serotonin receptor agonists are now used to treat anxiety disorders. Research has suggested two possible roles for the serotonin receptor HT$_{1A}$. During embryonic development, stimulation of HT$_{1A}$ receptors by serotonin may contribute to the development of normal brain circuitry necessary for normal anxiety responses. However, during adulthood, some serotonin reuptake inhibitors act through HT$_{1A}$ receptors to reduce anxiety responses.

Additional causes of anxiety disorders include medical conditions (anxiety disorder due to a general medical condition according to the *DSM-IV-TR*), psychiatric disorders, and substance abuse. Almost all major psychiatric illnesses may be associated with symptoms of anxiety (e.g., dementia, major depression, mania, schizophrenia). Anxiety related to substance abuse is categorized in the *DSM-IV-TR* as substance-induced anxiety disorder.

BOX 53.1 Anxiety Disorders

Generalized Anxiety Disorder

Major diagnostic criteria for generalized anxiety disorder (GAD) include worry about two or more circumstances and multiple symptoms for 6 months or longer and elimination of disease processes or drugs as possible causes. The frequency, duration, or intensity of the worry is exaggerated or out of proportion to the actual situation. Symptoms are related to motor tension (e.g., muscle tension, restlessness, trembling, fatigue), overactivity of the autonomic nervous system (e.g., dyspnea, palpitations, tachycardia, sweating, dry mouth, dizziness, nausea, diarrhea), and increased vigilance (feeling fearful, nervous, or keyed up; difficulty concentrating; irritability; insomnia).

Symptoms of anxiety occur with numerous disease processes, including medical disorders (e.g., hyperthyroidism, cardiovascular disease, cancer) and psychiatric disorders (e.g., mood disorders, schizophrenia, substance use disorders). They also frequently occur with drugs that affect the central nervous system (CNS). With CNS stimulants (e.g., nasal decongestants, antiasthma drugs, nicotine, caffeine), symptoms occur with drug administration; with CNS depressants (e.g., alcohol, benzodiazepines), symptoms are more likely to occur when the drug is stopped, especially if stopped abruptly.

When the symptoms are secondary to medical illness, they may decrease as the illness improves. However, most people with GAD experience little relief when one stressful situation or problem is resolved. Instead, they quickly move on to another worry. Additional characteristics of GAD include its chronicity, although the severity of symptoms fluctuates over time; its frequent association with somatic symptoms (e.g., headache, gastrointestinal complaints, including irritable bowel syndrome); and its frequent coexistence with depression, other anxiety disorders, and substance abuse or dependence.

Obsessive-Compulsive Disorder

An obsession involves an uncontrollable desire to dwell on a thought or a feeling; a compulsion involves repeated performance of some act to relieve the fear and anxiety associated with an obsession. Obsessive-compulsive disorder (OCD) is characterized by obsessions or compulsions that are severe enough to be time consuming (e.g., take more than an hour per day), cause marked distress, or impair the person's ability to function in usual activities or relationships. The compulsive behavior provides some relief from anxiety but is not pleasurable. The person recognizes that the obsessions or compulsions are excessive or unreasonable and attempts to resist them. When patients resist or are prevented from performing the compulsive behavior, they experience increasing anxiety and often abuse alcohol or antianxiety, sedative-type drugs in the attempt to relieve anxiety.

Panic Disorder

Panic disorder involves acute, sudden, recurrent attacks of anxiety, with feelings of intense fear, terror, or impending doom. It may be accompanied by such symptoms as palpitations, sweating, trembling, shortness of breath or a feeling of smothering, chest pain, nausea, or dizziness. Symptoms usually build to a peak over about 10 minutes and may require medication to be relieved. Afterward, the person is usually preoccupied and worried about future attacks.

A significant number (50%–65%) of patients with panic disorder are thought to also have major depression. In addition, some patients with panic disorder also develop agoraphobia, a fear of having a panic attack in a place or situation where one cannot escape or get help. Combined panic disorder and agoraphobia often involves a chronic, relapsing pattern of significant functional impairment and may require lifetime treatment.

Posttraumatic Stress Disorder

PTSD develops after seeing or being involved in highly stressful events that involve actual or threatened death or serious injury (e.g., natural disasters, military combat, violent acts such as rape or murder, explosions or bombings, serious automobile accidents). The person responds to such an event with thoughts and feelings of intense fear, helplessness, or horror and develops symptoms such as hyperarousal, irritability, outbursts of anger, difficulty sleeping, difficulty concentrating, and an exaggerated startle response. These thoughts, feelings, and symptoms persist as the traumatic event is relived through recurring thoughts, images, nightmares, or flashbacks in which the actual event seems to be occurring. The intense psychic discomfort leads people to avoid situations that remind them of the event; become detached from other people; have less interest in activities they formerly enjoyed; and develop other disorders (e.g., anxiety disorders, major depression, alcohol or other substance abuse).

The response to stress is highly individualized and the same event or type of event might precipitate PTSD in one person and have little effect in another. Thus, most people experience major stresses and traumatic events during their lifetimes, but many do not develop PTSD. This point needs emphasis because many people seem to assume that PTSD is the normal response to a tragic event and that intensive counseling is needed. For example, counselors converge on schools in response to events that are perceived to be tragic or stressful. Some authorities take the opposing view, however, that talking about and reliving a traumatic event may increase anxiety in some people and thereby increase the likelihood that PTSD will occur.

Social Anxiety Disorder

This disorder involves excessive concern about scrutiny by others, which may start in childhood and be lifelong. Affected people are afraid they will say or do something that will embarrass or humiliate them. As a result, they try to avoid certain situations (e.g., public speaking) or experience considerable distress if they cannot avoid them. They are often uncomfortable around other people or experience anxiety in many social situations. SAD may be inherited; there is a threefold increase in the occurrence of SAD in related family members.

Clinical Manifestations

Clinical manifestations of anxiety include motor tension, such as muscle tension, restlessness, trembling, and fatigue; they also include overactivity of the autonomic nervous system, such as dyspnea, palpitations, tachycardia, sweating, dry mouth, dizziness, nausea, and diarrhea. Other clinical manifestations include increased vigilance, such as feeling fearful, nervous, or keyed up; difficulty concentrating; irritability; and insomnia. Box 53.1 summarizes the clinical manifestations of specific anxiety disorders defined by the *DSM-IV-TR*.

TABLE 53.1

Drugs Administered to Reduce Anxiety and Produce Hypnosis

Drug Class	Prototype	Other Drugs in the Class
Benzodiazepines	Diazepam (Valium)	Alprazolam (Xanax, Xanax XR)
		Chlordiazepoxide (Librium)
		Clorazepate (Tranxene)
		Flurazepam (Dalmane)
		Lorazepam (Ativan)
		Midazolam (Versed)
		Oxazepam (Serax)
		Temazepam (Restoril)
		Triazolam (Halcion)
Sedative-hypnotics		Chloral hydrate (Aquachloral, Noctec)
		Eszopiclone (Lunesta)
		Ramelteon (Rozerem)
		Zaleplon (Sonata)
		Zolpidem (Ambien)

Drug Therapy

Benzodiazepines are widely used to treat anxiety disorders (Table 53.1). Benzodiazepines are useful in the short-term treatment symptoms of acute anxiety in response to stressful situations. Antidepressants (i.e., selective serotonin reuptake inhibitors, tricyclic antidepressants, and newer miscellaneous drugs) are preferred as first-line drugs for long-term treatment of most chronic anxiety disorders, with benzodiazepines considered second-line drugs. Chapter 54 discusses antidepressant medications in more detail.

The barbiturates, a historically important group of CNS depressants, are obsolete for most uses, including treatment of anxiety and insomnia. A few may find use as intravenous (IV) general anesthetics (see Chap. 50), as treatment for seizure disorders (phenobarbital; see Chap. 52), and as drugs or abuse (see Chap. 57).

Overview of Sleep and Insomnia

Sleep is a recurrent period of decreased mental and physical activity during which a person is relatively unresponsive to sensory and environmental stimuli. Normal sleep allows rest, renewal of energy for performing activities of daily living, and alertness on awakening.

Etiology

Insomnia, prolonged difficulty in going to sleep or staying asleep long enough to feel rested, is the most common sleep disorder. Occasional sleeplessness is a normal response to many stimuli and is not usually harmful. Insomnia is said to be chronic when it lasts longer than 1 month. As in anxiety, several neurotransmission systems are apparently involved in regulating sleep–wake cycles and producing insomnia.

Insomnia has many causes. Medical disorders, such as chronic pain syndromes and fibromyalgia, and neurologic disorders, such as movement disorders or headaches, may lead to sleep disturbances. Psychiatric conditions and substance abuse may also play a role. Other causes of insomnia include environmental factors (e.g., light, temperature, noise, uncomfortable mattress) or stress-related factors (e.g., stressful life events, deadlines, new job, personal losses). Certain medications, including stimulants such as caffeine, some antidepressants, beta-blockers, and over-the-counter (OTC) and herbal medications, can cause sleep difficulties. Evidence supports the genetic susceptibility to factors such as light and stress on sleep hygiene.

Also, research has demonstrated that patients with insomnia show evidence of increased brain arousal, higher day and night body temperatures, and increased levels of adrenocorticotropic hormone. In addition, patients with insomnia have higher rates of depression and anxiety.

Pathophysiology

When a person retires for sleep, there is an initial period of drowsiness or sleep latency, which lasts about 30 minutes. After the person is asleep, cycles occur approximately every 90 minutes during the sleep period. During each cycle, the sleeper progresses from drowsiness (stage I) to deep sleep (stages III and IV). These stages are characterized by depressed body functions, non–rapid eye movement (non-REM), and nondreaming, and they are thought to be physically restorative. Activities that occur during these stages include increased tissue repair, synthesis of skeletal muscle protein, and secretion of growth hormone. At the same time, there is decreased body temperature, metabolic rate, glucose consumption, and production of catabolic hormones. A period of 5 to 20 minutes of REM, dreaming, and increased physiologic activity follow stage IV.

Experts believe that REM sleep is mentally and emotionally restorative; REM deprivation can lead to serious psychological problems, including psychosis. It is estimated that people spend about 75% of sleeping hours in non-REM sleep and about 25% in REM sleep. However, older adults often have a different pattern, with less deep sleep, more light sleep, more frequent awakenings, and generally more disruptions.

Clinical Manifestations

Clinical manifestations of insomnia include fatigue, lack of energy, and irritability. Patients with insomnia report diminished work performance and decreased concentration. Generally, patients with insomnia do not complain of daytime sleepiness. They tend to be overconcerned about their inability to fall asleep; the more they try to sleep, the more agitated they become, and the less they are able to fall asleep.

Drug Therapy

The main drugs used to treat insomnia are the benzodiazepines and the nonbenzodiazepine hypnotics (see Table 53.1). However, it is important to note that drug companies market only a few benzodiazepines for the treatment of insomnia, although all are effective sedative–hypnotics. People also use OTC medications as sleep aids; these medications include antihistamines alone or in combination with pain relievers. Along with OTC medications, many herbal supplements are consumed to decrease stress, anxiety, and induce sleep. Box 53.2 summarizes herbal supplements that are commonly taken and may interact with other prescription medications administered for anxiety and sleep induction.

Clinical Application 53-1

- Mrs. Terrence's two sons come to visit her in the hospital. They complain to the nurse that their mother seems oversedated. In denial about her mental status, the sons request that their mother's medication be discontinued, but the nurses are concerned that if she is agitated, she may pull out her IV lines and Foley catheter as well as possibly strike out at staff. How does the nurse handle this situation while respecting the family's concerns, based on his or her knowledge and skills of patient-centered care according to the Quality and Safety Education for Nurses project (QSEN)?

BOX 53.2　Herbal Supplements Commonly Used to Reduce Anxiety and Produce Hypnosis

Kava

This supplement is derived from a shrub found in many South Pacific islands. It is claimed to be useful in numerous disorders, including anxiety, depression, insomnia, asthma, pain, rheumatism, muscle spasms, and seizures. It suppresses emotional excitability and may produce a mild euphoria. Effects include analgesia, sedation, diminished reflexes, impaired gait, and pupil dilation. Kava has been used or studied most often for treatment of anxiety, stress, and restlessness. It is thought to act similarly to the benzodiazepines by interacting with gamma-aminobutyric acid$_A$ (GABA$_A$) receptors on nerve cell membranes. This action and limited evidence from a few small clinical trials may support use of the herb in the treatment of anxiety, insomnia, and seizure disorders. However, additional studies are needed to delineate therapeutic and adverse effects, dosing recommendations, and drug interactions when used for these conditions.

Adverse effects include impaired thinking, judgment, motor reflexes, and vision. Serious adverse effects may occur with long-term, heavy use, including decreased plasma proteins, decreased platelet and lymphocyte counts, dyspnea, and pulmonary hypertension. Kava should not be taken concurrently with other central nervous system (CNS) depressant drugs (e.g., benzodiazepines, ethanol), antiplatelet drugs, or levodopa (increases Parkinson symptoms). In addition, it should not be taken by women who are pregnant or lactating or by children under 12 years of age. Finally, it should be used cautiously by patients with renal disease, thrombocytopenia, or neutropenia. Recently, the U.S. FDA issued a warning that products containing kava have been implicated in many cases of severe liver toxicity (e.g., hepatitis, cirrhosis, liver failure).

Melatonin

This hormone is produced by the pineal gland, an endocrine gland in the brain. Endogenous melatonin is derived from the amino acid tryptophan, which is converted to serotonin, which is then enzymatically converted to melatonin in the pineal gland. Exogenous preparations are produced synthetically and may contain other ingredients. Melatonin products are widely available. Recommended doses on product labels usually range from 0.3 to 5 mg.

Melatonin influences sleep–wake cycles; it is released during sleep, and serum levels are very low during waking hours. Prolonged intake of exogenous melatonin can reset the sleep–wake cycle. As a result, it is widely promoted for prevention and treatment of jet lag (considered a circadian rhythm disorder) and treatment of insomnia. It is thought to act similarly to the benzodiazepines in inducing sleep. In several studies of patients with sleep disturbances, those taking melatonin experienced modest improvement compared with those taking a placebo. Other studies suggest that melatonin supplements improve sleep in older adults with melatonin deficiency and decrease weight loss in people with cancer. Large, controlled studies are needed to determine the effects of long-term use and the most effective regimen when used for jet lag.

Melatonin supplements are contraindicated in patients with hepatic insufficiency because of reduced clearance. They are also contraindicated in people with a history of cerebrovascular disease, depression, or neurologic disorders. They should be used cautiously by people with renal impairment and those taking benzodiazepines or other CNS depressant drugs. Adverse effects include altered sleep patterns, confusion, headache, hypothermia, pruritus, sedation, and tachycardia.

Valerian

This herb is used mainly as a sedative–hypnotic. It apparently increases the amount of GABA in the brain, probably by inhibiting the transaminase enzyme that normally metabolizes GABA. Increasing GABA, an inhibitory neurotransmitter, results in calming, sedative effects.

There are differences of opinion about the clinical usefulness of valerian; some practitioners say that studies indicate the herb's effectiveness as a sleep aid and mild antianxiety agent, whereas others say that these studies were flawed by small samples, short durations, and poor definitions of patient populations. There is insufficient evidence to support the use of valerian for treating insomnia.

Adverse effects with acute overdose or chronic use include blurred vision, cardiac disturbance, excitability, headache, hypersensitivity reactions, insomnia, and nausea. There is a risk of hepatotoxicity from overdosage and from using combination herbal products containing valerian. Valerian should not be taken by people with hepatic impairment (risk of increased liver damage) or by pregnant or breast-feeding women (effects are unknown). The herb should not be taken concurrently with any other sedatives, hypnotics, alcohol, or CNS depressants because of the potential for additive CNS depression.

Nutritional and herbal supplements for anxiety and anxiety-related disorders

by S. LAKHAN, K. VIEIRA

Nutrition Journal
2010, 9(42), 1–14

Over the past several decades, complementary and alternative medications have increasingly become a part of everyday treatment. The lifetime prevalence of anxiety disorders is approximately 16% worldwide. Many people with these disorders consider the use of herbal and other natural treatments for the management of their psychological symptoms for various reasons, such as costs associated with prescriptions medications as well as the adverse effects associated with their use. This review included a total of 24 clinical studies published in English that used human subjects and examined the anxiolytic potential of dietary and herbal supplements.

The conclusion of this systematic review supports the use of nutritional and herbal supplements, such as kava, as an effective method for treating anxiety and anxiety-related conditions without the risk of serious adverse effects. However, more research is needed in this area due to potentially dangerous effects of over-consumption of supplements and adverse interactions with prescription and over-the-counter (OTC) medications.

IMPLICATIONS FOR NURSING PRACTICE: When caring for patients who are suffering from anxiety, it is imperative that nurses assess the patient's use of herbal and complementary supplements administered for the treatment of anxiety. The U.S. FDA does not regulate complementary and alternative medications, and they can place the patient at risk for adverse effects when administered with prescribed anxiolytics, sedatives, or hypnotics.

Benzodiazepines

Benzodiazepines are widely used for anxiety and insomnia and are also used for several other indications. These drugs have a wide margin of safety between therapeutic and toxic doses, and they are rarely fatal, even in overdose, unless combined with other CNS depressant drugs, such as alcohol. However, benzodiazepines are Schedule IV drugs under the Controlled Substances Act. Drugs of abuse, they may cause physiologic dependence; therefore, withdrawal symptoms occur if these drugs are stopped abruptly. To avoid withdrawal symptoms, it is necessary to taper benzodiazepines gradually before discontinuing them completely.

Although benzodiazepines are effective anxiolytics, long-term use is associated with concerns over tolerance, dependency, withdrawal, lack of efficacy for treating the depression that often accompanies anxiety disorders, and the need for multiple daily dosing with some agents. These drugs differ mainly in their plasma half-lives, production of active metabolites, and clinical uses. ℗ **Diazepam** (Valium) is the prototype benzodiazepine.

Pharmacokinetics

Diazepam has a long half-life (20–80 hours) and forms an active metabolite that tends to accumulate. The drug requires 5 to 7 days to reach steady-state serum levels. It is highly lipid soluble, widely distributed in body tissues, and highly bound to plasma proteins (85%–98%). The high lipid solubility allows the drug to easily enter the CNS and perform its actions. After IV injection, diazepam may act within 1 to 5 minutes. However, the duration of action of a single IV dose is short (30–100 minutes). Thus, the pharmacodynamic effects (e.g., sedation) do not correlate with plasma drug levels because the drugs move in and out of the CNS rapidly. This redistribution allows a patient to awaken even though the drug may remain in the blood and other peripheral tissues for days or weeks before it is completely eliminated.

Diazepam is mainly metabolized in the liver by the cytochrome P450 enzymes (CYP3A4 subgroup) and glucuronide conjugation. Metabolites are excreted through the kidneys.

Action

Diazepam enhances the inhibitory effect of GABA to relieve anxiety, tension, and nervousness and to produce sleep. The decreased neuronal excitability also accounts for its usefulness as a muscle relaxant, hypnotic, and anticonvulsant.

Use

Health care providers mainly use diazepam for antianxiety, hypnotic, and anticonvulsant purposes. They also give the drug for preoperative sedation; prevention of agitation and delirium tremens in acute alcohol withdrawal; and treatment of anxiety symptoms associated with depression, acute psychosis, or mania. Thus, patients often take it concurrently with antidepressants, antipsychotics, and mood stabilizers. However, use of diazepam contraindicates the use of some antidepressants. Experts do not advise using the drug for long periods, because it may cause excessive sedation and respiratory depression.

Investigators have extensively studied diazepam, and it has more approved uses than other drugs in its class. Table 53.2 gives route and dosage information for diazepam and the other benzodiazepines. Larger-than-usual doses may be necessary for patients who are severely anxious or agitated. Also, large doses are usually required to relax skeletal muscle; control muscle spasm; control seizures; and provide sedation before surgery, cardioversion, endoscopy, and angiography. When using benzodiazepines with opioid analgesics, it is important to reduce the analgesic dose initially and increase it gradually to avoid excessive CNS depression.

TABLE 53.2

DRUGS AT A GLANCE: Benzodiazepines

Drug	Pregnancy Category	Routes and Dosage Ranges	
		Adults	*Children*
Ⓟ Diazepam (Valium)	D	2–10 mg PO 2–4 times daily; 5–10 mg IM, IV; give IV slowly, no faster than 5 mg (1 mL)/min repeated in 3–4 h if necessary Older or debilitated adults, 2–5 mg PO once or twice daily, increased gradually if needed and tolerated	>6 mo: 1–2.5 mg PO 3–4 times daily, increased gradually if needed and tolerated
Alprazolam (Xanax, Xanax XR)	D	Anxiety: 0.25–0.5 mg PO 3 times daily; maximum 4 mg daily in divided doses; older or debilitated adults, 0.25 mg PO 2–3 times daily, increased gradually if necessary Panic disorder: 0.5 mg PO 3 times daily initially, gradually increase to 4–10 mg daily Xanax XR, 0.5–1 mg PO daily; gradually increase PRN to maximum dose of 3–6 mg daily	Dosage not established
Chlordiazepoxide (Librium)	D	15–100 mg PO daily, once at bedtime or in 3–4 divided doses 50–100 mg IM, IV; maximum 300 mg daily; older or debilitated adults, 5 mg PO 2–4 times daily; 25–50 mg IM, IV	>6 y: 5–10 mg PO 2–4 times daily <6 y: not recommended
Clonazepam (Klonopin, Klonopin wafers)	D	Seizure disorders: 0.5 mg PO 3 times daily, increased by 0.5–1 mg every 3 d until seizures are controlled or adverse effects occur; maximum 20 mg daily Panic disorder: 0.25 mg PO 2 times daily, increasing to 1 mg daily after 3 d	Up to 10 y or 30 kg: 0.01–0.03 mg/kg/d PO initially; not to exceed 0.05 mg/kg/d, in 2 or 3 divided doses; increase by 0.25–0.5 mg every third day until a daily dose of 0.1–0.2 mg/kg is reached
Clorazepate (Tranxene)	D	7.5 mg PO 3 times daily, increased by no more than 7.5 mg/wk; maximum 90 mg daily	9–12 y: 7.5 mg PO 2 times daily, increased by no more than 7.5 mg/wk; maximum 60 mg daily <9 y: not recommended
Flurazepam (Dalmane)	D	15–30 mg PO	Not for use in children <15 y of age
Lorazepam (Ativan)	D	2–6 mg/d PO in 2–3 divided doses; 0.05 mg/kg IM to a maximum of 4 mg; 2 mg IV, diluted with 2 mL of sterile water, sodium chloride, or 5% dextrose injection; do not exceed 2 mg/min; older or debilitated adults, 1–2 mg/d PO in divided doses	
Midazolam (Versed)	D	Preoperative sedation: 0.05–0.08 mg/kg IM ~1 h before surgery Prediagnostic test sedation: 0.1–0.15 mg/kg IV or up to 0.2 mg/kg IV initially; maintenance dose, ~25% of initial dose; reduce dose by 25%–30% if an opioid analgesic is also given Induction of anesthesia: 0.3–0.35 mg/kg IV initially, then reduce dose as above for maintenance; reduce initial dose to 0.15–0.3 mg/kg if a narcotic is also given	Preoperative or preprocedure sedation, induction of anesthesia: syrup 0.25–1 mg/kg PO; maximum of 20 mg as a single dose
Oxazepam (Serax)	D	10–30 mg PO 3–4 times daily; older or debilitated adults, 10 mg PO 3 times daily, gradually increased to 15 mg 3 times daily if necessary	
Temazepam (Restoril)	X	15–30 mg PO	Not for use in children <18 y of age
Triazolam (Halcion)	X	0.125–0.25 mg PO	Not for use in children <18 y of age

Use in Children

Prescribers often order diazepam for children with anxiety and sleep walking or night terrors. Use of the drug requires caution. Children may be more sensitive to its effects of this drug, namely mood and/or mental changes. They may have unanticipated or variable responses, including paradoxical CNS stimulation and excitement rather than CNS depression and calming. Children should take diazepam and other benzodiazepines only when clearly indicated, in the lowest effective dose, and for the shortest effective time. Diazepam should never be used in children younger than 6 months of age.

Use in Older Adults

In older adults, most benzodiazepines are metabolized more slowly, and half-lives are longer than in younger adults. Caution is necessary. The elderly may be sensitive to its effects, especially drowsiness, poor coordination, and mental and/or mood changes caused by the drug. Adverse effects may contribute to falls and other injuries unless patients are carefully monitored and safeguarded. It is important to make the initial dose of any antianxiety or sedative–hypnotic drug small and to increase doses gradually. Diazepam and other benzodiazepines may produce paradoxical excitement and aggression in adults older than 50 years of age who have a history of psychosis.

Use in Patients With Renal or Hepatic Impairment

In impaired renal excretion, active metabolites may accumulate, causing excessive sedation and respiratory depression. Hepatic impairment also rules out use of diazepam.

Use in Patients With Critical Illness

Antianxiety and sedative–hypnotic drugs are often useful in critically ill patients to relieve stress, anxiety, and agitation. Their calming effects decrease cardiac workload (e.g., heart rate, blood pressure, force of myocardial contraction, myocardial oxygen consumption) and respiratory effort. Additional benefits include improving tolerance of treatment measures (e.g., mechanical ventilation); keeping confused patients from harming themselves by pulling out IV catheters, feeding or drainage tubes, wound drains, and other treatment devices; and allowing more rest or sleep. In addition to sedation, the drugs often induce amnesia, which may be a desirable effect in the critically ill.

Caution is necessary with the use of diazepam in patients with critical illness. Patients should provide a comprehensive list of all medications to their health care provider, including antiretrovirals, certain antibiotics, and blood pressure medications. Use of many drugs is a contraindication to taking diazepam.

Use in Patients Receiving Home Care

Most patients take diazepam at home, and the home care nurse shares the responsibility for teaching patients how to use the drug effectively and how to recognize medication responses that should be reported to the health care provider. Accurate dosing is vitally important because underuse may cause the recurrence of the symptoms and overuse may cause toxicity, which may be life-threatening. The nurse tells the patient and any caregivers that if symptoms of withdrawal or overdose develop, it is necessary to seek medical attention immediately. The nurse also monitors the patient's response to the drug and any changes in the patient's condition.

Adverse Effects

Both therapeutic effects and adverse effects of diazepam are more likely to occur after 2 or 3 days of therapy than initially. Such effects accumulate with chronic usage and persist for several days after the drug is discontinued. Many of the adverse effects associated with diazepam are related to its CNS depressant effects. They include drowsiness, problems with memory, confusion, disinhibition, depressed mood with or without suicidal ideation, slurred speech, dizziness, shallow breathing, restlessness, irritability, loss of bladder control, and diminished sexual interest. Other effects may include new or worsening seizures, nausea, constipation, drooling or dry mouth, mild skin rash, and itching. Diazepam and other benzodiazepines exert effects on the GABA receptors and can lead to overdose. Signs of overdose include blurred or double vision, labored breathing, weakness, stupor, and coma. Flumazenil is a benzodiazepine agonist that interacts with the GABA receptors to reverse overdose (see Chap. 57).

Contraindications

Contraindications to diazepam include severe respiratory disorders, such as chronic obstructive pulmonary disease or sleep apnea, severe liver or kidney disease, hypersensitivity reactions, and a history of alcohol or other drug abuse. People with narrow-angle glaucoma or who are pregnant or breastfeeding should not take diazepam. Concurrent use of diazepam and any other CNS depressant warrants caution.

NCLEX Success

1. **A woman is receiving treatment for acute short-term anxiety with a benzodiazepine. The nurse should teach the patient which of the following?**

   A. Monitor serum glucose levels.
   B. Avoid alcohol when taking these medications.
   C. Take medications with food.
   D. Expect a delay in therapeutic effects of several weeks.

2. **Which baseline laboratory tests should a patient receive prior to starting the benzodiazepine?**

   A. blood glucose level
   B. liver enzymes
   C. lipid profile
   D. thyroid panel

Nursing Implications

Preventing Interactions

Smaller-than-usual doses of diazepam and other benzodiazepines may be necessary in patients receiving cimetidine or other drugs that decrease the hepatic metabolism of benzodiazepines.

Administering the Medication

There are various preparations of diazepam, for both oral and parenteral use. The nurse adheres to the following guidelines:

- Ensure that the patient has swallowed sustained-release tablets whole. It is important not to chew these tablets.
- Ensure that the patient consumes the entire dose of medication.
- Do not abruptly withdraw the medication. This places the patient at risk for alterations in mood.
- Administer the intramuscular preparation in a large muscle. Inject it slowly and rotate injection sites.
- Administer the IV form undiluted IV push at a rate of 5 mg/min. In children, inject it at a rate of 0.25 mg/kg over 3 minutes.

Assessing for Therapeutic Effects

The nurse observes for a relaxed, but easily aroused, appearance. The nurse interviews the patient to assess response to the medication. For example, the patient should verbalize that he or she feels less worried and more relaxed. Nonverbal behavior is important; response to the medication includes decreased heart rate and blood pressure and a relaxed posture. It is necessary to assess the level of drowsiness and sleep pattern.

Assessing for Adverse Effects

The nurse monitors the patient's blood pressure. It is necessary to make sure that the patient does not experience paradoxical responses, which include anger, aggression, and hallucinations, to the diazepam.

The nurse assesses for symptoms and symptoms of diazepam dependence, overdose, and withdrawal. The presence of withdrawal symptoms when the drug is stopped indicates physical dependence, which is associated with longer use and higher doses. Common signs and symptoms of withdrawal include increased anxiety, psychomotor agitation, insomnia, irritability, headache, tremor, and palpitations. Less common but more serious signs include confusion, abnormal perception of movement, depersonalization, psychosis, and seizures. Symptoms usually occur 4 to 5 days after stopping a long-acting drug such as diazepam. Relief requires administration of a benzodiazepine.

Patient Teaching

Box 53.3 identifies guidelines for teaching patients who are taking diazepam and other benzodiazepines for anxiety and insomnia.

Other Drugs in the Class

Alprazolam (Xanax, Xanax XR) is administered orally to reduce anxiety and panic disorders. Elderly patients are more sensitive to the effects of the drug and may experience ataxia and oversedation. The immediate-release preparations can be given sublingually if the patient cannot swallow. Alprazolam is preferred over diazepam due to its immediate onset of action. Calcium

---

BOX 53.3 Patient Teaching Guidelines for Benzodiazepines

- "Nerve pills" and "sleeping pills" can relieve symptoms temporarily, but they do not cure or solve the underlying problems. With rare exceptions, these drugs are recommended only for short-term use. For long-term relief, counseling or psychotherapy may be more beneficial because it can help you learn other ways to decrease your nervousness.
- Try to identify and avoid factors that cause nervousness, such as caffeine-containing beverages and stimulant drugs. This may prevent or decrease the severity of nervousness. If the drugs are used, these factors can cancel or decrease the drugs' effects. Stimulant drugs include asthma and cold remedies and appetite suppressants.
- Most pills to control anxiety belong to the same chemical group and have similar effects, including the ability to decrease nervousness, cause drowsiness, and cause dependence. Thus, there is no logical reason to take a combination of the drugs for anxiety, or to take one drug for daytime sedation and another for sleep. Xanax, Ativan, and Restoril are commonly used examples of this group, but there are several others as well.
- Inform all health care providers when taking a sedative-type medication, preferably by the generic and trade names. This helps avoid multiple prescriptions of drugs with similar effects and reduces the risk of serious adverse effects from overdose.

- Do not perform tasks that require alertness if drowsy from medication. The drugs often impair mental and physical functioning, especially during the first several days of use, and thereby make routine activities potentially hazardous. Avoid smoking, ambulating without help, driving a car, operating machinery, bathing and other potentially hazardous tasks. These activities may lead to falls or other injuries if undertaken while alertness is impaired.
- Avoid alcohol and other depressant drugs (e.g., over-the-counter [OTC] antihistamines and sleeping pills, narcotic analgesics, sedating herbs such as kava and valerian, and the dietary supplement melatonin) while taking any antianxiety or sedative–hypnotic drugs (except buspirone). An antihistamine that causes drowsiness is the active ingredient in OTC sleep aids (e.g., Compoz, Nytol, Sominex, Unisom) and in many pain reliever products with "PM" as part of their names (e.g., Tylenol PM). Because these drugs depress brain functioning when taken alone, combining them produces additive depression and may lead to excessive drowsiness, difficulty breathing, traumatic injuries, and other potentially serious adverse drug effects.
- Store drugs safely, out of reach of children and adults who are confused or less than alert. Accidental or intentional ingestion may lead to serious adverse effects. Also, do not keep the drug container at the bedside, because a person sedated by a previous dose may take additional doses.

(Continued on page 992)

channel blockers decrease the metabolism of alprazolam and other benzodiazepines, leading to increased adverse drug effects.

Chlordiazepoxide (Librium) is most commonly administered for the control of withdrawal symptoms related to acute alcoholism. It is important that this drug not be administered with grapefruit juice. The combination decreases drug metabolism and increase drug toxicity. Also, the herbs St. John's wort, kava, and valerian, if given in combination with chlordiazepoxide, increase CNS depression.

Clorazepate (Tranxene) has a longer onset of action than diazepam. This drug is commonly administered for anxiety, alcohol withdrawal, and epilepsy.

QSEN Safety Alert

It is important not to confuse clorazepate with clonazepam (Klonopin); both drugs are used to control seizure activity.

Flurazepam (Dalmane) is administered on a short-term basis for patients who suffer from insomnia. Patients should take it only at bedtime. It is necessary to observe the patient for dizziness and orthostatic hypotension.

Lorazepam (Ativan) is probably the benzodiazepine of first choice. The drug provides rapid tranquilization of patients experiencing agitation. Administered intravenously, it reduces nausea and vomiting as well as anxiety and induces procedural amnesia. Lorazepam has a slow onset of action (5–20 minutes) because of delayed brain penetration but an intermediate to prolonged duration. In addition, there is little accumulation and its elimination is not significantly affected by hepatic or renal disease.

QSEN Safety Alert

When administering prefilled Carpujects, it is essential to inspect and confirm the amount of medication visually.

In May of 2012, the U. S. Food and drug administration (FDA) issued a warning that one brand of cartridge actually contained twice the dosage of lorazepam, leading to possible overdose.

Midazolam (Versed) (see Chap. 50) provides preoperative sedation and mechanical ventilation. It is necessary to reduce the dosage 30% to 50% in the elderly population.

Oxazepam (Serax) is administered for alcohol withdrawal and for the reduction of anxiety. The management of simple partial seizures is an unlabeled use of the drug. It is completely absorbed, with 86% to 99% of the drug protein bound.

Temazepam (Restoril) appears to act at the subcortical levels of the CNS. The drug's main site of action is the limbic system and mesencephalic reticular formation. It potentiates the effects of GABA. Temazepam is eliminated by conjugation and excreted through the kidneys. Thus, it is the drug of choice for elderly patients, those patients who have liver disease, or those who take medications that interfere with hepatic drug-metabolizing enzymes. The adverse effects of temazepam are similar to those of other benzodiazepines. The most severe adverse effect is cardiovascular collapse.

Triazolam (Halcion) has a very rapid onset of action, and it is necessary to administer the drug while patients are in bed. Cirrhosis of the liver or hepatic insufficiency is a contraindication. If patients are receiving protracted therapy, diagnostic testing with routine complete blood counts, urinalysis, and blood chemistry is required because of possible decreases in the hematocrit level and development of blood dyscrasias. Patients should not combine triazolam with ketoconazole or itraconazole.

Clinical Application 53-2

Mrs. Terrence receives alprazolam 0.25 mg PO at 2:00 PM. Later, when the nurse brings in her supper tray, the patient seems relaxed. The supper tray contains roast beef, salad, chocolate pie, and hot tea. Visitors arrive at 5:00 PM and remark to the nurse that Mrs. Terrence is agitated and wringing her hands. She says that she is afraid to verbalize her anxiety to the nursing staff. The nurse prepares to give Mrs. Terrence another dose of medication.

- What does the nurse prepare and why?
- What foods on the supper tray contribute to the patient's anxiety?
- What patient teaching is necessary?

NCLEX Success

3. **Flumazenil is the treatment of choice for patients who have which of the following conditions?**

   A. severe agitation
   B. schizophrenia
   C. benzodiazepine overdose
   D. opioid dependence

4. **The nurse is conducting patient teaching for a patient who will be taking alprazolam for treatment of anxiety. Which of the following medications increases the amount of alprazolam in the body?**

   A. diltiazem (Cardizem)
   B. timolol (Istalol)
   C. albuterol inhaler
   D. bosentan (Tracleer)

5. **Benzodiazepines are thought to work by doing which of the following?**

   A. exciting the CNS
   B. stimulating the reticular activating system
   C. increasing inhibitory feelings
   D. enhancing the effects of GABA

6. **Which of the following medications can be administered to the elderly, accumulates to a small extent in the brain, and is not affected by diminished hepatic function?**

   A. diazepam
   B. lorazepam
   C. clonazepam
   D. chlordiazepoxide

7. **A patient is given chlordiazepoxide (Librium) for acute alcohol withdrawal. During the admission interview with the patient's family, the nurse asks if the patient has taken which of the following herbal supplements?**

   A. garlic
   B. ginger
   C. St. John's wort
   D. *gingko biloba*

Nonbenzodiazepine Sedative–Hypnotic Agents

The nonbenzodiazepine sedative–hypnotics produce sleep. People may receive them prior to diagnostic or surgical procedures or take them nightly. Table 53.1 lists the most commonly administered nonbenzodiazepines that produce sleep. This classification lacks a specific prototype, so each drug in the class will be discussed individually.

In general, people should use sedative–hypnotics only when insomnia causes significant distress and resists management by nonpharmacologic means. The drugs are not indicated for occasional sleeplessness. The goal of treatment is to relieve anxiety or sleeplessness without permitting sensory perception, responsiveness to the environment, or alertness to drop below

safe levels. The drugs of choice for most patients are the benzodiazepines and the nonbenzodiazepine hypnotics, eszopiclone, ramelteon, zaleplon, and zolpidem. However, for patients with insomnia associated with major depression, antidepressants are preferred (see Chap. 54).

Use of sedative–hypnotics every night should not occur unless absolutely necessary. Intermittent administration helps maintain drug effectiveness and decreases the risks of drug abuse and dependence. It also decreases disturbances of normal sleep patterns. For chronic insomnia, only eszopiclone is recommended for long-term treatment (less than or equal to 12 months). To restore the sleep-producing effect, administration of the hypnotic drug must be interrupted for 1 to 2 weeks. Table 53.3 gives route and dosage information for the sedative–hypnotics. Box 53.4 identifies guidelines for teaching patients who are taking sedative–hypnotics for anxiety and insomnia.

Chloral Hydrate

Chloral hydrate (Aquachloral, Noctec), the oldest sedative–hypnotic, is relatively safe, effective, and inexpensive in usual therapeutic doses. The drug produces cerebral depression without excessive decreases in blood pressure. It reportedly does not suppress REM sleep. Children commonly receive chloral hydrate before some diagnostic and therapeutic procedures. To mask the taste of the chloral hydrate, it is necessary to dilute the drug in chilled liquid. Other patients receive chloral hydrate for the relief of anxiety. The adult dose should not exceed 2 g in 24 hours. The most significant adverse effect of the drug is ataxia and generalized CNS depression. Tolerance develops after approximately 2 weeks of continual use. If the patient has been maintained on a high dose, it is important to withdraw the drug over 2 weeks to prevent delirium. Chloral hydrate is a drug of abuse and may cause physical dependence.

Eszopiclone

Eszopiclone (Lunesta) is the first oral nonbenzodiazepine hypnotic to receive FDA approval for long-term use (less than or equal to 12 months). During testing, researchers did not observe tolerance to the hypnotic benefits of the drug over a 6-month period. It increases total sleep time and reduces the amount of time needed to fall asleep. Studies show that eszopiclone does not reduce nighttime awakenings. The drug is a Schedule IV controlled substance.

Supposedly, the hypnotic effect of eszopiclone is due to interaction with the $GABA_A$ receptor at a location close to or coupled with the benzodiazepine receptors. The drug is rapidly absorbed after oral administration, reaching peak plasma levels 1 hour after administration. It has a half-life of 6 hours. It is metabolized in the liver and eliminated primarily by the renal system.

People should take eszopiclone immediately prior to going to bed due to its rapid onset of action.

QSEN Safety Alert

It is important to instruct patients not to engage in any activities following the administration of the medication.

TABLE 53.3

DRUGS AT A GLANCE: Sedative–Hypnotics

Drug	Pregnancy Category	Routes and Dosage Ranges	
		Adults	*Children*
Chloral hydrate (Aquachloral, Noctec)	C	Sedative: 250 mg PO, rectal suppository 3 times/d Hypnotic: 500–1000 mg PO, rectal suppository at bedtime; maximum dose 2 g/d	Sedative: 25 mg/kg PO, rectal suppository per day in 3 or 4 divided doses Hypnotic: 50 mg/kg PO, rectal suppository at bedtime; maximum single dose, 1 g
Eszopiclone (Lunesta)	C	2 mg PO at bedtime; may be increased to 3 mg if needed; debilitated patients, and those with hepatic impairment, 1 mg PO at bedtime; may be increased to 2 mg if needed	Not recommended
Ramelteon (Rozerem)	C	8 mg PO at bedtime	Not recommended
Zaleplon (Sonata)	C	10 mg PO at bedtime; 5 mg for adults who are elderly, of low weight, or have mild to moderate hepatic impairment	Dosage not established
Zolpidem (Ambien)	C	10 mg PO at bedtime; 5 mg for older adults and those with hepatic impairment	Not recommended

BOX 53.4   Patient Teaching Guidelines for Nonbenzodiazepine Sedative-Hypnotics

■ Sleeping pills, like antianxiety drugs, can relieve symptoms temporarily, but they do not cure or solve the underlying problems. With rare exceptions, these drugs are recommended only for short-term use. For long-term relief, counseling or psychotherapy may be more beneficial because it can help you learn other ways to decrease your difficulty in sleeping.

■ Avoid alcohol and other depressant drugs (e.g., over-the-counter [OTC] antihistamines and sleeping pills, narcotic analgesics, sedating herbs such as kava and valerian, and the dietary supplement melatonin) while taking sedative–hypnotic drugs. An antihistamine that causes drowsiness is the active ingredient in OTC sleep aids (e.g., Compoz, Nytol, Sominex, Unisom) and in many pain reliever products with "PM" as part of their names (e.g., Tylenol PM). Because these drugs depress brain functioning when taken alone, combining them produces additive depression and may lead to excessive drowsiness, difficulty breathing, traumatic injuries, and other potentially serious adverse drug effects.

■ Do not perform tasks that require alertness if drowsy from medication. The drugs often impair mental and physical functioning, especially during the first several days of use, and thereby make routine activities potentially hazardous. Avoid smoking, ambulating without help, driving a car, operating machinery, bathing and other potentially hazardous tasks. These activities may lead to falls or other injuries if undertaken while alertness is impaired.

■ Store drugs safely, out of reach of children and adults who are confused or less than alert. Accidental or intentional ingestion may lead to serious adverse effects. Also, do not keep the drug container at the bedside, because a person sedated by a previous dose may take additional doses.

■ Take nonbenzodiazepine hypnotics on an empty stomach, at bedtime, because fatty heavy meals delay onset of action.

■ Do not take herbal supplements with nonbenzodiazepine sedative–hypnotics.

■ Do not take most "sleeping pills" every night. Many sleeping pills lose their effectiveness in 2 to 4 weeks if taken nightly and cause sleep disturbances when stopped. If longer drug therapy for insomnia is needed, Lunesta and Rozerem are approved for long-term use.

■ Use nondrug measures to promote relaxation, rest, and sleep when possible. Physical exercise, reading, craft work, stress management, and relaxation techniques are safer than any drug.

■ Take sleeping pills just before going to bed so that you are lying down when the expected drowsiness occurs.

■ Do not take zolpidem concurrently with alcohol or other CNS depressant drugs because of increased risk of excessive sedation and respiratory depression.

■ Prime zolpidem oral spray prior to initial use. Compress the container five times, hold the container upright, and aim it directly into the mouth.

■ Report adverse effects such as hypersensitivity reactions, complex sleep-related behaviors, or thoughts of suicide to the prescriber.

Also, people should not take the medication following a high-fat meal, because the onset of action may be delayed by approximately 1 hour, or prior to bathing. In addition, geriatric people should not use the drug according to the Beers Criteria.

Adverse reactions to eszopiclone include behavioral changes such as reduced inhibition, aggression or bizarre behavior, worsening depression and suicidal ideation, hallucinations, and **anterograde amnesia** (short-term memory loss). A commonly reported reaction to the drug is an unpleasant taste. Contraindications include hypersensitivity reaction. Caution is necessary during pregnancy and lactation, in depression, and with impaired hepatic or respiratory function. Elderly patients, those with hepatic impairment or debilitating conditions, and those taking drugs that inhibit CYP3A4 enzymes (e.g., antidepressants, antifungals, erythromycin, grapefruit, protease inhibitors, others) require lower dosages to reduce adverse effects. People who take eszopiclone should not take alcohol or other CNS depressants to avoid additive effects.

Ramelteon

Ramelteon (Rozerem), the newest oral nonbenzodiazepine hypnotic, has received FDA approval for the long-term treatment of insomnia characterized by difficulty with sleep onset. Unlike other nonbenzodiazepine hypnotics, which bind to $GABA_A$ receptors, ramelteon binds to melatonin receptors in the CNS. Stimulation of melatonin receptors by ramelteon, like endogenous melatonin, is thought to play a role in the maintenance of the circadian rhythm, which helps regulate the normal sleep–wake cycle. Ramelteon does not appear to cause rebound insomnia post-treatment. Because it does not produce physical dependence, ramelteon is not classified as a controlled substance.

Ramelteon is rapidly absorbed orally, reaching peak plasma levels in about 45 minutes. Ramelteon is moderately protein bound (82%) and undergoes rapid hepatic first-pass metabolism by cytochrome P450 enzyme systems, including CYP3A4. Ramelteon is excreted primarily in the urine and does not accumulate in the body due to the short half-life of the drug (1–2.6 hours). Patients should avoid taking ramelteon with a high-fat meal because food may delay the onset of action.

Common adverse effects of ramelteon include headache, fatigue, dizziness, nausea, diarrhea, arthralgia/myalgia, and taste changes. The drug may affect endocrine hormones, resulting in decreased testosterone levels, increased prolactin levels, and decreased cortisol levels. Contraindications include severe hepatic impairment if combined with fluvoxamine. Caution is warranted in depression or impaired respiratory function. People should not take ramelteon with alcohol because of resulting excessive sedation and respiratory depression.

Zaleplon

Zaleplon (Sonata) is an oral, nonbenzodiazepine hypnotic approved for the short-term treatment (7–10 days) of insomnia. Overall, this drug is effective in helping people get to sleep and has several advantages as a hypnotic, including the rapid onset, absence of active metabolites, absence of clinically significant CYP450 drug interactions, rapid clearance from the body, and absence of major memory impairments. However, it may not increase total sleep time or decrease the number of awakenings during sleeping hours.

Zaleplon is well absorbed, but bioavailability is only about 30% because of extensive presystemic or first-pass hepatic metabolism. Onset of action is rapid, with a peak in 1 hour. A high-fat, heavy meal slows absorption and may reduce the drug's effectiveness in inducing sleep. It is 60% bound to plasma proteins, and its half-life is 1 hour. The drug is metabolized mainly in the liver to inactive metabolites. The metabolites and a small amount of unchanged drug are excreted in the urine.

Zaleplon apparently enhances the inhibitory effects of GABA, as do the benzodiazepines. A few studies indicate that it has abuse potential similar to that of the benzodiazepines; zaleplon is a Schedule IV controlled substance.

No dosage adjustment with zaleplon is necessary in mild to moderate renal impairment. However, to reduce the risk of adverse effects, it is necessary to decrease the dosage in mild to moderate hepatic impairment and avoid using the drug in severe hepatic impairment. It is also important to decrease the dosage in older adults.

Adverse effects associated with zaleplon include depression, drowsiness, nausea, dizziness, headache, hypersensitivity, impaired coordination, and short-term memory impairment. Contraindications include hypersensitivity reactions and lactation. Caution is warranted during pregnancy and in impaired hepatic or respiratory function.

Use of zaleplon with alcohol or other CNS depressant drugs should not occur because of the increased risk of excessive sedation and respiratory depression. There is also a risk of increased serum zaleplon levels if people take the hypnotic concurrently with cimetidine. It is very important that patients taking zaleplon be taught about this interaction because cimetidine is available without prescription, and the patient may not inform the health care provider who prescribes zaleplon about taking cimetidine.

Zolpidem

Zolpidem (Ambien, Ambien CR) is a nonbenzodiazepine hypnotic that differs structurally from the benzodiazepines but produces similar effects. This drug is a Schedule IV drug approved for short-term treatment (7–10 days) of insomnia. It is well absorbed with oral administration and has a rapid onset of action, usually within 20 to 30 minutes. The half-life of zolpidem is 2.5 hours, and its hypnotic effects last 6 to 8 hours. A newer controlled-release form (Ambien CR) contains a rapid-releasing layer, which promotes falling asleep, and a slow-releasing layer, which promotes sleep all night. The drug is metabolized to inactive metabolites in the liver; these are then eliminated by renal excretion.

Dosage reductions with zolpidem are not necessary in renal impairment, but this condition requires close monitoring. Increased bioavailability, peak plasma concentration, and half-life occur in older adults and in patients with impaired hepatic function. Thus, dosage reduction is essential for these groups. People should not take zolpidem concurrently with alcohol or other CNS depressant drugs because of the increased risk of excessive sedation and respiratory depression.

Adverse effects of zolpidem include daytime drowsiness, dizziness, nausea, diarrhea, and anterograde amnesia. Caution is necessary with signs and symptoms of major depression because of increased risk of intentional overdose. Rebound insomnia may occur for a night or two after stopping the drug, and withdrawal symptoms may occur if it is stopped abruptly after approximately a week of regular use.

NCLEX Success

8. **Zolpidem is the most appropriate choice for patients who have which of the following conditions?**

   A. difficulty in initiating and maintaining sleep
   B. early morning awakening
   C. agitation and violent outbursts
   D. obstructive sleep apnea and respiratory problems

9. **A 5-year-old child is scheduled for a sleep electroencephalogram (EEG). Which of the following medications is a drug of choice to be given prior to the diagnostic test?**

   A. diazepam
   B. lorazepam
   C. zolpidem
   D. choral hydrate

10. **A patient has received a prescription for Zolpidem (Ambien). Which of the following aspects of patient teaching is most important?**

    A. Take the medication with a high-fat meal.
    B. Only take the medication if Tylenol PM does not produce sleep.
    C. Go to bed immediately after taking the medication.
    D. Take the medication if nondrug relaxation has not produced sleep.

The Nursing Process

Assessment

- Ask the following questions: What is the patient's statement of the problem? Does the problem interfere with usual activities of daily living? If so, how much and for how long?
- Try to identify factors that precipitate anxiety or insomnia in the patient. Some common precursors are physical symptoms; feeling worried, tense, or nervous; factors such as illness, death of a friend or family member, divorce, or job stress; and excessive CNS stimulation from caffeine-containing beverages or drugs such as bronchodilators and nasal decongestants. In addition, excessive daytime sleep and too little exercise and activity may cause insomnia, especially in older patients.
- Observe for behavioral manifestations of anxiety, such as psychomotor agitation, facial grimaces, tense posture, and others.

- Observe for physiologic manifestations of anxiety. These signs may include increased blood pressure and pulse rate; increased rate and depth of respiration; increased muscle tension; and pale, cool skin.
- If behavioral or physiologic manifestations seem to indicate anxiety, try to determine whether this is actually the case. Because similar manifestations may indicate pain or other problems rather than anxiety, the observer's perceptions must be validated by the patient before appropriate action can be taken.
- If insomnia is reported, observe for signs of sleep deprivation such as drowsiness, slow movements or speech, and difficulty concentrating or focusing attention.
- Obtain a careful drug history, including the use of alcohol and sedative–hypnotic drugs, and assess the likelihood of drug abuse and dependence. People who abuse other drugs, including alcohol, are likely to abuse antianxiety and sedative–hypnotic drugs. Also, assess for use of CNS stimulants (e.g., appetite suppressants, bronchodilators, nasal decongestants, caffeine, cocaine) and herbs (e.g., ephedra).
- Identify coping mechanisms used in managing previous situations of stress, anxiety, and insomnia. These are very individualized. Reading, watching television, listening to music, or talking to a friend are examples. Some people are quiet and inactive; others participate in strenuous activity. Some prefer to be alone; others prefer being with a friend, family member, or group.
- After drug therapy for anxiety or insomnia is begun, assess the patient's level of consciousness and functional ability before each dose so that excessive sedation can be avoided.

Nursing Diagnoses

- Ineffective ndividual coping related to need for antianxiety or sedative–hypnotic drug
- Deficient knowledge: appropriate uses and effects of antianxiety or sedative–hypnotic drugs
- Deficient knowledge: nondrug measures for relieving anxiety and insomnia
- Noncompliance: overuse
- Risk for injury related to sedation, respiratory depression, impaired mobility, and other adverse effects
- Sleep pattern disturbance: insomnia related to one or more causes (e.g., anxiety, daytime sleep)

Planning/Goals

The patient will

- Feel more calm, relaxed, and comfortable with anxiety; experience improved quantity and quality of sleep with insomnia
- Be monitored for excessive sedation and impaired mobility to prevent falls or other injuries (in health care settings)
- Verbalize and demonstrate nondrug activities to reduce or manage anxiety or insomnia
- Demonstrate safe, accurate drug usage

- Notify a health care provider if he or she wants to stop taking a benzodiazepine; agree to not stop taking a benzodiazepine abruptly
- Avoid preventable adverse effects, including abuse and dependence

Nursing Interventions

The nurse will

- Use nondrug measures to relieve anxiety or to enhance the effectiveness of antianxiety drugs.
  - Assist patients to identify and avoid or decrease situations that cause anxiety and insomnia, when possible. In addition, help them to understand that medications do not solve underlying problems.
  - Support the patient's usual coping mechanisms when feasible. Provide the opportunity for reading, exercising, listening to music, or watching television; promote contact with significant others; or simply allow the patient to be alone and uninterrupted for a while.
  - Use interpersonal and communication techniques to help the patient manage anxiety. The degree of anxiety and the clinical situation largely determine which techniques are appropriate. For example, staying with the patient, showing interest, listening, and allowing him or her to verbalize concerns may be beneficial.
  - Provide information to the patient. This may be a therapeutic technique when anxiety is related to medical conditions. People vary in the amount and kind of information they want, but usually the following topics should be included
    - The overall treatment plan, including medical or surgical treatment, choice of outpatient care or hospitalization, expected length of treatment, and expected outcomes in terms of health and ability to function in activities of daily living
    - Specific diagnostic tests, including preparation; aftereffects, if any; and how the patient will be informed of results
    - Specific medication and treatment measures, including expected therapeutic results
    - What the patient must do to carry out the plan of treatment
  - When offering information and explanations, keep in mind that anxiety interferes with intellectual functioning. Thus, communication should be brief, clear, and repeated as necessary, because patients may misunderstand or forget what is said.

- Modify the environment to decrease anxiety-provoking stimuli. Modifications may involve altering temperature, light, and noise levels.
- Use measures to increase physical comfort. These may include a wide variety of activities, such as positioning, helping the patient bathe or ambulate, giving back rubs, or providing fluids of the patient's choice.
- Consult with other services and departments on the patient's behalf. For example, if financial problems were identified as a cause of anxiety, social services may be able to help.
- When a benzodiazepine is used with diagnostic tests or minor surgery, provide instructions for postprocedure care to the patient or to family members, preferably in written form.
- Implement measures to decrease the need for or increase the effectiveness of sedative–hypnotic drugs, such as the following:
  - Modify the environment to promote rest and sleep (e.g., reduce noise and light).
  - Plan care to allow uninterrupted periods of rest and sleep, when possible.
  - Relieve symptoms that interfere with rest and sleep. Drugs such as analgesics for pain or antitussives for cough are usually safer and more effective than sedative–hypnotic drugs. Nondrug measures, such as positioning, exercise, and back rubs, may be helpful in relieving muscle tension and other discomforts. Allowing the patient to verbalize concerns, providing information so that he or she knows what to expect, or consulting other personnel (e.g., social worker, chaplain) may be useful in decreasing anxiety.
  - Help the patient modify lifestyle habits to promote rest and sleep (e.g., limiting intake of caffeine-containing beverages, limiting intake of fluids during evening hours if nocturia interferes with sleep, avoiding daytime naps, having a regular schedule of rest and sleep periods, increasing physical activity, not trying to sleep unless tired or drowsy).
- Boxes 53.3 and 53.4 present patient guidelines for antianxiety and sedative–hypnotics.

Evaluation

- Decreased symptoms of anxiety or insomnia and increased rest and sleep are reported or observed.
- Excessive sedation and motor impairment are not observed.
- The patient reports no serious adverse effects.
- Monitoring of prescriptions (e.g., "pill counts") does not indicate excessive use.

Key Concepts

- Anxiety is a common disorder that occurs when a person perceives a situation as threatening to physical, emotional, social, or economic well-being.

- When anxiety is severe or prolonged and impairs the ability to function in usual activities of daily living, it is called an anxiety disorder. The American Psychiatric Association delineates anxiety disorders as medical diagnoses in the *DSM-IV-TR*.

- Examples of anxiety disorders include GAD, obsessive-compulsive disorder (OCD), panic disorder, posttraumatic stress disorder (PTSD), and social anxiety disorder (SAD) (see Box 53.1).

- Insomnia is a prolonged difficulty in going to sleep or staying asleep long enough to feel rested.

- Benzodiazepines are used as sedatives–hypnotics, antianxiety agents, muscle relaxants, and anticonvulsants.

- Benzodiazepines and some nonbenzodiazepine hypnotics are Schedule IV drugs under the Controlled Substance Act and can cause physical dependence and withdrawal syndromes.

- The choice of benzodiazepine for a particular purpose and patient depends on the pharmacokinetics of the drug. Benzodiazepines differ in terms of plasma half-life, production of active metabolites, and metabolism.

- Benzodiazepines and most nonbenzodiazepine hypnotics are indicated for short-term use only; tolerance develops after approximately 2 weeks. Eszopiclone, a nonbenzodiazepine hypnotic, is approved for use up to 12 months.

- Contraindications to most antianxiety and sedative–hypnotics include severe respiratory disorders, severe liver or kidney disease, hypersensitivity reaction, and a history of drug or alcohol abuse.

- Concurrent use of antianxiety or sedative–hypnotics with other CNS depressants should be avoided to prevent respiratory depression and excessive sedation.

- Generally, in older adults dosages of antianxiety and sedative–hypnotic drugs should be decreased.

Critical Thinking Questions

53-1. A 3-year-old child who is having a generalized tonic–clonic seizure is admitted to the emergency room of a large metropolitan children's hospital. The paramedics administer diazepam (Valium) 0.3 mg intravenously. In the emergency room, a nurse administers an additional 1 mg over 3 minutes. Following this dose, the child's seizure diminishes.

- What information does the nurse convey to the mother regarding the administration of diazepam?

- What assessments should the nurse make during and following the administration of diazepam?

53-2. The child in question 53.1 is admitted to the neurology unit, and a sleep EEG is scheduled for the morning. A neurologist has ordered chloral hydrate 50 mg/kg to be given 30 minutes before the sleep EEG. The child weighs 32 pounds. The choral hydrate elixir is 500 mg/1 mL.

- How much chloral hydrate does the nurse administer?

- What patient teaching does the nurse provide to the mother regarding the administration of chloral hydrate?

- How does the nurse administer the medication?

References and Resources

American Psychiatric Association (2000). *Diagnostic and statistical manual for mental disorders, text revision* (4th ed.). Washington, DC: American Psychiatric Association.

Anthony, M. (2011). Recent advances in the treatment of anxiety disorders. *Canadian Psychology, 52*(1), 1–9.

Davidson, J. (2009). Insomnia treatment options for women. *Obstetrics and Gynecology Clinics of North America, 36*(4), 831–846.

Dell'Osso, B., Buoli, M., Baldwin, D., & Altamura, C. (2010). Serotonin norepinephrine reuptake inhibitors (SNRIs) in anxiety disorders: a comprehensive review of their clinical efficacy. *Human Psychopharmacology: Clinical and Experimental, 25*(1), 17–29.

Drug facts and comparisons. (Updated monthly). St. Louis, MO: Facts and Comparisons.

Greenlee, A., Karp, J., Dew, M., Houck, P., Andreescu, C., & Reynolds, C. (2010). Anxiety impairs depression remission in partial responders during extended treatment in late-life. *Depression and Anxiety,* (27), 451–456.

Hausken, A., Furu, K., Skurtveit, S., Engeland, A., & Bramness, J. (2009). Starting insomnia treatment: The use of benzodiazepines versus z-hypnotics. A prescription database study of predictors. *European Journal of Clinical Pharmacology, 65*(1), 295–301.

Holdforeth, M., Wyss, T., Schulte, D., Trachsel, M., & Michalak, J. (2009). Some like it specific: the difference between treatment goals of anxious and depressed patients. *Psychology and Psychotherapy: Theory, Research and Practice, 82*(1), 279–290.

Katon, W., Unutzer, J., & Russo, J. (2010). Major depression: the importance of clinical characteristics and treatment response to prognosis. *Depression and Anxiety, 27*(1), 19–26.

Krakow, B., Ulibarri, V., & Romero, E. (2010). Patients with treatment-resistant insomnia taking nightly prescription medications for sleep: A retrospective assessment of diagnostic and treatment variables. *The Primary Care Companion to the Journal of Clinical Psychiatry, 12*(4), doi: 10.4088/PCC.09m00873bro.

Lakhan, S., & Vieira, K. (2010). Nutritional and herbal supplements for anxiety and anxiety-related disorders: Systematic review. *Nutrition Journal, 9*(42), 1–14.

Mark, T. (2010). For what diagnoses are psychotropic medications being prescribed? A nationally representative survey of physicians. *CNS Drugs, 24*(4), 319–326.

Mohlman, J. (2011). A community based survey of older adults' preferences for treatment of anxiety. *Psychology and Aging,* doi: 10.1037/a0023126.

Montgomery, P., & Shepard, L. (2010). Insomnia in older people. *Reviewers in Clinical Gerontology,* doi: 10.1017/S09525981000016X.

Pierse, J., & Dym, H. (2011). An update on treatments for sleep disorders. *The Clinical Advisor,* May, 49–56.

Roy-Byrne, P., Craske, M., Sullivan, G., Rose, R., Edlund, M., Lang, A., et al. (2010). Delivery of evidence-based treatment for multiple anxiety disorders in primary care. *The Journal of American Medical Association, 303*(19), 1921–1928.

Sarris, J., & Kavanaugh, D. (2009). Kava and St. John's Wort: current evidence for use in mood and anxiety disorders. *The Journal of Alternative and Complementary Medicine, 15*(8), 827–836.

Taylor, S., & Weiss, J. (2009). Review of insomnia pharmacology options for the elderly: Implications for managed care. *Population Health Management, 12*(6), 317–323.

Wittchen, H., & Gloster, A. (2009). Developments in the treatments of anxiety disorders. *Psychiatric Clinics of North America, 32*(3), xiii–xix.

Zammit, G. (2009). Comparative tolerability of newer agents for insomnia. *Drug Safety, 32*(9), 735–748.

54 Drug Therapy for Depression and Mood Stabilization

Clinical Application Case Study

While in the hospital, Carl Mehring, a 70-year-old man, receives a diagnosis of chronic depression secondary to chronic heart failure, hypertension, diabetes mellitus, and renal insufficiency. As his health has declined, so has his interest in his family, friends, and hobbies. His physician prescribes sertraline 50 mg orally at bedtime.

KEY TERMS

Antidepressant discontinuation syndrome: condition that occurs with sudden termination of most antidepressant drugs; typical symptoms may occur more rapidly and may be more intense with drugs that have a short half-life and/or are used for long periods

Bipolar disorder: mood disorder characterized by episodes of depression alternating with episodes of mania

Cyclothymia: mild type of bipolar disorder involving periods of hypomania and depression that do not meet the criteria for mania and major depression

Depression: most common mental illness, which is characterized by depressed mood, feelings of sadness, or emotional upset; occurs in people of all ages

Dysthymia: chronically depressed mood and at least two other symptoms of depression for 2 years

Enuresis: bedwetting or involuntary urination resulting from a physical or psychological disorder

Hypomania: persistent irritable mood but absence of psychotic symptoms characteristic of true mania

Mania: emotional disorder characterized by euphoria or irritability; usually occurs in bipolar disorder

Postnatal depression: major depressive episode occurring after the birth of a child

Seasonal affective disorder: depressive episode occurring in a certain season, usually the winter

Serotonin syndrome: serious and sometimes fatal reaction due to combined therapy with a selective serotonin reuptake inhibitor or serotonin–norepinephrine reuptake inhibitor and a monoamine oxidase inhibitor or another drug that potentiates serotonin neurotransmission

Introduction

Mood disorders include depression, dysthymia, bipolar disorder, and cyclothymia (Box 54.1). Major depressive disorder is relatively common in adults, and it also occurs in children and adolescents. This chapter focuses on depression and antidepressant drugs as well as bipolar disorder and mood-stabilizing drugs.

Overview of Depression

Depression is a mood disorder in which feelings of sadness, loss, anger, or frustration interfere with everyday life for several weeks or longer. The condition affects people of all ages. It is difficult to determine the overall incidence of depression in the United States, because only 50% of the people who meet the criteria for depression (see Box 54.1) seek help. Generally, major depression affects women twice as often as men. However, in older adults, at least one major study in older adults demonstrated showed overall incidence of depression to be the same in men and women (Steffens, Fisher, Langa, Potter, & Plassman, 2009). Depression has no particular racial affinity.

Etiology and Pathophysiology

Extensive study has demonstrated that depression results from interactions among several complex factors. Causes involve the immune system, monoamine neurotransmitter dysfunction, and neuroendocrine factors, as well as genetic and environmental factors.

Immune Factors

Immune cells (e.g., T lymphocytes, B lymphocytes) produce cytokines (e.g., interleukins, interferons, tumor necrosis factor), which affect neurotransmission. Possible mechanisms of cytokine-induced depression include increased corticotropin-releasing factor (CRF) and activation of the hypothalamic–pituitary–adrenal (HPA) axis, alteration of monoamine neurotransmitters in several areas of the brain, or cytokines functioning as neurotransmitters and exerting direct effects on brain function.

Monoamine Neurotransmitter Dysfunction

Depression is thought to result from a deficiency of norepinephrine and/or serotonin. This hypothesis has stemmed from studies demonstrating that antidepressant drugs increase the amounts of norepinephrine and/or serotonin in the central nervous system (CNS) synapse by inhibiting their reuptake into the presynaptic neuron. Serotonin helps regulate mood, sleep, appetite, energy level, and cognitive and psychomotor functions, which are disturbed in depression.

Emphasis shifted toward receptors because the neurotransmitter view did not explain why the amounts of neurotransmitter increased within hours after single doses of a drug, but relief of depression occurred only after weeks of drug therapy. Researchers identified desensitization in norepinephrine and serotonin receptors (downregulation) with chronic antidepressant drug therapy. Apparently, long-term administration of antidepressant drugs produces complex changes in the sensitivities of both presynaptic and postsynaptic receptor sites.

Overall, there is increasing awareness that balance, integration, and interactions among norepinephrine, serotonin, and possibly other neurotransmission systems (e.g., dopamine, acetylcholine) are probably more important etiologic factors than single neurotransmitter or receptor alterations.

Neuroendocrine Factors

In addition to monoamine neurotransmission systems, researchers have identified nonmonoamine systems that influence neurotransmission and are significantly altered in depression. A major nonmonoamine is CRF, whose secretion is increased in people with depression. CRF-secreting neurons are widespread in the CNS, and CRF apparently functions as a neurotransmitter and mediator of the endocrine, autonomic, immune, and behavioral responses to stress as well as a releasing factor for corticotropin. The subsequent increase in cortisol by the adrenal cortex (part of the normal physiologic response to stress) is thought to decrease the numbers or sensitivity of cortisol receptors (downregulation) and lead to depression. This alteration of cortisol receptors takes about 2 weeks, the approximate time interval required for the drugs to improve symptoms of depression. Extrahypothalamic CRF is also increased in depression. Secretion of both hypothalamic and extrahypothalamic CRF apparently returns to normal with recovery from depression.

Other Factors

Genetic factors are important because the link between genetics and depression suggests that a close relative of a depressed person is more likely to inherit the disease than the general population. Twin studies support this conclusion.

| BOX 54.1 | Types and Symptoms of Mood Disorders |

Depression

Depression, often described as the most common mental illness, is characterized by depressed mood, feelings of sadness, or emotional upset, and it occurs in all age groups. Mild depression occurs in everyone as a normal response to life stresses and losses and usually does not require treatment; severe or major depression is a psychiatric illness and requires treatment. Major depression also is categorized as unipolar, in which people of usually normal moods experience recurrent episodes of depression.

Major Depression

The American Psychiatric Association's *Diagnostic and Statistical Manual of Mental Disorders, 4th edition* (DSM-IV), lists criteria for a major depressive episode as a depressed mood plus at least five of the following symptoms for at least 2 weeks:

■ Loss of energy, fatigue

■ Indecisiveness

■ Difficulty thinking and concentrating

■ Loss of interest in appearance, work, and leisure and sexual activities

■ Inappropriate feelings of guilt and worthlessness

■ Loss of appetite and weight loss, or excessive eating and weight gain

■ Sleep disorders (hypersomnia or insomnia)

■ Somatic symptoms (e.g., constipation, headache, atypical pain)

■ Obsession with death or thoughts of suicide

■ Psychotic symptoms, such as hallucinations and delusions

Subtypes of depression recognized by the DSM-IV as "specifier" include

■ **Seasonal affective disorder** (SAD), which occurs during winter months, particularly in areas where there is a short period of natural sunlight. The person does not manifest a depressed mood during season of sunlight. The depression is thought to be associated with the decreased release of the neurohormone melatonin. SAD resolves in the spring, and treatment involves light therapy, antidepressants, and specifically timing the administration of melatonin.

■ **Postnatal depression** is defined as a depressive episode occurring within 1 to 6 months after delivery. Postnatal depression is common, affecting 12% to 15% of new mothers. For women with a history of postnatal depression, the risk of recurrence is 33%, and suicide is the main cause of maternal death within the first year of childbirth. Postnatal depression may resolve without treatment within 3 to 6 months; however, 25% of affected mothers will still be depressed 1 year after delivery. Treatment generally involves the use of psychotherapy and/or antidepressants; however, there is limited information available to guide the selection of the most efficacious antidepressants for treatment of postnatal depression.

Dysthymia

Dysthymia involves a chronically depressed mood and at least two other symptoms (e.g., anorexia, overeating, insomnia, hypersomnia, low energy, low self-esteem, poor concentration, feelings of hopelessness) for 2 years. Although the symptoms may cause significant social- and work-related impairments, they are not severe enough to meet the criteria for major depression.

Bipolar Disorder

Bipolar disorder involves episodes of depression alternating with episodes of mania. Mania is characterized by excessive central nervous system (CNS) stimulation with physical and mental hyperactivity (e.g., agitation, constant talking, constant movement, grandiose ideas, impulsiveness, inflated self-esteem, little need for sleep, poor concentration, racing thoughts, short attention span) for at least 1 week. Symptoms are similar to those of acute psychosis or schizophrenia. Hypomania involves the same symptoms, but they are less severe, indicate less CNS stimulation and hyperactivity, and last 3 or 4 days.

Cyclothymia

Cyclothymia is a mild type of bipolar disorder that involves periods of hypomania and depression that do not meet the criteria for mania and major depression. Symptoms must be present for at least 2 years. It does not usually require drug therapy.

Environmental factors include stressful life events, such as physical or sexual abuse in childhood, which apparently alter brain structure and function and contribute to the development of depression in some people. Experts have identified changes in CRF, the HPA axis, and the noradrenergic neurotransmission system, which are thought to cause a hypersensitive or exaggerated response to later stressful events, including mild stress or daily life events.

Clinical Manifestations

Box 54.1 outlines the clinical manifestations of depression. Behavioral changes, especially anxiety, agitation, panic attacks, insomnia, irritability, hostility, impulsivity, akathisia, hypomania, and mania, may indicate worsening depression or suicidality.

Drug Therapy

Antidepressant therapy may be indicated if depressive symptoms persist at least 2 weeks, impair social relationships or work performance, and occur independently of life events. Antidepressants are used to regulate mood specifically affecting serotonin, norepinephrine, and dopamine. Antidepressant effects are attributed to changes in receptors rather than changes in neurotransmitters. Although some of the drugs act more selectively on one neurotransmission system than another initially, this selectivity seems to be lost with chronic administration. Drugs used in the pharmacologic management of depressive disorders are derived from several chemical groups. Older antidepressants include the tricyclic antidepressants (TCAs) and the monoamine oxidase (MAO) inhibitors. Newer drugs include

TABLE 54.1

Drugs Administered for the Treatment of Depression

Drug Class	Prototype	Other Drugs in the Class
Antidepressants		
Tricyclic antidepressants	Imipramine (Tofranil)	Amitriptyline (Elavil) Clomipramine (Anafranil) Desipramine (Norpramin) Doxepin (Sinequan) Nortriptyline (Aventyl, Pamelor)
Selective serotonin reuptake inhibitors (SSRIs)	Fluoxetine (Prozac, Prozac Weekly, Sarafem)	Citalopram (Celexa) Escitalopram (Lexapro) Fluvoxamine (Luvox) Paroxetine (Paxil, Paxil CR) Sertraline (Zoloft) Vilazodone (Viibryd)
Serotonin–norepinephrine reuptake inhibitors (SNRIs)	Venlafaxine (Effexor, Effexor XR)	Duloxetine (Cymbalta)
Monoamine oxidase (MAO) inhibitors	Phenelzine (Nardil)	Isocarboxazid (Marplan) Tranylcypromine (Parnate)
Atypical antidepressants		Bupropion (Wellbutrin, Wellbutrin SR, Wellbutrin XL, Zyban) Mirtazapine (Remeron) Trazodone (Desyrel)
Mood-stabilizing agents	Lithium carbonate (Eskalith, Lithobid)	Aripiprazole (Abilify) Olanzapine (Zyprexa) Quetiapine (Seroquel) Olanzapine/fluoxetine (Symbyax) Risperidone (Risperdal) Ziprasidone (Geodon)

the selective serotonin reuptake inhibitors (SSRIs), the serotonin–norepinephrine reuptake inhibitors (SNRIs), and several adjuvant atypical antidepressant drugs that differ from TCAs and MAO inhibitors. As the name implies, reuptake inhibitors block the reuptake of certain neurotransmitters (serotonin with the SSRIs and serotonin and norepinephrine with the SNRIs). Table 54.1 lists the drugs used to treat depression.

General characteristics of antidepressants include the following:

- All are effective in relieving depression, but they differ in their adverse effects.
- People must take them for 2 to 4 weeks before depressive symptoms improve.
- Administration is oral. Absorbed from the small bowel, they enter the portal circulation and circulate through the liver, where they undergo extensive first-pass metabolism before reaching the systemic circulation.
- Metabolism is by the cytochrome P450 (CYP) enzymes in the liver. Thus, antidepressants may interact with each other and with a wide variety of drugs that are normally metabolized by the same subgroups of enzymes. Additionally, there is a documented ethnic variation in response to antidepressants (Box 54.2).

Because the available drugs have similar efficacy in treating depression, the choice of an antidepressant depends on the patient's age; medical condition; previous history of drug response, if any; and the specific drug's adverse effects. Cost is also a factor to consider. Although the newer drugs are much more expensive than the TCAs, they may be more cost-effective overall because TCAs are more likely to cause serious adverse effects, they require monitoring of plasma drug levels and electrocardiograms (ECGs), and patients are more likely to stop taking them.

It is important to note that sudden termination of most antidepressants results in **antidepressant discontinuation syndrome**. In general, symptoms, which include flu-like symptoms, insomnia, nausea, imbalance, sensory disturbances, and hyperarousal, develop more rapidly and may be more intense with drugs that have a short half-life and/or that are given for long periods. As with other psychotropic drugs, to avoid this syndrome, it is essential to taper the dosage of the antidepressant and discontinue it gradually, over 6 to 8 weeks, unless severe drug toxicity, anaphylactic reaction, or another life-threatening condition is present. The occurrence of withdrawal symptoms may indicate skipped doses or abrupt discontinuation of the drug.

| BOX 54.2 | Genetic and Ethnic Differences in Response to Antidepressant Drug Therapy |

Antidepressant therapy for nonwhite populations in the United States is based primarily on dosage recommendations, pharmacokinetic data, and adverse effects derived from white recipients. However, several studies document differences in drug effects in nonwhite populations mainly attributed to genetic or ethnic variations in the cytochrome P450 2D6 (CYP2D6) enzyme activity of the cytochrome P450 enzyme system. People are poor, intermediate, extensive or ultra fast metabolizers. Although all ethnic groups are genetically heterogeneous and individual members may respond differently, health care providers must consider potential differences in responses to drug therapy.

■ African Americans may be poor metabolizers and tend to have higher plasma drug levels for a given dose, respond more rapidly, experience a higher incidence of adverse effects, and metabolize tricyclic antidepressants (TCAs) more slowly than whites. With lithium, African Americans report more adverse reactions than whites and may need smaller doses.

■ Asians tend to metabolize antidepressant drugs slowly (poor metabolizers) and therefore have higher plasma drug levels for a given dose than whites. Most studies have used TCAs and a limited number of Asian subgroups. Thus, it cannot be assumed that all antidepressants and all people of Asian heritage respond similarly. With lithium, there are no apparent differences between effects in Asians and whites.

Information regarding the reaction of the Hispanic population to antidepressants is largely unknown. Few studies have been performed; some report a need for lower doses of TCAs and greater susceptibility to adverse effects, whereas others report no differences between Hispanics and whites.

Overview of Bipolar Disorder

Bipolar disorder is a condition in which people alternate between periods of depression and overexcitement. There are two subtypes of this disorder, which are defined by the presentation of the mood disorder. Bipolar disorder type I is characterized by episodes of major depression plus **mania** (euphoria or irritability) and occurs equally in men and women. Bipolar disorder type II is characterized by episodes of major depression plus episodes of **hypomania** (persistent irritable mood but absence of euphoria) and occurs more frequently in women. Bipolar spectrum disorder broadens the definition of bipolar disorder to include conditions such as **cyclothymia** (a mild type of bipolar disorder) and **dysthymia** (chronically depressed mood). Bipolar disorders may affect an estimated 5% of adults.

Etiology and Pathophysiology

Like depression, mania, and hypomania, the hallmarks of bipolar disorder have historically been associated with abnormal functioning of neurotransmitters or receptors, such as a relative excess of excitatory neurotransmitters (e.g., norepinephrine) or a relative deficiency of inhibitory neurotransmitters (e.g., gamma-aminobutyric acid [GABA]). Another more recent proposed etiology for bipolar disorder is alteration in neuronal growth and survival in areas of the brain (e.g., subgenual precortex, hippocampus) involved with mood and memory. Secondary causes of manic and hypomanic behavior include drugs that stimulate the CNS, CNS diseases and infections, and electrolyte or endocrine disorders.

Clinical Manifestations

Bipolar disorder manifests with unpredictable mood swings. In the manic phase, clinical manifestations include excessive happiness and energy, excitement, racing thoughts, restlessness, decreased need for sleep, high sex drive, and a tendency to make grandiose statements and unattainable plans. During a depressive episode, manifestations include sadness, lack of energy, increased need for sleep, uncontrollable crying, changes in appetite, and thoughts of suicide. Box 54.1 outlines additional symptoms.

Drug Therapy

Research has shown that mood-stabilizing drugs such as lithium stimulate neuronal growth and reduce brain atrophy in people with long-standing mood disorders. Table 54.1 lists some mood-stabilizing drugs.

Tricyclic Antidepressants

TCAs are the oldest antidepressants, although they are now second-line drugs for the treatment of depression. ⓟ**Imipramine** (Tofranil) is the prototype. A patient's previous response or susceptibility to adverse effects may be the basis for initial selection of TCAs. For example, if a patient (or a close family member) once responded well to a particular drug, that drug is probably the drug of choice for repeated episodes of depression. The response of family members to individual drugs may be significant because there is a strong genetic component to depression and drug response. If therapeutic effects do not occur within 4 weeks, it is probably necessary to discontinue or change the TCA, because some patients tolerate or respond better to one TCA than to another. For patients with suicidal tendencies, beginning an SSRI or another newer drug is preferred over a TCA due to the safety profile.

Pharmacokinetics

Imipramine is well absorbed after oral administration, and the drug is widely distributed in body tissues. Peak levels occur in 1 to 2 hours, and the duration of action is unknown. Its half-life is 8 to 16 hours. Imipramine is metabolized in the liver by CYP2D6 enzymes to active and inactive metabolites, and it is excreted primarily by the kidneys.

Action

Imipramine blocks the reuptake of norepinephrine and serotonin at the presynaptic nerve endings, increasing the action of both neurotransmitters. The drug's use in enuresis may be due to the fact that imipramine also blocks acetylcholine receptors.

Use

Imipramine may be useful in the treatment of depression. Prescribers may order it for children and adolescents in the management of **enuresis** (bedwetting or involuntary urination resulting from a physical or psychological disorder) after physical causes (e.g., urethral irritation, excessive intake of fluids) have been ruled out. Table 54.2 contains route and dosage information for imipramine and the other TCAs.

Use in Children

Imipramine or other TCAs are probably not the drugs of first choice for adolescents because TCAs are more toxic in overdose than other antidepressants, and suicide is a leading cause of death in adolescents. The U.S. Food and Drug Administration (FDA) has issued a **BLACK BOX WARNING** ◆ alerting health care providers to the increased risk of suicidal ideation in children, adolescents, and young adults 18 to 24 years of age who are taking antidepressants, including imipramine.

Use in Older Adults

Imipramine may cause or aggravate conditions common in older adults (e.g., cardiac conduction abnormalities, urinary retention, narrow-angle glaucoma). In addition, impaired compensatory mechanisms make older adults more likely to experience anticholinergic effects, confusion, orthostatic hypotension, and sedation. It is important to monitor vital signs, serum drug levels, and ECGs regularly.

Use in Patients With Hepatic Impairment

Hepatic impairment leads to higher plasma levels of imipramine. Thus, caution is necessary in patients with severe liver impairment.

TABLE 54.2

DRUGS AT A GLANCE: Tricyclic Antidepressants

Drug	Pregnancy Category	Routes and Dosage Ranges	
		Adults	*Children*
Ⓟ **Imipramine** (Tofranil)	D	75 mg PO daily in three divided doses, gradually increased to 200 mg daily if necessary; maintenance dose, 75–150 mg PO daily Older adults, PO 30–40 mg daily in divided doses, increased to 100 mg daily if necessary	Adolescents, 30–40 mg PO daily in divided doses, increased to 100 mg daily if necessary Children >6 y (enuresis), 25–50 mg PO 1 h before bedtime
Amitriptyline (Elavil)	C	50–100 mg PO once daily at bedtime, gradually increased to 150 mg daily if necessary; 80–120 mg IM daily in four divided doses Older adults, 10 mg PO 3 times daily and 20 mg at bedtime	Adolescents, 10 mg PO 3 times daily and 20 mg at bedtime
Clomipramine (Anafranil)	C	Obsessive–compulsive disorder: 25 mg PO daily, increased to 100 mg daily by end of 2 wk, in divided doses, with meals; give maintenance dose in a single dose at bedtime; max dose, 250 mg daily	Children and adolescents, 25 mg PO daily, increased to 3 mg/kg or 100 mg, whichever is smaller, over 2 wk; give maintenance dose in a single dose at bedtime; max dose 3 mg/kg or 200 mg, whichever is smaller
Desipramine (Norpramin)	C	100–200 mg PO daily in divided doses or as a single daily dose; give maintenance dose once daily; max dose 300 mg/d. Older adults, 25–100 mg PO daily in divided doses or as a single daily dose; max dose 150 mg/d	Adolescents, 25–100 mg PO daily in divided doses or as a single daily dose; max dose 150 mg/d
Doxepin (Sinequan)	C	75–150 mg daily PO in divided doses or a single dose at bedtime; max dose, 300 mg/d	Adolescents, 25–50 mg/d PO in single or divided doses; max dose 100 mg/d
Nortriptyline (Aventyl, Pamelor)	D	25 mg PO 3 or 4 times daily or in a single dose (75–100 mg) at bedtime; max dose, 150 mg/d Older adults, 30–50 mg/d PO in divided doses or a single dose once daily	Adolescents, 30–50 mg/d PO in divided doses or a single dose once daily

EVIDENCE-BASED PRACTICE

Outpatient Care of Young People after Emergency Treatment of Deliberate Self-Harm

by J. A. BRIDGE, S. C. MARCUS, & M. OLFSON

Journal of the American Academy of Child and Adolescent Psychiatry 2012, 51(2), 213–222

The authors completed a national retrospective longitudinal cohort analysis of Medicaid-extracted data for children and adolescents 10 to 19 years of age who presented to emergency departments after deliberate self-harm. They concluded that deliberate self-harm is the most common reason for an emergency department visit for people of this age and that nearly 90% of children and adolescents who deliberately harm themselves meet diagnostic criteria for at least one psychiatric disorder, usually related to mood. Also, they established that in this population, most children and adolescents who presented to emergency departments with deliberate self-harm were discharged to the community and did not receive inpatient care. Although some of these people could be low-risk patients, the researchers highlighted that deliberate self-harm is the major risk factor for suicide and that the greatest risk for suicide was immediately after a self-harm episode. Their findings indicated that staffing patterns and evaluation protocols may influence the decision to complete a mental health assessment in the emergency department more than the clinical characteristics of patients seeking help for a deliberate self-harm event.

IMPLICATIONS FOR NURSING PRACTICE: Nursing staff play a strategic role in influencing arrangements for a mental health assessment in the emergency department for all patients presenting with deliberate self-harm. Established evaluation protocols should include a mental health assessment with necessary referral for those at any age who inflict intentional self-harm. Identifying high-risk people who may commit suicide and providing appropriate mental health services can enhance suicide prevention.

Use in Patients With Critical Illness

Adverse effects common with imipramine use (e.g., confusion, dysrhythmias, tachycardia, orthostatic hypotension, urinary retention) are a concern and may further compromise patients who are critically ill. Antidepressants, including imipramine, warrant very cautious use perioperatively because of the risk of serious adverse effects and interactions with anesthetics and other commonly used drugs. It is necessary to discontinue imipramine several days before elective surgery and resume it several days after surgery.

Use in Patients Receiving Home Care

The nurse who sees a patient taking imipramine in the home setting should assess him or her for improvement of symptoms, appropriate administration of the drug, and management of adverse effects, particularly safety factors. A nurse visiting the home for other reasons should observe for signs of depression; health concerns may precipitate symptoms.

Adverse Effects

Adverse effects of imipramine include sedation, orthostatic hypotension, cardiac dysrhythmias, anticholinergic symptoms (e.g., blurred vision, dry mouth, constipation, urinary retention), and weight gain. Symptoms of TCA overdose occur 1 to 4 hours after drug ingestion. They consist primarily of CNS depression and cardiovascular effects (e.g., nystagmus, tremor, restlessness, seizures, hypotension, dysrhythmias, myocardial depression). Death usually results from cardiac, respiratory, and circulatory failure.

TCAs are associated with clearly defined withdrawal syndromes, and these drugs also have strong anticholinergic effects. When they are abruptly discontinued, cholinergic rebound may occur. Symptoms include hypersalivation, diarrhea, urinary urgency, abdominal cramping, and sweating.

Contraindications

Contraindications to imipramine include known sensitivity to the drug and immediately post–acute myocardial infarction.

Nursing Implications

Preventing Interactions

Several drugs interact with imipramine. The drug may inhibit the metabolism of other drugs, including antidepressants, phenothiazines, carbamazepine, flecainide, and propafenone. The use of imipramine and MAO inhibitors concurrently may have serious effects, including severe seizures and death. Alcohol may increase the sedative effects of imipramine. The herb St. John's wort may reduce the blood levels of imipramine and other TCAs.

Administering the Medication

People should take imipramine at bedtime to aid sleep and decrease daytime sedation. Overall, with TCAs, it is best to begin with small doses, which are increased to the desired dose over 1 to 2 weeks. Administration once or twice daily is possible because the drug has a long elimination half-life. Measurement of plasma levels is helpful in adjusting dosages.

Assessing for Therapeutic Effects

The nurse is aware of patient statements about feeling better or less depressed. He or she observes for increased appetite, physical activity, and interest in surroundings; improved sleep patterns; improved appearance; decreased anxiety; and decreased somatic complaints. Mood elevation may take 2 to 3 weeks.

Assessing for Adverse Effects

The nurse observes for CNS effects, gastrointestinal (GI) effects, cardiovascular effects, and other effects. Because imipramine may have adverse effects on the heart, especially in overdose, experts recommend baseline and follow-up ECGs for all patients. In addition, it is important to assess for suicidal thoughts or plans, especially at the beginning of therapy or when dosages are increased or decreased.

Patient Teaching

Box 54.3 presents patient teaching guidelines for the antidepressants, including the TCAs.

BOX 54.3　Patient Teaching Guidelines for Antidepressants

General Considerations

■ Take antidepressants as directed to maximize therapeutic benefits and minimize adverse effects. Do not alter doses when symptoms subside. Antidepressants are usually given for several months, perhaps years.

■ Therapeutic effects (relief of symptoms) may not occur for 2 to 4 weeks after drug therapy is started. As a result, it is very important not to think the drug is ineffective and stop taking it prematurely. Continue to take the drug even if you feel better to prevent the return of depression

■ Do not take other prescription or over-the-counter drugs, including cold remedies, without consulting a health care provider. Potentially serious drug interactions may occur.

■ Do not take the herbal supplement St. John's wort while taking a prescription antidepressant. Serious interactions may occur.

■ Inform any physician, surgeon, dentist, or nurse practitioner about the antidepressants being taken. Potentially serious adverse effects or drug interactions may occur if certain other drugs are prescribed.

■ Avoid activities that require alertness and physical coordination (e.g., driving a car, operating other machinery) until reasonably sure the medication does not make you drowsy or impair your ability to perform the activities safely.

■ Avoid alcohol and other central nervous system depressants (e.g., any drugs that cause drowsiness). Excessive drowsiness, dizziness, difficulty breathing, and low blood pressure may occur, with potentially serious consequences.

■ Learn the name and type of the prescribed antidepressant to help avoid undesirable interactions with other drugs or a physician prescribing other drugs with similar effects. There are several different types of antidepressants, with different characteristics and precautions for safe and effective usage.

■ Do not stop taking any antidepressant without discussing it with a health care provider. If a problem occurs, the type of drug, the dose, or other aspects may be changed to solve the problem and allow continued use of the medication.

■ Counseling, support groups, relaxation techniques, and other nonmedication treatments are recommended along with drug therapy.

■ Notify your physician if you become pregnant or intend to become pregnant during therapy with antidepressants.

Self- or Caregiver Administration

■ With a tricyclic antidepressant (e.g., amitriptyline), take at bedtime to aid sleep and decrease adverse effects.

Also, report urinary retention, fainting, irregular heartbeat, seizures, restlessness, and mental confusion. These are potentially serious adverse drug effects.

■ With a selective serotonin reuptake inhibitor, take the drug in the morning because it may interfere with sleep if taken at bedtime.

　■ In addition, notify a health care provider if a skin rash or other allergic reaction occurs. Allergic reactions are uncommon but may require that the drug be discontinued.

　■ Recognize the importance of follow-up and seeking professional help for the signs of dizziness or insomnia or other symptoms that negatively affect your life.

■ Realize that escitalopram (Lexapro) is a derivative of citalopram (Celexa). The two medications should not be taken concomitantly.

■ With venlafaxine (Effexor), take as directed or ask for instructions. This drug is often taken twice daily. Notify a health care provider if a skin rash or other allergic reaction occurs. An allergic reaction may require that the drug be discontinued.

■ With venlafaxine, use effective birth control methods while taking this drug. Pregnancy is a contraindication.

■ With duloxetine and desvenlafaxine, swallow the medication whole, do not crush, chew, or sprinkle capsule contents on food.

■ With phenelzine and other monoamine oxidase inhibitors, foods that contain tyramine or tyrosine may have to be avoided altogether to prevent the risk of hypertensive crisis. This includes aged cheeses, coffee, chocolate, wine, bananas, avocados, fava beans, and most fermented and pickled foods.

■ Bupropion is a unique drug prescribed for depression (brand name, Wellbutrin) and for smoking cessation (brand name, Zyban). It is extremely important not to increase the dose or take the two brand names at the same time (as might happen with different physicians or filling prescriptions at different pharmacies). Overdoses may cause seizures as well as other adverse effects. When used for smoking cessation, Zyban is recommended for up to 12 weeks if progress is being made. If significant progress is not made by approximately 7 weeks, it is considered unlikely that longer drug use will be helpful.

■ There are short-, intermediate-, and long-acting forms of bupropion that are taken three times, two times, or one time per day, respectively. Be sure to take your medication as prescribed by your physician.

■ Make sure that you and the people you live with are familiar with the signs and symptoms of worsening depression and know how to seek help for signs of overdose.

Other Drugs in the Class

Commonly used TCAs include amitriptyline (Elavil), clomipramine (Anafranil), desipramine (Norpramin), doxepin (Sinequan), and nortriptyline (Aventyl, Pamelor). Amitriptyline, desipramine, and nortriptyline are the TCAs most commonly prescribed to treat depression in children older than 12 years of age. The FDA has approved clomipramine for treatment of obsessive–compulsive disorder in children. In general, amitriptyline, clomipramine, desipramine, doxepin, and nortriptyline are similar to imipramine in terms of adverse effects. Amitriptyline and doxepin are more likely to cause weight gain. Desipramine is more likely to cause drowsiness. These TCAs are effective; however, antidepressants that produce fewer adverse effects are increasingly replacing them.

NCLEX Success

1. Which of the following adverse effects of the imipramine is considered the most serious?

   A. dry mouth
   B. constipation
   C. urinary retention
   D. orthostatic hypotension

2. A man has been taking imipramine (Tofranil) for 1 week for depression. He tells the nurse that he is going to stop taking this medication because it is not working. The best response is which of the following?

   A. "Contact your prescriber about taking a different antidepressant medication."
   B. "It may take up to 4 weeks before this medication makes you feel better."
   C. "You should slowly taper rather than suddenly discontinue this medication."
   D. "You should take an extra dose today to build up your blood level and get faster results."

Selective Serotonin Reuptake Inhibitors

SSRIs, of which Ⓟ **fluoxetine** (Prozac, Sarafem) is the prototype, produce fewer serious adverse effects than the TCAs. (SSRIs are called "selective" because they seem to primarily affect serotonin and not other neurotransmitters.) The drugs of first choice in the treatment of depression, SSRIs are effective and usually produce fewer and milder adverse effects than other antidepressants. There are no guidelines for choosing one SSRI over another.

Pharmacokinetics

Fluoxetine is well absorbed with oral administration, with a peak of action of 6 to 8 hours and a half-life of 24 to 72 hours; this may lead to accumulation with chronic administration. (An active metabolite has a half-life of 7–9 days.) Thus, steady-state blood levels are achieved slowly, over several weeks, and drug effects decrease slowly (over 2–3 months) when fluoxetine is discontinued. The drug is present in breast milk. Metabolism takes place in the liver, and excretion predominately occurs in the kidneys.

Action

Fluoxetine blocks the reabsorption of the neurotransmitter serotonin in the brain. This helps elevate mood.

Use

Uses for fluoxetine include the treatment of depression and its associated anxiety, obsessive–compulsive disorder, bulimia nervosa, and premenstrual dysphoric disorder. Table 54.3 gives the route and dosage information for fluoxetine and other SSRIs.

Use in Children

The FDA has issued a **BLACK BOX WARNING ◆** alerting health care providers to the increased risk of suicidal ideation in children, adolescents, and young adults 18 to 24 years of age when taking antidepressant medications, including fluoxetine.

Use in Older Adults

Fluoxetine and other SSRIs are the drugs of choice in older adults because they produce fewer sedative, anticholinergic, cardiotoxic, and psychomotor adverse effects than the TCAs and related antidepressants. Elimination may be slower, and smaller or less frequent doses may be prudent in older adults. Weight loss is often associated with SSRIs and may be undesirable in older adults. Use of maintenance antidepressant therapy is beneficial to prevent recurrence of depression in older adults.

Use in Patients With Hepatic Impairment

Hepatic impairment leads to reduced first-pass metabolism of fluoxetine and most antidepressant drugs, resulting in higher plasma levels. Thus, caution is warranted in severe liver impairment.

Use in Patients With Critical Illness

Patients who are critically ill may need a drug to combat the depression that often develops with major illness. The decision to start fluoxetine should involve a thorough assessment of the patient's condition, other drugs being given, and potential adverse drug effects.

Antidepressants, including imipramine, warrant caution perioperatively because of the risk of serious adverse effects and adverse interactions with anesthetics and other commonly used drugs.

Adverse Effects

Adverse effects of fluoxetine include a high incidence of GI symptoms (e.g., nausea, diarrhea, and weight loss) and sexual dysfunction (e.g., delayed ejaculation in men, impaired orgasmic ability in women). Most SSRIs also cause some degree of CNS stimulation (e.g., anxiety, nervousness, insomnia), which is most prominent with fluoxetine. These drugs are also associated with increased risk of GI bleeding. For patients with diabetes mellitus, SSRIs may have a hypoglycemic effect.

TABLE 54.3

DRUGS AT A GLANCE: Selective Serotonin Reuptake Inhibitors (SSRIs)

Drug	Pregnancy Category	Routes and Dosage Ranges	
		Adults	Children
Ⓟ **Fluoxetine** (Prozac, Prozac Weekly, Sarafem)	C	20 mg PO once daily in the morning, increased after several weeks if necessary; give doses larger than 20 mg once in the morning or in two divided doses, morning and noon; max daily dose 60 mg Prozac Weekly (delayed-release capsules), 90 mg PO once each week, starting 7 d after the last 20-mg dose	8–17 y for depression, 10 mg/d PO; may increase to 20 mg/d if necessary
Citalopram (Celexa)	C	20 mg PO once daily, morning or evening, increased to 40 mg daily in 1 wk, if necessary Elderly/hepatic impairment, 20 mg PO daily	Not approved for use in children and adolescents
Escitalopram (Lexapro)	C	10 mg PO once daily; may increase to max dose of 20 mg after minimum of 1 wk of therapy	12–17 y, 10 mg PO once daily; may increase to max dose of 20 mg if symptoms do not lessen within 3 wk of therapy
Paroxetine (Paxil, Paxil CR)	D	20 mg PO once daily in the morning, increased at 1 wk or longer intervals, if necessary; usual range, 20–50 mg/d; max dose 60 mg/d Controlled-release (CR) tablets, 25 mg PO once daily in the morning, increase up to 62.5 mg/d if necessary Elderly or debilitated adults, 10 mg PO once daily, increase if necessary; maximum dose, 40 mg Severe renal or hepatic impairment: same as for older adults	Not approved for use in children and adolescents
Sertraline (Zoloft)	C	Depression, OCD: 50 mg PO once daily morning or evening, increase at 1-wk or longer intervals to a max daily dose of 200 mg Panic disorder, PTSD: 25 mg PO once daily, increase after 1 wk to 50 mg once daily	OCD: 6–12 y, 25 mg PO once daily 13–17 y, 50 mg PO once daily

OCD, obsessive–convulsive disorder; PTSD, posttraumatic stress disorder

Serotonin syndrome, a serious and sometimes fatal reaction characterized by hypertensive crisis, hyperpyrexia, extreme agitation progressing to delirium and coma, muscle rigidity, and seizures, may occur due to combined therapy with an SSRI and an MAO inhibitor or another drug that potentiates serotonin neurotransmission. It is important not to take an SSRI or SNRI and an MAO inhibitor concurrently or within 2 weeks of each other. In most cases, if a patient taking an SSRI is transferred to an MAO inhibitor, it is necessary to discontinue the SSRI at least 14 days before starting the MAO inhibitor. However, the patient should discontinue fluoxetine at least 5 weeks before starting an MAO inhibitor due to the prolonged half-life.

As previous discussed, antidepressant discontinuation syndrome can occur with sudden termination of the SSRIs. Withdrawal symptoms include dizziness, GI upset, lethargy or anxiety/hyperarousal, dysphoria, sleep problems, and headache, which can last from several days to several weeks. More serious symptoms may include aggression, hypomania, mood disturbances, and suicidal tendencies. Fluoxetine, with its long half-life, has not been associated with withdrawal symptoms.

Contraindications

Contraindications to fluoxetine include known sensitivity to the drug as well as the use of MAO inhibitors or thioridazine.

QSEN Safety Alert

People of any age who have attempted suicide should not receive fluoxetine.

Nursing Implications

Preventing Interactions

Because fluoxetine and other SSRIs are highly bound to plasma proteins, they compete with endogenous compounds and other medications for binding sites, resulting in drug interactions. Several drugs increase the effects of fluoxetine (Box 54.4). Also, CYP2D6 enzymes metabolize fluoxetine; therefore, the drug may cause accumulation of other drugs using this enzyme system (e.g., amitriptyline, imipramine, desipramine, thioridazine).

BOX 54.4 Drug Interactions: Fluoxetine

Drugs That Increase the Effects of Fluoxetine

- Alcohol
  Increases the sedative effect
- Amiodarone, cimetidine, ciprofloxacin, cytochrome P450 2D6 inhibitors (e.g., opioid analgesics, beta adrenergic blockers, promethazine), macrolide antibiotics
  Increase the risk of toxicity
- Haloperidol
  Increases the risk of neurologic toxicity
- 5-Hydroxytryptophan
  Increases the risk of serotonin syndrome

QSEN Safety Alert ❗

In addition, fluoxetine can prevent the conversion of codeine to its active form, resulting in lack of pain relief when the drugs are used concurrently.

Administering the Medication

People typically take SSRIs, including fluoxetine, once daily in the morning to prevent interference with sleep. They may take the drug with food to avoid GI upset.

Assessing for Therapeutic Effects

The nurse assesses for statements of improved depression. He or she assesses improvement in appetite, physical activity, and interest in surroundings; improved sleep patterns; improved appearance; decreased anxiety; and reduced somatic complaints.

Assessing for Adverse Effects

The nurse assesses for dizziness, headache, nervousness, insomnia, nausea, diarrhea, dizziness, dry mouth, sedation, skin rash, and sexual dysfunction.

QSEN Safety Alert ❗

It is essential to assess for suicidal thoughts or plans, especially at the beginning of therapy or when dosages are increased or decreased.

Patient Teaching

Box 54.3 contains patient teaching guidelines for the antidepressants, including the SSRIs.

Other Drugs in the Class

Other SSRIs include citalopram (Celexa), escitalopram (Lexapro), paroxetine (Paxil), and sertraline (Zoloft).

Sertraline and citalopram also have active metabolites, but paroxetine, like fluoxetine, is more likely to accumulate. Escitalopram, paroxetine, and sertraline reach steady-state concentrations in 1 to 2 weeks. People may take the drugs in the morning or evening (but at the same time each day). An evening dose may interfere with sleep. The SSRIs are strong inhibitors

---

EVIDENCE-BASED PRACTICE

Antidepressant Prevention of Postnatal Depression

by L. M. HOWARD, S. HOFFBRAND, C. HENSHAW, L. BOATH, & E. BRADLEY

Cochrane Database of Systematic Reviews 2006, 2, CD004363

A randomized controlled trial evaluated the use of cognitive behavior therapy and fluoxetine and found that both were effective in treating postnatal depression. Sertraline, paroxetine, venlafaxine, and nortriptyline are reportedly safe for use by nursing mothers of healthy infants; however, fluoxetine is not recommended because it can cause irritability, sleep disturbances, and poor feeding in exposed breast-feeding infants. There appears to be no clear evidence to recommend antidepressant prophylaxis. Intrauterine exposure to fluoxetine and other selective serotonin reuptake inhibitors during the third trimester may result in a neonatal withdrawal syndrome, which shares some similarity to a mild serotonin syndrome. Common symptoms include irritability, prolonged crying, respiratory distress, rigidity, and possibly seizures. Care for neonatal withdrawal syndrome is supportive; symptoms usually abate within a few days.

IMPLICATIONS FOR NURSING PRACTICE: Women who receive antidepressants during pregnancy should be assessed for changes in feelings regarding the pregnancy and evaluated for postpartum depression during the first year of the child's life. Given the limited evidence available on the treatment of postnatal depression, further research is needed.

---

of the CYP enzyme system, which metabolizes many drugs. As a result, serum drug levels and risks of adverse effects are greatly increased. Most significantly, fluoxetine, paroxetine, and sertraline slow metabolism of bupropion, codeine, desipramine, dextromethorphan, flecainide, metoprolol, nortriptyline, phenothiazines, propranolol, risperidone, and timolol.

Paroxetine, which has a half-life of approximately 24 hours and does not produce active metabolites, may be associated with antidepressant discontinuation syndrome even when discontinued gradually, over 7 to 10 days. Symptoms may include a flu-like syndrome with nausea, vomiting, fatigue, muscle aches, dizziness, headache, and insomnia.

Clinical Application 54-1

- Mr. Mehring visits the physician again 2 weeks later. His wife complains that she sees no improvement in her husband's mood and that he is taking too many drugs. How should the nurse respond?

Serotonin–Norepinephrine Reuptake Inhibitors

Like the SSRIs, the SNRIs, of which ℗ **venlafaxine** (Effexor) is the prototype, inhibit the neuronal uptake of serotonin. In addition, they also inhibit the uptake of norepinephrine, increasing the activity of these neurotransmitters in the brain. The SNRIs are similar to SSRIs in terms of therapeutic effects.

Pharmacokinetics and Action

Venlafaxine is well absorbed, extensively metabolized in the liver, and excreted in urine. It crosses the placenta and may enter breast milk.

The drug increases the levels of serotonin and norepinephrine in the brain by preventing the reuptake of these neurotransmitters known to play an important part in mood. The drug also weakly inhibits dopamine reuptake.

Use

SNRIs are a standard first-line treatment for depression and anxiety disorders. Uses for venlafaxine include the treatment of depression, as well as generalized anxiety disorder, social phobia, and panic disorder. Table 54.4 gives route and dosage information of venlafaxine and the other SNRIs.

Use in Children

The FDA has issued a **BLACK BOX WARNING** ◆ alerting health care providers to the increased risk of suicidal ideation in children, adolescents, and young adults 18 to 24 years of age when taking antidepressant medications, including venlafaxine.

Use in Older Adults

Venlafaxine and other SNRIs are suitable for use in older people, although the weight loss often associated with these drugs may be undesirable. Authorities recommend using smaller initial doses and dosing increments.

Use in Patients With Renal Impairment

Venlafaxine is excreted by the kidneys. Thus, dosage adjustment is necessary in patients with renal impairment.

Use in Patients With Hepatic Impairment

Caution is warranted in patients with hepatic impairment. Prescribers should consider lower doses, longer intervals between doses, and slower dose increases than usual.

Use in Patients With Critical Illness

Patients who are critically ill may need a drug such as venlafaxine to combat the depression that often develops with major illness. It is necessary to make a thorough assessment of the patient's condition, other drugs being given, potential adverse drug effects, and other factors before starting the drug.

Adverse Effects

Adverse effects of venlafaxine, which may be greater than with the SSRIs, include the following:

- CNS effects: anxiety, dizziness, dreams, insomnia, nervousness, somnolence, and tremors
- GI effects: anorexia, weight loss, nausea, vomiting, constipation, and diarrhea
- Cardiovascular effects: hypertension, tachycardia, and vasodilation

TABLE 54.4

DRUGS AT A GLANCE: Serotonin–Norepinephrine Reuptake Inhibitors (SNRIs)

Drug	Pregnancy Category	Routes and Dosage Ranges	
		Adults	*Children*
℗ **Venlafaxine** (Effexor, Effexor XR)	C	Immediate-release tablets, initially 75 mg/d PO in two or three divided doses with food; increase by 75 mg/d (4 d or longer between increments) up to 225 mg/d if necessary Extended-release (XR) capsules, initially 37.5 or 75 mg/d PO in a single dose, morning or evening; increase by 75 mg/d (4 d or longer between increments) up to 225 mg/d if necessary Hepatic or renal impairment, reduce dose by 50% and increase very slowly	Not approved for use in children and adolescents
Desvenlafaxine (Pristiq)	C	50 mg PO once daily; increases >100 mg daily not recommended	Not approved for use in children and adolescents
Duloxetine (Cymbalta)	C	30–60 mg/d PO; increase by 30-mg increments every week up to a max daily dose of 120 mg/d Renal impairment, decrease doses	Not approved for use in children and adolescents

- Genitourinary effects: abnormal ejaculation, impotence, and urinary frequency. (The negative effect of venlafaxine on sexual function is less than that reported with the SSRIs.)
- Dermatologic effects: sweating, rash, and pruritus

Contraindications

Contraindications to venlafaxine include known sensitivity to the drug, use of an MAO inhibitor, and pregnancy.

Nursing Implications

Preventing Interactions

Venlafaxine and other SNRIs interact with MAO inhibitors, leading to increased serum levels and the risk of serotonin syndrome. It is necessary to discontinue the MAO inhibitor at least 14 days before starting venlafaxine.

Administering the Medication

People should take venlafaxine with food to decrease GI effects (e.g., nausea and vomiting).

Assessing for Therapeutic Effects

The nurse assesses for improvement in mood, including improvement in anxiety level, reduced agitation or irritability episodes, decreased number of panic attacks, and ability to sleep through the night.

Assessing for Adverse Effects

The nurse observes for dizziness, headache, nervousness, insomnia, nausea, diarrhea, dizziness, dry mouth, sedation, and skin rash. Also, it is necessary to assess for altered sexual function and provide options and resources for the patient and the significant other. In addition, the nurse evaluates for the occurrence of weight loss. Finally, it is important to monitor for signs of suicidal ideation and hostility.

Patient Teaching

Box 54.3 presents patient teaching guidelines for the antidepressants, including the SNRIs.

Other Drugs in the Class

The other SNRIs desvenlafaxine (Pristiq) and duloxetine (Cymbalta) also inhibit the neuronal uptake of serotonin. Duloxetine is commonly used in the treatment of neuropathic pain and relieves painful physical symptoms (e.g., overall pain, backache, shoulder pain) associated with depression, thereby reducing remission rates, and reduces depression-associated anxiety. The drug may result in hepatic toxicity, leading to increased liver transaminases and bilirubin. Use of alcohol with duloxetine increases the risk of liver damage, and thus it is not recommended for patients with significant alcohol use. Overall, the adverse effects of duloxetine and venlafaxine are similar. Significant drug interactions with SSRIs, MAO inhibitors, TCAs, lithium, St. John's wort, phenylpiperidine opioids, dextromethorphan, and tryptophan may potentiate the risk of serotonin syndrome with duloxetine.

Desvenlafaxine, a synthetic form of the major active metabolite of venlafaxine, is used to treat major depressive disorder in adults. The drug, which is metabolized by CYP3A4 and not CYP2D6 enzymes, is associated with fewer drug interactions than other SNRIs. It is generally well tolerated and is formulated as an extended-release product taken once a day. Adverse effects include constipation or diarrhea, decreased sexual desire, drowsiness, dry mouth, headache, and trouble sleeping.

Monoamine Oxidase Inhibitors

MAO inhibitors are third-line agents for the treatment of depression and are rarely used in clinical practice today, mainly because they may interact with some foods and drugs to produce severe hypertension and possible heart attack or stroke. Prescribers are most likely to order MAO inhibitors when a patient does not respond to other antidepressant drugs or when electroconvulsive therapy is refused or contraindicated. The prototype MAO inhibitor is ℗ **phenelzine** (Nardil).

Pharmacokinetics and Action

Phenelzine is well absorbed and widely distributed. The drug reaches peak levels in 2 to 4 hours, but mood elevation may take 2 to 8 weeks. It is metabolized in the liver and excreted by the kidneys.

The drug improves mood by binding irreversibly to MAO, increasing the concentrations of epinephrine, norepinephrine, serotonin, and dopamine in the CNS.

Use

Phenelzine is used to treat depression when other antidepressants have been unsuccessful in symptom management. Table 54.5 gives route and dosage information for this drug and other MAO inhibitors.

Use in Older Adults

Phenelzine and other MAO inhibitors may be more likely to cause hypertensive crises in older adults because their cardiovascular, renal, and hepatic functions are often diminished.

Use in Patients With Renal or Hepatic Impairment

Caution is necessary with phenelzine and other MAO inhibitors in people with renal or hepatic impairment.

Use in Patients With Critical Illness

Phenelzine interacts with numerous drugs and could potentially complicate the condition of patients with critical illness. If it is necessary to continue phenelzine, its use must be cautious and slow, careful monitoring of patients' responses is warranted; patients with critical illness are often frail and unstable, with multiple organ dysfunctions.

Adverse Effects

The most serious adverse effect associated with phenelzine is hypertensive crisis, which can be precipitated by intake of foods containing tyramine. Other reported effects include dysrhythmias, drowsiness, dizziness, sexual dysfunction, and orthostatic hypotension.

TABLE 54.5

DRUGS AT A GLANCE: Monoamine Oxidase (MAO) Inhibitors

Drug	Pregnancy Category	Routes and Dosage Ranges	
		Adults	Children
Ⓟ **Phenelzine** (Nardil)	C	15 mg PO 3 times daily; not to exceed 90 mg/d	Not approved for use in children and adolescents
Isocarboxazid (Marplan)	C	10 mg PO 2–4 times daily increase to 40 mg by the end of the first week, to a max daily dose of 60 mg/d	Not approved for use in children and adolescents
Tranylcypromine (Parnate)	C	30 mg PO daily in divided doses, not to exceed 60 mg/d	Younger than 16 y: not recommended 16 y of age or older, same as adults

Contraindications

Contraindications to phenelzine include known sensitivity to the drug. Patients should not have elective surgery requiring general anesthesia or spinal anesthesia or use local anesthesia containing sympathomimetic vasoconstrictors. Patients who take other MAO inhibitors or weight-reduction and over-the-counter cold or hay fever preparations containing vasoconstrictors should not take phenelzine.

Nursing Implications

Preventing Interactions

Phenelzine interacts with many drugs and some herbs and foods, increasing its effects (Boxes 54.5 and 54.6). It is important that SSRIs and phenelzine are not taken concurrently or close together because serious and fatal reactions may occur. Other

critical interactions occur with foods that contain tyramine, a monoamine precursor of norepinephrine. Normally, tyramine is deactivated in the GI tract and liver, so that large amounts do not reach the systemic circulation. When deactivation is blocked by MAO inhibitors, tyramine is absorbed systemically and transported to adrenergic nerve terminals, where it causes a sudden release of large amounts of norepinephrine.

Administering the Medication

Phenelzine is taken orally three times a day, which may require a reminder system for accurate administration. The drug may be crushed and mixed with fluids or food for patients with difficulty swallowing.

Assessing for Therapeutic and Adverse Effects

The nurse assesses for improvement in symptoms of depression, including improvement in anxiety level, reduced agitation or irritability episodes, decreased number of panic attacks, and ability to sleep through the night.

It is necessary to observe for blurred vision, constipation, dizziness, dry mouth, hypotension, urinary retention, and hypoglycemia.

Patient Teaching

Box 54.3 contains patient teaching guidelines for the antidepressants, including the MAO inhibitors.

BOX 54.5　Drug Interactions: Phenelzine

Drugs That Increase the Effects of Phenelzine
- Alcohol (red wine, beer)
  Increases central nervous system depression
- Altretamine
  Increases the risk of orthostatic hypotension
- Antidepressants (tricyclic antidepressants, selective serotonin reuptake inhibitors, serotonin–norepinephrine reuptake inhibitors), buspirone, carbamazepine, dextromethorphan, 5-hydroxytryptophan
  Increase the risk of serotonin syndrome
- Levodopa
  Increases the risk of hypertensive reactions
- Monoamine oxidase inhibitors
  Increase the risk of serotonin syndrome and hypertensive crisis
- Narcotic analgesics
  Increase the risk of hypotension, respiratory depression, or coma
- Selegiline, sibutramine, tramadol
  Increase the risk of hypertensive crisis

BOX 54.6　Herb and Dietary Interactions: Phenelzine

Herbs and Foods That Increase the Effects of Phenelzine
- Caffeine
- Kava kava
- Phenylalanine
- St. John's wort
- Tryptophan (e.g., game meats, soy products, seaweed, seafood, sesame seeds, aged cheeses and meats, brewer's yeast, sauerkraut, fava beans)
- Tyrosine (e.g., meat, seafood, wheat products, oatmeal)
- Valerian

TABLE 54.6

DRUGS AT A GLANCE: Atypical Antidepressants

Drug	Pregnancy Category	Routes and Dosage Ranges	
		Adults	Children
Bupropion (Wellbutrin, Wellbutrin SR, Wellbutrin XL, Zyban)	C	Immediate-release tablets, 150 mg PO twice daily, increase to 100 mg 3 times daily (at least 6 h apart) if necessary; max single dose, 450 mg Sustained-release (SR) tablets, 150 mg PO once daily in the morning, increase to 150 mg twice daily (at least 8 h apart); max daily dose, 400 mg. Wellbutrin XL: 150 mg PO once daily in the morning; may increase to target dose of 300 mg on or after 4th day of therapy; max single dose, 450 mg	Not recommended for use in children
Mirtazapine (Remeron)	C	15 mg/d PO, not to exceed 45 mg/d	Not recommended for use in children
Trazodone (Desyrel)	C	100–300 mg PO daily, increase to a max dose of 600 mg daily if necessary	Not recommended for use in children

Other Drugs in the Class

Isocarboxazid and tranylcypromine have the same adverse effects as phenelzine, and they interact with drugs and foods in the same way.

Atypical Antidepressants

Other drugs used to treat depression include bupropion, mirtazapine, and trazodone. Table 54.6 gives route and dosage information for these drugs. People also use the herbal preparation St. John's wort as an antidepressant (Box 54.7).

Bupropion

Bupropion (Wellbutrin, Zyban) inhibits the reuptake of dopamine, norepinephrine, and serotonin. After an oral dose, peak

---

BOX 54.7 | **Use of St. John's Wort as an Antidepressant**

St. John's wort (*Hypericum perforatum*) is an herb that is widely used for depression. However, evidence for the efficacy with St. John's wort is modest at best. Most authorities agree that there is insufficient evidence to support the use of St. John's wort for mild to moderate depression and that more studies are needed to confirm the safety and effectiveness of this herb.

Drug interactions may be extensive. People should not combine St. John's wort with alcohol, antidepressants, nasal decongestants or other over-the-counter cold and flu medications, bronchodilators, opioid analgesics, or amino acid supplements containing phenylalanine and tyrosine. All of these interactions may result in hypertension, possibly severe.

For patients who report use of St. John's wort, it is necessary to teach them to purchase products from reputable sources; to avoid taking antidepressant drugs, alcohol, and cold and flu medications while taking the herb; to avoid using the herb during pregnancy because effects are unknown; and to use sunscreen lotions and clothing to protect themselves from sun exposure.

plasma levels are reached in about 2 hours. The drug is metabolized in the liver and excreted primarily in the urine. Several metabolites are pharmacologically active. Bupropion is useful in the treatment of depression, and clinicians often add it to a drug regimen when an SSRI does not provide a complete response. (The drug is also effective as a long-term smoking cessation aid.) Acute episodes of depression usually require several months of drug therapy. It is necessary to reduce the dosage in patients with impaired hepatic or renal function.

Bupropion may have significant adverse effects. Seizures are likely to occur with doses above 450 mg/d and in patients known to have a seizure disorder. The drug has few adverse effects on cardiac function and does not cause orthostatic hypotension or sexual dysfunction. However, in addition to seizures, the drug has CNS stimulant effects (agitation, anxiety, excitement, increased motor activity, insomnia, restlessness) that may require a sedative during the first few days of administration. These effects may increase the risk of abuse. Other common adverse effects include dry mouth, headache, nausea and vomiting, and constipation.

Mirtazapine

Mirtazapine (Remeron), another atypical antidepressant, blocks presynaptic alpha$_2$-adrenergic receptors (which increase the release of norepinephrine), serotonin receptors, and histamine H$_1$ receptors. Consequently, the drug decreases anxiety, agitation, insomnia, and migraine headaches as well as depression.

Mirtazapine is well absorbed after oral administration, and it is metabolized in the liver, mainly to inactive metabolites. Common adverse effects include drowsiness (with accompanying cognitive and motor impairment), increased appetite, weight gain, dizziness, dry mouth, and constipation. The drug does not cause sexual dysfunction. Mirtazapine should not be taken concurrently with other CNS depressants (e.g., alcohol, benzodiazepine, antianxiety, or hypnotic agents) because of additive sedation. In addition, it should not be taken concurrently with an MAO inhibitor.

Trazodone

Trazodone (Desyrel) is used more often for sedation and sleep than for depression because high doses (greater than 300 mg/d) are required for antidepressant effects, and these amounts cause excessive sedation in many patients. The drug is often given concurrently with a stimulating antidepressant, such as bupropion, fluoxetine, sertraline, or venlafaxine.

Trazodone is well absorbed with oral administration, and it is metabolized in the liver and excreted primarily by the kidneys. Adverse effects include sedation, dizziness, edema, cardiac dysrhythmias, and priapism (prolonged and painful penile erection).

Mood-Stabilizing Agents: Drugs Used to Treat Bipolar Disorder

(P) **Lithium carbonate** (Eskalith), the prototype, is a naturally occurring metallic salt that is used in patients with bipolar disorder, mainly to treat and prevent manic episodes. When used therapeutically, lithium is effective in controlling mania in 65% to 80% of patients. When used prophylactically, the drug decreases the frequency and intensity of manic cycles.

Pharmacokinetics

Lithium is well absorbed after oral administration, with peak serum levels in 1 to 3 hours after a dose and steady-state concentrations in 5 to 7 days. The drug is not metabolized; it is entirely excreted by the kidneys.

Action

The exact mechanism of action of lithium is unknown. However, the drug is known to affect the synthesis, release, and reuptake of several neurotransmitters in the brain, including acetylcholine, dopamine, GABA, and norepinephrine. It also stabilizes postsynaptic receptor sensitivity to neurotransmitters, probably by competing with calcium, magnesium, potassium, and sodium ions for binding sites. Lithium may also stimulate neuronal growth, exerting a neuroprotective effect on areas of the brain involved with mood.

Use

Lithium is the drug of choice for use in the treatment of manic episodes of bipolar disorder and as a maintenance treatment to decrease the number and intensity of manic episodes. Long-term therapy is the usual practice because of the high recurrence rate of bipolar disorder if the drug is discontinued.

QSEN Safety Alert

Gradually tapering the dose over 2 to 4 weeks delays the recurrence of symptoms.

It is important to note that doses should be relatively low initially and may increase gradually according to regular measurements of serum drug levels. Dosage is based on serum drug levels, control of symptoms, and occurrence of adverse effects. Measurements of serum levels are required for two reasons: (1) therapeutic doses are only slightly lower than toxic doses, and (2) patients vary widely in rates of lithium absorption and excretion. Thus, a dose that is therapeutic in one patient may be toxic in another.

Table 54.7 gives route and dosage information for lithium and other mood-stabilizing drugs.

Use in Patients With Renal Impairment

Adequate renal function is a prerequisite for lithium therapy. The proximal renal tubules reabsorb approximately 80% of a lithium dose, and the amount of reabsorption depends on the concentration of sodium in the tubules. A sodium deficit causes more lithium to be reabsorbed and increases the risk of lithium toxicity. A sodium excess causes more lithium to be excreted

TABLE 54.7

DRUGS AT A GLANCE: Mood-Stabilizing Agents

Drug	Pregnancy Category	Routes and Dosage Ranges	
		Adults	*Children*
Ⓟ **Lithium carbonate** (Eskalith, Lithobid)	D	600 mg PO 3 times daily or 900 mg PO twice daily (slow-release forms); maintenance dose, PO 300 mg 3 or 4 times daily to maintain a serum lithium level of 0.6–1.2 mEq/L	6–11 y, initially 15–20 mg/kg/d PO 3 or 4 times daily >12 y, same as adults Maintenance dose, 15–60 mg/kg/d PO 3 or 4 times daily
Aripiprazole (Abilify)	C	30 mg PO daily	Mania: ≥10 y, 2 mg PO daily for 2 days, then 5 mg daily for 2 days to 10 mg daily, not to exceed 30 mg daily; not recommended for use in children with depression
Olanzapine (Zyprexa)	C	10–15 mg/d PO initially; may increase by 5 mg daily at no <24 intervals to max dose of 20 mg/d Elderly or debilitated adults, 5 mg/d PO	13–17 y, 2.5–5 mg/d PO initially; may increase by 2.5–5 mg daily to max dose of 20 mg/d
Quetiapine (Seroquel)	C	Acute mania: 50 mg PO twice daily on day 1; 100 mg PO twice daily on day 2; 150 mg PO twice daily on day 3; 200 mg PO twice daily on day 4; if needed, may continue to increase max dose 800 mg/d Depressive episodes: 50 mg PO at bedtime; may increase by 50 mg/d to max dose 600 mg at bedtime	13–17 y, 25 mg PO twice daily on day 1; 50 mg PO twice daily on day 2; 100 mg PO twice daily on day 3; 150 mg PO twice daily on day 4; 200 mg PO twice daily on day 5; if needed, may continue to increase in increments of no >100 mg/d to max dose 400–600 mg/d
Olanzapine/ fluoxetine (Symbyax)	C	Depressive episodes: 6/25 mg PO at bedtime; may increase to max 18/75 mg/d	Not approved for use in children
Risperidone (Risperdal)	C	Acute mania: 2–3 mg/d PO initially; may increase 1 mg/d to max dose of 6 mg/d Elderly or debilitated adults, 0.5 mg/d PO, may increase by 0.5–3 mg/d, then may increase by 1 mg/wk to max dose of 6 mg/d	10–17 y, 0.5 mg/d PO initially; titrate 0.5–1 daily to a target dose of 2.5 mg/d; dosage range 0.5–6 mg/d
Ziprasidone (Geodon)	C	Acute mania: 40 mg PO twice daily; may increase to max dose 80 mg twice daily	Not recommended for use in children with bipolar disorder

(i.e., lithium diuresis) and may lower serum lithium levels to nontherapeutic ranges.

Use in Patients With Hepatic Impairment

Caution is necessary when lithium is used in patients with hepatic impairment.

Use in Patients With Critical Illness

Lithium warrants caution in patients with critical illness. Lower doses are necessary in patients with conditions that impair lithium excretion (e.g., diuretic drug therapy, dehydration, low-salt diet, renal impairment, decreased cardiac output). It is necessary to discontinue lithium 1 to 2 days before surgery and resume it when full oral intake of food and fluids is allowed.

BOX 54.8 — Drug Interactions: Lithium

Drugs That Increase the Effects of Lithium

■ Alcohol, diuretics

Increase the risk of dehydration, increasing the risk of lithium toxicity

■ Angiotensin-converting enzyme inhibitors, angiotensin II receptor blockers, indomethacin and some other nonsteroidal anti-inflammatory drugs

Increase the serum level and the risk of toxicity

■ Selective serotonin reuptake inhibitors

Increase the risk of adverse effects such as confusion, drowsiness, and issues with coordination

Drugs That Decrease the Effects of Lithium

■ Theophylline

Increases renal excretion

Adverse Effects and Contraindications

Common adverse effects of lithium include metallic taste, hand tremors, nausea, polyuria, polydipsia, diarrhea, muscular weakness, fatigue, edema, and weight gain.

Contraindications include known sensitivity to the drug as well as pregnancy.

Preventing Interactions

Several drugs interact with lithium, increasing or decreasing its effects (Box 54.8). No herbal interactions exist.

Administering the Medication

Before beginning lithium therapy, it is important to obtain baseline studies of renal, cardiac, and thyroid status because adverse drug effects involve these organ systems. Baseline electrolyte studies are also necessary.

When lithium therapy begins, it is necessary to measure the serum drug concentration two or three times weekly in the morning, 12 hours after the last dose of the drug. For most patients, the therapeutic range of serum drug levels is 0.5 to 1.2 mEq/L (SI units, 0.5–1.2 mmol/L). Serum lithium levels should not exceed 1.5 mEq/L because of the risk of serious drug toxicity. Doses of lithium should decrease after mania is controlled. During long-term maintenance therapy, it is necessary to measure serum lithium levels at least every 3 months.

People should take lithium with food to decrease the risk of nausea and vomiting.

Assessing for Therapeutic and Adverse Effects

The nurse observes for decreases in manic behavior and stability in mood swings. Therapeutic effects do not occur until approximately 7 to 10 days after therapeutic serum drug levels are attained (1–1.5 mEq/L with acute mania; 0.6–1.2 mEq/L for maintenance therapy). In mania, a person usually takes a benzodiazepine or an antipsychotic drug to reduce agitation and control behavior until the lithium takes effect.

The nurse also observes for the presence of a metallic taste, hand tremors, nausea, polyuria, polydipsia, diarrhea, muscular weakness, fatigue, edema, and weight gain.

Patient Teaching

Box 54.9 contains patient teaching guidelines for lithium.

BOX 54.9 — Patient Teaching Guidelines for Lithium

General Considerations

■ Take lithium as directed to maximize therapeutic benefits and minimize adverse effects. Do not alter doses when symptoms subside. Lithium therapy may be lifelong.

■ Keep periodic office or clinic visits for blood tests. Regular measurements of blood lithium levels are necessary for safe and effective lithium therapy. Report for measurements of lithium blood levels as instructed and do not take the morning dose of lithium until the blood sample has been obtained. Accurate measurement of serum drug levels requires that blood be drawn approximately 12 hours after the previous dose of lithium.

■ Do not take diuretic medications without consulting a health care provider. Diuretics cause loss of sodium and water, which increases lithium toxicity.

■ Maintain a normal diet, including consistent salt and adequate fluid intake. Loss of salt in sweat increases the risk of adverse effects from lithium. Minimize activities that cause excessive perspiration, such as sweating during heavy exercise, sauna use, or outdoor activities during hot summer days. Loss of salt in sweat increases the risk of adverse effects from lithium.

■ Lithium can harm an unborn baby. If you are a woman of childbearing age, use an effective form of birth control during treatment, and notify your prescriber if you become pregnant.

■ If signs of overdose occur (e.g., vomiting, diarrhea, unsteady walking, tremor, drowsiness, muscle weakness), stop taking lithium and contact the prescriber or other health care provider.

Self- or Caregiver Administration

■ Take with food or milk or soon after a meal to decrease stomach upset.

■ Do not alter dietary salt intake. Decreased salt intake (e.g., low-salt diet) increases risk of adverse effects from lithium. Increased intake may decrease therapeutic effects.

■ Drink 8 to 12 glasses of fluids daily; avoid excessive intake of caffeine-containing beverages. Excessive intake of such beverages may decrease levels of lithium and reduce the effectiveness of the drug. Also, caffeine has a diuretic effect, and dehydration increases lithium toxicity.

Other Drugs in the Class

Atypical antipsychotics (see Chap. 55) are used to decrease dopamine activity in the treatment of the mania phase of bipolar disorder, including reducing acute mania, psychomotor agitation, and psychosis. Currently, aripiprazole, olanzapine (monotherapy or combination with fluoxetine), quetiapine, risperidone, and ziprasidone are approved by the FDA for this indication. Additionally, there is a potential risk for extrapyramidal signs and withdrawal symptoms in newborns whose mothers took these drugs during the third trimester of pregnancy.

Aripiprazole (Abilify) is used to treat acute manic and mixed bipolar disorder adults and in adolescents aged 10 to 17 years. The drug is well absorbed with oral administration, is highly protein-bound, metabolized in the liver, and is excreted in the urine and feces. Adverse effects include headache, somnolence, sedation, fatigue, dizziness, nausea, and vomiting.

Olanzapine (Zyprexa) is prescribed as monotherapy for the treatment of acute, mixed, or manic episodes associated with bipolar disorder and in combination with fluoxetine (Symbyax) for the treatment of depressive episodes associated with bipolar disorder. The drug is predominately excreted in the urine and feces. Reported adverse effects, which are dose dependent, include somnolence, extrapyramidal symptoms, dizziness, weight gain, constipation, and xerostomia.

Quetiapine (Seroquel) is an atypical antipsychotic used for the treatment of bipolar disorder and schizophrenia. The drug is excreted in the urine and feces. It may cause drowsiness, dizziness, decreased vision, fatigue, and weight gain.

Risperidone (Risperdal) is an atypical antipsychotic used alone or in combination with lithium or valproate for the treatment of acute mania or mixed episodes. The drug is approved by the FDA for use in adolescents aged 10 to 17 years with type I bipolar disorder. It is administered orally and intramuscularly and is well absorbed after oral administration. Risperidone is metabolized in the liver and predominately excreted in the urine. The drug enters breast milk. Adverse effects include significant weight gain, insomnia, sexual dysfunction, and photosensitivity. Neuroleptic malignant syndrome and tardive dyskinesia reportedly occur. Orthostatic hypotension may be present during the first few weeks of therapy.

Ziprasidone (Geodon) is another atypical antipsychotic used for the treatment of bipolar disorder in adults. The drug is well absorbed, is highly protein-bound, and is excreted in feces and urine. Adverse effects include dizziness, drowsiness, and lightheadedness.

Other Medications Used to Treat Bipolar Disorder

Anticonvulsants (see Chap. 52) are also used as mood-stabilizing agents in bipolar disorder because they modify nerve cell function. Carbamazepine (Tegretol), lamotrigine (Lamictal), and valproate (Depakene) are currently approved by the FDA for treating bipolar disorder. The drugs are typically used for patients who do not respond to lithium. Other anticonvulsants (e.g., gabapentin, topiramate, oxcarbazepine) are being studied and used off-label for their effects in bipolar disorder, but they do not have FDA approval for this use.

NCLEX Success

6. A nurse is teaching the importance of proper diet to a patient taking the MAO inhibitor tranylcypromine (Parnate) for depression. Which of the following food selections by the patient indicates that further teaching is needed?

   A. a tossed salad and a bowl of vegetable soup
   B. a salami and Swiss cheese sandwich and a banana
   C. a hamburger and French fries
   D. a cold plate with cottage cheese, chicken salad, and grapes

7. A patient taking lithium is having problems with coordination and unstable gait. The patient's lithium level is 2.3 mEq/L. The nurse should do which of the following?

   A. Continue to administer the lithium three times per day.
   B. Skip a dose of lithium and then resume the regular medication schedule.
   C. Administer an extra dose of lithium.
   D. Withhold the lithium and notify the prescriber of the lithium level.

8. A nurse practitioner plans to order lithium for a patient with bipolar disorder. Lithium is contraindicated in a patient with an impairment of which of the following systems?

   A. respiratory system
   B. cardiac system
   C. endocrine system
   D. renal system

9. A woman who is stable on lithium therapy for her bipolar disorder is shortly going to be receiving a drug for her hypertension. Which drug would be of greatest concern if added to the treatment regimen?

   A. a vasodilator
   B. an angiotensin-converting enzyme inhibitor
   C. a diuretic
   D. a calcium channel blocker

Clinical Application 54-2

- Mr. Mehring reports that he is having difficulty sleeping. What measures should the nurse initiate?

The Nursing Process

Assessment

- Identify patients at risk for current or potential depression. Areas to assess include health status, family and social relationship, and work status. Severe or prolonged illness, impaired interpersonal relationships, inability to work, and job dissatisfaction may precipitate depression. Depression also occurs without an identifiable cause.

- Observe for signs and symptoms of depression. Clinical manifestations are nonspecific and vary in severity. For example, fatigue and insomnia may be caused by a variety of disorders and range from mild to severe. When symptoms are present, try to determine their frequency, duration, and severity.
- When a patient appears depressed or has a history of depression, assess for suicidal thoughts and behaviors. Statements indicating a detailed plan, accompanied by the intent, ability, and method for carrying out the plan, place the patient at high risk for suicide.
- Identify the patient's usual coping mechanisms for stressful situations. Coping mechanisms vary widely, and behavior that may be helpful to one patient may not be helpful to another. For example, one person may prefer being alone or having decreased contact with family and friends, whereas another may find increased contact desirable.

Nursing Diagnoses

- Dysfunctional grieving related to loss (of health, ability to perform usual tasks, job, significant other, and so forth)
- Self-care deficit related to fatigue and self-esteem disturbance with depression or sedation with antidepressant drugs
- Sleep pattern disturbance related to mood disorder or drug therapy
- Risk for injury related to adverse drug effects
- Risk for violence: self-directed or directed at others
- Deficient knowledge: effects and appropriate use of antidepressant and mood-stabilizing drugs

Planning/Goals

The patient will

- Experience improvement of mood and depressive state
- Receive or self-administer the drugs correctly
- Be kept safe while sedated during therapy with the tricyclic antidepressants (TCAs) and related drugs

- Be assessed regularly for suicidal tendencies. If present, caretakers will implement safety measures
- Have needs met by staff in areas of nutrition, hygiene, exercise, and social interactions when unable to provide self-care
- Resume self-care and other usual activities
- Avoid preventable adverse drug effects

Nursing Interventions

The nurse will use general measures to prevent or decrease the severity of depression such as supportive psychotherapy and reduction of environmental stress. Specific measures include the following:

- Support the patient's usual mechanisms for handling stressful situations, when feasible. Helpful actions may involve relieving pain or insomnia, scheduling rest periods, and increasing or decreasing socialization.
- Call the patient by name, encourage self-care activities, allow him or her to participate in setting goals and making decisions, and praise efforts to accomplish tasks. These actions promote a positive self-image.
- When signs and symptoms of depression are observed, initiate treatment before depression becomes severe.

QSEN Safety Alert

Institute suicide precautions for patients at risk. These usually involve close observation, often on a one-to-one basis, and removal of potential weapons from the environment. For patients hospitalized on medical–surgical units, transfer to a psychiatric unit may be necessary.

- Provide patient teaching regarding drug therapy (see Boxes 54.3 and 54.9).

Evaluation

- Observe for behaviors indicating lessened depression.
- Interview regarding feelings and mood.
- Observe and interview regarding adverse drug effects.
- Observe and interview regarding suicidal thoughts and behaviors.

Key Concepts

- Major depression is associated with impaired ability to function in usual activities and relationships. Other types of depression include seasonal affective disorder and postnatal depression.
- Bipolar disorder is a mood disorder characterized by episodes of depression alternating with episodes of mania. There are two subtypes of this disorder, type I (characterized by a episodes of major depression plus mania) and type II (characterized by episodes of major depression plus episodes of hypomania).
- SSRIs are considered to be first-line medications in the treatment of depression because they have a more favorable side effect profile (e.g., GI symptoms, sexual dysfunction, CNS stimulation, and increased risk of GI bleeding).
- SNRIs are similar to SSRIs in terms of therapeutic effects but exhibit more anticholinergic, CNS sedation, and cardiac conduction abnormalities.

- TCAs, second-line medications in the treatment of depression, produce a high incidence of adverse effects (e.g., sedation, orthostatic hypotension, cardiac dysrhythmias, anticholinergic effects, and weight gain).

- MAO inhibitors are used in the treatment of depression only if other antidepressants are not effective; there is a high incidence of food and drug interactions that potentially lead to hypertensive crisis.

- Serotonin syndrome, a serious and sometimes fatal reaction characterized by hypertensive crisis, hyperpyrexia, extreme agitation progressing to delirium and coma, muscle rigidity, and seizures, may occur due to combined therapy with an SSRI or SNRI and an MAO inhibitor or other drug that potentiates serotonin neurotransmission. An SSRI or SNRI and an MAO inhibitor should not be given concurrently or within 2 weeks of each other. Fluoxetine, because of a long half-life, must be discontinued at least 5 weeks before starting an MAO inhibitor.

- Antidepressants must be taken for 2 to 4 weeks before depressive symptoms improve.

- Some antidepressant drugs are highly toxic and potentially lethal when taken in large doses.

- A **BLACK BOX WARNING** ◆ alerts health care providers to the increased risk of suicidal ideation in children, adolescents, and young adults 18 to 24 years of age when taking antidepressant medications.

- Antidepressant discontinuation syndrome has been reported with sudden termination of most antidepressant drugs.

- Most authorities agree that there is insufficient evidence to support the use of St. John's wort for treatment of depression.

- Lithium is the drug of choice to treat bipolar disorder. Lithium has a narrow therapeutic index, and dosage is determined by serum lithium levels, control of symptoms, and occurrence of adverse effects. Therapeutic range for serum lithium level is 0.5 to 1.2 mEq/L.

- Lithium is retained in the absence of sodium; thus, patients on a low-sodium diet are at greater risk of lithium toxicity.

- Other drugs useful in the treatment of bipolar disorder include atypical antipsychotics and some anticonvulsants.

Critical Thinking Questions

54-1. Ms. Greene, a 24-year-old woman, presents to the clinic complaining of feeling depressed. She has been taking St. John's wort, but it has not helped her symptoms. She says to a nurse practitioner, "A friend of mine was depressed and had good results with Prozac; could I get a prescription for that?"

- What questions does the nurse need to ask Ms. Greene to assess whether she meets the general indications for antidepressant drug therapy?

- What information does the nurse need to include in teaching Ms. Greene about fluoxetine (Prozac) if she receives a prescription for this drug?

References and Resources

American Psychiatric Association. (2000). *Diagnostic and statistical manual of mental disorders* (4th ed., text revision). Washington, DC: American Psychiatric Association.

Blier, P., Keller, M. B., Pollack, M. H., Thase, M. E., Zajecka, J. M., & Dunner, D. L. (2007). Preventing recurrent depression: Long-term treatment for major depressive disorder. *Journal of Clinical Psychiatry, 68*, e06.

Bridge, J. A., Marcus, S. C., & Olfson, M. (2012). Outpatient care of young people after emergency treatment of deliberate self-harm. *Journal of the American Academy of Child and Adolescent Psychiatry, 51*(2), 213–222.

Burgess, S., Geddes, J., Hawton, K., Townsend, E., Jamison, K., & Goodwin, G. (2007). Lithium for maintenance treatment of mood disorders. *Cochrane Database of Systematic Reviews, 3*, CD003013.

Cipriani, A., Brambilla, P., Furukawa, T., Geddes, J., Gregis, M., Hotopf, M., et al. (2007). Fluoxetine versus other types of pharmacotherapy for depression. *Cochrane Database of Systematic Reviews, 4*, CD004195.

Drug facts and comparisons. (Updated monthly). St. Louis, MO: Facts and Comparisons.

Gelenberg, A. J., Freeman, M. P., Markowitz, J. C., Rosenbaum, J. F., Thase, M. E., Trivedi, M. H., et al. (2010). *Guideline watch: Practice guideline for the treatment of patients with major depressive disorder* (3rd ed.). Arlington, VA: American Psychiatric Association.

Gelenberg, A. J., Freeman, M. P., Markowitz, J. C., Rosenbaum, J. F., Thase, M. E., & Trivedi, M. H. (2010). *Practice guideline for the treatment of patients with major depressive disorder* (3rd ed.). Arlington, VA: American Psychiatric Association.

Hirschfeld, R. M. A. (2005). *Guideline watch: Practice guideline for the treatment of patients with bipolar disorder* (2nd ed.). Arlington, VA: American Psychiatric Association.

Howard, L. (2005). Clinical evidence concise: Postnatal depression. A publication of BMJ Publishing Group. Reprinted in *American Family Physician*. Retrieved January 22, 2012, from http://www.aafp.org/afp/20051001/bmj.html

Howard, L. M., Hoffbrand, S., Henshaw, C., Boath, L., & Bradley, E. (2006). Antidepressant prevention of postnatal depression. *Cochrane Database of Systematic Reviews, 2,* CD004363.

Karch, A. M. (2013). *2013 Lippincott's nursing drug guide.* Philadelphia, PA: Lippincott Williams & Wilkins.

Kessler, R. C., Berglundy, P., Demler, O., Jin, R., Koretz, D., Merikangas, K. R., et al. (2003). The epidemiology of major depressive disorder: Results from the National Comorbidity Survey Replication CNCS-R. *JAMA: The Journal of the American Medical Association, 289,* 3095–3105.

Lacy, C. F., Armstrong, L. L., Goldman, M. P., & Lance, L. L. (2010). *Lexi-Comp's drug information handbook* (19th ed.). Hudson, OH: American Pharmaceutical Association.

Mottram, P., Wilson, K., & Strobl, J. (2007). Antidepressants for depressed elderly (Cochrane Review). *Cochrane Database of Systematic Reviews, 1,* CD003491.

Munoz, C., & Hilgenberg, C. (2005). Ethnopharmacology. *American Journal of Nursing, 105,* 40–48.

Steffens, D. C., Fisher, G. G., Langa, K. M., Potter, G. G., & Plassman, B. L. (2009). Prevalence of depression among older Americans: The aging, demographics and memory study. *International Psychogeriatrics, 21*(5), 879–888.

Warner, C. H., Bobo, W., Warner, C., Reid, S., & Rachal, J. (2006). Antidepressant discontinuation syndrome. *American Family Physician, 74,* 449–456. Retrieved February 16, 2012, from http://www.aafp.org/afp/20060801/449.html

55 Drug Therapy for Psychotic Disorders

LEARNING OBJECTIVES

After studying this chapter, you should be able to:

1 Discuss common manifestations of psychotic disorders, including schizophrenia.

2 Identify the prototype and describe the action, use, adverse effects, contraindications, and nursing implications for the phenothiazines.

3 Identify the prototype and describe the action, use, adverse effects, contraindications, and nursing implications for the typical antipsychotics.

4 Identify the prototype and describe the action, use, adverse effects, contraindications, and nursing implications for the atypical antipsychotics.

5 Compare characteristics of the "atypical" antipsychotics with those of the "typical" antipsychotics.

6 Implement the nursing process in the care of the patient being treated with antipsychotics.

Clinical Application Case Study

Caroline Jones, a 20-year-old college student, is brought to the university's mental health clinic by a friend. The friend says that Caroline has been talking to the television set and has complained that the voices from the television are telling her that she is ugly. In addition, she has become more withdrawn and reclusive. Caroline has not taken care of her personal hygiene for some time, and she looks disheveled. She receives a diagnosis of psychosis. The treatment plan involves supportive psychotherapy and haloperidol 10 mg twice daily.

KEY TERMS

Akathisia: motor restlessness and inability to be still, usually occurs in the first few months of treatment with antipsychotic agents

Anhedonia: lack of pleasure

Delusions: false beliefs that persist in the absence of reason or evidence

Drug-induced parkinsonism: loss of muscle movement, muscular rigidity and tremors, shuffling gait, masked facies, and drooling

Dystonia: uncoordinated, twisting, and repetitive movements

Extrapyramidal effects: movement disorders such as tardive dyskinesia, akathisia, dystonia, and drug-induced parkinsonism that may occur with usage of antipsychotic drugs

Hallucinations: sensory perceptions of people or objects that are not present in the external environment

Neuroleptics: antipsychotic drugs used to treat disorders that involve thought processes

Neuroleptic malignant syndrome: a rare but potentially fatal adverse effect; characterized by rigidity, severe hyperthermia, respiratory failure, and acute renal failure

Paranoia: belief that other people control their thoughts, feelings, and behaviors or seek to harm them

Psychosis: severe mental disorder characterized by disorganized thought processes, hallucinations, and delusions

Schizophrenia: variety of related psychotic disorders; symptoms include agitation, behavioral disturbances, delusions, disorganized speech, hallucinations, insomnia, and paranoia

Tardive dyskinesia: irreversible late extrapyramidal effect of some antipsychotic drugs

Introduction

This chapter introduces the pharmacological care of the patient who is experiencing psychosis. **Psychosis** is a severe mental disorder characterized by disorganized thought processes. Emotional responses may be blunted or inappropriate. Behavior may be bizarre and range from hypoactivity to hyperactivity with agitation, aggressiveness, hostility, and combativeness; it also may involve social withdrawal in which a person pays less-than-normal attention to the environment and other people, deterioration from previous levels of occupational and social functioning (poor self-care and interpersonal skills), hallucinations, and paranoid delusions. This chapter focuses primarily on schizophrenia as a chronic psychosis.

Several features are characteristic of psychosis. **Hallucinations** are sensory perceptions of people or objects that are not present in the external environment. More specifically, people see, hear, or feel stimuli that are not visible to external observers, and they cannot distinguish between these false perceptions and reality. Hallucinations occur in delirium, dementias, schizophrenia, and other psychotic states. In schizophrenia or bipolar affective disorder, they are usually auditory; in delirium, they are usually visual or tactile; and in dementia, they are usually visual. **Delusions** are false beliefs that persist in the absence of reason or evidence. Deluded people are often fearful and exhibit **paranoia**; they believe that other people control their thoughts, feelings, and behaviors or seek to harm them. Delusions indicate severe mental illness. Although they are commonly associated with schizophrenia, delusions also occur with delirium, dementias, and other psychotic disorders.

Overview of Psychosis

Psychosis may be acute or chronic. Acute episodes, also called confusion or delirium, have a sudden onset over hours to days and may be precipitated by physical disorders (e.g., brain damage related to cerebrovascular disease or head injury, metabolic disorders, infections); drug intoxication with adrenergics, antidepressants, some anticonvulsants, amphetamines, cocaine, and others; and drug withdrawal after chronic use (e.g., alcohol, benzodiazepine antianxiety or sedative-hypnotic agents). In addition, acute psychotic episodes may be superimposed on chronic dementias and psychoses, such as schizophrenia.

Etiology

Although **schizophrenia** is often referred to as a single disease, it includes a variety of related disorders. The lifetime prevalence of schizophrenia in the United States is approximately 1%. Males and females are equally affected; however, the disorder manifests itself earlier in males (early 20s for males as compared with late 20s to early 30s for females).

The etiology of schizophrenia is unknown. The neurodevelopmental model proposes that schizophrenia results when abnormal brain synapses are formed in response to an intrauterine insult during the second trimester of pregnancy, when neuronal migration is normally taking place. Intrauterine events such as upper respiratory infection, obstetric complications, and neonatal hypoxia have been associated with schizophrenia. The emergence of psychosis in response to the formation of these abnormal circuits in adolescence or early adulthood corresponds to the time period of neuronal maturation. Some studies of patients with schizophrenia have shown early neurologic abnormalities in infancy and early childhood, such as abnormal movements or motor developmental delays in infancy and psychological abnormalities as early as 4 years of age. This early onset of abnormalities coupled with emergence of schizophrenia in young adulthood suggests a neurodegenerative etiology for schizophrenia as well.

Genetics may play a role in the development of schizophrenia. Family studies identify increased risk if a first degree relative has the illness (10%), if a second degree relative has the illness (3%), if both parents have the illness (40%), and if a monozygotic twin has the illness (48%). Adoption studies of twins suggest that heredity rather than environment is a key factor in the development of schizophrenia.

Many genetic studies are underway to identify the gene or genes responsible for schizophrenia. Possible genes linked to schizophrenia include mutations in *WKL1* on chromosome 22, which may play a role in catatonic schizophrenia; mutations in *DISC1*, which causes delays in migration of brain neurons in mouse models; and mutation in the gene responsible for the glutamate receptor, which regulates the amount of glutamine in synapses.

Pathophysiology

There is evidence of abnormal neurotransmission systems in the brains of people with schizophrenia, especially in the dopaminergic, serotonergic, and glutamatergic systems. There is also evidence of extensive interactions among neurotransmission systems. In addition, illnesses or drugs that alter neurotransmission in one system are likely to alter neurotransmission in other systems. The dopaminergic, serotonergic, and glutamatergic systems have been the focus of the most studies.

Researchers have studied the dopaminergic system more extensively studied than other systems, because, historically, scientists have attributed schizophrenia to increased dopamine activity in the brain. Stimulation of dopamine can initiate psychotic symptoms or exacerbate an existing psychotic disorder. Two findings further support the importance of dopamine: (1) Antipsychotic drugs exert their therapeutic effects by decreasing dopamine activity (i.e., blocking dopamine receptors), and (2) drugs that increase dopamine levels in the brain (e.g., bromocriptine, cocaine, levodopa) can cause signs and symptoms of psychosis.

In addition to the increased amount of dopamine, dopamine receptor subtypes and their location also play a role. In general, authorities believe that overactivity of dopamine$_2$ (D_2) receptors in the basal ganglia, hypothalamus, limbic system, brainstem, and medulla accounts for the positive symptoms of schizophrenia, and these experts believe that underactivity of dopamine$_1$ (D_1) receptors in the prefrontal cortex accounts for the negative symptoms.

The serotonergic system, which is widespread in the brain, is mainly inhibitory in nature. In schizophrenia, serotonin apparently decreases dopamine activity in the part of the brain associated with negative symptoms, causing or aggravating these symptoms.

The glutamatergic neurotransmission system involves glutamate, the major excitatory neurotransmitter in the central nervous system (CNS). Glutamate receptors are widespread and possibly located on every neuron in the brain. They are also diverse, and their functions may vary according to subtypes and their locations in particular parts of the brain. When glutamate binds to its receptors, the resulting neuronal depolarization activates signaling molecules (e.g., calcium, nitric oxide) within and between brain cells. Thus, glutamatergic transmission may affect every CNS neuron and is considered essential for all mental, sensory, motor, and affective functions. Dysfunction of glutamatergic neurotransmission has been implicated in the development of psychosis.

In addition, the glutamatergic system interacts with the dopaminergic and gamma-aminobutyric acid (GABA) systems and possibly other neurotransmission systems. In people with schizophrenia, evidence indicates the presence of abnormalities in the number, density, composition, and function of glutamate receptors. In addition, glutamate receptors are genetically encoded and can interact with environmental factors (e.g., stress, alcohol and other drugs) during brain development. Thus, glutamatergic dysfunction may account for the roles of genetic and environmental risk factors in the development of schizophrenia as well as the cognitive impairments and negative symptoms associated with the disorder.

Clinical Manifestations

Symptoms of psychosis may begin gradually or suddenly, usually during adolescence or early adulthood. The American Psychiatric Association's *Diagnostic and Statistical Manual of Mental Disorders, 4th edition, Text Revision (DSM-IV-TR)* stipulates that characteristic psychotic symptoms must have been present during a 1-month period with presence of some overt psychotic symptoms for at least 6 months before schizophrenia can be diagnosed. Clinical manifestations of schizophrenia are categorized as positive and negative symptoms. Positive, or excess, symptoms are characterized by CNS stimulation and include agitation, behavioral disturbances, delusions, disorganized speech, hallucinations, insomnia, and paranoia. Negative, or deficit, symptoms are characterized by **anhedonia** (lack of pleasure), lack of motivation, blunted affect, poor grooming and hygiene, poor social skills, poverty of speech, and social withdrawal. Antipsychotic drugs are generally more effective in treating positive symptoms than negative symptoms.

Drug Therapy

Overall, the goal of drug treatment is to relieve symptoms with minimal or tolerable adverse effects. In patients with acute psychosis, the goal during the first week of treatment is to decrease symptoms (e.g., aggression, agitation, combativeness, hostility) and normalize patterns of sleeping and eating. The next goals may be increased ability for self-care and increased socialization. Therapeutic effects usually occur gradually, over 1 to 2 months. Long-term goals include increasing the patient's ability to cope with the environment, promoting optimal functioning in self-care and activities of daily living, and preventing acute episodes and hospitalizations. With drug therapy, patients often can participate in psychotherapy, group therapy, or other treatment modalities; return to community settings; and return to their preillness level of functioning.

Table 55.1 summarizes the drugs used in the treatment of psychosis, which are also known as **neuroleptics**. These drugs may be broadly categorized as first-generation or "typical" agents and second-generation or "atypical" agents. First-generation drugs include the phenothiazines and older nonphenothiazines, such as haloperidol. Second-generation drugs or newer nonphenothiazines include clozapine and other related drugs listed in Table 55.1. Most of these drugs bind to D_2 dopamine receptors and block the action of dopamine (Fig. 55.1). However, binding to the receptors does not account for antipsychotic effects because binding occurs within a few hours after a drug dose, and antipsychotic effects may not occur until the drugs have been given for a few weeks.

Prescribers caring for patients with psychosis have a greater choice of drugs than ever before. Some general factors to consider include the patient's age and physical condition, the severity and duration of illness, the frequency and severity of adverse effects produced by each drug, the patient's use of and response to antipsychotic drugs in the past, the supervision available, and the physician's experience with a particular drug.

Duration of Treatment

People with schizophrenia usually need to take antipsychotics for years because there is a high rate of relapse (acute psychotic episodes) when drug therapy is discontinued, most often by patients who become unwilling or unable to continue taking their medication. With wider use of maintenance therapy and the newer, better-tolerated antipsychotic drugs, patients may experience fewer psychotic episodes and hospitalizations.

TABLE 55.1

Drugs Administered for the Treatment of Psychosis

Drug Class	Prototype	Other Drugs in the Class
(Typical) phenothiazines	Chlorpromazine (Thorazine)	Fluphenazine (Prolixin) Perphenazine (Trilafon) Prochlorperazine (Compazine) Thioridazine (Mellaril) Trifluoperazine (Stelazine)
Typical antipsychotics	Haloperidol (Haldol)	Thiothixene (Navane)
Atypical antipsychotics	Clozapine (Clozaril)	Aripiprazole (Abilify) Asenapine (Saphris) Iloperidone (Fanapt) Lurasidone (Latuda) Olanzapine (Zyprexa) Paliperidone (Invega) Quetiapine (Seroquel) Risperidone (Risperdal, Risperdal Consta) Ziprasidone (Geodon)

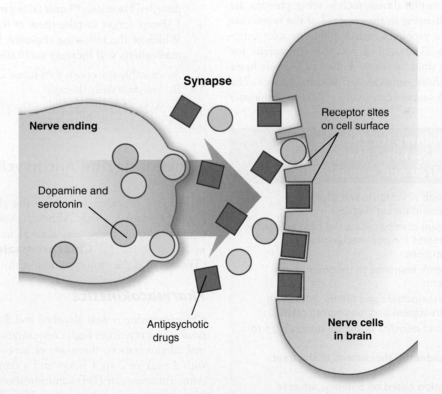

Figure 55.1 Antipsychotic drugs prevent dopamine and serotonin from occupying receptor sites on neuronal cell membranes and exerting their effects on cellular functions. This action leads to changes in receptors and cell functions that account for therapeutic effects (i.e., relief of psychotic symptoms). Other neurotransmitters and receptors may also be involved.

Most antipsychotics are available in oral formulations. Patients who are unable or unwilling to take daily doses of an antipsychotic may receive periodic injections of a long-acting form of fluphenazine, haloperidol, risperidone, or paliperidone. Extrapyramidal symptoms may be more problematic with depot injections of antipsychotics.

Treatment in Children

Schizophrenia in children is often characterized by more severe symptoms and a more chronic course than in adults. Drug therapy in children is largely empiric, because few studies have been conducted in young people. Dosage regulation is difficult because children may require lower plasma levels for therapeutic effects, but they also metabolize antipsychotic drugs more rapidly than adults. It is not clear which antipsychotics are safest and most effective in children and adolescents.

The American Academy of Child and Adolescent Psychiatry has established practice guidelines that advocate for high-quality assessment of the child or adolescent with the administration of antipsychotic medications. The purpose of the practice guidelines is to promote the appropriate use of antipsychotic medications and to enhance safety in the pediatric population. Box 55.1 lists major recommendations.

Drug Use in Home Care

People with chronic mental illness, such as schizophrenia, are among the most challenging in the caseload of the home care nurse. Major recurring problems include failure to take antipsychotic medications as prescribed and the concurrent use of alcohol and other drugs of abuse. Either problem is likely to lead to acute psychotic episodes and hospitalizations. The nurse must assist and support caregivers' efforts to administer medications and manage adverse effects, other aspects of daily care, and follow-up psychiatric care. In addition, the nurse may need to coordinate the efforts of several health and social service agencies or providers.

Clinical Application 55-1

- Describe the positive and negative symptoms that Caroline is experiencing.
- What neurotransmitter system is involved in Caroline's psychosis?
- How do antipsychotic drugs decrease the Caroline's psychotic symptoms?

NCLEX Success

1. A man is diagnosed with schizophrenia. He exhibits anhedonia, which is defined as which of the following?
   A. seizure activity
   B. lack of pleasure
   C. worm-like movements
   D. depression

2. A man is hospitalized due to a relapse of his psychotic disorder. He states, "I quit taking my medicines because I always forget to take them at least one time a day." Which of the following regimens for his antipsychotic medications will increase medication adherence?
   A. monthly injections by a home care nurse
   B. low-dose daily therapy
   C. daily visits to the clinic to receive his medications
   D. once-a-week drug therapy

Phenothiazine Antipsychotics

Health care providers have used the phenothiazines to treat psychosis since the 1950s. Although these drugs are historically significant, their usage and clinical importance have waned in recent years. Ⓟ **Chlorpromazine hydrochloride** (Thorazine) is the prototype drug of this class.

Pharmacokinetics

Chlorpromazine is well absorbed and distributed to most body tissues, and it reaches high concentrations in the brain. After oral administration, the onset of action is 30 to 60 minutes, with a peak of 2 to 4 hours and a duration of 4 to 6 hours. After intramuscular (IM) administration, the onset of action is 10 to 15 minutes, with a peak at 15 to 20 minutes and a duration of 4 to 6 hours. The half-life is 2 to 30 hours. The drug is metabolized in the liver and excreted in urine.

Action

The mechanism of action of chlorpromazine is not fully understood. When the drug produces antipsychotic effects, it blocks the postsynaptic dopamine receptors in the brain.

BOX 55.1	Guidelines for the Use of Antipsychotic Medications in Children and Adolescents

- Conduct a thorough psychiatric and physical examination before initiating therapy.
- Develop a treatment plan based on the best evidence and include strategies for pharmacological and psychosocial treatment.
- Monitor the patient's response to treatment both short and long term.
- Communicate to the patient and family, educating them about the treatment and monitoring plan.
- Explain all risks and benefits of the treatment plan to the parents.
- Document the consent of the parents to the treatment plan.
- Choose a medication based on potency, adverse effects, and the patient's medication response.
- Inform the patient and family of the use of medication combinations and the plan for monitoring the response of the medication combination.

From Walkup, J. and the Work Group on Quality Issues. (2009). Practice parameter on the use of psychotropic medication in children and adolescents. *Journal of the American Academy of Child and Adolescent Psychiatry, 48*(9), 961–973. Retrieved December 22, 2011 from www.jaacap.com. Used with permission from Elsevier.

Use

The major clinical indication for chlorpromazine and other phenothiazine antipsychotics is schizophrenia. Other uses include treatment of psychotic symptoms associated with brain impairment induced by head injury, tumor, stroke, alcohol withdrawal, overdoses of CNS stimulants, and other disorders.

It is necessary to individualize the dosage and route of administration of chlorpromazine according to the patient's condition and response; in some cases, prescribers may exceed the recommended maximum dosage approved by the U.S. Food and Drug Administration (FDA). Table 55.2 gives route and dosage information for the phenothiazine antipsychotics.

Use in Older Adults

Chlorpromazine should be administered cautiously to older adults. The dosage of chlorpromazine should be started at one fourth to one third of the level for younger adults. Older adults are more likely to have problems for which chlorpromazine and other antipsychotic agents are contraindicated (e.g., severe cardiovascular disease, liver damage, Parkinson's disease) or must be used very cautiously (diabetes mellitus, glaucoma, prostatic hypertrophy, peptic ulcer disease, chronic respiratory disorders).

Use in Children

Chlorpromazine is not routinely administered to children under the age of 6 months. Chlorpromazine is administered for the treatment of psychosis. It is also used preoperatively for

TABLE 55.2

DRUGS AT A GLANCE: Phenothiazine Antipsychotics

Drug	Pregnancy Category	Routes and Dosage Ranges	
		Adults	*Children*
ⓟ **Chlorpromazine** (Thorazine)	C	Excessive anxiety, agitation in psychiatric patients: 25 mg IM; may repeat in 1 h; increase dosage gradually in inpatients up to 400 mg every 4–6 h; max daily dosage 2000 mg/d; as soon as possible, switch to an oral dosage of 25–50 mg PO 3 times/d Initial oral dosage: 10 mg PO 3–4 times/d or 25 mg PO 2–3 times/d; increase daily dose by 20–50 mg semiweekly until optimum dosage is reached; dosages of 200–800 mg can be administered in discharged mental patients	Generally not used in children younger than 6 mo Psychiatric outpatients: 0.5 mg/kg PO every 4–6 h, 1 mg/kg rectally every 6–8 h not to exceed 40 mg/d (up to 5 y) or 75 mg/d (5–12 y) Psychiatric inpatients: 50–100 mg PO per day; max dosage 40 mg IM per day for children up to 5 y; 75 mg/d IM for children 5–12 y
Fluphenazine (Prolixin)	C	2.5–10 mg PO initially, gradually reduced to maintenance dose of 1–5 mg (doses above 3 mg are rarely necessary) Acute psychosis: 1.25 mg initially, increased gradually to 2.5–10 mg daily in 3–4 divided doses	5–12 y, 0.75–10 mg PO daily; no IM dosage established
Perphenazine (Trilafon)	C	Outpatients: 4–8 mg PO 3 times/d; reduce dose as soon as possible to minimum effective dosage; max dosage 64 mg/d Inpatients: 8–16 mg PO 2–4 times/d; max dosage 64 mg/d	4 mg PO 2–4 times/d; max dosage 16 mg/d
Prochlorperazine (Compazine)	C	5–10 mg PO 3–4 times daily, increased gradually (usual daily dose, 100–150 mg); 10–20 mg IM; may be repeated in 2–4 h; switch to oral form as soon as possible	2.5 mg PO, rectal 2–3 times daily
Thioridazine (Mellaril) Trifluoperazine (Stelazine)	C	Outpatients: 2–4 mg PO daily in divided doses Inpatients: 4–10 mg PO daily in divided doses Acute psychosis: 1–2 mg IM every 4–5 h; max of 10 mg daily	Children 6 y and older: 1–2 mg daily PO, IM; max daily dose 15 mg

the control of restlessness and apprehension. Chlorpromazine is administered rectally or intramuscularly for the control of nausea and vomiting.

Use in Patients With Renal Impairment

Excretion of chlorpromazine takes place in the kidneys, and therefore caution is necessary when using the drug in patients with impaired renal function. It is necessary to monitor renal function periodically during long-term therapy and lower the dosage or discontinue the drug altogether if test results (e.g., blood urea nitrogen) become abnormal.

Use in Patients With Hepatic Impairment

Chlorpromazine undergoes extensive hepatic metabolism, which means that caution is warranted in patients with hepatic impairment. In the presence of liver disease (e.g., cirrhosis, hepatitis), metabolism may be slowed and drug elimination half-lives prolonged, with resultant accumulation and increased risk of adverse effects.

Adverse Effects

Chlorpromazine has several adverse effects, including

- CNS effects: excessive sedation, with drowsiness, lethargy, fatigue, slurred speech, impaired mobility, and impaired mental processes. **Extrapyramidal effects** may also occur. Symptoms include movement disorders such as tardive dyskinesia, akathisia, dystonia, and drug-induced parkinsonism.
  - **Tardive dyskinesia** occurs as the result of long-term chlorpromazine use. Patients may experience lip smacking, tongue protrusion, and facial grimaces and may have choreic movements of trunk and limbs. This condition is usually irreversible, and there is no effective treatment.
  - **Akathisia**, the most common extrapyramidal reaction, may occur about 5 to 60 days from the start of drug therapy.
  - **Dystonias** are uncoordinated bizarre movements of the neck, face, eyes, tongue, trunk, or extremities. These adverse effects may occur suddenly 1 to 5 days after drug therapy is started and may be misinterpreted as seizures or other disorders.
  - **Drug-induced parkinsonism** is loss of muscle movement (akinesia), muscular rigidity and tremors, shuffling gait, masked facies, and drooling.
  - **Neuroleptic malignant syndrome** is a rare but potentially fatal reaction, which may occur hours to months after initial drug use. Symptoms of fever, muscle rigidity, respiratory failure, and confusion develop rapidly.
- Cardiovascular effects: prolonged QT and PR interval, T-wave blunting, and depression of the ST interval
- Hematologic effects: agranulocytosis and pancytopenia
- Other effects: antiadrenergic effects, such as hypotension, dizziness, fatigue, and faintness, as well as respiratory depression; endocrine effects; photosensitivity; and difficulty with temperature regulation

Contraindications

Because of wide-ranging adverse effects, chlorpromazine may cause or aggravate a number of conditions. Contraindications include liver damage, coronary artery disease, cerebrovascular disease, parkinsonism, bone marrow depression, severe hypotension or hypertension, coma, and severely depressed states. Caution is warranted in seizure disorders, diabetes mellitus, glaucoma, prostatic hypertrophy, peptic ulcer disease, and chronic respiratory disorders, as well as in pregnancy, especially during the first trimester.

Nursing Implications

Preventing Interactions

Many medications interact with chlorpromazine, increasing or decreasing its effects (Box 55.2). The combination of the herbal supplement with kava results in increased dystonia.

Administering the Medication

For acute psychotic episodes, therapy with chlorpromazine may require IM administration and hospitalization. Control of symptoms usually occurs within 48 to 72 hours, after which the person takes the oral drug. It is necessary to obtain a baseline electrocardiogram (ECG) prior to administering the drug, because of associated risk of alterations in the cardiac rhythm. The nurse needs to check doses carefully, especially when starting or stopping an antipsychotic drug or substituting one for another. The dosages are often changed during the course of treatment. When the drug is started, it is usually necessary to titrate initial doses upward over days or weeks and then reduce them for maintenance. Discontinuation of the drug requires a gradual reduction in dosage.

BOX 55.2   Drug Interactions: Chlorpromazine

Drugs That Increase the Effects of Chlorpromazine

- Anesthetic barbiturates, central nervous system (CNS) depressants, narcotics
  Produce additive CNS depression and hypotension
- Anticholinergic drugs
  Increase anticholinergic effects such as decreased secretions and urinary retention
- Beta blockers
  Produce tachycardia
- Epinephrine, norepinephrine
  Produce hypotension

Drugs That Decrease the Effects of Chlorpromazine

- Antacids
  Decrease absorption
- Anticholinergic drugs
  Decrease antipsychotic effects

For IM administration, the nurse adheres to the following guidelines:

- Determine the dose, which is approximately half of an oral dose. IM doses avoid first-pass metabolism and produce serum drug levels approximately double those of oral doses.
- Change the needle after filling the syringe with the injectable medication.
- Give the injection in the ventrogluteal muscle with a 1½-inch needle.
- Have the patient lie down for 30 to 60 minutes after the injection to prevent orthostatic hypotension.
- Watch for idiopathic edema and muscle necrosis, which may occur with IM administration.

For oral administration, the nurse adheres to the following guidelines:

- Give doses 1 to 2 hours before bedtime; peak sedation occurs in about 2 hours.
- Mix liquid concentrations with at least 60 mL of fruit juice. Avoid contact with skin because the liquid forms can cause contact dermatitis.
- Administer the oral preparation with food to reduce gastric upset.
- Use divided doses.

Assessing for Therapeutic Effects

With acute psychotic episodes, the nurse observes for decreased agitation, combativeness, and psychomotor activity. The sedative effects of chlorpromazine, considered to be therapeutic, occur within 48 to 72 hours. With acute or chronic psychosis, the nurse observes for decreased psychotic behaviors, such as decreased hallucinations and delusions.

Assessing for Adverse Effects

The nurse assesses the fluid and electrolyte status for a possible fluid volume deficit. It is also necessary to measure the patient's weight daily and assess for signs of dehydration. In addition, the nurse assesses for increased anticholinergic effects, such as diminished fluid status and urinary retention.

The nurse assesses for aspiration related to depressed cough reflex. It is important to monitor renal and hepatic function along with the complete blood count. A depression in white blood cell count requires discontinuation of the medication.

The nurse monitors for increased CNS depression that could result in falls or altered safety. He or she assesses for extrapyramidal effects such as dystonia, tardive dyskinesia, and akathisia.

Patient Teaching

Box 55.3 identifies patient teaching guidelines for chlorpromazine.

NCLEX Success

3. **The nurse should administer chlorpromazine (Thorazine) in which of the following ways?**
   A. intramuscularly into the deltoid muscle
   B. subcutaneously into the abdomen
   C. intramuscularly in the ventrogluteal muscle
   D. subcutaneously in the small of the back

4. **In monitoring the status of a patient on a long-term course of a phenothiazine antipsychotic, the nurse needs to be most aware that an adverse effect of long-term use of phenothiazine antipsychotics is the development of which of the following?**
   A. glaucoma
   B. tardive dyskinesia
   C. hypertension
   D. diabetes

5. **A man is taking chlorpromazine (Thorazine). He develops a high fever, respiratory depression, and diminished level of consciousness. What condition has the patient developed?**
   A. neuroleptic malignant syndrome
   B. dystonia
   C. anhedonia
   D. akathisia

6. **A 68-year-old man is seen by a home care nurse. He has been taking chlorpromazine (Thorazine) since 1969 for schizophrenia. Which of the following adverse effects are most commonly seen after use of chlorpromazine for long periods?**
   A. lethargy
   B. amnesia
   C. tardive dyskinesia
   D. dystonia

Nonphenothiazines

Nonphenothiazines include the first-generation "typical" antipsychotics, which are similar to phenothiazines in many ways. They were introduced approximately 50 years ago and

---

BOX 55.3 **Patient Teaching Guidelines for Chlorpromazine**

- Take the medication as prescribed.
- Do not combine the medication with over-the-counter medications or alcohol.
- Be sure to drink enough fluids, especially during hot weather.
- If you go outdoors, wear protective clothing and use sunscreen.
- Use caution when changing positions. It may be necessary to lie down for approximately an hour after taking your medication, because faintness and dizziness may occur.
- Do not overexercise and reduce body fluids.
- Do not drive a car or operate dangerous machinery. Dizziness or decreased mental alertness may occur.
- Report dark urine, pale stools, and yellowing of the eyes or skin to a health care provider.
- If you are a woman of childbearing age and intend to become pregnant, discuss chlorpromazine use with a health care provider.

are effective in treating acute psychosis, chronic psychotic disorders, and other psychiatric conditions. The second-generation "atypical" antipsychotics have a broader range of action due to their effects on the serotonergic, noradrenergic, and dopaminergic systems. They are effective in treating both psychotic disorders and nonpsychotic depression.

FIRST-GENERATION "TYPICAL" ANTIPSYCHOTICS

ⓟ **Haloperidol** (Haldol) is the prototype "typical" nonphenothiazine. This butyrophenone is a frequently used, long-acting antipsychotic.

Pharmacokinetics

Haloperidol is well absorbed after oral or IM administration. For the oral drug, the onset of action is 2 hours, with a peak of 2 to 6 hours and a duration of 8 to 12 hours. For the IM drug, the onset of action is 20 to 30 minutes, with a peak of 30 to 45 minutes and a duration of 4 to 8 hours. The half-life of the drug is 21 to 24 hours. It is metabolized in the liver and is excreted in urine and bile.

Action

The mechanism of action of haloperidol is not fully understood, but experts believe that the drug produces antipsychotic effects by blocking the postsynaptic dopamine receptors in the brain.

Use

Prescribers order haloperidol to control the symptoms of schizophrenia and psychotic disorders. Table 55.3 presents route and dosage information for haloperidol and some other nonphenothiazine antipsychotics.

Use in Children

The FDA has issued a **BLACK BOX WARNING** ◆ regarding extrapyramidal and withdrawal symptoms in newborns who have been exposed to haloperidol. Withdrawal symptoms occur in newborns born to women who take haloperidol during the third trimester of pregnancy.

Use in Older Adults

It is important to note that the FDA has not approved haloperidol for treatment of dementia-related psychosis. A **BLACK BOX WARNING** ◆ alerts health care practitioners that

TABLE 55.3

DRUGS AT A GLANCE: Typical Antipsychotics

Drug	Pregnancy Category	Routes and Dosage Ranges	
		Adults	*Children*
ⓟ **Haloperidol** (Haldol)	C	Acute psychosis: 1–15 mg PO daily initially in divided doses; gradually increase to 100 mg daily, if necessary; usual maintenance dose, 2–8 mg daily; 2–10 mg IM every 1–8 h until symptoms are controlled (usually within 72 h) Chronic schizophrenia: 6–15 mg PO daily; max 100 mg daily; dosage is reduced for maintenance, usually 15–20 mg daily Haloperidol decanoate IM, initial dose up to 100 mg, depending on previous dose of oral drug, then titrated according to response; usually given every 4 wk Mental retardation with hyperkinesia: 80–120 mg PO daily; gradually reduce to a maintenance dose of ~60 mg/d; 20 mg IM daily in divided doses, gradually increase to 60 mg/d if necessary; oral administration should be substituted after symptoms are controlled Elderly or debilitated adults: same as for children <12 y	Acute psychosis: 3–12 y, 0.05–0.15 mg/kg/d PO in 2–3 divided doses Acute psychosis, chronic refractory schizophrenia, Tourette's syndrome, mental retardation with hyperkinesia: 13 y and older, same as adults Chronic refractory schizophrenia: dosage not established Tourette's syndrome: 1.5–6 mg PO daily initially in divided doses; usual maintenance dose, 1.5 mg daily Mental retardation with hyperkinesia: 1.5 mg PO initially, in divided doses, gradually increase to a max of 15 mg daily, if necessary; when symptoms are controlled, dosage is gradually reduced to the minimum effective level; IM dosage not established
Thiothixene (Navane)	C	6–10 mg PO daily in divided doses; max 60 mg daily Acute psychosis: 8–16 mg IM daily in divided doses; max 30 mg daily Elderly or debilitated adults, PO, IM one third to one half the usual adult dosage	<12 y, dosage not established 12 y and older, same as adults

older patients who suffer from dementia and dementia-related psychosis and receive haloperidol have an increased risk of death compared with those patients who receive a placebo. (The deaths were related to cardiovascular or infectious diseases.)

Use in Patients With Renal Impairment

Excretion of haloperidol takes place in the kidneys, and therefore caution is necessary when using the drug in patients with impaired renal function. It is necessary to monitor renal function periodically during long-term therapy and lower the dosage or discontinue the drug altogether if test results (e.g., blood urea nitrogen) become abnormal.

Use in Patients With Hepatic Impairment

Haloperidol undergoes extensive hepatic metabolism. In the presence of liver disease (e.g., cirrhosis, hepatitis), metabolism may be slower, with resultant accumulation and increased risk of adverse effects. Thus, caution is necessary.

Use in Patients With Critical Illness

Haloperidol has relatively weak sedative effects and does not cause respiratory depression. However, it can cause hypotension in patients who are volume depleted or receiving antihypertensive drugs. It can also cause cardiac dysrhythmias, including life-threatening torsade de pointes, in patients who are receiving large doses (greater than 50 mg/d) or who have abnormal serum electrolyte levels (e.g., calcium, potassium, magnesium). Patients should be on a cardiac monitor, and it is necessary to check the ECG for a prolonged QT interval.

Adverse Effects

Haloperidol has several adverse effects, including

- Cardiovascular effects: abnormal T waves, prolonged ventricular depolarization, QT prolongation, torsade de pointes, tachycardia, and sudden death
- CNS effects: akathisia, hyperthermia, dystonia, extrapyramidal symptoms, neuroleptic malignant syndrome, parkinsonism, seizures, and vertigo
- Dermatologic effects: photosensitivity, hyperpigmentation, contact dermatitis, and alopecia
- Genitourinary effects: anticholinergic adverse effects such as urinary retention, sexual dysfunction, amenorrhea, breast engorgement and galactorrhea (women), and priapism and gynecomastia (men)
- Metabolic effects: hyperglycemia, hypoglycemia, and hyponatremia
- Respiratory effects: bronchospasm or laryngospasm

Contraindications

Contraindications to haloperidol include Parkinson's disease, seizure disorders, and severe mental depression.

Nursing Implications

Preventing Interactions

Many medication and herbs interact with haloperidol (Boxes 55.4 and 55.5), increasing or decreasing its effects.

BOX 55.4 Drug Interactions: Haloperidol

Drugs That Increase the Effects of Haloperidol

- Alcohol, central nervous system depressants, anticholinergic drugs, antidepressants, antihistamines
  Increase sedation and anticholinergic effects
- Nonsteroidal anti-inflammatory drugs
  Increase drowsiness and confusion
- Propranolol and angiotensin-converting enzyme inhibitors, lithium
  Enhance neurotoxic effect of antipsychotics and increase extrapyramidal symptoms

Drugs That Decrease the Effects of Haloperidol

- Antacids
  Inhibit absorption

Administering the Medication

Oral administration of haloperidol tablets requires taking the tablets with a full glass of water or milk. People should take them with food to decrease gastric upset. IM administration of haloperidol decanoate requires that the nurse gives the drug intramuscularly deep in the ventrogluteal muscle. (The amount injected should not exceed 3 mL.) During administration of the IM preparation, the patient should be in the recumbent position and remain recumbent for 1 hour following the administration. It is necessary to keep the preparation in a light-protected container.

When discontinuing haloperidol, it is essential to taper the dosage to prevent extrapyramidal symptoms. If the medication is abruptly discontinued, the patient is at risk for this condition.

Assessing for Therapeutic Effects

When haloperidol is given for acute psychotic episodes, the nurse observes for sedation, decreased agitation, combativeness, and psychomotor activity. When the drug is given for acute or chronic psychosis, he or she observes for decreased psychotic behaviors, such as decreased hallucinations and delusions.

Assessing for Adverse Effects

The nurse assesses the ECG for tachycardia and other abnormalities. Also, he or she assesses the patient's temperature for the onset of neuroleptic malignant syndrome. In addition, the nurse assesses for laryngospasm. Finally, it is necessary to monitor

---

BOX 55.5 Herb and Dietary Interactions: Haloperidol

Herbs and Foods That Increase the Effects of Haloperidol

- Kava
- Gotu kola
- St. John's wort
- Valerian

BOX 55.6   Patient Teaching Guidelines for Haloperidol

- Take the medication as prescribed.
- Report sore throat or fever to the prescriber.
- Notify the prescriber of any adverse effects such as tardive dyskinesia, dystonia, or akathisia.
- Do not drive a car or operate dangerous machinery. Dizziness or decreased mental alertness may occur.
- If you go outdoors, wear protective closing and use sun screen.
- Maintain adequate hydration.
- Use lozenges to counteract anticholinergic effects.
- Realize that dark-colored urine (pink or red-brown) is normal.
- If you are a woman of childbearing age and intend to become pregnant, discuss haloperidol use with a health care provider.

for the development of parkinsonism and extrapyramidal signs and symptoms, most notably tardive dyskinesia.

Patient Teaching

Box 55.6 identifies patient teaching guidelines for haloperidol.

Other Drugs in the Class

Thiothixene (Navane), another high-potency drug, is used only for its antipsychotic effects. Compared with haloperidol, thiothixene is more likely to produce orthostatic hypotension. Thiothixene can be given orally or parenterally.

Clinical Application 55-2

- After 6 weeks of therapy, Caroline has far fewer symptoms. She has withdrawn from her university classes to focus on her treatment and recovery. However, her friends observe that she has a gradual loss of muscle movement and a shuffling gait. What adverse reaction is likely to be occurring?
- Caroline has decided that she no longer wants to take the medication because of the adverse effects, despite experiencing a decrease in psychotic thinking. How would the nurse handle this situation?

NCLEX Success

7. An elderly woman with dementia is receiving haloperidol (Haldol). What adverse effect is this woman at increased risk for developing?

    A. anorexia
    B. increased temperature
    C. infection
    D. tardive dyskinesia

8. A patient is receiving haloperidol decanoate 100 mg intramuscularly. What assessment should the nurse make before and after the administration of the medication?

    A. pulse rate
    B. respiratory rate
    C. blood pressure
    D. mental status

9. A patient is taking thiothixene (Navane). Which of the following outcomes is desirable with this medication?

    A. decreased heart rate and diminished agitation
    B. blood pressure within normal limits and diminished psychosis
    C. heart rate of 60 beats/min with increased pulse pressure
    D. a widened QT complex and normal ST segment

SECOND-GENERATION "ATYPICAL" ANTIPSYCHOTICS

The "atypical" antipsychotics are the drugs of choice, especially for patients who are newly diagnosed with schizophrenia. These drugs may be more effective in relieving some symptoms, they usually produce milder adverse effects, and patients seem to take them more consistently. Better adherence to the drug regimen helps prevent acute episodes of psychosis and repeated hospitalizations, thereby reducing the overall cost of health care, according to studies. A major drawback is the high cost of these drugs, which may preclude their use in some patients. **Clozapine** (Clozaril), which is chemically different from the older antipsychotics, is the prototype "atypical" antipsychotic.

Pharmacokinetics

Clozapine is an oral drug. Its onset of action is unknown, with a peak of 1 to 6 hours and a duration of weeks. The half-life is 12 hours. Clozapine crosses the placenta and enters the breast milk. The drug is metabolized in the liver, and it is excreted in the urine and in the feces.

Action

The mechanism of action of clozapine is not clearly understood. Apparently, the drug blocks the dopamine receptors in the brain, depressing the reticular activating system. It also blocks the serotonin and glutamate receptors. In addition, clozapine has anticholinergic, antihistamine, and alpha-adrenergic blocking activity.

Use

Clinicians consider clozapine and other "atypical" antipsychotics to be first-line therapy for schizophrenia. Prescribers use the drug to manage patients with severe schizophrenia who have not responded to standard antipsychotic medications. Other uses in psychosis include reducing the risk of recurrent suicidal behavior in patients with schizophrenia or with schizoaffective disorder. Table 55.4 presents route and dosage information for atypical antipsychotics, including clozapine.

TABLE 55.4

DRUGS AT A GLANCE: Atypical Antipsychotics

Drug	Pregnancy Category	Routes and Dosage Ranges	
		Adults	*Children*
P Clozapine (Clozaril)	B	12.5 mg PO once or twice daily; increase by 25–50 mg daily every 3–7 d up to a max dose of 900 mg daily	<16 y, safety not established 16 y, 12.5–25 mg PO daily; increase to a target dose of 25–400 mg/d
Aripiprazole (Abilify) (Abilify Discmelt)	C	5–10 mg PO daily initially; given once daily at bedtime; increase over several weeks to 20 mg daily, if necessary Older adults: 12.5–25 mg PO daily, increase in 2.5-mg increments to desired response	Safety and efficacy not established
Asenapine (Saphris)	C	Schizophrenia: 5 mg SL 2 times/d Bipolar disorder: 10 mg SL 2 times/d; may be decreased to 5 mg/d as needed	Safety and efficacy not established
Iloperidone (Fanapt)	C	12–24 mg PO daily; titrate based on orthostatic hypotension tolerance; initially 1 mg PO 2 times/d then 2, 4, 6, 8, 10, and 12 mg PO 2 times/d on days 2, 3, 4, 5, 6, and 7, respectively	Safety and efficacy not established
Lurasidone (Latuda)	C	Starting dose is 40 mg PO once daily; max recommended dose is 80 mg/d; take with food (350 calories) Elderly: do not give to older patients with dementia-related psychosis (Black Box Warning)	Safety and efficacy not established
Olanzapine (Zyprexa)	C	5–10 mg PO initially once daily at bedtime; increase over several weeks to 20 mg daily, if necessary	<18 y, safety not established
Paliperidone (Invega)	C	6 mg PO daily in the morning; may be increased over several weeks to max of 12 mg daily	Safety and efficacy not established
Quetiapine (Seroquel)	C	25 mg PO 2 times/d initially; increase by 25–50 mg 2 or 3 times daily on 2nd and 3rd days, as tolerated, to 300–400 mg, in two or three divided doses on the 4th day; additional increments or decrements can be made at 2-day intervals; max dose 800 mg/d Elderly or debilitated adults: use lower initial doses and increase more gradually, to a lower target dose than for other adults Hepatic impairment: same as for elderly or debilitated adults	Safety and efficacy not established
Risperidone (Risperdal)	C	1 mg twice daily PO, initially; increase to 2 mg/d twice daily on the 2nd day; increase to 3 mg twice daily on the 3rd day, if necessary; usual maintenance dose, 4–8 mg/d; after initial titration, dosage increases or decreases should be made at a rate of 1 mg/wk Elderly or debilitated adults: initially 0.5 mg twice daily; increase in 0.5-mg increments to 1.5 mg twice daily Renal or hepatic impairment: same as for elderly or debilitated adults	13–17 y, initially 0.5 mg/d PO; increase 1–2 mg/d for a target dose of 3 mg/d; dosage range is 1–6 mg/d
Risperidone (Risperdal Consta)	C	25 mg IM every 2 wk; max dose not to exceed 50 mg/2 wk; oral Risperdal should be continued for first 3 wk of therapy to ensure adequate blood levels are maintained.	<18 y, dosage not established
Ziprasidone (Geodon)	C	20 mg PO twice daily with food, initially; gradually increased up to 80 mg twice daily, if necessary Acute agitation in schizophrenia: 10–20 mg IM every 4 h up to a max of 40 mg/d, not to exceed 3 d	Safety not established

EVIDENCE-BASED PRACTICE

Antipsychotic Medication for Elderly People With Schizophrenia

by MARRIOTT, R., NEIL, W., WADDINGHAM, S.

The Cochrane Collaboration, published by John Wiley & Sons. 2010, 1–46

An important consideration is the most appropriate choice for elderly patients with schizophrenia. The objective of this review was to find and assimilate good evidence of antipsychotic medication for the treatment of schizophrenia in people older than 65 years of age. An increasing number of elderly patients suffer from schizophrenia, and these patients have health concerns other than psychiatric disorders that may complicate treatment and recovery. However, studies of young adults largely form the basis for recommendations for pharmacologic treatment options in older patients. This review examined 252 elderly patients in three relevant randomized controlled trials. The conclusions were somewhat disappointing; despite wide use of antipsychotic medications with the elderly, little robust data are available to guide clinicians about the most appropriate medication to prescribe. It is important to consider the possible adverse effects of antipsychotic medications in relation to patients' preexisting health concerns. There are black box warnings for certain antipsychotic medications for use in the elderly with dementia.

IMPLICATIONS FOR NURSING PRACTICE: When caring for an elderly patient who has been prescribed antipsychotic medications for the treatment of schizophrenia, the nurse should assess the patient for adverse effects, impaired safety, and the presence of symptoms associated with black box warnings.

Use in Older Adults

The FDA has issued a **BLACK BOX WARNING** ◆ related to the administration of clozapine to elderly patients with dementia. The risk of death is increased in these patients. The FDA has not approved the drug for use in dementia.

Adverse Effects

Clozapine has several adverse effects, including

- Cardiovascular effects: orthostatic hypotension, tachycardia, ECG changes, and increased risk of myocarditis (greatest during the first month of treatment). The patient is also at risk for myocardial infarction, pericarditis, cardiomyopathy, mitral insufficiency, heart failure, and pericardial effusion.
- CNS effects: increased risk of seizures in patients with a known seizure disorder. An FDA-issued **BLACK BOX WARNING** ◆ alerts users of clozapine that the drug increases the risk of seizure activity as the dose increases.

BOX 55.7 Drug Interactions: Clozapine

Drugs That Increase the Effects of Clozapine

- Alcohol
  Increases central nervous system depression
- Cimetidine, caffeine, other cytochrome P450 inhibitors
  Increase the risk of toxicity

Drugs That Decrease the Effects of Clozapine

- Phenytoin, ethotoin, other cytochrome P450 inducers
  Decrease the serum concentration

- Hematologic effects: agranulocytosis. The FDA has issued a **BLACK BOX WARNING** ◆ regarding the potential risk of fatal agranulocytosis in patients who take clozapine.
- Metabolic effects: hyperglycemia and weight gain. The FDA has issued a **BLACK BOX WARNING** ◆ regarding the risk of hyperglycemia in patients who take clozapine. (In some extreme cases, there have been reports of ketoacidosis, hyperosmolar coma, and death.)

Contraindications

Contraindications to clozapine include a known allergy to the drug, a history of clozapine-induced agranulocytosis or severe granulocytopenia, CNS depression, and a history of seizure disorders. Caution is warranted in cardiovascular disease and narrow-angle glaucoma. Conditions that rule out drug use include pregnancy, especially the first trimester, and immunosuppression.

Nursing Implications

Preventing Interactions

Many medications and herbs interact with clozapine, increasing or decreasing its effects (Boxes 55.7 and 55.8).

Administering the Medication

Prior to beginning the administration of clozapine, it is necessary to obtain a baseline white blood cell count and neutrophil count. Also, it is important to monitor the blood glucose level regularly for hyperglycemia, especially if signs and symptoms of diabetes mellitus or risk factors are present.

BOX 55.8 Herb and Dietary Interactions: Clozapine

Herbs and Foods That Increase the Effects of Clozapine

- Gotu kola
- Kava
- St. John's wort
- Valerian

If clozapine is to be discontinued, gradual tapering over a 2-week period is essential. If the drug is discontinued abruptly, the nurse monitors for symptoms of acute psychosis.

Assessing for Therapeutic Effects

When clozapine is given for acute psychotic episodes, the nurse observes for sedation, decreased agitation, combativeness, and psychomotor activity. When the drug is given for acute or chronic psychosis, the nurse observes for decreased psychotic behaviors, such as decreased hallucinations and delusions.

Assessing for Adverse Effects

The nurse implements a thorough assessment of the cardiovascular and cardiopulmonary status to check for orthostatic hypotension, heart failure, and cardiovascular adverse events. It is essential to monitor the complete blood count due to the risk of fatal agranulocytosis. Also, it is necessary to monitor the intraocular pressure for increased pressure and potential development of glaucoma.

Patient Teaching

Box 55.9 identifies patient teaching guidelines for clozapine.

Clinical Application 55-3

- Caroline's family has read some literature about the newer atypical antipsychotic medications and the success they have had in treating patients with positive and negative symptoms of schizophrenia. Consequently, her physician has prescribed clozapine 12.5 mg twice daily. What safety patient teaching should the nurse conduct?

BOX 55.9   Patient Teaching Guidelines for Clozapine

- Obtain weekly blood tests to determine the safe and effective dosage.
- Keep appointments for white blood cell count monitoring.
- Keep counseling appointments.
- Be aware that only 1 week of medication will be dispensed at a time.
- Do not drive a car or operate dangerous machinery. Dizziness or decreased mental alertness may occur.
- Do not stop the medication abruptly.
- You may experience drowsiness, dizziness, and decreased alertness.
- If you are a woman of childbearing age and intend to become pregnant or are pregnant, discuss clozapine use with a health care provider.
- Notify the prescriber of increased heart rate.
- Report lethargy, weakness, or flu-like symptoms to the prescriber.

Other Drugs in the Class

Aripiprazole (Abilify) is approved for the treatment of schizophrenia and acute mania associated with bipolar disorder. The drug is well absorbed orally, with or without food. It is 99% protein bound. Aripiprazole is metabolized in the liver and has an active metabolite. Generally, no dosage adjustment for the drug is necessary on the basis of hepatic or renal impairment. It may cause neuroleptic malignant syndrome, tardive dyskinesia, weight gain, hyperglycemia, and diabetes mellitus.

Olanzapine (Zyprexa) is indicated for treatment of schizophrenia and the acute phase of bipolar disorder. The drug is well absorbed after oral administration; its absorption is not affected by food. After approximately 1 week of once-daily administration, a steady-state concentration is reached. Olanzapine is metabolized in the liver and excreted in urine and feces. The drug's therapeutic effects are similar to those of clozapine, but its adverse effects may be different. Compared with clozapine, olanzapine is more likely to cause extrapyramidal effects and less likely to cause agranulocytosis. Compared with the typical antipsychotics, olanzapine reportedly causes less sedation, extrapyramidal symptoms, anticholinergic effects, and orthostatic hypotension. However, the drug has been associated with weight gain, hyperglycemia, and initiation or aggravation of diabetes mellitus.

Quetiapine (Seroquel) relieves both positive and negative symptoms of psychosis and is also indicated for the acute manic phase of bipolar disorder. After oral administration, quetiapine is well absorbed and may be taken without regard to meals. It is extensively metabolized in the liver and excreted in the feces and urine. Common adverse effects include drowsiness, headache, orthostatic hypotension, and weight gain.

Risperidone (Risperdal), a first-choice drug that is usually well tolerated, also relieves both positive and negative symptoms of psychosis as well as the acute manic phase of bipolar disorder. It is frequently prescribed. Risperidone is well absorbed with oral administration. Peak blood levels occur in 1 to 2 hours, but therapeutic effects are delayed for 1 to 2 weeks. Risperidone is metabolized mainly in the liver and produces an active metabolite. Effects are attributed approximately equally to the drug and the metabolite. It is excreted in urine and in feces.

Adverse effects of risperidone include agitation, anxiety, headache, insomnia, dizziness, and hypotension. The drug may also cause parkinsonism and other movement disorders, especially at higher doses, but is less likely to do so than the typical antipsychotic drugs.

Paliperidone (Invega) is the major active metabolite of risperidone. Administration is oral, and the drug reaches peak blood levels 24 hours after administration. The drug is eliminated by the renal system. Adverse effects include akathisia, extrapyramidal effects, QT prolongation, orthostatic hypotension, syncope, hyperprolactinemia, and hyperglycemia.

Ziprasidone (Geodon) is another atypical agent used to treat schizophrenia and the acute manic phase of bipolar disorder. This drug is effective in suppressing many negative symptoms such as blunted affect, lack of motivation, and social withdrawal. It is metabolized in the liver and excreted in the urine. Adverse effects include cardiac dysrhythmias, drowsiness, headache, and nausea. Because ziprasidone may prolong

56 Drug Therapy to Stimulate the Central Nervous System

LEARNING OBJECTIVES

After studying this chapter, you should be able to:

1. Understand the etiology, pathophysiology, and clinical manifestations of attention deficit hyperactivity disorder.

2. Understand the etiology, pathophysiology, and clinical manifestations of narcolepsy.

3. Describe general characteristics of central nervous system stimulants.

4. Identify the prototypes and discuss the action, use, adverse effects, contraindications, and nursing implications for the stimulants used in the treatment of attention deficit hyperactivity disorder and narcolepsy.

5. Identify sources and effects of caffeine.

6. Implement the nursing process in the care of patients who take central nervous stimulants.

Clinical Application Case Study

Brian Connor received a diagnosis of attention deficit hyperactivity disorder at 7 years of age. He is now 9 years old. As a result of taking methylphenidate (Ritalin) 15 mg daily and receiving individual counseling, his attention span and school performance have improved. However, his most recent physical examination shows that his height and weight are less than normal for his age and that he has lost weight since his examination last year. The school nurse talks with Brian's teachers, who report that he seems more restless in class after lunch. He has had more difficulty getting along with his classmates due to his impulsive behaviors.

KEY TERMS

Attention deficit hyperactivity disorder: relatively common disorder of childhood onset characterized by inattention, impulsiveness, and overactivity

Narcolepsy: sleep disorder in which a person goes to sleep at any place or at any time

Introduction

This chapter introduces the pharmacological care of attention deficit hyperactivity disorder (ADHD) and narcolepsy. Clinicians use drugs that stimulate the central nervous system (CNS) to treat these disorders.

Overview of Attention Deficit Hyperactivity Disorder

To adequately understand the pharmacologic treatment of **attention deficit hyperactivity disorder**, or ADHD, it is important to understand the causes, pathophysiology, and clinical manifestations of ADHD. This condition is characterized by persistent hyperactivity, short attention span, difficulty completing assigned tasks or schoolwork, restlessness, and impulsiveness.

Etiology and Pathophysiology

ADHD is the most common psychiatric or neurobehavioral disorder in children. Although the cause is not fully understood, evidence suggests that subtle dysfunction in the frontal lobe and functionally related subcortical structures plays an essential role in the core symptoms of ADHD. Research has suggested that ADHD is a highly heritable, neurobiological disorder partially attributed to dopamine and norepinephrine transport dysfunction in the brain.

ADHD is usually diagnosed between 3 and 7 years of age and may affect as many as 8% of school-age children. Children with ADHD find it difficult to get along with others (e.g., family members, peer groups, teachers) and to function in situations requiring controlled behavior (e.g., classrooms). Approximately 10% to 20% of children with ADHD also have a diagnosed learning disability, causing further academic and emotional difficulties.

ADHD continues into adolescence and adulthood in approximately 50% of cases and may affect 4% of adults in the United States. In adolescents and adults, hyperactivity is not prominent, but impulsiveness, inattention, and difficulties in structured settings such as school or work may continue. Some studies indicate that children with ADHD are more likely to have mood disorders and substance abuse disorders as adolescents and adults. A major criterion for diagnosing later ADHD is a previous diagnosis of ADHD by 7 years of age. Some authorities believe this age limit is too restrictive. The diagnosis of ADHD in adults has greatly increased in recent years, with a concomitant increase in the use of prescribed CNS stimulants for its treatment.

Clinical Manifestations

Clinical manifestations of ADHD usually occur in various or multiple environments in a child's life, including school, home, church, or recreational activities. The level of problems typically varies, but symptoms generally worsen in situations that require sustained attention, such as listening to teacher, performing repetitive tasks, or reading lengthy materials.

Hyperactivity in children presents as fidgeting or squirming in their seats, excessive running or climbing when it is dangerous or inappropriate, disruptive playing during quiet activities, and demonstrating a driven verbal or motor quality. Impulsivity manifests as impatience, blurting out answers, and frequently interrupting others. Inattention manifests as messy work, careless mistakes, and appearance of daydreaming. Based on the behaviors associated with ADHD, affected people also may have low self-esteem and strained peer relations. Early diagnosis and treatment are essential. Evidence suggests that behavior management combined with pharmacotherapy yields the best outcomes.

Drug Therapy

Drug therapy is indicated when symptoms are moderate to severe; are present for several months; and interfere in social, academic, or behavioral functioning. Counseling and psychotherapy (e.g., parental counseling, family therapy) are recommended along with drug therapy for effective treatment and realistic expectations of outcomes. Young children may not require treatment until starting school. Then, the goal of drug therapy is to control symptoms, facilitate learning, and promote social development. Table 56.1 summarizes the drugs used in the treatment of ADHD. Treatment is based on individual signs and symptoms.

TABLE 56.1

Drugs Administered for the Treatment of Attention Deficit Hyperactivity Disorder and Narcolepsy

Drug Class	Prototype	Other Drugs in the Class
Amphetamines	Dextroamphetamine (Dexedrine, DextroStat)	Dextroamphetamine and amphetamine (Adderall XR, Adderall) Lisdexamfetamine (Vyvanse) Methamphetamine (Desoxyn)
Amphetamine-related central nervous system stimulants	Methylphenidate (Ritalin, Ritalin LA, Ritalin SR, Concerta, Daytrana, Metadate CD, Metadate ER)	Dexmethylphenidate (Focalin, Focalin XR)
Selective norepinephrine reuptake inhibitors	Atomoxetine (Strattera)	
Sympatholytics	Guanfacine (Intuniv)	
Stimulants	Modafinil (Provigil)	

Overview of Narcolepsy

To adequately understand the pharmacologic treatment of the chronic sleep disorder **narcolepsy**, it is important to understand the causes, pathophysiology, and clinical manifestations of narcolepsy. This condition is characterized by excessive sleepiness and sleep attacks at inappropriate times, such as at work.

Etiology and Pathophysiology

Narcolepsy is a neurological sleep disorder, not the result of mental illness or psychological problems. It is most likely due to a number of genetic abnormalities that affect specific biologic factors in the brain, combined with an environment trigger, such as exposure to a virus, during the brain's development. The exact cause is unknown, and sleep studies are required for an accurate diagnosis. People with narcolepsy often have a reduced number of protein-producing neurons in the brain that are responsible for controlling appetite and sleep patterns.

Narcolepsy affects men and women equally and usually begins during the teenage or young adult years. When people with narcolepsy fall asleep, they generally experience the rapid eye movement (REM) stage of sleep within 10 minutes, whereas most people experience REM sleep after 1 hour of sleep.

Clinical Manifestations

People with narcolepsy often experience disturbed nocturnal sleep and an abnormal daytime sleep pattern; it is important not to confuse this pattern with insomnia. Excessive daytime drowsiness (even after an adequate night's sleep) and fatigue are characteristic. People are likely to become drowsy or fall asleep or just be very tired. The hazards of drowsiness during normal waking hours and suddenly going to sleep in unsafe environments restrict activities of daily living.

Other signs and symptoms of narcolepsy include cataplexy, hypnagogic hallucinations, disturbances of nighttime sleep patterns, and sleep paralysis. Cataplexy is an episodic condition featuring the loss of muscle function, ranging from slight weakness to complete body collapse. These episodes may be triggered by emotional reactions such as laughter, anger, or fear, lasting from a few seconds to minutes. Hypnagogic hallucinations are vivid, often frightening, dream-like experiences that occur while dozing, falling asleep, or awakening. Sleep paralysis is the temporary inability to move or talk on waking.

Drug Therapy

Treatment of narcolepsy is based on individual symptoms and therapeutic response. In addition to drug therapy, prevention of sleep deprivation, regular sleeping and waking times, avoiding shift work, and short naps may be helpful in reducing daytime sleepiness. However, even adequate amounts of nighttime sleep do not produce full alertness. Table 56.1 summarizes the medications used in the treatment of narcolepsy.

Stimulants

CNS stimulants act by facilitating initiation and transmission of nerve impulses that excite other cells. The drugs are somewhat selective in their actions at lower doses but tend to involve the entire CNS at higher doses. In ADHD, the drugs improve academic performance, behavior, and interpersonal relationships. In narcolepsy, stimulants improve the performance of daily activities by 70% to 80% of normal (Burgess & Scammell, 2012). Major groups of stimulants are amphetamines, amphetamine-related drugs, and xanthines.

The main goal of therapy with CNS stimulants is to relieve symptoms of the disorders for which they are given. A secondary goal is to have patients use the drugs appropriately. Misuse and abuse of stimulants often occurs when people who want to combat fatigue and delay sleep, such as long-distance drivers, students, and athletes, take the drugs. College students reportedly use stimulants as study aids; this is not justified. These drugs are dangerous for drivers and those involved in similar activities, and they have no legitimate use in athletics.

When a prescriber orders a CNS stimulant, the dose starts low and then increases as necessary, usually at weekly intervals, until the drug becomes effective or the dose reaches a maximum. It is also necessary to limit the number of doses that can be obtained with one prescription. This action reduces the likelihood of drug dependence or diversion (use by people for whom the drug is not prescribed).

Overdoses may occur with acute or chronic ingestion of large amounts of a single stimulant, combinations of stimulants, or concurrent ingestion of a stimulant and another drug that slows the metabolism of the stimulant. Signs of toxicity may include severe agitation, cardiac dysrhythmias, combativeness, confusion, delirium, hallucinations, high body temperature, hyperactivity, hypertension, insomnia, irritability, nervousness, panic states, restlessness, tremors, seizures, coma, circulatory collapse, and death.

AMPHETAMINES

Amphetamines produce mood elevation or euphoria, increasing mental alertness and capacity for work, decreasing fatigue and drowsiness, and prolonging wakefulness. Large doses can lead to signs of excessive CNS stimulation (e.g., agitation, confusion, hyperactivity, difficulty concentrating on tasks, hyperactivity, nervousness, restlessness) and sympathetic nervous system stimulation (e.g., increased heart rate and blood pressure, pupil dilation, slowed gastrointestinal [GI] motility, and other symptoms). Overdoses can result in psychosis, convulsions, stroke, cardiac arrest, and death. Amphetamines are schedule II drugs under the Controlled Substances Act; they have a high potential for drug abuse and dependence. Widely sold on the street, they are commonly abused. ℗ **Dextroamphetamine** (Dexedrine, DextroStat) is the prototype amphetamine.

Pharmacokinetics

Dextroamphetamine has a rapid absorption and onset of action. The drug reaches its peak in 1 to 5 hours, and the duration is between 8 and 10 hours. It is metabolized by the liver and excreted in the urine. Dextroamphetamine may cross the placenta and has been found in breast milk.

Action

Dextroamphetamine acts in the CNS to release norepinephrine from nerve terminals and increases the amounts of norepinephrine, dopamine, and possibly serotonin in the brain. Dopamine is released in higher doses. Dextroamphetamine suppresses appetite, increases alertness, elevates mood, and improves physical performance. The drug's effectiveness and efficacy in ADHD is paradoxical, and its action is not well understood.

Use

The clinical indications for use of dextroamphetamine include the management of ADHD and narcolepsy. Amphetamines are useful in both acute and chronic conditions. Table 56.2 summarizes the route and dosage information for dextroamphetamine and other amphetamines.

Use in Children

Parents need to monitor their children's use of medications for ADHD, and it is necessary to titrate the dosage carefully to avoid excessive CNS stimulation, anorexia, and insomnia. Suppression of weight and height (e.g., less than the estimated average of 2 inches per year) may occur, and the nurse ensures that growth is monitored during drug therapy. In children with psychosis or Tourette's syndrome, CNS stimulants may exacerbate symptoms. In children and adolescents with preexisting heart disease, usual doses of dextroamphetamine may cause sudden death.

In ADHD, careful documentation of baseline symptoms over approximately 1 month is necessary to establish the diagnosis and evaluate outcomes of treatment. This may involve videotapes of behavior; observations and ratings by clinicians familiar with the condition; and by interviewing the child, parents, or caretakers. Some authorities believe that ADHD is overdiagnosed and that stimulant drugs are prescribed unnecessarily.

Use in Older Adults

The use of dextroamphetamine warrants caution in older adults. As with most other drugs, slowed metabolism and excretion increase the risks of accumulation and toxicity. Older adults are likely to experience anxiety, confusion, insomnia, and nervousness from excessive CNS stimulation. In addition, older adults often have cardiovascular disorders (e.g., angina, dysrhythmias, hypertension) that may be aggravated by the cardiac-stimulating effects of the drug. In general, reduced doses are safer in older adults.

Use in Patients With Renal or Hepatic Impairment

Dextroamphetamine is excreted in the urine after being metabolized in the liver. Thus, caution is necessary in patients with renal and/or hepatic impairment. The nurse monitors such patients for adverse effects and helps ensure that lower doses are used.

Adverse Effects

Dextroamphetamine has several adverse effects.

- Cardiovascular effects: tachycardia, other dysrhythmias, and hypertension. A **BLACK BOX WARNING ◆** makes users aware of the drug's high abuse potential; misuse may cause sudden death or serious cardiovascular events. It is essential to obtain a baseline electrocardiogram (ECG) and blood pressure reading.
- CNS effects: excessive CNS stimulation; possible anxiety, hyperactivity, nervousness, insomnia, tremors, convulsion, and psychotic behavior may occur. These reactions are more likely with larger doses.
- GI effects: gastritis, nausea, diarrhea, and constipation
- Other effects: anorexia and weight loss

Contraindications

Contraindications to dextroamphetamine include cardiovascular disorders (e.g., angina, dysrhythmias, hypertension), which are likely to be aggravated by the drug. Other contraindications

TABLE 56.2

DRUGS AT A GLANCE: Amphetamines

Drug	Pregnancy Category	Routes and Dosage Ranges	
		Adults	*Children*
Ⓟ **Dextroamphetamine** (Dexedrine, DextroStat)	C	Narcolepsy: start with 10 mg/d PO in divided doses, increase in increments of 10 mg/d at weekly intervals; reduce dose if adverse effects occur; usual dose is 5–60 mg/d PO in divided doses; long-acting forms can be given once daily	ADHD: 3–5 y, start with 2.5 mg/d PO; increase in increments of 2.5 mg/d at weekly intervals until optimal response is obtained 6 y and older, start with 5 mg PO twice daily; increase in increments of 5 mg/d until optimal response is obtained; dosage will rarely exceed 40 mg/d; long-acting forms may be used once a day Narcolepsy: 6–12 y, start with 5 mg/d PO; increase in increments of 5 mg at weekly intervals until optimal response is obtained 12 y and older, same as adults
Dextroamphetamine and amphetamine (Adderall XR, Adderall)	C	Narcolepsy: 10 mg/d PO initially, increased if necessary ADHD: extended-release, 20 mg/d	ADHD: 3–5 y, 2.5 mg/d PO, increased if necessary 6 y and older, 5 mg PO 1–2 times daily, increase if necessary; max dose 40 mg/d in 1–3 divided doses; extended-release, 5–10 mg/d PO, increase at weekly intervals if necessary; max dose, 30 mg/d 13–17 y, 10 mg PO once daily, increase to 20 mg if necessary
Lisdexamfetamine (Vyvanse)	C		ADHD: 6–12 y, 30 mg PO once daily, increased if necessary; max dose, 70 mg/d
Methamphetamine (Desoxyn)	C		5 mg/d PO initially, increased if necessary; usual dose 20–25 mg/d, in 2 divided doses

ADHD, attention deficit hyperactivity disorder.

include anxiety or agitation, glaucoma, and hyperthyroidism, as well as a history of drug abuse, pregnancy, or lactation.

Nursing Implications

Preventing Interactions

Many medications and herbs interact with dextroamphetamine, increasing or decreasing its effects (Boxes 56.1 and 56.2).

Administering the Medication

People should take the first dose of dextroamphetamine on awakening or early in the day and the last dose at least 6 hours before bedtime. Children with ADHD should take the drug 30 to 45 minutes before meals to minimize the appetite-suppressing effects. It is important not to crush, chew, or bite the long-acting form; this destroys the extended-release feature and may result in an overdose. For young children who have difficulty swallowing pills, the capsules may be opened and taken with pudding or ice cream.

Dextroamphetamine often causes loss of appetite, and the health care provider may stop the medication during the months when the child is not in school. A drug holiday, as this is called, helps decrease weight loss and growth suppression. It may not be appropriate for every child.

Assessing for Therapeutic Effects

For patients with ADHD, the nurse assesses for improved behavior and performance of cognitive and psychomotor tasks. For patients with narcolepsy, the nurse assesses for fewer sleep attacks, increased mental alertness, and decreased mental fatigue.

Assessing for Adverse Effects

The nurse assesses for signs and symptoms of excessive CNS stimulation as evidenced by an inability to complete tasks due to nervousness and hyperactivity. It is necessary to check the patient's cardiovascular status for tachycardia and elevation in blood pressure. The nurse assesses the patient's diet for inability to eat and the patient for loss of weight. It is also important to assess the GI system for constipation or diarrhea.

BOX 56.1 Drug Interactions: Dextroamphetamine

Drugs That Increase the Effects of Dextroamphetamine

■ Albuterol, pseudoephedrine, tricyclic antidepressants

Increase stimulant effects of dextroamphetamine

■ Antacids

Decrease the excretion of amphetamines

■ Monoamine oxidase inhibitors

Enhance the hypertensive effects of amphetamines

Drugs That Decrease the Effects of Dextroamphetamine

■ Ammonium chloride

Decreases the serum concentration of dextroamphetamine

■ Antipsychotics, lithium, alcohol

Diminish the stimulant effect of dextroamphetamine

■ Gastrointestinal acidifying agents

Decrease the serum concentration of dextroamphetamine

Patient Teaching

Box 56.3 identifies patient teaching guidelines for drugs used in ADHD or narcolepsy.

Clinical Application 56-2

Brian has been taking methylphenidate ER every morning for 2 months, and the teachers have noticed that his concentration and his behavior have improved after lunch. However, his appetite has decreased dramatically and he has lost 4 pounds. The teachers have noticed that he does not eat his lunch and skips his afternoon snack. His parents are concerned and schedule a visit to the health care provider. The health care provider is hesitant to change Brian's medication regimen since his behavior at school has improved. What patient teaching can the school nurse provide to Brian and his parents to increase his weight?

BOX 56.2 Herbs and Dietary Interactions: Dextroamphetamine

Herbs and Foods That Increase the Effects of Dextroamphetamine

■ Ephedra

Herbs and Foods That Decrease the Effects of Dextroamphetamine

■ Acidic foods and juices, caffeine

EVIDENCE-BASED PRACTICE

Homeopathy for Attention Deficit-Hyperactivity Disorder or Hyperkinetic Disorder

by DEAN, H

The Cochrane Collaboration
2009, 1–30.

The objective of this review was to assess the safety and efficacy of homeopathy as a treatment for attention deficit hyperactivity disorder (ADHD) or hyperkinetic disorder. Homeopathy is a form of complementary/alternative medicine that is promoted as being a safe and effective form of treatment for children and adults. Because there are an increasing number of children and adults receiving homeopathic treatments for ADHD, it is important to review the safety and efficacy of such treatments. Four studies (n = 168) were included for review and the results of the studies were synthesized. Overall, there was no difference found between homeopathic treatment and placebo. Therefore, the results do not indicate a significant benefit of homeopathic treatment for ADHD. Patients and their families need to learn about available pharmacological treatment options for ADHD that have been proven to be effective.

IMPLICATIONS FOR NURSING PRACTICE: The nurse must be knowledgeable about the proven treatments for ADHD. He or she must educate the patient and family about effective treatment options. Based on this research, the nurse should instruct patients and their families to contact the primary health care provider before taking any homeopathic treatments for ADHD.

NCLEX Success

3. A prescriber has ordered a central nervous system stimulant for a child. What is the expected outcome of this medication?

A. increased behavioral problems
B. improved performance in schoolwork
C. decreased ability to complete a task
D. increased hyperactivity

4. The nurse is caring for a child who is receiving a central nervous system stimulant for attention deficit hyperactivity disorder. It is most important to monitor for which of the following?

A. liver function
B. weight loss
C. fever
D. seizure activity

5. A clinician prescribes dextroamphetamine for a patient. Which of the following is an adverse effect of this medication?

   A. increased appetite
   B. respiratory depression
   C. sedation
   D. cardiac dysrhythmias

6. A 10-year-old child diagnosed with attention deficit hyperactivity disorder has been taking amphetamine sulfate (Adderall) for the past 2 years. Which of the following are normal adverse effects of the drug? (Choose all that apply.)

   A. weight loss
   B. anorexia
   C. dry mouth
   D. bradycardia

7. A physician has prescribed a central nervous system stimulant for a 7-year-old child, who is already of short stature. Which of the following interventions will promote growth?

   A. administer growth hormone.
   B. encourage daily exercise.
   C. maintain a 2200-calorie diet.
   D. drug holidays when on school breaks

AMPHETAMINE-RELATED DRUGS

Amphetamine-related drugs, which resemble amphetamines, have essentially the same effects as the amphetamines and are also schedule II drugs. **Ⓟ Methylphenidate** (Ritalin, others) is the prototype. This drug, marketed under generic and trade names, is available in several dosage forms, including immediate-release and chewable tablets, extended-release capsules, and a transdermal patch. These dosage forms are not interchangeable.

The U.S. Food and Drug Administration (FDA) has issued a **BLACK BOX WARNING** ◆ regarding the risk of drug dependence with amphetamine-related drugs. Methylphenidate has become a drug of abuse, and its nonmedical use, alone or with other drugs, has increased visits for emergency departments by adolescents and young adults.

Pharmacokinetics

Methylphenidate is well absorbed after oral administration. Depending on the formulation, the onset of action varies, with a peak in 1 to 8 hours and a duration of 3 to 12 hours (longer for transdermal preparation). The drug is mostly metabolized in the liver and excreted in the urine.

Action

Methylphenidate is a mild cortical stimulant that acts on the CNS-like amphetamines. The drug suppresses appetite, increases alertness, elevates mood, and improves physical

---

BOX 56.3   **Patient Teaching Guidelines for Drugs Used in Attention Deficit Hyperactivity Disorder and Narcolepsy**

General Considerations

- When diagnosed with attention deficit hyperactivity disorder (ADHD) and before taking any medication for it, adult patients and parents of affected children should inform the health care provider about any other stimulant drugs being taken, involvement in strenuous activities of any kind, any heart disease, or any family history of sudden cardiac death. All drugs for ADHD stimulate the heart and blood vessels. The effects are usually a faster heartbeat and increased blood pressure, but cardiac arrest, stroke, or sudden death may occur.

- Use caution while driving or performing other tasks requiring alertness. These drugs may mask symptoms of fatigue, impair physical coordination, and cause dizziness or drowsiness.

- Notify a health care provider of nervousness, insomnia, heart palpitations, vomiting, fever, or skin rash. These are adverse drug effects and dosage may need to be reduced.

- Avoid other stimulants, including caffeine.

- Record weight at least weekly; report excessive losses.

- The drugs may cause weight loss; caloric intake (of nutritional foods) may need to be increased, especially in children.

- Take stimulant drugs only as prescribed.

  - Accurate dosing is important because underuse may cause the recurrence of symptoms and overuse may cause toxicity.

  - Do not increase the dosage without consulting with your health care provider. These drugs have a

high potential for abuse. The risks of serious health problems and drug dependence are lessened if they are taken correctly. The likelihood of medical problems is greatly increased when ADHD medication is used improperly or in combination with other drugs.

- Get adequate rest and sleep. Do not take stimulant drugs to delay fatigue and sleep; these are normal, necessary resting mechanisms for the body.

- Keep these medications away from children, preferably in a locked cabinet. Parents (or a school nurse) need to dispense each dose and to be sure the drug is taken only by the child for whom it was prescribed.

Self- or Parental Administration

- Take (or give) regular tablets approximately 30 to 45 minutes before meals.

- Take (or give) the last dose of the day in the afternoon, before 6:00 PM, to avoid interference with sleep.

- Ensure that long-acting/extended-release central nervous system stimulants are swallowed whole, without crushing or chewing.

- Apply the Daytrana skin patch to hip area as prescribed. Patch should be removed after 9 hours; alternate hips. See the manufacturer's instructions for opening, applying, removing, and disposing of the skin patch.

- If excessive weight loss, nervousness, or insomnia develops, ask the prescribing physician if the dose can be reduced or taken on a different schedule to relieve these adverse effects.

TABLE 56.3

DRUGS AT A GLANCE: Amphetamine-Related Central Nervous System Stimulants

Drug	Pregnancy Category	Routes and Dosage Ranges	
		Adults	*Children*
Ⓟ **Methylphenidate** (Ritalin, Ritalin LA, Ritalin SR, Concerta, Daytrana, Metadate CD, Metadate ER)	C	10–60 mg/d PO 2 or 3 times daily, preferably 30–45 min before meals; if insomnia is a problem, drug should be taken before 6:00 PM; timed-release tablets (duration of 8 h) may be used ER forms, 18 mg PO daily in the morning; may be increased by 18 mg/d at 1-wk intervals to a max of 54 mg/d (Concerta); increments of 10–20 mg/d to a max of 60 mg/d (Metadate CD, Ritalin LA)	6–12 y, start with 5 mg PO before breakfast and lunch with gradual increase 13–17 y, start with 18 mg/d in the morning without regard to food; titrate to a max of 72 mg/d; do not exceed 2 mg/kg/d Transdermal patch (Daytrana), 10–30 mg/d; apply patch 2 h before effect needed and remove after 9 h in increments of 5–10 mg/wk; daily dosage exceeding 60 mg/d is not recommended; discontinue use after 1 mo if no improvement ER forms, use adult dosage
Dexmethylphenidate (Focalin, Focalin XR)	C	5–10 mg/d PO, increased if necessary; max dose, 20 mg/d	6 y and older, 2.5–5 mg/d PO, increased if necessary; max dose 20 mg/d

performance. The efficacy in ADHD is paradoxical and not well understood.

Use

The clinical indications for use of methylphenidate include the management of ADHD and narcolepsy. The drug may be useful for treatment of both acute and chronic conditions. Table 56.3 gives route and dosage information for methylphenidate and other amphetamine-related drugs.

Use in Children and in Older Adults

The use of methylphenidate in both children and older adults is similar to that for dextroamphetamine. This information is available in Amphetamines, Use.

Use in Patients With Renal or Hepatic Impairment

Methylphenidate is excreted in the urine after being metabolized by the liver. Thus, it is necessary to use the drug with caution in patients with renal or hepatic impairment. The nurse should help ensure that lower doses are used.

Adverse Effects

Methylphenidate has several adverse effects.

- Cardiovascular effects: tachycardia, other dysrhythmias, and hypertension. It is necessary to obtain a baseline ECG and blood pressure.
- CNS effects: excessive CNS stimulation as well as anxiety, hyperactivity, nervousness, insomnia, tremors,

convulsion, and possibly psychotic behavior. These reactions are more likely with larger doses of medication.
- GI effects: gastritis, nausea, diarrhea, and constipation
- Dermatologic effects: rash, exfoliative dermatitis, and loss of scalp hair
- Hematologic effects: leukopenia and anemia. It is important to obtain a baseline complete blood count and platelet count.
- Other effects: anorexia and weight loss

It is important to note that in recent years, warnings have been added to all drugs used to treat ADHD and narcolepsy about the associated risks of sudden death, serious cardiovascular problems (e.g., heart attack, hypertension), and psychiatric illnesses (e.g., psychosis, aggression, mania).

Contraindications

Contraindications to methylphenidate include cardiovascular conditions (e.g., angina, dysrhythmias, hypertension) that are likely to be aggravated by the drug. Other contraindications are anxiety or agitation, glaucoma, or hyperthyroidism. Conditions such as a history of drug abuse or pregnancy or lactation usually preclude use of the drug. Caution is necessary with seizure disorders.

Nursing Implications

Preventing Interactions

Methylphenidate may increase effects of phenytoin, tricyclic antidepressants, selective serotonin reuptake inhibitors, and oral anticoagulants. Also, methylphenidate may decrease effects of antihypertensive drugs.

Administering the Medications

People should take the first dose of methylphenidate on awakening or early in the day, and they should take the last dose at least 6 hours before bedtime. Children with ADHD should take the drug 30 to 45 minutes before meals to minimize the appetite-suppressive effects. It is important not to crush, chew, or bite the long-acting form of methylphenidate; this destroys the extended-release feature and may result in an overdose.

Like dextroamphetamine, methylphenidate often causes loss of appetite. Thus, the health care provider may stop the medication during the months when the child is not in school. A drug holiday, as this is called, helps decrease weight loss and growth suppression. It may not be appropriate for every child.

Assessing for Therapeutic Effects

For patients with ADHD, the nurse assesses for improved behavior and performance of cognitive and psychomotor tasks. For patients with narcolepsy, the nurse assesses for fewer sleep attacks, as well as for increased mental alertness and decreased mental fatigue.

Assessing for Adverse Effects

The nurse assesses the blood pressure and pulse for hypertension and tachycardia related to the stimulant effects. It is necessary to assess the patient's CNS response for increased anxiety and hyperactivity that impairs the ability to perform activities of daily living. The nurse checks the patient's sleep patterns and inability to sleep restfully. It is also important to assess the patient's GI status for reflux and pain leading to gastritis. In addition, the nurse checks the complete blood count and platelet count for the onset of anemia.

Patient Teaching

Box 56.3 identifies patient teaching guidelines for medications administered for the treatment of ADHD or narcolepsy.

Clinical Application 56-3

Brian has been maintaining his weight with his current dosage of methylphenidate and continues to drink two nutritional supplement drinks per day. It is now late spring, and his health care provider wants to try a drug holiday in the summer. Brian's parents are concerned about their son's being able to function at summer camp without any pharmacologic intervention. They voice their worries to the school nurse. What information should the school nurse provide to Brian's parents?

XANTHINES

Xanthines stimulate the cerebral cortex, increasing mental alertness and decreasing drowsiness and fatigue. ℗ **Caffeine** is the prototype for this class. Caffeine is a frequently consumed CNS stimulant worldwide, mostly from dietary sources (e.g., coffee, tea, soft drinks). What determines the caffeine content of coffee or tea is the particular coffee bean or tea leaf and the method of preparation. Caffeine is an ingredient in about 70% of the soft drinks ingested in the United States. In addition, many people, especially teenagers and young adults, like so-called energy drinks. These products contain large amounts of caffeine, and most contain large amounts of sugar.

Caffeine is the active ingredient in nonprescription stimulant (antisleep) preparations. Also, the drug is an ingredient in some nonprescription analgesic preparations. In addition, it is available by prescription in combination with an ergot alkaloid to treat migraine headaches (e.g., Cafergot) (Chap. 51).

Because of the widespread ingestion of caffeine-containing beverages and the wide availability of over-the-counter products that contain caffeine, toxicity may result from concomitant consumption of caffeine from several sources. Some authorities recommend that normal, healthy, nonpregnant adults consume no more than 250 mg of caffeine daily. Table 56.4 lists common sources and amounts of caffeine.

Pharmacokinetics

Caffeine is well absorbed from the GI tract and reaches a peak blood level within 30 to 45 minutes of oral ingestion. It readily crosses the blood–brain barrier and has a half-life of 3.5 to 5 hours. It is extensively metabolized, mainly in the liver, and excreted mainly in urine.

Action

In low to moderate amounts, caffeine increases alertness, wakefulness, and capacity for work; decreases fatigue; and delays sleep. Large amounts cause anxiety, agitation, diarrhea, hyperactivity, insomnia, irritability, nausea, nervousness, premature ventricular contractions, restlessness, tachycardia, tremors, and vomiting. Toxic amounts may cause delirium and seizures.

Use

Caffeine is an ingredient in many drinks (see Table 56.4). It is also found in nonprescription analgesics and stimulants that promote wakefulness (e.g., NoDoz).

Use in Children

A combination of caffeine and sodium benzoate is occasionally used as a respiratory stimulant in neonates. Caffeine is generally not recommended for use in young children.

Use in Patients With Renal or Hepatic Impairment

Caffeine is excreted in the urine after being metabolized by the liver. Thus, it is necessary to use the drug with caution in patients with renal or hepatic impairment. The nurse should help ensure that lower doses are used.

Adverse Effects

Adverse effects of caffeine include insomnia, restlessness, excitement, tinnitus, headaches, and muscular tremors. Cardiovascular effects include hypertension and palpitations;

TABLE 56.4

Sources of Caffeine

Source	Amount (oz)	Caffeine (mg)	Comments
Coffee			
Brewed, regular	5–8	40–180	Caffeine content varies with product and preparation.
Instant		30–120	
Espresso	12	120	
Starbucks (regular)	12	58–279	
	16	116–372	
Tea			
Brewed, leaf or bag	8	80	Caffeine content varies with product and preparation.
Instant	8	50	
Iced	12	70	
Soft Drinks			
Coke, Diet Coke	12	45	Most other cola drinks contain 35–45 mg/12 oz.
Pepsi, Diet Pepsi	12	38	
Mountain Dew	12	54	
Energy Drinks			
Amp	8.4	75	Sugar 31 g (6 tsp)
Full Throttle	16	141	Sugar 58 g (12 tsp)
Monster	16	140	Sugar 54 g (11 tsp)
Red Bull	8	80	Sugar 39 g (8 tsp)
Rockstar	16	160	Sugar 60 g (12 tsp)
SoBe Adrenaline Rush	8.3	79	Sugar 35 g (7 tsp)
SoBe No Fear	16	66	Sugar 66 g (13 tsp)
Tab Energy	10.5	95	Sugar 0 g
OTC Analgesics			
Anacin, Vanquish	1 tablet or caplet	30	
APAP-Plus, Excedrin, Midol	1 tablet, caplet, or gel tab	60–65	
OTC Antisleep Products			
Caffedrine, NoDoz, Vivarin	1 tablet or capsule	200	
OTC Diuretic			
Aqua-Ban	1 tablet	100	2 tablets PO 3 times daily
Prescription Drugs			
Cafergot	1 tablet	100	Also contains ergotamine; 2 tablets PO at onset of migraine, then 1 tablet every hour if needed, up to 6 tablets per attack or 2 suppositories per attack
	1 rectal suppository	100	
Fiorinal	1 capsule	40	Also contains a barbiturate and is a schedule III controlled drug; 1–2 capsules PO every 4 h, up to 6 capsules in 24 h

OTC, over the counter.

myocardial stimulation leads to increased cardiac output and heart rate. Some patients experience nausea, vomiting, diarrhea, and stomach pain. There may be increased secretion of pepsin and hydrochloric acid. Patients also experience increased diuresis.

Large doses of caffeine can impair mental and physical functions by producing agitation, anxiety, cardiac dysrhythmias, insomnia, and nervousness. Some authorities have implicated caffeine as a causative or aggravating factor in cardiovascular disease (hypertension, dysrhythmias), GI disorders (esophageal reflux, peptic ulcers), reproductive disorders, osteoporosis (may increase loss of calcium in urine), psychiatric disturbances, and drug abuse liability.

Caffeine produces tolerance to its stimulating effects, and physical dependence occurs. Abstinence produces withdrawal symptoms, including drowsiness, fatigue, headache, and irritability, within 18 to 24 hours after stopping caffeine intake.

BOX 56.4　Patient Teaching Guidelines for Caffeine

General Considerations

■ There are numerous sources of caffeine, including coffee, cocoa, tea, most soft drinks, and several over-the-counter medications. In addition, "energy drinks" (e.g., Red Bull, Monster, many others) containing high amounts of caffeine and sugar are popular with teenagers and young adults. They are aggressively marketed to this population for weight loss, increased endurance and wakefulness, decreased fatigue, and legal "highs." Parents may think the drinks will help their children in school; coaches may think the drinks will help athletic performance. There is no evidence for these claims, and the risks of excessive caffeine intake are high. There are increasing visits to hospital emergency rooms and calls to poison centers for teens who become ill from excessive caffeine.

　■ Some of the drinks also contain B vitamins, which can cause rapid heartbeat, heart palpitations, and numbness and tingling in the hands and feet when taken in large doses, and some are being mixed with alcoholic beverages. Two large companies produce "energy beers," and a drink containing a mixture of Red Bull and vodka has been popular for several years. There is a great potential for traumatic injuries and alcohol poisoning with these products.

■ In general, authorities recommend no more than 250 mg of caffeine per day for healthy adults and little to none for people with heart disease. Signs and symptoms of excess caffeine intake (e.g., anxiety, agitation, heart palpitations, insomnia, nausea, nervousness, tremors) usually occur with ingestion of 500 mg/d or more.

■ Prevent nervousness, anxiety, tremors, and insomnia from excessive intake by decreasing consumption of caffeinated beverages or by drinking decaffeinated coffee, tea, and cola. Sprite and 7 UP have no caffeine.

■ Supervise and possibly limit children's intake of caffeinated beverages, especially energy drinks. If children do consume such products, their parents should discuss the consequences of drinking too much.

■ Caution high school and college students that caffeine, in any form, is not a substitute for adequate rest and sleep. Being tired and sleepy are normal and necessary resting mechanisms for the body.

Self-Administration

■ Limit intake of caffeinated beverages and read labels of over-the-counter stay-awake products and multi-ingredient pain reliever products so that you do not develop trouble sleeping as well as brain, heart, and stomach problems from excessive caffeine intake.

Contraindications

Contraindications to caffeine include cardiac dysrhythmias, history of stroke, peptic ulcer disease, bipolar mood disorder, and schizophrenia. Caution is necessary within pregnancy, depression, or cardiovascular disease.

Nursing Implications

Preventing Interactions

Several medications increase the effects of caffeine; these include cimetidine, oral contraceptives, disulfiram, ciprofloxacin, and mexiletine. Caffeine increases the effects of theophylline and clozapine. There is decreased absorption of iron if it is taken within 1 hour after caffeine. Patients who take caffeine should avoid other alternative medications that have stimulant effects to prevent potentiation of drug.

Administering the Medication

People should take the first dose of therapeutic caffeine on awakening or early in the day. They should take the last dose at least 6 hours before bedtime.

Assessing for Therapeutic Effects

The nurse assesses the therapeutic effects of the medication. Caffeine increases alertness, wakefulness, and capacity for work; decreases fatigue; and delays sleep.

Assessing for Adverse Effects

The nurse assesses the patient's intake of caffeinated foods and liquids. It is necessary to assess the patient's blood pressure and pulse rate due to the vasoconstrictive action of caffeine. The nurse assesses the patient's sleep patterns. It is also important to interview the patient regarding feelings of fatigue or excitement and ask if he or she has experienced gastric upset or reflux.

Patient Teaching

Box 56.4 identifies patient teaching guidelines for caffeine.

NCLEX Success

8. Patient teaching for children taking methylphenidate for attention deficit hyperactivity disorder should include which of the following?

A. Give the child the drug at bedtime.
B. Drowsiness may be a side effect.
C. If necessary, the child may take over-the-counter cold products without problems.
D. Provide for periodic drug-free holidays.

9. A boy comes to the school nurse's office and states, "I did not take my Ritalin today." Which of the following is the most appropriate nursing intervention?

A. Call the child's parent or guardian to try to find out if the boy has taken his medicine.
B. Give the child his morning dose since it is in the office.
C. Send him back to class and tell him it is not necessary to take the medication.
D. Call the child's physician to obtain a one-time dose of methylphenidate.

TABLE 56.5

DRUGS AT A GLANCE: Other Drugs Administered for Attention Deficit Hyperactivity Disorder

Drug	Pregnancy Category	Routes and Dosage Ranges	
		Adults	*Children*
Selective Norepinephrine Reuptake Inhibitors			
℗ **Atomoxetine** (Strattera)	C	Adults and children more than 70 kg, start with 40 mg/d PO, increase after a minimum of 3 d to a target daily dose of 80 mg PO daily given as a single dose in the morning or 2 evenly divided doses during the day; dosage may be increased to 100 mg/d after 2–4 wk if needed	32 kg or less, start with 0.5 mg/kg/d PO and increase after a minimum of 3 d to a target daily dose of ~1.2 mg/kg/d as a single daily dose in the morning; may be given in 2 evenly divided doses throughout the day; do not exceed 1.4 mg/kg/d or 100 mg/d, whichever is less
Sympatholytics			
℗ **Guanfacine** (Intuniv)	B		6–17 y, 1 mg/kg/d PO in ER tablet; increase by 1 mg/d/wk to a max of 4 mg/d.
Stimulants			
℗ **Modafinil** (Provigil)	C	Narcolepsy: 200 mg PO daily given as a single dose; up to 400 mg/d may be given as a single dose	Safety and efficacy not established

Other Medications Used to Treat Attention Deficit Hyperactivity Disorder and Narcolepsy

Three other drugs are commonly administered for the treatment of ADHD or narcolepsy. These drugs include the selective norepinephrine reuptake inhibitor atomoxetine, the antihypertensive drug guanfacine, and the stimulant modafinil. Table 56.5 gives route and dosage information for these medications.

℗ **Atomoxetine** (Strattera), a second-line drug for the treatment of ADHD in children and adults, acts to inhibit reuptake of norepinephrine in nerve synapses. It has a low risk of abuse and dependence compared with the other drugs used for ADHD and is not a controlled drug. Atomoxetine is rapidly absorbed with oral administration, with peak plasma levels in 1 to 2 hours. Atomoxetine is metabolized in the liver and is excreted mainly in urine. People may take the drug with or without food. Common adverse effects include abdominal pain, anorexia, cough, dry mouth, headache, insomnia, nausea, and vomiting. A **BLACK BOX WARNING** ◆ advises that suicidal ideation may occur in children and adolescents who take atomoxetine.

℗ **Guanfacine** (Intuniv), an antihypertensive drug, has recently received FDA approval as extended-release tablets for the treatment of ADHD in children 6 to 17 years of age. Its onset of action is 2 hours, and its duration of action is 24 hours. It is metabolized by the liver and excreted by the urine. Guanfacine crosses the placenta and enters breast milk.

Adverse effects include sedation, weakness, dizziness, vision disturbance, and headache, as well as cardiovascular conditions (bradycardia and hypotension) and GI problems (dry mouth, constipation, and abdominal pain). Caution is necessary in cardiovascular disease, hepatic and renal insufficiency, and in pregnancy or lactation.

℗ **Modafinil** (Provigil) is used to treat narcolepsy and to improve wakefulness in other sleep disorders (e.g., obstructive sleep apnea/hypopnea syndrome, shift work sleep disorder). The drug is also used to decrease the fatigue associated with multiple sclerosis and other disorders. Its ability to promote wakefulness is similar to that of amphetamines and methylphenidate, but its mechanism of action is unknown. Like other CNS stimulants, modafinil has psychoactive effects that alter mood, perception, and thinking; it is a schedule IV controlled drug. The drug is rapidly absorbed and reaches peak plasma levels in 2 to 4 hours. It is metabolized by the liver to metabolites that are then excreted in the urine. Adverse effects include anxiety, chest pain, dizziness, dyspnea, dysrhythmias, headache, nausea, palpitations, and nervousness. Modafinil should not be used in patients with a history of left ventricular hypertrophy or ischemic changes on ECGs.

Herbal and Dietary Supplements

Caffeine is in important ingredient in guarana, made from the seeds of a South American plant. Box 56.5 presents more information about guarana.

BOX 56.5   Guarana as Source of Caffeine

The seeds of the South American shrub guarana contain more caffeine than coffee beans or dried tea leaves. Guarana is widely used as a source of caffeine by soft drink manufacturers. It is also used as a flavoring agent and is an ingredient in herbal stimulant and weight-loss products, energy drinks, vitamin supplements, candies, and chewing gums. The product, which may also contain theophylline and theobromine, is also available in teas, extracts, elixirs, capsules, and tablets of various strengths. In general, the caffeine content of a guarana product is unknown, and guarana may not be listed as an ingredient. As a result, consumers may not know how much caffeine they are ingesting in products containing guarana.

As with caffeine from other sources, guarana may cause excessive nervousness and insomnia. It is contra-indicated during pregnancy and lactation and should be used cautiously, if at all, in people who are sensitive to the effects of caffeine or who have cardiovascular disease. Overall, the use of guarana as a central nervous system stimulant and weight-loss aid is not recommended and should be discouraged.

NCLEX Success

10. Which of the following groups are most commonly used for drug management of the hyperactive child?

   A. central nervous system (CNS) depressants
   B. CNS stimulants
   C. anticonvulsants
   D. major tranquilizers

11. Which of the following groups are most commonly used for drug management of the patient with narco-lepsy?

   A. central nervous system (CNS) depressants
   B. CNS stimulants
   C. anticonvulsants
   D. major tranquilizers

12. Which of the following statements indicate the patient is in need of further patient teaching regarding medi-cation for attention deficit hyperactivity disorder?

   A. I should not crush my tablets.
   B. I can skip doses when I am feeling good.
   C. I should not change my dosage without consulting my health care provider.
   D. I should consult with my health care provider before taking any new medications.

The Nursing Process

Assessment

- Assess use of stimulant and depressant drugs (prescribed, over-the-counter, or street drugs).
- Assess caffeine intake as a possible cause of anxiety, nervousness, insomnia, or tachycardia, alone or in combination with other CNS stimulants. Heavy users of caffeine may also be taking other psychoactive medications, especially CNS depressants such as antianx-iety and sedative–hypnotic drugs.

- Try to identify potentially significant sources of caffeine intake.
- Assess for conditions that are aggravated by CNS stimu-lants.
- For a child with possible ADHD, assess behavior as specifically and thoroughly as possible.
- For any patient receiving amphetamines or methyl-phenidate, assess behavior for signs of tolerance and abuse.

Nursing Diagnoses

- Sleep pattern disturbance related to hyperactivity, ner-vousness, and insomnia
- Risk for injury: adverse drug effects (excessive cardiac and CNS stimulation, drug dependence)
- Deficient knowledge: drug effects on children and adults
- Noncompliance: overuse of drug

Planning/Goals

The patient will

- Take CNS stimulants safely and accurately
- Improve attention span and task performance (children and adults with ADHD) and decrease hyperactivity (chil-dren with ADHD)
- Have fewer sleep episodes during normal waking hours (for patients with narcolepsy)

Nursing Interventions

The nurse will

- For a child receiving a CNS stimulant, assist parents in scheduling drug administration to increase beneficial effects and help prevent drug dependence and stunted growth. In addition, ask parents to control drug distribu-tion and monitor the number of pills or capsules avail-able and the number prescribed. The goals are to prevent overuse by the child for whom the drug is prescribed and to prevent the child from sharing his medication with other children who wish to take the drug for nonmedical purposes.
- Record weight at least weekly.
- Promote nutrition to avoid excessive weight loss.
- Provide information about the condition for which a stimulant drug is being given and the potential conse-quences of overusing the drug.

Evaluation

- Ask parents and teachers of children with ADHD to report on behavior and academic performance.
- For adolescents and adults with ADHD, ask the patient or family about the patient's ability to function in work, school, or social environments.
- Assess for decreased inappropriate sleep episodes in patients with narcolepsy.

NCLEX Success

13. An 8-year-old boy has been taking dexmethylphenidate 5 mg daily for 3 months. His mother is concerned that this dosage is not adequately treating his symptoms of attention deficit hyperactivity disorder. Which of the following behaviors would support the mother's concerns?

    A. increased concentration during school
    B. weight gain of 8 pounds over the past 3 months
    C. increased activity
    D. bradycardia

14. A mother calls the clinic to report that her son has recently started medication to treat attention deficit hyperactivity disorder (ADHD). The mother fears her son is experiencing side effects of the medication. Which of the following side effects are typically related to medications used for ADHD?

    A. poor appetite
    B. frequency of urination
    C. weight gain
    D. sedation

Key Concepts

- ADHD is characterized by hyperactivity, impulsivity, and a short attention span.
- ADHD usually starts in childhood and may persist through adulthood.
- CNS stimulants improve behavior and attention in patients with ADHD.
- Narcolepsy is characterized by daytime drowsiness and unpredictable "sleep attacks."
- Prescribed CNS stimulants are also abused and used for nonmedical purposes.
- All of the CNS stimulants, including caffeine, can cause life-threatening health problems with excessive intake.
- A **BLACK BOX WARNING** ◆ makes users aware of dextroamphetamine's high abuse potential; misuse may cause sudden death or serious cardiovascular events.
- A **BLACK BOX WARNING** ◆ states that there is a the risk of drug dependence with amphetamine-related drugs.
- A **BLACK BOX WARNING** ◆ advises that suicidal ideation may occur in children and adolescents who take atomoxetine.

Critical Thinking Questions

56-1. The health care provider has prescribed methylphenidate (Ritalin) for a 7-year-old boy diagnosed with attention deficit hyperactivity disorder (ADHD). The nurse is conducting some patient teaching with the child and his parents.

- What are the major adverse effects of central nervous system (CNS) stimulants, and how is it possible to minimize them?
- What information does the nurse provide about drug holidays? Are drug-free periods appropriate for all children taking CNS stimulants for ADHD?

References and Resources

Brams, M., Moon, E., Pucci, M., & Lopez, F. (2010). Duration of effect of long-acting stimulant medications for ADHD throughout the day. *Current Medical Research and Opinion*, 26(8), 1809–1825.

Burgess, C. R. & Scammell, T. E. (2012). Narcolepsy: neural mechanisms of sleepiness and cataplexy. *The Journal of Neuroscience: The Official Journal of the Society of Neuroscience*, 32(36), 12305–12311.

Epstein, J., Langberg, J., Lichtenstein, P., Kolb, R., & Stark, L. (2010). Sustained improvement in pediatricians' ADHD practice behaviors in the context of a community-based quality improvement initiative. *Children's Health Care*, 39, 296–311.

Faraone, S., & Giatt, S. (2010). A comparison of the efficacy of medications for adult attention-deficit/hyperactivity disorder using meta-analysis of effect sizes. *Journal of Clinical Psychiatry*, 71(6), 754–763.

Knutson, K., & O'Malley, M. (2010). Adult attention-deficit/hyperactivity disorder: A survey of diagnosis and treatment process. *Journal of the American Academy of Nurse Practitioners*, 22, 593–601.

List, B., & Barzman, D. (2011). Evidence-based recommendations for the treatment of aggression in pediatric patients with attention-deficit/hyperactivity disorder. *The Psychiatric Quarterly*, 82(1), 33–42.

May, D., & Kratochvil, C. (2010). Attention-deficit/hyperactivity disorder: Recent advances in paediatric pharmacotherapy. *Drugs*, 70(1), 15–40.

Mikami, A., Cox, D., Davis, M., Wilson, H., Merkel, R., & Burket R. (2009). Sex differences in effectiveness of extended-release stimulant medications among adolescents with attention-deficit/hyperactivity disorder. *The Cochrane Controlled Trials Register. In: The Cochrane Library*, Issue 1.

Poulton, A. (2009). Stimulant medications and growth. *Journal of the American Academy of Child and Adolescent Psychiatry, 48*(8), 574–576.

Roman, M. (2010). Newly approved once-daily formulations of medications for the treatment of attention-deficit(hyperactivity) disorder (ADHD) in children and adolescents. *Issues in Mental Health Nursing, 31,* 548–549.

Silva, R., Skimming, J., & Muniz, R. (2010). Cardiovascular safety of stimulant medications for pediatric attention-deficit hyperactivity disorder. *Clinical Pediatrics, 49*(9), 840–851.

Singh, I., Kendall, T., Taylor, C., Mears, A., Hollis, C., Batty, M., et al. (2010). Young people's experience of ADHD stimulant medication: A qualitative study for the NICE guidelines. *Child and Adolescent Mental Health, 14*(4), 186–192.

Swanson, J., & Volkow, N. (2009). Psychopharmacology: Concepts and opinions about the use of stimulant medication. *The Journal of Child Psychology and Psychiatry, 50*(1–2), 180–193.

Vaughan, B., Roberts, H., & Needelman, H. (2009). Current medications for the treatment of attention-deficit/hyperactivity disorder. *Psychology in the Schools, 46*(9), 846–856.

57 Drug Therapy for Substance Abuse Disorders

Clinical Application Case Study

Bryan Wilson is a 24-year-old man who regularly uses marijuana, alcohol, and tobacco. He was involved in a physical altercation at a local nightclub, and the owner called the police. The police brought Mr. Wilson to the emergency department, where he received a diagnosis of acute alcohol intoxication. He is admitted for treatment of alcohol withdrawal.

KEY TERMS

Intoxication: development of a reversible substance-specific syndrome caused by the recent ingestion of or exposure to a substance

Physical dependence: cluster of cognitive, behavioral, and physiological symptoms, indicating a person continues to use a substance of abuse despite significant substance-related problems

Psychological dependence: overwhelming desire to repeat the use of a particular drug to produce pleasure or avoid discomfort

Substance abuse: maladaptive pattern of substance use manifested by recurrent and significant adverse consequences related to repeated use of the substance

Tolerance: need for increasingly larger or more frequent doses of a substance to obtain the desired effects originally produced by a lower dose

Withdrawal: development of a substance-specific maladaptive behavioral change, with physiological and cognitive concomitants due to the cessation of or reduction in heavy and prolonged substance use

Introduction

This chapter introduces the pharmacological care of the patient who is experiencing substance abuse and substance dependence. It describes commonly abused substances, characteristics of substance-related disorders, and drugs used to treat substance-related disorders. **Substance abuse** is a maladaptive pattern of substance use, leading to clinically significant impairment or distress. This abuse involves self-administration of a drug for prolonged periods or in excessive amounts. It produces physical or psychological dependence, impairs functions of body organs, reduces the ability to function in usual activities of daily living, and decreases the ability and motivation to function as a productive member of society.

Substance abuse is a significant health, social, economic, and legal problem. It is often associated with substantial damage to the abuser and society (e.g., crime, child and spouse abuse, traumatic injury, chronic health problems, death).

Overview of Substance Abuse and Dependence

Most drugs of abuse are those that affect the central nervous system (CNS) and alter the state of consciousness. Commonly abused drugs include CNS depressants (e.g., alcohol, antianxiety and sedative–hypnotic agents, opioid analgesics), CNS stimulants (e.g., cocaine, methamphetamine, methylphenidate, nicotine), and other mind-altering drugs (e.g., marijuana, "ecstasy"). The overwhelming desire to repeat the use of a particular drug to produce pleasure or avoid discomfort is known as substance dependence. Many of these commonly abused drugs have clinical usefulness and are discussed elsewhere: anxiolytics and sedative–hypnotics (see Chap. 53), opioids (see Chap. 48), and CNS stimulants (see Chap. 56). Although they produce different effects, they are associated with feelings of pleasure, positive reinforcement, and compulsive self-administration.

Psychological dependence involves feelings of satisfaction and pleasure from taking a drug. These feelings, perceived as extremely desirable by the drug-dependent person, contribute to acute **intoxication** (symptoms caused by recent ingestion of a substance), development and maintenance of drug-abuse patterns, and return to drug-taking behavior after periods of abstinence.

Physical dependence involves physiologic adaptation to chronic use of a drug so that **withdrawal**, or unpleasant symptoms, occur when the drug is stopped, when its action is antagonized by another drug, or when its dosage is decreased. Withdrawal or abstinence produces specific manifestations according to the type of drug and does not occur as long as adequate dosage is maintained. Attempts to avoid withdrawal symptoms reinforce psychological dependence and promote continuing drug use.

Characteristics of drug dependence include craving a drug, often with unsuccessful attempts to decrease its use; compulsive drug-seeking behavior; physical dependence; and continuing to take a drug despite adverse consequences (e.g., drug-related illnesses, mental or legal problems, job loss or decreased ability to function in an occupation, impaired family relationships). Box 57.1 describes other characteristics of substance abuse.

Tolerance, which may be associated with many drugs if used repeatedly, is often an element of drug dependence. Increasing doses are required to obtain psychological effects or avoid physical withdrawal symptoms. The body "adjusts" to the drugs, and higher doses are needed to achieve feelings of

---

BOX 57.1   Characteristics of Substance Abuse and Dependence

■ Substance abuse involves all socioeconomic levels and affects all age groups. It is especially prevalent among adolescents and young adults. Patterns of abuse may vary by age group. For example, adolescents and young adults are more likely to use illicit drugs and older adults are more likely to abuse alcohol and prescription drugs. Health care professionals (e.g., physicians, pharmacists, nurses) are also considered at high risk for development of substance abuse disorders, at least partly because of easy access.

■ A person who abuses one drug is likely to abuse others.

■ Multiple drugs are often abused concurrently. Alcohol, for example, is often used with other drugs of abuse, probably because it is legal and readily available. In addition, alcohol, marijuana, opioids, and sedatives are often used to combat the anxiety and nervousness induced by cocaine, methamphetamine, and other CNS stimulants.

■ Abusers of alcohol and other drugs are not reliable sources of information about the types or amounts of drugs used. Most abusers understate the amount and frequency of substance use; heroin addicts may overstate the amount used in attempts to obtain higher doses of methadone. In addition, those who use illegal street drugs may not know what they have taken because of varying purity, potency, additives, contaminants, names, and substitutions of one drug for another.

■ Substance abusers rarely seek health care unless circumstances force the issue. Thus, most substance abuse comes to the attention of health care professionals when the abuser experiences a complication such as acute intoxication, withdrawal, or serious medical problems resulting from chronic drug overuse, misuse, or abuse.

■ Smoking or inhaling drug vapors is a preferred route of administration for cocaine, marijuana, and nicotine because the drugs are rapidly absorbed from the large surface area of the lungs. Then, they rapidly circulate to the heart and brain without dilution by the systemic circulation or metabolism by enzymes.

■ Substance abusers who inject drugs intravenously are prey to serious problems because they use impure drugs of unknown potency, contaminated needles, poor hygiene, and other dangerous practices. Specific problems include overdoses, death, and numerous infections (e.g., hepatitis, human immunodeficiency virus [HIV] infection, endocarditis, phlebitis, cellulitis at injection sites).

pleasure ("reward") or to stave off withdrawal symptoms ("punishment"). Both reward and punishment serve to reinforce continued substance abuse.

Etiology

Researchers have identified a number of factors in the predisposition to substance abuse and dependence. Biological factors include genetics. This is evident with many substances, especially with alcohol. Studies indicate that children of alcoholics are three times more likely than other children to become alcoholics themselves, even if reared away from the abusing parent. In addition, certain personality traits are thought to contribute to addictive behavior. Personality characteristics, such as low self-esteem, depression, and the inability to delay gratification, have been found in people with substance abuse and dependence.

Other factors important in developing drug dependence include the specific drug; the amount, frequency, and route of administration; and environmental or circumstantial characteristics. The environment in which a person uses a substance may contribute to the reinforcement. Moreover, the pleasurable effect of the substance itself may encourage the user to repeat it.

Cultural and ethnic influences may also play a role in substance abuse and dependence, related to patterns of consumption of substance and cultural acceptance of substance use. Lastly, peer pressure is often an important factor in initial and continuing drug ingestion. Although patterns of drug abuse vary in particular populations and in geographic areas, continuing trends seem to include increased use of methamphetamines, "club drugs," prescription drugs, and using multiple drugs at the same time. Internet web sites have become an important source of the drugs, and in some instances, instructions for manufacturing particular drugs are available.

Pathophysiology

Many drugs of abuse activate the pleasure or reward system in the brain by altering neurotransmission systems. Prolonged drug-abuse damages nerve cells in the brain and alters brain functions. The damage is long lasting.

Drug dependence is a complex phenomenon. Although the cause is unknown, one theory is that drugs stimulate or inhibit neurotransmitters in the brain to produce pleasure and euphoria or to decrease unpleasant feelings such as anxiety. For example, dopaminergic neurons in the limbic system are associated with the brain's reward system and are thought to be sites of action of alcohol, amphetamines, cocaine, nicotine, and opiates. These major drugs of abuse increase dopaminergic transmission and the availability of dopamine. These actions are believed to stimulate the brain's reward system and lead to compulsive drug administration and abuse.

The noradrenergic neurotransmission system, which uses norepinephrine as its neurotransmitter, is often involved as well as the dopaminergic system. Noradrenergic neurons innervate the limbic system and cerebral cortex and are important in setting mood and affect. Drugs that alter noradrenergic transmission have profound effects on mood and affect. Amphetamines and cocaine increase noradrenergic transmission, as with dopaminergic transmission, by promoting the release of norepinephrine and/or inhibiting its reuptake. Increased norepinephrine leads to mood elevation and euphoria, which promotes continued drug abuse. Increased norepinephrine also leads to major adverse effects of amphetamines and cocaine, including myocardial infarction, severe hypertension, and stroke, as well as profound mood swings from euphoria to depression.

Clinical Manifestations

Drug effects vary according to the type of substance being abused, the amount, route of administration, duration of use, and phase of substance abuse (e.g., acute intoxication, withdrawal syndromes, organ damage, medical illness). Thus, acute intoxication often produces profound behavioral changes, and chronic abuse often leads to serious organ damage and impaired ability to function in work, family, or social settings. Withdrawal symptoms are characteristic of particular types of drugs and are usually opposite to the effects originally produced. For example, withdrawal symptoms of alcohol and sedative-type drugs are mainly agitation, nervousness, and hyperactivity.

Therapy
General Approach

The major goals of treatment for substance abuse are detoxification, initiation of abstinence, and prevention of relapse. Patients who are likely to benefit from treatment are those who recognize that substance abuse is negatively influencing their problems and causing significant problems in their ability to function. Despite advances in treatment and the many adverse consequences of substance abuse, relapses to drug-taking behavior are common among people who have been detoxified or even abstinent for varying periods of time.

Treatments for substance abuse are limited but increasing, and more treatment facilities are needed. For most health professionals, contact with substance abusers is more likely to occur in acute situations, such as with intoxication or overdose, withdrawal syndromes, or various medical–surgical illnesses associated with the substance abuse. In general, treatment depends on the type, extent, and duration of drug-taking behavior and the particular situation for which treatment is needed.

Psychological rehabilitation efforts should be part of any treatment program for a drug-dependent person. Several approaches may be useful, including inpatient and outpatient psychotherapy, voluntary self-help groups (e.g., Alcoholics Anonymous, Narcotics Anonymous), and other types of emotional support and counseling. Box 57.2 gives sources of information about substance abuse.

Use of Drugs

Drug therapy for treatment of drug dependence is limited for several reasons. First, specific antidotes are available only for benzodiazepines (flumazenil) and opioid narcotics (naltrexone). Second, there is a high risk of substituting one abused drug for another. Third, there are significant drawbacks to giving CNS stimulants to reverse effects of CNS depressants and vice versa. Fourth, there is often inadequate information about the types and amounts of drug taken. Two of the more successful drug therapy regimens are methadone administration for heroin dependence and nicotine replacement (or other drugs [e.g., bupropion or varenicline]) for nicotine dependence. With

<table>
<tr><td colspan="2">

BOX 57.2 Sources of Information About Substance Abuse

</td></tr>
</table>

- The National Institute on Drug Abuse (NIDA) of the National Institutes of Health supports most of the world's research on the health aspects of drug abuse and addiction.
  6001 Executive Blvd.
  Bethesda, MD 20892-9561
  (301) 443-1124
  www.drugabuse.gov
  www.nida.nih.gov

- Substance Abuse and Mental Health Services Administration (SAMHSA)
  PO Box 2345
  Rockville, MD 20847-2345
  (877) 726-4727
  www.samhsa.org
  - SAMHSA's National Clearinghouse for Alcohol and Drug Information (NCADI): http://ncadi.samhsa.gov

- The National Institute on Alcohol Abuse and Alcoholism (NIAAA) conducts and supports research on the causes, consequences, prevention, and treatment of alcohol abuse and disseminates research findings to general, professional, and academic audiences. Publications and research information are available at www.niaaa.nih.gov.

both treatments, however, a combination of drug therapy and counseling is more effective than either method alone.

Treatment programs for substance abuse and dependence emphasize sobriety, which is complete abstinence from substance use. Combined with psychotherapy, there are pharmacological interventions that can assist the patient with sobriety. Table 57.1 lists the specific drugs that may be used treat substance-related disorders.

NCLEX Success

1. The nurse who is caring for a patient who has been abusing alcohol may expect to see what symptom as the patient enters withdrawal?

   A. sleep
   B. muscle relaxation
   C. euphoria
   D. agitation

2. The nurse is taking care of an adolescent male with a history of compulsive drug use. His parents have questioned him about the reasons behind such drug use. What factor is attributed to compulsive drug use?

   A. drug stimulation of the "reward" center in the brain
   B. a belief that the drugs are not harmful
   C. parental pressure to do well in school
   D. a permissive attitude toward taking drugs by parents and society

TABLE 57.1

Drugs Administered for the Treatment of Substance Abuse and Dependence

Drug Class	Prototype	Other Drugs in the Class
Antialcoholic drug; enzyme inhibitor	Disulfiram (Antabuse)	
Benzodiazepine	Chlordiazepoxide (Librium)	Lorazepam (Ativan)
Centrally acting alpha-agonist antihypertensive	Clonidine (Catapres)	
Benzodiazepine receptor antagonist	Flumazenil (Romazicon)	
Opioid antagonist	Naloxone (Narcan)	
Opioid antagonist	Naltrexone (ReVia, Vivitrol)	
Opioid agonist–antagonist analgesic	Buprenorphine (Buprenex, Subutex)	Naltrexone-buprenorphine (Suboxone)
Opioid agonist analgesic	Methadone (Methadone, Methadose)	
Antipsychotic; dopamine blocker	Haloperidol (Haldol)	
Nicotine receptor agonist	Varenicline (Chantix)	
Atypical antidepressant; smoking deterrent	Bupropion (Zyban)	
Smoking deterrent	Nicotine (Nicorette Gum, NicoDerm CQ, Nicotrol Inhaler)	

Central Nervous System Depressant Abuse and Dependence: Drug Therapy

CNS depressants are drugs that slow down or "depress" brain activity. These drugs are capable of inducing varying degrees of CNS depression ranging from tranquilizing relief of anxiety to anesthesia, coma, and even death. Effects produced by these substances depend on the size of dose and potency of the drug administered. They include alcohol, benzodiazepines (antianxiety drugs), and opioids. Box 57.3 summarizes information about these drugs.

BENZODIAZEPINES FOR TREATMENT OF ALCOHOL WITHDRAWAL

Benzodiazepines are the drugs of choice for treating withdrawal from alcohol and other CNS depressants. Ⓟ **Chlordiazepoxide** (Librium), the prototype benzodiazepine for treatment of such substance abuse, provides adequate sedation and has a significant anticonvulsant effect. The drug may also make it easier for the patient to participate in rehabilitation programs and allow for the gradual reduction and discontinuation of the abused substance.

BOX 57.3   Central Nervous System Depressants of Abuse

Alcohol (Ethanol)

Alcohol is commonly abused around the world. It is legal and readily available, and its use is accepted in most societies. Excessive amounts and long-term abuse damages essentially all organ systems of the body. Alcohol is thought to exert its effects on the central nervous system (CNS) mainly by enhancing the activity of gamma-aminobutyric acid, an inhibitory neurotransmitter, or by inhibiting the activity of glutamate, an excitatory neurotransmitter.

The clinical manifestations of acute alcohol intoxication include impaired thinking, judgment, and psychomotor coordination, which may lead to poor work performance and accidents. There is a loss of conscious control of behavior, and exhibitionism and aggressiveness often result. Chronic ingestion may cause severe organ damage and mental problems.

Psychological dependence, physical dependence, tolerance, and cross-tolerance with other CNS depressants may occur with chronic alcohol consumption. People who are alcohol dependent are unlikely to seek treatment for alcohol abuse unless an acute illness or other situation forces the issue. However, they are likely to seek treatment for other disorders, such as agitation and anxiety. Delirium tremens, the most serious form of alcohol withdrawal, is characterized by confusion, disorientation, delusions, visual hallucinations, and other signs of acute psychosis. Treatment with psychological counseling, referral to a self-help group such as Alcoholics Anonymous, and drug therapy with disulfiram or naltrexone may be useful.

Benzodiazepines

Benzodiazepines, commonly used for their anxiolytic and sedative-hypnotic effects (see Chap. 53), are also widely abused, mainly by people who also abuse alcohol and/or other drugs. Benzodiazepines rarely cause respiratory depression or death, even in overdose, unless taken with alcohol or other drugs. However, they may cause oversedation, memory impairment, poor motor coordination, and confusion. Withdrawal reactions can be extremely uncomfortable. Unfortunately, abusers often combine drugs in their quest for a greater "high" or to relieve the unpleasant effects of CNS stimulants and other street drugs.

With mild benzodiazepine overdose, the patient usually sleeps off the effects of the drug. More severe overdoses cause respiratory depression and coma.

Flumazenil (Romazicon) is a specific antidote that can reverse benzodiazepine-induced sedation, coma, and respiratory depression. The drug competes with benzodiazepines for benzodiazepine receptors. It has a short duration of action, and repeated intravenous injections are usually necessary. Close observation is required, because symptoms of overdose may recur when the effects of a dose of flumazenil subside and because the drug may precipitate acute withdrawal symptoms (e.g., agitation, confusion, seizures).

Opioids

Opioids are potent analgesics extensively used in pain management (see Chap. 48). They are also commonly abused. Legal opioid analgesics are increasingly being diverted from their appropriate use and bought and sold as street drugs. The focus here is on heroin, a common drug of abuse. A Schedule I drug in the United States, it is not used therapeutically. Heroin produces the same effects as naturally occurring endorphins and other opioid drugs. The drug rapidly enters the brain, where it is converted to morphine. Morphine stimulates opioid receptors in the reward system of the brain, which causes greater amounts of dopamine to be released.

Opioids produce tolerance and high degrees of psychological and physical dependence. Most other drugs that produce dependence do so with prolonged usage of large doses, but morphine-like drugs produce dependence with repeated administration of small doses. Medical usage of these drugs produces physical dependence and tolerance but rarely leads to use or abuse for mind-altering effects. Thus, "addiction" should not be an issue when the drugs are needed for pain management in patients with cancer or other severe illnesses.

Treatment may be needed for overdose or withdrawal syndromes. Overdose may produce severe respiratory depression and coma. Insertion of an endotracheal tube and mechanical ventilation may be necessary. Drug therapy consists of an opioid antagonist, such as naloxone, to reverse opioid effects. In addition to profound respiratory depression, pulmonary edema, hypoglycemia, pneumonia, cellulitis, and other infections often accompany opioid overdose and require specific treatment measures.

Pharmacokinetics

The oral form of chlordiazepoxide has a rapid onset of action, with a peak of 1 hour. The intramuscular (IM) form has an onset of action within 10 to 15 minutes and peaks within 15 to 30 minutes. The intravenous (IV) form has an immediate onset of action and peaks within 30 minutes. For all forms, the duration is 48 to 72 hours. Metabolism occurs in the liver, and excretion is in the urine.

Action

The exact mechanism of action of chlordiazepoxide is not understood; however, the drug acts mainly at the subcortical levels of the CNS. The main sites of action may be the limbic system and reticular formation.

Use

Prescribers may order chlordiazepoxide for acute alcohol withdrawal as well as for the management of anxiety disorders. The drug is useful in symptomatic relief of acute agitation, tremors, and delirium tremens. Treatment with chlordiazepoxide for alcohol withdrawal should begin as soon as the clinician identifies that the patient needs it. Table 57.2 gives route and dosage information for chlordiazepoxide and other drugs used to treat substance abuse.

Use in Patients With Renal or Hepatic Impairment

Chlordiazepoxide is excreted in the urine after being metabolized in the liver. Thus, caution is warranted in patients with renal or hepatic impairment.

	TABLE 57.2

DRUGS AT A GLANCE: Drugs Used to Treat Substance Abuse and Dependence

Drug	Pregnancy Category	Routes and Dosage Ranges	
		Adults	Children
Ⓟ **Chlordiazepoxide** (Librium)	D	Parenteral form may be used initially, or 50–100 mg PO followed by repeated doses up to 300 mg/d IM or IV, repeated every 2–4 h; up to 300 mg may be given in 6 h; subsequent doses are reduced to maintenance levels of 25 mg orally up to 3 times a day Older adults, 5 mg PO twice a day up to 4 times a day, or 25–50 mg IM or IV	Not recommended in children younger than 6 y Older than 6 y, 5 mg PO 2 to 4 times daily; may be increased to 10 mg PO 2 to 4 times daily
Ⓟ **Disulfiram** (Antabuse)	C	Initially, 500 mg/d PO (maximum) in a single dose for 1–2 wk Maintenance, 125–500 mg PO daily	Safety and efficacy in patients younger than 18 y not established
Buprenorphine (Buprenex, Subutex)	C	Subutex, 12–16 mg/d SL; use as induction with switch to Suboxone for maintenance (same dosage)	Ages 2–12 y, 2–6 mcg/kg of body weight IM or slow IV injection every 4–6 h
Bupropion (Zyban) Smoking cessation	C	150 mg PO once daily for 3 d, then increase to 150 mg twice daily, at least 8 h apart; maximum dose, 300 mg/d; treat for 7–12 wk	Safety and efficacy in patients younger than 18 y not established
Clonidine (Catapres)	C	Alcohol withdrawal: 0.3–0.6 mg PO every 6 h Opiate withdrawal: 2 mcg/kg PO 3 times daily for 7–10 d (up to 17 mcg/kg/d)	Safety and efficacy in patients younger than 18 y not established
Flumazenil (Romazicon)	C	0.2 mg IV over 30 s; repeat with 0.3 mg IV every 30 s to maximum dose of 3 mg	Safety and efficacy in patients younger than 18 y not established
Haloperidol (Haldol)	C	0.5–2 PO mg 2 to 3 times daily with moderate symptoms, 3–5 mg PO 2 to 3 times daily for more resistant patients; 2–5 mg IM daily every 60 min or 4–8 h as needed	Ages 3–12 y or 15–40 kg, 0.5 mg/d (25–50 mcg/kg/d) as initial dose; may increase in 0.5-mg increments
Lorazepam (Ativan)	D	Agitation: IM every 30 min to 6 h as needed Alcohol withdrawal hallucinations or seizures: 2 mg IM, repeat if necessary Benzodiazepine withdrawal: 2 mg PO every 6–8 h initially, then tapered over 1–2 wk	Should not be used in children young than 12 y

TABLE 57.2

DRUGS AT A GLANCE: Drugs Used to Treat Substance Abuse and Dependence (Continued)

Drug	Pregnancy Category	Routes and Dosage Ranges	
		Adults	Children
Methadone	C	Withdrawal: 20–30 mg daily initially PO or parenteral; increase dose to suppress withdrawal signs; 40 mg/d in single or divided doses is an adequate stabilizing dose; gradually reduce dosage every day after 2–3 d of stabilization dose Maintenance, 20–120 mg PO daily	Not recommended for pain relief in children due to insufficient documentation
Naloxone (Narcan)	C	Initial dose, 0.4–2 mg IV; additional doses may be repeated at 2–3-min intervals; if no response after 10 mg, question the diagnosis; IM or subcutaneous routes may be used if IV route is unavailable	Initial dose, 0.01 mg/kg IV; additional 0.1 mg/kg may be administered as needed; may be given IM or SC in divided doses
Naltrexone (ReVia, Vivitrol)	C	Alcoholism: 50 mg PO daily or 380 mg IM every 4 wk Opioid dependence: initial dose, 25 mg PO; observe for 1 h; if no signs or symptoms are seen, complete dose with 25 mg PO; usual maintenance dose is 50 mg/24 h; flexible dosing can include 100 mg PO every other day or 150 mg PO every 3 d	Safety and efficacy in patients younger than 18 y not established
Nicotine	D	Topical, apply system 5–21 mg, once every 24 h; dosage based on response and stage of withdrawal Nicotrol chewing gum, 1 piece every 1–2 h for wk 1–6; 1 piece every 2–4 h for wk 7–9; 1 piece every 4–8 h for wk 10–12 Nasal spray, 1 spray in each nostril, 1–2 doses each hour, up to 4 doses/h and 40 doses/d Nasal inhaler, 1 spray in each nostril, 1–2 doses each hour, up to 4 doses/h and 40 doses/d	Safety and efficacy in patients younger than 18 y who smoke not established
Varenicline (Chantix)	C	Patient should pick a date to stop smoking and begin drug therapy 1 wk before that date; d 1–3, 0.5 mg/d PO; d 4–7, 0.5 mg PO twice daily; d 8 until the end of treatment, 1 mg PO twice daily; treatment should last 12 wk	Not recommended for children younger than 18 y

Use in Patients With Critical Illness

Patients who abuse alcohol or other CNS depressants often have comorbid critical illnesses. Thus, chlordiazepoxide requires caution in patients with critical illness.

Use in Patients Receiving Home Care

Alcohol detoxification through pharmacological means generally takes place in a hospital setting but may occur in the home. The home care nurse shares the responsibility for teaching patients how to use chlordiazepoxide effectively and how to recognize medication responses that should be reported to the health care provider. The nurse instructs the patient and/or caregivers to recognize signs and symptoms of alcohol withdrawal and reviews the pharmacological treatment regimen

with them. Also, the nurse monitors the patient's response to the drug. If the patient is unable to take the medication for any reason or is not responding to current dosage, it is essential to notify the health care provider.

Adverse Effects

CNS adverse effects of chlordiazepoxide include sedation, depression, lethargy, disorientation, and delirium. Patients taking high dosages may experience paradoxical excitatory reactions during the first few weeks of treatment. Other adverse effects include alterations in pulse and blood pressure, urticaria, constipation, diarrhea, dry mouth, jaundice, changes in libido, and blood dyscrasias.

Contraindications

Contraindications to chlordiazepoxide include hypersensitivity to benzodiazepines, psychosis, acute narrow-angle glaucoma, shock, coma, acute alcoholic intoxication with depression of vital signs, pregnancy, labor and delivery, and lactation.

Nursing Implications

Preventing Interactions

Some medications and herbs interact with chlordiazepoxide, increasing its effects (Boxes 57.4 and 57.5).

Administering the Medication

Chlordiazepoxide is available in capsule form for oral use and powder form for parenteral use. For adults, the dosage is individualized, and it is necessary to increase it carefully to avoid adverse effects. The nurse gives IM injections slowly in the upper outer quadrant of the gluteus muscle. He or she should take the patient's vital signs regularly during this period, especially when giving the IV form of the drug, as well as observe and document subjective and objective reports by the patient. It is important to taper the drug gradually based on the patient's response to treatment.

Assessing for Therapeutic Effects

The nurse assesses the patient's vital signs; they should stabilize to within normal parameters. Also, the nurse observes for the presence of cognitive impairment and/or thought disturbances and assesses for signs and symptoms of agitation and/or restlessness. The patient should not appear restless or confused and should not complain of thought disturbances.

Assessing for Adverse Effects

The nurse assesses the patient for signs and symptoms of CNS depression. It is necessary to check the blood pressure

for fluctuations from hypertension to hypotension. The nurse assesses the skin for redness, itching, and signs of bruising as well as the skin and sclera for jaundice. It is also necessary to interview the patient regarding the following:

- Frequency and amount of bowel movements
- Desire for sexual intercourse

Patient Teaching

With chlordiazepoxide, it is necessary to instruct the patient and/or caregiver to

- Take the drug as prescribed and not to stop taking it without consulting the health care provider
- Understand what adverse effects are associated with use of the drug

In addition, it is important that females do not become pregnant while taking chlordiazepoxide.

ENZYME INHIBITORS FOR MAINTENANCE OF ALCOHOL SOBRIETY

Drug therapy for maintenance of sobriety is limited, mainly because of poor adherence. One of the drugs approved for this purpose is Ⓟ **disulfiram** (Antabuse).

Pharmacokinetics and Action

Disulfiram is quickly absorbed in the gastrointestinal tract. It has a slow onset of action, with a peak of up to 12 hours and a duration of 1 to 2 weeks. The medication is deposited in fat. It is metabolized slowly by the liver and excreted by the lungs and in the feces.

Disulfiram inhibits the enzyme aldehyde dehydrogenase to block the oxidation of alcohol. This allows acetaldehyde to accumulate in the blood to concentrations that are 5 to 10 times higher than normally achieved during alcohol metabolism. This accumulation of acetaldehyde produces an unpleasant reaction when disulfiram is consumed with alcohol.

Use

Prescribers order disulfiram for people with chronic alcoholism to maintain a state of sobriety. Table 57.2 gives route and dosage information for disulfiram and other drugs used to treat substance abuse.

Use in Patients With Hepatic Impairment

Hepatitis and hepatic failure may occur with disulfiram. This reaction may be severe, resulting in death in patients with hepatic impairment.

Adverse Effects

The combination of disulfiram with alcohol may result in headaches, confusion, seizures, chest pain, flushing, palpitations, hypotension, sweating, blurred vision, nausea, vomiting, and a garlic-like aftertaste. More severe effects (with alcohol) include dysrhythmias, cardiovascular collapse, heart failure, myocardial infarction, and death.

Contraindications

Contraindications to disulfiram include use with alcohol, metronidazole, or paraldehyde, as well as multiple drug dependence. A **BLACK BOX WARNING** ◆ states that the drug should not be given to a patient who has consumed alcohol in the past 12 hours. It is important that disulfiram never be administered to patients with myocardial disease, coronary occlusion, or psychosis. Also, patients who are known to be allergic to the drug should not take it.

Nursing Implications

Preventing Interactions

Nitroglycerin, paraldehyde, metronidazole, and cotrimoxazole produce a reaction similar to that of alcohol; the accumulation of acetaldehyde produces an unpleasant reaction accompanied by nausea and vomiting. Isoniazid and disulfiram produce neurologic effects such as changes in behavior and coordination. Warfarin, paraldehyde, and phenytoin combined with disulfiram result in increased serum blood levels of the drugs.

Administering the Drug

Administration of disulfiram at bedtime allows the patient to sleep, because the drug has a sedative effect.

Assessing Therapeutic and Adverse Effects

The nurse determines whether the patient has remained sober. In the event disulfiram is consumed with alcohol, the nurse assesses for cardiovascular effects. In a patient who presents with a severe reaction, it is essential to monitor for shock and hypokalemia.

Patient Teaching

With disulfiram, it is necessary to instruct the patient to

- Take the medication daily—at bedtime if dizziness and drowsiness occur
- Never consume alcohol in any form, including liniments, mouthwash, over-the-counter cough and cold aids, vinegars, sauces, and colognes
- Have periodic liver function tests
- Wear a medical alert bracelet

NCLEX Success

3. A patient is admitted to the chemical dependence unit. The nurse receives an order to administer flumazenil (Romazicon). Clinicians use flumazenil to treat overdoses with which of the following?

   A. alcohol
   B. benzodiazepines
   C. opioids
   D. amphetamines

4. A patient is admitted to the chemical dependence unit with chronic alcohol abuse. For which of the following symptoms does the nurse assess during alcohol withdrawal?

   A. euphoria, hyperactivity, and insomnia
   B. depression, suicidal ideation, and hypersomnia
   C. diaphoresis, nausea, vomiting, and tremors
   D. unsteady gait, nystagmus, and profound disorientation

5. Which of the following medications is the health care provider most likely to prescribe for a patient who is experiencing alcohol withdrawal?

   A. haloperidol (Haldol)
   B. chlordiazepoxide (Librium)
   C. propoxyphene (Darvon)
   D. phenytoin (Dilantin)

Clinical Application 57-2

Mr. Wilson is scheduled to be discharged after completing an alcohol withdrawal protocol for several days. After discharge, he is scheduled to attend outpatient chemical dependency treatment. His health care provider has prescribed disulfiram (Antabuse) for the patient to take on an outpatient basis.

- Is this an appropriate treatment choice for the patient?
- What symptoms will Mr. Wilson have if he drinks alcohol and takes disulfiram?
- What patient teaching should the nurse provide to Mr. Wilson regarding his treatment plan with disulfiram?

OPIOID AGONISTS AND ANTAGONISTS FOR TREATMENT OF OPIOID ABUSE

Ideally, the goal of treatment for opioid abuse is abstinence from further opioid use. However, because opioid users rarely meet this goal, long-term drug therapy may be used to treat heroin dependence.

The first option uses opioid substitutes to prevent withdrawal symptoms and improve a lifestyle that revolves around obtaining, using, and recovering from a drug. The substitute is methadone, an agonist at specific opioid receptors in the CNS. This drug has long been used as a detoxification and/or as maintenance therapy for opioid addiction, usually given in a single, daily oral dose at an outpatient methadone clinic. The FDA has issued a **BLACK BOX WARNING** ◆ concerning methadone stating that it should be part of an approved program for opioid addiction. Deaths have been reported during the initiation of treatment. It is essential that emergency services be on standby. Another **BLACK BOX WARNING** ◆ for methadone stipulates that monitoring for QT interval prolongation is necessary.

Proponents say that methadone blocks the euphoria produced by heroin, acts longer, and reduces preoccupation with drug use. This effect allows a more normal lifestyle for the patient and reduces morbidity and mortality associated with the use of illegal and injected drugs. Opponents say that methadone maintenance only substitutes one type of drug dependence for another. In addition, a substantial percentage of those people receiving methadone maintenance therapy abuse other drugs, including cocaine.

A second option uses naltrexone (ReVia), a pure opioid antagonist that blocks opioids from occupying receptor sites, thereby preventing their physiologic effects. (This drug is also used to combat alcohol abuse.) Used to maintain opioid-free states in the opioid addict, it is recommended for use in conjunction with psychological counseling to promote patient motivation and adherence. If the patient taking naltrexone has mild or moderate pain, he or she should receive a nonopioid analgesic (e.g., acetaminophen or a nonsteroidal anti-inflammatory drug). If the patient has severe pain and requires an opioid, administration of the naltrexone should occur in a setting staffed and equipped for cardiopulmonary resuscitation because respiratory depression may be deeper and more prolonged than usual. The FDA has issued a **BLACK BOX WARNING** ◆ about naltrexone and the risk of hepatocellular injury. It is necessary to obtain periodic liver function tests during therapy and discontinue the drug at signs of increasing hepatic impairment.

A third option is buprenorphine, an opioid agonist-antagonist analgesic that is occasionally injected therapeutically to relieve pain. The drug is given sublingually (Subutex) to treat opioid dependence. It is essential that the patient let the pill dissolve under the tongue and does not swallow the pill. Serious and potentially deadly adverse effects may occur if a patient combines this drug with other CNS depressant medications. Suboxone, a buprenorphine–naloxone

EVIDENCE-BASED PRACTICE

Opiate Antagonists for Alcohol Dependence
by ROSNER, S., HACKL-HERRWERTH, A., LEUCHT, S., VECCHI, S., SRISURAPANONT, M., & SOYKA, M.

Database of Systematic Reviews
2010, Issue 12.

The treatment of alcohol dependence is a complex therapeutic process, and research on its effectiveness meets with many challenges because of the high drop-out rates in clinical trials for treatment of this disease. The objective of this meta-analysis of 50 randomized controlled trials was to determine the effectiveness and tolerability of opioid antagonists in the treatment of alcohol dependence. A total of 7793 patients were included in the 50 studies that compared the effects of naltrexone (ReVia) or nalmefene (Revex) with placebo or active control on drinking-related outcomes. The data indicated that naltrexone appears to be an effective and safe strategy in alcoholism treatment; more patients who took this drug were able to reduce the amount and frequency of their drinking.

IMPLICATIONS FOR NURSING PRACTICE: Treatment of substance dependence should be comprehensive and include psychosocial strategies, both in individual and in group formats, as well as pharmacological interventions. The low levels of adherence to drug regimens and the high drop-out rates from programs for addiction treatment may hinder therapeutic effects.

combination, is used for maintenance therapy for opioid addiction. Physicians who prescribe the drug for outpatient use must meet several restrictions and are required to have 8 hours of special training.

Central Nervous System Stimulant Abuse and Dependence: Drug Therapy

CNS stimulants are identified by the behavioral stimulation and psychomotor agitation that they produce. The amount of CNS stimulation caused by a certain drug depends on both the area in the brain or spinal cord that is affected by the drug and the cellular mechanism fundamental to the increased excitability. CNS stimulants include amphetamines and related drugs, caffeine (discussed in Chap. 56), cocaine, and nicotine. Box 57.6 discusses these substances in more detail. For the most part, few proven pharmacological treatments are effective in the treatment of CNS stimulant abuse and dependence, because most of the cravings patients experience are psychological in nature.

NCLEX Success

6. A construction worker sees the company's occupational health nurse. He inquires about smoking-cessation medications. Which of the following drug products can be used to aid smoking cessation?

   A. naltrexone (ReVia)
   B. disulfiram (Antabuse)
   C. bupropion (Zyban)
   D. dronabinol (Marinol)

7. The nurse who is caring for a patient admitted with an acute overdose of cocaine. What physiologic response should the nurse expect?

   A. severe lung damage
   B. anaphylaxis
   C. myocardial infarction
   D. hypotension

8. A teenager is taking a central nervous system (CNS) stimulant. Which of the following is a common effect of CNS stimulant medications?

   A. Hypotension
   B. Anorexia
   C. Sedation
   D. Hypouricemia

9. What is the most common cause of death from opioids?

   A. hypertension
   B. central nervous system stimulation
   C. respiratory depression
   D. myocardial infarction

10. A nurse working in the emergency department is caring for a patient who has been brought in with suspected opioid overdose. What is the appropriate treatment to administer?

    A. disulfiram (Antabuse)
    B. naloxone (Narcan)
    C. amitriptyline (Elavil)
    D. chlordiazepoxide (Librium)

Psychoactive Substance Abuse and Dependence: Drug Therapy

Other psychoactive substances include marijuana, hallucinogens, "club" and "date-rape" drugs, and inhalants. Box 57.7 contains information about these substances. Few proven pharmacological treatments are effective in the treatment of psychoactive substance abuse and dependence.

BOX 57.6   Central Nervous System Stimulants of Abuse

Amphetamines

Amphetamines and related drugs (see Chap. 56) are used therapeutically for narcolepsy and attention deficit-hyperactivity disorder (ADHD). However, amphetamines are more important as drugs of abuse than therapeutic agents. These drugs may be part of a pattern of polydrug use in which central nervous system (CNS) depressants such as alcohol or sedative-type drugs ("downers") are alternated with CNS stimulants, such as amphetamines ("uppers").

Amphetamines and related drugs produce stimulation and euphoria. Small amounts produce mental alertness, wakefulness, and increased energy for a few hours. Tolerance develops rapidly. Methamphetamine is a commonly abused drug that is often manufactured in illegal "meth labs." Inhalation or intravenous injection produces a pleasurable sensation that lasts only a few minutes. Methylphenidate (Ritalin, others), a prescription drug used to treat ADHD, is increasingly being used for nonmedical purposes. The pattern of abuse is similar to that of other CNS stimulants, with episodes of binge use followed by severe depression and continued use despite serious adverse consequences.

Symptomatic treatment includes sedation, lowering of body temperature, and administration of an antipsychotic drug. Sedative-type drugs must be used with great caution, however, because depression and sleep usually follow amphetamine use, and these after-effects can be aggravated by sedative administration.

Cocaine

Cocaine is a popular drug of abuse. It produces strong CNS stimulation by preventing reuptake of catecholamine neurotransmitters (e.g., dopamine, norepinephrine), which increases and prolongs neurotransmitter effects. The two main drug forms are cocaine hydrochloride powder and "crack." In addition to intense euphoria, acute use of cocaine produces increased energy and alertness, sexual arousal, tachycardia, increased blood pressure, and restlessness. High doses can cause cardiac dysrhythmias, convulsions, myocardial infarction, respiratory failure, stroke, and death. Cocaine is not thought to produce physical dependence. However, it may lead to psychological dependence.

Drug therapy of cocaine dependence is largely symptomatic. Thus, agitation and hyperactivity may be treated with a benzodiazepine antianxiety agent, psychosis may be treated with haloperidol (Haldol) or another antipsychotic agent, cardiac dysrhythmias may be treated with usual antidysrhythmic drugs, myocardial infarction may be treated by standard methods, and so forth. Initial detoxification and long-term treatment are best accomplished in centers or units that specialize in substance-abuse disorders.

Nicotine

Nicotine, one of many active ingredients in tobacco products, is the ingredient that promotes compulsive use, abuse, and dependence. Inhaling smoke from a cigarette produces CNS stimulation in a few seconds. Nicotine produces its effects by increasing levels of dopamine and other substances in the brain.

Nicotine dependence is characterized by compulsive use and the development of tolerance and physical dependence, including mental depression. Cigarette smokers may smoke to obtain the perceived pleasure of nicotine's effects, avoid the discomfort of nicotine withdrawal, or both. Evidence indicates a compulsion to smoke when blood levels of nicotine become low. Abstinence from

(Continued on page 1066)

BOX 57.6	**Central Nervous System Stimulants of Abuse** (Continued)

smoking leads to signs and symptoms of withdrawal (e.g., anxiety, irritability, difficulty concentrating, restlessness, headache, increased appetite, weight gain, sleep disturbances).

Most tobacco users who quit do so on their own. For those who are strongly dependent and unable or unwilling to quit on their own, there are two main methods of treatment. One method is nicotine replacement therapy with drug formulations of nicotine. The other method involves smoking-cessation drugs for nicotine dependence.

Nicotine is available in a transdermal patch, chewing gum, an oral inhaler, and a nasal spray. Nicotine products are intended to be used for limited periods of 3 to 6 months, with tapering of dosage and discontinuation. They are effective in helping smokers achieve abstinence, but many users resume smoking.

Drugs include the antidepressant bupropion (see Chap. 54); the smoking-cessation formulation is Zyban, a sustained-release tablet. Varenicline (Chantix) blocks some nicotine receptors and thereby decreases the ability of nicotine to stimulate dopamine activity in the brain (the "reward" system). It also stimulates some other nicotine receptors and thereby decreases symptoms of nicotine withdrawal (the "punishment" system). Both medications are generally well tolerated. The most common adverse effects are insomnia with bupropion and nausea with varenicline. A **BLACK BOX WARNING** ◆ alerts practitioners about the risk of serious mental health events, including changes in behavior, depressed mood, hostility, and suicidal thoughts, with the administration of varenicline. It is necessary to monitor the patient accordingly.

BOX 57.7	**Other Psychoactive Medications of Abuse**

Marijuana

Marijuana and other cannabis preparations are obtained from *Cannabis sativa*, the hemp plant, which grows in most parts of the world, including the entire United States. Marijuana and hashish are the two cannabis preparations used in the United States. Delta-9-tetrahydrocannabinol (THC) is the main psychoactive ingredient.

Use of marijuana results in a dose-dependent impairment of memory, thought, concentration, time and depth perception, and coordinated movement. THC may cause serious cardiovascular (e.g., hypertension, bradycardia, vasoconstriction; hypotension may occur with high doses) as well as respiratory effects (e.g., chronic bronchitis with cough and wheezing, respiratory infections, possibly increased risk of lung cancer).

Most cannabis preparations are illegal and not used therapeutically in the United States as more effective legal treatments are available with less abuse potential. However, dronabinol (Marinol) is used to treat nausea and vomiting associated with anticancer drugs and to stimulate appetite in patients with acquired immunodeficiency syndrome (AIDS).

Hallucinogens

Hallucinogenic drugs include a variety of substances that cause mood changes, anxiety, distorted sensory perceptions, hallucinations, delusions, depersonalization, pupil dilation, elevated body temperature, and elevated blood pressure.

Dextromethorphan is a cough suppressant found in many over-the-counter multisymptom cold and cough remedies. It is a central nervous system (CNS) depressant but is usually classified as a hallucinogen because of dissociative effects similar to those of phencyclidine and ketamine (see below) when it is taken in the high doses characteristic of abuse. Adverse effects include blurred vision, brain damage, confusion, dizziness, drowsiness, excessive sweating, hallucinations, impaired breathing, impaired judgment and mental functioning, loss of consciousness, loss of physical coordination, muscle twitches, nausea and vomiting, paranoia, rapid and irregular heartbeat, seizures, slurred speech, and death.

Lysergic acid diethylamide, or LSD, is a synthetic, potent derivative of a naturally occurring compound. The exact mechanism of action is unknown, and effects cannot be predicted accurately. LSD alters sensory perceptions and thought processes; impairs most intellectual functions; distorts perception of time and space; and produces sympathomimetic reactions,

including increased blood pressure, heart rate, and body temperature, as well as pupil dilation. Adverse reactions include self-injury and possibly suicide, violent behavior, psychotic episodes, "flashbacks," and possible chromosomal damage.

Mescaline is an alkaloid of the peyote cactus. It is the least active of the commonly used psychotomimetic agents but produces effects similar to those of LSD.

Phencyclidine, or PCP, produces excitement, delirium, hallucinations, and other profound psychological and physiologic effects; altered sensory perceptions; impaired thought processes; impaired motor skills; psychotic reactions; sedation and analgesia; nystagmus and diplopia; and pressor effects that can cause hypertensive crisis, cerebral hemorrhage, convulsions, coma, and death. Tolerance develops, but there is no apparent physical dependence or abstinence syndrome. Psychological dependence probably occurs but is usually not intense.

"Club" and "Date-Rape" Drugs

"Ecstasy" (3,4 methylenedioxy-methamphetamine; MDMA) is an illegal, Schedule I derivative of amphetamine. Structurally similar to methamphetamine and mescaline, it produces stimulant and hallucinogenic effects. MDMA first became popular with adolescents and young adults at "raves," but its use has spread to a variety of settings and age groups. Users report increased energy and perception, euphoria, and feelings of closeness to others. MDMA is extremely dangerous, and usage is decreasing as users become more aware of serious adverse effects. Adverse effects include acute psychiatric symptoms (e.g., anxiety, panic, depression, paranoid thinking), cardiac dysrhythmias, coma, dehydration, delirium, hypertension, hyperthermia, hyponatremia, rhabdomyolysis, seizures, tachycardia, and death. These effects have occurred with a single use. MDMA is not thought to cause dependence or withdrawal syndromes.

Flunitrazepam (Rohypnol) is a benzodiazepine that is a Schedule I drug that produces dependence; the drug has never been approved for any therapeutic use. In addition to intentional use, it has reportedly been added to punch and other drinks at fraternity parties and other social events, leading to its designation as a "date-rape" drug. In relatively low doses, flunitrazepam can cause muscle relaxation, general sedative and hypnotic effects, and the appearance of intoxication. It also leads to confusion, dizziness, drowsiness, hypotension, memory impairment, and visual disturbances. Combining the drug with alcohol increases its adverse effects.

BOX 57.7 Other Psychoactive Medications of Abuse (Continued)

Gamma-hydroxybutyrate (GHB) is a Schedule I controlled drug only approved in the United States for research. A CNS depressant, this drug is structurally related to the inhibitory neurotransmitter gamma-aminobutyric acid. Usage of GHB has increased in recent years, mainly in the party or dance-club setting, and is increasingly involved in poisonings, overdoses, date rapes, visits to hospital emergency departments, and fatalities. GHB is also sometimes used by body builders for alleged anabolic effects. Effects of GHB include drowsiness, respiratory depression, seizures, unconsciousness, vomiting, hypoxia, and death. With chronic use, GHB reportedly induces tolerance and produces dependence.

Ketamine is an anesthetic that is chemically related to PCP and used mainly by veterinarians. The drug is a Schedule III controlled substance. It has become a "recreational" drug, with effects similar to those of PCP and LSD (e.g., distorted senses and perceptions, dissociative reactions). These effects produce a high risk of injuries.

Inhalants

These drugs include volatile solvents such as acetone, toluene, and gasoline, substances that produce chemical vapors that can be inhaled to induce mind-altering effects. These solvents may be constituents of some types of glues, plastic cements, aerosol sprays, butane lighters, spray paints, degreasers or cleaning fluids, paint thinners and removers, felt-tip marker fluids, and other products. Some general inhalation anesthetics, such as nitrous oxide, have also been abused to the point of dependence. Volatile solvents are most often abused by preadolescents and adolescents who squeeze glue into a plastic bag, for example, and sniff the fumes. Suffocation sometimes occurs when the sniffer loses consciousness while the bag covers the face.

Inhalants produce symptoms comparable with those of acute alcohol intoxication, including initial mild euphoria followed by ataxia, confusion, and disorientation. Some substances in gasoline and toluene also may produce symptoms similar to those produced by the hallucinogens, including euphoria, hallucinations, recklessness, and loss of self-control. These substances can harm the brain, liver, heart, kidneys, and lungs, and abuse of any drug during adolescence may interfere with brain development. Inhalants can also produce psychological dependence, and some produce tolerance. There is some question about whether physical dependence occurs.

The Nursing Process

Assessment

- Interview the patient regarding alcohol and other drug use to help determine immediate and long-term nursing care needs.
- Assess behavior that may indicate drug abuse, such as alcohol on the breath, altered speech patterns, staggering gait, and other signs of excessive CNS depression or stimulation.
- Assess for disorders that may be caused by substance abuse. These disorders may include infections, liver disease, accidental injuries, and psychiatric problems of anxiety or depression.
- Assess liver function, complete blood count (hypocalcemia, hypomagnesemia, and acidosis are common in alcoholics), and alcohol and drug levels in the blood.

Nursing Diagnoses

- Ineffective coping related to reliance on alcohol or other drugs
- Risk for injury: adverse effects of abused drug(s)
- Disturbed thought processes related to use of psychoactive drugs
- Risk for other- or self-directed violence related to disturbed thought processes, impaired judgment, and impulsive behavior
- Imbalanced nutrition: less than body requirements related to drug effects and drug-seeking behavior
- Dysfunctional family processes: alcoholism
- Risk for injury: infection, hepatitis, or acquire immunodeficiency syndrome (AIDS) related to use of contaminated needles and syringes for IV drugs

Planning/Goals

The patient will

- Maintain safety if impaired by alcohol and drug abuse
- Remain current on information regarding drug effects and treatment resources
- Maintain efforts toward stopping drug usage be recognized and reinforced

Nursing Interventions

The nurse will

- Decrease environmental stimuli for the person undergoing drug withdrawal
- Record vital signs; cardiovascular, respiratory, and neurologic functions; mental status; and behavior at regular intervals
- Support use of resources for stopping drug abuse (psychotherapy, treatment programs)
- Request patient referrals to psychiatric/mental health physicians, nurse clinical specialists, or self-help programs when indicated
- Use therapeutic communication skills to discuss alcohol or other drug-related health problems, health-related benefits of stopping substance use or abuse, and available services or treatment options
- Teach nondrug techniques for coping with stress and anxiety
- Provide positive reinforcement for efforts toward quitting substance abuse
- Inform smokers with young children in the home that cigarette smoke can precipitate or aggravate asthma and upper respiratory disorders in children
- Inform smokers with nonsmoking spouses or other members of the household that secondhand smoke can increase the risks of cancer and lung disease in the nonsmokers as well as in the smoker

- For smokers who are concerned about weight gain if they quit smoking, emphasize that the health benefits of quitting far outweigh the disadvantages of gaining a few pounds and discuss ways to control weight without smoking

Evaluation

- Observe for improved behavior (e.g., less impulsiveness, improved judgment and thought processes, commits no injury to self or others).

- Observe for use or avoidance of nonprescribed drugs while hospitalized.
- Interview to determine the patient's insight into personal problems stemming from drug abuse.
- Verify enrollment in a treatment program.
- Observe for appropriate use of drugs to decrease abuse of other drugs.

Key Concepts

- Substance abuse is a maladaptive pattern of substance use, leading to clinically significant impairment or distress.
- Commonly abused drugs include CNS depressants (e.g., alcohol, antianxiety and sedative-hypnotic agents, opioid analgesics), CNS stimulants (e.g., cocaine, methamphetamine, methylphenidate, nicotine), and other mind-altering drugs (e.g., marijuana, "ecstasy").
- CNS depressants are drugs that slow down or "depress" brain activity. These types of drugs are capable of inducing varying degrees of CNS depression, ranging from tranquilizing relief of anxiety to anesthesia, coma, and even death. They include alcohol, antianxiety and sedative-hypnotic agents, and opiates.
- Benzodiazepines are the drugs of choice for treating alcohol withdrawal and withdrawal from other CNS depressant drugs. Chlordiazepoxide is the prototype.
- Methadone acts as an agonist at specific opioid receptors in the CNS to produce analgesia, euphoria, and sedation. This drug has long been used as a detoxification and/or as maintenance therapy for opioid addiction, usually given in a single, daily oral dose at an outpatient methadone clinic.
- A **BLACK BOX WARNING** ◆ states that methadone used for treatment of opioid addiction should be part of an approved program. Deaths have been reported during the initiation of treatment. The nurse ensures that emergency services are on standby. Another **BLACK BOX WARNING** ◆ states that it is necessary to monitor the patient taking methadone for QT interval prolongation, especially with higher doses.
- A **BLACK BOX WARNING** ◆ states that it is necessary to obtain periodic liver function tests during naltrexone therapy and discontinue therapy at signs of increasing hepatic impairment.
- Drug therapy for maintenance of sobriety is limited, mainly because of poor adherence. The drugs approved for this purpose include disulfiram (Antabuse) and naltrexone (ReVia, Vivitrol).
- A **BLACK BOX WARNING** ◆ states that it is essential never to administer the disulfiram to a patient who has consumed alcohol in the past 12 hours.
- Treatment for nicotine dependence involves nicotine products and certain drugs.

Critical Thinking Questions

57-1. A 32-year-old woman was found unresponsive by paramedics in an alley. Her friends reported that she had been drinking vodka and taking pills all night long. The paramedics found an empty bottle of oxycodone hydrochloride in her purse. Based on the date on the prescription bottle, they estimated that she has ingested 25 20-mg capsules. The patient is transported to the local emergency department with a diagnosis of opioid and alcohol overdose.

- What is the treatment protocol for opioid overdose?
- What other nursing interactions should the nurse perform?

57-2. A 66-year-old man has recently undergone a quadruple coronary artery bypass graft; he suffers from cardiovascular disease. Part of his cardiac rehabilitation program includes exercise training, nutrition counseling, and smoking cessation. He has smoked for 30 years—two packs a day. He is motivated to try to stop smoking, but he has failed every time he has tried to quit using tobacco.

- What are some possible treatment options to help the patient with smoking cessation?

References and Resources

Deitz, D., Cook, R., & Hendrickson, A. (2011). Preventing prescription drug misuse: Field test of the SmartRxWeb program. *Substance Use and Misuse, 45*(5), 678–686.

Ferri, M., Davoli, M., & Perucci, C. (2011). *Cochrane Database of Systematic Reviews,* Issue 12.

Friedmann, P., Jiang, L., & Alexander, J. (2010). Top manager effects on buprenorphine adoption in outpatient substance abuse treatment programs. *Journal of Behavioral Health Sciences and Research, 37*(3), 322–335.

Hays, J., & Ebbert, J. (2010). Adverse effects and tolerability of medications for the treatment of tobacco use and dependence. *Drugs, 70*(18), 2357–2372.

Herrin, D., Rush, C., & Grabowski, J. (2010). Agonist-like pharmacotherapy for stimulant dependence: Preclinical, human laboratory, and clinical studies. *Annals of New York Academy of Sciences, 1187,* 76–100.

Hollands, G., McDermontt, M., Parsons, A., & Aveyard, P. (2011) Interventions to increase adherence to medications for tobacco dependence. *The Cochrane Database of Systematic Reviews,* Issue 6.

Karch, A. (2011). *2011 Lippincott's nursing drug guide.* Philadelphia, PA: Lippincott Williams & Wilkins.

Merlo, L., Arana, J., & Stone, A. (2010). Pharmacological trials for the treatment of substance use disorders. In: M. Hertzman & L. Adler (Eds.). *Clinical trials in pharmacology: A better brain* (2nd ed.). New Jersey: Wiley-Blackwell.

Pani, P., Trogu, E., Vecchi, S., & Amato, L. (2011). Antidepressants for cocaine dependence and problematic cocaine use. *The Cochrane Database of Systematic Reviews,* Issue 12.

Saber-Tehrani, A., Bruce, R., & Altice, F. (2011). Pharmacokinetic drug interactions and adverse consequences between psychotropic medications and pharmacotherapy for the treatment of opioid dependence. *The American Journal of Drug and Alcohol Abuse, 37,* 1–11.

Up-To-Date. (2012) *Disulfiram: Drug information.* Lexi-Comp, Inc.

Vandrey, R., & Haney, M. (2009). Pharmacotherapy for cannabis dependence. *CNS Drugs, 23*(7), 543–553.

Weinstein, A., & Gorelick, D. (2011). Pharmacological treatment of cannabis dependence. *Current Pharmaceutical Design, 17*(14), 1351–1358.

SECTION **11**

Drugs Affecting the Eye, Ear, and Skin

Drugs Affecting the Eye, Ear, and Skin

CHAPTER OUTLINE

58 Drug Therapy for Disorders of the Eye

LEARNING OBJECTIVES

After studying this chapter, you should be able to:

1 Describe the basic structures and functions of the eye.

2 Understand the pathophysiology of glaucoma as well as ocular infections and inflammation.

3 Identify the prototypes and describe the action, use, adverse effects, contraindications, and nursing implications for medications administered for diagnosis and treatment of ocular disorders.

4 Identify the prototypes and describe the action, use, adverse effects, contraindications, and nursing implications for medications administered for glaucoma.

5 Identify the prototypes and describe the action, use, adverse effects, contraindications, and nursing implications for medications administered for ocular infections and inflammation.

6 Understand how to implement the nursing process in the care of the patient with an ocular disorder.

Clinical Application Case Study

Irene Molnar is a 75-year-old woman who has open-angle glaucoma. Her physician has prescribed the following: acetazolamide (Diamox), 250 mg orally, every 6 hours; timolol (Timoptic), one drop in each eye, twice daily; and pilocarpine (Isopto-Carpine), one drop of 2% solution in each eye, three times daily. You are a home care nurse visiting Mrs. Molnar.

KEY TERMS

Conjunctiva: mucous membrane lining the eyelids

Glaucoma: group of diseases characterized by optic nerve damage and changes in visual fields, which is characterized by increased intraocular pressure (IOP) (greater than 22 mm Hg), although it may also occur with normal IOP (less than 21 mm Hg); one of the leading causes of blindness in the United States

Intraocular pressure (IOP): pressure inside the eye; normally less than 21 mm Hg (average 15–16 mm Hg)

Keratitis: inflammation of the cornea

Lacrimation: production of tears

Miosis: pupil constriction

Mydriasis: pupil dilation

Nasolacrimal occlusion: application of pressure to the tear duct

Refraction: deflection of light rays in various directions according to the density of the ocular structures through which they pass

Tonometry: diagnostic test to measure the pressure inside the eye to determine if glaucoma is present

Introduction

This chapter introduces the eye and its disorders. It addresses the drug therapy implemented to enhance visualization of the eye for eye examination and the drug therapy for ocular disorders, including glaucoma, ocular infection, and ocular inflammation.

Basic Structure and Function of the Eye

The eye is the major sensory organ through which a person receives information about the external environment. Extensive discussion of vision and ocular anatomy is beyond the scope of this chapter, but some characteristics and functions are described to facilitate understanding of ocular drug therapy.

The eyelids and lacrimal system function to protect the eye. The eyelid is a barrier to the entry of foreign bodies, strong light, dust, and other potential irritants. The **conjunctiva** is the mucous membrane lining the eyelids. The canthi (singular, canthus) are the angles where the upper and lower eyelids meet. The lacrimal system produces a fluid that constantly moistens and cleanses the anterior surface of the eyeball. The fluid drains through two small openings in the inner canthus and flows through the nasolacrimal duct into the nasal cavity. When the conjunctiva is irritated or certain emotions are experienced (e.g., sadness), the lacrimal gland produces more fluid than the drainage system can accommodate. The excess fluid overflows the eyelids and becomes tears. Production of tears is known as **lacrimation**.

The eyeball is a spherical structure composed of the sclera, cornea, choroid, and retina, plus special refractive tissues. The sclera is a white, opaque, fibrous tissue that covers the posterior five sixths of the eyeball. The cornea is a transparent, special connective tissue that covers the anterior sixth of the eyeball. It contains no blood vessels. The choroid, composed of blood vessels and connective tissue, continues forward to form the iris. The iris is composed of pigmented cells, the opening called the pupil, and muscles that control the size of the pupil by contracting or dilating in response to stimuli. Pupil constriction is called **miosis**, and pupil dilation is called **mydriasis**. The retina is the innermost layer of the eyeball.

For vision to occur, light rays must enter the eye through the cornea; travel through the pupil, lens, and vitreous body (discussed below); and be focused on the retina. Light rays do not travel directly to the retina. Instead, they are deflected in various directions according to the density of the ocular structures through which they pass. This process, called **refraction**, is controlled by the aqueous humor, lens, and vitreous body.

The optic disk is the area of the retina where ophthalmic blood vessels and the optic nerve enter the eyeball.

The structure and function of the eyeball are further influenced by the lens, aqueous humor, and vitreous body. The lens is an elastic, transparent structure; its function is to focus light rays to form images on the retina. It is located behind the iris and is held in place by ligaments attached to the ciliary body. The aqueous humor is a clear fluid produced by capillaries in the ciliary body. Most of the fluid flows through the pupil into the anterior chamber (between the cornea and the lens and anterior to the iris). A small amount flows into a passage called Schlemm's canal, from which it enters the venous circulation. Normally, production and drainage of aqueous humor are approximately equal, and the **intraocular pressure (IOP)** is normal. Impaired drainage of aqueous humor causes increased IOP. The vitreous body is a transparent, jelly-like mass located in the posterior portion of the eyeball. It functions to refract light rays and maintain the normal shape of the eyeball.

Overview of Disorders of the Eye

The eye is subject to many disorders that threaten its structure, function, or both. Some disorders in which ophthalmic drugs play a prominent role are discussed in this section.

Specific Disorders of the Eye

Refractive Errors

Refractive errors include myopia (nearsightedness), hyperopia (farsightedness), presbyopia, and astigmatism. These conditions impair vision by interfering with the eye's ability to focus light rays on the retina. Ophthalmic drugs are used only in the diagnosis of the conditions; treatment involves prescription of eyeglasses or contact lenses.

Glaucoma

Glaucoma is one of the leading causes of blindness in the United States and the most common cause of blindness in African Americans. It is a group of diseases characterized by optic nerve damage and changes in visual fields. It is often characterized by increased IOP (above 22 mm Hg) but may also occur with normal IOP (below 21 mm Hg; average 15–16 mm Hg). Diagnostic tests for glaucoma include ophthalmoscopic examination of the optic disk; measurement of IOP, or **tonometry**; and testing of visual fields.

Ocular Infections and Inflammation

Ocular infections may result from foreign bodies, contaminated hands, contaminated eye medications, or infections in contiguous structures (e.g., nose, face, sinuses). Ocular inflammation may be caused by bacteria, viruses, allergic reactions, or irritating chemicals. These conditions include the following:

- Conjunctivitis, which is inflammation of the conjunctiva
- Blepharitis, which is a chronic infection of glands and lash follicles on the margins of the eyelids
- **Keratitis**, which is inflammation of the cornea
- Corneal ulcers
- Fungal infections

Etiology

Refractive errors of the eye result in impaired vision. Light rays cannot focus sharply on the retina if the eyeball is lengthened or shortened. When the distance to the eyeball is shortened, the visual image is focused at the front of the retina, resulting in myopia. If the focus is beyond the retina, the result is hyperopia. The most common cause of refractive errors is astigmatism or an irregular curve of the cornea.

The cause of open-angle glaucoma is unknown, but contributing factors include advanced age; family history of glaucoma and elevated IOP; diabetes mellitus; hypertension; myopia; long-term use of corticosteroid drugs; and previous eye injury, inflammation, or infection. The incidence of glaucoma in African Americans is about three times higher than in non–African Americans. Closed-angle glaucoma may occur when pupils are dilated and the outflow of aqueous humor is blocked. Inflammatory or infectious conditions may be caused by several factors.

Conjunctivitis, a common eye disorder, may be caused by allergens (e.g., airborne pollens), bacterial or viral infections, or physical or chemical irritants. Bacterial conjunctivitis is often caused by *Staphylococcus aureus*, *Streptococcus pneumoniae*, or *Haemophilus influenzae*. Conjunctivitis with a purulent discharge is caused by *Neisseria gonorrhoeae* infection. Neonates are infected as they pass through the birth canal of infected mothers. Neonates can also develop keratoconjunctivitis if mothers are infected with *Chlamydia trachomatis*. Blepharitis, a chronic ocular condition, refers to a family of inflammatory disease processes of the eyelid(s). The condition usually results from seborrhea and staphylococcal infections. Keratitis results from infection with microorganisms, trauma, allergy, ischemia, and drying of the cornea (e.g., from inadequate lacrimation).

Corneal ulcers may be bacterial, fungal, or viral. Bacterial ulcers most often occur because of infections with pneumococci and staphylococci. Pseudomonal ulcers are less common. Fungal ulcers may follow topical corticosteroid therapy or injury with plant matter, such as a tree branch. Viral ulcers are usually caused by the herpesvirus. Other fungal infections may often be attributed to frequent use of ophthalmic antibiotics and corticosteroids.

Pathophysiology

As previously stated, refractive errors impair vision by interfering with the eye's ability to focus light rays on the retina. When the dimension of the eyeball is too short, near images are blurred. Conversely, if the eyeball dimension is too long, distant objects will be blurred.

Glaucoma is characterized by increased IOP, possibly damaging the optic nerve, which transmits images to the brain. If damage to the optic nerve from high IOP continues, glaucoma leads to loss of vision. The most common type of glaucoma is open-angle glaucoma, which is characterized by IOP. In this type of glaucoma, there is no obstruction at the iridocorneal angle. This form of open-angle glaucoma most commonly occurs due to an abnormality of the trabecular meshwork that controls the flow of aqueous humor into the canal of Schlemm. A secondary form of open-angle glaucoma occurs with the formation of red cell fragments after trauma or iris pigment epithelial granules clogging the trabecular mesh. Closed-angle glaucoma is usually an acute situation requiring emergency surgery. It may occur when pupils are dilated and the outflow of aqueous humor is blocked.

Inflammatory or infectious conditions may lead to conjunctivitis, blepharitis, keratitis, bacterial corneal ulcers, or fungal infections of the eye. Conjunctivitis typically is a self-limited process. However, depending on the immune status of the patient and the etiology, conjunctivitis can progress to more severe and sight-threatening infections. Blepharitis involves bacterial colonization of the eyelids, which results in direct microbial invasion of tissues, immune system–mediated damage, or damage caused by the production of bacterial toxins, waste products, and enzymes. Keratitis may not initially affect vision. However, if the condition is not treated effectively, corneal ulceration, scarring, and impaired vision may result. In nonulcerative keratitis, the layers of the epithelium are affected but remain intact. Ulcerative keratitis affects the epithelium, stroma, or both. Chronic ulcerative keratitis will result in deformities of the eyelid, paralysis of the lid muscles, or severe exophthalmos.

Clinical Manifestations

Refractive errors are manifested by loss of near or far vision. Glaucoma is characterized by blurred vision, halos around lights, difficulty focusing, difficulty adjusting to low lighting, loss of peripheral vision, headache, and aching around the eye. Conjunctivitis involves redness, tearing, itching, edema, and burning or gritty sensations. Blepharitis is an inflammation of the anterior or posterior structures of the eyelids. Anterior blepharitis presents with burning, redness, and itching of the anterior eyelids. Posterior blepharitis is eyelid inflammation with inflammation of the meibomian glands. An infected sebaceous gland is noted as a hordeolum or stye-producing pain, redness, and swelling of the site. Keratitis is characterized by irritation, increased tear production, and photophobia. Corneal ulcers and fungal infections also produce eye pain, discharge, changes in vision, swelling, and redness.

Clinical Application 58-1

- Mrs. Molnar has been diagnosed with open-angle glaucoma. What is the pathophysiology of this disease?
- If untreated, what is the outcome of this disease?

Drug Therapy

Drug therapy of ophthalmic conditions is unique because of the location, structure, and function of the eye. Many systemic drugs are unable to cross the blood–eye barrier and achieve therapeutic concentrations in ocular structures. In general, penetration is greater if the drug achieves a high concentration in the blood, is fat soluble, is poorly bound to serum proteins, and if inflammation is present.

Because of the difficulties associated with systemic therapy, various methods of administering drugs locally have been developed. The most common and preferred method is topical application of ophthalmic solutions or suspensions (eye drops) to the conjunctiva. Drugs are distributed through the tear film covering the eye and may be used for superficial disorders (e.g., conjunctivitis) or for relatively deep ocular disorders (e.g., glaucoma). Topical ophthalmic ointments may also be used. In addition, ophthalmologists may inject medications (e.g., antibiotics, corticosteroids, local anesthetics) into or around various eye structures. A major use of topical ophthalmic drugs in children is to dilate the pupil and paralyze accommodation for ophthalmoscopic examination. As a general rule, practitioners prefer the short-acting mydriatics and cycloplegics (e.g., cyclopentolate, tropicamide) because they cause fewer systemic adverse effects than atropine and scopolamine. In addition, children usually receive lower drug concentrations (given empirically) because of their smaller size and the potential risk of systemic adverse effects.

Drug Therapy for the Diagnosis and Treatment of Ocular Disorders

Drugs used to diagnose or treat ophthalmic disorders represent numerous therapeutic classifications, most of which are discussed in other chapters. This chapter describes the major classes of drugs used in ophthalmology. Later, the chapter discusses drugs used in the treatment of glaucoma. Table 58.1 summarizes the medications used to diagnose and treat some ocular disorders. Ocular medications are administered topically with limited systemic effects.

ANTICHOLINERGIC DRUGS

Anticholinergic drugs dilate the pupil to provide greater observation of the inner aspect of the eye. The prototype of this class is Ⓟ **atropine sulfate** (ophthalmic).

Pharmacokinetics and Action

The onset of action of atropine (ophthalmic) is 5 to 10 minutes, with a peak of action in 30 to 40 minutes and a duration of action of 7 to 14 days. Metabolism occurs in the liver, and excretion takes place in the urine.

Atropine (ophthalmic) blocks the effects of acetylcholine in the central nervous system (CNS). It produces mydriatic effects by relaxing the pupil of the eye and prevents accommodation of near vision.

TABLE 58.1

Drugs Administered for Diagnosis and Treatment of Ocular Disorders

Drug Class	Prototype	Other Drugs in the Class
Anticholinergic drugs	Atropine sulfate (ophthalmic)	Cyclopentolate (AK-Pentolate, Cyclogyl) Homatropine (Isopto Homatropine) Scopolamine (Isopto-Hyoscine) Tropicamide (Mydriacyl, Opticyl, Tropicacyl)
Adrenergic agonists	Phenylephrine hydrochloride (AK-Dilate, Altafrin, Mydfrin, Neofrin)	
Local anesthetic drugs	Lidocaine (Akten)	Proparacaine (Alcaine) Tetracaine (Altacaine, Tetcaine)

Use

Diagnostic use of atropine (ophthalmic) involves production of mydriasis and cycloplegia-pupillary dilation in acute and inflammatory conditions of the iris and uveal tract. Other uses include measurement of refractive errors and treatment of uveitis. Table 58.2 presents route and dosage information for atropine and related drugs in adults and children.

Adverse Effects and Contraindications

Atropine (ophthalmic) may cause local transient stinging. The systemic effects of this medication depend on the amount of medication absorbed and rarely lead to an inhibition of vagal stimulation affecting the heart or diminished bronchial or gastric secretions.

Contraindications to atropine (ophthalmic) include the presence of glaucoma or the tendency to this condition.

TABLE 58.2

DRUGS AT A GLANCE: Drugs for the Diagnosis and Treatment of Ocular Disorders

Drug	Pregnancy Category	Routes and Dosage Ranges	
		Adults	Children
Anticholinergic Drugs			
Ⓟ **Atropine sulfate** (ophthalmic)	C	Prior to evaluation: 1–2 drops During minor surgical procedures: repeat dose every 5–10 min for 3 doses During major surgical procedures: repeat dose every 5–10 min for 5 doses	<1 y, 1 drop of 0.25% solution 3 times per day for 3 d before procedure 1–5 y, 1 drop of 0.5% solution 3 times per day for 3 d before procedure >5 y, 1 drop of 1% solution three times per day for 3 d before procedure
Cyclopentolate (AK-Pentolate, Cyclogyl)	C	1 drop of 1% followed by another drop in 5 min; instill 2% in heavily pigmented iris	1 drop of 0.5%, 1%, or 2% followed by 1 drop of 0.5 or 1% in 5 min
Homatropine (Isopto Homatropine)	C	1–2 drops in 1 h before refraction Uveitis: 1–2 drops up to 4 times per day	Procedure: 1 drop of 2% solution immediately before Uveitis: 1–2 drops 2% solution 2–3 times per day
Scopolamine (Isopto-Hyoscine)	C	Procedure: 1–2 drops of 0.25% 1 h before	Procedure: 1 drop of 0.25% to eye twice daily for 2 d before
Tropicamide (Mydriacyl, Opticyl, Tropicacyl)	C	Examination: 1–2 drops 15–20 min before; may repeat every 30 min as needed	Examination: 1–2 drops 15–20 min before; may repeat every 30 min as needed
Adrenergic Agonists			
Ⓟ **Phenylephrine** (AK-Dilate, Altafrin, Mydfrin, Neofrin)	C	Before ophthalmoscopy or refraction: 1 drop of 2.5% or 10% solution Before surgery: 1 drop of 2.5% or 10% solution 30–60 min After surgery: 1 drop of 10% solution once or twice daily	Refraction: 1 drop of 2.5% solution
Local Anesthetic Drugs			
Ⓟ **Lidocaine**	B	2 drops to ocular surface in the area of procedure	Refer to drug insert for pediatric specifications of dosage
Proparacaine	C	Ophthalmic surgery: 1 drop of 0.5% solution in the eye every 5–10 min for 5–7 doses Tonometry, gonioscopy, suture removal: 1 drop of 0.5% solution in eye prior to procedure	Same as adult dosage
Tetracaine	C	Short-term anesthesia: 1–2 drops in the affected eye before examination Minor surgical procedure: 1–2 drops every 5–10 min for up to 3 doses Prolonged surgical procedure: 1–2 drops every 5–10 min for up to 5 doses	Safety and efficacy not established

BOX 58.1	General Nursing Guidelines for the Administration of Topical Ophthalmic Medications

- Topical application is the most common route of administration for ophthalmic drugs, and correct administration is essential for optimal therapeutic effects.
- Systemic absorption of eye drops can be decreased by closing the eye and applying pressure over the tear duct (nasolacrimal occlusion) for 3 to 5 minutes after instillation.
- When multiple eye drops are required, there should be an interval of 5 to 10 minutes between drops because of limited eye capacity and rapid drainage into tear ducts.
- Absorption of eye medications is increased in eye disorders associated with hyperemia and inflammation.
- Many ophthalmic drugs are available as eye drops (solutions or suspensions) and ointments. Ointments are administered less frequently than drops and often produce higher concentrations of drug in target tissues. However, they also cause blurred vision,

which limits their daytime use, at least for ambulatory patients. For some patients, drops may be used during waking hours and ointments at bedtime.

- Topical ophthalmic medications should not be used after the expiration date; cloudy, discolored solutions should be discarded.
- Topical eye medications contain a number of inactive ingredients, such as preservatives, buffers, tonicity drugs, antioxidants, and so on. Some contain sulfites, to which some people may have an allergic reaction.
- Some eye drops contain benzalkonium hydrochloride, a preservative, which is absorbed by soft contact lenses. The medications should not be applied while wearing soft contacts and should be instilled 15 minutes or longer before inserting soft contacts.
- To increase safety and accuracy of ophthalmic drug therapy, the labels and caps of eye medications are color coded.

Nursing Implications

Administering the Medication

For uveitis, it is necessary to instill one to two drops of atropine (ophthalmic) in the eye 1 hour prior to examination or three times per day to decrease inflammation of the iris and uveal tract. The nurse uses **nasolacrimal occlusion** to prevent the systemic absorption of the ophthalmic medication. He or she applies finger pressure over the lacrimal sac for 1 to 2 minutes after instillation to decrease the risk of absorption and systemic effects. Box 58.1 presents general nursing guidelines for the topical administration of eye medications.

Assessing for Therapeutic and Adverse Effects

One hour following administration, the ophthalmologist uses an ophthalmic scope to assess the ability to visualize the inner aspect of the eye. In the treatment of uveitis, the nurse assesses for diminished blurred vision and diminished photophobia.

It is necessary to assess for pain and stinging. In addition, the nurse assesses for blurred vision and sensitivity to light. These effects should diminish and are reversible over time.

Patient Teaching

The nurse instructs patients about the effects of the medication such as photophobia and stinging on administration. It is essential to tell patients not to drive if their vision is impaired. The nurse should tell them to wear sunglasses. Box 58.2 presents additional patient teaching guidelines for ophthalmic medications, including atropine.

Other Drugs in the Class

Cyclopentolate (Cyclogyl) is useful when given prior to ophthalmic examinations that involve diagnostic testing. It increases the papillary size so the fundus of the eye can be thoroughly examined. Five minutes before the examination, the ophthalmologist or nurse administers the drug (2% solution) to patients who have a heavily pigmented iris. To avoid excessive

systemic absorption, it is necessary to use nasolacrimal occlusion during and for 1 to 2 minutes following administration. Patients who have uveitis should receive cyclopentolate in combination with atropine (ophthalmic). Caution is important in the elderly due to increased IOP. Psychotic reactions and behavioral disturbances have occurred in children. It is important to withhold infant feeding for 4 hours after ophthalmic examination due to feeding intolerance.

NCLEX Success

3. A nurse is administering cyclopentolate (Cyclogyl) to a patient with uveitis. What is the most important nursing intervention when administering the medication?

   A. Touch the inner canthus of the eye with the medication applicator.
   B. Evaluate the redness and inflammation prior to administering the medication.
   C. Ask the patient to blink to enhance absorption of the medication.
   D. Apply pressure to the lacrimal sac for 2 minutes after medication administration.

4. An elderly patient is receiving cyclopentolate (Cyclogyl) for visualization of the eye. What is the patient at risk for developing?

   A. cataracts
   B. retinal detachment
   C. increased intraocular pressure
   D. cerebral edema

ADRENERGIC AGONIST

Ⓟ **Phenylephrine**, the prototype ophthalmic adrenergic agonist, is used for its mydriatic effects. Unlike anticholinergic drugs, it does not produce cycloplegic effects.

Pharmacokinetics and Action

The mydriatic effects of phenylephrine (ophthalmic) occur 15 to 30 minutes after administration. Peak plasma effects occur in less than 20 minutes, and the duration of action is 1 to 3 hours. Systemic absorption is minimal.

Phenylephrine (ophthalmic) causes contraction of the dilator muscles of the pupil. It produces mydriasis, vasoconstriction, and increased outflow of aqueous humor.

Use

Uses of phenylephrine (ophthalmic) include mydriasis prior to ophthalmic procedures and therapy of wide-angle glaucoma. It can also provide relief of redness with eye irritation. Table 58.2 presents route and dosage information for phenylephrine.

Adverse Effects and Contraindications

With phenylephrine (ophthalmic), systemic adverse effects are rare, but dysrhythmia, hypertension, myocardial infarction, syncope, and subarachnoid bleeding may occur. Ocular effects are reversible and include burning, irritation, visual changes, floaters, and rebound miosis.

Contraindications include hypersensitivity reactions, hypertension, ventricular tachycardia, and narrow-angle glaucoma.

Nursing Implications

Preventing Interactions

Phenylephrine combined with atomoxetine enhances the effects of hypertension and tachycardia. Taking phenylephrine with monoamine oxidase (MAO) inhibitors and sympathomimetic drugs also contributes to the effects of hypertension.

Administering the Medication

Box 58.1 lists general nursing guidelines for the administration of ophthalmic medications. Patients should take phenylephrine for no longer than 72 hours. To administer the ophthalmic solution, the nurse has the patient lie down with the head tilted back. Then he or she takes the following steps:

- Holds the dropper above the eye and drops the medication inside the lower lid, without touching the dropper to the eye
- Has the patient keep the eye open and avoid blinking for 30 seconds
- Applies pressure to the inside corner of the eye for 1 minute

Assessing for Therapeutic and Adverse Effects

The nurse assesses whether the inner aspect of the eye can be visualized 15 minutes after administration.

The nurse measures the blood pressure and the heart rate and checks for hypertension for dysrhythmia. He or she also asks the patient about visual floaters. In addition, it is necessary to assess for burning and irritation of the eye.

Patient Teaching

Box 58.2 presents patient teaching guidelines for topical ophthalmics, including phenylephrine.

LOCAL ANESTHETIC DRUGS

Ⓟ **Lidocaine** (Atken) is the prototype local anesthetic drug for ophthalmic use.

Pharmacokinetics and Action

The onset of action of lidocaine is 20 seconds to 5 minutes, with a median onset of 40 seconds. The duration of action is 5 to 30 minutes, with a median of 15 minutes.

Lidocaine blocks the initiation and conduction of nerve impulses. It decreases the neuronal membrane's permeability to sodium ions, resulting in an inhibition of depolarization and blocking of conduction.

Use

Lidocaine produces local anesthesia of the ocular surface during ophthalmic procedures such as surgery, tonometry, and gonioscopy. Table 58.2 presents route and dosage information for lidocaine and other ophthalmic local anesthetics.

Adverse Effects

Local adverse effects of lidocaine include burning. Specific ocular effects include conjunctival hyperemia, corneal epithelial changes, diplopia, and changes in vision.

Nursing Implications

Administering the Medication

It is important not to administer solution if it is crystallized. The nurse is certain not to touch the eye with the tip of the applicator.

BOX 58.2 📋 **Patient Teaching Guidelines for Topical Eye Medications**

General Considerations

■ Prevent eye disorders, when possible. For example, try to avoid long periods of reading and computer work; minimize exposure to dust, smog, cigarette smoke, and other eye irritants; and wash hands often and avoid touching the eyes to decrease risk of infection. Use protective eyewear when indicated.

■ Do not use nonprescription eye drops (e.g., Murine, Visine) on a regular basis for longer than 48 to 72 hours. Report persistent eye irritation and redness to a health care provider.

■ Have regular eye examinations and testing for glaucoma after 40 years of age.

■ Eye-drop preparations often contain sulfites, which can cause allergic reactions in some people.

■ If you have glaucoma, do not take any drugs without your ophthalmologist's knowledge and consent. Many drugs given for purposes other than eye disorders may cause or aggravate glaucoma. Also, wear a medical alert bracelet or carry identification that states you have glaucoma. This helps avoid administration of drugs that aggravate glaucoma or to maintain treatment of glaucoma, in emergencies.

■ If you have an eye infection, wash your hands before and after contact with the infected eye to avoid spreading the infection to the unaffected eye or to other people. Also, avoid touching the unaffected eye.

■ If you wear contact lenses, wash your hands before inserting them and follow instructions for care (e.g., cleaning, inserting, or removing, and duration of wear). Improper or infrequent cleaning may lead to infection. Overwearing is a common cause of corneal abrasions and should be avoided to prevent the development of ulcers.

■ If you wear soft contact lenses, do not use any eye medication without consulting a specialist in eye care. Some eye drops contain benzalkonium hydrochloride, a preservative, which is absorbed by soft contacts. The medication should not be applied while wearing soft contacts and should be instilled 15 minutes or longer before inserting soft contacts.

■ Never use eye medications used by someone else and never allow your eye medications to be used by anyone else. These preparations should be used by one person only, and they are dispensed in small amounts

for this purpose. Single-person use minimizes cross-contamination and risks of infection.

■ Many eye drops and ointments cause temporary blurring of vision. Do not use such medications just before driving or operating potentially hazardous machinery.

■ Avoid straining at stool (use laxatives or stool softeners if necessary), heavy lifting, bending over, coughing, and vomiting when possible. These activities increase intraocular pressure, which may cause eye damage in glaucoma and after eye surgery.

Self-Administration

■ If using more than one eye medication, be sure to administer the correct one at the correct time. Benefits depend on accurate administration.

■ Check expiration dates; do not use any eye medication after the expiration date and do not use any liquid medication that has changed colors or contains particles.

■ Shake the container if instructed on the label to do so. Suspensions should be shaken well to ensure the drug is evenly dispersed in the liquid and not settled in the bottom of the container.

■ Wash hands thoroughly.

■ Tilt the head back or lie down and look up.

■ Pull the lower lid down to expose the conjunctiva (mucous membrane).

■ Place the dropper directly over the eye. Avoid contact of the dropper with the eye, finger, or any other surface. Such contact contaminates the solution and may cause eye infections and serious damage to the eye, with possible loss of vision.

■ Look up just before applying a drop; look down for several seconds after applying the drop.

■ Release the eyelid, close the eyes, and press the inside corner of the eye with a finger for 3 to 5 minutes. Closing the eyes and blocking the tear duct helps the medication be more effective by slowing its drainage out of the eye.

■ Do not blink for 30 seconds after the administration of eye medications and during the eye examination.

■ Do not rub the eye; do not rinse the dropper.

■ If more than one eye drop is ordered, wait 10 minutes before instilling the second medication.

■ Use the same basic procedure to insert eye ointments.

Assessing for Therapeutic and Adverse Effects

The physician performing the procedure assesses for adequate anesthesia. The nurse may assess for opacity of the lens and loss of vision with prolonged use.

Drug Therapy for the Treatment of Glaucoma

For chronic open-angle glaucoma, the goal of drug therapy is to slow disease progression by reducing IOP. The first-line drugs are topical beta blockers. Health care providers commonly use

these drugs either alone or in combination with other antiglaucoma drugs. Table 58.3 lists drugs administered for the treatment of chronic open-angle glaucoma.

BETA-BLOCKING DRUGS

The purpose of the administration of beta-blocking drugs is to decrease the IOP. Although the prototype medication in this class is propranolol (see Chap. 28), it is not formulated in an ophthalmic preparation. The drug ⓟ **timolol maleate** (Timoptic, Timoptic-XE) was the first drug developed in this class for the treatment of open-angle glaucoma.

TABLE 58.3

Drugs Administered for the Treatment of Open-Angle Glaucoma

Drug Class	Prototype	Other Drugs in the Class
Beta-blocking drugs	Timolol maleate (Timoptic, Timoptic-XE)	Betaxolol (Betoptic) Carteolol Levobunolol (Betagen) Metipranolol (OptiPranolol)
Alpha$_2$-adrenergic agonists	Brimonidine (Alphagan P)	Apraclonidine hydrochloride (Iopidine)
Cholinergic drugs	Pilocarpine (Isopto Carpine) Pilocarpine Ocular System (Ocusert Pilo-20 or Pilo-40)	
Carbonic anhydrase inhibitors	Acetazolamide (Diamox)	Brinzolamide (Azopt) Dorzolamide (Trusopt)
Osmotic drugs	Mannitol (Osmitrol)	Glycerin (Osmoglyn) Isosorbide (Ismotic)
Prostaglandin analogs	Bimatoprost (Lumigan)	Latanoprost (Xalatan) Travoprost (Travatan)

Pharmacokinetics and Action

The onset of action of timolol is 30 minutes, with a peak action in 1 to 2 hours. The duration of action for intraocular effects is 24 hours.

Timolol blocks the beta$_1$- and beta$_2$-adrenergic receptors to reduce the IOP by reducing aqueous humor production and increasing outflow.

Use

Uses for timolol include chronic open-angle glaucoma, aphakic glaucoma, secondary glaucoma, and ocular hypertension. Table 58.4 presents route and dosage information for timolol and other beta-blocking drugs.

Adverse Effects and Contraindications

The most common adverse effects associated with timolol are burning and stinging. Most adverse effects of systemic beta blockers may also occur with ophthalmic preparations, and patients with respiratory or cardiac disease may not be able to take them.

Contraindications include asthma and chronic obstructive pulmonary disease, as well as heart failure, bradycardia, atrioventricular block, left ventricular dysfunction, and cardiogenic shock. Known hypersensitivity to timolol is also a contraindication.

Nursing Implications

Preventing Interactions

Many medications and herbs interact with timolol maleate, increasing its effects (Boxes 58.3 and 58.4).

Administering the Medication

Administration of the ophthalmic form of timolol necessitates the following:

- Have patients who wear contact lenses remove the lenses prior to administration.
- When administering more than one ophthalmic medication, wait 10 minutes between each medication.
- Use good hand hygiene before administering ophthalmic drugs.
- Always invert the bottle of timolol and shake it before use.
- Have the patient tilt the head back. Use the index finger of one hand to pull the lower lid down to form a pocket for the eye drop. Place the dispenser tip close to the eye and gently squeeze the bottle to administer one drop.
- Have patients who wear contact lenses wait 15 minutes before inserting them. The product can contain benzalkonium chloride, which can be absorbed into the soft contact lens.

Assessing for Therapeutic and Adverse Effects

The nurse helps ensure that the patient keeps regularly scheduled appointments with the ophthalmologist to assess the IOP. In addition, the nurse asks the patient about stinging and burning of the eyes.

Patient Teaching

Box 58.2 contains additional patient teaching information for topical ophthalmic medications, including timolol.

TABLE 58.4

DRUGS AT A GLANCE: Antiglaucoma Drugs

Drug	Pregnancy Category	Routes and Dosage Ranges	
		Adults	*Children*
Beta-blocking Drugs			
℗ **Timolol maleate** (Timoptic, Timoptic-XE)	C	Solution, 1 drop in twice daily Gel, 1 drop once daily	Same as adults
Betaxolol (Betoptic)	C	1 or 2 drops twice daily	1 drop twice daily
Carteolol	C	1 drop twice daily	Safety and efficacy not established
Levobunolol (Betagen)	C	1 or 2 drops once or twice daily	Same as adults
Metipranolol (OptiPranolol)	C	1 drop twice daily	Same as adults
Alpha₂-Adrenergic Agonists			
℗ **Brimonidine** (Alphagan B)	B	1 drop 3 times daily, every 8 h	Same as adult dose for children 2 y and older
Apraclonidine hydrochloride (Iopidine)	C	Open-angle glaucoma: 1 drop 0.5% solution every 12 h Intraoperative and postoperative increased IOP: 1 drop 1% solution 1 h before surgery and immediately after surgery	
Cholinergic Drugs			
℗ **Pilocarpine** (Isopto Carpine)			
Pilocarpine Ocular System (Ocusert Pilo-20 or Pilo-40)	B	Glaucoma: solution (1% or 2%), 1 drop in each eye 3 or 4 times daily; gel, 0.5-inch ribbon into lower conjunctival sac once daily at bedtime Miosis (Pilocarpine Ocular System): one system in conjunctival sac per wk	Same as adults
Carbonic Anhydrase Inhibitors			
℗ **Acetazolamide** (Diamox)	C	Glaucoma: 250 mg PO every 6 h; sustained-release capsules, PO 500 mg every 12 h Preoperatively: 5–10 mg/kg/d IV, IM in divided doses, every 6 h	Glaucoma: 10–15 mg/ kg/d PO every 6–8 h Preoperatively: 5–10 mg/ kg IV, IM every 6 h
Brinzolamide (Azopt)	C	1 drop 3 times daily	Safety and efficacy not established
Dorzolamide (Trusopt)	C	1 drop 3 times daily	Same as adults
Osmotic Drugs			
℗ **Mannitol** (Osmitrol)	B	1.5–2 g/kg as a 20% solution over 30–60 min	Same as adults
Isosorbide (Ismotic)	B	Emergency reduction of IOP: 1.5 g/kg PO up to 4 times daily	
℗ **Glycerin** (Osmoglyn)	C	Reduction of IOP: 1–1.8 g/kg PO, 1–1½ h before surgery Reduction of corneal edema: 1–2 drops prior to examination	Same as adults

TABLE 58.4

DRUGS AT A GLANCE: Antiglaucoma Drugs (Continued)

Drug	Pregnancy Category	Routes and Dosage Ranges	
		Adults	Children
Prostaglandin Analogs			
Ⓟ **Bimatoprost** (Latisse, Lumigan)	C	Glaucoma: 1 drop at bedtime Hypotrichosis of eyelashes: 1 drop applied evenly along the skin of the upper eyelid at the base of the eyelashes at bedtime	Not recommended under age of 16 due to hyperpigmentation
Latanoprost (Xalatan)	C	1 drop at bedtime	
Travoprost (Travatan)	C*	1 drop at bedtime	

*Contact with contents of vial should be avoided by women who are pregnant or are trying to become pregnant. In case of accidental exposure to skin, wash the exposed area thoroughly with soap and water.

EVIDENCE-BASED PRACTICE

Pharmacotherapy Compliance in Patients with Ocular Hypertension or Primary Open-Angle Glaucoma

by CARLO E. TRAVERSO, JOHN G. WALT, LEE S. STERN, & MARGARTIA DOLGITSER

Journal of Ocular Pharmacology and Therapeutics
November 1, 2009, 25, 77–82.
Retrieved October 21, 2011

The aim of this study was to compare the rates of pharmacotherapy coverage in patients with ocular hypertension (OH) and patients with primary open-angle glaucoma (POAG). A retrospective cohort study analysis of a multimanager health plan database included 4818 medicated patients with OH and 52,985 patients with POAG. OH is characterized by an elevated intraocular pressure, and POAG is a chronic debilitating eye disease. It causes progressive damage of the retinal ganglion cells and the optic nerve, eventually leading to loss of nerve fibers, decreased visual fields, and possible blindness. Adherence to treatment to OH can prevent the development of POAG. The results of this study revealed that patients with POAG were significantly more likely to be adherent to pharmacotherapy than those with OH.

IMPLICATIONS FOR NURSING PRACTICE: In the case management arena, the nurse should lobby for coverage of pharmacotherapies to treat OH and POAG. The nurse should also provide patient education on medication adherence in OH to prevent the development of the more debilitating POAG.

Clinical Application 58-2

- Mrs. Molnar has received prescriptions for timolol and pilocarpine eye drops. What patient teaching regarding these medications should the nurse provide?
- What is the action of timolol?

ALPHA₂-ADRENERGIC AGONISTS

Alpha₂-adrenergic agonists are administered when a patient's IOP is not lowered adequately with a beta blocker or when a beta blocker is contraindicated. Ⓟ **Brimonidine** (Alphagan P) is the prototype. Practitioners, who consider this group of medications to be as effective as timolol, use it in conjunction with other antiglaucoma drugs such as beta blockers or carbonic anhydrase inhibitors when multiple drugs are required.

Pharmacokinetics and Action

Brimonidine has a rapid onset of action, with a half-life of 2 hours. Extensive metabolism occurs in the liver. The drug reduces aqueous humor production and increases uveoscleral outflow.

BOX 58.3 | Drug Interactions: Timolol

Drugs That Increase the Effect of Timolol
■ Amifostine, amiodarone, antihypertensives, beta blockers, calcium channel blockers, cardiac glycosides, monoamine oxidase inhibitors, reserpine
Increase hypotensive and bradycardic effects

BOX 58.4　Herbal and Dietary Interactions: Timolol

Herbs and Foods That Increase the Effects of Timolol

- Garlic
- Ginger
- Ginseng
- Goldenseal
- Nettle

BOX 58.5　Drug Interactions: Brimonidine

Drugs That Increase the Effects of Brimonidine

- Hypotensive drugs, monoamine oxidase inhibitors
  Increase hypotensive effects
- Hydroxyzine, selective serotonin reuptake inhibitors, central nervous system (CNS) depressants
  Increase CNS depression

Use

Brimonidine is used to lower IOP in patients with open-angle glaucoma or ocular hypertension. Table 58.4 presents route and dosage information for brimonidine and the other alpha$_2$-adrenergic agonists.

Use in Children

Administration to children can result in a higher risk of adverse effects. Children are at greatest risk for CNS depression from brimonidine, with somnolence and diminished alertness.

Adverse Effects

Several adverse effects may occur with brimonidine use. Cardiovascular effects include hypertension, bradycardia, hypotension, and tachycardia. CNS effects include headache, dizziness, somnolence, diminished attention and alertness, and insomnia. Respiratory effects are bronchitis, cough, dyspnea, sinusitis, nasal dryness, and apnea. Local reactions such as stinging and burning of the eye may occur. Other ocular effects are blepharitis, conjunctival edema, conjunctival hemorrhage, dryness, irritation, and eye pain. In addition, allergic conjunctivitis, hyperemia, and pruritus affect approximately 10% to 20% of patients.

Contraindications

Contraindications to brimonidine include known hypersensitivity to the drug or use within 14 days of an MAO inhibitor. Caution is warranted in patients with advanced cardiovascular disease.

Nursing Implications

Preventing Interactions

Many medications and herbs interact with brimonidine, increasing or decreasing its effects (Boxes 58.5 and 58.6).

Administering the Medication

Box 58.1 lists general guidelines for the administration of topical ophthalmic medications.

Assessing for Therapeutic and Adverse Effects

It is necessary to assess the IOP.

The nurse monitors the blood pressure and assesses for hypertension and hypotension, and he or she checks the heart rate and monitors for bradycardia or tachycardia. The nurse also assesses the CNS for depressive effects such as dizziness, somnolence, and diminished alertness. In addition, the nurse assesses the respiratory status for cough and dyspnea and checks for nasal dryness, sinus infection, and sinusitis. It is necessary to assess for hypersensitivity reactions as well.

Patient Teaching

The nurse ensures that the patient keeps regularly scheduled appointments with the ophthalmologist to assess the IOP. Box 58.2 contains additional patient teaching information for the topical ophthalmic medications, including brimonidine.

CHOLINERGIC DRUGS

Ophthalmic cholinergic drugs increase the outflow of aqueous humor to reduce IOP. The prototype of this class is ℗ **pilocarpine** (Isopto Carpine, Pilocar), which is administered for glaucoma and as a miotic drug.

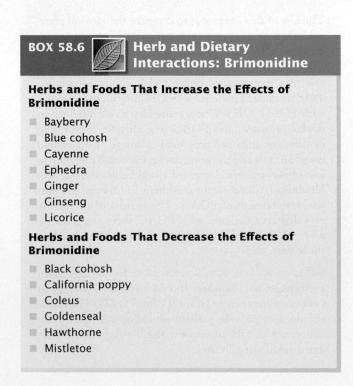

BOX 58.6　Herb and Dietary Interactions: Brimonidine

Herbs and Foods That Increase the Effects of Brimonidine

- Bayberry
- Blue cohosh
- Cayenne
- Ephedra
- Ginger
- Ginseng
- Licorice

Herbs and Foods That Decrease the Effects of Brimonidine

- Black cohosh
- California poppy
- Coleus
- Goldenseal
- Hawthorne
- Mistletoe

Pharmacokinetics and Action

Following administration of pilocarpine, miosis begins in 10 to 30 minutes, with reduction in IOP in 1 hour. The miotic duration of action is 4 to 8 hours. Metabolism occurs in the liver.

Pilocarpine stimulates the cholinergic receptors in the eye, causing miosis, loss of accommodation, and lowering of the IOP.

Use

Pilocarpine is used for chronic simple glaucoma as well as for chronic and acute angle-closure glaucoma. Table 58.4 gives route and dosage information for pilocarpine.

Adverse Effects

Several adverse effects may occur with pilocarpine. Ocular conditions include burning, ciliary spasm, conjunctival vascular congestion, lacrimation, lens opacity, retinal detachment, myopia, and diminished visual acuity. CNS problems may include headache. Cardiopulmonary manifestations are hypertension, tachycardia, bronchial spasm, and pulmonary edema. Gastrointestinal (GI) effects include nausea, vomiting, diarrhea, and increased salivation.

Contraindications

Contraindications include known hypersensitivity to the drug or acute inflammation of the anterior chamber of the eye.

Nursing Implications

Preventing Interactions

Acetylcholinesterase inhibitors may enhance the adverse effects of pilocarpine.

Administering the Medication

If the solution and gel have been prescribed together, it is necessary to administer the solution first and then give the gel 5 minutes later. Following the administration of the solution, the nurse or patient should provide pressure on the lacrimal sac for 1 to 2 minutes. Box 58.1 lists general guidelines for the administration of topical ophthalmic medications.

Assessing for Therapeutic and Adverse Effects

It is necessary to check the IOP.

Assessing for Adverse Effects

The nurse assesses for ocular burning, lens opacity, diminished visual acuity, and headache over the affected eye. He or she monitors the patient's blood pressure and heart rate and assesses for signs of hypertension and tachycardia. The nurse also assesses for bronchial spasm and pulmonary edema as well as for nausea, vomiting, diarrhea, and increased salivation.

Patient Teaching

The nurse helps ensure that the patient keeps regularly scheduled appointments with the ophthalmologist to assess the IOP. Box 58.2 provides patient teaching information for pilocarpine.

NCLEX Success

7. A patient with Parkinson's disease is taking selegiline hydrochloride (L-Deprenyl). He receives a diagnosis of increased IOP. His ophthalmologist prescribes brimonidine (Alphagan P) drops. What recommendation does the nurse make to the prescriber?
   A. Stop the selegiline hydrochloride (L-Deprenyl) for 2 weeks before starting the brimonidine (Alphagan P).
   B. Suggest that because administration of brimonidine (Alphagan P) increases blood pressure, another alpha₂ adrenergic agonist should be prescribed.
   C. Ask the prescriber whether levobunolol (Betagen) would be more stable and cause fewer adverse effects.
   D. Increase the selegiline hydrochloride (L-Deprenyl) to prevent the increase in Parkinson's-related symptoms.

8. A patient with glaucoma is receiving pilocarpine (Pilocar). What patient teaching does the nurse provide to decrease the possible cardiac adverse effects?
   A. Administer the medication at bedtime.
   B. Apply pressure to the lid after application.
   C. Apply pressure to the lacrimal sac after application.
   D. Administer the medication every 3 hours.

CARBONIC ANHYDRASE INHIBITORS

Ⓟ **Acetazolamide** (Diamox), the prototype ocular carbonic anhydrase inhibitor, is an oral drug. Prescribers use it for the management of glaucoma.

Pharmacokinetics and Action

Oral acetazolamide has an onset of action in 1 hour. Absorption occurs in the GI tract. Intravenous administration has an onset of action of 15 minutes. Distribution takes place throughout the body, concentrating in the red blood cells, plasma, and kidneys. Elimination is in the urine.

Acetazolamide inhibits carbonic anhydrase in the eye to reduce the rate of aqueous humor formation and lower the IOP.

Use

Uses for acetazolamide include open-angle glaucoma and secondary glaucoma. Practitioners also use it preoperatively for the treatment of acute closed-angle glaucoma. Table 58.4 presents route and dosage information for acetazolamide and other carbonic anhydrase inhibitors.

Adverse Effects

The major adverse effects associated with acetazolamide are Stevens-Johnson syndrome, flaccid paralysis, agranulocytosis, hemolytic anemia, aplastic anemia, leukopenia, pancytopenia, and metabolic acidosis.

BOX 58.7 — Drug Interactions: Acetazolamide

Drugs That Increase the Effect of Acetazolamide

- Alcohol, central nervous system (CNS) depressants, droperidol, hydroxyzine, selective serotonin reuptake inhibitors
  Enhance CNS depression
- Alfuzosin, amifostine, antihypertensives, diazoxide, pentoxifylline, phosphodiesterase 5 inhibitors (sildenafil), prostacyclin analogs (treprostinil)
  Enhance antihypertensive effects
- Salicylates
  Act by unknown mechanism

Contraindications

Contraindications to acetazolamide include known hypersensitivity to carbonic anhydrase inhibitors, renal and hepatic disease, and Addison's disease, as well as electrolyte imbalance. Caution is necessary in older adults. Specialists do not recommend the drug for the treatment of chronic noncongestive angle-closure glaucoma.

Nursing Implications

Preventing Interactions

Many medications and herbs interact with acetazolamide, increasing its effects (Boxes 58.7 and 58.8).

Administering the medication

To reduce GI upset, it is necessary to administer acetazolamide with food or meals. Patients should not crush or chew sustained-release preparations.

Assessing Therapeutic and Adverse Effects

It is necessary to assess the IOP.

The nurse assesses the patient's skin for signs of redness, blisters, or swelling that may indicate Stevens-Johnson syndrome. In addition, he or she checks the complete blood count for signs of anemia and the electrolytes for signs of acidosis.

Patient Teaching

The nurse helps ensure that the patient keeps regularly scheduled appointments with the ophthalmologist to assess the IOP. Box 58.9 presents patient teaching guidelines for acetazolamide.

BOX 58.8 — Herbal and Dietary Interactions: Acetazolamide

Herbs and Foods That Increase the Effects of Acetazolamide

- Garlic
- Ginger
- Ginseng
- Goldenseal
- Nettle

BOX 58.9 — Patient Teaching Guidelines for Acetazolamide

- Maintain regularly scheduled medical appointments to monitor laboratory values and intraocular pressure.
- Maintain a fluid intake of 1.5 to 2.5 L per 24 hours as well as a diet high in potassium. Good sources of potassium are milk and other dairy products, meat, poultry, fish, eggs, and nuts.
- Report numbness, tingling, burning, drowsiness, and visual disturbances to the prescriber.

Other Drugs in the Class

Brinzolamide (Azopt) reduces IOP in patients with ocular hypertension or open-angle glaucoma. The drug is contraindicated in patients with a known hypersensitivity to brinzolamide, sulfonamides, or any component of the formulation. It reaches peak effect in 2 hours and has an 8- to 12-hour duration of action. It can be absorbed in the systemic circulation and accumulates in the red blood cells. It is excreted unchanged in the urine.

Dorzolamide hydrochloride (Trusopt) is a carbonic anhydrase inhibitor administered for increased IOP or open-angle glaucoma. One drop is inserted into each eye three times per day. It decreases the aqueous humor secretion by slowing bicarbonate ions to reduce sodium and fluid transport, thus reducing IOP. Adverse reactions are bitter taste, ocular burning and stinging, photophobia, and superficial punctuate keratitis.

OSMOTIC DRUGS

In Chapter 32, mannitol (Osmitrol) is the prototype osmotic diuretic. However, (P) **glycerin** (Osmoglyn) is more commonly administered to reduce IOP in glaucoma, and it is discussed as the prototype in this section.

Pharmacokinetics and Action

After oral administration, glycerin begins to work in 10 to 30 minutes. Absorption is good. The drug reaches its peak of action in 60 to 90 minutes and has a 4- to 8-hour duration of action. Glycerin reduces the IOP by creating an osmotic gradient in between the plasma and ocular fields.

Use

Glycerin temporarily reduces IOP in acute attacks of glaucoma. Prescribers also order it for reduction of IOP prior to surgery. Table 58.4 contains route and dosage information for glycerin and other osmotic drugs.

Adverse Effects and Contraindications

Adverse effects of glycerin relate to decreased fluid volume. The most serious of these conditions is hyperosmolar nonketotic coma. Other adverse effects include confusion, headache, syncope, cardiac dysrhythmias, nausea, vomiting, and severe dehydration.

Contraindications include severe dehydration, abdominal pain, appendicitis, pulmonary edema, and severe cardiac decompensation.

Nursing Implications

Assessing for Therapeutic and Adverse Effects

It is important to check for therapeutic effects, indicated by a reduction in IOP. In addition, the nurse checks fluid and electrolytes and assesses for signs and symptoms of dehydration. He or she monitors blood pressure, pulse, and respirations. The nurse assesses for hyperglycemia, adventitious breath sounds, and pupillary reflexes. It is also necessary to assess for hypersensitivity to glycerin.

Patient Teaching

The nurse instructs the patient about the importance of keeping regularly scheduled medical appointments to check IOP. In addition, the nurse reminds the patient to report severe headache, chest pain, confusion, rapid respirations, and violent diarrhea to his or her prescriber. Box 58.2 contains additional patient teaching information for the ophthalmologic medications.

PROSTAGLANDIN ANALOGS

Of the prostaglandin analogs, Ⓟ **bimatoprost** (Latisse, Lumigan) is the prototype.

Pharmacokinetics

The onset of action of bimatoprost is approximately 4 hours, with maximum reduction of IOP in 8 to 12 hours. It is 88% protein bound and undergoes oxidation, *N*–de-ethylation, and glucuronidation after reaching systemic circulation to form metabolites. Excretion is primarily in the urine, with 25% excreted in the feces.

Action

Bimatoprost produces ocular hypotensive effects to decrease IOP and to increase outflow of aqueous humor. In the Latisse formulation, it can increase the percent and duration of hairs in the growth phase to increase eyelash growth.

Use

In patients with open-angle glaucoma and ocular hypertension, health care providers use bimatoprost to reduce IOP. Hypotrichosis of the eyelashes is another use. Table 58.4 contains route and dosage information for bimatoprost and other prostaglandin analogs.

Adverse Effects and Contraindications

Ocular adverse effects of bimatoprost include conjunctival hyperemia and ocular pruritus. Use of the Latisse formulation may result in erythema of the eyelid, allergic conjunctivitis, blepharitis, burning, cataract formation, conjunctival edema, iris pigmentation, pain, photophobia, tearing, and visual disturbances.

Contraindications include hypersensitivity.

Nursing Implications

Administering the Medication

When applying Latisse to the eyelid, have the patient who is wearing contacts remove them; in addition, it is necessary to remove makeup and wash the face thoroughly with soap and water. The nurse applies the medication with a sterile applicator and uses a new applicator for each eye. It is important to not reinsert contacts for 15 minutes.

Assessing for Therapeutic and Adverse Effects

It is important to assess IOP. In patients taking the medication for hypertrichosis of the eyelashes, the nurse assesses for increased growth of eyelashes.

The nurse assesses for ocular changes, including pruritus, blepharitis, and visual disturbances.

Patient Teaching

The nurse instructs the patient about the importance of keeping regularly scheduled medical appointments to check IOP. Box 58.2 contains additional patient teaching information.

Other Drugs in the Class

Other prostaglandin analogs include latanoprost (Xalatan) and travoprost (Travatan). Like bimatoprost, they act to lower IOP.

NCLEX Success

9. A patient's physician has prescribed glycerin (Osmoglyn) orally for the treatment of glaucoma. Which of the following aspects of patient teaching will provide the patient with information about the action of the medication?

   A. It competitively blocks the effects of acetylcholine.
   B. It selectively binds to serotonin receptors to block the release of serotonin.
   C. It stimulates the alpha$_2$-adrenergic receptors to reduce intraocular pressure (IOP).
   D. It reduces the IOP by creating an osmotic gradient in between the plasma and ocular fields.

10. A 14-year-old girl visits the school nurse's office. She has seen a commercial for Latisse and wants longer eyelashes. What information should the school nurse provide the girl regarding brimapost?

   A. "This medication is only given to patients with glaucoma."
   B. "This medication is not recommended for anyone under the age of 16."
   C. "You do not need this medication—your eyelashes are long enough."
   D. "You should talk to your guidance counselor about ways to build your self-esteem."

Drug Therapy for Ocular Infections and Inflammation

Previous chapters have presented information about the medications administered to treat viral, fungal, and bacterial infections and the inflammation that often accompanies an infection. This section of the chapter addresses the anti-infective medications administered for the treatment of ocular infections and the anti-inflammatory drugs used to decrease inflammation. The nonsteroidal anti-inflammatory drugs (NSAIDs) and corticosteroids are administered to decrease the inflammatory response. Table 58.5 lists the drugs administered to treat ocular infections and to reduce ocular inflammation.

ANTIBACTERIAL DRUGS

Various antibacterial drugs have ophthalmic uses. The most common prescribed drug is the prototype fluoroquinolone Ⓟ **ciprofloxacin** (Ciloxan).

Pharmacokinetics and Action

The amount of ciprofloxacin absorbed by the body is so small that its pharmacokinetic properties are inconsequential. Ciprofloxacin ophthalmic inhibits DNA gyrase and the relaxation of supercoiled DNA, which promotes breakage of double-stranded DNA in the target bacteria.

Use

Uses of ciprofloxacin include the treatment of corneal ulcer and bacterial conjunctivitis. It is essential that contact lenses not be worn during drug therapy. Table 58.6 presents route and dosage information about ciprofloxacin and other antibacterial ophthalmic drugs.

Adverse Effects

Ciprofloxacin ophthalmic has adverse effects that include hypersensitivity reactions and superinfection. When ciprofloxacin ophthalmic is administered concurrently with any of the quinolones, hypersensitivity reactions, tendon inflammation, and tendon rupture may occur. There have been reports of superinfections with prolonged use, with possible fungal or bacterial infections.

Contraindications

Patients with a known hypersensitivity to ciprofloxacin or any quinolone should not receive the drug.

Nursing Implications

Preventing Interactions

The only interaction identified with ciprofloxacin ophthalmic is anaphylaxis when administered with quinolones.

TABLE 58.5

Drugs Administered for the Treatment of Ocular Infections and Inflammation

Drug Class	Prototype	Other Drugs in the Class
Antibacterial drugs	Ciprofloxacin Ophthalmic (Ciloxan)	Erythromycin 5% ointment (Ilotycin) Gatifloxacin (Zymar) Gentamicin 3 mg/mL solution or 3 mg/g ointment (Garamycin) Levofloxacin 5 mg/mL solution (Quixin) Moxifloxacin (Vigamox) Ofloxacin 3 mg/mL solution (Ocuflox) Sulfacetamide 10% solution or ointment (Bleph-10), 15% solution (Isopto Cetamide), 10% and 30% solution, 10% ointment (Sodium Sulamyd) Sulfisoxazole 4% solution (Gantrisin) Tobramycin (0.3% solution and 3 mg/g ointment) (Tobrex)
Antiviral drugs	Trifluridine 1% solution (Viroptic)	
Antifungal drugs	Natamycin 5% suspension (Natacyn)	
Antiallergic drugs	Cromolyn (Crolom, Opticrom)	Azelastine (Optivar) Emedastine (Emadine) Epinastine (Elestat) Ketotifen (Zaditor) Lodoxamide (Alomide) Olopatadine (Patanol)
Corticosteroids	Dexamethasone (Decadron, Maxidex)	Fluorometholone (FML) Loteprednol (Lotemax, Alrex) Prednisolone (Econopred, others) Rimexolone (Vexol)
Anti-inflammatory drugs	Diclofenac (Voltaren)	Flurbiprofen (Ocufen) Ketorolac (Acular)
Immunosuppressants	Cyclosporine emulsion (Restasis)	

TABLE 58.6

DRUGS AT A GLANCE: Antimicrobial Drugs

Drug	Pregnancy Category	Routes and Dosage Ranges	
		Adults	*Children*
Antibacterial Drugs			
℗ **Ciprofloxacin Ophthalmic** (Ciloxan)	C	Corneal ulcer: d 1, 2 drops every 15 min for 6 h, then every 30 min for rest of day; d 2, 2 drops every hour; d 3–14, 2 drops every 4 h Conjunctivitis: 1 or 2 drops every 2 h while awake for 2 d, then 1 or 2 drops every 4 h while awake for 5 d	Safety and efficacy not established in infants <1 y
Erythromycin 5% Ointment (Ilotycin)	B		Prevention of neonatal gonococcal or chlamydial conjunctivitis: 0.5–1 cm in each eye
Gatifloxacin (Zymar)	C	1 drop every 2 h while awake, up to 8 times daily for 2 d, then 1 drop up to 4 times daily while awake for 5 d	Dosage not established
Gentamicin 3 mg/mL solution or 3 mg/g ointment (Garamycin)	D	Solution, 1 drop every 1–4 h Ointment, apply 2 or 3 times daily	Same as adults
Levofloxacin 5 mg/mL solution (Quixin)	C	1 or 2 drops every 2 h up to 8 doses/d for 1 or 2 d, then every 4 h up to 4 doses/d for 5 d	Dosage not established
Moxifloxacin (Vigamox)	C	1 drop 3 times daily for 7 d	Children >1 y, same as adults
Ofloxacin 3 mg/mL solution (Ocuflox)	C	Conjunctivitis: 1 or 2 drops every 2–4 h while awake for 2 d, then 4 times daily for 3–5 d Corneal ulcer: 1 or 2 drops every 30 min while awake, every 4–6 h during sleep for 1–2 d, then every hour while awake for 4–6 d, then every 4 h while awake until healed	Children >1 y, same as adults
Sulfacetamide 10% solution or ointment (Bleph-10), 15% solution (Isopto Cetamide), 10% and 30% solution, 10% ointment (Sodium Sulamyd)	C	Conjunctivitis, corneal ulcers, or other superficial infections caused by susceptible organisms: 1 or 2 drops every 4 h or 0.5-inch ointment 3 or 4 times daily for 7–10 d	Safety and efficacy not established; contraindicated in infants <2 mo of age
Sulfisoxazole 4% solution (Gantrisin)	C	1 or 2 drops 3 or more times daily	Safety and efficacy not established; contraindicated in infants <2 mo of age
Tobramycin (0.3% solution and 3 mg/g ointment) (Tobrex)	D	1 or 2 drops 2–6 times daily or ointment 2 or 3 times daily	See manufacturer's instructions
Antiviral Drugs			
℗ **Trifluridine 1% solution** (Viroptic)	C	Keratoconjunctivitis or corneal ulcers caused by herpes simplex virus: 1 drop every 2 h while awake (maximum, 9 drops/d) until corneal ulcer heals, then 1 drop every 4 h (minimum, 5 drops/d), for 7 d	>6 y, same as adults
Antifungal Drugs			
℗ **Natamycin 5% suspension** (Natacyn)	C	1 drop every 1–2 h for 3–4 d, then every 3–4 h for 14–21 d	Safety and efficacy not established

Administering the Medication

Ciprofloxacin ophthalmic is for topical use only. It is important not to contaminate the tip of the applicator.

Assessing for Therapeutic Effects

The nurse assesses for decreased conjunctival redness and eye drainage.

Patient Teaching

Box 58.2 contains patient teaching information for topical ophthalmic medications.

Other Drugs in the Class

An ophthalmic form of erythromycin (Ilotycin) can produce edema, urticaria, dermatitis, and angioneurotic edema. Long-term topical use may lead to superinfection, and patients with viral, fungal, or mycobacterial infections of the eye should not use this drug.

ANTIVIRAL DRUGS

The prototype Ⓟ **trifluridine** (Viroptic) is the most commonly administered antiviral ophthalmic drug. A locally active drug, it is available as an ophthalmic ointment. Another antiviral drug may be useful. In 2009, the Centers for Disease Control and Prevention (CDC) identified an unlabeled use of intravitreal ganciclovir plus systemic foscarnet for the treatment of progressive outer retinal necrosis in patients with human immunodeficiency virus.

Pharmacokinetics and Action

Systemic absorption of trifluridine is negligible. The drug does not affect liver or kidney function.

Trifluridine interferes with viral replication. It incorporates viral DNA in place of thymidine to inhibit thymidylate synthetase, causing formation of defective viral proteins.

Use

Uses of trifluridine include treatment of primary keratoconjunctivitis and recurrent epithelial keratitis caused by herpes simplex virus types 1 and 2. Table 58.6 presents route and dosage information for trifluridine.

Adverse Effects and Contraindications

The most common adverse effects associated with trifluridine are burning and stinging. Rare adverse effects include epithelial keratopathy, increased IOP, palpebral edema, and stromal edema.

Contraindications include known hypersensitivity to trifluridine or its components.

Nursing Implications

Administering the Medication

Trifluridine is a hazardous drug, and it is important to wear gloves when administering the medication. If trifluridine is being used with other ophthalmic medications, it is necessary to wait several minutes between applications. Storage of the medication in the refrigerator at 2 to 8°C or 36 to 48°F is required. Disposal in accordance with biohazard procedures should occur.

Assessing for Therapeutic and Adverse Effects

It is necessary to assess for decreased erythema of the conjunctiva. Complete healing of the corneal ulcer should occur in 1 to 2 weeks.

The nurse assesses for transient burning, stinging, and irritation of the eye. He or she also assesses for photophobia, increased IOP, epithelial keratopathy, keratitis, palpebral edema, and stromal edema.

Patient Teaching

The nurse provides instruction to the patient on medication administration, including safe handling of the drug. He or she also teaches the patient about the importance of keeping regularly scheduled medical appointments for eye examinations. In addition, the nurse tells the patient that herpetic eye infections often recur and, if not treated, lead to damage of the cornea. Box 58.2 contains additional patient teaching information.

NCLEX Success

11. **A male college student receives a diagnosis of bacterial conjunctivitis. His physician orders ciprofloxacin (Ciloxan) to be instilled every 4 hours for 5 days. On day 3, the student visits to the campus health center. He states, "My tongue is swollen." He is having trouble speaking clearly. What is the possible cause of the swollen tongue?**

    A. He is allergic to a food.
    B. He has a bacterial infection of the mouth.
    C. He is having a hypersensitivity reaction.
    D. He has a fungal or bacterial superinfection.

12. **Which of the following is the most important aspect of patient teaching with the administration of trifluridine (Viroptic)?**

    A. Tell the patient to instill the medication by pulling the upper lid toward the forehead.
    B. Tell the patient that he or she will be cured of herpetic eye infections.
    C. Tell the patient to use safe handling of the drug and wear gloves when administering.
    D. Tell the patient not to take acetazolamide due to a drug interaction.

ANTIFUNGAL DRUGS

Ⓟ **Natamycin** (Natacyn) is the prototype ophthalmic antifungal drug.

Pharmacokinetics and Action

Approximately 2% of natamycin administered topically is absorbed systemically. It is distributed by adhering to the cornea and is retained in the conjunctival fornices. It does not affect intraocular fluid concentrations.

Natamycin increases cellular permeability to susceptible fungi.

Use

Uses of natamycin include the treatment of blepharitis, conjunctivitis, and keratitis. It is effective against common fungi such as *Aspergillus*, *Candida*, *Cephalosporium*, *Fusarium*, and *Penicillium*. Table 58.6 presents route and dosage information for natamycin.

Adverse Effects

Reported adverse effects of natamycin may be numerous. These conditions may include hypersensitivity and allergic reactions, chest pain, opacity of the cornea, eye pain, edema, dyspnea, hyperemia, irritation, foreign body sensation of the eye, paresthesia, tearing, and alteration in visual acuity.

Contraindications

Patients who have exhibited a hypersensitivity reaction to natamycin should not take the drug.

Nursing Implications

Administering the Medication

It is important that contact lenses are not worn when signs and symptoms of the fungal infection are visible. In any case, the natamycin solution contains benzalkonium chloride, which can be absorbed by the lens; thus, it is necessary to remove the lenses prior to administration of the medication. Reinsertion of the lenses should not occur for 15 minutes. The nurse shakes the medication well and then administers it without touching the applicator tip to the eye.

Assessing for Therapeutic and Adverse Effects

The nurse assesses for decreased eye pain, redness, and tearing. Also, the patient should also have increased visual acuity with a decrease in blurring and cloudiness.

It is also necessary to assess for signs and symptoms of a hypersensitivity reaction such as hyperemia, dyspnea, edema, or chest pain. The nurse also assesses for paresthesia and visual changes.

Patient Teaching

The nurse tells the patient to discontinue wearing contacts during the acute phase of the fungal infection. Also, the nurse emphasizes that even when the patient is wearing contacts, he or she should not reinsert them for 15 minutes after instillation of the medication. In addition, it is important to maintain good hand hygiene and prevent contamination of the applicator tip. Box 58.2 contains additional patient teaching information.

ANTIALLERGIC DRUGS

Ⓟ **Cromolyn sodium** (Crolom) is the prototype antiallergic ophthalmic drug.

Pharmacokinetics and Action

The onset of action varies. The half-life of the drug is 80 to 90 minutes. Cromolyn is excreted unchanged in the urine and feces with small amounts in exhaled gases.

Cromolyn reduces the release of leukotrienes, thus decreasing or stopping the body's reaction to an allergen.

Use

Uses of cromolyn include the treatment of vernal keratitis, vernal conjunctivitis, and vernal keratoconjunctivitis. Table 58.7 presents route and dosage information for cromolyn and other ophthalmic antiallergy medications.

Adverse Effects and Contraindications

Cromolyn is associated with several adverse effects, including hypersensitivity reactions. Eye effects include edema, dryness, irritation, itching, puffiness, rash, and tearing. Styes may also develop.

Contraindications include a known hypersensitivity to the drug or its formulations.

Nursing Implications

Assessing for Therapeutic Effects

The nurse assesses for a reduction in allergic conjunctivitis, keratitis, or keratoconjunctivitis. Response to treatment with cromolyn may occur in a few days. However, treatment for up to 6 weeks is routinely necessary.

Assessing for Adverse Effects

The nurse assesses for hypersensitivity response to the medication as well as ocular effects that include edema, dryness, irritation, itching, swelling, rash, or tearing. It is necessary to ask the patient about feelings of a foreign body, which could indicate a stye. Withdrawal may result in the exacerbation of symptoms.

Patient Teaching

Box 58.2 contains additional patient teaching information.

Corticosteroids

The prototype corticosteroid ophthalmic drug is Ⓟ **dexamethasone** (Decadron, Maxidex, Ozurdex).

Pharmacokinetics

The onset of action of dexamethasone ophthalmic drops is unknown. The half-life and duration of action are unknown. The onset of action of the implant is 20% to 30% within the first 2 months following intravitreal injection. The duration of action is 1 to 3 months.

Action

Dexamethasone decreases inflammation by suppressing the migration of neutrophils and decreasing the production of the mediators of inflammation. It reverses the increase in capillary permeability and suppresses the normal immune response.

TABLE 58.7

DRUGS AT A GLANCE: Anti-inflammatory Drugs

Drug	Pregnancy Category	Routes and Dosages Ranges	
		Adults	*Children*
Antiallergic Drugs			
Ⓟ **Cromolyn sodium** (Crolom)	B	1–2 drops in each eye 4–6 times per day	>4 y, same as adults
Azelastine (Optivar)	C	1 drop every 2 h while awake (maximum dose 9 drops per day) until reepithelialization of corneal ulcer occurs, then 1 drop every 4 h for 7 d; do not exceed 21 d of treatment	Same as adults
Emedastine (Emadine)	C	1 drop 4 times per day	>3 y, same as adults
Epinastine (Elestat)	C	1 drop 2 times per day even when symptoms subside	>3 y, same as adults
Ketotifen (Zaditor)	C	1 drop 2 times a day at least 8 h apart	>3 y, same as adults
Lodoxamide (Alomide)	B	1–2 drops 4 times a day for 3 mo	>2 y, same as adults
Olopatadine (Patanol)	C	1 drop 2 times per day at least 6 h between doses	>3 y, same as adults
Corticosteroids			
Ⓟ **Dexamethasone** (Decadron, Maxidex, Ozurdex)	C	Ophthalmic solution, 1–2 drops into conjunctival sac every hour during the day and night; gradually reduce dose to every 3–4 h then to 3–4 times per day Ophthalmic suspension, 1–2 drops into conjunctival sac 4–6 times per day; may use hourly in severe disease; taper dose during discontinuation Macular edema or noninfective uveitis: Ophthalmic injection, ocular implant with Ozurdex, intravitreal 0.7-mg implant injected in affected eye	Ophthalmic solution, 1–2 drops into conjunctival sac every hour during the day and every other hour during the night; gradually reduce dose to every 3–4 h, then 3–4 times per day Ophthalmic suspension, 1–2 drops into conjunctival sac up to 4–6 times per day; may use hourly in severe disease in older children; taper dose during discontinuation; Following strabismus surgery: 2–4 times per day
Fluorometholone (FML)	C	Ointment, 1/2-inch ribbon to conjunctival sac 1–3 times/d; may increase to every 4 h during the initial 24–48 h Suspension, 1 drop into the conjunctival sac 2–4 times per day	>2 y of age, same as adults
Loteprednol (Lotemax, Alrex)	C	Seasonal allergic conjunctivitis: 0.2% suspension 1 drop 4 times per day Inflammatory conditions: 0.5% suspension 1–2 drops into the conjunctival sac 4 times per day; during the first week the dose may be increased by 1 drop every hour; do not discontinue therapy prematurely; if signs and symptoms do not improve in 2 d, the patient should be reevaluated Postoperative inflammation: 0.5% suspension 1–2 drops into the conjunctival sac 4 times per day beginning 24 h after surgery and continue for 2 wk	Safety and efficacy not established

TABLE 58.7

DRUGS AT A GLANCE: Anti-inflammatory Drugs (Continued)

Drug	Pregnancy Category	Routes and Dosages Ranges	
		Adults	Children
Prednisolone (Econopred, others)	C	1–2 drops into conjunctival sac every hour during the day and every 2 h at night; when a favorable response is obtained, use 1 drop every 4 h	Same as adults
Rimexolone (Vexol)	C	Anti-inflammatory: 1–2 drops into conjunctival sac 4 times per day beginning 24 h after surgery and continuing through the first 2 wk of the postoperative period Anterior uveitis: 1–2 drops into conjunctival sac every hour during waking hours for the first week, then 1 drop every 2 h during waking hours of the second week, and then taper until uveitis is resolved	Safety and efficacy not established
Anti-inflammatory Drugs			
Ⓟ **Diclofenac** (Voltaren)	C	Cataract surgery: 1 drop 4 times per day beginning 24 h after surgery and continuing for 2 wk Corneal refractive surgery: 1–2 drops within the hour prior to surgery and continuing for 2 wk	Safety and efficacy not established
Flurbiprofen (Ocufen)	C	1 drop every 30 min starting 2 h prior to surgery (total of 4 drops to each affected eye)	Same as adults
Ketorolac (Acular)	C	Seasonal allergic conjunctivitis: 1 drop 4 times per day Postoperative inflammation: 1 drop 4 times per day starting 24 h after cataract surgery and through 14 d after surgery Postoperative pain: 1 drop 4 times per day as needed up to 4 d after corneal refractive surgery Postoperative pain and photophobia: 1 drop 4 times per day as needed for up to 3 d after incisional refractive surgery	>3 y, same as adults
Immunosuppressants			
Ⓟ **Cyclosporine emulsion** (Restasis)	C	1 drop every 12 h	>16 y, same as adults

Use

Uses of dexamethasone include a decrease of symptoms of allergic conjunctivitis, iritis, and cyclitis. It is a treatment of corneal injury from chemical, radiation, and thermal burns or penetrating foreign bodies. Dexamethasone in the form of an intravitreal implant (Ozurdex) is used for the treatment of macular edema following retinal vein occlusion or central retinal vein occlusion, as well as for noninfective uveitis. Table 58.7 presents dosage information for the corticosteroid ophthalmic drugs.

Adverse Effects

Ocular adverse effects associated with dexamethasone include blurred vision, increased IOP, photophobia, vitreous detachment, conjunctival edema, corneal edema, eye pain, dryness, irritation, and eye discharge.

Contraindications

Contraindications to dexamethasone include corneal or conjunctival viral disease caused by herpes simplex, vaccina, or varicella.

Also, other contraindications are mycobacterial and fungal infection of the eye as well as advanced glaucoma and hypersensitivity to corticosteroids. In addition, patients who are taking corticorelin, a synthetic hormone that is administered to diagnose Cushing's disease, should not receive ophthalmic forms of dexamethasone.

Nursing Implications

Preventing Interactions

The dexamethasone decreases the therapeutic effects of corticorelin. If patients who are taking the chelating drug deferasirox combine it with corticosteroids, there is an increased risk of GI ulceration, irritation, and bleeding.

Administering the Medication

QSEN Safety Alert

It is important to double check medications before administration. The nurse should not confuse medications with similar names. For example, it is easy to confuse dexamethasone (Maxidex) with triamterene/hydrochlorothiazide (Maxzide).

The solution and suspension contain benzalkonium chloride. Thus, a nurse may administer dexamethasone solutions and suspensions, but an ophthalmologist gives the implant (Ozurdex) under aseptic conditions. Prior to the administration of Ozurdex, a broad-spectrum bactericidal drug is administered prior to the injection. If administered to both eyes, a different applicator is used for each application. Box 58.1 lists general guidelines for the administration of topical ophthalmic medications.

Assessing for Therapeutic Effects

The nurse assesses for decreased pain, irritation, redness, and eye drainage. An ophthalmologist evaluates patients who have received Ozurdex for decreased macular edema and inflammation of the uveal tract.

Assessing for Adverse Effects

The nurse assesses for eye pain, blurred vision, photophobia, increased IOP, photophobia, vitreous detachment, conjunctival edema, eye dryness, or eye discharge.

Patient Teaching

For patients who use the ophthalmic implant (Ozurdex), it is important to instruct them about the sterile procedure for administration and the rationale for the implant. Box 58.2 contains additional patient teaching information.

ANTI-INFLAMMATORY DRUGS

The prototype ophthalmic NSAID is Ⓟ**diclofenac** (Voltaren), an analgesic, non-narcotic drug.

Pharmacokinetics and Action

Very little systemic absorption of diclofenac occurs. Mainly, it has local effects.

This cyclooxygenase 1 and 2 inhibitor decreases the formation of prostaglandin, thus resulting in an anti-inflammatory action.

Use

Diclofenac reduces inflammation following cataract extraction. It is administered to relieve pain and photophobia associated with corneal refractive surgery. Table 58.7 provides route and dosage information about diclofenac and other NSAIDs.

Adverse Effects

Diclofenac may produce facial edema, dizziness, fever, headache, pain, and insomnia. Associated ocular adverse effects are burning, stinging, increased IOP, keratitis, and lacrimation. Less frequently occurring ocular conditions include disturbances in vision, inflammation, corneal deposits and edema, corneal lesions or opacity, discharge, swelling, iritis, itching, and allergy. In addition, rhinitis, muscle pain and weakness, abdominal pain, nausea, vomiting, and viral infection may follow use.

Contraindications

Contraindications to diclofenac include hypersensitivity to any NSAID.

Nursing Implications

Preventing Interactions

Any ophthalmic NSAID combined with latanoprost diminishes the therapeutic effect of latanoprost.

Administering the Medication

As with other ophthalmic medications, it is necessary to prevent contamination of the applicator tip. In addition, it is important to wait at least 5 minutes before administering any other eye drops.

Assessing for Therapeutic and Adverse Effects

The nurse assesses for decreased inflammation and pain related to surgery.

In addition, the nurse assesses for tearing, inflammation, and pain or discomfort of the eye, as well as for facial edema and rhinitis. It is necessary to assess for increased IOP. Also, the nurse assesses for GI conditions and viral infections.

Patient Teaching

Box 58.2 contains patient teaching information.

IMMUNOSUPPRESSANTS

The prototype ophthalmic immunosuppressant drug is Ⓟ **cyclosporine emulsion** (Restasis).

Pharmacokinetics and Action

No systemic concentrations of cyclosporine are detected in blood samples.

The drug increases tear production.

Use

Cyclosporine emulsion increases tear production in keratoconjunctivitis sicca, which is an ocular inflammation. Table 58.7 presents route and dosage information for the cyclosporine emulsion.

Adverse Effects and Contraindications

The adverse effects of cyclosporine emulsion are burning, hyperemia, ocular pain, and pruritus.

Contraindications include active eye infections or hypersensitivity to the medication.

Nursing Implications

Administering the Medication

It is important to invert the medication bottle to mix the emulsion adequately prior to administration. In addition, patients should remove contact lenses before administration and not reinsert them for 15 minutes. The instillation of other ocular medications should occur at 15-minute intervals.

Assessing for Therapeutic and Adverse Effects

The nurse interviews the patient to determine if the dryness of the eye has resolved.

In addition, the nurse assesses for discomfort of the eye, pruritus, and hyperemia.

Patient Teaching

It is important to instruct the patient about medication administration, including inversion of the bottle to mix the medication, removal of contacts, and waiting 15 minutes between the administration of other ocular medications. Box 58.2 contains additional patient teaching information.

The Nursing Process

Assessment

- Determine whether the patient has impaired vision and, if so, the extent of the impairment. Minimal assessment includes the vision-impaired patient's ability to participate in activities of daily living, including safe ambulation. Maximal assessment depends on the nurse's ability and working situation. Some nurses do vision testing and ophthalmoscopic examinations.
- Identify risk factors for eye disorders. These include trauma, allergies, infection in one eye (a risk factor for infection in the other eye), use of contact lenses, infections of facial structures or skin, and occupational exposure to chemical irritants or foreign bodies.
- Signs and symptoms vary with particular disorders:
  - Pain is usually associated with corneal abrasions or inflammation. Sudden, severe pain may indicate acute glaucoma, which requires immediate treatment to lower IOP and minimize damage to the optic nerve.
  - Signs of inflammation (redness, edema, heat, tenderness) are especially evident with infection or inflammation of external ocular structures, such as the eyelids

and conjunctiva. A watery or mucoid discharge also often occurs.
  - Pruritus is most often associated with allergic conjunctivitis.
  - Photosensitivity commonly occurs with keratitis.

Nursing Diagnoses

- Disturbed sensory perception: visual, related to eye disorders
- Risk for injury: blindness related to inadequately treated glaucoma or ophthalmic infections
- Deficient knowledge related to prevention and treatment of ocular disorders

Planning/Goals

The patient will

- Take ophthalmic medications as prescribed
- Follow safety precautions to protect eyes from trauma and disease
- Experience improvement in signs and symptoms (e.g., decreased drainage with infections, decreased eye pain with glaucoma)
- Avoid injury from impaired vision (e.g., falls)
- Avoid systemic effects of ophthalmic drugs
- Have regular eye examinations to monitor effects of antiglaucoma drugs

Nursing Interventions

The nurse will

- Implement measures to minimize ocular disorders:
  - Promote regular eye examinations in all patient populations, but most importantly in middle-aged and older adults. Patients older than 40 years of age should be tested annually for glaucoma.
  - Instruct patients who have glaucoma not to take any medications without a physician's knowledge. Many drugs given for purposes other than eye disorders may cause or aggravate glaucoma. Also, suggest that patients wear a medical alert bracelet stating that they have glaucoma.
- Assess for adverse drug effects
- Assist patients at risk of eye damage from IOP (e.g., those with glaucoma; those who have had intraocular surgery, such as cataract removal) to avoid straining at stool (use laxatives or stool softeners if needed), heavy lifting, bending over, coughing, and vomiting when possible
- Promote handwashing and keeping hands away from eyes to prevent eye infections
- Cleanse contact lenses or assist patients in lens care, when needed
- Treat eye injuries appropriately:
  - For chemical burns, irrigate the eyes with copious amounts of water as soon as possible (i.e., near the area where the injury occurred). Do not wait for transport to a first-aid station, hospital, or other health care facility. Damage continues as long as the chemical is in contact with the eye.

- For thermal burns, apply cold compresses to the area.
- Superficial foreign bodies may be removed by irrigation with water. Foreign bodies embedded in ocular structures must be removed by a health care provider.
- Consider applying warm, wet compresses, they are often useful in ophthalmic inflammation or infections. They relieve pain and promote healing by increasing the blood supply to the affected area.
- Instruct patient who wear contact lenses to wash their hands before inserting the lenses and follow instructions for care of the lenses (e.g., cleaning, inserting or removing, and duration of wear). Improper or infrequent cleaning may lead to infection. Overwearing is a common

cause of corneal abrasion and may cause corneal ulceration. Encourage lens wearers to consult an ophthalmologist when eye pain occurs. Antibiotics are often prescribed for corneal abrasions to prevent development of ulcers.

Evaluation

- Observe and interview for compliance with instructions regarding drug therapy and follow-up care.
- Observe and interview for relief of symptoms.
- Observe for systemic adverse effects of ophthalmic drugs (e.g., tachycardia and dysrhythmias with adrenergics; bradycardia or bronchoconstriction with beta blockers).

Key Concepts

- Drug therapy for eye disorders is unique because of the location, structure, and function of the eye.
- Eye medications represent several different drug classes.
- Most eye medications are administered as drops.
- Therapeutic effects of eye drops depend on accurate administration.
- Eye medications should be kept sterile to avoid infection.
- Local eye medications may cause systemic effects.
- Systemic drugs may affect eye function.

Critical Thinking Questions

58-1. A 33-year-old woman is scheduled for an ophthalmological examination next week. An elementary school teacher, she stops by the nurse's office to inquire about the eye examination; she has not had one before. The school nurse instructs the woman about the administration of mydriatic drugs.

- What is a mydriatic drug and why is it administered?
- What is the onset of action of ophthalmic atropine sulfate and why is it administered?
- What is the purpose of applying pressure to the nasolacrimal region of the eye?

58-2. A 75-year-old woman is being treated for open-angle glaucoma. She has received a prescription for timolol (Timoptic).

- What is open-angle glaucoma?
- What type of medication is timolol (Timoptic)?
- What is the action of timolol (Timoptic)?
- What are the nursing responsibilities when administering timolol (Timoptic)?

References and Resources

Byas, P., Naik, U., & Gangaiah, J. B. (2011). Efficacy of bimatoprost 0.03% in reducing intraocular pressure in patients with 360° synechial angle-closure glaucoma: A preliminary study. *Indian Journal of Ophthalmology*, 59(1), 13–16.

Jacobs, D. S. (2011). *Open-angle glaucoma.* Up-To-Date. (Retrieved: October 21, 2011).

Karch, A. M. (2010). *2010 Lippincott's nursing drug guide.* Philadelphia, PA: Lippincott Williams & Wilkins.

Keane, P., Khan, M., Saeed, A., Stack, J., Tormey, P., Hayes, P., et al. (2009). The impact of available anti-glaucoma

therapy on the volume and age profile of patients undergoing glaucoma filtration surgery. *Eye*, 23, 1675–1680.

Lin, A. P., Orengo-Nania, S., & Braun, U. K. (2009). Management of chronic open-angle glaucoma in the aging US population. *Geriatrics*, 64(7), 20–28.

Nguyen, Q. H., & Earl, M. (2009). Fixed-combination brimonidine/timolol as adjunctive therapy to a prostaglandin analog: A 3 month, open-label replacement study in glaucoma patients. *J Ocul Pharmacol Ther*, 25(6), 541–544.

Nursing 2011 Drug Handbook. (2011). Philadelphia, PA: Lippincott Williams & Wilkins.

Olitsky, S. E., & Reynolds, J. D. (2011). *Primary infantile glaucoma.* Up-To-Date. Retrieved October 23, 2011.

Porth, C. M., & Matfin, (2009). *Pathophysiology concepts of altered health states.* Philadelphia, PA: Lippincott Williams & Wilkins.

Smeltzer, S. C., Bare, B. G., Hinkle, J. H., & Cheever, K. H. (2010). *Brunner & Suddarth's textbook of medical-surgical nursing* (12th ed.). Philadelphia, PA: Lippincott Williams & Wilkins.

Traverso, C. E., Walt, J. G., Sterne, L. S., & Dolgitser, M. (2009). Pharmacotherapy compliance in patients with ocular hypertension or primary open-angle glaucoma. *J Ocul Pharmacol Ther, 25*(10), 77–82.

Up-To-Date. (2011). *Atropine: drug information.* Retrieved October 21, 2011.

Up-To-Date. (2011). *Atropine: pediatric drug information.* Retrieved October 21, 2011.

Up-To-Date. (2011). *Bimatoprost: drug information.* Retrieved October 24, 2011.

Up-To-Date. (2011). *Brinzolamide: drug information.* Retrieved October 24, 2011.

Up-To-Date. (2011). *Brinzolamide and timolol: drug information.* Retrieved October 24, 2011).

Up-To-Date. (2011). *Brimonidine: pediatric drug information.* Retrieved October 23, 2011.

Up-To-Date. (2011). *Ciprofloxacin: drug information.* Retrieved October 27, 2011.

Up-To-Date. (2011). *Cromolyn sodium (ophthalmic): drug information.* Retrieved October 28, 2011.

Up-To-Date. (2011). *Cyclopentolate: drug information.* Retrieved October 21, 2011.

Up-To-Date. (2011). *Cyclosporine (ophthalmic): drug information.* Retrieved November 6, 2011.

Up-To-Date. (2011). *Dexamethasone: drug information.* Retrieved October 21, 2011.

Up-To-Date. (2011). *Dorzolamide and timolol: drug information.* Retrieved October 24, 2011.

Up-To-Date. (2011). *Diclofenac (ophthalmic): drug information.* Retrieved October 27, 2011.

Up-To-Date. (2011). *Diclofenac (ophthalmic): pediatric drug information.* Retrieved October 27, 2011.

Up-To-Date. (2011). *Glycerin: drug information.* Retrieved October 24, 2011.

Up-To-Date. (2011). *Homatropine: drug information.* Retrieved October 21, 2011.

Up-To-Date. (2011). *Homatropine: pediatric drug information.* Retrieved October 21, 2011.

Up-To-Date. (2011). *Latanoprost: drug information.* Retrieved October 24, 2011.

Up-To-Date. (2011). *Lidocaine (ophthalmic): drug information.* Retrieved October 21, 2011.

Up-To-Date. (2011). *Natamycin: drug information.* Retrieved October 27, 2011.

Up-To-Date. (2011). *Phenylephrine: drug information.* Retrieved October 22, 2011).

Up-To-Date. (2011). *Pilocarpine (ophthalmic): drug information.* Retrieved October 21, 2011.

Up-To-Date. (2011). *Proparacaine: drug information.* Retrieved October 21, 2011.

Up-To-Date. (2011). *Scopolamine: pediatric drug information.* Retrieved October 21, 2011.

Up-To-Date. (2011). *Tetracaine: drug information.* Retrieved October 21, 2011.

Up-To-Date. (2011). *Timolol: drug information.* Retrieved October 23, 2011.

Up-To-Date. (2011). *Travoprost: drug information.* Retrieved October 24, 2011.

Up-To-Date. (2011). *Trifluridine: drug information.* Retrieved October 27, 2011.

Up-To-Date. (2011). *Tropicamide: pediatric drug information.* Retrieved October 21, 2011.

Watson, S. (2010). Improving care of chronic open-angle glaucoma. *Nursing Older People, 22*(8), 18–23.

White, J. (2011). Diagnosis and management of acute angle-closure glaucoma. *Emergency Nurse, 19*(3), 27.

59 Drug Therapy for Disorders of the Ear

LEARNING OBJECTIVES

After studying this chapter, you should be able to:

1. Understand the etiology, pathophysiology, and clinical manifestations of both acute otitis externa and necrotizing otitis externa.

2. Identify the prototype and describe the action, use, adverse effects, contraindications, and nursing implications for topical medications used to treat otitis externa.

3. Identify the prototype and describe the action, use, adverse effects, contraindications, and nursing implications for systemic medications used to treat necrotizing otitis externa.

4. Identify the prototype and describe the action, use, adverse effects, contraindications, and nursing implications for systemic medications used to treat otitis media.

5. Identify the adjuvant drugs used to treat otitis externa and otitis media.

6. Implement the nursing process in the care of the patient with otitis externa or otitis media.

Clinical Application Case Study

Derrick Washington is a member of the high school swim team. He has been swimming two times per day for the past 3 months. The swim team has been very successful this season; it has qualified for the state finals. One morning well before the state meet, Derrick awakens with a severe earache. His mother makes an appointment with a pediatric nurse practitioner, who diagnoses acute otitis externa (swimmer's ear). The nurse prescribes polymyxin B–neomycin–hydrocortisone suspension (Cortisporin Otic).

KEY TERMS

Otalgia: ear pain

Otic: relating to the ear

Otitis externa: inflammation of the external ear that occurs as a mild allergic dermatitis or as a severe cellulitis

Otitis media: inflammation of the middle ear

Otorrhea: purulent ear drainage

Introduction

This chapter discusses some ear-related disorders and their pharmacological treatment. Infections, whether bacterial or fungal, or allergic reactions, result in ear pain-related inflammation. **Otitis externa** is a disorder of the external ear that produces inflammation. This condition, most commonly known as swimmer's ear, is more likely to occur in the summer months. People whose ears are frequently exposed to moisture are more prone to the development of this disorder. Malignant necrotizing otitis externa most commonly affects elderly patients with diabetes mellitus and patients with the human immunodeficiency virus. **Otitis media** is an acute infection or inflammation of the middle ear. Acute otitis media is the most common ailment for which anti-infective agents are prescribed in children.

The pharmacological therapy of choice for disorders of the ear is **otic** preparations. These medications, which are discussed elsewhere in this book, have special uses in the treatment of ear conditions.

Overview of Disorders of the Ear

Etiology

Otitis Externa

Causes of otitis externa include moisture in the ear canal, allergic reactions such as psoriasis, or trauma of the ear canal related to itching or scratching. *Pseudomonas aeruginosa, Proteus,* and *Staphylococcus aureus* are bacteria that may play a causal role. *Aspergillus* is the fungus that thrives in the most ear canal.

Otitis Media

Otitis media is more common in children than adults. The causative pathogens include *Haemophilus influenzae, Streptococcus pneumoniae,* and *Moraxella catarrhalis.* They enter the middle ear as a result of an alteration in the eustachian tube. This can be caused by upper respiratory congestion, inflammation, or an allergic reaction. Bacteria may enter the middle ear from the contaminated secretions of the nasopharynx or perforation of the tympanic membrane of the middle ear.

Pathophysiology

Otitis Externa

Otitis externa involves the presence of moisture in the external ear canal, leading to the development of inflammation of the pinna and canal. The canal becomes itchy, red, and tender, and increased swelling makes it narrower. Ear pain occurs with movement because of the inflammation. There may be watery or purulent drainage, and intermittent hearing loss may result (Porth & Matfin, 2009).

Necrotizing otitis externa is a soft tissue infection of the external auditory canal. The epidermis becomes thickened and inflamed and the underlying dermis exhibits chronic inflammation. Involvement of the osseous portion of the external auditory canal can lead to temporal bone osteomyelitis. The infection is progressive causing rapid debilitation. If the infection spreads to the base of the skull, it can be fatal.

Otitis Media

In otitis media, infection causes an obstruction of the eustachian tube, resulting in fluid retention and suppuration of retained secretions. This infection is more common in children because the eustachian tube is straighter, allowing the pathogen to enter the ear more easily.

Clinical Manifestations

Otitis Externa

In acute otitis externa, the patient complains of ear pain and discharge from the external auditory canal. The discharge may be yellow or green, possessing a foul odor. The patient may also report a feeling of "fullness" in the ear, decreased hearing, and pruritus.

In necrotizing otitis externa, the presenting symptoms are **otalgia,** or ear pain, and **otorrhea,** or purulent drainage. The pain is primarily experienced at night and may extend to the temporomandibular joint when chewing. The advancement of the infection results in osteomyelitis of the skull and temporomandibular joint.

Otitis Media

In acute otitis media, marked fluid and inflammation in the mucosa lining the middle ear space are present (Fig. 59.1). Otalgia and diminished hearing occur. Fever may or may not be present. An upper respiratory tract infection or seasonal allergic rhinitis commonly precedes acute otitis media. Changes in equilibrium may occur. If the tympanic membrane ruptures, patients report a reduction or relief of ear pain.

Drug Therapy

Table 59.1 lists the various drugs used to treat ear disorders.

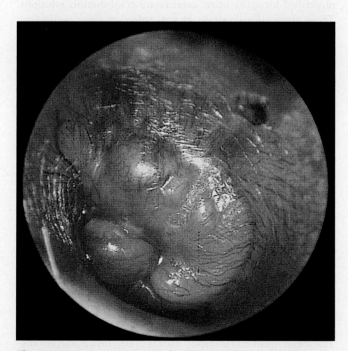

Figure 59.1 Acute otitis media. (From Weber, J. & Kelly, J. H. (2010). *Health assessment in nursing.* (4th ed.). Philadelphia, PA: Wolters Kluwer Health | Lippincott Williams & Wilkins.)

TABLE 59.1

Drugs Administered for the Treatment of Disorders of the Ear

Drug Class	Prototype	Other Drugs in the Class
Acute otitis externa Anti-infective, anti-septic, glucocorticoid, and acidifying agents	Neosporin–polymyxin B–hydrocortisone (Cortisporin Otic)	Coly-Mycin S Otic Cipro HC Otic Ofloxacin (Floxin Otic)
Necrotizing otitis externa Fluoroquinolones	Ciprofloxacin (Cipro)	
Acute otitis media Penicillin	Amoxicillin (Ampicillin)	

Otitis Externa

For acute otitis externa, use of topical agents, as opposed to systemic agents, is more common. Systemic medications are indicated only if a deep tissue infection develops outside the external canal or if immunocompromised status is an issue. Topical drugs are more effective because they deliver higher concentrations of medication to the infected, inflamed tissue. The use of these agents also reduces adverse effects.

When the infection extends to the pinna, prescribers order oral anti-infective agents. For necrotizing otitis externa, the primary treatment is systemic antipseudomonal antimicrobial agents. Ciprofloxacin is the drug of choice for adults, whereas cephalexin (Keflex) is the preferred drug for children (see Chaps. 16 and 17). The otic solutions most commonly prescribed for acute otitis externa are combination solutions. These medications contain an anti-infective agent, antiseptic, glucocorticoid, and acidifying agent.

Otitis Media

Oral amoxicillin (Amoxil) is the drug of choice for the treatment of acute otitis media (see Table 59.3). Patients who are allergic to penicillins may take cephalosporins.

Anti-Infective, Antiseptic, Glucocorticoid, and Acidifying Agents

Health care providers use the combination drug Ⓟ**neomycin-polymyxin B–hydrocortisone** (Cortisporin Otic) for the treatment of acute external otitis media. Neomycin and polymyxin B are antibiotics, which combat bacterial infections. Hydrocortisone is a steroid, which reduces the actions of chemicals in the body that cause inflammation, redness, and swelling.

Pharmacokinetics

The metabolism and transport effects of polymyxin and neomycin are unknown. Hydrocortisone is metabolized in the liver, and excretion occurs in the urine.

Action

Each component of Cortisporin Otic has its own mechanism of action. Neomycin, an aminoglycoside, inhibits bacterial protein synthesis by irreversibly binding to the 30S ribosome of the susceptible bacteria. Polymyxin B, a miscellaneous anti-infective agent, binds to the lipid phosphates in the bacterial cell membrane, which changes the membrane permeability to prevent leakage of cytoplasm from the bacterial cell wall, contributing to cell death. Hydrocortisone, a steroid, decreases inflammation by stabilizing the leukocyte lysosome membrane, inhibiting phagocytosis and release of allergic substances.

Use

Health care providers use Cortisporin Otic for the treatment of acute otitis externa caused by *P. aeruginosa*, *Proteus*, and *S. aureus*. Table 59.2 presents route and dosage information for Cortisporin Otic.

Use in Children

Authorities recommend Cortisporin Otic in children only for bacterial infections of the external auditory canal due to the adverse effect of ototoxicity. The hydrocortisone may cause suppression of the hypothalamic-pituitary-adrenal axis in younger children.

Adverse Effects and Contraindications

Adverse effects of Cortisporin Otic include burning, stinging, and ototoxicity.

Contraindications include a known hypersensitivity to the drug's components. Prescribers should not order it for viral, fungal, or mycobacterial infections.

Nursing Implications

Preventing Interactions

Cortisporin Otic is associated with no significant drug or herbal interactions.

TABLE 59.2

DRUGS AT A GLANCE: Anti-Infective, Antiseptic, Glucocorticoid, and Acidifying Drugs

Drug	Pregnancy Category	Routes and Dosage Ranges	
		Adults	Children
Ⓟ **Neomycin–polymyxin B–hydrocortisone** (Cortisporin Otic)	C	Instill 4 drops 3–4 times daily for no more than 10 d	6 mo and older, 3 drops into affected ear 3–4 times daily
Coly-Mycin S Otic	C	4 drops in affected ear 3–4 times daily	3 drops in affected ear 3–4 times daily
Ciprofloxacin–hydrocortisone (Cipro HC Otic)	C	3 drops in affected ear twice daily for 7 d	1 y and older, 3 drops in affected ear twice daily for 7 d
Ofloxacin (Floxin Otic)	C	10 drops into affected ear twice daily for 14 d	6 mo–13 y, 5 drops into affected ear twice daily for 10 d; 13 y and older, same as adult

EVIDENCE-BASED PRACTICE

Pseudomonas aeruginosa *Isolated from Otitis Externa Associated with Recreational Waters in some Public Swimming Pools in Tehran*

by MOHAMMAD HAJJARTABAR

Iranian Journal of Clinical Infectious Diseases
2010, 5(3), 142–151

Pseudomonas aeruginosa, the most significant bacteria in swimming pools, is the most common bacteria in otitis externa. This study analyzed the bacteriological quality of 11 public outdoor and indoor swimming pools in east and northeast Tehran. It isolated *P. aeruginosa* from 81.8% of the pools as well as from ear swabs of 79.3% of swimming pool users. The study results revealed that otitis externa was strongly related to the swimming pools contaminated with *P. aeruginosa*. Based on this study, the public pools in the city enacted strict standards for bathing prior to swimming and policies to prevent overuse of the pools.

IMPLICATIONS FOR NURSING PRACTICE: Although this study is international, it has implications for nursing practice in the United States. Nurses in schools and in the public health sector should ensure the maintenance of strict standards for bathing prior to using public pools; this practice can reduce the rate of otitis externa in the general population. Nurses should be at the forefront of establishment and enforcement of public health initiatives.

Administering the Medication

Administration of Cortisporin Otic is directly in the external ear canal. Prior to administering the otic suspension, it is necessary to shake the medication well. In addition, if cerumen is present, cleaning of the ear canal with a cotton swab is important.

QSEN Safety Alert

It is necessary to assess the tympanic membrane with an otoscope before inserting Cortisporin Otic. If the tympanic membrane is torn, then the medication is absorbed directly by the inner ear, leading to hearing loss.

The proper administration of ear drops requires tilting the head toward the opposite shoulder, pulling the superior aspect of the auricle upward, and instilling the ear drops into the ear canal. The patient should then lie on the side opposite the side of administration for 20 minutes. To maximize medication absorption, the patient should have a cotton ball placed in the ear canal.

Assessing for Therapeutic and Adverse Effects

The nurse assesses for decreased ear pain and itching as well as for decreased drainage from the ear canal.

It is also necessary to assess for signs of hearing loss due to ototoxicity. He or she also assesses for burning and stinging.

Patient Teaching

Box 59.1 lists patient teaching guidelines for Cortisporin.

Other Drugs in the Class

The otic drug Coly-Mycin, a combination of neomycin, colistin, hydrocortisone, and thonzonium, is an antibiotic and corticosteroid administered for ear inflammation and infection. Contraindications include a known hypersensitivity to aminoglycosides as well as the presence of herpes simplex, vaccinia,

BOX 59.1 Patient Teaching Guidelines for Cortisporin Otic

■ Use the ear drops properly. Put them directly in the ear canal. Prior to administering the otic suspension, it is necessary to shake the medication well. If any ear wax is present, use a cotton swab to remove it.

  ■ Tilt your head toward the opposite shoulder, pull the top of your outer ear upward, and put the ear drops into the ear canal.

  ■ Then lie on the side opposite the side of administration for 20 minutes. To maximize medication absorption, place a cotton ball in your ear for that time.

■ Refrain from inserting anything in the ear canal.

■ Do not let water enter the ear canal during the treatment period. If you swim, use ear plugs, shake the ear dry after swimming, and use a blow dryer on the low setting 12 inches away to dry the ear canal.

■ Stop using the medication after 10 days.

■ Have a follow-up assessment in 1 to 2 weeks.

or varicella. The neomycin may cause cutaneous sensitization, with itching, redness, edema, and diminished healing.

The combination drug Cipro HC contains ciprofloxacin and hydrocortisone. Its twice-daily administration makes it more convenient for parents with young children.

Ofloxacin (Floxin Otic), which health care providers use for treatment of otitis externa and otitis media, is suitable for administration to a patient with a perforated tympanic membrane. This medication does not contain neomycin; therefore, there is no risk of ototoxicity.

Clinical Application 59-1

- What does the nurse tell Derrick and his mother about the pathophysiology of otitis externa?
- What is the reason for the development of otitis externa in this case?
- With what signs and symptoms of otitis externa does the nurse expect Derrick to present?

NCLEX Success

1. Which of the following patients are at risk for the development of otitis externa?

   A. a patient who wears ear plugs while swimming
   B. a patient who has hearing loss
   C. a patient who wears a hearing aid
   D. a patient with labyrinthitis

2. What is the duration of therapy for neomycin–polymyxin B–hydrocortisone (Cortisporin Otic)?

   A. 5 days
   B. 8 days
   C. 10 days
   D. 14 days

3. Which of the following medications is administered for otitis externa and otitis media?

   A. ofloxacin (Floxin Otic)
   B. Burow's solution
   C. benzoyl alcohol
   D. acetic acid as VoSoL Otic

4. Which of the following nursing actions should be implemented when instilling ear drops?

   A. Tilt the head toward the opposite shoulder.
   B. Lay on the affected ear after instillation.
   C. Apply the medication on a cotton ball and insert in the outer auricle.
   D. Apply ear plugs after instilling ear drops.

5. Which nursing action should be implemented prior to instilling ear drops?

   A. Evaluate the patient's pain level.
   B. Assess the amount of hearing loss.
   C. Instruct the patient to lie on the affected ear.
   D. Assess if cerumen is visible.

Clinical Application 59-2

- What patient teaching does the nurse need to provide to Derrick and his mother?
- The state swim meet is in 2 weeks. Will Derrick be able to participate?
- What does the school nurse need to teach the swim coach to prevent further outbreaks of otitis externa?

Fluoroquinolone: Ciprofloxacin

The fluoroquinolone Ⓟ **ciprofloxacin** (Cipro) is the drug of choice for necrotizing otitis externa. Initially, administration is intravenous, until symptoms decrease; then it is oral.

Pharmacokinetics

The intravenous preparation has an onset of action in 10 minutes, with a peak of action in 30 minutes and duration of 4 to 5 hours. Onset of action for the oral preparation varies, with a peak of action in 60 to 90 minutes, and the same duration of action. The intravenous and oral preparations are absorbed rapidly and distributed to the kidneys, gallbladder, liver, lungs, gynecological or prostate tissue, and the cerebrospinal fluid. It is 20% to 40% protein bound, and partial metabolism takes place in the liver. The serum half-life is 3 to 5 hours with normal renal function. The excretion of the drug occurs in the urine and feces.

Action

Ciprofloxacin inhibits DNA gyrase in susceptible organisms and inhibits the supercoiled DNA, promoting breakage of the double-stranded DNA.

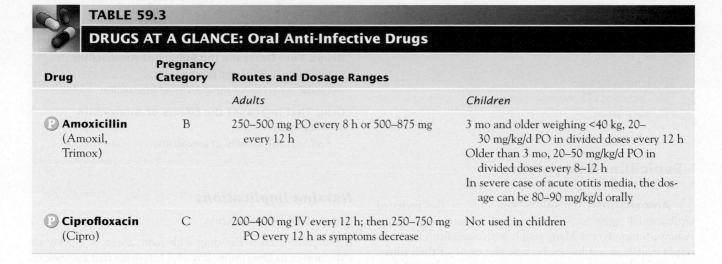

TABLE 59.3

DRUGS AT A GLANCE: Oral Anti-Infective Drugs

Drug	Pregnancy Category	Routes and Dosage Ranges	
		Adults	Children
℗ **Amoxicillin** (Amoxil, Trimox)	B	250–500 mg PO every 8 h or 500–875 mg every 12 h	3 mo and older weighing <40 kg, 20–30 mg/kg/d PO in divided doses every 12 h Older than 3 mo, 20–50 mg/kg/d PO in divided doses every 8–12 h In severe case of acute otitis media, the dosage can be 80–90 mg/kg/d orally
℗ **Ciprofloxacin** (Cipro)	C	200–400 mg IV every 12 h; then 250–750 mg PO every 12 h as symptoms decrease	Not used in children

Use

Health care providers use ciprofloxacin for the treatment of *P. aeruginosa* in patients with necrotizing otitis externa. The cure rate with fluoroquinolones is approximately 90% (Gandis & Yu, 2011). (If the causative agent is *Aspergillus*, amphotericin B is the drug of choice [see Chap. 22].) Table 59.3 gives route and dosage information for ciprofloxacin and other oral anti-infective drugs.

Use in Patients with Renal Impairment

Dosage adjustment is necessary for patients with renal impairment (see Chap. 17).

Adverse Effects

Patients generally tolerate ciprofloxacin well. The most frequent adverse effects are gastrointestinal (GI) and include nausea, vomiting, and abdominal discomfort. Dizziness and mild headache may occur. There are reports of allergic and skin reactions. Photosensitivity can occur while taking ciprofloxacin with exposure to direct or indirect sunlight. Artificial light or sun lamps may also precipitate photosensitivity reactions. Patients older than 60 years of age are at risk for tendonitis or tendon rupture.

Contraindications

Patients with a known sensitivity to ciprofloxacin should not receive the drug or any other fluoroquinolone. Administration of ciprofloxacin with tizanidine is contraindicated.

Nursing Implications

Preventing Interactions

Many medications, herbs, and foods interact with ciprofloxacin, increasing or decreasing its effects (see Boxes 17.2 and 17.3).

Administering the Medication

Parenteral administration of ciprofloxacin should occur over 60 minutes. If signs and symptoms of hypersensitivity develop, it is important to discontinue the medication. Patients may take the oral preparation with food to reduce GI upset. However,

they should not take it within 2 hours of eating dairy products, calcium-fortified juices, antacids, zinc, or iron.

Assessing for Therapeutic and Adverse Effects

The nurse assesses for diminished pain with chewing, otalgia, and otorrhea.

The nurse assesses the patient's renal function during the course of treatment. It is also important to assess for any signs or symptoms of hypersensitivity to the medication.

Patient Teaching

Patient teaching guidelines for ciprofloxacin are listed in the Box 59.2.

NCLEX Success

6. A woman is taking oral ciprofloxacin for necrotizing otitis externa. When she takes the ciprofloxacin, which of the following foods should be eliminated from her diet?

   A. cranberry juice
   B. calcium-enriched orange juice
   C. bread
   D. turkey

BOX 59.2   Patient Teaching Guidelines for Ciprofloxacin

- Avoid exposure to sunlight and apply sunscreen during the course of drug treatment.
- Do not operate machinery or drive if experiencing dizziness or lightheadedness occurs.
- Stay well hydrated during the course of treatment.
- Do not drink calcium-fortified juices or dairy products while taking the drug.
- Do not take antacids, zinc, or iron supplements during the course of drug treatment.
- Report tendon pain to the primary care provider.
- Report nausea, vomiting, or diarrhea.

7. A 70-year-old man has been diagnosed with necrotizing otitis media. What is the patient at risk for developing while being treated with ciprofloxacin?

A. edema
B. tendon rupture
C. decreased QT interval
D. chest pain

Penicillin: Amoxicillin

Ⓟ **Amoxicillin** (Amoxil), a penicillin, is the preferred antibacterial agent for the treatment of acute otitis media. Administration is oral. Many people with acute otitis media do not benefit from antibiotics because the cause of their illness is viral, not bacterial, or the infection resolves without the use of a drug.

Pharmacokinetics

Amoxicillin has a variable onset of action; it reaches a peak in 1 hour. The duration of action is 6 to 8 hours. The therapeutic half-life is 1 to 1.4 hours. Metabolism occurs in the liver, and excretion of unchanged drug is in the urine. Amoxicillin crosses the placenta and enters the breast milk, which is a consideration because penicillin agents are often given during pregnancy.

Action

Amoxicillin has bactericidal properties. It inhibits cell wall synthesis of sensitive organisms, resulting in cell death.

Use

Amoxicillin is administered for the treatment of acute otitis media. It is active against *Staphylococcus pneumoniae*, *H. influenzae*, *Streptococcus pyogenes*, and *Moraxella catarrhalis*.

Adverse Effects

The most common adverse effect is hypersensitivity to the medication, with the development of a rash or severe reactions with anaphylaxis. The most common GI adverse effects are glossitis, stomatitis, gastritis, sore throat, nausea, vomiting, abdominal pain, and diarrhea. Other adverse effects include the development of superinfections.

Contraindications

Contraindications to use of amoxicillin include a known hypersensitivity to penicillin, cephalosporin, or other allergens. In the event of a penicillin allergy without urticaria or anaphylaxis, the patient is prescribed cefdinir, cefpodoxime, or cefuroxime. See Chapter 16.

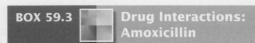

BOX 59.3 Drug Interactions: Amoxicillin

Drugs That Decrease the Effects of Amoxicillin
■ Chloramphenicol, tetracycline
   Cause inhibition of the activity of amoxicillin

Drug That Increases the Effects of Amoxicillin
■ Probenecid
   Prolongs the activity of amoxicillin

Nursing Implications

Preventing Interactions

If the patient takes the drug with food, there is a delay or reduction in its absorption. Box 59.3 lists drugs that increase or decrease the effect of amoxicillin.

Administering the Medication

It is necessary to take amoxicillin orally in divided doses around the clock. The patient should take the full course of antibiotics and not discontinue them, even if the otitis media seems to be improving.

Assessing for Therapeutic Effects

The nurse assesses for otalgia and otorrhea. Both pain and drainage should decrease with antibiotic therapy. It is also necessary to assess the patient's hearing. As the fullness of the tympanic membrane decreases, the patient reports improvement in hearing. The nurse inspects the tympanic membrane for bulging (see Fig. 59.1). As the infection resolves, the tympanic membrane becomes shiny gray with a visible cone of light from the otoscope (Fig. 59.2).

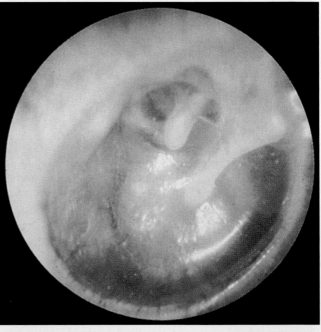

Figure 59.2 Normal tympanic membrane, after resolution of otitis media. (From Moore, K. L., Agur, A. M. R., & Dalley, A. F. (2011). *Essential clinical anatomy.* (4th ed.). Philadelphia, PA: Wolters Kluwer Health | Lippincott Williams & Wilkins.)

<table>
<tr><td>

BOX 59.4 **Patient Teaching Guidelines for Amoxicillin**

■ Self- or Caregiver Administration
■ Ensure that the child takes the entire course of the drug.
■ Administer the drug around the clock.
■ Take the medication on an empty stomach to enhance the drug's effectiveness.
■ Report ear pain or diminished hearing.

</td></tr>
</table>

Assessing for Adverse Effects

The nurse assesses the patient for signs and symptoms of hypersensitivity, with symptoms of wheezing, rash, or difficulty breathing. It is also important to assess for GI adverse effects such as nausea, vomiting, stomatitis, mouth irritation, sore throat, abdominal pain, and diarrhea. In addition, the nurse assesses for signs of superinfection.

Patient Teaching

Box 59.4 lists patient teaching guidelines for amoxicillin.

NCLEX Success

8. A child receives a diagnosis of acute otitis media. His physician orders amoxicillin (Amoxil). Which of the following adverse effects warrants the discontinuation of the medication?

A. onset of diarrhea
B. onset of abdominal pain
C. onset of diminished appetite
D. onset of wheezing

9. Which of the following assessment findings reveals that the amoxicillin (Amoxil) is decreasing the symptoms of acute otitis media?

A. retracted tympanic membrane
B. otalgia
C. otorrhea
D. visible cone of light

10. A 76-year-old woman is receiving amoxicillin (Amoxil) for acute otitis media. She also has gout. Which of the following antigout medications increases the effect of amoxicillin?

A. allopurinol
B. probenecid
C. aspirin
D. acetaminophen

Adjuvant Medications to Treat Pain and Fever Related to Infections of the Ear

Infections of the ear produce pain and may result in fever. The adjuvant medications most commonly administered for relief of pain and fever include agents such as aspirin, acetaminophen (Tylenol), or ibuprofen (Motrin) (see Chap. 14).

Salicylates

Ⓟ Aspirin is the prototype of the salicylates. Children should not take this drug. Aspirin has the ability to inhibit prostaglandin synthesis (a cause of the inflammatory effect). Its role in fever reduction, or antipyretic action, is not understood. Experts believe that aspirin acts on the thermoregulatory center of the hypothalamus, blocking the effects of the endogenous pyrogens and inhibiting the synthesis of prostaglandins. Administration is oral or rectal. To prevent gastric irritation, it is necessary to take the oral preparation with food.

Nonnarcotic Analgesic Antipyretic

Ⓟ Acetaminophen is equivalent to aspirin in analgesic and antipyretic effects. This drug is safe for children. It acts directly on the hypothalamus to increase vasodilation and sweating. Its mechanism of action to reduce pain is not known. Acetaminophen is oral or rectal. Alternating acetaminophen and ibuprofen every 4 hours over a 3-day period to control fever in young children (ages 6–36 months) has been shown to be more effective than monotherapy with either agent.

Propionic Acid Derivatives

Ⓟ Ibuprofen (Motrin, Advil) is a nonsteroidal anti-inflammatory agent that inhibits prostaglandin synthesis in both the central and peripheral nervous systems. There are two forms of cyclooxygenase, COX-1 and COX-2. Ibuprofen blocks prostaglandin synthesis and modulates T-cell production, inhibiting the chemotaxis of the inflammatory cells and increasing their destruction. The drug blocks COX-1 and COX-2 and is more selective with COX-1. It is administered to reduce pain, inflammation, and fever. Ibuprofen is administered orally or intravenously. For treatment of otalgia and fever, the drug is administered orally.

The Nursing Process

Assessment

- Assess for diminished hearing and signs of ear infection.
  - Inspect the external ear and palpate the auricle and surrounding tissue.
  - Inspect for alterations in skin integrity of the outer ear.
  - Inspect the tympanic membrane with an otoscope.
  - Assess for fluid in the ear drum and absence of the cone of light.
- Interview the patient related to fullness of the ear, diminished hearing, or pain.
- Assess temperature.

Nursing Diagnoses

- Pain related to inflammation and infection of the external or middle ear
- Impaired skin integrity related to auricle lesion
- Infection related to ear moisture, trauma, or organism invasion
- Impaired hearing related to fluid in the middle ear

Planning/Goals

The patient will

- Take the entire course of anti-infective agents safely and accurately
- Take anti-inflammatory/antipyretic agents as ordered to reduce pain and fever
- Not insert any items in the ear
- Use earplugs when swimming
- Dry the ear carefully following bathing or swimming

Nursing Interventions

The nurse will

- Instruct the patient on the administration of ear drops
- Instruct on the medication regime, and to administer anti-infective agents around the clock

- Assess the tympanic membrane for signs of infection
- Assess the lesion of the external ear for signs of healing
- Instruct parents to never let a baby sleep drinking a bottle (this promotes the development of otitis media)
- Administer pain and fever reducers as needed
- Assess for ear drainage

Evaluation

- Interview the patient for relief of symptoms with the completion of the course of anti-infective agents.
- Interview the patient regarding compliance with the medication regime.
- Assess the external and middle ear for signs of infection or inflammation.

Key Concepts

- Otitis externa is a disorder of the external ear that produces inflammation.
- Malignant necrotizing otitis externa occurs in elderly patients with diabetes or in patients who are immunocompromised. The causative agent is *P. aeruginosa*.
- Anti-infective, antiseptic, glucocorticoid, and acidifying agents such as Cortisporin Otic are administered to treat otitis externa.
- Antipseudomonal antimicrobial agents are the primary therapy for malignant necrotizing otitis externa.
- Otitis media is inflammation of the middle ear and is most common in children but can also occur in adults.
- Oral amoxicillin (Amoxil) is the drug of choice for the treatment of acute otitis media.
- Infections of the ear produce pain and may result in fever. The adjuvant medications most commonly administered for relief of pain and fever include agents such as aspirin, acetaminophen (Tylenol), and ibuprofen (Motrin)

Critical Thinking Questions

59-1. A 76-year-old woman with a history of type 1 diabetes mellitus since age 22 is experiencing severe ear pain that extends into the temporomandibular joint. The patient experiences pain primarily at night. When she chews, this pain sometimes extends to the temporomandibular joint. She has called to schedule an appointment at the diabetic acute care clinic.

- Based on her symptoms, from what condition does the nurse suspect that this woman is suffering?
- The woman's physician prescribes ciprofloxacin. What is the action of ciprofloxacin?
- What patient teaching is more appropriate related to the woman's medication regimen?
- What adverse effects of ciprofloxacin is this woman prone to developing?

59-2. A mother calls the pediatric division at the local children's hospital seeking information. She says her 3-month-old child has been up all night crying and pulling on her right ear. She thinks the baby may have a fever, but she does not have a thermometer.

- What information does the nurse convey to the mother?
- What does the nurse suspect is wrong with the baby?
- What patient teaching should the emergency department nurse provide to the mother regarding the administration of amoxicillin (Amoxil), as well as acetaminophen (Tylenol) and ibuprofen (Motrin, Advil)?

References and Resources

Carpenito-Moyet, L. J. (2010). *Nursing diagnosis application to clinical practice* (13th ed.). Philadelphia, PA: Lippincott Williams & Wilkins.

Gandis, J. R., & Yu, V. L. (2011). *Malignant (necrotizing) external otitis*. Up-To-Date. Retrieved November 27, 2011.

Glynn, F., & Walsh, R. M. (2009). Necrotizing otitis externa: A new trend? Report of 6 atypical cases. *Ear, Nose, & Throat Journal, 88*(12), 1261–1263.

Goguen, L. A. (2011). *External otitis media*. Up-To-Date. Retrieved November 25, 2011.

Hajjartabar, M. (2010). *Pseudomonas aeruginosa* isolated from otitis externa associated with recreational waters in some public swimming pools in Tehran. *Iranian Journal of Clinical Infectious Disease, 5*(3), 142–151.

Karch, A. M. (2013). *2013 Lippincott's nursing drug guide*. Philadelphia, PA: Lippincott Williams & Wilkins.

Limb, C. J., Lustig, L. R., & Klein, J. O. (2011). *Acute otitis media in adults (suppurative and serous)*. Up-To-Date. Retrieved November 25, 2011.

Mayo Clinic Health Letter. (2011).*Outer ear infection don't delay care*. www.HealthLetter.MayoClinic.com. Retrieved November 22, 2011.

Morbidity and Mortality Weekly Report. (May 20, 2011). Estimated burden of acute otitis externa—United States, 2003–2007, 60(19), 605–609.

Porth, C. M., & Matfin, (2009). *Pathophysiology concepts of altered health states*. Philadelphia, PA: Lippincott Williams & Wilkins.

Smeltzer, S. C., Bare, B. G., Hinkle, J. H., & Cheever, K. H. (2010). *Brunner & Suddarth's textbook of medical-surgical nursing* (12th ed.). Philadelphia, PA: Lippincott Williams & Wilkins.

Stedman's. (2012). *Medical dictionary for the health professions and nursing* (7th ed.). Philadelphia, PA: Lippincott Williams & Wilkins.

Up-To-Date. (2011). *Ciprofloxacin (systemic): Drug information*. Retrieved November 26, 2011.

Up-To-Date. (2011). *Ciprofloxacin and hydrocortisone: Drug information*. Retrieved November 26, 2011.

Up-To-Date. (2011). *Common drugs for external otitis*. Retrieved November 25, 2011.

Up-To-Date. (2011). *Neomycin, polymyxin B, and hydrocortisone*. Retrieved November 26, 2011.

Up-To-Date. (2011). *Ofloxacin (otic): Pediatric drug information*. Retrieved November 27, 2011.

60 Drug Therapy for Disorders of the Skin

LEARNING OBJECTIVES

LEARNING OBJECTIVES

After studying this chapter, you should be able to:

1. Identify the disorders of the skin.

2. Identify drug therapy for the treatment of acne vulgaris and drug therapy for other skin disorders.

3. Identify the prototype and describe the action, use, adverse effects, contraindications, and nursing implications for the retinoids.

4. Implement the nursing process in the care of the patient with disorders of the skin.

Clinical Application Case Study

Gerard Aylward is a 16-year-old high school sophomore who has a history of asthma. As a child, he received allergy shots on a weekly basis. He now has a severe case of acne vulgaris. He has been taking tetracycline hydrochloride 500 mg orally every 12 hours. His acne remains severe, and his dermatologist has decided to discontinue the tetracycline and start isotretinoin 35 mg orally two times per day for 15 weeks.

KEY TERMS

Acne vulgaris: common disorder characterized by excessive production of sebum and obstruction of hair follicles, which normally carry sebum to the skin surface

Dermatitis: general term denoting an inflammatory response of the skin to injuries, irritants, allergens, or trauma; also referred to as eczema

Emollient: lubricant used to relieve pruritus and dryness of the skin

Erythema: redness of the skin

Pruritus: itching

Psoriasis: scaling, dry, erythematous skin eruptions on the elbows, knees, scalp, and trunk

Rosacea: chronic disease characterized by erythema, telangiectases (fine, red, superficial blood vessels), and acne-like lesions of facial skin

Tinea pedis: common type of ringworm infection; also called athlete's foot

Urticaria: inflammatory response characterized by a skin lesion called a wheal, a raised edematous area with a pale center and red border, which itches intensely; also known as hives

Introduction

This chapter discusses the disorders of the skin. In addition, it introduces acne vulgaris and the drugs administered for their treatment.

Disorders of the Skin

Dermatologic disorders may be primary (i.e., originate in the skin or mucous membranes) or secondary (i.e., result from a systemic condition, such as measles or adverse drug reactions).

Inflammatory Disorders

Dermatitis

Dermatitis, also called eczema, is a general term denoting an inflammatory response of the skin to injuries from irritants, allergens, or trauma. Whatever the cause, dermatitis is usually characterized by **erythema** (redness), **pruritus** (itching), and skin lesions. It may be acute or chronic.

Atopic dermatitis is a common disorder characterized by dry skin, pruritus, and lesions that vary according to the extent of inflammation, stages of healing, and scratching. Scratching damages the skin and increases the risk of secondary infection. Acute lesions are reddened skin areas containing papules and vesicles; chronic lesions are often thick, fibrotic, and nodular. The cause is uncertain but may involve allergic, hereditary, or psychological elements. Exposure to possible causes or exacerbating factors such as allergens, irritating chemicals, foods, and emotional stress are factors to consider.

Contact dermatitis results from direct contact with irritants (e.g., soaps, detergents) or allergens (e.g., clothing materials or dyes, jewelry, cosmetics) that stimulate inflammation. Irritants cause tissue damage and dermatitis in anyone with sufficient contact or exposure. Allergens cause dermatitis only in sensitized or hypersensitive people. The location of the dermatitis may indicate the cause (e.g., facial dermatitis may indicate an allergy to cosmetics).

Seborrheic dermatitis is a disease of the sebaceous glands characterized by excessive production of sebum. It may occur on the scalp, face, or trunk. A simple form involving the scalp is dandruff, which is characterized by flaking and itching of the skin. More severe forms are characterized by greasy, yellow scales or crusts with variable amounts of erythema and itching.

Drug-induced skin reactions can occur with virtually any drug and can resemble the signs and symptoms of virtually any skin disorder. Topical drugs usually cause a localized, contact dermatitis–type of reaction and systemic drugs cause generalized skin lesions. Skin manifestations of serious drug reactions include erythema, facial edema, pain, blisters, necrosis, and urticaria. Systemic manifestations may include fever, enlarged lymph nodes, joint pain or inflammation, shortness of breath, hypotension, and leukocytosis. Drug-related reactions usually occur within the 1st or 2nd week of drug administration and subside when the drug is discontinued.

Urticaria

Urticaria (hives) is an inflammatory response characterized by a skin lesion called a wheal, a raised edematous area with a pale center and red border, which itches intensely. Histamine, the most common mediator of urticaria, causes vasodilation, increased vascular permeability, and pruritus. Mast cells and basophils release histamine as a result of both allergic (e.g., insect bites, foods, drugs) and nonallergic (e.g., radiocontrast media, opiates, heat, cold, pressure, ultraviolet [UV] light) stimuli. An important difference between allergic and nonallergic reactions is that many allergic reactions require prior exposure to the stimulus, whereas nonallergic reactions can occur with the first exposure.

Psoriasis

Psoriasis is a chronic, inflammatory disorder attributed to activated T lymphocytes, which produce cytokines that stimulate abnormal growth of affected skin cells and blood vessels. The abnormal growth results in excessively rapid turnover of epidermal cells. Instead of 30 days from formation to elimination of normal epidermal cells, epidermal cells involved in psoriasis are abnormal in structure and have a lifespan of about 4 days. Skin lesions of psoriasis are erythematous, dry, and scaling. The lesions may occur anywhere on the body but commonly involve the skin covering bony prominences, such as the elbows and knees. Skin lesions may be tender, but they do not usually cause severe pain or itching. However, the lesions are unsightly and usually cause embarrassment and mental distress.

This skin disease is characterized by remissions and exacerbations. Exacerbating factors include infections, winter weather, some drugs (e.g., beta blockers, lithium), and possibly stress, obesity, and alcoholism.

Rosacea

Rosacea is a chronic disease characterized by erythema, telangiectases (fine, red, superficial blood vessels), and acne-like lesions of facial skin. Hyperplasia of the nose (rhinophyma) eventually develops. The disorder usually occurs in middle-aged and older people, and it is more common in men. The etiology is thought to be excessive production of certain inflammatory proteins. Spicy foods, heat, alcohol, and embarrassment can worsen the condition.

Dermatologic Infections

Bacterial Infections

Bacterial infections of the skin are common; they are most often caused by streptococci or staphylococci.

- Cellulitis is characterized by erythema, tenderness, and edema, which may spread to subcutaneous tissue. Generalized malaise, chills, and fever may occur.
- Folliculitis is an infection of the hair follicles that most often occurs on the scalp or bearded areas of the face.
- Furuncles and carbuncles are infections usually caused by staphylococci. Furuncles (boils) may result from folliculitis and tend to recur. They usually occur in the neck, face, axillae, buttocks, thighs, and perineum. Carbuncles involve many hair follicles and include multiple pustules. Carbuncles may cause fever, malaise, leukocytosis, and bacteremia. Healing of carbuncles often produces scar tissue.
- Impetigo is a superficial skin infection caused by streptococci or staphylococci.

Fungal Infections

Fungal infections of the skin and mucous membranes are most often caused by *Candida albicans*.

- Oral candidiasis (thrush) involves mucous membranes of the mouth. It often occurs as a superinfection after the use of broad-spectrum systemic antibiotics.
- Candidiasis of the vagina and vulva occurs with systemic antibiotic therapy and in women with diabetes mellitus.
- Intertrigo involves skin folds or areas where two skin surfaces are in contact (e.g., groin, pendulous breasts).
- Tinea infections (ringworm) are caused by fungi (dermatophytes). These infections may involve the scalp (tinea capitis), the body (tinea corporis), the foot (tinea pedis), and other areas of the body. **Tinea pedis**, commonly called athlete's foot, is a type of ringworm infection.

Viral Infections

Viral infections of the skin include verrucae (warts) and herpes infections. There are two types of herpes simplex infections: type 1 usually involves the face or neck (e.g., fever blisters or cold sores on the lips) and type 2 involves the genitalia. Other herpes infections include varicella (chickenpox) and herpes zoster (shingles).

Trauma

Trauma refers to a physical injury that disrupts the skin. When the skin is broken, it may not be able to function properly. The major problem associated with skin wounds is infection. Common wounds include lacerations (cuts or tears), abrasions (shearing or scraping of the skin), puncture wounds, surgical incisions, and burns.

Ulcerations

Cutaneous ulcerations are usually caused by trauma and impaired circulation. They may become inflamed or infected.

- Pressure ulcers (also called decubitus ulcers) may occur anywhere on the body when external pressure decreases blood flow. Older adults often have thin, dry skin and are at risk of pressure ulcers. Pressure ulcers are most likely to develop in patients who are immobilized, incontinent, malnourished, and debilitated. Common sites include the sacrum, trochanters, ankles, and heels. In addition, abraded skin is susceptible to infection and ulcer formation.
- Venous stasis ulcers, which usually occur on the legs, result from impaired venous circulation. Other signs of venous insufficiency include edema, varicose veins, stasis dermatitis, and brown skin pigmentation. Bacterial infection may occur in the ulcer.

Anorectal Disorders

Hemorrhoids and anal fissures are common anorectal disorders characterized by pruritus, bleeding, and pain. Inflammation and infection may occur.

Acne

Acne is a common disorder characterized by excessive production of sebum and obstruction of hair follicles, which normally carry sebum to the skin surface. As a result, hair follicles expand and form comedones (blackheads and whiteheads). Acne lesions vary from small comedones to **acne vulgaris**, the most severe form, in which follicles become infected and irritating secretions leak into surrounding tissues to form inflammatory pustules, cysts, and abscesses. Most patients have a variety of lesion types at one time. At least four pathologic events take place within acne-infected hair follicles: (1) androgen-mediated stimulation of sebaceous gland activity, (2) abnormal keratinization leading to follicular plugging (comedone formation), (3) proliferation of the bacterium *Propionibacterium acnes* within the follicle, and (4) inflammation.

Acne occurs most often on the face, upper back, and chest because there are large numbers of sebaceous glands in these areas. One etiologic factor is increased secretion of male hormones (androgens), which occurs at puberty in both sexes. This leads to increased production of sebum and proliferation of *P. acnes*, which depend on sebum for survival. *P. acnes* bacteria contain lipase enzymes that break down free fatty acids and produce inflammation in acne lesions. Other causative factors may include medications (e.g., phenytoin, corticosteroids) and stress (i.e., the stress mechanism may involve stimulation of androgen secretion). There is no evidence that certain foods (e.g., chocolate) or lack of cleanliness causes acne.

NCLEX Success

1. **What role do androgens play in the development of acne vulgaris?**
   A. increased production of testosterone
   B. increased production of estrogen
   C. increased production of sebum
   D. increased production of facial oil

2. **A patient is taking dexamethasone for increased pain and inflammation in her right heel. She states that she has developed acne. What is the best response to this patient's statement?**
   A. Dexamethasone should decrease acne, not cause it.
   B. Dexamethasone may cause acne.
   C. Dexamethasone has no effect on acne or contact dermatitis.
   D. Dexamethasone should be combined with tetracycline to prevent acne.

3. **A 30-year-old man has been asthmatic since age 2 years. Which of the following dermatological disorders is this man prone to developing?**
   A. rosacea
   B. atopic dermatitis
   C. external otitis media
   D. impetigo

4. **Which of the following foods contributes to the development of rosacea?**
   A. milk
   B. high-protein foods
   C. alcohol
   D. ice creams

Drug Therapy

Many different drugs are used to prevent or treat dermatologic disorders. General treatment goals for many skin disorders are to relieve symptoms (e.g., dryness, pruritus, inflammation, infection), eradicate or improve lesions, promote healing and repair, restore skin integrity, and prevent recurrence. Specific goals often depend on the condition being treated. With acne, for example, goals are to reduce the number of lesions.

Topical drugs are used primarily for local effects of skin and mucous membranes, and systemic absorption is undesirable. Major factors that increase systemic absorption of topical medications include damaged or inflamed skin; high concentrations of drug; and application of drug to the face or mucous membranes, to large areas of the body, or for prolonged periods. With topical medications, cautious use is recommended with infants and young children due to the fact they have more permeable skin and are more likely to absorb the topical drugs. Box 60.1 presents general patient teaching information for topical medications for skin disorders.

General Guidelines

Most of the drugs used to treat dermatologic disorders fit into one or more of the following categories:

- Antimicrobials are used to treat infections caused by bacteria, fungi, and viruses (see Chaps. 13–23). When used in dermatologic infections, antimicrobials may be administered locally (topically) or systemically (orally or parenterally). Topical antibacterials are used to treat superficial skin disorders such as acne and skin infections. Systemic antibacterials (e.g., cephalosporins) are used for soft tissue infections such as cellulitis and postoperative wound infections. Tetracyclines are used for acne and rosacea; fluoroquinolones (e.g., ciprofloxacin) may be used to treat soft tissue infections caused by gram-negative organisms.
- Antiseptics kill or inhibit the growth of bacteria, viruses, or fungi. They are used primarily to prevent infection. Skin surfaces should be clean before application of antiseptics.
- Corticosteroids (see Chap. 15) are used to treat the inflammation present in many dermatologic conditions. They are most often applied topically but also may be given orally or parenterally. The choice of a corticosteroid depends on the acuity, severity, location, and extent of the condition being treated.
- **Emollients** and moisturizers (e.g., lanolin) are used to relieve dry skin and pruritus.
- Enzymes may be used to débride burn wounds, decubitus ulcers, and venous stasis ulcers. They promote healing by removing necrotic tissue.
- Immunosuppressants (see Chap. 11) may be used to treat inflammatory skin disorders. Two topical agents, tacrolimus (Protopic) ointment and pimecrolimus (Elidel) cream, are used for moderate to severe atopic dermatitis. However, both tacrolimus and pimecrolimus have **BLACK BOX WARNINGS** ◆ about a possible increased risk of skin cancer and lymphoma. Precautions include using the drugs only when other drugs are ineffective and avoiding long-term use. Several systemic drugs, including alefacept (Amevive), efalizumab (Raptiva), etanercept (Enbrel), and infliximab (Remicade), are used for the treatment of severe psoriasis. The U.S. Food and Drug Administration (FDA) has issued **BLACK BOX WARNINGS** ◆ for these drugs concerning the increased risks of infection, and their long-term effects are unknown.
- Keratolytics are used to treat keratin-containing skin conditions. Alpha hydroxy acids (e.g., glycolic acid) are used to treat wrinkles and sun-damaged skin. These acids are a component of many "antiaging" cosmetics and other products. Salicylic acid is used to remove warts, corns, and calluses.
- Sunscreens are used to protect the skin from the damaging effects of UV radiation, thereby decreasing skin cancer and signs of aging, including wrinkles. Dermatologists recommend sunscreen preparations that block both UVA and UVB and have a "sun protection factor" (SPF) value of 30 or higher.

Tables 60.1 and 60.2 list antimicrobial drugs as well as other drugs used in the therapy of skin disorders, including acne vulgaris.

Herbal Preparations

Many supplements are promoted for use in skin conditions. Most of these formulations have not been tested adequately to ensure effectiveness. At the same time, however, topical use rarely causes serious adverse effects or drug interactions. Two topical agents for which there is some support of safety and effectiveness are aloe and oat preparations (Box 60.2).

NCLEX Success

5. A patient has been diagnosed with atopic dermatitis. She receives a prescription for pimecrolimus (Elidel) cream. What is she at increased risk for developing?

    A. skin cancer
    B. infection
    C. papilledema
    D. joint pain

6. A 22-year-old man has developed a soft tissue cellulitis on his right heel. He has been swimming in the ocean and been in the hotel hot tub. It is cultured as a gram-negative organism. Which anti-infective agent will he receive?

    A. fluconazole
    B. acetazolamide
    C. ampicillin
    D. ciprofloxacin

Acne Vulgaris

Several prescription and nonprescription antiacne products are available for acne vulgaris.

Antimicrobial drugs include both topical and systemic agents. Topical drugs are indicated for mild to moderate acne,

BOX 60.1 Patient Teaching Guidelines for Topical Medications for Skin Disorders

General Considerations

- Promote healthy skin by a balanced diet, personal hygiene measures, avoiding excessive exposure to sunlight, avoiding skin injuries, and lubricating dry skin. Healthy skin is less susceptible to inflammation, infections, and other disorders. It also heals more rapidly when disorders or injuries occur.

- Prevent actinic keratosis and skin cancer by minimizing sun exposure, wearing sun-protective clothing, and using sunscreen. Such measures should begin in early childhood.

- Common symptoms of skin disorders are inflammation, infection, and itching, and the goal of most drug therapy is to relieve these symptoms and promote healing. Systemic medications (e.g., oral antihistamines, antibiotics, and corticosteroids) may be used for severe disorders, at least initially, but most medications are applied directly to the skin. There is a wide array of topical products, both prescription and over-the-counter.

- It is important to use the correct topical medication and the correct amount for the condition being treated. Topical corticosteroids, for example, come in many vehicles (e.g., creams, lotions, ointments) that cannot be used interchangeably. In addition, they should not be covered with occlusive dressings unless instructed to do so.

- Adverse effects of topical medications may involve the skin (e.g., irritation, infection) where the drug is applied or the entire body, when the drug is absorbed into the bloodstream. Systemic absorption is increased when the drug is highly potent; applied to inflamed skin, over a large surface area, or frequently; or covered with an occlusive dressing (e.g., plastic wrap). Systemic absorption is of most concern with corticosteroid preparations.

- Some ways to prevent or decrease skin disorders include the following:
  - Identifying and avoiding, when possible, substances that cause skin irritation and inflammation (e.g., harsh cleaning products, latex gloves, cosmetics, pet dander)
  - Bathing in warm water with a mild cleanser (e.g., Cetaphil), patting skin dry, and applying lotions or oils (e.g., Eucerin, mineral oil) to lubricate skin and decrease dryness
  - Avoiding scratching, squeezing, or rubbing skin lesions. These behaviors cause additional skin damage and increase risks of infection. Fingernails should be cut short; cotton gloves can be worn at night.
  - Maintaining a cool environment; preventing sweating
  - Applying cold compresses to inflamed, itchy skin
  - Using baking soda or colloidal oatmeal (Aveeno) in bath water to relieve itching

- If you are taking an oral antihistamine to relieve itching, take it on a regular schedule, around the clock, for greater effectiveness.

- Unavoidable skin lesions or scars can often be hidden or rendered less noticeable with makeup or clothing.

- Women can wear cosmetics over most topical medications. If unclear, ask a health care provider whether makeup is permissible. With acne, use noncomedogenic makeup, moisturizers, and sunscreens.

Self-Administration

- Use topical medications only as prescribed or according to the manufacturer's instructions (for over-the-counter products). Use the correct preparation for the intended area of application (i.e., skin, ear, vagina).

- For topical application to skin lesions, cleanse the skin and remove previously applied medication to promote drug contact with the affected area of the skin.

- Wash the skin and pat it dry.

- Apply a small amount of the drug preparation and rub it in well. A thin layer of medication is effective and decreases the incidence and severity of adverse effects. With acne and rosacea, preventing skin lesions is easier than eliminating lesions that are already present. As a result, topical medications should be applied to the general area of involvement rather than individual lesions.

- Wash hands before and after application. Wash before to avoid infection; wash afterward to avoid transferring the drug to the face or eyes and causing adverse reactions.

- With azelaic acid (Azelex) for acne, use for the full prescribed period, do not use occlusive dressings or wrappings, and keep away from mouth, eyes, and other mucous membranes (if it gets into eyes, wash eyes with a large amount of water).

- With benzoyl peroxide for acne:
  - With cleansing solutions, wash affected areas once or twice daily. Wet skin areas to be treated before applying the cleanser. Rinse thoroughly and pat dry. Reduce use if excessive drying or peeling occurs.
  - With other dosage forms, apply once daily initially and gradually increase to two or three times daily if needed. Cleanse skin, let dry completely, and apply a small amount over the affected area. Reduce dosage if excessive drying, redness, or discomfort occurs. If excessive stinging or burning occurs after any single application, remove with mild soap and water and resume use the next day. Keep away from eyes, mouth, and inside of nose. Rinse with water if contact occurs with these areas. Avoid other sources of skin irritation (e.g., sunlight, sunlamps, other topical acne medications).

often in combination with a topical retinoid to maximize reduction in severity and number of lesions. Azelaic acid (Azelex) has antibacterial activity against *P. acnes* and is reportedly as effective as benzoyl peroxide or topical erythromycin. Benzoyl peroxide is an effective topical agent that is available in numerous preparations (e.g., gel, lotion, cream, wash) and concentrations (e.g., 2.5%–10%). Lotion and cream preparations are the least irritating. Clindamycin and erythromycin are also available in topical dosage forms. These drugs reduce *P. acnes* and are equally effective. Combination

TABLE 60.1

DRUGS AT A GLANCE: Antimicrobial Drugs for Skin Disorders

Drug	Pregnancy Category	Indications	Route and Dosage Ranges
Antibacterial Drugs			
Azelaic acid (Azelex, Finacea)	B	Acne Rosacea	To lesions, twice daily
Bacitracin	C	Bacterial skin infections	To affected area, 1–3 times daily
Benzoyl peroxide	C	Acne	To affected areas, once or twice daily
Clindamycin (Cleocin T)	C	Acne	To affected areas, twice daily
Erythromycin (Akne-Mycin)	C	Acne	To affected areas, twice daily
Gentamicin (Garamycin)	D if significantly absorbed systemically with topical application	Skin infections caused by susceptible organisms	To infected areas, 3–4 times daily
Metronidazole (MetroGel, Noritate)	B	Rosacea	To affected area, once or twice daily
Mupirocin (Bactroban)	B	Impetigo caused by *Staphylococcus aureus*, beta-hemolytic streptococci, or *Streptococcus pyogenes* Eradication of nasal colonization with methicillin-resistant *S. aureus*	Impetigo: ointment, to affected areas, 3 times daily Other skin lesions: cream, 3 times daily for 10 d Eradication of nasal colonization: ointment from single-use tube, one half in each nostril, morning and evening for 5 d
Retapamulin (Altabax)	B	Impetigo	To affected area, twice daily for 5 d
Silver sulfadiazine (Silvadene)	B	Prevent or treat infection in burn wounds caused by *Pseudomonas* and many other organisms	To affected area, once or twice daily, using sterile technique
Combination Products			
Bacitracin and polymyxin B (Polysporin)	C	Bacterial skin infections	To lesions, 1–3 times daily
Erythromycin/benzoyl peroxide (Benzamycin)	C	Acne	To affected areas, twice daily
Neomycin, polymyxin B, and bacitracin (Neosporin)	C	Bacterial skin infections	To lesions, 2 or 3 times daily
Antifungal Drugs			
Butenafine (Mentax)	C	Tinea pedis	To affected area, once daily for 2–4 wk
Ciclopirox (Loprox)	B	Tinea infections Cutaneous candidiasis	To affected area, twice daily for 2–4 wk
Clotrimazole (Lotrimin)	B	Tinea infections Cutaneous candidiasis	To affected areas, twice daily for 2–4 wk
Econazole (Spectazole)	C	Tinea infections Cutaneous candidiasis	To affected areas, once daily for tinea infections, twice daily for candidiasis
Ketoconazole (Nizoral)	C	Tinea infections Cutaneous candidiasis Seborrheic dermatitis	Tinea infections and candidiasis: to affected areas, once daily for 2–4 wk Seborrheic dermatitis: twice daily for 4 wk

(Continued on page 1114)

TABLE 60.1

DRUGS AT A GLANCE: Antimicrobial Drugs for Skin Disorders (Continued)

Drug	Pregnancy Category	Indications	Route and Dosage Ranges
Miconazole (Micatin)	B	Tinea infections Cutaneous candidiasis	To affected area, once daily for 2–4 wk
Naftifine (Naftin)	B	Tinea infections	To affected areas, once daily with cream, twice daily with gel
Nystatin (Mycostatin)	A: vaginal C: topical	Candidiasis of skin and mucous membranes	To affected areas, 2 or 3 times daily until healed
Oxiconazole (Oxistat)	B	Tinea infections	To affected areas, once or twice daily for 2–4 wk
Terbinafine (Lamisil)	A	Tinea infections	To affected areas, twice daily for 1–4 wk
Tolnaftate (Tinactin)	A	Tinea infections	To affected areas, twice daily for 2–4 wk
Antiviral Drugs Acyclovir (Zovirax)	B	Herpes genitalis Herpes labialis in immu-nosuppressed patients	To lesions, every 3 h 6 times daily for 7 d
Penciclovir (Denavir)	B	Herpes labialis	To lesions, every 2 h while awake for 4 d

TABLE 60.2

DRUGS AT A GLANCE: Other Drugs Used for Skin Disorders

Drug	Pregnancy Category	Indications	Route and Dosage Ranges
Enzymes Trypsin (Granulex)	B	Débridement of infected wounds (e.g., decubitus and varicose ulcers)	Topically by spray twice daily
Immunomodulators Pimecrolimus (Elidel)	C	Atopic dermatitis	Topically to affected skin, twice daily
Tacrolimus (Protopic)	C	Atopic dermatitis	Topically to affected skin, twice daily
Retinoids Ⓟ **Isotretinoin** (Accutane, others)	X	Severe cystic acne Disorders characterized by excessive keratinization (e.g., pityriasis, ichthyosis) Mycosis fungoides	1–2 mg/kg/d PO, in 2 divided doses, for 15–20 wk
Acitretin (Soriatane)	X	Severe psoriasis	25–50 mg/d PO
Adapalene (Differin)	C	Acne vulgaris	Topically to skin lesions once daily
Tazarotene (Tazorac)	X	Acne Psoriasis	Topically to skin, after cleansing, once daily in the evening
Tretinoin (Retin-A)	D	Acne vulgaris	Topically to skin lesions once daily
Other Drugs Becaplermin (Regranex)	C	Diabetic skin ulcers	Topically to ulcer; amount calculated according to size of the ulcer
Calcipotriene (Dovonex)	C	Psoriasis	Topically to skin lesions twice daily

TABLE 60.2

DRUGS AT A GLANCE: Other Drugs Used for Skin Disorders (Continued)

Drug	Pregnancy Category	Indications	Route and Dosage Ranges
Capsaicin (Zostrix)	B	Relief of pain associated with rheumatoid arthritis, osteoarthritis, and neuralgias	Topically to affected area, up to 3 or 4 times daily
Coal tar (Balnetar, Zetar, others)	A	Psoriasis Dermatitis	Topically to skin, in various concentrations and preparations
Colloidal oatmeal (Aveeno)	A	Pruritus	Topically as a bath solution (1 cup in bathtub of water)
Dextranomer (Debrisan)	B	Cleansing of ulcers (e.g., venous stasis, decubitus) and wounds (e.g., burn, surgical, traumatic)	Apply to a clean, moist wound surface every 12 h initially, then less often as exudate decreases
Fluorouracil (Efudex)	X	Actinic keratoses Superficial basal cell carcinomas	Topically to skin lesions twice daily for 2–6 wk
Masoprocol (Actinex)	B	Actinic keratoses	Topically to skin lesions morning and evening for 28 d
Salicylic acid	C	Removal of warts, corns, calluses Superficial fungal infections Seborrheic dermatitis Acne Psoriasis	Topically to skin lesions
Selenium sulfide (Selsun)	C	Dandruff Tinea versicolor	Topically to scalp as shampoo once or twice weekly

products of topical clindamycin or erythromycin and benzoyl peroxide are more effective than antibiotics alone. Best results require 8 to 12 weeks of therapy, and maintenance therapy is usually required. Adverse effects of topical antibiotics include erythema, peeling, dryness, and burning as well as development of resistant strains of *P. acnes*. Recommendations for reducing drug resistance include using topical retinoids or benzoyl peroxide or both when using topical antibiotics. It is important to avoid long-term use of topical or oral antibiotics when feasible. Benzoyl peroxide can also cause an irritant dermatitis and bleach hair, clothes, and bed linens.

Oral antimicrobials are first-line treatment for patients with moderate to severe inflammatory acne. These drugs have both antimicrobial and anti-inflammatory effects. They reduce *P. acnes* organisms and thereby inhibit production of *P. acnes*–induced inflammatory cytokines. Commonly used oral antibiotics include tetracycline, doxycycline, minocycline, and erythromycin. Tetracycline and erythromycin suppress leukocyte chemotaxis and bacterial lipase activity; minocycline and doxycycline inhibit cytokines and proteinase enzymes that contribute to inflammation and tissue breakdown. Resistance to the tetracyclines is less common than to erythromycin and

BOX 60.2   Herbal Preparations Used in Skin Conditions

■ Aloe is often used as a topical remedy for minor burns and wounds (e.g., sunburn, cuts, abrasions) to decrease pain, itching, and inflammation and to promote healing. Its active ingredients are unknown. Wound healing is attributed to moisturizing effects and increased blood flow to the area. Reduced inflammation and pain may result from inhibition of arachidonic acid metabolism and formation of inflammatory prostaglandins. Reduced itching may result from inhibition of histamine production.

  Commercial products are available for topical use, but fresh gel from the plant may be preferred. When used for this purpose, a clear, thin, gel-like liquid can be squeezed directly from a plant leaf onto the burned or injured area several times daily if needed.

■ Oats, a cereal, a good source of dietary fiber, and a well-documented cholesterol-lowering product, is used topically to treat minor skin irritation and pruritus associated with common skin disorders. They contain gluten, which forms a sticky mass that has emollient effects and holds moisture in the skin when it is mixed with a liquid. Oats are contained in bath products, cleansing bars, and lotions (e.g., Aveeno products) that can be used topically once or twice daily. They should not be used near the eyes or on inflamed skin. After use, it is important to wash bath products off with water.

is least with minocycline. All oral antibiotics require at least 6 to 8 weeks of use. Although there are no established guidelines for duration of use, some clinicians encourage using the drugs for shorter periods and avoiding long-term use as maintenance therapy, to decrease the development of resistant *P. acnes*.

Retinoids, in both systemic and topical forms, may be used for moderate to severe acne. All topical retinoids (isotretinoin, adapalene, tazarotene) reduce acne lesions, usually within 12 weeks. Isotretinoin is often used with other products.

NCLEX Success

7. **A 15-year-old girl receives a prescription for tetracycline twice daily for an outbreak of acne. How does tetracycline decrease the girl's acne?**

   A. It suppresses the cell membrane.
   B. It suppresses leukocyte cytokines.
   C. It blocks the development of sebum.
   D. It produces isotonic changes in the cell.

8. **The mother of a boy being treated for acne vulgaris asks a nurse why her son is being treated with doxycycline and a topical benzoyl peroxide agent. Which of the following is the best response the nurse can make to the patient's mother?**

   A. "Benzoyl peroxide cannot be administered without doxycycline."
   B. "Doxycycline should be administered only until the acne vulgaris improves."
   C. "If your son's acne does not improve in 2 weeks, then one of the two agents will be stopped."
   D. "Doxycycline orally and benzoyl peroxide topically will provide better treatment of the acne vulgaris."

Clinical Application 60-1

- Gerard first took tetracycline for his acne vulgaris. How does tetracycline work against this disorder?
- What are some topical applications that he could use to assist in clearing his acne vulgaris?

Retinoids

Retinoids are vitamin A derivatives that are active in proliferation and differentiation of skin cells. These drugs are commonly used to treat acne, psoriasis, aging and wrinkling of skin from sunlight exposure, and skin cancers. The prototype drug in this class is **℗ isotretinoin** (Accutane, Amnesteem, Claravis, Sotret).

Pharmacokinetics

Isotretinoin dissolves slowly in the gastrointestinal (GI) tract, and the drug is then absorbed rapidly. It crosses the placenta. Isotretinoin is metabolized in the liver and excreted in equal amounts in the feces and urine.

Action

The anti-acne effects of isotretinoin include suppression of sebum production, inhibition of comedone formation, and inhibition of inflammation. The drug normalizes keratinization, reversibly decreases the size of sebaceous glands, and makes sebum less viscous and less likely to plug follicles. The decrease in sebum results in the inhibition of the sebum-dependent bacterium *P. acnes*, which is a key promoter of inflammation in acne vulgaris (Owen, 2011). Researchers have often found that isotretinoin also decreases cell proliferation and induces differentiation in neuroblastoma.

Use

Uses of isotretinoin include treatment of severe recalcitrant nodular acne that is unresponsive to other treatments in adolescents and adults. Unlabeled uses are treatment of moderate acne in adolescents and adults and treatment of high-risk neuroblastoma in children and adolescents.

Adverse Effects

Isotretinoin has several adverse effects. They include

- Dermatologic effects (most common): dryness and swelling of the lips (cheilitis), dry skin and mucous membranes, nasal dryness, epistaxis, dry mouth, conjunctivitis, peeling skin, skin fragility, rash, and pruritus
- GI effects (potential): nausea, vomiting and, rarely, inflammatory bowel disease and pancreatitis
- Musculoskeletal effects (common): arthralgia, myalgia (particularly with vigorous exercise), weakness, increased creatine phosphokinase (CPK), and back pain in some children; as well as bone abnormalities, decreased bone mineral density, premature epiphyseal closure
- Metabolic effects: hyperlipidemia (elevated triglycerides in 45% of patients, elevated total cholesterol, and low-density lipoprotein in 30% of patients: usually transient elevations)
- Psychiatric effects (serious): depression, psychosis, aggressive or violent behavior, and changes in mood; rarely, suicidal thoughts and actions have been reported. It is important to observe closely all patients for symptoms of depression or suicidal thoughts; it may be necessary to discontinue therapy and make appropriate referrals to mental health professionals.
- Other effects: decreased night vision, corneal opacities, hepatotoxicity, and bone marrow suppression

Contraindications

Contraindications to isotretinoin include hypersensitivity to the drug, parabens (used as a preservative), vitamin A, or other retinoids, as well as pregnancy. The FDA has issued a **BLACK BOX WARNING ◆** stating that isotretinoin, in pregnancy category X, causes both spontaneous abortions and severe life-threatening congenital malformations. In addition, women of childbearing potential should not take isotretinoin unless they have had two negative pregnancy test results before beginning therapy, will begin drug therapy on the 2nd or 3rd day of the next menstrual period, and will comply with stringent contraceptive measures for 1 month before therapy, during therapy, and for 1 month after therapy. Box 60.3 describes the measures put in place by

---

BOX 60.3   iPLEDGE Program

- The iPLEDGE program requires that:
- All female patients who are able to become pregnant must use two forms of birth control for at least 1 month prior to starting therapy, during therapy, and for 1 month after therapy. Patients are allowed to avoid the contraceptive requirements if they agree to abstain completely from sex; this commitment must be made in writing.
- All female patients who are able to become pregnant must have two negative blood or urine pregnancy tests before receiving the initial prescription. It is essential that the second pregnancy test be conducted in a certified laboratory. During each month of therapy and 1 month after completing therapy, patients must see their health care provider for evaluation, counseling,

and education. They must also have a negative pregnancy test in a certified laboratory monthly and 1 month after completing therapy.

- Every month, prescribers must document in the iPLEDGE system the results of the pregnancy test and the two forms of birth control in use. The prescriber must also document the counseling and education. All patients, even if not able to become pregnant, must be counseled about the iPLEDGE program and the risk of birth defects.
- Health care providers can prescribe only a maximum 30-day supply at each monthly visit.
- Physicians must certify their expertise in the diagnosis and treatment of acne.

---

the iPLEDGE program developed by the FDA. The FDA has established a computer-based Risk Evaluation and Mitigation Strategy (REMS) to prevent fetal exposure to isotretinoin.

QSEN Safety Alert ❗

All patients receiving isotretinoin, as well as all prescribers, dispensing pharmacies, and wholesale distributors of the medication, are required to register with the iPLEDGE program and strictly follow its requirements.

Cautious use is also advisable with a history of mental illness or a family history of psychiatric disorders. Other conditions that warrant caution are asthma, liver disease, diabetes, heart disease, osteoporosis, history of childhood osteoporosis, genetic predisposition for age-related osteoporosis, weak bones, anorexia nervosa, osteomalacia, and other disorders of bone metabolism.

Nursing Implications

Preventing Interactions

Many medications interact with isotretinoin, increasing its effects (Box 60.4). Isotretinoin may decrease the therapeutic effect of estrogen and progestin contraceptives. Microdosed progesterone-only preparations, in particular, may be ineffective.

BOX 60.4   Drug Interactions: Isotretinoin

Drugs That Increase the Effects of Isotretinoin
- Alcohol
  Increases triglycerides
- Corticosteroids
  Increase the risk of osteoporosis
- Phenytoin
  Increases the risk of osteomalacia
- Tetracycline
  Increases the risk of cerebri pseudotumor
- Vitamin A
  Produces toxic effects associated with isotretinoin

Administering the Medication

Before starting isotretinoin, it is necessary to perform a complete blood cell count (CBC), a fasting lipid profile, and liver function tests to obtain a baseline. People should take the drug with or shortly after a meal to improve absorption. It is necessary to swallow capsules whole with a full glass of liquid. The contents of the capsule may irritate the esophagus if removed from the capsule. Women should avoid coming in contact with the contents of the capsules because the drug is teratogenic.

Assessing for Therapeutic Effects

The nurse assesses for a decrease in total cyst count. The ideal value is a 70% decrease.

Assessing for Adverse Effects

With oral retinoids the nurse observes for hypervitaminosis. Nausea and vomiting; headache; blurred vision, eye irritation, and conjunctivitis; skin disorders; musculoskeletal pain (any evidence of osteoporosis, osteopenia, or fractures); and depression and suicidal ideation are common signs of hypervitaminosis. Although adverse effects commonly occur with usual doses, they are more severe with higher doses. Most adverse effects can be managed without stopping the drug.

Also, the nurse monitors laboratory tests. It is important to conduct repeat tests (CBC, lipid profile, liver function tests) at 4 and 8 weeks. If the repeat tests are normal and the dose is stable, monitoring is no longer necessary.

Patient Teaching

Box 60.5 identifies patient teaching guidelines for isotretinoin.

Clinical Application 60-2

- How does isotretinoin work to reduce acne vulgaris?
- Isotretinoin may cause severe psychiatric adverse effects, such as depression, psychosis, or violent behavior. What are some strategies the nurse can teach Gerard's parents about looking for psychosocial abnormalities?

EVIDENCE-BASED PRACTICE

Neuromuscular Adverse Effects Associated with Systemic Retinoid Dermatotherapy Monitoring and Treatment Algorithm for Clinicians

by ELISABETH CRHONI, ALEXANDRA MONASTRIRLI, & DIONYSIOS TSAMBAOS.

Drug Safety
2010, 33(1), 25–34

Neuromuscular adverse effects have been reported with the administration of systemic retinoid therapy. There is also a potential of neuromuscular toxicity of vitamin A with retinoids. The most common neuromuscular adverse effect associated with isotretinoin is headache with benign intracranial hypertension, nausea, and visual changes. The patient may also experience seizures, myalgia, and generalized muscle stiffness. The authors have developed an algorithm for monitoring patients treated with oral retinoids. Patients who have previous neuromuscular symptoms and have been initiated on retinoid therapy should be monitored closely for central nervous system (CNS) and peripheral nervous system (PNS) adverse effects. If these adverse effects occur, the patient should be withdrawn from the medication.

IMPLICATIONS FOR NURSING PRACTICE: When educating patients about the adverse effects of retinoids, the nurse should pay particular attention to the risk of CNS- and PNS-related adverse effects associated with retinoid therapy. The nurse should stress the importance of these effects to both the patient and family. They should report the onset of headache to the primary health care provider immediately.

NCLEX Success

9. A 13-year-old girl has developed a mild case of acne vulgaris. Which of the following medications will be prescribed?

   A. doxycycline
   B. benzoyl peroxide
   C. isotretinoin
   D. fluconazole

10. A 17-year-old boy is seen in the school nurse's office. He has been taking isotretinoin (Accutane) for 6 months. He is complaining of nausea and visual changes. What should the nurse suspect the symptoms may be related to?

    A. He has an adverse effect of the medication.
    B. The patient may have a pseudotumor cerebri.
    C. He has developed the flu.
    D. He may have developed migraine headaches..

BOX 60.5   Patient Teaching Guidelines for Isotretinoin

■ Understand that acne is not caused by dirt, that washing does not improve acne, and that vigorous scrubbing may worsen acne lesions. There is also no evidence that acne is caused by eating chocolate or other foods.

■ If you are a woman of childbearing age, it is essential that you adhere to all requirements of the iPLEDGE program.

  ■ Use two forms of birth control.

  ■ Adhere to mandatory pregnancy testing requirements.

■ Take the drug with or shortly after meals.

■ Report bone, muscle, or joint pain or visual disturbances immediately, as well as persistent headaches or gastrointestinal pain.

■ Report depression or suicidal thoughts immediately.

■ Do not take oral vitamin A supplements.

■ Avoid using abrasives, medicated soaps and cleansers, acne preparations containing peeling drugs, and topical products containing alcohol (e.g., cosmetics, aftershave). These products will exacerbate skin dryness and irritation.

■ Avoid prolonged sun exposure. Use sun block.

■ Do not donate blood during therapy and up to 1 month after therapy.

The Nursing Process

Assessment

• When a skin rash is present, inspect the area and interview the patient to determine the following:
  • Appearance of individual lesions
  • Location or distribution
  • Accompanying symptoms
  • Historic development
  • Etiologic factors. In many instances, appropriate treatment is determined by the cause. Some etiologic factors include the following:
    • Drug therapy. Many commonly used drugs may cause skin lesions, including antibiotics (e.g., penicillins, sulfonamides, tetracyclines), narcotic analgesics, and thiazide diuretics. Skin rashes due to drug therapy are usually generalized and appear abruptly.
    • Irritants or allergens that may cause contact dermatitis. For example, dermatitis involving the hands may be caused by soaps, detergents, or various other cleansing agents. Dermatitis involving the trunk may result from allergic reactions to clothing.
    • Communicable diseases (e.g., measles, chickenpox), which cause characteristic skin rashes and systemic signs and symptoms.
• When assessing the skin, consider the age of the patient. Infants are likely to have "diaper" dermatitis, miliaria (heat rash), and tinea capitis (ringworm infection of the scalp). School-aged children have a relatively high incidence of measles, chickenpox, and tinea infections. Adolescents often have acne. Older adults are more likely

to have dry skin, actinic keratoses (lesions on sun-exposed skin formerly thought to be premalignant but now considered early-stage squamous cell cancer), and skin cancer.

- Assess for skin neoplasms. Basal cell carcinoma, the most common type, may initially appear as a pale nodule, most often on the head and neck. Squamous cell carcinomas may appear as actinic keratoses or ulcerated areas. Malignant melanoma is the most serious skin cancer. It involves melanocytes, the pigment-producing cells of the skin. Malignant melanoma may occur in pigmented nevi (moles) or previously normal skin. In nevi, malignant melanoma may be manifested by enlargement and ulceration. In previously normal skin, lesions appear as irregularly shaped pigmented areas.

Nursing Diagnoses

- Disturbed body image related to visible skin lesions
- Anxiety related to potential for permanent scarring or disfigurement
- Pain related to skin lesions and pruritus
- Risk for injury: infection related to entry of microbes through damaged skin

Planning/Goals

The patient will

- Apply topical drugs correctly
- Experience relief of symptoms
- Use techniques to prevent or minimize skin damage and disorders
- Avoid scarring and disfigurement when possible
- Be encouraged to express concerns about acute and chronic body-image changes

Nursing Interventions

The nurse will

- Use measures to prevent or minimize skin disorders, including good personal hygiene.
- Use general measures to promote health and increase resistance to disease (i.e., maintain nutrition, rest, and exercise).

- Practice safety measures to avoid injury to the skin. Any injury, especially one that disrupts the integrity of the skin (e.g., lacerations, puncture wounds, scratching of skin lesions) increases the likelihood of skin infections.
- Avoid known irritants or allergens.
- Use measures to relieve dry skin and pruritus. Measures to decrease skin dryness include the following:
  - Alternating complete and partial baths
  - Liberal use of lubricating creams, and lotions. Creams and lotions may be applied several times daily.
- Prevent pressure ulcers by avoiding trauma to the skin and prolonged pressure on any part of the body. In patients at high risk for development of pressure ulcers, major preventive measures include frequent changes of position and correct lifting techniques. Various pressure-relieving devices (e.g., special beds and mattresses) also are useful. Daily inspection of the skin is needed for early detection and treatment of beginning pressure ulcers.
- Avoid excessive exposure to sunlight and other sources of UV light.
- Apply sunscreen daily.
- When skin rashes are present, cool, wet compresses or baths are often effective in relieving pruritus. Water or normal saline may be used alone or with additives, such as colloidal oatmeal (e.g., Aveeno) or baking soda. A cool environment also tends to decrease pruritus. The patient's fingernails should be cut short and kept clean to avoid skin damage and infection from scratching.
- For severe itching, a systemic antihistamine may be needed.

Evaluation

- Observe and interview regarding use of dermatologic drugs.
- Observe for improvement in skin lesions and symptoms.
- Interview regarding use of measures to promote healthy skin and prevent skin disorders.

Key Concepts

- Many dermatologic medications are applied topically to skin and mucous membranes. The drugs may improve barrier function, soften and remove scaly lesions, alter inflammation in the skin, alter blood flow, exert antimicrobial effects, or affect proliferating cells.

- Immunosuppressants such as tacrolimus and pimecrolimus are used for moderate to severe atopic dermatitis. The drugs have **BLACK BOX WARNINGS** ◆ about a possible increased risk of skin cancer and lymphoma. Several systemic biologic drugs, alefacept, efalizumab, etanercept, and infliximab, are used for the treatment of severe psoriasis. **BLACK BOX WARNINGS** ◆ for these drugs alert clinicians about increased risks of developing infections and their unknown long-term effects.

- Acne is a common disorder characterized by excessive production of sebum and obstruction of hair follicles, which normally carry sebum to the skin surface. As a result, hair follicles expand and form comedones (blackheads and whiteheads). Acne lesions vary from small comedones to acne vulgaris, the most severe form, in which follicles become infected and irritating secretions leak into surrounding tissues to form inflammatory pustules, cysts, and abscesses.

- Retinoids are vitamin A derivatives that are active in proliferation and differentiation of skin cells. These drugs are commonly used to treat acne, psoriasis, aging and wrinkling of skin from sunlight exposure, and skin cancers. The prototype drug in this class is isotretinoin.

- Isotretinoin should not be prescribed to women who are or are likely to become pregnant while using the drug. A **BLACK BOX WARNING** ◆ warns that isotretinoin causes both spontaneous abortions and severe life-threatening congenital malformations.

Critical Thinking Questions

60-1. A 17-year-old girl has a severe case of acne vulgaris. She has received a prescription for isotretinoin.

- When providing patient teaching to the girl and her parents, the nurse needs to address iPLEDGE. What is iPLEDGE?
- What hygienic practices decrease acne vulgaris?
- When taking isotretinoin, what is important about its administration?

References and Resources

Chroni, E., Monastirli, A., & Tsambaos, D. (2010). Neuromuscular adverse effects associated with systemic retinoid dermatotherapy monitoring and treatment of algorithm for clinicians. *Drug Safety, 33*(1), 25–34.

iPLEDGE: Committed to Pregnancy Prevention. U. S. Food and Drug Administration–approved program for use of isotretinoin. Program accessed at ww.ipledgeprogram.com

Karch, A. M. (2010). *2010 Lippincott's nursing drug guide.* Philadelphia, PA: Lippincott Williams & Wilkins.

Lippincott Williams & Wilkins. (2012). *Nursing drug handbook.* Philadelphia, PA: Wolters Kluwer Publishers.

Porth, C. M., & Matfin, G. (2009). *Pathophysiology concepts of altered health states.* Philadelphia, PA: Lippincott Williams & Wilkins.

Owen, C. (2011). *Oral isotretinoin therapy for acne vulgaris.* Up-To-Date, Lexi-Comp, Inc.

Smeltzer, S. C., Bare, B. G., Hinkle, J. H., & Cheever, K. H. (2008). *Brunner & Suddarth's textbook of medical-surgical nursing* (11th ed.). Philadelphia, PA: Lippincott Williams & Wilkins.

Up-To-Date. (2012). *Isotretinoin: Drug information.* Lexi-Comp, Inc.

Index

(Note: Page numbers followed by "f" indicate figures; "t", tables; "b", boxes)